American
DRUG INDEX

44th Edition

American DRUG INDEX

2000

44th Edition

NORMAN F. BILLUPS, RPh, MS, PhD

Dean and Professor of Pharmacy
College of Pharmacy
The University of Toledo

Associate Editor

SHIRLEY M. BILLUPS, RN, LPC, MEd

Oncology Nurse
Licensed Professional Counselor

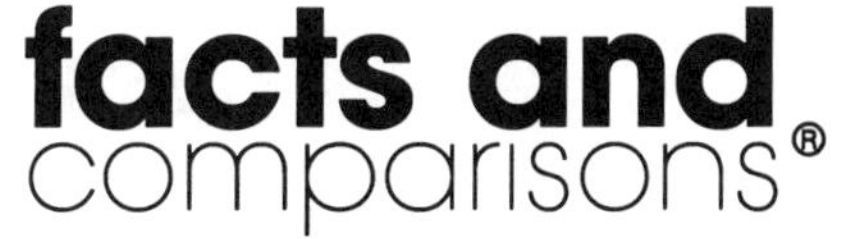

A **Wolters Kluwer** Company

Facts and Comparisons® Staff

Michael R. Riley
president and publisher

Steven K. Hebel, BS Pharm
director, editorial/production

Bernie R. Olin, PharmD
director of drug information

Heidi L. Meredith
business development

Noël A. Shamleffer
managing editor

Julie A. Scott
quality control editor

Kimberly A. Faulhaber
Sophia J. Oh
Orlando L. Thomas
Adrienne N. Wartts
assistant editors

ISBN 1-57439-051-1

Library of Congress Catalog Card Number 55-6286

Printed in the United States of America

Published by
Facts and Comparisons®
A **Wolters Kluwer** Company
111 West Port Plaza, Suite 300
St. Louis, Missouri 63146-3098

Preface

The 44th Edition of the *American Drug Index (ADI)* has been prepared for the identification, explanation, and correlation of the many pharmaceuticals available to the medical, pharmaceutical, and allied health professions. The need for this index has become even more acute as the variety and number of drugs and drug products have continued to multiply. Hence, *ADI* should be useful to pharmacists, nurses, health care administrators, physicians, medical transcriptionists, dentists, sales personnel, students, and teachers in the fields incorporating pharmaceuticals.

Special note to medical transcriptionists: All generic names are in lowercase and all trade names are in upper/lowercase as appropriate to facilitate transcription. (Tradenames which happen to start with a lowercase letter have been set in uppercase for consistency.) The names for officially designated products (eg, *United States Pharmacopeia* or U.S.P.) are preceded by a bullet (•) and should appear in lowercase in transcription.

The organization of *ADI* falls into 21 major sections:

- Monographs of Drug Products
- Standard Medical Abbreviations
- Calculations
- Common Systems of Weights and Measures
- Approximate Practical Equivalents
- International System of Units
- Normal Laboratory Values
- Trademark Glossary
- Medical Terminology Glossary
- Container Requirements for U.S.P. 23 Drugs
- Container and Storage Requirements for Sterile U.S.P. 23 Drugs
- Oral Dosage Forms that Should Not Be Crushed or Chewed
- Drug Names that Look Alike and Sound Alike
- Recommended Childhood Immunization Schedule
- FDA Pregnancy Categories
- Controlled Substances Summary
- Radio-Contrast Media
- Radio-Isotopes
- Agents for Imaging
- Pharmaceutical Company Labeler Code Index
- Pharmaceutical Manufacturer and Drug Distributor Listing

MONOGRAPHS: The organization of the monograph section of *ADI* is alphabetical with extensive cross-indexing. Names listed are generic (also called nonproprietary, public name, or common name); brand (also called trademark, proprietary, or specialty); and chemical. Synonyms that are in general use also are included. All names used for a pharmaceutical appear in alphabetical order with the pertinent data given under the brand name by which it is made available.

The monograph for a typical brand name product appears in upper/lowercase as appropriate, and consists of the manufacturer, generic name, composition and strength, pharmaceutical dosage forms available, package size and use, and appropriate legend designation (eg, *Rx, otc, c-v).*

Generic names appear in lowercase in alphabetical order, followed by the pronunciation and the corresponding recognition of the drug to the U.S.P. (*United States Pharmacopeia*), N.F. (*National Formulary*), and USAN (*USP Dictionary of United States Adopted Names and International Drug Names*). Each of these official generic names is preceded by a bullet (•) at the beginning of each entry. The information is in accord with the U.S.P. 23 and N.F. 18 which became official on January 1, 1995; Supplement 1 which became official on January 1, 1995 through Supplement 9 which became official November 15, 1998; and the 1998 USP Dictionary of USAN and International Drug Names.

Pronunciations have been included for many of the generic drugs. However, not every drug will have a corresponding pronunciation. Some of the most common pronunciations are not listed for every drug. The following list is included as a guide to very common names.

Acetate	ASS-eh-tate	Lactobionate	LACK-toe-BYE-oh-nate
Besylate	BESS-ih-late	Maleate	MAL-ee-ate
Borate	BOE-rate	Mesylate	MEH-sih-LATE
Bromide	BROE-mide	Monosodium	MAHN-oh-SO-dee-uhm
Butyrate	BYOO-tih-rate	Nitrate	NYE-trate
Calcium	KAL-see-uhm	Pendetide	PEN-deh-TIDE
Chloride	KLOR-ide	Pentetate	PEN-teh-tate
Citrate	SIH-trate	Phosphate	FOSS-fate
Dipotassium	die-poe-TASS-ee-uhm	Potassium	poe-TASS-ee-uhm
Disodium	die-SO-dee-uhm	Propionate	PRO-pee-oh-nate
Edetate	eh-deh-TATE	Sodium	SO-dee-uhm
Fosfatex	foss-FAH-tex	Succinate	SUCK-sih-nate
Fumarate	FEW-mah-rate	Sulfate	SULL-fate
Hydrobromide	HIGH-droe-BROE-mide	Tartrate	TAR-trate
Hydrochloride	HIGH-droe-KLOR-ide	Trisodium	try-SO-dee-uhm
Iodide	EYE-oh-dide		

Because of the multiplicity of brand names used for the same therapeutic agent or the same combination of therapeutic agents, it was apparent that some correlation could be done. As an example of this, please turn to tetracycline HCl. Here under the generic name are listed the various brand names. Following are combinations of tetracycline HCl organized in a manner to point out relationships among the many products. Reference then is made to the brand name or names having the indicated composition. Under the brand name are given manufacturer, composition, available forms, sizes, dosage, and use.

The multiplicity of generic names for the same therapeutic agent has complicated the nomenclature of these agents. Examples of multiple generic names for the same chemical substance are: (1) parabromdylamine, brompheniramine; (2) acetaminophen, p-hydroxy acetanilid, N-acetyl-p-aminophenol; (3) guaifenesin, glyceryl guaiacolate, glyceryl guaiacol ether, guaianesin, guaifylline, guaiphenesin, guayanesin, methphenoxydiol; (4) pyrilamine, pyranisamine, pyranilamine, pyraminyl, anisopyradamine.

The cross-indexing feature of *ADI* permits the finding of drugs or drug combinations when only one major ingredient is known. For example, a combination of aluminum hydroxide gel and magnesium trisilicate is available. This combination can be found by looking under the name of either of the two ingredients, and in each case the brand names are given. A second form of cross-indexing lists drugs under various therapeutic and pharmaceutical classes (ie, antacids, antihistamines, diuretics, laxatives, etc.).

ABBREVIATIONS: The listing of Standard Medical Abbreviations is included as an aid in interpreting medical orders. The Latin or Greek word and abbreviation are given with the meaning.

CALCULATIONS: A listing of common formulas used to calculate weight, creatinine clearance, ideal body weight, body surface area, and approximate surface area of children; and convert temperature between celsius and farenheit. The suggested adult weight table is also included.

WEIGHTS AND MEASURES: Tables containing the Common Systems of Weights and Measures are included to aid the practitioner in calculating dosages in the metric, apothecary, and avoirdupois systems, as well as the International System of Units.

CONVERSION FACTORS: A listing of Approximate Practical Equivalents is added as an aid in calculating and converting dosages among the metric, apothecary, and avoirdupois systems.

INTERNATIONAL SYSTEM OF UNITS: A modernized version of the metric system listed in tables for rapid reference.

NORMAL LABORATORY VALUES: Tables containing normal reference values for commonly requested laboratory tests are included as a guideline for the health care practitioner.

TRADEMARK GLOSSARY: An alphabetical listing of trademarked dosage forms and package types is included to aid in the identification of drug products listed in *ADI.*

MEDICAL TERMINOLOGY GLOSSARY: Commonly used terms are listed and defined as an aid in interpreting the use given for drug monographs included in *ADI.*

CONTAINER AND STORAGE REQUIREMENTS FOR U.S.P. 23 DRUGS AND STERILE DRUGS: These sections on container and storage requirements specified by the U.S.P. 23 for compendial drugs have been added to aid the practitioner in storing and dispensing.

ORAL DOSAGE FORMS THAT SHOULD NOT BE CRUSHED OR CHEWED: This section has been added to alert the health care practitioner about oral dosage forms that should not be crushed, and to serve as an aid in consulting with patients. Examples of products falling into the "non-crush" category are extended-release, enteric-coated, encapsulated beads, wax matrix, sublingual dosage forms, and encapsulated liquid formulations.

DRUG NAMES THAT LOOK ALIKE AND SOUND ALIKE: A listing of common drugs that look alike and sound alike. Familiarity with this list may save the prescriber from making a dispensing error.

RECOMMENDED CHILDHOOD IMMUNIZATION SCHEDULE: This section contains dosing and scheduling information for routine childhood vaccines.

FDA PREGNANCY CATEGORIES: This table summarizes each of the pregnancy categories established by the FDA.

CONTROLLED SUBSTANCES SUMMARY: A brief summary explanation of the key points of the Controlled Substances Act of 1970.

RADIO-CONTRAST MEDIA AND ISOTOPES: These tables provide the generic and trade names, dose form and packaging, and manufacturer information as an aid to the health care provider.

AGENTS FOR IMAGING: This table provides the generic and trade names, dose form and packaging, and manufacturer information as an aid to the health care provider.

PHARMACEUTICAL COMPANY LABELER CODE INDEX: The Pharmaceutical Labeler Code Index is presented to aid in the identification of drug products. The codes are listed in numerical order followed by the name of the manufacturer.

MANUFACTURER ADDRESSES: The name, address, and zip code of virtually every American pharmaceutical manufacturer and drug distributor are listed in alphabetical order in this section. Additionally, a pharmaceutical labeler code number appears before the address of each company as a further aid in identifying drug products.

Special appreciation and acknowledgment are given to my wife, Shirley, who served again this year as my Associate Editor – and to Dr. Bernie R. Olin, Director of Drug Information of Facts and Comparisons, for compiling the monograph section of this volume. Special thanks are also extended to the manufacturers who supplied product information, to Dr. Kenneth S. Alexander for organizing the Container and Storage Requirements information, and to Dr. John F. Mitchell for the table on Oral Dosage Forms that Should Not Be Crushed or Chewed.

Correspondence or communication with reference to a drug or drug products listed in *ADI* should be directed to Editorial/Production, Attn: ADI, Facts and Comparisons, 111 West Port Plaza, Suite 300, St. Louis, Missouri 63146, or call 1-800-223-0554.

Norman F. Billups, RPh, MS, PhD

Contents

[•] Denotes official name: Generic name or chemical name recognized by the U.S.P., N.F., or USAN.

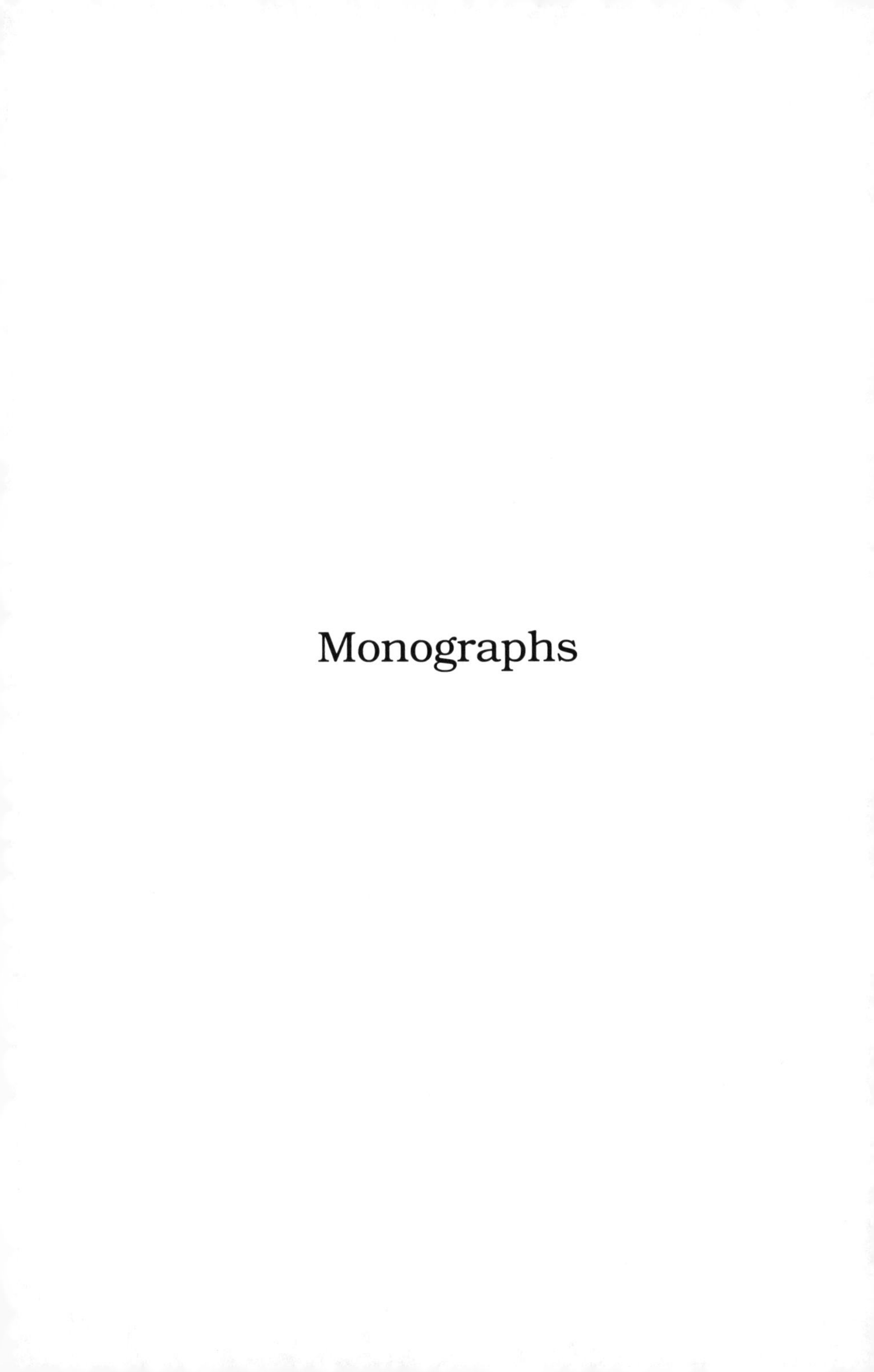

Monographs

A

AA-HC Otic. (Schein Pharmaceutical, Inc.) Hydrocortisone 1%, acetic acid glacial 2%, propylene glycol diacetate 3%, benzethonium Cl 0.02%, sodium acetate 0.015%, citric acid 0.2%. Soln. Bot. 10 ml. *Rx.*
Use: Otic.

A and D Ointment. (Schering-Plough Corp.) Fish liver oil, cholecalciferol. Tube 1.5 oz, 4 oz. Jar lb. *otc.*
Use: Emollient.

A & D Tablets. (Barth's) Vitamins A 10,000 IU, D 400 IU/Tab. Bot. 100s, 500s. *otc.*
Use: Vitamin supplement.

•**abacavir succinate.** (ab-ah-KAV-ear SUCK-sih-nate) USAN.
Use: Antiviral.

abacavir sulfate.
Use: Antiviral.
See: Ziagen (GlaxoWellcome).

•**abafilcon a.** (ab-ah-FILL-kahn) USAN.
Use: Contact lens material (hydrophilic).

•**abamectin.** (abe-ah-MEK-tin) USAN.
Use: Antiparasitic.

•**abarelix.** (ab-ah-RELL-ix) USAN.
Use: Gonad-stimulating principle antagonist, antineoplastic, infertility therapy adjunct, antiendometriotic agent.

Abbokinase. (Abbott Laboratories) Urokinase 250,000 IU/5 ml. Lyophilized pow. Vial 5 ml. *Rx.*
Use: Thrombolytic.

Abbokinase Open-Cath. (Abbott Laboratories) Urokinase for catheter clearance 5000 IU/ml. Univial 1 ml. *Rx.*
Use: Thrombolytic.

Abbott AFP-EIA. (Abbott Diagnostics) Enzyme immunoassay for the quantitative measurement of alpha-fetoprotein (AFP) in human serum and amniotic fluid. Test kits 100s.
Use: Diagnostic aid.

Abbott AFP-EIA Monoclonal. (Abbott Diagnostics) Enzyme immunoassay for the quantitative measurement of alpha-fetoprotein (AFP) in human serum and amniotic fluid.
Use: Diagnostic aid.

Abbott Anti-Delta. (Abbott Diagnostics) Radioimmunoassay for the detection of antibody to hepatitis delta antigen (HDAg) in human serum or plasma.
Use: For research only. Not for use in diagnostic procedures.

Abbott Anti-Delta EIA. (Abbott Diagnostics) Enzyme immunoassay for the detection of antibody to hepatitis delta antigen (HDAg) in human serum or plasma.
Use: For research only. Not for use in diagnostic procedures.

Abbott β-HCG 15/15. (Abbott Diagnostics) Enzyme immunoassay for the quantitative determination of human chorionic gonadotropin (hCG) in human serum.
Use: Diagnostic aid.

Abbott CA125-EIA. (Abbott Diagnostics) Enzyme immunoassay for the quantitative measurement of cancer antigen (CA) 125 in human serum.
Use: For research only. Not for use in diagnostic procedures.

Abbott CEA-EIA Monoclonal. (Abbott Diagnostics) Enzyme immunoassay for the quantitative measurement of carcinoembryonic antigen (CEA) in human serum or plasma to aid in the management of cancer patients and assessing prognosis.
Use: Diagnostic aid.

Abbott CEA-RIA. (Abbott Diagnostics) Solid phase radioimmunoassay for the quantitative measurement of carcinoembryonic antigen (CEA) in human serum or plasma to aid in the management of cancer patients and assessing prognosis.
Use: Diagnostic aid.

Abbott CMV Total AB EIA. (Abbott Diagnostics) Enzyme immunoassay for the detection of antibody to cytomegalovirus in human serum, plasma, and whole blood. Test kits 100s.
Use: Diagnostic aid.

Abbott Diagnostic Reagents. (Abbott Diagnostics) A series of diagnostic tests for cancer, cardiovascular, hepatitis, infectious disease and immunology, metabolic and digestive disease, OB/GYN, rubella, and thyroid.
Use: Diagnostic aid.

Abbott ER-EIA Monoclonal. (Abbott Diagnostics) Enzyme immunoassay for the quantitative measurement of human estrogen receptor in tissue cytosol.
Use: For research only. Not for use in diagnostic procedures.

Abbott ER-ICA Monoclonal. (Abbott Diagnostics) Immunoassay for the detection of estrogen receptor.
Use: For research only. Not for use in diagnostic procedures.

Abbott-HB EIA. (Abbott Diagnostics) Enzyme immunoassay for the detection of hepatitis Be antigen or antibody to

hepatitis Be antigen.
Use: Diagnostic aid.

Abbott-HBe Test. (Abbott Diagnostics) Radioimmunoassay or enzyme immunoassay for detection of hepatitis Be antigen or antibody to hepatitis Be antigen. Test kits 100s.
Use: Diagnostic aid.

Abbott HIVAB HIV-1 EIA. (Abbott Diagnostics) Enzyme immunoassay for the antibody to human immunodeficiency virus type 1 (HIV-1) in serum or plasma. Test kits 100s, 1000s.
Use: Diagnostic aid.

Abbott HIVAG-1. (Abbott Diagnostics) Enzyme immunoassay for the human immunodeficiency virus type 1 (HIV-1) antigens in serum or plasma. Test kits 100s, 1000s.
Use: Diagnostic aid.

Abbott HTLV I EIA. (Abbott Diagnostics) To detect antibody to Human T-Lymphotropic Virus Type I in serum or plasma. Test kits 100s.
Use: Diagnostic aid.

Abbott HTLV III Antigen EIA. (Abbott Diagnostics) Enzyme immunoassay for the detection of Human T-Lymphotropic Virus Type III (HIV) antigens. For research only. Not for use in diagnostic procedures.

Abbott HTLV III Confirmatory EIA. (Abbott Diagnostics) Enzyme immunoassay for confirmation of specimens found to be positive to antibody to HTL VIII. Test kits 100s.
Use: Diagnostic aid.

Abbott HTLV III EIA. (Abbott Diagnostics) Enzyme immunoassay for the detection of antibody to Human T-Lymphotropic Virus Type III (HIV) in human serum or plasma. Test kits 1s.
Use: Diagnostic aid.

Abbott IGE EIA. (Abbott Diagnostics) Enzyme immunoassay for quantitative determination of IgE in human serum and plasma. Test kits 100s.
Use: Diagnostic aid.

Abbott PAP-EIA. (Abbott Diagnostics) Enzyme immunoassay for the measurement of prostatic acid phosphatase (PAP) in serum or plasma.
Use: Diagnostic aid.

Abbott RSV-EIA. (Abbott Diagnostics) Enzyme immunoassay for the detection of respiratory syncytial virus (RSV) in nasopharyngeal washes and aspirates.
Use: Diagnostic aid.

Abbott SCC-RIA. (Abbott Diagnostics) Radioimmunoassay for the quantitative measurement of squamous cell carcinoma-associated antigen in human serum. For research only. Not for use in diagnostic procedures.

Abbott TdT EIA. (Abbott Diagnostics) Enzyme immunoassay for the quantitative measurement of terminal deoxynucleotidyl transferase (TdT), in extracts of human whole blood or isolated mononuclear cells.
Use: Diagnostic aid.

Abbott Testpack hCG-Serum. (Abbott Diagnostics) Monoclonal antibody, enzyme immunoassay for the qualitative determination of human chorionic gonadotropin (hCG) in serum. No instrumentation required.
Use: Diagnostic aid.

Abbott Testpak hCG-Urine. (Abbott Diagnostics) Monoclonal antibody, enzyme immunoassay for the qualitative determination of human chorionic gonadotropin (hCG) in urine. No instrumentation required.
Use: Diagnostic aid.

Abbott Testpack-Strep A. (Abbott Diagnostics) A rapid screening and confirmatory test for the detection of group A beta-hemolytic streptococci from throat swabs. No instrumentation required.
Use: Diagnostic aid.

Abbott Toxo-G EIA. (Abbott Diagnostics) Enzyme immunoassay for the qualitative and quantitative determination of IgG antibody to toxoplasma gondii in human serum and plasma.
Use: Diagnostic aid.

Abbott Toxo-M EIA. (Abbott Diagnostics) Enzyme immunoassay for the qualitative determination of IgM antibody to toxoplasma gondii in human serum.
Use: Diagnostic aid.

ABC to Z. (NBTY, Inc.) Iron 18 mg, Vitamins A 5000 IU, D 400 IU, E 30 IU, B_1 1.5 mg, B_2 1.7 mg, B_3 20 mg, B_5 10 mg, B_6 2 mg, B_{12} 6 mcg, C 60 mg, folic acid 0.4 mg, biotin 30 mcg, Ca, P, I, Mg, Cu, Mn, K, Cl, Cr, Mo, Se, Ni, Si, Sn, V, B, vitamin K, Zn 15 mg/Tab. Bot. 100s. *otc.*
Use: Mineral, vitamin supplement.

•**abciximab.** (ab-SICK-sih-mab) USAN.
Use: Monoclonal antibody (antithrombotic).
See: ReoPro (Eli Lilly and Co.).

Abelcet. (Liposome Co.) Amphotericin B 100 mg/20 ml (as lipid complex)/Susp. for Inj. Single-use Vial w/5-micron filter needles. *Rx.*
Use: Invasive fungal infections. [Orphan Drug]

Abitrexate. (International Pharm) Methotrexate sodium 25 mg/ml. Vial 2 ml, 4 ml, 8 ml. *Rx.*
Use: Antineoplastic.

•**ablukast.** (ab-LOO-kast) USAN.
Use: Antiasthmatic (leukotriene antagonist).

•**ablukast sodium.** (ab-LOO-kast) USAN.
Use: Antiasthmatic (leukotriene antagonist).
See: Ulpax (Roche Laboratories).

abortifacients.
See: Hemabate, Inj. (Pharmacia & Upjohn).
Prostin E_2, Supp. (Pharmacia & Upjohn).

absorbable cellulose cotton or gauze.
See: Oxidized Cellulose (Various Mfr.).

absorbable dusting powder.
Use: Lubricant.

absorbable gelatin film.
Use: Hemostatic, topical.
See: Gelfilm (Pharmacia & Upjohn).
Gelfilm Ophthalmic (Pharmacia & Upjohn).

absorbable gelatin powder.
Use: Hemostatic, topical.
See: Gelfoam, Pow. (Pharmacia & Upjohn).

absorbable gelatin sponge.
Use: Hemostatic.
See: Gelfoam (Pharmacia & Upjohn).

absorbable surgical suture.
Use: Surgical aid.

Absorbase. (Carolina Medical Products) Petrolatum, mineral oil, ceresin wax, wool wax, alcohol. Oint. Tube 114 g, 454 g. *otc.*
Use: Pharmaceutical aid, emollient base.

absorbent gauze.
Use: Surgical aid.

Absorbent Rub Relief Formula. (De-Witt) Green soap 11.64%, camphor 1.63%, menthol 1.63%, pine tar soap 0.87%, wintergreen oil 0.71%, sassafras oil 0.54%, benzocaine 0.48%, capsicum 0.03%, wormwood oil 0.6%, isopropyl alcohol 75%. Bot. 2 oz. *otc.*
Use: Analgesic, topical.

Absorbine Arthritis Strength Liquid with Capsaicin. (W.F. Young, Inc.) Natural menthol 4%, capsaicin 0.025%, acetone, calendula plant extracts, echinacea, wormwood. Liq. *otc.*
Use: Liniment.

Absorbine Athlete's Foot Cream. (W.F. Young, Inc.) Tolnaftate 1%, parabens. Cream Tube. 21.3 g. *otc.*
Use: Antifungal, topical.

Absorbine FootCare. (W.F. Young, Inc.) Tolnaftate 1%, menthol, acetone, chloroxylenol, wormwood oil. Spray Liq. Bot. 59.2 ml, 118.3 ml. *otc.*
Use: Antifungal, topical.

Absorbine Foot Powder. (W.F. Young, Inc.) Zinc stearate, parachloroxylenol, aluminum chlorhydroxy, allantonate, benzethonium Cl, menthol. Plastic bot. 3 oz w/shaker top. *otc.*
Use: Antifungal, topical.

Absorbine, Jr. (W.F. Young, Inc.) Wormwood, thymol, chloroxylenol, menthol, acetone, zinc stearate, parachloroxylenol, aluminum chlorhydroxy, allantonate, benzethonium Cl, menthol. Liq. Bot. 1oz, 2 oz, 4 oz, 12 oz w/applicator. *otc.*
Use: Analgesic; antifungal, topical.

Absorbine Jr. Extra Strength Liniment. (W.F. Young, Inc.) Natural menthol 4%, plant extracts of calendula, echinacea and wormwood, acetone, chloroxylenol iodine, potassium iodide, thymol, wormwood oil. Lot. Bot. 59 ml, 118 ml. *otc.*
Use: Liniment.

Absorbine Jr. Extra Strength Liquid. (W.F. Young, Inc.) Menthol 4%. Liq. Bot. 59 ml, 118 ml. *otc.*
Use: Rub or liniment.

Absorbine Jr. Liniment. (W.F. Young, Inc.) Menthol 1.27%, plant extracts of calendula, echinacea and wormwood, iodine, potassium iodide, thymol, acetone, chloroxylenol. Lot. Bot. 60 ml, 120 ml. *otc.*
Use: Liniment.

Abuscreen. (Roche Laboratories) An immunological and radiochemical assay for morphine and morphine glucuronide in nanogram levels. Utilizes I-125 labeled morphine requiring gamma scintillation equipment. Tests 100s.
Use: Diagnostic aid.

•**acacia.** (ah-KAY-shah) N.F. 18.
Use: Pharmaceutic aid (suspending, viscosity agent).

•**acadesine.** (ack-AH-dess-een) USAN.
Use: Platelet aggregation inhibitor.

•**acarbose.** (A-car-bose) USAN.
Use: Inhibitor (α-glucosidase).
See: Precose, Tab. (Bayer Corp. (Consumer Div.)).

Accolate. (Zeneca Pharmaceuticals) Zafirlukast 20 mg/Tab. Bot. 60s, 100s. *Rx.*
Use: Treatment of asthma.

Accupep HPF. (Sherwood Davis & Geck) Hydrolyzed lactalbumin, maltodextrin, MCT oil, corn oil, mono- and diglycerides, vitamins A, B_1, B_2, B_3, B_5, B_6,

B_{12}, C, D, E, K, Ca, Cl, Cu, Fe, I, Mg, Mn, P, Zn, biotin, and choline. Pks. 128 g. *otc.*
Use: Nutritional supplement.

Accupril. (Parke-Davis) Quinapril 5 mg, 10 mg, 20 mg, 40 mg/Tab. Bot. Lactose. 90s and UD 100s. *Rx.*
Use: Antihypertensive.

Accurbron. (Hoechst Marion Roussel) Theophylline, anhydrous 10 mg/ml. Bot. Pt. *Rx.*
Use: Bronchodilator.

Accusens T Taste Function Kit. (Westport Pharmaceuticals, Inc.) Test for ability to distinguish among salty, sweet, sour, and bitter tastants. Kit contains 15 bottles (60 ml) tastants and 30 taste record forms.
Use: Diagnostic aid.

Accutane. (Roche Laboratories) Isotretinoin 10 mg, 20 mg, or 40 mg/Cap. Bot. UD 100s. *Rx.*
Use: Dermatologic, acne.

Accuzyme. (Healthpoint Medical) Papain 1.1×10^4 IU/g, urea 10% in a hydrophilic ointment base. Oint. Tube 30 g. *Rx.*
Use: Enzyme combination, topical.

A-C-D Solution. Sodium citrate, citric acid, and dextrosein sterile pyrogen-free solution. (Baxter Pharmaceutical Products, Inc.). 600 ml bot. with 70 ml, 120 ml, 300 ml Soln.; 1000 ml Bot. with 500 ml Soln. (Bayer Biological). 500 ml Bot. with 75 ml, 120 ml Soln.; 650 ml bot. with 80 ml, 130 ml Soln. (The Diamond Co.). 250 ml, 500 ml (Abbo-Vac). *Rx.*
Use: Anticoagulant for preparation of plasma or whole blood.

A-C-D Solution Modified. (Bristol-Myers Squibb) Acid citrate dextrose anticoagulant solution modified. *Rx.*
Use: Anticoagulant, radiolabeled.

•**acebutolol.** (ass-cee-BYOO-toe-lahl) USAN.
Use: Antiadrenergic (β-receptor).
See: Sectral, Cap. (Wyeth-Ayerst Laboratories).

•**acebutolol hydrochloride.** (ass-cee-BYOO-toe-lahl) U.S.P. 23.
Use: Antiadrenergic (β-receptor).
See: Sectral, Cap. (Wyeth-Ayerst Laboratories).

acebutolol hydrochloride. (ass-cee-BYOO-toe-lahl) (Mylan Pharmaceuticals) 200, 400 mg/Cap. Bot. 100s. *Rx.*
Use: Antiadrenergic.

•**acecainide hydrochloride.** (ASS-eh-CANE-ide) USAN.
Use: Cardiovascular agent.
See: NAPA (Medco Research, Inc.; Parke-Davis).

•**aceclidine.** (ass-ECK-lih-DEEN) USAN.
Use: Cholinergic.

•**acedapsone.** (ASS-eh-DAP-sone) USAN.
Use: Antimalarial; antibacterial (leprostatic).

Acedoval. (Pal-Pak, Inc.) Dover's powder 15 mg, ipecac 1.5 mg, aspirin 162 mg, caffeine anhydrous 8.1 mg/Tab. Bot. 1000s, 5000s. *otc.*
Use: Analgesic, antispasmodic, antiperistaltic.

•**aceglutamide aluminum.** (AH-see-GLUE-tah-mide ah-LOO-min-uhm) USAN.
Use: Antiulcerative.

Acel-Imune. (ESI Lederle Generics) Diphtheria toxoid 7.5 Lf units, tetanus toxoid 5 Lf units, acellular pertussis vaccine 300 hemagglutinating units and aluminum ≤ 0.85 mg/0.5 ml. With formaldehyde ≤ 0.02%, thimerosal final concentration of 1:10,000. Aluminum hydroxide and phosphate, thimerosal, gelatin, glycine, polysorbate 80.5 ml/ Vial for Inj. *Rx.*
Use: Immunization.

•**acemannan.** (ah-see-MAN-an) USAN.
Use: Antiviral; immunomodulator.
See: Carrisyn (Carrington Labs).

Aceon. (Ortho McNeil Pharmaceutical) Perindopril erbumine 2 mg, 4 mg, or 8 mg. Tab. Bot. 100s and UD blister packs. *Rx.*
Use: Antihypertensive.

Acephen. (G & W Laboratories) **Adult:** Acetaminophen 650 mg/Supp. Box 12s, 100s. **Pediatric:** Acetaminophen 120 mg/Supp. Box 12s, 100s. *otc.*
Use: Analgesic.

acepromazine. (ASS-ee-PRO-mah-zeen) (Wyeth-Ayerst Laboratories) *Rx.*
Use: Anxiolytic.

Acerola-C. (Barth's) Vitamin C 300 mg/ Wafer. Bot. 30s, 90s, 180s, 360s. *otc.*
Use: Vitamin supplement.

Acerola-Plex. (Barth's) Vitamin C 100 mg, bioflavonoids 50 mg/Tab. Bot. 100s, 500s. *otc.*
Use: Vitamin supplement.

Aceta. (Century Pharmaceuticals, Inc.) Acetaminophen 325 mg or 500 mg/ Tab. Bot. 100s, 1000s. *otc.*
Use: Analgesic.

Aceta w/Codeine. (Century Pharmaceuticals, Inc.) Acetaminophen 300 mg, codeine phosphate 30 mg/Tab. Bot. 100s. *c-III.*

Use: Analgesic combination-narcotic.

Aceta Elixir. (Century Pharmaceuticals, Inc.) Acetaminophen 160 mg/5 ml, alcohol 7%. Elix. Bot. 120 ml, 1 gal. *otc.*
Use: Analgesic.

Aceta-Gesic. (Rugby Labs, Inc.) Acetaminophen 325 mg, phenyltoloxamine citrate 30 mg/Tab. Bot. 100s, 1000s. *otc.*
Use: Analgesic, antihistamine.

•**acetaminophen.** (ass-cet-ah-MEE-noe-fen) U.S.P. 23. APAP.
Use: Analgesic, antipyretic.
See: Acephen, Supp. (G & W Laboratories).
Aceta, Tab., Elix., Supp. (Century Pharmaceuticals, Inc.).
Acetaminophen Uniserts, Supp. (Upsher-Smith Labs, Inc.).
Actamin, Tab. (Buffington).
Actamin Extra, Tab. (Buffington).
Aminodyne, Elix. (Jones Medical Industries, Inc.).
Anexsia 5/500, Tab. (Mallinckrodt).
Anexsia 7.5/650, Tab. (Mallinckrodt).
Anexsia 10/660, Tab. (Mallinckrodt).
Apap, Cap., Tab. (Various Mfr.).
Children's Dynafed Jr., Chew. Tab. (BDI Pharmaceuticals, Inc.).
Dapa, Tab. (Ferndale Laboratories, Inc.).
Dorcol, Prods. (Novartis Pharmaceutical Corp.).
Dynafed Jr., Children's, Chew. Tab. (BDI Pharmaceuticals, Inc.).
Extra Strength Dynafed E.X., Tab (BDI Pharmaceuticals, Inc.).
G-1 (Roberts Pharmaceuticals).
Genapap, Chew. Tab. (Zenith Goldline Pharmaceuticals).
Genebs, Tab., Cap. (Zenith Goldline Pharmaceuticals).
Halenol, Tab., Elix. (Halsey Drug Co.).
Liquiprin, Soln. (SmithKline Beecham Pharmaceuticals).
Meda Cap, Cap. (Circle Pharmaceuticals, Inc.).
Meda Tab, Tab. (Circle Pharmaceuticals, Inc.).
Neopap, Supp. (PolyMedica Pharmaceuticals).
Panadol, Cap., Chew. Tab., Tab., Liq. Drops (Bayer Corp. (Consumer Div.)).
Panex, Tab. (Roberts Pharmaceuticals).
Parten, Tab. (Parmed Pharmaceuticals, Inc.).
Phenaphen, Cap., Tab. (Wyeth-Ayerst Laboratories).
Proval, Cap., Elix., Drops, Tab. (Solvay Pharmaceuticals).
Suppap-120, 325, 650, Supp. (Raway Pharmacal, Inc.).
Temetan, Elix., Tab. (Nevin).
Tempra, Drops, Syr. (Bristol-Myers Squibb).
Ty-Caplets, Tab. (Major Pharmaceuticals).
Ty-Caps, Cap. (Major Pharmaceuticals).
Tylenol, Drops, Elix., Liq., Tab., Chew. Tab. (Ortho McNeil Pharmaceutical).
Tylenol Extra-Strength, Tab., Cap. (Ortho McNeil Pharmaceutical).
Ty-Pap, Supp., Elix. (Major Pharmaceuticals).
Ty-Tabs, Tab. (Major Pharmaceuticals).

acetaminophen w/combinations.
See: Aceta w/Codeine, Tab. (Century Pharmaceuticals, Inc.).
Acid-X, Tab. (BDI Pharmaceuticals, Inc.).
Actifed Plus, Tab. (GlaxoWellcome).
Actifed Sinus Daytime/Nighttime, Capl. (GlaxoWellcome).
Allerest Headache Strength, Tab. (Novartis Pharmaceutical Corp.).
Allergy-Sinus Comtrex, Capl., Tab. (Bristol-Myers Squibb).
Alumadrine, Tab. (Fleming & Co.).
Amaphen, Cap. (Trimen Laboratories, Inc.).
Anexsia, Tab. (Mallinckrodt).
Anodynos Forte, Tab. (Buffington).
Anoquan, Cap. (Roberts Pharmaceuticals).
Apap w/Codeine, Tab. (Schwarz Pharma, Inc.).
Aspirin Free Anacin P.M., Tab. (Wyeth-Ayerst Laboratories).
Aspirin-Free Bayer Select Head & Chest Cold, Capl. (Bayer Corp. (Allergy Div.)).
Axocet, Cap. (Savage Laboratories).
Bayer Select Flu Relief, Capl. (Bayer Corp. (Consumer Div.)).
Bayer Select Head Cold, Capl. (Bayer Corp. (Consumer Div.)).
Bayer Select Night Time Cold, Capl. (Bayer Corp. (Consumer Div.)).
Bromo Seltzer, Gran. (Warner Lambert).
Bupap, Tab. (ECR Pharmaceuticals).
Capital and Codeine, Susp. (Carnrick Laboratories, Inc.).
Children's Cepacol, Liq. (JB Williams).
Children's Dynafed Jr., Chew. Tab. (BDI Pharmaceuticals, Inc.).
Children's Tylenol Cold Plus Cough, Chew. Tab. (Ortho McNeil Pharmaceutical).

Codimal, Tab. (Schwarz Pharma, Inc.).
Comtrex Caplets (Bristol-Myers Squibb).
Comtrex Liquid (Bristol-Myers Squibb).
Comtrex Liqui-Gels (Bristol-Myers Squibb).
Comtrex Tablets (Bristol-Myers Squibb).
Contac Day & Night Allergy/Sinus Caplets (SmithKline Beecham Pharmaceuticals).
Contac Day & Night Cold & Flu Caplets (SmithKline Beecham Pharmaceuticals).
Coricidin, Tab. (Schering-Plough Corp.).
Coricidin D, Tab. (Schering-Plough Corp.).
Coricidin Sinus Headache, Tab. (Schering-Plough Corp.).
Darvocet-N 100, Tab. (Eli Lilly and Co.).
DHC Plus, Cap. (Purdue Frederick Co.).
Dristan Cold Multi-Symptom Formula, Tab. (Whitehall Robins Laboratories).
Drixoral Cold & Flu, Tab. (Schering-Plough Corp.).
Drixoral Cough & Sore Throat, Liquid caps. (Schering-Plough Corp.).
Endolor, Cap. (Keene).
Esgesic, Cap., Tab. (Gilbert).
Esgesic-Plus, Tab. (Forest Pharmaceutical, Inc.).
Excedrin Aspirin Free, Cap. (Bristol-Myers Squibb).
Excedrin Extra Strength, Geltab. (Bristol-Myers Squibb).
Excedrin Sinus, Capl., Tab. (Bristol-Myers Squibb).
Extra Strength Dynafed E.X., Tab. (BDI Pharmaceuticals, Inc.).
Femcet, Cap. (Russ).
Fem-1, Tab. (BDI Pharmaceuticals, Inc.).
Fioricet, Tab. (Novartis Pharmaceutical Corp.).
Fiorpap, Tab. (Creighton).
Flextra-DS (Poly Pharm).
Hycomine Compound, Tab. (DuPont Merck Pharmaceutical Co.).
Hydrocet, Cap. (Carnrick Laboratories, Inc.).
Hy-Phen, Tab. (B.F. Ascher and Co.).
Isocet, Tab. (Rugby Labs, Inc.).
Liquiprin, Soln. (Menley & James Labs, Inc.).
Lortab, Elix. (UCB Pharmaceuticals, Inc.).
Lortab 10/500, Tab. (UCB Pharmaceuticals, Inc.).
Mapap CF, Tab. (Major Pharmaceuticals).
Margesic, Cap. (Major Pharmaceuticals).
Maximum Strength Arthriten, Tab. (Alva/Amco Pharmacal Cos. Inc.).
Medigesic, Cap. (US Pharm).
Midol Maximum Strength, Tab. (Bayer Corp. (Consumer Div.)).
Midol Teen, Cap. (Bayer Corp. (Consumer Div.)).
Midrin, Cap. (Carnrick Laboratories, Inc.).
Multi-Symptom Tylenol Cough, Liq. (Ortho McNeil Pharmaceutical).
Multi-Symptom Tylenol Cough with Decongestant (Ortho McNeil Pharmaceutical).
Naldegesic, Tab. (Bristol-Myers Squibb).
N-D Gesic, Tab. (Hyrex Pharmaceuticals).
Norco (Watson Labs).
Nyquil, Liq. (Procter & Gamble Pharm.).
Ornex (Menley & James Labs, Inc.).
Ornex Maximum Strength, Cap. (Menley & James Labs, Inc.).
Pamprin Prods. (Chattem Consumer Products).
Percocet, Tab. (DuPont Merck Pharmaceutical Co.).
Percogesic, Tab. (DuPont Merck Pharmaceutical Co.).
Phenaphen #2, #3, #4 (Robins).
Phrenilin, Tab. (Carnrick Labs.).
Prominol, Tab. (MCR American Pharm.).
Propacet 100, Tab. (Teva USA).
Proval No. 3, Tab. (Solvay).
Quiet World, Tab. (Whitehall Robins).
Renpap, Tab. (Wren).
Repan, Tab. (Everett Laboratories).
Repan CF, Tab. (Everett Laboratories).
Robitussin Night Relief (Whitehall Robins).
Saleto, Tab. (Roberts Pharm.).
Saleto D, Tab. (Roberts Pharm.).
Sedapap, Tab. (Merz).
Sinarest, Tab. (Novartis).
Sine-Aid Maximum Strength, Cap., Tab. (McNeil Consumer Products).
Sine-Off Maximum Strength No Drowsiness Formula, Capl. (SmithKline Beecham Pharmaceuticals).
Sine-Off Sinus Medicine, Capl. (SmithKline Beecham Pharmaceuticals).

Sinulin, Tab. (Carnrick Labs.).
Sinutab, Prods. (Warner Lambert).
St. Joseph Cold Tablets for Children, Tab. (Schering Plough).
Sudafed Cold & Cough, Liq. Cap. (GlaxoWellcome).
Sudafed Severe Cold, Tab. (GlaxoWellcome).
Supac, Tab. (Mission Pharmacal).
Talacen, Cap. (Sanofi Winthrop).
Tencon (Inter Ethical Labs).
Triad, Cap. (UAD).
Triaminic Sore Throat Formula, Liq. (Novartis).
Triaprin, Cap. (Dunhall Pharmaceuticals).
Two-Dyne, Tab. (Hyrex).
Tylenol Children's Chewable Tablets (Ortho McNeil Pharmaceutical).
Tylenol Children's Cold Tablets (Ortho McNeil Pharmaceutical).
Tylenol Children's Suspension (Ortho McNeil Pharmaceutical).
Tylenol Cold, Liq., Cap., Tab. (Ortho McNeil Pharmaceutical).
Tylenol Cold & Flu No Drowsiness, Pow. (Ortho McNeil Pharmaceutical).
Tylenol Cold Night Time, Liq. (Ortho McNeil Pharmaceutical).
Tylenol Cold No Drowsiness, Capl., Gelcap. (Ortho McNeil Pharmaceutical).
Tylenol Cough, Liq. (Ortho McNeil Pharmaceutical).
Tylenol Extended Relief, Capl. (Ortho McNeil Pharmaceutical).
Tylenol w/Codeine, Tab. (Ortho McNeil Pharmaceutical).
Tylenol, Preps. (Ortho McNeil Pharmaceutical).
Tylox, Cap. (Ortho McNeil Pharmaceutical).
Vanquish, Tab. (Bayer Corp.).
Vicks NyQuil Multi-Symptom Cold and Flu Relief, Liq. (Procter & Gamble).
Vicodin, Tab. (Knoll Pharmaceuticals).
Vicodin HP, Tab. (Knoll Pharmaceuticals).
Viro-Med, Tab. (Whitehall Robins).
Wygesic, Tab. (Wyeth-Ayerst).
Zydone, Cap. (DuPont Merck Pharmaceuticals).

acetaminophen and aspirin tablets.
Use: Analgesic.

acetaminophen and caffeine.
Use: Analgesic.
See: Excedrin Extra Strength (Bristol-Myers Squibb).

acetaminophen, aspirin, and caffeine. Cap.,Tab.
Use: Analgesic.

Acetaminophen w/Codeine. (ass-cet-ah-MEE-noe-fen) (Various Mfr.) **Tab.:** Codeine phosphate 15 mg, acetaminophen 300 mg/Tab. Bot. 100s, 500s, 1000s. Codeine phosphate 30 mg, acetaminophen 300 mg/Tab. Bot. 100s, 500s, 1000s, UD 100s, RN 100s. Codeine phosphate 60 mg, acetaminophen 300 mg/Tab. Bot. 100s, 500s, 1000s. *c-iii.* **Soln.:** Codeine phosphate 12 mg, acetaminophen 120 mg/5 ml. Bot. 120 ml, 500 ml, Pt, gal, UD 5 ml, 12.5 ml, 15 ml. *c-v.*
Use: Analgesic combination-narcotic.

acetaminophen and butalbital.
Use: Analgesic.
See: Axocet (Savage Labs).
Bupap, Tab. (ECR Pharmaceuticals).
Margesic (Marnel).
Prominol (MCR AMerican Pharm).
Repan CF (Everett).
Tencon (Inter. Ethical Labs).
Triad (UAD).

acetaminophen and codeine phosphate oral solution.
Use: Analgesic.

acetaminophen and diphenhydramine citrate.
Use: Analgesic, antihistamine.
See: Excedrin PM, Prods. (Bristol-Myers Squibb).
Legatrin PM, Capl. (Columbia Laboratories, Inc.).
Midol PM, Capl. (Bayer Corp. (Consumer Div.)).

acetaminophen and pamabrom tablets.
Use: Analgesic.
See: Fem-1, Tab. (BDI Pharmaceuticals, Inc.).

acetaminophen and pseudoephedrine hydrochloride tablets.
Use: Analgesic, decongestant.
See: Allerest No Drowsiness, Tab. (Ciba Vision).
Coldrine, Tab. (Roberts Pharmaceuticals).
Maximum Strength Dynafed Plus, Tab. (BDI Pharmaceuticals, Inc.).
Ornex No Drowsiness, Tab. (Menley & James Labs, Inc.).
Sinus Relief, Tab. (Major Pharmaceuticals).

acetaminophen oral solution.
Use: Analgesic.

acetaminophen oral suspension.
Use: Analgesic.

acetaminophen suppositories.
Use: Analgesic.

acetaminophen uniserts. (Upsher-

Smith Labs, Inc.) Acetaminophen **120 mg or 325 mg/Supp.:** Ctn. 12s, 50s. **650 mg/Supp.:** Ctn. 12s, 50s, 500s. *otc.*
Use: Analgesic.

acetaminophenol.
See: Acetaminophen.

acetanilid. (Various Mfr.) (Acetylaminobenzene, acetylaniline, antifebrin).
Use: Analgesic (former use).

Acetasol.
See: Acetarsone.

Acetasol HC Otic. (Zenith Goldline Pharmaceuticals) Hydrocortisone 1%, acetic acid 2%. Bot. 10 ml. *Rx.*
Use: Anti-infective; corticosteroid, otic.

Acetasol Otic. (Zenith Goldline Pharmaceuticals) Acetic acid (non-aqueous) 2%. Bot. 5 ml. *Rx.*
Use: Anti-infective, otic.

•**acetazolamide.** (uh-seet-uh-ZOLE-uh-mide) U.S.P. 23.
Use: Carbonic anhydrase inhibitor.
See: Diamox (ESI Lederle Generics).

acetazolamide. (Various Mfr.) **Tab.:** 125 mg, Bot. 100s; 250 mg, Bot. 100s, 1000s, UD 100s. **Pow.:** 500 mg/vial.
Use: Carbonic anhydrase inhibitor.

•**acetazolamide sodium, sterile.** (uh-seet-uh-ZOLE-uh-mide) U.S.P. 23.
Use: Carbonic anhydrase inhibitor.

acet-dia-mer-sulfonamide. Sulfacetamide, sulfadiazine, and sulfamerazine, Susp. *Rx.*
Use: Antibacterial, sulfonamide.

Acetest Reagent. (Bayer Corp. (Consumer Div.)) Sodium nitroprusside, disodium phosphate, aminoacetic acid, lactose. Tab. Bot. 100s, 250s.
Use: Diagnostic aid.

•**acetic acid.** (ah-SEE-tick) N.F. 18.
Use: Pharmaceutic aid (acidifying agent).
See: Borofair Otic (Major).
Otic Domeboro, Soln. (Bayer Corp. (Consumer Div.)).
Vosol Otic Solution (Wallace Laboratories).

•**acetic acid, glacial.** U.S.P. 23.
Use: Pharmaceutic aid (acidifying agent).
See: Aci-Jel (Ortho McNeil Pharmaceutical).

acetic acid irrigation. (Abbott Laboratories) 0.25% soln. 250 ml glass cont.; 250 ml, 1000 ml.
Use: Irrigating solution.

Acetic Acid Otic. (Various Mfr.) Acetic acid 2% with propylene glycol diacetate 3%, benzethonium chloride 0.02%, and sodium acetate 0.015%. Soln. Bot. 15 ml, 30 ml, 60 ml. *Rx.*
Use: Otic preparation.

acetic acid, potassium salt. Potassium Acetate, U.S.P. 23.

•**acetohexamide.** (uh-seet-toe-HEX-uh-mide) U.S.P. 23.
Use: Antidiabetic.
See: Dymelor, Tab. (Eli Lilly).

acetohexamide. (Various Mfr.) 250 or 500 mg/Tab. Bot. 100s. *Rx.*
Use: Antidiabetic.

•**acetohydroxamic acid.** (ass-EE-toe-high-drox-AM-ik) U.S.P. 23.
Use: Enzyme inhibitor (urease).
See: Lithostat (Mission Pharmacal Co.).

acetomeroctol.
Use: Antiseptic, topical.

•**acetone.** (ASS-eh-tone) N.F. 18.
Use: Pharmaceutic aid (solvent).

acetone or diacetic acid test.
See: Acetest, Tab. (Bayer Corp. (Consumer Div.)).

acetophenetidin.
Use: Analgesic, antipyretic.
See: Phenacetin, Ethoxyacetanilide.

•**acetosulfone sodium.** (ah-SET-oh-SULL-fone) USAN.
Use: Antibacterial (leprostatic).

acetoxyphenylmercury.
See: Phenylmercuric acetate.

n-acetyl-p-aminophenol. Acetaminophen.

acetylaniline.
See: Acetanilid (Various Mfr.).

acetyl-bromo-diethylacetyl-carbamide.
See: Acetylcarbromal (Various Mfr.).

acetylcarbromal. Acetyladalin, acetylbromodiethylacetylcarbamide. Pow. for manufacturing.
Use: Sedative.
See: Paxarel, Tab. (Circle Pharmaceuticals, Inc.).

•**acetylcholine chloride.** (ah-SEH-till-KOE-leen KLOR-ide) U.S.P. 23.
Use: Cardiovascular agent; cholinergic; miotic; vasodilator (peripheral).
See: Miochol Ophthalmic (Ciba Vision).
Miochol-E (Ciba Vision).

acetylcholine-like therapeutic agents.
See: Cholinergic agents.

•**acetylcysteine.** (ASS-cee-till-SIS-teen) U.S.P. 23.
Use: Mucolytic. [Orphan Drug]
See: Acetylcysteine (Various Mfr.).
Mucosil (Dey Laboratories, Inc.).
Mucomyst, Soln. (Bristol-Myers Squibb).

acetylcysteine. (Various Mfr.) Soln: 10%, in 4, 10, and 30 ml vials; 20%, in 4, 10,

30, and 100 ml vials. *Rx.*
Use: Mucolytic.

acetylcysteine. (ASS-cee-till-sis-teen)
Use: Treatment for severe acetaminophen overdose. [Orphan Drug]
See: Mucomyst (Apothecon, Inc.).
Mucomyst 10 IV (Apothecon, Inc.).

acetylcysteine and isoproterenol hydrochloride inhalation solution.
Use: Mucolytic.

acetylin.
See: Acetylsalicylic Acid (Various Mfr.).

acetylphenylisatin. *Rx.*
See: Oxyphenisatin Acetate.

acetylprocainamide-n.
Use: Cardiovascular agent.
See: acecainide, NAPA.

acetylsalicylic acid. Aspirin.
Use: Analgesic; antipyretic; antirheumatic.
See: Aspirin Preps. (Various Mfr.).

n[1]-acetylsulfanilamide.
Use: Sulfonamide therapy.

acetyl sulfisoxazole.
See: Sulfisoxazole Acetyl.

acetyltannic acid. Tannic acid acetate.
Use: Antiperistaltic.

AC Eye Drops. (Walgreen Co.) Tetrahydrozoline HCl 0.05%, zinc sulfate 0.25%. Bot. 0.75 oz. *otc.*
Use: Decongestant combination, ophthalmic.

achlorhydria therapy.
See: Glutamic Acid HCl (Various Mfr.).

Achol. (Enzyme Process) Vitamin A 4000 units, ketocholanic acids 62 mg/Tab. Bot. 100s, 250s. *otc.*
Use: Vitamin supplement.

acid acriflavine.
See: Acriflavine HCl (Various Mfr.).

acid citrate dextrose anticoagulant solution modified.
See: A-C-D Solution Modified (Bristol-Myers Squibb).

acid citrate dextrose solution.
See: A-C-D Solution (Various Mfr.).

acidifiers.
See: Ammonium Cl (Various Mfr.).
K-Phos M.F. (Beach Pharmaceuticals).

Acid Mantle. (Doak Dermatologics) Water, cetearyl alcohol, sodium lauryl sulfate, sodium cetearyl sulfate, petrolatum, glycerin, synthetic beeswax, mineral oil, methlyparaben, aluminum sulfate, calcium acetate, white potato dextrin. Cream. Jar 4 oz. *otc.*
Use: Ointment, lotion base.

Acid Mantle. (Novartis Pharmaceutical Corp.) Aluminum sulfate, calcium acetate, cetearyl alcohol, glycerin, light mineral oil, methylparaben, sodium lauryl sulfate, synthetic beeswax, white petrolatum, ammonium hydroxide, citric acid. Cream. Jar 120 g. *otc.*
Use: Pharmaceutic aid, emollient base.

Acid Mantle Creme. (Novartis Pharmaceutical Corp.) Aluminum acetate in specially prepared water-soluble hydrophilic cream at pH 4.2. Tube 1 oz, Jar 4 oz, lb. *otc.*
Use: Ointment, lotion base.

acidophilus.
See: Bacid (Medeva Pharmaceuticals, Inc.).
Lactinex (Becton Dickinson & Co.).
More Dophilus (Freeda Vitamins, Inc.).

acidophilus w/pectin. (Barth's) *Lactobacillus acidophilus* w/natural citrus pectin 100 mg/Cap. Bot. 100s. *otc.*
Use: Antidiarrheal.

acid trypaflavine.
See: Acriflavine HCl. (Various Mfr.).

Acidulated Phosphate Fluoride. (Scherer Laboratories, Inc.) Fluoride ion 0.31% in 0.1 molar phosphate. Soln. Bot. 64 oz. (Office Product).
Use: Dental caries agent.

Acid-X. (BDI Pharmaceuticals, Inc.) Acetaminophen 500 mg, calcium carbonate 250 mg/Tab. Bot. 36s. *otc.*
Use: Antacid.

•**acifran.** (ACE-ih-FRAN) USAN.
Use: Antihyperlipoproteinemic.

Aci-jel. (Ortho McNeil Pharmaceutical) Glacial acetic acid 0.921%, ricinoleic acid 0.7%, oxyquinoline sulfate 0.025%, glycerin 5%. Propylparaben. Vag. jelly Tube 85 g w/dose applicator. *Rx.*
Use: Vaginal agent.

•**acitretin.** (ASS-ih-TREH-tin) USAN.
Use: Antipsoriatic.
See: Soriatane, Cap. (Roche Laboratories).

•**acivicin.** (ace-ih-VIH-sin) USAN.
Use: Antineoplastic.

•**aclarubicin.** (ack-lah-ROO-bih-sin) USAN. *Formerly Aclacinomycin A.*
Use: Antineoplastic.

Aclophen. (Nutripharm Laboratories, Inc.) Phenylephrine HCl 40 mg, chlorpheniramine maleate 8 mg, acetaminophen 500 mg/S.R. tab. Dye free. Bot. 100s. *Rx.*
Use: Analgesic, antihistamine, decongestant.

Aclovate. (GlaxoWellcome) Alclometasone dipropionate 0.05%. Cream or Oint. Tube 15 g, 45 g. *Rx.*
Use: Anti-inflammatory, topical.

A.C.N. (Person and Covey, Inc.) Vitamin A 25,000 IU, ascorbic acid 250 mg, niacinamide 25 mg/Tab. Bot. 100s. *otc.*
Use: Vitamin supplement.

Acnaveen. (Rydelle Laboratories)
See: Aveenobar Medicated (Rydelle Laboratories).

Acna-Vite. (Cenci, H.R. Labs, Inc.) Vitamins A 10,000 IU, C 250 mg, hesperidin 50 mg, niacinamide 25 mg/Cap. Bot. 75s. *otc.*
Use: Dermatologic, acne; vitamin supplement.

Acne-5. (Various Mfr.) Benzoyl peroxide 5%. Mask 30 ml. *otc.*
Use: Dermatologic, acne.

Acne-10. (Various Mfr.) Benzoyl peroxide 10%. Bot. 30 ml. *otc.*
Use: Dermatologic, acne.

Acno Cleanser. (Baker Cummins Dermatologicals, Inc.) Isopropyl alcohol 60%, laureth-23, tetrasodium EDTA. Bot. 240 ml. *otc.*
Use: Dermatologic, acne.

Acno Lotion. (Baker Cummins Dermatologicals, Inc.) Micronized sulfur 3%. Bot. 120 ml. *otc.*
Use: Dermatologic, acne.

Acnomel. (Menley & James Labs, Inc.) Resorcinol 2%, sulfur 8%, alcohol 11%. Cream Tube 28 g. *otc.*
Use: Dermatologic, acne.

Acnotex. (C & M Pharmacal, Inc.) Sulfur 8%, resorcinol 2%, isopropyl alcohol 20%, acetone. In lotion base. Bot. 60 ml. *otc.*
Use: Dermatologic, acne.

•**acodazole hydrochloride.** (ah-KOE-dah-ZOLE) USAN.
Use: Antineoplastic.

aconiazide. (Lincoln Diagnostics)
Use: Antituberculous. [Orphan Drug]

Acotus. (Whorton Pharmaceuticals, Inc.) Phenylephrine HCl 5 mg, guaiacol glyceryl ether 100 mg, menthol 1 mg, alcohol by volume 10%/5 ml. Bot. 4 oz, 12 oz, gal. *otc.*
Use: Antitussive, decongestant.

ACR. (Western Research) Ammonium Cl 7.5 gr/Tab. Handicount 28s (36 bags of 28 tab.). *Rx.*
Use: Diuretic.

acriflavine. (Eli Lilly and Co.) 1.5 gr/Tab. Bot. 100s.
Use: Antiseptic.

acriflavine hydrochloride. (Various Mfr.) Hydrochloride form of acriflavine. Acid acriflavine, acid trypaflavine, flavine, trypaflavine. National Aniline-Pow., Bot. (1 g, 5 g, 10 g, 25 g, 50 g). Tab. (1.5 gr). Bot. 50s, 100s. *Rx.*
Use: Anti-infective.

•**acrisorcin.** (ACK-rih-sahr-sin) USAN, U.S.P. XXII.
Use: Antifungal.
See: Akrinol (Schering-Plough Corp.).

•**acrivastine.** (ACK-rih-VASS-teen) USAN.
Use: Antihistamine.
See: Semprex-D, Cap. (Glaxo-Wellcome).

•**acronine.** (ACK-row-neen) USAN.
Use: Antineoplastic.

ACT. Dactinomycin, U. S. P. 23.
Use: Antineoplastic.
See: Actinomycin D.

ACT. (J & J Merck Consumer Pharm.) **Rinse:** 0.02% (from 0.05% sodium fluoride). **Mint:** Tartrazine, alcohol 8%. **Cinnamon:** Alcohol 7%. Bot. 360 ml, 480 ml. *otc.*
Use: Dentrifice.

A-C. (Century Pharmaceuticals, Inc.) Aspirin 6 gr, caffeine 0.5 gr/Tab. Bot. 100s, 1000s. *otc.*
Use: Analgesic.

Actacin-C. (Vangard Labs, Inc.) Codeine phosphate 10 mg, triprolidine HCl 2 mg, pseudoephedrine HCl 20 mg, guaifenesin 100 mg/5 ml. Syrup. Bot. Pt, gal. *c-v.*
Use: Antihistamine, antitussive, decongestant, expectorant.

Actacin Tablets. (Vangard Labs, Inc.) Triprolidine HCl 2.5 mg, pseudoephedrine HCl 60 mg. Bot. 100s, 1000s. *Rx-otc.*
Use: Antihistamine, decongestant.

Actagen Syrup. (Zenith Goldline Pharmaceuticals) Triprolidine HCl 1.25 mg, pseudoephedrine HCl 30 mg/5 ml. Bot. 118 ml. *otc.*
Use: Antihistamine, decongestant.

Actagen Tablets. (Zenith Goldline Pharmaceuticals) Triprolidine HCl 2.5 mg, pseudoephedrine HCl 60 mg. Bot. 100s, 1000s. *otc.*
Use: Antihistamine, decongestant.

Actagen-C Cough. (Zenith Goldline Pharmaceuticals) Triprolidine HCl 1.25 mg, pseudoephedrine HCl 30 mg, codeine phosphate 10 mg/5 ml, alcohol 4.3%. Syrup. Bot. 120 ml, Pt, gal. *c-v.*
Use: Antihistamine, antitussive, decongestant.

Actal Plus Tablets. (Sanofi Winthrop Pharmaceuticals) Aluminum hydroxide, magnesium hydroxide. *otc.*
Use: Antacid.

Actal Suspension. (Sanofi Winthrop Pharmaceuticals) Aluminum hydroxide. *otc.*

Use: Antacid.

Actal Tablets. (Sanofi Winthrop Pharmaceuticals) Aluminum hydroxide. *otc.*
Use: Antacid.

Actamin. (Buffington) Acetaminophen 325 mg/Tab. Dispens-A-Kit 100s, 200s, 500s. *otc.*
Use: Analgesic.

Actamin Extra. (Buffington) Acetaminophen 500 mg/Tab. Bot. 100s, 200s, 500s. *otc.*
Use: Analgesic.

Actamin Super. (Buffington) Acetaminophen 500 mg, caffeine. Sugar, salt, and lactose free. Tab. Dispens-A-Kit 500s, Medipak 200s. *otc.*
Use: Analgesic.

Actamine. (H.L. Moore Drug Exchange, Inc.) **Tab.:** Pseudoephedrine HCl 60 mg, triprolidine HCl 2.5 mg. Bot. 100s, 1000s. **Syr.:** Pseudoephedrine HCl 30 mg, triprolidine HCl 1.25 mg/5 ml. Bot. 120 ml, Pt, gal. *Rx-otc.*
Use: Antihistamine, decongestant.

ACTH-Actest Gel. (Forest Pharmaceutical, Inc.) Repository corticotropin 40 units or 80 units/ml. Vial 5 ml. *Rx.*
Use: Corticosteroid.

ACTH. Adrenocorticotrophic hormone. Adrenocorticotropin. *Rx.*
Use: Corticosteroid.
See: Corticotropin, U.S.P.
40 units/ml, 5 ml (Roberts Pharmaceuticals).
40 units or 80 units/ml, 5 ml (Forest Pharmaceutical, Inc.).
25 units/vial; 40 units/vial (Parke-Davis).
40 units or 80 units/ml, 5 ml (Pharmex).

ACTH Gel, Purified. (Arcum) 40 or 80 units/ml, vial 5 ml (Conal). 40 or 80 units/ml, vial 5 ml (Heart Health & Safety). 40 units/ml, vial 5 ml (Jones Medical Industries, Inc.). Adrenocorticotrophic hormone 40 units, aqueous gelatin 16%, phenol 0.5%/ml. Vial 5 ml. *Rx.*
Use: Repository corticotropin.
See: 40 or 80 units/ml, 5 ml (Arcum).
40 or 80 units/ml, 5 ml (Bell).
40 units/ml, 5 ml (Jones Medical Industries, Inc.).
40 or 80 units/ml, 5 ml (Hyrex Pharmaceuticals).
40 or 80 units/ml, 5 ml (Jenkins).
40 or 80 units/ml, vial 5 ml (Wesley Pharmacal Co, Inc.).
40 or 80 units/ml or Tubex (Wyeth-Ayerst Laboratories).

Acthar. (Centeon) Corticotropin for inj. (Lyophilized w/gelatin). 40 units/vial. Vial 25 units. *Rx.*
Use: Corticosteroid.

ActHIB. (Pasteur Merieux Connaught) Purified capsular polysaccharide of *Haemophilus influenzae* type b 10 mcg, tetanus toxoid 24 mcg/0.5 ml, sucrose 8.5%. Pow. for Inj. Vial with 7.5 ml vials of diphtheria and tetanus toxoids and pertussis vaccine as diluents. *Rx.*
Use: Vaccine against *Haemophilus influenzae* type b.

ActHIB/DTP. (Pasteur Merieux Connaught) Diphtheria and tetanus toxoids and pertussis and *Haemophilus influenzae* type b vaccines. One package consists of one 7.5 ml vial of Connaught's DTwP and 10 single-dose vials of ActHIB vaccine. *Rx.*
Use: Immunization.

Acthrel. (Ferring Pharmaceuticals, Inc.) Corticorelin ovine triflutata 100 mcg. Cake, lyophilized. 5 ml single-dose vial w/diluent. *Rx.*
Use: Diagnostic aid.

ActiBath. (The Andrew Jergens Co.) Colloidal oatmeal 20%. Tab. Effervescent. Pkg. 4s. *otc.*
Use: Emollient.

Acticin. (Alpharma USPD Inc.) Permethrin 5%. Cream. Tube 60 g. *Rx.*
Use: Scabicide.

Acticort 100 Lotion. (Baker Cummins Dermatologicals, Inc.) Hydrocortisone 1%. Bot. 60 ml. *Rx.*
Use: Corticosteroid, topical.

Actidose. (Paddock Laboratories) Activated charcoal. Soln. 25 g/120 ml or 50 g/240 ml. *otc.*
Use: Antidote.

Actidose-Aqua. (Paddock Laboratories) Activated charcoal. Aqueous susp. 25 g/120 ml or 50 g/240 ml. *otc.*
Use: Antidote.

Actidose w/Sorbitol. (Paddock Laboratories) Activated charcoal. Liq: 25 g in 120 ml susp. w/sorbitol, 50 g in 240 ml susp. w/sorbitol. *otc.*
Use: Antidote.

Actifed. (Warner Lambert Consumer Healthcare) **Tab.:** Triprolidine HCl 2.5 mg, pseudoephedrine HCl 60 mg/Tab. Pkg. 12s. Bot. 24s, 48s, 100s. *otc.*
Cap.: Triprolidine HCl 2.5 mg, pseudoephedrine HCl 60 mg/Cap. Box 10s, 20s. *otc.*
Use: Antihistamine, decongestant.

Actifed Allergy. (Warner Lambert Consumer Healthcare) **Daytime:** Pseudoephedrine 30 mg. **Nighttime:** Pseudoephedrine 30 mg, diphenhydramine

HCl 25 mg/Capl. Pkg. 24 daytime, 8 nighttime. *otc.*
Use: Antihistamine, decongestant.

Actifed 12-Hour. (GlaxoWellcome) Triprolidine HCl 5 mg, pseudoephedrine HCl 120 mg/Cap. Box 10s, 20s. *otc.*
Use: Antihistamine, decongestant.

Actifed Plus. (Warner Lambert Consumer Healthcare) Pseudoephedrine HCl 30 mg, triprolidine HCl 1.25 mg, acetaminophen 500 mg/Tab. or Cap. Bot. 20s, 40s. *otc.*
Use: Analgesic, antihistamine, decongestant.

Actifed Sinus Daytime/Nighttime. (Warner Lambert Consumer Healthcare) **Daytime:** Pseudoephedrine HCl 30 mg, acetaminophen 500 mg/Capl. Pk. 18s. **Nighttime:** Pseudoephedrine HCl 30 mg, diphenhydramine HCl 25 mg, acetaminophen 500 mg/Capl. Pkg. 6s. *otc.*
Use: Analgesic, antihistamine, decongestant.

Actigall. (Novartis Pharmaceutical Corp.) Ursodiol (Ursodeoxycholic acid) 300 mg/Cap. Bot. 100s. *Rx.*
Use: Urolithic.

Actimmune. (Genentech, Inc.) Interferon gamma-1b 100 mcg (3 million units)/vial. *Rx.*
Use: Anti-infective.

Actinex. (Schwarz Pharma, Inc.) Masoprocol 10%, isostearyl and stearyl alcohol, light mineral oil, parabens, polyethylene glycol 400, propylene glycol and sodium metabisulfite. Cream Tube 30 g. *Rx.*
Use: Antineoplastic.

actinomycin c. Name previously used for Cactinomycin.

actinomycin d. Dactinomycin, U.S.P. 23. *Rx.*
Use: Antineoplastic.
See: Cosmegen (Merck & Co.).

•**actinoquinol sodium.** (ack-TIN-oh-kwih-nole) USAN.
Use: Ultraviolet screen.

actinospectocin. Name previously used for Spectinomycin.

Actiq. (Abbott Laboratories) Fentanyl transmucosal system 200 mcg, 400 mcg, 600 mcg, 800 mcg, 1200 mcg, 1600 mcg. Loz. on a stick. Box 24s. *c-II.*
Use: Analgesic, narcotic.

Actisite. (Alza Corp.) Tetracycline HCl 12.7 mg/23 cm. Fiber. Pkg. 10s. *Rx.*
Use: Mouth and throat preparation.

•**actisomide.** (ackt-EYE-so-MIDE) USAN.
Use: Cardiovascular agent.

Activase. (Genentech, Inc.) Alteplase recombinant. Inj. Vial 20 mg, 50 mg, 100 mg. *Rx.*
Use: Thrombolytic.

activated attapulgite. *otc.*
Use: Dermatologic, acne.
W/Aluminum hydroxide, magnesium carbonate coprecipitate, compressed gel.
See: Hykasil, Cream (Roxane Laboratories, Inc.).
W/Polysorbate 80, colloidal sulfur, salicylic acid, propylene glycol.
See: Sebasorb Lotion (Summers Laboratories, Inc.).

activated charcoal tablets. (Cowley) 5 gr/Tab. Bot. 1000s. *otc.*
Use: Antidote.

activated charcoal powder. (Various Mfr.) 15, 30, 40, 120, and 140 g. *otc.*
Use: Antidote.

activated charcoal liquid. (Various Mfr.) 12.5 g or 25 g with propylene glycol. 60 ml (12.5 g), 120 ml (25 g). *otc.*
Use: Antidote.

activated 7-dehydrocholesterol.
See: Vitamin D-3 (Various Mfr.).

activated ergosterol.
See: Calciferol

•**actodigin.** (ACK-toe-dihj-in) USAN.
Use: Cardiovascular agent.

Actonel. (Procter & Gamble Pharm.) Risedronate sodium 30 mg, lactose/Tab. 30s. *Rx.*
Use: Bone resorption inhibitor.

actoquinol sodium.
Use: Ultraviolet screen.

Acucron. (Seatrace Pharmaceuticals, Inc.) Acetaminophen 300 mg, salicylamide 200 mg, phenyltoloxamine 20 mg/Tab. Bot. 100s, 1000s, 5000s. *otc.*
Use: Analgesic, antihistamine.

Acu-Dyne. (Acme United Corp.) **Douche:** Povidone-iodine. Pkt. 240 ml. **Oint.:** Povidone-iodine. Jar. lb. Pkt. 1.2 g, 2.7 g (100s). **Perineal wash conc.:** Available iodine 1%. Bot. 40 ml. **Prep. Soln.:** Povidone-iodine. Bot. 240 ml, Pt, qt, gal. Pkt. 30 ml, 60 ml. **Skin Cleanser:** Povidone-iodine. Bot. 60 ml, 240 ml, Pt, qt, gal. **Soln, prep. swabs:** Available iodine 1%. Bot. 100s. **Soln, swabsticks:** Povidone-iodine. Pkt. 1 or 3 in 25s. **Whirlpool conc.:** Available iodine 1%. Bot. gal. *otc.*
Use: Antiseptic, antimicrobial.

Acular. (Allergan, Inc.) Ketorolac tromethamine 0.5% Ophth. Soln. Drop. Bot. 3 ml, 5 ml, 10 ml. *Rx.*
Use: NSAID, ophthalmic.

AcuTrim Diet Gum. (Heritage Consumer Products) Phenylpropanolamine HCl

7.5 mg/piece, aspartame, glycerin, menthol, sorbitol, phenylalanine 1.7 mg. Gum. Pkg. 30s. *otc.*
Use: Diet aid.

Acutrim Maximum Strength. (Novartis Consumer Health) Phenylpropanolamine HCl 75 mg/Tab. Precision release Bot. 20s, 40s. *otc.*
Use: Dietary aid.

Acutrim II, Maximum Strength. (Novartis Consumer Health) Phenylpropanolamine HCl 75 mg/Tab. Precision release Bot. 20s, 40s. *otc.*
Use: Dietary aid.

Acutrim 16 Hour. (Novartis Consumer Health) Phenylpropanolamine HCl 75 mg/Tab. Precision release Bot. 20s, 40s. *otc.*
Use: Dietary aid.

•**acyclovir.** (A-SIKE-low-vir) U.S.P. 23.
Use: Antiviral.
See: Zovirax Cap., Oint., Tab., Susp. (GlaxoWellcome).

acyclovir. (Various Mfr.) Acyclovir 400 mg, 800 mg/Tab. Bot. 100s, 500s, 1000s (400 mg only). Acyclovir 200 mg/Cap. Bot. 100s. *Rx.*
Use: Antiviral.

•**acyclovir sodium.** (A-SIKE-low-vir) USAN.
Use: Antiviral.
See: Zovirax Sterile Powder (GlaxoWellcome).

acyclovir sodium. (A-SIKE-low-vir) (Bedford Laboratories) 50 mg/ml. Inj. Cartons of 10. *Rx.*
Use: Antiviral.

Adagen. (Enzon, Inc.) Pegademase bovine 250 units/ml. Vial 1.5 ml. *Rx.*
Use: Enzyme (ADA) replacement therapy.

Adalat. (Bayer Corp (Consumer Div.)) Nifedipine 10 mg or 20 mg/Cap. Bot. 100s, 300s, UD 100s. *Rx.*
Use: Calcium channel blocker.

Adalat CC. (Bayer Corp (Consumer Div.)) Nifedipine 30 mg, 60 mg, or 90 mg. ER Tab. Bot. 100s, 1000s. *Rx.*
Use: Calcium channel blocker.

adamantanamine hydrochloride.
See: Amantadine HCl.
Symmetrel, Cap., Syr. (DuPont Merck Pharmaceutical Co.).

•**adapalene.** (ADE-ah-PALE-een) USAN.
Use: Dermatologic, acne.
See: Differin (Galderma Laboratories, Inc.).

Adapettes. (Alcon Laboratories, Inc.) Povidone and other water-soluble polymers, sorbic acid, EDTA. Soln. Bot. 15 ml. *otc.*
Use: Contact lens care.

Adapettes for Sensitive Eyes. (Alcon Laboratories, Inc.) Povidone and other water-soluble polymers, EDTA, sorbic acid. Pkg. 15 ml. *otc.*
Use: Contact lens care.

Adapin. (Lotus Biochemical) Doxepin HCl **10 mg, 75 mg, 100 mg:** Cap. Bot. 100s, 1000s, UD 100s. **25 mg, 50 mg:** Cap. Bot. 100s, 1000s, 5000s, UD 100s. **150 mg:** Cap. Bot. 50s, 100s. *Rx.*
Use: Antidepressant.

•**adaprolol maleate.** (ad-AH-prole-ole) USAN.
Use: Antihypertensive (β-blocker, ophthalmic).

Adapt. (Alcon Laboratories, Inc.) Povidone, EDTA 0.1%, thimerosal 0.004%. Bot. 15 ml. *otc.*
Use: Contact lens care.

Adapt Wetting Solution. (Alcon Laboratories, Inc.) Adsorbobase with thimerosal 0.004%, EDTA 0.1%. Soln. Bot. 15 ml. *otc.*
Use: Contact lens care.

•**adatanserin hydrochloride.** (ahd-at-AN-ser-in) USAN.
Use: Antidepressant, anxiolytic.

AdatoSil 5000. (Escalon Ophthalmics, Inc.) Polydimethylsiloxane oil. Inj. Vial 10 ml, 15 ml. *Rx.*
Use: Ophthalmic.

Adavite. (Hudson Corp.) Vitamins A 5000 IU, D 400 IU, E 30 mg, B_1 3 mg, B_2 3.4 mg, B_3 30 mg, B_5 10 mg, B_6 3 mg, B_{12} 9 mcg, C 90 mg, folic acid 0.4 mg, biotin 35 mcg, beta-carotene 1250 IU/Tab. Bot. 130s. *otc.*
Use: Mineral, vitamin supplement.

Adavite. (NBTY, Inc.) Vitamins A 5500 IU, D 400 IU, E 30 mg, B_1 3 mg, B_2 3.4 mg, B_3 30 mg, B_5 10 mg, B_6 3 mg, B_{12} 9 mcg, C 120 mg, folic acid 0.4 mg, biotin 15 mcg. Tab. Bot. 100s. *otc.*
Use: Vitamin supplement.

Adavite-M. (Hudson Corp.) Iron 27 mg, Vitamins A 5000 IU, D 400 IU, E 30 mg, B_1 3 mg, B_2 3.4 mg, B_3 20 mg, B_5 10 mg, B_6 3 mg, B_{12} 9 mcg, C 190 mg, folic acid 0.4 mg, Ca, Cl, Cr, Cu, I, K, Mg, Mn, Mo, P, Se, Zinc 15 mg, biotin 30 mcg/Tab. Bot. 130s. *otc.*
Use: Mineral, vitamin supplement.

ADC with Fluoride. (Various Mfr.) Fluoride 0.5 mg, vitamins A 1500 IU, D 400 IU, C 35 mg, methylparaben/ml. Drops. Bot. 50 ml. *Rx.*
Use: Mineral, vitamin supplement.

Adderall. (Richwood Pharmaceuticals) **5 mg:** Dextroamphetamine saccharate

1.25 mg, amphetamine aspartate 1.25 mg, dextroamphetamine sulfate 1.25 mg, amphetamine sulfate 1.25 mg/Tab. Bot. 100s. **10 mg:** Dextroamphetamine sulfate 2.5 mg, dextroamphetamine saccharate 2.5 mg, amphetamine aspartate 2.5 mg, amphetamine sulfate 2.5 mg/Tab. Bot. 100s. **20 mg:** Dextroamphetamine sulfate 5 mg, dextroamphetamine saccharide 5 mg, amphetamine aspartate 5 mg, amphetamine sulfate 5 mg/Tab. Bot. 100s. **30 mg:** Dextroamphetamine saccharate 7.5 mg, amphetamine aspartate 7.5 mg, dextroamphetamine sulfate 7.5 mg, amphetamine sulfate 7.5 mg/Tab. Bot. 100s. *c-II.*
Use: CNS stimulant.

Adeecon. (CMC) Vitamins A 5000 IU, D 1000 IU/Cap. Bot. 1000s. *otc.*
Use: Vitamin supplement.

Adeflor M Tablets. (Kenwood Laboratories) Vitamins A 6000 IU, D 400 IU, B_1 1.5 mg, B_2 2.5 mg, C 100 mg, B_3 20 mg, B_5 10 mg, B_6 10 mg, B_{12} 2 mcg, fluoride 1 mg, calcium 250 mg, iron 30 mg, sorbitol, sucrose/Tab. Bot. 100s, 500s. *Rx.*
Use: Dental caries agent, vitamin supplement.

•**adefovir.** (ah-DEF-fah-vihr) USAN.
Use: Antiviral.

•**adefovir dipivoxil.** (ah-DEF-fah-vihr) USAN.
Use: Antiviral (treatment of HIV and HBV infections).

ADEKs. (Scandipharm, Inc.) Vitamins A 4000 IU, D 400 IU, E 150 IU, vitamin K, C 60 mg, B_1 1.2 mg, B_2 1.3 mg, B_3 10 mg, B_6 1.5 mg, B_{12} 12 mcg, B_5 10 mg, folic acid 0.2 mg, biotin 50 mcg, beta-carotene 3 mg, Zn 1.1 mg, fructose. Tab. Bot. 60s. *otc.*
Use: Mineral, vitamin supplement.

ADEKs Pediatric. (Scandipharm, Inc.) Vitamin A 1500 IU, D 400 IU, E 40 IU, K_1 0.1 mg, C 45 mg, B_1 0.5 mg, B_2 0.6 mg, B_3 6 mg, B_5 3 mg, B_6 0.6 mg, B_{12} 4 mcg, biotin 15 mcg, Zn 5 mg, beta-carotene 1 mg per ml. Drops. Bot. 60 ml. *otc.*
Use: Vitamin supplement.

•**adenine.** U.S.P. 23.
Use: Vitamin.

adeno-associated viral-based vector cystic fibrosis gene therapy. (Targeted Genetics Corp.)
Use: Cystic fibrosis. [Orphan Drug]

Adenocard. (Fujisawa USA, Inc.) Adenosine 6 mg/2 ml. NaCl 9 mg/ml. Preservative free. Inj. Vial 2 ml, 5 ml. *Rx.*
Use: Antiarrhythmic.

Adenolin Forte. (Lincoln Diagnostics) Adenosine-5-monophosphate 25 mg, methionine 25 mg, niacin 10 mg/ml. Vial 15 ml. *Rx.*
Use: Anti-inflammatory.

Adenoscan. (Fujisawa USA, Inc.) Adenosine 3 mg/ml. Inj. Vial 30 ml. *Rx.*
Use: Diagnostic aid.

•**adenosine.** (ah-DEN-oh-seen) USAN.
Use: Cardiovascular agent.
See: Adenocard, Inj. (Fujisawa USA, Inc.).
Adenoscan, Inj. (Fujisawa USA, Inc.).

adenosine. (ah-DEN-oh-seen) (Medco Research, Inc.)
Use: Antineoplastic. [Orphan Drug]

adenosine in gelatin. (Forest Pharmaceutical, Inc.) **Forte:** Adenosine-5-monophosphate 50 mg/ml. **Super:** Adenosine-5-monophosphate 100 mg/ml. *Rx.*
Use: Varicosity.

•**adenosine phosphate.** (ah-DEN-oh-seen) USAN. Adenosine monophosphate, AMP.
Use: Nutritional supplement.

adenosine phosphate. (Various Mfr.) 25 mg/ml. May contain benzyl alcohol. 10 ml, 30 ml/Inj. *Rx.*
Use: Treatment of statis dermatitis.

Adeno Twelve Gel Injection. (Forest Pharmaceutical, Inc.) Adenosine-5-monophosphate 25 mg, methionine 25 mg, niacin 10 mg/ml. Vial 10 ml. *Rx.*
Use: Anti-inflammatory.

adenovirus vaccine type 4. (Wyeth-Ayerst Laboratories) Adenovirus vaccine live type 4. At least 32,000 $TCID_{50}$/Tab. Bot. 100s. *Rx.*
Use: Immunization.

adenovirus vaccine type 7. (Wyeth-Ayerst Laboratories) Adenovirus vaccine live type 7. At least 32,000 $TCID_{50}$/Tab. Bot. 100s. *Rx.*
Use: Immunization.

adepsine oil.
See: Petrolatum Liquid (Various Mfr.)

AdGVCFTR 10. (GenVec, Inc.)
Use: Cystic fibrosis. [Orphan Drug]

•**adinazolam.** (AHD-in-AZE-oh-lam) USAN.
Use: Antidepressant, hypnotic, sedative.

•**adinazolam mesylate.** (AHD-in-AZE-oh-lam) USAN.
Use: Antidepressant.

Adipex-P. (Teva Pharmaceuticals USA) **Cap.:** Phentermine HCl 37.5 mg. Bot.

100s, 400s. **Tab.:** Phentermine HCl 37.5 mg. Bot. 100s, 400s, 1000s. *c-iv.*
Use: Anorexiant.

•**adiphenine hydrochloride.** (ah-DIH-feh-neen) USAN.
Use: Muscle relaxant.

Adipost. (Jones Medical Industries, Inc.) Phendimetrazine tartrate 105 mg/SR Cap. 100s. *c-iii.*
Use: Anorexiant.

Adisol. (Major Pharmaceuticals) Disulfiram. **250 mg/Tab:** Bot. 100s. **500 mg/Tab:** Bot. 50s. *Rx.*
Use: Antialcoholic.

Adlerika. (Last) Magnesium sulfate 4 g/15 ml. Bot. 12 oz. *otc.*
Use: Laxative.

Adlone. (Forest Pharmaceutical, Inc.) Methylprednisolone acetate 40 mg, 80 mg/Inj. Vial 5 ml. *Rx.*
Use: Corticosteroid, topical.

Adolph's Salt Substitute. (Adolphs) Potassium Cl 2480 mg/5 g, silicon dioxide, tartaric acid. Gran. Bot. 99.2 g. *otc.*
Use: Salt substitute.

Adolph's Seasoned Salt Substitute. (Adolphs) Potassium Cl 1360 mg/5 g, silicon dioxide, tartaric acid. Gran. Bot. 92.1 g. *otc.*
Use: Salt substitute.

Adonidine. (City Chemical Corp.) Bot. g. *Rx.*
Use: Cardiovascular agent.

•**adozelesin.** (ADE-oh-ZELL-eh-sin) USAN.
Use: Antineoplastic.

Adprin-B. (Pfeiffer Co.) Aspirin 325 mg, calcium carbonate, magnesium carbonate, magnesium oxide. Tab. Bot. 130s. *otc.*
Use: Analgesic.

Adprin-B, Extra Strength. (Pfeiffer Co.) Aspirin 500 mg w/calcium carbonate, magnesium carbonate, magnesium oxide/Tab. Bot. 130s. *otc.*
Use: Analgesic.

ADR.
Use: Antineoplastic.
See: Doxorubicin HCl

adrenalin (e).
See: Epinephrine. (Various Mfr.).

Adrenalin Chloride. (Parke-Davis) **Soln. for Inh.:** Epinephrine HCl 1:100, benzetonium chloride, sodium bisulfite 0.2%. Bot. 7.5 ml. Epinephrine HCl 1:1000, chlorobutanol, sodium bisulfite 0.15%. Bot. 30 ml. **Inj.:** Epinephrine HCl 1:1000 (1 mg/ml), Amp. 1 ml, sodium bisulfite. Steri-vial 30 ml, sodium bisulfite, chlorobutanol. Soln. *Rx.*
Use: Bronchodilator, sympathomimetic.

adrenaline hydrochloride.
See: Epinephrine Hydrochloride. (Various Mfr.).

•**adrenalone.** (ah-DREN-ah-lone) USAN.
Use: Adrenergic (ophthalmic).

adrenamine.
See: Epinephrine (Various Mfr.).

adrenergic agents.
See: Sympathomimetic agents.

adrenergic-blocking agents.
See: Sympatholytic agents.

adrenine.
See: Epinephrine (Various Mfr.).

adrenocorticotrophic hormone. ACTH acts by stimulating the endogenous production of cortisone. *Rx.*
See: ACTH.
Corticotropin, U.S.P.

Adrenomist Inhalant and Nebulizers. (Nephron Pharmaceuticals Corp.) Epinephrine 1%, Bot. 0.5 oz, 1.25 oz. *Rx-otc.*
Use: Bronchodilator.

Adrenucleo. (Enzyme Process) Vitamin C 250 mg, d-calcium pantothenate 12.5 mg, bioflavonoids 62.5 mg/Tab. Bot. 100s, 250s. *otc.*
Use: Vitamin supplement.

Adriamycin. (Pharmacia & Upjohn) Doxorubicin HCl 20 mg. Inj. Vial. *Rx.*
Use: Antineoplastic.

Adriamycin PFS. (Pharmacia & Upjohn) Doxorubicin HCl 2 mg/ml. Preservative free. Inj. Vial. 5 ml, 10 ml, 25 ml, 100 ml. *Rx.*
Use: Antibiotic.

Adriamycin RDF. (Pharmacia & Upjohn) Doxorubicin HCl 10 mg, 20 mg, 50 mg, 150 mg. Pow. for Inj., lyophilized. Vial. Rapid dissolution formula. *Rx.*
Use: Antibiotic.

Adrucil. (Pharmacia & Upjohn) Fluorouracil 50 mg/10 ml. Amp. 10 ml. *Rx.*
Use: Antineoplastic.

Adsorbocarpine. (Alcon Laboratories, Inc.) Pilocarpine HCl 1%, 2%, or 4%. Bot. 15 ml. *Rx.*
Use: Miotic.

Adsorbonac Ophth. Solution. (Alcon Laboratories, Inc.) Sodium Cl 2% or 5%. Vial 15 ml. *otc.*
Use: Hyperosmolar preparation.

Adsorbotear. (Alcon Laboratories, Inc.) Hydroxyethylcellulose 0.4%, povidone 1.67%, water-soluble polymers, thimerosal 0.004%, EDTA 0.1%. Soln. Bot. dropper 15 ml. *otc.*
Use: Artificial tears.

Advance. (Ross Laboratories) **Ready-to-Feed infant formula:** (16 cal/fl oz). Can 13 fl oz. **Conc. liq:** 32 fl oz. *otc.*

Use: Nutritional supplement.

Advance Pregnancy Test. (Advanced Care Products) Can be used as early as 3 days after a missed period. Gives results in 30 min. Test kit 1s.
Use: Diagnostic aid.

Advanced Care Cholesterol Test. (Johnson & Johnson)
Use: At home cholesterol test.

Advanced Formula Centrum Liquid. (ESI Lederle Generics) Vitamins A 2500 IU, E 30 IU, C 60 mg, B_1 1.5 mg, B_2 1.7 mg, B_3 20 mg, B_5 10 mg, B_6 2 mg, B_{12} 6 mcg, D 400 IU, iron 9 mg, biotin 300 mcg, I, Zn 3 mg, Mn, Cr, Mo, alcohol 6.7%, sucrose. Bot. 236 ml. *otc.*
Use: Mineral, vitamin supplement.

Advanced Formula Centrum Tablets. (ESI Lederle Generics) Iron 18 mg, vitamins A 5000 IU, D 400 IU, E 30 IU, B_1 1.5 mg, B_2 1.7 mg, B_3 20 mg, B_5 10 mg, B_6 2 mg, B_{12} 6 mcg, C 60 mg, folic acid 0.4 mg, biotin 30 mcg, B, Ca, Cl, Cr, Cu, I, K, Mg, Mn, Mo, Ni, P, Se, Si, Sn, V, Zn 15 mg, vitamin K. Bot. 60s, 130s, 200s. *otc.*
Use: Mineral, vitamin supplement.

Advanced Formula Oxy Sensitive. (SmithKline Beecham Pharmaceuticals) Benzoyl peroxide 2.5%, diazolidinyl urea, EDTA. Gel. 30 g. *otc.*
Use: Dermatologic, acne.

Advanced Formula Plax. (Pfizer US Pharmaceutical Group) Tetrasodium pyrophosphate, alcohol, saccharin. Mouthwash. In 120 ml, 240 ml, 473 ml, 720 ml, 1740 ml. *otc.*
Use: Anti-infective.

Advanced Formula Tegrin. (Block Drug Co., Inc.) Coal tar solution 7%, alcohol 7%, hydroxypropyl methylcellulose, parabens. Shampoo. Bot. 207 ml. *otc.*
Use: Antiseborrheic.

Advanced Formula Zenate. (Solvay Pharmaceuticals) Fe 65 mg, vitamins A 3000 IU, D 400 IU, E 10 IU, C 70 mg, folic acid 1 mg, B_1 1.5 mg, B_2 1.6 mg, B_3 17 mg, B_6 2.2 mg, B_{12} 2.2 mcg, Ca 200 mg, I 175 mcg, Mg 100 mg, Zn 15 mg. Tab. UD 30s. *Rx.*
Use: Mineral, vitamin supplement.

Advantage 24. (Women's Health Institute) Nonoxynol 93.5%. Gel. 1.5 g (3s, 6s). *otc.*
Use: Contraceptive, spermicide.

Advera. (Ross) Protein 14.2 g, fat 5.4 g, carbohydrate 51.2 g, l-carnitine 30 mg, taurine 50 mg, vitamins A 2550 IU, D 80 IU, E 9 IU, K 24 mcg, C 90 mg, folic acid 120 mcg, B, 0.75 mg, B_2 0.68 mg, B_6 9.5 mg, B_{12} 12 mcg, niacin 6 mg, choline 50 mg, biotin 50 mcg, B_5 3 mg, sodium 250 mg, potassium 670 mg, chloride 350 mg, Ca 260 mg, Ph 260 mg, Mg 50 mg, I 30 mcg, Mn 1.3 mg, Cu 0.5 mg, Zn 2 mg, Fe 4.5 mg, Se 14 mcg, chromium 17 mcg, Md 54 mcg/240 ml. 1.28 calories/ml. Vanilla flavor. Liq. Bot. 273 ml. *otc.*
Use: Nutritional supplement, enteral.

Advil. (Whitehall Robins Laboratories) Ibuprofen 200 mg, sucrose (Tab.), parabens (Capl.). In 8s, 24s, 50s, 100s, 165s, 250s (Tab.). *otc.*
Use: Analgesic, NSAID.

Advil, Children's. (Whitehall Robins Laboratories) Ibuprofen 100 mg per 5 ml. Fruit flavor, sorbitol, sucrose, EDTA. Susp. Bot. 199 ml, 473 ml. *Rx.*
Use: Analgesic, NSAID.

Advil Cold & Sinus. (Whitehall Robins Laboratories) Pseudoephedrine HCl 30 mg, ibuprofen 200 mg/Tab. Pkg. 20s. Bot. 40s, 75s. *otc.*
Use: Analgesic, decongestant.

Advil Liqui-Gels. (Whitehall Robins Laboratories) Ibuprofen 200 mg, sorbitol. Cap. Bot. 4s, 20s, 40s, 80s. *otc.*
Use: Analgesic.

A.E.R. (Birchwood Laboratories, Inc.) Hamamelis water (witch hazel) 50%, glycerin 12.5%, methylparaben, benzalkonium chloride. Pads. Jar 40s. *otc.*
Use: Dermatologic.

Aerdil. (Econo Med Pharmaceuticals) Triprolidine HCl 1.25 mg, pseudoephedrine HCl 30 mg/5 ml. Bot. Pt, gal. *otc.*
Use: Antihistamine, decongestant.

Aeroaid. (Graham Field) Thimerosal 1:1000, alcohol 72%. Spray bot. 90 ml.
Use: Antiseptic.

AeroBid. (Forest Pharmaceutical, Inc.) Flunisolide in an inhaler system ≈ 250 mcg/actuation. Canister 100 metered inhalations. *Rx.*
Use: Corticosteroid.

AeroBid-M. (Forest Pharmaceutical, Inc.) Flunisolide in an inhaler system ≈ 250 mcg/actuation. Canister. 100 metered inhalations. Menthol flavor. *Rx.*
Use: Corticosteroid.

AeroCaine. (Health & Medical Techniques) Benzocaine 13.6%, benzethonium Cl 0.5%. Spray bot. 0.5 oz, 2.5 oz. *otc.*
Use: Local anesthetic, topical.

Aerocell. (Health & Medical Techniques) Exfoliative cytology fixative spray. Bot. 3.5 oz.
Use: Exfoliative cytology fixative spray.

Aerodine. (Health & Medical Techniques) Povidone-iodine. Bot. 3 oz.

Use: Antiseptic.

Aerofreeze. (Graham Field) Trichloromonofluoromethane and dichlorodifluoromethane. 240 ml/Aerosol spray. Cont. 8 oz. (12s). *otc.*
Use: Anesthetic, local.

Aerolate-III. (Fleming & Co.) Theophylline 65 mg/TD Cap. Bot. 100s, 1000s. *Rx.*
Use: Bronchodilator.

Aerolate Sr. & Jr. (Fleming & Co.) **Cap.:** Theophylline 4 gr for Sr., 2 gr for Jr./Cap. Bot. 100s, 1000s. **Syr.:** 160 mg/15 ml. Bot. Pt, gal. *Rx.*
Use: Bronchodilator.

Aeropin. Heparin, 2-0-desulfated.
Use: Cystic fibrosis. [Orphan Drug]

Aeropure. (Health & Medical Techniques) Isopropanol 7.8%, triethylene glycol 3.9%, essential oils 3%, methyldodecyl benzyl trimethyl ammonium Cl 0.12%, methyldodecylxylene bis (trimethyl ammonium Cl) 0.03%, inert ingredients, 85.15%. Bot. 0.8 oz, 4.5 oz.
Use: Antiseptic, deodorant.

Aerosan. (Ulmer Pharmacal Co.) Aerosol 16.6 oz.
Use: Antiseptic, deodorant.

Aeroseb-Dex. (Allergan, Inc.) Dexamethasone 0.01%, alcohol 65.1%. Aerosol 58 g. *Rx.*
Use: Corticosteroid, topical.

Aerosil. (Health & Medical Techniques) Dimethylpolysiloxane. Bot. 4.5 oz.
Use: Lubricant, protectant.

aerosol ot.
See: Docusate Sodium, U.S.P.

aerosol talc, sterile. (Bryan Corp.)
Use: Malignant pleural effusion. [Orphan Drug]

Aerosolv. (Health & Medical Techniques) Isopropyl alcohol, methylene Cl, silicone. Aerosol 5.5 oz.
Use: Adhesive remover.

AeroTherm. (Health & Medical Techniques) Benzethonium Cl 0.5%, benzocaine 13.6%. Spray bot. 5 oz. *otc.*
Use: Anesthetic, local.

AeroZoin. (Health & Medical Techniques) Benzoin compound tincture 30%, isopropyl alcohol 44.8%. Spray bot. 3.5 oz. *otc.*
Use: Dermatologic, protectant.

Afaxin Capsules. (Sanofi Winthrop Pharmaceuticals) Vitamin A Palmitate 10,000 IU or 50,000 IU/Cap. *Rx-otc.*
Use: Vitamin supplement.

A-Fil. (Medicis Dermatologicals, Inc.) Methyl anthranilate 5%, titanium dioxide 5% in vanishing cream base. Tube 45 g. Neutral or dark. *otc.*
Use: Sunscreen.

Afko-Lube. (APC) Docusate sodium 100 mg/Cap. Bot. 100s. *otc.*
Use: Laxative.

Afko-Lube Lax. (APC) Docusate sodium 100 mg, casanthranol 30 mg/Cap. Bot. 100s. *otc.*
Use: Laxative.

•**afovirsen sodium.** (aff-oh-VEER-sen SO-dee-uhm) USAN.
Use: Antiviral.

Afrikol. (Citroleum) Bot. 4 oz.
Use: Sunscreen.

Afrin. (Schering-Plough Corp.) Oxymetazoline HCl 0.05%. **Nose Drops:** Drop. Bot. 20 ml. **Nasal Spray:** Reg.: Bot. 15 ml, 30 ml; Menthol: Bot. 15 ml. **Children's Nose Drops:** Oxymetazoline HCl 0.025%. Drop. Bot. 20 ml. *otc.*
Use: Decongestant.

Afrin Moisturizing Saline Mist. (Schering-Plough Corp.) Sodium chloride 0.64%, benzalkonium chloride, EDTA. Soln. Bot. 30 ml. *otc.*
Use: Decongestant.

Afrin Sinus. (Schering-Plough Corp.) Oxymetazoline HCl 0.05%, benzyl alcohol. Spray. Bot. 15 ml. *otc.*
Use: Decongestant.

Afrinol Repetabs. (Schering-Plough Corp.) Pseudoephedrine sulfate 120 mg/Repeat Action Tab. Box 12s. Bot. 100s, dispensary pack 48s. *otc.*
Use: Decongestant.

After Bite. (Tender) Ammonium hydroxide 3.5% in aqueous solution. Pen-like dispenser. *otc.*
Use: Analgesic; antipruritic, topical.

After Burn. (Tender) Lidocaine 0.5% in aloe vera 98% solution. *otc.*
Use: Anesthetic, local.

•**agar.** (AH-gahr) N.F. 18.
Use: Pharmaceutical aid (suspending agent).
W/Mineral oil.
See: Agoral, Emulsion (Parke-Davis).

Agenerase. (GlaxoWellcome) Amprenavir. **Cap.:** 50 mg, 150 mg. Bot. 480s (50 mg only), 240s (150 mg only). **Oral Soln.:** 15 mg/ml. Bot. 240 ml. *Rx.*
Use: Antiviral.

Aggrastat. (Merck & Co.) Tirofiban 250 mcg/ml, preservative free. Inj. for Soln. Vial 50 ml. Tirofiban 50 mcg/ml, preservative free. Inj. Single-dose *IntraVia-cont.* 500 ml. *Rx.*
Use: Antiplatelet.

aglucerase injection. (Genzyme Corp)
Use: Treatment of Type II and III Gaucher's disease. [Orphan Drug]

Agoral. (Parke-Davis) Phenolphthalein

0.2 g, mineral oil 4.2 g/15 ml in an emulsion containing agar, tragacanth, egg-albumin, acacia, glycerin. Raspberry flavor. Bot. 240 ml, 480 ml. *otc.*
Use: Laxative.

Agrylin. (Roberts Pharmaceuticals) Anagrelide HCl 0.5 mg and 1 mg. Lactose/Cap. Bot. 100s. *Rx.*
Use: Thrombocythemia; polycythemia vera; essential thrombocythemia; thrombocytosis in chronic myelogenous leukemia. [Orphan Drug]

A/G-Pro. (Miller Pharmacal Group, Inc.) Protein hydrolysate 50 gr w/essential and nonessential amino acids 45%, l-lysine 300 mg, methionine 75 mg, Vitamins C, B_6, Fe, Cu, I, Mn, K, Zn, Mg/6 Tab. Bot. 180s. *otc.*
Use: Nutritional supplement.

agurin.
See: Theobromine Sodium Acetate (Various Mfr.).

AH-Chew. (WE Pharmaceuticals, Inc.) Chlorpheniramine maleate 2 mg, phenylephrine HCl 10 mg, methscopolamine nitrate 1.25 mg. Chew. Tab. 100s. *Rx.*
Use: Antihistamine, decongestant.

AH-Chew D. (WE Pharmaceuticals, Inc.) Phenylephrine 10 mg/Tab. Chewable. Bot. 100s. *Rx.*
Use: Decongestant.

AHF.
See: Antihemophilic factor.

A-Hydrocort. (Abbott Hospital Products) Hydrocortisone sodium succinate. 100 mg or 250 mg/2 ml Univial, with benzyl alcohol; 500 mg/4 ml Univial with benzyl alcohol; 1000 mg/8 ml Univial with benzyl alcohol. *Rx.*
Use: Corticosteroid.

AIDS vaccine. (Various Mfr.) Phase I to III AIDS, HIV prophylaxis and treatment. *Rx.*
Use: Immunization.

Airet. (Medeva Pharmaceuticals, Inc.) Albuterol sulfate 0.083%. Soln. for Inhalation. Vial. *Rx.*
Use: Bronchodilator, sympathomimetic.

•**air, medical.** U.S.P. 23.
Use: Gas, medicinal.

AI-RSA. (AutoImmune, Inc.)
Use: Autoimmune uveitis. [Orphan Drug]

air & surface disinfectant. (Health & Medical Techniques) Aerosol 16 oz.
Use: Antiseptic, deodorant.

Akarpine. (Akorn, Inc.) Pilocarpine HCl 1%, 2%, or 4%. Soln. Bot. 15 ml. *Rx.*
Use: Miotic.

AKBeta. (Akorn, Inc.) Levobunolol HCl 0.25%, 0.5%. Ophth. Soln. Bot. 2 ml, 5 ml, 10 ml, 15 ml. *Rx.*
Use: Antiglaucoma.

AK-Chlor. (Akorn, Inc.) **Oint.:** Chloramphenicol 10 mg/g. Tube 3.5 g. **Soln.:** Chloramphenicol 5 mg/ml. Bot. 7.5 ml, 15 ml. *Rx.*
Use: Anti-infective, ophthalmic.

AK-Cide. (Akorn, Inc.) **Susp.:** Prednisolone acetate 0.5%, sulfacetamide sodium 10%. Dropper bot. 5 ml. **Oint.:** Prednisolone acetate 0.5%, sodium sulfacetamide 10%. Tube 3.5 g. *Rx.*
Use: Anti-infective; corticosteroid, ophthalmic.

AK-Con. (Akorn, Inc.) Naphazoline HCl 0.1%. Soln. Bot. 15 ml. *Rx.*
Use: Mydriatic, vasoconstrictor.

AK-Con-A. (Akorn, Inc.) Naphazoline HCl 0.025%, pheniramine maleate 0.3%, benzalkonium Cl 0.01%, EDTA. Soln. Bot. 15 ml. *Rx.*
Use: Antihistamine; decongestant, ophthalmic.

AK-Dex. (Akorn, Inc.) Dexamethasone phosphate (as sodium phosphate). Ophth. Soln. 0.1%. Bot. 5 ml. *Rx.*
Use: Corticosteroid, ophthalmic.

AK-Dilate. (Akorn, Inc.) Phenylephrine HCl 2.5% or 10%. Bot. 2 ml, 5 ml (10%), 15 ml (2.5%). *Rx.*
Use: Mydriatic, vasoconstrictor.

AK-Fluor. (Akorn, Inc.) Fluorescein sodium. **10%:** Amp. 5 ml, Vial 5 ml. **25%:** Amp. 2 ml, Vial 2 ml.
Use: Diagnostic aid, ophthalmic.

Akineton. (Knoll Pharmaceuticals) Biperiden HCl 2 mg/Tab. Bot. 100s, 1000s. *Rx.*
Use: Antiparkinsonian.

Akineton Lactate. (Knoll Pharmaceuticals) Biperiden lactate 5 mg in aqueous 1.4% sodium lactate soln/ml. Amp. 1 ml. Box 10s. *Rx.*
Use: Antiparkinsonian.

AK-Mycin. (Akorn, Inc.) Erythromycin 5 mg/g with white petrolatum, mineral oil. Oint. Tube 3.75 g. *Rx.*
Use: Anti-infective, ophthalmic.

AK-NaCl. (Akorn, Inc.) **Oint.:** Sodium Cl hypertonic 5%. Tube 3.5 g. **Soln.:** Sodium Cl, hypertonic 5%. Bot. 15 ml. *otc.*
Use: Ophthalmic.

Akne Drying Lotion. (Alto Pharmaceuticals, Inc.) Zinc oxide 12%, urea 10%, sulfur 6%, salicylic acid 2%, benzalkonium Cl 0.2%, isopropyl alcohol 70%, in a base containing menthol, silicon dioxide, iron oxide, perfume. Bot. ¾ oz, 2.25 oz. *otc.*

Use: Dermatologic, acne.

AK-Nefrin. (Akorn, Inc.) Phenylephrine HCl. Soln. Bot. 15 ml. *otc.*
Use: Mydriatic, vasoconstrictor.

Akne-Mycin. (Hermal Pharmaceutical Labs) Erythromycin. **Oint.:** 2%. Tube 25 g. **Soln.:** 2%. Bot. 60 ml. *Rx.*
Use: Dermatologic, acne.

AK-Neo-Dex. (Akorn, Inc.) Dexamethasone sodium phosphate 0.1% and neomycin sulfate 0.35%. Ophth. Soln. 5 ml. *Rx.*
Use: Anti-infective; corticosteroid, ophthalmic.

Akne Scrub. (Alto Pharmaceuticals, Inc.) Povidone-iodine with polyethylene granules. Bot. 3/4 oz. *otc.*
Use: Dermatologic, acne.

AK-Pentolate. (Akorn, Inc.) Cyclopentolate HCl 1%, benzalkonium Cl 0.01%, EDTA. Soln. Bot. 2 ml, 15 ml. *Rx.*
Use: Cycloplegic, mydriatic.

AK-Poly-Bac. (Akorn, Inc.) Polymyxin B sulfate 10,000 units, bacitracin zinc 500 units/g. Oint. Tube 3.5 g. *Rx.*
Use: Anti-infective, ophthalmic.

AK-Pred. (Akorn, Inc.) Prednisolone sodium phosphate 0.125% or 1%. Ophth. Soln. Bot. 5 ml, 10 ml, and 15 ml (1% only). *Rx.*
Use: Corticosteroid, ophthalmic.

AKPro. (Akorn, Inc.) Dipivefrin HCl 0.1%. Liq. Bot. 2, 5, 10, 15 ml. *Rx.*
Use: Antiglaucoma agent.

AK-Ramycin. (Akorn, Inc.) Doxycycline hyclate 100 mg/Cap. Bot. 50s, 100s, 200s, 250s, 500s, UD 100s. *Rx.*
Use: Anti-infective, tetracycline.

AK-Ratabs. (Akorn, Inc.) Doxycycline hyclate 100 mg/Tab. Bot. 50s. *Rx.*
Use: Anti-infective, tetracycline.

Akrinol. (Schering-Plough Corp.) Acrisorcin.
Use: Antifungal.

AK-Rinse. (Akorn, Inc.) Sodium carbonate, potassium Cl, boric acid, EDTA, benzalkonium Cl 0.01%. Soln. Bot. 30 ml, 118 ml. *otc.*
Use: Irrigant, ophthalmic.

AK-Spore. (Akorn, Inc.) **Oint.:** Polymyxin B sulfate 10,000 units, neomycin (as sulfate) 3.5 mg, bacitracin zinc 400 units/g. Tube 3.5 g. **Soln.:** Polymyxin B sulfate 10,000 units, neomycin sulfate 1.75 mg, gramicidin 0.025 mg/ml. Soln. Dropper bot. 2 ml, 10 ml. *Rx.*
Use: Anti-infective, ophthalmic.

AK-Spore H.C. ophthalmic. (Akorn, Inc.) **Susp.:** Hydrocortisone 1%, neomycin sulfate 0.35%, polymyxin B sulfate 10,000 units. Soln. Bot. 7.5 ml. **Oint.:** Hydrocortisone 1%, neomycin sulfate 0.35%, bacitracin zinc 400 units, polymyxin B sulfate 10,000 units. Tube 3.5 g. *Rx.*
Use: Corticosteroid, anti-infective.

AK-Spore H.C. Otic. (Akorn, Inc.) **Susp.:** Hydrocortisone 1%, neomycin sulfate 5 mg, polymyxin B sulfate 10,000 units/ml. Bot. w/dropper 10 ml. **Soln.:** Hydrocortisone 1%, neomycin sulfate 5 mg, polymyxin B sulfate 10,000 units/ml. Bot. w/dropper 10 ml. *Rx.*
Use: Corticosteroid, anti-infective.

AK-Sulf. (Akorn, Inc.) **Soln.:** Sodium sulfacetamide 10%. Dropper Bot. 2 ml, 5 ml, 15 ml. **Oint.:** Sodium sulfacetamide 10%. Tube 3.5 g. *Rx.*
Use: Anti-infective, ophthalmic.

AK-Taine. (Akorn, Inc.) Proparacaine HCl 0.5%, glycerin, chlorobutanol, benzalkonium Cl. Dropper bot. 2 ml, 15 ml. *Rx.*
Use: Anesthetic, ophthalmic.

AK-Tate. (Akorn, Inc.) Prednisolone acetate 1%, benzalkonium Cl, EDTA, polysorbate 80, polyvinyl alcohol, hydroxyethyl cellulose. Susp. Dropper bot. 5 ml, 10 ml, 15 ml. *Rx.*
Use: Corticosteroid, ophthalmic.

AKTob. (Akorn, Inc.) Tobramycin 0.3%. Soln. Bot. 5 ml. *Rx.*
Use: Anti-infective, ophthalmic.

AK-Tracin. (Akorn, Inc.) Bacitracin 500 units/g. Oint. Tube 3.5 g. *Rx.*
Use: Anti-infective, ophthalmic.

AK-Trol. (Akorn, Inc.) **Susp.:** Dexamethasone 0.1%, neomycin sulfate equivalent to 0.35% neomycin base, polymyxin B sulfate 10,000 units. Bot. 5 ml. **Oint.:** Dexamethasone 0.1%, neomycin sulfate equivalent to 0.35% neomycin base, polymyxin B sulfate 10,000 units. Tube 3.5 g. *Rx.*
Use: Anti-infective; corticosteroid, ophthalmic.

Akwa Tears. (Akorn, Inc.) **Soln.:** Polyvinyl alcohol 1.4%, sodium Cl, sodium phosphate, benzalkonium Cl 0.01%, EDTA. Bot. 15 ml. **Oint.:** White petrolatum, mineral oil, lanolin. Tube 3.5 g. *otc.*
Use: Artificial tears.

AL-721. (Matrix Laboratories) Phase I/II AIDS, ARC, HIV positive.
Use: Antiviral.

Ala-Bath. (Del-Ray Laboratory, Inc.) Bath oil. Bot. 8 oz. *otc.*
Use: Emollient.

Ala-Cort. (Del-Ray Laboratory, Inc.) Hydrocortisone 1%. **Cream:** Tube 1 oz, 3 oz. **Lot.:** Bot. 4 oz. *Rx.*

Use: Corticosteroid, topical.

Ala-Derm. (Del-Ray Laboratory, Inc.) Lot. Bot. 8 oz, 12 oz.
Use: Emollient.

Aladrine. (Scherer Laboratories, Inc.) Ephedrine sulfate 8.1 mg, secobarbital sodium 16.2 mg/Tab. Bot. 100s. *c-II.*
Use: Decongestant, hypnotic, sedative.

Alamag. (Alpharma USPD Inc.) Magnesium-aluminum hydroxide gel. Susp. Bot. Pt. *otc.*
Use: Antacid.

Alamag Suspension. (Zenith Goldline Pharmaceuticals) Aluminum hydroxide 225 mg, magnesium hydroxide 200 mg, sorbitol, sucrose, parabens. Bot. 355 ml. *otc.*
Use: Antacid.

Alamag Plus Antacid. (Zenith Goldline Pharmaceuticals) Magnesium hydroxide 200 mg, aluminum hydroxide 225 mg, simethicone 25 mg/5 ml. Bot. 355 ml. *otc.*
Use: Antacid.

•**alamecin.** (al-ah-MEE-sin) USAN.
Use: Anti-infective.

•**alanine.** (AL-ah-NEEN) U.S.P. 23.
Use: Amino acid.

•**alaproclate.** (AL-ah-PRO-klate) USAN.
Use: Antidepressant.

Ala-Quin 0.5%. (Del-Ray Laboratory, Inc.) Hydrocortisone, iodochlorhydroxyquinoline cream. Tube 1 oz. *Rx-otc.*
Use: Corticosteroid, topical.

Ala-Scalp HP 2%. (Del-Ray Laboratory, Inc.) Hydrocortisone Lot. Bot. 1 oz. *Rx.*
Use: Corticosteroid, topical.

Ala-Seb Shampoo. (Del-Ray Laboratory, Inc.) Bot. 4 oz, 12 oz. *otc.*
Use: Antiseborrheic.

Ala-Seb T Shampoo. (Del-Ray Laboratory, Inc.) Bot. 4 oz, 12 oz. *otc.*
Use: Antiseborrheic.

Alasulf. (Major Pharmaceuticals) Sulfanilamide 15%, aminacrine HCl 0.2%, allantoin 2%. Vaginal Cream Tube w/applicator 120 g. *Rx.*
Use: Anti-infective, vaginal.

Alatone. (Major Pharmaceuticals) Spironolactone 25 mg/Tab. Bot. 100s, 250s, 500s, 1000s, UD 100s. *Rx.*
Use: Antihypertensive.

•**alatrofloxacin mesylate.** (al-at-row-FLOX-ah-sin) USAN.
Use: Anti-infective.
See: Trovan, Inj. (Pfizer US Pharmaceutical Group).

Alaxin. (Delta Pharmaceutical Group) Oxyethlene oxypropylene polymer 240 mg/Cap. Bot. 100s. *otc.*
Use: Laxative.

Al-Ay. (Jones Medical Industries, Inc.) **Green Oblong Tube:** Phenylephrine HCl 5 mg, chlorpheniramine maleate 2 mg, aspirin 162 mg, caffeine 15 mg, aminoacetic acid 162 mg/Tab. Bot. 100s, 1000s. **Dark Green S.C.:** Phenylephrine HCl 5 mg, chlorpheniramine maleate 2 mg, acetaminophen 160 mg, caffeine 15 mg/Tab. Bot. 100s, 1000s. *otc.*
Use: Analgesic, antihistamine, decongestant.

alazanine trichlorphate. *Rx.*
Use: Anthelmintic.

Alazide Tabs. (Major Pharmaceuticals) Spironolactone w/hydrochlorothiazide. Bot. 250s, 1000s. *Rx.*
Use: Antihypertensive, diuretic.

Alazine Tabs. (Major Pharmaceuticals) Hydralazine 10 mg, 25 mg, or 50 mg/Cap. Bot. 100s, 1000s. *Rx.*
Use: Antihypertensive.

Albalon. (Allergan, Inc.) Naphazoline HCl 0.1%. Bot. 15 ml. *Rx.*
Use: Vasoconstrictor, ophthalmic.

Albamycin. (Pharmacia & Upjohn) Novobiocin sodium 250 mg/Cap. Bot. 100s. *Rx.*
Use: Anti-infective.

Albay. (Bayer Corp. (Consumer Div.)) Freeze-dried venom and venom protein. Vials of 550 mcg for each of honeybee, white-faced hornet, yellow hornet, yellow jacket, or wasp. Vials of 1650 mcg for mixed vespids (white-faced hornet, yellow hornet, yellow jacket). 10 ml/Inj. *Rx.*
Use: Antivenin.

•**albendazole.** (AL-BEND-ah-zole) U.S.P. 23.
Use: Anthelmintic.
See: Zentel (SmithKline Beecham Pharmaceuticals).

albendazole. (SmithKline Beecham Pharmaceuticals) 200 mg/Tab. Bot. 112s. *Rx.*
Use: Anthelmintic. Hydatid disease. [Orphan Drug]
See: Albenza, Tab. (SmithKline Beecham Pharmaceuticals).

Albenza. (SmithKline Beecham Pharmaceuticals) Albendazole 200 mg/Tab. Bot. 112s. *Rx.*
Use: Anthelmintic. Hydatid disease. [Orphan Drug]

Albolene Cream. (SmithKline Beecham Pharmaceuticals) Unscented or scented. Jar 6 oz, 12 oz.

Albuconn 25% Solution. (Cryosan) Normal serum albumin (human) 12.5 g in

50 ml solution for IV administration. Vial 50 ml. *Rx.*
Use: Treatment of plasma or blood volume deficit, acute hypoproteinemia, oncotic deficit.

•**albumin, aggregated.** (al-BYOO-min AGG-reh-GAY-tuhd) USAN.
Use: Diagnostic aid (lung-imaging).
See: Technescan MAA.

•**albumin, aggregated iodinated I 131 injection.** (al-BYOO-min AGG-reh-GAY-tuhd) U.S.P. 23.
Use: Radiopharmaceutical.

•**albumin, aggregated iodinated I 131 serum.** (al-BYOO-min AGG-reh-GAY-tuhd) USAN. Blood serum aggregates of albumin labeled with iodine-131.
Use: Radiopharmaceutical.
See: Albumotopel-131 (Squibb).

•**albumin, chromated cr 51 serum.** USAN. Blood serum albumin labeled with chromium-51.
Use: Radiopharmaceutical.

•**albumin human.** (al-BYOO-MIN human) U.S.P. 23. *Formerly Albumin, Normal Human Serum.*
Use: Plasma protein fraction.; blood volume supporter.
See: Albunex, Inj. (Mallinckrodt).
Albutein 5%, Inj. (Alpha Therapeutic Corp.).
Albutein 25%, Inj. (Alpha Therapeutic Corp.).
Buminate, Soln. (Baxter Pharmaceutical Products, Inc.).
Plasbumin-5 (Bayer Corp. (Consumer Div.)).
Plasbumin-25 (Bayer Corp. (Consumer Div.)).

albumin human, 5%. (al-BYOO-MIN human) (Baxter Healthcare Corp.) Normal serum albumin 5%. Inj. Vial 250 ml. *Rx.*
Use: Plasma protein fraction.
See: Albuminar-5, Inj. (Centeon).
Albutein 5%, Inj. (Alpha Therapeutic Corp.).
Buminate 5%, Inj. (Baxter Pharmaceutical Products, Inc.).
Plasbumin-5, Inj. (Bayer Corp. (Consumer Div.)).

albumin human, 25%. (al-BYOO-MIN human) (Baxter Healthcare Corp.) Normal serum albumin 25%. Inj. Vial 10 ml, 50 ml. *Rx.*
Use: Plasma protein fraction.
See: Albuminar 5 and Albuminar-25, Inj. (Centeon).
Albutein 25%, Inj. (Alliance Pharmaceuticals).
Buminate 25%, Inj. (Baxter Pharmaceutical Products, Inc.).
Plasbumin-25, Inj. (Bayer Corp. (Consumer Div.)).

•**albumin, iodinated I 125 injection.** U.S.P. 23. Albumin labeled with iodine-125.
Use: Diagnostic aid (blood volume determination); radiopharmaceutical.

•**albumin, iodinated I 125 serum.** USAN. U.S.P. XIX.
Use: Diagnostic aid (blood volume determination); radiopharmaceutical.

•**albumin, iodinated I 131 injection.** U.S.P. 23. Albumin labeled with iodine-131. Inj.
Use: Diagnostic aid (blood volume determination; intrathecal imaging); radiopharmaceutical.

albumin, iodinated I 131 serum. USAN. U.S.P. XIX.
Use: Diagnostic aid (blood volume determination, intrathecal imaging); radioactive agent.

albumin, normal serum 5%. (Baxter Healthcare Corp.) Albumin human 5%. Inj. Vial 120 ml. *Rx.*
Use: Plasma protein fraction.

albumin, normal serum 25%. (Baxter Healthcare Corp.) Albumin human 25%. Inj. Vial 10 ml, 50 ml. *Rx.*
Use: Plasma protein fraction.

albumin-saline diluent. (Bayer Corp. (Consumer Div.)) Dilute allergenic extracts and venom products for patient testing and treating. Pre-measured vials 1.8 ml, 4 ml, 4.5 ml, 9 ml, 30 ml. Vial 2 ml, 5 ml, 10 ml, 30 ml.
Use: Pharmaceutical necessity, diluent.

Albuminar-5 and Albuminar-25. (Centeon) Albumin, (human) U.S.P. 5%: solution with administration set. Bot. 50 ml, 250 ml, 500 ml, 1000 ml. 25%: solution. Vial 20 ml, 50 ml, 100 ml with administration set. *Rx.*
Use: Plasma protein fraction.

Albumotope I-131. (Bristol-Myers Squibb) Albumin, Iodinated I-131 Serum (50 uCi).
Use: Diagnostic aid.

Albunex. (Mallinckrodt) Albumin (human) 5%, sonicated. Sodium acetyl tryptophanate 0.08 mmol, sodium caprylate 0.08 mmol/g albumin. Inj. Vial. 5 ml, 10 ml, 20 ml. Pkg. 6s. *Rx.*
Use: Plasma protein fraction.

Albustix Reagent Strips. (Bayer Corp. (Consumer Div.)) Firm paper reagent strips impregnated with tetrabromphenol blue, citrate buffer and a protein-

adsorbing agent. Bot. 50s, 100s.
Use: Diagnostic aid.

Albutein 5%. (Alpha Therapeutic Corp.) Normal serum albumin 5%. Inj. Vial w/ IV set: 250 ml, 500 ml. *Rx.*
Use: Plasma protein fraction.

Albutein 25%. (Alpha Therapeutic Corp.) Normal serum albumin 25%. Inj. Vial w/ IV set: 50 ml. *Rx.*
Use: Plasma protein fraction.

•**albuterol.** (al-BYOO-ter-ahl) U.S.P. 23.
Use: Bronchodilator.
See: Proventil (Schering-Plough Corp.).
Ventolin (GlaxoWellcome).

albuterol. (Various Mfr.) Albuterol 90 mcg per actuation. Inh. Aer. Can. 17 g (≥ 200 inhalations). *Rx.*
Use: Bronchodilator.

•**albuterol sulfate.** (al-BYOO-teh-rahl) U.S.P. 23.
Use: Bronchodilator.
See: Airet, Inhalation soln. (Medeva Pharmaceuticals, Inc.).
Proventil (Schering-Plough Corp.).
Ventolin (GlaxoWellcome).
Volmax, ER Tab. (Muro Pharmaceutical, Inc.).

albuterol sulfate. (al-BYOO-ter-al SULL-fate) (Various Mfr.) **Tab.:** 2 mg, 4 mg. Bot. 100s, 500s, 600s, 1000s, UD 100s, 600s. **Syr.:** 2 mg/5 ml. Bot. 480 ml. **Inh. Soln.:** 0.083%, 0.5%. UD 3 ml (0.083% only), Bot. 20 ml (0.5% only). *Rx.*
Use: Bronchodilator, sympathomimetic.

albuterol sulfate and ipratropium bromide. (al-BYOO-ter-ahl and IH-pruh-TROE-pee-uhm)
Use: Chronic obstructive pulmonary disease (COPD).
See: Combivent, Aerosol (Boehringer Ingelheim, Inc.).

•**albutoin.** (al-BYOO-toe-in) USAN.
Use: Anticonvulsant.

Alcaine. (Alcon Laboratories, Inc.) Proparacaine HCl 0.5%, glycerin, sodium Cl, benzalkonium Cl. Bot. 15 ml. *Rx.*
Use: Anesthetic, ophthalmic.

Alcare. (SmithKline Beecham Pharmaceuticals) Ethyl alcohol 62%. Foam Bot. 210 ml, 300 ml, 600 ml. *otc.*
Use: Antiseptic.

Alclear Eye Lotion. (Walgreen Co.) Sterile isotonic fluid. Bot. 8 oz. *otc.*
Use: Anti-irritant, ophthalmic.

•**alclofenac.** (al-KLOE-feh-nak) USAN.
Use: Analgesic, anti-inflammatory.
See: Mervan (Continental Pharma, Belgium).

•**alclometasone dipropionate.** (al-kloe-MEH-tah-zone die-PRO-pee-oh-nate) U.S.P. 23.
Use: Anti-inflammatory, topical.
See: Aclovate, Cream, Oint. (GlaxoWellcome).

•**alcloxa.** (al-KLOX-ah) USAN.
Use: Astringent, keratolytic.

Alco-Gel. (Tweezerman) Ethyl alcohol 60%. Tube 60 g, 480 g. *otc.*
Use: Dermatologic, cleanser.

•**alcohol.** U.S.P. 23. Ethanol, ethyl alcohol.
Use: Anti-infective, topical; pharmaceutic aid (solvent).
See: Anbesol, Gel, Liq. (Whitehall Robins Laboratories).
Anbesol Maximum Strength, Gel. Liq. (Whitehall Robins Laboratories).
Ru-Tuss Expectorant (Knoll Pharmaceuticals).
Ru-Tuss w/ Hydrocodone (Knoll Pharmaceuticals).
Ru-Tuss Liquid (Knoll Pharmaceuticals).

alcohol, dehydrated.
Use: Solvent, vehicle.

•**alcohol, diluted.** N.F. 18.
Use: Pharmaceutic aid (solvent).

•**alcohol, rubbing.** U.S.P. 23.
Use: Rubefacient.
See: Lavacol (Parke-Davis).

Alcohol 5% and Dextrose 5%. (Abbott Hospital Products) Alcohol 5 ml, dextrose 5 g/100 ml. Bot. 1000 ml. *Rx.*
Use: Nutritional supplement, parenteral.

Alcojet. (Alconox) Biodegradable machine washing detergent and wetting agent. Ctn. 9 × 4 lb, 25 lb, 50 lb, 100 lb, 300 lb. *otc.*
Use: Detergent, wetting agent.

Alcolec. (American Lecithin Company) Lecithin w/choline base, cephalin, lipositol. Cap. 100s. Gran. 8 oz, lb. *otc.*
Use: Nutritional supplement.

Alconefrin 12 and 50. (PolyMedica Pharmaceuticals) Phenylephrine HCl 0.16% w/benzalkonium Cl. Dropper bot. 30 ml. *otc.*
Use: Decongestant.

Alconefrin 25. (PolyMedica Pharmaceuticals) Phenylephrine HCl 0.25% w/ benzalkonium Cl. Dropper bot. 30 ml. Spray Pkg. 30 ml. *otc.*
Use: Decongestant.

Alcon Enzymatic Cleaning Tablets for Extended Wear. (Alcon, Vision Care) Pancreatin. Tab. Pkg. 12s. *otc.*
Use: Contact lens care.

Alcon Lens Case. (Alcon, Vision Care) Two lens cases. Ctn. 12s. *otc.*

Use: Contact lens care.

Alcon Opti-Pure Sterile Saline Solution. (Alcon, Vision Care) Sterile unpreserved saline solution. Aerosol 8 oz. *otc.*
Use: Contact lens care.

Alcon Saline Solution for Sensitive Eyes. (Alcon, Vision Care) Sodium Cl, edetate disodium, borate buffer system, sorbic acid. Bot. 360 ml. *otc.*
Use: Contact lens care.

Alconox. (Alconox) Biodegradable detergent and wetting agent. Box 4 lb, Container 25 lb, 50 lb, 100 lb, 300 lb. *otc.*
Use: Contact lens care, detergent; wetting agent.

Alcotabs. (Alconox) Tab. Box 6s, 100s.
Use: Cleanser.

•**alcuronium chloride.** (al-cure-OH-nee-uhm) USAN. Diallyldinortoxiferin dichloride.
Use: Muscle relaxant.

Aldactazide. (Searle) Spironolactone and hydrochlorothiazide. **25 mg/25 mg:** Bot. 100s, 500s, 1000s, 2500s, UD 100s. **50 mg/50 mg:** Bot. 100s, UD 32s, UD 100s. Tab. *Rx.*
Use: Antihypertensive, diuretic.

Aldactone. (Searle) Spironolactone. **25 mg/Tab.:** Bot. 100s, 500s, 1000s, UD 100s. **50 mg/Tab.:** Bot. 100s, UD 100s. **100 mg/Tab.:** Bot. 100s, UD 100s. *Rx.*
Use: Antihypertensive.

Aldara. (3M Pharm) Imiquimod 5%. Cream Box. 12s (250 mg single-use packets). *Rx.*
Use: Treatment of external genital and perianal warts/condyloma.

•**aldesleukin.** (al-dess-LOO-kin) USAN. Recombinant form of interleukin-2.
Use: Biological response modifier; antineoplastic; immunostimulant.
See: Proleukin, Pow for Inj. (Chiron Therapeutics).

aldesleukin. (al-dess-LOO-kin)
Use: Metastatic renal cell carcinoma/melanoma; primary immunodeficiency disease associated with T-cell defects.
See: Proleukin, Pow. for Inj. (Chiron).

•**aldioxa.** (al-DIE-ox-ah) USAN. Aluminum dihydroxy allantoinate.
Use: Astringent, keratolytic.

Aldoclor 150. (Merck & Co.) Methyldopa 250 mg, chlorothiazide 150 mg/Tab. Bot. 100s. *Rx.*
Use: Antihypertensive.

Aldoclor 250. (Merck & Co.) Methyldopa 250 mg, chlorothiazide 250 mg/Tab. Bot. 100s. *Rx.*
Use: Antihypertensive.

Aldomet. (Merck & Co.) Methyldopa. **125 mg/Tab.:** Bot. 100s. **250 mg/Tab.:** Bot. 100s, 1000s, UD 100s, Unit-of-use 100s. **500 mg/Tab.:** Bot. 100s, 500s, UD 100s, Unit-of-use 60s, 100s. *Rx.*
Use: Antihypertensive.
W/Chlorothiazide.
See: Aldoclor, Tab. (Merck & Co.).
W/Hydrochlorothiazide.
See: Aldoril, Tab. (Merck & Co.).

Aldomet Ester Hydrochloride. (Merck & Co.) Methyldopate HCl 250 mg/5 ml, citric acid anhydrous 25 mg, sodium bisulfite 16 mg, disodium edetate 2.5 mg, monothioglycerol 10 mg, sodium hydroxide to adjust pH, methylparaben 0.15%, propylparaben 0.02% w/water for inj. q.s. to 5 ml. Vial 5 ml. *Rx.*
Use: Antihypertensive.

Aldomet Oral Suspension. (Merck & Co.) Methyldopa 250 mg/5 ml, alcohol 1%, benzoic acid 0.1%, sodium bisulfite 0.2%. Bot. 473 ml. *Rx.*
Use: Antihypertensive.

Aldoril-15. (Merck & Co.) Methyldopa 250 mg, hydrochlorothiazide 15 mg/Tab. Bot. 100s, 1000s. *Rx.*
Use: Antihypertensive.

Aldoril-25. (Merck & Co.) Methyldopa 250 mg, hydrochlorothiazide 25 mg/Tab. Bot. 100s, 1000s, UD 100s. *Rx.*
Use: Antihypertensive.

Aldoril D30 & D50. (Merck & Co.) Methyldopa 500 mg, hydrochlorothiazide 30 mg or 50 mg. Tab. Bot. 100s. *Rx.*
Use: Antihypertensive.

Aldosterone RIA Diagnostic Kit. (Abbott Diagnostics) Test kits 50s.
Use: Diagnostic aid.

ALEC. (Forum Products, Inc.) Dipalmitoyl phosphatidylcholine/phosphatidylglycerol.
Use: Neonatal respiratory distress syndrome. [Orphan Drug]

•**alendronate sodium.** (al-LEN-droe-nate) USAN.
Use: Bone resorption inhibitor.
See: Fosamax, Tab. (Merck & Co.).

Alenic Alka Liquid. (Rugby Labs, Inc.) Aluminum hydroxide 31.7 mg, magnesium carbonate 137.3 mg, sodium alginate, EDTA, sodium 13 mg. Bot. 355 ml. *otc.*
Use: Antacid.

Alenic Alka Tablets. (Rugby Labs, Inc.) Aluminum Hydroxide 80 mg, magnesium trisilicate 20 mg, sodium bicarbonate, calcium stearate, sugar. Chew. Tab. Bot. 100s. *otc.*

Use: Antacid.

Alenic Alka Tablets, Extra Strength. (Rugby Labs, Inc.) Aluminum hydroxide 160 mg, magnesium carbonate 105 mg, sodium 29.9 mg. Chew. Tab. Bot. 100s. *otc.*
Use: Antacid.

•**alentemol hydrobromide.** (al-EN-teh-mole) USAN.
Use: Antipsychotic; dopamine agonist.

Alersule. (Misemer Pharmaceuticals, Inc.) Chlorpheniramine maleate 8 mg, phenylephrine HCl 20 mg/Cap. Bot. 100s. *Rx-otc.*
Use: Antihistamine, decongestant.

Alert-Pep. (Health for Life Brands, Inc.) Caffeine 200 mg/Cap. Bot. 16s. *otc.*
Use: CNS stimulant.

Alesse-21. (Wyeth-Ayerst Laboratories) Levonorgestrel 0.1 mg, ethinyl estradiol 0.02 mg, lactose/Tab. Pkg. 21s. *Rx.*
Use: Contraceptive.

Alesse-28. (Wyeth-Ayerst Laboratories) Levonorgestrel 0.1 mg, ethinyl estradiol 0.02 mg, lactose/Tab. Pkg. 21s. Lactose/Inactive Tab. 7s. *Rx.*
Use: Contraceptive.

•**aletamine hydrochloride.** (al-ETT-ah-meen) USAN.
Use: Antidepressant.

Aleve. (Procter & Gamble Pharm.) Naproxen sodium 220 mg (naproxen base 200 mg with sodium 20 mg) Tab. Bot. 24s, 50s, 100s. *otc.*
Use: NSAID.

•**alexidine.** (ah-LEX-ih-DEEN) USAN.
Use: Anti-infective.

alfa interferon-2a.
See: Roferon A (Roche Laboratories).

alfa interferon-2b.
See: Intron A (Schering-Plough Corp.).

Alfenta. (Taylor) Alfentanil HCl 500 mcg/ml. Inj. Amp. 2 ml, 5 ml, 10 ml, 20 ml. *c-II.*
Use: Analgesic, anesthetic-narcotic.

•**alfentanil hydrochloride.** (al-FEN-tuh-NILL) USAN.
Use: Analgesic, anesthetic-narcotic.
See: Alfenta, Inj. (Taylor).

•**alfuzosin hydrochloride.** (al-FEW-zoe-sin) USAN.
Use: Antihypertensive (α-blocker).

Algel. (Faraday) Magnesium trisilicate 0.5 g, aluminum hydroxide 0.25 g/Tab. Bot. 100s. Susp. Bot. gal. *otc.*
Use: Antacid.

•**algeldrate.** (AL-jell-drate) USAN.
Use: Antacid.

Algemin. (Thurston) Macrocystis pyrifera alga. Pow. Jar 8 oz. Tab. Bot. 300s. *otc.*
Use: Dietary aid.

Algenic Alka Improved Tablets. (Rugby Labs, Inc.) Aluminum hydroxide 240 mg, magnesium hydroxide 100 mg/Chew. Tab. Bot. 100s, 500s. *otc.*
Use: Antacid.

Algenic Alka Liquid. (Rugby Labs, Inc.) Aluminum hydroxide 31.7 mg/ml, magnesium carbonate 137 mg/ml, sodium alginate, sorbitol. Bot. 355 ml. *otc.*
Use: Antacid.

•**algestone acetonide.** (al-JESS-tone ah-SEE-toe-nide) USAN.
Use: Anti-inflammatory.

•**algestone acetophenide.** (al-JESS-tone ah-SEE-toe-FEN-ide) USAN.
Use: Hormone, progestin.

Algex. (Health for Life Brands, Inc.) Menthol, camphor, methylsalicylate, eucalyptus. Liniment Bot. 4 oz. *otc.*
Use: Analgesic, topical.

algin.
See: Sodium Alginate, N.F. 18.

Algin-All. (Barth's) Sodium alginate from kelp. Tab. Bot. 100s, 500s.

•**alginic acid.** (al-JIN-ik) N.F. 18.
Use: Pharmaceutic aid (tablet binder, emulsifying agent).

alginic acid. W/Aluminum hydroxide dried gel, magnesium trisilicate, sodium bicarbonate. *otc.*
Use: Antacid.
See: Gaviscon Foamtabs (Hoechst Marion Roussel).

alginic acid combinations. (al-JIN-ik)
See: Pretts Diet-Aid, Chew. Tab. (Mi-Lance).

•**alglucerase.** (al-GLUE-ser-ACE) USAN.
Formerly Macrophage-targeted β-glucocerebrosidase.
Use: Enzyme replenisher (glucocerebrosidase). [Orphan Drug]
See: Ceredase, Inj. (Genzyme Corp.).

alglucerase. (al-GLUE-ser-ACE) Inj.
Use: Replacement therapy in Gaucher's disease Type I, II, III. [Orphan Drug]
See: Ceredase, Inj. (Genzyme Corp.).

alidine dihydrochloride or phosphate. Anileridine, N.F.

•**aliflurane.** (al-IH-flew-rane) USAN.
Use: Anesthetic (inhalation).

Alikal Powder. (Sanofi Winthrop Pharmaceuticals) Sodium bicarbonate, tartaric acid powder. *otc.*
Use: Antacid.

Alimentum. (Ross Laboratories) Casein hydrolysate, sucrose, tapioca starch, MCT (fractionated coconut oil), safflower oil, soy oil. Qt. Ready-to-use. *otc.*
Use: Nutritional supplement-enteral.

•**alipamide.** (al-IH-pam-ide) USAN.
Use: Antihypertensive, diuretic.

alisobumal.
See: Butalbital, U.S.P. 23.

•**alitame.** (AL-ih-TAME) USAN.
Use: Sweetener.

alitretinoin.
Use: Antineoplastic.
See: Panretin, Gel (Ligand Pharmaceuticals, Inc.).

alkalinizers, minerals and electrolytes.
See: Polycitra (Baker Norton Pharmaceuticals, Inc.).
Oracit (Carolina Medical Products).
Bicitra (Baker Norton Pharmaceuticals, Inc.).

alkalinizers urinary tract products.
See: Sodium Bicarbonate (Various Mfr.).
Urocit-K (Mission Pharmacal Co.).
Citrolith (Beach Pharm).
Polycitra (Baker Norton Pharmaceuticals, Inc.).
Bicitra (Baker Norton Pharmaceuticals, Inc.).

Alkalol. (Alkalol) Thymol, eucalyptol, menthol, camphor, benzoin, potassium alum, potassium chlorate, sodium bicarbonate, sodium Cl, sweet birch oil, spearmint oil, pine and cassia oil, alcohol 0.05%. Bot. Pt. Nasal douche cup pkg. 1s. *otc.*
Use: Eyes, nose, throat, and all inflamed mucous membranes.

Alka-Med Liquid. (Halsey Drug Co.) Aluminum hydroxide 200 mg, magnesium hydroxide 200 mg/5 ml. Bot. 8 oz. *otc.*
Use: Antacid.

Alka-Med Tablets. (Halsey Drug Co.) Magnesium hydroxide, aluminum hydroxide. Bot. 60s. *otc.*
Use: Antacid.

Alka-Mints. (Bayer Corp. (Consumer Div.)) Calcium carbonate 850 mg/Chew. Tab. Carton 30s. *otc.*
Use: Antacid.

Alka-Seltzer. (Bayer Corp. (Consumer Div.)) Heat treated sodium bicarbonate 1916 mg, citric acid 1000 mg, aspirin 325 mg, sodium 567 mg/Tab. Bot. 36s. *otc.*
Use: Analgesic, antacid.

Alka-Seltzer, Advanced Formula. (Bayer Corp. (Consumer Div.)) Heat treated sodium bicarbonate 465 mg, citric acid 900 mg, acetaminophen 325 mg, potassium bicarbonate 300 mg, calcium carbonate 280 mg/Tab. Foil pack 36s. *otc.*
Use: Analgesic, antacid.

Alka-Seltzer Effervescent, Gold Tablets. (Bayer Corp. (Consumer Div.)) Heat treated sodium bicarbonate 958 mg, citric acid 832 mg, potassium bicarbonate 312 mg, sodium 311 mg/Tab. Bot. 20s, 36s. *otc.*
Use: Analgesic, antacid.

Alka-Seltzer, Extra Strength. (Bayer Corp (Consumer Div.)) Aspirin 500 mg, heat treated sodium bicarbonate 1985 mg, citric acid 1000 mg, sodium 588 mg/Tab. Bot. 12s, 24s. *otc.*
Use: Analgesic, antacid.

Alka-Seltzer Flavored Effervescent Antacid-Analgesic. (Bayer Corp. (Consumer Div.)) Aspirin 325 mg, sodium bicarbonate 1700 mg, citric acid 1000 mg, phenylalanine 9 mg, sodium 506 mg, aspartame, lemon-lime flavor. Tab. Bot. 24s. *otc.*
Use: Analgesic, antacid.

Alka-Seltzer Plus. (Bayer Corp. (Consumer Div.)) Chlorpheniramine maleate 2 mg, phenylpropanolamine bitartrate 24 mg, aspirin 324 mg, sodium 506 mg/Tab. Foil pack 20s, 36s. *otc.*
Use: Analgesic, antihistamine, decongestant.

Alka-Seltzer Plus Allergy Liqui-Gels. (Bayer Corp. (Consumer Div.)) Pseudoephedrine HCl 30 mg, brompheniramine maleate 2 mg, acetaminophen 500 mg/Tab. Pkg. 12s. *otc.*
Use: Analgesic, antihistamine, decongestant.

Alka-Seltzer Plus Cold and Cough Liqui-Gels. (Bayer Corp. (Consumer Div.)) Dextromethorphan HBr 10 mg, pseudoephedrine HCl 30 mg, chlorpheniramine maleate 2 mg, acetaminophen 250 mg/Cap. Pkg. 12s, 20s. *otc.*
Use: Analgesic, antihistamine, antitussive, decongestant.

Alka-Seltzer Plus Cold & Cough Tablets. (Bayer Corp. (Consumer Div.)) Phenylpropanolamine bitartrate 20 mg, chlorpheniramine maleate 2 mg, dextromethorphan HBr 10 mg, aspirin 325 mg, phenylalanine 11.2 mg/Tab. 12s, 20s, 36s. *otc.*
Use: Analgesic, antitussive, antihistamine, decongestant.

Alka-Seltzer Plus Cold Liqui-Gels. (Bayer Corp. (Consumer Div.)) Chlorpheniramine maleate 2 mg, pseudoephedrine HCl 30 mg, acetaminophen 250 mg/Cap. Pkg. 12s, 20s. *otc.*
Use: Analgesic, antihistamine, decongestant.

Alka-Seltzer Plus Cold Medicine. (Bayer Corp. (Consumer Div.)) Phenylpropanolamine bitartrate 20 mg, chlor-

pheniramine maleate 2 mg, aspirin 325 mg/Tab. 12s, 20s, 36s, 48s. *otc.*
Use: Analgesic, antihistamine, decongestant.

Alka-Seltzer Plus Cold & Sinus. (Bayer Corp. (Consumer Div.)) **Cap.:** Pseudoephedrine HCl 30 mg, acetaminophen 325 mg, sorbitol. Pkg. 12s, 20s. **Effervescent Tab.:** Aspirin 325 mg, phenylpropanolamine bitartrate 20 mg, aspartame, phenylalanine 12 mg. Pkg. 20s. *otc.*
Use: Decongestant combination.

Alka-Seltzer Plus Cold Tablets. (Bayer Corp. (Consumer Div.)) Phenylpropanolamine bitartrate 24.08 mg, chlorpheniramine maleate 2 mg, aspirin 325 mg/Tab. Pkg. 12s, 20s. Bot. 36s, 48s. *otc.*
Use: Analgesic, antihistamine, decongestant.

Alka-Seltzer Plus Flu & Body Aches Non-Drowsy Liqui-Gels. (Bayer Corp. (Consumer Div.)) Pseudoephedrine HCl 30 mg, dextromethorphan HBr 10 mg, acetaminophen 250 mg/Tab. Pkg. 12s. *otc.*
Use: Analgesic, antitussive, decongestant.

Alka-Seltzer Plus Nighttime Cold Liqui-Gels. (Bayer Corp. (Consumer Div.)) Pseudoephedrine HCl 30 mg, dextromethorphan HBr 10 mg, doxylamine succinate 6.25 mg, acetaminophen 250 mg/Cap. Pkg. 20s. *otc.*
Use: Antihistamine, antitussive, decongestant.

Alka-Seltzer Plus Night-Time Cold Tablets. (Bayer Corp. (Consumer Div.)) Phenylpropanolamine bitartrate 20 mg, doxylamine succinate 6.25 mg, dextromethorphan HBr 15 mg, aspirin 500 mg, phenylalanine 16.2 mg/Tab. Bot. 12s, 20s, 36s. *otc.*
Use: Analgesic, antihistamine, decongestant.

Alka-Seltzer Plus Sinus. (Bayer Corp. (Consumer Div.)) Phenylpropanolamine bitartrate 20 mg, aspirin 325 mg, aspartame, phenylalanine 8.98 mg/Tab. Pkg. 20s. *otc.*
Use: Analgesic, decongestant.

Alka-Seltzer Plus Sinus Allergy. (Bayer Corp. (Consumer Div.)) Phenylpropanolamine bitartrate 24.08 mg, brompheniramine maleate 2 mg, aspirin 500 mg, aspartame, phenylalanine 9 mg/Tab. Bot. 16s, 32s. *otc.*
Use: Analgesic, antihistamine, decongestant.

Alka-Seltzer Special Effervescent Antacid. (Bayer Corp. (Consumer Div.)) Heat treated sodium bicarbonate 958 mg, citric acid 832 mg, potassium bicarbonate 312 mg, sodium 284 mg/Tab. Foil pack 12s, 20s, 36s. *otc.*
Use: Effervescent antacid.

Alka-Seltzer Tablets. (Bayer Corp. (Consumer Div.)) Aspirin 325 mg, citric acid 1000 mg, phenylalanine 9 mg, sodium 506 mg/Tab. Bot. 24s. *otc.*
Use: Analgesic, antacid.

Alka-Seltzer w/Aspirin. (Bayer Corp. (Consumer Div.)) Sodium bicarbonate 1916 mg, citric acid 1000 mg, aspirin 325 mg, and sodium 567 mg. 17.2 mEq acid neutralizing capacity. Foil pack 8s, 12s, 24s, 26s, and 36s. *otc.*
Use: Analgesic, antacid.

Alkeran. (GlaxoWellcome) Melphalan; 50 mg/Pow. for Inj. Single-use vial w/ 10 ml of sterile diluent. *Rx.*
Use: Antineoplastic.

Alkets. (Roberts Pharmaceuticals) Calcium carbonate 500 mg, dextrose, peppermint flavor. Chew. Tab. Bot. 36s, 96s, 150s. *otc.*
Use: Antacid.

alkylbenzyldimethylammonium chloride. Benzalkonium Cl, N.F. 18.

•**alkyl (C12-15) benzoate, N.F. 18.**
Use: Pharmaceutical aid (oleaginous vehicle emollient).

•**allantoin.** (al-AN-toe-in) USAN.
Use: Vulnerary (topical).
See: Cutemol (Summers Laboratories, Inc.).
W/Aminacrine, sulfanilamide.
See: Par Cream (Parmed Pharmaceuticals, Inc.).
Balmex Med. Lot. (Block Drug Co., Inc.).
W/p-Chloro-m-xylenol.
See: Cebum, Shampoo (Dermik Laboratories, Inc.).
W/Coal tar extract, hexachlorophene, glycerin, lanolin.
See: Pso-Rite, Cream (DePree).
W/Coal tar in cream base.
See: Tegrin Cream (Block Drug Co., Inc.).
W/Coal tar solution, isopropyl myristate, psorilan.
See: Psorelief, Soln. (Quality Formulations, Inc.).
W/Dienestrol, sulfanilamide, aminacrine HCl.
See: Tackle, Gel. (Colgate Oral Pharmaceuticals).
W/Salicylic acid, sulfur.
See: Neutrogena Disposables (Neutrogena).

W/Sulfanilamide, 9-aminoacridine HCl.
See: Nil Vaginal Cream (Century Pharmaceuticals, Inc.).
Vagisan Creme (Sandia).
Sebical Shampoo (Schwarz Pharma, Inc.).

Allay. (LuChem Pharmaceuticals, Inc.) Acetaminophen 650 mg, hydrocodone bitartrate 7.5 mg/ Cap. Bot. 100s. *c-III.*
Use: Analgesic combination, narcotic.

Allbee C-800. (Wyeth-Ayerst Laboratories) Vitamins E 45 IU, C 800 mg, B_1 15 mg, B_2 17 mg, B_3 100 mg, B_5 25 mg, B_{12} 12 mcg/Tab. Bot. 60s. *otc.*
Use: Vitamin supplement.

Allbee C-800 Plus Iron. (Wyeth-Ayerst Laboratories) Vitamins E 45 IU, C 800 mg, B_1 15 mg, B_2 17 mg, niacin 100 mg, B_6 25 mg, B_{12} 12 mcg, pantothenic acid 25 mg, iron 27 mg, folic acid 0.4 mg/Tab. Bot. 60s. *otc.*
Use: Mineral, vitamin supplement.

Allbee w/C. (Wyeth-Ayerst Laboratories) Vitamins B_1 15 mg, B_6 5 mg, B_2 10.2 mg, B_3 50 mg, B_5 10 mg, C 300 mg/ Cap. Bot. 30s. *otc.*
Use: Vitamin supplement.

Allbee-T. (Wyeth-Ayerst Laboratories) Vitamins B_1 15.5 mg, B_2 10 mg, B_6 8.2 mg, B_5 23 mg, B_3 100 mg, C 500 mg, B_{12} 5 mcg/Tab. Bot. 100s, 500s. *otc.*
Use: Vitamin supplement.

Allbex. (Health for Life Brands, Inc.) Vitamins B_1 5 mg, B_2 2 mg, B_6 0.25 mg, calcium pantothenate 3 mg, niacinamide 20 mg, ferrous sulfate 194.4 mg, inositol 10 mg, choline 10 mg, B_{12} (concentrate) 3 mcg/Cap. Bot. 100s, 1000s. *otc.*
Use: Mineral, vitamin supplement.

All-Day-C. (Barth's) Vitamin C 200 mg/ Cap. or 500 mg/Tab. with rose hip extract. Bot. 30s, 90s, 180s, 360s. *otc.*
Use: Vitamin supplement.

All-Day Iron Yeast. (Barth's) Iron 20 mg, Vitamins B_1 2 mg, B_2 4 mg, niacin 0.57 mg/Cap. Bot. 30s, 90s, 180s. *otc.*
Use: Mineral, vitamin supplement.

All-Day-Vites. (Barth's) Vitamins A 10,000 IU, D 400 IU, B_1 3 mg, B_2 6 mg, niacin 1 mg, C 120 mg, B_{12} 10 mcg, E 30 IU/Cap. Bot. 30s, 90s, 180s, 360s. *otc.*
Use: Vitamin supplement.

Allegra. (Hoechst Marion Roussel) Fexofenadine HCl 60 mg, lactose/Cap. Bot. 60s, 100s, 500s, UD 100s. *Rx.*
Use: Antihistamine.

Allegra-D. (Hoechst Marion Roussel) Fexofenadine 60 mg, pseudoephedrine HCl 120 mg/ER Tab. Bot. 60s, 100s, 500s, UD 100s. *Rx.*
Use: Antihistamine.

allegron. Nortriptyline.
Use: Antidepressant.

Allent. (B.F. Ascher and Co.) Pseudoephedrine HCl 120 mg, brompheniramine maleate 12 mg. SR Cap. Bot. 100s. *Rx.*
Use: Antihistamine, decongestant.

Allerben Injection. (Forest Pharmaceutical, Inc.) Diphenhydramine 10 mg/ ml. Vial 30 ml. *Rx.*
Use: Antihistamine.

Allerchlor. (Forest Pharmaceutical, Inc.) Chlorpheniramine maleate 10 mg/ml. Inj. Vial 30 ml. *Rx.*
Use: Antihistamine.

Aller-Chlor. (Rugby Labs, Inc.) Chlorpheniramine maleate. **Tab.:** 4 mg. Bot. 100s. **Syr.:** 2 mg/5 ml. Alcohol 5%, menthol, parabens, sugar. Bot. 118 ml. *otc.*
Use: Antihistamine.

Allercon. (Parmed Pharmaceuticals, Inc.) Pseudoephedrine HCl 60 mg, triprolidine HCl 2.5 mg/Tab. Bot. 24s, 100s, and 1000s. *otc.*
Use: Antihistamine, decongestant.

Allercreme Skin Lotion. (Galderma Laboratories, Inc.) Mineral oil, petrolatum, lanolin, lanolin oil, lanolin alcohols, glycerin, triethanolamine, cetyl alcohol, stearic acid, parabens. Lot. Bot. 240 ml. *otc.*
Use: Emollient.

Allercreme Ultra Emollient. (Galderma Laboratories, Inc.) Mineral oil, petrolatum, lanolin, lanolin alcohol, lanolin oil, glycerin, glyceryl stearate, PEG-100 stearate, squalane, cetyl alcohol, sorbitan laurate, quaternium-15, parabens. Cream Bot. 60 g. *otc.*
Use: Emollient.

Allerdec Capsules. (Towne) Phenylpropanolamine HCl 25 mg, chlorpheniramine maleate 1 mg, pyrilamine maleate 5 mg/Cap. Bot. 25s, 50s. *otc.*
Use: Antihistamine, decongestant.

Allerest. (Novartis Consumer Health) **Tab.:** Phenylpropanolamine HCl 18.7 mg, chlorpheniramine maleate 2 mg/ Tab. Sleeve Pack 24s, 48s. Bot. 72s. **Chew. Tab. for Children:** Phenylpropanolamine HCl 9.4 mg, chlorpheniramine maleate 1 mg/Tab. Sleeve Pack 24s. **Eye Drops:** Naphazoline HCl 0.012%. Bot. 0.5 oz. **Headache Strength Tab.:** Acetaminophen 325 mg, pseudoephedrine HCl 30 mg, chlorpheniramine maleate 2 mg/Tab. Pkg. 24s. **Nasal Spray:** Oxymetazoline HCl 0.05%. Bot. 0.5 oz. *otc.*

Use: Analgesic (Headache Strength Tab. only), antihistamine, decongestant.

Allerest 12-Hour. (Novartis Pharmaceutical Corp.) Phenylpropanolamine HCl 75 mg, chlorpheniramine maleate 8 mg/Cap. Sleevepak 10s. *otc.*
Use: Antihistamine, decongestant.

Allerest, Children's. (Novartis Pharmaceutical Corp.) Phenylpropanolamine HCl 94 mg, chlorpheniramine maleate 6 mg. Chew. Tab. Bot. 24s. *otc.*
Use: Antihistamine, decongestant.

Allerest Maximum Strength. (Medeva Pharmaceuticals, Inc.) Pseudoephedrine 30 mg, chlorpheniramine maleate 2 mg/Tab. Bot. 24s, 48s, 72s. *otc.*
Use: Antihistamine, decongestant.

Allerest Maximum Strength 12-Hour Caplets. (Novartis Pharmaceutical Corp.) Phenylpropanolamine HCl 75 mg, chlorpheniramine maleate 12 mg/Capl. Pkg. 10s. *otc.*
Use: Antihistamine, decongestant.

Allerest No Drowsiness. (Novartis Pharmaceutical Corp.) Pseudoephedrine 30 mg, acetaminophen 325 mg/Tab. Bot. 20s. *otc.*
Use: Analgesic, decongestant.

Allerest Sinus Pain Formula. (Novartis Pharmaceutical Corp.) Acetaminophen 500 mg, pseudoephedrine HCl 30 mg, chlorpheniramine maleate 2 mg/Tab. Pkg. 20s. *otc.*
Use: Analgesic, antihistamine, decongestant.

Allerfrim. (Rugby Labs, Inc.) **Tab.:** Pseudoephedrine HCl 60 mg, triprolidine HCl 2.5 mg. Bot. 24s, 100s, 1000s. **Syr.:** Pseudoephedrine HCl 30 mg, triprolidine HCl 1.25 mg. Bot. 118 ml, 473 ml. *otc.*
Use: Antihistamine, decongestant.

Allerfrin OTC Syrup. (Rugby Labs, Inc.) Pseudoephedrine 30 mg, triprolidine 1.25 mg. Syr. Bot. Pt. *otc.*
Use: Antihistamine, decongestant.

Allerfrin w/Codeine. (Rugby Labs, Inc.) Pseudoephedrine HCl 30 mg, triprolidine HCl 1.25 mg, codeine phosphate 10 mg, alcohol 4.3%. Syr. Bot. 120 ml, Pt, gal. *c-v.*
Use: Antihistamine, antitussive, decongestant.

Allergan Enzymatic. (Allergan, Inc.) Papain, sodium Cl, sodium carbonate, sodium borate, edetate disodium. Kits 12s, 24s, 36s, 48s. *otc.*
Use: Contact lens care.

Allergan Hydrocare Cleaning & Disinfecting Solution. (Allergan, Inc.) tris (2-hydroxyethyl) tallow ammonium Cl 0.013%, thimerosal 0.002%, bis (2-hydroxyethyl) tallow ammonium Cl, sodium bicarbonate, dibasic, monobasic and anhydrous sodium phosphate, hydrochloric acid, propylene glycol, polysorbate 80, special soluble polyhema. Bot. 4 oz, 8 oz, 12 oz. *otc.*
Use: Contact lens care.

Allergan Hydrocare Preserved Saline Solution. (Allergan, Inc.) Sodium Cl, sodium hexametaphosphate, sodium hydroxide, boric acid, sodium borate, EDTA 0.01%, thimerosal 0.001%. Bot. 8 oz, 12 oz. *otc.*
Use: Contact lens care.

Allergen Ear Drops. (Zenith Goldline Pharmaceuticals) Benzocaine 1.4%, antipyrine 5.4%, glycerin, oxyquinoline sulfate. Bot. 0.5 oz. *Rx.*
Use: Otic.

Allergen Patch Test Kit. (Hermal Pharmaceutical Labs) Box of tubes of semisolid pastes or solutions. Allergens are either suspended in 4.5 g petrolatum, USP, or dissolved in 5.5 g water. Kit includes 20 reclosable syringes for topical use only (not for injection), each exuding sufficient allergen to test 150 patients, housed in a plastic case with two drawers. Allergens include benzocaine, mercaptobenzothiazole, colophony, p-phenylenediamine, imidazolidinyl urea (Germall115), cinnamon aldyhyde, lanolin alcohol (woolwax alcohols), carbarubber mix, neomycin sulfate, thiuram rubber mix, formaldehyde, ethylenediamine dihydrochloride, epoxyresin, quaternium 15, p-tert-butylphenol formalde hyderesin, mercapto rubber mix, black rubber p-phenylenediamine mix, potassium dichromate, balsam of Peru and nickel sulfate.

allergen test patches.
Use: Diagnostic aid, allergic dermatitis.
See: T.R.U.E. Test (GlaxoWellcome).

Allergenic Extracts. (Various Mfr.) Allergenic extracts of pollen, mold, housedust, inhalants, epidermals, insects in saline 0.9% and phenol 0.4% up to 1:10 w/v or 40,000 PNU/ml insets or vials up to 30 ml.
Use: Diagnostic aid, allergens.

Allergenic Extracts. (Bayer Corp. (Consumer Div.)) Allergenic extracts of pollens, foods, inhalants, epidermals, fungi, insects, miscellaneous antigens.
Use: Diagnostic aid, allergens.

allergenic extracts, alum-precipitated.
See: Allpyral (Bayer Corp. (Consumer Div.)).

Center-Al (Center Laboratories).

Allergex. (Bayer Corp. (Consumer Div.)) Silicones, polyethylene and triethylene glycol, antioxidants, mineral oil concentrate. Bot. Pt. Aerosol pt.
Use: Antiallergic.

Allergy. (Major Pharmaceuticals) Chlorpheniramine maleate 4 mg, lactose/Tab. Bot. 24s, 100s. *otc.*
Use: Antihistamine.

Allergy Drops. (Bausch & Lomb Pharmaceuticals) Naphazoline HCl 0.012%. Bot. 15 ml. *otc.*
Use: Mydriatic, vasoconstrictor.

allergy preparations.
See: Antihistamine Preparations.

allergy relief medicine.
Use: Antihistamine, decongestant.
See: A.R.M. Caplets (SmithKline Beecham Pharmaceuticals).

Allergy-Sinus Comtrex. (Bristol-Myers Squibb) Pseudoephedrine HCl 30 mg, chlorpheniramine maleate 2 mg, acetaminophen 500 mg/Capl. or Tab. Bot. 50s, UD 24s. *otc.*
Use: Analgesic, antihistamine, decongestant.

Allergy Tablets. (Weeks & Leo) Phenylpropanolamine HCl 37.5 mg, chlorpheniramine 4 mg/Tab. Bot. 30s. *otc.*
Use: Antihistamine, decongestant.

AllerMax. (Pfeiffer Co.) Diphenhydramine HCl 50 mg, lactose/Capl. Pkg. 24s. *otc.*
Use: Antihistamine.

AllerMax Allergy & Cough Formula. (Pfeiffer Co.) Diphenhydramine HCl 6.25 mg/5 ml, alcohol 0.5%, raspberry flavor, menthol, sucrose, glucose, saccharin, sorbitol. 118 ml. *otc.*
Use: Antihistamine.

Allerphed. (Great Southern Laboratories) Pseudoephedrine HCl 30 mg, triprolidine HCl 1.25 mg/5 ml. Syr. Bot. 118 ml. *otc.*
Use: Antihistamine, decongestant.

Allersone. (Roberts Pharmaceuticals) Hydrocortisone 0.5%, diperodon HCl 0.5%, zinc oxide 5%, sodium lauryl sulfate, propylene glycol, cetyl alcohol, petrolatum, methyl- and propylparabens. Oint. Tube 15 g. *Rx-otc.*
Use: Corticosteroid, topical.

Allersule Forte. (Misemer Pharmaceuticals, Inc.) Phenylephrine HCl 20 mg, chlorpheniramine maleate 8 mg, methscopolamine nitrate 2.5 mg/Cap. Bot. 100s. *Rx-otc.*
Use: Anticholinergic, antihistamine, decongestant.

All-Nite Cold Formula. (Major Pharmaceuticals) Pseudoephedrine HCl 10 mg, doxylamine succinate 1.25 mg, dextromethorphan HBr 5 mg, acetaminophen 167 mg/5 ml. Liq. Bot. 177 ml. *otc.*
Use: Analgesic, antihistamine, antitussive, decongestant.

•**allobarbital.** (AL-low-BAR-bih-tal) USAN.
Formerly Diallybarbituric acid.
Use: Hypnotic, sedative.
W/Acetaminophen, salicylamide, caffeine.
See: Allylvon, Cap. (Zeneca Pharmaceuticals).
W/Aspirin, acetaminophen, aluminum aspirin.
See: Allylgesic, Tab. (Zeneca Pharmaceuticals).

•**allopurinol.** (AL-oh-PURE-ee-nahl) U.S.P. 23.
Use: Antigout, xanthine oxidase inhibitor.
See: Lopurin, Tab. (Knoll Pharmaceuticals).
Zyloprim, Tab. (GlaxoWellcome).

allopurinol riboside.
Use: Antiprotozoal.

allopurinol sodium. (AL-oh-PURE-ee-nal) Inj.
Use: Ex vivo preservation of cadaveric kidneys for transplantation; antineoplastic. [Orphan Drug]
See: Zyloprim, Inj. (GlaxoWellcome).

Allpyral. (Bayer Corp. (Consumer Div.)) Allergenic extracts, alum-precipitated. For subcutaneous inj. pollens, molds, epithelia, house dust, other inhalants, stinging insects.
Use: Diagnostic aid, allergens.

allylbarbituric acid. Allylisobutylbarbituric acid, butalbital. Tab. (Various Mfr.).
Use: Sedative.
W/A.P.C.
See: Anti-Ten, Tab. (Century Pharmaceuticals, Inc.).
Fiorinal, Cap., Tab. (Novartis Pharmaceutical Corp.).
Tenstan (Standex).
W/Acetaminophen, homatropine methylbromide.
See: Panitol H.M.B., Tab. (Wesley Pharmacal Co., Inc.).
W/Acetaminophen, salicylamide, caffeine.
See: Renpap, Tab. (Wren).

allyl-isobutylbarbituric acid.
See: Allylbarbituric Acid.

allylisopropylmalonyl urea.
See: Aprobarbital.

•**allyl isothiocyanate.** U.S.P. 23.
Use: Counterirritant in neuralgia.

Almacone. (Rugby Labs, Inc.) **Chew tab.:** Aluminum hydroxide 200 mg,

magnesium hydroxide 200 mg, simethicone 20 mg/Bot. 100s, 1000s. **Liq.:** Aluminum hydroxide 200 mg, magnesium hydroxide 200 mg, simethicone 20 mg, sodium 0.75 mg/5 ml. Bot. 360 ml, gal. *otc.*
Use: Antacid.

Almacone II Double Strength Liquid. (Rugby Labs, Inc.) Aluminum hydroxide 400 mg, magnesium hydroxide 400 mg, simethicone 40 mg/5 ml. Bot. 360 ml, gal. *otc.*
Use: Antacid.

•**almadrate sulfate.** (AL-ma-drate) USAN. Aluminum magnesium hydroxide-oxide-sulfate-hydrate.
Use: Antacid.

•**almagate.** (AL-mah-gate) USAN.
Use: Antacid.

almagucin. Gastric mucin, dried aluminum hydroxide gel, magnesium trisilicate. *otc.*
Use: Antacid.

Almebex Plus B_{12}. (Dayton Laboratories, Inc.) Vitamins B_1 1 mg, B_2 2 mg, B_3 5 mg, B_6 0.4 mg, B_{12} 5 mcg, choline 33 mg/5 ml. 473 ml (with B_{12} in separate container). *otc.*
Use: Vitamin supplement.

•**almond oil.** N.F. 18.
Use: Pharmaceutic aid (emollient, oleaginous vehicle, perfume).

Almora. (Forest Pharmaceutical, Inc.) Magnesium gluconate 0.5 g/Tab. Pkg. 100s. *otc.*
Use: Mineral supplement.

•**almotriptan.** (al-moe-TRIP-tan) USAN.
Use: Antimigraine.

•**alniditan dihydrochloride.** (al-nih-DIH-tan die-HIGH-droe-KLOR-ide) USAN.
Use: Antimigraine.

Alnyte. (Mayer Lab) Scopolamine aminoxide HBr 0.2 mg, salicylamide 250 mg/Tab. Pkg. 16s. *Rx.*
Use: Analgesic, anticholinergic.

Alocass Laxative. (Western Research) Aloin 0.25 gr, cascara sagrada 0.5 gr, rhubarb 0.5 gr, ginger 1/32 gr, powdered extract of belladonna gr/Tab. Bot. 1000s. Pak 28s. *otc.*
Use: Laxative.

Alodopa-15. (Major Pharmaceuticals) Hydrochlorothiazide 15 mg, methyldopa 250 mg. Tab. Bot. 100s. *Rx.*
Use: Antihypertensive.

Alodopa-25. (Major Pharmaceuticals) Hydrochlorothiazide 25 mg, methyldopa 250 mg. Tab. Bot. 100s. *Rx.*
Use: Antihypertensive.

•**aloe.** U.S.P. 23.
Use: See Compound Benzoin Tincture.

Aloe Grande Creme. (Gordon Laboratories) Aloe, vitamins E 1500 IU, A 100,000 units/oz in cream base. Jar 2.5 oz. *otc.*
Use: Emollient.

Aloe Vesta Perineal. (SmithKline Beecham Pharmaceuticals) Solution of sodium C14-16 olefin sulfonate, propylene glycol, aloe vera gel, hydrolyzed collagen. Bot. 118 ml, 236 ml, gal. *otc.*
Use: Perianal hygiene.

•**alofilcon a.** (AL-oh-FILL-kahn) USAN.
Use: Contact lens material (hydrophilic).

aloin. (Baker, J.T.) A mixture of crystalline pentosides from various aloes. Bot. oz. *otc.*
Use: Laxative.

Alomide. (Alcon Laboratories, Inc.) Lodoxamide tromethamine 0.1%. Soln. Drop-tainers 10 ml. *Rx.*
Use: Antiallergic, ophthalmic.

•**alonimid.** (ah-LAHN-ih-mid) USAN.
Use: Hypnotic, sedative.

Alor 5/500. (Atley Pharmaceuticals, Inc.) Hydrocodone bitartrate 5 mg, aspirin 500 mg/Tab. Bot. 100s. *c-III.*
Use: Analgesic, narcotic.

Alora. (Procter & Gamble Pharm.) Estradiol 1.5 mg (0.05 mg/day), 2.3 mg (0.075 mg/day), and 3 mg (0.1 mg/day)/Patch. Calendar packs 8 and 24 systems. *Rx.*
Use: Estrogen.

•**alosetron hydrochloride.** (al-OH-seh-trahn) USAN.
Use: Antiemetic.

Alotone. (Major Pharmaceuticals) Triamcinolone 4 mg/Tab. Bot. 100s. *Rx.*
Use: Corticosteroid.

•**alovudine.** (al-OHV-you-deen) USAN.
Use: Antiviral.

•**alpertine.** (al-PURR-teen) USAN.
Use: Antipsychotic.

l-alpha-acetyl-methadol (LAAM). (Bio Development Corp.) *Rx.*
Use: Treatment of heroin addicts.

•**alpha amylase.** (AL-fah AM-ih-lace) USAN. A concentrated form of alpha amylase produced by a strain of non-pathogenic bacteria.
Use: Digestive aid; anti-inflammatory.
See: Kutrase, Cap. (Schwarz Pharma, Inc.).
Ku-Zyme, Cap. (Schwarz Pharma, Inc.).

alpha-amylase w-100. W/Proteinase W-300, cellase W-100, lipase, estrone, testosterone, vitamins, minerals. *Rx.*

Use: Digestive aid.

alpha-1-adrenergic blockers.
Use: Antihypertensive.
See: Cardura (Roerig).

alpha-1-antitrypsin (recombinant DNA origin).
Use: Supplementation therapy for alpha$_1$-antitrypsin deficiency in the ZZ phenotype population. [Orphan Drug]

alpha/beta-adrenergic blocker.
See: Normodyne (Schering-Plough Corp.).
Trandate (GlaxoWellcome).

alpha-chymotrypsin.
See: Alpha Chymar, Vial (Centeon).

Alphaderm. (Teva Pharmaceuticals USA) Hydrocortisone 1%. Cream 30 g, 100 g. *Rx-otc.*
Use: Corticosteroid, topical.

alpha-d-galactosidase.
Use: Antiflatulent.

Alpha-E. (Barth's) d-Alpha tocopherol. **50 IU or 100 IU:** Cap. Bot. 100s, 500s, 1000s. **200 IU:** Cap. Bot. 100s, 250s. **400 IU:** Cap. Bot. 100s, 250s, 500s. *otc.*
Use: Vitamin supplement.

alpha-estradiol. Known as beta-estradiol.
See: Estradiol (Various Mfr.).

alpha-estradiol benzoate.
See: Estradiol benzoate (Various Mfr.).

Alpha Fast. (Eastwood) Bath oil. Bot. 16 oz. *otc.*
Use: Emollient.

alpha-fetoprotein w/tc-99m. USAN.
Use: Diagnostic aid.

•**alphafilcon a.** (al-fah-FILL-kahn) USAN.
Use: Contact lens material (hydrophilic).

alpha-galactosidase.
See: Aspergillus niger enzyme.

alpha-galactosidase a.
Use: Fabry's disease. [Orphan Drug]

alpha-galactoside a. USAN.
Use: Treatment of Fabry's disease.

Alphagan. (Allergan, Inc.) Brimonidine tartrate 0.2%, polyvinyl alcohol/Soln. Dropper Bot. 5 ml, 10 ml. *Rx.*
Use: Agent for glaucoma.

alpha-hypophamine.
See: Oxytocin Inj.

alpha interferon-2a.
See: Roferon-A (Roche Laboratories).

alpha interferon-2b.
See: Intron A (Schering-Plough Corp.).

Alpha-Keri. (Westwood Squibb Pharmaceuticals) **Therapeutic Bath:** Mineral oil, lanolin oil, PEG-4-dilaurate, benzophenone-3, D&C green #6, fragrance. Bot. 4 oz, 8 oz, 16 oz. **Cleansing Bar:** Bar containing sodium tallowate, sodium cocoate, water, mineral oil, fragrance, PEG-75, glycerin, titanium dioxide, lanolin oil, sodium Cl, BHT, EDTA, D&C green #5, D&C yellow #10. 120 g. *otc.*
Use: Emollient.

alpha-methyldopa. Name previously used for Methyldopa.

Alphanate. (Alliance Pharmaceuticals) ≥ 10 IU FVIII: C/mg total protein. 0.05 to 1 g albumin (human), ≤ 10 mmol Ca/ml, ≥ 750 mcg glycine/IU FVIII: C, ≤ 2 IU heparin/ml, ≤ 300 mmol arginine/L, ≤ 2.5mg PEG, 80/IU FVIII: C, ≤ 10 mEq Na/vial after reconstitution. Pow., lyophilized. Single-dose vials with diluent. *Rx.*
Use: Antihemophilic, treatment for von Willebrand's disease. [Orphan Drug]

AlphaNine. (Alpha Therapeutic Corp.) Purified heat-treated/solvent preparation of coagulation Factor IX from human plasma. With ≥ 50 units Factor IX per mg protein, < 5 units each Factor II (prothrombin) and Factor VII (proconvertin) per 100 IU Factor IX and < 20 units Factor X (Stuart-Power Factor) per 100 IU Factor IX. In single-dose vials with diluent, double-ended needle, and microaggregated filter. Pow. for Inj. *Rx.*
Use: Antihemophilic.

Alphanine SD. (Alpha Therapeutic Corp.) ≥ 150 IU Factor IX/mg. Pow., lyophilized. Single-dose vial with 10 ml diluent, double-ended needle, filter. *Rx.*
Use: Antihemophilic.

alpha-1-antitrypsin (recombinant DNA origin). (Chiron)
Use: Treatment of alpha-1-antitrypsin deficiency. [Orphan Drug]

alpha-1-proteinase inhibitor.
Use: Treatment of alpha-1-antitrypsin deficiency. [Orphan Drug]
See: Prolastin (Bayer Corp. (Biological and Pharmaceutical Div.))

alphasone acetophenide. Name previously used for Algestone acetonide.

alpha-tocopherol.
See: Tocopherol, Alpha (Various Mfr.).

Alphatrex. (Savage Laboratories) **Cream and Oint.:** Betamethasone dipropionate 0.05%. Tube 15 g, 45 g. **Lot.:** Betamethasone dipropionate 0.05%. Bot. 60 ml. *Rx.*
Use: Corticosteroid, topical.

Alpha Vee-12. (Schlicksup) Hydroxocobalamin 1000 mcg/ml. Vial 10 ml. *Rx.*
Use: Vitamin supplement.

Alphosyl. (Schwarz Pharma, Inc.) Allantoin 1.7%, special crude coal tar extracts 5%. **Lot.:** Bot. 8 fl oz. **Cream:** 2

oz. *otc.*
Use: Antipruritic.

•**alpidem.** (AL-PIH-dem) USAN.
Use: Antianxiety (anxiolytic).

•**alprazolam.** (al-PRAY-zoe-lam) U.S.P. 23.
Use: Hypnotic, sedative.
See: Xanax, Tab. (Pharmacia & Upjohn).

alprazolam. (Various Mfr.) Alprazolam **0.25 mg, 0.5 mg, 1 mg:** Tab. Bot. 30s, 100s, 500s, 1000s, UD 100s. **2 mg:** Tab. Bot. 100s, 500s. *c-IV.*
Use: Management of anxiety disorders.

alprazolam. (Roxane Laboratories, Inc.) **Oral Soln.:** Alprazolam 0.5 mg/5 ml, sorbitol, saccharin, fruit-mint flavor. Bot. 500 ml, UD 2.5 ml, UD 5 ml, UD 10 ml. **Intensol Soln.:** Alprazolam 1 mg/ml. Dropper. Bot. 30 ml. *c-IV.*
Use: Anxiolytic.

•**alprenolol hydrochloride.** (al-PREH-no-lole) USAN.
Use: Antiadrenergic (β-receptor).

•**alprenoxime hydrochloride.** (al-PREN-ox-eem) USAN.
Use: Antiglaucoma agent.

•**alprostadil.** (al-PRAHST-uh-dill) U.S.P. 23. *Formerly Prostaglandin E_1, PGE_1.*
Use: Vasodilator, anti-impotence agent, arterial patency agent.
See: Caverject (Pharmacia & Upjohn).
Edex, Inj. (Schwarz Pharma, Inc.).
Prostin VR, Inj. (Pharmacia & Upjohn).
Prostin VR Pediatric, Inj. (Pharmacia & Upjohn).

alprostadil. (al-PRAHST-uh-dill) (Schwarz Pharma, Inc.)
Use: Severe peripheral arterial occlusive disease. [Orphan Drug]

Alramucil. (Alra Laboratories, Inc.) Psyllium hydrophilic mucilloid 3.6 g, citric acid, sucrose, saccharin, potassium bicarbonate, sodium bicarbonate, 4 calories and < 0.01 g sodium per packet. Pow. effervescent. Pkg. 30s. *otc.*
Use: Laxative.

Alredase. (Wyeth-Ayerst Laboratories) Tolrestat. *Rx.*
Use: Aldose reductase inhibitor.

•**alrestatin sodium.** (AHL-reh-STAT-in) USAN.
Use: Enzyme inhibitor (aldose reductase).

Alrex. (Bausch & Lomb Pharmaceuticals) Loteprednol etabonate 0.2%, benzalkonium chloride 0.01%, EDTA. Ophth. Susp. Bot. 5 ml, 10 ml. *Rx.*
Use: Corticosteroid, ophthalmic.

Alsorb Gel. (Standex) Magnesium and aluminum hydroxide. Colloidal Susp. *otc.*
Use: Antacid.

Alsorb Gel, C.T. (Standex) Calcium carbonate 2 gr, glycine 3 gr, magnesium trisilicate 3 gr/Tab. *otc.*
Use: Antacid.

Altace. (Monarch) Ramipril 1.25 mg, 2.5 mg, 5 mg, or 10 mg/Cap. Bot. 100s, UD 100s. *Rx.*
Use: Antihypertensive; congestive heart failure.

•**altanserin tartrate.** (AL-TAN-ser-in) USAN.
Use: Serotonin antagonist.

•**alteplase.** (AL-teh-PLACE) U.S.P. 23.
Use: Plasminogen activator.
See: Activase, Inj. (Genentech, Inc.).

AlternaGEL. (J & J Merck Consumer Pharm.) Aluminum hydroxide 600 mg/5 ml. Liq. Bot. 150 ml, 360 ml. *otc.*
Use: Antacid.

•**althiazide.** (al-THIGH-azz-ide) USAN.
Use: Antihypertensive; diuretic.

Altracin. (Alpharma USPD Inc.) Bacitracin.
Use: Antibiotic. [Orphan Drug]

•**altretamine.** (ahl-TRETT-uh-meen) USAN.
Use: Antineoplastic. [Orphan Drug]
See: Hexalen (US Bioscience).

altretamine. (ahl-TRETT-uh-meen)
Use: Antineoplastic. [Orphan Drug]
See: Hexalen (US Bioscience).

Alu-Cap. (3M Pharm) Aluminum hydroxide gel 400 mg/Cap. Bot. 100s. *otc.*
Use: Antacid.

Al-U-Creme. (MacAllister) Aluminum hydroxide equivalent to 4% aluminum oxide. Susp. Bot. Pt, gal. *otc.*
Use: Antacid.

Aludrox. (Wyeth-Ayerst Laboratories) Aluminum hydroxide gel 307 mg, magnesium hydroxide 103 mg/5 ml. Susp. Bot. 355 ml. *otc.*
Use: Antacid.

alukalin. Activated kaolin.
Use: Antidiarrheal.

Alulex. (Lexington) Magnesium trisilicate 3.25 gr, aluminum hydroxide gel 3.5 gr, phenobarbital ⅛ gr, homatropine methylbromide gr/Tab. Bot. 100s. *Rx.*
Use: Agent for peptic ulcer.

alum. Sulfuric acid, aluminum ammonium salt (2:1:1), dodecahydrate. Sulfuric acid, aluminum potassium salt (2:1:1), dodecahydrate.
Use: Astringent.

•**alum, ammonium.** U.S.P. 23.

Use: Astringent.

•**alum, potassium.** U.S.P. 23.
Use: Astringent.

alum-precipitated allergenic extracts.
See: Allpyral (Bayer Corp. (Consumer Div.)).
Center-Al (Center Laboratories).

Alumadrine. (Fleming & Co.) Acetaminophen 500 mg, phenylpropanolamine HCl 25 mg, chlorpheniramine maleate 4 mg/Tab. Bot. 100s, 1000s. *Rx.*
Use: Analgesic, antihistamine, decongestant.

Alumate-HC. (Dermco) Hydrocortisone 0.125%, 0.25%, 0.5%, or 1%/Cream. Pkg. 0.5 oz, 1 oz, 4 oz. *otc.*
Use: Corticosteroid, topical.

Alumate Mixture. (Schlicksup) Aluminum hydroxide gel, milk of magnesia/5 ml. Bot. 12 oz, gal. *otc.*
Use: Antacid.

alumina hydrated powder. W/Activated attapulgite, pectin. *otc.*
Use: Antidiarrheal.

alumina, magnesia, and calcium carbonate tablets.
Use: Antacid.

alumina, magnesia, calcium carbonate, and simethicone tablets.
Use: Antacid.

alumina, magnesia, and calcium chloride oral suspension.
Use: Antacid.

alumina and magnesia oral suspension.
Use: Antacid.

alumina and magnesia tablets.
Use: Antacid.

alumina, magnesia, and simethicone.
Use: Antacid, antiflatulent.

alumina, magnesia, and simethicone suspension. (Roxane Laboratories, Inc.) Aluminum hydroxide 213 mg, magnesium hydroxide 200 mg, simethicone 20 mg, parabens, sorbitol/5 ml. Susp. Bot. UD 15, 30 ml. *otc.*
Use: Antacid.

alumina and magnesium carbonate oral suspension.
Use: Antacid.

alumina, magnesium carbonate, and magnesium oxide tablets.
Use: Antacid.

alumina and magnesium trisilicate oral suspension.
Use: Antacid.

alumina and magnesium trisilicate tablets.
Use: Antacid.

Aluminostomy. (Richards Pharm) Aluminum pow. 18%, zinc oxide, zinc stearate in a bland water repellent ointment. Jar 2 oz, 6 oz, lb.
Use: Dermatologic, protectant.

aluminum. (uh-LOO-min-uhm)
See: Aluminostomy (Richards Pharm).

aluminum acetate.
Use: Astringent.
See: Acid Mantle Creme (Novartis Pharmaceutical Corp.).
Buro-Sol, Pow., Sol. (Doak Dermatologics).

•**aluminum acetate topical solution.** U.S.P. 23.
Use: Astringent.
See: Bluboro Powder (Allergan, Inc.).
Buro-Sol (Doak Dermatologics).
Domeboro, Pow., Tab. (Bayer Corp. (Consumer Div.)).
Domeboro Otic, Soln. (Bayer Corp. (Consumer Div.)).

aluminum aminoacetate, dihydroxy.
See: Dihydroxy aluminum aminoacetate (Various Mfr.).

aluminum carbonate basic.
Use: Antacid.
See: Basaljel, Susp. (Wyeth-Ayerst Laboratories).

aluminum carbonate, dried basic, gel. Cap., Tab.
Use: Antacid.

•**aluminum carbonate, basic.** USAN. U.S.P. XXII.
Use: Antacid.
See: Basaljel, Susp., Cap., Tab. (Wyeth-Ayerst Laboratories).

aluminum chlorhydroxy allantoinate.
See: Alcloxa (Schuylkill).

•**aluminum chloride.** U.S.P. 23. Aluminum Cl hexahydrate.
Use: Astringent.
See: Drysol (Person and Covey, Inc.).
Xerac AC (Person and Covey, Inc.).

aluminum chloride hexahydrate.
Use: Astringent.
See: Drysol (Person and Covey, Inc.).

•**aluminum chlorohydrate.** (ah-LOO-min-uhm) U.S.P. 23. *Formerly Aluminum chlorhydroxide, aluminum hydroxychloride.*
Use: Anhidrotic.
See: Ostiderm, Lot., Roll-On (Pedinol Pharmacal, Inc.).

•**aluminum chlorohydrex.** (ah-LOO-min-uhm) USAN. *Formerly Aluminum chlorhydroxide alcohol soluble complex, aluminum chlorohydrol propylene glycol complex.*
Use: Astringent.

•**aluminum chlorohydrex polyethylene glycol.** U.S.P. 23.

Use: Anhidrotic.

•**aluminum chlorohydrex propylene glycol.** U.S.P. 23.
Use: Anhidrotic.

•**aluminum dichlorohydrate.** U.S.P. 23.
Use: Anhidrotic.

•**aluminum dichlorohydrex polyethylene glycol.** U.S.P. 23.
Use: Anhidrotic.

•**aluminum dichlorohydrex propylene glycol.** U.S.P. 23.
Use: Anhidrotic.

aluminum dihydroxyaminoacetate.
See: Dihydroxy Aluminum Aminoacetate, U.S.P. 23. (Various Mfr.).

aluminum glycinate, basic.
See: Dihydroxy Aluminum Aminoacetate, U.S.P. 23
W/Aspirin, magnesium carbonate.
See: Bufferin, Tab. (Bristol-Myers Squibb).

•**aluminum hydroxide gel.** U.S.P. 23.
Use: Antacid.
See: AlternaGEL, Liq. (J & J Merck Consumer Pharm.).
Alu-Cap, Cap. (3M Pharm).
Al-U-Creme, Susp. (MacAllister).
Alu-Tab, Tab. (3M Pharm).
Amphojel, Susp., Tab. (Wyeth-Ayerst Laboratories).
Maalox HRF, Liq. (Rhone-Poulenc Rorer Pharmaceuticals, Inc.).
Maalox Plus, Tab. (Rhone-Poulenc Rorer Pharmaceuticals, Inc.).
Nutrajel (Cenci, H.R. Labs, Inc.).
W/Aminoacetic acid, magnesium trisilicate.
See: Maracid-2, Tab. (Marlin Industries).
W/Belladonna extract, magnesium hydroxide.
See: Trialka, Liq., Tab. (Del Pharmaceuticals, Inc.).
W/Calcium carbonate.
See: Alkalade, Susp., Tab. (DePree).
W/Calcium carbonate, magnesium carbonate, magnesium trisilicate.
See: Marblen, Susp., Tab. (Fleming & Co.).
W/Clioquinol, methylcellulose, atropine sulfate, hyoscine HBr, hyoscyamine sulfate.
See: Enterex, Tab. (Person and Covey, Inc.).
W/Dicyclomine HCl, magnesium hydroxide, methylcellulose.
See: Triactin Liq., Tab. (Procter & Gamble Pharm.).
W/Gastric mucin, magnesium glycinate.
See: Mucogel, Liq., Tab. (Inwood).
W/Kaolin, pectin.
See: Metropectin, Liq. (Medeva Pharmaceuticals, Inc.).
W/Magnesium carbonate.
See: Algicon, Tab. (Rhone-Poulenc Rorer Pharmaceuticals, Inc.)
Estomul-M Liq., Tab. (3M Pharm).
W/Magnesium carbonate, calcium carbonate, amino-acetic acid.
See: Glycogel Tab., Susp. (Schwarz Pharma, Inc.).
W/Magnesium hydroxide.
See: Alsorb Gel (Standex).
Aludrox, Susp., Tab. (Wyeth-Ayerst Laboratories).
Delcid, Liq. (Hoechst Marion Roussel).
Gas Ban DS, Liq. (Roberts Pharmaceuticals).
Kolantyl, Gel, Wafer (Hoechst Marion Roussel).
Maalox, Susp. (Rhone-Poulenc Rorer Pharmaceuticals, Inc.).
Mylanta, Tab. (Zeneca Pharmaceuticals).
Mylanta II, Tab. (Zeneca Pharmaceuticals).
Neutralox, Susp. (Teva USA).
WinGel, Liq., Tab. (Sanofi Winthrop).
W/Magnesium hydroxide, aspirin.
See: Ascriptin, Tab. (Rhone-Poulenc Rorer Pharmaceuticals, Inc.).
Ascriptin Extra Strength, Tab. (Rhone-Poulenc Rorer Pharmaceuticals, Inc.).
Calciphen, Tab. (Westerfield).
Cama, Tab. (Novartis Pharmaceutical Corp.).
Cama Inlay-Tab. (Novartis Pharmaceutical Corp.).
W/Magnesium hydroxide, calcium carbonate.
See: Camalox, Susp. (Rhone-Poulenc Rorer Pharmaceuticals, Inc.).
W/Magnesium hydroxide, simethicone.
See: Di-Gel, Liq. (Schering-Plough Corp.).
Gas-Ban DS (Roberts Med.).
Maalox Plus, Susp. (Rhone-Poulenc Rorer Pharmaceuticals, Inc.).
Mylanta, Liq. (Zeneca Pharmaceuticals).
Mylanta-II, Liq. (Zeneca Pharmaceuticals).
Silain-Gel, Liq., Tab. (Robins).
Simeco, Liq. (Wyeth-Ayerst).
W/Magnesium trisilicilate.
See: Antacid G, Tab. (Walgreen Co.).
Antacid Tablets, Tab. (Panray).
Arcodex Antacid, Tab. (Arcum).
Gacid, Tab. (Arcum).

Malcogel, Susp. (Pharmacia & Upjohn).
Malcotabs (Pharmacia & Upjohn).
Manalum, Tab. (Paddock).
W/Phenindamine tartrate, phenylephrine HCl, aspirin, caffeine, magnesium carbonate.
See: Dristan, Tab. (Whitehall Robins).
W/Phenol, zinc oxide, camphor, eucalyptol, ichthammol.
See: Almophen, Oint. (Jones Medical Industries).
W/Prednisolone.
See: Fernisolone-B (Ferndale Laboratories).
Predoxine, Tab. (Roberts Pharm).
W/Sodium salicylate, acetaminophen, vitamin C.
See: Gaysal-S., Tab. (Roberts Pharm).

aluminum hydroxide gel. (Various Mfr.) 320 mg/5 ml. Susp. Bot. 360 ml, 480 ml, UD 15 and 30 ml. *otc.*
Use: Antacid.

aluminum hydroxide gel, concentrated. (Various Mfr.) 600 mg/5 ml. Liq. Bot. 30 ml, 180 ml, 480 ml. *otc.*
Use: Antacid.

aluminum hydroxide gel, concentrated. (Roxane Laboratories, Inc.) Susp. **450 mg/5 ml:** Bot. 500 ml, UD 30 ml; **675 mg/5 ml:** Bot. 180 ml, 500 ml, UD 20 ml and 30 ml. *otc.*
Use: Antacid.

•**aluminum hydroxide gel, dried.** U.S.P. 23.
Use: Antacid.
See: AlternaGEL, Liq. (J & J Merck Consumer Pharm.).
Alu-Cap, Cap. (3M Pharm).
Amphojel, Tab. (Wyeth-Ayerst Laboratories).
Ascriptin, Tab. (Rhone-Poulenc Rorer Pharmaceuticals, Inc.).
Di-Gel, Liq. (Schering-Plough Corp.).
Mylanta, Liq, Tab. (J & J Merck Consumer Pharm.).

aluminum hydroxide gel, dried w/combinations.
Use: Antacid.
See: Aludrox, Susp., Tab. (Wyeth-Ayerst Laboratories).
Alurex, Tab. (Rexall Group).
Banacid, Tab. (Buffington).
Delcid, Liq. (Hoechst Marion Roussel).
Eulcin, Tab. (Leeds).
Gaviscon, Foamtab (Hoechst Marion Roussel).
Maalox, Tab. (Rhone-Poulenc Rorer Pharmaceuticals, Inc.).
Maalox Plus, Tab. (Rhone-Poulenc Rorer Pharmaceuticals, Inc.)
Mylanta, Tab, Liq. (Zeneca Pharmaceuticals).
Mylanta II, Tab, Liq. (Zeneca Pharmaceuticals).
Presalin, Tab. (Roberts Pharmaceuticals).

aluminum hydroxide glycine.
See: Dihydroxyaluminum aminoacetate.

aluminum hydroxide magnesium carbonate.
Use: Antacid.
See: Aloxine (Forest Pharmaceutical, Inc.).
Di-Gel, Tab. (Schering-Plough Corp.).
Eugel, Tab., Liq. (Solvay Pharmaceuticals).
W/Dicyclomine HCl, magnesium trisilicate, methylcellulose.
See: Triactin, Liq., Tab. (Procter & Gamble Pharm.).

•**aluminum monostearate.** N.F. 18.
Use: Pharmaceutic necessity for preparation of penicillin G procaine w/aluminum stearate suspension.
See: Penicillin G procaine w/aluminum stearate suspension.

Aluminum Paste. (Paddock Laboratories) Metallic aluminum 10%. Oint. Jar lb. *otc.*
Use: Dermatologic, protectant.

•**aluminum phosphate gel.** U.S.P. 23.
Use: Antacid.

•**aluminum sesquichlorohydrate.** (ah-LOO-min-uhm sess-kwih-KLOR-oh-HIGH-drate) U.S.P. 23.
Use: Anhidrotic.

•**aluminum sesquichlorohydrex polyethylene glycol.** U.S.P. 23.
Use: Anhidrotic.

•**aluminum sesquichlorohydrex propylene glycol.** U.S.P. 23.
Use: Anhidrotic.

aluminum sodium carbonate hydroxide.
See: Dihydroxyaluminum sodium carbonate.

•**aluminum subacetate topical solution.** U.S.P. 23.
Use: Astringent.

•**aluminum sulfate.** U.S.P. 23.
Use: Pharmaceutic necessity for preparation of aluminum subacetate solution.
See: Aluminum Subacetate, Soln.
Bluboro, Pow. (Allergan, Inc.).
Ostiderm, Roll-on (Pedinol Pharmacal, Inc.).

•**aluminum zirconium octachlorohydrate.** U.S.P. 23.
Use: Anhidrotic.

•**aluminum zirconium octachlorohydrex gly.** U.S.P. 23.
Use: Anhidrotic.

•**aluminum zirconium pentachlorohydrate.** U.S.P. 23.
Use: Anhidrotic.

•**aluminum zirconium pentachlorohydrex gly.** U.S.P. 23.
Use: Anhidrotic.

•**aluminum zirconium tetrachlorohydrate.** U.S.P. 23.
Use: Anhidrotic.

•**aluminum zirconium tetrachlorohydrex gly.** (ah-LOO-min-uhm zihr-KOE-nee-uhm teh-trah-KLOR-oh-HIGH-drex Gly) U.S.P. 23.
Use: Anhidrotic.

•**aluminum zirconium trichlorohydrate.** U.S.P. 23.
Use: Anhidrotic.

•**aluminum zirconium trichlorohydrex gly.** (ah-LOO-min-uhm zihr-KOE-nee-uhm try-KLOR-oh-HIGH-drex Gly) U.S.P. 23.
Use: Anhidrotic.

Alupent. (Boehringer Ingelheim, Inc.) Metaproterenol sulfate. **Aer.:** 75 mg (0.65 mg/dose). Inhaler 5 ml. 150 mg (0.65 mg dose). Inhaler 10 ml, refill 10 ml. **Syr.:** 10 mg/5 ml. Bot. 480 ml. **Inhalant Soln.: 0.4%:** 2.5 ml UD vial. **0.6%:** 2.5 ml UD vial. **5%:** Bot. 10 ml, 30 ml. *Rx.*
Use: Bronchodilator.

Alurate. (Roche Laboratories) Aprobarbital 40 mg/5 ml. Alcohol 20%. Elix. Bot. Pt. *c-III.*
Use: Hypnotic, sedative.

Alurex. (Rexall Group) Magnesium-aluminum hydroxide. **Susp.:** (200 mg-150 mg/5 ml) Bot. 12 oz. **Tab:** (400 mg-300 mg) Box 50s. *otc.*
Use: Antacid.

Alu-Tab. (3M Pharm) Aluminum hydroxide gel 500 mg/Tab. Bot. 250s. *otc.*
Use: Antacid.

Alvedil. (Luly-Thomas) Theophylline 4 gr, pseudoephedrine HCl 50 mg, butabarbital 15 mg/Cap. Bot. 100s. *Rx.*
Use: Bronchodilator, decongestant, hypnotic, sedative.

•**alverine citrate.** (AL-ver-een) USAN. N.F. XIII.
Use: Anticholinergic.

•**alvircept sudotox.** (AL-vihr-sept SOOD-ah-tox) USAN.
Use: Antiviral.

Alzapam. (Major Pharmaceuticals) Lorazepam 0.5 mg, 1 mg, or 2 mg/Tab. Bot. 100s, 500s. *c-IV.*
Use: Antianxiety.

Ama. (Wampole Laboratories) Antimitochondrial antibodies test by IFA. Test 48s.
Use: Diagnostic aid.

amacetam sulfate.
Use: Cognition adjuvant.

•**amadinone acetate.** (aim-AD-ih-nohn) USAN.
Use: Hormone, progestin.

•**amantadine hydrochloride.** (uh-MAN-tuh-deen) U.S.P. 23.
Use: Antiviral.

amantadine hydrochloride. (uh-MAN-tuh-deen) (Various Mfr.) **Cap.:** 100 mg. Bot. 100s, 250s, 500s, UD 100s. **Syrup:** 50 mg/5 ml Bot. Pt. *Rx.*
Use: Antiviral, treatment of Parkinson's disease.
See: Symmetrel, Cap., Syr. (DuPont Merck Pharmaceutical Co.).

Amaphen. (Trimen Laboratories, Inc.) Acetaminophen 325 mg, caffeine 40 mg, butalbital 50 mg/Cap. Bot. 100s. *Rx.*
Use: Analgesic, hypnotic, sedative.

amaranth.
Use: Color (Not for internal use).

Amaryl. (Hoechst Marion Roussel) Glimepiride 1, 2, or 4 mg, lactose/Tab. Bot. 100s, UD 100s (except 1 mg). *Rx.*
Use: Antidiabetic.

Amatine. (Roberts Pharmaceuticals) Midodrine HCl.
Use: Orthostatic hypotension. [Orphan Drug]

ambenonium chloride.
Use: Cholinergic for treatment of myasthenia gravis.
See: Mytelase, Cap. (Sanofi Winthrop Pharmaceuticals).

Ambenyl Cough. (Forest Pharmaceutical, Inc.) Codeine phosphate 10 mg, bromodiphenhydramine HCl 12.5 mg/5 ml, alcohol 5%. Syr. Bot. 4 oz, Pt, gal. *c-v.*
Use: Antihistamine, antitussive.

Ambenyl-D. (Forest Pharmaceutical, Inc.) Guaifenesin 100 mg, pseudoephedrine HCl 30 mg, dextromethorphan HBr 15 mg/10 ml, alcohol 9.5%. Liq. Bot. 4 oz. *otc.*
Use: Antitussive, decongestant, expectorant.

Amberlite. (Rohm and Haas) I.R.P.-64. Polacrilin.

Amberlite. (Rohm and Haas) I.R.P.-88. Polacrilin potassium.

Ambi 10 Cream. (Kiwi Brands, Inc.) Benzoyl peroxide 10%, parabens. Cream. Tube 28.3 g. *otc.*
Use: Antiacne.

Ambi 10 Soap. (Kiwi Brands, Inc.) Triclosan, sodium tallouate, PEG-20, titanium dioxide. Soap, Bar 99 g. *otc.*
Use: Antiacne.

Ambien. (Searle) Zolpidem tartrate 5 mg, 10 mg/Tab. Bot. 100s, 500s, UD 100s. *c-iv.*
Use: Hypnotic, sedative.

Ambi Skin Tone. (Kiwi Brands, Inc.) Hydroquinone, padimate O, sodium metabisulfite, parabens, EDTA, vitamin E. Cream. Tube 57 g, 28.4 g. *otc.*
Use: Dermatologic.

•**ambomycin.** (AM-boe-MY-sin) USAN. Isolated from filtrates of *Streptomyces ambofaciens.*
Use: Antineoplastic.

•**ambruticin.** (am-brew-TIE-sin) USAN.
Use: Antifungal.

ambucaine. Ambutoxate HCl.

•**ambuphylline.** (AM-byoo-fill-in) USAN. *Formerly Bufylline.*
Use: Diuretic, muscle relaxant.

•**ambuside.** (AM-buh-SIDE) USAN.
Use: Diuretic.

ambutonium bromide.
Use: Antispasmodic.

AMC. (Schlicksup) Ammonium Cl 7.5 gr/ Tab. Bot. 1000s. *Rx.*
Use: Diuretic, expectorant.

Amcill. (Parke-Davis) **Cap.:** Ampicillin trihydrate 250 mg or 500 mg/Cap. Bot. 100s, 500s, UD 100s. **Oral Susp.:** 125 mg or 250 mg/5 ml. Bot. 100 ml, 200 ml.
Use: Anti-infective, penicillin.

•**amcinafal.** (am-SIN-ah-fal) USAN.
Use: Anti-inflammatory.

•**amcinafide.** (am-SIN-ah-fide) USAN.
Use: Anti-inflammatory.

•**amcinonide.** (am-SIN-oh-nide) U.S.P. 23.
Use: Corticosteroid, topical.
See: Cyclocort, Cream, Oint. (ESI Lederle Generics).

Amcort. (Keene Pharmaceuticals, Inc.) Triamcinolone diacetate 40 mg/ml. Vial 5 ml. *Rx.*
Use: Corticosteroid.

•**amdinocillin.** (am-DEE-no-SILL-in) U.S.P. 23.
Use: Anti-infective.

•**amdinocillin pivoxil.** (am-DEE-no-SILL-in pihv-OX-ill) USAN.
Use: Anti-infective.

ameban.
See: Carbarsone.

amebicides.
See: Acetarsone (Various Mfr.).
Aralen HCl, Inj. (Sanofi Winthrop Pharmaceuticals).
Aralen Phosphate, Tab. (Sanofi Winthrop Pharmaceuticals).
Carbarsone, Pulv., Tab. (Eli Lilly and Co.).
Chiniofon, Tab. (Various Mfr.).
Chloroquine Phosphate, Tab. (Various Mfr.).
Diiodohydroxyquin (Various Mfr.).
Emetine HCl (Various Mfr.).
Flagyl, Tab. (Searle).
Humatin, Kapseal, Syr. (Parke-Davis).
Yodoxin, Tab. (Glenwood, Inc.).

Amechol.
Use: Diagnostic aid.
See: Methacholine Cl.

•**amedalin hydrochloride.** (ah-MEH-dah-lin) USAN.
Use: Antidepressant.

•**ameltolide.** (AH-mell-TOE-lide) USAN.
Use: Anticonvulsant.

Amen. (Carnrick Laboratories, Inc.) Medroxyprogesterone acetate 10 mg, lactose/Tab. Bot. 50s, 100s, 1000s. *Rx.*
Use: Hormone, progestin.

Amerge. (GlaxoWellcome) Naratriptan HCl 1 mg, 2.5 mg, lactose/Tab. Blister pack 9s. *Rx.*
Use: Antimigraine.

Americaine. (Novartis Pharmaceutical Corp.) Benzocaine 20%. Spray Bot. 60 ml. *otc.*
Use: Anesthetic, local.

Americaine Anesthetic Lubricant. (Fisions) Benzocaine 20%, benzethonium chloride 0.1%. Gel Tube 30 g, UD 2.5 g. *Rx.*
Use: Anesthetic, local, topical.

Americaine First Aid Burn Ointment. (Novartis Pharmaceutical Corp.) Benzocaine 20%, benzethonium Cl 0.1% in a water-soluble polyethylene glycol base. Tube 0.75 oz. *otc.*
Use: Anesthetic, local.

Americaine Hemorrhoidal Ointment. (Novartis Pharmaceutical Corp.) Benzocaine 20%. Tube 22.5 g w/rectal applicator. *otc.*
Use: Anesthetic, local.

Americaine Otic. (Novartis Pharmaceutical Corp.) Benzethonium Cl 0.1%, benzocaine 20% in a water-soluble base of 1% (w/w) glycerin, polyethylene glycol 300. Bot. 0.5 oz. *Rx.*
Use: Otic.

Ames Dextro System Lancets. (Bayer Corp. (Consumer Div.)) Sterile dispos-

able lancet. Box 100s.
Use: Diagnostic aid.

•**amesergide.** (am-eh-SIR-jide) USAN.
Use: Serotonin antagonist.

•**ametantrone acetate.** (am-ETT-an-TRONE) USAN.
Use: Antineoplastic.

A-Methapred Univial. (Abbott Hospital Products) Methylprednisolone sodium succinate. **40 mg/ml:** Pkg. 1s, 25s, 50s, 100s; 125 mg/2 ml Pkg. 1s, 5s, 25s, 50s, 100s; **500 mg/4 ml:** Pkg. 1s, 5s, 25s, 100s; **1000 mg/8 ml:** Pkg. 1s, 5s, 25s, 100s. *Rx.*
Use: Corticosteroid.

amethocaine hydrochloride.
Use: Anesthetic, local.
See: Tetracaine HCl.

amethopterin.
Use: Antineoplastic.
See: Methotrexate (ESI Lederle Generics).

•**amfenac sodium.** (AM-fen-ack SO-dee-uhm) USAN.
Use: Anti-inflammatory.

•**amfilcon a.** (AM-FILL-kahn A) USAN.
Use: Contact lens material (hydrophilic).

•**amflutizole.** (am-FLEW-tih-zole) USAN.
Use: Treatment of gout.

amfodyne.
See: Imidecyl iodine.

•**amfonelic acid.** (am-fah-NEH-lick Acid) USAN.
Use: Central nervous system stimulant.

Amgenal Cough. (Zenith Goldline Pharmaceuticals) Bromodiphenhydramine HCl 12.5 mg, codeine phosphate 10 mg/5 ml, alcohol 5%. Syr. Bot. 120 ml, Pt, gal. *c-v.*
Use: Antihistamine, antitussive.

amibiarson.
See: Carbarsone (Various Mfr.).

Amicar. (Immunex Corp.) **Tab.:** Aminocaproic acid 500 mg. In 100s. **Syr.:** Aminocaproic acid 250 mg/ml, sorbitol, saccharin. In 480 ml. **Inj.:** Aminocaproic acid 250 mg/ml, benzyl alcohol 0.9%. In 20 or 96 ml. *Rx.*
Use: Hemostatic, systemic.

•**amicycline.** (AM-ee-SIGH-kleen) USAN.
Use: Anti-infective.

Amidate. (Abbott Hospital Products) Etomidate 2 mg/ml, propylene glycol 35%. Single-dose Amp 20 mg/10 ml or 40 mg/20 ml; Abboject syringe 40 mg/20 ml. *Rx.*
Use: Anesthetic, general.

•**amidephrine mesylate.** (AM-ee-DEH-frin MEH-sih-LATE) USAN.
Use: Adrenergic.

amidofebrin.
See: Aminopyrine (Various Mfr.).

amidone hydrochloride.
Use: Analgesic, narcotic.
See: Methadone HCl (Various Mfr.).

amidopyrazoline.
See: Aminopyrine (Various Mfr.).

amidotrizoate, sodium.
See: Diatrizoate sodium.

•**amifloxacin.** (am-ih-FLOX-ah-SIN) USAN.
Use: Anti-infective.

•**amifloxacin mesylate.** (am-ih-FLOX-ah-SIN MEH-sih-LATE) USAN.
Use: Anti-infective.

•**amifostine.** (am-ih-FOSS-teen) USAN.
Formerly Ethiofos.
Use: Protectant (topical); radioprotector.
See: Ethyol (Alza/US Bioscience).

amifostine. (am-ih-FOSS-teen)
Use: Chemoprotective. [Orphan Drug]
See: Ethyol (US Bioscience).

Amigen. (Baxter Pharmaceutical Products, Inc.) Protein hydrolysate. **5%:** Bot. 500 ml, 1000 ml; **10%:** Bot. 500 ml, 1000 ml. **5% w/dextrose 5%:** Bot. 500 ml, 1000 ml. **5% w/dextrose 5%, alcohol 5%:** Bot. 1000 ml. **5% w/fructose 10%:** Bot. 1000 ml. **5% w/fructose 12.5%, alcohol 2.4%:** Bot. 1000 ml. *Rx.*
Use: Nutritional supplement.

Amigesic. (Amide Pharmaceuticals, Inc.) Salsalate 500 mg/Cap or Tab. Salsalate 75 mg/Capl. Bot. 100s, 500s. *Rx.*
Use: Analgesic.

•**amikacin.** (am-ih-KAE-sin) U.S.P. 23.
Use: Anti-infective.

amikacin. (Bedford Laboratories) Amikacin sulfate 250 mg, sodium metabisulfite 0.66%, sodium citrate dihydrate 2.5%/ml. Inj. Vial 2 ml, 4 ml. *Rx.*
Use: Anti-infective.

amikacin. (Various Mfr.) 50 mg (as sulfate) per ml, sodium metabisulfite 0.13%, sodium citrate dihydrate 0.5%. Inj. Vial 2, 4 ml. 10s. *Rx.*
Use: Anti-infective.

•**amikacin sulfate.** (am-ih-KAE-sin) U.S.P. 23.
Use: Anti-infective.

amikacin sulfate injection. (Various Mfr.) Amikacin sulfate 50 mg/ml. Vial 2 ml, 4 ml (10s).
Use: Anti-infective.
See: Amikin, Inj. (Bristol-Myers Squibb).

Amikin. (Bristol-Myers Squibb) Amikacin sulfate. Inj. Vial 100 mg, 500 mg, 1 g, disposable syringes 500 mg. *Rx.*

Use: Anti-infective, aminoglycoside.
•**amiloride hydrochloride.** (uh-MILL-oh-ride) U.S.P. 23.
Use: Diuretic.
See: Midamor, Tab. (Merck & Co.).
amiloride hydrochloride solution for inhalation. (GlaxoWellcome)
Use: Cystic fibrosis. [Orphan Drug]
amiloride hydrochloride and hydrochlorothiazide tablets.
Use: Antihypertensive, diuretic.
See: Moduretic, Tab. (Merck & Co.).
Amina-21. (Miller Pharmacal Group, Inc.) L-form amino acids 600 mg/Cap. Bot. 100s, 300s.
Use: Dermatologic, wound therapy.
aminacrine. F.D.A. 9-Aminoacridine.
Use: Anti-infective, topical.
•**aminacrine hydrochloride.** (ah-MEE-nah-kreen) USAN.
Use: Anti-infective, topical.
W/Dienestrol, sulfanilamide, allantoin.
See: AVC, Cream, Supp. (Hoechst Marion Roussel).
aminarsone.
See: Carbarsone (Various Mfr.).
amine resin.
See: Polyamine Methylene Resin.
Aminess. (Clintec Nutrition) Essential amino acids. 10 Tab. = adult amino acid MDR. Jar 300s. *Rx.*
Use: Parenteral nutritional supplement.
Aminess 5.2%. (Clintec Nutrition) Amino acids and electrolytes, Inj. *Rx.*
Use: Nutritional supplement, parenteral.
Aminicotin.
Use: Vitamin supplement.
See: Nicotinamide (Various Mfr.).
aminoacetic acid. Glycerine, U.S.P. 23. (Various Mfr.) (Glycine, glycocoll) available as elix., pow., tab.
Use: Myasthenia gravis, irrigant.
W/Aluminum hydroxide, magnesium hydroxide, calcium carbonate.
See: Eugel, Tab., Liq. (Solvay Pharmaceuticals).
W/Calcium carbonate.
See: Antacid pH, Tab. (Towne).
Eldamint, Tab. (Zeneca Pharmaceuticals).
W/Calcium carbonate, aluminum hydroxide, magnesium carbonate.
See: Glytabs, Tab. (Pharmics, Inc.).
W/Calcium carbonate, magnesium carbonate, bismuth subcarbonate, dried aluminum hydroxide gel.
See: Buffer-Tabs (Forest Pharmaceutical, Inc.).
W/Magnesium trisilicate, aluminum hydroxide.
See: Maracid-2, Tab. (Marlin Industries).
W/Phenylephrine HCl, pyrilamine maleate, acetylsalicylic acid, caffeine.
See: Al-Ay, Tab. (Jones Medical Industries, Inc.).
W/Phenylephrine HCl, chlorpheniramine maleate, acetaminophen, caffeine.
See: Codimal, Tab. (Schwarz Pharma, Inc.).
aminoacetic acid & calcium carbonate.
amino acid & protein prep.
See: Aminoacetic Acid, U.S.P. 23.
Glutamic Acid.
Histidine HCl.
Lysine.
Phenylalanine.
Thyroxine.
amino acids.
Use: Amino acid supplement.
See: Aminosyn, Soln. (Abbott Laboratories).
W/Estrone, testosterone, vitamins, minerals.
See: Stuart Amino Acids and B_{12}, Tab. (Zeneca Pharmaceuticals).
amino acid combinations.
See: Dequasine (Miller Pharmacal Group, Inc.).
A/G-Pro (Miller Pharmacal Group, Inc.).
Jets (Freeda Vitamins, Inc.).
PDP Liquid Protein (Wesley Pharmacal Co., Inc.).
Amino-Min-D. (Tyson & Associates, Inc.) Ca 250 mg, D 100 IU, Fe 7.5 mg , Zn 5.6 mg, Mg, I, Mn, Cu, K, Cr, Se, betaine HCl, glutamic acid HCl. Cap. Bot. 100s. *otc.*
Use: Mineral, vitamin supplement.
aminoacridine. (ah-MEE-no-ACK-rih-deen)
Use: Bacteriostatic agent.
See: 9-aminoacridine
9-aminoacridine hydrochloride. (9-ah-MEE-no-ACK-rih-deen) (Various Mfr.) Aminacrine HCl.
Use: Anti-infective, vaginal.
See: Vagisec Plus (Durex).
W/Hydrocortisone acetate, tyrothricin, phenylmercuric acetate, polysorbate 80, urea, lactose.
See: Aquacort, Vaginal Supp. (Poly-Medica Pharmaceuticals).
W/Iodoquinol.
See: Vagitric, Oint. (Zeneca Pharmaceuticals).
W/Phenylmercuric acetate, tyrothricin, urea, lactose.
See: Trinalis, Vaginal Supp. (Poly-Medica Pharmaceuticals).
W/Polyoxyethylene nonyl phenol, sodium edetate, docusate sodium.

See: Vagisec Plus, Supp. (Durex).
W/Pramoxine HCl, acetic acid, parachlorometa-xylenol, methyl-dodecylbenzyltrimethyl ammonium Cl.
See: Drotic No. 2, Drops (B.F. Ascher and Co.).
W/Sulfanilamide, allantoin.
See: AVC Cream, Supp. (Hoechst Marion Roussel).
Nil Vaginal Cream (Century Pharmaceuticals, Inc.).
Par Cream (Parmed Pharmaceuticals, Inc.).
Vagisan, Creme (Sandia).

p-aminobenzene-sulfonylacetylimide.
See: Sulfacetamide.

•**aminobenzoate potassium.** (ah-MEE-no-BEN-zoe-ate) U.S.P. 23.
Use: Analgesic.
See: Potaba, Pow., Tab. (Glenwood, Inc.).
W/Hydrocortisone, ammonium salicylate, ascorbic acid.
See: Neocylate sodium free, Tab. (Schwarz Pharma, Inc.).
W/Potassium salicylate.
See: Pabalate-SF, Tab. (Wyeth-Ayerst Laboratories).

•**aminobenzoate sodium.** U.S.P. 23.
Use: Analgesic.
See: PABA sodium, Tab. (Various Mfr.).
W/Phenobarbital, colchicine salicylate, Vitamin B_1, aspirin.
See: Doloral, Tab. (Alamed).
W/Salicylamide, sodium salicylate, ascorbic acid, butabarbital sodium.
See: Bisalate, Tab. (Allison Lab).
W/Sodium salicylate.
See: Pabalate, Tab. (Wyeth-Ayerst Laboratories).

•**aminobenzoic acid.** U.S.P. 23. *Formerly Para-aminobenzoic acid.*
Use: Ultraviolet screen.
See: Pabanol, Lot. (Zeneca Pharmaceuticals).
W/Mephenesin, salicylamide.
See: Sal-Phenesin, Tab. (Hoechst Marion Roussel).

•**aminocaproic acid.** (uh-mee-no-kuh-PRO-ik) U.S.P. 23.
Use: Hemostatic.
See: Amicar, Syr., Tab., Vial (Immunex Corp.).

aminocaproic acid. (uh-mee-no-kuh-PRO-ik) (Orphan Medical, Inc.)
Use: Topical treatment of traumatic hyphema of the eye.

aminocaproic acid. (Various Mfr.) 250 mg/ml. 20 ml/Inj. *Rx.*
Use: Antifibrinolytic.

aminocardol.
Use: Bronchodilator.
See: Aminophylline (Various Mfr.).

Amino-Cerv pH 5.5. (Milex Products, Inc.) Urea 8.34%, sodium propionate 0.5%, methionine 0.83%, cystine 0.35%, inositol 0.83%, benzalkonium Cl, water miscible base. Tube with applicator 82.5 g. *Rx.*
Use: Vaginal agent.

Aminodyne Compound. (Jones Medical Industries, Inc.) Acetaminophen 2.5 gr, aspirin 3.5 gr, caffeine 0.5 gr/Tab. Bot. 100s, 1000s. *otc.*
Use: Analgesic combination.

2-aminoethanethiol. USAN.
Use: Urinary tract agent.

amino-ethyl-propanol.
See: Aminoisobutanol.
W/Bromotheophyllin
See: Pamabrom (Various Mfr.).

Aminofen. (Dover Pharmaceuticals) Acetaminophen 325 mg/Tab. Sugar, lactose, and salt free. UD Box 500s. *otc.*
Use: Analgesic.

Aminofen Max. (Dover Pharmaceuticals) Acetaminophen 500 mg/Tab. Sugar, lactose, and salt free. UD Box 500s. *otc.*
Use: Analgesic.

aminoform.
Use: Anti-infective, urinary.
See: Methenamine (Various Mfr.).

Aminogen. (Christina) Vitamin B complex, folic acid. Amp. 2 ml Box 12s, 24s, 100s. Vial 10 ml. *Rx.*
Use: Vitamin supplement.

•**aminoglutethimide.** (ah-MEE-no-glue-TETH-ih-mide) U.S.P. 23.
Use: Treatment of Cushing's syndrome; adrenocortical suppressant; antineoplastic.
See: Cytadren, Tab. (Novartis Pharmaceutical Corp.).

aminohippurate sodium. (Merck & Co.) 0.2 g/10 ml. Amp 10 ml, 50 ml.
Use: IV, diagnostic aid for renal plasma flow and function determination.

•**aminohippurate sodium injection.** (ah-MEE-no-HIP-your-ate) U.S.P. 23.
Use: Diagnostic aid (renal function determination).

•**aminohippuric acid.** (ah-MEE-no-hip-YOUR-ik) U.S.P. 23.
Use: Component of aminohippurate sodium (Inj.); diagnostic aid (renal function determination).

aminoisobutanol.
See: Butaphyllamine.
Pamabrom for combinations

aminoisometradine.

See: Methionine.

•**aminolevulinic acid hydrochloride.** (ah-MEE-no-lev-you-LIN-ik ASS-id HIGH-droe-KLOR-ide) USAN.
Use: Antineoplastic.

Aminonat. Protein hydrolysates (oral).

aminonitrozole. N- (5-Nitro-2-thiazolyl) acetamide.
Use: Antitrichomonal.

Amino-Optic-C. (Tyson & Associates, Inc.) Lemon bioflavonoids 250 mg, rutin, hesperidin, vitamin C, and rose hips powder 1000 mg/SR Tab. Bot. 100s. *otc.*
Use: Vitamin supplement.

Amino-Opti-E. (Tyson & Associates, Inc.) Vitamin E 165 mg/Cap. Bot. 100s. *otc.*
Use: Vitamin supplement.

aminopentamide sulfate.
Use: Anticholinergic.

Aminophyllin. (Searle) Trademark for Aminophylline. **100 mg/Tab.:** Bot. 100s, 1000s, UD 100s. **200 mg/Tab.:** Bot. 100s, 1000s, UD 100s. *Rx.*
Use: Bronchodilator.

Aminophyllin Injection. (Searle) Trademark for Aminophylline. Amp. **250 mg:** 10 ml; 25s, 100s. **500 mg:** 20 ml; 25s, 100s. *Rx.*
Use: Bronchodilator.

•**aminophylline.** (am-in-AHF-ih-lin) U.S.P. 23. *Formerly Theophylline ethylenediamine.*
Use: Muscle relaxant.
See: Phyllocontin, Tab. (Purdue Frederick Co.).

aminophylline combinations.
See: Amesec, Cap. (GlaxoWellcome).
Amphedrine Compound, Cap. (Lannett Co., Inc.).
Asminorel, Tab. (Solvay Pharmaceuticals).
B.M.E., Elix. (Brothers).
Mudrane GG-2, Tab. (ECR Pharmaceuticals).
Orthoxine and Aminophylline, Cap. (Pharmacia & Upjohn).
Quinamm, Tab. (Hoechst Marion Roussel).
Quinite, Tab. (Solvay Pharmaceuticals).
Strema, Cap. (Foy Laboratories).

aminophylline injection. (Abbott Laboratories) Amp. 250 mg/10 ml, 500 mg/20 ml; Flip top vial 10 mg/20 ml, 20 mg/50 ml.
Use: Bronchodilator.

aminophylline injection. Theophylline ethylenediamine. Amp. 3¾ gr, 7.5 gr (Various Mfr.).
Use: Muscle relaxant.

aminophylline suppositories. (Various Mfr.) 3⅜ gr, 7.5 gr.
Use: Muscle relaxant.

aminophylline tablets. Plain or enteric coated 1.5 gr, 3 gr (Various Mfr.).
Use: Muscle relaxant.

aminophylline with phenobarbital combinations.
See: Amodrine, Tab. (Searle).
Mudrane, Tab. (ECR Pharmaceuticals).
Mudrane GG, Tab. (ECR Pharmaceuticals).

Aminoprel. (Taylor Pharmaceuticals) L-lysine 60 mg, dl-methionine 15 mg, hydrolyzed protein 750 mg, iron 2 mg, Cu, I, K, Mg, Mn, Zn. Cap. Bot. 180s.
Use: Nutritional supplement.

aminopromazine. (I.N.N.) Proquamezine.

4-aminopyridine.
Use: Relief of symptoms of multiple sclerosis. [Orphan Drug]

aminopyrine.
Use: Antipyretic, analgesic.
See: Dipyrone, Vial (Maurry).

4-aminoquinoline derivatives.
Use: Antimalarial.
See: Aralen HCl (Sanofi Winthrop Pharmaceuticals).
Chloroquine Phosphate (Various Mfr.).
Plaquenil Sulfate (Sanofi Winthrop Pharmaceuticals).

8-aminoquinoline derivatives.
Use: Antimalarial.
See: Primaquine Phosphate, U.S.P.
Primaquine Phosphate (Sanofi Winthrop Pharmaceuticals).

•**aminorex.** (am-EE-no-rex) USAN.
Use: Anorexic.

aminosalicylate calcium. (Dumas-Wilson) U.S.P. XXI. 7.5 gr, Bot. 1000s.
Use: Tuberculosis therapy.

aminosalicylate potassium. Monopotassium 4-aminosalicylate.
Use: Antibacterial, tuberculostatic.

•**aminosalicylate sodium.** (uh-MEE-no-suh-LIS-ih-LATE) U.S.P. 23.
Use: Anti-infective, tuberculostatic.

aminosalicylate sodium. (uh-MEE-no-suh-LIS-ih-LATE) (Syncom Pharmaceuticals, Inc.)
Use: Crohn's disease. [Orphan Drug]

• **aminosalicylic acid.** (ah-MEE-no-sal-ih-SILL-ik) U.S.P. 23.
Use: Anti-infective, tuberculostatic.

aminosalicylic acid. (ah-MEE-no-SAL-ih-sill-ik)
Use: Tuberculosis infection treatment.
See: Paser, Gran. (Jacobus Pharmaceutical Co.).

4-aminosalicylic acid.
Use: Treatment of ulcerative colitis in patients intolerant to sulfasalazine. [Orphan Drug]

5-aminosalicylic acid.
See: Mesalamine.

p-aminosalicylic acid salts.
See: Aminosalicylate Calcium
Aminosalicylate Potassium
Aminosalicylate Sodium

aminosidine.
Use: Mycobacterium avium complex; tuberculosis; visceral leishmaniasis (KALA-AZAR). [Orphan Drug]
See: Gabbromicina
Paromomycin

Aminosyn. (Abbott Hospital Products) Crystalline amino acid solution. **3.5%:** 1000 ml; **5%:** Container 250 ml, 500 ml, 1000 ml; **7%:** 500 ml; 7% kit (cs/3); **8.5%:** Single-dose container 500 ml, 1000 ml. **10%:** 500 ml, 1000 ml. W/ Electrolytes. **7%:** 500 ml. **8.5%:** 500 ml. *Rx.*
Use: Nutritional supplement, parenteral

Aminosyn (pH6). (Abbott Laboratories) Crystalline amino acid infusion. 10%: 500 ml, 1000 ml. *Rx.*
Use: Nutritional supplement, parenteral.

Aminosyn-HBC 7%. (Abbott Laboratories) Crystalline amino acid infusion for high metabolic stress. 500 ml, 1000 ml. *Rx.*
Use: Nutritional supplement, parenteral.

Aminosyn M 3.5%. (Abbott Laboratories) Crystalline amino acid infusion with electrolytes. 1000 ml. *Rx.*
Use: Nutritional supplement, parenteral.

Aminosyn-PF. (Abbott Laboratories) Crystalline amino acid infusions for pediatric use. **7%:** 250 ml, 500 ml; **10%:** 1000 ml. *Rx.*
Use: Nutritional supplement, parenteral.

Aminosyn-RF. (Abbott Laboratories) Crystalline amino acid infusion for renal failure patients. **5.2%:** 300 ml. *Rx.*
Use: Nutritional supplement, parenteral.

Aminosyn II. (Abbott Laboratories) Crystalline amino acid infusion. **3.5%:** 1000 ml. **5%:** 1000 ml. **7%:** 500 ml. **8.5%:** 500 ml, 1000 ml. **10%:** 500 ml, 1000 ml. W/Dextrose: **3.5% in 5% dextrose:** 1000 ml. **3.5% in 25% dextrose:** 1000 ml. **5% in 25% dextrose:** 1000 ml. W/ Dextrose and electrolytes: **3.5% in 5% dextrose:** 1000 ml. **3.5% in 25% dextrose:** 1000 ml. **4.25% in 10% dextrose:** 1000 ml. **4.25% in 25% dextrose:** 1000 ml.W/Electrolytes: **7%:** 1000 ml. **8.5%:** 1000 ml. **10%:** 1000 ml. *Rx.*
Use: Nutritional supplement, parenteral.

Aminosyn II M. (Abbott Laboratories) Crystalline amino acid infusion with maintenance electrolytes, 10% dextrose. Soln. 1000 ml. *Rx.*
Use: Nutritional supplement, parenteral.

Amino-Thiol. (Marcen) Sulfur 10 mg, casein 50 mg, sodium citrate 5 mg, phenol 5 mg, benzyl alcohol 5 mg/ml. Vial 10 ml, 30 ml. *Rx.*
Use: Treatment of arthritis, neuritis.

aminotrate phosphate. Trolnitratephosphate.
See: Triethanolamine, Preps.

aminoxytropine tropate hydrochloride. Atropine-N-oxide HCl.

Amio-Aqueous. (Academic Pharmaceuticals, Inc.) Amiodarone.
Use: Antiarrhythmic. [Orphan Drug]

•**amiodarone.** (A-MEE-oh-duh-rone) USAN.
Use: Cardiovascular agent (antiarrhythmic, ventricular).

amiodarone hydrochloride. (Copley) Amiodarone HCl 200 mg, lactose. Tab. Bot. 60s, 100s, 250s. *Rx.*
Use: Antiarrhythmic.
See: Amio-Aqueous (Academic Pharmaceuticals, Inc.).
Cordarone, Tab., Inj. (Wyeth-Ayerst Laboratories).
Pacerone (Upsher-Smith).

Amipaque. (Sanofi Winthrop Pharmaceuticals) Metrizamide 18.75%/20 ml Vial.
Use: Radiopaque agent.

•**amiprilose hydrochloride.** (ah-MIH-prih-LOHS) USAN.
Use: Anti-infective, antifungal, anti-inflammatory, antineoplastic, antiviral, immunomodulator.

•**amiquinsin hydrochloride.** (AM-ih-KWIN-sin) USAN. Under study.
Use: Antihypertensive.

Ami-Tex LA. (Amide Pharmaceuticals, Inc.) Phenylpropanolamine HCl 75 mg, guaifenesin 400 mg/tab. Bot. 100s, 500s, 1000s. *Rx.*
Use: Decongestant, expectorant.

Amitin. (Thurston) Vitamin C 200 mg, lemon bioflavonoid 100 mg, niacinamide 60 mg, methionine 100 mg/Tab. Bot. 100s, 500s. *Rx.*
Use: Vitamin supplement.

Amitone. (Menley & James Labs, Inc.) Calcium carbonate 350 mg/Chew. Tab. Bot. 100s. *otc.*
Use: Antacid.

•**amitraz.** (AM-ih-trazz) U.S.P. 23.
Use: Scabicide.

•**amitriptyline hydrochloride.** (am-ee-TRIP-tih-leen) U.S.P. 23.
Use: Antidepressant.
See: Amitril, Tab. (Parke-Davis).
Elavil HCl, Tab., Inj. (Merck & Co.).
Emitrip, Tab. (Major Pharmaceuticals).
Endep, Tab. (Roche Laboratories).
W/Chlordiazepoxide.
See: Limbitrol, Tab. (Roche Laboratories).
W/Perphenazine.
See: Etrafon, Prods. (Schering-Plough Corp.).

AmLactin. (Upsher-Smith Labs, Inc.) Ammonium lactate 12%/Cream, Lot. 140 g, 225 g, 400 g. *otc.*
Use: Emollient.

•**amlexanox.** (am-LEX-an-ox) USAN.
Use: Treatment of mouth ulcers; antiallergic.
See: Aphthasol.

•**amlintide.** (AM-lin-tide) USAN.
Use: Treatment of type I diabetes mellitus; antidiabetic.

amlodipine. (am-LOW-dih-PEEN)
Use: Calcium channel blocker.
See: Norvasc (Pfizer US Pharmaceutical Group).

amlodipine and benazepril HCl. (am-LOW-dih-PEEN and BEN-AZE-eh-prill)
See: Lotrel, Cap. (Novartis Pharmaceutical Corp.).

•**amlodipine besylate.** (am-LOW-dih-PEEN) USAN.
Use: Antianginal; antihypertensive.
See: Norvasc (Pfizer US Pharmaceutical Group).

•**amlodipine maleate.** (am-LOW-dih-PEEN) USAN.
Use: Antianginal, antihypertensive.

Ammens Medicated Powder. (Bristol-Myers Squibb) Boric acid 4.55%, zinc oxide 9.10%, talc, starch. Can 6.25 oz, 11 oz. *otc.*
Use: Dermatologic, protectant.

ammoidin. Methoxsalen.
Use: Psoralen.

•**ammonia N 13 injection.** (ah-MOE-nee-ah N13) U.S.P. 23.
Use: Diagnostic aid (cardiac imaging, liver imaging); radiopharmaceutical.

•**ammonia solution, strong.** (ah-MOE-nee-ah) N.F. 18.
Use: Pharmaceutic aid (solvent; source of ammonia).

•**ammonia spirit, aromatic.** (ah-MOE-nee-ah) U.S.P. 23.
Use: Respiratory.

ammoniated mercury. (Various Mfr.)
Use: Anti-infective, topical.
See: Mercuronate 5% Oint. (Jones Medical Industries, Inc.).
W/Salicylic acid.
See: Emersal, Lot. (Medco Research, Inc.).

•**ammonio methacrylate copolymer.** (ah-MOE-nee-oh meth-ah-KRILL-ate koe-PAHL-ih-mer) N.F. 18.
Use: Pharmaceutic aid (coating agent).

ammonium benzoate.
Use: Antiseptic, urinary.

ammonium biphosphate, sodium biphosphate, and sodium acid pyrophosphate.
Use: Genitourinary.

•**ammonium carbonate.** (ah-MOE-nee-uhm) N.F. 18.
Use: Pharmaceutic aid (source of ammonia).

•**ammonium chloride.** (ah-MOE-nee-uhm) U.S.P. 23.
Use: Acidifier; diuretic.

ammonium chloride. (Various Mfr.) **Delayed Release Tab.:** Plain or E.C. 5 gr, 7.5 gr. (Bayer Corp. (Consumer-Div.)). **Inj.:** 120 mEq/30 ml. Vial.
Use: Acidifier; diuretic; expectorant; alkalosis.

Ammonium Chloride, Enseals. (Eli Lilly and Co.) Ammonium Cl. Tab. Enseal 7.5 gr. Bot. 100s. *Rx.*
Use: Acidifier, urinary.

•**ammonium lactate.** (ah-MOE-nee-uhm LACK-tate) USAN.
Use: Antipruritic (topical).
See: AmLactin, Cream, Lot. (Upsher-Smith Labs, Inc.).
Lac-Hydrin, Lot. (Westwood Squibb).

ammonium mandelate. Ammonium salt of mandelic acid. Syr. 8 g/fl oz. Bot. Pt, gal.
Use: Urinary antiseptic, oral.

•**ammonium molybdate.** (ah-MOE-nee-uhm) U.S.P. 23.

ammonium nitrate.
See: Reditemp-C, Cold Pack (Wyeth-Ayerst Laboratories).

•**ammonium phosphate.** (ah-MOE-nee-uhm) N.F. 18. Phosphoric acid diammonium salt. Diammonium phosphate.
Use: Pharmaceutic aid.

ammonium tetrathiomolybdate.
Use: Treatment of Wilson's disease. [Orphan Drug]

ammonium valerate.
Use: Sedative.

ammophyllin.
Use: Bronchodilator.
See: Aminophylline, U.S.P. 23. (Various Mfr.).

amobarbital. (am-oh-BAR-bih-tahl) (Various Mfr.) Tab. Elix.
Use: Hypnotic of intermediate duration.
See: Amytal, Elix., Pulv. (Eli Lilly and Co.).

•**amobarbital sodium.** (am-oh-BAR-bih-tahl) U.S.P. 23.
Use: Hypnotic, sedative.

amobarbital sodium. (Various Mfr.) Cap. **1 gr:** Bot. 100s, 500s; **3 gr:** Bot. 100s, 500s, 1000s. (Various Mfr.) Tab. **30 mg:** Bot. 100s; **50 mg:** Bot. 100s; **100 mg:** Bot. 100s. (Eli Lilly and Co.) Vial 250 mg, 500 mg. (Eli Lilly and Co.).
Use: Sedative, hypnotic.
See: Amytal sodium (Eli Lilly and Co.).
W/Ephedrine HCl, theophylline, chlorpheniramine maleate.
See: Theo-Span, Cap. (Scrip).
W/Secobarbital sodium.
See: Dusotal, Cap. (Harvey).
Tuinal, Cap. (Eli Lilly and Co.).

•**amodiaquine.** (am-oh-DIE-ah-kwin) U.S.P. 23.
Use: Antiprotozoal.

•**amodiaquine hydrochloride.** U.S.P. 23.
Use: Antimalarial.

Amodopa. (Major Pharmaceuticals) Methyldopa 125 mg, 250 mg, or 500 mg. **125 mg:** 100s, UD 100s. **250 mg:** 100s, 1000s, UD 100s. **500 mg:** 100s, 500s, UD 100s. *Rx.*
Use: Antihypertensive.

AMO Endosol. (Allergan, Inc.) Sodium chloride 0.64%, potassium chloride 0.075%, calcium chloride dihydrate 0.048%, magnesium chloride hexahydrate 0.03%, sodium acetate trihydrate 0.39%, sodium citrate dihydrate 0.17%. Preservative free. Soln. Bot. 18 ml, 500 ml. *Rx.*
Use: Physiological irrigating solution.

AMO Endosol Extra. (Allergan, Inc.) **Part I:** Water for injection with sodium chloride 7.14 mg, potassium chloride 0.38 mg, calcium chloride dihydrate 0.154 mg, magnesium chloride hexahydrate 0.2 mg, dextrose 0.92 mg, sodium hydroxide or hydrochloric acid/ml. Soln. Bot. 515 ml. **Part II:** Sodium bicarbonate 1081 mg, dibasic sodium phosphate anhydrous 216 mg, glutathione disulfide 95 mg. Soln. Bot. 60 ml. *Rx.*
Use: Ophthalmic irrigation solution.

Amol. (Mono-n-amyl-hydroquinone ether.)
See: B-F-I, Pow. (SmithKline Beecham Pharmaceuticals).

Amoline. (Major Pharmaceuticals) Aminophylline 100 mg or 200 mg/Tab. Bot. 100s, 1000s, UD 100s. *Rx-otc.*
Use: Bronchodilator.

amopyroquin hydrochloride.
See: Propoquin.

•**amorolfine.** (am-OH-role-feen) USAN.
Use: Antimycotic.

Amosan. (Oral-B Laboratories, Inc.) Sodium perborate, saccharin. 1.76 g single-dose packet box. 20s, 40s. *otc.*
Use: Mouth and throat preparation.

Amotriphene. *Rx.*
Use: Coronary vasodilator.

AMO Vitrax. (Allergan, Inc.) Sodium hyaluronate 30 mg/ml. Inj. Disp. syringe 0.65 ml. *Rx.*
Use: Viscoelastic, ophthalmic.

•**amoxapine.** (am-OX-uh-peen) U.S.P. 23.
Use: Antidepressant.
See: Asendin, Tab. (ESI Lederle Generics).

amoxapine tablets.
Use: Antidepressant.

•**amoxicillin.** (a-MOX-ih-sil-in) U.S.P. 23.
Use: Anti-infective.
See: Amoxil, Preps. (SmithKline Beecham Pharmaceuticals).
Trimox (Apothecon).
Wymox (Wyeth-Ayerst).

amoxicillin and potassium clavulanate. (a-MOX-ih-sil-in and poe-TASS-ee-uhm CLAV-you-lon-ate)
Use: Anti-infective, penicillin.
See: Augmentin (SmithKline Beecham Pharmaceuticals).

amoxicillin intramammary infusion.
Use: Anti-infective, penicillin.

•**amoxicillin sodium.** USAN.
Use: Antibiotic.

amoxicillin trihydrate. (a-MOX-ih-sil-in) (Various Mfr.) **Chew. Tab.:** 125 mg, 250 mg. Bot. 30s (250 mg only), 40s, 60s, 100s, 500s. **Cap.:** 250 mg, 500 mg. Bot. 21s, 30s, 50s (500 mg only), 100s, 250s, 500s, 1000s (250 mg only), UD 45s, UD 100s. **Pow. for Oral Susp.:** 125 mg/5 ml, 250 mg/ml when reconstituted. Bot. 80 ml, 100 ml, 150 ml, 200 ml. *Rx.*
Use: Anti-infective, penicillin.

Amoxil. (SmithKline Beecham Pharmaceuticals) Amoxicillin trihydrate. **Chew. Tab.:** 125 mg, 250 mg. Bot. 30s (250 mg only), 60s (125 mg only), 100s (250 mg only). **Cap.:** 250 mg, 500 mg Bot. 100s, 500s, UD 100s. **Pow. for Oral Susp.:** 125 mg/5 ml, 250 mg/5 ml. Bot. 80 ml, 100 ml, 150 ml, UD 5 ml. *Rx.*
Use: Anti-infective, penicillin.

Amoxil Pediatric Drops. (SmithKline

Beecham Pharmaceuticals) Amoxicillin trihydrate 50 mg/ml when reconstituted. Bot. 15 ml, 30 ml. *Rx.*
Use: Anti-infective, penicillin.

d-AMP. (Dunhall Pharmaceuticals, Inc.) Ampicillin trihydrate 500 mg. Cap. Bot. 100s. *Rx.*
Use: Anti-infective, penicillin.

AMP. Adenosine Phosphate, USAN.
Use: Nutrient.

amperil. (Armenpharm Ltd.) Ampicillin trihydrate 250 mg or 500 mg/Cap. Bot. 100s, 500s. *Rx.*
Use: Anti-infective, penicillin.

•**amphecloral.** (AM-feh-klahr-ahl) USAN.
Use: Sympathomimetic; anorexic.

amphenidone.
Use: CNS stimulant.

amphetamine aspartate combinations. (am-FET-uh-meen)
See: Adderall (Richwood Pharmaceuticals).

amphetamine hydrochloride. (am-FET-uh-meen) **Amp:** 20 mg/ml, 1 ml (Various Mfr.). **Cap:** (Various Mfr.). *Rx.*
Use: Vasoconstrictor, CNS stimulant.

amphetamine, levo.
Use: CNS stimulant.

amphetamine phosphate.
Use: CNS stimulant.

amphetamine phosphate, dextro. Tab. Dextroamphetamine phosphate. (Various Mfr.).
Use: CNS stimulant.

amphetamine phosphate, dibasic. (Various Mfr.) Racemic amphetamine phosphate. **Cap:** 5 mg or 10 mg. **Tab:** 5 mg or 10 mg. *Rx.*
Use: CNS stimulant.

amphetamines.
See: Amphetamine Sulfate, Tab. (Lannett Co., Inc.).
Desoxyn, Tab. (Abbott Laboratories).
Desoxyn Gradumets, Long-acting Tab. (Abbott Laboratories).
Dexedrine, Elix., Tab., S.R. Cap. (SmithKline Beecham Pharmaceuticals).
Dextroamphetamine Sulfate, Tab., S.R Cap. (Various Mfr.).

•**amphetamine sulfate.** U.S.P. 23.
Use: CNS stimulant.

amphetamine sulfate. (Various Mfr.) 5 mg, 10 mg/Cap. Tab; 20 mg/ml Vial.
Use: CNS stimulant.

amphetamine sulfate combinations. (am-FET-uh-meen)
See: Adderall. (Richwood Pharmaceuticals).

amphetamine sulfate, dextro.
Use: CNS stimulant.
See: Dextroamphetamine Sulfate, U.S.P. 23.

amphetamine with dextroamphetamine as resin complexes.
Use: Appetite depressant.

Amphocaps. (Halsey Drug Co.) Ampicillin 250 mg or 500 mg/Cap. Bot. 100s. *Rx.*
Use: Anti-infective, penicillin.

Amphojel. (Wyeth-Ayerst Laboratories) Aluminum hydroxide gel. **Susp.:** 320 mg/5 ml. Bot. 355 ml; **Tab.:** 300 mg or 600 mg. Bot. 100s. *otc.*
Use: Antacid.

•**amphomycin.** (AM-foe-MY-sin) USAN. An antibiotic produced by *Streptomyces canus.*
Use: Anti-infective.

Amphotec. (Sequus Pharmaceuticals, Inc.) Amphotericin B (as cholesteryl) 50 mg and 100 mg/Pow. for Inj. Vial 20 ml, 50 ml. *Rx.*
Use: For treatment of certain fungal infections.

amphotericin.
Use: Antifungal.
See: Fungizone, Preps. (Bristol-Myers Squibb).

•**amphotericin b.** (am-foe-TER-ih-sin B) U.S.P. 23.
Use: Antifungal.
See: Abelcet, Susp. for Inj. (Liposome Co.).
Amphotec, Pow. for Inj. (Sequus Pharmaceuticals, Inc.).
Amphotericin B (PharmaTek).
Fungizone, Preps. (Bristol-Myers Squibb).

amphotericin B. (Pharmos Corp.) 50 mg as desoxycholate/Inj. Vial. *Rx.*
Use: Antifungal.

amphotericin B lipid complex. (Bristol-Myers Squibb)
Use: Anti-infective.

amphotericin b lipid complex. (am-foe-TER-ih-sin B)
Use: Invasive fungal infections. [Orphan Drug]
See: Abelcet, Inj. (Liposome Co.).

•**ampicillin.** (am-pih-SILL-in) U.S.P. 23.
Use: Anti-infective.
See: Marcillin, Cap. (Marnel).
Omnipen, Preps. (Wyeth-Ayerst Laboratories).
Polycillin, Preps. (Bristol-Myers Squibb).
Principen, Preps. (Apothecon).
Totacillin, Preps. (SmithKline Beecham Pharmaceuticals).
W/Probenecid.

See: Principen w/Probenecid Cap. (Bristol-Myers Squibb).

ampicillin with probenecid. Cap.,Oral Susp.
Use: Anti-infective, penicillin.
See: Principen w/Probenecid (Bristol-Myers Squibb).

•**ampicillin sodium.** (am-pih-SILL-in) U.S.P. 23.
Use: Anti-infective.
See: Omnipen-N, Pow. for Inj. (Wyeth-Ayerst Laboratories).

ampicillin sodium. (Various Mfr.) Ampicillin sodium 150 mg, 250 mg, 500 mg, 1 g, 2 g, 10 g bulk. Vials, piggyback vials (500 mg, 1 g, 2 g only). *Rx.*
Use: Anti-infective.
See: Omnipen-N, Pow. for Inj. (Wyeth-Ayerst Laboratories).

ampicillin sodium and sulbactam sodium. (am-pih-SILL-in and sull-BAK-tam)
Use: Anti-infective, penicillin.
See: Unasyn, Pow. for Inj. (Roerig).

ampicillin trihydrate. (Various Mfr.) Ampicillin (as trihydrate) 250 mg, 500 mg. Cap. Bot. 16s (500 mg only), 20s, 28s (500 mg only), 30s (250 mg only), 40s, 100s, 500s, 1000s, UD 100s, 125 mg/5 ml, 250 mg/5 ml. Pow. for oral susp. Bot. 80, 100, 150, 200 ml. *Rx.*
Use: Anti-infective, penicillin.
See: Amcill, Cap., Susp. (Parke-Davis).
D-Amp, Cap., Susp. (Dunhall Pharmaceuticals, Inc.).
Marcillin, Cap. (Marnel Pharmaceuticals, Inc.).
Omnipen, Cap., Pow. for Oral Susp. (Wyeth-Ayerst Laboratories).
Polycillin Preps. (Apothecon).
Principen, Cap, Susp. (Bristol-Myers Squibb).
Totacillin, Cap, Pow. for Oral Susp. (SmithKline Beecham Pharmaceuticals).

Amplicor. (Roche Laboratories) Kits 10s, 96s, 100s. *Rx.*
Use: Diagnostic aid, chlamydia.

Amplicor HIV-1 Monitor. (Roche Laboratories) Reagent kit for plasma HIV-1 tests. Kit. 24 tests.
Use: Diagnostic aid.

Ampligen. (HEM Research) Poly I: Poly C12U. Phase II/III HIV.
Use: Immunomodulator.

amprenavir.
Use: Antiviral.
See: Agenerase (GlaxoWellcome).

•**ampyzine sulfate.** (AM-pih-zeen) USAN.
Use: Central nervous system stimulant.

•**amquinate.** (am-KWIN-ate) USAN.
Use: Antimalarial.

•**amrinone.** (AM-rih-nohn) U.S.P. 23.
Use: Cardiovascular agent.
See: Inocor Lactate Inj. (Sanofi Winthrop Pharmaceuticals).

amrinone lactate. (AM-rih-nohn LAK-tate)
See: Inocor (Sanofi Winthrop Pharmaceuticals).

•**amsacrine.** (AM-sah-KREEN) USAN.
Use: Antineoplastic. [Orphan Drug]

Am-Tuss Elixir. (T.E. Williams Pharmaceuticals) Codeine phosphate 10 mg, phenylephrine HCl 10 mg, phenylpropanolamine HCl 5 mg, prophenpyridamine maleate 12.5 mg, guaifenesin 44 mg, fluid extract of ipecac 0.17 min., citric acid 60 mg, sodium citrate 197 mg/5 ml, alcohol 5%. Bot. Pt, gal. *c-v.*
Use: Antihistamine, antitussive, decongestant, expectorant.

Amvisc. (Chiron Therapeutics) **Inj.:** Sodium hyaluronate 12 mg/ml. Disp. syringe 0.5 ml, 0.8 ml. *Rx.*
Use: Viscoelastic.

Amvisc Plus. (Chiron Therapeutics) **Inj.:** Sodium hyaluronate 16 mg/ml. Disp. syringe: 0.5 ml, 0.8 ml. *Rx.*
Use: Viscoelastic.

Am-Wax. (Amlab) Urea, benzocaine, propylene glycol, glycerin. Bot. 10 ml. *otc.*
Use: Otic.

amyl. Phenyl phenol, phenyl mercuric nitrate.
See: Lubraseptic Jelly (Guardian Laboratories).

•**amyl nitrite.** (A-mill NYE-trite) U.S.P. 23.
Use: Vasodilator.

amyl nitrite. Isoamyl nitrite. Isopentylnitrite. (GlaxoWellcome). Vaporole 0.18 ml or 0.3 ml. Box 12s. (Eli Lilly and Co.). Aspirols 0.3 ml. Box 12s.
Use: Inhalation, coronary vasodilator in angina pectoris.
W/Sodium nitrite, sodium thiosulfate.
See: Cyanide Antidote Pkg. (Eli Lilly and Co.).

α**amylase.**
W/Calcium carbonate, glycine, belladonna extract.
See: Trialka, Tab. (Del Pharmaceuticals, Inc.).
W/Pancreatin, protease, lipase.
See: Dizymes, Cap. (Recsei Laboratories).
W/Pepsin, homatropine methyl bromide, lipase, protease, bile salts.
See: Gourmase, Cap. (Solvay Pharmaceuticals).

•**amylene hydrate.** (AM-ih-leen HIGH-drate) N.F. 18.
Use: Pharmaceutic aid (solvent).

amylolytic enzyme.
W/Butabarbital sodium, belladonna extract, cellulolytic enzyme, proteolytic enzyme, lipolytic enzyme, iron ox bile.
See: Butibel-Zyme, Tab. (Ortho McNeil Pharmaceutical).
W/Calcium carbonate, glycine, proteolytic and cellulolytic enzymes.
See: Converspaz, Tab. (B.F. Ascher and Co.).
W/Lipase, proteolytic, cellulolytic enzymes, phenobarbital, hyoscyamine sulfate, atropine sulfate.
See: Arco-Lipase Plus, Tab. (Arco Pharmaceuticals, Inc.).
W/Proteolytic, cellulolytic, lipolytic enzymes, iron, ox bile.
See: Ku-Zyme, Cap. (Schwarz Pharma, Inc.).
W/Proteolytic, cellulolytic, lipolytic enzymes.
See: Arco-Lase, Tab. (Arco Pharmaceuticals, Inc.)

Amytal Sodium. (Eli Lilly and Co.) Amobarbital sodium. Pow. for Inj. Vial. 250 mg, 500 mg. *c-II.*
Use: Hypnotic, sedative.

Ana. (Wampole Laboratories) Antinuclear antibodies test by IFA. Test 54s.
Use: Diagnostic aid.

Ana Hep-2. (Wampole Laboratories) Antinuclear antibodies test by IFA. Tests 60s.
Use: Diagnostic aid.

anabolic agents. These agents stimulate constructive processes leading to retention of nitrogen and increasing the body protein.
See: Adroyd, Tab. (Parke-Davis).
Anabolin-IM, Vial (Alto Pharmaceuticals, Inc.).
Anadrol, Tab. (Roche Laboratories).
Anavar, Tab. (Searle).
Android, Tab. (Zeneca Pharmaceuticals).
Androlone, Vial (Keene Pharmaceuticals, Inc.).
Deca-Durabolin, Amp., Vial (Organon Teknika Corp.).
Di Genik, Vial (Savage Laboratories).
Drolban, Vial (Eli Lilly and Co.).
Durabolin, Amp., Vial (Organon Teknika Corp.).
Halotestin, Tab. (Pharmacia & Upjohn).
Hybolin, Vial (Hyrex Pharmaceuticals).
Maxibolin, Elix, Tab. (Organon Teknika Corp.).
Nandrobolic, Vial (Forest Pharmaceutical, Inc.).
Ora-Testryl, Tab. (Bristol-Myers Squibb).
Winstrol, Tab. (Sanofi Winthrop Pharmaceuticals).

Anabolin. (Alto Pharmaceuticals, Inc.) Nandrolone phenpropionate 50 mg, benzyl alcohol 2%, sesame oil q.s./ml. Vial 2 ml. *Rx.*
Use: Anabolic steroid.

Anabolin-IM. (Alto Pharmaceuticals, Inc.) Nandrolone phenpropionate 50 mg, benzyl alcohol 2%, sesame oil q.s./ml. Vial 2 ml. *Rx.*
Use: Anabolic steroid.

Anabolin LA-100. (Alto Pharmaceuticals, Inc.) Nandrolone decanoate 100 mg/ml. Vial 2 ml. *Rx.*
Use: Anabolic steroid.

Anacaine. (Gordon Laboratories) Benzocaine 10%. Jar oz, lb. *otc.*
Use: Anesthetic, local.

Anacin Tablets. (Whitehall Robins Laboratories) Aspirin 400 mg, caffeine 32 mg. **Tab.:** Tin 12s, bot. 30s, 50s, 100s, 200s. **Cap.:** Bot. 30s, 50s, 100s. *otc.*
Use: Analgesic.

Anacin Maximum Strength. (Whitehall Robins Laboratories) Aspirin 500 mg, caffeine 32 mg/Tab. Bot. 12s, 20s, 24s, 40s, 72s, 75s, 150s. *otc.*
Use: Analgesic.

Anadrol-50. (Roche Laboratories) Oxymetholone 50 mg/Tab. Bot. 100s. *c-III.*
Use: Anabolic steroid.

anafebrina.
See: Aminopyrine (Various Mfr.).

Anafranil. (Novartis Pharmaceutical Corp.) Clomipramine HCl 25 mg, 50 mg, or 75 mg/Cap. Bot. 100s, UD 100s. *Rx.*
Use: Antidepressant.

•**anagestone acetate.** (AN-ah-JEST-ohn) USAN.
Use: Hormone, progestin.

anagrelide. (AN-AGG-reh-lide)
Use: Polycythemia vera; essential thrombocythemia; thrombocytosis in chronic myelogenous leukemia. [Orphan Drug]
See: Agrylin, Cap. (Roberts Pharmaceuticals).

•**anagrelide hydrochloride.** (AN-AGG-reh-lide) USAN.
Use: Antithrombotic.
See: Agrylin, Cap. (Roberts Pharmaceuticals).

Ana-Guard. (Bayer Corp. (Consumer Div.)) Epinephrine 1:1000. Syr. 1 ml. *Rx.*
Use: Bronchodilator, sympathomimetic.

•**anakinra.** (an-ah-KIN-rah) USAN. Interleukin-1 receptor antagonist (recombinent).
Use: Anti-inflammatory (nonsteroidal); suppressant (inflammatory bowel disease).

Ana-Kit. (Bayer Corp (Consumer Div.)) Syringe, epinephrine 1:1000 in 1 ml; four (each 2 mg) chlorpheniramine maleate; two sterilized swabs, tourniquet, instructions/kit. *Rx.*
Use: Anaphylactic therapy.

Analbalm Improved Formula. (Schwarz Pharma, Inc.) Methyl salicylate 10%, menthol 1.25%, camphor 3%. Liq. Bot. **Green:** 4 oz, gal. **Pink:** 4 oz, Pt, gal. *otc.*
Use: Counterirritant.

analeptics. Usually a term applied to agents with stimulant action, particularly on the central nervous system. See also central nervous system stimulants.
See: Amphetamine salts (Various Mfr.).
Caffeine (Various Mfr.).
Cylert, Tab. (Abbott Laboratories).
Dextroamphetamine salts (Various Mfr.).
Dopram, Vial (Wyeth-Ayerst Laboratories).
Ephedrine Salts (Various Mfr.).
Methamphetamine salts (Various Mfr.).
Ritalin HCl, Tab. (Novartis Pharmaceutical Corp).
Sodium Succinate (Various Mfr.).

Analgesia Creme. (Rugby Labs, Inc.) Trolamine sulfate 10%. Cream, Tube 85 g. *otc.*
Use: Liniment.

analgesic balm. (Various Mfr.) Menthol w/methylsalicylate in a suitable base. *otc.*
Use: Counterirritant.
See: A.P.C., 1.5 oz, lb.
Lilly, oz.
Musterole (Schering-Plough Corp).

Analgesic Liquid. (Weeks & Leo) Triethanolamine salicylate 20% in an alcohol base. Bot. 4 oz. *otc.*
Use: Analgesic, topical.

Analgesic Lotion. (Weeks & Leo) Methyl nicotinate 1%, methyl salicylate 10%, camphor 0.1%, menthol 0.1%. Bot. 4 oz. *otc.*
Use: Analgesic, topical.

Analpram-HC. (Ferndale Laboratories, Inc.) Hydrocortisone acetate 1% or 2%, pramoxine HCl 1%. Cream Tube 30 g. *Rx.*
Use: Anesthetic; corticosteroid, local.

Analval. (Pal-Pak, Inc.) Aspirin 227 mg, acetaminophen 162 mg, caffeine 32 mg/Tab. Bot. 1000s. *otc.*
Use: Analgesic combination.

Anamine. (Merz Pharmaceuticals) Pseudoephedrine HCl 30 mg, chlorpheniramine maleate 2 mg/5 ml. Syr. Bot. 473 ml. *Rx.*
Use: Antihistamine, decongestant.

Anamine HD. (Merz Pharmaceuticals) Phenylephrine HCl 5 mg, chlorpheniramine maleate 2 mg, hydrocodone bitartrate 1.67 mg. 10 ml tid or qid. Syr. *c-III.*
Use: Antihistamine, antitussive, decongestant.

Anamine TD. (Merz Pharmaceuticals) Chlorpheniramine maleate 8 mg, pseudoephedrine HCl 120 mg/TD Cap. Bot. 100s. *Rx.*
Use: Antihistamine, decongestant.

Ananain, Comosain.
Use: Burn therapy. [Orphan Drug]
See: Vianain (Genzyme Corp.).

Anaplex. (ECR Pharmaceuticals) Pseudoephedrine HCl 30 mg, chlorpheniramine maleate 2 mg/5 ml. Syr. Bot. 473 ml. *Rx.*
Use: Antihistamine, decongestant.

Anaplex HD. (ECR Pharmaceuticals) Hydrocodone bitartrate 1.7 mg, phenylephrine HCl 5 mg, chlorpheniramine maleate 2 mg. Syr. Bot. 120 ml, 480 ml. *c-III.*
Use: Antihistamine, antitussive, decongestant.

Anaprox. (Roche Laboratories) Naproxen sodium 275 mg (naproxen base 250 mg with sodium 25 mg), lactose/ Tab. Bot. 100s, 500s. UD 100s. *Rx.*
Use: NSAID.

Anaprox DS. (Roche Laboratories) Naproxen sodium 550 mg (naproxen base 500 mg with sodium 50 mg)/Tab. Bot. 100s, 500s, UD 100s. *Rx.*
Use: NSAID.

anarel. Guanadrel sulfate.

•**anaritide acetate.** (an-NAR-ih-TIDE) USAN.
Use: Antihypertensive, diuretic.

anaritide acetate. (an-NAR-ih-TIDE)
Use: Improvement of early renal allograft function following renal transplantation; acute renal failure.
See: Auriculin (Scios Nova, Inc.).

Anaspaz. (B.F. Ascher and Co.) l-Hyoscyamine sulfate 0.125 mg/Tab. Bot. 100s, 500s. *Rx.*
Use: Anticholinergic, antispasmodic.

•**anastrozole.** (an-ASS-troe-zole) USAN.
Use: Antineoplastic.
See: Arimidex, Tab. (Zeneca Pharmaceuticals).

Anatrast. (Lafayette Pharmaceuticals, Inc.) GI contrast agent, 100% paste. Tube 500 g.

Anatuss DM. (Mayrand) **Syr.:** Guaifenesin 100 mg, pseudoephedrine HCl 30 mg, dextromethorphan HBr 10 mg/5 ml. Bot. 480 ml. **Tab.:** Guaifenesin 400 mg, pseudoephedrine HCl 60 mg, dextromethorphan HBr 20 mg. Bot. 100s. *otc.*
Use: Antitussive, decongestant, expectorant.

Anatuss LA. (Merz Pharmaceuticals) Guaifenesin 400 mg, pseudoephedrine HCl 120 mg. Tab. Bot. 100s. *Rx.*
Use: Decongestant, expectorant.

Anatuss Syrup. (Merz Pharmaceuticals) Dextromethorphan HBr 15 mg, phenylpropanolamine HCl 25 mg, guaifenesin 100 mg/10 ml. Bot. 120 ml, 480 ml. *otc.*
Use: Antitussive, decongestant, expectorant.

Anatuss Tabs. (Merz Pharmaceuticals) Guaifenesin 100 mg, acetaminophen 325 mg, dextromethorphan HBr 15 mg, phenylpropanolamine HCl 25 mg/Tab. Bot. 100s, 500s. *Rx.*
Use: Analgesic, antitussive, decongestant, expectorant.

Anatuss w/Codeine. (Merz Pharmaceuticals) **Syr.:** Phenylpropanolamine HCl 25 mg, codeine phosphate 10 mg, guaifenesin 100 mg/5 ml. Bot. 120 ml, 480 ml. *c-v.* **Tab.:** Phenylpropanolamine HCl 25 mg, codeine phosphate 10 mg, guaifenesin 100 mg, acetaminophen 300 mg. Bot. 100s. *c-iii.*
Use: Analgesic (Tab. only), antitussive, decongestant, expectorant.

Anavar. (Searle) Oxandrolone 2.5 mg/Tab. Bot. 100s. *Rx.*
Use: Anabolic steroid.

anayodin.
See: Chiniofon.

•**anazolene sodium.** (an-AZZ-oh-leen) USAN. Sodium Anoxynaphthonate.
Use: Diagnostic aid (blood volume, cardiac output determination).

Anbesol Baby Gel. (Whitehall Robins Laboratories) Benzocaine 7.5%. Tube 0.25 oz. *otc.*
Use: Anesthetic, local.

Anbesol Gel. (Whitehall Robins Laboratories) Benzocaine 6.3%, phenol 0.5%, alcohol 70%. Tube 7.5 g. *otc.*
Use: Anesthetic, topical combination.

Anbesol Liquid. (Whitehall Robins Laboratories) Benzocaine 6.3%, phenol 0.5%, povidone-iodine 0.04%, alcohol 70%. Bot. 9 ml, 22 ml. *otc.*
Use: Anesthetic combination, topical.

Anbesol Maximum Strength. (Whitehall Robins Laboratories) **Gel:** Benzocaine 20%, alcohol 60%, carbomer 934P, polyethylene glycol, saccharin. Tube 7.2 g. **Liq.:** Benzocaine 20%, alcohol 60%, saccharin, polyethylene glycol. Bot. 9 ml. *otc.*
Use: Anesthetic, local.

Ancef. (SmithKline Beecham Pharmaceuticals) Cefazolin sodium. **Vial:** Equivalent to 500 mg or 1 g of cefazolin. **Multi Pack:** 500 mg or 1 g/Pack. 25s. **Bulk Vial:** 5 g, 10 g. **Piggyback Vial:** 500 mg or 1 g/100 ml. **Minibag:** 500 mg/50 ml, 1 g/50 ml w/5% dextrose inj. (D5W). 500 mg/50 ml D5W. *Rx.*
Use: Anti-infective, cephalosporin.

•**ancestim.** (an-SESS-tim) USAN.
Use: Treatment of anemia; hematopoietic adjuvant (stem call factor).

Ancid Tablet and Suspension. (Sheryl) Calcium aluminum carbonate, di-amino acetate complex. Tab. 100s. Susp. pt. *otc.*
Use: Antacid.

Ancobon. (Roche Laboratories) Flucytosine 250 mg or 500 mg/Cap. Bot. 100s. *Rx.*
Use: Anti-infective.

•**ancrod.** (AN-krahd) USAN. An active principle obtained from the venom of the Malayan pit viper *Agkistrodonrhodostoma.*
Use: Anticoagulant.

ancrod. (AN-krahd) (Knoll Pharmaceuticals)
Use: Antithrombotic in patients with heparin-induced thrombocytopenia orthrombosis who require immediate and continued anticoagulation.

Andesterone Suspension. (Lincoln Diagnostics) Estrone 2 mg, testosterone 6 mg/ml. Vial 15 ml. **Forte:** Estrone 1 mg, testosterone 20 mg/ml. Inj. Vial 15 ml. *Rx.*
Use: Androgen, estrogen combination.

Andrest 90-4. (Seatrace Pharmaceuticals, Inc.) Testosterone enanthate 90 mg, estradiol valerate 4 mg/ml. Vial 10 ml. *Rx.*
Use: Androgen, estrogen combination.

Andro 100. (Forest Pharmaceutical, Inc.) Testosterone 100 mg/ml. Vial 10 ml. *c-III.*
Use: Androgen.

Andro-Cyp 100. (Keene Pharmaceuticals, Inc.) Testosterone cypionate 100 mg/ml. Vial 10 ml. *c-III.*
Use: Androgen.

Andro-Cyp 200. (Keene Pharmaceuti-

cals, Inc.) Testosterone cypionate 200 mg/ml. Vial 10 ml. *c-III.*
Use: Androgen.

Androderm. (SmithKline Beecham) Testosterone 2.5 mg, 5 mg/patch. Pkg. 30s, 60s. *c-III.*
Use: Hormone, testosterone.

Andro-Estro 90-4. (Rugby Labs, Inc.) Estradiol valerate 4 mg, testosterone enanthate 90 mg/ml with chlorobutanol in sesame oil. Inj. Vial. 10 ml. *Rx.*
Use: Androgen, estrogen combination.

Androgel. (Unimed) Testosterone.
Use: AIDS. [Orphan Drug]

Androgel-DHT. (Unimed) Dihydrotestosterone.
Use: AIDS. [Orphan Drug]

androgens. Substances which possess masculinizing activities.
See: Methyltestosterone.
Testosterone.
Testosterone cyclopentylpropionate.
Testosterone enanthate.
Testosterone heptanoate.
Testosterone phenylacetate.
Testosterone propionate.

androgen-estrogen therapy.
See: Dienestrol with Methyltestosterone.
Estradiol Esters with Methyltestosterone.
Estradiol Esters with Testosterone.
Estrogenic Substance, Conjugated with Methyltestosterone.
Estrogenic Substance Mixed with Methyltestosterone.
Estrogenic Substance Mixed with Testosterone.
Estrone with Testosterone.

androgen hormone inhibitor.
See: Proscar (Merck & Co.).

Android-10 and 25. (Zeneca Pharmaceuticals) Methyltestosterone 5 mg/ Buccal Tab., 10 mg/Tab. or 25 mg/Tab. Bot. 60s. *c-III.*
Use: Androgen.

Andro L.A. 200. (Forest Pharmaceutical, Inc.) Testosterone enanthate 200 mg/ ml. Inj. Vial 10 ml. *c-III.*
Use: Androgen.

Androlin. (Lincoln Diagnostics) Testosterone 100 mg/ml. Vial 10 ml. *c-III.*
Use: Androgen.

Androlone. (Keene Pharmaceuticals, Inc.) Nandrolone phenpropionate 25 mg/ml in sesame oil. Vial 5 ml. *c-III.*
Use: Anabolic steroid.

Androlone-D 200. (Keene Pharmaceuticals, Inc.) Nandrolone decanoate w/ benzyl alcohol, 200 mg/ml. Inj. Vial 1 ml. *c-III.*
Use: Anabolic steroid.

Andronaq-50. (Schwarz Pharma, Inc.) Testosterone 50 mg/ml, sodium carboxymethylcellulose, methylcellulose, povidone, DSS, thimerosal. Inj. Vial. 10 ml. *c-III.*
Use: Androgen.

Andronaq LA. (Schwarz Pharma, Inc.) Testosterone cypionate 100 mg, benzyl alcohol 0.9% in cottonseed oil. Vial 10 ml. Bot. 12s. *c-III.*
Use: Androgen.

Andronate 100. (Taylor Pharmaceuticals) Testosterone cypionate 100 mg/ml with benzyl alcohol in cottonseed oil. Vial 10 ml. *c-III.*
Use: Androgen.

Andronate 200. (Taylor Pharmaceuticals) Testosterone cypionate 200 mg/ml with benzyl alcohol, benzyl benzoate in cottonseed oil. Vial 10 ml. *c-III.*
Use: Androgen.

Andropository 200. (Rugby Labs, Inc.) Testosterone enanthate 200 mg/ml in sesame oil with chlorobutanol. Inj. Vial 10 ml. *c-III.*
Use: Androgen.

androstanazole.
See: Stanozolol.

androstanolone. (I.N.N.) Stanolone.

androstenopyrazole. Anabolic steroid; pending release.

Androtest P.
See: Testosterone propionate.

Androvite. (Optimox Corp.) Tab.: Iron 3 mg, vitamins A 4167 IU, D 67 IU, E 67 IU, B_1 8.3 mg, B_2 8.3 mg, B_3 8.3 mg, B_5 16.7 mg, B_6 16.7 mg, B_{12} 20.8 mcg, C 167 mg, folic acid 0.06 mg, PABA, inositol, biotin, betaine, B, Cr, Cu, I, Mg, Mn, Se, Zn 8.3 mg, pancreatin, hesperidin, rutin. Bot. 180s. *otc.*
Use: Mineral, vitamin supplement.

Andryl 200. (Keene Pharmaceuticals, Inc.) Testosterone enanthate 200 mg/ ml. Vial 10 ml. *c-III.*
Use: Androgen.

Andylate Forte. (Vita Elixir) Acetaminophen 3 gr, salicylamide 3 gr, caffeine 0.25 gr/Tab. *otc.*
Use: Analgesic combination.

Andylate Rub. (Vita Elixir) Methylnicotinate, methyl salicylate, camphor, dipropylene glycol salicylate, oil of cassia, oleo resin of capsicum, oleo resin of ginger. *otc.*
Use: Analgesic, topical.

Andylate Tablets. (Vita Elixir) Sodium salicylate 10 gr/Tab. *otc.*
Use: Analgesic.

•**anecortave acetate.** (an-eh-CORE-tave ASS-eh-tate) USAN.
Use: Angiostatic steroid.

Anectine. (GlaxoWellcome) Succinylcholine Cl. Soln. 20 mg/ml. Multidose Vial 10 ml. Sterile Pow. Flo-Pak 500 mg or 1000 mg. Box 12s. *Rx.*
Use: Muscle relaxant.

Anefrin Nasal Spray, Long Acting. (Walgreen Co.) Oxymetazoline HCl 0.05%. Bot. 0.5 oz. *otc.*
Use: Decongestant.

Anergan 50. (Forest Pharmaceutical, Inc.) Promethazine HCl 50 mg/ml EDTA, phenol. Vial 10 ml. *Rx.*
Use: Antihistamine.

anergy testing.
Use: Diagnostic aid.
See: Multitest CMI (Pasteur-Merieux Connaught).

anertan.
See: Testosterone propionate.

Anestacon. (PolyMedica Pharmaceuticals) Lidocaine HCl 20 mg/ml. Jelly 15 ml, 240 ml. *Rx.*
Use: Anesthetic, local.

Anesthesin. (Ethyl-p-aminobenzoate.)
Use: Anesthetic, local.
See: Benzocaine, U.S.P. 23.

anethaine.
See: Tetracaine HCl.

•**anethole.** (AN-eh-thole) N.F. 18.
Use: Pharmaceutic aid (flavor).

aneurine hydrochloride.
See: Thiamine HCl, Preps. (Various Mfr.).

Anexsia 5/500. (Mallinckrodt) Hydrocodone bitartrate 5 mg, acetaminophen 500 mg/Tab. Bot. 100s. *c-III.*
Use: Analgesic combination, narcotic.

Anexsia 7.5/650. (Mallinckrodt) Hydrocodone bitartrate 7.5 mg, acetaminophen 650 mg/Tab. Bot. 100s. *c-III.*
Use: Analgesic combination, narcotic.

Anexsia 10/660. (Mallinckrodt) Hydrocodone bitartrate 10 mg, acetaminophen 660 mg/Tab. Bot. 100s, 1000s. *c-III.*
Use: Analgesic combination, narcotic.

Angel Sweet. (Garrett) Vitamins A and D_2. Cream 90 g. *otc.*
Use: Dermatologic, protectant.

Angen. (Davis & Sly) Estrone 2 mg, testosterone 25 mg/ml Aqueous Susp. Vial 10 ml. *Rx.*
Use: Androgen, estrogen combination.

Angerin. (Kingsbay) Nitroglycerin 1 mg/Cap. Bot. 60s. *Rx.*
Use: Coronary vasodilator.

Angex. (Janssen Pharmaceutical, Inc.) Lidoflazine. *Rx.*
Use: Coronary vasodilator.

Angio-Conray. (Mallinckrodt) Iothalamate sodium 80% (48% iodine), EDTA. Inj. Vial 50 ml.
Use: Radiopaque agent.

•**angiotensin amide.** (an-JEE-oh-TEN-sin AH-mid) USAN. N.F. XIII.
Use: Vasoconstrictor.

angiotensin-converting enzyme inhibitors.
Use: Antihypertensive; congestive heart failure.
See: Accupril, Tab. (Parke-Davis).
Altace, Cap. (Hoechst Marion Roussel).
Capoten, Tab. (Bristol-Myers Squibb).
Lotensin, Tab. (Novartis Pharmaceutical Corp.).
Monopril, Tab. (Bristol-Myers Squibb).
Prinivil, Tab. (Merck & Co.).
Univasc, Tab. (Schwarz Pharma, Inc.).
Vasotec, Tab. (Merck & Co.).
Vasotec IV, Inj. (Merck & Co.).
Zestril, Tab. (Zeneca Pharmaceuticals).

Angiovist 282. (Berlex Laboratories, Inc.) Diatrizoate meglumine 60% (iodine 28%). Vial 50 ml, 100 ml, 150 ml. Box 10s.
Use: Radiopaque agent.

Angiovist 292. (Berlex Laboratories, Inc.) Diatrizoate meglumine 52%, diatrizoate sodium 8% (iodine 29.2%). Vial 30 ml, 50 ml, or 100 ml. Box 10s.
Use: Radiopaque agent.

Angiovist 370. (Berlex Laboratories, Inc.) Diatrizoate meglumine 66%, diatrizoate sodium 10%, (iodine 37%). Vial 50 ml, 100 ml, 150 ml, or 200 ml. Box 10s.
Use: Radiopaque agent.

anhydrohydroxyprogesterone. Ethisterone.

•**anidoxime.** (AN-ih-DOX-eem) USAN.
Use: Analgesic.

A-Nil. (Vangard Labs, Inc.) Codeine phosphate 10 mg, bromodiphenhydramine HCl 3.75 mg, diphenhydramine HCl 8.75 mg, ammonium Cl 80 mg, potassium guaiacolsulfonate 80 mg, menthol 0.5 mg/5 ml, alcohol 5%. Bot. Pt. gal. *c-v.*
Use: Antitussive, expectorant.

•**anileridine.** (an-ih-LURR-ih-deen) U.S.P. 23.
Use: Analgesic (narcotic).

•**anileridine hydrochloride.** U.S.P. 23.
Use: Analgesic (narcotic).

•**anilopam hydrochloride.** (AN-ih-low-

pam) USAN.
Use: Analgesic.

Animal Shapes. (Major Pharmaceuticals) Vitamin A 2500 IU, D 400 IU, E 15 IU, C 60 mg, B_1 1.05 mg, B_2 1.2 mg, B_3 13.5 mg, B_6 1.05 mg, B_{12} 4.5 mcg, folic acid 0.3 mg. Chew. Tab. Bot. 100s, 250s. *otc.*
Use: Vitamin supplement.

Animal Shapes + Iron. (Major Pharmaceuticals) Vitamin A 2500 IU, D 400 IU,E 15 IU, C 60 mg, B_1 1.05 mg, B_2 1.2 mg, B_3 13.5 mg, B_6 1.05 mg, B_{12} 4.5 mcg, folic acid 0.3 mg, iron 15 mg. Chew. Tab. Bot. 100s, 250s. *otc.*
Use: Mineral, vitamin supplement.

anion exchange resins.
See: Polyamine-Methylene Resin.

•**aniracetam.** (AN-ih-RASS-eh-tam) USAN.
Use: Mental performance enhancer.

•**anirolac.** (ah-NIH-role-ACK) USAN.
Use: Analgesic, anti-inflammatory.

anise oil. N.F. XVI.
Use: Flavoring.

anisindione.
See: Miradon (Schering-Plough Corp.).

anisopyradamine.
See: Pyrilamine Maleate.

anisotropine. F.D.A. Tropine 2-propylvalerate.

•**anisotropine methylbromide.** (ah-NIH-so-TROE-peen meth-ill-BROE-mide) USAN.
Use: Anticholinergic.

•**anistreplase.** (uh-NISS-truh-place) USAN.
Use: Fibrinolytic, thrombolytic.
See: Eminase (SmithKline Beecham Pharmaceuticals).

•**anitrazafen.** (AN-ih-TRAY-zaff-en) USAN.
Use: Anti-inflammatory, topical.

anodynon.
See: Ethyl Cl.

Anodynos. (Buffington) Aspirin 420.6 mg, salicylamide 34.4 mg caffeine 34.4 mg/Tab. Sugar, lactose, and salt free. Dispens-A-Kit 500s, Bot. 100s, 500s, Medipak 200s. *otc.*
Use: Analgesic combination.

Anodynos-DHC. (Forest Pharmaceutical, Inc.) Hydrocodone bitartrate 5 mg, acetaminophen 500 mg/Tab. Bot. 100s. *c-III.*
Use: Analgesic combination, narcotic.

Anodynos Forte. (Buffington) Chlorpheniramine maleate, phenylephrine HCl, salicylamide, acetaminophen, caffeine/Tab. Sugar, lactose, and salt free. Dispens-A-Kit 500s, Bot. 100s. *Rx.*
Use: Analgesic, antihistamine, decongestant.

Anoquan. (Roberts Pharmaceuticals) Butalbital 50 mg, caffeine 40 mg, acetaminophen 325 mg/Cap. Bot. 100s, 1000s. *Rx.*
Use: Analgesic, hypnotic, sedative.

Anorex. (Dunhall Pharmaceuticals, Inc.) Phendimetrazine 35 mg/Tab. Bot. 100s. *c-III.*
Use: Anorexiant.

anorexigenic agents. Appetite suppressants.
See: Amphetamine Preps.
Didrex, Tab. (Pharmacia & Upjohn).
Sanorex, Tab. (Novartis Pharmaceutical Corp.).
Tenuate (Hoechst Marion Roussel).
Tepanil, Tab. (3M Pharm).
Wilpo, Tab. (Novartis Pharmaceutical Corp).

anovlar. Norethindrone plus ethinyl estradiol. *Rx.*
Use: Contraceptive.

•**anoxomer.** (an-OX-ah-MER) USAN.
Use: Pharmaceutic aid (antioxidant); food additive.

anoxynaphthonate sodium. Anazolene sodium.

Ansaid. (Pharmacia & Upjohn) Flurbiprofen 50 mg or 100 mg. Tab. 100s, 500s, UD 100s. *Rx.*
Use: Analgesic, NSAID.

Anspor. (SmithKline Beecham Pharmaceuticals) Cephradine (a semisynthetic cephalosporin) **Cap.:** 250 mg. Bot. 100s, UD 100s; 500 mg. Bot. 20s, 100s, UD 100s. **Oral Susp.:** 125 mg or 250 mg/5 ml. Bot. 100 ml.
Use: Anti-infective, cephalosporin.

Answer. (Carter Wallace) Reagent in-home pregnancy test kit for urine testing. Test kit box 1s.
Use: Diagnostic aid.

Answer 2. (Carter Wallace) Reagent in-home pregnancy test kit for urine testing. Test kit box 2s.
Use: Diagnostic aid.

Answer Ovulation. (Carter Wallace) Home test to predict time of ovulation. In 6 day test kits.
Use: Diagnostic aid, ovulation.

Answer Plus. (Carter Wallace) Reagent in-home pregnancy test kit for urine testing. Test kit box 1s.
Use: Diagnostic aid.

Answer Plus 2. (Carter Wallace) Reagent in-home pregnancy test kit for urine testing. Test kit box 2s.
Use: Diagnostic aid.

Answer Quick & Simple. (Carter Wallace) Reagent in-home kit for urine testing. Test kit box 1s.
Use: Diagnostic aid.

Antabuse. (Wyeth-Ayerst Laboratories) Disulfiram. **250 mg/Tab.:** Bot. 100s; **500 mg/Tab.:** Bot. 50s, 1000s. *Rx.*
Use: Antialcoholic.

Antacid. (Walgreen Co.) Calcium carbonate 500 mg/Tab. Bot. 75s. *otc.*
Use: Antacid.

Antacid #2. (Global Source) Calcium carbonate 5.5 gr, magnesium carbonate 2.5 gr/Tab. Bot. 100s. *otc.*
Use: Antacid.

Antacid M Liquid. (Walgreen Co.) Aluminum oxide 225 mg, magnesium hydroxide 200 mg/5 ml. Bot. 12 oz, 26 oz. *otc.*
Use: Antacid.

Antacid No. 6. (Jones Medical Industries, Inc.) Calcium carbonate 0.42 g, glycine 0.18 g/Tab. Bot. 100s. *otc.*
Use: Antacid.

Antacid Relief Tablets. (Walgreen Co.) Dihydroxyaluminum sodium carbonate 334 mg/Tab. Bot. 75s. *otc.*
Use: Antacid.

antacids. Drugs that neutralize excess gastric acid.
See: Alka-Seltzer, Tab. (Bayer Corp. (Consumer Div.)).
Alka-Seltzer Plus, Tab. (Bayer Corp. (Consumer Div.)).
Alka-Seltzer Special Effervescent Antacid, Tab. (Bayer Corp. (Consumer Div.)).
Aluminum Hydroxide Gel (Various Mfr.).
Aluminum Hydroxide Gel w/Combinations (Various Mfr.).
Aluminum Hydroxide Gel Dried (Various Mfr.).
Aluminum Hydroxide Gel Dried w/ Combinations (Various Mfr.).
Aluminum Hydroxide Magnesium Carbonate, Tab. (Various Mfr.).
Aluminum Phosphate Gel (Wyeth-Ayerst Laboratories).
Aluminum Proteinate, Tab. (Solvay Pharmaceuticals).
Amitone, Tab. (SmithKline Beecham).
Calcium Carbonate, Precipitated (Various Mfr.).
Calcium Carbonate Tab. (Various Mfr.).
Ceo-Two, Supp. (Beutlich, Inc.).
Chooz, Gum Tab. (Schering-Plough Corp.).
Citrocarbonate, Liq. (Pharmacia & Upjohn).
Dicarbosil, Tab. (Arch).
Di-Gel, Liq., Tab. (Schering-Plough Corp.).
Dihydroxyaluminum Aminoacetate (Various Mfr.).
Dihydroxyaluminum Sodium Carbonate Tab. (Warner Lambert).
Magaldrate, Tab, Susp. (Wyeth-Ayerst Laboratories).
Magnesium Carbonate (Various Mfr.).
Magnesium Glycinate, Tab. (Various Mfr.).
Magnesium Hydroxide (Various Mfr.).
Magnesium Oxide, Tab., Cap. (Various Mfr.).
Magnesium Trisilicate (Various Mfr.).
Rolaids, Tab. (Warner Lambert).
Romach, Tab. (RPR Pharmacal).
Sodium Bicarbonate, Inj., Tab. (Various Mfr.).
Tums, Tab. (SmithKline Beecham).

Antacid Suspension. (Geneva Pharmaceuticals) Aluminum hydroxide 225 mg, magnesium hydroxide 200 mg/5 ml. Bot. 360 ml. *otc.*
Use: Antacid.

Antacid Tablets. (Zenith Goldline Pharmaceuticals) Calcium carbonate 500 mg/Chew. Tab. Bot. 150s. *otc.*
Use: Antacid.

Antacid Extra Strength. (Various Mfr.) Calcium carbonate 750 mg/Tab. Bot. 96s. *otc.*
Use: Antacid.

Anta-Gel. (Halsey Drug Co.) Aluminum hydroxide 200 mg, magnesium hydroxide 200 mg, simethicone 20 mg/5 ml. Bot. 12 oz. *otc.*
Use: Antacid, antiflatulent.

antagonists of curariform drugs.
See: Neostigmine Methylsulfate.
Tensilon Cl (Roche Laboratories).

antastan.
See: Antazoline Hydrochloride, U.S.P. 23.

antazoline hydrochloride. Antastan.

•**antazoline phosphate.** U.S.P. 23.
Use: Antihistamine.

W/Naphazoline, boric acid, phenylmercuric acetate, sodium Cl, sodium carbonate anhydrous.
See: Vasocon-A Ophthalmic, Soln. (Smith, Miller & Patch).

Antazoline-V. (Rugby Labs, Inc.) Naphazoline HCl 0.05%, antazoline phosphate 0.5%, PEG 8000, polyvinyl alcohol, EDTA, benzalkonium chloride 0.01%. Soln. Drop. Bot. 5 ml, 15 ml. *Rx.*
Use: Ophthalmic decongestant combination.

anterior pituitary.

See: Pituitary, anterior.
anthelmintic. A remedy for worms.
See: Antiminth, Susp. (Roerig).
Betanaphthol Benzoate (Various Mfr.).
Biltricide, Tab. (Bayer Corp. (Consumer Div.)).
Carbon Tetrachloride (Various Mfr.).
Gentian Violet (Various Mfr.).
Mintezol, Tab., Susp. (Merck & Co.).
Piperazine Preps. (Various Mfr.).
Terramycin (Various Mfr.).
Tetrachlorethylene.
Vansil, Cap. (Pfizer).
Vermox, Chew Tab., Oral Susp. (Merck & Co.).

•**anthelmycin.** (AN-thell-MY-sin) USAN.
Use: Anthelmintic.

Anthelvet. Tetramisole HCl.

•**anthralin.** (AN-thrah-lin) U.S.P. 23.
Use: Antipsoriatic.
See: Dritho-Scalp, Cream (Dermik Laboratories, Inc.).
Miconal (Bioglan Pharma).

•**anthramycin.** (an-THRAH-MY-sin) USAN.
Use: Antineoplastic.

anthraquinone of cascara.
See: Cascara Sagrada, Prods.

anthrax vaccine. (Michigan Biological Products Institute) Vial 5 ml. *Rx.*
Use: Immunization.

anti-a blood grouping serum.
Use: Diagnostic aid (blood in vitro).

anti-b blood grouping serum.
Use: Diagnostic aid (blood in vitro).

Antiacid. (Hillcrest North) Aluminum hydroxide, magnesium trisilicate, calcium carbonate/Tab. Bot. 100s. *otc.*
Use: Antacid.

Antialcoholic.
See: Disulfiram (Various Mfr.).
Antabuse (Wyeth-Ayerst Laboratories).

Anti-Allergy. (Walgreen Co.) Phenylpropanolamine HCl 18.7 mg, chlorpheniramine maleate 2 mg/Tab. Bot. 24s. *otc.*
Use: Antihistamine, decongestant.

antiandrogen.
See: Eulexin (Schering-Plough Corp.).

antiasthmatic combinations.
See: Cromolyn Sodium, Cap. (Various Mfr.).
Decadron Respihaler, Aerosol. (Merck & Co.).
Ephedrine HCl (Various Mfr.).
Ephedrine Sulfate (Various Mfr.).
Isoephedrine HCl (Various Mfr.).
Isoetharine (Sanofi Winthrop Pharmaceuticals).
Isoetharine HCl (Sanofi Winthrop Pharmaceuticals).
Isoetharine Mesylate (Sanofi Winthrop Pharmaceuticals).
Isoproterenol HCl (Various Mfr.).
Isoproterenol Sulfate (Various Mfr.).
Methoxyphenamine HCl (Various Mfr.).
Phenylephrine HCl (Various Mfr.).
Phenylpropanolamine HCl (Various Mfr.).
Pseudoephedrine HCl (Various Mfr.).
Racephedrine HCl (Various Mfr.).

antiasthmatic inhalant.
See: AsthmaHaler (SmithKline Beecham).
AsthmaNefrin, Soln. (SmithKline Beecham).

antibacterial antibodies.
See: Botulinum antitoxin.
Diphtheria antitoxin.
Immune globulin IM.
Immune globulin IV.
Tetanus immune globulin.

antibason.
See: Methylthiouracil. (Various Mfr.).

Antibiotic. (Parnell Pharmaceuticals, Inc.) **Otic susp.:** Polymyxin B sulfate 10,000 units, neomycin (as sulfate) 3.5 mg, hydrocortisone 10 mg/ml, thimerosal 0.01%. Bot. 10 ml w/dropper. **Otic soln.:** Polymyxin B sulfate 10,000 units, neomycin (as sulfate) 3.5 mg, hydrocortisone 10 mg/ml. Bot. 10 ml w/ dropper. *Rx.*
Use: Anti-infective, anti-inflammatory.

antibiotics/anti-infectives.
See: Amebicides, general.
Amikacin Sulfate, Vial (Various Mfr.).
Amoxicillin (Various Mfr.).
Amoxicillin and Potassium Clavulanate (SmithKline Beecham Pharmaceuticals).
Amoxicillin w/Comb. (Various Mfr.).
Ampicillin (Various Mfr.).
Ampicillin w/Comb. (Various Mfr.).
Anthelmintic agents, general.
Antimalarial agents, general.
Antiprotozoal agents, general.
Antituberculosis agents, general.
Antiviral agents, general.
Azithromycin, Caps. (Pfizer US Pharmaceutical Group).
Aztreonam, Vial (Bristol-Myers Squibb).
Bacampicillin HCl (Roerig).
Bacitracin (Various Mfr.).
Carbenicillin (Various Mfr.).
Cefaclor (Various Mfr.).
Cefadroxil (Various Mfr.).
Cefamandole Nafate (Eli Lilly and Co.).
Cefazolin Sodium, Vial (Various Mfr.).

Cefixime (ESI Lederle Generics).
Cefmetazole Sodium (Pharmacia & Upjohn).
Cefonicid Sodium, Vial (SmithKline Beecham Pharmaceuticals).
Cefoperazone Sodium, Vial (Roerig).
Cefotaxime Sodium, Vial (Hoechst Marion Roussel).
Cefotetan Disodium, Vial (Zeneca Pharmaceuticals).
Cefoxitin Sodium, Vial (Merck & Co.).
Cefpodoxime Proxetil (Pharmacia & Upjohn).
Cefprozil (Bristol-Myers Squibb).
Ceftazidime, Vial (Various Mfr.).
Ceftizoxime Sodium, Vial (Fujisawa USA, Inc.).
Ceftriaxone Sodium, Vial (Roche Laboratories).
Cefuroxime (Various Mfr.).
Cephalexin (Various Mfr.).
Cephalexin Monohydrate, Pulv., Susp. (Various Mfr.).
Cephalothin, Sodium, Vial (Various Mfr.).
Cephradine (Various Mfr.).
Chloramphenicol (Various Mfr.).
Ciprofloxacin (Bayer Corp. (Consumer Div.)).
Clarithromycin (Abbott Laboratories).
Clindamycin (Various Mfr.).
Clofazimine, Cap. (Novartis Pharmaceutical Corp.).
Cloxacillin Sodium (Various Mfr.).
Colistimethate Sodium, Inj. (Parke-Davis).
Colistin Sulfate (Various Mfr.).
Dapsone, Tab. (Jacobus Pharmaceutical Co.).
Demeclocycline (ESI Lederle Generics).
Dicloxacillin, Cap., Susp. (Various Mfr.).
Doxycycline (Various Mfr.).
Enoxacin, Tab. (Rhone-Poulenc Rorer Pharmaceuticals, Inc.).
Erythromycin (Various Mfr.).
Erythromycin w/Comb. (Various Mfr.).
Fungicides, general.
Furazolidone (Procter & Gamble Pharm.).
Gentamicin Sulfate (Various Mfr.).
Kanamycin Sulfate (Various Mfr.).
Lincomycin (Various Mfr.).
Lomefloxacin HCl, Tab. (Searle).
Lorcarbef (Eli Lilly and Co.).
Methacycline HCl, Cap., Syr. (Wallace Laboratories).
Methenamine (Various Mfr.).
Methenamine w/Comb. (Various Mfr.).
Methicillin Sodium, Vial, Pow. (Various Mfr.).
Methylene Blue, Tab. (Various Mfr.).
Metronidazole (Various Mfr.).
Mezlocillin Sodium, Vial (Bayer Corp. (Consumer Div.)).
Minocycline (ESI Lederle Generics).
Nafcillin Sodium, Vial, Cap., Pow. (Wyeth-Ayerst Laboratories).
Nalidixic Acid (Sanofi Winthrop Pharmaceuticals).
Netilmicin Sulfate, Vial (Schering-Plough Corp.).
Neomycin Sulfate, Vial (Various Mfr.).
Nitrofurantoin (Various Mfr.).
Norfloxacin, Tab. (Roberts Pharmaceuticals).
Novobiocin (Various Mfr.).
Ofloxacin (Ortho McNeil Pharmaceutical).
Oxacillin, Sodium (Various Mfr.).
Oxytetracycline (Various Mfr.).
Paromomycin, Cap., Syr. (Parke-Davis).
Penicillin G Benzathine (Various Mfr.).
Penicillin G Benzathine w/Comb. (Various Mfr.).
Penicillin G Potassium (Various Mfr.).
Penicillin G Potassium w/Comb. (Various Mfr.).
Penicillin G Procaine (Various Mfr.).
Penicillin G Procaine w/Comb. (Various Mfr.).
Penicillin G Sodium (Various Mfr.).
Penicillin V Potassium (Various Mfr.).
Pentamidine Isethionate (Fujisawa).
Phenoxymethyl Penicillin (Various Mfr.).
Piperacillin Sodium, Vial (ESI Lederle Generics).
Piperacillin Sosium w/Comb. (Various Mfr.).
Polymyxin B Sulfate (Various Mfr.).
Spectinomycin, Vial (Pharmacia & Upjohn).
Spectinmycin Sulfate (Various Mfr.).
Sulfadiazine (Various Mfr.).
Sulfamethizole, Tab. (Wyeth-Ayerst Laboratories).
Sulfamethoxazole (Various Mfr.).
Sulfamethoxazole w/Comb. (Various Mfr.).
Sulfasalazine (Various Mfr.).
Sulfasalazine w/Comb. (Various Mfr.).
Sulfisoxazole (Various Mfr.).
Tetracycline HCl (Various Mfr.).
Ticarcillin w/Comb. (Various Mfr.).
Ticarcillin Disodium, Vial (SmithKline Beecham Pharmaceuticals).
Tobramycin Sulfate (Various Mfr.).
Triacetyloleandomycin (Various Mfr.).
Trimethoprim (Various Mfr.).
Trimethoprim w/Comb. (Various Mfr.).

Trimetrexate Glucuronate, Vial (US Bioscience).
Troleandomycin, Cap. (Roerig).
Vancomycin HCl (Eli Lilly).

anticholinergic agents. Parasympatholytic agents.
See: Akineton (Knoll Pharmaceuticals).
Artane HCl (ESI Lederle Generics).
Atropine Preps.
Atrovent, Spray (Boehringer Ingelheim, Inc.).
Banthine Bromide (Searle).
Belladonna Preps.
Cantil Preps. (Hoechst Marion Roussel).
Cogentin (Merck & Co.).
Dicyclomine HCl (Various Mfr.).
Homatropine methylbromide.
Kemadrin, Tab. (GlaxoWellcome).
Norflex, Inj, Tab. (3M Pharm).
Pamine Bromide, Tab., Soln. (Pharmacia & Upjohn).
Panparnit HCl
Pathilon (ESI Lederle Generics).
Pro-Banthine Bromide, Preps. (Searle).
Robinul, Tab, Inj. (Wyeth-Ayerst Laboratories).
Scopolamine methylbromide
Scopolamine methylbromide HBr
Tral, Preps. (Abbott Laboratories).
Trihexyphenidyl HCl (Various Mfr.).

•**anticoagulant citrate dextrose solution.** U.S.P. 23.
Use: Anticoagulant (for storage of whole blood).
See: A-C-D Solution. (Various Mfr.).

•**anticoagulant citrate phosphate dextrose adenine solution.** U.S.P. 23.
Use: Anticoagulant (for storage of whole blood).

•**anticoagulant citrate phosphate dextrose solution.** U.S.P. 23.
Use: Anticoagulant (for storage of whole blood).

•**anticoagulant heparin solution.** U.S.P. 23.
Use: Anticoagulant (for storage of whole blood).

anticoagulants.
See: Anisindione.
Coumadin, Amp., Tab. (DuPont Merck Pharmaceutical Co.).
Dalteparin Sodium.
Diphenadione.
Enoxaparin Sodium.
Ethyl Biscoumacetate, Tab.
Fragmin (Pharmacia & Upjohn).
Heparin, Calcium.
Heparin, Sodium (Various Mfr.).
Lovenox, Inj. (Rhone-Poulenc Rorer Pharmaceuticals, Inc.).
Miradon, Tab. (Schering-Plough Corp.).
ReoPro (Eli Lilly and Co).
Warfarin (Various Mfr.).

•**anticoagulant sodium citrate solution.** U.S.P. 23.
Use: Anticoagulant (for plasma and blood fractionation).

anticonvulsants.
See: Acetazolamide, Tab. (Various Mfr.).
Amytal Sodium, Amp. (Eli Lilly and Co.).
Carbamazepine, Tab. (Various Mfr.)
Celontin Kapseals (Parke-Davis).
Clorazepate, Tab. (Various Mfr.).
Depakene (Abbott Laboratories).
Diamox, Tab., Inj. (ESI Lederle Generics).
Diazepam, Tab., Soln. (Various Mfr.).
Diazepam Intensol, Soln. (Roxane Laboratories, Inc.).
Dilantin, Preps. (Parke-Davis).
Epitol, Tab. (Teva Pharmaceuticals USA).
Felbatol, Tab., Susp. (Wallace Laboratories).
Gen-Xene, Tab. (Alra Laboratories, Inc.).
Klonopin, Tab. (Roche Laboratories).
Lamictal, Tab. (GlaxoWellcome).
Magnesium sulfate (Various Mfr.).
Mephobarbital, Tab. (Sanofi Winthrop Pharmaceuticals).
Mesantoin, Tab. (Novartis Pharmaceutical Corp.).
Milontin, Kapseals (Parke-Davis).
Mysoline, Tab., Susp. (Wyeth-Ayerst Laboratories).
Neurontin, Cap. (Parke-Davis).
Peganone, Tab. (Abbott Laboratories).
Phenobarbital (Various Mfr.).
Phenytoin, Susp., Tab. (Various Mfr.).
Phenytoin Sodium, Cap. (Various Mfr.).
Primidone, Tab. (Various Mfr.)
Tegretol, Tab. (Novartis Pharmaceutical Corp.).
Tranxene, Tab. (Abbott Laboratories).
Tranxene-SD, Tab. (Abbott Laboratories).
Tranxene-T, Tab. (Abbott Laboratories).
Tridione (Abbott Laboratories).
Valium, Tab. (Roche Laboratories).
Zarontin, Cap., Syr. (Parke-Davis).

anticytomegalovirus monoclonal antibodies.

Use: Treatment of cytomegalovirus.

antidepressants.

See: Adapin, Cap. (Lotus Biochemical).
Amitriptyline HCl (Various Mfr.).
Amoxapine, Tab. (Various Mfr.).
Anafranil, Cap. (Novartis Pharmaceutical Corp.).
Asendin, Tab. (ESI Lederle Generics).
Aventyl HCl, Pulv., Liq. (Eli Lilly and Co.).
Desipramine HCl, Cap., Tab. (Various Mfr.).
Desyrel, Tab. (Bristol-Myers Squibb).
Effexor, Tab. (Wyeth-Ayerst Laboratories).
Elavil Tab., Inj. (Merck & Co.).
Endep, Tab. (Roche Laboratories).
Imipramine HCl, Amp., Tab. (Various Mfr.).
Imipramine Pamoate, Cap. (Novartis Pharmaceutical Corp.).
Janimine, Tab. (Abbott Laboratories).
Ludiomil, Tab. (Novartis Pharmaceutical Corp.).
Luvox, Tab. (Solvay Pharmaceuticals).
Maprotiline HCl, Tab. (Various Mfr.).
Monoamine oxidase inhibitors.
Nardil, Tab. (Parke-Davis).
Norpramin, Preps. (Hoechst Marion Roussel).
Pamelor, Cap., Liq. (Novartis Pharmaceutical Corp.).
Parnate Sulfate, Tab. (SmithKline Beecham Pharmaceuticals).
Paxil, Tab. (SmithKline Beecham Pharmaceuticals).
Protriptyline HCl (Merck & Co.).
Prozac, Liq., Pulv. (Eli Lilly and Co.).
Serzone, Tab. (Bristol-Myers Squibb).
Sinequan, Cap. (Pfizer US Pharmaceutical Group).
Surmontil, Cap. (Wyeth-Ayerst Laboratories).
Tofranil, Amp., Tab. (Novartis Pharmaceutical Corp.).
Tofranil-PM, Cap. (Novartis Pharmaceutical Corp.).
Trazodone HCl, Tab. (Various Mfr.).
Vivactil, Tab. (Merck & Co.).
Wellbutrin, Tab. (GlaxoWellcome).
Zoloft, Tab. (Roerig).

antidiarrheals.

See: Attapulgite, Activated (Various Mfr.).
Cantil, Liq., Tab. (Hoechst Marion Roussel).
Coly-Mycin S, Oral Susp. (Parke-Davis).
Diasorb, Liq., Tab. (Columbia Laboratories, Inc.).
Diphenoxylate HCl w/Atropine sulfate, Tab., Liq. (Various Mfr.).
Donnagel, Chew. Tab., Liq., Susp. (Wyeth-Ayerst Laboratories).
Furoxone Liq., Tab. (Eaton Medical Corp.).
Imodium, Cap. (Janssen Pharmaceutical, Inc.).
Imodium A-D, Tab., Liq. (McNeil Consumer Products Co.).
Kaodene Non-Narcotic, Liq. (Pfeiffer Co.).
Kaolin (Various Mfr.).
Kaolin Colloidal (Various Mfr.).
Kaopectate, Prods. (Pharmacia & Upjohn).
Kao-Spen, Susp. (Century Pharmaceuticals, Inc.).
Kapectolin (Various Mfr.).
K-C, Susp. (Century Pharmaceuticals, Inc.).
K-Pek, Susp. (Rugby Labs, Inc.).
Lactinex, Tab., Gran. (Becton Dickinson & Co.).
Lactobacillus acidophilus & bulgaricus mixed culture, Tab. (Becton Dickinson & Co.).
Lactobacillus acidophilus, viable culture (Various Mfr.).
Logen, Tab. (Zenith Goldline Pharmaceuticals).
Lomanate, Liq. (Various Mfr.).
Lomotil, Liq., Tab. (Searle).
Lonox, Liq. (Geneva Pharmaceuticals).
Loperamide, Cap., Liq. (Various Mfr.).
Maalox Antidiarrheal, Capl. (Rhone-Poulenc Rorer Pharmaceuticals, Inc.).
Milk of Bismuth (Various Mfr.).
Motofen, Tab. (Carnrick Laboratories, Inc.).
Mycifradin Sulfate, Soln., Tab. (Pharmacia & Upjohn).
Pepto-Bismol, Liq., Tab. (Procter & Gamble Pharm.).
Pepto Diarrhea Control, Liq. (Procter & Gamble Pharm.)
Pink Bismuth, Liq. (Various Mfr.).
Rheaban Maximum Strength, Capl. (Pfizer US Pharmaceutical Group).

antidiuretics.

See: Pitressin, Amp. (Parke-Davis).
Pitressin Tannate In Oil, Amp. (Parke-Davis).
Pituitary Post. Inj. (Various Mfr.).

antiemetic/antivertigo agents.

See: Antivert, Tab. (Roerig).
Antrizine, Tab. (Major Pharmaceuticals).
Atarax, Tab., Syr. (Roerig).

Bonine, Tab. (Pfizer US Pharmaceutical Group).
Bucladin-S, Softab Tab. (Zeneca Pharmaceuticals).
Compazine, Preps. (SmithKline Beecham Pharmaceuticals).
Dimenhydrinate, Tab., Inj., Liq. (Various Mfr.).
Dinate, Inj. (Seatrace Pharmaceuticals, Inc.).
Dizmiss, Tab. (Jones Medical Industries, Inc.).
Dramamine, Preps. (Searle).
Dramanate, Inj. (Taylor Pharmaceuticals).
Dymenate, Inj. (Keene Pharmaceuticals, Inc.).
Emetrol, Liq. (Rhone-Poulenc Rorer Pharmaceuticals, Inc.).
Hydrate, Inj. (Hyrex Pharmaceuticals).
Kytril, Tab., Inj. (SmithKline Beecham Pharmaceuticals).
Marezine, Tab. (GlaxoWellcome).
Marinol, Cap. (Roxane Laboratories, Inc.).
Maxolon, Tab. (SmithKline Beecham Pharmaceuticals).
Meclizine HCl, Tab. (Various Mfr.).
Meni-D, Cap. (Seatrace Pharmaceuticals, Inc.).
Mepergan, Inj. (Wyeth-Ayerst Laboratories).
Metoclopramide, Tab. (Various Mfr.).
Naus-A-Tories, Supp. (Table Rock).
Nausetrol, Syr. (Medical Chemicals).
Octamide, Tab. (Pharmacia & Upjohn).
Phenergan, Preps. (Wyeth-Ayerst Laboratories).
Prochlorperazine, Supp. (Various Mfr.).
Reclomide, Tab. (Major Pharmaceuticals).
Reglan, Inj., Syr., Tab. (Wyeth-Ayerst Laboratories).
Tebamide, Supp. (G & W Laboratories).
T-Gen, Supp. (Zenith Goldline Pharmaceuticals).
Thorazine, Preps. (SmithKline Beecham Pharmaceuticals).
Ticon, Inj. (Roberts Pharmaceuticals).
Tigan, Preps. (SmithKline Beecham Pharmaceuticals).
Torecan Amp., Supp., Tab. (Novartis Pharmaceutical Corp.).
Transderm-Scop, Transdermal Therapeutic System (Novartis Pharmaceutical Corp.).
Trilafon, Preps. (Schering-Plough Corp.).
Trimazide, Cap., Supp. (Major Pharmaceuticals).
Trimethobenzamide HCl, Cap., Inj., Supp. (Various Mfr.).
Triptone, Capl. (Del Pharmaceuticals, Inc.).
Vesprin, Inj. (Bristol-Myers Squibb).
Vistaril, Cap., Susp., Soln. (Pfizer US Pharmaceutical Group).
Zofran, Inj., Tab. (GlaxoWellcome).

antiepilepsirine.
Use: Treatment for drug-resistant generalized tonic-clonic epilepsy. [Orphan Drug]

antiepileptic agents.
See: Anticonvulsant.

antiestrogen. Tamoxifen citrate.
Use: Hormone for cancer therapy.
See: Nolvadex (Zeneca Pharmaceuticals).
Tamoxifen (Barr Laboratories, Inc.).

antifebrin.
See: Acetanilid (Various Mfr.).

antiflatulents.
See: Di-Gel, Prods. (Schering-Plough Corp.).
Simethicone Prods.

Antifoam A Compound. (Hoechst Marion Roussel)
Use: Antiflatulent.
See: Simethicone, U.S.P. 23.

antifolic acid.
See: Methotrexate, Tab. (ESI Lederle Generics).

Antiformin. Sodium hypochlorite in sodium hydroxide 7.5%, available chlorine 5.2%; may be colored with meta cresol purple.
Use: Antiseptic, antimicrobial.

antifungal agents.
See: Fungicides.

•**antihemophilic factor.** U.S.P. 23.
Use: Antihemophilic.

antihemophilic factor. (Baxter & Alpha Therapeutic Corp.) Antihemophilic Factor, human. Method for Syringe Administration 10 ml 450 A.H.F. or 300 A.H.F. units/Pkg. W/Syringe 30 ml or 900 A.H.F. units/Pkg.
Use: Antihemophilic.
See: Alphanate, Inj. (Alpha Therapeutic Corp.).
Bioclate, Inj. (Centeon).
Helixate, Inj. (Centeon).
Hemofil, Vial (Baxter Pharmaceutical Products, Inc.).
Humate-P, Inj. (Centeon).
Koate HP, Inj. (Bayer Corp. (Consumer Div.)).
KOGENATE, Inj. (Bayer Corp. (Consumer Div.)).

Monoclate-P, Inj. (Centeon).
Recombinate, Inj. (Baxter Pharmaceutical Products, Inc.).

antihemophilic factor, human.
Use: Treatment of von Willebrand's disease. [Orphan Drug]
See: Alphanate (Alpha Therapeutic Corp.).
Humate P (Behringwerke Aktiengesellschaft).

Antihemophilic Factor (Porcine) Hyate: C. (Speywood Pharmaceuticals, Inc.) Freeze-dried concentrate of Antihemophilic Factor, 400 to 700 porcine units of Factor VIII: C. Pow. for Inj. Vials. *Rx.*
Use: Antihemophilic.

antihemophilic factor (recombinant).
Use: Prophylaxis/treatment of bleeding in hemophilia A. [Orphan Drug]
See: Kogenate (Bayer Corp. (Biological and Pharmaceutical Div.)).

antiheparin.
See: Protamine Sulfate.

Antihist-D. (Zenith Goldline) Clemastine fumarate (immediate release) 1.34 mg, phenylpropanolamine (extended release) 75 mg, lactose/Tab. Pkg. 16s. *otc.*
Use: Antihistamine, decongestant.

Antihist-1. (Various Mfr.) Clemastine fumarate 1.34 mg/Tab. Pkg. 16s. *otc.*
Use: Antihistamine.

Antihistamine Cream. (Towne) Methapyrilene HCl 10 mg, pyrilamine maleate 5 mg, allantoin 2 mg, diperodon HCl 2.5 mg, benzocaine 10 mg, menthol 2 mg/g. Cream Jar 2 oz. *otc.*
Use: Antihistamine, topical.

antihistamines.
See: Aller-Chlor, Syr., Tab. (Rugby Labs, Inc.).
AllerMax, Capl. (Pfeiffer Co.).
Anergan, Inj. (Forest Pharmaceutical, Inc.).
Astelin, Nasal Spray (Wallace Laboratories).
Allegra, Cap. (Hoechst Marion Roussel).
Benadryl, Preps. (Parke-Davis).
Benahist, Inj. (Keene Pharmaceuticals, Inc.).
Benylin Cough, Syr. (Parke-Davis).
Brompheniramine, Tab., Elix. (Various Mfr.).
Bromphen, Elix. (Various Mfr.).
Bydramine, Syr. (Major Pharmaceuticals).
Chlo-Amine, Tab. (Bayer Corp. (Consumer Div.)).
Chlorpheniramine Maleate (Various Mfr.).
Chlor-Pro, Inj. (Schein Pharmaceutical, Inc.).
Chlor-Trimeton, Inj., Syr., Tab. (Schering-Plough Corp.).
Claritin, Tab. (Schering-Plough Corp.).
Co-Pyronil 2, Pulv., Susp. (Eli Lilly and Co.).
Cyproheptadine HCl, Syr., Tab. (Various Mfr.).
Dexchlor, Tab. (Schein Pharmaceutical, Inc.).
Dexchlorpheniramine Maleate, Tab. (Various Mfr.).
Dimetane, Preps. (Wyeth-Ayerst Laboratories).
Diphen Cough, Syr. (Rosemont Pharmaceutical Corp.).
Diphenhydramine HCl (Various Mfr.).
Disophrol, Prods. (Schering-Plough Corp.).
Doxylamine Succinate (Various Mfr.).
Drixoral, Prods. (Schering-Plough Corp.).
Diphen Cough, Syr. (Rosemont Pharmaceutical Corp.).
Genahist, Cap., Tab., Elix. (Zenith Goldline Pharmaceuticals).
Hismanal, Tab. (Janssen Pharmaceutical, Inc.).
Hyrexin-50, Inj. (Hyrex Pharmaceuticals).
Nasahist B, Inj. (Keene Pharmaceuticals, Inc.).
ND Stat, Inj. (Hyrex Pharmaceuticals).
Nolahist, Tab. (Carnrick Laboratories, Inc.).
Optimine, Tab. (Schering-Plough Corp.).
Oraminic, Inj. (Vortech Pharmaceuticals).
PBZ, Tab. (Novartis Pharmaceutical Corp.).
PBZ-SR, Tab. (Novartis Pharmaceutical Corp.).
Pentazine, Inj. (Century Pharmaceuticals, Inc.).
Periactin, Syr., Tab. (Merck & Co.).
Pfeiffer's Allergy, Tab. (Pfeiffer Co.).
Phenameth, Tab. (Major Pharmaceuticals).
Phendry, Prods. (HN Norton).
Phenergan, Prods. (Wyeth-Ayerst Laboratories).
Poladex, Tab. (Major Pharmaceuticals).
Polaramine, Syr., Tab. (Schering-Plough Corp.).
Poly-Histine, Elix. (Sanofi Winthrop Pharmaceuticals).
Promethazine HCl (Various Mfr.).
Prophenpyridamine Maleate (Various Mfr.).

Pyrilamine Maleate (Various Mfr.).
Tacaryl, Tab., Syr. (Westwood Squibb Pharmaceuticals).
Tavist, Tab., Syr. (Novartis Pharmaceutical Corp.).
Telachlor, Cap. (Major Pharmaceuticals).
Teldrin, Cap. (SmithKline Beecham Pharmaceuticals).
Tripelennamine HCl (Various Mfr.).
Triprolidine HCl (Various Mfr.).
Tusstat, Syr. (Century Pharmaceuticals, Inc.).
Wehydryl, Inj. (Roberts Pharmaceuticals).

antihyperlipidemics.
See: Atromid-S, Cap. (Wyeth-Ayerst Laboratories).
Choloxin, Tab. (Knoll Pharmaceuticals).
Clofibrate, Cap. (Various Mfr.).
Mevacor, Tab. (Merck & Co.).
Niacin, Prods. (Various Mfr.).
Pravachol, Tab. (Bristol-Myers Squibb).
Questran, Prods. (Bristol-Myers Squibb).
Zocor, Tab. (Merck & Co.).

antihypertensives.
See: Accupril, Tab. (Parke-Davis).
Acebutolol hydrochloride.
Aceon, Tab. (Ortho McNeil Pharmaceutical).
Adaprolol maleate.
Alazide, Tab. (Major Pharmaceuticals).
Alazine, Tab. (Major Pharmaceuticals).
Aldactazide, Tab. (Searle).
Aldactone, Tab. (Searle).
Aldoclor 250, Tab. (Merck & Co.).
Aldomet, Tab. (Merck & Co.).
Aldoril, Tab. (Merck & Co.).
Alfuzosin hydrochloride.
$Alpha_1$-adrenergic blockers.
Altace, Cap. (Hoechst Marion Roussel, Pharmacia & Upjohn).
Althiazide.
Amiquinsin hydrochloride.
Amlodipine besylate.
Amlodipine maleate.
Amodopa (Major Pharmaceuticals).
Anaritide acetate.
ACE inhibitors.
Apresazide, Cap. (Novartis Pharmaceutical Corp.).
Apresodex, Tab. (Rugby Labs, Inc.).
Apresoline, Amp., Tab. (Novartis Pharmaceutical Corp.).
Aprozide, Cap. (Major Pharmaceuticals).
Arcum R-S, Tab. (Arcum).
Arlix (Hoechst Marion Roussel).
Artarau, Tab. (Archer-Taylor).
Atenolol/chlorthalidone, Tab. (Various Mfr.).
Atiprosin maleate.
Belfosdil.
Bendacalol mesylate.
Bendroflumethiazide.
Benzthiazide.
Betaxolol hydrochloride.
Bethanidine sulfate.
Bevantolol hydrochloride.
Biclodil hydrochloride.
Bisoprolol fumarate.
Bucindolol hydrochloride.
Cam-Ap-Es, Tab. (Camall Co., Inc.).
Candoxatril.
Candoxatrilat.
Capoten, Tab. (Bristol-Myers Squibb).
Capozide, Tab. (Bristol-Myers Squibb).
Captopril.
Cardura, Tab. (Roerig).
Carvedilol.
Catapres, Tab. (Boehringer Ingelheim, Inc.).
Ceronapril.
Chlorothiazide sodium.
Chlorthalidone, Tab. (Various Mfr.).
Cicletanine.
Cilazapril.
Cithal, Cap. (Table Rock).
Citrin, Cap. (Table Rock).
Clentiazem maleate.
Clonidine.
Clonidine hydrochloride.
Clonidine hydrochloride and Chlorthalidone, Tab. (Various Mfr.).
Clopamide.
Combipres, Tab. (Boehringer Ingelheim, Inc.).
Coreg, Tab. (SmithKline Beecham Pharmaceuticals).
Cyclothiazide.
Debrisoquin sulfate.
Delapril hydrochloride.
Demser, Cap. (Merck & Co.).
De Serpa, Tab. (de Leon).
Diaserp, Tab. (Major Pharmaceuticals).
Diazoxide.
Diazoxide parenteral.
Dibenzyline, Cap. (SmithKline Beecham Pharmaceuticals).
Dilevalol hydrochloride.
Diovan, Cap. (Novartis Pharmaceutical Corp.).
Ditekiren.
Diucardin, Tab. (Wyeth-Ayerst Laboratories).

Diulo, Tab. (Searle).
Diurigen w/Reserpine, Tab. (Zenith Goldline Pharmaceuticals).
Diuril, Tab., Susp. (Merck & Co.).
Diuril sodium, I.V. (Merck & Co.).
Diutensen-R, Tab. (Wallace Laboratories).
Doxazosin mesylate.
Elserpine, Tab. (Canright).
Enalapril maleate.
Enalaprilat.
Enalkiren.
Endralazine mesylate.
Enduronyl, Tab. (Abbott Laboratories).
Enduronyl Forte, Tab. (Abbott Laboratories).
Eprosartan.
Eprosartan mesylate.
Eserdine, Tab. (Major Pharmaceuticals).
Eserdine Forte, Tab. (Major Pharmaceuticals).
Esidrix, Tab. (Novartis Pharmaceutical Corp.).
Esimil, Tab. (Novartis Pharmaceutical Corp.).
Exna, Tab. (Wyeth-Ayerst Laboratories).
Fenoldopam mesylate.
Flavodilol maleate.
Flolan, Pow. for Inj. (GlaxoWellcome).
Flordipine.
Flosequinan.
Forasartan.
Fosinopril.
Fosinopril sodium.
Fosinoprilat.
Guanabenz.
Guanabenz acetate.
Guanacline sulfate.
Guanadrel sulfate.
Guancydine.
Guanethidine monosulfate.
Guanethidine sulfate.
Guanfacine hydrochloride.
Guanisoquin.
Guanisoquin sulfate.
Guanoclor sulfate.
Guanocitine hydrochloride.
Guanoxabenz.
Guanoxan sulfate.
Guanoxyfen sulfate.
Harbolin, Tab. (Arcum).
H.H.R., Tab. (Geneva Pharm).
Hiwolfia, Tab. (Jones Medical Industries, Inc.).
Hydralazine, Inj. (Solopak).
Hydralazine hydrochloride, Tab. (Various Mfr.).
Hydralazine polistirex.
Hydrap-ES, Tab. (Parmed).
Hydraserp, Tab. (Zenith Goldline).
Hydrazide, Cap. (Zenith Goldline).
Hydra-Zide, Cap. (Par Pharm).
Hydrochloroserpine, Tab. (Freeport).
Hydrochlorothiazide/Hydralazine, Cap. (Various Mfr.).
Hydroflumethiazide.
Hydromox-R, Tab. (ESI Lederle Generics).
Hydropine, Tab. (Rugby).
Hydropine H.P., Tab. (Rugby).
Hydropres-50, Tab. (Merck & Co.).
Hydroserp, Tab. (Zenith Goldline).
Hydroserp-50, Tab. (Freeport).
Hydroserpine #1, #2 (Various Mfr.).
Hydrosine 25, 50, Tab. (Major).
Hydrotensin-50, Tab. (Merz).
Hydroxyisoindolin.
Hylorel, Tab. (Hyrex).
Hyperstat, I.V. Inj. (Schering-Plough).
Hytrin, Tab., Cap. (Abbott Laboratories).
Hyzaar, Tab. (Merck & Co.).
Indacrinone.
Indapamide.
Inderide, Tab. (Wyeth-Ayerst Laboratories).
Inderide LA, Cap. (Wyeth-Ayerst Laboratories).
Indolapril hydrochloride.
Indoramin.
Indoramin hydrochloride.
Indorenate hydrochloride.
Ingadine, Tab. (Major).
Inhibace (Roche/GlaxoWellcome).
Inversine, Tab. (Merck & Co.).
Irbesartan.
Ismelin, Tab. (Novartis).
Labetalol hydrochloride.
Leniquinsin.
Levcromakalim.
Lexxel, ER Tab. (Astra Merck).
Lofexidine hydrochloride.
Loniten, Tab. (Pharmacia & Upjohn).
Lopressor HCT, Tab. (Novartis).
Losartan potassium.
Losulazine hydrochloride.
Lotensin, Tab. (Novartis).
Lotrel, Cap. (Novartis).
Lozol, Tab. (Rhone-Poulenc Rorer).
Marpres, Tab. (Marnel).
Mavik, Tab. (Knoll Pharmaceuticals).
Maxzide, Tab. (ESI Lederle Generics).
Mebutamate.
Mecamylamine hydrochloride.
Medroxalol.
Medroxalol hydrochloride.
Metatensin, Tab. (Hoechst Marion Roussel).
Methalthiazide.

Methyclodine, Tab. (Rugby).
Methylclothiazide.
Methyldopa.
Methyldopa and Chlorothiazide, Tab.
Methyldopa and Hydrochlorothiazide, Tab. (Various Mfr.).
Methyldopate hydrochloride, Inj. (Fujisawa).
Metipranolol.
Metipranolol hydrochloride.
Metolazone.
Metoprolol fumarate.
Metoprolol succinate.
Metoprolol tartrate and Hydrochlorothiazide.
Metyrosine.
Midamor, Tab. (Merck & Co.).
Minipress, Cap. (Pfizer).
Minizide, Cap. (Pfizer).
Minoxidil, Tab. (Rugby).
Moduretic, Tab. (Merck & Co.).
Moexipril hydrochloride.
Monopril, Tab. (Bristol-Myers Squibb).
Muzolimine.
Nadolol, Tab. (Various Mfr.).
Nadolol and Bendroflumethiazide.
Natrico, Pulvoid (Drug Products).
Nebivolol.
Nitrendipine.
Nitropress, Vial (Abbott Laboratories).
Nitroprusside sodium.
Normodyne, Inj., Tab. (Schering-Plough).
Normotensin, Inj. (Marcen).
Pargyline hydrochloride.
Pelanserin hydrochloride.
Pentina, Tab. (Freeport).
Pentolinium tartrate.
Perindopril erbumine.
Pheniprazine hydrochloride.
Phenoxybenzamine hydrochloride.
Phentolamine hydrochloride.
Pinacidil.
Pivopril.
Prazosin hydrochloride, Cap. (Various Mfr.).
Prinivil, Tab. (Merck & Co.).
Prinzide, Tab. (Merck & Co.).
Priscoline, Vial (Novartis).
Prizidilol hydrochloride.
Propanolol hydrochloride and Hydrochlorothiazide, Tab. (Various Mfr.).
Quinapril hydrochloride.
Quinaprilat.
Quinazosin hydrochloride.
Quinelorane hydrochloride.
Quinuclium bromide.
Ramipril.
Rauneed, Tab. (Hanlon).
Raunescine (Penick).
Raurine, Tab., Cap. (New England Pharmacy Co.).
Rautina, Tab. (Fellows).
Rauval, Tab. (Pal-Pak).
Rauwolfia/Bendroflumethiazide, Tab. (Various Mfr.).
Rauwolfia serpentina.
Rauwolscine.
Rauzide, Tab. (Bristol-Myers Squibb).
Rawfola, Tab. (Foy).
Regroton, Tab. (Rhone-Poulenc Rorer).
Regroton Demi, Tab. (Rhone-Poulenc Rorer).
Renese, Tab. (Pfizer).
Renese-R, Tab. (Pfizer).
Reserpaneed, Tab. (Hanlon).
Reserpine.
Reserpine and Chlorothiazide, Tab.
Reserpine and Hydrochlorothiazide, Tab. (Various Mfr.).
Reserpine, hydralazine hydrochloride, and Hydrochlorothiazide, Tab. (Various Mfr.).
R-HCTZ-H, Tab. (ESI Lederle Generics).
Salazide, Tab. (Major).
Salazide-Demi, Tab. (Major).
Salutensin, Tab. (Roberts Pharm.).
Salutensin-Demi, Tab. (Bristol-Myers Squibb).
Saprisartan potassium.
Saralasin acetate.
Sectral, Cap. (Wyeth-Ayerst Laboratories).
Ser-A-Gen, Tab. (Zenith Goldline).
Ser-Ap-Es, Tab. (Novartis).
Serpasil-Apresoline, Tab. (Novartis).
Serpasil-Esidrix, Tab. (Novartis).
Serpazide, Tab. (Major).
Sertabs, Tab. (Table Rock).
Sertina, Tab. (Fellows).
Sodium nitroprusside, Pow. for Inj. (ESI Lederle Generics).
Sulfinalol hydrochloride.
Tarka, Tab. (Knoll Pharmaceuticals).
Teludipine hydrochloride.
Temocapril hydrochloride.
Tenex, Tab. (Robins).
Tenoretic, Tab. (Zeneca).
Tenormin, Amp., Tab. (Zeneca).
Terazosin hydrochloride.
Tiamenidine hydrochloride.
Ticrynafen.
Timolide 10-25, Tab. (Merck & Co.).
Timolol maleate.
Timolol maleate and Hydrochloride, Tab.
Tinabinol.
Tipentosin hydrochloride.
Tolazoline hydrochloride.
Toprol XL, Tab. (Astra USA).
Trandate, Tab., Inj. (Allen & Hanburys).

Trandate hydrochlorothiazide, Tab. (Allen & Hanburys).
Tri-Hydroserpine, Tab. (Rugby).
Trimazosin hydrochloride.
Trimethamide.
Trimethaphan camsylate.
Trimoxamine hydrochloride.
T-Sert, Tab. (Tennessee Pharmaceutic).
Univasc, Tab. (Schwarz Pharma).
Valsartan.
Vaseretic, Tab. (Merck & Co.).
Vasotec, Tab., Inj. (Merck & Co.).
Visken, Tab. (Novartis).
Xipamide.
Zankiren hydrochloride.
Zepine, Tab. (Foy).
Zestoretic, Tab. (Zeneca).
Zestril, Tab. (Zeneca).
Ziac, Tab. (ESI Lederle Generics).
Zofenoprilat arginine.

anti-infectives.
See: Antibiotics/Anti-infectives.

anti-inhibitor coagulant complex.
Use: Antihemophilic.
See: Autoplex T. (Baxter Pharmaceutical Products, Inc.).
Feiba VH. (Baxter Healthcare Corp.).

Anti-Itch Cream. (Rugby Labs, Inc.) Burow's solution 5%, phenol 0.5%, menthol 0.5%, camphor 1% in washable base. Tube oz. *otc.*
Use: Antipruritic, counterirritant.

Antilerge. (Metz) Chlorpheniramine maleate 8 mg, phenylephrine HCl 12 mg/Tab. Bot. 30s. *otc.*
Use: Antihistamine, decongestant.

antileukemia.
See: Antineoplastic agents.

Antilirium. (Forest Pharmaceutical, Inc.) Physostigmine salicylate 1 mg/ml, benzyl alcohol 2%, sodium bisufite 0.1%. 2 ml. *Rx.*
Use: Antidote. [Orphan Drug]

antimalarial agents.
See: Amodiaquine HCl.
Aralen HCl, Inj. (Sanofi Winthrop Pharmaceuticals).
Aralen Phosphate. (Sanofi Winthrop Pharmaceuticals).
Aralen Phosphate w/Primaquine. (Sanofi Winthrop Pharmaceuticals).
Chloroguanide HCl.
Daraprim Tab. (GlaxoWellcome).
Hydroxychloroquine Sulfate.
Plaquenil Sulfate, Tab. (Sanofi Winthrop Pharmaceuticals).
Plasmochin Naphthoate.
Primaquine Phosphate, Tab. (Sanofi Winthrop Pharmaceuticals).
Pyrimethamine.
Quinine Salts. (Various Mfr.).
Quinine Sulfate. (Various Mfr.).
Totaquine, Pow.

Antiminth. (Pfizer US Pharmaceutical Group) Pyrantel pamoate 250 mg/5 ml. Oral susp. Bot. 60 ml. *otc.*
Use: Anthelmintic.

•**antimony potassium tartrate.** U.S.P. 23.
Use: Antischistosomal, leishmaniasis, expectorant, emetic.
W/Cocillana, euphorbia pilulifera, squill, senega.
See: Cylana, Syr. (Jones Medical Industries, Inc.).
W/Guaifenesin, codeine phosphate.
See: Cheracol, Syr. (Pharmacia & Upjohn).
W/Guaifenesin, dextromethorphan HBr.
See: Cheracol D, Syr. (Pharmacia & Upjohn).

antimony preparations.
See: Antimony Potassium Tartrate. (Various Mfr.).
Antimony Sodium Thioglycollate. (Various Mfr.).
Tartar Emetic. (Various Mfr.).

•**antimony sodium tartrate.** U.S.P. 23.
Use: Antischistosomal.

antimony sodium thioglycollate. (Various Mfr.). *Rx.*
Use: Schistosomiasis, leishmaniasis, filariasis.

•**antimony trisulfide colloid.** USAN.
Use: Pharmaceutic aid.

anti-my9-blocked ricin.
Use: Leukemia treatment.

antinauseants.
See: Antiemetic, antivertigo.

antineoplastic agents.
See: Adriamycin, Vial (Pharmacia & Upjohn).
Alkeran, Tab. (GlaxoWellcome).
Amsacrine.
Azacitidine.
Blenoxane, Amp. (Bristol-Myers Squibb).
Cosmegen, Inj. (Merck & Co.).
Elspar, Inj. (Merck & Co.).
Emcyt, Cap. (Pharmacia & Upjohn).
Estinyl, Tab. (Schering-Plough Corp.).
FUDR, Vial (Roche Laboratories).
Hexalen (US Bioscience).
Hydrea, Cap. (Bristol-Myers Squibb).
Idamycin (Pharmacia & Upjohn).
Leukeran, Tab. (GlaxoWellcome).
Lysodren, Tab. (Bristol-Myers Oncology/Immunology).
Matulane, Cap. (Roche Laboratories).
Medroxyprogesterone Acetate Tab., Vial (Various Mfr.).

Megace, Tab. (Bristol-Myers Squibb).
Mercaptopurine, Tab.
Methotrexate, Tab. (ESI Lederle Generics).
Methotrexate Sodium, Vial (ESI Lederle Generics).
Mithracin, Vial (Pfizer US Pharmaceutical Group).
Mustargen, Inj. (Merck & Co.).
Myleran, Tab. (GlaxoWellcome).
Nolvadex, Tab. (Zeneca Pharmaceuticals).
Oncovin, Amp. (Eli Lilly and Co.).
Purinethol, Tab. (GlaxoWellcome).
Tamoxifen, Tab. (Barr Laboratories, Inc.).
Thioguanine, Tab. (GlaxoWellcome).
Thio Tepa, Vial (ESI Lederle Generics).
Velban, Amp. (Eli Lilly and Co.).

antiobesity agents.
See: Acutrim, Prods. (Novartis Pharmaceutical Corp.).
Adderall (Richwood Pharmaceuticals).
Adipex-P, Tab., Cap. (Teva Pharmaceuticals USA).
Amphetamine Preps. (Various Mfr.).
Anorex, Cap. (Dunhall Pharmaceuticals, Inc.).
Bontril, Prods. (Carnrick Laboratories, Inc.).
Control, Cap. (Thompson Medical Co.).
Dexatrim Pre-Meal, Cap. (Thompson Medical Co.).
Dextroamphetamine Preps. (Various Mfr.).
Didrex, Tab. (Pharmacia & Upjohn).
Diethylpropion HCl.
Dieutrim T.D., Cap. (Legere Pharmaceuticals, Inc.).
Fastin, Cap. (SmithKline Beecham Pharmaceuticals).
Ionamin, Cap. (Medeva Pharmaceuticals, Inc.).
Levo-Amphetamine.
Maximum Strength Dexatrim, Cap. (Thompson Medical Co.).
Mazanor, Tab. (Wyeth-Ayerst Laboratories).
Methamphetamine Preps. (Various Mfr.).
Obe-Nix 30, Cap. (Holloway).
Phendimetrazine Tartrate, Cap., Tab. (Various Mfr.).
Phentermine HCl, Tab., Cap. (Various Mfr.).
Phentermine Resin, Cap. (Various Mfr.).
Prelu-2, Cap. (Boehringer Ingelheim, Inc.).
Sanorex, Tab. (Novartis Pharmaceutical Corp.).
Tenuate, Tab. (Hoechst Marion Roussel).
Tenuate Dospan, Tab. (SmithKline Beecham Pharmaceuticals).
Tepanil, Tab. (3M Pharm).
Trimstat, Tab. (Laser, Inc.).
Wehless Timecelles, Cap. (Roberts Pharmaceuticals).
Xenical, Cap. (Roche Laboratories).

Antiox. (Mayrand) Vitamin C 120 mg, vitamin E 100 IU, beta-carotene 25 mg. Cap. Bot. 60s. *otc.*
Use: Vitamin supplement.

Anti-Pak Compound. (Lowitt) Phenylephrine HCl 5 mg, salicylamide 0.23 g, acetophenetidin 0.15 gr, caffeine 0.03 g, ascorbic acid 50 mg, hesperidin complex 50 mg, chlorprophenpyridamine maleate 2 mg/Tab. Bot. 30s, 100s. *otc.*
Use: Analgesic, antihistamine, decongestant combination.

antiparasympathomimetics.
See: Parasympatholytic agents.

antipellagra vitamin.
See: Nicotinic acid.

antipernicious anemia principle.
See: Vitamin B_{12}.

Antiphlogistine. (Denver Chemical [Puerto Rico] Inc.) Medicated poultice. Jar 5 oz, lb. Tube 8 oz. Can 5 lb.

antiplatelet antibodies.
See: ReoPro (Eli Lilly and Co.).

antiprotozoal agents.
See: Antimony Preps.
Arsenic Preps.
Bismuth Preps.
Chiniofon (Various Mfr.).
Diiodohydroxyquinoline.
Emetine HCl (Various Mfr.).
Furazolidone.
Levofuraltadone.
Ornidyl (Hoechst Marion Roussel).
Quinoxyl.
Suramin Sodium

•**antipyrine.** U.S.P. 23.
Use: Analgesic, antipyretic.
W/Benzocaine, chlorobutanol.
See: G.B.A., Drops (Scrip).
W/Carbamide, benzocaine, cetyldimethylbenzylammonium HCl.
See: Auralgesic, Liq. (ICN Pharmaceuticals, Inc.).
W/Phenylephrine HCl, benzocaine.
See: Tympagesic, Liq. (Pharmacia & Upjohn).

antipyrine and benzocaine otic solution.
Use: Anesthetic, local.

See: Auro Ear Drops. (Del Pharmaceuticals, Inc.).
antipyrine, benzocaine, and phenylephrine hydrochloride otic solution.
Use: Anesthetic, local; decongestant eardrop.
•**antirabies serum.** U.S.P. 23.
Use: Immunization.
antirickettsial agents.
See: p-Aminobenzoic Acid. (Various Mfr.).
Aureomycin, Preps. (ESI Lederle Generics).
Chloromycetin, Preps. (Parke-Davis).
Terramycin, Preps. (Pfizer US Pharmaceutical Group).
antiscorbutic vitamin.
See: Ascorbic Acid.
antiseptic, chlorine, active.
See: Antiseptic, N-Chloro Compounds, Hypochlorite Preps.
antiseptic, dyes.
See: Acriflavine (Various Mfr.).
Aminoacridine HCl.
Bismuth Violet, Preps. (Table Rock).
Crystal Violet.
Fuchsin.
Gentian Violet. (Various Mfr.).
Methylrosaniline Cl (Various Mfr.).
Methyl Violet.
Pyridium, Tab. (Parke-Davis).
antiseptic, mercurials.
See: Merthiolate, Preps. (Eli Lilly and Co.).
Phenylmercuric Acetate (Various Mfr.).
Phenylmercuric Borate (Various Mfr.).
Phenylmercuric Nitrate (Various Mfr.).
Phenylmercuric Picrate (Various Mfr.).
Thimerosal.
antiseptic, n-chloro compounds.
See: Chloramine-T (Various Mfr.).
Chlorazene, Pow., Tab. (Badger).
Dichloramine T (Various Mfr.).
Halazone, Tab. (Abbott Laboratories).
antiseptic, phenols.
See: Anthralin (Various Mfr.).
Bithionol.
Coal Tar Products (Various Mfr.).
Creosote (Various Mfr.).
Guaiacol (Various Mfr.).
Hexachlorophene (Various Mfr.).
Hexylresorcinol (Various Mfr.).
Methylparaben (Various Mfr.).
o-Phenylphenol (Various Mfr.).
Oxyquinoline Salts (Various Mfr.).
Parachlorometaxylenol (Various Mfr.).
Phenol (Various Mfr.).
Picric Acid (Various Mfr.).
Propylparaben (Various Mfr.).
Pyrogallol (Various Mfr.).
Resorcinol (Various Mfr.).
Resorcinol Monoacetate (Various Mfr.).
Thymol (Various Mfr.).
Trinitrophenol (Various Mfr.).
antiseptics.
See: Furacin, Preps. (Eaton Medical Corp.).
Iodine Products.
Phenols.
antiseptic, surface-active agents.
See: Bactine, Preps. (Bayer Corp. (Consumer Div.)).
Benzalkonium Cl (Various Mfr.).
Benzethonium Cl (Various Mfr.).
Ceepryn (Hoechst Marion Roussel).
Cepacol Preps. (Hoechst Marion Roussel).
Cetylpyridinium Cl (Various Mfr.).
Diaparene Cl, Preps. (Bayer Corp (Consumer Div.)).
Methylbenzethonium Cl (Various Mfr.).
Zephiran Cl, Preps. (Sanofi Winthrop Pharmaceuticals).
Antispas. (Keene Pharmaceuticals, Inc.) Dicyclomine HCl 10 mg/ml. Vial 10 ml. *Rx.*
Use: Antispasmodic.
antispasmodics. Parasympatholytic agents.
See: Anticholinergic Agents.
Spasmolytic Agents.
Antispasmodic Capsules. (Teva Pharmaceuticals USA) Phenobarbital 16.2 mg, hyoscyamine sulfate 0.1037 mg, atropine sulfate 0.0194 mg, scopolamine HBr 0.0065 mg/Cap. Bot. 1000s. *Rx.*
Use: Anticholinergic, antispasmodic, hypnotic, sedative.
Antispasmodic Elixir. (Various Mfr.) Atropine sulfate 0.0194 mg, scopolamine HBr 0.0065 mg, hyoscyamine HBr or SO_4 0.1037 mg, phenobarbital 16.2 mg/ml w/alcohol 23%. Elix. Bot. 120 ml, Pt, gal, and UD 5 ml. *Rx.*
Use: Anticholinergic, antispasmodic, hypnotic, sedative.
antistreptolysin-O.
Use: Titration procedure.
antisterility vitamin.
See: Vitamin E.
anti-t lymphocyte immunotoxin xmmly-h65-rta. (Xoma)
See: Anti Pan T Lymphocyte Monoclonal Antibody.
Anti-Tac, Humanized. (Roche Laboratories)
Use: Prevention of acute renal allograft rejection. [Orphan Drug]

Anti-Ten. (Century Pharmaceuticals, Inc.) Allylisobutylbarbituric acid ¾ gr, aspirin 3 gr, phenacetin 2 gr, caffeine gr/Tab. Bot. 100s, 1000s. *Rx.*
Use: Analgesic, sedative, stimulant.

antithrombin III concentrate IV.
Use: Prophylaxis/treatment of thromboembolic episodes in AT-III deficiency. [Orphan Drug]

antithrombin III human.
Use: Thromboembolic.
See: Thrombate III (Bayer Corp. (Biological and Pharmaceutical Div.)).

antithrombin III human. (Red Cross)
Use: Thromboembolic. [Orphan Drug]

antithymocyte globulin.
Use: Immunosuppressant. [Orphan Drug]

Nashville Rabbit Antithymocyte. (Applied Medical Research) Antithymocyte serum.
Use: Immunosuppressant.

antithyroid agents.
See: Iothiouracil Sodium.
Methimazole.
Methylthiouracil (Various Mfr.).
Propylthiouracil (Various Mfr.).
Tapazole, Tab. (Eli Lilly and Co.).

antitoxins.
See: Botulism Antitoxin.
Diphtheria Antitoxin.
Tetanus Immune Globulin.

antitrypsin, alpha 1.
See: alpha-1-antitrypsin.

antituberculosis agents.
See: Benzoylpas Calcium (Various Mfr.).
Capastat Sulfate, Amp. (Eli Lilly and Co.).
Cycloserine.
Dihydrostreptomycin (Various Mfr.).
Isoniazid (Various Mfr.).
Myambutol, Tab. (ESI Lederle Generics).
Pyrazinamide, Tab. (ESI Lederle Generics).
Rifadin, Cap., Inj. (Hoechst Marion Roussel).
Rimactane, Cap. (Novartis Pharmaceutical Corp.).
Seromycin, Pulv. (Eli Lilly and Co.).
Streptomycin (Various Mfr.).
Trecator SC, Tab. (Wyeth-Ayerst Laboratories).

Anti-Tuss. (Century Pharmaceuticals, Inc.) Guaifenesin 100 mg/5 ml. Bot. 4 oz, gal. *otc.*
Use: Expectorant.

Anti-Tuss D.M. (Century Pharmaceuticals, Inc.) Guaifenesin 100 mg, dextromethorphan HBr 15 mg/5 ml. Bot. 4 oz, Pt, gal. *otc.*
Use: Antitussive, expectorant.

Anti-Tussive. (Canright) Dextromethorphan HBr 10 mg, potassium guaiacol sulfonate 125 mg, terpin hydrate 100 mg, phenylpropanolamine HCl 12.5 mg, pyrilamine maleate 12.5 mg/Tab. Bot. 60s. *otc.*
Use: Antihistamine, antitussive, decongestant, expectorant.

Antitussive Cough Syrup. (Weeks & Leo) Chlorpheniramine 2 mg, phenylephrine HCl 5 mg, dextromethorphan 15 mg, ammonium Cl 50 mg/5 ml. *otc.*
Use: Antihistamine, antitussive, decongestant, expectorant.

Antitussive Cough Syrup with Codeine. (Weeks & Leo) Chlorpheniramine maleate 2 mg, phenylephrine HCl 5 mg, codeine phosphate 10 mg, ammonium Cl 50 mg/5 ml. Bot. 4 oz. *c-v.*
Use: Antihistamine, antitussive, decongestant, expectorant.

antitussive-decongestant.
See: St. Joseph Cough Syrup for Children (Schering-Plough Corp.).
Tussend, Tab., Liq. (Hoechst Marion Roussel).

•**antivenin (latrodectus mactans).** U.S.P. 23. *Formerly Widow spider species antivenin (Latrodectus mactans).*
Use: Immunization.

antivenin (latrodectus mactans). Black widow spider antivenin. Each vial contains not less than 6000 antivenin units. Thimerosal (mercury derivative) 1:10,000 added as preservative. Vial 2.5 ml of Sterile Water for Injection and a 1 ml vial of normal horse serum for sensitivity testing.
Use: Treatment of black widow spider bites.

•**antivenin (micrurus fulvius).** U.S.P. 23.
Use: Immunization.

antivenin (micrurus fulvius). North American coral snake antivenin. Lyophilized antivenin of animal origin (*Micrurus fulvius*) with phenol 0.25% and thimerosal 0.005% as preservatives. Bacteriostatic water w/phenylmercuric nitrate 1:100,000 as preservative. Combination package. Vial 10 ml.
Use: Bites of North American coral snake and Texas coral snake.

antivenin Centruroides sculpturatus. (Arizona State University) Available in Arizona only. 5 ml vials.
Use: Antivenin.

•**antivenin (crotalidae) polyvalent.**

U.S.P. 23.
Use: Immunization.

antivenin (crotalidae) polyvalent. (Wyeth-Ayerst Laboratories) Rattlesnake, copperhead, and cottonmouth moccasin antitoxic serum. One vial lyophilized serum with 0.25% phenol and 0.005% thimerosal. One vial, 10 ml of bacteriostatic water for inj. w/phenylmercuric nitrate 0.001%; one vial normal horse serum 1:10, as sensitivity testing material w/thimerosal 0.005% and phenol 0.35%.
Use: Bites of crotalid snakes of North, Central, and South America.

antivenin, polyvalent crotalid (ovine) fab.
Use: Bites of North American crotalid snakes. [Orphan Drug]
See: Crotab. (Therapeutic Antibodies, Inc.).

antivenom (crotalidae) purified (avian). (Ophidian Pharmaceuticals,Inc.)
Use: Bites of snakes of the crotalidae family. [Orphan Drug]

Antivert. (Roerig) Meclizine HCl 12.5 mg, 25 mg or 50 mg/Tab. **12.5 mg:** Bot. 100s, 1000s, UD 100s; **25 mg:** Bot. 100s, 1000s, UD 100s. **50 mg:** Bot. 100s. *Rx.*
Use: Antiemetic, antivertigo.

antiviral agents.
See: Cytovene, Inj. (Roche Laboratories).
Famvir, Tab. (SmithKline Beecham Pharmaceuticals).
Foscavir, Inj. (Astra Pharmaceuticals, L.P.).
Hivid, Tab. (Roche Laboratories).
Retrovir, Preps. (GlaxoWellcome).
Symmetrel, Cap., Syr. (DuPont Merck Pharmaceutical Co.).
Vira-A, Inj. (Parke-Davis).
Virazole, Pow for Reconstitution for aerosol. (ICN Pharmaceuticals, Inc).
Zerit, Cap. (Bristol-Myers Squibb).
Zovirax, Cap., Inj. (GlaxoWellcome).

antiviral antibodies.
See: Cytomegalovirus immune globulin.
Immune globulin IM.
Immune globulin IV.
Hepatitis B immune globulin.
Rabies immune globulin.
Vaccinia immune globulin.
Varicella-zoster immune globulin.

antixerophthalmic vitamin.
See: Vitamin A.

Antizol. (Orphan Medical, Inc.) Fomepizole 1 g/ml. Preservative free. Inj. Conc. Vial 1.5 ml. *Rx.*
Use: Antidote.

Antril. (Amgen, Inc.) Interleukin-1 receptor antagonist (human recombinant).
Use: Arthritis, organ rejection. [Orphan Drug]

Antrizine Tabs. (Major Pharmaceuticals) Meclizine 12.5 mg, 25 mg, or 50 mg/Tab. **12.5 mg:** 100s, 500s, 1000s. **25 mg:** 100s, 500s, 1000s, UD 100s. **50 mg:** 100s. *Rx.*
Use: Antiemetic, antivertigo.

Antrocol. (ECR Pharmaceuticals) Atropine sulfate 0.195 mg, phenobarbital 16 mg, alcohol 20%/5 ml. Sugar free. Elix. Bot. Pt. *Rx.*
Use: Anticholinergic, antispasmodic, hypnotic, sedative.

Antrypol. Suramin. *Rx.*
Use: CDC anti-infective agent.

Anturane. (Novartis Pharmaceutical Corp.) Sulfinpyrazone, U.S.P. **100 mg/Tab.:** Bot 100s. **200 mg/Cap.:** Bot. 100s. *Rx.*
Use: Antigout agent.

Anucaine. (Calvin) Procaine 50 mg, butyl-p-aminobenzoate 200 mg, benzyl alcohol 265 mg in sweet almond oil/5 ml. Amp. 5 ml. Box 6s, 24s, 100s. *otc.*
Use: Anorectal preparation.

Anucort-HC. (G & W Laboratories) Hydrocortisone acetate 25 mg in a hydrogenated vegetable oil base. Supp. Box 12s, 24s, 100s. *Rx.*
Use: Anorectal preparation.

Anuject. (Roberts Pharmaceuticals) Procaine. Soln. Vial 5 ml or 10 ml. *Rx.*
Use: Anorectal preparation.

Anumed. (Major Pharmaceuticals) Bismuth subgallate 2.25%, bismuth resorcin compound 1.75%, benzyl benzoate 1.2%, zinc oxide 11%, balsam Peru 1.8% in a hydrogenated vegetable oil base. Supp. Box 12s. *otc.*
Use: Anorectal preparation.

Anumed HC. (Major Pharmaceuticals) Hydrocortisone acetate 10 mg. Supp. Box 12s. *Rx.*
Use: Anorectal preparation.

Anuprep HC. (Great Southern Laboratories) Hydrocortisone acetate 25 mg. Supp. Box 12s.
Use: Anorectal preparation.

Anuprep Hemorrhoidal. (Great Southern Laboratories) Bismuth subgallate 2.25%, bismuth resorcin compound 1.75%, benzyl benzoate 1.2%, peruvian balsam 1.8%, and zinc oxide 11% in a hydrogenated vegetable oil base. Supp. Box 12s, 24s. *Rx.*
Use: Anorectal preparation.

Anusol. (GlaxoWellcome) Topical starch 51%, benzyl alcohol, soybean oil, tocopheryl acetate. Supp. Pkg. 12s. *otc.*
Use: Anorectal preparation.

Anusol-HC 2.5%. (Monarch Pharmaceuticals) Hydrocortisone 2.5%. Cream Tube 30 g. *Rx.*
Use: Corticosteroid, topical.

Anusol-HC-1. (Monarch Pharmaceuticals) Hydrocortisone 1%, diazolidinyl urea, parabens, mineral oil, sorbitan sesquioleate, white petrolatum. Oint. Tube 21 g. *otc.*
Use: Corticosteroid, topical.

Anusol Ointment. (Monarch Pharmaceuticals) Pramoxine HCl 1% and zinc oxide 12.5%/g, benzyl benzoate 1.2%, pramoxine HCl 1% in a mineral oil and cocoa butter. Tube 30 g. *otc.*
Use: Anorectal preparation.

Anzemet. (Hoechst Marion Roussel) Dolasetron mesylate 50 mg, 100 mg, lactose/Tab. 5s, UD 5s, 10s. Dolasetron mesylate 20 mg/ml, mannitol 38.2 mg/ml/Inj. Single-use Amp. 0.625 ml, single-use Vial 5 ml. *Rx.*
Use: Antiemetic.

AOSEPT. (Ciba Vision) Hydrogen peroxide 3%, sodium Cl 0.85%, phosphonic acid, phosphate buffer. Soln. Bot. 120 ml, 240 ml, 360 ml. *otc.*
Use: Contact lens care.

Apacet. (Parmed Pharmaceuticals, Inc.) Acetaminophen 80 mg/Chew. Tab. Bot. 100s. *otc.*
Use: Analgesic.

•**apafant.** (APP-ah-fant) USAN.
Use: Platelet activating factor antagonist; antiasthmatic.

•**apalcillin sodium.** (APE-al-SIH-lin) USAN.
Use: Anti-infective.

APAP.
See: Acetaminophen.

Apatate w/Fluoride. (Kenwood Laboratories) Vitamins B_1 15 mg, B_6 0.5 mg, B_{12} 25 mcg, F 0.5 mg/5 ml. Liq. Bot. 120 ml. *Rx.*
Use: Mineral, vitamin supplement.

Apatate Liquid. (Kenwood Laboratories) Vitamins B_1 15 mg, B_{12} 25 mcg, B_6 0.5 mg/5 ml. Liq. Bot. 120 ml, 240 ml. *otc.*
Use: Vitamin supplement.

Apatate Tablets. (Kenwood Laboratories) Vitamins B_1 15 mg, B_{12} 25 mcg, B_6 0.5 mg/Tab. Bot. 50s. *otc.*
Use: Vitamin supplement.

•**apaxifylline.** (A-pock-SIH-fih-leen) USAN.
Use: Selective adenosine A_1 antagonist.

•**apazone.** (APP-ah-zone) USAN.
Use: Anti-inflammatory.

A.P.C. (Various Mfr.) Aspirin, phenacetin, caffeine. Cap., Tab.
Use: Analgesic combination.
See: A.S.A. Compound, Preps. (Eli Lilly and Co.).
Pan-APC, Tab. (Panray).
Phensal, Tab. (Hoechst Marion Roussel).
W/Codeine phosphate. (Various Mfr.).
See: Anexsia w/Codeine, Tab. (SmithKline Beecham Pharmaceuticals).
Anexsia D, Tab. (SmithKline Beecham Pharmaceuticals).

A.P.C. w/gelsemium combinations.
See: Valacet, Tab. (Pal-Pak, Inc.).

Apcogesic. (Apco) Sodium salicylate 5 gr, colchicine 1/320 gr, calcium carbonate 65 mg, dried aluminum hydroxide gel 130 mg, phenobarbital ⅛ gr/Tab. Bot. 100s. *Rx.*
Use: Antigout agent, hypnotic, sedative.

Apcohist. (APC) Phenylpropanolamine HCl 25 mg, chlorpheniramine maleate 1 mg/Tab. Bot. 100s. *otc.*
Use: Antihistamine, decongestant.

Apcoretic. (APC) Caffeine anhydrous 100 mg, ammonium Cl 325 mg/Tab. Bot. 90s. *Rx.*
Use: Diuretic.

Ap Creme. (T.E. Williams Pharmaceuticals) Hydrocortisone 0.5%, iodochlorhydroxyquin 3%. Tube. *Rx-otc.*
Use: Antifungal; corticosteroid, topical.

Apetil. (Kenwood Laboratories) B_1 1.7 mg, B_2 0.3 mg, B_3 6.7 mg, B_6 2.5 mg, B_{12} 5 mcg, Zn 14.6 mg, Mg, Mn, l-lysine. Liq. Bot. 237 ml. *otc.*
Use: Mineral, vitamin supplement.

APF. (Whitehall Robins Laboratories)
Use: Analgesic.
See: Arthritis Pain Formula (Whitehall Robins Laboratories).

Aphco Hemorrhoidal Combination. (APC) Combination package of Aphco Hemorrhoidal Ointment 1.5 oz tube, Aphco Hemorrhoidal Supp. Box 12s, 1000s. *otc.*
Use: Anorectal preparation.

Aphen Tabs. (Major Pharmaceuticals) Trihexyphenidyl 2 mg or 5 mg/Tab. Bot. 250s, 1000s. *Rx.*
Use: Antiparkinsonian.

Aphrodyne. (Star Pharmaceuticals, Inc.) Yohimbine HCl 5.4 mg/Tab. Bot. 100s, 1000s. *Rx.*
Use: Alpha-adrenergic blocker.

Aphthasol. (Block Drug Co., Inc.) Amlexanox 5%, benzyl alcohol, glyceryl

monostearate, mineral oil, petrolatum/ Paste. Tube. 5 g. *Rx.*
Use: Treatment of mouth ulcers.

Apicillin. D-(-)-α-Aminobenzyl penicillin.
See: Ampicillin.

A.P.L. (Wyeth-Ayerst Laboratories) Chorionic Gonadotropin for Injection. 5000 units, 10,000 units, or 20,000 units, sterile diluent, w/benzyl alcohol, phenol, lactose. *Rx.*
Use: Hormone, chorionic gonadotropin.

APL 400-020. (Apollon, Inc.)
Use: Treatment of cutaneous t-cell lymphoma. [Orphan Drug]

Aplisol. (Parke-Davis) Tuberculin purified protein derivative diluted 5 units/ 0.1 ml, polysorbate 80, potassium and sodium phosphates, phenol. Vial 1 ml (10 tests), 5 ml (50 tests). *Rx.*
Use: Diagnostic aid.

Aplitest. (Parke-Davis) Purified tuberculin protein derivative buffered with potassium and sodium phosphates, phenol 0.5%/single-use, multipuncture unit. 25s. *Rx.*
Use: Diagnostic aid.

•**apomorphine hydrochloride.** (ah-poh-MORE-feen) U.S.P. 23.
Use: Treatment of Parkinson's disease; emetic.

apomorphine hydrochloride. (ah-poh-MORE-feen) (Forum Products, Inc.; Pentech Pharmaceuticals)
Use: Treatment of Parkinson's disease.

aporphine-10, 11-diol hydrochloride.
See: Apomorphine HCl.

appetite-depressants.
See: Anorexiant agents.

APPG.
See: Penicillin G, Procaine, Aqueous.

•**apraclonidine hydrochloride.** (app-rah-KLOE-nih-deen) U.S.P. 23.
Use: Adrenergic (α_2-agonist).
See: Iopidine (Alcon Laboratories, Inc.).

•**apramycin.** (APP-rah-MY-sin) USAN.
Use: Anti-infective.

Aprazone. (Major Pharmaceuticals) Sulfinpyrazone. **Tab.:** 100 mg. Bot. 100s. *Rx.*
Use: Antigout agent.

Apresazide. (Novartis Pharmaceutical Corp.) **25/25:** Hydralazine HCl 25 mg, hydrochlorothiazide 25 mg/Cap. **50/50:** Hydralazine HCl 50 mg, hydrochlorothiazide 50 mg/Cap. **100/50:** Hydralazine 100 mg, hydrochlorothiazide 50 mg/Cap. Bot. 100s. *Rx.*
Use: Antihypertensive.

Apresodex. (Rugby Labs, Inc.) Hydrochlorothiazide 15 mg, hydralazine HCl 25 mg. Tab. Bot. 100s, 1000s. *Rx.*
Use: Antihypertensive.

Apresoline. (Novartis Pharmaceutical Corp.) Hydralazine HCl. **Amp.:** 20 mg w/propylene glycol, methyl and propyl parabens/ml. Pkg. 5s. **Tab.:** 10 mg Bot. 100s, 1200s; 25 mg or 50 mg Bot. 100s, 1000s; 100 mg Bot. 100s. Consumer pack 100s. *Rx.*
Use: Antihypertensive.
W/Serpasil.
See: Serpasil Prods., Preps. (Novartis Pharmaceutical Corp.).

Apresoline-Esidrix. (Novartis Pharmaceutical Corp.) Hydralazine HCl 25 mg, hydrochlorothiazide 15 mg/Tab. Bot. 100s. *Rx.*
Use: Antihypertensive.

•**aprindine.** (APE-rin-deen) USAN.
Use: Cardiovascular agent.

•**aprindine hydrochloride.** (APE-rin-deen) USAN.
Use: Cardiovascular agent.

aprobarbital. Pow. *c-III.*
Use: Hypnotic, sedative.
See: Alurate, Elix. (Roche Laboratories).

Aprobee w/C. (Health for Life Brands, Inc.) Vitamins B_1 15 mg, B_2 10 mg, B_6 5 mg, niacinamide 50 mg, calcium pantothenate 10 mg, C 250 mg/Cap. or Tab. **Cap.:** Bot. 100s, 1000s. **Tab.:** Bot. 50s, 100s, 1000s. *otc.*
Use: Mineral, vitamin supplement.

Aprodine. (Major Pharmaceuticals) **Tab.:** Pseudoephedrine HCl 60 mg, triprolidine HCl 2.5 mg. Bot. 24s, 100s, 1000s, UD 100s. **Syr.:** Pseudoephedrine HCl 30 mg, triprolidine HCl 1.25 mg/5 ml. Bot. 120 ml, pt. *otc.*
Use: Antihistamine, decongestant.

Aprodine w/Codine. (Major Pharmaceuticals) Pseudoephedrine HCl 30 mg, triprolidine HCl 1.25 mg, codeine phosphate 10 mg. Syr. Bot. Pt, gal. *c-v.*
Use: Antihistamine, decongestant.

•**aprotinin.** (app-row-TIE-nin) USAN.
Use: Enzyme inhibitor (proteinase).
See: Trasylol, Inj. (Bayer Corp. (Consumer Div.)).

aprotinin. (app-row-TIE-nin)
Use: Blood loss prophylaxis and homologous blood transfusion in coronary artery bypass graft surgery (CABG).
See: Trasylol (Bayer Corp. (Biological and Pharmaceutical Div.)).

Aprozide 25/25. (Major Pharmaceuticals) Hydralazine 25 mg, hydrochlorothiazide 25 mg/Cap. Bot. 100s, 250s. *Rx.*
Use: Antihypertensive.

Aprozide 50/50. (Major Pharmaceuticals) Hydrochlorothiazide 50 mg, hydralazine 50 mg/Cap. Bot. 100s, 250s. *Rx.*
Use: Antihypertensive.

A.P.S. Aspirin, phenacetin, and salicylamide.

•**aptazapine maleate.** (app-TAZZ-ah-PEEN MAL-ee-ate) USAN.
Use: Antidepressant.

•**aptiganel hydrochloride.** (app-tih-GAN-ehl) USAN.
Use: Stroke and traumatic brain injury treatment (NMDA ion channel blocker).

APSAC. Thrombolytic enzyme.
See: Eminase (SmithKline Beecham Pharmaceuticals).

apyron.
See: Magnesium acetylsalicylate.

AQ-4B. (Western Research) Trichlormethiazide 4 mg/Tab. Bot. 1000s. *Rx.*
Use: Diuretic.

Aqua-Ban. (Thompson Medical Co.) Caffeine 100 mg, ammonium Cl 325 mg/Tab. Bot. 60s. *otc.*
Use: Diuretic.

Aqua-Ban, Maximum Strength.
See: Maximum Strength Aqua-Ban, Tab. (Thompson Medical Co.).

Aqua-Ban Plus. (Thompson Medical Co.) Ammonium Cl 650 mg, caffeine 200 mg, iron 6 mg/Tab. Bot. 30s. *otc.*
Use: Diuretic, mineral supplement.

Aquabase. (Pal-Pak, Inc.) Cetyl alcohol, propylene glycol, sodium lauryl sulfate, white wax, purified water. Jar lb. *otc.*
Use: Pharmaceutic aid, ointment base.

Aquacare Cream. (Allergan, Inc.) Urea 2%, benzyl alcohol, carbomer 934, cetyl esters wax, fragrance, glycerin, oleth-3 phosphate, petrolatum, phenyldimethicone, water, sodium hydroxide. Tube 2.5 oz. *otc.*
Use: Emollient.

Aquacare/HP. (Allergan, Inc.) Urea 10%, benzyl alcohol. **Cream:** Tube 2.5 oz. **Lot.:** Bot. 8 oz, 16 oz. *otc.*
Use: Emollient.

Aquacare Lotion. (Allergan, Inc.) Benzyl alcohol, oleth-3 phosphate, phenyldimethicone, fragrance. Bot. 8 oz. *otc.*
Use: Emollient.

Aquachloral. (PolyMedica Pharmaceuticals) Chloral hydrate, polyethylene glycol, spreading agent. Supp. 5 gr, 10 gr. Strip 12s. *c-iv.*
Use: Hypnotic, sedative (rectal).

Aquacillin G. (Armenpharm Ltd.) Penicillin G. *Rx.*
Use: Anti-infective, penicillin.

Aquacycline. (Armenpharm Ltd.) Tetracycline HCl. *Rx.*
Use: Anti-infective, tetracycline.

Aquaderm. (C & M Pharmacal, Inc.) Purified water, glycerin 25%, salicylic acid 0.1%, octoxynol-9 0.03%, FD&C; Red #40 0.0001%. Bot. 2 oz. *otc.*
Use: Emollient.

Aquaderm. (Baker Norton Pharmaceuticals, Inc.) Octyl methoxycinnamate 7.5%, oxybenzone 6%. SPF 15. Cream 105 g. *otc.*
Use: Sunscreen.

Aquaflex Ultrasound Gel Pad. (Parker) Clear, solid, flexible, moist, standoff gel pad for use where transducer movement is impeded by bony or irregular body surfaces. 2 cm × 9 cm.
Use: Ultrasound aid.

Aquafuren. (Armenpharm Ltd.) Nitrofurantoin. *Rx.*
Use: Anti-infective, urinary.

Aquagen. (ALK Laboratories, Inc.) Allergenic extracts. Vials.

aquakay.
See: Menadione. (Various Mfr.).

Aqua Lacten Lotion. (Allergan) Demineralized water, urea, petrolatum, propylene glycol monostearate, sorbitan monostearate, lactic acid. Bot. 8 oz. *otc.*
Use: Emollient.

AquaMEPHYTON Injection. (Merck & Co.) Phytonadione 2 mg/ml or 10 mg/ml, vitamin K_{-1}, w/polyoxyethylated fatty acid derivative 70 mg, dextrose 37.5 mg, benzyl alcohol 0.9%, water for injection q.s. to 1 ml. Inj. Amp. 1 mg/0.5 ml Box 25s; 10 mg/1 ml Box 6s, 25s. Vial 10 mg/ml 2.5 ml, 5 ml. *Rx.*
Use: Coagulant.

Aqua Mist. (Faraday) Nasal spray. Squeeze Bot. 20 ml.

Aquamycin. (Armenpharm Ltd.) Erythromycin. *Rx.*
Use: Anti-infective, erythromycin.

Aquanil. (Sigma-Tau Pharmaceuticals, Inc.) Mersalyl 100 mg, theophylline (hydrate) 50 mg, methylparaben 0.18%, propylparaben 0.02%. Vial 10 ml. *otc.*
Use: Bronchodilator, diuretic.

Aquanil Cleanser. (Person and Covey, Inc.) Glycerin, cetyl, stearyl, and benzyl alcohol, sodium laureth sulfate, xanthan gum. Lipid free. Lot. Bot. 240 ml, 480 ml. *otc.*
Use: Dermatologic, cleanser.

Aquanine. (Armenpharm Ltd.) Quinine HCl. *Rx.*
Use: Antimalarial.

Aquaoxy. (Armenpharm Ltd.) Oxytetracycline HCl. *Rx.*
Use: Anti-infective, tetracycline.

Aquaphenicol. (Armenpharm Ltd.) Chloramphenicol. *Rx.*
Use: Anti-infective.

Aquaphilic Ointment. (Medco Lab, Inc.) Hydrated hydrophilic oint. Jar 16 oz. *otc.*
Use: Emollient, ointment base.

Aquaphilic Ointment with Carbamide 10% and 20%. (Medco Lab, Inc.) Stearyl alcohol, white petrolatum, sorbitol, propylene glycol, sodium lauryl sulfate, lactic acid, methylparaben, propylparaben.
Use: Prescription compounding, emollient.

Aquaphor Natural Healing. (Beiersdorf, Inc.) Petrolatum, mineral oil, mineral wax, wool wax alcohol, panthenol, glycerin, chamomile essence. Oint. Tube 52.5 g. *otc.*
Use: Emollient.

Aquaphor. (Beiersdorf, Inc.) Cholesterolized anhydrous petrolatum ointment base. Tube 1.75 oz, 3.25 oz, 16 oz, Jar 5 lb, Bar 3 oz. *otc.*
Use: Pharmaceutic aid, ointment base.
See: Eucerin, Emulsion (Duke).

Aquaphor Antibiotic. (Beiersdorf, Inc.) 10,000 units polymyxin B sulfate and 500 units bacitracin zinc/g in a cholesterolized ointment base. Oint. Tube 15 g. *otc.*
Use: Anti-infective, topical.

Aquaphyllin Syrup. (Ferndale Laboratories, Inc.) Theophylline anhydrous 80 mg/15 ml UD pk. 15 ml, 30 ml. Bot. 16 oz, gal. *Rx.*
Use: Bronchodilator.

Aquapool Concentrate. (Parker) Color additive for hydrotherapy to control foaming. Bot. Pt, gal.

AquaSite. (Ciba Vision) PEG-400 0.2%, dextran 70, polycarbophil, NaCl, EDTA, sodium hydroxide. Preservative free. Soln. Single-use vials 0.6 ml, 15 ml. *otc.*
Use: Artificial tears.

Aquasol A. (Astra Pharmaceuticals, L.P.) Water-miscible Vitamin A. Chlorobutanol 0.5%, polysorbate 80, butylated hydroxyanisole, butylated hydroxytoluene. **Inj.:** 50,000 U.S.P. units/ml. Vial 2 ml Box 10s. **Cap.:** 25,000 U.S.P. units/Cap. Bot. 100s. 50,000 U.S.P. units/Cap. Bot. 100s, 500s. **Drops:** 5000 U.S.P. units/0.1 ml. Bot. 30 ml w/dropper. *Rx-otc.*
Use: Vitamin supplement.

Aquasol E. (Astra Pharmaceuticals, L.P.) Vitamin E. **Cap.:** 73.5 mg Bot. 100s; 400 IU Bot. 30s. **Drops:** 50 mg/ml Bot. 12 ml, 30 ml w/dropper. *otc.*
Use: Vitamin supplement.

Aquasonic 100. (Parker) Water-soluble, viscous, contact medium gel for ultrasonic transmission. Bot. 250 ml, 1 L, 5 L.
Use: Ultrasound aid.

Aquasonic 100 sterile. (Parker) Water-soluble, sterile gel for ultrasonic transmission. Overwrapped Foil Pouches 15 g, 50 g.
Use: Ultrasound aid.

Aquasulf. (Armenpharm Ltd.) Triple sulfa tablet. *Rx.*
Use: Anti-infective.

Aquatensen. (Wallace Laboratories) Methyclothiazide 5 mg/Tab. Bot. 100s, 500s. *Rx.*
Use: Antihypertensive, diuretic.

Aquavite. (Armenpharm Ltd.) Soluble multivitamin.
Use: Vitamin supplement.

Aquavite-E. (Cypress Pharmaceutical, Inc.) Dl-alpha tocopheryl acetate 15 IU/0.3 ml. Sol., Oral. Bot. 30 ml. *Rx.*
Use: Vitamin supplement.

Aquazide. (Western Research) Trichlormethiazide 4 mg/Tab. Bot. 100s. *Rx.*
Use: Antihypertensive, diuretic.

Aquazide H. (Western Research) Hydrochlorothiazide 50 mg/Tab. Bot. 1000s. *Rx.*
Use: Diuretic.

Aquazol. (Armenpharm Ltd.) Sulfisoxazole.
Use: Anti-infective.

Aqueous Allergens. (Bayer Corp. (Consumer Div.))
Use: Antiallergic.

aquinone.
See: Menadione, U.S.P. 23.

Aquol Bath Oil. (Lamond) Vegetable oil, olive oil. Bot. 4 oz, 6 oz, 16 oz, qt, gal. *otc.*
Use: Antipruritic, emollient.

AR-121. (Argus Pharmaceuticals, Inc.) Phase I/II HIV. *Rx.*
Use: Antiviral.

ARA-A.
See: Vidarabine.

ARA-C.
See: Cytarabine.

Aralen Hydrochloride. (Sanofi Winthrop Pharmaceuticals) Chloroquine HCl 50 mg/ml. Inj. Amp. 5 ml. *Rx.*
Use: Amebicide, antimalarial.

Aralen Phosphate. (Sanofi Winthrop Pharmaceuticals) Chloroquine phosphate 500 mg/Tab. Bot. 25s. *Rx.*
Use: Amebicide, antimalarial.

Aralis. (Sanofi Winthrop Pharmaceuticals) Glycobiarsol, chloroquine phos-

phate. Tab. *Rx.*
Use: Amebicide.

Aramine. (Merck & Co.) Metaraminol bitartrate 10 mg/ml, methylparaben 0.15%, propylparaben 0.02%, sodium bisulfite 0.2%. Inj. Vial 10 ml. *Rx.*
Use: Antihypotensive.

•**aranotin.** (AR-ah-NO-tin) USAN.
Use: Antiviral.

Arava. (Hoechst Marion Roussel) Leflunomide 10 mg, 20 mg, 100 mg. Tab. Bot. 30s, 100s. Blister pack 3 count (100 mg only). *Rx.*
Use: Antiarthritic.

•**arbaprostil.** (ahr-bah-PRAHST-ill) USAN.
Use: Antisecretory (gastric).

Arbolic. (Burgin-Arden) Methandriol dipropionate 50 mg/ml. Vial 10 ml. *Rx.*
Use: Anabolic steroid.

Arbutal. (Arcum) Butalbital ¾ gr, phenacetin 2 gr, aspirin 3 gr, caffeine gr/Tab. Bot. 100s, 1000s. *Rx.*
Use: Analgesic, hypnotic, sedative.

•**arbutamine hydrochloride.** (ahr-BYOO-tah-meen) USAN.
Use: Cardiovascular agent.
See: GenESA, Inj. (Gensia Automedics).

Arcet. (Econo Med Pharmaceuticals) Butalbital 50 mg, acetaminophen 325 mg, caffeine 40 mg/Tab. Bot. 100s. *Rx.*
Use: Analgesic, hypnotic, sedative.

•**arcitumomab.** (ahr-sigh-TOO-moe-mab) USAN.
Use: Monoclonal antibody.
See: CEA-Scan. (Immunomedics, Mallinckrodt).

arcitumomab. (ahr-sigh-TOO-moe-mab)
Use: Diagnosis and localization of thyroid carcinoma.
See: CEA-Scan. (Immunomedics).

•**arclofenin.** (AHR-kloe-FEN-in) USAN.
Use: Diagnostic aid for hepatic function determination.

Arcoban. (Arcum) Meprobamate 400 mg/Tab. Bot. 50s, 1000s. *Rx.*
Use: Anxiolytic.

Arcobee w/C. (NBTY, Inc.) Vitamins B_1 15 mg, B_2 10.2 mg, B_3 50 mg, B_5 10 mg, B_6 5 mg, C 300 mg, tartrazine. Cap. Box 100s. *otc.*
Use: Vitamin supplement.

Arcodex Antacid. (Arcum) Magnesium trisilicate 500 mg, aluminum hydroxide 250 mg/Tab. Bot. 100s, 1000s. *otc.*
Use: Antacid.

Arco-Lase. (Arco Pharmaceuticals, Inc.) Trizyme 38 mg (amylase 30 mg, protease 6 mg, cellulase 2 mg), lipase 25 mg/Tab. Bot. 50s. *Rx.*
Use: Digestive aid.

Arcosterone. (Arcum) Methyltestosterone. **Oral:** 10 mg or 25 mg/Tab. Bot. 100s, 1000s. **Sublingual:** 10 mg/Tab. Bot. 100s, 1000s. *Rx.*
Use: Androgen.

Arco-Thyroid. (Arco Pharmaceuticals, Inc.) Thyroid 1.5 gr/Tab. Bot. 1000s. *Rx.*
Use: Hormone, thyroid.

Arcotrate. (Arcum) Pentaerythritol tetranitrate 10 mg/Tab. **No. 2:** Pentaerythritol tetranitrate 20 mg/Tab. **No. 3:** Pentaerythritol tetranitrate 20 mg, phenobarbital ⅛ gr/Tab. Bot. 100s, 1000s. *Rx.*
Use: Antianginal.

Arcoval Improved. (Arcum) Vitamin A palmitate 10,000 IU, D 400 IU, thiamine mononitrate 15 mg, B_2 10 mg, nicotinamide 150 mg, B_6 5 mg, calcium pantothenate 10 mg, B_{12} 5 mcg, C 150 mg, E 5 IU/Cap. Bot. 100s, 1000s. *otc.*
Use: Mineral, vitamin supplement.

Arcum R-S. (Arcum) Reserpine 0.25 mg/Tab. Bot. 100s, 1000s. *Rx.*
Use: Antihypertensive.

Arcum V-M. (Arcum) Vitamin A palmitate 5000 IU, D 400 IU, B_1 2.5 mg, B_2 2.5 mg, B_6 0.5 mg, B_{12} 2 mcg, C 50 mg, niacinamide 20 mg, calcium pantothenate 5 mg, iron 18 mg/Cap. Bot. 100s, 1000s. *otc.*
Use: Mineral, vitamin supplement.

A-R-D. (Birchwood Laboratories, Inc.) Anatomically shaped dressing. Dispenser 24s.
Use: Antipruritic; counterirritant, rectal.

Ardeben. (Burgin-Arden) Diphenhydramine HCl 10 mg, chlorobutanol 0.5%. Inj. Vial 30 ml. *Rx.*
Use: Antihistamine.

Ardecaine 1%. (Burgin-Arden) Lidocaine HCl 1%. Inj. Vial 30 ml. *Rx.*
Use: Anesthetic, local.

Ardecaine 2%. (Burgin-Arden) Lidocaine HCl 2%. Inj. Vial 30 ml. *Rx.*
Use: Anesthetic, local.

Ardecaine 1% w/Epinephrine. (Burgin-Arden) Lidocaine HCl 1%, epinephrine. Inj. Vial 30 ml. *Rx.*
Use: Anesthetic, local.

Ardecaine 2% w/Epinephrine. (Burgin-Arden) Lidocaine HCl 2%, epinephrine. Inj. Vial 30 ml. *Rx.*
Use: Anesthetic, topical.

Ardefem 10. (Burgin-Arden) Estradiol valerate 10 mg/ml. Vial 10 ml. *Rx.*
Use: Estrogen.

Ardefem 20. (Burgin-Arden) Estradiol valerate 20 mg/ml. Vial 10 ml. *Rx.*

Use: Estrogen.

Ardefem 40. (Burgin-Arden) Estradiol valerate 40 mg/ml. Vial 10 ml. *Rx.*
Use: Estrogen.

•**ardeparin sodium.** (ahr-dee-PA-rin) USAN.
Use: Anticoagulant.
See: Normiflo, Inj. (Wyeth-Ayerst Laboratories).

Ardepred Soluble. (Burgin-Arden) Prednisolone 20 mg, niacinamide 25 mg, disodium edetate 0.5 mg, sodium bisulfite 1 mg, phenol 5 mg/ml. Vial 10 ml. *Rx.*
Use: Corticosteroid combination.

Arderone 100. (Burgin-Arden) Testosterone enanthate 100 mg/ml. Vial 10 ml. *c-III.*
Use: Androgen.

Arderone 200. (Burgin-Arden) Testosterone enanthate 200 mg/ml. Vial 10 ml. *c-III.*
Use: Androgen.

Ardevila tablets. (Sanofi Winthrop Pharmaceuticals) Inositol hexanicotinate. *Rx.*
Use: Vasodilator.

Ardiol 90/4. (Burgin-Arden) Testosterone enanthate 90 mg, estradiol valerate 4 mg/ml. Vial 10 ml. *Rx.*
Use: Androgen, estrogen combination.

Arduan. (Organon Teknika Corp.) Pipecuronium Br 10 mg/10 ml. Vial. *Rx.*
Use: Neuromuscular blocker.

Aredia. (Novartis Pharmaceutical Corp.) Pamidronate disodium 30 mg (470 mg mannitol), 60 mg (400 mg mannitol), 90 mg (375 mg mannitol). Pow. for Inj., lyophilized. Vial. *Rx.*
Use: Antihypercalcemic.

•**argatroban.** (ahr-GAT-troe-ban) USAN.
Use: Anticoagulant.

Argesic. (Econo Med Pharmaceuticals) Methyl salicylate and triethanolamine in a nongreasy vanishing cream base. Jar 60 g. *otc.*
Use: Analgesic, topical.

Argesic-SA. (Econo Med Pharmaceuticals) Disalicylic acid 500 mg/Tab. Bot. 100s. *Rx.*
Use: Analgesic, topical.

•**arginine.** (AHR-jih-neen) U.S.P. 23.
Use: Ammonia detoxicant; diagnostic aid (pituitary function determination).

arginine butyrate. (AHR-jih-neen)
Use: Sickle cell disease, beta-thalassemia. [Orphan Drug]

arginine glutamate. (AHR-jih-neen GLUE-tah-mate) USAN.
Use: Ammonia detoxicant.

arginine hydrochloride. (AHR-jih-neen)
Use: Diagnostic aid.
See: R-Gene 10, Inj. (Pharmacia & Upjohn).

•**arginine hydrochloride.** (AHR-jih-neen) U.S.P. 23.
Use: Ammonia detoxicant.

8-arginine-vasopressin.
See: Vasopressin.

•**argipressin tannate.** (AHR-JIH-press-in TAN-ate) USAN.
Use: Antidiuretic.

argyn.
See: Mild Silver Protein. (Various Mfr.).

Aricept. (Eisai; Pfizer US Pharmaceutical Group) Donepezil HCl 5 mg and 10 mg/Tab. Blisterpack. 30s and 100s. *Rx.*
Use: Treatment of mild to moderate dementia associated with Alzheimer's disease.

Aridol. (MPL) Pamabrom 52 mg, pyrilamine maleate 30 mg, homatropine methylbromide 1.2 mg, hyoscyamine sulfate 0.10 mg, scopolamine HBr 0.02 mg, methamphetamine HCl 1.5 mg/Tab. Bot. 100s. *Rx.*
Use: Anticholinergic, antispasmodic, diuretic, stimulant.

•**arildone.** (AR-ill-dohn) USAN.
Use: Antiviral.

Arimidex. (Zeneca Pharmaceuticals) Anastrozole 1 mg, lactose/Tab. 30s. *Rx.*
Use: Aromatase inhibitor.

•**aripiprazole.** (A-rih-PIP-ray-zole) USAN.
Use: Antipsychotic, antischizophrenic.

Aris Phenobarbital Reagent Strips. (Bayer Corp. (Consumer Div.)) Box 25s.
Use: Diagnostic aid.

Aris Phenytoin Reagent Strips. (Bayer Corp. (Consumer Div.)) Box 25s.
Use: Diagnostic aid.

Aristocort. (ESI Lederle Generics) Triamcinolone. **Tab.:** 1 mg Bot. 50s; 2 mg Bot. 100s; 4 mg Bot. 30s, 100s; 8 mg Bot. 50s. **Syr.:** Diacetate (w/methylparaben 0.08%, propylparaben 0.02%) 2 mg/5 ml. Bot. 4 oz. *Rx.*
Use: Corticosteroid.

Aristocort A Cream. (Fujisawa USA, Inc.) Triamcinolone acetonide w/emulsifying wax, isopropyl palmitate, glycerin, sorbitol, lactic acid, benzyl alcohol. **0.025% w/Aquatain:** Tube 15 g, 60 g. **0.1%:** Tube 15 g, 60 g, Jar 240 g. **0.5%:** Tube 15 g. *Rx.*
Use: Corticosteroid, topical.

Aristocort Acetonide, Sodium Phosphate Salt. (ESI Lederle Generics)
Use: Corticosteroid, topical.

See: Aristocort Preps.
Sodium Phosphate Triamcinolone Acetonide.

Aristocort A Ointment. (Fujisawa USA, Inc.) Triamcinolone acetonide 0.1%. Tube 15 g, 60 g. *Rx.*
Use: Corticosteroid, topical.

Aristocort Cream. (Fujisawa USA, Inc.) Triamcinolone acetonide w/emulsifying wax, polysorbate 60, mono and diglycerides, squalane, sorbitol soln., sorbic acid, potassium sorbate. **LP: 0.025%:** Tube 15 g, 60 g, Jar 240 g, 480 g; **R: 0.1%:** Tube 15 g, 60 g, Jar 240 g, 480 g; **HP: 0.5%:** Tube 15 g, Jar 240 g. *Rx.*
Use: Corticosteroid, topical.

Aristocort Forte. (ESI Lederle Generics) Triamcinolone diacetate 40 mg/ml. Vial 1 ml, 5 ml. *Rx.*
Use: Corticosteroid.

Aristocort Intralesional. (ESI Lederle Generics) Triamcinolone diacetate 25 mg/ml. Vial 5 ml. *Rx.*
Use: Corticosteroid.

Aristocort Ointment. (Fujisawa USA, Inc.) Triamcinolone acetonide. **R: 0.1%:** Tube 15 g, 60 g, Jar 240 g. **HP: 0.5%:** Tube 15 g, Jar 240 g. *Rx.*
Use: Corticosteroid, topical.

Aristo-Pak. (ESI Lederle Generics) Triamcinolone 4 mg/Tab. 16s. *Rx.*
Use: Corticosteroid.

Aristospan Intra-articular. (ESI Lederle Generics) Triamcinolone hexacetonide 20 mg/ml micronized susp., polysorbate 80 0.4% w/v, sorbitol soln. 64% w/v, water q.s., benzyl alcohol 0.9% w/v. Vial 1 ml, 5 ml. *Rx.*
Use: Corticosteroid.

Aristospan Intralesional. (ESI Lederle Generics) Triamcinolone hexacetonide 5 mg/ml, polysorbate 80 0.2% w/v, sorbitol soln. 64% w/v, water q.s., benzyl alcohol 0.9% w/v. Vial 5 ml. *Rx.*
Use: Corticosteroid.

Arlacel 83. (Zeneca Pharmaceuticals) Sorbitan Sesquioleate.
Use: Surface active agent.

Arlacel 165. (Zeneca Pharmaceuticals) Glyceryl monostearate, PEG-100 stearate nonionic self-emulsifying.
Use: Surface active agent.

Arlacel C. (Zeneca Pharmaceuticals) Sorbitan Sesquioleate. Mixture of oleate esters of sorbitol and its anhydrides.
Use: Surface active agent.

Arlamol E. (Zeneca Pharmaceuticals) Polyoxypropylene (15), stearyl ether, BHT 0.1%.
Use: Emollient.

Arlatone 507. (Zeneca Pharmaceuticals) Padimate O. *otc.*
Use: Sunscreen.

Arlix. (Hoechst Marion Roussel) Piretanide HCl. *Rx.*
Use: Antihypertensive, diuretic.

Arm-a-Med Metaproterenol Sulfate. (Centeon) Soln. for nebulization: Metaproterenol sulfate 0.4% or 0.6% with sodium Cl, EDTA. Vial UD 2.5 ml for use with IPPB device. *Rx.*
Use: Bronchodilator.

Arm-a-Vial. (Centeon) Sterile water, sodium Cl 0.45% or 0.9%. Box 100s. Plastic vial 3 ml, 5 ml.
Use: Electrolyte supplement.

A.R.M.. (Menley & James Labs, Inc.) Chlorpheniramine maleate 4 mg, phenylpropanolamine HCl 25 mg/Capl. Pkg. 20s, 40s. *otc.*
Use: Antihistamine, decongestant.

Arnica Tincture. (Eli Lilly and Co.) Arnica 20% in alcohol 66%. Bot. 120 ml, 480 ml. *otc.*
Use: Analgesic, topical.

•**arofylline.** (ah-ROE-fih-lin) USAN.
Use: Bronchodilator; asthma prophylactic.

Aromatic Ammonia Vaporole. (GlaxoWellcome) Inhalant. Vial 5 min. Box 10s, 12s, 100s. *Rx.*
Use: Respiratory.

•**aromatic elixir.** N.F. 18.
Use: Pharmaceutic aid (vehicle; flavored, sweetened).

aromatic elixir. (Eli Lilly and Co.) Alcohol 22%. Bot. 16 fl. oz.
Use: Pharmaceutic aid, flavoring.

•**arprinocid.** (ahr-PRIN-oh-sid) USAN.
Use: Coccidiostat.

arseclor.
See: Dichlorophenarsine HCl. (Various Mfr.).

arsenic compounds.
Use: Rarely employed in modern medicine; there are no longer any official compounds.
See: Acetarsone.
Arsphenamine.
Carbarsone (Various Mfr.).
Dichlorophenarsine HCl.
Ferric Cacodylate.
Glycobiarsol.
Neoarsphenamine.
Oxophenarsine HCl.
Sodium Cacodylate (Various Mfr.).
Tryparsamide.

arsenobenzene.
See: Arsphenamine.

arsenphenolamine.
See: Arsphenamine.

Arsobal. Melarsoprol (Mel B).
Use: CDC anti-infective agent.

arsphenamine. Arsenobenzene, arsenobenzol, arsenophenolamine, Ehrlich 606, salvarsan.
Use: Formerly used as antisyphilitic.

arsthinol. Cyclic.
Use: Antiprotozoal.

Artane. (ESI Lederle Generics) Trihexyphenidyl HCl. **Elix.:** 2 mg/5 ml w/methylparaben 0.08%, propylparaben 0.02%, Bot. Pt. **Tab.:** 2 mg or 5 mg, Bot. 100s, 1000s, UD 10 × 10 in 10s. **Sequel:** 5 mg Bot. 60s, 500s. *Rx.*
Use: Antiparkinsonian.

Artarau. (Archer-Taylor) Rauwolfia serpentina 50 mg or 100 mg/Tab. Bot. 100s, 1000s. *Rx.*
Use: Antihypertensive.

Arta-Vi-C. (Archer-Taylor) Multivitamins with Vitamin C 100 mg/Tab. Bot. 100s. *otc.*
Use: Vitamin supplement.

Artazyme. (Archer-Taylor) Bot. 13 ml.
Use: Autolyzed proteolytic enzyme.

•**arteflene.** (AHR-teh-fleen) USAN.
Use: Antimalarial.

•**artegraft.** (AHR-teh-graft) USAN. Arterial graft composed of a section of bovine carotid artery that has been subjected to enzymatic digestion with ficin and tanned with dialdehyde starch.
Use: Prosthetic aid (arterial).

arterenol.
See: Norepinephrine bitartrate.

Artha-G. (T.E. Williams Pharmaceuticals) Salsalate 750 mg/Tab. Bot. 120s. *Rx.*
Use: Analgesic.

Arthralgen. (Wyeth-Ayerst Laboratories) Salicylamide 250 mg, acetaminophen 250 mg/Tab. Bot. 30s, 100s, 500s. *otc.*
Use: Analgesic combination.

Arthricare Daytime Formula. (Del Pharmaceuticals, Inc.) Menthol 1.25%, methyl nicotinate 0.25%, capsaicin 0.025%, with aloe vera gel, carbomer 940, DMDM hydantoin, glyceryl stearate SE, myristyl propionate, propylparaben, triethanolamine. Cream Jar 90 g. *otc.*
Use: Analgesic, topical.

ArthriCare Double Ice. (Del Pharmaceuticals, Inc.) Menthol 4%, camphor 3.1%, with aloe vera gel, carbomer 940, dioctyl sodium sulfosuccinate, propylene glycol, triethanolamine. Gel. Jar 90 g. *otc.*
Use: Analgesic, topical.

ArthriCare Odor Free Rub. (Del Pharmaceuticals, Inc.) Menthol 1.25%, methyl nicotinate 0.25%, capsaicin 0.025%, aloe vera gel, carbomer 940, DMDM hydantoin, emulsifying wax, glyceryl stearate SE, isopropyl alcohol, myristyl propionate, propylparaben, triethanolamine. Oint. Jar 90 g. *otc.*
Use: Liniment.

ArthriCare Triple Medicated. (Del Pharmaceuticals, Inc.) Methyl salicylate 30%, menthol 1.25%, methyl nicotinate 0.7%, dioctyl sodium sulfosuccinate, hydroxypropyl methylcellulose, isopropyl alcohol, propylene glycol. Gel. Tube 3 oz. *otc.*
Use: Analgesic, topical.

Arthritic Pain Lotion. (Walgreen Co.) Triethanolamine salicylate 10%. Bot. 6 oz. *otc.*
Use: Analgesic, topical.

Arthriten, Maximum Strength. (Alva/Amco Pharmacal Cos. Inc.) Acetaminophen 250 mg, magnesium salicylate 250 mg, caffeine anhydrous 32.5 mg. Buffered with magnesium carbonate, magnesium oxide, calcium carbonate. 40s. *otc.*
Use: Analgesic.

Arthritis Bayer Timed Release Aspirin. (Bayer Corp. (Consumer Div.)) Aspirin 650 mg/TR Tab. Bot. 30s, 72s, 125s. *otc.*
Use: Analgesic.

Arthritis Hot Creme. (Thompson Medical Co.) Methyl salicylate 15%, menthol 10%, glyceryl stearate, carbomer 934, lanolin, PEG-100 stearate, propylene glycol, trolamine, parabens. Cream Jar 90 g. *otc.*
Use: Liniment.

Arthritis Pain Formula. (Whitehall Robins Laboratories) Aspirin 486 mg, aluminum hydroxide gel 20 mg, magnesium hydroxide 60 mg/Tab. Bot. 40s, 100s, 175s. *otc.*
Use: Analgesic combination.

Arthritis Pain Formula, Aspirin Free. (Whitehall Robins Laboratories) Acetaminophen 500 mg/Tab. Bot. 30s, 75s. *otc.*
Use: Analgesic.

Arthropan. (Purdue Frederick Co.) Choline salicylate 870 mg/5 ml. Liq. Bot. 8 oz, 16 oz. *Rx.*
Use: Analgesic.

Arthrotec. (Searle) Diclofenac sodium 50 mg/misoprostol 200 mcg or diclofenac sodium 75 mg/misoprostol 200 mcg, lactose/Tab. Bot. 60s, 90s. *Rx.*
Use: Analgesic.

Arthrotrin Tablets. (Whiteworth Towne) Enteric-coated aspirin 325 mg/Tab. Bot. 100s.

Use: Analgesic.

Articulose L.A. (Seatrace Pharmaceuticals, Inc.) Triamcinolone diacetate 40 mg/ml. Vial 5 ml. *Rx.*
Use: Corticosteroid.

artificial tanning agent.
See: Sudden Tan, Prods. (Schering-Plough Corp.).

artificial tear insert.
See: Lacrisert. (Merck & Co.).

artificial tears. (Various Mfr.) Benzalkonium Cl 0.01%. May also contain EDTA, NaCl, polyvinyl alcohol, hydroxypropyl methylcellulose Soln. Bot. 15 ml, 30 ml. *otc.*
Use: Lubricant, ophthalmic.

Artificial Tears. (Rugby Labs, Inc.) White petrolatum, anhydrous liquid lanolin, mineral oil. Ophth. Oint. Tube 3.5 g. *otc.*
Use: Lubricant, ophthalmic.

artificial tear solutions.
Use: Lubricant, ophthalmic.
See: Akwa Tears, Soln. (Akorn).
Aquasite, Soln. (Ciba Vision).
Artificial Tears, Soln. (Various Mfr.).
Artificial Tears Plus, Soln. (Various Mfr.).
Celluvisc, Soln. (Allergan).
Comfort Tears, Soln. (Allergan).
Dry Eyes, Soln. (Bausch & Lomb).
Preservative Free Moisture Eyes, Soln. (Bausch & Lomb).
Puralube Tears, Soln. (Fougera).
Refresh Plus, Soln. (Allergan).
Teargen, Soln. (Zenith Goldline).

Artificial Tears Plus. (Various Mfr.) Polyvinyl alcohol 1.4%, povidone 0.6%, chlorobutanol 0.5%, NaCl. Soln. Bot. 15 ml. *otc.*
Use: Lubricant, ophthalmic.

•**artilide fumarate.** (AHR-tih-lide) USAN.
Use: Cardiovascular agent.

Artra Beauty Bar. (Schering-Plough Corp.) Triclocarban 1% in soap base. Cake 3.6 oz. *otc.*
Use: Dermatologic, cleanser.

Artra Skin Tone Cream. (Schering-Plough Corp.) Hydroquinone 2%. Oint. Tube 1 oz (normal only), 2 oz, 4 oz.
Use: Dermatologic.

AS-101. (Wyeth-Ayerst Laboratories) Phase I/II ARC, AIDS. *Rx.*
Use: Immunomodulator.

5-asa. Mesalamine.
See: Asacol (Procter & Gamble Pharm.).
Rowasa (Solvay Pharmaceuticals).

ASA. (Wampole Laboratories) Anti-skin antibodies test by IFA. Test 48s.
Use: Diagnostic aid.

A.S.A. (Eli Lilly and Co.) Aspirin. Acetylsalicylic acid. **Enseal:** 5 gr or 10 gr. Bot. 100s, 1000s. **Supp.:** 5 gr or 10 gr. Pkg. 6s, 144s. *otc.*
Use: Analgesic.

Asacol. (Procter & Gamble Pharm.) Mesalamine 400 mg/Tab. DR Bot. 100s. *Rx.*
Use: Anti-inflammatory.

asafetida, emulsion of. Milk of Asafetida.

Asaped Tablets. (Sanofi Winthrop Pharmaceuticals) Acetylsalicylic acid. *otc.*
Use: Analgesic.

Asawin Tablets. (Sanofi Winthrop Pharmaceuticals) Acetylsalicylic acid. *otc.*
Use: Analgesic.

A.S.B. (Femco) Calcium carbonate, magnesium carbonate, bismuth subcarbonate, sodium bicarbonate, kaolin. Pow., Can 3 oz. Tabs. 50s. *otc.*
Use: Antacid.

Asclerol. (Spanner) Liver injection crude (2 mcg/ml) 50%, Vitamins B_1 20 mg, B_2 3 mg, B_6 1 mg, B_{12} 30 mcg, niacinamide 100 mg, panthenol 2.8 mg, choline Cl 20 mg, inositol 10 mg/ml. Multiple dose vial 10 ml. *Rx.*
Use: Vitamin supplement.

ascorbate sodium. Antiscorbutic vitamin.

•**ascorbic acid.** (ASS-kor-bik) U.S.P. 23.
Use: Vitamin (antiscorbutic); acidifier (urinary).

ascorbic acid. (ASS-kor-bik) (Various Mfr.) Antiscorbutic vitamin; Vitamin C. **Cap.:** 25 mg, 100 mg, 250 mg, 500 mg. **Inj.:** Amp. (100 mg/ml) 1 ml, 2 ml, 5 ml; (200 mg/ml) 5 ml, (500 mg) 2 ml, 5 ml, 10 ml, 30 ml, (250 mg/ml) 10 ml; (1000 mg/ml) 10 ml. **Tab.:** 50 mg, 100 mg, 250 mg, 500 mg. **Chew. Tab.:** 100 mg, 250 mg, 500 mg. **SR Tab.:** 500 mg, 1500 mg. **SR Cap.:** 500 mg. **Pow.:** 4 g/5 ml. **Soln.:** 35 mg/0.6 ml or 100 mg/ml.
Use: Vitamin supplement.
See: Ascorbicap, Cap. (ICN Pharmaceuticals, Inc.).
Ascorbineed, Cap. (Hanlon).
Cecon, Soln. (Abbott Laboratories).
Cenolate, Amp. (Abbott Laboratories).
Cevalin, Tab., Amp. (Eli Lilly and Co.).
Cevi-Bid, Cap. (Roberts Pharmaceuticals).
Ce-Vi-Sol, Drops. (Bristol-Myers Squibb).
Neo-Vadrin, Preps. (Scherer Laboratories, Inc.).
Sunkist Vitamin C, Capl., Chew. Tab. (Novartis Pharmaceutical Corp.).

ascorbic acid injection.
Use: Vitamin supplement.
See: Cevalin, Amp. (Eli Lilly and Co.).

ascorbic acid salts.
See: Bismuth Ascorbate.
Calcium Ascorbate.
Sodium Ascorbate.

Ascorbicap. (ICN Pharmaceuticals, Inc.) Ascorbic acid 500 mg/S.R. Cap. Bot. 50s. *otc.*
Use: Vitamin supplement.

Ascorbin/11. (Taylor Pharmaceuticals) Lemon bioflavonoids 110 mg, Vitamin C 1 g, rosehips powder 50 mg, rutin 25 mg/S.R. Tab. Bot. 100s. *otc.*
Use: Vitamin supplement.

Ascorbineed. (Hanlon) Vitamin C 500 mg/T-Cap. Bot. 100s. *otc.*
Use: Vitamin supplement.

Ascorbocin Powder. (Paddock Laboratories) Vitamin C 500 mg, niacin 500 mg, B_1 50 mg, B_6 50 mg, d-α-tocopheryl, polyethylene glycol 1000 succinate 50 IU, lactose/3 g. Bot. lb. *otc.*
Use: Vitamin supplement.

•**ascorbyl palmitate.** (ah-SCORE-bill PAL-mih-tate) N.F. 18.
Use: Preservative; pharmaceutic aid (antioxidant).

Ascorvite S.R. (Eon Labs Manufacturing, Inc.) Vitamin C 500 mg/S.R. Cap. *otc.*
Use: Vitamin supplement.

Ascriptin. (Rhone-Poulenc Rorer Pharmaceuticals, Inc.) Aspirin 325 mg, magnesium hydroxide 50 mg, aluminum hydroxide 50 mg/Tab. Bot. 50s, 100s, 225s, 500s. *otc.*
Use: Analgesic, antacid.

Ascriptin A/D. (Rhone-Poulenc Rorer Pharmaceuticals, Inc.) Acetylsalicylic acid 325 mg with magnesium hydroxide 75 mg, aluminum hydroxide and calcium carbonate 75 mg/Capsule shape coated tabs. Bot. 225s. *otc.*
Use: Analgesic, antacid.

Ascriptin Extra Strength. (Rhone-Poulenc Rorer Pharmaceuticals, Inc.) Aspirin 500 mg with magnesium hydroxide 80 mg, aluminum hydroxide and calcium carbonate 80 mg. Capsule shape coated tabs. Bot. 50s. *otc.*
Use: Analgesic, antacid.

Asendin. (ESI Lederle Generics) Amoxapine. Tab.: **25 mg:** Bot. 100s; **50 mg:** Bot. 100s, 500s, UD 100s; **100 mg:** Bot. 100s, UD 100s; **150 mg:** Bot. 30s. *Rx.*
Use: Antidepressant.

aseptichrome.
See: Merbromin. (Various Mfr.).

Aslum. (Drug Products) Carbolic acid 1%, aluminum acetate, ichthammol, zinc oxide, aromatic oils in a petrolatum-stearin base. Tube oz. Jar lb.
Use: Astringent.

Asma. (Wampole Laboratories) Anti-smooth muscle antibody test by IFA. Test 48.
Use: Diagnostic aid.

Asmalix. (Century Pharmaceuticals, Inc.) Theophylline 80 mg, alcohol 20%/15 ml. Bot. qt, gal. *Rx.*
Use: Bronchodilator.

Asma-Tuss. (Halsey Drug Co.) Phenobarbital 4 mg, theophylline 15 mg, ephedrine sulfate 12 mg, guaifenesin 50 mg/5 ml. Bot. 4 oz. *Rx.*
Use: Bronchodilator.

Asolectin. (Associated Concentrates) Chemical lecithin 25%, chemical cephalin 22%, inositol phosphatides 16%, soybean oil 2.5%, other miscellaneous sterols and lipids 34.5%. *otc.*
Use: Diet supplement.

•**asparaginase.** (ass-PAR-uh-jin-aze) USAN.
Use: Antineoplastic.
See: Elspar, Inj. (Merck & Co.).

•**aspartame.** (ass-PAR-tame) N.F. 18.
Use: Sweetener.

•**aspartic acid.** (ass-PAR-tick Acid) USAN. Aspartic acid; aminosuccinic acid.
Use: Management of fatigue; amino acid.

•**aspartocin.** (ass-PAR-toe-sin) USAN.
Use: Anti-infective.

A-Spas. (Hyrex Pharmaceuticals) Dicyclomine HCl 10 mg/ml. Vial 10 ml. *Rx.*
Use: Antispasmodic.

A-Spas S/L. (Hyrex Pharmaceuticals) Hyoscyamine sulfate 0.125 mg/Tab., sublingual. Bot. 100s. *Rx.*
Use: Antispasmodic.

Aspercreme. (Thompson Medical Co.) Triethanolamine salicylate 10% in cream base. *otc.*
Use: Analgesic, topical.

aspergillus niger enzyme. Alpha-galactosidase. *otc.*
See: Beano, Tab. (AK-Pharma).

aspergillus oryzae enzyme. Diastase.

Aspergum. (Schering-Plough Corp.) Aspirin 227.5 mg/1 Gum. Tab. Orange or Cherry flavor. Box 16s, 40s. *otc.*
Use: Analgesic.

asperkinase. Proteolytic enzyme mixture derived from aspergillus oryzae.

•**asperlin.** (ASS-per-lin) USAN.
Use: Anti-infective, antineoplastic.

Aspermin. (Buffington) Aspirin 325 mg/Tab. Sugar, caffeine, lactose, and salt

free. Dispens-A-Kit 500s. *otc.*
Use: Analgesic.

Aspermin Extra. (Buffington) Aspirin 500 mg/Tab. Sugar, caffeine, lactose, and salt free. Dispens-A-Kit 500s. *otc.*
Use: Analgesic.

•**aspirin.** (ASS-pihr-in) U.S.P. 23.
Use: Analgesic, antipyretic, antirheumatic. Prophylactic to reduce risk of death or non-fatal MI in patients with a previous infarction or unstable angina pectoris.
See: A.S.A., Preps. (Eli Lilly and Co.)
Aspergum, Gum, Tab. (Schering-Plough Corp.)
Asprimox (Invamed).
Bayer Buffered Aspirin (Bayer Corp. (Consumer Div.)).
Bayer Children's Aspirin, Tab. (Bayer Corp. (Consumer Div.)).
Bayer, 8-Hour Timed-Release, Tab. (Bayer Corp. (Consumer Div.)).
Bayer Low Adult Strength (Bayer Corp. (Consumer Div.)).
Easprin, Tab. (Parke-Davis).
Ecotrin, Tab. (SmithKline Beecham Pharmaceuticals).
Ecotrin Adult Low Strength (SmithKline Beecham Pharmaceuticals).
Ecotrin Maximum Strength, Capl., Tab. (SmithKline Beecham Pharmaceuticals).
Genprin, Tab. (Zenith Goldline Pharmaceuticals).
Genuine Bayer Aspirin, Tab., Capl. (Bayer Corp. (Consumer Div.)).
Halfprin 81, EC Tab. (Kramer Laboratories, Inc.).
Heartline, Tab. Enteric Coated. (BDI Pharmaceuticals, Inc.).
Maximum Bayer Aspirin, Tab, Capl. (Bayer Corp. (Consumer Div.)).
Norwich Aspirin, Tab. (Procter & Gamble Pharm.).
St Joseph, Prods. (Schering-Plough Corp.).
ZORprin, Tab. (Knoll Pharmaceuticals).

aspirin, alumina, and magnesia tablets.
Use: Analgesic, antacid.

aspirin, alumina, and magnesium oxide tablets.
Use: Analgesic, antacid.

aspirin-barbiturate combinations.
Use: Analgesic, sedative, hypnotic.
See: BAC, Tab. (Merz Pharmaceuticals).
Butalbital, Tab., Cap. (Various Mfr.).
Fiorinal, Cap., Tab. (Novartis Pharmaceutical Corp.).
Fiortal, Cap. (Geneva Pharmaceuticals).
Lanorinal, Cap, Tab. (Lannett Co, Inc.).

aspirin, caffeine, and dihydrocodeine bitartrate capsules.
Use: Analgesic.

aspirin w/codeine no. 3. (Various Mfr.) Codeine phosphate 30 mg, aspirin 325 mg. Tab. Bot. 100s, 1000s. *c-III.*
Use: Analgesic combination, narcotic.

aspirin w/codeine no. 4. (Various Mfr.) Codeine phosphate 60 mg, aspirin 325 mg Tab. Bot. 100s, 500s, 1000s. *c-III.*
Use: Analgesic combination, narcotic.

aspirin, codeine, phosphate alumina, and magnesia tablets.
Use: Analgesic.

aspirin and codeine phosphate tablets.
Use: Analgesic.

aspirin delayed-release capsules.
Use: Analgesic.

aspirin delayed-release tablets.
Use: Analgesic.
See: Bayer Low Adult Strength. (Bayer Corp. (Consumer Div.)).

aspirin, enteric coated.
Use: Analgesic.
See: A.S.A., Preps. (Eli Lilly and Co.).
Ecotrin, Tab. (SmithKline Beecham Pharmaceuticals).

Aspirin Free Anacin Maximum Strength. (Whitehall Robins Laboratories) Acetaminophen 500 mg. **Capl., Gel Capl.:** Bot. 100s; **Tab.:** Bot. 60s. *otc.*
Use: Analgesic.

Aspirin Free Anacin P.M. (Wyeth-Ayerst Laboratories) Diphenhydramine HCl 25 mg, acetaminophen 500 mg/Tab. Bot. 20s. *otc.*
Use: Sleep aid.

Aspirin-Free Bayer Select Allergy Sinus. (Bayer Corp. (Consumer Div.)) Pseudoephedrine HCl 30 mg, chlorpheniramine maleate 2 mg, acetaminophen 500 mg/Cap. Pkg. 16s. *otc.*
Use: Analgesic, antihistamine, decongestant.

Aspirin-Free Bayer Select Head & Chest Cold. (Bayer Corp. (Consumer Div.)) Pseudoephedrine HCl 30 mg, dextromethorphan HBr 10 mg, guaifenesin 100 mg, acetaminophen 325 mg. Capl. Bot. 16s. *otc.*
Use: Analgesic, decongestant, expectorant.

Aspirin-Free Bayer Select Headache. (Bayer Corp. (Consumer Div.)) Acetaminophen 500 mg, caffeine 65 mg. Cap.

Bot. 50s. *otc.*
Use: Analgesic combination.

Aspirin Free Excedrin. (Bristol-Myers Squibb) Acetaminophen 500 mg, caffeine 65 mg/Tab., Capl. Bot. 20s, 40s, 80s. *otc.*
Use: Analgesic combination.

Aspirin-Free Excedrin Dual. (Bristol-Myers Squibb) Acetaminophen 500 mg, calcium carbonate 111 mg, magnesium carbonate 64 mg, magnesium oxide 30 mg/Capl. Bot. 100s. *otc.*
Use: Analgesic combination.

Aspirin Free Pain Relief. (Hudson Corp.) Acetaminophen 325 mg/Tab. Bot. 100s. *otc.*
Use: Analgesic.

aspirin-narcotic combinations.
See: Alor 5/500, Tab. (Atley Pharmaceuticals, Inc.).

aspirin w/otc combinations.
See: Adprin-B, Tab. (Pfeiffer Co.).
Alka Seltzer, Tab. (Bayer Corp. (Consumer Div.)).
Alka Seltzer Plus, Tab. (Bayer Corp. (Consumer Div.)).
Anacin, Cap., Tab. (Whitehall Robins Laboratories).
A.P.C., Tab., Cap. (Various Mfr.).
Arthritis Foundation Pain Reliever, Tab. (McNeil-PPC).
Arthritis Strength BC Powder. (Block Drug Co., Inc.).
Ascriptin, Tab. (Rhone-Poulenc Rorer Pharmaceuticals, Inc.).
Ascriptin A/D, Tab. (Rhone-Poulenc Rorer Pharmaceuticals, Inc.).
Ascriptin, Extra Strength, Tab. (Rhone-Poulenc Rorer Pharmaceuticals, Inc.).
Asprimox Extra Protection for Arthritis Pain, Capl. (Invamed, Inc.).
Bayer Aspirin Preps. (Bayer Corp. (Consumer Div.)).
Bayer Buffered Aspirin, Tab. (Bayer Corp. (Consumer Div.)).
Bayer Low Adult Strength, DR Tab. (Bayer Corp. (Consumer Div.)).
BC, Powder, Tab. (Block Drug Co., Inc.).
Buffaprin, Tab. (Buffington).
Buffets, Tab. (Jones Medical Industries, Inc.).
Cama, Tab. (Novartis Pharmaceutical Corp.).
Cama Arthritis Pain Reliever (Novartis Pharmaceutical Corp.).
Cope, Tab. (Mentholatum Co., Inc.).
Ecotrin Adult Low Strength, EC Tab. (SmithKline Beecham).
Excedrin, Cap., Tab. (Bristol-Myers Squibb).
Extra Strength Adprin-B (Pfeiffer).
Extra Strength Bayer Plus (Bayer Corp. (Consumer Div.)).
4-Way, Tab., Spray. (Bristol-Myers Squibb).
Gelpirin, Tab. (Alra Laboratories, Inc.).
Gensan, Tab. (Zenith Goldline Pharmaceuticals).
Goody's Headache Powders (Goody's Manufacturing Corp.).
Halfprin 81, EC Tab. (Kramer Laboratories, Inc).
Heartline, EC Tab. (BDI Pharmaceuticals, Inc).
Midol, Cap, Spray. (Bayer Corp. (Consumer Div.)).
Momentum, Cap. (Whitehall Robins Laboratories).
Night-Time Effervescent, Tab. (Zenith Goldline Pharmaceuticals).
Pain Reliever, Tab. (Rugby Labs, Inc).
Presalin, Tab. (Roberts Pharmaceuticals).
St. Joseph Adult Chewable Aspirin, Chew. Tab. (Schering-Plough Corp).
Saleto, Preps. (Roberts Pharmaceuticals).
Salocol, Tab. (Roberts Pharmaceuticals).
Sine-Off, Tab. (Menley & James Labs, Inc.).
St. Joseph Cold Tablets For Children (Schering-Plough Corp.).
Supac, Tab. (Mission Pharmacal Co.).
Vanquish, Cap. (Bayer Corp. (Consumer Div.)).

aspirin & oxycodone. (Various Mfr.) Oxycodone HCl 4.5 mg, oxycodone terephthalate 0.38 mg, aspirin 325 mg/Tab. Bot. 100s, 500s, 1000s, UD 25s. *c-II.*
Use: Analagesic combination, narcotic.

Aspirin Plus. (Walgreen Co.) Aspirin 400 mg, caffeine 32 mg/Tab. Bot. 100s. *otc.*
Use: Analgesic combination.

aspirin salts.
See: Calcium Acetylsalicylate.

aspirin tablets, buffered.
Use: Analgesic.

Aspirin Uniserts. (Upsher-Smith Labs, Inc.) Aspirin 125 mg, 300 mg, or 650 mg/supp. Ctn. 12s, 50s. *otc.*
Use: Analgesic.

Aspirtab. (Dover Pharmaceuticals) Aspirin 325 mg/Tab. Sugar, lactose, and salt free. UD Box 500s. *otc.*
Use: Analgesic.

Aspirtab Max. (Dover Pharmaceuticals) Aspirin 500 mg/Tab. Sugar, lactose, and salt free. UD Box 500s. *otc.*

Use: Analgesic.

Aspogen. Dihydroxyaluminum aminoacetate.

Asprimox. (Invamed, Inc.) Aspirin 325 mg (buffered). Capl. Bot. 100s, 500s. *otc.*
Use: Analgesic.

Asprimox Extra Protection for Arthritis Pain. (Invamed, Inc.) Aspirin 325 mg, aluminum hydroxide gel (dried) 75 mg, magnesium hydroxide 75 mg, calcium carbonate. Capl. Bot. 100s, 500s. *otc.*
Use: Analgesic.

Astaril tablets. (Sanofi Winthrop Pharmaceuticals) Theophylline anhydrous, ephedrine sulphate. *Rx.*
Use: Bronchodilator.

Astelin. (Wallace Laboratories) Azelastine HCl 125 mcg, benzalkonium chloride, EDTA/Spray. Bot. 17 mg (100 actuations) per bottle. 2s. *Rx.*
Use: Antihistamine.

•**astemizole.** (ASS-TEM-ih-zole) USAN.
Use: Antihistamine; antiallergic.

asterol.
Use: Antifungal.

AsthmaHaler Mist. (Menley & James) Epinephrine bitartrate 0.3 mg/ml. Oral inhaler 15 ml with mouthpiece; 15 ml refills. *otc.*
Use: Bronchodilator, sympathomimetic.

Asthmalixir. (Reese Pharmaceutical Co. Inc.) Theophylline 45 mg, ephedrine sulfate 36 mg, guaifenesin 150 mg, phenobarbital 12 mg/15 ml. Alcohol 19%. Bot. *Rx.*
Use: Bronchodilator, expectorant, hypnotic, sedative.

AsthmaNefrin. (Numark) Racepinephrine HCl 2.25%. Soln. for Inh. Bot. 15 ml. *otc.*
Use: Sympathomimetic.

AsthmaNefrin Solution & Nebulizer. (SmithKline Beecham Pharmaceuticals) Racepin (racemic epinephrine) as HCl equivalent to epinephrine base 2.25%, chlorobutanol 0.5%. Bot. 0.5 fl oz. With sodium bisulfite. Bot. 1 fl oz. *otc.*
Use: Bronchodilator.

•**astifilcon a.** (ASS-tih-FILL-kahn) USAN.
Use: Contact lens material (hydrophilic).

Astramorph PF. (Astra Pharmaceuticals, L.P.) Morphine sulfate 0.5 mg/ml or 1 mg/ml, preservative free. Inj. Amp. 2 ml, 10 ml. Vial 10 ml. *c-II.*
Use: Analgesic, narcotic.

Astroglide. (BioFilm, Inc.) Purified water, glycerin, propylene glycol, and parabens. Vaginal gel. Bot 66.5 ml. Travel pks. 5 ml. *otc.*
Use: Lubricant.

•**astromicin sulfate.** (ASS-troe-MY-sin) USAN.
Use: Anti-infective.

Astro-Vites. (Faraday) Vitamins A 3500 IU, D 400 IU, C 60 mg, B_1 0.8 mg, B_2 1.3 mg, niacinamide 14 mg, B_6 1 mg, B_{12} 2.5 mcg, folic acid 0.05 mg, pantothenic acid 5 mg, iron 12 mg/Tab. Bot. 100s, 250s. *otc.*
Use: Mineral, vitamin supplement.

AST/SGOT Reagent Strips. (Bayer Corp. (Consumer Div.)) Seralyzer reagent strip. A quantitative strip test for aspartate transaminase/serum glutamic oxaloacetic transaminase in serum or plasma. Bot. Strip 25s.
Use: Diagnostic aid.

Asupirin. (Suppositoria Laboratories, Inc.) Aspirin 60 mg, 120 mg, 200 mg, 300 mg, 600 mg, or 1.2 g/Supp. Box 12s, 100s, 1000s. *otc.*
Use: Analgesic.

A.T. 10.
See: Dihydrotachysterol.

Atabee TD. (Defco) Vitamins C 500 mg, B_1 15 mg, B_2 10 mg, B_6 2 mg, nicotinamide 50 mg, calcium pantothenate 10 mg/Cap. Bot. 30s, 1000s. *otc.*
Use: Vitamin supplement.

Atacand. (Astra Merck) Candesartan cilexetil 4 mg, 8 mg, 16 mg, 32 mg. Tab. Bot. 30s, UD 100s (only 16 mg and 32 mg). *Rx.*
Use: Antihypertensive.

Atarax. (Pfizer US Pharmaceutical Group) Hydroxine HCl. **Tab.:** 10 mg or 25 mg Bot. 100s, 500s, UD 100s, 40s; 50 mg Bot. 100s, 250s, 500s, 1000s, UD 100s. **Syr.:** 10 mg/5 ml, alcohol 0.5%. Bot. Pt. *Rx.*
Use: Anxiolytic.

W/Ephedrine sulfate, theophylline.
See: Marax, Tab., Syr. (Roerig).

Atarax 100. (Pfizer US Pharmaceutical Group) Hydroxyzine HCl 100 mg, lactose/Tab. Bot. 100s, UD 100s. *Rx.*
Use: Antihistamine.

atarvet. Acepromazine.

•**atenolol.** (ah-TEN-oh-lahl) U.S.P. 23.
Use: Beta-adrenergic blocker.
See: Tenormin, Tab. (Zeneca Pharmaceuticals).

atenolol/chlorthalidone. ((ah-TEN-oh-lahl/klor-THAL-ih-dohn)) (Various Mfr.) Atenolol 50 mg or 100 mg, chlorthalidone 25 mg/Tab. Bot. 50s, 100s, 250s, 500s, 1000s. *Rx.*
Use: Antihypertensive.

•**atevirdine mesylate.** (at-TEH-vihr-DEEN) USAN.
Use: Antiviral.

Atgam. (Pharmacia & Upjohn) Lymphocyte immune globulin, antithymocyte globulin 250 mg protein (50 mg/ml). Amp. 5 ml. *Rx.*
Use: Immunosuppressant.

Athlete's Foot Ointment. (Walgreen Co.) Zinc undecylenate 20%, undecylenic acid 5%. Tube 1.5 oz. *otc.*
Use: Antifungal, topical.

•**atipamezole.** (AT-ih-pam-EH-zole) USAN.
Use: Antagonist (α_2-receptor).

•**atiprimod dihydrochloride.** (at-TIH-prih-mahd) USAN.
Use: Antiarthritic (immunomodulator, suppressor cell inducing agent), anti-inflammatory, antirheumatic (disease-modifying).

•**atiprimod dimaleate.** USAN.
Use: Antiarthritic; anti-inflammatory; immunomodulator; antirheumatic (disease-modifying).

•**atiprosin maleate.** (ah-TIH-pro-SIN) USAN.
Use: Antihypertensive.

Ativan Injection. (Wyeth-Ayerst Laboratories) Lorazepam in 2 mg/ml or 4 mg/ml. Vial 1 ml, 10 ml/2 ml Tubex (w/1 ml fill). Pkg. 10s. *c-IV.*
Use: Anxiolytic.

Ativan Tablets. (Wyeth-Ayerst Laboratories) Lorazepam 0.5 mg, 1 mg, or 2 mg/Tab. Bot. 100s, 500s, 1000s, Redipak 25s. *c-IV.*
Use: Anxiolytic.

•**atlafilcon a.** (at-LAH-FILL-kahn A) USAN.
Use: Contact lens material (hydrophilic).

ATnativ. (Bayer Corp. (Biological and Pharmaceutical Div.)) Antithrombin III (human), lyophilized powder/500 IU. Inj. Bot. 50 ml w/10 l sterile water. *Rx.*
Use: Thromboembolic. [Orphan Drug]

atolide. (ATE-oh-lide) USAN. Under study.
Use: Anticonvulsant.

Atolone. (Major Pharmaceuticals) Triamcinolone 4 mg/Tab. Bot. 100s, Uni-Pak 16s. *Rx.*
Use: Corticosteroid.

•**atorvastatin calcium.** USAN.
Use: HMG-CoA reductase inhibitor; antihyperlipidemic.
See: Lipitor, Tab. (Parke-Davis).

•**atosiban.** (at-OH-sih-ban) USAN.
Use: Antagonist, oxytocin.

•**atovaquone.** (uh-TOE-vuh-KWONE) USAN.
Use: Antipneumocystic.
See: Mepron. (GlaxoWellcome).

atovaquone. (uh-TOE-vuh-KWONE)
Use: Treatment and prevention of AIDS-associated *Pneumocystis carinii* pneumonia (PCP), and *toxoplasma gondii encephalitis.*
See: Mepron. (GlaxoWellcome).

Atozine Tabs. (Major Pharmaceuticals) Hydroxyzine HCl 10 mg, 25 mg, or 50 mg/Tab; **10 and 25 mg:** Bot. 100s, 250s, 1000s, UD 100s; **50 mg:** Bot. 100s, 250s, 500s, UD 100s. *Rx.*
Use: Anxiolytic.

Atpeg. (Zeneca Pharmaceuticals) Polyethylene glycol available as 300, 400, 600, or 4000.
Use: Humectant, surfacant.

•**atracurium besylate.** (AT-rah-CUE-ree-uhm BESS-ih-late) USAN.
Use: Neuromuscular blocker; muscle relaxant.
See: Tracrium. (GlaxoWellcome).

Atragen. (Hannan Ophthalmic Marketing Services, Inc.) Tretinoin.
Use: Antineoplastic. [Orphan Drug]

•**atreleuton.** (at-reh-LOO-tuhn) USAN.
Use: Antiasthmatic.

Atretol. (Athena Neurosciences, Inc.) Carbamazepine 200 mg, lactose/Tab. 100s. *Rx.*
Use: Antiepileptic.

Atridine. (Henry Schein, Inc.) Triprolidine 2.5 mg, pseudoephedrine HCl 60 mg/Tab. Bot. 100s, 1000s. *otc.*
Use: Antihistamine, decongestant.

Atrocap. (Freeport) Atropine sulfate 0.06 mg, hyoscyamine sulfate 0.3 mg, hyoscine hydrobromide 0.02 mg, phenobarbital 50 mg/T.R. Cap. Bot. 1000s. *Rx.*
Use: Anticholinergic, antispasmodic, hypnotic, sedative.

Atrocholin. (GlaxoWellcome) Dehydrocholic acid 130 mg/Tab. Bot. 100s. *otc.*
Use: Laxative.

Atrofed. (Genetco, Inc.) Pseudoephedrine HCl 60 mg, triprolidine HCl 2.5 mg. Tab. Bot. 24s, 100s, 1000s. *otc.*
Use: Antihistamine, decongestant.

Atrohist LA. (Medeva Pharmaceuticals, Inc.) Pseudoephedrine HCl 120 mg, brompheniramine maleate 4 mg, phenyltoloxamine citrate 50 mg/SR Tab with atropine sulfate 0.0242 mg available for immediate release. Bot. 100s. *Rx.*
Use: Antihistamine, decongestant.

Atrohist Pediatric Capsules. (Medeva

Pharmaceuticals, Inc.) Chlorpheniramine maleate 4 mg, pseudoephedrine HCl 60 mg/SR Cap. Bot. 100s. *Rx.*
Use: Antihistamine, decongestant.

Atrohist Pediatric Suspension. (Medeva Pharmaceuticals, Inc.) Phenylephrine tannate 5 mg, chlorpheniramine tannate 2 mg, pyrilamine tannate 12.5 mg. Susp. Bot. 473 ml. Unit-of-use 118 ml. *Rx.*
Use: Antihistamine, decongestant.

Atrohist Plus. (Medeva Pharmaceuticals, Inc.) Phenylephrine HCl 25 mg, phenylpropanolamine HCl 50 mg, chlorpheniramine maleate 8 mg, hyoscyamine sulfate 0.19 mg, atropine sulfate 0.04 mg, scopolamine HBr 0.01 mg/SR Tab. Bot. 100s. *Rx.*
Use: Anticholinergic, antihistamine, decongestant.

Atrohist Sprinkle. (Medeva Pharmaceuticals, Inc.) Pseudoephedrine HCl 120 mg, brompheniramine maleate 2 mg, phenytoloxamine citrate 25 mg/SR Cap. Bot. 100s. *Rx.*
Use: Antihistamine, decongestant.

Atromid-S. (Wyeth-Ayerst Laboratories) Clofibrate 500 mg/Cap. Bot. 100s. *Rx.*
Use: Antihyperlipidemic.

AtroPen Auto-Injecter. (Survival Technology, Inc.) Atropine sulfate, phenol 2 mg. In prefilled automatic injection device. *Rx.*
Use: Antidote, cholinergics.

•**atropine.** (AT-troe-peen) U.S.P. 23.
Use: Anticholinergic.

Atropine-1. (Optopics Laboratories, Corp) Atropine sulfate 1% soln. Bot. 2, 5, 15 ml. *Rx.*
Use: Cycloplegic, mydriatic.

Atropine Care. (Akorn, Inc.) Atropine sulfate 1%. Soln. Bot. 2 ml, 5 ml, 15 ml. *Rx.*
Use: Cycloplegic, mydriatic.

atropine and demerol injection. (Sanofi Winthrop Pharmaceuticals) Atropine sulfate 0.4 mg, meperidine HCl 50 mg or 75 mg/Carpuject. *c-II.*
Use: Sedative.

atropine-hyoscine-hyoscyamine combinations. *(See also Belladonna Products).*
See: Barbella, Tab., Elix. (Forest Pharmaceutical, Inc.).
Barbeloid, Tab. (Pal-Pak, Inc.).
Belbutal No. 2 Kaptabs. (Churchill).
Brobella-P.B., Tab. (Brothers).
Donnagel, Susp. (Wyeth-Ayerst Laboratories).
Donnatal, Cap., Elix., Tab. (Wyeth-Ayerst Laboratories).
Donnatal #2, Tab. (Wyeth-Ayerst Laboratories).
Donnatal Extentabs, Tab. (Wyeth-Ayerst Laboratories).
Donnazyme, Tab. (Wyeth-Ayerst Laboratories).
Nilspasm, Tab. (Parmed Pharmaceuticals, Inc.).
Sedamine, Tab. (Dunhall Pharmaceuticals, Inc.).
Sedapar, Tab. (Parmed Pharmaceuticals, Inc.).
Spabelin, Elix. (Arcum).
Spasmolin, Tab. (Bell).
Urogesic, Tab. (Edwards Pharmaceuticals, Inc.).

atropine methylnitrate. (Various Mfr.) dl-Hyoscyamine methylnitrate.
See: Harvatrate, Tab. (Forest Pharmaceutical, Inc.)
W/Hyoscine HBr, hyoscyamine sulfate, amobarbital sodium.
See: Amocine, Tab. (Roberts Pharmaceuticals).

atropine-n-oxide hydrochloride.
See: Atropine Oxide HCl.

•**atropine oxide hydrochloride.** (AT-row-peen OX-ide) USAN.
Use: Anticholinergic.
See: X-Tro (Xttrium Laboratories, Inc.).

•**atropine sulfate.** (AT-row-peen) U.S.P. 23.
Use: Anticholinergic (ophthalmic).

atropine sulfate. (Various Mfr.). **Pediatric Inj.:** 0.05 mg/ml 5 ml Abboject. **Tab, Hypodermic:** 0.3 mg, 0.4 mg, and 0.6 mg/Tab. Bot. 100s. **Inj.:** 0.1 mg/ml 5 ml and 10 ml Abboject 0.3 mg/ml. Vial 1 ml; 0.4 mg/ml. Amp. 1 ml, vial 20 ml; 0.8 mg/ml. Amp. 1 ml, dosette 0.5 ml; 1mg/ml. Amp., vial 1 ml, syringe 10 ml; 1.2 mg/ml. Vial 1 ml syringe. **Lyophilized:** Lyopine (Hyrex Pharmaceuticals). **Ophth. Oint:** 1%. Tube 3.5 g., UD 1 g. **Ophth. Soln:** 1%. Bot. UD 1 ml, 2 ml, 5 ml, 15 ml; 2%. Bot. 2 ml.
Use: Anticholinergic (ophthalmic).
See: Atropine-1, Soln. (Optopics Laboratories,Corp.).
Atropine Care, Soln. (Akorn, Inc.).
Atropine Sulfate S.O.P., Oint. (Allergan, Inc.).
Atropisol, Soln. (Ciba Vision).
Isopto-Atropine (Alcon Laboratories, Inc.).
Lyopine, Inj. (Hyrex Pharmaceuticals).
Parasympatholytic and antispasmodic.
Sal-Tropine, Tab. (Hope Pharmaceuticals).

atropine sulfate and edrophonium

chloride. Anticholinesterase muscle stimulant.
See: Enlon-Plus. (Ohmeda Pharmaceuticals).

atropine sulfate and meperidine hcl.
See: Atropine and Demerol. (Sanofi Winthrop Pharmaceuticals).

atropine sulfate and morphine sulfate.
See: Morphine and Atropine Sulfates (SmithKline Beecham Pharmaceuticals).

atropine sulfate S.O.P. (Allergan, Inc.) 0.5%, 1%. Oint. Tube 3.5 g. *Rx.*
Use: Cycloplegic, mydriatic.

atropine sulfate combinations.
See: Bellatal, Tab. (Richwood Pharmaceuticals).

atropine sulfate w/phenobarbital.
See: Antrocol, Tab., Cap. (ECR Pharmaceuticals).
Arco-Lase Plus, Tab. (Arco Pharmaceuticals, Inc.).
Barbeloid, Tab. (Pal-Pak, Inc.).
Brobella-P.B., Tab. (Brothers).
Donnatal, Cap., Extentab, Tab., Elix. (Wyeth-Ayerst Laboratories).
Donnatal #2, Tab. (Wyeth-Ayerst Laboratories).
Palbar No. 2, Tab. (Roberts Pharmaceuticals).
Spabelin, Elix. (Arcum).

Atropisol. (Ciba Vision) Atropine sulfate 1%. Soln. Dropperette 1 ml. *Rx.*
Use: Cycloplegic, mydriatic.

Atrosed. (Freeport) Atropine sulfate 0.0195 mg, hyoscine HBr 0.0065 mg, hyoscyamine sulfate 0.104 mg, phenobarbital 0.25 gr/Tab. Bot. 1000s, 5000s. *Rx.*
Use: Anticholinergic, antispasmodic, hypnotic, sedative.

Atrosept. (Geneva Pharmaceuticals) Methenamine 40.8 mg, phenylsalicylate 18.1 mg, atropine sulfate 0.03 mg, hyoscyamine 0.03 mg, benzoic acid 4.5 mg, methylene blue 5.4 mg/Tab. Bot. 100s, 1000s. *Rx.*
Use: Anti-infective, urinary.

Atrovent. (Boehringer Ingelheim, Inc.) Ipratropium bromide. **Aerosol:** 18 mcg/dose. Metered dose inhaler 14 g (200 inhalations). **Soln.:** 0.02% (500 mcg/vial). Preservative free. Unit-dose Vial 25s. **Nasal Spray:** 0.03% (21 mcg/spray). Bot. 30 ml (345 sprays); 0.06% (42 mcg/spray). Bot. 15 ml (165 sprays). *Rx.*
Use: Bronchodilator.

A/T/S. (Hoechst Marion Roussel) Erythromycin 2%. Gel. Tube 30 g. *Rx.*
Use: Dermatologic, acne.

A/T/S Topical Solution. (Hoechst Marion Roussel) Erythromycin 2% topical soln. Bot. 60 ml. *Rx.*
Use: Dermatologic, acne.

AT-Solution. (Sanofi Winthrop Pharmaceuticals) Dihydrotachysterol solution.
Use: Antihypocalcemic.

Attain Liquid. (Sherwood Davis & Geck) Sodium caseinate, calcium caseinate, maltodextrin, corn oil, soy lecithin. Can 250 ml and 1000 ml closed system. *otc.*
Use: Nutritional supplement.

•**attapulgite, activated.** (at-ah-PULL-gyte) U.S.P. 23.
Use: Antidiarrheal; pharmaceutic aid (suspending agent).
See: Kaopectate Advanced Formula (Pharmacia & Upjohn).
W/Pectin, hydrated alumina powder.
See: Sebasorb Lot. (Summers Laboratories, Inc.).

Attenuvax. (Merck & Co.) Measles virus vaccine, live, attenuated w/neomycin 25 mcg/Vial. Single-dose vial w/diluent. Pkg. 1s, 10s. *Rx.*
Use: Immunization.
W/Meruvax.
See: M-R-Vax-II, Vial. (Merck & Co.).
W/Mumpsvax, Meruvax.
See: M-M-R II, Vial (Merck & Co.).

Atuss DM. (Atley Pharmaceuticals, Inc.) Dextromethorphan 15 mg, phenylephrine HCl 5 mg, chlorpheniramine maleate 2 mg, sucrose, saccharin, menthol, methylparaben, strawberry flavor/Syr. Bot. 480 ml. *Rx.*
Use: Antihistamine, antitussive, decongestant.

Atuss EX. (Atley Pharmaceuticals, Inc.) Hydrocodone bitartrate 5 mg, guaifenesin 100 mg/5 ml, parabens, menthol, saccharin, sorbitol, cherry flavor/Syr. Bot. 473 ml. *c-III.*
Use: Expectorant, narcotic.

Atuss G. (Atley Pharmaceuticals, Inc.) Hydrocodone bitartrate 2 mg, phenylephrine HCl 10 mg, guaifenesin 100 mg/5 ml, sucrose, saccharin, grape flavor/Syr. Bot. 480 ml. *c-III.*
Use: Narcotic decongestant expectorant.

Atuss HD. (Atley Pharmaceuticals, Inc.) Hydrocodone bitartrate 2.5 mg, phenylephrine HCl 5 mg, chlorpheniramine maleate 2 mg/5 ml. Menthol, sucrose, alcohol, cherry flavor. Liq. Bot. 480 ml. *Rx.*
Use: Antihistamine, antitussive, decongestant.

Augmented Betamethasone Dipropionate.

Use: Corticosteroid, topical.
See: Diprolene. (Schering-Plough Corp.).

Augmentin Chewable Tablets. (SmithKline Beecham Pharmaceuticals) **125:** Amoxicillin 125 mg, clavulanic acid 31.25 mg, saccharin/Tab. Bot. 30s. **200:** Amoxicillin 200 mg, clavulanic acid 28.5 mg, saccharin, aspartame/Tab. Bot. 20s. **250:** Amoxicillin 250 mg, clavulanic acid 62.5 mg, saccharin/Tab. Bot. 30s. **400:** Amoxicillin 400 mg, clavulanic acid 57 mg, saccharin, aspartame/Tab. Bot. 20s. *Rx.*
Use: Anti-infective, penicillin.

Augmentin Powder for Oral Suspension. (SmithKline Beecham Pharmaceuticals) **125:** Amoxicillin 125 mg, clavulanic acid 31.25 mg/5 ml. Pow. for Oral Susp. Bot. 75 ml, 100 ml, 150 ml. **200:** Amoxicillin 200 mg, clavulanic acid 28.5 mg/5 ml, saccharin, aspartame. Pow. for Oral Susp. Bot. 50 ml, 75 ml, 100 ml. **250:** Amoxicillin 250 mg, clavulanic acid 62.5 mg/5 ml. Pow. for Oral Susp. Bot. 75 ml, 100 ml, 150 ml. **400:** Amoxicillin 400 mg, clavulanic acid 57 mg/5 ml, saccharin, aspartame. Pow. for Oral Susp. Bot. 50 ml, 75 ml, 100 ml. *Rx.*
Use: Anti-infective, penicillin.

Augmentin Tablets. (SmithKline Beecham Pharmaceuticals) Amoxicillin trihydrate 250 mg, 500 mg, or 875 mg, clavulanic acid 125 mg/Tab. Bot. 20s, 30s (250 mg only), UD 100s. *Rx.*
Use: Anti-infective, penicillin.

Auralgan Otic Solution. (Wyeth-Ayerst Laboratories) Antipyrine 54 mg, benzocaine 14 mg/ml w/oxyquinoline sulfate in dehydrated glycerin (contains not more than 0.6% moisture). Bot. Dropper 15 ml. *Rx.*
Use: Otic.

Auralgesic. (Wesley Pharmacal Co., Inc.) Carbamide 10%, antipyrine 5%, benzocaine 2.5%, cetyldimethylbenzylammonium HCl 0.2%. Bot. 0.5 oz. *Rx.*
Use: Otic.

•**auranofin.** (or-RAIN-oh-fin) USAN.
Use: Antirheumatic.
See: Ridaura, Cap. (SmithKline Beecham Pharmaceuticals).

aureomycin preparations. (Storz Ophthalmics) Chlortetracycline HCl. **Ophth. Oint.:** 1% (10 mg/g) Tube 0.125 oz. **Topical Oint.:** 3% (30 mg/g) in white petrolatum, anhydrous lanolin base. Tube 0.5 oz, 1 oz. *Rx.*
Use: Anti-infective.

Aureoquin Diamate. Name previously used for Quinetolate.

Auriculin. (Scios Nova, Inc.) Anaritide acetate.
Use: Improvement of early renal allograft function following renal transplantation; acute renal failure.

Aurinol Ear Drops. (Various Mfr.) Chloroxylenol and acetic acid, w/benzalkonium chloride and glycerin. Soln. Bot. 15 ml. *Rx.*
Use: Otic.

Aurocein. (Christina) Gold naphthyl sulfhydryl derivative. 5% or 12.5% Amp. 10 ml. *Rx.*
Use: Antirheumatic.

Auro-Dri. (Del Pharmaceuticals, Inc.) Boric acid 2.75% in isopropyl alcohol. Bot. oz. *otc.*
Use: Otic.

Auro Ear Drops. (Del Pharmaceuticals, Inc.) Carbamide peroxide 6.5% in a specially prepared base. Bot. 15 ml. *otc.*
Use: Otic.

Aurolate. (Taylor Pharmaceuticals) Gold sodium thiomalate 50 mg, benzyl alcohol 0.5%/ml. Inj. Vial 2 ml, 10 ml. *Rx.*
Use: Antirheumatic.

aurolin.
See: Gold sodium thiosulfate.

auropin.
See: Gold sodium thiosulfate.

aurosan.
See: Gold sodium thiosulfate.

•**aurothioglucose.** (or-oh-THIGH-oh-GLUE-kose) U.S.P. 23.
Use: Antirheumatic.

aurothioglucose injection.
See: Sterile aurothioglucose suspension.

aurothiomalate, sodium.
See: Gold Sodium Thiomalate, U.S.P. 23.

Auroto Otic. (Alpharma USPD Inc.) Benzocaine 1.4%, antipyrine 5.4%, glycerin and oxyquinoline sulfate/Soln. Bot. 15 ml w/dropper. *Rx.*
Use: Otic preparation.

Ausab. (Abbott Diagnostics) Radioimmunoassay or enzyme immunoassay for detection of antibody to hepatitis B surface antigen. Test kit 100s.
Use: Diagnostic aid.

Ausab EIA. (Abbott Diagnostics) Enzyme immunoassay for the detection of antibody to hepatitis B surface antigen.
Use: Diagnostic aid.

Auscell. (Abbott Diagnostics) Reverse passive hemagglutination test for hepatitis B surface antigen. Test kit 110s, 450s, 1800s.
Use: Diagnostic aid.

Ausria II-125. (Abbott Diagnostics) Radioimmunoassay for detection of hepatitis B surface antigen. Test kit 100s, 500s, 600s, 700s, 800s, 900s, 1000s.
Use: Diagnostic aid.

Auszyme II. (Abbott Diagnostics) Enzyme immunoassay for detection of hepatitis B surface antigen (HBsAg) in human serum or plasma. Test kit 100s, 500s.
Use: Diagnostic aid.

Auszyme Monoclonal. (Abbott Diagnostics) Qualitative third generation enzyme immunoassay for the detection of hepatitis B surface antigen (HBsAg) in human serum or plasma.
Use: Diagnostic aid.

Autoantibody Screen. (Wampole Laboratories) Autoantibody screening system. To screen serum for the presence of a variety of autoantibodies. Test 48s.
Use: Diagnostic aid.

Autolet Kit. (Bayer Corp. (Consumer Div.)) Automatic bloodletting spring-loaded device to obtain capillary blood samples from fingertips, ear lobes, or heels.
Use: Diagnostic aid.

autolymphocyte therapy; ALT. (Cellcor, Inc.)
Use: Treatment of renal cancer. [Orphan Drug]

Autoplex. (Baxter Pharmaceutical Products, Inc.) Anti-inhibitor coagulant complex prepared from pooled human plasma. Vial 30 ml.
Use: Diagnostic aid.

Autoplex T. (Baxter Pharmaceutical Products, Inc.) Dried anti-inhibitor coagulant complex. With a maximum of heparin 2 units and polyethylene glycol 2 mg per ml reconstituted material. Inj. Vial with diluent and needles. *Rx.*
Use: Diagnostic aid.

Autrinic. Intrinsic factor concentrate. *Rx.*
Use: To increase absorption of Vitamin B_{12}.

Auxotab Enteric 1 & 2. (Colab) Rapid identification of enteric bacteria and *Pseudomonas.* Test contains capillary units with selective biochemical reagents.
Use: Diagnostic aid.

Avail. (Menley & James Labs, Inc.) Iron 18 mg, vitamin A 5000 IU, D 400 IU, E 30 mg, B_1 2.25 mg, B_2 2.55 mg, B_3 20 mg, B_6 3 mg, B_{12} 9 mcg, C 90 mg, folic acid 0.4 mg, Ca, Cr, I, Mg, Se, and zinc 22.5 mg/Tab. Bot. 60s. *otc.*
Use: Mineral, vitamin supplement.

Avalgesic Lotion. (Various Mfr.) Methyl salicylate, menthol, camphor, methylnicotinate, dipropylene glycol salicylate, oil of cassia, oleoresins capsicum, and ginger. Bot. 120 ml, Pt, gal. *otc.*
Use: Analgesic, topical.

A-Van. (Stewart-Jackson Pharmacal, Inc.) Dimenhydrinate 50 mg/Cap. Bot. 100s.
Use: Antivertigo.

Avapro. (Sanofi Winthrop Pharmaceuticals) Irbesartan 75 mg, 150 mg, 300 mg, lactose/Tab. Bot. 30s, 90s, 500s, UD 100s. *Rx.*
Use: Antihypertensive.

•**avasimibe.** (av-ASS-ih-mibe) USAN.
Use: Antiatherosclerotic; hypolipidemic (acylCoA: Cholesterol acyltransferase [ACAT] inhibitor).

AVC Cream. (Hoechst Marion Roussel) Sulfanilamide 15% in a water-miscible base of propylene glycol, stearic acid, diglycol stearate to acid pH. Tube 4 oz. w/applicator. *Rx.*
Use: Anti-infective, vaginal.

AVC Suppositories. (Hoechst Marion Roussel) Sulfanilamide 1.05 g in a base made from polyethylene glycol 400, polysorbate 80, polyethylene glycol 3350, glycerin, inert glycerin-gelatin covering. Box 16s w/inserter. *Rx.*
Use: Anti-infective, vaginal.

Aveeno Anti-Itch. (Rydelle Laboratories) Calamine 3%, pramoxine HCl, camphor 0.3% in a base of glycerin, distearyldimonium chloride, petrolatum, oatmeal flour, isopropyl palmitate, cetyl alcohol, dimethicone, and sodium chloride. Cream 30 g, Lotion 120 ml. *otc.*
Use: Antipruritic.

Aveenobar Medicated. (Rydelle Laboratories) Aveeno colloidal oatmeal 50%, sulfur 2%, salicylic acid 2%, in soap-free cleansing bar. *Formerly Acnaveen.* Bar 3.5 oz. *otc.*
Use: Antipruritic.

Aveenobar Oilated. (Rydelle Laboratories) Vegetable oils, lanolin derivative, glycerine 29%, aveeno colloidal oatmeal 30% in soap-free base. Formerly Emulave. Bar. 3 oz. *otc.*
Use: Emollient.

Aveenobar Regular. (Rydelle Laboratories) Colloidal oatmeal 50%, an ionic sulfonate, hypo-allergenic lanolin. Formerly Aveeno Bar. Bar 3.2 oz., 4.4 oz. *otc.*
Use: Dermatologic, cleanser.

Aveeno Bath. (Rydelle Laboratories) Colloidal oatmeal. Box 1 lb, 4 lb. *otc.*

Use: Emollient.

Aveeno Cleansing for Acne Prone Skin. (Rydelle Laboratories) Sulfur 2%, salicylic acid 2%, colloidal oatmeal 50%, glycerin, titanium dioxide. Soap Bar 90 g. *otc.*
Use: Antiacne.

Aveeno Cleansing Bar. (Rydelle Laboratories) **Combination Skin:** Soap free. Colloidal oatmeal 51%, sodium cocoyl isethionate, glycerin, lactic acid, sodium lactate, petrolatum, magnesium aluminum silicate, potassium sorbate, titanium dioxide, PEG 14M. Bar 90 g. **Dry Skin:** Soap free. Colloidal oatmeal 51%, sodium cocoyl isethionate, vegetable oil and shortening, glycerin, PEG-75, lauramide DEA, lactic acid, sodium lactate, sorbic acid, titanium dioxide. Bar 90 g. *otc.*
Use: Dermatologic, cleanser.

Aveeno Colloidal Oatmeal. (Rydelle Laboratories) Colloidal oatmeal. Box 1 lb, 4 lb. *otc.*
Use: Emollient.

Aveeno Dry. (Rydelle Laboratories) Dry skin formula, soap free, emollient colloidal oatmeal, vegetable oils, lanolin derivative, and glycerin 29% in mild surfactant base. Cleansing bar 90 g. *otc.*
Use: Dermatologic, cleanser.

Aveeno Lotion. (Rydelle Laboratories) Colloidal oatmeal 1%, glycerin, petrolatum, dimethicone, phenylcarbinol. Bot. 354 ml. *otc.*
Use: Emollient.

Aveeno Moisturizing Cream. (Rydelle Laboratories) Colloidal oatmeal, glycerin, petrolatum, dimethicone, phenylcarbinol. Cream Tube 120 g. *otc.*
Use: Emollient.

Aveeno Normal. (Rydelle Laboratories) Normal to oily skin formula, soap free. Colloidal oatmeal 50%, lanolin derivative and mild surfactant. Cleansing bar 96 g, 132 g. *otc.*
Use: Dermatologic, cleanser.

Aveeno Oilated. (Rydelle Laboratories) Aveeno colloidal oatmeal impregnated with 35% liquid petrolatum, refined olive oil. Box 8 oz, 2 lb. *otc.*
Use: Emollient.

Aveeno Shave. (Rydelle Laboratories) Oatmeal flour. Gel. Can 210 g. *otc.*
Use: Emollient.

Aveeno Shower & Bath. (Rydelle Laboratories) Colloidal oatmeal, 5% mineral oil, laureth-4, silica benzaldehyde. Oil. Bot. 240 ml. *otc.*
Use: Emollient.

Aventyl Hydrochloride. (Eli Lilly and Co.) Nortriptyline HCl. **Liq.:** Equivalent to 10 mg base/5 ml in alcohol 4%. Bot. 16 fl. oz. **Pulv.:** Equivalent to 10 mg base or 25 mg base/Cap. Bot. 100s, 500s, Blister pak 10 × 10s. *Rx.*
Use: Antidepressant.

Avertin. Tribromoethanol. (Various Mfr.).

•**avilamycin.** (ah-VILL-ah-MY-sin) USAN.
Use: Anti-infective.

Avinar. Uredepa.
Use: Antineoplastic.

Avita. (DPT Laboratories, Inc.) Tretinoin 0.025%. Cream Tube 20 g, 45 g. *Rx.*
Use: Dermatologic, acne.

Avitene Hemostat. (Davol) Hydrochloric acid salt of purified bovine corium collagen. **Fibrous Form:** Jar 1 g, 5 g. **Web Form:** Blister Pak. Sheets of 70 mm × 70 mm, 70 mm × 35 mm, 35 mm × 35 mm. *Rx.*
Use: Hemostatic, topical.

•**avitriptan fumarate.** (av-ih-TRIP-tan FEW-mah-rate) USAN.
Use: Antimigraine.

•**avobenzone.** (AV-ah-BENZ-ohn) USAN.
Use: Sunscreen.

avobenzone w/combinations. (AV-ah-BENZ-ohn)
See: PreSun Ultra, Lot., Clear Gel (Westwood Squibb Pharmaceuticals).

Avonex. (Biogen) Interferon Beta-1a 33 mcg (6.6 million IU) albumin human 15 mg, sodium chloride and sodium phosphates. Pow. for inj. Vials. Single-use vial w/10 ml vial of diluent, swabs, syringe, access pin, needle, and bandage. *Rx.*
Use: Multiple sclerosis agent, hepatitis, brain tumor. [Orphan Drug]

Avonique. (Armenpharm Ltd.) Vitamins A 4000 IU, D 400 IU, B_1 1 mg, B_2 1.2 mg, B_6 2 mg, B_{12} 2 mcg, calcium pantothenate 5 mg, B_3 10 mg, C 30 mg, calcium 100 mg, phosphorus 76 mg, iron 10 mg, manganese 1 mg, magnesium 1 mg, zinc 1 mg. *otc.*
Use: Mineral, vitamin supplement.

•**avoparcin.** (AVE-oh-PAR-sin) USAN.
Use: Anti-infective.

•**avridine.** (AV-rih-deen) USAN.
Use: Antiviral.

Awake. (Walgreen Co.) Caffeine 100 mg/Tab. Bot. 36s. *otc.*
Use: CNS stimulant.

axerophthol.
See: Vitamin A.

Axid. (Eli Lilly and Co.) Nizatidine 150 mg or 300 mg/Cap. Bot. 30s, 60s. *Rx.*

Use: H_2 antagonist.

Axid AR. (Whitehall Robins Laboratories) Nizatidine 75 mg/Tab. Bot. 6s, 12s, 18s, 30s. *otc.*
Use: Gastrointestinal.

Axocet. (Savage Laboratories) Butalbital 50 mg, acetaminophen 650 mg, parabens/Cap. Bot. 100s. *Rx.*
Use: Analgesic, hypnotic, sedative.

Axsain.
See: Zostrix (Medicis Dermatologicals, Inc.).

Aygestin. (ESI Lederle Generics) Norethindrone acetate 5 mg, lactose/Tab. Bot. 50s. *Rx.*
Use: Hormone, progestin.

Ayr Saline Nasal Drops. (B.F. Ascher and Co.) Sodium Cl 0.65% adjusted with phosphate buffers to proper tonicity and pH to prevent nasal irritation. **Drops:** Bot. 20 ml. **Mist:** Bot. 50 ml. *otc.*
Use: Dermatologic, moisturizer.

•**azabon.** (AZE-ah-bahn) USAN.
Use: CNS stimulant.

•**azacitidine.** (AZE-ah-SIGH-tih-deen) USAN. *Formerly Ladakamycin.*
Use: Antineoplastic.

•**azaclorzine hydrochloride.** (AZE-ah-KLOR-zeen) USAN. *Formerly Nonachlazine.*
Use: Coronary vasodilator.

•**azaconazole.** (AZE-ah-CONE-ah-zole) USAN. *Formerly Azoconazole.*
Use: Antifungal.

AZA-CR. NCI Investigational agent.
See: Azacitidine.

Azactam. (Bristol-Myers Squibb) Aztreonam 500 mg, 1 g, 2 g (≈ 780 mg L-arginine/g of aztreonam). Pow. for Inj. (lyophilized cake). Single-dose vial 15 ml (500 mg, 1 g), 30 ml (2 g only); Single-dose infusion bot. 100 ml (1 g and 2 g). *Rx.*
Use: Anti-infective.

5-aza-2 deoxycytidine.
Use: Treatment of acute leukemia.

•**azalanstat dihydrochloride.** (aze-ah-LAN-stat die-HIGH-droe-KLOR-ide) USAN.
Use: Hypolipidemic.

Azaline. (Major Pharmaceuticals) Sulfasalazine 500 mg/Tab. Bot. 100s, 500s, 1000s.
Use: Anti-inflammatory.

•**azaloxan fumarate.** (aze-ah-LOX-ahn) USAN.
Use: Antidepressant.

azamethonium bromide. (Novartis Pharmaceutical Corp.) *Rx.*
Use: Ganglionic blocking.

•**azanator maleate.** (AZE-an-nay-tore) USAN.
Use: Bronchodilator.

•**azanidazole.** (AZE-ah-NIH-dah-zole) USAN.
Use: Antiprotozoal.

•**azaperone.** (AZE-app-eh-RONE) U.S.P. 23.
Use: Antipsychotic.

•**azaribine.** (aze-ah-RYE-bean) USAN.
Use: Dermatologic.

•**azarole.** (AZE-ah-role) USAN.
Use: Immunoregulator.

•**azaserine.** (AZE-ah-SER-een) USAN.
Use: Antifungal.

•**azatadine maleate.** (aze-AT-ad-EEN) U.S.P. 23.
Use: Antihistamine.
See: Optimine, Tab. (Key Pharmaceuticals).
Trinalin, Tab. (Schering-Plough Corp.).

•**azathioprine.** (AZE-uh-THIGH-oh-preen) U.S.P. 23.
Use: Immunosuppressant.
See: Imuran, Inj., Tab. (Glaxo-Wellcome).

azathioprine sodium. (Various Mfr.) 100 mg. Pow. for Inj. Vial. 20 ml. *Rx.*
Use: Antileukemic.

•**azathioprine sodium for injection.** (AZE-uh-THIGH-oh-preen) U.S.P. 23.
Use: Immunosuppressant.

5-azc.
See: Azacitidine.

Azdone. (Schwarz Pharma, Inc.) Hydrocodone bitartrate 5 mg, aspirin 500 mg/Tab. Bot. 100s, 1000s. *c-III.*
Use: Analgesic combination, narcotic.

•**azelaic acid.** (aze-eh-LAY-ik) USAN.
Use: Dermatologic, acne.
See: Azelex, cream. (Allergan, Inc.).

•**azelastine hydrochloride.** (ah-ZELL-ass-teen) USAN.
Use: Antiallergic, antiasthmatic.
See: Astelin, Nasal Spray. (Wallace Laboratories).

Azelex. (Allergan, Inc.) Azelaic acid 20%, glycerin, cetearyl alcohol, benzoic acid. Cream 30 g. *Rx.*
Use: Dermatologic, acne.

•**azepindole.** (AZE-eh-PIN-dole) USAN.
Use: Antidepressant.

•**azetepa.** (AZE-eh-teh-pah) USAN.
Use: Antineoplastic.

•**3-azido-2, 3 dideoxyuridine.** USAN.
Use: Antiviral, HIV.

azidothymidine.
See: Zidovudine.

Azidouridine. (Berlex Laboratories, Inc.) Phase I HIV-positive symptomatic, ARC, AIDS. *Rx.*
Use: Antiviral.

•**azimilide dihydrochloride.** (azz-IM-ih-lide die-HIGH-droe-KLOR-ide) USAN.
Use: Cardiovascular agent.

•**azipramine hydrochloride.** (aze-IPP-RAH-meen) USAN.
Use: Antidepressant.

•**azithromycin.** (UHZ-ith-row-MY-sin) U.S.P. 23.
Use: Anti-infective.
See: Zithromax, Tab. (Pfizer US Pharmaceutical Group).

Azlin. (Bayer Corp. (Consumer Div.)) Azlocillin sodium. Vial 2 g, 3 g, 4 g.
Use: Anti-infective, penicillin.

•**azlocillin.** (AZZ-low-SILL-in) USAN.
Use: Anti-infective.
See: Azlin, Inj. (Bayer Corp. (Consumer Div.)).

•**azlocillin sodium.** (AZZ-low-SILL-in) U.S.P. 23.
Use: Anti-infective.

Azma-Aid. (Purepac Pharmaceutical Co.) Theophylline 118 mg, ephedrine 24 mg, phenobarbital 8 mg/Tab. Bot. 100s, 250s, 1000s. *Rx.*
Use: Bronchodilator.

Azmacort. (Rhone-Poulenc Rorer Pharmaceuticals, Inc.) Triamcinolone acetonide in an inhaler system ≈ 100 mcg/actuation. Canister 20 g (240 metered doses). *Rx.*
Use: Corticosteroid.

AZO-100. (Scruggs) Phenylazodiaminopyridine HCl 100 mg/Tab. Bot. 100s, 1000s. *otc.*
Use: Analgesic, urinary.

azoconazole.
Use: Antifungal.

Azodyne Hydrochloride.
See: Pyridium, Tab. (Parke-Davis).

•**azolimine.** (aze-OLE-ih-meen) USAN.
Use: Diuretic.

AZO Negacide Tablets. (Sanofi Winthrop Pharmaceuticals) Nalidixic acid, phenazopyridine HCl. *Rx.*
Use: Anti-infective, urinary.

Azopt. (Alcon Laboratories, Inc.) Brinzolamide 1%/Ophth. Susp. Drop-Tainers 2.5 ml, 5 ml, 10 ml, 15 ml. *Rx.*
Use: Glaucoma treatment.

•**azosemide.** (AZE-oh-SEH-mide) USAN.
Use: Diuretic.

AZO-Standard. (PolyMedica Pharmaceuticals) Phenazopyridine HCl 100 mg/Tab. Bot. 360s. *otc.*
Use: Analgesic, urinary.

Azostix Reagent Strips. (Bayer Corp (Consumer Div.)) Bromthymol blue, urease, buffers. Colorimetric test for blood urea nitrogen level. Bot 25 strips.
Use: Diagnostic aid.

azo-sulfisoxazole. (Various Mfr.) Sulfisoxazole 500 mg, phenazopyridine HCl 50 mg/Tab. Bot. 100s, 1000s. *Rx.*
Use: Anti-infective, urinary.

•**azotomycin.** (aze-OH-toe-MY-sin) USAN. Antibiotic isolated from broth filtrates of *Streptomyces ambofaciens.*
Use: Antineoplastic.

Azovan Blue.
See: Evans Blue Dye, Amp. (City Chemical; Harvey).

AZO Wintomylon. (Sanofi Winthrop Pharmaceuticals) Nalidixic acid, phenazopyridine HCl. *Rx.*
Use: Anti-infective, urinary.

AZT.
See: Zidovudine.

AZT-P-ddi. (Baker Norton Pharmaceuticals, Inc.) Phase I AIDS.
Use: Antiviral.

•**aztreonam.** (AZZ-TREE-oh-nam) U.S.P. 23.
Use: Antimicrobial.
See: Azactam, Pow. for Inj. (Bristol-Myers Squibb).

Azulfidine. (Pharmacia & Upjohn) Sulfasalazine. 500 mg/Tab. Bot. 100s, 300s, UD 100s. *Rx.*
Use: Anti-inflammatory.

Azulfidine EN-tabs. (Pharmacia & Upjohn) Sulfasalazine. Enteric coated. 500 mg/Tab. Bot. 100s, 300s. *Rx.*
Use: Anti-inflammatory.

•**azumolene sodium.** (AH-ZUH-moe-leen) USAN.
Use: Muscle relaxant.

B

B_1. Thiamine HCl.
B_2. Riboflavin.
B_3. Niacin, nicotinamide.
B_5. Calcium pantothenate.
B_6. Pyridoxine HCl.
B_6 50. (Western Research) Vitamin B_6 50 mg/Tab. Bot. 1000s. *otc.*
Use: Vitamin supplement.
B_{12}. Cyanocobalamin. *otc.*
B-50. (NBTY, Inc.) Vitamins B_1 50 mg, B_2 50 mg, B_3 50 mg, B_5 50 mg, B_6 50 mg, B_{12} 50 mcg, folic acid 0.1 mg, d-biotin 50 mcg, PABA, choline bitartrate, inositol/Tab. Bot. 50s, 100s. *otc.*
Use: Mineral, vitamin supplement.
B-50 Time Release. (NBTY, Inc.) Vitamins B_1 50 mg, B_2 50 mg, B_3 50 mg, B_5 50 mg, B_6 50 mg, B_{12} 50 mcg, folic acid 0.1 mg, d-biotin 50 mcg, PABA 50 mg, choline bitartrate 50 mg, inositol 50 mg, lecithin/Tab. Bot. 100s. *otc.*
Use: Mineral, vitamin supplement.
B 100. (Fibertone) B_1 100 mg, B_2 100 mg, B_3 100 mg, B_5 100 mg, B_6 100 mg, B_{12} 100 mcg, FA 0.4 mg, biotin 50 mcg, PABA 100 mg, choline bitartrate 100 mg, inositol 100 mg/SR Tab. Bot. 100s. *otc.*
Use: Vitamin supplement.
B-100. (NBTY, Inc.) Vitamins B_1 100 mg, B_2 100 mg, B_3 100 mg, B_5 100 mg, B_6 100 mg, B_{12} 100 mcg, folic acid 0.1 mg, d-biotin 100 mcg, PABA 100 mg, choline bitartrate, inositol, lecithin. Tab. Bot. 50s, 100s. *otc.*
Use: Mineral, vitamin supplement.
B125. (NBTY, Inc.) Vitamins B_1 125 mg, B_2 125 mg, B_3 125 mg, B_5 125 mg, B_6 125 mg, B_{12} 125 mcg, folic acid 0.1 mg, d-biotin 125 mcg, PABA 125 mg, choline bitartrate 125 mg, inositol 125 mg, lecithin. Tab. Bot. 100s. *otc.*
Use: Mineral, vitamin supplement.
B150. (NBTY, Inc.) Vitamins B_1 150 mg, B_2 150 mg, B_3 150 mg, B_5 150 mg, B_6 150 mg, B_{12} 150 mcg, folic acid 0.1 mg, d-biotin 150 mcg, PABA 150 mg, choline bitartrate 150 mg, inositol 150 mg, lecithin. Tab. Bot. 100s. *otc.*
Use: Mineral, vitamin supplement.
B & A. (Eastern Research) Sodium bicarbonate, potassium, aluminum, borax. Hygienic pow. Jar. 8 oz, 5 lb. *Rx.*
Use: Vaginal agent.
B.A. Gradual. (Federal) Theophylline 260 mg, pseudoephedrine HCl 50 mg, butabarbital 15 mg/Gradual. Bot. 50s, 1000s. *Rx.*
Use: Bronchodilator, decongestant, hypnotic, sedative.
Babee Teething. (Pfeiffer Co.) Benzocaine 2.5%, cetalkonium Cl 0.02%, alcohol, eucalyptol, menthol, camphor. Soln. Bot. 15 ml. *otc.*
Use: Anesthetic, local.
Baby Anbesol. (Whitehall Robins Laboratories) Benzocaine 7.5%, saccharin. Gel Tube 7.2 g. *otc.*
Use: Mouth and throat preparation.
Baby Cough Syrup. (Towne) Ammonium Cl 300 mg, sodium citrate 600 mg/oz w/citric acid. Bot. 4 oz.
Use: Antitussive.
Baby Orajel. (Del Pharmaceuticals, Inc.) Benzocaine 7.5%, saccharin, sorbitol, alcohol free. Gel Tube 9.45 g. *otc.*
Use: Mouth and throat preparation.
Baby Orajel Nighttime Formula. (Del Pharmaceuticals, Inc.) Benzocaine 10%, saccharin, sorbitol, alcohol free. Gel Tube 6 g. *otc.*
Use: Mouth and throat preparation.
Baby Oragel Teeth & Gum Cleanser. (Del Pharmaceuticals, Inc.) Poloxamer 407 2%, simethicone 0.12%, parabens, saccharin, sorbitol. Gel Tube 14.2 g. *otc.*
Use: Mouth and throat preparation.
Baby Vitamin Drops. (Zenith Goldline Pharmaceuticals) Vitamins A 1500 IU, D 400 IU, E 5 IU, B_1 0.5 mg, B_2 0.6 mg, B_3 8 mg, B_6 0.4 mg, B_{12} 2 mcg, C 35 mg/ml/Drop. Bot. 50 ml. *otc.*
Use: Vitamin supplement.
Baby Vitamin Drops with Iron. (Zenith Goldline Pharmaceuticals) Iron 10 mg, vitamins A 1500 IU, D 400 IU, E 5 IU, B_1 0.5 mg, B_2 0.6 mg, B_3 8 mg, B_6 0.4 mg, C 35 mg/ml. Bot. 50 ml. *otc.*
Use: Mineral, vitamin supplement.
BAC. Benzalkonium Cl.
•**bacampicillin HCl.** (BACK-am-PIH-sill-in) U.S.P. 23.
Use: Anti-infective.
See: Spectrobid, Tab. (Roerig).
Bacco-Resist. (Vita Elixir) Lobeline sulfate 1/64 gr.
Use: Smoking deterrent.
Bacid. (Novartis Nutrition Corp.) A specially cultured strain of human *Lactobacillus acidophilus*, sodium carboxymethylcellulose 100 mg, sodium 0.5 mEq/Cap. Bot. 50s, 100s. *otc.*
Use: Antidiarrheal, nutritional supplement.
Baciguent Antibiotic Ointment. (Pharmacia & Upjohn) Bacitracin 500 units/g. Oint. Tube 0.5 oz, 1 oz, 4 oz. *otc.*
Use: Anti-infective, topical.
Bacillus Calmette-Guerin.
See: BCG Vaccine.

bacitracin. (Various Mfr.) An antibiotic produced by a strain of *Bacillus subtilis.* Diagnostic Tabs. Oint., Ophthalmic Oint. 500 units/g. Tube 3.5 g, 3.75 g. Soluble Tab., Systemic Use, Vial., Topical Use, Vial., Troche. Vaginal Tab.
Use: Anti-infective. [Orphan Drug]

•**bacitracin.** (bass-ih-TRAY-sin) U.S.P. 23.
Use: Anti-infective.
See: AK-Tracin, Oint. (Akorn, Inc.).
Altracin (Alpharma USPD Inc.).
Baciguent, Oint. (Pharmacia & Upjohn).
W/Neomycin sulfate.
See: Bacimycin, Oint. (Hoechst Marion Roussel).
Bacitracin-Neomycin, Oint., Ophth. Oint. (Various Mfr.).
W/Neomycin, polymyxin B sulfate.
See: BPN Ointment (Procter & Gamble Pharm.).
Mycitracin, Oint., Ophth. Oint. (Pharmacia & Upjohn).
Neosporin, Oint., Ophth. Oint., Aerosol, Pow. (GlaxoWellcome).
Neo-Thrycex, Oint. (Del Pharmaceuticals, Inc.).
Tigo, Oint. (Burlington).
Tri-Biotic, Oint. (Burgin-Arden, Standex).
Triple Antibiotic Oint. (Towne).
W/Neomycin sulfate, polymyxin B sulfate, diperodon HCl.
See: Polysporin, Oint., Ophth. Oint. (GlaxoWellcome).
W/Polymyxin B Sulfate, neomycin sulfate, lidocaine.
See: Clomycin, Oint. (Roberts Pharmaceuticals).
Triliotic Plus, Oint. (Thompson Medical Co).
W/Polymyxin B sulfate and neomycin sulfate.
See: Trimixin, Oint (Hance).
W/Polymyxin B sulfate, neomycin sulfate, and hydrocortisone-free alcohol.
See: Biotic-Ophth (Scrip).
HC, Oint. (GlaxoWellcome).

bacitracin-neomycin ointment. (Various Mfr.) Neomycin sulfate equivalent to 3.5 mg base, bacitracin 500 units/g. Topical Oint. Tube 0.5 oz, 1 oz, Ophth. Oint. ⅛ oz. *otc.*
Use: Anti-infective, topical.

bacitracin/neomycin/polymyxin B ointment. (Various Mfr.) Polymyxin B sulfate 10,000 units/g, neomycin sulfate 3.5 mg/g, bacitracin zinc 400 units/g. Tube 3.5 g. *Rx.*
Use: Anti-infective, ophthalmic.

bacitracin and polymyxin b sulfate. Topical Aerosol.
Use: Anti-infective, topical.
See: Polysporin Oint., Pow. (GlaxoWellcome).

bacitracin zinc. (Pharmacia & Upjohn) Sterile pow. 10,000 units, 50,000 units/Vial.
Use: Anti-infective.

•**bacitracin zinc.** U.S.P. 23.
Use: Anti-infective.
W/Neomycin sulfate, polymyxin B sulfate.
See: AK-Spore Ophth. Oint. (Akorn, Inc.).
See: Neomixin, Oint. (Roberts Pharmaceuticals).
Neosporin, Prods. (GlaxoWellcome).
Neotal, Oint. (Roberts Pharmaceuticals).
Ocutricin Ophth. Oint. (Bausch & Lomb Pharmaceuticals).
Triple Antibiotic Ophth. Oint. (Various Mfr.).
W/Neomycin sulfate, polymyxin B, benzalkonium Cl.
See: Coracin, Oint. (Roberts Pharmaceuticals).

bacitracin zinc/neomycin sulfate/polymyxin B sulfate/hydrocortisone. (Various Mfr.) Hydrocortisone 1%, neomycin sulfate 0.35%, bacitracin zinc 400 units, polymyxin B sulfate 10,000 units. Tube 3.5 g *Rx.*
Use: Anti-infective, corticosteroid ophthalmic.

bacitracin zinc ointment. Bacitracin zinc isan anhydrous ointment base. (Alpharma USPD Inc.) Polymyxin B sulfate 10,000 units, bacitracin zinc 500 units. Tube 3.5 g.
Use: Anti-infective, topical.

Bacit White. (Whiteworth Towne) Bacitracin. Oint. Tube 0.5 oz, 1 oz. *otc.*
Use: Anti-infective, topical.

Backache Maximum Strength Relief. (Bristol-Myers Squibb) Magnesium salicylate anhydrous (as tetrahydrate) 467 mg. Capl. Bot. 24s, 50s. *otc.*
Use: Analgesic.

baclofen. (BACK-low-fen) **Tab.:** Bot. 10 mg, 20 mg. 100s, UD 100s; **Intrathecal.:** 10 mg/20 ml, 10 mg/5 ml. Single-use amps 1 amp refill kit (10 mg/20 ml), 2 or 4 amp refill kit (10 mg/5 ml).
Use: Muscle relaxant.

•**baclofen.** U.S.P. 23.
Use: Muscle relaxant.
See: Baclofen, Tab. (Eon Labs Manufacturing, Inc.).
Lioresal, Tab., Intrathecal. (Novartis Pharmaceutical Corp.).

baclofen, l-baclofen. *Rx.*

Use: Treatment of muscle spasticity. [Orphan Drug]

Bacmin. (Marnel Pharmaceuticals, Inc.) Iron 27 mg, Vitamin A 5000 IU, E 30 IU, C 500 mg, B_1 20 mg, B_2 20 mg, B_3 100 mg, B_5 25 mg, B_6 25 mg, B_{12} 50 mcg, biotin 0.15 mg, folic acid 0.8 mg, Cr, Cu, Mg, Mn, Zn 22.5 mg/Tab. Bot. 100s. *Rx.*
Use: Mineral, vitamin supplement.

Bac-Neo-Poly Ointment. (Burgin-Arden) Bacitracin 400 units, neomycin sulfate 5 mg, polymyxin B sulfate 5000 units/g. Tube 5 oz. *otc.*
Use: Anti-infective, topical.

Bactal Soap. (Whittaker General) Triclosan 0.5% and anhydrous soap 10%. Liq. 240 ml, 1/2 gal. *otc.*
Use: Antiseptic, cleaner.

bacteriostatic sodium chloride. (Various Mfr.) Sodium Cl 0.9%. Also contains benzyl alcohol or parabens. Inj. Bot. 10 ml, 20 ml, 30 ml. *Rx.*
Use: Parenteral diluent.

bacteriostatic water for injection. U.S.P. 23. (Abbott Laboratories) 30 ml. Multiple-dose Fliptop vial (plastic).
Use: Pharmaceutic aid for diluting and dissolving drugs for injection.

bacteriuria tests. In vitro diagnostic aids.
See: Isocult for bacteriuria (SmithKline Diagnostics).
Microstix-3 strips (Bayer Corp.(Consumer Div)).
Uricult (Orion Diagnostica).

Bacti-Cleanse. (Pedinol Pharmacal, Inc.) Benzalkonium Cl, mineral oil, isopropyl palmitate, cetyl alcohol, glycerine, glyceryl stearate, PEG-100 stearate, dimethicone, diazolidinyl urea, parabens, DMDM hydantion, EDTA. Liq. Bot. 453.6 g. *otc.*
Use: Dermatolgic cleanser.

Bacticort. (Rugby Labs, Inc.) Hydrocortisone 1%, neomycin sulfate equivalent to 0.35% neomycin base, polymyxin B sulfate 10,000 units/ml, benzalkonium Cl, cetyl alcohol, glyceryl monostearate, mineral oil, polyoxyl 40 stearate, propylene glycol. Ophth. Soln. Bot. 7.5 ml. *Rx.*
Use: Anti-infective, corticosteroid, ophthalmic.

Bactigen Group A Streptococcus. (Wampole Laboratories) Latex agglutination slide test for the qualitative detection of group A streptococcal antigen directly from throat swabs. Test kit 60s.
Use: Diagnostic aid.

Bactigen Group A Streptococcus with Gast Trak Slides. (Wampole Laboratories) Latex agglutination slide test for qualitative detection of group A streptococcal antigen directly from throat swabs. Test 24s. Test kit 48s.
Use: Diagnostic aid.

Bactigen H. Influenzae. (Wampole Laboratories) Rapid latex agglutination slide test for the qualitative detection of *Haemophilus influenzae* type b antigen in cerebrospinal fluid, serum, and urine. Test kit 15s, 30s.
Use: Diagnostic aid.

Bactigen Meningitis Panel. (Wampole Laboratories) Rapid latex agglutination slide test for the qualitative detection of *Haemophilus influenzae* type b, *Neisseria meningitidis* A/B/C/Y/W135, and *Streptococcus pneumoniae* antigens in cerebrospinal fluid, serum, and urine. Test kit 18.
Use: Diagnostic aid.

Bactigen N. Meningitidis. (Wampole Laboratories) Rapid latex agglutination slide test for the qualitative detection of *Neisseria meningitidis*, serogroups A/B/C/Y/W135 antigens in cerebrospinal fluid, serum, and urine. Test kit 15s, 30s.
Use: Diagnostic aid.

Bactigen Salmonella-Shigella. (Wampole Laboratories) Latex agglutination slide test for the qualitative detection of *Salmonella* or *Shigella* from cultures. 96s.
Use: Diagnostic aid.

Bactine Antiseptic/Anesthetic First Aid Spray. (Bayer Corp. (Consumer Div.)) Benzalkonium Cl 0.13%, lidocaine 2.5%. **Squeeze Bot.:** 2 oz, 4 oz. **Liq.:** 16 oz. **Aerosol:** 3 oz. *otc.*
Use: Anesthetic, antiseptic, topical.

Bactine First Aid Antibiotic. (Bayer Corp. (Consumer Div.)) Polymyxin B sulfate 5000 units, bacitracin 500 units, neomycin sulfate 5 mg/g in mineral oil, white petrolatum. Oint. Tube 15 g. *otc.*
Use: Anti-infective, topical.

Bactine First Aid Antibiotic Plus Anesthetic. (Bayer Corp. (Consumer Div.)) Polymyxin B sulfate 5000 units, neomycin 3.5 mg/g, bacitracin 400 units, diperodon HCl 10 mg, in mineral oil and white petrolatum. Oint. Tube 15 g. *otc.*
Use: Anti-infective, topical.

Bactine Hydrocortisone Skin Cream. (Bayer Corp. (Consumer Div.)) Hydrocortisone 0.5%. Tube 0.5 oz. *otc.*
Use: Corticosteroid, topical.

Bactine Maximum Strength. (Bayer Corp. (Consumer Div.)) Hydrocortisone 1%, glycerin, mineral oil, methylpara-

ben, white petrolatum. Cream Tube 30 g. *otc.*
Use: Corticosteroid, topical.

Bactocill. (SmithKline Beecham Pharmaceuticals) Oxacillin sodium. 500 mg, 1 g, 2 g, 4 g, 10 g. Pow. for Inj. Vial (except 10 g); piggyback and *ADD-Vantage* vial (only 1 g and 2 g); Bulk vial (10 g only). *Rx.*
Use: Anti-infective; penicillin.

Bacto Shield Foam. (Steris Laboratories, Inc.) Chlorhexidine gluconate 4%, isopropyl alcohol 4%. Foam. Aerosol. 180 ml. *otc.*
Use: Dermatologic, cleanser.

Bacto Shield Solution. (Steris Laboratories, Inc.) Chlorhexidine gluconate 4%, isopropyl alcohol 4%. Soln. Bot. 960 ml. *otc.*
Use: Dermatologic, cleanser.

Bacto Shield 2. (Steris Laboratories, Inc.) Chlorhexidine glyconate 2%, isopropyl alcohol 4%. Soln. Bot. 960 ml. *otc.*
Use: Preoperative skin preparation/cleanser.

Bactrim. (Roche Laboratories) Sulfamethoxazole 400 mg, trimethoprim 80 mg/Tab. Bot. 100s. *Rx.*
Use: Anti-infective.

Bactrim DS. (Roche Laboratories) Trimethoprim 160 mg, sulfamethoxazole 800 mg/Tab. Bot. 100s, 200s, 500s. *Rx.*
Use: Anti-infective.

Bactrim IV Infusion. (Roche Laboratories) Sulfamethoxazole 400 mg, trimethoprim 80 mg/5 ml. Multidose vials. 10 ml, 30 ml. *Rx.*
Use: Anti-infective.

Bactrim Pediatric Suspension. (Roche Laboratories) Trimethoprim 40 mg, sulfamethoxazole 200 mg/5 ml. Bot. 480 ml. *Rx.*
Use: Anti-infective combination.

Bactrim Suspension. (Roche Laboratories) Sulfamethoxazole 200 mg, trimethoprim 40 mg/5 ml. Bot. 16 oz. *Rx.*
Use: Anti-infective.

Bactroban. (SmithKline Beecham Pharmaceuticals) Mupirocin 2% in a polyethylene glycol base. Topical Oint. Tube 15 g. Mupirocin calcium 2%. Intranasal Oint. Tube 1 g. Mupirocin Calcium 2%, alcohols. Cream Tube 15 g, 30 g. *Rx.*
Use: Anti-infective, topical; anti-infective used in adult patients and health care workers during institutional outbreaks (intranasal).

Bactroban Cream. (SmithKline Beecham) Mupirocin calcium 2%; benzyl, cetyl, steryl alcohols. Cream Tube 15 g, 30 g. *Rx.*
Use: Anti-infective, topical.

Bacturcult. (Wampole Laboratories) A urinary bacteria culture medium diagnostic urine culture system for urine collection, bacteriuria screening, and presumptive bacterial identification. Test kit 10s, 100s.
Use: Diagnostic aid.

Bain de Soleil All Day For Kids SPF 30. (Procter & Gamble Pharm.) Ethylhexyl p-methoxycinnamate, 2-ethyl hexyl 2-cyano-3, 3 diphenyl acrylate, oxybenzone, titanium dioxide, stearyl alcohol, tocopheryl acetate, EDTA. PABA free. Waterproof. Lot. Bot. 120 ml. *otc.*
Use: Sunscreen.

Bain de Soleil All Day Waterproof Sunblock. (Procter & Gamble Pharm.) SPF 15, 30. Ethylhexyl p-methoxycinnamate, 2-ethylhexyl 2-cyano-3, 3-diphenyl acrylate, oxybenzone, titanium dioxide, stearyl alcohol, vitamin E, EDTA. Lot. Bot. 120 ml. *otc.*
Use: Sunscreen.

Bain de Soleil All Day Waterproof Sunfilter. (Procter & Gamble Pharm.) SPF 4, 8. 2-ethylhexyl 2-cyano-3, 3 diphenyl acrylate, ethylhexyl p-methoxycinnamate, titanium dioxide, stearyl alcohol, vitamin E, EDTA. Lot. Bot. 120 ml. *otc.*
Use: Sunscreen.

Bain de Soleil Body Silkening Creme. (Procter & Gamble Pharm.) Padimate O, ethylhexyl p-methoxycinnamate, oxybenzone, benzyl alcohol. Waterproof cream. Bot. 94 g. *otc.*
Use: Sunscreen.

Bain de Soleil Body Silkening Spray. (Procter & Gamble Pharm.) Padimate O, oxybenzone, ethylhexyl p-methoxycinnamate. Waterproof lotion. Bot. 240 ml. *otc.*
Use: Sunscreen.

Bain de Soleil Body Silkening Stick. (Procter & Gamble Pharm.) Padimate O, ethylhexyl p-methoxycinnamate, oxybenzone, dioxybenzone. Stick 53 g. *otc.*
Use: Sunscreen.

Bain de Soleil Face Creme. (Procter & Gamble Pharm.) Padimate O, ethylhexyl p-methoxycinnamate, oxybenzone. Waterproof cream. Bot. 60 g. *otc.*
Use: Sunscreen.

Bain de Soleil Kids Sport. (Procter & Gamble Pharm.) SPF 25. Ethylhexyl-p-methoxycinnamate, 2-ethylhexyl 2-cyano-3, 3-diphenyl acrylate, titanium

dioxide, PVP/eicosene copolymer, dimethicone, cyclomethicone, triethanolamine, glyceryl tribehenate, tocopheryl acetate, carbomer, EDTA, DMDM hydantoin. PABA free. Waterproof, all day protection. Lot. Bot. 120 ml. *otc.*
Use: Sunscreen.

Bain de Soleil Lip Protecteur. (Procter & Gamble Pharm.) Ethylhexyl p-methoxycinnamate, oxybenzone, 2-ethylhexyl salicylate, oleyl alcohol, petrolatum. PABA free lip balm, 3 g. *otc.*
Use: Sunscreen.

Bain de Soleil Megatan. (Procter & Gamble Pharm.) Ethylhexyl p-methoxycinnamate, 2-ethylhexyl salicylate, lanolin, cocoa butter, palm oil, aloe, DMDM hydantoin, xanthan gum, shea butter, EDTA. Lot. Bot. 120 ml. *otc.*
Use: Sunscreen.

Bain de Soleil Orange Gelee SPF 4. (Procter & Gamble Pharm.) Ethylhexyl p-methoxycinnamate, 2-ethylhexyl salicylate. PABA free. Gel Tube 93.75 g. *otc.*
Use: Sunscreen.

Bain de Soleil SPF 8 + Color. (Procter & Gamble Pharm.) Octyl methoxycinnamate, octocrylene, mineral oil, cetyl alcohol, EDTA. Lot. Bot. 118 ml. *otc.*
Use: Sunscreen.

Bain de Soleil SPF 15+ Color. (Procter & Gamble Pharm.) Octyl methoxycinnamate, octocrylene, oxybenzone, mineral oil, cetyl alcohol, EDTA. Lot. Bot. 118 ml. *otc.*
Use: Sunscreen.

Bain de Soleil SPF 30 + Color. (Procter & Gamble Pharm.) Octocrylene, octyl methoxycinnamate, oxybenzone, mineral oil, cetyl alcohol, EDTA. Lot. Bot. 118 ml. *otc.*
Use: Sunscreen.

Bain de Soleil Sport. (Procter & Gamble Pharm.) SPF 15. 2-ethylhexyl 2-cyano-3, 3 diphenylacrylate, ethylhexyl-p-methoxycinnamate, titanium dioxide, dimethicone, cyclomethicone, panthenol, tocopheryl acetate, carbomer, EDTA, DMDM hydantoin. PABA free. Waterproof, sweatproof, all day protection. Lot. Bot. 180 ml. *otc.*
Use: Sunscreen.

Bain de Soleil Tropical Deluxe SPF 4. (Procter & Gamble Pharm.) Ethylhexyl p-methoxycinnamate, 2-ethylhexyl salicylate, cetyl alcohol, EDTA. PABA free. Waterproof. Lot. Bot. 240 ml. *otc.*
Use: Sunscreen.

Bain de Soleil Under Eye. (Procter & Gamble Pharm.) Ethylhexyl p-methoxycinnamate, oxybenzone, 2-ethylhexyl salicylate. Stick 1.5 g. *otc.*
Use: Sunscreen.

Bakers Best. (Scherer Laboratories, Inc.) Water, alcohol 38%, propylene glycol, extract of capsicum, glycerin, boric acid, Tween 80, diethylphthalate, rose oil, pyrilamine maleate, glacial acetic acid, Uvinul MS 40, hexetidine, benzalkonium Cl 50%, sodium hydroxide 76%. Bot. 8 oz. *otc.*
Use: Antipruritic, antiseborrheic, topical.

•**balafilcon A.** (ba-lah-FILL-kahn A) USAN.
Use: Contact lens material (hydrophilic).

Balanced B_{100}. (Fibertone) Vitamins B_1 100 mg, B_2 100 mg, B_3 100mg,B_5 100 mg, B_6 100 mg, B_{12} 100 mcg, folic acid 0.1 mg, PABA 100 mg, inositol 100 mg, d-biotin 100 mcg/SR Tab. Bot. 50s.
Use: Mineral, vitamin supplement.

Balanced Salt Solution. (Various Mfr.) Sodium Cl 0.64%, potassium Cl, 0.075%, calcium Cl 0.048%, magnesium Cl 0.03%, sodium acetate 0.39%, sodium citrate 0.17%, sodium hydroxide or hydrochloric acid. Soln. Droptainer 18 ml, 500 ml.
Use: Irrigant, ophthalmic.

Baldex Ophthalmic Ointment. (Bausch & Lomb Pharmaceuticals) Dexamethasone phosphate 0.05%. 3.75 g. *Rx.*
Use: Corticosteroid, ophthalmic.

Baldex Ophthalmic Solution. (Bausch & Lomb Pharmaceuticals) Dexamethasone phosphate 0.01%. Dropper Bot. 5 ml. *Rx.*
Use: Corticosteroid, ophthalmic.

BAL in Oil. (Becton Dickinson & Co.) 2, 3-dimercaptopropanol 100 mg, benzylbenzoate 210 mg, peanut oil 680 mg/ml. Amp. 3 ml Box 10s. *Rx.*
Use: Antidote.

Balmex Baby Powder. (Block Drug Co., Inc.) Specially purified balsam Peru, zinc oxide, starch, calcium carbonate. Shaker top can. 4 oz. *otc.*
Use: Adsorbent, emollient.

Balmex Ointment. (Block Drug Co., Inc.) Specially purified balsam Peru, Vitamins A and D, zinc oxide, bismuth subnitrate in a base w/silicone. Tube 1 oz, 2 oz, 4 oz. Jar lb. *otc.*
Use: Emollient.

Balneol Perianal Cleansing. (Solvay Pharmaceuticals) Mineral oil, lanolin oil, methylparaben. Bot. 120 ml. *otc.*
Use: Anorectal preparation.

Balnetar. (Westwood Squibb Pharmaceuticals) Tar equivalent to 2.5% coal

tar, U.S.P. 23. Bot. 8 oz. *otc.*
Use: Dermatologic.

•**balsalazide disodium.** (bahl-SAL-ah-zide) USAN.
Use: Anti-inflammatory (gastrointestinal).

Balsan. Specially purified balsam Peru.
See: Balmex Prods. (Block Drug Co., Inc.).

•**bambermycins.** (BAM-ber-MY-sinz) USAN.
Use: Anti-infective.

•**bamethan sulfate.** (BAM-eth-an) USAN.
Use: Vasodilator.

•**bamifylline hydrochloride.** (BAM-ih-FILL-in) USAN.
Use: Bronchodilator.

•**bamnidazole.** (bam-NIH-DAH-zole) USAN.
Use: Antiprotozoal (trichomonas).

Banacid Tablets. (Buffington) Magnesium trisilicate 220 mg. Bot. 100s, 200s, 500s. *otc.*
Use: Antacid.

Banadyne-3. (Norstar Consumer Products, Inc.) Lidocaine 4%, menthol 1%, alcohol 45%. Soln. Bot. 7.5 ml. *otc.*
Use: Mouth and throat preparation.

Banalg. (Forest Pharmaceutical, Inc.) Methyl salicylate 4.9%, camphor 2%, menthol 1%. Lot. Bot. 60 ml, 480 ml. *otc.*
Use: Analgesic, topical.

Banalg Hospital Strength Liniment. (Forest Pharmaceutical, Inc.) Methyl salicylate 14%, menthol 3%. Bot. 60 ml. *otc.*
Use: Analgesic, topical.

Bancap HC. (Forest Pharmaceutical, Inc.) Acetaminophen 500 mg, hydrocodone bitartrate 5 mg/Cap. Bot. 100s, 500s. *c-III.*
Use: Analgesic combination, narcotic.

•**bandage, adhesive.** U.S.P. 23.
Use: Surgical aid.

•**bandage, gauze.** U.S.P. 23.
Use: Surgical aid.

Banex Capsules. (LuChem Pharmaceuticals, Inc.) Phenylpropanolamine HCl 45 mg, phenylephrine HCl 5 mg, guaifenesin 200 mg. Bot. 100s, 500s. *otc.*
Use: Decongestant, expectorant.

Banex-LA Tablets. (LuChem Pharmaceuticals, Inc.) Phenylpropanolamine HCl 75 mg, guaifenesin 400 mg. Bot. 100s, 500s. *otc.*
Use: Decongestant, expectorant.

Banflex. (Forest Pharmaceutical, Inc.) Orphenadrine citrate 30 mg/ml. Inj. Vial 10 ml. *Rx.*
Use: Muscle relaxant.

Bangesic. (H.L. Moore Drug Exchange, Inc.) Menthol, camphor, methyl salicylate, eucalyptus oil in nongreasy base. Bot. 2 oz, gal. *otc.*
Use: Analgesic, topical.

Banocide.
See: Diethylcarbamazine Citrate, U.S.P. 23.

Banophen. (Major Pharmaceuticals) Diphenhydramine HCl. **Cap.:** 25 mg, lactose, parabens. Bot. 100s. **Elixir:** 12.5 mg, alcohol 5.6%, EDTA, saccharin, sugar. Bot. 118 ml, 240 ml. *otc.*
Use: Antihistamine.

Banophen Decongestant. (Major Pharmaceuticals) Diphenhydramine 25 mg, pseudoephedrine 60 mg. Cap. Bot. 24s. *otc.*
Use: Antihistamine, decongestant.

Bansmoke. (Thompson Medical Co.) Benzocaine 6 mg, corn syrup, dextrose, lecithin, sucrose. Gum, Pack 24s. *otc.*
Use: Smoking deterrent.

Banthine. (Schiapparelli Searle) Methantheline bromide 50 mg/Tab. Bot. 100s. *Rx.*
Use: Anticholinergic.

Barbased. (Major Pharmaceuticals) **Tab.:** Butabarbital 0.25 gr or 0.5 gr/Tab. Bot. 1000s. **Elix.:** Butabarbital 30 mg/5 ml, alcohol 7%. Bot. 480 ml. *Rx.*
Use: Hypnotic, sedative.

Barbatose No. 2 Tablets. (Pal-Pak, Inc.) Barbital 64.8 mg/Tab. w/hyoscyamus sulfate, passiflora, valerian. Bot. 1000s. *Rx.*
Use: Sedative.

Barbella Elixir. (Forest Pharmaceutical, Inc.) Phenobarbital 0.25 gr, hyoscyamine sulfate 0.1037 mg, atropine sulfate 0.0194 mg, scopolamine HBr 0.0065 mg, alcohol 23%/5 ml. Bot. 4 oz, gal. *Rx.*
Use: Anticholinergic, antispasmodic, hypnotic, sedative.

Barbella Tablets. (Forest Pharmaceutical, Inc.) Phenobarbital 16.2 mg, atropine sulfate 0.0194 mg, hyoscyamine sulfate 0.1037 mg, hyoscine HBr 0.0065 mg/Tab. Bot. 100s, 1000s, 5000s. *Rx.*
Use: Anticholinergic, antispasmodic, hypnotic, sedative.

Barbeloid. (Pal-Pak, Inc.) Phenobarbital 16.2 mg, hyoscyamine sulfate 0.1037 mg, atropine sulfate 0.0194 mg, scopolamine HBr 0.0065 mg/Tab. Bot. 100s, 1000s. *Rx.*
Use: Anticholinergic, antispasmodic, hypnotic, sedative.

Barbenyl.
See: Phenobarbital.

Barbidonna. (Wallace Laboratories) Phenobarbital 16 mg, hyoscyamine sulfate 0.1286 mg, atropine sulfate 0.025 mg, scopolamine HBr 0.0074 mg, lactose. Tab. Bot. 100s, 500s. *Rx.*
Use: Anticholinergic, antispasmodic, hypnotic, sedative.

Barbidonna No. 2. (Wallace Laboratories) Phenobarbital 32 mg, hyoscyamine sulfate 0.1286 mg, atropine sulfate 0.025 mg, scopolamine HBr 0.0074 mg, lactose. Tab. Bot. 100s. *Rx.*
Use: Anticholinergic, antispasmodic, hypnotic, sedative.

Barbiphenyl.
See: Phenobarbital.

barbital. Barbitone, Deba, Dormonal, Hypnogene, Malonal, Sedeval, Uronal, Veronal, Vesperal, diethylbarbituric acid, diethylmalonylurea.
Use: Hypnotic, sedative.

barbital sodium. Barbitone Sodium, diethylbarbiturate monosodium, diethylmalonylurea sodium, Embinal, Medinal, Veronal Sodium.
Use: Hypnotic, sedative.

barbitone.
See: Barbital.

barbitone sodium.
See: Barbital Sodium.

barbiturate-aspirin combinations.
See: Aspirin-Barbiturate Combinations.

barbiturates, intermediate duration.
See: Butabarbital (Various Mfr.).
Butethal (Various Mfr.).

barbiturates, long duration.
See: Barbital (Various Mfr.).
Mebaral, Tab. (Sanofi Winthrop Pharmaceuticals).
Mephobarbital (Various Mfr.).
Phenobarbital (Various Mfr.).
Phenobarbital Sodium (Various Mfr.).

barbiturates, short duration.
See: Amobarbital (Various Mfr.).
Amobarbital Sodium (Various Mfr.).
Butalbital (Various Mfr.).
Butallylonal (Various Mfr.).
Cyclobarbital (Various Mfr.).
Pentobarbital Salts (Various Mfr.).
Sandoptal.
Secobarbital (Various Mfr.).

barbiturates, ultrashort duration.
See: Hexobarbital.
Neraval.
Pentothal Sodium, Amp. (Abbott Laboratories).
Thiopental Sodium (Various Mfr.).

Barc Gel. (Del Pharmaceuticals, Inc.) Pyrethrins 0.18%, piperonyl butoxide technical 2.2%, petroleum distillate 4.8% in gel base. Tube oz. *otc.*
Use: Pediculicide.

Barc Non-Body Lice Control Spray. (Del Pharmaceuticals, Inc.) Spray can 5 oz. *otc.*
Use: Pediculicide.

Baricon. (Lafayette Pharmaceuticals, Inc.) Barium sulfate 98% Pow. for Susp. UD 340 g. *Rx.*
Use: Radiopaque agent, gastrointestinal.

Baridium. (Pfeiffer Co.) Phenazopyridine HCl 100 mg/Tab. Bot. 32s. *otc.*
Use: Analgesic, urinary.

Bari-Stress M. (Alpharma USPD Inc.) Vitamins B_1 10 mg, B_2 10 mg, niacinamide 100 mg, C 300 mg, B_6 2 mg, B_{12} 4 mcg, folic acid 1.5 mg, calcium pantothenate 20 mg/Cap. or Tab. **Cap.:** Bot. 30s, 100s, 1000s. **Tab.:** Bot. 100s, 1000s. *Rx.*
Use: Mineral, vitamin supplement.

•**barium hydroxide lime.** (BA-ree-uhm) U.S.P. 23.
Use: Carbon dioxide absorbent.

•**barium sulfate.** U.S.P. 23.
Use: Diagnostic aid (radiopaque medium).
See: Anatrast, Paste (Lafayette).
Baricon, Pow. for Susp. (Lafayette).
Barobag, Susp. (Lafayette).
Baro-cat, Susp. (Lafayette).
Barosperse, Pow. for Susp. (Lafayette).
Bear-E-Yum CT, Susp. (Lafayette).
Bear-E-Yum GI, Susp. (Lafayette).
Enecat, Conc. Susp. (Lafayette).
Enhancer, Susp. (Lafayette).
Entrobar, Susp. (Lafayette).
Epi-C, Susp. (Lafayette).
Flo-Coat, Susp. (Lafayette).
HD 85, Susp. (Lafayette).
HD 200 Plus, Pow. for Susp. (Lafayette).
Imager ac, Susp. (Lafayette).
Intropaste, Paste (Lafayette).
Liqui-Coat HD, Susp. (Lafayette).
Liquid Barosperse, Susp. (Lafayette).
Medebar Plus, Susp. (Lafayette).
Medescan, Susp. (Lafayette).
Novopaque, Susp. (LPI Diagnostics).
Pediatric Bear-E-Bag, Susp. (Lafayette).
Prepcat, Susp. (Lafayette).
Quick AC Enema Kit, Susp. (LPI Diagnostics).
Tomocat, Conc. Susp. (Lafayette).
Tonopaque, Pow. for Susp. (Lafayette).

barium sulfate. (Various Mfr.) Pow. for

Susp. Pkg. 1 lb. *Rx.*
Use: Radiopaque agent.
barium sulfate preparation.
See: Fleet.
Barlevite. (Barth's) Vitamins B_6 0.6 mg, B_{12} 3 mcg, pantothenic acid 0.6 mg, D 3 IU, l-lysine 20 mg/0.6 ml. 100-day supply. *otc.*
Use: Vitamin/mineral supplement.
•**barmastine.** (BAR-mast-een) USAN.
Use: Antihistamine.
BarnesHind Cleaning and Soaking Solution. (PBH Wesley Jessen) Cleaning and buffering agents, benzalkonium Cl 0.01%, disodium edetate 0.2%. Bot. 1.2 oz, 4 oz. *otc.*
Use: Contact lens care.
BarnesHind Saline for Sensitive Eyes. (PBH Wesley Jessen) Potassium sorbate 0.13%, EDTA 0.025%. Soln. Bot. 360 ml (2s). *otc.*
Use: Contact lens care.
BarnesHind Wetting & Soaking Solution. (PBH Wesley Jessen) Polyvinyl alcohol, povidone, hydroxyethyl cellulose, octylphenoxy (oxyethylene) ethanol, benzalkonium Cl, edetate disodium. Bot. 4 oz. *otc.*
Use: Contact lens care.
BarnesHind Wetting Solution. (PBH Wesley Jessen) Polyvinyl alcohol, edetate disodium 0.02%, benzalkonium Cl 0.004%. Bot. 35 ml, 60 ml. *otc.*
Use: Contact lens care.
Barobag. (Lafayette) Barium sulfate 97%. Susp. Kit 340 g, 454 g. *Rx.*
Use: Radiopaque agent.
Baro-cat. (Lafayette Pharmaceuticals, Inc.) Barium sulfate 1.5% Susp. Bot. 300 ml, 900 ml, 1900 ml. *Rx.*
Use: Radiopaque agent, gastrointestinal.
Baros. (Lafayette Pharmaceuticals, Inc.) Sodium bicarbonate 460 mg (sodium 126 mg) and tartaric acid 420 mg/g with simethicone. Granules, effervescent. Plastic amp. 3 g. *Rx.*
Use: Diagnostic aid.
Baroset. (Lafayette Pharmaceuticals, Inc.) Air contrast stomach. Unit-of-use kit. Case 12s.
Use: Radiopaque agent.
barosmin.
See: Diosmin.
Barosperse. (Lafayette Pharmaceuticals, Inc.) Barium sulfate 95%. Pow. for Susp. UD 225 g, 340 g, 900 g. Kit 454 g. Bulk 25 lb. *Rx.*
Use: Radiopaque agent.
Basa. (Freeport) Acetylsalicylic acid 324 mg/Tab. Bot. 1000s. *otc.*
Use: Analgesic.
Basaljel. (Wyeth-Ayerst Laboratories) Aluminum carbonate gel. **Susp.:** Equivalent to aluminum hydroxide 400 mg/5 ml. Bot. 355 ml. **Cap.:** Equivalent to 608 mg dried aluminum hydroxide gel or 500 mg aluminum hydroxide. Bot. 100s, 500s. **Tab.:** Equivalent to 608 mg dried aluminum hydroxide gel or 500 mg aluminum hydroxide. Bot. 100s. *otc.*
Use: Antacid.
basic aluminum aminoacetate.
See: Dihydroxyaluminum Aminoacetate.
basic aluminum carbonate.
See: Basaljel, Susp. (Wyeth-Ayerst Laboratories).
basic aluminum glycinate.
See: Dihydroxyaluminum aminoacetate.
basic bismuth carbonate.
See: Bismuth Subcarbonate.
basic bismuth gallate.
See: Bismuth Subgallate (Various Mfr.).
basic bismuth nitrate.
See: Bismuth Subnitrate (Various Mfr.).
basic bismuth salicylate.
See: Bismuth Subsalicylate.
basic fuchsin.
See: Carbol-Fuchsin Topical Soln., U.S.P. 23.
•**basifungin.** (bass-ih-FUN-jin) USAN.
Use: Antifungal.
basiliximab.
Use: Immunosuppressant.
See: Simulect, Pow. for Inj. (Novartis).
Basis, Glycerin Soap. (Beiersdorf, Inc.) **Bar:** Tallow, coconut oil, glycerin. **Sensitive:** Bar 90 g, 150 g. **Normal to dry:** Bar 90 g, 150 g. *otc.*
Use: Dermatologic, cleanser.
Basis, Superfatted Soap. (Beiersdorf, Inc.) **Bar:** Sodium tallowate, sodium cocoate, petrolatum, glycerin, zinc oxide, sodium Cl, titanium dioxide, lanolin, alcohol, beeswax, BHT, EDTA. Bar 99 g, 225 g. *otc.*
Use: Dermatologic, cleanser.
•**batanopride hydrochloride.** (bah-TAN-oh-pride) USAN.
Use: Antiemetic.
•**batelapine maleate.** (bat-EH-lap-EEN) USAN.
Use: Antipsychotic.
•**batimastat.** (bat-IM-ah-stat) USAN.
Use: Antineoplastic.
Baycol. (Bayer Corp. (Allergy Div.)) Cerivastatin sodium 0.2 mg, 0.3 mg, mannitol. Tab. Bot. 100s. *Rx.*

Use: Antihyperlipidemic.

Bayer 8-Hour Timed-Release Aspirin. (Bayer Corp. (ConsumerDiv.)) Aspirin 10 gr (650 mg)/TR Tab. Bot. 30s, 72s, 125s. *otc.*
Use: Analgesic.

Bayer Aspirin, Genuine. (Bayer Corp. (Consumer Div.)) Aspirin 325 mg/Tab. Bot. 50s, 100s, 200s, 300s. Pkg. 12s, 24s. *otc.*
Use: Analgesic.

Bayer Aspirin, Maximum. (Bayer Corp. (Consumer Div.)) Aspirin 500 mg/Tab. Bot. 30s, 60s, 100s. *otc.*
Use: Analgesic.

Bayer Buffered Aspirin. (Bayer Corp. (Consumer Div.)) Buffered aspirin 325 mg. Tab. Bot. 100s. *otc.*
Use: Analgesic.

Bayer Children's Chewable Aspirin. Bayer Corp. (Consumer Div.) Aspirin 1.25 gr (81 mg)/Tab. Bot. 30s. *otc.*
Use: Analgesic.

Bayer Children's Cold Tablets. (Bayer Corp. (Consumer Div.)) Phenylpropanolamine HCl 3.125 mg, aspirin 1.25 gr (81 mg)/Tab. Bot. 30s. *otc.*
Use: Analgesic, decongestant.

Bayer Cough Syrup for Children. (Bayer Corp. (Consumer Div.)) Phenylpropanolamine HCl 9 mg, dextromethorphan HBr 7.5 mg/5 ml w/alcohol 5%. Bot. 3 oz. *otc.*
Use: Antitussive, decongestant.

Bayer Enteric 500 Aspirin, Extra Strength. (Bayer Corp. (Consumer Div.)) Aspirin 500 mg. Tab. Enteric coated. Bot. 60s. *otc.*
Use: Analgesic.

Bayer Enteric Coated Caplets, Regular Strength. (Bayer Corp. (Consumer Div.)) Aspirin 325 mg. Tab. Enteric coated. Bot. 50s, 100s. *otc.*
Use: Analgesic.

Bayer Low Adult Strength. (Bayer Corp. (Consumer Div.)) Aspirin 81 mg, lactose. DR Tab. Bot. 120s. *otc.*
Use: Analgesic.

Bayer Plus Extra Strength. (Bayer Corp. (Consumer Div.)) Aspirin 500 mg buffered with calcium carbonate, magnesium carbonate, magnesium oxide. Cap. Bot. 30s, 60s. *otc.*
Use: Analgesic.

Bayer Select Chest Cold. (Bayer Corp. (Consumer Div.)) Dextromethorphan HBr 15 mg, acetaminophen 500 mg. Capl. Pkg. 16s. *otc.*
Use: Analgesic, antitussive.

Bayer Select Flu Relief. (Bayer Corp. (Consumer Div.)) Acetaminophen 500 mg, pseudoephedrine HCl 30 mg, dextromethorphan HBr 15 mg, chlorpheniramine maleate 2 mg. Capl. Blisterpack 16s. *otc.*
Use: Analgesic, antihistamine, antitussive, decongestant.

Bayer Select Head Cold. (Bayer Corp. (Consumer Div.)) Pseudoephedrine HCl 30 mg, acetaminophen 500 mg. Capl. Pkg. 16s. *otc.*
Use: Analgesic, decongestant, expectorant.

Bayer Select Maximum Strength Backache. (Bayer Corp. (Consumer Div.)) Magnesium salicylate tetrahydrate 580 mg. Capl. Bot. 24s, 50s. *otc.*
Use: Analgesic.

Bayer Select Maximum Strength Headache. (Bayer Corp. (Consumer Div.)) Acetaminophen 500 mg, caffeine 65 mg/Cap. Bot. 36s. *otc.*
Use: Analgesic combination.

Bayer Select Maximum Strength Menstrual. (Bayer Corp. (Consumer Div.)) Acetaminophen 500 mg, pamabrom 25 mg/Capl. Bot. 24s, 50s. *otc.*
Use: Analgesic, diuretic.

Bayer Select Maximum Strength Night Time Pain Relief. (Bayer Corp. (Consumer Div.)) Acetaminophen 500 mg, diphenhydramine HCl/Tab. Bot. 24s, 50s. *otc.*
Use: Antihistamine.

Bayer Select Maximum Strength Sinus Pain Relief. (Bayer Corp. (Consumer Div.)) Acetaminophen 500 mg, pseudoephedrine HCl 30 mg/Tab. Bot. 50s. *otc.*
Use: Analgesic, decongestant.

Bayer Select Night Time Cold. (Bayer Corp. (Consumer Div.)) Acetaminophen 500 mg, pseudoephedrine HCl 30 mg, dextromethorphan HBr 15 mg, triprolidine HCl 1.25 mg. Capl. Blister-pack 16s. *otc.*
Use: Analgesic, antihistamine, antitussive, decongestant.

BayHep B. (Bayer Corp. (Consumer Div.)) Hepatitis B immune globulin (Human). Vial 250 unit, prefilled syringe 250 unit. Vial 1 ml. *Rx.*
Use: Immunization.

Baylocaine 2% Viscous. (Bay Labs) Lidocaine 2% w/sodium carboxymethylcellulose. Soln. Bot. 100 ml. *otc.*
Use: Local anesthetic, topical.

Baylocaine 4%. (Bay Labs) Lidocaine 4% w/methylparaben. Soln. Bot. 50 ml, 100 ml.
Use: Anesthetic, local.

Baypress. *Rx.*

Use: Type II calcium channel blocking agent.
See: Nitrendipine.

Bayrab. (Bayer Corp. (Consumer Div.)) Rabies immune globulin (Human) 150 IU/ml. Vial 2 ml, 10 ml. *Rx.*
Use: Immunization.

BayRho D. (Bayer Corp. (Consumer Div.)) Rh_o(D) immune globulin (Human). Prefilled single-dose syringe. Single-dose syringe. Single-dose vial. Pkg. *Rx.*
Use: Immunization.

Baytet. (Bayer Corp. (Consumer Div.)) Tetanus immune globulin (Human). Vial 250 units, Disp. Syringe 250 units. *Rx.*
Use: Immunization.

BC-1000. (Solvay Pharmaceuticals) Vitamins B_1 50 mg, B_2 5 mg, B_{12} 1000 mcg, B_6 5 mg, d-panthenol 6 mg, niacinamide 125 mg, ascorbic acid 50 mg, benzyl alcohol 1%/ml. Vial 10 ml. *otc.*
Use: Vitamin supplement.

BC Arthritis Strength. (Block Drug Co., Inc.) Aspirin 742 mg, salicylamide 222 mg, caffeine 36 mg/Pow. Bot. 6s, 24s, 50s. *otc.*
Use: Analgesic combination.

B-C-Bid. (Roberts Pharmaceuticals) Vitamins B_1 15 mg, B_2 10 mg, B_3 50 mg,B_5 10 mg, B_6 5 mg, vitamin C 300 mg, B_{12} 5 mcg /Cap. Bot. 30s, 100s, 500s. *otc.*
Use: Mineral, vitamin supplement.

B-C Bid Caplets. (Roberts Pharmaceuticals) Vitamin C 300 mg, B_1 15 mg, B_2 10.2 mg, B_3 50 mg, B_5 10 mg B_6 5 mg/Cap. Bot. 100s. *otc.*
Use: Vitamin supplement.

BC Cold-Sinus-Allergy Powder. (Block Drug Co., Inc.) Phenylpropanolamine HCl 25 mg, chlorpheniramine maleate 4 mg, aspirin 650 mg, lactose. Pow. Pck. 6s, 24s. *otc.*
Use: Analgesic, antihistamine, decongestant.

BC Cold-Sinus Powder. (Block Drug Co., Inc.) Phenylpropanolamine HCl 25 mg, aspirin 650 mg, lactose. Pkg. 6s. *otc.*
Use: Decongestant combination.

•**bcg vaccine.** U.S.P. 23.
Use: Immunization.

BCG vaccine. (Organon, Inc.) Prepared from Tice strain of BCG bacillus. Amp. 2 ml. *Rx.*
Use: Immunization against tuberculosis, active.
See: Tice BCG (Organon, Inc.).

BCG for Intravesicular Use.
Use: Antineoplastic.
See: TheraCys (Pasteur Merieux Connaught).
TICE BCG, Pow. for Susp. (Organon, Inc.).

BCNU.
Use: Antineoplastic.
See: BiCNU, Inj. (Bristol-Myers Squibb).

BCO. (Western Research) Vitamins B_1 10 mg, B_2 2 mg, B_6 1.5 mg, B_{12} 25 mcg, niacinamide 50 mg/Tab. Bot. 1000s. *otc.*
Use: Vitamin supplement.

B-Com. (Century Pharmaceuticals, Inc.) Vitamins B_1 3 mg, B_2 3 mg, B_6 0.5 mg, niacinamide 20 mg, calcium pantothenate 5 mg, B_{12} 1 mcg, desiccated liver (undefatted) 60 mg, debittered brewer's dried yeast 60 mg/Cap. Bot. 100s, 1000s. *otc.*
Use: Mineral, vitamin supplement.

B-Complex 25-25 Inj. (Forest Pharmaceutical, Inc.) Niacinamide 100 mg, Vitamins B_1 25 mg, B_2 1 mg, B_6 2 mg, pantothenic acid 2 mg/ml. Vial 30 ml. *Rx.*
Use: Vitamin supplement.

B-Complex "50". (Vitaline Corp.) Vitamins B_1 50 mg, B_2 50 mg, B_3 50 mg, B_4 50 mg, B_5 50 mg, B_6 50 mg, B_{12} 50 mcg, FA 0.1 mg, PABA 30 mg, inositol 50 mg, biotin 50 mcg, choline bitartrate 50 mg. Reg. or TR tabs. Bot. 90s, 1000s. *otc.*
Use: Vitamin supplement.

B-Complex-50. (Nion Corp.) Vitamins B_1 50 mg, B_2 50 mg, B_3 50 mg, B_5 50 mg, B_6 50 mg, B_{12} 50 mcg, FA 0.4 mg, biotin 50 mcg, PABA 50 mg, choline bitartrate 50 mg, inositol 50 mg/SR Tab. Bot. 100s. *otc.*
Use: Mineral, vitamin supplement.

B-Complex#100. (Medical Chem) Vitamins B_1 100 mg, B_2 2 mg, B_6 4 mg, d-panthenol 4 mg, niacinamide 100 mg/ml. Vial 30 ml. *Rx.*
Use: Vitamin supplement.

B-Complex 100. (Rabin-Winters) Vitamins B_1 100 mg, B_2 2 mg, B_6 2 mg, niacinamide 125 mg, panthenol 10 mg/ml. Vial 30 ml. *Rx.*
Use: Vitamin supplement.

B-Complex 100/100. (Sandia) Vitamins B_1 100 mg, B_2 2 mg, B_6 2 mg, niacinamide 100 mg/ml. Inj. Vial 30 ml. *Rx.*
Use: Vitamin supplement.

B-Complex-150. (Nion Corp.) Vitamins B_1 150 mg, B_2 150 mg, B_3 150 mg, B_5 150 mg, B_6 150 mg, B_{12} 1 mcg, FA 0.4 mg, biotin 150 mcg, PABA 100 mg, choline bitartrate 150 mg, inositol 150 mg. SR Tab. Bot. 30s. *otc.*
Use: Mineral, vitamin supplement.

B-Complex and B_{12}. (NBTY, Inc.) Vitamins B_1 7 mg, B_2 14 mg, B_3 4.5 mg,

B_{12} 25 mcg, protease 10 mg/Tab. Bot. 90s. *otc.*
Use: Vitamin supplement.

B-Complex with B-12. (Zenith Goldline Pharmaceuticals) B_1 1.5 mg, B_2 1.7 mg, B_3 20 mg, B_5 10 mg, B_6 2 mg, B_{12} 6 mcg, FA 0.4 mg/Tab. Bot. 100s *otc.*
Use: Mineral, vitamin supplement.

B-Complex Capsules. (Arcum) Vitamins B_1 1.5 mg, B_2 2 mg, niacinamide 10 mg, B_6 0.1 mg, calcium pantothenate 1 mg, desiccated liver 70 mg, dried yeast 100 mg/Cap. Bot. 100s, 1000s. *otc.*
Use: Mineral, vitamin supplement.

B-Complex Capsules J.F. (Bryant) Vitamins B_1 1 mg, B_2 0.3 mg, nicotinic acid 0.3 mg, B_6 0.25 mg, desiccated liver 0.15 g, yeast powder, dried 0.15 g/Cap. Bot. 100s, 1000s. *otc.*
Use: Mineral, vitamin supplement.

B-Complex Elixir. (Nion Corp.) B_1 2.3 mg, B_2 1 mg, B_3 6.7 mg, B_6 0.3 mg, alcohol 10%. Elix. Bot. 240 ml, 480 ml. *otc.*
Use: Mineral, vitamin supplement.

B-Complex Injection with Vitamin C.
Use: Vitamin supplement.
See: Cplex Cap. (Arcum).

B Complex with B_{12} Capsules. (Bryant) Vitamins B_1 2 mg, B_2 2 mg, B_6 0.5 mg, niacinamide 10 mg, B_{12} 2 mcg, biotin 10 mcg, calcium pantothenate 1.5 mg, choline dihydrogen citrate 40 mg, inositol 30 mg, desiccated liver 1 gr, brewer's yeast 3 gr/Cap. Bot. 100s, 1000s. *otc.*
Use: Mineral, vitamin supplement.

B-Complex/Vitamin C Caplets. (Geneva Pharmaceuticals) Vitamins B_1 15 mg, B_2 10.2 mg, B_3 50 mg, B_5 10 mg, B_6 5 mg, C 300 mg/Capl. Bot. 100s. *otc.*
Use: Vitamin supplement.

B-Complex with Vitamin C and B_{12}-10,000. (Fujisawa USA, Inc.) Vitamins B_1 20 mg, B_2 3 mg, B_3 75 mg, B_5 5 mg, B_6 5 mg, B_{12} 1000 mcg, C 100 mg. Covial. 10 ml multiple dose. *Rx.*
Use: Vitamin supplement.

B Complex + C. (Various Mfr.) Vitamins B_1 15 mg, B_2 10 mg, B_3 100 mg, B_5 20 mg, B_6 5 mg, B_{12} 10 mcg, C 500 mg/Tab. Bot. 100s. *otc.*
Use: Vitamin supplement.

B-Complex + C. (NBTY, Inc.) Vitamins C 200 mg, B_1 10 mg, B_2 10 mg, B_3 50 mg, B_5 10 mg, B_6 5 mg/Tab. Bot. 100s. *otc.*
Use: Vitamin supplement.

B Complex with C and B-12 Injection. (Zenith Goldline Pharmaceuticals) Vitamins B_1 50 mg, B_2 5 mg, B_3 125 mg, B_5 6 mg, B_6 5 mg, B_{12} 1000 mcg, C 50 mg/Inj. 10 ml. *Rx.*
Use: Vitamin supplement.

BC Powder. (Block Drug Co., Inc.) Aspirin 650 mg, salicylamide 145 mg, caffeine 32 mg/Pow. Pkg. 2s, 6s, 24s, 50s. *otc.*
Use: Analgesic combination.

BC Powder, Arthritis Strength. (Block Drug Co., Inc.) Aspirin 742 mg, salicylamide 222 mg, caffeine 36 mg/Powder. Pkg. 6s, 24s, 50s. *otc.*
Use: Analgesic combination.

BC Tablets. (Block Drug Co., Inc.) Aspirin 325 mg, salicylamide 95 mg, caffeine 16 mg/Tab. Pkg. 4s. Bot. 50s, 100s. *otc.*
Use: Analgesic combination.

B-C with Folic Acid. (Geneva Pharmaceuticals) Vitamins B_1 15 mg, B_2 15 mg, B_3 100 mg, B_5 18 mg, B_6 4 mg, B_{12} 5 mcg, C 500 mg, folic acid 0.5 mg/Tab. Bot. 100s. *Rx.*
Use: Mineral, vitamin supplement.

B-C w/Folic Acid Plus. (Geneva Pharmaceuticals) Fe 27 mg, vitamins A 5000 IU, E 30 IU, B_1 20 mg, B_2 20 mg, B_3 100 mg, B_5 25 mg, B_6 25 mg, B_{12} 50 mcg, C 500 mg, FA 0.8 mg, biotin 0.15 mg, Cr, Cu, Mg, Mn, Zn 22.5 mg. Tab. Bot. 100s. *Rx.*
Use: Mineral, vitamin supplement.

B-Day Tablets. (Barth's) Vitamins B_1 7 mg, B_2 14 mg, niacin 4.67 mg, B_{12} 5 mcg/Tab. Bot. 100s, 500s. *otc.*
Use: Vitamin supplement.

B-D Glucose. (Becton Dickinson & Co.) Glucose 5 g. Chew. Tab. Bot. 36s. *otc.*
Use: Hyperglycemic.

B Dozen. (Standex) Vitamin B_{12} 25 mcg Tab. Bot. 1000s. *otc.*
Use: Vitamin supplement.

B-Dram w/C Computabs. (Dram) Vitamins B_1 5 mg, B_2 10 mg, B_6 5 mg, nicotinamide 50 mg, calcium pantothenate 20 mg/Tab. Bot. 100s. *otc.*
Use: Mineral, vitamin supplement.

Beano. (AK Pharma, Inc.) Alpha-D-galactosidase derived from *Aspergillus niger*, a fungal source in carrier of water and glycerol. Liq. Bot. 75 serving size at 5 drops per dose. Tab. Pkg. 12s. Bot. 30s, 100s. *otc.*
Use: Antiflatulent.

Bear-E-Yum CT. (Lafayette) Barium sulfate 1.5%. Susp. Bot. 200 ml, 1900 ml. *Rx.*
Use: Radiopaque agent.

Bear-E-Yum GI. (Lafayette) Barium sulfate 60%. Susp. Bot. 200 ml, 1900 ml. *Rx.*

Use: Radiopaque agent.

Bebatab No. 2. (Freeport) Belladonna 1/6 gr, phenobarbital 0.25 gr/Tab. Bot. 1000s. *Rx.*
Use: Anticholinergic, antispasmodic, hypnotic, sedative.

•**becanthone hydrochloride.** (BEE-kan-thone) USAN.
Use: Antischistosomal.

•**becaplermin.** (beh-kah-PLER-min) USAN.
Use: Chronic dermal ulcers treatment.
See: Regranex, Gel (Ortho McNeil Pharmaceutical).

Beceevite Capsules. (Halsey Drug Co.) Vitamins C 300 mg, B_1 15 mg, B_2 10 mg, niacin 50 mg, B_6 5 mg, pantothenic acid 10 mg/Tab. Bot. 100s. *otc.*
Use: Vitamin supplement.

•**beclomethasone dipropionate.** (BEK-low-METH-uh-zone die-PRO-peo-uh-NATE) U.S.P. 23.
Use: Corticosteroid, topical.
See: Beclovent Inhalation Aerosol (GlaxoWellcome).
Beconase (GlaxoWellcome).
Vancenase (Schering-Plough Corp.).
Vanceril (Schering-Plough Corp.).

beclomycin dipropionate.
Use: Corticosteroid.

Beclovent Inhalation Aerosol. (Glaxo-Wellcome) Beclomethasone dipropionate 42 mcg/actuation. Canister 6.7 g (80 metered doses), 16.8 g (200 metered doses), adapter. Refill canister 16.8 g. *Rx.*
Use: Corticosteroid.

Becomp-C. (Cenci, H.R. Labs, Inc.) Vitamins C 250 mg, B_1 25 mg, B_2 10 mg, nicotinamide 50 mg, B_6 2 mg, calcium pantothenate 10 mg, hesperidin complex 50 mg/Cap. Bot. 100s, 500s. *otc.*
Use: Mineral, vitamin supplement.

Beconase. (GlaxoWellcome) Beclomethasone dipropionate 42 mcg/actuation. Canister 6.7 g (80 metered doses), 16.8 g (200 metered doses). *Rx.*
Use: Corticosteroid.

Beconase AQ. (GlaxoWellcome) Beclomethasone dipropionate 0.042%. Spray. Pump aerosol bot. 25 g (G 200 metered inhalations). *Rx.*
Use: Corticosteroid.

Becotin-T. (Eli Lilly and Co.) Vitamins B_1 15 mg, B_2 10 mg, B_6 5 mg, niacinamide 100 mg, pantothenic acid 20 mg, B_{12} 4 mcg, C 300 mg/Tab. Bot. 100s, 1000s, Blister pkg. 10 × 10s. *otc.*
Use: Vitamin supplement.

•**bectumomab.** (beck-TYOO-moe-mab) USAN.
Use: Monoclonal antibody (diagnosis of non-Hodgkin's lymphoma and detection of AIDS-related lymphoma).

Bedoce. (Lincoln Diagnostics) Crystalline anhydrous vitamin B_{12} 1000 mcg/ml. Vial 10 ml. *Rx.*
Use: Vitamin supplement.

Bedoce-Gel. (Lincoln Diagnostics) Vitamin B_{12} 1000 mcg/ml in 17% gelatin soln. Vial 10 ml. *Rx.*
Use: Vitamin supplement.

Bedside Care. (Sween) Bot. 8 oz, gal.
Use: Dermatologic.

Beeceevites Capsules. (Halsey Drug Co.)
Use: Vitamin supplement.

beechwood creosote.
See: Creosote, N.F.

Bee-Forte w/C. (Rugby Labs, Inc.) Vitamins B_1 25 mg, B_2 12.5 mg, B_3 50 mg, B_5 10 mg, B_6 3 mg, B_{12} 2.5 mcg, C 250 mg/Cap. Bot. 100s. *otc.*
Use: Vitamin supplement.

beef peptones. (Sandia) Water-soluble peptones derived from beef 20 mg/2 ml. Inj. Vial 30 ml. *Rx.*
Use: Nutritional supplement, parenteral.

Beelith. (Beach Pharmaceuticals) Pyridoxine HCl 20 mg, magnesium oxide 600 mg/Tab. Bot. 100s. *otc.*
Use: Mineral, vitamin supplement.

Beepen-VK. (SmithKline Beecham Pharmaceuticals) Penicillin V. **Tab.:** 250 mg. Bot. 1000s; 500 mg. Bot. 500s. **Pow. for Oral Soln.:** 125 mg/5 ml; 250 mg/5 ml Bot. 100 ml, 200 ml. *Rx.*
Use: Anti-infective; penicillin.

Bee-Thi. (Burgin-Arden) Cyanocobalamin 1000 mcg, thiamine HCl 100 mg in isotonic soln. of sodium Cl/ml. Vial 10 ml, 20 ml. *Rx.*
Use: Vitamin supplement.

Bee-Twelve 1000. (Burgin-Arden) Cyanocobalamin 1000 mcg /ml. Vial 10 ml, 30 ml. *Rx.*
Use: Vitamin supplement.

Bee-Zee. (Rugby Labs, Inc.) Vitamins E 45 mg, B_1 15 mg, B_2 10.2 mg, B_3 100 mg, B_5 25 mg, B_6 10 mg, B_{12} 6 mcg, C 600 mg, zinc 5.2 mg/Tab. Bot. 60s. *otc.*
Use: Mineral, vitamin supplement.

Behepan.
See: Vitamin B_{12}.

Belatol No. 1; No. 2. (Cenci, H.R. Labs, Inc.) **No. 1:** Belladonna leaf extract 1/8 gr, phenobarbital 0.25 gr/Tab. 100s, 1000s. **No. 2:** Belladonna leaf extract gr, phenobarbital 0.5 gr/Tab. Bot. 100s,

1000s. *Rx.*
Use: Anticholinergic, antispasmodic, hypnotic, sedative.

Belatol Elixir. (Cenci, H.R. Labs, Inc.) Phenobarbital 20 mg, belladonna 6.75 min/5 ml w/alcohol 45%. Elix. Bot. Pt, gal. *Rx.*
Use: Anticholinergic, antispasmodic, hypnotic, sedative.

Belbutal No. 2 Kaptabs. (Churchill) Phenobarbital 32.4 mg, hyoscyamine sulfate 0.1092 mg, atropine sulfate 0.0215 mg, hyoscine HBr 0.0065 mg/Tab. Bot. 100s. *Rx.*
Use: Anticholinergic, antispasmodic, hypnotic, sedative.

Beldin. (Halsey Drug Co.) Diphenhydramine HCl 12.5 mg/5 ml w/alcohol 5%. Bot. gal. *otc.*
Use: Antihistamine.

Belexal. (Pal-Pak, Inc.) Vitamins B_1 1.5 mg, B_2 2 mg, B_6 0.167 mg, calcium pantothenate 1 mg, niacinamide 10 mg/Tab. w/brewer's yeast. Bot. 1000s, 5000s. *otc.*
Use: Mineral, vitamin supplement.

Belexon Fortified Improved. (APC) Liver fraction No. 2, 3 gr, yeast extract 3 gr, vitamins B_1 5 mg, B_2 6 mg, niacinamide 10 mg, calcium pantothenate 2 mg, cyanocobalamin 1 mcg, iron 10 mg/Cap. Bot. 100s. *otc.*
Use: Mineral, vitamin supplement.

Belfer. (Forest Pharmaceutical, Inc.) Vitamins B_1 2 mg, B_2 2 mg, B_{12} 10 mcg, B_6 2 mg, C 50 mg, iron 17 mg/Tab. Bot. 100s. *otc.*
Use: Mineral, vitamin supplement.

•**belfosdil.** (bell-FOSE-dill) USAN.
Use: Antihypertensive (calcium channel blocker).

Belganyl. CDC anti-infective agent. *Rx.*
See: Suramin.

belladonna alkaloids.
Use: Anticholinergic, antispasmodic.
W/Combinations.
See: Fitacol Stankaps (Standex).
Nilspasm, Tab. (Parmed Pharmaceuticals, Inc.).
Urised, Tab. (PolyMedica Pharmaceuticals).
Wigraine, Tab., Supp. (Organon Teknika Corp).
Wyanoids, Supp. (Wyeth-Ayerst Laboratories).

belladonna alkaloids w/phenobarbital. (Various Mfr.) Atropine sulfate 0.0194 mg, scopolamine HBr 0.0065 mg, hyoscyamine HBr or SO_4 0.1037 mg, phenobarbital 16.2 mg/Tab. Bot. 20s, 1000s, UD 100s. *Rx.*
Use: Anticholinergic, antispasmodic, hypnotic, sedative.

•**belladonna extract.** U.S.P. 23.
Use: Antispasmodic.

belladonna extract. (Eli Lilly and Co.) 15 mg (0.187 mg belladonna)/Tab.
Use: Antispasmodic.

belladonna extract combinations.
Use: Anticholinergic, antispasmodic.
See: B & O Supprettes (PolyMedica Pharmaceuticals).
Butibel, Tab., Elix. (Ortho McNeil Pharmaceutical).

belladonna leaf.
Use: Antispasmodic.

belladonna leaf, phenobarbital and benzocaine.
Use: Anticholinergic.

belladonna products and phenobarbital combinations.
Use: Anticholinergic, antispasmodic, hypnotic, sedative.
See: Atrocap, Cap. (Freeport).
Atrosed, Tab. (Freeport).
Bebatab, Tab. (Freeport).
Belatol, Tab., Elix. (Cenci, H.R. Labs, Inc.).
Bellergal, Tab., Spacetab. (Novartis Pharmaceutical Corp.).
Chardonna, Tab. (Rhone-Poulenc Rorer Pharmaceuticals, Inc.).
Donnatal, Tab., Extentab, Cap., Elix. (Wyeth-Ayerst Laboratories).
Donnatal #2, Tab. (Wyeth-Ayerst Laboratories).
Donnazyme, Tab. (Wyeth-Ayerst Laboratories).
Phenobarbital and Belladonna, Tab. (Eli Lilly and Co).
Sedapar, Tab. (Parmed Pharmaceuticals, Inc).
Spabelin, Tab. (Arcum).
Spabelin No 2, Tab. (Arcum).

belladonna tincture. (Eli Lilly and Co.) Bot. 4 oz, 16 oz.
Use: Antispasmodic.

Bellaneed. (Hanlon) Belladonna, phenobarbital 16 mg/Cap. Bot. 100s. *Rx.*
Use: Anticholinergic, antispasmodic, hypnotic, sedative.

Bell/ans. (C. S. Dent & Co. Division) Sodium bicarbonate 520 mg, sodium content 144 mg/Tab. Bot. 30s, 60s. *otc.*
Use: Antacid.

Bellastal. (Wharton) Atropine sulfate 0.0194 mg, scopolamine HBr 0.0065 mg, hyoscyamine HBr or SO_4 0.1037 mg, phenobarbital 16.2 mg Cap. Bot. 1000s. *Rx.*
Use: Anticholinergic, antispasmodic.

Bellatal. (Richwood Pharmaceuticals)

Phenobarbital 16.2 mg (hyoscyamine sulfate 0.1037 mg, atropine sulfate 0.0194 mg, scopolamine HBr 0.0065 mg), lactose/Tab. Bot. 100s, 500s. *Rx.*
Use: Hypnotic, sedative.

Bellergal-S. (Novartis Pharmaceutical Corp.) Ergotamine tartrate 0.6 mg, bellafoline 0.2 mg, phenobarbital 40 mg, tartrazine, lactose, sucrose. SR Tab. Bot. 100s. *Rx.*
Use: Anticholingergic, antispasmodic, hypnotic, sedative.

•**beloxamide.** (bell-OX-ah-mid) USAN.
Use: Antihyperlipoproteinemic.

•**beloxepin.** (beh-LOX-eh-pin) USAN.
Use: Antidepressant.

Bel-Phen-Ergot SR. (Zenith Goldline Pharmaceuticals) Phenobarbital 40 mg, ergotamine tartrate 0.6 mg, l-alkaloids of belladonna 0.2 mg. Tab. Bot. 100s. *Rx.*
Use: Anticholingergic.

Bel-Phen-Ergot SR. (Zenith Goldline Pharmaceuticals) l-alkaloids of belladonna 0.2 mg, phenobarbital 40 mg, ergotamine tartrate 0.6 mg, lactose/SR Tabs. Bot. 100s. *Rx.*
Use: Anticholinergic.

•**bemarinone hydrochloride.** (BEH-mah-rih-NOHN) USAN.
Use: Cardiovascular agent (positive inotropic, vasodilator).

•**bemesetron.** (beh-meh-SET-rone) USAN.
Use: Antiemetic.

Beminal 500. (Whitehall Robins Laboratories) Vitamins B_1 25 mg, B_2 12.5 mg, B_3 100 mg, B_6 10 mg, B_5 20 mg, C 500 mg, B_{12} 5 mcg/Tab. Bot. 100s. *otc.*
Use: Vitamin supplement.

Beminal Forte w/Vit. C. (Wyeth-Ayerst Laboratories) Vitamins B_1 25 mg, B_2 12.5 mg, niacinamide 50 mg, B_6 3 mg, calcium pantothenate 10 mg, C 250 mg, B_{12} 2.5 mcg/Cap. Bot. 100s. *otc.*
Use: Mineral, vitamin supplement.

Beminal Stress Plus Iron. (Wyeth-Ayerst Laboratories) Vitamins B_1 25 mg, B_2 12.5 mg, B_3 100 mg, B_5 20 mg, B_6 10 mg, B_{12} 25 mcg, folic acid 400 mcg, C 700 mg, E 45 IU, iron 27 mg. Dye-free. Tab. Bot. 60s. *otc.*
Use: Mineral, vitamin supplement.

Beminal Stress Plus Zinc. (Wyeth-Ayerst Laboratories) Vitamins B_1 25 mg, B_2 12.5 mg, B_3 100 mg, B_5 20 mg, B_6 10 mg, B_{12} 25 mcg, C 700 mg, E 45 IU, zinc 45 mg/Tab. Bot. 60s, 250s. *otc.*
Use: Mineral, vitamin supplement.

•**bemitradine.** (beh-MIH-trah-DEEN) USAN.
Use: Antihypertensive, diuretic.

•**bemoradan.** (beh-MOE-rah-DAN) USAN.
Use: Cardiovascular agent.

Benacen. (Cenci, H.R. Labs, Inc.) Probenecid 0.5 g/Tab. Bot. 100s, 1000s. *Rx.*
Use: Anitgout.

Benacol. (Cenci, H.R. Labs, Inc.) Dicyclomine HCl 20 mg/Tab. Bot. 100s, 1000s. *Rx.*
Use: Anticholinergic, antispasmodic.

benactyzine hydrochloride. 2-Diethylaminoethyl benzilate HCl.
Use: Anxiolytic.

benactyzine/meprobamate. Psychotherapeutic combination.

Benadryl. (Parke-Davis) Diphenhydramine HCl. **Cream:** 1%. Tube 1 oz. **Elix. (w/alcohol 14%):** 12.5 mg/5 ml. Bot. 4 oz, pt, gal, UD 5 ml 100s. **Spray:** 1%. Bot. 2 oz. **Tab.:** 25 mg. Bot. 100s. *otc.*
Use: Antihistamine.

Benadryl Allergy. (Warner Lambert Consumer Healthcare) Diphenhydramine HCl, phenylalanine 4. **Chew. Tab.:** 12.5 mg/Tab. Pkg. 24s. **Liq.:** 6.25 mg/5 ml. Liq. Bot. 118 ml. *otc.*
Use: Antihistamine.

Benadryl Allergy Decongestant Liquid. (Warner Lambert Consumer Healthcare) Pseudoephedrine HCl 30 mg, diphenhydramine HCl 12.5 mg/5 ml. Liq. Bot. 118 ml. *otc.*
Use: Antihistamine, decongestant.

Benadryl Allergy/Sinus Headache Caplets. (Warner Lambert Consumer Healthcare) Pseudoephedrine HCl 30 mg, diphenhydramine HCl 12.5 mg, acetaminophen 500 mg/Capl. Bot. 24s. *otc.*
Use: Analgesic, antihistamine, decongestant.

Benadryl Allergy Ultratabs. (Warner Lambert Consumer Healthcare) Diphenhydramine HCl 25 mg. Tab. 24s, 48s. *otc.*
Use: Antihistamine.

Benadryl Cold Liquid. (Parke-Davis) Pseudoephedrine HCl 10 mg, diphenhydramine HCl 8.3 mg, acetaminophen 167 mg, alcohol 10%, saccharin. Liq. Bot. 180 ml. *otc.*
Use: Antihistamine, decongestant.

Benadryl Cough Preparation.
See: Benylin Cough Syrup (Parke-Davis).

Benadryl Decongestant Allergy. (Warner Lambert Consumer Healthcare) Diphenhydramine HCl 25 mg,

pseudoephedrine HCl 60 mg/Cap. Box 24s. *otc.*
Use: Antihistamine, decongestant.

Benadryl Dye Free. (Warner Lambert Consumer Healthcare) Diphenhydramine HCl 6.25 mg/5 ml. Liq. 236 ml. *otc.*
Use: Antihistamine.

Benadryl Dye-Free Allergy Liqui Gels. (Parke-Davis) Diphenhydramine HCl 25 mg, sorbitol/Softgel Cap. Bot. 24s. *otc.*
Use: Antihistamine.

Benadryl Dye Free LiquiGels. (Glaxo-Wellcome) Diphenhydramine HCl 25 mg/Cap. Pkg. 24s. *otc.*
Use: Antihistamine.

Benadryl Elixir. (Parke-Davis) Diphenhydramine HCl 12.5 mg/5 ml w/alcohol 14%. Bot. 4 oz, pt, gal, UD (5 ml) 100s. *otc.*
Use: Antihistamine.

Benadryl Injection. (Parke-Davis) Diphenhydramine HCl. 50 mg/ml Inj. Amp. 1 ml, Steri-Vials 10 ml, Steri-dose syringe 1 ml. *Rx.*
Use: Antihistamine.

Benadryl Itch Relief. (GlaxoWellcome) Diphenhydramine HCl 1%, zinc acetate 0.1%, alcohol 73.6%, aloe vera. Spray. Bot. 59 ml. *otc.*
Use: Antihistamine.

Benadryl Itch Relief Children's. (Glaxo-Wellcome) **Cream:** Diphenhydramine HCl 1%, zinc acetate 0.1%, aloe vera, cetyl alcohol, parabens. Jar 14.2 g. **Spray:** Diphenhydramine HCl 1%, zinc acetate 0.1%, alcohol 73.6%, aloe vera, povidone. Can. 59 ml. *otc.*
Use: Antihistamine.

Benadryl Itch Relief, Maximum Strength. (GlaxoWellcome) **Cream:** Diphenhydramine HCl 2%, zinc acetate 0.1%, parabens, aloe vera. Tube 14.2 g. **Stick:** Diphenhydramine HCl 2%, zinc acetate 0.1%, alcohol 73.5%, aloe vera. Tube 14 ml.

Benadryl Itch Stopping Gel Children's Formula. (GlaxoWellcome) Diphenhydramine HCl 1%, zinc acetate 1%, camphor, parabens. Gel Tube 118 ml. *otc.*
Use: Antihistamine.

Benadryl Itch Stopping Gel Maximum Strength. (GlaxoWellcome) Diphenhydramine HCl 2%, zinc acetate 1%, camphor, parabens. Tube 118 g. *otc.*
Use: Antihistamine.

Benadryl Maximum Strength. (Parke-Davis) **Cream:** Diphenhydramine HCl 2% and parabens in a greaseless base in 15 g. **Non-aerosol spray:** Diphenhydramine HCl 2%, alcohol 85% in 60 ml. *otc.*
Use: Dermatologic.

Benadryl Plus. (Parke-Davis) Pseudoephedrine 30 mg, diphenhydramine 12.5 mg, acetaminophen 500 mg/Tab. 24s. *otc.*
Use: Analgesic, antihistamine, decongestant.

Benadryl Plus Nighttime. (Parke-Davis) Pseudoephedrine 30 mg, diphenhydramine 25 mg, acetaminophen 500 mg/5 ml. 180 ml, 300 ml. *otc.*
Use: Analgesic, antihistamine, decongestant.

Benahist 10. (Keene Pharmaceuticals, Inc.) Diphenhydramine 10 mg/ml. Vial 30 ml. *Rx.*
Use: Antihistamine.

Benahist 50. (Keene Pharmaceuticals, Inc.) Diphenhydramine 50 mg/ml. Vial 10 ml. *Rx.*
Use: Antihistamine.

benanserin hydrochloride.
Use: Serotonin antagonist.

Benaphen Caps. (Major Pharmaceuticals) Diphenhydramine 25 mg or 50 mg/Cap. Bot. 100s, 1000s. *otc.*
Use: Antihistamine.

•**benapryzine hydrochloride.** (BEN-ah-PRY-zeen) USAN.
Use: Anticholinergic.

Benase. (Ferndale Laboratories, Inc.) Proteolytic enzymes extracted from Carica papaya 20,000 units enzyme activity. Tab. Bot. 1000s. *Rx.*
Use: Reduction of edema, relief of episiotomy.

Benat-12. (Roberts Pharmaceuticals) Cyanocobalamin 30 mcg, liver injection 0.5 ml, vitamins B_1 10 mg, B_2 2 mg, niacinamide 50 mg, d-panthenol 1 mg, B_6 1 mg/ml, benzyl alcohol 4%, phenol 0.5%. Vial 10 ml. *Rx.*
Use: Mineral, vitamin supplement.

benazepril and amlodipine.
Use: Antihypertensive.
See: Lotrel (Novartis).

•**benazepril hydrochloride.** (BEN-AZE-eh-prill) USAN.
Use: ACE inhibitor.
See: Lotensin (Novartis Pharmaceutical Corp.).

•**benazeprilat.** (BEN-AZE-eh-prill-at) USAN.
Use: ACE inhibitor.

•**bendacalol mesylate.** (ben-DACK-ah-LOLE) USAN.
Use: Antihypertensive.

•**bendazac.** (BEN-dah-ZAK) USAN.

Use: Anti-inflammatory.

•**bendroflumethiazide.** U.S.P. 23.
Use: Antihypertensive, diuretic.
See: Naturetin, Tab. (Bristol-Myers Squibb).
W/Potassium Cl.
See: Naturetin W-K, Tab. (Bristol-Myers Squibb).
W/Rauwolfia serpentina.
See: Rauzide, Tab. (Bristol-Myers Squibb).

BeneFix. (Genetics Institute) Non-pyrogenic lyophilized powder preparation. Purified protein produced by recombinant DNA. Single-dose vial with diluent needle, filter, infusion set and alcohol swabs. 250, 500, and 1000 IU. *Rx.*
Use: For use in therapy of Factor IX deficiency.

Benemid. (Merck & Co.) Probenecid 0.5 g/Tab. Bot. 100s, 1000s, UD 100s. *Rx.*
Use: Antigout.

Benephen Antiseptic Medicated Powder. (Halsted) Methylbenzethonium Cl 1:1800, magnesium carbonate in corn starch base. Shaker can 3.56 oz. *otc.*
Use: Antiseptic, deodorant.

Benephen Antiseptic Ointment w/Cod Liver Oil. (Halsted) Methylbenzethonium Cl 1:1000, water-repellent base of zinc oxide, corn starch. Tube 1.5 oz, jar lb. *otc.*
Use: Antiseptic.

Benephen Antiseptic Vitamin A & D Cream. (Halsted) Methylbenzethonium Cl 1:1000, cod liver oil w/vitamins A and D in petrolatum and glycerin base. Tube 2 oz, jar lb. *otc.*
Use: Antiseptic.

Benepro Tabs. (Major Pharmaceuticals) Probenecid 500 mg/Tab. Bot. 100s, 1000s. *Rx.*
Use: Antigout.

bengal gelatin.
See: Agar.

Ben-Gay Children's Vaporizing Rub. (Pfizer US Pharmaceutical Group) Camphor, menthol, w/oils of turpentine, eucalyptus, cedar leaf, nutmeg, thyme in stainless white base. Jar 1. 125 oz. *otc.*
Use: Analgesic, topical.

Ben-Gay Extra Strength Balm. (Pfizer US Pharmaceutical Group) Methyl salicylate 30%, menthol 8%. Jar 3.75 oz. *otc.*
Use: Analgesic, topical.

Ben-Gay Extra Strength Sports Balm. (Pfizer US Pharmaceutical Group) Methyl salicylate 28%, menthol 10%. Tube 1.25 oz, 3 oz. *otc.*
Use: Analgesic, topical.

Ben-Gay Gel. (Pfizer US Pharmaceutical Group) Methyl salicylate 15%, menthol 7%, alcohol 40%. Tube 1.25 oz, 3 oz. *otc.*
Use: Analgesic, topical.

Ben-Gay Greaseless Ointment. (Pfizer US Pharmaceutical Group) Methyl salicylate 18.3%, menthol 16%. Tube 1.25 oz, 3 oz, 5 oz. *otc.*
Use: Analgesic, topical.

Ben-Gay Lotion. (Pfizer US Pharmaceutical Group) Methyl salicylate 15%, menthol 7% in lotion base. Bot. 2 oz, 4 oz. *otc.*
Use: Analgesic, topical.

Ben-Gay Ointment. (Pfizer US Pharmaceutical Group) Methyl salicylate 15%, menthol 10% in ointment base. Tube 1.25 oz, 3 oz, 5 oz. *otc.*
Use: Analgesic, topical.

Ben-Gay Original. (Pfizer US Pharmaceutical Group) Methyl salicylate 18.3% and menthol 16%. Oint. Tube. 37.5 g, 90 g, 150 g. *otc.*
Use: Analgesic, topical.

Ben-Gay SPA. (Pfizer US Pharmaceutical Group) Menthol 10%. Cream Tube 2 oz. *otc.*
Use: Liniment.

Ben-Gay Sportsgel. (Pfizer US Pharmaceutical Group) Methyl salicylate, menthol, alcohol 40%. Tube 1.25 oz, 3 oz. *otc.*
Use: Analgesic, topical.

Benoquin. (ICN Pharmaceuticals, Inc.) Monobenzone 20% in cream base. Tube 35 g, 453.6 g. *Rx.*
Use: Dermatologic.

•**benorterone.** (bee-NAHR-ter-ohn) USAN.
Use: Antiandrogen.

•**benoxaprofen.** (ben-OX-ah-PRO-fen) USAN.
Use: Anti-inflammatory, analgesic.

•**benoxinate hydrochloride.** (ben-OX-ih-nate) U.S.P. 23.
Use: Anesthetic (topical).
See: Flurate, Soln. (Bausch & Lomb Pharmaceuticals).
Fluress (PBH Wesley Jessen).

Benoxyl Lotion. (Stiefel Laboratories, Inc.) Benzoyl peroxide 5% or 10% in mild lotion base. Bot. 30 ml, 60 ml. *otc.*
Use: Antiacne.

•**benperidol.** (BEN-peh-rih-dahl) USAN.
Use: Antipsychotic.

bensalan. (BEN-sal-an) USAN. Under study.
Use: Disinfectant.

Bensal HP. (7 Oaks Pharmaceutical Corp.) Benzoic acid 6%, salicyclic acid 3%, extract of oak bark. Oint. Tube 15 g, 30 g. Jar 30 g, 60 g. *Rx.*
Use: Anti-infective, topical.

•**benserazide.** (ben-SER-ah-zide) USAN.
Use: Inhibitor (decarboxylase); antiparkinson.

Bensulfoid. (ECR Pharmaceuticals) Sulfur 8%, resorcinol 2%, alcohol 12%. Cream Tube 15 g. *otc.*
Use: Antiacne.

•**bentazepam.** (BEN-tay-zeh-pam) USAN.
Use: Hypnotic, sedative.

Bentical. (Lamond) Bentonite, zinc oxide, zinc carbonate, titanium dioxide. Bot. 4 oz, 6 oz, 8 oz, 16 oz, 32 oz, 0.5 gal, gal.
Use: Emollient.

•**bentiromide.** (ben-TIRE-oh-mide) USAN.
Use: Diagnostic aid (pancreas function determination).
See: Chymex, Soln. (Pharmacia & Upjohn).

•**bentonite.** N.F. 18.
Use: Pharmaceutic aid (suspending agent).

bentonite magma.
Use: Pharmaceutic aid (suspending agent).

bentonite, purified.
Use: Pharmaceutic aid.

•**bentoquatam.** (BEN-toe-KWAH-tam) USAN.
Use: Barrier for prevention of allergic contact dermatitis.

Bentyl. (SmithKline Beecham Pharmaceuticals) Dicyclomine HCl. **Cap.:** 10 mg. Bot. 100s, 500s, UD 100s. **Tab.:** 20 mg. Bot. 100s, 500s, 1000s, UD 100s. **Syr.:** 10 mg/5 ml. Bot. Pt. **Inj.:** 10 mg/ml. Amp. 2 ml, syringe 2 ml. Vial 10 ml (also contains chlorobutanol). *Rx.*
Use: Anticholinergic, antispasmodic.

•**benurestat.** (BEN-YOU-reh-stat) USAN.
Use: Enzyme inhibitor (urease).

Benylin Adult. (GlaxoWellcome) Dextromethorphan HBr 15 mg/5 ml, saccharin, sorbitol, alcohol free. Liq. Bot. 118 ml. *otc.*
Use: Antitussive.

Benylin DM Cough Syrup. (Parke-Davis) Dextromethorphan HBr 10 mg/5 ml, alcohol 5%. Bot. 4 oz, 8 oz. *otc.*
Use: Antitussive.

Benylin DME. (Parke-Davis) **Liq.:** Dextromethorphan HBr 5 mg, guaifenesin 100 mg, alcohol 5%, saccharin, menthol. Bot. 240 ml. *otc.*
Use: Antitussive, expectorant.

Benylin Expectorant. (GlaxoWellcome) Dextromethorphan HBr 5 mg, guaifenesin 100 mg, saccharin, menthol, sucrose, alcohol free. Bot. Liq. 118, 236 ml. *otc.*
Use: Antitussive, expectorant.

Benylin Multi-Symptom. (GlaxoWellcome) Dextromethorphan HBr 5 mg, pseudoephedrine HCl 15 mg, guaifenesin 100 mg/5 ml. Liq. Bot. 118 ml. *otc.*
Use: Antitussive, decongestant, expectorant.

Benylin Pediatric. (GlaxoWellcome) Dextromethorphan HBr 7.5 mg/5 ml, saccharin, sorbitol, alcohol free. Liq. Bot. 118 ml. *otc.*
Use: Antitussive.

Benza. (Century Pharmaceuticals, Inc.) Benzalkonium Cl 1:5000 and 1:750. Bot. 2 oz, 4 oz.
Use: Antimicrobial, antiseptic.

Benzac 5 & 10. (Galderma Laboratories, Inc.) Benzoyl peroxide 5% or 10%, alcohol 12%. Tube 60 g, 90 g. *Rx.*
Use: Antiacne.

Benzac w/2.5, 5 & 10. (Galderma Laboratories, Inc.) Benzoyl peroxide 2.5%, 5%, 10%. Tube 60 g, 90 g. *Rx.*
Use: Antiacne.

Benzac AC 2.5, 5, & 10. (Galderma Laboratories, Inc.) Benzoyl peroxide 2.5%, 5%, or 10%, glycerine and EDTA in water base. Gel Tube. 60 g, 90 g. *Rx.*
Use: Antiacne.

Benzac AC Wash 2.5, 5, & 10. (Galderma Laboratories, Inc.) Benzoyl peroxide 2.5%, 5%, 10%, glycerin. Liq. Bot. 240 ml. *Rx.*
Use: Antiacne.

Benzac W Wash 5 & 10. (Galderma Laboratories, Inc.) Benzoyl peroxide 5% or 10%. **5%:** Bot. 120 ml, 240 ml. **10%:** Bot. 240 ml. *Rx.*
Use: Antiacne.

5- & 10-Benzagel. (Dermik Laboratories, Inc.) Benzoyl peroxide 5% or 10% in gel base of water, alcohol 14%, laureth-46% (10% only). Tube 42.5 g, 85 g. *Rx.*
Use: Antiacne.

benzalkonium chloride. (benz-al-KOE-nee-uhm) N.F. 18.
Use: Surface antiseptic; pharmaceutical aid (preservative).
See: Bacti-Cleanse, Liq. (Pedinol Pharmacal, Inc.).
Benz-All, Liq. (Xttrium Laboratories, Inc.).

Econopred, Susp. (Alcon Laboratories, Inc.).
Eye-Stream (Alcon Laboratories, Inc.).
Germicin, Soln. (Consolidated Mid.).
Hyamine 3500 (Rohm and Haas).
Mycocide NS, Soln. (Woodward Laboratories, Inc.).
Ony-Clear, Soln. (Pedinol Pharmacal, Inc.).
Otrivin Spray (Novartis Pharmaceutical Corp.).
Ultra Tears (Alcon Laboratories, Inc.).
Zephiran Chloride Preps. (Sanofi Winthrop Pharmaceuticals).

W/Aluminum Cl, oxyquinoline sulfate.
See: Alochor Styptic, Liq. (Gordon Laboratories).

W/Bacitracin zinc, polymyxin B, neomycin sulfate.
See: Aerocaine, Oint. (Graham Field).

W/Benzocaine, orthohydroxyphenyl-mercuric Cl, parachlorometaxylenol.
See: Unguentine, Aerosol (Procter & Gamble Pharm.).

W/Berberine HCl, sodium borate, phenylephrine HCl, sodium Cl, boric acid.
See: Ocusol, Eye Lotion, Drops (Procter & Gamble Pharm.).

W/Boric acid, potassium Cl, sodium carbonate anhydrous, disodium edetate.
See: Swim-Eye, Drops (Savage Laboratories).

W/Chlorophyll.
See: Mycomist, Spray Liq. (Gordon Laboratories).

W/Hydrocortisone.
See: Barseb Thera-Spray, Soln. (PBH Wesley Jessen).

W/Diperodon HCl, carbolic acid, ichthammol, thymol, camphor, juniper tar.
See: Boro, Oint. (Scrip).

W/Disodium edetate, potassium Cl, isotonic boric acid.
See: Dacriose (Smith, Miller & Patch).

W/Epinephrine.
See: Epinal, Soln. (Alcon Laboratories, Inc.).

W/Epinephrine bitartrate, pilocarpine HCl, mannitol.
See: E-Pilo Ophth., Preps. (Smith, Miller & Patch).

W/Ethoxylated lanolin, methylparaben, hamamelis water, glycerin.
See: Medicone, clothwipes. (Medicore).

W/Gentamicin sulfate disodium phosphate, monosodium, phosphate, sodium Cl.
See: Garamycin Ophth. Soln., Preps. (Schering-Plough Corp.).

W/Hydroxypropyl methylcellulose.
See: Isopto Plain & Tears (Alcon Laboratories, Inc.).

W/Hydroxypropyl methylcellulose, disodium edetate.
See: Goniosol (Smith, Miller & Patch).

W/Isopropyl alcohol, methyl salicylate.
See: Cydonol Massage Lotion (Gordon Laboratories).

W/Lidocaine, phenol.
See: Unguentine, Spray (Procter & Gamble Pharm.).

W/Methylcellulose.
See: Tearisol (Smith, Miller & Patch).

W/Oxyquinoline sulfate, distilled water.
See: Oxyzal Wet Dressing, Soln. (Gordon Laboratories).

W/Phenylephrine, pyrilamine maleate, antipyrine.
See: Prefrin-A, Ophth. (Allergan, Inc.).

W/Pilocarpine HCl, epinephrine bitartrate, mannitol.
See: E-Pilo Ophth., Preps. (Smith, Miller & Patch).

W/Polymyxin B, neomycin sulfate, zinc bacitracin.
See: Ionax, Aerosol Can (Galderma Laboratories, Inc.).

•**benzbromarone.** (BENZ-brome-ah-rone) USAN.
Use: Uricosuric.

•**benzethonium chloride.** (benz-eth-OH-nee-uhm) U.S.P. 23.
Use: Anti-infective, topical, pharmaceutic aid (preservative).

•**benzetimide hydrochloride.** (benz-ETT-ih-mide HIGH-droe-klor-ide) USAN.
Use: Anticholinergic.

•**benzilonium bromide.** (BEN-zill-oh-nih-uhm-BROE-mide) USAN.
Use: Anticholinergic.

•**benzindopyrine hydrochloride.** (BENZ-in-doe-pie-reen HIGH-droe-KLOR-ide) USAN.
Use: Antipsychotic.

benzoate and phenylacetate.
Use: Treatment of hyperammonemia. [Orphan Drug]

Benzo-C. (Freeport) Benzocaine 5 mg, cetalkonium Cl 5 mg, ascorbic acid 50 mg/Troche. Bot. 1000s, cello-packed boxes 1000s. *otc.*
Use: Anesthetic, local.

•**benzocaine.** U.S.P. 23. Ethyl-p-aminobenzoate. Anesthesin, orthesin, parathesin.
Use: Anesthetic, topical.
See: BanSmoke, Gum (Thompson Medical Co.).
Cepacol Maximum Strength, Loz.

(J.B. Williams).
SensoGARD, Gel (Block).
Trocaine, Loz. (Roberts Pharmaceuticals).
W/Combinations.
See: Aerocaine, Oint. (Graham Field).
Aerotherm, Oint. (Graham Field).
Americaine, Oint., Aerosol (Du Pont Merck Pharmaceutical Co.).
Anacaine, Oint. (Gordon Laboratories).
Auralgan, Otic Drops (Wyeth-Ayerst Laboratories).
Auralgesic, Liq. (ICN Pharmaceuticals, Inc.).
Benzo-C, Troche (Freeport)
Benzodent, Oint. (Procter & Gamble Pharm.).
Bicozene, Cream. (Novartis Pharmaceutical Corp.).
Boil-Ease Anesthetic, Oint. (Del Pharmaceuticals, Inc.).
Bowman Drawing Paste, Oint. (Jones Medical Industries, Inc.).
Calamatum, Preps. (Blair Laboratories).
Cepacol, Troches (Hoechst Marion Roussel).
Cetacaine, Preps. (Cetylite Industries, Inc.).
Chiggerex, Oint. (Scherer Laboratories, Inc.).
Chigger-Tox, Liq. (Scherer Laboratories, Inc.).
Chloraseptic Children's Lozenges (Procter & Gamble Pharm.).
Culminal, Cream (Culminal).
Dent's Dental Poultice (C.S. Dent & Co. Division).
Dent's Lotion, Jel (C.S. Dent & Co. Division).
Dent's Toothache Gum (C.S. Dent & Co. Division).
Derma Medicone (Medicore).
Derma Medicone-HC (Medicore).
Dermoplast, Lot. (Wyeth-Ayerst Laboratories).
Detane, Gel (Del Pharmaceuticals, Inc.).
Foille, Preps. (Carbisulphoil).
Foille, Spray (Blistex, Inc.).
Foille Medicated First Aid, Oint, Spray. (Blistex, Inc.).
Foille Plus, Spray (Blistex, Inc).
Formula 44 Cough Control Discs, Loz. (Procter & Gamble Pharm).
GBA (Scrip).
Hurricaine, Liq, Spray, or Gel (Beutlich, Inc.).
Jiffy, Drops (Block Drug Co, Inc.).
Lanacane, Spray, Cream (Whitehall Robins Laboratories).
Listerine Cough Control Lozenges (Warner Lambert Consumer Health Products).
Maximum Strength Anbesol, Liq, Gel (Whitehall Robins Laboratories).
Medicone Dressing (Medicore).
Off-Ezy Corn Remover, Liq. (Del Pharmaceuticals, Inc.).
Orabase Gel (Colgate-Palmolive Co.).
Orajel Mouth-Aid, Liq., Gel (Del Pharmaceuticals, Inc.).
Pazo, Oint., Supp. (Bristol-Myers Squibb).
Pyrogallic Acid, Oint. (Gordon Laboratories).
Rectal Medicone (Medicore).
Rectal Medicone-HC, Supp. (Medicore).
Rectal Medicone Unguent (Medicore).
Solarcaine, Lot., Spray (Schering-Plough Corp.).
Spec-T Sore Throat-Cough Suppressant, Loz. (Bristol-Myers Squibb).
Spec-T Sore Throat-Decongestant, Loz. (Bristol-Myers Squibb).
Sucrets Cold Control, Loz. (SmithKline Beecham Pharmaceuticals).
Sucrets Cold Decongestant, Loz. (SmithKline Beecham Pharmaceuticals).
Tanac, Liq. (Del Pharmaceuticals).
Toothache, Gel (Roberts Pharmaceuticals).
Tympagesic, Liq. (Pharmacia & Upjohn).
Unguentine, Aerosol (Procter & Gamble Pharm.).
Vicks Cough Silencers, Loz. (Procter & Gamble Pharm.).
Vicks Formula 44 Cough Control Discs, Loz. (Procter & Gamble Pharm.).
Vicks Medi-Trating Throat Lozenges, Loz. (Procter & Gamble Pharm.).
Vicks Oracin, Loz. (Procter & Gamble Pharm.).
Zilactin-B Medicated, Gel (Zila Pharmaceuticals, Inc.).

benzochlorophene sodium. Sodium salt of ortho-benzyl-para-chlorophenol.

•**benzoctamine hydrochloride.** (benz-OCK-tah-meen) USAN.
Use: Hypnotic, muscle relaxant, sedative.

Benzodent. (Procter & Gamble Pharm.) Benzocaine 20%. Tube 30 g. *otc.*
Use: Anesthetic, local.

•**benzodepa.** (BEN-zoe-DEH-pah) USAN.
Use: Antineoplastic.

benzoic acid. (Various Mfr.) Pkg. 0.25

lb, 1 lb. *otc.*
Use: Antifungal, fungistatic.

•**benzoic acid.** (ben-ZOE-ik) U.S.P. 23.
Use: Pharmaceutic aid (antifungal).
W/Boric acid, zinc oxide, zinc stearate.
See: Whitfield's Oint. (Various Mfr.).

benzoic acid, 2-hydroxy. Salicylic Acid.

benzoic and salicylic acids ointment.
Use: Antifungal, topical.
See: Whitfield's Oint. (Various Mfr.).

•**benzoin.** (BEN-zoyn) U.S.P. 23.
Use: Topical protectant, expectorant.
See: Methagual, Oint. (Gordon Laboratories).
W/Podophyllum resin.
See: Podoben, Liq. (Maurry).
W/Polyoxyethylene dodecanol, aromatics.
See: Vicks Vaposteam, Liq. (Procter & Gamble Pharm).

Benzoin Spray. (Morton International) Benzoin, tolu balsam, styrax, alcohol w/propellant. Aerosol Can 7 oz. *otc.*
Use: Skin protectant.

benzol. Usually refers to benzene.

Benzo-Menth. (Pal-Pak, Inc.) Benzocaine 2.2 mg/Tab. Bot. 1000s. *otc.*
Use: Anesthetic, topical.

•**benzonatate.** (ben-ZOE-nah-tate) U.S.P. 23.
Use: Antitussive.
See: Tessalon, Perles (Du Pont Merck Pharmaceutical Co.).

benzonatate softgels. (Various Mfr.) Benzonatate 100 mg. Cap. Bot. 100s, 500s, 1000s. *Rx.*
Use: Antitussive.

benzophenone.
See: Pan Ultra, Lot., Lipstick (Baker Norton Pharmaceuticals, Inc.).
W/Oxybenzone, dioxybenzone.
See: Solbar, Lot. (Person and Covey, Inc.).

benzoquinonium chloride. (Various Mfr.) *Rx.*
Use: Muscle relaxant.

benzosulfimide.
See: Saccharin, N.F. 18.

benzosulphinide sodium. Name previously used for Saccharin Sodium.

•**benzoxiquine.** (benz-OX-ee-kwine) USAN.
Use: Disinfectant.

•**benzoylpas calcium.** (benz-oe-ILL-pass) USAN.
Use: Anti-infective (tuberculostatic).

benzoyl peroxide, hydrous. (BEN-zoyl per-OX-ide) (Various Mfr.) Peroxide, dibenzoyl. **Mask:** 5%. In 30 ml. **Lotion:** 5%, 10%. Bot. 30 ml. **Gel:** 5%, 10%. 45 g, 90 g (10% only).
Use: Keratolytic.

•**benzoyl peroxide, hydrous.** (BEN-zoyl per-OX-ide) U.S.P. 23.
Use: Keratolytic.
See: Benoxyl, Lot. (Stiefel Laboratories, Inc.).
Benzac AC, Gel, Liq. (Galderma Laboratories, Inc.).
Benzagel-5 & 10, Oint. (Dermik Laboratories, Inc.).
Brevoxyl, Gel (Stiefel Laboratories, Inc.).
Clearasil Acne Treatment, Cream (Procter & Gamble Pharm.).
Clearasil Antibacterial Acne Lotion (Procter & Gamble Pharm.).
Dermoxyl, Gel (Zeneca Pharmaceuticals).
Exact, Cream (Advanced Polymer Systems).
Oxy Wash Antibacterial Skin Wash (SmithKline Beecham Pharmaceuticals).
Panoxyl, Bar (Stiefel Laboratories, Inc.).
Peroxin A5, A10, Gel (Dermol Pharmaceuticals, Inc.).
Persadox, Cream, Lot. (Ortho McNeil Pharmaceutical).
Persadox HP, Cream, Lot. (Galderma Laboratories, Inc.).
Persa-Gel, Gel (Ortho McNeil Pharmaceutical).
Theroxide, Liq, Lot. (Medicis Dermatologicals, Inc).
Triaz, Gel (Medicis Dermatologics).
W/Chlorhydroxyquinoline, hydrocortisone.
See: Vanoxide-HC, Lot. (Dermik Laboratories, Inc).
W/Polyoxyethylene lauryl ether.
See: Benzac 5 & 10, Gel (Galderma Laboratories, Inc).
Desquam-X, Gel (Westwood Squibb Pharmaceuticals).
W/Sulfur.
See: Sulfoxyl, Lot. (Stiefel Laboratories, Inc).

Benzoyl Peroxide Wash, 5% & 10%. (Glades Pharmaceuticals) Benzoyl peroxide 5%. Liq. Bot. 120 ml, 150 ml, 240 ml. 10%. Liq. Bot. 150 ml, 240 ml. *Rx.*
Use: Keratolytic.

n'-benzoylsulfanilamide.
See: Sulfabenzamide.
W/Sulfacetamide, sulfathiazole, urea.
See: Sultrin, Tab., Cream (Ortho McNeil Pharmaceutical).

benzphetamine hydrochloride. (benz-FET-uh-meen)

Use: Anorexiant.
See: Didrex, Tab. (Pharmacia & Upjohn).

•**benzquinamide.** (benz-KWIN-ah-mid) USAN.
Use: Antiemetic.

•**benzthiazide.** (benz-THIGH-ah-zide) U.S.P. 23.
Use: Antihypertensive, diuretic.
See: Exna, Tab. (Wyeth-Ayerst Laboratories).

•**benztropine mesylate.** (BENZ-troe-peen) U.S.P. 23.
Use: Parasympatholytic, antiparkinsonian.
W/Sodium Cl.
See: Cogentin, Tab., Amp. (Merck & Co.).

benztropine methanesulfonate.
See: Benztropine mesylate.

•**benzydamine hydrochloride.** (ben-ZIH-dah-meen) USAN.
Use: Analgesic, anti-inflammatory, antipyretic.

benzydroflumethiazide.
See: Bendroflumethiazide.

•**benzyl alcohol.** N.F. 18. Phenylcarbinol.
Use: Anesthetic, antiseptic, topical, pharmaceutic aid (antimicrobial).
See: Topic, Gel (Ingram).
Vicks Blue Mint, Regular, & Wild Cherry Medicated Cough Drops (Procter & Gamble Pharm.).

•**benzyl benzoate.** U.S.P. 23.
Use: Pharmaceutical necessity for Dimercaprol Inj.

benzyl benzoate saponated. Triethanolamine 20 g, oleic acid 80 g, benzyl benzoate q.s. 1000 ml.

benzyl carbinol.
See: Phenylethyl Alcohol, U.S.P. 23.

benzylpenicillin, benzylpenicilloic, benzylpenilloic acid. (Kremers Urban)
Use: Assessment of penicillin sensitivity. [Orphan Drug]
See: Pre-Pen/MDM.

benzyl penicillin-C-14. (Nuclear-Chicago) Carbon-14 labelled penicillin. Vacuum-sealed glass vial 50 microcuries, 0.5 millicuries.
Use: Radiopharmaceutical.

benzyl penicillin G potassium.
See: Penicillin G Potassium.

benzyl penicillin G sodium.
See: Penicillin G Sodium.

•**benzylpenicilloyl polylysine concentrate.** U.S.P. 23.
Use: Diagnostic aid (penicillin sensitivity).
See: Pre-Pen (Kremers Urban).

bepanthen.
See: Panthenol.

bephedin. Benzyl ephedrine.

bephenium hydroxynaphthoate. U.S.P. XXI.
Use: Anthelmintic (hookworms).

•**bepridil hydrochloride.** USAN.
Use: Vasodilator.
See: Vascor (Ortho McNeil Pharmaceutical).

•**beractant.** (ber-ACT-ant) USAN.
Use: Lung surfactant. [Orphan Drug]
See: Survanta (Ross Laboratories).

beractant intrathecal suspension.
Use: Lung surfactant. [Orphan Drug]
See: Survanta.

•**beraprost.** USAN.
Use: Platelet aggregation inhibitor, improves ischemic syndromes.

•**beraprost sodium.** (BEH-reh-prahst) USAN.
Use: Platelet aggregation inhibitor, improves ischemic action.

berberine.
W/Hydrastine, glycerin
See: Murine, Ophth. Soln.

berberine hydrochloride.
W/Borax, sodium Cl, boric acid, camphor water, cherry laurel water, rose water, thimerosal.
See: Lauro, eye irrigator and drops (Otis Clapp & Son, Inc.).

•**berefrine.** (BEH-reh-FREEN) USAN. Formerly Burefrine.
Use: Mydriatic.

Ber-Ex. (Dolcin) Calcium succinate 2.8 gr, acetyl salicylic acid 3.7 gr/Tab. Bot. 100s, 500s. *otc.*
Use: Antiarthritic, antirheumatic.

Berinert P. (Behringwerke Aktiengesellschaft) C1-Esterase-inhibitor, human, pasteurized.
Use: Hereditary angioedema. [Orphan Drug]

Berocca Plus. (Roche Laboratories) Vitamins A 5000 IU, E 30 IU, C 500 mg, B_1 20 mg, B_2 20 mg, B_3. Tab. Bot. 100s. *Rx.*
Use: Iron, vitamin supplement.

•**berythromycin.** (beh-RITH-row-MY-sin) USAN.
Use: Antiamebic, anti-infective.

Beserol. (Sanofi Winthrop Pharmaceuticals) Acetaminophen, chlormezanone. Tab. *Rx.*
Use: Analgesic, tranquilizer, muscle relaxant.

•**besipirdine hydrochloride.** (beh-SIH-pihr-deen) USAN.
Use: Cognition enhancer (Alzheimer's disease).

Besta. (Roberts Pharmaceuticals) Vitamins B_1 20 mg, B_2 15 mg, niacinamide 100 mg, calcium pantothenate 20 mg, E 50 IU, magnesium sulfate 70 mg, zinc 18.4 mg, B_{12} 4 mcg, B_6 25 mg, C 300 mg/Cap. Bot. 100s. *otc.*
Use: Vitamin/mineral supplement.

Best C. (Roberts Pharmaceuticals) Ascorbic acid 500 mg/TR Cap. Bot. 100s. *otc.*
Use: Vitamin supplement.

Bestrone. (Bluco Inc./Med. Discnt. Outlet) Estrone in aqueous susp. 2 mg or 5 mg/ml. Inj. Vial 10 ml. *Rx.*
Use: Hormone, estrogen.

Beta-2. (Nephron Pharmaceuticals Corp.) Isoetharine HCl 1% with glycerin, sodium bisulfite, parabens. Liq. Bot. 10 ml, 30 ml. *Rx.*
Use: Respiratory product.

beta-adrenergic blockers.
See: Blocadren, Tab. (Merck & Co.).
Brevibloc, Inj. (Du Pont Merck Pharmaceutical Co.).
Cartrol, Tab. (Abbott Laboratories).
Corgard, Tab. (Bristol-Myers Squibb).
Inderal, Tab., Inj. (Wyeth-Ayerst Laboratories).
Inderal LA, Sustained-Release Cap. (Wyeth-Ayerst Laboratories).
Kerlone, Tab. (Searle).
Levatol, Tab. (Schwarz Pharma, Inc.).
Lopressor, Tab., Inj. (Novartis Pharmaceutical Corp.).
Nadolol, Tab. (Various Mfr.).
Propranolol HCl, Tab. (Various Mfr.).
Propranolol HCl, Inj. (SoloPak Pharmaceuticals, Inc.).
Sectral, Cap. (Wyeth-Ayerst Laboratories).
Tenormin, Tab. (ICI Pharm).
Timolol, Tab. (Various Mfr.).
Visken, Tab. (Novartis Pharmaceutical Corp).

beta-adrenergic blockers, ophthalmic.
See: Betagan Liquifilm, Soln. (Allergan, Inc.).
Betoptic, Soln. (Alcon Laboratories, Inc.).
Ocupress, Soln. (Otsuka).
OptiPranolol, Soln. (Bausch & Lomb Pharmaceuticals).
Timoptic in Ocudose, Soln. (Merck & Co).
Timoptic, Soln. (Merck & Co.).

beta alethine.
Use: Antineoplastic. [Orphan Drug]
See: Betathine (Dovetail Technologies, Inc.).

•**beta carotene.** (BAY-tah CARE-oh-teen) U.S.P. 23.
Use: Ultraviolet screen.

Betachron E-R. (Inwood Laboratories, Inc.) Propranolol HCl 60 mg, 80 mg, 120 mg, 160 mg. ER Cap. Bot. 100s. *Rx.*
Use: Beta-adrenergic blockers.

•**beta cyclodextrin.** (BAY-tah-sigh-kloe-DEX-trin) N.F. 18.
See: Betadex.

•**betadex.** (BAY-tah-dex) USAN. *Formerly beta cyclodextrin.*
Use: Pharmaceutical aid.

Betadine. (Purdue Frederick Co.) Povidone-iodine. **Available as:** Aerosol Spray, Bot. 3 oz. Antiseptic Gz. Pads 3″ × 9″. Box 12s. Antiseptic Lubricating Gel, Tube 5 g. Disposable Medicated Douche, concentrated packette w/cannula and 6 oz water. Douche, Bot. 1 oz, 4 oz, 8 oz. Douche Packette, 0.5 oz (6 per carton). Helafoam Solution Canister 250 g. Mouthwash/Gargle, Bot. 6 oz. Oint. Tube 1 oz. Jar 1 lb, 5 lb. Oint., Packette. Perineal Wash Conc. Kit, Bot. 8 oz w/dispenser. Skin Cleanser, Bot. 1 oz, 4 oz. Skin Cleanser Foam, Canister 6 oz. Solution, 0.5 oz, 8 oz, 16 oz, 32 oz, gal. Solution Packette, oz. Solution Swab Aid, 100s. Solution Swabsticks, 1s Box 200s; 3s Box 50s. Surgical Scrub, Bot. Pt w/dispenser, qt, gal, packette 0.5 oz. Surgiprep Sponge-Brush 36s. Vaginal Suppositories, Box 7s w/vaginal applicator. Viscous Formula Antiseptic Gauze Pads: 3″ × 9″, 5″ × 9″. Box 12s. Whirlpool Concentrate, Bot gal. *otc.*
Use: Antiseptic

Betadine Antiseptic. (Purdue Frederick Co.) Povidone-iodine 10%. Vaginal gel. 18 g with applicator. *otc.*
Use: Vaginal agent.

Betadine Cream. (Purdue Frederick Co.) Povidone-iodine 5% mineral oil, polyoxyethylene stearate, polysorbate, sorbitan monostearate, white petrolatum. Cream Tube 14 g. *otc.*
Use: Antimicrobial, antiseptic.

Betadine First Aid Antibiotics & Moisturizer. (Purdue Frederick Co.) Polymyxin B sulfate 10,000 IU, bacitracin zinc 500 IU. Oint. 14 g. *otc.*
Use: Anti-infective, topical.

Betadine 5% Sterile Ophthalmic Prep Solution. (Akorn, Inc.) Povidone-iodine 5%. Soln. Bot. 50 ml. *Rx.*
Use: Antiseptic, ophthalmic.

Betadine Medicated Disposable Douche. (Purdue Frederick Co.) Povidone-iodine 10% Soln. (0.3% when diluted). Vial 5.4 ml with 180 ml bot.

Sanitized water. 1 and 2 packs. *otc.*
Use: Vaginal agent.

Betadine Medicated Douche. (Purdue Frederick Co.) Povidone-iodine 10% (0.3% when diluted). Soln. In 15 ml (6s) packettes and 240 ml. *otc.*
Use: Vaginal agent.

Betadine Medicated Premixed Disposable Douche. (Purdue Frederick Co.) Povidone-iodine 10% soln (0.3% when diluted). Bot. 180 ml.1s, 2s. *otc.*
Use: Vaginal agent.

Betadine Medicated Vaginal Gel and Suppositories. (Purdue Frederick Co.) **Gel:** Povidone-iodine 10%. Tube 18 g, 85 g w/applicator. **Supp:** Povidone-iodine 10%. In 7s w/applicator. *otc.*
Use: Vaginal agent.

Betadine Plus First Antibiotics and Pain Reliever. (Purdue Frederick Co.) Polymyxin B sulfate 10,000 IU, bacitracin zinc 500 IU, pramoxine 10 mg/g. Oint.
Use: Anti-infective, topical.

Betadine Shampoo. (Purdue Frederick Co.) Povidone-iodine 7.5%. Shampoo Bot. 118 ml. *otc.*
Use: Antiseborrheic.

beta-estradiol.
See: Estradiol, U.S.P. 23

beta eucaine hydrochloride. Name previously used for Eucaine HCl.

Betagen. (Enzyme Process) Vitamins B_1 1 mg, B_2 1.2 mg, niacin 15 mg, B_6 18 mg, pantothenic acid 18 mg, choline 1.8 g, betaine 96 mg/6 Tab. Bot. 100s, 250s. *otc.*
Use: Mineral, vitamin supplement.

Betagan Liquiflim. (Allergan, Inc.) Levobunolol HCl 0.25% or 0.5%. Bot. 2 ml (0.5%), 5 ml, 10 ml (0.25%) w/ B.I.D. C Cap and Q.D. C Cap (0.5%). *Rx.*
Use: Beta-adrenergic blocker.

Betagen Ointment. (Zenith Goldline Pharmaceuticals) Povidone-iodine. Oint. Tube oz. Jar lb. *otc.*
Use: Antiseptic.

Betagen Solution. (Zenith Goldline Pharmaceuticals) Povidone-iodine. Bot. Pt, gal. *otc.*
Use: Antiseptic.

Betagen Surgical Scrub. (Zenith Goldline Pharmaceuticals) Povidone-iodine. Bot. Pt, gal. *otc.*
Use: Antiseptic.

•**betahistine hydrochloride.** (BEE-tah-HISS-teen) USAN.
Use: Vasodilator. Meniere's disease. A diamine oxidase inhibitor. Increase microcirculation.

beta-hypophamine.
See: Vasopressin.

betaine anhydrous. (Orphan Medical, Inc.)
Use: Treatment of homocystinuria. [Orphan Drug]
See: Cystadane (Orphan Medical, Inc.).

•**betaine hydrochloride.** (BEE-tane) U.S.P. 23. Acidol HCl, lycine HCl.
Use: Replenisher adjunct (electrolyte).

W/Ferrous fumarate, docusate sodium, desiccated liver, vitamins, minerals.
See: Hemaferrin, Tab. (Western Research).

Betalin S. (Eli Lilly and Co.) Thiamine HCl 50 mg or 100 mg. Tab. Bot. 100s. *otc.*
Use: Vitamin supplement.

•**betamethasone.** (BAY-tuh-METH-uh-zone) U.S.P. 23.
Use: Corticosteroid, topical.
See: Celestone, Inj., Syr., Tab. (Schering-Plough Corp.).

•**betamethasone acetate.** (BAY-tuh-METH-uh-zone) U.S.P. 23.
Use: Corticosteroid, topical.

•**betamethasone dipropionate.** (BAY-tah-METH-ah-zone die-PRO-pee-oh-nate) U.S.P. 23.
Use: Corticosteroid, topical.
See: Alphatrex Prods. (Savage Laboratories).
Diprolene Prods. (Schering-Plough Corp.).
Diprosone Prods. (Schering-Plough Corp.).
Psorion Cream (Zeneca Pharmaceuticals).

•**betamethasone sodium phosphate.** (BAY-tah-METH-ah-zone) U.S.P. 23.
Use: Corticosteroid, topical.
See: Celestone Phosphate Inj. (Schering-Plough Corp.).

betamethasone sodium phosphate and betamethasone acetate suspension, sterile.
See: Celestone Soluspan (Schering-Plough Corp.).

•**betamethasone valerate.** (BAY-tah-METH-ah-zone VAL-eh-rate) U.S.P. 23.
Use: Corticosteroid, topical.
See: Betatrex Prods. (Savage Laboratories).
Beta-Val Prods. (Teva Pharmaceuticals USA).
Valisone Prods. (Schering-Plough Corp.).
Valnac Prods. (Schering-Plough Corp.).

•**betamicin sulfate.** (bay-tah-MY-sin) USAN.

Use: Anti-infective.

betanaphthol. 2-Naphthol.
Use: Parasiticide.

Betapace. (Berlex Laboratories, Inc.) Sotalol HCl 80 mg, 120 mg, 160 mg, 240 mg/Tab. Bot. 100s, UD 100s. *Rx.*
Use: Beta-adrenergic blocker.

Betapen-VK. (Bristol-Myers Squibb) Penicillin V potassium. **Oral Soln.:** 125 mg/ml Bot. 100 ml. 250 mg/5 ml Bot. 100 ml, 200 ml. **Tab.:** 250 mg/Tab. Bot. 100s, 1000s; 500 mg/Tab. Bot. 100s. *Rx.*
Use: Anti-infective, penicillin.

beta-phenyl-ethyl-hydrazine. Phenelzine dihydrogen sulfate.
See: Nardil, Tab. (Parke-Davis).

beta-pyridyl-carbinol. Nicotinyl alcohol. Alcohol corresponding to nicotinic acid.

BetaRx. (VivoRx, Inc.) Encapsulated porcine islet preparation.
Use: Type I diabetic patients already on immunosuppression. [Orphan Drug]

Betasept. (Purdue Frederick Co.) Chlorhexidine gluconate 4%, isopropyl 4%, alcohol/Liq. Bot. 946 ml. *otc.*
Use: Dermatologic.

Betaseron. (Berlex Laboratories, Inc.) Interferon beta 1b 0.3 mg, (9.6 million IU per vial) albumin human 15 mg, dextrose 15 mg. Pow. for Inj. Single-use Vial w/ 2 ml vial of diluent. *Rx.*
Use: Multiple sclerosis agent.

Betathine. (Dovetail Technologies, Inc.) Beta alethine.
Use: Antineoplastic. [Orphan Drug]

Betatrex. (Savage Laboratories) Betamethasone valerate 0.1%. Cream, Oint. Tube 15 g, 45 g; Lot. Bot. 60 ml. *Rx.*
Use: Corticosteroid, topical.

Beta-Val Cream. (Teva Pharmaceuticals USA) Betamethasone valerate equivalent to 0.1% betamethasone base in cream base. Tube 15 g, 45 g. *Rx.*
Use: Corticosteroid, topical.

•**betaxolol hydrochloride.** (BAY-TAX-oh-lahl) U.S.P. 23.
Use: Antianginal, antihypertensive.
See: Betoptic, Soln. (Alcon Laboratories, Inc.).
Betoptic S, Susp. (Alcon Laboratories, Inc.).
Kerlone (Searle).

betaxolol ophthalmic solution.
Use: Beta-adrenergic blocker.

•**bethanechol chloride.** (beth-AN-ih-kole) U.S.P. 23.
Use: Cholinergic.
See: Duvoid, Tab. (Procter & Gamble Pharm.).
Myotonachol, Tab., Amp. (Glenwood, Inc.).
Urabeth, Tab. (Major Pharmaceuticals).
Urecholine, Tab., Amp. (Merck & Co.).

bethanidine.
Use: Hypotensive.

•**bethanidine sulfate.** (beth-AN-ih-deen) USAN.
Use: Antihypertensive.

Bethaprim. (Major Pharmaceuticals) Trimethoprim 40 mg, sulfamethoxazole 200 mg/5 ml, alcohol 0.26%, saccharin and sorbitol. Susp. *Rx.*
Use: Anti-infective.

Bethaprim DS Tabs. (Major Pharmaceuticals) Trimethoprim 160 mg, sulfamethoxazole 800 mg/Tab. Bot. 100s, 500s, UD 100s. *Rx.*
Use: Anti-infective.

Bethaprim SS Tabs. (Major Pharmaceuticals) Trimethoprim 80 mg, sulfamethoxazole 400 mg/Tab. Bot. 100s, 500s. *Rx.*
Use: Anti-infective.

•**betiatide.** (BEH-tie-ah-tide) USAN.
Use: Pharmaceutic aid.

Betimol. (Ciba Vision) Timolol maleate 0.25% or 0.5%, benzalkonium Cl 0.01%/Soln. Bot. 2.5 ml, 5 ml, 10 ml, 15 ml. *Rx.*
Use: Antiglaucoma agent.

Betoptic. (Alcon Laboratories, Inc.) Betaxolol HCl 0.5%. Soln. Bot. 2.5 ml, 5 ml, 10 ml, 15 ml. *Rx.*
Use: Beta-adrenergic blocking agent, ophthalmic.

Betoptic S. (Alcon Laboratories, Inc.) Betaxolol HCl 0.25%. Susp. Bot. 2.5 ml, 5 ml, 10 ml, 15 ml. *Rx.*
Use: Beta-adrenergic blocking agent, ophthalmic.

•**bevantolol hydrochloride.** (beh-VAN-toe-LOLE) USAN.
Use: Antianginal, antihypertensive, cardiac depressant (antiarrhythmic).

•**bexarotene.** (bex-AIR-oh-teen) USAN.
Use: Antineoplastic; antidiabetic.

Bexomal-C. (Roberts Pharmaceuticals) Vitamins B_1 6 mg, B_2 7 mg, B_3 80 mg, B_5 10 mg, B_6 5 mg, B_{12} 6 mcg, C 250 mg/Tab. Bot. 50s. *otc.*
Use: Vitamin supplement.

•**bezafibrate.** (BEH-zah-FIE-brate) USAN.
Use: Antihyperlipoproteinemic.

Bezon. (Whittier) Vitamins B_1 5 mg, B_2 3 mg, niacinamide 20 mg, pantothenic acid 3 mg, B_6 0.5 mg, C 50 mg, B_{12} 1 mcg/Cap. Bot. 30s, 100s. *otc.*
Use: Vitamin supplement.

Bezon Forte. (Whittier) Vitamins B_1 25 mg, B_2 12.5 mg, niacinamide 50 mg, pantothenic acid 10 mg, B_6 5 mg, C 250 mg/Cap. Bot. 30s, 100s. *otc.*
Use: Vitamin supplement.

B-F-I Powder. (SmithKline Beecham Pharmaceuticals) Bismuth-formic-iodide, zinc phenolsulfonate, bismuth subgallate, amol, potassium alum, boric acid, menthol, eucalyptol, thymol, and inert diluents. Can 0.25 oz, 1.25 oz, 8 oz. *otc.*
Use: Antiseptic, topical.

B.G.O. (Calotabs) Iodoform, salicylic acid, sulfur, zinc oxide, phenol (liquefied) 1%, calamine, menthol, petrolatum, lanolin, mineral oil, undecylenic acid 1%. Jar ⅞ oz, Tube 1 oz. *otc.*
Use: Antifungal, topical, antiseptic.

•**bialamicol hydrochloride.** (bye-AH-lam-IH-KAHL) USAN.
Use: Antiamebic.

•**biapenem.** (bye-ah-PEN-en) USAN.
Use: Anti-infective.

biaphasic insulin injection. A suspension of insulin crystals in a solution of insulin buffered at pH 7. Insulin Novo Rapitard.

Biavax-II. (Merck & Co.) Rubella and mumps virus vaccine, live. See details under Meruvax-II and Mumps vax. Single-dose vial w/diluent. Pkg. 1s, 10s. *Rx.*
Use: Immunization.

Biaxin. (Abbott Laboratories) Clarithromycin 250 mg, 500 mg. Tab. Bot. 60s, UD 100s. Clarithromycin 125 mg/5 ml and 250 mg/5 ml. Gran for Oral Susp. Bot. 50 ml, 100 ml. Sucrose, fruit punch flavor. *Rx.*
Use: Anti-infective, erythromycin.

•**bibapcitide.** (bib-APP-sih-tide) USAN.
Use: Radionuclide carrier; detection and localization of deep vein thrombosis.

•**bicalutamide.** (bye-kah-LOO-tah-mide) USAN.
Use: Antineoplastic.
See: Casodex, Tab. (Zeneca Pharmaceuticals)

•**bicifadine hydrochloride.** (bye-SIGH-fah-deen) USAN.
Use: Analgesic.

Bicillin. (Wyeth-Ayerst Laboratories) Penicillin G benzathine 200,000 units/Tab. Bot. 36s. *Rx.*
Use: Anti-infective, penicillin.

Bicillin C-R. (Wyeth-Ayerst Laboratories) Penicillin G benzathine 150,000 U, penicillin G procaine 150,000 U. Vial 10 ml. Penicillin G benzathine 300,000 U, penicillin G procaine 300,000 U. Tubex 1 ml. Penicillin G benzathine 600,000, penicillin G procaine 600,000 U. Tubex 2 ml. Penicillin G benzathine 1,200,000 U, penicillin G procaine 1,200,000 U. Syr. 4 ml. Parabens, lechithin, povidone. Inj. *Rx.*
Use: Anti-infective, penicillin.

Bicillin C-R 900/300. (Wyeth-Ayerst Laboratories) Penicillin G benzathine 900,000 units, penicillin G procaine 300,000 units with parabens, lecithin, and povidone/Inj. Tubex. 2 ml. *Rx.*
Use: Anti-infective, penicillin.

Bicillin L-A. (Wyeth-Ayerst Laboratories) Penicillin G benzathine 300,000 units/ml w/lecithin, povidone, methyl- and propylparabens. 300,000 units/ml. Vial 10 ml. 600,000 units/Tubex. 1,200,000 units/2 ml Tubex. 2,400,000 units/4 ml single-dose syringe. *Rx.*
Use: Anti-infective, penicillin.

•**biciromab.** (bye-SIH-rah-mab) USAN.
Use: Monoclonal antibody (antifibrin).

Bicitra. (Baker Norton Pharmaceuticals, Inc.) Sodium citrate dihydrate 500 mg, citric acid monohydrate 334 mg, 5 mEq sodium ion/5 ml. Shohl's Solution. Bot. 4 oz, pt, gal, Unit-dose 15 ml, 30 ml. *Rx.*
Use: Systemic alkalinizer.

•**biclodil hydrochloride.** (BYE-kloe-DILL) USAN.
Use: Antihypertensive (vasodilator).

BiCNU. (Bristol-Myers Oncology/Immunology) Carmustine (BCNU) 100 mg, sterile diluent 3 ml Pow. for Inj. Vial. *Rx.*
Use: Antineoplastic.

Bicozene Cream. (Novartis Pharmaceutical Corp.) Benzocaine 6%, resorcinol 1.66% in cream base/Cream. Tube 30 g. *otc.*
Use: Anesthetic, topical.

Bicycline. (Knight) Tetracycline HCl 250 mg/Cap. Bot. 100s.
Use: Anti-infective.

•**bidisomide.** (bye-DIH-so-mide) USAN.
Use: Cardiovascular agent (antiarrhythmic).

•**bifonazole.** (BYE-FONE-ah-zole) USAN.
Use: Antifungal.

bile acids, oxidized. Note also dehydrocholic acid.

W/Atropine methyl nitrate, ox and hog bile extract, phenobarbital.
See: G.B.S., Tab. (Forest Pharmaceutical, Inc.).

W/Bile whole (desiccated), desiccated whole pancreas, homatropine methylbromide.

See: Pancobile, Tab. (Solvay Pharmaceuticals).
bile acid suquestrants.
See: Questran (Bristol-Myers Squibb).
Questran Light (Bristol-Myers Squibb).
Colestid (Pharmacia & Upjohn).
bile extract. (Various Mfr.) Pow. 0.25 lb, 1 lb.
W/Cascara sagrada, dandelion root, podophyllin, nux vomica.
See: Neocholan, Tab. (Hoechst Marion Roussel).
bile extract, ox. Purified ox gall. (Eli Lilly and Co.) Enseal 5 gr, Bot. 100s, 500s, 1000s. (C.D. Smith) Tab. 5 gr, Bot. 1000s. (Stoddard) Tab. 3 gr, Bot. 100s, 500s, 1000s.
W/Cellulase, pepsin, glutamic acid HCl, pancreatin.
See: Kanumodic, Tab. (Novartis Pharmaceutical Corp.).
W/Dehydrocholic acid, homatropine methylbromide, phenobarbital.
See: Bilamide, Tab. (Norgine).
W/Dehydrocholic acid, pepsin, homatropine methylbromide.
See: Biloric, Cap. (Arcum).
W/Desoxycholic acid, oxidized bile acids, pancreatin.
See: Bilogen, Tab. (Organon Teknika Corp.).
W/Enzyme concentrate, pepsin, dehydrocholic acid, belladonna extract.
See: Konzyme, Tab. (Brunswick).
bilein. Bile salts obtained from ox bile.
bile-like products. bile products
See: Bile Salts.
Dehydrocholic Acid.
bile salts. Sodium glycocholate and taurocholate. Note also Bile Extract, Ox, and oxidized bile acids. (Eli Lilly and Co.) Enseal Bot. 100s.
See: Bilein.
Bisol, Tab. (Paddock Laboratories).
Ox Bile Extract.
Oxidized Bile Acids.
W/Cascara sagrada, phenolphthalein, capsicum oleoresin, peppermint oil.
See: Torocol, Tab. (Plessner)
W/Cellulase, calcium carbonate, pancrelipase.
See: Progestive, Tab. (NCP).
W/Pancrelipase, cellulase.
See: Torocol Compound, Tab. (Plessner).
W/Pepsin, homatropine, methylbromide, amylase, lipase, protease.
See: Bile Anthus Compound, Cap. (Scrip).
bile salts and belladonna. Belladonna, nux vomica compound bile salts 60 mg, belladonna leaf extract 5 mg, nux vomica extract 2 mg, phenolphthalein 30 mg, sodium salicylate 15 mg, aloin 15 mg/Tab. Bot.1000s.
Use: Laxative, antispasmodic.
bile, whole desiccated.
W/Pancreatin, mycozyme diastase, pepsin, nux vomica extract.
See: Enzobile, Tab. (Roberts Pharmaceuticals).
Bili-Labstix Reagent Strips. (Bayer Corp. (Consumer Div.)) Reagent strips. Test for pH, protein, glucose, ketones, bilirubin and blood in urine. Bot. 100s.
Use: Diagnostic aid.
Bili-Labstix SG Reagent Strips. (Bayer Corp. (Consumer Div.)) Urinalysis reagent strip test for specific gravity, pH, protein, glucose, ketone, bilirubin, and blood. Bot. 100s.
Use: Diagnostic aid.
Bilirubin Reagent Strips. (Bayer Corp. (Consumer Div.)) Seralyzer reagent strip. Quantitative strip test for total bilirubinin serum or plasma. Bot. 25s.
Use: Diagnostic aid.
Bilirubin Test.
See: Ictotest. (Bayer Corp. (Consumer Div.)).
Bilivist. (Berlex Laboratories, Inc.) Ipodate sodium 500 mg/Cap. Bot. 120s. *Rx.*
Use: Radiopaque agent.
Bilopaque. (Nycomed) Tyropanoate sodium 750 mg, iodine 430.5 mg, benzyl alcohol. Cap. 4s. *Rx.*
Use: Radiopaque agent.
Biloric. (Arcum) Pepsin 9 mg, ox bile 160 mg/Cap. Bot. 100s, 1000s. *otc.*
Use: Antispasmodic.
Bilstan. (Standex) Bile salts 0.5 gr, cascara sagrada powder extract 0.5 gr, phenolphthalein 0.5 gr, aloin 1/8 gr, podophyllin gr/Tab. Bot. 100s. *otc.*
Use: Laxative.
Biltricide. (Bayer Corp. (Consumer Div.)) Praziquantel 600 mg/Tab. Bot. 6s. *Rx.*
Use: Anthelmintic.
•**bindarit.** (BIN-dah-rit) USAN.
Use: Antirheumatic.
•**biniramycin.** (bih-NEER-ah-MY-sin) USAN.
Use: Anti-infective.
•**binospirone mesylate.** (bih-NO-spy-rone) USAN.
Use: Anxiolytic.
Bintron Tablets. (Madland) Liver fraction 4.6 gr, ferrous sulfate 5 gr, vitamins B_1 3 mg, B_2 0.5 mg, B_6 0.15 mg,

C 20 mg, calcium pantothenate 0.3 mg, niacinamide 10 mg/Tab. Bot. 100s, 1000s. *otc.*
Use: Mineral, vitamin supplement.

Bio-Acerola C Complex. (Solgar Co., Inc.) Vitamin C 500 mg, citrus bioflavonoids 10 mg, rutin 5 mg in a natural base of acerola, rose hips, buckwheat, black currant, and green pepper concentrate powders, cherry flavored. Wafers. Bot. 50s, 100s. *otc.*
Use: Vitamin supplement.

Biobrane. (Sanofi Winthrop Pharmaceuticals) Temporary skin substitute available in various sizes. *otc.*
Use: Dermatologic.

Biocal 250. (Bayer Corp. (Consumer Div.)) Calcium 250 mg/Chew. Tab. Bot. 75s. *otc.*
Use: Calcium supplement.

Biocal 500. (Bayer Corp. (Consumer Div.)) Calcium 500 mg/Tab. Bot. 75s. *otc.*
Use: Mineral supplement.

Biocef. (International Ethical Labs) Cephalexin monohydrate 500 mg/Cap. Bot. 100s. Cephalexin monohydrate 125 mg/ml and 250 mg/ml. Pow. for susp. Bot. 100 ml. *Rx.*
Use: Anti-infective, cephalosporin.

Bioclate. (Centeon) Concentrated recombinant hemophilic factor. After reconstitution, also contains albumin (human) 12.5 mg/ml, PEG-3350 1.5 mg/ml, sodium 180 mEq/L, histidine 55 mM, polysorbate 801.5 mcg/AHF IU, calcium 0.2 mg/ml. Bot. IU 250, 500, 1000. *Rx.*
Use: Antihemophilic.

Biocult-GC. (Orion Diagnostica) Swab test for gonorrhea. For endocervical, urethral, rectal, and pharyngeal cultures. Box 1 test per kit.
Use: Diagnostic aid.

biodegradable polymer implant containing carmustine.
Use: Antineoplastic. [Orphan Drug]
See: Biodel Implant/BCNU.

Biodel Implant/BCNU. (Scios Nova, Inc.) Biodegradable polymer implant containing carmustine. *Rx.*
Use: Antineoplastic.

Biodine. (Major Pharmaceuticals) Iodine 1%. Soln. Bot. Pt, gal. *otc.*
Use: Antimicrobial, antiseptic.

bio-flavonoid compound, citrus. W/Vitamin C.
See: Peridin-C, Tab. (Beutlich, Inc.).

bio-flavonoid compounds. Vitamin P.

Biogastrone.
See: Carbenoxolone.

Biohist-LA. (Wakefield Pharmaceuticals, Inc.) Carbinoxamine maleate 8 mg, pseudoephedrine HCl 120 mg/TR Tab. Bot. 100s. *Rx.*
Use: Antihistamine, decongestant.

•**biological indicator for dry-heat sterilization, paper strip.** U.S.P. 23.
Use: Biological indicator, sterilization.

•**biological indicator for ethylene oxide sterilization, paper strip.** U.S.P. 23.
Use: Biological indicator, sterilization.

•**biological indicator for steam sterilization, paper strip.** U.S.P. 23.
Use: Biological indicator, sterilization.

•**biological indicator for steam sterilization, self-contained.** U.S.P. 23.
Use: Biological indicator, sterilization.

Bion Tears. (Alcon Laboratories, Inc.) Dextran 70 0.1%, hydroxypropyl methylcellulose 2910 0.3%, NaCl, KCl, sodium bicarbonate. Preservative free. Soln. In single-use 0.45 ml containers (28s). *otc.*
Use: Artificial tears.

Bionate 50-2. (Seatrace Pharmaceuticals, Inc.) Testosterone cypionate 50 mg, estradiol cypionate 2 mg/ml. Vial 10 ml. *Rx.*
Use: Androgen, estrogen combination.

Bioral.
See: Carbenoxolone.

Bio-Rescue. (Biomedical Frontiers, Inc.) Dextran and deferoxamine.
Use: Acute iron poisoning. [Orphan Drug]

Bios I.
See: Inositol.

Biosynject. (Chembiomed, Inc.) Trisaccharides A and B.
Use: Hemolytic disease of the newborn. [Orphan Drug]

Bio-Tab. (International Ethical Labs) Doxycycline hyclate 100 mg. Tab. Bot. 50s, 100s, 500s. *Rx.*
Use: Anti-infective, tetracycline.

Biotel Diabetes. (Biotel Corp.) In vitro diagnostic test for diabetes and other metabolic disorders by screening for glucose in the urine. Test Kit 12s.
Use: Diagnostic aid.

Biotel Kidney. (Biotel Corp.) In vitro diagnostic test for early detection of diseases of the kidneys, bladder, and urinary tract by screening for hemoglobin, red blood cells, and albumin in the urine. Test Kit 12s.
Use: Diagnostic aid.

Biotel U.T.I. (Biotel Corp.) In vitro diagnostic home test to detect urinary tract infections by screening fornitrate in urine. Test Kit 12s.

Use: Diagnostic aid.

Biotexin.
See: Novobiocin.

Biothesin. (Pal-Pak, Inc.) Phosphorated carbohydrate solution ceriumoxalate 120 mg, bismuth subnitrate 120 mg, benzocaine 15 mg, aromatics/Tab. 1000s. *otc.*
Use: Antiemetic antivertigo.

Bio-Tytra. (Health for Life Brands, Inc.) Neomycin sulfate 2.5 mg, gramicidin 0.25 mg, benzocaine 10 mg/Troche. Box 10s. *Rx.*
Use: Anti-infective.

•**bipenamol hydrochloride.** (bye-PEN-ah-MAHL) USAN.
Use: Antidepressant.

•**biperiden.** (by-PURR-ih-den) U.S.P. 23.
Use: Anticholinergic; antiparkinson.

•**biperiden hydrochloride.** (by-BURR-ih-den) U.S.P. 23.
Use: Anticholinergic, antiparkinson.

biperiden hydrochloride and lactate.
Use: Anticholinergic, antiparkinson.
See: Akineton, Amp., Tab. (Knoll Pharmaceuticals).

•**biperiden lactate, injection.** (by-PURR-ih-den) U.S.P. 23.
Use: Anticholinergic, antiparkinsonian.

•**biphenamine hydrochloride.** (bye-FEN-ah-meen) USAN.
Use: Anesthetic, local, anti-infective, antimicrobial.

Bipole-S. (Spanner) Testosterone 25 mg, estrone 2 mg/ml. Inj. Vial. 10 ml. *Rx.*
Use: Androgen, estrogen combination.

bisacetoxphenyl oxindol.
See: Oxyphenisatin.

•**bisacodyl.** (BISS-uh-koe-dill) U.S.P. 23.
Use: Laxative.
See: Bisacodyl Uniserts, Supp. (Upsher-Smith Labs, Inc.).
Correctol, Tab. (Schering-Plough).
Dacodyl, Tab. Supp. (Major Pharmaceuticals).
Deficol, Tab., Supp. (Vangard Labs, Inc.).
Delco-Lax, Tab. (Delco).
Dulcagen, Tab., Supp. (Zenith Goldline Pharmaceuticals).
Dulcolax, Tab. Supp. (Novartis Self-Medication).
Feen-a-mint, Tab. (Schering-Plough).
Fleet Bisacodyl, Tab Supp. (CB Fleet Co.).

•**bisacodyl tannex.** (BISS-uh-koe-dill) USAN. Water-soluble complex of bisacodyl and tannic acid.
Use: Laxative.
See: Clysodrast, packet (PBH Wesley Jessen).

Bisacodyl Uniserts. (Upsher-Smith Labs, Inc.) Bisacodyl 5 mg and 10 mg/Supp. Pack. 12, 50s, 500s. *otc.*
Use: Laxative.

Bisalate. (Allison) Sodium salicylate 5 gr, salicylamide 2.5 gr, sodium paraminobenzoate 5 gr, ascorbic acid 50 mg, butabarbital sodium ⅛ gr/Tab. Bot. 100s and 1000s. *Rx.*
Use: Antirheumatic.

•**bisantrene hydrochloride.** (BISS-an-TREEN HIGH-droe-KLOR-ide) USAN.
Use: Antineoplastic.

bisatin.
See: Oxyphenisatin.

bishydroxycoumarin.
See: Dicumarol, U.S.P. 23.

Bismapec. (Pal-Pak, Inc.) Bismuth hydroxide 137.7 mg, colloidal kaolin 648 mg, citrus pectin 129.6 mg/Tab. Bot. 1000s. *otc.*
Use: Antidiarrheal.

Bismu-Kino. (Denver Chemical (Puerto Rico) Inc.) Bismuth oxycarbonate 10 gr, eucalyptus gum 6 gr, phenyl salicylate, camphor, menthol, carminative oils of nutmeg, and clove in soothing, demulcent base w/alcohol 2%/fl oz. Bot. 4 oz, pt. *otc.*
Use: Gastrointestinal.

•**bismuth aluminate.** (BISS-muth) USAN. Aluminum bismuth oxide.

•**bismuth carbonate.** (BISS-muth) USAN.
Use: Protectant, topical.

bismuth glycolylarsanilate. (BISS-muth)
Use: Antiamebic.
See: Glycobiarsol, N.F. 18.

bismuth hydroxide.
See: Bismuth, Milk of, U.S.P. 23.

bismuth, insoluble products.
See: Bismuth Subgallate (Various Mfr.).
Bismuth Subsalicylate (Various Mfr.).
Bismuth Tribromophenate (N.Y. Quinine).

bismuth, magma. Name previously used for Milk of Bismuth.

•**bismuth, milk of.** (BISS-muth) U.S.P. 23.
Formerly Bismuth Magma.
Use: Astringent, antacid.

bismuth oxycarbonate.
See: Bismuth Subcarbonate.

bismuth potassium tartrate. Basic bismuth potassium bismuthotartrate. (Brewer) 25 mg/ml Amp. 2 ml. (Miller Pharmacal Group, Inc.) 0.016 g/ml Amp. 2 ml, Box 12s, 100s; Bot. 30 ml, 60 ml. (Raymer) 2.5% Amp. 2 ml, Box 12s, 100s. *Rx.*
Use: Agent for syphilis.

bismuth resorcin compound.
W/Bismuth subgallate, balsam Peru, benzocaine, zinc oxide, boric acid.
See: Bonate, Supp. (Suppositoria Laboratories, Inc.).
W/Bismuth subgallate, balsam Peru, zinc oxide, boric acid.
See: Versal, Supp. (Suppositoria Laboratories, Inc.).
bismuth sodium tartrate. (BISS-muth)
Use: I.M., syphilis.
bismuth subbenzoate. (BISS-muth)
Use: Dusting powder for wounds.
•**bismuth subcarbonate.** (BISS-muth) U.S.P. 23.
Use: Protectant (topical).
bismuth subcarbonate. (BISS-muth)
Use: Gastroenteritis, diarrhea.
W/Benzocaine, zinc oxide, boric acid.
See: Aracain Rectal Supp. (Del Pharmaceuticals, Inc.).
W/Calcium carbonate, magnesium carbonate, aminoacetic acid, dried aluminum hydroxide gel.
See: Buffertabs, Tab. (Forest Pharmaceutical, Inc.).
W/Charcoal and ginger.
See: Harv-a-carbs, Tab. (Forest Pharmaceutical, Inc.).
W/Hydrocortisone acetate, belladonna extract, ephedrine sulfate, zinc oxide, boric acid, balsam Peru, cocoa butter.
See: K-C, Liq. (Century Pharmaceuticals, Inc.).
W/Pectin, kaolin, opium powder.
See: Bismuth, salol, zinc compound (Jones Medical Industries, Inc.).
W/Phenyl salicylate, chloroform, eucalyptus gum, camphor.
See: Bismu-Kino, Liq. (Denver Chem.).
W/Ephedrine sulfate, belladonna extract, zinc oxide, boric acid, bismuth oxyiodide, balsam Peru.
See: Wyanoids, Preps. (Wyeth-Ayerst Laboratories).
bismuth subgallate. (BISS-muth) (Various Mfr.) Dermatol.
Use: Topically for skin conditions; orally as an antidiarrheal.
See: Devrom, Tab. (Parthenon Co., Inc.).
W/Benzocaine, resorcin, cod liver oil, lanolin, zinc oxide.
See: Biscolan, Supp. (Lannett Co., Inc.).
W/Benzocaine, zinc oxide, boric acid, balsam Peru.
See: Bonate, Supp. (Suppositoria Laboratories, Inc.).
W/Bismuth resorcin compound, balsam Peru, benzocaine, zinc oxide, boric acid.
See: Bonate, Supp. (Suppositoria Laboratories, Inc.).
W/Bismuth resorcin compound, zinc oxide, boric acid, balsam Peru.
See: Versal, Supp. (Suppositoria Laboratories, Inc.).
W/Cod liver oil, benzocaine, lanolin, zinc oxide, resorcin, balsam Peru, hydrocortisone.
See: Anusol-HC, Supp. (Parke-Davis).
W/Diethylaminoacet-2, 6-xylidide, zinc oxide, aluminum subacetate, balsam Peru.
See: Xylocaine Suppositories (Astra Pharmaceuticals, L.P.).
W/Kaolin, colloidal.
See: Diastop, Liq. (ICN Pharmaceuticals, Inc.).
W/Kaolin colloidal, calcium carbonate, magnesium trisilicate, papain, atropine sulfate.
See: Kaocasil, Tab. (Jenkins).
W/Kaolin, opium, zinc phenolsulfonate, pectin.
See: Cholactabs, Tab. (Roxane Laboratories, Inc.).
W/Kaolin, pectin, zinc phenolsulfonate, opium powder.
See: Diastay, Tab. (ICN Pharmaceuticals, Inc.).
W/Opium powder, pectin, kaolin, zinc phenolsulfonate.
See: Bismuth, Pectin, Paregoric (Teva Pharmaceuticals USA).
W/Zinc oxide, bismuth resorcin compound, balsam Peru, benzyl benzoate.
See: Anusol, Supp., Oint. (Parke-Davis).
bismuth subiodide.
See: Bismuth oxyiodide.
•**bismuth subnitrate.** (BISS-muth) U.S.P. 23.
Use: Pharmaceutic necessity, gastroenteritis, amebic dysentery, locally for wounds.
W/Calcium carbonate, magnesium carbonate.
See: Antacid No. 2, Tab. (Jones Medical Industries, Inc.).
•**bismuth subsalicylate.** (BISS-muth) U.S.P. 23. Basic bismuth salicylate. Agent for syphilis. Used in combination with metronidazole and tetracycline HCl to treat active duodenal ulcer associated with *H. pylori* infection.
Use: Anitdiarrheal, antacid, antiulcerative.
W/Calcium carbonate, glycocoll.
See: Pepto-Bismol, Tab. (Procter & Gamble Pharm.).
W/Pectin, salol, kaolin, zinc sulfocarbo-

late, aluminum hydroxide.
See: Pepto-Bismol, Liq. (Procter & Gamble Pharm.).

bismuth tannate. (BISS-muth) (Various Mfr.) Tan bismuth. *otc.*
Use: Astringent and protective in GI disorders.

bismuth tribromophenate. (BISS-muth)
Use: Intestinal antiseptic.

bismuth violet. (BISS-muth) (Table Rock) Bismuth Violet. **Oint.:** 1%. Jar oz, lb. **Soln.:** 0.5%. Bot. 0.5 oz, 6 oz, pt, gal. **Tr.:** 0.5%. Bot. 6 oz, pt, also 1% w/ benzoic and salicylic acid. Bot. 0.5 oz, 6 oz, pt. *otc.*
Use: Anti-infective, topical.

bismuth, water-soluble products.
See: Bismuth Potassium Tartrate (Various Mfr.).

•**bisnafide dimesylate.** (BISS-nah-fide die-MEH-sih-late) USAN.
Use: Antineoplastic.

•**bisobrin lactate.** (BISS-oh-brin LACK-tate) USAN.
Use: Fibrinolytic.

•**bisoprolol.** (bih-SO-pro-lahl) USAN.
Use: Antihypertensive (β-blocker).

•**bisoprolol fumarate.** USAN.
Use: Antihypertensive (β-blocker).
See: Zebeta (ESI Lederle Generics).
Ziac, Tab. (ESI Lederle Generics).

•**bisoxatin acetate.** (biss-OX-at-in) USAN.
Use: Laxative.

bispecific antibody 520C9x22. (Medarex)
Use: Antineoplastic, serotherapy. [Orphan Drug]

bisphosphonates.
Use: Antihypercalcomic, bone resorption inhibitor.
See: Actonel, Tab. (Procter & Gamble Pharm.).
Aredia, Inj. (Novartis Pharmaceutical Corp.)
Aredia, Pow. for Inj. (Novartis Pharmaceutical Corp.).
Didronel (Procter & Gamble Pharm.).
Didronel, IV (MGI Pharma, Inc)
Fosamax, Tab. (Merck & Co.).
Skelid, Tab. (Sanofi Winthrop Pharmaceuticals).

•**bispyrithione magsulfex.** (BISS-PIHR-ih-thigh-ohn mag-sull-fex) USAN.
Use: Antidandruff, anti-infective, antimicrobial.

bis-tropamide. Tropicamide.
See: Mydriacyl, Soln. (Alcon Laboratories, Inc.)

Bite & Itch Lotion. (Weeks & Leo) Pramoxine HCl 1%, pyrilamine maleate 2%, pheniramine maleate 0.2%, chlorpheniramine maleate 0.2%. Bot. 4 oz. *otc.*
Use: Dermatologic, topical.

•**bithionolate, sodium.** (bye-THIGH-oh-noe-late) USAN.
Use: Topical anti-infective.

Bitin. CDC Anti-infective agent.
See: Bithionol.

•**bitolterol mesylate.** (by-TOLE-tor-ole) USAN.
Use: Bronchodilator.
See: Tornalate (Dura Pharmaceuticals).

Bitrate. (Arco Pharmaceuticals, Inc.) Phenobarbital 15 mg, pentaerythritol tetranitrate 20 mg/Tab. Bot. 100s. *Rx.*
Use: Antianginal, hypnotic, sedative.

•**bivalirudin.** (bye-VAL-ih-ruh-din) USAN.
Use: Anticoagulant, antithrombotic.

•**bizelesin.** (bye-ZELL-eh-sin) USAN.
Use: Antineoplastic.

B-Ject-100. (Hyrex Pharmaceuticals) Vitamins B_1 100 mg, B_2 2 mg, B_3 100 mg, B_5 2 mg, B_6 2 mg/ml. Inj. Vial 10 ml, 30 ml. *Rx.*
Use: Vitamin supplement.

Black and White Bleaching Cream. (Schering-Plough Corp.) Hydroquinone 2%. Tube 0.75 oz, 1.5 oz. *Rx.*
Use: Dermatologic.

Black and White Ointment. (Schering-Plough Corp.) Resorcinol 3%. Tube 0.62 oz, 2.25 oz.
Use: Antiseptic, dermatologic, topical.

Black-Draught. (Chattem Consumer Products) Powdered senna extract. **Tab.:** 600 mg. Bot. 30s. **Gran.:** 1.65 g/ 0.5 tsp. Jar 22.5 g. *otc.*
Use: Laxative.

Black-Draught Syrup. (Chattem Consumer Products) Casanthranol 90 mg w/senna, rhubarb, anise, methyl salicylate, ginger, peppermint oil, spearmint oil, menthol, alcohol 5%, tartrazine/15 ml. Bot. 2 oz, 5 oz. *otc.*
Use: Laxative.

black widow spider, antivenin.
See: Antivenin (*Lactrodectus mactens*), Inj. (Merck & Co.).

Blairex Hard Contact Lens Cleaner. (Blairex Labs, Inc.) Anionic detergent. Liq. Bot. 60 ml. *otc.*
Use: Contact lens care.

Blairex Lens Lubricant. (Blairex Labs, Inc.) Isotonic. Sorbic acid 0.25%, EDTA 0.1%, borate buffer, NaCl, hydroxypropyl methylcellulose, glycerin. Soln. Bot. 15 ml. *otc.*
Use: Contact lens care.

Blairex Sterile Saline Solution. (Blairex Labs, Inc.) Sodium Cl, boric acid, so-

dium borate. Aerosol. 90 ml, 240 ml, 360 ml. *otc.*
Use: Contact lens care.

Blairex System. (Blairex Labs, Inc.) Sodium Cl 135 mg/Tab. 200s, 365s w/15 ml bot. *otc.*
Use: Contact lens care.

Blairex System II. (Blairex Labs, Inc.) Sodium Cl 250 mg/Tab. 90s, 180s w/ 27.7 ml bot. *otc.*
Use: Contact lens care.

Blaud Strubel. (Strubel) Ferrous sulfate 5 gr/Cap. Bot. 100s. *otc.*
Use: Mineral supplement.

Blefcon. (Madland) Sodium sulfacetamide 30%. Oint. Tube ⅛ oz. *Rx.*
Use: Anti-infective, ophthalmic.

Blenoxane. (Bristol-Myers Oncology/Immunology) Bleomycin sulfate 15 units, 30 unites Pow. for Inj. Vial. *Rx.*
Use: Antineoplastic.

•**bleomycin sulfate, sterile.** (BLEE-oh-MY-sin) U.S.P. 23. Antibiotic obtained from cultures of *Streptomyces verticillus.*
Use: Antineoplastic.
See: Blenoxane, Inj. (Bristol-Myers Squibb).

Bleph-10. (Allergan, Inc.) Sulfacetamide sodium 10%. Dropper Bot. 2.5 ml, 5 ml, 15 ml. *Rx.*
Use: Anti-infective, ophthalmic.

Bleph-10 Sterile Ophthalmic Ointment. (Allergan, Inc.) Sulfacetamide sodium 10%. Tube 3.5 g. *Rx.*
Use: Anti-infective, ophthalmic.

Blephamide. (Allergan, Inc.) Sulfacetamide sodium 10%, prednisolone acetate 0.2%. Bot. 2.5 ml, 5 ml, 10 ml. *Rx.*
Use: Anti-inflammatory, anti-infective, ophthalmic.

Blephamide Ophthalmic Ointment. (Allergan, Inc.) Prednisolone acetate 0.2%, sulfacetamide sodium 10%. Tube 3.5 g. *Rx.*
Use: Anti-inflammatory, anti-infective, ophthalmic.

Blinx. (Akorn, Inc.) Sodium Cl, potassium Cl, sodium phosphate, benzalkonium Cl 0.005%, EDTA 0.02%. Soln. Bot. 120 ml. *otc.*
Use: Irrigant, ophthalmic.

Blis. (Del Pharmaceuticals, Inc.) Boric acid 47.5%, salicylic acid 17%. Bot. 7 oz. *otc.*
Use: Antifungal, topical.

BlisterGard. (Medtech Laboratories, Inc.) Alcohol 6.7%, pyroxylin solution, oil of cloves, B-hydroxyquinolone. Liq. Bot. 30 ml. *otc.*
Use: Dermatologic, protectant.

Blistex. (Blistex, Inc.) Camphor 0.5%, phenol 0.5%, allantoin 1%, lanolin, mineral oil. Tube 4.2 g, 10.5 g. *otc.*
Use: Lip protectant.

Blistex Lip Balm. (Blistex, Inc.) SPF 10. Camphor 0.5%, phenol 0.5%, allantoin 1%, dimethicone 2%, pamidate 0.25%, oxybenzone, parabens, petrolatum. Tube. 4.5 g. *otc.*
Use: Lip protectant.

Blistex Ultra Protection. (Blistex, Inc.) Octyl methoxycinnamate, oxybenzone, octylsalicylate, menthylanthranilate, homosalate, dimethicone. Tube 4.2 g. *otc.*
Use: Lip protectant.

Blistik. (Blistex, Inc.) Padimate O 6.6%, oxybenzone 2.5%, dimethicone 2%. Lipbalm stick 4.5 g. *otc.*
Use: Lip protectant.

Blis-To-Sol. (Chattem Consumer Products) **Liq.:** Tolnaftate 1%. Bot. 30 ml. **Pow.:** Zinc undecylenate 12%. Bot. 60 g. **Soln:** Tolnaftate 1% Bot. 30 ml, 55.5 ml. *otc.*
Use: Antifungal, topical.

BLM.
See: Bleomycin sulfate.

Blocadren. (Merck & Co.) Timolol maleate 5 mg, 10 mg, or 20 mg/Tab. **5 mg:** Bot. 100s; **10 mg:** Bot. 100s, UD 100s; **20 mg:** Bot. 100s. *Rx.*
Use: Beta-adrenergic blocker.

Block Out By Sea & Ski. (Carter Wallace) Padimate O, octyl methoxycinnamate, oxybenzone. Cream. Tube 120 g. *otc.*
Use: Sunscreen.

Block Out Clear By Sea & Ski. (Carter Wallace) Padimate O, octyl methoxycinnamate, octyl salicylate, SD alcohol 40. Lot. Bot. 120 ml. *otc.*
Use: Sunscreen.

blood, anticoagulants.
See: Anticoagulants.

•**blood cells, red.** U.S.P. 23. *Formerly Blood cells, human red.*
Use: Blood replenisher.

blood coagulation.
See: Hemostatics.

blood fractions.
See: Albumin (Human) Salt-Poor (Armour Pharmaceutical; Baxter).

blood glucose concentrator.
See: Glucagon (Eli Lilly and Co.).

blood glucose test.
See: Chemstrip bG Strips. (Boehringer Mannheim Pharmaceuticals).
Dextrostix Reagent Strips (Bayer Corp. (Consumer Div.)).

First Choice, Strips (Polymer Technology, Int.).
Glucostix Strips (Bayer Corp. (Consumer Div.)).

•**blood grouping serum, anti-A.** U.S.P. 23.
Use: Diagnostic aid (blood, in vitro).

•**blood grouping serum, anti-B.** U.S.P. 23.
Use: Diagnostic aid (blood, in vitro).

•**blood grouping serums anti-D, anti-C, anti-E, anti-c, anti-e.** U.S.P. 23. *Formerly Anti-Rh typing serums.*
Use: Diagnostic aid (blood, in vitro).

•**blood group specific substances a, b and ab.** U.S.P. 23. *Formerly Blood Grouping specific substances A and B.*
Use: Blood neutralizer.

•**blood, whole.** U.S.P. 23. *Formerly Blood, whole human.*
Use: Blood replenisher.

Blu-12 100. (Bluco Inc./Med. Discnt. Outlet) Cyanocobalamin 100 mcg/ml. Vial 30 ml. *Rx.*
Use: Vitamin supplement.

Blu-12 1000. (Bluco Inc./Med. Discnt. Outlet) Cyanocobalamin 1000 mcg/ml. Vial 30 ml. *Rx.*
Use: Vitamin supplement.

Bluboro Powder. (Allergan, Inc.) Aluminum sulfate 53.9%, calcium acetate 43% w/boric acid, FD&C Blue 1. Packet 1.9 g. Box 12s. *otc.*
Use: Astringent.

Bludex. (Burlington) Methenamine 40.8 mg, methylene blue 5.4 mg, phenylsalicylate 18.1 mg, atropine sulfate 0.03 mg, hyoscyamine 0.03 mg, benzoic acid 4.5 mg/Tab. Bot. 100s, 1000s. *Rx.*
Use: Antiseptic, antispasmodic, urinary.

Blue. (Various Mfr.) Pyrethrins 0.3%, piperonyl butoxide 3%, petroleum distillate 1.2%. Gel Bot. 30 g, 480 g. *otc.*
Use: Pediculicide.

Blue Gel Muscular Pain Reliever. (Rugby Labs, Inc.) Menthol in a specially formulated base. Gel Tube 240 g. *otc.*
Use: Liniments.

Blue Star Ointment. (McCue Labs.) Salicylic acid, benzoic acid, methyl salicylate, camphor, lanolin, petrolatum. Jar 2 oz. *otc.*
Use: Dermatologic, counterirritant.

B-Major. (Barth's) Vitamins B_1 7 mg, B_2 14 mg, niacin 2.35 mg, B_{12} 7.5 mcg, B_6 0.15 mg, pantothenic acid 0.37 mg, choline 85 mg, inositol 6 mg, biotin, folic acid, aminobenzoic acid/Cap. Bot. 1s, 3s, 6s, 12s. *Rx-otc.*
Use: Mineral, vitamin supplement.

B.M.E. (Brothers) Aminophylline 32 mg, ephedrine sulfate 8 mg, phenobarbital 8 mg, chlorpheniramine maleate 2 mg, alcohol 15%/5 ml. Bot. Pt. *Rx.*
Use: Antihistamine, bronchodilator, decongestant, hypnotic, sedative.

B-N. (Eric, Kirk & Gary) Bacitracin 500 units, neomycin sulfate 5 mg. Oint. Tube 0.5 oz. *otc.*
Use: Anti-infective, topical.

b-naphthyl salicylate. Betol, Naphthosalol, Salinaphthol.
Use: G.I. & G.U., antiseptic.

B-Nutron. (Nion Corp.) Vitamins B_1 2 mg, niacinamide 18 mg, B_2 3 mg, B_6 2.2 mg, cyanocobalamin 3 mcg, folic acid 0.4 mg, iron 6 mg, pantothenic acid 3.3 mg, B complex as provided by 150 mg Brewer's yeast/Tab. Bot. 100s, 500s. *otc.*
Use: Mineral, vitamin supplement.

B and O Supprettes No. 15A & No. 16A. (PolyMedica Pharmaceuticals) Opium 30 mg or 60 mg, belladonna extract 16.2 mg/Supp. Jar 12s. *c-II.*
Use: Analgesic, antispasmodic, narcotic.

Bobid. (Boyd) Phenylpropanolamine HCl 50 mg, chlorpheniramine maleate 8 mg, methscopolamine bromide 2.5 mg/Cap. Bot. 100s. *otc.*
Use: Antihistamine, anticholinergic, decongestant.

Bo-Cal. (Fibertone) Calcium 250 mg, magnesium 125 mg, vitamin D_3 100 IU, boron 0.75 mg/Tab. Bot. 120s. *otc.*
Use: Mineral, vitamin supplement.

Boil-Ease Salve. (Del Pharmaceuticals, Inc.) Benzocaine 20%, camphor, eucalyptus oil, menthol, petrolatum, phenol. Oint. 30 g. *otc.*
Use: Anesthetic drawing salve.

BoilnSoak. (Alcon Laboratories, Inc.) Sodium Cl 0.7%, boric acid, sodium borate, thimerosal 0.001%, disodium edetate 0.1%. Bot. 8 oz, 12 oz. *otc.*
Use: Contact lens care.

•**bolandiol dipropionate.** (bole-AN-die-ole die-PRO-pee-oh-nate) USAN.
Use: Anabolic.

•**bolasterone.** (BOLE-ah-STEE-rone) USAN.
Use: Anabolic.

Bolax. (Boyd) Docusate sodium 240 mg, phenolphthalein 30 mg, dihydrocholic acid. ¾ gr. Cap. Bot. 100s. *otc.*
Use: Laxative.

•**boldenone undecylenate.** (BOLE-deen-ohn uhn-deh-sih-LEN-ate) USAN. Parenabol. Under study.

Use: Anabolic.

•**bolenol.** (BOLE-ee-nahl) USAN.
Use: Anabolic.

•**bolmantalate.** (BOLE-MAN-tah-late) USAN.
Use: Anabolic.

Bonacal Plus. (Kenwood Laboratories) Vitamins A 5000 IU, D 400 IU, C 100 mg, B_1 3 mg, B_2 3 mg, B_6 10 mg, B_{12} 4 mcg, niacinamide 20 mg, d-calcium pantothenate 3.3 mg, iron 42 mg, calcium 350 mg, manganese 0.33 mg, zinc 0.1 mg, magnesium 1.67 mg, potassium 1.67 mg/Tab. Bot. 100s. *otc.*
Use: Mineral, vitamin supplement.

Bonamil Infant Formula with Iron. (Wyeth-Ayerst Laboratories) Protein 2.3 g (from nonfat milk, taurine), fat 5.4 g (from soybean and coconut oils, soy lecithin), carbohydrate 10.7 g (from lactose), linoleic acid 1300 mg, vitamin A 300 IU, D 60 IU, E 2.85 IU, K 8 mcg, $B_1$100 mcg, B_2 150 mcg, B_6 63 mcg, B_{12} 0.2 mcg, B_3 750 mcg, folic acid 7.5 mcg, B_5 315 mcg, biotin 2.2 mcg, vitamin C 8.3 mg, choline 15 mg, Ca 69 mg, P 54 mg, Mg 6 mg, Fe 1.8 mg, Zn 0.75 mg, Mn 15 mcg, Cu 70 mcg, I 5 mcg, Na 27 mg, K 93 mg, Cl 63 mg/100 cal (5.3 cal/g). Conc., Liq. Bot. 453 g Conc. 384 ml. Ready-to-feed liq. 946 ml. *otc.*
Use: Nutritional supplement, enteral.

Bonate. (Suppositoria Laboratories, Inc.) Bismuth subgallate, balsam Peru, benzocaine, zinc oxide/Supp. Box 12s, 100s, 1000s. *otc.*
Use: Anorectal preparation.

Bonefos. (Leiras Pharmaceuticals, Inc.) Disodium Clodronate tetrahydrate.
Use: Bone resorption inhibitor. [Orphan Drug]

Bone Meal w/ Vitamin D. (Natures Bounty, Inc.) Calcium 220 mg, vitamin D 100 IU, phosphorus 100 mg, iron 0.45 mg, copper 3.25 mg, zinc 20 mcg, manganese 2.75 mcg, magnesium 0.925 mg. Tab. Bot. 100s, 250s. *otc.*
Use: Mineral, vitamin supplement.

Bonine. (Pfizer US Pharmaceutical Group) Meclizine HCl 25 mg/Chew. tab. Pkg. 8s, 48s. *otc.*
Use: Antiemetic, antivertigo.

Bontril PDM. (Schwarz Pharma, Inc.) Phendimetrazine tartrate 35 mg/3 layer Tab. Bot. 100s, 1000s. *c-III.*
Use: Anorexiant.

Bontril Slow Release. (Schwarz Pharma, Inc.) Phendimetrazine tartrate 105 mg/Cap. Bot. 100s, 1000s *c-III.*
Use: Anorexiant.

Boost. (Mead Johnson) Protein 10 mg, fat 7 g, carbohydrate 35 g, sodium 130 mg, potassium 400 mg, vitamins A, C, D, E, B_1, B_2, B_3, B_5, B_6, B_9, B_{12}, biotin, Ca, P, I, Mg, Zn, Cu, sugar, corn syrup. Liq. Bot. 237 ml. *otc.*
Use: Nutritional supplement, enteral.

Boost Nutritional Pudding. (Mead Johnson Nutritionals) Protein 7 g, fat 9 g, carbohydrate 32 g, sodium 120 mg, potassium 320 mg, calories 240/serving, vitamins A, C, D, E, K, B_6, B_{12}, B_1, B_2, B_3, B_5, Ca, Fe, folic acid, biotin, P, I, Mg, Zn, Se, Cu, Mn, Cr, Mo, sugar. Pudding Cont. 142 g. *otc.*
Use: Nutritional supplement.

Bopen-VK. (Boyd) Potassium phenoxymethyl penicillin 400,000 units/Tab. Bot. 100s.
Use: Anti-infective, penicillin.

borax. Sodium Borate, N.F. 18.

•**boric acid.** N.F. 18.
Use: Antiseptic, pharmaceutic necessity.
See: Borofax, Oint. (GlaxoWellcome).
W/Combinations.
See: Saratoga Ointment (Blair Laboratories).

boric acid ointment. (Various Mfr.) Topical ointment 5% or 10%. Tube, Jar 30 g, 52.5 g, 60 g, 120 g, 454 g. Ophth. oint. 0.5% or 10%. Tube, Jar. 3.5 g, 3.75 g, 30 g, 60 g, 480 g. *Rx-otc.*
Use: Dermatologic, counterirritant.

2-bornanone. Camphor, U.S.P. 23.

•**bornelone.** (BORE-neh-LONE) USAN.
Use: Ultraviolet screen.

•**bornyl acetate.** USAN.

•**borocaptate sodium 10.** (bore-oh-CAP-tate) USAN.
Use: Antineoplastic, radiopharmaceutical.

Borocell. (Neutron Technology Corp.) Sodium monomercaptoundecahdrocloso-dodecaborate.
Use: Boron neutron capture therapy (BNCT) in glioblastoma multiforme.

Borofair Otic. (Major Pharmaceuticals) Acetic acid 2% in aluminum acetate. Soln. Bot. 60 ml. *Rx.*
Use: Otic preparation.

Borofax Skin Protectant. (Warner Lambert Consumer Healthcare) Zinc oxide 15%, petrolatum 68.6%, lanolin, mineral oil. Oint. Tube 50 g. *otc.*
Use: Dermatologic, counterirritant.

Boroglycerin. Glycerol borate. (Emerson Laboratories) Bot. Pt.

boroglycerin glycerite. Boric acid 31 parts, glycerin 96 parts.

Use: Agent for dermatitis.

Boropak Powder. (Glenwood, Inc.) Aluminum sulfate and calcium acetate. One packet dissolved in a pint of water yields a 1:40 dilution. Pcks 2.4 g. 100s. *otc.*
Use: Anti-inflammatory, topical.

borotannic complex. Boric acid 31 mg, tannic acid 50 mg.

•**bosentan.** (boe-SEN-tan) USAN.
Use: Antagonist (endothelin receptor).

Boston Advance Cleaner. (Polymer Technology International) Concentrated homogenous surfactant with friction-enhancing agents. Soln. Bot. 30 ml. *otc.*
Use: Contact lens care.

Boston Advance Comfort Formula. (Polymer Technology International) Buffered, slightly hypertonic. Polyaminopropyl biguanide 0.00015%, EDTA 0.05%, cationic cellulose derivative polymer. Soln. Bot. 120 ml. *otc.*
Use: Contact lens care.

Boston Advance Conditioning Solution. (Polymer Technology International) Sterile, buffered, slightly hypertonic. Polyaminopropyl biguanide 0.0015%, EDTA 0.05%. Bot.120 ml or with cleaner in a convenience pack. *otc.*
Use: Contact lens care.

Boston Advance Rewetting Drops. (Polymer Technology International) Buffered, slightly hypertonic. Polyaminopropyl biguanide 0.0015%, EDTA 0.05%. Bot. 10 ml. *otc.*
Use: Contact lens care.

Boston Cleaner. (Polymer Technology International) Concentrated homogenons surfactant with friction-enhancing agents, sodium Cl. Soln. Bot. 30 ml. *otc.*
Use: Contact lens care.

Boston Conditioning Solution. (Polymer Technology International) Sterile, buffered, slightly hypertonic, low viscosity. EDTA 0.05%, chlorhexidine gluconate 0.006%. Bot. 120 ml. *otc.*
Use: Contact lens care.

Boston Reconditioning Drops. (Polymer Technology International) Hydrophilic polyelectrolyte, polyvinyl alcohol, hydroxyethylcellulose, chlorhexidine gluconate, EDTA. Soln. Bot. 120 ml. *otc.*
Use: Contact lens care.

Boston Rewetting Drops. (Polymer Technology International) Buffered, slightly hypertonic. Chlorhexidine gluconate 0.006%, EDTA 0.05%, cationic cellulose derivative polymer. Soln. Bot. 10 ml. *otc.*
Use: Contact lens care.

Botox. (Allergan, Inc.) Botulinum toxin type A 100 units, albumin 0.05 mg, sodium chloride 0.9 mg. Pow. for Inj. (lyophilized). Vials. *Rx.*
Use: Ophthalmic.

Bottom Better. (InnoVisions) Petrolatum 49%, lanolin 15.5%, beeswax, sodium borate, lanolin alcohols, methyl salicylate, sorbitan sesquioleate, parabens, oxyquinolone, EDTA. Oint. Pkg. 18s. *otc.*
Use: Diaper rash preparation.

botulinum toxin type A.
Use: Ophthalmic. [Orphan Drug]
See: Botox (Allergan, Inc.).

botulinum toxin type B. (Athena Neurosciences, Inc.)
Use: Cervical dystonia. [Orphan Drug]

botulinum toxin type F. (Porton Product Limited)
Use: Cervical dystonia; essential blepharospasm. [Orphan Drug]

• **botulism antitoxin.** U.S.P. 23.
Use: Prophylaxis and treatment of the toxins of C botulinum, Types A or B; passive immunizing agent.

botulism immune globulin.
Use: Infant botulism. [Orphan Drug]

Bounty Bears. (NBTY, Inc.) Vitamins A 2500 IU, D 400 IU, E 15 IU, C 60 mg, B_1 1.05 mg, B_2 1.2 mg, B_3 13.5 mg, B_6 1.05 mg, B_{12} 4.5 mcg, folic acid 0.3 mg/Tab. Bot. 100s. *otc.*
Use: Mineral, vitamin supplement.

Bounty Bears Plus Iron. (NBTY, Inc.) Vitamins A 2500 IU, D 400 IU, E 15 IU, C 60 mg, B_1 1.05 mg, B_2 1.2 mg, B_3 13.5 mg, B_6 1.05 mg, B_{12} 4.5 mcg, folic acid 0.3 mg, iron 15 mg/Tab. Bot. 100s. *otc.*
Use: Mineral, vitamin supplement.

bourbonal.
See: Ethyl Vanillin, N.F. 18.

bovine colostrum.
Use: AIDS-related diarrhea. [Orphan Drug]

bovine immunoglobulin concentrate, cryptosporidium parvum.
Use: Anti-infective. [Orphan Drug]

bovine whey protein concentrate.
Use: Treatment of cryptosporidiosis. [Orphan Drug]
See: Immuno-C (Biomune Systems, Inc.).

Bowman Cold Tabs. (Jones Medical Industries, Inc.) Acetaminophen 324 mg, phenylpropanolamine HCl 24.3 mg, caffeine 16.2 mg/Tab. Bot. 1000s, 5000s. *otc.*
Use: Analgesic, decongestant.

Bowman's Poison Antidote Kit. (Jones

Medical Industries, Inc.) Syrup of ipecac 1 oz, 1 bottle; activated charcoal liquid 2 oz, 3 bottles. *otc.*
Use: Antidote.

Bowsteral. (Jones Medical Industries, Inc.) Isopropanol 60%. Bot. Pt, gal.
Use: Disinfectant.

•**boxidine.** (BOX-ih-deen) USAN.
Use: Adrenal steroid blocker, antihyperlipoproteinemic.

Boylex. (Health for Life Brands, Inc.) Diperodon, hexachlorophene, rosin cerate, ichthammol, carbolic acid, thymol, camphor, juniper tar. Tube oz. *otc.*
Use: Drawing salve.

B-Pap. (Wren) Acetaminophen 120 mg, sodium butabarbital 15 mg/5 ml. Bot. Pt, gal. *Rx.*
Use: Analgesic, sedative.

b-pas.
See: Calcium Benzoyl PAS.

B-Plex. (Zenith Goldline Pharmaceuticals) Vitamins B_1 15 mg, B_2 15 mg, B_3 100 mg, B_5 18 mg, B_6 4 mg, B_{12} 5 mcg, C 500 mg, folic acid 0.5 mg/Tab. Bot. 100s. *Rx.*
Use: Mineral, vitamin supplement.

BP-Papaverine. (Burlington) Papaverine HCl 150 mg/SR Cap. Bot. 50s. *Rx.*
Use: Vasodilator.

BP Cold Tablets. (Bristol-Myers Squibb) Acetaminophen 325 mg, phenylpropanolamine HCl 12.5 mg, chlorpheniramine maleate 2 mg/Tab. Card 16s, Bot. 16s, 30s, 50s. *otc.*
Use: Analgesic, antihistamine, decongestant.

Brace. (SmithKline Beecham Pharmaceuticals) Denture adhesive. Tube 1.4 oz, 2.4 oz.

Bradosol Bromide. (Novartis Pharmaceutical Corp.) Domiphen bromide.

BranchAmin 4%. (Baxter Pharmaceutical Products, Inc.) Isoleucine 1.38 g, leucine 1.38 g, valine 1.25 g, phosphate 31.6 mOsm/100 ml. Bot. 500 ml. *Rx.*
Use: Adjunct to regular TPN therapy for highly stressed or traumatized patients.

branched chain amino acids.
Use: Nutritional supplement; amyotrophic lateral sclerosis agent. [Orphan Drug]

Brasivol Fine, Medium, and Rough. (Stiefel Laboratories, Inc.) Aluminum oxide scrub particles in a surfactant cleansing base. **Fine:** Jar 153 g. **Medium:** Jar 180 g. **Rough:** Jar 195 g. *otc.*
Use: Scrub cleanser.

Breacol Decongestant Cough Medication. (Bayer Corp. (Consumer Div.)) Dextromethorphan HBr 10 mg, phenylpropanolamine HCl 37.5 mg, alcohol 10%, chlorpheniramine maleate 4 mg/5 ml. Bot. 3 oz, 6 oz. *otc.*
Use: Antihistamine, antitussive, decongestant.

Breatheasy. (Pascal Co. Inc.) Racemic epinephrine HCl Soln. 2.2% inhaled by use of nebulizer. Bot. 0.25 oz, 0.5 oz, 1 oz. *otc.*
Use: Bronchodilator.

Breezee Mist. (Pedinol Pharmacal, Inc.) Aluminum chlorhydrate, undecylenic acid, menthol. Aerosol Bot. 4 oz. *otc.*
Use: Antifungal, deodorant, antiperspirant, foot powder.

Breezee Mist Antifungal. (Pedinol Pharmacal, Inc.) Miconazole nitrate 2%, isobutane, talc, aluminum chlorhydrate, cyclomethicone, isopropyl myristate, propylene carbonate, menthol. Pow. Tube. 113 g. *otc.*
Use: Anti-infective, topical.

Breezee Mist Antifungal. (Pedinol Pharmacal, Inc.) Tolnaftate 1%, talc, menthol crystals. Pow. Tube 113 g. *otc.*

Breezee Mist Foot Powder. (Pedinol Pharmacal, Inc.) Isobutane, talc, aluminium chlorhydrate, cyclomethicone, isopropyl myristate, propylene carbonate, stearalkonium hectorite, undecylenic acid, fragrance, menthol. Pow. Tube 113 g. *otc.*
Use: Antifungal, topical.

Breonesin. (Sanofi Winthrop Pharmaceuticals) Guaifenesin 200 mg/Cap. Bot. 100s. *otc.*
Use: Expectorant.

•**brequinar sodium.** (BREh-kwih-NAHR) USAN.
Use: Antineoplastic.

•**bretazenil.** (bret-AZZ-eh-nill) USAN.
Use: Anxiolytic.

Brethaire. (Novartis Pharmaceutical Corp.) Terbutaline sulfate 0.2 mg/actuation. Aer. Canister 10.5 g (≥ 300 inhalations). *Rx.*
Use: Bronchodilator.

Brethancer. (Novartis Pharmaceutical Corp.) Inhaler (complete unit to be used with Brethaire).

Brethine. (Novartis Pharmaceutical Corp.) Terbutaline sulfate. **Tab.:** 2.5 mg, 5 mg. Bot. 100s, 1000s, UD 100s, Gy-Pak 100s. **Inj.:** 1 mg/ml Amp. 2 ml w/ 1 ml fill. *Rx.*
Use: Bronchodilator.

•**bretylium tosylate.** (bre-TILL-ee-uhm TAH-sill-ate) U.S.P. 23.

Use: Hypotensive, antiadrenergic, cardiovascular agent (antiarrhythmic).

bretylium tosylate in 5% dextrose. (Various Mfr.) Bretylium tosylate 500 mg or 1000 mg. Inj. Vial 250 ml. *Rx.*
Use: Antiarrhythmic.

Brevibloc. (Ohmeda Pharmaceuticals) Esmolol HCl 10 mg/ml or 250 mg/ml, propylene glycol 25%. Inj. **10 mg/ml:** Vial 10 ml. **250 mg/ml:** Amp 10 ml. *Rx.*
Use: Beta-adrenergic blocker.

Brevicon. (Roche Laboratories) Norethindrone 0.5 mg, ethinyl estradiol 0.035 mg/Tab. 21 and 28 day (7 inert tabs) Wallette. *Rx.*
Use: Contraceptive.

Brevital Sodium. (Eli Lilly and Co.) Methohexital sodium. **Vial:** 500 mg/50 ml, 500 mg/50 ml w/diluent, 2.5 g/250 ml, 5 g/500 ml. **Amp.:** 2.5 g, 5 g. *Rx.*
Use: Anesthetic, general.

Brevoxyl. (Stiefel Laboratories, Inc.) Benzoyl peroxide 4%, cetyl and stearyl alcohol. Gel Tube 42.5 g, 90 g. *Rx.*
Use: Antiacne.

brewer's yeast. (NBTY, Inc.) Vitamins B_1 0.06 mg, B_2 0.02 mg, B_3 0.2 mg/Tab. Bot. 250s. *otc.*
Use: Vitamin supplement.

Brexin EX Liquid. (Savage Laboratories) Pseudoephedrine HCl 30 mg, guaifenesin 200 mg/5 ml. *otc.*
Use: Decongestant, expectorant.

Brexin EX Tablet. (Savage Laboratories) Pseudoephedrine HCl 60 mg, guaifenesin 400 mg/Tab. Bot. 100s. *otc.*
Use: Decongestant, expectorant.

Brexin L.A. (Savage Laboratories) Chlorpheniramine maleate 8 mg, pseudoephedrine HCl 120 mg/LA Cap. Bot. 100s. *otc.*
Use: Antihistamine, decongestant.

Bricanyl. (Hoechst Marion Roussel) Terbutaline sulfate. **Tab.:** 2.5 mg, 5 mg. Bot. 100s. **Inj.:** 1 mg/ml. Amp. 2 ml w/1 ml fill. *Rx.*
Use: Bronchodilator.

•**brifentanil hydrochloride.** (brih-FEN-tah-NILL) USAN.
Use: Analgesic, narcotic.

Brigen-G. (Grafton) Chlordiazepoxide 5 mg, 10 mg, or 25 mg/Tab. Bot. 500s. *c-iv.*
Use: Anxiolytic.

Brij 96 and 97. (ICI Americas) Polyoxyl 10 oleyl ether available as 96 and 97.
Use: Surface active agent.

Brij-721. (ICI Americas) Polyoxyethylene 21 stearyl ether (100% active).
Use: Surface active agent.

•**brimonidine tartrate.** (brih-MOE-nih-DEEN) USAN.
Use: Adrenergic (ophthalmic).
See: Alphagan (Allergan, Inc.).

•**brinolase.** (BRIN-oh-laze) USAN. Fibrinolytic enzyme produced by *Aspergillus oryzae.*
Use: Fibrinolytic.

•**brinzolamide.** (brin-ZOE-lah-mide) USAN.
Use: Antiglaucoma agent.
See: Azopt, Ophth. Susp. (Alcon Laboratories, Inc.).

Bristoject. (Bristol-Myers Squibb) Prefilled disposable syringes w/needle. **Available with:** Aminophylline: 250 mg/10 ml. Atropine Sulfate: 5 mg/5 ml or 1 mg/ml. 10s. Calcium Cl: 10%. 10 ml. 10s. Dexamethasone: 20 mg/5 ml. Dextrose: 50%. 50 ml. 10s. Diphenhydramine: 50 mg/5 ml. Dopamine HCl: 200 mg/5 ml, 400 mg/10 ml. Ephedrine: 50 mg/10 ml. Epinephrine: 1:10,000. 10 ml. 10s. Lidocaine HCl: 1%: 5 ml, 10 ml; 2%: 5 ml; 4%: 25 ml, 50 ml; 20%: 5 ml, 10 ml. Magnesium Sulfate: 5 g/10 ml 10s. Metaraminol: 1% 10 ml. Sodium Bicarbonate: 75%: 50 ml; 84%: 50 ml. 10s.
Use: Medical device.

british anti-lewisite. Dimercaprol.
See: BAL.

Brobella-P.B. (Brothers) Atropine sulfate 0.0195 mg, hyoscine HBr 0.0065 mg, hyoscyamine sulfate 0.1040 mg, phenobarbital 0.25 gr/Tab. Bot. 100s, 1000s. *Rx.*
Use: Anticholinergic, antispasmodic, hypnotic, sedative.

•**brocresine.** (broe-KREE-seen) USAN.
Use: Histidine decarboxylase inhibitor.

•**brocrinat.** (BROE-krih-NAT) USAN.
Use: Diuretic.

Brocycline. (Brothers) Tetracycline HCl 250 mg/Cap. Bot. 100s, 1000s. *Rx.*
Use: Anti-infective, tetracycline.

Brofed. (Marnel Pharmaceuticals, Inc.) Pseudoephedrine HCl 30 mg, brompheniramine maleate 4 mg/5 ml. Elix. Bot. 473 ml. *otc.*
Use: Antihistamine, decongestant.

•**brofoxine.** (BROE-fox-een) USAN.
Use: Antipsychotic.

Brolade. (Brothers) Chlorpheniramine maleate 8 mg, phenylephrine HCl 20 mg, methscopolamine nitrate 2.5 mg/Cap. Bot. 50s, 500s. *Rx.*
Use: Anticholinergic, antihistamine, decongestant.

Brolene. (Bausch & Lomb Pharmaceuti-

cals) Propamidine isethionate 0.1% Ophth. Soln.
Use: Acanthamoeba Keratitis. [Orphan Drug]

Bromadine-DM. (Cypress Pharmaceutical, Inc.) Brompheniramine maleate 2 mg, dextromethorphan HBr 10 mg/5 ml, cherry flavor, Syr. Bot. 473 ml. *Rx.*
Use: Antihistamine, antitussive, decongestant.

•**bromadoline maleate.** (BROE-mah-DOE-leen) USAN.
Use: Analgesic.

bromaleate.
See: Pamabrom.

Bromaline. (Rugby Labs, Inc.) Phenylpropanolamine HCl 12.5 mg, brompheniramine maleate 2 mg, alcohol 2.3%. Elix. Bot. 118 ml, 473 ml, gal. *otc.*
Use: Antihistamine, decongestant.

Bromaline Plus. (Rugby Labs, Inc.) Phenylpropanolamine HCl 12.5 mg, brompheniramine maleate 2 mg, acetaminophen 500 mg. Captabs. Bot. 24s. *otc.*
Use: Analgesic, antihistamine, decongestant.

Bromalix. (Century Pharmaceuticals, Inc.) Brompheniramine maleate 4 mg, phenylephrine HCl 5 mg, phenylpropanolamine HCl 5 mg, alcohol 2.3%/5 ml. Liq. Bot. 4 oz, pt, gal. *otc.*
Use: Antihistamine, decongestant.

Bromanate DC Cough Syrup. (Various Mfr.) Phenylpropanolamine HCl 12.5 mg, brompheniramine maleate 2 mg, codeine phosphate 10 mg, alcohol 0.95%. Syr. Bot. 120 ml, pt, gal. *c-v.*
Use: Antihistamine, antitussive, decongestant.

Bromanate Elixir. (Alpharma USPD Inc.) Phenylpropanolamine HCl 12.5 mg, brompheniramine maleate 2 mg/5 ml. Elix. Bot. 118 ml, 237 ml, 473 ml, gal. *otc.*
Use: Antihistamine, decongestant.

Bromanyl. (Various Mfr.) Bromodiphenhydramine HCl 12.5 mg, codeine phosphate 10 mg, alcohol 5%. Syr. Bot. Pt, gal. *c-v.*
Use: Antihistamine, antitussive.

Bromarest DX. (Warner Chilcott Laboratories) Pseudoephedrine HCl 30 mg, brompheniramine maleate 2 mg, dextromethorphan HBr 10 mg, alcohol 0.95%. Butterscotch flavor. Syr. Bot. 480 ml. *Rx.*
Use: Antihistamine, antitussive, decongestant.

Bromatane D.C. Cough Syrup. (Zenith Goldline Pharmaceuticals) Brompheniramine maleate, phenylpropanolamine HCl, codeine phosphate. Bot. Gal. *c-v.*
Use: Antihistamine, antitussive, decongestant.

Bromatane DX Cough Syrup. (Zenith Goldline Pharmaceuticals) Pseudoephedrine HCl 3 0 mg, brompheniramine maleate 2 mg, dextromethorphan HBr 10 mg. Bot. 480 ml. *Rx.*
Use: Antihistamine, antitussive, decongestant.

Bromatap Elixir. (Zenith Goldline Pharmaceuticals) Brompheniramine maleate 2 mg, phenylephrine HCl 12.5 mg, alcohol 2.3%/5 ml. Liq. Bot. 4 oz, 8 oz, pt, gal. *otc.*
Use: Antihistamine, decongestant.

Bromatapp Tablets. (Copley Pharmaceutical, Inc.) Brompheniramine maleate 12 mg, phenylpropanolamine HCl 75 mg/Tab. Bot. 100s. *otc.*
Use: Antihistamine, decongestant.

bromauric acid. Hydrogen tetrabromoaurate.

•**bromazepam.** (broe-MAY-zeh-pam) USAN.
Use: Anxiolytic.

Brombay Elixir. (Rosemont Pharmaceutical Corp.) Brompheniramine maleate 2 mg/5 ml, alcohol 3%. Bot. 4 oz, pt, gal. *otc.*
Use: Antihistamine.

•**bromchlorenone.** (brome-KLOR-ee-nohn) USAN.
Use: Anti-infective, topical.

•**bromelains.** (BROE-meh-lanes) USAN.
Use: Anti-inflammatory.
See: Dayto-Anase, Tab. (Dayton Laboratories, Inc.).

Bromenzyme. (Barth's) Bromelains 40 mg/Tab. Bot. 100s, 250s, 500s. *Rx-otc.*
Use: Digestive aid.

Bromezyme. (Barth's) Bromelains 40 mg, papaya fruit, papain enzyme/Tab. Bot. 100s, 250s, 500s. *Rx-otc.*
Use: Digestive aid.

bromethol.
See: Avertin.

Bromfed Capsules. (Muro Pharmaceutical, Inc.) Brompheniramine maleate 12 mg, pseudoephedrine HCl 120 mg/TR Cap. Bot. 100s, 500s. *Rx.*
Use: Antihistamine, decongestant.

Bromfed-DM Syrup. (Muro Pharmaceutical, Inc.) Brompheniramine maleate 2 mg, pseudoephedrine HCl 30 mg, dextromethorphan HBr 10 mg/5 ml. Bot. 120 ml, 240 ml, 480 ml. *Rx.*
Use: Antihistamine, antitussive, decongestant.

Bromfed-PD Capsules. (Muro Pharmaceutical, Inc.) Brompheniramine maleate 6 mg, pseudoephedrine HCl 60 mg/TR Cap. Bot. 100s, 500s. *Rx.*
Use: Antihistamine, decongestant.

Bromfed Syrup. (Muro Pharmaceutical, Inc.) Brompheniramine maleate 2 mg, pseudoephedrine HCl 30 mg/5 ml. Bot. 120 ml, 473 ml. *otc.*
Use: Antihistamine, decongestant.

Bromfed Tablets. (Muro Pharmaceutical, Inc.) Brompheniramine maleate 4 mg, pseudoephedrine HCl 60 mg/Tab. Bot. 100s. *Rx.*
Use: Antihistamine, decongestant.

Bromfenex. (Ethex Corp.) Brompheniramine maleate 12 mg, pseudoephedrine HCl 120 mg/ER Cap. Bot. 100s. *Rx.*
Use: Antihistamine, decongestant.

Bromfenex PD. (Ethex Corp.) Brompheniramine maleate 6 mg, pseudoephedrine HCl 60 mg, sucrose/ER Cap. Bot. 100s, 500s. *Rx.*
Use: Antihistamine, decongestant.

•**bromhexine hydrochloride.** (brome-HEX-een) USAN.
Use: Expectorant, mucolytic.

bromhexine. (Boehringer Ingelheim, Inc.)
Use: Mild/moderate keratoconjunctivitis sicca. [Orphan Drug]

bromides.
See: Peacock's Bromides, Liq. (Natcon).

bromide salts.
See: Calcium Bromide.
Ferrous Bromide.
Potassium Bromide.
Sodium Bromide.
Strontium Bromide.

Bromi-Lotion. (Gordon Laboratories) Aluminum hydroxychloride 20%, emollient base. Bot. 1.5 oz, 4 oz. *otc.*
Use: Antiperspirant.

•**bromindione.** (BROME-in-die-ohn) USAN.
Use: Anticoagulant.

Bromi-Talc. (Gordon Laboratories) Potassium alum, bentonite, talc. Shaker can 3.5 oz, 1 lb, 5 lb. *otc.*
Use: Bromidrosis, hyperhidrosis.

•**bromocriptine.** (BROE-moe-KRIP-teen) USAN.
Use: Enzyme inhibitor (prolactin).

•**bromocriptine mesylate.** (BROE-moe-KRIP-teen) U.S.P. 23.
Use: Enzyme inhibitor (prolactin).
See: Parlodel, Tab. (Novartis Pharmaceutical Corp.).

bromodeoxyuridine. (NeoPharm, Inc.)
Use: Radiation sensitizer in treatment of primary brain tumors. [Orphan Drug]

bromodiethylacetylurea.
See: Carbromal.

•**bromodiphenhydramine hydrochloride.** (BROE-moe-die-feu-HIGH-drahmeen) U.S.P. 23.
Use: Antihistamine.

bromodiphenhydramine hydrochloride/codeine phosphate. (Rosemont Pharmaceutical Corp.) Bromodiphenhydramine HCl 12.5 mg, codeine phosphate 10 mg. Syr. Bot. 480 ml. *c-v.*
Use: Antitussive combination.

bromofrom. Tribromomethane.

bromoisovaleryl urea. Alpha, bromoisovaleryl urea.

Bromophen T.D. (Rugby Labs, Inc.) Phenylpropanolamine HCl 15 mg, phenylephrine HCl 15 mg, brompheniramine maleate 12 mg/Tab. Bot. 100s, 1000s. *Rx.*
Use: Antihistamine, decongestant.

Bromophin.
See: Apomorphine HCl (Various Mfr.).

Bromo Seltzer. (Warner Lambert) Acetaminophen 325 mg, sodium bicarbonate 2.78 g, citric acid 2.22 g (when dissolved, forms sodium citrate 2.85 g)/ Dose. Large (2 5/8 oz), King (4.25 oz), Giant (9 oz), Foil pack, single-dose 48s. *otc.*
Use: Antacid, analgesic.

bromotheophyllinate aminoisobutanol.
See: Pamabrom.

bromotheophyllinate pyranisamine.
See: Pyrabrom.

bromotheophyllinate pyrilamine.
See: Pyrabrom.

8-bromotheophylline.
See: Pamabrom.

Bromotuss W/Codeine. (Rugby Labs, Inc.) Bromodiphenhydramine HCl 12.5 mg, codeine phosphate 10 mg, alcohol 5%. Syr. Bot. 120 ml, pt, gal. *c-v.*
Use: Antihistamine, antitussive.

•**bromoxanide.** (broe-MOX-ah-nide) USAN.
Use: Anthelmintic.

•**bromperidol.** (brome-PURR-ih-dahl) USAN.
Use: Antipsychotic.

•**bromperidol decanoate.** (brome-PURR-ih-dole deh-KAN-oh-ate) USAN.
Use: Antipsychotic.

Bromphen DC w/Codeine Cough Syrup. (Various Mfr.) Phenylpropanolamine HCl 12.5 mg, brompheniramine

maleate 2 mg, codeine phosphate 10 mg, alcohol 0.95%. Syr. Bot. 120 ml, pt, gal. *c-v.*
Use: Antihistamine, antitussive, decongestant.

Bromphen DX. (Rugby Labs, Inc.) Pseudoephedrine HCl 30 mg, brompheniramine maleate 2 mg, dextromethorphan HBr 10 mg, alcohol 0.95%. Syr. Bot. 480 ml. *Rx.*
Use: Antihistamine, antitussive, decongestant.

Bromphen Expectorant. (Various Mfr.) Phenylpropanolamine HCl 5 mg, phenylephrine HCl 5 mg, brompheniramine maleate 2 mg, guaifenesin 100 mg, alcohol 3.5%. Liq. Bot. 120 ml, pt, gal. *otc.*
Use: Antihistamine, decongestant, expectorant.

Brompheniramine Cough Syrup. (Geneva Pharmaceuticals) Pseudoephedrine HCl 30 mg, brompheniramine maleate 2 mg, dextromethorphan HBr 10 mg, alcohol 0.95%. Bot. 480 ml. *Rx.*
Use: Antihistamine, antitussive, decongestant.

Brompheniramine DC. (Geneva Pharmaceuticals) Phenylpropanolamine HCl 12.5 mg, brompheniramine maleate 2 mg, codeine phosphate 10 mg, alcohol 0.95%. Syr. Bot. 120 ml. *c-v.*
Use: Antihistamine, antitussive, decongestant.

•**brompheniramine maleate.** (brome-fen-AIR-uh-meen) U.S.P. 23.
Use: Antihistamine.
See: Dimetane, Tab., Elix., Inj. (Wyeth-Ayerst Laboratories).
Dimetapp Allergy, Liquigels (A.H. Robins).

brompheniramine maleate. (Various Mfr.) Brompheniramine maleate 10 mg/ml, parabens. Inj. Multi-dose vial 10 ml. *Rx.*
Use: Antihistamine.

brompheniramine maleate w/combinations.
See: Bromadine-DM, Syr. (Cypress Pharmaceutical, Inc.)
Bromfenex, ER Cap. (Ethex Corp.).
Bromfenex PD, ER Cap. (Ethex Corp.).
Cortane, Preps. (Standex).
Cortapp, Elix. (Standex).
Dimetane Decongestant, Tab., Elix. (Wyeth-Ayerst Laboratories).
Dimetane Expectorant, Liq. (Wyeth-Ayerst Laboratories).
Dimetane Expectorant-DC, Liq. (Wyeth-Ayerst Laboratories).
Dimetapp Extentabs, Elix. (Wyeth-Ayerst Laboratories).
Iofed, ER Cap. (Iomed).
Iofed PD, ER Cap. (Iomed).
Iohist DM, Syr. (Iomed).
Liqui-Histine DM, Syr. (Liquipharm).
Rondec, Chew. Tab. (Dura).
Siltapp with Dextromethorphan HBr Cold & Cough, Elix. (Silarx).

Brompton's Cocktail. Heroin or morphine 10 mg, cocaine 10 mg, alcohol, chloroform water, syrup. *c-II.*
Use: Analgesic, narcotic.

Bromtapp. (Halsey Drug Co.) Brompheniramine maleate 4 mg, phenylephrine HCl 5 mg, phenylpropanolamine HCl 5 mg/5 ml. Bot. 16 oz, gal. *otc.*
Use: Antihistamine, decongestant.

Bronchial Capsules. (Various Mfr.) Theophylline 150 mg, guaifenesin 90 mg. Cap. Bot. 100s, 1000s. *Rx.*
Use: Antiasthmatic, expectorant.

Broncholate Capsules. (Sanofi Winthrop Pharmaceuticals) Ephedrine HCl 12.5 mg, guaifenesin 200 mg/Cap. Bot. 100s, 1000s. *Rx.*
Use: Bronchodilator, expectorant.

Broncholate Softgels. (Sanofi Winthrop Pharmaceuticals) Ephedrine HCl 12.5 mg, guaifenesin 200 mg. Cap. Bot. 100s. *Rx.*
Use: Bronchodilator, expectorant.

Broncholate Syrup. (Sanofi Winthrop Pharmaceuticals) Ephedrine HCl 6.25 mg, guaifenesin 100 mg/5 ml. Bot. Pt. *Rx.*
Use: Bronchodilator, expectorant.

Broncho Saline. (Blairex Labs, Inc.) Sodium Cl 0.9%. Aer. 90 ml, 240 ml w/ metered dispensing valve. *otc.*
Use: Diluent.

Brondecon. (Parke-Davis) **Tab.:** Oxtriphylline 200 mg, guaifenesin 100 mg/ Tab. Bot. 100s. **Elix.:** Oxtriphylline 100 mg, guaifenesin 50 mg/5 ml w/alcohol 20%. Bot. 8 oz, 16 oz. *Rx.*
Use: Bronchodilator, expectorant.

Brondelate. (Various Mfr.) Oxtriphylline 300 mg, guaifenesin 150 mg/5 ml. Elix. Bot. 480 ml, gal. *Rx.*
Use: Bronchodilator, expectorant.

Bronitin. (Whitehall Robins Laboratories) Theophylline hydrous 120 mg, guaifenesin 100 mg, ephedrine HCl 24.3 mg, pyrilamine maleate 16.6 mg/ Tab. Bot. 24s, 60s. *otc.*
Use: Bronchodilator.

Bronitin Mist. (Whitehall Robins Laboratories) Epinephrine bitartrate in inhalation aerosol. Each spray releases 0.3 mg epinephrine bitartrate equivalent to

0.16 mg epinephrine base. Bot 15 ml or 15 ml refills. *otc.*
Use: Bronchodilator.

Bronkaid Dual Action. (Bayer Corp. (Consumer Div.)) Ephedrine sulfate 25 mg, guaifenesin 400 mg. Capl. Bot. 24s. *otc.*
Use: Bronchodilator, expectorant.

Bronkodyl. (Sanofi Winthrop Pharmaceuticals) Theophylline 100 mg or 200 mg/Cap. Bot. 100s. Theophylline 300 mg/SR Cap. Bot. 100s. *Rx.*
Use: Bronchodilator.

Bronkometer. (Sanofi Winthrop Pharmaceuticals) Isoetharine mesylate 0.61%, saccharin, menthol, alcohol 30%. Metered dose of 340 mcg isoetharine in fluorohydrocarbon propellant. Bot. w/ nebulizer 10 ml, 15 ml. Refill 10 ml, 15 ml. *Rx.*
Use: Bronchodilator.

Bronkosol. (Sanofi Winthrop Pharmaceuticals) Isoetharine HCl 1% w/glycerin, sodium bisulfite, parabens for oral inhalation. Bot. 10 ml, 30 ml. *Rx.*
Use: Bronchodilator.

Bronkotuss. (Hyrex Pharmaceuticals) Chlorpheniramine maleate 4 mg, guaifenesin 100 mg, ephedrine sulfate 8.216 mg, hydriodic acid syrup 1.67 mg/5 ml w/alcohol 5%. Bot. Pt, gal. *Rx.*
Use: Antihistamine, decongestant, expectorant.

Brontex Liquid. (Procter & Gamble Pharm.) Codeine phosphate 2.5 mg, guaifenesin 75 mg/5 ml, methylparaben, saccharin, sucrose/Liq. Bot. 473 ml. *c-v.*
Use: Antitussive expectorant, narcotic.

Brontex Tablets. (Procter & Gamble Pharm.) Codeine phosphate 10 mg, guaifenesin 300 mg/Tab. Bot. 100s. *c-III.*
Use: Antitussive expectorant, narcotic.

•**broperamole.** (BROE-PURR-ah-mole) USAN.
Use: Anti-inflammatory.

•**bropirimine.** (broe-PIE-rih-MEEN) USAN.
Use: Antineoplastic, antiviral.

Broserpine. (Brothers) Reserpine 0.25 mg/Tab. Bot. 250s, 100s.
Use: Antihypertensive.

Brotane Expectorant. (Halsey Drug Co.) Guaifenesin 100 mg, brompheniramine maleate 2 mg, phenylephrine HCl 5 mg, phenylpropanolamine HCl 5 mg/5 ml, alcohol 3.5%. Bot. 16 oz. *otc.*
Use: Antihistamine, decongestant, expectorant.

•**brotizolam.** (broe-TIE-zoe-LAM) USAN.
Use: Hypnotic, sedative.

Bro-T's. (Brothers) Bromisovalum 0.12 g, carbromal 0.2 g/Tab. Bot. 100s, 1000s. *Rx.*
Use: Sedative, anxiolytic.

Bro-Tuss. (Brothers) Dextromethorphan HBr 15 mg, chlorpheniramine maleate 2 mg, phenylephrine HCl 5 mg, ammonium Cl 100 mg, sodium citrate 150 mg, vitamin C 30 mg/10 ml. Bot. 4 oz, pt, gal. *otc.*
Use: Antihistamine, antitussive, decongestant, expectorant.

Bro-Tuss A.C. (Brothers) Acetaminophen 120 mg, codeine phosphate 10 mg, phenylephrine HCl 5 mg, chlorpheniramine maleate 2 mg, menthol 1 mg, alcohol 10%/5 ml. Bot. Pt, gal. *c-v.*
Use: Analgesic, antihistamine, antitussive, decongestant.

Bryrel Syrup. (Sanofi Winthrop Pharmaceuticals) Piperazine citrate anhydrous 110 mg/ml. Bot. Oz. *Rx.*
Use: Anthelmintic.

B-Salt Forte. (Akorn, Inc.) **Part I:** Sodium Cl 7.14 mg, potassium Cl 0.38 mg, calcium chloride dihydrate 0.154 mg, magnesium chloride hexahydrate 0.2 mg, dextrose 0.92 mg, hydrochloric acid or sodium hydroxide/ml. Soln. Bot. 515 ml. **Part II:** Sodium bicarbonate 1081 mg, dibasic sodium phosphate (anhydrous) 216 mg, glutathione disulfide 95 mg/Vial. Soln. Bot. 60 ml. *Rx.*
Use: Irrigant, ophthalmic.

B-Scorbic. (Pharmics, Inc.) Vitamins C 300 mg, B_1 25 mg, B_2 10 mg, calcium pantothenate 10 mg, niacinamide 50 mg, lemon flavored complex 200 mg/ Tab. Bot. 100s, 1000s. *otc.*
Use: Mineral, vitamin supplement.

BSS. (Alcon Laboratories, Inc.) Sodium Cl 0.64%, potassium Cl 0.075%, magnesium Cl 0.03%, calcium Cl 0.048%, sodium acetate 0.39%, sodium citrate 0.17%, sodium hydroxide or hydrochloric acid. Bot. 15 ml, 30 ml, 250 ml, 500 ml. *Rx.*
Use: Irrigant, ophthalmic.

BSS Plus. (Alcon Laboratories, Inc.) **Part I:** Sodium Cl 7.44 mg, potassium Cl 0.395 mg, dibasic sodium phosphate 0.433 mg, sodium bicarbonate 2.19 mg, hydrochloric acid, or sodium hydroxide/ml. Soln. Bot. 240 ml. **Part II:** Calcium chloride dihydrate 3.85 mg, magnesium chloride hexahydrate 5 mg, dextrose 23 mg, glutathione disulfide 4.5 mg/ml. Soln. Bot. 10 ml. *Rx.*
Use: Irrigant, ophthalmic.

BTA Rapid Urine Test. (Bard) Reagent kit for detection of bladder tumor associated analytes in urine to aid in management of bladder cancer. Kits of 15 and 30 tests. *Rx.*
Use: Diagnostic aid.

•**bucainide maleate.** (byoo-CANE-ide) USAN.
Use: Cardiovascular agent (antiarrhythmic).

Bucet. (Forest Pharmaceutical, Inc.) Butalbital 50 mg, acetaminophen 650 mg. Cap. Bot. 100s. *Rx.*
Use: Analgesic.

buchu.
See: Barosmin.

•**bucindolol hydrochloride.** (BYOO-SIN-doe-lole) USAN.
Use: Investigative, antihypertensive.

Bucladin-S. (Zeneca Pharmaceuticals) Buclizine HCl 50 mg. Softab. Tab. Bot. 100s. *Rx.*
Use: Antiemetic, antivertigo.

•**buclizine hydrochloride.** (BYOO-klih-zeen) USAN.
Use: Antiemetic, antinauseant.
See: Bucladin-S, Tab. (Zeneca Pharmaceuticals).

•**bucromarone.** (byoo-KROE-mah-rone) USAN.
Use: Cardiovascular agent (antiarrhythmic).

•**bucrylate.** (BYOO-krih-late) USAN.
Use: Surgical aid (tissue adhesive).

•**budesonide.** (BYOO-DESS-oh-nide) USAN.
Use: Anti-inflammatory.
See: Pulmicort Turbuhaler, Pow. for Inhalation (Astra Pharmaceuticals, L.P.).
Rhinocort, Aer. (Astra Pharmaceuticals, L.P.).

Buf Acne Cleansing Bar. (3M Pharmaceuticals) Salicylic acid 1%, sulfur 1% in detergent cleansing bar. 3.5 oz. *otc.*
Use: Antiacne.

Buf-Bar. (3M Pharmaceuticals) Sulphur 3% and titanium dioxide. Bar 105 g. *otc.*
Use: Antiacne.

Buf Body Scrub. (3M Pharmaceuticals) Round cleansing sponge on plastic handles. *otc.*
Use: Cleansing sponge.

Buff-A. (Merz Pharmaceuticals) Aspirin acid 5 gr. buffered w/magnesium hydroxide, aluminum hydroxide dried gel. Tab. Bot. 100s, 1000s. *otc.*
Use: Analgesic, antacid.

Buffaprin. (Buffington) Aspirin 325 mg. buffered with magnesium oxide. Sugar, caffeine, lactose, salt free. Tab. Dispens-A-Kit 500s. *otc.*
Use: Analgesic.

Buffasal. (Dover Pharmaceuticals) Aspirin 325 mg/Tab. w/ magnesium oxide. Sugar, lactose, salt free. UD Box 500s. *otc.*
Use: Analgesic.

Buffasal Max. (Dover Pharmaceuticals) Aspirin 500 mg/Tab w/magnesium oxide. Sugar, lactose, salt free. *otc.*
Use: Analgesic.

Bufferin AF Nite Time. (Bristol-Myers Squibb) Acetaminophen 500 mg, diphenhydramine citrate 38 mg, simethicone. Tab. Bot. 24s and 50s. *otc.*
Use: Analgesic, sedative.

Buffered Aspirin. (Various Mfr.) Aspirin 325 mg with buffers. Tab. Bot. 100s, 500s, 1000s, and UD 100s and 200s. *otc.*
Use: Analgesic.

buffered intrathecal electrolyte/dextrose injection.
Use: Diluent. [Orphan Drug]
See: Elliot's B Solution.

Buffets II. (Jones Medical Industries, Inc.) Aspirin 227 mg, acetaminophen 162 mg, caffeine 32.4 mg, aluminum hydroxide 50 mg/Tab. Bot. 1000s. *otc.*
Use: Analgesic combination.

Buffex. (Roberts Pharmaceuticals) Aspirin 325 mg w/dihydroxyaluminum aminoacetate. Tab. Bot. 1000s, Sanipack 1000s. *otc.*
Use: Analgesic.

Buf Foot Care Kit. (3M Pharmaceuticals) Cleansing system for the feet. *otc.*
Use: Foot preparation.

Buf Foot Care Lotion. (3M Pharmaceuticals) Moisturizing lotion for feet. *otc.*
Use: Foot preparation.

Buf Foot Care Soap. (3M Pharmaceuticals) Bar 3.5 oz. *otc.*
Use: Foot preparation.

•**bufilcon a.** (BYOO-fill-kahn A) USAN.
Use: Contact lens material (hydrophilic).

Buf Kit for Acne. (3M Pharmaceuticals) Cleansing sponge, cleansing bar. 3.5 oz w/booklet, holding tray. *otc.*
Use: Antiacne.

Buf Lotion. (3M Pharmaceuticals) Moisturizing lotion. *otc.*
Use: Emollient.

•**buformin.** (BYOO-FORE-min) USAN.
Use: Antidiabetic.

Bufosal. (Table Rock) Sodium salicylate 15 gr/dram w/calcium carbonate, sodium bicarbonate as granulated effervescent powder. Bot. 4 oz. *otc.*

Use: Analgesic, antacid.

Buf-Ped Non Medicated Cleansing Sponge. (3M Pharmaceuticals) Abrasive cleansing sponge. *otc.*
Use: Cleansing skin on feet.

Buf-Puf Bodymate. (3M Pharmaceuticals) Oval two-sided cleansing sponge. Abrasive/gentle. *otc.*
Use: Cleansing all areas of the body.

Buf-Puf Medicated. (3M Pharmaceuticals) Water-activated. Salicylic acid 0.5% (reg. strength), alcohols, benzoate, EDTA, triethanolamine and vitamin E acetate. Salicylic acid 2% (max. strength). Pads. Jar 30s. *otc.*
Use: Antiacne.

Buf-Puf Non-Medicated Cleansing Sponge. (3M Pharmaceuticals) Abrasive cleansing sponge. *otc.*
Use: Skin cleansing.

Buf-Sul Tablets and Suspension. (Sheryl) Sulfacetamide 167 mg, sulfadiazine 167 mg, sulfamerazine 167 mg. Tab. 100s. Susp. Pt. *Rx.*
Use: Anti-infective, sulfonamide.

Buf-Tabs. (Halsey Drug Co.) Aspirin 5 gr/Tab. w/aluminum hydroxide, glycine magnesium carbonate. Bot. 100s. *otc.*
Use: Analgesic, antacid.

Bugs Bunny Chewable Vitamins and Minerals. (Bayer Corp. (Consumer Div.)) Vitamins A 5000 IU, D 400 IU, E 30 IU, C 60 mg, folic acid 0.4 mg, B_1 1.5 mg, B_2 1.7 mg, niacin 20 mg, B_6 2 mg, B_{12} 6 mcg, biotin 40 mcg, pantothenic acid 10 mg, iron 18 mg, calcium 100 mg, phosphorus 100 mg, iodine 150 mcg, magnesium 20 mg, copper 2 mg, zinc 15 mg/Tab. Bot 60s. *otc.*
Use: Mineral, vitamin supplement.

Bugs Bunny Complete. (Bayer Corp. (Consumer Div.)) Ca 100 mg, iron 18 mg, vitamins A 5000 IU, D 400 IU, E 30 mg, B_1 1.5 mg, B_2 1.7 mg, B_3 20 mg, B_5 10 mg, B_6 2 mg, C 60 mg, folic acid 0.4 mg, biotin 40 mcg, Cu, I, Mg, P, aspartame, phenylalanine, Zn 15 mg/Tab. Bot 60s. *otc.*
Use: Mineral, vitamin supplement.

Bugs Bunny Plus Iron. (Bayer Corp. (Consumer Div.)) Vitamins A 2500 IU, E 15 IU, C 60 mg, folic acid 0.3 mg, B_1 1.05 mg, B_2 1.2 mg, niacin 13.5 mg, B_6 1.05 mg, B_{12} 4.5 mcg, D 400 IU, iron 15 mg/Chew. tab. Bot. 60s. *otc.*
Use: Mineral, vitamin supplement.

Bugs Bunny With Extra C. (Bayer Corp. (Consumer Div.)) Vitamins A 2500 IU, D 400 IU, E 15 IU, C 250 mg, folic acid 0.3 mg, B_1 1.05 mg, B_2 1.2 mg, niacin 13.5 mg, B_6 1.05 mg, B_{12} 4.5 mcg/Tab. Bot. 60s. *otc.*
Use: Mineral, vitamin supplement.

bulkogen. A mucin extracted from the seeds of *Cyanopsis tetragonaloba.*

Bullfrog. (Chattem Consumer Products) Benzophenone-3, octyl methoxycinnamate, isostearyl alcohol, aloe, hydrogenated vegetable oil, vitamin E. Waterproof. Stick 16.5 g. *otc.*
Use: Sunscreen.

Bullfrog Extra Moisturizing Gel. (Chattem Consumer Products) Benzophenone-3, octocrylene, octyl methoxycinnamate, vitamin E, aloe. SPF 18. Tube 90 g. *otc.*
Use: Sunscreen.

Bullfrog for Kids. (Chattem Consumer Products) SPF 18. Octocrylene, octyl methoxycinnamate, octyl salicylate, vitamin E, aloe, alcohols, benzoate. Gel Tube 60 g. *otc.*
Use: Sunscreen.

Bullfrog Sport Lotion. (Chattem Consumer Products) SPF 18. Benzophenone-3, octocrylene, octyl methoxycinnamate, octyl salicylate, titanium dioxide, diazolidinyl urea, EDTA, parabens, vitamin E, aloe. Bot. 120 ml. *otc.*
Use: Sunscreen.

Bullfrog Sunblock. (Chattem Consumer Products) SPF 18, 36. Benzophenone-3, octocrylene, octyl methoxycinnamate, aloe, vitamin E, isostearyl alcohol. PABA free. Waterproof. Gel Tube 120 g. *otc.*
Use: Sunscreen.

•**bumetanide.** (BYOO-MET-uh-hide) U.S.P. 23.
Use: Diuretic.
See: Bumex, Inj., Tab. (Roche Laboratories).

bumetanide. (BYOO-MET-uh-nide) (Various Mfr.) **Tab:** 0.5 mg, 1 mg, 2 mg/Tab. Bot. 100s. (Various Mfr.) **Inj.:** 0.25 mg/ml. Amp. 2 ml. Vial 2 ml, 4 ml, 10 ml; 4 ml fill in 5 ml. *Rx.*
Use: Diuretic.

•**bumetrizole.** (BYOO-meh-TRY-zole) USAN.
Use: Ultraviolet screen.

Bumex. (Roche Laboratories) Bumetanide 0.5 mg, 1 mg, or 2 mg/Tab. 0.5 mg and 1 mg Bot. 100s, 500s, UD 100s. 2 mg Bot. 100s, UD 100s. Inj. Amp 2 ml, 0.25 mg/ml. Box 10s. Vial 2 ml, 4 ml, or 10 ml, 0.25 mg/ml. Box 10s. *Rx.*
Use: Diuretic.

Buminate. (Baxter Pharmaceutical Products, Inc.) Normal serum albumin (human). **25%:** soln. in 20 ml w/o administration set; 50 ml and 100 ml w/admin-

istration set. **5%:** soln. in 250 ml and 500 ml w/administration set. *Rx.*
Use: Albumin replacement.

•**bunamidine hydrochloride.** (BYOO-NAM-ih-deen) USAN.
Use: Anthelmintic.

bunamiodyl sodium.
Use: Diagnostic aid (radiopaque medium).

•**bunaprolast.** (BYOO-nah-PROLE-ast) USAN.
Use: Antiasthmatic.

•**bunolol hydrochloride.** (BYOO-no-lole) USAN.
Use: Antiadrenergic (β-receptor).

Bun Reagent Strips. (Bayer Corp. (Consumer Div.)) Seralyzer reagent strips. A quantitative strip test for BUN in serum or plasma. Bot. 25s.
Use: Diagnostic aid.

Bupap. (ECR Pharmaceuticals) Butalbital 50 mg, acetaminophen 650 mg. Tab. Bot. 100s. *Rx.*
Use: Analgesic.

Buphenyl. (Ucyclyd Pharma, Inc.) Sodium phenylbutyrate 500 mg/Tab. Bot. 250s, 500s. 3.2 g (3 g sodium phenylbutyrate)/tsp. and 9.1 g (8.6 g sodium phenylbutyrate)/tsp. Pow. for Inj. Bot. 500 ml and 950 ml. *Rx.*
Use: Antihyperammonemic.

•**bupicomide.** (byoo-PIH-koe-mide) USAN.
Use: Antihypertensive.

bupivacaine and epinephrine injection.
Use: Anesthetic, local.
See: Marcaine w/Epinephrine, Inj. (Sanofi Winthrop Pharmaceuticals).

bupivacaine HCl. (Abbott Laboratories) Bupivacaine 0.25%. Inj. Vial. 20 ml, 50 ml. Bupivacaine HCl 0.5%. Inj. Vial. 20 ml, 30 ml. Bupivacaine HCl 0.75%. Inj. Vial. 20 ml. *Rx.*
Use: Anesthetic, local.

•**bupivacaine hydrochloride.** (byoo-PIH-vah-cane) U.S.P. 23.
Use: Anesthetic, local.

bupivacaine hydrochloride.
Use: Anesthetic, local.
See: Bupivacaine HCl, Inj. (Abbott Laboratories).
Marcaine, Inj. (Astra Pharmaceuticals, L.P.).
Marcaine Spinal, Inj. (Astra Pharmaceuticals, L.P.).
Marcaine w/Epinephrine, Inj. (Cook-Waite Laboratories, Inc.).
Sensorcaine, Inj. (Astra Pharmaceuticals, L.P.).
Sensorcaine MPF, Inj. (Astra Pharmaceuticals, L.P.).
Sensorcaine MPF Spinal, Inj. (Astra Pharmaceuticals, L.P.).

bupivacaine in dextrose injection.
Use: Anesthetic, local.

Buprenex Injection. (Reckitt & Colman) Buprenorphine HCl 0.3 mg/ml w/50 mg anhydrous dextrose. Amp. 1 ml. *c-v.*
Use: Analgesic, narcotic.

•**buprenorphine hydrochloride.** (BYOO-preh-NAHR-feen) U.S.P. 23.
Use: Analgesic.

bupropion hydrochloride. (Reckitt and Coleman)
Use: Treatment of opiate addiction. [Orphan Drug]

•**bupropion hydrochloride.** (byoo-PRO-pee-ahn) USAN.
Use: Antidepressant; smoking deterrent.
See: Wellbutrin, Tab. (GlaxoWellcome).
Wellbutrin SR, SR Tab. (GlaxoWellcome).
Zyban, SR Tab. (GlaxoWellcome).

•**buramate.** (BYOO-rah-mate) USAN.
Use: Anticonvulsant, antipsychotic, anxiolytic.

Burdeo. (Hill Dermaceuticals, Inc.) Aluminum subacetate 100 mg, boric acid 300 mg/oz. Bot. 3 oz. Roll-on 8 oz. *otc.*
Use: Deodorant.

Burn-a-Lay. (Ken-Gate) Chlorobutanol 0.75%, oxyquinoline benzoate 0.025%, zinc oxide 2%, thymol 0.5%. Cream. Tube oz. *otc.*
Use: Burn therapy.

Burnate. (Burlington) Vitamins A 4000 IU, D-2 400 IU, thiamine HCl 3 mg, riboflavin 2 mg, niacinamide 10 mg, pyridine HCl 2 mg, cyanocobalamin 5 mcg, calcium pantothenate 0.5 mg, folic acid 0.4 mg, ascorbic acid 50 mg, ferrous fumarate 300 mg, calcium 200 mg, iodine 0.15 mg, copper 1 mg, magnesium 5 mg, zinc 1.5 mg/Tab. Bot. 100s. *otc.*
Use: Mineral, vitamin supplement.

Burn-Quel. Halperin aerosol dispenser. 1 oz, 2 oz.
Use: Burn therapy.

burn therapy.
See: Americaine, Preps. (Du Pont Merck Pharmaceutical Co.).
Burn-A-Lay, Cream (Ken-Gate).
Burn-Quel, Aerosol (Halperin).
Butesin Picrate, Oint. (Abbott Laboratories).
Foille, Preps. (Carbisulphoil).
Nupercainal, Oint. (Novartis Pharmaceutical Corp.).

Silvadene, Cream (Hoechst Marion Roussel).
Solarcaine, Preps. (Schering-Plough Corp).
Sulfamylon, Cream (Sanofi Winthrop Pharmaceuticals).
Unguentine, Preps. (Procter & Gamble Pharm.).

Buro-Sol. (Doak Dermatologics) Aluminum acetate 0.23%. Soln. Pkt. 12s. *otc.*
Use: Astringent.

Buro-Sol Antiseptic Powder. (Doak Dermatologics) Contents make a diluted Burow's Solution. Aluminum acetate topical soln. plus benzethonium Cl. Pkg. (2.36 g) 12s, 100s. Bot. Pow. 4 oz, 1 lb, 5 lb. *otc.*
Use: Astringent.

Bursul. (Burlington) Sulfamethizole 500 mg/Tab. Bot. 100s. *Rx.*
Use: Anti-infective; sulfonamide.

Bur-Tuss. (Burlington) Chlorpheniramine maleate 2 mg, phenylephrine HCl 5 mg, phenylpropanolamine HCl 5 mg, guaifenesin 100 mg, alcohol 2.5%/5 ml. Bot. Pt, gal. *otc.*
Use: Antihistamine, decongestant, expectorant.

Bur-Zin. (Lamond) Aluminum acetate solution 2%, zinc oxide 10%. Bot. 4 oz, 8 oz, pt, qt, gal. Also w/o lanolin. *otc.*
Use: Antipruritic, counterirritant.

•**buserelin acetate.** (BYOO-seh-REH-lin ASS-eh-tate) USAN.
Use: Gonad-stimulating principle.

BuSpar. (Bristol-Myers Squibb) Buspirone HCl 5 mg or 10 mg/Tab. *Rx.*
Use: Anxiolytic.

•**buspirone hydrochloride.** (byoo-SPY-rone) U.S.P. 23.
Use: Anxiolytic.
See: BuSpar, Tab. (Bristol-Myers Squibb).

•**busulfan.** (byoo-SULL-fate) U.S.P. 23.
Use: Alkylating agent.
See: Busulfex, Inj. (Orphan Medical, Inc.).
Myleran, Tab. (GlaxoWellcome).

Busulfex. (Orphan Medical, Inc.) Busulfan 6 mg/ml. Inj. Single-use amp 10 ml w/syr. filters. *Rx.*
Use: Alkylating agent.

•**butabarbital.** (byoo-tah-BAR-bih-tahl) U.S.P. 23.
Use: Hypnotic, sedative.
See: BBS, Tab. (Solvay Pharmaceuticals).
Butisol, Prods. (Wallace Laboratories).
Da-Sed, Tab. (Sheryl).
Expansatol, Cap. (Merit).
Medarsed, Elix., Tab. (Medar).

W/Acetaminophen.
See: Sedapap, Elix. (Merz Pharmaceuticals).
Sedapap-10, Tab. (Merz Pharmaceuticals).

W/Acetaminophen, codeine phosphate.
See: T-Caps, Cap. (Burlington).

W/Acetaminophen, salicylamide, phenyltoloxamine citrate.
See: Aludrox, Susp., Tab. (Wyeth-Ayerst Laboratories).

W/Aminophylline, phenylpropanolamine HCl, chlorpheniramine maleate, aluminum hydroxide, magnesium trisilicate.
See: Asmacol, Tab. (Pal-Pak, Inc.).

W/Carboxyphen.
See: Bontril Timed No. 2, Tab. (G. W. Carnrick).

W/Chlorpheniramine maleate, hyoscine HBr.
See: Pedo-Sol, Tab., Elix. (Warren Pharmacal).

W/Dihydroxypropyl theophylline, ephedrine HCl.
See: Airet R, Tab. (Baylor).

W/Ephedrine HCl, theophylline, guaifenesin
See: Quibron Plus, Cap., Elix. (Bristol-Myers Squibb).

W/Ephedrine sulfate, theophylline.
See: Airet Y, Tab., Elix. (Baylor).

W/Ephedrine sulfate, theophylline, guaifenesin.
See: Broncholate, Cap., Elix. (Sanofi Winthrop Pharmaceuticals).

W/l-Hyoscyamine.
See: Cystospaz-SR, Cap. (PolyMedica Pharmaceuticals).

W/Hyoscyamine sulfate, atropine sulfate, hyoscine HBr, homatropine methylbromide.
See: Butabell HMB, Tab., Elix. (Saron).

W/Hyoscyamine sulfate, scopolamine methylnitrate, atropine sulfate.
See: Banatil, Cap., Elix. (Trimen Laboratories, Inc.).

W/Nitroglycerin.
See: Petn Plus (Saron).

W/Pentobarbital, phenobarbital.
See: Quiess, Tab. (Forest Pharmaceutical, Inc.).

W/Phenazopyridine, hyoscyamine HBr.
See: Pyridium Plus, Tab. (Parke-Davis).

W/Phenazopyridine, scopolamine HBr, atropine sulfate, hyoscyamine sulfate.
See: Dapco, Tab. (Mericon Industries, Inc.).

W/Secobarbital.

See: Monosyl, Tab. (Arcum).
W/Secobarbital, pentobarbital, phenobarbital.
See: Quad-Set, Tab. (Kenyon).

•**butabarbital sodium.** (byoo-tah-BAR-bih-tahl) U.S.P. 23.
Use: Hypnotic, sedative.
See: BBS, Tab. (Solvay Pharmaceuticals).
Butalan, Elix. (Lannett Co., Inc.).
Butisol Sodium, Elix., Tab. (Wallace Laboratories).
Expansatol, Cap. (Merit).
Quiebar, Spantab, Tab. (Nevin).
Renbu, Tab. (Wren).
W/Acetaminophen.
See: Amino-Bar, Tab. (Jones Medical Industries, Inc.).
Minotal, Tab. (Schwarz Pharma, Inc.).
W/Acetaminophen, aspirin, caffeine.
See: Dolor Plus, Tab. (Roberts Pharmaceuticals).
W/Acetaminophen, caffeine.
See: Dularin-TH, Tab. (Donner).
Phrenilin, Tab. (Schwarz Pharma, Inc.).
W/Acetaminophen, mephenesin, codeine phosphate.
See: Bancaps-C, Cap. (Westerfield).
W/Acetaminophen, salicylamide.
See: Banesin Forte, Tab. (Westerfield).
Indogesic, Tab. (Century Pharmaceuticals, Inc.).
W/d-Amphetamine sulfate.
See: Bontril, Tab. (Schwarz Pharma, Inc.).
W/Ascorbic acid, sodium p-aminobenzoate, salicylamide, sodium salicylate.
See: Bisalate, Tab. (Allison).
W/Atropine sulfate, hyoscyamine HBr, alcohol, hyoscine HBr.
See: Hyonatol, Tab., Hyonatol B, Elix., Hexett, Tab. (Jones Medical Industries, Inc.).
W/Belladonna extract.
See: Butibel,Tab., Elix. (Ortho McNeil Pharmaceutical).
Quiebel, Elix., Cap. (Nevin).
W/Dehydrocholic acid, belladonna extract.
See: Decholin-BB, Tab. (Bayer Corp. (Consumer Div.)).
W/Methscopolamine bromide, aluminum hydroxide gel, dried, magnesium trisilicate.
See: Eulcin, Tab. (Leeds).
W/Pentobarbital sodium, phenobarbital sodium.
See: Trio-Bar, Tab. (Jenkins).
W/Salicylamide, mephenesin.
See: Metrogesic, Tab. (Lexis Laboratories).
W/Secobarbital sodium.
See: Monosyl, Tab. (Arcum).
W/Secobarbital sodium, pentobarbital sodium, phenobarbital.
See: Nidar, Tab. (Centeon).
W/Simethicone, hyoscyamine sulfate, atropine sulfate, hyoscine HBr.
See: Sidonna, Tab. (Schwarz Pharma, Inc.).

butabarbital sodium. Tab.: 15 mg. Bot. 1000s; 30 mg Bot. 100s, 1000s. **Elixir:** 30 mg/5 ml Bot. Pt.
Use: Sedative, hypnotic.

butacaine.
Use: Anesthetic, local.

•**butacetin.** (byoot-ASS-ih-tin) USAN.
Use: Analgesic, antidepressant.

•**butaclamol hydrochloride.** (byoo-tah-KLAM-ole) USAN.
Use: Antipsychotic.

Butagen Caps. (Zenith Goldline Pharmaceuticals) Phenylbutazone 100 mg/Cap. Bot. 100s, 500s. *Rx.*
Use: Antirheumatic; hypnotic; sedative.

•**butalbital.** (BYOO-TAL-bih-tuhl) U.S.P. 23. *Formerly Allybarbituric acid.*
Use: Hypnotic, sedative.
See: Buff-A-Comp #3 (Merz Pharmaceuticals).
Sandoptal, Preps. (Novartis Pharmaceutical Corp.).
W/Acetaminophen.
See: Axocet, Cap. (Savage Laboratories).
Bupap, Tab. (ECR Pharmaceuticals).
Phrenilin, Tab. (Schwarz Pharma, Inc.).
Phrenilin Forte, Cap. (Schwarz Pharma, Inc.).
Prominol, Tab. (MCR American Pharmaceuticals).
Repan CF, Tab. (Everett).
Tencon, Cap. (International Ethical Labs).
W/Acetaminophen, caffeine.
See: Arbutal, Tab. (Arcum).
Buff-A-Comp, Tab., Cap. (Merz Pharmaceuticals).
Esgic, Tab. (Gilbert).
Cefinal, Tab. (Alto Pharmaceuticals, Inc.).
Margesic, Cap. (Marnel).
Protension, Tab. (Blaine Co., Inc.).
Repan, Tab. (Everett Laboratories, Inc.).
Triad, Cap. (UAD).
W/Acetaminophen, codeine.
See: Phrenilin w/Codeine, Cap. (Schwarz Pharma, Inc.).
W/Aspirin, caffeine.

See: Duogesic, Cap. (Western Research).
Fiorinal, Cap., Tab. (Novartis Pharmaceutical Corp.).
W/Aspirin, caffeine, codeine phosphate.
See: Buff-A-Comp, Tab. w/Codeine (Merz Pharmaceuticals).
Fiorinal With Codeine, Cap. (Novartis Pharmaceutical Corp.).

butalbital, acetaminophen, and caffeine. (BYOO-TAL-bih-tuhl, us-seet-uh-min-oh-fen and kaff-EEN) (Various Mfr.) Acetaminophen 325 mg, caffeine 40 mg, butalbital 50 mg, Tab. Bot. 100s, 500s. *Rx.*
Use: Analgesic.
See: Esgic-Plus, Tab. (Forest Pharmaceutical, Inc.).
Fiorpap, Tab. (Creighton).
Isocet, Tab. (Rugby Labs, Inc.).
Margesic, Cap. (Marnell).
Triad, Cap. (Forest Pharmaceutical, Inc.).

butalbital and aspirin tablets.
Use: Analgesic, sedative.

butalbital, aspirin, & caffeine. (BYOO-TAL-bih-tuhl, ass-pihr-in, and kaff-EEN) (Various Mfr.) **Tab.:** Aspirin 325 mg, caffeine 40 mg, butalbital 50 mg. Bot. 20s, 30s, 50s, 100s, 500s, 1000s, UD 100s. **Cap.:** Aspirin 325 mg, caffeine 40 mg, butalbital 50 mg. Bot. 100s, 1000s. *c-III.*
Use: Analgesic combination.

butalbital compound. (Various Mfr.) Tab., Cap. Bot. 15s, 30s, 100s, 500s, 1000s. *c-III.*
Use: Analgesic.
W/Acetaminophen, butalbital.
See: Phrenilin (Schwarz Pharma, Inc.).
Bancap (Forest Pharmaceutical, Inc.).
Bucet, Cap. (Forest Pharmaceutical, Inc.).
Sedapap-10 (Merz Pharmaceuticals).
Tencon, Cap. (International Ethical Labs).
See: Arcet, Tab. (Econo Med Pharmaceuticals).
Amaphen (Trimen Laboratories, Inc.).
Endolor (Keene Pharmaceuticals, Inc.).
Esgic (Forest Pharmaceutical, Inc.).
Esgic-Plus, Tab. (Forest Pharmaceutical, Inc.).
Fioricet (Novartis Pharmaceutical Corp.).
G-1 (Roberts Pharmaceuticals).
Isocet, Tab. (Rugby Labs, Inc.).
Margesic, Cap. (Marnel Pharmaceuticals, Inc.).
Medigesic Plus (US Pharmaceutical Corp.).
Phrenilin Forte (Schwarz Pharma, Inc).
Repan (Everett Laboratories, Inc).
Sedapap-10 (Merz Pharmaceuticals).
Triad, Cap. (Forest Pharmaceutical, Inc.).
W/Aspirin, butalbital. Aspirin 325 mg, caffeine 40 mg, butalbital 50 mg.
See: Axotal (Pharmacia & Upjohn).
W/Aspirin, caffeine, butalbital.
See: Fiorinal (Novartis Pharmaceutical Corp.).
Lanorinal (Lannett Co, Inc.).
Lorprn (UCB Pharmaceuticals, Inc.).
BAC (Merz Pharmaceuticals).

Butalan. (Lannett Co., Inc.) Sodium butabarbital 0.2 g/30 ml. Elix. Bot. Pt, gal.
Use: Hypnotic, sedative.

butalgin.
See: Methadone HCl (Various Mfr.).

butallylonal. (Pernocton)
Use: Hypnotic.

•**butamben.** (BYOO-tam-ben) U.S.P. 23.
Formerly Butyl aminobenzoate.
Use: Anesthetic, local.

• **butamben picrate.** (BYOO-tam-ben PIC-rate) USAN.
Use: Anesthetic, local.
See: Butesin Picrate, Oint. (Abbott Laboratories).

•**butamirate citrate.** (byoo-tah-MY-rate SIH-trate) USAN.
Use: Antitussive.

•**butane.** N.F. 18.
Use: Aerosol propellant.

•**butaperazine.** (BYOO-tah-PURR-ah-zeen) USAN.
Use: Antipsychotic.

•**butaperazine maleate.** USAN.
Use: Antipsychotic.

butaphyllamine. Ambuphylline. Theophylline aminoisobutanol. Theophylline with 2-amino-2-methyl-1-propanol.

Butapro Elixir. (Health for Life Brands, Inc.) Butabarbital sodium 0.2 g/30 ml. Bot. Pt, gal. *c-v.*
Use: Hypnotic, sedative.

•**butaprost.** (BYOO-tah-PRAHST) USAN.
Use: Bronchodilator.

Butazone. (Major Pharmaceuticals) Phenylbutazone. **Cap.:** 100 mg. Bot. 100s, 500s. **Tab.:** 100 mg. Bot. 500s. *Rx.*
Use: Antirheumatic.

•**butedronate tetrasodium.** (BYOO-teh-DROE-nate TET-rah-SO-dee-uhm) USAN.
Use: Diagnostic aid (bone imaging).

butelline.
See: Butacaine Sulfate (Various Mfr.).

•**butenafine hydrochloride.** (byoo-TEN-ah-feen) USAN.
Use: Antifungal.

butenafine hydrochloride. (Penederm, Inc.)
Use: Treatment of interdigital tinea pedis (athlete's foot).
See: Mentax (Penederm, Inc.).

•**buterizine.** (byoo-TER-ih-ZEEN) USAN.
Use: Vasodilator (peripheral).

Butesin Picrate. (Abbott Laboratories) n-Butyl-p-aminobenzoate. Lidocaine 1%, lanolin, parabens, mineral oil. Oint. Jar. 28.4 g. *otc.*
Use: Anesthetic, local.

Butesin Picrate Ointment. (Abbott Laboratories) Butamben picrate 1%. Tube Oz. *otc.*
Use: Anesthetic, local.

butethal. (Various Mfr.) *Rx.*
Use: Hypnotic, sedative.

butethanol.
See: Tetracaine.

•**buthiazide.** (byoo-THIGH-azz-IDE) USAN.
Use: Antihypertensive, diuretic.

Butibel. (Wallace Laboratories) Butabarbital sodium 15 mg, belladonna extract 15 mg/Tab. or 5 ml. **Tab.:** Bot. 100s. **Elix.:** (w/alcohol 7%) Bot. Pt. *Rx.*
Use: Anticholinergic, antispasmodic, hypnotic, sedative.

•**butikacin.** (BYOO-tih-KAY-sin) USAN.
Use: Anti-infective.

•**butilfenin.** (BYOO-till-FEN-in) USAN.
Use: Diagnostic aid (hepatic function determination).

•**butirosin sulfate.** (byoo-TIHR-oh-sin) USAN. A mixture of the sulfates of the A and B forms of an antibiotic produced by *Bacillus circularis.*
Use: Anti-infective.

Butisol Sodium. (Wallace Laboratories) Butabarbital sodium. **Elix.:** 30 mg/5 ml. Bot. Pt, gal. **Tab.:** 15 mg, 30 mg. Bot. 100s, 1000s. 50 mg or 100 mg. Bot. 100s. *c-III.*
Use: Hypnotic, sedative.
See: Buticaps, Cap. (Wallace Laboratories).
W/Belladonna extract.
See: Butibel (Wallace Laboratories).

•**butixirate.** (BYOO-TIX-ih-rate) USAN.
Use: Analgesic, antirheumatic.

•**butoconazole nitrate.** (BYOO-toe-KOE-nuh-zole) U.S.P. 23.
Use: Antifungal.
See: Femstat, Cream (Procter-Syntex).
Femstat 3, Cream (Procter-Syntex).

butolan. Benzylphenyl carbamate.

•**butonate.** (BYOO-tahn-ate) USAN.
Use: Anthelmintic.

•**butopamine.** (BYOO-TOE-pah-meen) USAN.
Use: Cardiovascular agent.

•**butoprozine hydrochloride.** (byoo-TOE-pro-ZEEN) USAN.
Use: Cardiovascular agent (antiarrhythmic), antianginal.

butopyronoxyl. (Indalone) Butylmesityl oxide.
Use: Insect repellant.

•**butorphanol.** (BYOO-TAR-fan-ahl) USAN.
Use: Analgesic, antitussive.

•**butorphanol tartrate.** (BYOO-TAR-fan-ahl) U.S.P. 23.
Use: Analgesic, antitussive.
See: Stadol, Inj. (Bristol-Myers Squibb).

•**butoxamine hydrochloride.** (byoo-TOX-ah-meen) USAN.
Use: Antidiabetic, antihyperlipoproteinemic.

•**butriptyline hydrochloride.** (BYOO-TRIP-till-een) USAN.
Use: Antidepressant.

•**butyl alcohol.** N.F. 18. Butyl alcohol is n-butyl alcohol.
Use: Pharmaceutic aid (solvent).

butyl aminobenzoate. n-Butyl p-Aminobenzoate. Scuroforme.
Use: Anesthetic, local.
W/Benzocaine, tetracaine HCl.
See: Cetacaine, Preps. (Cetylite Industries, Inc.).
W/Benzyl alcohol, phenylmercuric borate, benzocaine.
See: Dermathyn, Oint. (Davis & Sly).
W/Procaine, benzyl alcohol, in sweet almond oil.
See: Anucaine, Amp. (Calvin).
W/Tetracaine.
See: Pontocaine, Oint. (Sanofi Winthrop Pharmaceuticals).

•**butylated hydroxyanisole.** N.F. 18.
Use: Pharmaceutic aid (antioxidant).

•**buylated hydroxytoluene.** N.F. 18.
Use: Pharmaceutic aid (antioxidant).

•**butylparaben.** (byo-till-PAR-ah-ben) N.F. 18.
Use: Pharmaceutic aid (antifungal).

butylphenylsalicylamide.
See: Butylphenamide.

butyrophenone. Class of antipsychotic agents. *Rx.*
See: Haloperidol.

butyrylcholinesterase. (Pharmavene, Inc.)

Use: Treat cocaine overdose; post-surgical apnea. [Orphan Drug]

B vitamins, parenteral.
See: B-Ject-100 (Hyrex Pharmaceuticals).

B vitamins with vitamin C, parenteral.
See: Key-Plex Injection (Hyrex Pharmaceuticals).
Neurodep Injection (Medical Products Panamericana).
Vicam Injection (Keene Pharmaceuticals, Inc.).

B-Vite Injection. (Bluco Inc./Med. Discnt. Outlet) Vitamins B_1 50 mg, B_2 5 mg, B_6 5 mg, niacinamide 125 mg, B_{12} 1000 mcg, dexpanthenol 6 mg, C 50 mg/10 ml. Mono vial w/benzyl alcohol 1% in water for injection. *Rx.*
Use: Vitamin supplement.

Byclomine w/Phenobarbital. (Major Pharmaceuticals) **Cap.:** Dicyclomine HCl 10 mg, phenobarbital 15 mg. Bot. 250s, 1000s **Tab.:** Dicyclomine HCl 20 mg, phenobarbital 15 mg. Bot. 100s, 250s, 1000s. *Rx.*
Use: Antispasmodic, sedative, hypnotic.

Bydramine. (Major Pharmaceuticals) Diphenhydramine HCl 12.5 mg/5 ml, alcohol 5%. Syr. Bot. 118 ml, pt, gal. *otc.*
Use: Antihistamine.

C

c1-esterase-inhibitor, human, pasteurized. (Alpha Therapeutic Corp.)
Use: Prevention/treatment of angioedema. [Orphan Drug]

c1-esterase-inhibitor, human, pasteurized.
Use: Prevention/treatment of angioedema.
See: Berinert P (Behringwerke Aktiengesellschaft)

c1-inhibitor. (Osterreichisches)
Use: Treatment of angioedema. [Orphan Drug]

c1-inhibitor (human) vapor heated. (Immuno Therapy Co.)
Use: Treatment of angioedema. [Orphan Drug]

c vitamin.
See: Ascorbic Acid, Prep.

•**cabergoline.** (cab-ERR-go-leen) USAN.
Use: Antidyskinetic; antihyperprolactinemic; antiparkinsonian; dopamine agonist; hyperprolactinemic disorders treatment.
See: Dostinex, Tab. (Pharmacia & Upjohn).

•**cabufocon a.** USAN.
Use: Contact lens material (hydrophobic).

•**cabufocon b.** (cab-YOU-FOE-kahn B) USAN.
Use: Contact lens material.

Cachexon. (Telluride Pharm. Corp.) L-Glutathione.
Use: AIDS-associated cachexia. [Orphan Drug]

cacodylic acid salts.
See: Ferric Salt.
Iron Salt.
Sodium Salt.

•**cactinomycin.** (KACK-tih-no-MY-sin) USAN. Antibiotic produced by *Streptomyces chrysomallus. Formerly Actinomycin c.*
Use: Antineoplastic.

cade oil.
See: Juniper Tar.

•**cadexomer iodine.** (kad-EX-oh-mer) USAN.
Use: Antiseptic, antiulcerative.

C & E Softgels. (NBTY, Inc.) E 400 mg, C 500 mg/Cap. Bot. 50s.
Use: Vitamin supplement.

Cafatine Suppositories. (Major Pharmaceuticals) Ergotamine tartrate 2 mg, caffeine 100 mg. Supp. Box 12s. *Rx.*
Use: Antimigraine.

Cafatine-PB. (Major Pharmaceuticals) Ergotamine tartrate 2 mg, caffeine 100 mg, belladonna alkaloids 0.25 mg, pentobarbital 60 mg/Supp. Box foil 10s. *Rx.*
Use: Antimigraine.

Cafenol. (Sanofi Winthrop Pharmaceuticals) Aspirin, caffeine. *otc.*
Use: Analgesic combination.

Cafergot P-B Suppositories. (Novartis Pharmaceutical Corp.) Ergotamine tartrate 2 mg, caffeine 100 mg, bellafoline 0.25 mg, pentobarbital 60 mg/Supp. Box 12s. *Rx.*
Use: Antimigraine.

Cafergot P-B Tablets. (Novartis Pharmaceutical Corp.) Ergotamine tartrate 1 mg, caffeine 100 mg, bellafoline 0.125 mg, pentobarbital sodium 30 mg/Tab. SigPak dispensing pkg. of 90s, 250s. *c-iv.*
Use: Antimigraine.

Cafergot Suppositories. (Novartis Pharmaceutical Corp.) Ergotamine tartrate 2 mg, caffeine 100 mg in cocoa butter base. Supp. Box 12s. *Rx.*
Use: Antimigraine.

Cafergot Tablets. (Novartis Pharmaceutical Corp.) Ergotamine tartrate 1 mg, caffeine 100 mg/SC Tab. Bot. 250s. SigPak dispensing pkg. of 90s. *Rx.*
Use: Antimigraine.

Caffedrine. (Thompson Medical Co.) Caffeine 200 mg, lactose. Tab. Pkg. 16s.
Use: CNS stimulant.

•**caffeine.** U.S.P. 23.
Use: CNS stimulant; apnea of prematurity. [Orphan Drug]
See: Caffedrine, Tab. (Thompson Medical Co.).
Enerjets, Loz. (Chilton Laboratories).
NoDoz, Tab. (Bristol-Myers Squibb).
Quick Pep, Tab. (Thompson Medical Co.).
Stim 250, Cap. (Scrip).
Vivarin, Tab. (J.B. Williams Company Inc.).

caffeine citrated.
Use: CNS stimulant.

caffeine sodio-benzoate.
See: Caffeine sodium benzoate.

caffeine and sodium benzoate injection. Caffeine and sodium benzoate 250 mg/ml (121. 25 mg caffeine, 128.75 mg sodium benxoate). Inj. Amp. 2 ml. *Rx.*
Use: Oral, IM CNS stimulant.

caffeine sodium salicylate. (Various Mfr.) Bot. 1 oz; Pkg. 0.25 lb, 1 lb. *otc.*
Use: See caffeine.

Cagol. (Harvey) Guaiacol 0.1 g, eucalyp-

tol 0.08 g, iodoform 0.2 g, camphor 0.05 g/2 ml in olive oil. Vial 30 ml. *Rx*.
Use: Expectorant.

Caladryl. (Parke-Davis) Calamine 8%, pramoxine HCl 1%, alcohol 2.2%, camphor, diazolidinyl urea, parabens. Lot. Bot. 180 ml. *otc*.
Use: Antipruritic-topical.

Caladryl Clear. (Parke-Davis) Pramoxine HCl 1%, zinc acetate 0.1%, alcohol 2%, camphor, diazolidinyl urea, parabens. Lot. Bot. 180 ml. *otc*.
Use: Antipruritic, topical.

Caladryl for Kids. (Parke-Davis) Calamine 8%, pramoxine HCl 1%, camphor, cetyl alcohol, diazolidinyl urea, parabens. Cream Tube 45 g. *otc*.
Use: Antipruritic, topical.

Calaformula. (Eric, Kirk & Gary) Ferrous gluconate 130 mg, calcium lactate 130 mg, vitamins A 1000 IU, D 400 IU, B_1 2 mg, B_2 2 mg, niacinamide 5 mg, ascorbic acid 20 mg, folic acid 0.13 mg, Mg 0.25 mg, Cu 0.25 mg, Zn 0.25 mg, Mn 0.25 mg, K 0.075 mg/Cap. Bot. 50s, 100s, 500s, 1000s, 5000s. *otc*.
Use: Mineral, vitamin supplement.

Calaformula F. (Eric, Kirk & Gary) Calaformula plus fluorine 0.333 mg/Tab. Bot. 100s. *Rx*.
Use: Mineral, vitamin supplement, dental caries agent.

Cala-Gen. (Zenith Goldline Pharmaceuticals) Diphenhydramine HCl 1%, camphor, alcohol 2%. Lot. Bot. 178 ml. *otc*.
Use: Antipruritic-topical.

Calahist Lotion. (Walgreen Co.) Diphenhydramine HCl 1%, calamine 8.1%, camphor 0.1%. Lot. Bot. 6 oz. *otc*.
Use: Antipruritic, topical.

Calamatum. (Blair Laboratories) **Lot.:** Calamine, zinc oxide, phenol, camphor, benzocaine 3%, nongreasy base. Bot. 1125 ml. **Oint.:** Calamine, zinc oxide, phenol, camphor, benzocaine. Tube 45 g. *otc*.
Use: Dermatologic, counterirritant.

Calamatum Aerosol Spray. (Blair Laboratories) Benzocaine 3%, zinc oxide, calamine, phenol, camphor. Spray can 3 oz. *otc*.
Use: Anesthetic, local.

•**calamine.** U.S.P. 23.
Use: Protectant, topical.
See: Caladryl, Prods. (Parke-Davis).

calamine. (Various Mfr.) Calamine 8%, zinc oxide 8%, glycerin 2%, bentonite magma, calcium hydroxide soln. Lot. Bot. 120 ml, 240 ml, pt, gal.
Use: Antiseptic, astringent.

Calamine, Phenolated. (Humco Holding Group, Inc.) Calamine 8%, zinc oxide 8%, glycerin 2%, bentonite magma and phenol 1% in calcium hydroxide solution. Lot. Bot. 120 ml, 240 ml. *otc*.
Use: Antiseptic, astringent.

Calamox. (Roberts Pharmaceuticals) Prepared calamine 0.17 g. Oint. Tube 60 g. *otc*.
Use: Antiseptic, astringent.

Calamycin. (Pfeiffer Co.) Pyrilamine maleate, zinc oxide 10%, calamine 10%, benzocaine, chloroxylenol, zirconium oxide, isopropyl alcohol 10%. Lot. Bot. 120 ml. *otc*.
Use: Antipruritic, topical.

Calan. (Searle) Verapamil HCl 40 mg, 80 mg or 120 mg/Tab. Bot. 100s, 500s, 1000s, UD 100s. *Rx*.
Use: Calcium channel blocker.

Calan SR. (Searle) Verapamil HCl. **120 mg, 180 mg/SR Tab.:** Bot. 100s, UD 100s. **240 mg/SR Tab.:** Bot. 100s, 500s, UD 100s. *Rx*.
Use: Calcium channel blocker.

Cal-Bid. (Roberts Pharmaceuticals) Elemental calcium 250 mg, ascorbic acid 100 mg, vitamin D 125 IU/Tab. Bot. 100s. *otc*.
Use: Mineral, vitamin supplement.

Cal Carb-HD. (Konsyl Pharmaceuticals) Calcium 6.5 g per packet, simethicone. Pow. 7 g packets, Bot. 210 g. *otc*.
Use: Antacid.

Calcet. (Mission Pharmacal Co.) Elemental calcium 153 mg, vitamin D 100 units/Tab. Bot. 100s. *otc*.
Use: Mineral, vitamin supplement.

Calcet Plus. (Mission Pharmacal Co.) Elemental calcium 152.8 mg, elemental iron 18 mg, vitamins A 5000 IU, D 400 IU, E 30 mg, B_1 2.25 mg, B_2 2.55 mg, B_3 30 mg, B_5 15 mg, B_6 3 mg, B_{12} 9 mcg, C 500 mg, folic acid 0.8 mg, zinc 15 mg, sugar/Tab. Bot 60s. *otc*.
Use: Mineral, vitamin supplement.

Calcibind. (Mission Pharmacal Co.) Inorganic phosphate content 34%, sodium content 11%. Packets: Cellulose sodium phosphate 25 g. Single-dose 90 packets, 300 g bulk pack. *Rx*.
Use: Genitourinary.

CalciCaps. (Nion Corp.) Calcium (dibasic calcium phosphate, calcium gluconate, calcium carbonate) 125 mg, vitamin D 67 IU, phosphorus 60 mg/Tab. Bot. 100s, 500s. *otc*.
Use: Mineral, vitamin supplement.

CalciCaps with Iron. (Nion Corp.) Calcium 125 mg, phosphorus 60 mg, vitamin D 67 IU, ferrous gluconate 7 mg, tartrazine/Tab. Bot. 100s, 500s. *otc*.

Use: Mineral, vitamin supplement.

CalciCaps M-Z. (Nion Corp.) Ca 400 mg, Mg 133 mg, Zn 5 mg, vitamin A 1667 mg, D 133 IU, Se. Tab. Bot. 90s. *otc.*
Use: Mineral, vitamin supplement.

CalciCaps, Super. (Nion Corp.) Calcium 400 mg, phosphorus 41.7 mg, vitamin D 100 IU/Tab. Bot. 90s. *otc.*
Use: Mineral, vitamin supplement.

Calci-Chew. (R & D Laboratories, Inc.) Calcium carbonate 1.25 g (500 mg calcium)/Chew. Tab. Bot. 100s. *otc.*
Use: Mineral supplement.

Calciday-667. (NBTY, Inc.) Calcium carbonate 667 mg (266.8 mg calcium)/ Tab. Bot. 60s. *otc.*
Use: Calcium supplement.

Calcidrine syrup. (Abbott Laboratories) Codeine 8.4 mg, calcium iodide anhydrous 152 mg, alcohol 6%/5 ml. Bot. 120 ml, 480 ml. *c-v.*
Use: Antitussive, expectorant.

•**calcifediol.** (KAL-sih-feh-DIE-ahl) U.S.P. 23.
Use: Calcium regulator.
See: Calderol (Organon Teknika Corp.).

calciferol. Ergosterol. (Vitamin D_2) **Liq.:** 8000 IU/ml. Bot. 60 ml. **Tab.:** 50,000 IU. Bot. 100s. **Inj.:** 500,000 IU/ml. Amp. 1 ml. *Rx-otc.*
Use: Refractory rickets, familial hypophosphatemia, hypoparathyroidism.

Calcijex. (Abbott Laboratories) Calcitriol 1 mcg or 2 mcg/ml. Inj. Amp. 1 ml. *Rx.*
Use: Antihypocalcemic, antihypoparathyroid.

Calcimar Injection, Synthetic. (Rhone-Poulenc Rorer Pharmaceuticals, Inc.) Calcitonin solution (salmon origin), phenol/200 IU/ml. Vial 2 ml. *Rx.*
Use: Treatment of Paget's disease.

Calci-Mix. (R & D Laboratories, Inc.) Calcium carbonate 1250 mg. Cap. Bot. 100s. *otc.*
Use: Mineral supplement.

•**calcipotriene.** (kal-sih-POE-try-een) USAN.
Use: Antipsoriatic.
See: Dovonex, Prods. (Westwood Squibb Pharmaceuticals).

•**calcitonin.** (kal-sih-TOE-nin) USAN.
Use: Treatment of Paget's disease, calcium regulator.
See: Calcimar (Rhone-Poulenc Rorer Pharmaceuticals, Inc.).
Cibacalcin (Novartis Pharmaceutical Corp.).
Miacalcin (Novartis Pharmaceutical Corp.).

calcitonin-human for injection. (kal-sih-TOE-nin human) Hormone from thyroid gland.
Use: Plasma hypocalcemic hormone; symptomatic Paget's disease of bone. [Orphan Drug]
See: Cibacalcin (Novartis Pharmaceutical Corp.).

calcitonin-salmon. (kal-sih-TOE-nin salmon)
Use: Antihypercalcemic.
See: Calcimar (Rhone-Poulenc Rorer Pharmaceuticals, Inc.).
Miacalcin (Novartis Pharmaceutical Corp.).
Osteocalcin, Inj. (Arcola Laboratories).

calcitonin salmon nasal spray.
Use: Symptomatic Paget's disease of bone. [Orphan Drug]
See: Miacalcin (Novartis Pharmaceutical Corp.).

•**calcitriol.** (KAL-sih-TRY-ole) USAN.
Use: Antihypocalcemic; calcium regulator.
See: Calcijex, Inj. (Abbott Laboratories).
Rocaltrol, Cap. (Roche Laboratories).

Calcium-600. (Schein Pharmaceutical, Inc.) Calcium 600 mg. Tab. Bot. 60s. *otc.*
Use: Mineral supplement.

Calcium 600/Vitamin D. (Schein Pharmaceutical, Inc.) Ca 600 mg, D 125 IU. Tab. Bot. 60s. *otc.*
Use: Mineral, vitamin supplement.

•**calcium acetate.** (KAL-see-uhm) U.S.P. 23.
Use: Pharmaceutic aid (buffering agent). Hyperphosphatemia. [Orphan Drug]

calcium acetate mineral/electrolytes.
See: Calphron, Tab. (Nephro-Tech, Inc.).
Phos-Ex 62.5 Mini-Tabs (Vitaline Corp.).
PhosLo (Braintree Laboratories, Inc.).

calcium acetylsalicylate. Kalmopyrin, kalsetal, soluble aspirin, tylcalsin.
Use: Analgesic.

calcium aluminum carbonate. W/DI-Amino acetate complex.
See: Ancid Tab., Susp. (Sheryl).

calcium aminosalicylate. N.F. 18. Aminosalicylate calcium.

calcium amphomycin.
See: Amphomycin.

calcium and magnesium carbonates tablets.
Use: Antacid.

•**calcium ascorbate.** U.S.P. 23.
Use: Nutritional supplement.

calcium ascorbate. (Freeda Vitamins, Inc.) **Tab.:** Calcium ascorbate 610 mg (equivalent to 500 mg ascorbic acid). Bot. 100s, 250s, 500s. **Pow.:** Calcium ascorbate 1 g (equivalent to 826 mg ascorbic acid) per ¼ tsp. Bot. 120 g, 448 g. *otc.*
Use: Mineral supplement.

calcium 4-benzamidosalicylate. Calcium Aminacyl B-PAS. Benzoylpas Calcium.
See: Benzopas, Pow., Tab. (Novartis).

calcium benzoyl-p-aminosalicylate.
See: Benzoylpas calcium.

calcium benzoylpas.
See: Benzoylpas calcium.

calcium bis-dioctyl sulfosuccinate.
See: Dioctyl calcium.

calcium carbimide. Calcium cyanamide. Sulfosuccinate.
See: Alka-Mints (Bayer Corp. (Consumer Div.)).
Amitone, Tab. (Menley & James Labs, Inc.).
Antacid Tab. (Zenith Goldline Pharmaceuticals).
Chooz (Schering-Plough Corp.).
Dicarbosil, Tab. (SmithKline Beecham Pharmaceuticals).
Extra Strength Antacid (Various Mfr.).
Maalox Antacid (Rhone-Poulenc Rorer Pharmaceuticals, Inc.).
Mallamint, Tab. (Roberts Pharmaceuticals).
Mylanta (J & J Merck Consumer Pharm.).
Tums (SmithKline Beecham Pharmaceuticals).

•**calcium carbonate.** U.S.P. 23. *Formerly calcium carbonate, precipitated.*
Use: Antacid.
See: Extra Strength Alkets Antacid, Chew. Tab. (Roberts Pharmaceuticals).
Tums 500, Chew. Tab. (SmithKline Beecham).

calcium carbonate. (Various Mfr.) Precipitated chalk; carbonic acid, calcium salt (1:1).
Use: Antacid.

calcium carbonate.
Use: Hyperphosphatemia. [Orphan Drug]
See: R&D Calcium Carbonate/600 (R&D).

calcium carbonate. (Various Mfr.) 500 mg/Tab. 100s, 120s, UD 100s; 600 mg/Tab. 60s, 72s, 150s, UD 100s; 650 mg/Tab. 100s, 1000s. *otc.*
Use: Antacid, calcium supplement.

calcium carbonate. (Roxane Laboratories, Inc.) **Tab.:** 1250 mg. Bot. 100s, UD 100s. **Susp.:** 1250 mg/5 ml. Bot. 500 ml, UD 5 ml. *otc.*
Use: Antacid, calcium supplement.

calcium carbonate, aromatic. (Eli Lilly and Co.) Calcium carbonate 10 gr/Tab. Bot. 100s, 1000s. *otc.*
Use: Antacid.

calcium carbonate w/combinations.
See: Acid-X, Tab. (BDI).
Alkets, Tab. (Pharmacia & Upjohn).
Ca-Plus, Tab. (Miller Pharmacal Group, Inc.).
Gas Ban, Tab. (Roberts Pharmaceuticals).
Lactocal, Tab. (Laser, Inc.).
Natabec, Prep. (Parke-Davis).
Titralac, Liq., Tab. (3M Pharmaceuticals).

Calcium Carbonate 600 mg + Vitamin D. (Major Pharmaceuticals) Ca 600 mg, D 125 IU. Tab. Bot. 60s. *otc.*
Use: Mineral, vitamin supplement.

calcium caseinate.
See: Casec, Pow. (Bristol-Myers Squibb).

calcium channel blockers.
Use: Angina pectoris, vasospastic and unstable angina.
See: Adalat, Cap. (Bayer Corp. (Consumer Div.)).
Calan, Inj., Tab. (Searle).
Calan SR, SR Cap. (Searle).
Cardene, Cap. (Roche Laboratories).
Cardene SR, SR Cap. (Roche Laboratories).
Cardene IV, Inj. (Du Pont Merck Pharmaceutical Co.).
Cardizem, Tab. (Hoechst Marion Roussel).
Diltiazem HCl, ER Cap. (Various Mfr.).
DynaCirc, Cap. (Novartis Pharmaceutical Corp.).
Isoptin, Inj., Tab. (Knoll Pharmaceuticals).
Isoptin SR, SR Cap. (Knoll Pharmaceuticals).
Nimotop, Cap. (Bayer Corp. (Consumer Div.)).
Plendil, SR Tab. (Merck & Co.).
Procardia, Cap. (Pfizer US Pharmaceutical Group).
Vascor, Tab. (Ortho McNeil Pharmaceutical).
Verapamil HCl, Inj., Tab. (Various Mfr.).

Calcium Chel 330. (Novartis Pharmaceutical Corp.)
Use: Antidote, heavy metals.
See: Calcium Trisodium Pentetate.

•**calcium chloride.** U.S.P. 23.
Use: Electrolyte, calcium replenisher.

•**calcium chloride Ca 45.** USAN.
Use: Radiopharmaceutical.

•**calcium chloride Ca 47.** USAN.
Use: Radiopharmaceutical.

calcium chloride injection. (Pharmacia & Upjohn) 1 g Amp. 10 ml, 25s. (Torigian) 1 g Amp. 10 ml 12s, 25s, 100s. (Trent) 10% Amp. 10 ml. (Bayer Corp. (Consumer Div.)) 13.6 mEq/10 ml Vial.
Use: Antihypocalcemic.

•**calcium citrate.** U.S.P. 23.
Use: Mineral supplement.

calcium cyclamate. Calcium cyclohexanesulfamate.

calcium cyclobarbital.
Use: Central depressant.

calcium cyclohexanesulfamate.
See: Calcium Cyclamate.

Calcium 600 + D. (NBTY, Inc.) Calcium 600 mg, vitamin D 125 IU. Film coated. Tab. Bot. 60s. *otc.*
Use: Mineral, vitamin supplement.

calcium dl-pantothenate. U.S.P. 23. Calcium Pantothenate, Racemic.

calcium dioctyl sulfosuccinate. U.S.P. 23. Docusate Calcium.
See: Surfak (Hoechst Marion Roussel).

calcium disodium edathamil. U.S.P. 23.
See: Edetate Calcium Disodium.

calcium disodium edetate. (KAL-see-uhm die-SO-dee-uhm ed-deh-TATE) U.S.P. 23. Edetate Calcium Disodium.
Use: Antidote for acute and chronic lead poisoning, lead encephalopathy.
See: Calcium Disodium Versenate (3M Pharmaceuticals).

calcium disodium versenate. (3M Pharmaceuticals) Calcium Disodium Edetate U.S.P. Inj. 200 mg/ml. Amp 5 ml. *Rx.*
Use: IV or IM for lead poisoning and lead encephalopathy.

calcium edetate sodium.
See: Calcium Disodium Edetate.

calcium EDTA.
See: Calcium Disodium Versenate, Amp. (3M Pharmaceuticals).

calcium glubionate syrup. (KAL-see-uhm glue-BYE-oh-nate) U.S.P. 23.
Use: Calcium replenisher.
See: Neo-Calglucon (Novartis Pharmaceutical Corp.).

calcium gluceptate. (KAL-see-uhm GLUE-sep-tate) U.S.P. 23.
Use: Calcium replenisher.
See: Calcium Gluceptate (Abbott Laboratories).
Calcium Gluceptate (I.M.S.).
Calcium Gluceptate (Eli Lilly and Co.).

calcium gluceptate. (Various Mfr.) 1.1 g (5 ml) contains 90 mg (4.5 mEq) calcium. Inj. 1.1 g/5 ml; Amp. 5 ml; Vial 50 ml.
Use: Calcium electrolyte replacement.

calcium glucoheptonate. (Various Mfr.) Cal. D-glucoheptonate O. *otc.*
Use: Nutritional supplement.

•**calcium gluconate.** U.S.P. 23.
Use: Calcium replenisher.

calcium gluconate gel 2.5%. (LTR Pharmaceuticals, Inc.)
Use: Topical treatment of hydrogen fluoride burns. [Orphan Drug]
See: H-F Gel (Paddock Laboratories).

calcium glycerophosphate. Neurosin. (Various Mfr.)

•**calcium hydroxide.** U.S.P. 23.
Use: Astringent; pharmaceutic necessity for calamine lotion.

calcium hydroxide powder. (Eli Lilly and Co.) Powder 4 oz/Bot.
Use: Lime water.

calcium hypophosphite. (N.Y. Quinine & Chem. Works)

calcium iodide.
W/Codeine phosphate.
See: Calcidrine Syr. (Abbott Laboratories).
W/Chloral hydrate, ephedrine HCl.
See: Iophen, Syr. (Marsh Labs).

calcium iodized.
See: Cal-Lime-1, Tab. (Scrip).
W/Calcium creosote.
See: Niocrese, Tab. (PJ, Noyes, Co., Inc.).

calcium iodobehenate. Calioben. (Various Mfr.).

calcium ipodate. U.S.P. 23. Ipodate Calcium.
See: Oragrafin Calcium, Granules (Bristol-Myers Squibb).

calcium kinate gluconate. Kinate is hexahydrotetrahydroxybenzoate. Calcium Quinate.

•**calcium lactate.** U.S.P. 23.
Use: Calcium replenisher.
W/Calcium glycerophosphate.
See: Calphosan, Amp., Vial (Carlton).
W/Calcium glycerophosphate, phenol, sodium Cl solution.
See: Calpholac, Vial (Century Pharmaceuticals, Inc.).
Calphosan, Inj. (Zeneca Pharmaceuticals).
W/Niacinamide, folic acid, ferrous gluconate, vitamins.
See: Pergrava No. 2, Cap. (Arcum).
W/Theobromine sodium salicylate, phenobarbital.

See: Zinc-220, Cap. (Alto Pharmaceuticals, Inc.).

•**calcium lactobionate.** U.S.P. 23.
Use: Mineral supplement.

calcium lactophosphate. Lactic acid hydrogen phosphate calcium salt.

calcium leucovorin. Leucovorin Calcium. Inj. Tab. Powder for Oral. Susp. Powder for Inj. *Rx.*
Use: For overdosage of folic acid antagonists; megalobastic anemias.
See: Leucovorin Calcium (ESI Lederle Generics).
Wellcovorin (GlaxoWellcome).

•**calcium levulinate.** (KAL-see-uhm LEV-you-lih-nate) U.S.P. 23.
Use: Calcium replenisher.

Calcium Magnesium Chelated. (NBTY, Inc.) Ca 500 mg, Mg 250 mg/Tab. Bot. 50s, 100s. *otc.*
Use: Mineral supplement.

Calcium Magnesium Zinc. (NBTY, Inc.) Ca 333 mg, Mg 133 mg, Zn 8.3 mg/Tab. Bot. 100. *otc.*
Use: Mineral supplement.

calcium novobiocin. Calcium salt of an antibacterial substance produced by *Streptomyces niveus.*
Use: Anti-infective.

calcium oxytetracycline. N.F. 18. Oxytetracycline Calcium.

•**calcium pantothenate.** (KAL-see-uhm pan-toe-THEH-nate) U.S.P. 23.
Use: Pantothenic acid (B_5) deficiency, coenzyme A precursor, vitamin (enzyme co-factor).
See: Calcium Pantothenate (Freeda Vitamins, Inc.).
Calcium Pantothenate (Fibertone).

W/Ascorbic acid, niacinamide, vitamins B_1, B_2, B_6, B_{12}, A, D, E.
See: Tota-Vi-Caps Gelatin, Cap. (Zeneca Pharmaceuticals).

W/Calcium carbonate.
See: Ilomel, Pow. (Warren-Teed).

W/Calcium carbonate, ferrous fumarate, niacinamide.
See: Prenatag, Tab. (Solvay Pharmaceuticals).

W/Danthron.
See: Modane, Tab., Liq. (Warren-Teed).
Parlax, Tab. (Parmed Pharmaceuticals, Inc.).

W/Docusate sodium.
See: Pantyl, Tab. (McGregor Pharmaceuticals, Inc.).

W/Methoscopolamine nitrate, mephobarbital.
See: Ilocalm, Tabs. (Warren-Teed).

W/Niacinamide and vitamins.
See: Allbee C-800, Prods. (Wyeth-Ayerst Laboratories).
Allbee T, Cap. (Wyeth-Ayerst Laboratories).
Allbee with C, Cap. (Wyeth-Ayerst Laboratories).
Ferrovite, Tab. (Laser, Inc.).
Fumatinic, Tab. (Laser, Inc.).
Maintenance Vitamin Formula, Tab. (Burgin-Arden).
Mulvidren, Tab. (Zeneca Pharmaceuticals).
OB-Tabs, Tab. (Laser, Inc.).
Probec, Tab. (Zeneca Pharmaceuticals).
Probec-T, Tab. (Zeneca Pharmaceuticals).
Stuart Hematinic, Tab. (Zeneca Pharmaceuticals).
Stuart Therapeutic Multivitamin, Tab. (Zeneca Pharmaceuticals).

W/Niacinamide, vitamins B_1, B_2, B_6.
See: Noviplex Capsules, Cap. (Zeneca Pharmaceuticals).

W/Vitamins B_1, B_2, B_6, B_{12}, niacinamide, choline Cl, inositol, dl-methionine, testosterone, estrone, procaine.
See: Geriatric Vitamin Formula, Tab. (Burgin-Arden).

W/Vitamins A, E, C, zinc sulfate, magnesium sulfate, niacinamide, B_1, B_2, manganese Cl, B_6, folic acid, B_{12}.
See: Vicon Forte, Cap. (GlaxoWellcome).

W/Vitamin C, niacin, zinc sulfate, vitamins E, B_1, B_2, B_6, B_{12}.
See: Z-Bec, Tab. (Wyeth-Ayerst Laboratories).

W/Vitamin complex, iron.
See: Vita-iron, Tab. (Century Pharmaceuticals, Inc.).

W/Vitamins, minerals, niacinamide.
See: Arcum-VM, Cap. (Arcum).
Capre, Tab. (Hoechst Marion Roussel).
Orovimin, Tab. (Solvay Pharmaceuticals).
Os-Cal Forte, Tab. (Hoechst Marion Roussel).
Os-Vim, Tab. (Hoechst Marion Roussel).
Stuartinic, Tab. (Zeneca Pharmaceuticals).
Theramin, Tab. (Arcum).
Uplex, Cap. (Arcum).

W/Vitamins, minerals, methyl testosterone, ehtinyl estradiol, niacinamide.
See: Geritag, Cap. (Solvay Pharmaceuticals).

W/Vitamin C, niacinamide, zinc sulfate, magnesium sulfate, vitamins B_1, B_2, B_6.

See: Vicon-C, Cap. (GlaxoWellcome).
W/Zinc sulfate, niacinamide, magnesium sulfate, manganese sulfate, vitamin complex.
See: Vicon Plus, Cap. (GlaxoWellcome).

•**calcium pantothenate, racemic.** U.S.P. 23.
Use: Vitamin B (enzyme cofactor).

•**calcium phosphate, dibasic.** U.S.P. 23.
Use: Calcium replenisher, pharmaceutic aid (tablet base).
W/Dicalcium Phosphate.
See: Diostate D, Tab. (Pharmacia & Upjohn).

calcium phosphate, monocalcium.
See: Dicalcium Phosphate.

•**calcium phosphate, tribasic.** N.F. 18.
Use: Calcium replenisher.
See: Posture (Wyeth-Ayerst Laboratories).

calcium-phosphorus-free.
See: Fosfree, Tab. (Mission Pharmacal Co.).

•**calcium polycarbophil.** (KAL-see-uhm PAHL-ee-CAR-boe-fill) U.S.P. 23.
Use: Laxative.
See: Equalactin, Chew. Tab. (Numark Laboratories, Inc.).
Fibercon, Tab. (ESI Lederle Generics).
FiberNorm, Tab. (G & W).
Konsyl Fiber, Tab. (Konsyl Pharmaceuticals).

calcium polysulfide.
Use: Wet dressing, soak.
See: Vlemasque, Cream. (Dormik).

calcium quinate.
See: Calcium Kinate Gluconate.

•**calcium saccharate.** U.S.P. 23.
Use: Pharmaceutic aid, sweetener (stabilizer).

calcium saccharin. Saccharin Calcium.
Use: Pharmaceutic aid, sweetener.

calcium salts of sennosides A & B.
Use: Laxative.
See: Gentle Nature, Tab. (Novartis Pharmaceutical Corp.).

•**calcium silicate.** N.F. 18.
Use: Pharmaceutic aid (tablet excipient).

•**calcium stearate.** N.F. 18.
Use: Pharmaceutic aid (tablet and capsule lubricant).

calcium succinate.
W/Apsirin.
See: Ber-Ex, Tab. (Dolcin).
Dolcin, Tab. (Dolcin).

•**calcium sulfate.** N.F. 18.
Use: Pharmaceutic aid (tablet and capsule diluent).

calcium thiosulfate.
Use: Wet dressing, soak.
See: Vlemasque Cream (Dermik Laboratories, Inc.).

calcium trisodium pentetate. (KAL-see-uhm try-SO-dee-uhm PEN-teh-tate)
Use: Antidote, heavy metals.
See: Calcium Chel 330 (Novartis Pharmaceutical Corp.).

•**calcium undecylenate.** U.S.P. 23.
Use: Antifungal.

calcium undecylenate. 10% calcium undecylenate Powder.
Use: Antifungal, topical.
See: Cruex Squeeze Pow. (Novartis Pharmaceutical Corp.).

calcium with vitamin D tablets.
Use: Mineral, vitamin supplement.

Calcium with Vitamin D. (Schein Pharmaceutical, Inc.) Calcium 600 mg, vitamin D 125 IU Bot. 60s. *otc.*
Use: Mineral, vitamin supplement.

Caldecort Spray. (Novartis Pharmaceutical Corp.) Hydrocortisone 0.5%. Aerosol Can 1.5 oz. *otc.*
Use: Corticosteroid, topical.

Calderol. (Organon Teknika Corp.) Calcifediol 20 mcg or 50 mcg/Cap. Bot. 60s. *Rx.*
Use: Antihypocalcemia.

•**caldiamide sodium.** (KAL-DIE-ah-MIDE) USAN.
Use: Pharmaceutic aid.

Cal-D-Mint. (Enzyme Process) Ca 800 mg, Mg 150 mg, Fe 18 mg, iodine 0.1 mg, Cu 2 mg, vitamin D 200 IU/2 Tab. Bot. 100s, 250s. *otc.*
Use: Mineral, vitamin supplement.

Cal-D-Phos. (Archer-Taylor) Dicalcium phosphate 4.5 gr, calcium gluconate 3 gr, vitamin D/Tab. Bot. 1000s. *otc.*
Use: Mineral, vitamin supplement.

calfactant.
Use: Lung surfactant.
See: Infasurf, Susp. (Forest Pharmaceuticals).

Cal-Guard. (Rugby Labs, Inc.) Calcium carbonate 50 mg. Softgel Cap. Bot. 60s. *otc.*
Use: Mineral supplement.

Calicylic Creme. (Gordon Laboratories) Salicylic acid 10%, mineral oil, cetyl alcohol, propylene glycol, white wax, sodium lauryl sulfate, oleic acid, methyl- and propylparabens, triethanolamine. 60 g. *otc.*
Use: Keratolytic.

Cal-Im. (Standex) Calcium glycerophosphate 1%, calcium levulinate 1.5%. Vial 30 ml. *Rx.*
Use: Mineral supplement.

Calinate-FA. (Solvay Pharmaceuticals) Ca 250 mg, vitamins A 4000 IU, D 400 IU, B_1 3 mg, B_2 3 mg, B_6 5 mg, B_{12} 1 mcg, folic acid 1 mg, C 50 mg, B_3 (niacinamide) 20 mg, B_5 (d-panthenol) 1 mg, Fe 60 mg, I 0.02 mg, Mn 0.2 mg, Mg 0.2 mg, Zn 0.1 mg, Cu 0.15 mg/Tab. Bot. 100s. *Rx.*
Use: Mineral, vitamin supplement.

calioben.
See: Calcium Iodobehenate.

Calivite. (Apco) Calcium carbonate 885 mg, ferrous sulfate 199 mg, vitamins A 3600 IU, D 400 IU, C 75 mg, B_1 1.5 mg, B_2 1.95 mg, B_6 0.75 mg, nicotinic acid 15 mg, B_{12} activity 0.025 mcg, choline 1500 mcg, inositol 2500 mcg, pantothenic acid 75 mcg, folic acid 25 mcg, p-aminobenzoic acid 12 mcg, K 10 mg, Mg 1 mg, Zn 0.075 mg, Mn 0.02 mg, Cu 0.01 mg, cobalt 0.02 mcg/Tab. Bot. 100s. *otc.*
Use: Mineral, vitamin supplement.

Cal-Lime-1. (Scrip) Calcium iodized 1 gr/ Tab. Bot. 1000s.

Calmol 4. (Mentholatum Co., Inc.) **Supp.:** Cocoa butter 80%, zinc oxide 10%, parabens. Box 12s, 24s. *otc.*
Use: Anorectal preparation.

Calmosin. (Spanner) Calcium gluconate, strontium bromide. Amp. 10 ml. 100s.

Cal-Nor. (Vortech Pharmaceuticals) Calcium glycerophosphate 100 mg, calcium levulinate 150 mg/10 ml. Inj. Vial 100 ml. *Rx.*
Use: Mineral supplement.

Calocarb. (Pal-Pak, Inc.) Calcium carbonate 648 mg/Tab. w/cinnamon flavor. Bot. 1000s. *otc.*
Use: Antacid.

calomel. Mercurous Cl.
Use: Cathartic.

Calotabs. (Calotabs) Reformulated. Docusate sodium 100 mg, casanthranol 30 mg/Tab. Box 10s. *otc.*
Use: Laxative.

caloxidine (iodized calcium).
See: Calcium Iodized.

Calphosan. (Glenwood, Inc.) Calcium glycerophosphate 50 mg, calcium lactate 50 mg/10 ml sodium Cl solution. Contains calcium 0.08 mEq/ml. Inj. Amp. 10 ml, Vial 60 ml. *Rx.*
Use: Mineral supplement.

Calphron. (Nephro-Tech, Inc.) Calcium acetate 667 mg/Tab. Bot. 200s. *otc.*
Use: Mineral supplement.

Cal-Plus. (Roberts Pharmaceuticals) Calcium carbonate 1500 mg/Tab. Bot. 100s. *otc.*
Use: Mineral supplement.

Calsan. (Burgin-Arden) Calcium glycerophosphate 10 mg, calcium levulinate 15 mg, chlorobutanol 0.5% ml. Inj. Vial 100 ml. *Rx.*
Use: Calcium supplement.

Cal Sup Instant 1000. (3M Personal Care Products) Elemental calcium 1000 mg, vitamins D 400 IU, C 60 mg. Pow. Packet 12s. *otc.*
Use: Mineral, vitamin supplement.

Cal Sup 600 Plus. (3M Personal Care Products) Elemental calcium 600 mg, vitamins D 200 IU, C 30 mg/Tab. Bot. 60s. *otc.*
Use: Mineral, vitamin supplement.

•**calteridol calcium.** (KAL-TER-ih-dahl KAL-see-uhm) USAN.
Use: Pharmaceutic aid.

Caltrate 600. (ESI Lederle Generics) Calcium carbonate 1.5 g (calcium 600 mg). Bot. 60s, 120s. *otc.*
Use: Mineral supplement.

Caltrate 600 + D. (ESI Lederle Generics) Vitamin D 200 IU, Ca 600 mg. Sugar free. Tab. Bot. 60s. *otc.*
Use: Mineral, vitamin supplement.

Caltrate 600 + Iron. (ESI Lederle Generics) Calcium carbonate 600 mg, iron 18 mg, vitamin D 125 IU/Tab. Bot. 60s. *otc.*
Use: Mineral, vitamin supplement.

Caltrate Jr. (ESI Lederle Generics) Calcium carbonate 750 mg (300 mg calcium)/Chew. Tab. Bot. 60s. *otc.*
Use: Mineral supplement.

Caltrate Plus. (ESI Lederle Generics) Vitamin D 200 IU, Ca 600 mg, Zn 7.5 mg, Mg, Cu, Mn, B. Sugar free. Tab. Bot. 60s. *otc.*
Use: Mineral, vitamin supplement.

Caltro. (Geneva Pharmaceuticals) Elemental calcium 250 mg, vitamin D 125 IU/Tab. Bot. 100s, 1000s. *otc.*
Use: Mineral, vitamin supplement.

•**calusterone.** USAN.
Use: Antineoplastic.

Cama Arthritis Pain Reliever. (Novartis Pharmaceutical Corp.) Aspirin 500 mg, magnesium oxide 150 mg, aluminum hydroxide 125 mg, methylparaben. Tab. Bot. 100s. *otc.*
Use: Analgesic, antacid.

Cam-Ap-Es. (Camall Co., Inc.) Hydrochlorothiazide 15 mg, reserpine 0.1 mg, hydralazine HCl 25 mg/Tab. Bot. 100s. *Rx.*
Use: Antihypertensive.

•**cambendazole.** (kam-BEND-ah-zole) USAN.
Use: Anthelmintic.

Camellia. (O'Leary) Moisturizer for face, hands and body. For normal to oily skin. Lot. Bot. 4 oz. *otc.*
Use: Emollient.

Cameo Oil. (Medco Lab, Inc.) Mineral oil, isopropyl myristate, lanolin oil, PEG-8-Dioleate. Plastic Bot. 8 oz, 16 oz, 32 oz. *otc.*
Use: Emollient.

•**camiglibose.** (kah-mih-GLIE-bose) USAN.
Use: Antidiabetic (glucohydrolase inhibitor).

Camouflage Crayon. (O'Leary) Coverup for minor skin discolorations, under eye concealer, lipstick fixer. Available in 6 shades. Crayon 0.05 oz. *otc.*
Use: Skin coverup.

Campho-Phenique. (Sanofi Winthrop Pharmaceuticals) Camphor 10.8%, phenol 4.7%. **Liq.:** 22.5 ml, 45 ml, 120 ml. **Gel:** 6.9 g, 15 g. *otc.*
Use: Analgesic, antiseptic, local.

Campho-Phenique Antibiotic Plus Pain Reliever. (Sanofi Winthrop Pharmaceuticals) Bacitracin 500 units, neomycin 3.5 mg, polymyxin B 5000 units/g, lidocaine 40 mg. **Oint.:** Tube 5 g. *otc.*
Use: Anti-infective, topical.

•**camphor.** U.S.P. 23.
Use: Topical antipruritic; anti-infective; pharmaceutic necessity for camphorated phenol, paregoric and flexible collodion, antitussive, expectorant, local counterirritant, nasal decongestant.
See: Vicks Inhaler (Procter & Gamble Pharm.).
Vicks Regular and Wild Cherry Medicated Cough Drops (Procter & Gamble Pharm.).
Vicks Medi-Trating Throat Lozenges (Procter & Gamble Pharm.).
Vicks Sinex, Nasal Spray (Procter & Gamble Pharm.).
Vicks Vaporub, Oint. (Procter & Gamble Pharm.).
Vicks Vaposteam, Liq. (Procter & Gamble Pharm.).
Vicks Va-Tro-Nol, Nose Drops (Procter & Gamble Pharm.).

camphorated, parachlorophenol.
Use: Anti-infective (dental).

camphoric acid ester. Ester of p-Tolylmethylcarbinal as Diethanolamine Salt.

Camptosar. (Pharmacia & Upjohn) Irinotecan HCl 20 mg/ml, sorbitol/Inj. Vial. 5 ml. *Rx.*
Use: Antineoplastic.

•**candesartan.** (Kan-deh-SAHR-tan) USAN.
Use: Antagonist, angiotensin II receptor, antihypertensive.

•**candesartan cilexetil.** (kan-deh-SAHR-tan sigh-LEX-eh-till) USAN.
Use: Antagonist, angiotension II receptor, antihypertensive.
See: Atacand, Tab. (Astra Merck).

•**candicidin.** (KAN-dih-SIDE-in) U.S.P. 23. An antifungal antibiotic derived from *Strep. griseus.*
Use: Antifungal.

candida albicans skin test antigen.
Use: Diagnostic aid.
See: Candin, Inj. (Allermed, ALK Laboratories).

candida test. (SmithKline Diagnostics) Culture test for *Candida.* Box 4s.
Use: Diagnostic aid.

Candin. (Allermed, ALK Laboratories) *Candida albicans* skin test antigen prepared from the culture filtrate and cells of two strains of *Candida albicans.* Vial 1 ml. *Rx.*
Use: Evaluation of cell-mediated immunity; diagnostic aid.

•**candoxatril.** (kan-DOXE-at-trill) USAN.
Use: Antihypertensive.

•**candoxatrilat.** (kan-DOXE-at-trill-at) USAN.
Use: Antihypertensive.

Candycon. (Allison) Chlorprophenpyridamine maleate 2 mg, phenylephrine HCl 5 mg/Tab. Bot. 50s. *otc.*
Use: Antihistamine, decongestant.

cannabinoids. Antiemetic/Antivertigo agent.
See: Dronabinol.

cannabis. Antiemetic, antivertigo.
See: Dronabinol.

•**canrenoate potassium.** (kan-REN-oh-ate) USAN.
Use: Aldosterone antagonist.

•**canrenone.** (kan-REN-ohn) USAN.
Use: Aldosterone antagonist.

cantharidin.
Use: Keratolytic.

Cantil. (Hoechst Marion Roussel) Mepenzolate bromide 25 mg/Tab. Bot. 100s. *Rx.*
Use: Anticholinergic, antispasmodic.

Ca-Orotate. (Miller Pharmacal Group, Inc.) Calcium (as calcium orotate) 50 mg/Tab. Bot. 100s. *otc.*
Use: Mineral supplement.

C-A-P. (Eastman Kodak Co.) Cellulose acetate phthalate.

Capahist-DMH. (Freeport) Chlorpheniramine maleate 8 mg, phenylpropanolamine HCl 50 mg, atropine sulfate 1/180

gr, dextromethorphan HBr 20 mg/T.R. Cap. *Rx.*
Use: Anticholinergic, antihistamine, antispasmodic, antitussive, decongestant.

Capastat Sulfate. (Dura Pharmaceuticals) Capreomycin sulfate 1 g/10 ml. Vial 10 ml. *Rx.*
Use: Antituberculosal.

•**capecitabine.** (cap-eh-SITE-ah-bean) USAN.
Use: Antineoplastic.
See: Xeloda, Tab. (Roche Laboratories).

Capital with Codeine. (Carnrick Laboratories, Inc.) Acetaminophen 120 mg, codeine phosphate 12 mg/5 ml. Susp. Bot. 473 ml. *c-v.*
Use: Analgesic combination, narcotic.

Capital with Codeine. (Carnrick Laboratories, Inc.) Codeine phosphate 30 mg, acetaminophen 325 mg, Tab. Bot. 100s. *c-III.*
Use: Analgesic combination, narcotic.

Capitrol Cream Shampoo. (Westwood Squibb Pharmaceuticals) Chloroxine 2%. Shampoo Bot. 120 ml. *Rx.*
Use: Antiseborrheic.

Ca-Plus-Protein. (Miller Pharmacal Group, Inc.) Calcium (as contained in a calcium-protein complex made with specially isolated soy protein) 280 mg/Tab. Bot. 100s. *otc.*
Use: Mineral supplement.

Capnitro. (Freeport) Nitroglycerin 6.5 mg/TR Cap. Bot. 100s. *Rx.*
Use: Antianginal agent.

•**capobenate sodium.** (CAP-oh-BEN-ate) USAN.
Use: Cardiovascular agent (antiarrhythmic).

•**capobenic acid.** (CAP-oh-BEN-ik) USAN.
Use: Cardiovascular agent (antiarrhythmic).

Capoten. (Bristol-Myers Squibb) Captopril 12.5 mg, 25 mg, 50 mg, or 100 mg, lactose. Tab. Bot 100s, 1000s (except 100 mg), UD 100s. *Rx.*
Use: Antihypertensive.

Capozide. (Bristol-Myers Squibb) Captopril/hydrochlorothiazide 25/15 mg, 25/25 mg, 50/15 mg, 50/25 mg/Tab. Bot. 100s. *Rx.*
Use: Antihypertensive.

•**capreomycin sulfate, sterile.** (CAP-ree-oh-MY-sin) U.S.P. 23. An antibiotic derived from *Streptomyces capreolus.* Caprocin.
Use: Anti-infective (tuberculostatic).
See: Capastat Sulfate, Pow. for Inj. (Dura).

•**capromab pendetide.** (CAP-row-mab PEN-deh-TIDE) USAN.
Use: Monoclonal antibody.
See: Prostascint (Cytogen).

caprylate, salts.
See: Sodium Caprylate.
Zinc Caprylate.

caprylate sodium, injection. (Ingram) Amp. 33%, 1 ml Pkg. 12s, 25s, 100s.
Use: Antifungal.
See: Sodium Caprylate Preps.

•**capsaicin.** (kap-SAY-uh-sin) U.S.P. 23.
Use: Analgesic, topical; antineuralgic, specific pain syndromes, topical.
See: Capsin, Lot. (Fleming & Co.).
Capzasin-P, Cream (Thompson Medical Co.).
Dolorac, Cream (Medicis Dermatologicals, Inc.).
No Pain-HP, Roll-on (Young Again Products).
Pain Doctor, Cream (Fougera).
Pain-X, Gel (B.F. Ascher and Co.).
R-Gel (Healthline Laboratories, Inc.).
Zostrix Cream (Medicis Dermatologicals, Inc.).

•**capsicum.** (CAP-sih-kum) U.S.P. 23.
Use: Carminative; counterirritant (external), stomachic.

•**capsicum oleoresin.** U.S.P. 23.
Use: Carminative; counterirritant (external); stomachic.

Capsin. (Fleming & Co.) Capsaicin 0.025% or 0.075%, benzyl alcohol, propylene glycol, denatured alcohol. Lot. Bot. 59 ml. *otc.*
Use: Analgesic, topical.

capsules, empty gelatin. (Eli Lilly and Co.) Lilly markets clear empty gelatin capsules in sizes 000, 00, 0, 1, 2, 3, 4, 5.

•**captamine hydrochloride.** (CAP-tam-een) USAN.
Use: Depigmentor.

•**captopril.** (KAP-toe-prill) U.S.P. 23.
Use: Antihypertensive, enzyme inhibitor (angiotensin-converting).
See: Capoten, Tab. (Bristol-Myers Squibb).

captopril. (Various Mfr.) Captopril 12.5 mg, 25 mg, 50 mg. 100 mg. Tab. Bot. 100s, 500s; 1000s, 5000s (except 100 mg); UD 100s (12.5 mg and 25 mg only). *Rx.*
Use: Antihypertensive, enzyme inhibitor (angiotensin-converting).

•**capuride.** (CAP-you-ride) USAN.
Use: Hypnotic, sedative.

Capzasin-P. (Thompson Medical Co.) Capsaicin 0.025%, benzyl and cetyl alcohol. Cream Tube 42.5 g. *otc.*
Use: Analgesic, topical.

Caquin. (Forest Pharmaceutical, Inc.) Hydrocortisone 1%, iodochlorhydroxyquin 3%, hydrophilic base. Cream. Tube 20 g. *Rx-otc.*
Use: Corticosteroid, topical.

•**caracemide.** (car-ASS-eh-MIDE) USAN.
Use: Antineoplastic.

Carafate. (Hoechst Marion Roussel) **Tab.:** Sucralfate 1 g. Bot. 100s, 120s, 500s, UD 100s. **Susp.:** Sucralfate 1 g/10 ml. Bot. 420 ml. *Rx.*
Use: Antiulcerative.

•**caramel.** N.F. 18.
Use: Pharmaceutic aid (color).

caramiphen ethanedisulfonate.
W/Phenylephrine HCl, phenindamine tartrate.
See: Dondril, Tab. (Whitehall Robins Laboratories).

caramiphen hydrochloride.
Use: Proposed antiparkinson.

caraway. N.F. 18.
Use: Flavoring.

•**carbachol.** (CAR-bah-kole) U.S.P. 23.
Use: Parasympathomimetic, cholinergic, ophthalmic.
See: Carbastat, Soln. (Ciba Vision).
Miostat Intraocular, Soln. (Alcon Laboratories, Inc.).
Murocarb, Soln. (Muro Pharmaceutical, Inc.).
W/Methylcellulose.
See: Isopto Carbachol, Soln. (Alcon Laboratories, Inc.).

carbacrylamine resins.
Use: Cation-exchange resin.

•**carbadox.** (CAR-bah-dox) USAN.
Use: Anti-infective.

•**carbamazepine.** (KAR-bam-AZE-uh-peen) U.S.P. 23.
Use: Analgesic, anticonvulsant.
See: Atretol, Tab. (Athena Neurosciences, Inc.).
Carbamazepine (Rugby Labs, Inc.).
Carbatrol, ER Cap. (Athena Neurosciences, Inc.).
Epitol, Tab. (Teva Pharmaceuticals USA).
Tegretol, Tab. (Novartis Pharmaceutical Corp.).

carbamazepine. (KAR-bam-AZE-uh-peen) (Various Mfr.) **Chew. Tab.:** 100 mg. Bot. 25s, 100s, UD 100s. **Tab.:** 200 mg. Bot. 25s, 100s, 1000s, UD 100s, 300s. *Rx.*
Use: Treatment of epilepsy and trigeminal neuralgia.

carbamide. (Various Mfr.) Urea. Cream, Lot.
Use: Emollient.
See: Aquacare (Allergan, Inc.).
Carmol 20 (Roche Laboratories).
Nutraplus (Galderma Laboratories, Inc.).
Rea-Lo (Whorton Pharmaceuticals, Inc.).
Ultra Mide Moisturizer (Baker Cummins Dermatologicals, Inc.).
Ureacin-20 (Pedinol Pharmacal, Inc.).

carbamide compounds.
See: Acetylcarbromal (Various Mfr.).
Carbromal (Various Mfr.).

•**carbamide peroxide.** (CAR-bah-mide per-ox-ide) U.S.P. 23. Urea compound w/hydrogen peroxide (1:1).
Use: Anti-infective, topical (dental); anti-inflammatory; analgesic.
See: Gly-Oxide (Hoechst Marion Roussel).
Orajel Brace-aid Rinse (Del Pharmaceuticals, Inc.).
Orajel Perioseptic, Liq. (Del Pharmaceuticals, Inc.).
Proxigel (Schwarz Pharma, Inc.).

carbamide peroxide 6.5% in glycerin.
Use: Otic.
See: Murine Ear Drops (Abbott Laboratories).
Murine Ear Wax Removal System (Abbott Laboratories).

carbamylcholine chloride.
See: Carbachol.

carbamylmethylcholine chloride.
See: Urecholine, Tab., Inj. (Merck & Co.).

•**carbantel lauryl sulfate.** (CAR-ban-tell LAH-ruhl) USAN.
Use: Anthelmintic.

carbarsone. (Various Mfr.) N-carbamoylarsanilic acid. Amabevan, ameban, amibiarson, arsambide, fenarsone, leucarsone, aminarsone, amebarsone. p-Ureidobenzenearsonic acid. Caps.
Use: Acute and chronic amebiasis and trichomoniasis.

•**carbaspirin calcium.** USAN.
Use: Analgesic.

Carbastat. (Ciba Vision) Carbachol 0.1%, sodium Cl 0.64%, potassium Cl 0.075%, calcium Cl dihydrate 0.048%, magnesium Cl hexahydrate 0.03%, sodium acetate trihydrate 0.39%, sodium citrate dihydrate 0.17%. Soln. Vial 1.5 ml. *Rx.*
Use: Antiglaucoma.

Carbatrol. (Athena Neurosciences, Inc.) Carbamazepine 200 mg, 300 mg, lac-

tose, talc. ER Cap. Bot. 120s. *Rx.*
Use: Anticonvulsant.

•**carbazeran.** (CAR-BAY-zeh-ran) USAN.
Use: Cardiovascular agent.

•**carbenicillin disodium, sterile.** (CAR-ben-ih-SILL-in die-SO-dee-uhm) U.S.P. 23.
Use: Anti-infective.
See: Geopen, Vial (Roerig).

•**carbenicillin indanyl sodium.** (car-BEN-ih-SILL-in IN-duh-nil) U.S.P. 23.
Use: Anti-infective.
See: Geocillin, Tab. (Roerig).

•**carbenicillin phenyl sodium.** (CAR-ben-ih-SILL-in FEN-ill) USAN.
Use: Anti-infective.

•**carbenicillin potassium.** (CAR-ben-ih-SILL-in) USAN.
Use: Anti-infective.

•**carbenoxolone sodium.** (CAR-ben-ox-ah-lone) USAN.
Use: Corticosteroid, topical.

carbetapentane citrate.
Use: Antitussive.
W/Codeine phosphate, chlorpheniramine maleate, guaifenesin.
See: Tussar-2, Syr. (Rhone-Poulenc Rorer Pharmaceuticals, Inc.).
Tussar SF, Liq. (Rhone-Poulenc Rorer Pharmaceuticals, Inc.).

•**carbetimer.** (car-BEH-tih-MER) USAN.
Use: Antineoplastic.

Carbex. (Du Pont Pharma.) Selegiline HCl 5 mg, lactose/Tab. Bot. 60s. *Rx.*
Use: Used in combination with levodopa/carbidopa for treatment of Parkinson's disease.

•**carbidopa.** (CAR-bih-doe-puh) U.S.P. 23.
Use: Decarboxylase inhibitor.
See: Lodosyn, Tab. (Merck & Co.).
W/Levodopa.
See: Sinemet, Tab. (Du Pont Pharma.).

carbidopa and levodopa tablets.
Use: Antiparkinsonian.
See: Sinemet (Du Pont Pharma.).

carbidopa & levodopa. (Various Mfr.) Carbidopa 10 mg, levodopa 100 mg; carbidopa 25 mg, levodopa 100 mg; carbidopa 25 mg, levodopa 250 mg. Tab. Bot. 100s, 500s, 1000s. *Rx.*
Use: Antiparkinsonian.

carbinoxamine compound syrup. (Rosemont Pharmaceutical Corp.) Pseudoephedrine HCl 60 mg, dextromethorphan HBr 15 mg, carbinoxamine maleate 4 mg. Grape flavor. Syr. Bot. 120 ml, pt, gal. *Rx.*
Use: Antihistamine, antitussive, decongestant.

carbinoxamine drops. (Morton Grove Pharmaceuticals, Inc.) Carbinoxamine maleate 2 mg, pseudoephedrine HCl 25 mg/ml, sorbitol, parabens, alcohol free, raspberry, fruit flavors. Drops. Bot. 30 ml w/calibrated dropper. *Rx.*
Use: Antihistamine, decongestant.

carbinoxamine maleate and pseudophedrine HCl.
See: Biohist-LA, TR Tab. (Wakefield Pharmaceuticals, Inc.).
Carbinoxamine Preps. (Morton Grove Pharmaceuticals, Inc.).

carbinoxamine maleate, pseudoephedrine HCl, dextromethorphan HBr. (Cypress) **Syr.:** Carbinoxamine maleate 4 mg, pseudoephedrine HCl 60 mg, dextromethorphan HBr 15 mg/5 ml. Bot. 120 ml, pt., gal. **Drops:** Carbinoxamine maleate 2 mg, pseudoephedrine HCl 25 mg, dextromethorphan HBr 4 mg/ml. Bot. 30 ml w/dropper. *Rx.*
Use: Antihistamine, decongestant, antitussive.

carbinoxamine maleate w/combinations.
See: Sildec-DM, Ped. Drops (Silarx Pharmaceuticals, Inc.).

carbinoxamine syrup. (Morton Grove Pharmaceuticals, Inc.) Carbinoxamine maleate 4 mg, pseudoephedrine HCl 60 mg/5 ml, sorbitol, parabens, alcohol free, raspberry, fruit flavors. Syr. Bot. 118 ml, 237 ml, 473 ml. *Rx.*
Use: Antihistamine, decongestant.

•**carbiphene hydrochloride.** (CAR-bih-FEEN) USAN.
Use: Analgesic.

Carbiset Tablets. (Nutripharm Laboratories, Inc.) Pseudoephedrine 60 mg, carbinoxamine maleate 4 mg/Tab. Bot. 100s, 500s. *Rx.*
Use: Antihistamine, decongestant.

Carbiset-TR. (Nutripharm Laboratories, Inc.) Pseudoephedrine HCl 120 mg, carbinoxamine maleate 8 mg/Tab. Bot. 100s. *Rx.*
Use: Antihistamine, decongestant.

Carbocaine. (Cook-Waite Laboratories, Inc.) Mepivacaine HCl 3%. Inj. Dental cartridge 1.8 ml. *Rx.*
Use: Anesthetic, local.

Carbocaine. (Sanofi Winthrop Pharmaceuticals) Mepivacaine HCl. **1%:** Vial 30 ml, 50 ml. **1.5%:** Vial 30 ml. **2%:** Vial 20 ml, 50 ml. *Rx.*
Use: Anesthetic, local.

Carbocaine-Neo-Cobefrin. (Cook-Waite Laboratories, Inc.) Mepivacaine HCl 2% with levonorefrin 1:20,000. Inj. Dental cartridge 1.8 ml. *Rx.*
Use: Anesthetic, local.

•**carbocloral.** (CAR-boe-KLOR-uhl) USAN.
Use: Hypnotic, sedative.
See: Chloralurethane.

•**carbocysteine.** (car-boe-SIS-teen) USAN.
Use: Mucolytic.

Carbodec. (Rugby Labs, Inc.) Pseudoephedrine HCl 60 mg, carbinoxamine maleate 4 mg/5 ml. Syr. Bot. 473 ml. *Rx.*
Use: Antihistamine, decongestant.

Carbodec DM Products. (Rugby Labs, Inc.) **Syr.:** Pseudoephedrine HCl 60 mg, carbinoxamine maleate 4 mg, dextromethorphan HBr 15 mg, alcohol < 0.6%/5 ml. Bot. 30 ml, 120 ml, pt, gal. **Drops (Pediatric Pharmaceuticals):** Pseudoephedrine HCl 25 mg, carbinoxamine maleate 2 mg, dextromethorphan HBr 4 mg, alcohol 0.6%/ml. Bot. 30 ml. *Rx.*
Use: Antihistamine, antitussive, decongestant.

Carbodec Tablets. (Rugby Labs, Inc.) Pseudoephedrine HCl 60 mg, carbinoxamine maleate 4 mg/Tab. Bot. 100s. *Rx.*
Use: Antihistamine, decongestant.

Carbodec TR. (Rugby Labs, Inc.) Pseudoephedrine HCl 120 mg, carbinoxamine maleate 8 mg/Tab. Bot. 100s. *Rx.*
Use: Antihistamine, decongestant.

carbol-fuchsin paint. Original fuchsin formula known as Castellani's Paint. Basic Fuchsin 0.3%, phenol 4.5%, resorcinol 10%, acetone 5%, alcohol 10%. Bot. 30 ml, 120 ml, 480 ml.
Use: Antifungal, topical.
See: Castellani's Paint (Various Mfr.).

•**carbol-fuchsin, topical solution.** (CAR-buhl-FOOK-sin) U.S.P. 23.
Use: Antifungal.

carbomer. (CAR-boe-mer) A polymer of acrylic acid, crosslinked with a polyfunctional agent.
Use: Pharmaceutic aid (emulsifying, suspending agent).

•**carbomer 910.** (CAR-boe-mer 910) N.F. 18.
Use: Pharmaceutic aid (emulsifying, suspending agent).

•**carbomer 934.** (CAR-boe-mer 934) N.F. 18.
Use: Pharmaceutic aid (emulsifying, suspending agent).

•**carbomer 934p.** (CAR-boe-mer 934) N.F. 18. *Formerly carpolene.*
Use: Pharmaceutic aid (emulsifying, suspending, viscosity, thickening agent).

•**carbomer 940.** (CAR-boe-mer 940) N.F. 18.
Use: Pharmaceutic aid (emulsifying, suspending agent).

•**carbomer 941.** (CAR-boe-mer 941) N.F. 18.
Use: Pharmaceutic aid (emulsifying, suspending agent).

•**carbomer 1342.** (CAR-boe-mer 1342) N.F. 18.
Use: Pharmaceutic aid (emulsifying, suspending agent).

carbomycin. An antibiotic from *Streptomyces halstedii.*
Use: Anti-infective.

•**carbon dioxide.** U.S.P. 23.
Use: Inhalation, respiratory.
See: Ceo-Two, Supp. (Beutlich, Inc.).

•**carbon monoxide c 11.** (CAR-bahn moe-NOX-ide C11) U.S.P. 23.
Use: Diagnostic aid (blood volume determination), radiopharmaceutical.

carbonic acid, dilithium salt. U.S.P. 23. Lithium Carbonate.

carbonic acid, disodium salt. N.F. 18. Sodium Carbonate.

carbonic acid, monosodium salt. U.S.P. 23. Sodium Bicarbonate.

carbonic anhydrase inhibitors.
See: Acetazolamide, Tab. (Various Mfr.).
Daranide, Tab. (Merck & Co.).
Dazamide, Tab. (Major Pharmaceuticals).
Diamox, Tab., Sequel, Vial (ESI Lederle Generics).
Neptazane, Tab. (ESI Lederle Generics).

Carbonis Detergens, Liquor.
See: Coal Tar Solution.

carbonyl diamide.
See: Chap Cream (Ar-Ex).

carbon tetrachloride. N.F. 18. Benzinoform. (Various Mfr.).
Use: Pharmaceutic aid (solvent).

•**carboplatin.** (car-boe-PLATT-in) U.S.P. 23.
Use: Antineoplastic.
See: Paraplatin Pow. for Inj. (Bristol-Myers Oncology/Immunology).

•**carboprost.** (CAR-boe-prahst) USAN.
Use: Oxytocic.

•**carboprost methyl.** (CAR-boe-prahst METH-ill) USAN.
Use: Oxytocic.

•**carboprost tromethamine.** (CAR-boe-prahst troe-METH-ah-meen) U.S.P. 23.
Use: Oxytocic.
See: Prostin, Amp. (Pharmacia & Upjohn).

Carboptic. (Optopics Laboratories, Corp.) Carbachol 3%. Soln. Bot. 15 ml. *Rx.*
Use: Ophthalmic.

carbose d.
See: Carboxymethylcellulose sodium, Prep.

carbovir. (GlaxoWellcome)
Use: Antiviral, HIV. [Orphan Drug]

carbowax. 300, 400, 1540, 4000. Polyethylene glycol 300, 400, 1540, 4000.

carboxymethylcellulose.
Use: Ocular lubricant.
See: Refresh Tears (Allergan).

•**carboxymethylcellulose calcium.** N.F. 18.
Use: Pharmaceutic aid (tablet disintegrant).

carboxymethylcellulose salt of dextroamphetamine. Carboxyphen.
See: Bontril Timed Tab. (Carnrick Laboratories, Inc.).

•**carboxymethylcellulose sodium.** (car-BOX-ee-meth-ill-SELL-you-lohs) U.S.P. 23.
Use: Pharmaceutic aid (suspending agent, tablet excipient), viscosity-increasing; cathartic.
W/Belladonna extract, kaolin, pectin, zinc phenosulfonate.
See: Foxalin, Cap. (Standex).
W/Docusate sodium.
See: Dialose, Cap. (Zeneca Pharmaceuticals).
W/Docusate sodium, casanthranol.
See: Dialose Plus, Cap. (Zeneca Pharmaceuticals).
Tri-Vac, Cap. (Rhode).
W/Docusate sodium, oxyphenisatin acetate.
See: Dialose Plus, Cap. (Zeneca Pharmaceuticals).
W/Methylcellulose.
See: Ex-Caloric, Wafer (Eastern Research).

•**carboxymethylcellulose sodium 12.** N.F. 18.
Use: Pharmaceutic aid (suspending, viscosity-increasing agent); mucolytic agent.

carboxyphen.
W/Butabarbital.
See: Bontril, Timed Tab. (Carnrick Laboratories, Inc.).

Carbromal. (Various Mfr.) Bromodiethylacetylurea, bromadel, nyctal, planadalin, uradal. *Rx.*
Use: Sedative, hypnotic.
W/Bromisovalum (Bromural).
See: Bro-T's, Tab. (Brothers).

carbutamide.
Use: Hypoglycemic.

•**carbuterol hydrochloride.** (car-BYOO-ter-ole) USAN.
Use: Bronchodilator.

cardamon. Oil, seed, Cpd. Tincture.
Use: Flavoring.

Cardec DM Drops. (Various Mfr.) Carbinoxamine maleate 2 mg, pseudoephedrine HCl 25 mg, dextromethorphan HBr 4 mg, alcohol < 0.6%/ml. Drop. Bot. 30 ml. *Rx.*
Use: Antihistamine, antitussive, decongestant.

Cardec DM Pediatric Syrup. (Schein Pharmaceutical, Inc.) Pseudoephedrine HCl 60 mg, dextromethorphan HBr 15 mg, carbinoxamine maleate 4 mg, < 0.6% alcohol. Bot. pt. *Rx.*
Use: Antihistamine, antitussive, decongestant.

Cardec DM Syrup. (Various Mfr.) Carbinoxamine maleate 4 mg, pseudoephedrine HCl 60 mg, dextromethorphan HBr 15 mg, alcohol g 0.6%/5 ml. Bot. 30 ml, 120 ml, pt, gal. *Rx.*
Use: Antihistamine, antitussive, decongestant.

Cardec-S. (Alpharma USPD Inc.) Pseudoephedrine HCl 60 mg, carbinoxamine maleate 4 mg/5 ml. Syr. Bot. 473 ml. *Rx.*
Use: Antihistamine, decongestant.

Cardene. (Roche Laboratories) Nicardipine 20 mg or 30 mg/Cap. Bot. 100s, 500s, UD 100s. *Rx.*
Use: Calcium channel blocker.

Cardene IV. (Wyeth-Ayerst Laboratories) Nicardipine HCl 2.5 ml, sorbitol 48 mg/ml. Inj. 10 ml Amp. *Rx.*
Use: Calcium channel blocker.

Cardene SR. (Roche Laboratories) Nicardipine HCl 30 mg, 45 mg, 60 mg/SR Cap. Bot. 60s, 200s, UD 100s. *Rx.*
Use: Calcium channel blocker.

Cardenz. (Miller Pharmacal Group, Inc.) Vitamins C 25 mg, E 5 mg, inositol 30 mg, p-aminobenzoic acid 9 mg, A 2000 IU, B_6 1.5 mg, B_{12} 1 mcg, D 100 IU, niacinamide 20 mg, Mg 23 mg, I 0.05 mg, K 8 mg/Tab. Bot. 100s. *otc.*
Use: Mineral, vitamin supplement.

Cardilate. (GlaxoWellcome) Erythrityl tetranitrate 10 mg/Tab. Bot. 100s.
Use: Antianginal.

Cardio-Green (CG). (Becton Dickinson & Co.) Indocyanine Green 25 mg, 50 mg. Inj. Amps 10 ml (2s).
Use: Diagnostic aid.

Cardio-Green Disposable Unit. (Becton Dickinson & Co.) Cardio-Green 10 mg.

Vial. Amp. Aqueous solvent and calibrated syringe.
Use: Diagnostic aid.

Cardi-Omega 3. (Thompson Medical Co.) EPA 180 mg, DHA 120 mg, cholesterol 5 mg, < 2% RDA of vitamins A, B_1, B_2, B_3, C, D, Fe, Ca/Cap. Bot. 60s. *otc.*
Use: Mineral, vitamin supplement.

cardioplegic solution.
Use: During open heart surgery.
See: Plegisol, Soln. (Abbott Laboratories).

Cardioquin. (Purdue Frederick Co.) Quinidine polygalacturonate 275 mg equivalent to quinidine sulfate 200 mg/Tab. Bot. 100s, 500s. *Rx.*
Use: Antiarrhythmic.

Cardiotrol-CK. (Roche Laboratories) Lyophilized human serum containing three CK isoenzymes from human tissue source. 10 × 2 ml.
Use: Diagnostic aid, quality control.

Cardiotrol-LD. (Roche Laboratories) Lyophilized human serum containing all LD isoenzymes from human tissue source. 10 × 1 ml.
Use: Diagnostic aid, quality control.

Cardizem. (Hoechst Marion Roussel) Diltiazem HCl **30 mg/Tab.:** Bot. 100s, 500s, UD 100s. **60 mg/Tab.:** Bot. 90s, 100s, 500s, UD 100s. **90 mg/Tab.:** Bot 90s, 100s, UD 100s. **120 mg/Tab.:** Bot. 100s and UD 100s. *Rx.*
Use: Calcium channel blocker.

Cardizem CD. (Hoechst Marion Roussel) Diltiazem HCl 120 mg, 180 mg, 240 mg, 300 mg/ER Cap. Bot. 30s, 90s, 5000s, and UD 100s. *Rx.*
Use: Calcium channel blocker.

Cardizem Injection. (Hoechst Marion Roussel) **25 mg (5 mg/ml)/Inj.:** Diltiazem HCl, 3.75 mg citric acid, 3.25 mg sodium citrate dihydrate, 357 mg sorbitol solution. Vial 5 ml. **50 mg (5 mg/ml)/Inj.:** Diltiazem HCl, 7.5 mg citric acid, 6.5 mg sodium citrate dihydrate, 714 mg sorbitol solution. Vial 10 ml. *Rx.*
Use: Calcium channel blocker.

Cardizem SR. (Hoechst Marion Roussel) Diltiazem HCl 60 mg, 90 mg or 120 mg/SR Cap. Bot. 100s, UD 100s. *Rx.*
Use: Calcium channel blocker.

Cardophyllin.
See: Aminophylline. (Various Mfr.).

Cardoxin. (Vita Elixir) Digoxin 0.25 mg/Tab. *Rx.*
Use: Cardiovascular agent.

Cardura. (Roerig) Doxazosin mesylate 1 mg, 2 mg, 4 mg, 8 mg/Tab. Bot. 100s, UD 100s. *Rx.*
Use: Antihypertensive.

carena.
See: Aminophylline. (Various Mfr.).

•**carfentanil citrate.** (car-FEN-tah-NILL SIH-trate) USAN.
Use: Analgesic, narcotic.

Cargentos.
See: Silver Protein, Mild.

•**carisoprodol.** (car-eye-so-PRO-dole) U.S.P. 23.
Use: Muscle relaxant.
See: Rela, Tab. (Schering-Plough Corp.).
Soma, Tab. (Wallace Laboratories).

carisoprodol. (Various Mfr.) 350 mg. Tab. Bot. 30s, 60s, 100, 500s, 1000s, UD 100s.
Use: Muscle relaxant.

carisoprodol and aspirin tablets.
Use: Analgesic, muscle relaxant.
See: Soma Compound, Tab. (Wallace Laboratories).

carisoprodol, aspirin, and codeine phosphate tablets.
Use: Analgesic, muscle relaxant.
See: Soma Compound w/Codeine, Tab. (Wallace Laboratories).

Carisoprodol Compound. (Various Mfr.) Carisoprodol 200 mg, aspirin 325 mg/Tab. Bot. 15s, 30s, 40s, 100s, 500s, 1000s. *Rx.*
Use: Analgesic, muscle relaxant.

Cari-Tab. (Jones Medical Industries, Inc.) Fluoride 0.5 mg, vitamins A 2000 IU, D 200 IU, C 75 mg/Softab. Bot. 100s. *Rx.*
Use: Vitamin supplement, dental caries agent.

•**carmantadine.** (car-MAN-tah-deen) USAN.
Use: Antiparkinsonian.

Carmol 10. (Doak Dermatologics) Urea (carbamide) 10% in hypoallergenic water-washable lotion base. Bot. 6 fl oz. *otc.*
Use: Emollient.

Carmol 20. (Doak Dermatologics) Urea (carbamide) 20% in hypoallergenic vanishing cream base. Tube 3 oz, Jar lb. *otc.*
Use: Emollient.

Carmol HC Cream 1%. (Doak Dermatologics) Micronized hydrocortisone acetate 1%, urea 10% in water-washable base. Tube 1 oz, Jar 4 oz. *Rx.*
Use: Corticosteroid, topical.

•**carmustine (BCNU).** (CAR-muss-teen) USAN.
Use: Antineoplastic.
See: BiCNU, Inj. (Bristol-Myers Oncology/Immunology).

Gliadel, Wafer (Rhone-Poulenc Rorer Pharmaceuticals, Inc.).

Carnation Follow-Up. (Carnation) Protein (from non-fat milk) 18 g, carbohydrate (from lactose and corn syrup) 89.2 g, fat 27.7 g, vitamins A, D, E, K, C, B_1, B_2, B_3, B_6, B_{12}, B_5, biotin, choline, Ca, P, Cl, Mg, I, Mn, Cu, Zn, Fe 13 mg, inositol, cholesterol 11.4 mg, taurine, Na 264 mg, K 913 mg. Pow. 360 g. Conc. 390 ml. *otc.*
Use: Nutritional supplement.

Carnation Good-Start. (Carnation) Protein 16 g, carbohydrate 74.4 g, fat 34.5 g, vitamins A, D, E, K, B_1, B_2, B_3, B_5, B_6, B_{12}, C, biotin, choline, inositol, cholesterol 68 mg, taurine, Ca, P, Mg, Fe 10 mg, Zn, Mn, Cu, I, Cl, Na 162 mg, K 663 mg. Pow 360 g. Conc. 390 ml. *otc.*
Use: Nutritional supplement.

Carnation Instant Breakfast. (Carnation) Non-fat instant breakfast containing 280 K calories w/15 g protein and 8 oz whole milk. Pkt. 35 g, Ctn. 6s. Six flavors. *otc.*
Use: Nutritional supplement.

•**carnidazole.** (car-NIH-dah-zole) USAN. Methyl-nitro-imidazole.
Use: Antiparasitic, antiprotozoal.

Carnitor. (Sigma-Tau Pharmaceuticals, Inc.) Levocarnitine. **Liq.:** 100 mg/ml. Bot. 10 ml. **Tab.:** 330 mg. Bot. 90s. **Inj.:** 1 g/5 ml. Single-dose amps 5 ml. *Rx.*
Use: Vitamin supplement.

•**caroxazone.** (car-OX-ah-zone) USAN.
Use: Antidepressant.

•**carphenazine maleate.** (car-FEN-azz-een) USAN. U.S.P XXII.
Use: Antipsychotic.

•**carprofen.** (car-PRO-fen) USAN.
Use: Analgesic, NSAID.
See: Rimadyl (Roche Laboratories).

•**carrageenan.** (ka-rah-GEE-nan) N.F. 18.
Use: Pharmaceutic aid; (suspending, viscosity-increasing agent).

Carrisyn. (Carrington Labs) Phase I AIDS, ARC. *Rx.*
Use: Antiviral, immunomodulator.

•**carsatrin succinate.** (car-SAT-rin) USAN.
Use: Cardiovascular agent.

•**cartazolate.** (car-TAZZ-oh-late) USAN.
Use: Antidepressant.

•**carteolol hydrochloride.** (CAR-tee-oh-lahl) U.S.P. 23.
Use: Antiadrenergic (β-receptor).
See: Ocupress, Ophth. Soln. (Otsuka America Pharmaceutical, Inc.).

Carter's Little Pills. (Carter Wallace) Bisacodyl 5 mg. Pill. Bot. 30s, 85s. *otc.*
Use: Laxative.

Cartrol. (Abbott Laboratories) Carteolol 2.5 mg, 5 mg/Tab. Bot. 100s. *Rx.*
Use: Beta-adrenergic blocker.

Cartucho Cook with Ravocaine. (Sanofi Winthrop Pharmaceuticals) Ravocaine, novacaine, levophed or neocobefrin. *Rx.*
Use: Anesthetic.

•**carubicin hydrochloride.** (kah-ROO-bih-sin) USAN. *Formerly carminomycin hydrochloride.*
Use: Antineoplastic.

•**carumonam sodium.** (kah-roo-MOE-nam) USAN.
Use: Anti-infective.

•**carvedilol.** (CAR-veh-DILL-ole) USAN.
Use: Antianginal, antihypertensive.
See: Coreg, Tab. (SmithKline Beecham).

Car-Vit. (Mericon Industries, Inc.) Ascorbic acid 60 mg, vitamins A acetate 4000 IU, D-2 400 IU, ferrous fumarate 90 mg (elemental iron 30 mg), oyster shell 600 mg (calcium 230 mg)/Cap. Bot. 90s, 1000s. *otc.*
Use: Mineral, vitamin supplement.

•**carvotroline hydrochloride.** (car-VAH-trah-leen) USAN.
Use: Antipsychotic.

•**carzelesin.** (car-ZELL-eh-sin) USAN.
Use: Antineoplastic (site-selective DNA binding).

carzenide.
Use: Carbonic anhydrase inhibitor.

casa-dicole. (Halsey Drug Co.) Docusate sodium 100 mg, casanthrol 30 mg/Cap. Bot. 100s. *otc.*
Use: Laxative.

•**casanthranol.** (kass-AN-thrah-nole) U.S.P. 23. A purified mixture of the anthranol glycosides derived from *Cascara sagrada.*
Use: Laxative.
See: Black Draught, Prods. (Chattem Consumer Products).

W/Docusate sodium.
See: Bu-Lax-Plus, Cap. (Ulmer Pharmacal Co.).
Calotabs, Tab. (Calotabs).
Comfolax-Plus, Cap. (Rhone-Poulenc Rorer Pharmaceuticals, Inc.).
Comfolax-Plus, Cap. (Searle).
Comfula-Plus (Searle).
Constiban, Cap. (Quality Formulations, Inc.).
Diolax, Cap. (Century Pharmaceuticals, Inc.).
Dio-Soft (Standex).
Disulans, Cap. (PJ, Noyes, Co., Inc.).

Easy-Lax Plus, Cap. (Walgreen Co.).
Genericace, Cap. (Forest Pharmaceutical, Inc.).
Neo-Vardin D-S-S-C, Cap. (Scherer Laboratories, Inc.).
Nuvac, Cap. (LaCrosse).
Peri-Colace, Cap, Syr. (Bristol-Myers Squibb).

W/Docusate sodium, sodium carboxymethylcellulose.
See: Dialose Plus, Cap. (Zeneca Pharmaceuticals).
Silace-C, Syr. (Silarx).
Tri-Vac, Cap. (Rhode).

Cascara. (Eli Lilly and Co.) Cascara 150 mg/Tab. Bot. 100s. *otc.*

cascara fluid extract, aromatic.
Use: Laxative.

cascara glycosides.
Use: Laxative.

•**cascara sagrada.** (kass-KA-rah sah-GRAH-dah) U.S.P. 23.
Use: Cathartic.
W/Bile salts, papain, phenolphthalein, capsicum oleoresin.
See: Torocol Compound, Tab. (Plessner).
W/Bile salts, phenolphthalein, capsicum oleoresin, peppermint oil.
See: Torocol, Tab. (Plessner).
W/Ox bile (desiccated), phenolphthalein, aloin, podophyllin.
See: Bocresin, Liq. (Scrip).

cascara sagrada. (Various Mfr.) 325 mg/Tab. Bot. 100s, 1000s.
Use: Cathartic.

cascara sagrada fluid extract. (Parke-Davis) Alcohol 18%/5 ml. Bot. Pt, gal, UD 5 ml.
Use: Laxative. [Orphan Drug]
See: Bilstan (Standex).

cascara sagrada fluid extract aromatic. Aromatic Cascara Fluid extract. Liq. Alcohol ≈ 18%/5 ml. Bot. 60 ml, 120 ml, pt, gal, UD 5 ml.
Use: Laxative.

cascarin.
See: Casanthranol (Various Mfr.).

Casec. (Bristol-Myers Squibb) Calcium caseinate (derived from skim milk curd and calcium carbonate). Pow. Can 2.5 oz. *otc.*
Use: Mineral supplement.

Casodex. (Zeneca Pharmaceuticals) Bicalutamide 50 mg, lactose/Tab. In 100s and UD 30s. *Rx.*
Use: Antineoplastic.

•**caspofungin acetate.** (KASS-poe-FUN-jin ASS-eh-tate) USAN.
Use: Antifungal.

CAST. (Biomerica, Inc.) Reagent test for immunoglobulin E in serum. Tube Kit 25s.
Use: Diagnostic aid.

Castellani Paint Modified. (Pedinol Pharmacal, Inc.) Basic fuchsin, phenol resorcinol, acetone, alcohol. Bot. 30 ml, 120 ml, 480 ml. Also available as colorless solution without basic fuchsin. Bot. 30 ml, 120 ml, 480 ml. *Rx.*
Use: Antifungal, topical.

Castellani's Paint. (Penta) Carbol-fuchsin solution. Fuchsin 0.3%, phenol 4.5%, resorcinol 10%, acetone 1.5%, alcohol 13%. Bot. 1 oz, 4 oz, pt. *Rx.*
Use: Antifungal, topical.

•**castor oil.** (KASS-ter oil) U.S.P. 23.
Use: Laxative, pharmaceutic aid (plasticizer).
See: Neoloid (ESI Lederle Generics).
Purge (Fleming & Co.).

castor oil. (KASS-ter oil) Aromatic Caps. Liq. emulsion. Liq. Bot. 60 ml, 120 ml, pt.
Use: Laxative, pharmaceutic aid (plasticizer).

castor oil emulsion.
Use: Cathartic.
See: Emulsoil (Paddock Laboratories).
Fleet Flavored (C.B. Fleet Co.).

castor oil, hydrogenated.
Use: Laxative.

Cataflam. (Novartis Pharmaceutical Corp.) Diclofenac 50 mg (as potassium), sucrose. Tab. Bot. 100s, UD 100s. *Rx.*
Use: Analgesic, NSAID.

Catapres. (Boehringer Ingelheim, Inc.) Clonidine HCl 0.1 mg, 0.2 mg, 0.3 mg/Tab. Bot. 100s, 1000s, UD 100s (except 0.3 mg). *Rx.*
Use: Antihypertensive.

Catapres-TTS. (Boehringer Ingelheim, Inc.) Clonidine 2.5 mg, 5 mg, 7.5 mg/Transdermal patch. Pkg. 4s, 12s. *Rx.*
Use: Antihypertensive.

Catatrol. (Zeneca Pharmaceuticals) Viloxazine.
Use: Antidepressant.

cathomycin calcium. Calcium novobiocin.
Use: Anti-infective.

cathomycin sodium. Novobiocin sodium.
Use: Anti-infective.

cationic resins.
See: Resins, Sodium-Removing.

Caverject. (Pharmacia & Upjohn) Alprostadil 11.9 mcg (10 mcg/ml) or 23.2 mcg (20 mcg/ml). Lyophilized pow. for inj. Vials with diluent syringes. *Rx.*
Use: Anti-impotence agent.

Cav-X Fluoride Treatment. (Palisades Pharmaceuticals, Inc.) Stannous fluoride 0.4% gel. Bot. 121.9 g. *Rx.*
Use: Dental caries agent.

C-Bio. (Barth's) Vitamin C 150 mg, citrus bioflavonoid complex 100 mg, rutin 50 mg/Tab. Bot. 100s, 500s, 1000s. *otc.*
Use: Vitamin supplement.

C-B Time Liquid. (Arco Pharmaceuticals, Inc.) Vitamins C 300 mg, B_1 15 mg, B_2 10 mg, B_3 100 mg, B_5 20 mg, B_6 5 mg, B_{12} 5 mcg. Liq. Bot. 120 ml. *otc.*
Use: Vitamin supplement.

CCD 1042. (Cocensys, Inc.)
Use: Treatment of infantile spasms. [Orphan Drug]

CC-Galactosidase. Alpha-galactosidase A.
Use: Fabry's disease. [Orphan Drug]

CCNU. Lomustine.
Use: Antineoplastic.
See: CeeNu, Tab. (Bristol-Myers Squibb).

C-Crystals. (NBTY, Inc.) Vitamin C 5000 mg/tsp. Crystals. Bot. 180 g. *otc.*
Use: Vitamin supplement.

CD4 human truncated 369 AA polypeptide. *Rx.*
Use: Antiviral, HIV.

CD4, recombinant soluble human (rCD4).
Use: Antiviral, HIV. [Orphan Drug]

CD-45 monoclonal antibodies.
Use: Prevent graft rejection in organ transplants. [Orphan Drug]

CDDP.
Use: Antineoplastic.
See: Cisplatin.

C.D.P. (Zenith Goldline Pharmaceuticals) Chlordiazepoxide HCl 5 mg, 10 mg, 25 mg/Cap. Bot. 100s, 500s, 1000s. *c-iv.*
Use: Anxiolytic.

Cea. (Abbott Diagnostics) Radioimmunoassay or enzyme immunoassay for quantitative measurement of carcinoembryonic antigen in human serum or plasma. Test Kit 100s.
Use: Diagnostic aid.

Cea-Roche. (Roche Laboratories) Radioimmunoassay capable of detecting and measuring plasma levels of CEA in the nanogram range. Sensitivity-0.5 ng/ml of CEA.
Use: Diagnostic aid.

Cea-Roche Test Kit. (Roche Laboratories) Carcinoembryonic antigen, a glycoprotein which is a constituent of the glycocalyx of embryonic entodermal epithelium. Test Kit.
Use: Diagnostic aid.

CEA-Scan. (Immunomedics, Mallinckrodt) Arcitumomab 1.25 mg. Reconstitute with Tc 99m sodium pertechnetate in NaCl for Inj. Inj. Single-dose Vial. *Rx.*
Use: For detection of recurrent or metastatic colorectal carcinoma of the liver, extrahepatic abdomen and pelvis; radioimmunoscintigraphy.

Cebid Timecelles. (Roberts Pharmaceuticals) Ascorbic acid 500 mg/Cap. Bot. 100s. *otc.*
Use: Vitamin supplement.

Ceb Nuggets. (Scott/Cord) Vitamins B_1 15 mg, B_2 15 mg, B_6 5 mg, B_{12} 5 mcg, C 600 mg, niacinamide 100 mg, E 40 IU, calcium pantothenate 20 mg, folic acid 0.1 mg/Nugget. Bot. 60s. *otc.*
Use: Mineral, vitamin supplement.

Cebo-Caps. (Forest Pharmaceutical, Inc.) Placebo capsules. *otc.*

C & E Capsules. (NBTY, Inc.) Vitamins C 500 mg, E 400 mg/Cap. Bot. 50s, 100s. *otc.*
Use: Vitamin supplement.

Ceclor. (Eli Lilly and Co.) **Pulv.:** Cefaclor 250 mg or 500 mg. Bot. 15s, 30s, 100s, UD 100s. **Oral Susp.:** Cefaclor 125 mg, 187 mg, 250 mg, 375 mg/5 ml. Bot. 50 ml, 75 ml, 100 ml, 150 ml. 375 mg/5 ml.
Use: Anti-infective, cephalosporin.

Ceclor CD. (Eli Lilly and Co.) Cefaclor anhydrous 375 mg, 500 mg, mannitol/ER Tab. Bot. 60s. *Rx.*
Use: Anti-infective.

Cecon Solution. (Abbott Laboratories) Ascorbic acid 10% in propylene glycol. Each drop from enclosed dropper supplies 2.5 mg ascorbic acid; contains 100 mg/ml. Bot. w/dropper 50 ml. *otc.*
Use: Vitamin supplement.

Cedax. (Schering-Plough Corp.) **Cap.:** Ceftibuten 400 mg, parabens/Bot 20s, 100s, UD 40s. **Susp.:** Ceftibuten 90 or 180 mg/5 ml, sucrose/Bot 30 ml, 60 ml, 90 ml, 120 ml. *Rx.*
Use: Anti-infective, cephalosporin.

•**cedefingol.** (seh-deh-FIN-gole) USAN.
Use: Antineoplastic, adjunct; antipsoriatic.

•**cedelizumab.** (sed-eh-LIE-zoo-mab) USAN.
Use: Monoclonal antibody, immunosuppressant.

Ceebevim. (NBTY, Inc.) Vitamins B_1 15 mg, B_2 10.2 mg, B_3 50 mg, B_5 10 mg, B_6 5 mg, C 300 mg/Cap. Bot. 100s, 300s. *otc.*
Use: Vitamin supplement.

CeeNu. (Bristol-Myers Oncology/Immunology) Lomustine (CCNU) 10 mg, 40

mg, 100 mg/Cap. Dose pk. of two cap. each of all three strengths. *Rx.*
Use: Antineoplastic.

Ceepa. (Geneva Pharmaceuticals) Theophylline 130 mg, ephedrine HCl 24 mg, phenobarbital 8 mg/Tab. Bot. 100s, 1000s. *Rx.*
Use: Bronchodilator, decongestant, hypnotic, sedative.

Ceepryn. Cetylpyridinium Cl. *otc.*
Use: Antiseptic.
See: Cepacol Lozenges, Soln., Troches (J.B. Williams Company Inc.).

Cee with Bee. (Wesley Pharmacal Co., Inc.) Vitamins B_1 15 mg, B_2 10.2 mg, B_3 50 mg, B_5 10 mg, B_6 5 mg, C 300 mg, tartrazine. Bot. 100s, 1000s. *otc.*
Use: Vitamin supplement.

•**cefaclor.** (SEFF-uh-klor) U.S.P. 23.
Use: Anti-infective, cephalosporin.
See: Ceclor, Prods. (Eli Lilly and Co.).

cefaclor. (Various Mfr.) **Cap.:** 250 mg, 500 mg. Bot. 15s (500 mg), 30s (250 mg), 100s, 500s (250 mg), 1000s (250 mg), UD 100s (500 mg). **Pow. for Oral Susp.:** 125 mg/5 ml, 187 mg/5 ml, 250 mg/5 ml, 375 mg/5 ml, Bot. 50 ml, 75 ml, 100 ml, 150 ml. *Rx.*
Use: Anti-infective.

•**cefadroxil.** (SEFF-uh-DROX-ill) U.S.P. 23.
Use: Anti-infective, cephalosporin.
See: Duricef, Cap., Tab., Susp. (Bristol-Myers Squibb).

cefadroxil. (Various Mfr.) Cefadroxil **Cap.:** 500 mg/Bot 100s. **Tab.:** 1 g/Bot 24s, 50s, 100s, 500s. *Rx.*
Use: Anti-infective, cephalosporin.

•**cefamandole.** (SEFF-ah-MAN-dole) USAN.
Use: Anti-infective.

•**cefamandole nafate for injection.** (SEFF-uh-MAN-dahl NA-fate) U.S.P. 23.
Use: Anti-infective, cephalosporin.
See: Mandol, Amp. (Eli Lilly and Co.).

•**cefamandole sodium for injection.** U.S.P. 23.
Use: Anti-infective, cephalosporin.

Cefanex. (Apothecon, Inc.) Cephalexin monohydrate 250 mg, 500 mg/Cap. Bot. 100s. *Rx.*
Use: Anti-infective, cephalosporin.

•**cefaparole.** (SEFF-ah-pah-ROLE) USAN.
Use: Anti-infective.

•**cefatrizine.** (SEFF-ah-TRY-zeen) USAN.
Use: Anti-infective, cephalosporin.

•**cefazaflur sodium.** (seff-AZE-ah-flure) USAN.
Use: Anti-infective, cephalosporin.

•**cefazolin.** (seff-AH-zoe-lin) U.S.P. 23.
Use: Anti-infective (systemic), cephalosporin.

•**cefazolin sodium, injection.** (seff-uh-zoe-lin) U.S.P. 23.
Use: Anti-infective (systemic), cephalosporin.
See: Ancef, Vial (SmithKline Beecham Pharmaceuticals).
Kefzol, Amp. (Eli Lilly and Co.).

cefazolin sodium. (Apothecon, Inc.) Cefazolin sodium 250 mg/Vial; 500 mg, 1 g/Vial, piggyback vial; 5 g, 10 g, 20 g/bulk pkg.
Use: Anti-infective (systemic), cephalosporin.

•**cefbuperazone.** (SEFF-byoo-PURR-ah-zone) USAN.
Use: Anti-infective, cephalosporin.

•**cefdinir.** (SEFF-dih-ner) USAN.
Use: Anti-infective, cephalosporin.
See: Omnicef, Cap., Oral Susp. (Parke-Davis).

•**cefepime.** (SEFF-eh-pim) USAN.
Use: Anti-infective.

•**cefepime hydrochloride.** (SEFF-eh-pim) USAN.
Use: Anti-infective.
See: Maxipime, Pow. for Inj. (Dura).

•**cefetecol.** (seff-EH-teh-kahl) USAN.
Use: Antibacterial, cephalosporin.

Cefinal II. (Alto Pharmaceuticals, Inc.) Salicymide 150 mg, acetaminophen 250 mg, doxylamine succinate 25 mg/Tab. Bot. 100s. *otc.*
Use: Analgesic combination.

•**cefixime.** (SEFF-IKS-eem) U.S.P. 23.
Use: Antibacterial, cephalosporin.
See: Suprax (ESI Lederle Generics).

Cefizox. (SmithKline Beecham) Ceftizoxime sodium. **Pow. for Inj.:** 500 mg (single-dose fliptop vials 10 ml); 1 g, 2 g (vial 20 ml, piggyback vial 100 ml); 10 g (bulk pkg). **Inj.:** 1 g, 2 g. Frozen, premixed, single-dose plastic containers 50 ml. *Rx.*
Use: Anti-infective, cephalosporin.

•**cefmenoxine hydrochloride, sterile.** (SEFF-men-ox-eem) U.S.P. 23.
Use: Anti-infective, cephalosporin.

•**cefmetazole.** (seff-MET-ah-zole) U.S.P. 23.
Use: Anti-infective, cephalosporin.

•**cefmetazole sodium.** (seff-MET-ah-zole) U.S.P. 23.
Use: Anti-infective, cephalosporin.
See: Zefazone (Pharmacia & Upjohn).

Cefobid. (Roerig) Cefoperazone sodium.

Pow. for Inj.: 1 g or 2 g. Piggyback unit. **Inj.:** 1 g, 2 g. Premixed, frozen, 50 ml plastic container 10 g Pharmacy bulk package. *Rx.*
Use: Anti-infective, cephalosporin.

Cefol Filmtab. (Abbott Laboratories) Vitamins B_1 15 mg, B_2 10 mg, B_6 5 mg, B_{12} 6 mcg, C 750 mg, E 30 mg, B_5 20 mg, B_3 100 mg, folic acid 0.5 mg/Tab. Bot. 100s. *otc.*
Use: Mineral, vitamin supplement.

•**cefonicid monosodium.** (seh-FAHN-ih-SID MAHN-oh-SO-dee-uhm) USAN.
Use: Anti-infective, cephalosporin.

•**cefonicid sodium, sterile.** (seh-FAHN-ih-SID) U.S.P. 23.
Use: Anti-infective, cephalosporin.
See: Monocid, Pow. for Inj. (SmithKline Beecham).

•**cefoperazone sodium.** (SEFF-oh-PUR-uh-zone) U.S.P. 23.
Use: Anti-infective, cephalosporin.
See: Cefobid, Inj. (Roerig).

•**ceforanide for injection.** (seh-FAR-ah-NIDE) U.S.P. 23.
Use: Anti-infective, cephalosporin.

Cefotan. (Zeneca Pharmaceuticals) Cefotetan disodium. **Pow. for Inj.:** 1 g, 2 g (*ADD-Vantage* and piggyback vials); 10 g (vial 100 ml). **Inj.:** 1 g/50 ml, 2 g/50 ml, dextrose. Frozen, iso-osmotic, premixed single-dose *Galaxy* containers 50 ml. *Rx.*
Use: Anti-infective, cephalosporin.

•**cefotaxime sodium.** (seff-oh-TAX-eem) U.S.P. 23.
Use: Anti-infective, cephalosporin.
See: Claforan, Inj. (Hoechst Marion Roussel).

•**cefotetan.** (SEFF-oh-tee-tan) U.S.P. 23.
Use: Anti-infective, cephalosporin.

•**cefotetan disodium.** (SEFF-oh-tee-tan die-SO-dee-uhm) U.S.P. 23.
Use: Anti-infective.
See: Cefotan (Zeneca Pharmaceuticals).

•**cefotiam hydrochloride sterile.** (SEFF-oh-TIE-am) U.S.P. 23.
Use: Anti-infective, cephalosporin.

•**cefoxitin.** (seff-OX-ih-tin) USAN.
Use: Anti-infective, cephalosporin.
See: Mefoxin, Inj. (Merck & Co.).

•**cefoxitin sodium.** (seff-OX-ih-tin) U.S.P. 23.
Use: Anti-infective, cephalosporin.

•**cefpimizole.** (seff-PIH-mih-zole) USAN.
Use: Anti-infective, cephalosporin.

•**cefpimizole sodium.** (seff-PIH-mih-zole) USAN.
Use: Anti-infective, cephalosporin.
See: Mefoxin, Inj., Pow. for Inj. (Merck & Co.).

•**cefpiramide.** (SEFF-PIHR-am-ide) U.S.P. 23.
Use: Anti-infective, cephalosporin.

•**cefpiramide sodium.** (SEFF-PIHR-am ide) USAN.
Use: Anti-infective, cephalosporin.

•**cefpirome sulfate.** (SEFF-pihr-ome) USAN.
Use: Anti-infective, cephalosporin.

•**cefpodoxime proxetil.** (SEFF-pode-OX-eem PROX-uh-til) USAN.
Use: Anti-infective, cephalosporin.
See: Vantin, Gran. for Susp., Tab. (Pharmacia & Upjohn).

•**cefprozil.** (SEFF-pro-zill) U.S.P. 23.
Use: Anti-infective, cephalosporin.
See: Cefzil Pow. for Susp., Tab. (Bristol Labs).

•**cefroxadine.** (SEFF-ROX-ah-deen) USAN.
Use: Anti-infective, cephalosporin.

•**cefsulodin sodium.** (SEFF-SULL-oh-din) USAN.
Use: Anti-infective, cephalosporin.

•**ceftazidime.** (seff-TAZE-ih-deem) U.S.P. 23.
Use: Anti-infective, cephalosporin.
See: Ceptaz, Inj. (GlaxoWellcome).
Fortaz, Inj. (GlaxoWellcome).
Tazicef, Inj. (Abbott Laboratories).
Tazidime, Inj. (Eli Lilly and Co.).

•**ceftibuten.** (seff-TIE-byoo-ten) USAN.
Use: Anti-infective.
See: Cedax, Cap., Susp. (Schering-Plough Corp.).

Ceftin. (GlaxoWellcome) Cefuroxime axetil. **Tab.:** 125 mg, 250 mg, or 500 mg/Tab. Bot. 20s, 60s, UD 50s, 100s. **Susp.:** 125 mg/5 ml, 250 mg/5 ml, sucrose/Bot. 50 ml, 100 ml. *Rx.*
Use: Anti-infective, cephalosporin.

•**ceftizoxime sodium.** (SEFF-tih-ZOX-eem) U.S.P. 23.
Use: Anti-infective, cephalosporin.
See: Cefizox, Pow. for Inj. (Fujisawa USA, Inc.).

•**ceftriaxone sodium.** (SEFF-TRY-AXE-own) U.S.P. 23.
Use: Anti-infective, cephalosporin.
See: Rocephin, Inj. (Roche Laboratories).

•**cefuroxime.** (SEFF-yur-OX-eem) USAN.
Use: Anti-infective, cephalosporin.
See: Ceftin, Tab. (GlaxoWellcome).

•**cefuroxime axetil.** (SEFF-your-OX-eem ACK-seh-TILL) USAN.

Use: Anti-infective, cephalosporin.
See: Ceftin, Tab. (GlaxoWellcome).

•**cefuroxime pivoxetil.** (SEFF-your-OX-eem pih-VOX-eh-till) USAN.
Use: Anti-infective, cephalosporin.

•**cefuroxime sodium.** U.S.P. 23.
Use: Anti-infective, cephalosporin.
See: Kefurox, Pow. for Inj. (Eli Lilly and Co.).
Zinacef, Inj., Pow. for Inj. (Glaxo-Wellcome).

cefuroxime sodium. (Various Mfr.) **Pow. for Inj.:** 750, 1.5 g in 10 ml (750 mg only), 20 ml (1.5 g only), 100 ml piggyback vials; 7.5 g/vial pharmacy bulk package. *Rx.*
Use: Anti-infective, cephalosporin.

cefuroxime sodium, sterile.
Use: Anti-infective, cephalosporin.
See: Kefurox, Inj. (Eli Lilly and Co.).
Zinacef, Inj. (GlaxoWellcome).

Cefzil. (Bristol-Myers Squibb) Cefprozil. **Tab.:** 250 mg, 500 mg. Bot. 50s, 100s, and UD 100s. **Pow. for Oral Susp.:** 125 mg/5 ml, 250 mg/5 ml. Sucrose, aspartame, phenylalanine 28 mg/5 ml. Bot. 50 ml, 75 ml, 100 ml. *Rx.*
Use: Anti-infective, cephalosporin.

Celebrex. (Searle) Celecoxib 100 mg, 200 mg. Cap. Bot. 100s, UD 100s. *Rx.*
Use: Nonsteroidal anti-inflammatory agent.

Celecoxib.
Use: Nonsteroidal anti-inflammatory agent.
See: Celebrex, Cap. (Searle).

Celestone. (Schering-Plough Corp.) **Tab.:** Betamethasone 0.6 mg. Bot. 100s, 500s, UD 21s. **Syr.:** Betamethasone 0.6 mg/5 ml, alcohol < 1%. Bot. 120 ml. *Rx.*
Use: Corticosteroid.

Celestone Phosphate Injection. (Schering-Plough Corp.) Betamethasone sodium phosphate 4 mg/ml equivalent to betamethasone alcohol 3 mg/ml. Vial 5 ml. *Rx.*
Use: Corticosteroid.

Celestone Soluspan. (Schering-Plough Corp.) Betamethasone sodium phosphate 3 mg, betamethasone acetate 3 mg, dibasic sodium phosphate 7.1 mg, monobasic sodium phosphate 3.4 mg, edetate disodium 0.1 mg, benzalkonium Cl 0.2 mg/ml. Vial 5 ml. *Rx.*
Use: Corticosteroid.

Celexa. (Forest Pharmaceuticals) Citalopram hydrobromide 20 mg, 40 mg. Tab. Bot. 30s, 100s, 500s, UD 100s. *Rx.*
Use: Antidepressant.

•**celgosivir hydrochloride.** (sell-GO-sih-vihr) USAN.
Use: Antiviral; inhibitor (α-glucoside).

•**celiprolol hydrochloride.** (SEE-lih-PRO-lahl) USAN.
Use: Anti-adrenergic (β-receptor).

Cellaburate. (Eastman Kodak Co.) Cellulose acetate butyrate.
Use: Pharmaceutic aid (plastic filming agent).

cellacefate.
Use: Pharmaceutic aid (tablet coating agent).
See: Cellulose acetate phthalate.

CellCept. (Roche Laboratories) Mycophenolate mofetil. **Cap.:** 250 mg. Bot. 100s, 500s. **Tab.:** 500 mg, alcohols. Bot. 100s, 500s. **Pow. for Inj.:** 500 mg (as HCl). Vial 20 ml. *Rx.*
Use: Immunosuppressant.

Cellepacbin. (Arthrins) Vitamins A 1200 IU, B_1 1.5 mg, B_2 1.5 mg, B_6 0.75 mg, niacinamide 7.5 mg, panthenol 3 mg, C 20 mg, B_{12} 2 mcg, E 1 IU/Cap. Bot. 180s. *otc.*
Use: Vitamin supplement.

Cellothyl. (Numark Laboratories, Inc.) Methylcellulose 0.5 g/Tab. Bot. 100s, 1000s. *otc.*
Use: Laxative.

•**cellulase.** (SELL-you-lace) USAN. A concentrate of cellulose-splitting enzymes derived from *Aspergillus niger* and other sources.
Use: Enzyme (digestive adjunct).
W/Bile salts, mixed conjugated, pancrelipase.
See: Zylase, Tab. (Eon Labs Manufacturing, Inc.).
W/Mylase, prolase, lipase.
See: Ku-Zyme, Cap. (Kremers Urban).

cellulose. (SELL-you-lohs)
W/Hexachlorophene.
See: Zeasorb, Pow. (Stiefel Laboratories, Inc.).

•**cellulose acetate.** (SELL-you-lohs) N.F. 18.
Use: Pharmaceutic aid (coating agent), polymer membrane (insoluble).

•**cellulose acetate phthalate.** (SELL-you-lohs) N.F. 18.
Use: Pharmaceutic aid (tablet coating agent).
See: Cellacefate.

cellulose, carboxymethyl, sodium salt. (SELL-you-lohs) U.S.P. 23. Carboxymethylcellulose Sodium.

cellulose, hydroxypropyl methyl ether. U.S.P. 23. Hydroxypropyl Methylcellulose.

cellulose methyl ether. (SELL-you-lohs)
See: Methylcellulose, Prep. (Various Mfr.).

•**cellulose microcrystalline.** (SELL-you-lohs) N.F. 18.
Use: Pharmaceutic aid (tablet and capsule diluent).

cellulose, nitrate. Pyroxylin.

•**cellulose, oxidized.** (SELL-you-lohs) U.S.P. 23.
Use: Hemostatic.

•**cellulose, oxidized regenerated.** (SELL-you-lohs) U.S.P. 23.
Use: Hemostatic.

cellulose, powdered. (SELL-you-lohs)
Use: Tablet and capsule diluent.

•**cellulose sodium phosphate.** U.S.P. 23.
Use: Antiurolithic.
See: Calcibind (Mission Pharmacal Co.).

cellulosic acid.
See: Oxidized Cellulose. (Various Mfr.).

cellulolytic enzyme.
See: Cellulase (Various Mfr.).
W/Amylolytic, proteolytic enzymes, lipase, phenobarbital, hyoscyamine sulfate, atropine sulfate.
See: Arco-Lipase Plus, Tab. (Arco Pharmaceuticals, Inc.).
W/Amylolytic enzyme, proteolytic enzyme, lipolytic enzyme, butisol sodium, belladonna.
See: Butibel-zyme, Tab. (Ortho McNeil Pharmaceutical).
W/Calcium carbonate, glycine, amylolytic and proteolytic enzymes.
See: Ku-Zyme, Cap. (Kremers Urban).

Celluvisc. (Allergan, Inc.) Carboxymethylcellulose 1%, NaCl, KCl, sodium lactate. Ophth. Soln. Single-use containers 0.3 ml (UD 30s). *otc.*
Use: Artificial tears.

Celontin. (Parke-Davis) Methsuximide 150 mg, 300 mg/Kapseal. Bot. 100s. *Rx.*
Use: Anticonvulsant.

Cel-U-Jec. (Roberts Pharmaceuticals) Betamethasone sodium phosphate 4 mg (equivalent to betamethasone alcohol 3 mg)/ml. Soln. Inj. Vial 5 ml. *Rx.*
Use: Corticosteroid.

Cenafed. (Century Pharmaceuticals, Inc.) **Tab.:** Pseudoephedrine HCl 30 mg, 60 mg. Bot. 100s, 1000s. **Syr.:** Pseudoephedrine HCl 30 mg/5 ml. Bot. 120 ml, pt, gal. *otc.*
Use: Decongestant.

Cenafed Plus. (Century Pharmaceuticals, Inc.) Pseudoephedrine HCl 60 mg, triprolidine HCl 2.5 mg/Tab. Bot. 100s. *otc.*
Use: Antihistamine, decongestant.

Cena-K. (Century Pharmaceuticals, Inc.) Potassium and Cl 20 mEq/15 ml (10% KCl), saccharin. Bot. Pt, gal. *Rx.*
Use: Electrolyte supplement.

Cenalax. (Century Pharmaceuticals, Inc.) Bisacodyl. **Tab.:** 5 mg. Bot. 100s, 1000s. **Supp.:** 10 mg. Pkg. 12s, 1000s. *otc.*
Use: Laxative.

Cenestin. (Duramed) Synthetic conjugated estrogen A 0.625 mg, 0.9 mg, lactose. Tab. Bot. 30s, 100s, 1000s. *Rx.*
Use: Estrogen.

Cenolate. (Abbott Hospital Products) Sodium ascorbate 562.5 mg/ml (equivalent to 500 mg/ml ascorbic acid), sodium hydrosulfate 0.5%. Inj. Amp. 1 ml, 2 ml. *Rx.*
Use: Vitamin supplement.

Centeon Thyroid. (Rhone-Poulenc Rorer Pharmaceuticals, Inc.) Desiccated animal thyroid glands (active thyroid hormones) T-4 thyroxine, T-3 thyronine 0.25 gr, 0.5 gr, 1 gr, 1.5 gr, 2 gr, 3 gr, 4 gr, or 5 gr/Tab. Bot. 100s, 1000s. Handy Hundreds, Carton Strip 100s. *Rx.*
Use: Hormone, thyroid.

Center-Al. (Center Laboratories) Allergenic extracts, alum precipitated 10,000 PNU/ml or 20,000 PNU/ml. Vial 10 ml, 30 ml. *Rx.*
Use: Antiallergic.

Centoxin. (Centocor, Inc.) Nebacumab.
Use: Antibacterial. [Orphan Drug]

Centrafree. (NBTY, Inc.) Iron 27 mg, vitamins A 5000 IU, D 400 IU, E 30 IU, B_1 2.25 mg, B_2 2.6 mg, B_3 20 mg, B_5 10 mg, B_6 3 mg, B_{12} 9 mcg, C 90 mg, folic acid 0.4 mg, biotin 45 mcg, Ca, Cl, Cr, Cu, I, K, Mg, Mn, Mo, P, Se, Zn/Tab. Bot. 100s. *otc.*
Use: Mineral, vitamin supplement.

central nervous system depressants.
See: Sedative/hypnotic agents.

central nervous system stimulants.
See: Amphetamine (Various Mfr.).
Anorexigenic agents.
Caffeine (Various Mfr.).
Desoxyephedrine HCl, Tab. (Various Mfr.).
Desoxyn HCl, Tab. Gradumet (Abbott Laboratories).
Dexedrine, Preps. (SmithKline Beecham Pharmaceuticals).
Methamphetamine HCl (Various Mfr.).
Ritalin HCl, Tab., Inj. (Novartis Pharmaceutical Corp.).

Centrovite Advanced Formula. (Rugby

Labs, Inc.) Fe 18 mg, A 5000 IU, D 400 IU, E 30 IU, B_1 1.5 mg, B_2 1.7 mg, B_3 20 mg, B_5 10 mg, B_6 2 mg, B_{12} 6 mcg, C 60 mg, Fa 0.4 mg, biotin 30 mcg, Ca, Cl, Cr, Cu, I, vitamin K, Mg, Mn, Mo, Ni, P, Se, Si, Sn, V, Zn, K. Tab. Bot. 100s. *otc.*
Use: Miineral, vitamin supplement.

Centrovite Jr. (Rugby Labs, Inc.) Iron 18 mg, vitamins A 5000 IU, D 400 IU, E 15 IU, B_1 1.5 mg, B_2 1.7 mg, B_3 20 mg, B_5 10 mg, B_6 2 mg, B_{12} 6 mcg, C 60 mg, folic acid 0.4 mg, biotin 45 mcg, Cr, Cu, I, Mg, Mn, Mo, Zn/Chew. Tab. Bot. 60s. *otc.*
Use: Mineral, vitamin supplement.

Centrum. (ESI Lederle Generics) Vitamins A 5000 IU, E 30 IU, C 90 mg, folic acid 400 mcg, B_1 2.25 mg, B_2 2.6 mg, B_6 3 mg, niacinamide 20 mg, B_{12} 9 mcg, D 400 IU, biotin 45 mcg, pantothenic acid 10 mg, Ca 162 mg, P 125 mg, I 150 mcg, Fe 27 mg, Mg 100 mg, K 30 mg, Mn 5 mg, chromium 25 mcg, Se 25 mcg, Mo 25 mcg, Zn 15 mg, Cu 2 mg, vitamin K 25 mcg, Cl 27.2 mg/Tab. *otc.*
Use: Mineral, vitamin supplement.

Centrum, Advanced Formula. (ESI Lederle Generics) Vitamins A 2500 IU, E 30 IU, C 60 mg, B_1 1.5 mg, B_2 1.7 mg, B_3 20 mg, B_5 10 mg, B_6 2 mg, B_{12} 6 mcg, D_2 400 IU, Fe 9 mg, biotin 300 mcg per 15 ml. With I, Zn, Mn, Cr, Mo, alcohol. 6.6%. Liq. Bot. 236 ml. *otc.*
Use: Mineral, vitamin supplement.

Centrum Jr. (ESI Lederle Generics) Vitamins A 5000 IU, D 400 IU, E 30 IU, C 60 mg, folic acid 400 mcg, B_1 1.5 mg, B_6 2 mg, B_{12} 6 mcg, riboflavin 1.7 mg, niacinamide 20 mg, Fe 18 mg, Mg 25 mg, Cu 2 mg, Zn 10 mg, biotin 45 mcg, panthothenic acid 10 mg, Mo 20 mcg, chromium 20 mcg, I 150 mcg, Mn 1 mg/Chew. Tab. Bot. 60s. *otc.*
Use: Mineral, vitamin supplement.

Centrum Jr. + Extra C. (ESI Lederle Generics) Vitamins A 5000 IU D 400 IU, E 30 IU, C 300 mg, folic acid 400 mcg, biotin 45 mcg, B_1 1.5 mg, B_5 10 mg, B_2 1.7 mg, B_3 20 mg, B_6 2 mg, B_{12} 6 mcg, K, Fe 18 mg, Mg, I, Cu, P, Ca 108 mg, Zn 15 mg, Mn, Mo, Cr, biotin 45 mcg, sugar, lactose/Chew. Tab. Bot. 60s. *otc.*
Use: Mineral, vitamin supplement.

Centrum Jr. + Extra Calcium. (ESI Lederle Generics) Calcium 160 mg, iron 18 mg, vitamins A 5000 IU, D 400 IU, E 30 mg, B_1 1.5 mg, B_2 1.7 mg, B_3 20 mg, B_5 10 mg, B_6 2 mg, B_{12} 6 mcg, C 60 mg, folic acid 400 mcg, Cr, Cu, I, Mn, Mg, Mo, P, Zn 15 mg, vitamin K, biotin 45 mcg, sugar/Chew. Tab. Bot. 60s. *otc.*
Use: Mineral, vitamin supplement.

Centrum Jr. + Iron. (ESI Lederle Generics) Iron 18 mg, vitamins A 5000 IU, D 400 IU, E 30 IU, B_1 1.5 mg, B_2 1.7 mg, B_3 20 mg, B_5 10 mg, B_6 2 mg, B_{12} 6 mcg, C 60 mg, folic acid 0.4 mg, Ca, Cr, Cu, I, Mg, Mn, Mo, P, Zn 15 mg, biotin 45 mcg, vitamin K/Chew. Tab. Bot. 60s. *otc.*
Use: Mineral, vitamin supplement.

Centrum Silver. (ESI Lederle Generics) Tab. Vitamin A 5000 IU, D 400 IU, E 45 IU, B_1 1.5 mg, B_2 1.7 mg, B_3 20 mg, B_5 10 mg, B_6 3 mg, B_{12} 25 mcg, C 60 mg, Fe 4 mg, folic acid 0.4 mg, Ca 200 mg, Zn 15 mg, biotin 30 mcg, vitamin K, Cu, I, Mg, P, Cl, Cr, Mn, Mo, Ni, Se, Si, V. Bot. 60s, 100s, 180s. *otc.*
Use: Mineral, vitamin supplement.

Centrum Silver Gel-Tabs. (ESI Lederle Generics) Vitamins A 6000 IU, D 400 IU, E 45 IU, B_1 1.5 mg, B_2 1.7 mg, B_3 20 mg, B_5 10 mg, B_6 3 mg, B_{12} 25 mcg, C 60 mg, K 10 mcg, biotin 30 mcg, folic acid 200 mcg, Fe 9 mg. With Ca 200 mg, Cu, I, Mg, P, Zn, Cl, Cr, Mn, Mo, Ni, K, Se, Si, V. Tab. Bot. 60s. *otc.*
Use: Mineral, vitamin supplement.

Centurion A-Z. (Mission Pharmacal Co.) Fe 27 mg, A 5000 IU, D 400 IU, E 30 IU, B_1 2.25 mg, B_2 2.6 mg, B_3 20 mg, B_5 10 mg, B_6 3 mg, B_{12} 9 mcg, C 90 mg, FA 0.4 mg, biotin 0.45 mg, Ca, Cl, Cr, Cu, I, K, Mg, Mn, Mo, P, Se, Zn, vitamin K. Tab. Bot. 130s. *otc.*
Use: Vitamin/mineral supplement.

Ceo-Two. (Beutlich, Inc.) Potassium bitartrate, sodium bicarbonate in polyethylene glycol base/Supp. 10s. *otc.*
Use: Laxative.

Cepacol. (J.B. Williams Company Inc.) Cetylpyridinium Cl 0.05%, alcohol 14%, tartrazine, saccharin. Liq. Bot. 360 ml, 540 ml, 720 ml, 960 ml. *otc.*
Use: Antiseptic.

Cepacol Anesthetic Lozenges. (J.B. Williams Company Inc.) Benzocaine 10 mg, cetylpyridinium Cl 0.07%, tartrazine. Pkg. 18s, 24s. *otc.*
Use: Anesthetic, local.

Cepacol Maximum Strength. (J.B. Williams Company Inc.) Benzocaine 10 mg, menthol, cool mint, cherry flavors. Loz. Pkg. 16s. *otc.*
Use: Mouth and throat product.

Cepacol Throat Lozenges. (J.B. Williams Company Inc.) Cetylpyridinium Cl 0.07%, benzyl alcohol 0.3%, tartrazine.

Pkg. 27s, 40s. *otc.*
Use: Antiseptic.

Cepastat Cherry Lozenges. (SmithKline Beecham Pharmaceuticals) Phenol 14.5 mg, menthol, sorbitol, saccharin. Sugar free. Box 18s. *otc.*
Use: Anesthetic.

Cepastat Extra Strength. (SmithKline Beecham Pharmaceuticals) Phenol 29 mg, menthol, sorbitol, eucalyptus oil. Sugar free. Loz. Pkg. 18s. *otc.*
Use: Anesthetic.

•**cephacetrile sodium.** (SEFF-ah-seh-TRILE) USAN. U.S.P. XX.
Use: Anti-infective, cephalosporin.

•**cephalexin.** (SEFF-ah-LEX-in) U.S.P. 23.
Use: Anti-infective, cephalosporin.
See: Biocef, Cap., Pow. (International Ethical Labs).
Keflex, Cap., Susp. (Eli Lilly and Co.).

Cephalexin. (Various Mfr.) **Cap.:** 250 mg, 500 mg. Bot. 100s, 250s (500 mg), 500s, 1000s, UD 20s, 100s. **Tab.:** 250 mg, 500 mg, 1 g. Bot. 20s, 100s, 500s. Pkg. 24s (1 g only). **Pow. for Oral Susp.:** 125 mg/5 ml, 250 mg/5 ml. Bot. 100 ml, 200 ml. *Rx.*
Use: Anti-infective, cephalosporin.

•**cephalexin hydrochloride.** (SEFF-ah-LEX-in) U.S.P. 23.
Use: Anti-infective, cephalosporin.
See: Keftab, Tab. (Eli Lilly and Co.).

cephalexin monohydrate. (SEFF-ah-LEX-in)
Use: Anti-infective, cephalosporin.
See: Biocef, Cap., Pow. (International Ethical Labs).
Keflex, Cap., Susp. (Eli Lilly and Co.).

cephalin.
W/Lecithin with choline base, lipositol.
See: Alcolec, Cap., Gran. (American Lecithin Company).

•**cephaloglycin.** (SEFF-ah-low-GLIE-sin) USAN. U.S.P. XX.
Use: Anti-infective.

•**cephaloridine.** (SEFF-ah-lor-ih-deen) USAN. U.S.P. XX.
Use: Anti-infective, cephalosporin.

•**cephalothin sodium.** (seff-AY-low-thin) U.S.P. 23.
Use: Anti-infective, cephalosporin.

•**cephapirin benzathine.** U.S.P. 23.
Use: Anti-infective.

•**cephapirin sodium, sterile.** (SEFF-uh-PIE-rin) U.S.P. 23.
Use: Anti-infective, cephalosporin.

cephazolin sodium.
See: Cefazolin.

•**cephradine.** (SEFF-ruh-deen) U.S.P. 23.
Use: Anti-infective, cephalosporin.
See: Velosef, Cap., Inj., Susp. (Bristol-Myers Squibb).

cephradine. (Various Mfr.) **Cap.:** 250 mg, 500 mg. Bot. 24s, 40s, 100s, 500s, UD 100s. **Pow. for Oral Susp.:** 125 mg/5 ml, 250 mg/5 ml when reconstituted. Bot. 100 ml, 200 ml. *Rx.*
Use: Anti-infective, cephalosporin.

Cephulac. (Hoechst Marion Roussel) Lactulose syrup 10 g/15 ml (< galactose 2.2 g, lactose 1.2 g, other sugars 1.2 g). Bot. 473 ml, 1890 ml, UD 15 ml, 30 ml. Box 100s. *Rx.*
Use: Laxative.

Ceptaz. (GlaxoWellcome) Ceftazidime pentahydrate with L-arginine 1 g, 2 g, 10 g. Vial. Infusion packs (1 g, 2 g). Pharmacy bulk packages (10 g). *Rx.*
Use: Anti-infective, cephalosporin.

ceramide trihexosidase/alpha-galactosidase a. (Genzyme Corp.)
Use: Fabry's disease. [Orphan Drug]

Cerapon. (Purdue Frederick Co.) Triethanolamine Polypeptide Oleate Condensate.
See: Cerumenex, Drops (Purdue Frederick Co.).

Cerebyx. (Parke-Davis) Fosphenytoin 150 mg (100 mg phenytoin sodium) in 2 ml vials and 750 mg (500 mg phenytoin sodium) in 10 ml vials. *Rx.*
Use: Treatment of certain types of seizures.

Ceredase. (Genzyme Corp.) Alglucerase 10 U/ml, 80 U/ml. Inj. Bot. 50 U with 5 ml fill volume (10 U). 400 U with 5 ml fill volume (80 U). *Rx.*
Use: Enzyme replacement for Gaucher's disease.

cerelose.
See: Glucose (Various Mfr.).

Ceretex. (Enzyme Process) Iron 15 mg, vitamins B_{12} 10 mcg, B_1 2 mg, B_6 1 mg, niacinamide 1 mg, pantothenic acid 0.15 mg, B_2 2 mg, iodine 15 mg/2 ml. Bot. 60 ml, 240 ml. *otc.*
Use: Mineral, vitamin supplement.

Cerezyme. (Genzyme Corp.) Imiglucerase 212 units (equiv. to a withdrawal dose of 200 units). Pow. for Inj. Vials. *Rx.*
Use: Treatment for Gaucher's disease.

•**cerivastatin sodium.** (seh-RIHV-ah-stat-in) USAN.
Use: Antihyperlipidemic; inhibitor.
See: Baycol, Tab. (Bayer Corp. (Allergy Div.)).

•**ceronapril.** (seh-ROW-nap-rill) USAN.
Use: Antihypertensive.

Cerose. (Wyeth-Ayerst Laboratories) Dextromethorphan HBr 15 mg, chlor-

pheniramine maleate 4 mg, phenylephrine HCl 10 mg/5 ml, alcohol 2.4%, saccharin. Sugar free. Liq. Bot. 120 ml, 480 ml. *otc.*
Use: Antihistamine, antitussive, decongestant.

Cerovite. (Rugby Labs, Inc.) Iron 18 mg, vitamins A 5000 IU, D 400 IU, E 30 IU, B_1 1.5 mg, B_2 1.7 mg, B_3 20 mg, B_5 10 mg, B_6 2 mg, B_{12} 6 mcg, C 60 mg, folic acid 0.4 mg, Ca, Cl, Cr, Cu, I, Mg, Mn, Mo, Ni, P, Se, Si, SN, V, biotin 30 mcg, vitamin K, Zn 15 mg/Tab. Bot. 130s. *otc.*
Use: Mineral, vitamin supplement.

Cerovite Advanced Formula. (Rugby Labs, Inc.) Iron 18 mg, A 5000 IU, D 400 IU, E 30 IU, B_1 1.5 mg, B_2 1.7 mg, B_3 20 mg, B_5 10 mg, B_6 2 mg, B_{12} 6 mcg, C 60 mg, folic acid 0.4 mg, biotin 30 mcg, Ca, P, I, Mg, Cu, Mn, K, Cl, Cr, Mo, Se, Ni, Si, Sn, V, vitamin K, Zn 15 mg/Tab. Bot. 130s, 200s. *otc.*
Use: Iron with vitamin supplement.

Cerovite Jr. (Rugby Labs, Inc.) Iron 18 mg, vitamins A 5000 IU, D 400 IU, E 15 IU, B_1 1.5 mg, B_2 1.7 mg, B_3 20 mg, B_5 10 mg, B_6 2 mg, B_{12} 6 mcg, C 60 mg, folic acid 0.4 mg, Cu, I, Mg, Zn, Mn, Mo, biotin 45 mcg, Cr, sugar/Tab. Bot. 60s. *otc.*
Use: Mineral, viatmin supplement.

Cerovite Senior. (Rugby Labs, Inc.) Vitamins A 6000 IU, D 400 IU, E 45 IU, B_1 1.5 mg, B_2 1.7 mg, B_3 20 mg, B_5 10 mg, B_6 3 mg, B_{12} 25 mcg, C 60 mg, iron 9 mg, folic acid 0.2 mg, Ca 200 mg, Zn 15 mg, biotin 30 mcg, Cu, I, Mg, P, Cl, Cr, Mn, Mo, Ni, Se, Si, V, vitamin K. Tab. Bot. 60s. *otc.*
Use: Mineral, viatmin supplement.

Certagen. (Zenith Goldline Pharmaceuticals) Iron 18 mg, A 5000 IU, D 400 IU, E 30 IU, B_1 1.5 mg, B_2 1.7 mg, B_3 20 mg, B_5 10 mg, B_6 2 mg, B_{12} 6 mcg, C 60 mg, folic acid 0.4 mg, biotin 30 mcg, Ca, P, I, Mg, Cu, Mn, K, Cl, Cr, Mo, Se, Ni, Si, Sn, V, vitamin K, Zn 15 mg/Tab. Bot. 130s, 1000s. *otc.*
Use: Mineral, vitamin supplement.

Certagen Liquid. (Zenith Goldline Pharmaceuticals) Vitamins A 2500 IU, B_1 1.5 mg, B_2 1.7 mg, B_3 20 mg, B_5 10 mg, B_6 2 mg, B_{12} 6 mcg, C 60 mg, D_3 400 IU, E 30 IU, biotin 300 mcg, iron 9 mg, Zn 3 mg, Cr, I, Mn, Mo/15 ml. Alcohol 6.6%. Liq. Bot. 237 ml. *otc.*
Use: Mineral, vitamin supplement.

Certagen Senior. (Zenith Goldline Pharmaceuticals) Vitamin A 6000 IU, B_1 1.5 mg, B_2 1.7 mg, B_6 3 mg, B_{12} 25 mcg, C 60 mg, D 400 IU, E 45 IU, vitamin K, biotin 30 mcg, folic acid 200 mcg, B_3 20 mg, B_5 10 mg, Ca 80 mg, Cl, Cr, Cu, I, Fe 3 mg, Mg, Mn, Mo, Ni, P, K, Se, Si, V, Zn 15 mg/Tab. Bot. 60s. *otc.*
Use: Mineral, vitamin supplement.

Certa-Vite. (Major Pharmaceuticals) Vitamin A 5000 IU, D 400 IU, E 30 IU, K_1, C 60 mg, B_1 1.5 mg, B_2 1.7 mg, B_3 20 mg, B_6 2 mg, B_{12} 6 mcg, B_5 10 mg, folic acid 0.4 mg, biotin 30 mcg, Fe 18 mg, Ca, P, I, Mg, Cu, Zn, Mn, K, Cl, Cr, Mo, Se, Ni, Si, V, B. Tab. Bot. 130s, 300s. *otc.*
Use: Mineral, vitamin supplement.

Certa-Vite Golden. (Major Pharmaceuticals) Vitamin A 6000 IU, D 400 IU, E 45 IU, B_1 1.5 mg, B_2 1.7 mg, B_3 20 mg, B_5 10 mg, B_6 3 mg, B_{12} 25 mcg, C 60 mg, vitamin K, Ca 200 mg, Zn 15 mg, biotin 30 mcg, Cl, Cr, Cu, I, K, Mg, Mn, Mo, Ni, P, Se, Si, V. Tab. Bot. 60s. *otc.*
Use: Mineral, vitamin supplement.

Certiva. (Ross Pediatrics) Diphtheria toxoid 15 Lf, tetanus toxoid 6 Lf, pertussis toxoid 40 mcg, aluminum 0.5 mg, thimerosal 0.01%/0.5 ml dose. Inj. Vial 7.5 ml. *Rx.*
Use: Toxoid.

•**ceruletide.** (seh-ROO-leh-tide) USAN.
Use: Stimulant (gastric secretory).

•**ceruletide diethylamine.** (seh-ROO-leh-tide die-ETH-ill-ah-meen) USAN.
Use: Stimulant (gastric secretory).

Cerumenex Drops. (Purdue Frederick Co.) Triethanolamine polypeptide oleate-condensate 10%, chlorobutanol in propylene glycol 0.5%. Liq. Dropper bot. 6 ml, 12 ml. *Rx.*
Use: Otic.

cervical ripening agents.
See: Prepidil (Pharmacia & Upjohn).

Cervidil. (Forest Pharmaceutical, Inc.) Dinoprostone 10 mg. Insert. 1s. *Rx.*
Use: Cervical ripening.

Ces. (ICN Pharmaceuticals, Inc.) Conjugated estrogens 0.625 mg, 1.25 mg, 2.5 mg/Tab. *Rx.*
Use: Estrogen.

•**cesium chloride Cs 131.** (SEE-zee-uhm KLOR-ide) USAN.
Use: Radiopharmaceutical agent.

Ceta. (C & M Pharmacal, Inc.) Soap-free. Propylene glycol, hydroxyethylcellulose, cetyl and cetearyl alcohols, sodium lauryl sulfate, parabens. Liq. Bot. 240 ml. *otc.*
Use: Dermatologic cleanser.

Ceta-Plus. (Seatrace Pharmaceuticals, Inc.) Hydrocodone bitartrate 5 mg,

acetaminophen 500 mg/Cap. Bot. 100s. *c-III.*
Use: Analgesic combination, narcotic.

•**cetaben sodium.** (SEE-tah-ben) USAN.
Use: Antihyperlipoproteinemic.

Cetacaine. (Cetylite Industries, Inc.) Benzocaine 14%, butyl aminobenzoate 2%, tetracaine HCl 2%, benzalkonium Cl 0.5%, cetyl dimethyl ethyl ammonium bromide 0.005%. **Aerosol Spray:** 56 g. **Liq.:** 56 g. **Oint.:** Jar 37 g, flavored. **Hosp. Gel:** 29 g. *Rx.*
Use: Anesthetic, local.

Cetacort. (Galderma Laboratories, Inc.) Hydrocortisone in concentrations of 0.25%, 0.5%, 1% w/cetyl alcohol, propylene glycol, stearyl alcohol, sodium lauryl sulfate, butylparaben, methylparaben, propylparaben, purified water. Bot. 120 ml (0.25% only), 60 ml (0.5%, 1%). *Rx.*
Use: Corticosteroid, topical.

cetalkonium. (SEET-al-KOE-nee-uhm) F.D.A. Benzylhexadecyldimethylammonium ion.

•**cetalkonium chloride.** (SEET-al-KOE-nee-uhm) USAN.
Use: Anti-infective, topical.
W/Phenylephrine, pyrilamine maleate, thimerosal.
See: Anti-B Mist (DePree).

Cetamide. (Alcon Laboratories, Inc.) Sulfacetamide sodium 10%. Sterile ophthalmic oint. Tube 3.5 g. *Rx.*
Use: Anti-infective, ophthalmic.

•**cetamolol hydrochloride.** (SEET-AM-oh-lahl) USAN.
Use: Anti-adrenergic (β-receptor).

Cetaphil. (Galderma Laboratories, Inc.) **Cream, Lot.:** Cetyl alcohol, stearyl alcohol, propylene glycol (cream only), sodium lauryl sulfate, methylparaben, propylparaben, butylparaben. Bot. 480 g (cream), 120 ml, 240 ml, 480 ml (lotion). **Antibacterial Bar:** Triclosan, petrolatum. Soap-free. 127 g. **Bar:** Petrolatum. Soap-free. 127 g. **Cleanser:** Cetyl alcohol, stearyl alcohol, parabens. Bot. 236 ml. *otc.*
Use: Dermatologic cleanser.

Cetapred. (Alcon Laboratories, Inc.) Sulfacetamide sodium 10%, prednisolone acetate 0.25%. Ophth. Oint. Tube 3.5 g. *Rx.*
Use: Anti-infective, ophthalmic.

Cetazol. (Professional Pharmacal) Acetazolamide 250 mg/Tab. Bot. 100s. *Rx.*
Use: Anticonvulsant, diuretic.

•**cetiedil citrate.** (see-TIE-eh-DILL SIH-trate) USAN.
Use: Vasodilator (peripheral).

•**cetirizine hydrochloride.** (seh-TIH-rih-zeen) USAN.
Use: Antihistamine.
See: Zyrtec, Syr., Tab. (Pfizer US Pharmaceutical Group).

•**cetocycline hydrochloride.** (SEE-toe-SIGH-kleen) USAN. *Formerly cetotetrine HCl.*
Use: Anti-infective.

•**cetophenicol.** (see-toe-FEN-ih-kole) USAN.
Use: Antibacterial.

•**cetostearyl alcohol.** N.F. 18.
Use: Pharmaceutic aid (emulsifying agent).

•**cetraxate hydrochloride.** (seh-TRAX-ate) USAN.
Use: Antiulcerative (gastrointestinal).

•**cetyl alcohol.** (SEE-till) N.F. 18.
Use: Pharmaceutic aid (emulsifying and stiffening agent).

Cetylcide Solution. (Cetylite Industries, Inc.) Cetyldimethylethyl ammonium bromide 6.5%, benzalkonium Cl 6.5%, isopropyl alcohol 13%. Inert ingredients 74%, including sodium nitrite. Bot. 16 oz, 32 oz.
Use: Disinfectant.

cetyldimethyl benzyl ammonium chloride.
W/Benzocaine, ascorbic acid.
See: Locane, Troches (Solvay Pharmaceuticals).

•**cetyl esters wax.** N.F. 18. *Formerly synthetic spermacet.*
Use: Pharmaceutic aid (stiffening agent).

•**cetylpyridinium chloride.** (SEE-till-pihr-ih-DIH-nee-uhm) U.S.P. 23.
Use: Anti-infective (topical), pharmaceutic aid (preservative).
See: Bactalin (LaCrosse).
W/Benzocaine.
See: Axon Throat Loz. (McKesson Drug Co.).
Cepacol, Throat Loz. (J.B. Williams Co. Inc.).
Coirex, Preps. (Solvay Pharmaceuticals).
Semets, Troches (SmithKline Beecham Pharmaceuticals).
Spec-T Sore Throat Loz. (Bristol-Myers Squibb).
Vicks Medi-Trating Throat Loz. (Procter & Gamble Pharm.).
W/Benzocaine.
See: Cepacol Antiseptic, Loz. (J.B. Williams Co. Inc.).
W/Benzocaine, menthol, camphor, eucalyptus oil.

See: Vicks Medi-Trating Throat, Loz. (Procter & Gamble Pharm.).

W/d-Methorphan HBr, phenyltoloxamine dihydrogen citrate, sodium citrate.
See: Exo-Kol, Cough Syrup, Spray, Tab. (Inwood Laboratories, Inc.).

W/Phenylephrine HCl, methapyrilene HCl, menthol, eucalyptol, camphor, methyl salicylate.
See: Vicks Sinex Nasal Spray (Procter & Gamble Pharm.).

cetyltrimethyl ammonium bromide. (Bioline Labs, Inc.) Cetrimide B.P., Cetavlon, CTAB.
Use: Antiseptic.

Cevalin. (Eli Lilly and Co.) Ascorbic acid 100 mg, 500 mg/ml. Inj. Amp. 10 ml (100 mg), 1 ml (500 mg). *Rx.*
Use: Vitamin supplement.

Cevi-Bid. (Roberts Pharmaceuticals) Ascorbic acid 500 mg/TR Caps. Bot. 30s, 100s, 500s. *otc.*
Use: Vitamin supplement.

Cevi-Fer. (Roberts Pharmaceuticals) Ascorbic acid 300 mg, ferrous fumarate 20 mg, folic acid 1 mg/TR Cap. Bot. 30s, 100s. *Rx.*
Use: Mineral, vitamin supplement.

•**cevimeline hydrochloride.** (seh-vih-MEH-leen) USAN.
Use: Treatment of Alzheimer's disease, adjunct.

Ce-Vi-Sol. (Bristol-Myers Squibb) Ascorbic acid 35 mg/0.6 ml, alcohol 5%. Bot. w/dropper 50 ml. *otc.*
Use: Vitamin supplement.

cevitamic acid.
See: Ascorbic acid.

cevitan.
See: Ascorbic acid.

Cewin Tablets. (Sanofi Winthrop Pharmaceuticals) Ascorbic acid. *otc.*
Use: Vitamin supplement.

ceylon gelatin.
See: Agar.

Cezin. (Forest Pharmaceutical, Inc.) Vitamins B_1 20 mg, B_2 10 mg, B_3 100 mg, B_5 20 mg, B_6 5 mg, C 300 mg, magnesium sulfate 70 mg, zinc sulfate 80 mg. Cap. Bot. 100s. *otc.*
Use: Vitamin supplement.

Cezin-S. (Forest Pharmaceutical, Inc.) Vitamins A 10,000 IU, D 50 IU, E 50 IU, B_1 10 mg, B_2 5 mg, B_3 50 mg, B_5 10 mg, B_6 2 mg, C 200 mg, folic acid 0.5 mg, Zn 18 mg, Mg, Mn/Cap. Bot. 100s. *Rx.*
Use: Vitamin supplement.

C Factors "1000" Plus. (Solgar Co., Inc.) Vitamins C with rosehips 1000 mg, citrus bioflavonoids 250 mg, rutin 50 mg, hesperidin complex 25 mg. Tab. Bot. 50s, 100s, 250s. *otc.*
Use: Vitamin supplement.

C.G. (Sigma-Tau Pharmaceuticals, Inc.) Chorionic gonadotropin (lyophilized) 10,000 units, mannitol 100 mg, supplied with diluent. Univial 10 ml. *Rx.*
Use: Hormone, chorionic gonadotropin.

CG Disposable Unit.
See: Cardio Green, Vial (Becton Dickinson & Co.).

CG Ria. (Abbott Diagnostics) Radioimmunoassay for the quantitative measurement of total circulating serum cholylglycine.
Use: Diagnostic aid.

Chap Cream. (Ar-Ex) Carbonyl diamide. Tube 1.5 oz, 3.25 oz. Jar 4 oz, 9 oz, 18 oz. *otc.*
Use: Emollient.

Chapoline Cream Lotion. (Wade) Glycerin, boric acid, chlorobutanol 0.5%, alcohol 10%. Bot. 4 oz, pt, gal. *otc.*
Use: Emollient.

Chapstick Medicated Lip Balm. (Wyeth-Ayerst Laboratories) **Jar:** Petrolatum 60%, camphor 1%, menthol 0.6%, phenol 0.5%, microcrystalline wax, mineral oil, cocoa butter, lanolin, paraffin wax, parabens 7 g. **Squeezable tube:** Petrolatum 67%, camphor 1%, menthol 0.6%, phenol 0.5%, microcrystalline wax, mineral oil, cocoa butter, lanolin, parabens 10 g. **Stick:** Petrolatum 41%, camphor 1%, menthol 0.6%, phenol 0.5%, paraffin wax, mineral oil, cocoa butter, 2-octyl dodecanol, arachydil propionate, polyphenyl methylsiloxane 556, white wax, oleyl alcohol, isopropyl lanolate, carnuba wax, isopropyl myristate, lanolin, cetyl alcohol, parabens. 4.2 g. *otc.*
Use: Mouth and throat preparation.

Chapstick Sunblock 15. (Wyeth-Ayerst Laboratories) Padimate O 0.7%, oxybenzone 3%. Stick 4.25 g. *otc.*
Use: Lip protectant.

Chapstick Sunblock 15 Petroleum Jelly Plus. (Wyeth-Ayerst Laboratories) White petrolatum 89%, padimate O 7%, oxybenzone 3%, aloe, lanolin. Stick 10 g. *otc.*
Use: Lip protectant.

CharcoAid. (Requa, Inc.) Activated charcoal 15 g/120 ml, 30 g/150 ml, sorbitol/Susp. Bot. *otc.*
Use: Antidote.

CharcoAid 2000. (Requa, Inc.) Activated charcoal 15 g/120 ml, 50 g/240 ml with and without sorbitol/Liq. 15 g/240 ml. Granules. Bot. *otc.*
Use: Antidote.

charcoal. (CHAR-kole) (Various Mfr.) Cap., Tab. *otc.*
Use: Antiflatulent.
See: Charcoal (Paddock Laboratories).
Charcoal (Rugby Labs, Inc.).

•**charcoal, activated.** (CHAR-kole) U.S.P. 23.
Use: Antidote (general purpose), pharmaceutic aid (adsorbent).
See: Actidose-Aqua, Liq. (Paddock Laboratories).
CharcoAid, Susp. (Requa, Inc.).
Charcoal Plus, EC Tab. (Kramer Laboratories, Inc.).
Liqui-Char, Liq. (Jones Medical Industries, Inc.).
W/Nux vomica, bismuth subgallate, pepsin, berberis, diastase, pancreatin, hydrastis, papain.
See: Charcocaps, Cap. (Requa, Inc.).

Charcoal Plus. (Kramer Laboratories, Inc.) Activated charcoal 250 mg, sugar. EC Tab. Bot. 120s. *otc.*
Use: Antiflatulent.

charcoal and simethicone. Antiflatulent.
See: Charcoal Plus, EC Tab. (Kramer Laboratories, Inc.).
Flatulex (Dayton Laboratories, Inc.).

CharcoCaps. (Requa, Inc.) Activated charcoal 260 mg/Cap. Bot. 36s. *otc.*
Use: Antiflatulent.

Chardonna-2. (Kremers Urban) Belladonna extract 15 mg, phenobarbital 15 mg/Tab. Bot. 100s. *Rx.*
Use: Anticholinergic, antispasmodic, hypnotic, sedative.

Charo Scatter-Paks. (Requa, Inc.) Activated charcoal 5 g/Packet.
Use: Odor absorbent.

Chaz Scalp Treatment Dandruff Shampoo. (Revlon) Zinc pyrithione 1% in liquid shampoo. *otc.*
Use: Antiseborrheic.

Chealamide Injection. (Vortech Pharmaceuticals) Disodium edetate 150 mg/ml. Vial 20 ml. *Rx.*
Use: Chelating agent.

Checkmate. (Oral-B Laboratories, Inc.) Acidulated phosphate fluoride 1.23%. Bot. 2 oz, 16 oz. *Rx.*
Use: Dental caries agent.

Chek-Stix Urinalysis Control Strips. (Bayer Corp. (Consumer Div.)) Bot. 25s.
Use: Diagnostic aid.

chelafrin.
See: Epinephrine.

Chelated Calcium Magnesium. (NBTY, Inc.) Ca^{++} 500 mg, Mg 250 mg/Tab. Protein coated. Bot. 50s. *otc.*
Use: Mineral supplement.

Chelated Calcium Magnesium Zinc. (NBTY, Inc.) Ca^{++} 333 mg, Mg 133 mg, Zn 8.3 mg/Tab. Bot. 100s. *otc.*
Use: Mineral supplement.

Chelated Magnesium. (Freeda Vitamins, Inc.) Magnesium amino acids chelate 500 mg (magnesium 100 mg)/Tab. Bot. 100s, 250s, 500s. *otc.*
Use: Vitamin supplement.

Chelated Manganese. (Freeda Vitamins, Inc.) Manganese 20 mg or 50 mg/Tab. Bot. 100s, 250s, 500s. *otc.*
Use: Mineral supplement.

chelating agent.
See: BAL, Amp. (Becton Dickinson & Co.).
Calcium Disodium Versenate, Amp., Tab. (3M Pharmaceuticals).
Desferal, Amp. (Novartis Pharmaceutical Corp.).
Endrate Disodium, Amp. (Abbott Laboratories).

chelen.
See: Ethyl Chloride.

Chemet. (Sanofi Winthrop Pharmaceuticals) Succimer 100 mg. Cap. Bot. 100s. *Rx.*
Use: Chelating agent.

Chemipen. Potassium phenethicillin.
Use: Anti-infective, penicillin.

Chemovag Suppositories. (Forest Pharmaceutical, Inc.) Sulfisoxazole 0.5 g/Supp. Bot. 12s w/applicators. *Rx.*
Use: Anti-infective, sulfonamide.

Chemozine. (Tennessee Pharmaceutic) Sulfadiazine, 0.167 g, sulfamerazine 0.167 g, sulfamethazine 0.167 g/Tab. Bot. 100s, 1000s. Susp. Bot. Pt, gal. *Rx.*
Use: Anti-infective, sulfonamide.

Chemstrip 6. (Boehringer Mannheim Pharmaceuticals) Broad range test for glucose, protein, pH, blood, ketones, leukocytes. Strip Bot. 100s.
Use: Diagnostic aid.

Chemstrip 7. (Boehringer Mannheim Pharmaceuticals) Broad range test for glucose, protein, pH, blood, ketones, bilirubin, leukocytes. Strip Bot. 100s.
Use: Diagnostic aid.

Chemstrip 8. (Boehringer Mannheim Pharmaceuticals) Broad range urine test for glucose, protein, pH, blood, ketones, bilirubin, urobilinogen, leukocytes. Strip Bot. 100s.
Use: Diagnostic aid.

Chemstrip 9. (Boehringer Mannheim Pharmaceuticals) Broad range test for glucose, protein, pH, blood, ketones, bilirubin, urobilinogen, nitrite, leukocytes in urine. Strip Bot. 100s.
Use: Diagnostic aid.

Chemstrip 10 SG. (Boehringer Mannheim Pharmaceuticals) Broad range test for glucose, protein, pH, blood, ketones, bilirubin, urobilinogen, nitrite, leukocytes in urine. Strip Bot. 100s.
Use: Diagnostic aid.

Chemstrip 4 the OB. (Boehringer Mannheim Pharmaceuticals) Broad range test for glucose, protein, blood, leukocytes in urine. Strip Bot. 100s.
Use: Diagnostic aid.

Chemstrip bG. (Boehringer Mannheim Pharmaceuticals) Reagent strips for testing blood sugar. Strip Bot. 50s.
Use: Diagnostic aid.

Chemstrip 2 GP. (Boehringer Mannheim Pharmaceuticals) Broad range test for glucose and protein. Strip Bot. 100s.
Use: Diagnostic aid.

Chemstrip-K. (Boehringer Mannheim Pharmaceuticals) Reagent papers for ketones in urine. Paper Bot. 25s, 100s.
Use: Diagnostic aid.

Chemstrip 2 LN. (Boehringer Mannheim Pharmaceuticals) Broad range test for nitrite and leukocytes. Strip Bot. 100s.
Use: Diagnostic aid.

Chemstrip Micral. (Boehringer Mannheim Pharmaceuticals) In vitro reagent strips to detect albumin in urine. Strip Pkg. 5s, 30s.
Use: Diagnostic aid.

Chemstrip Mineral. (Boehringer Mannheim Pharmaceuticals) In vitro reagent strips used to detect albumin in urine. Strip Pkg. 5s, 30s.
Use: In vitro diagnostic aid.

Chemstrip uG. (Boehringer Mannheim Pharmaceuticals) Reagent strips for glucose in urine. Strip Bot. 100s.
Use: Diagnostic aid.

Chemstrip uGK. (Boehringer Mannheim Pharmaceuticals) Broad range test for glucose and ketones. Strip Bot. 50s, 100s.
Use: Diagnostic aid.

Chenatal. (Miller Pharmacal Group, Inc.) Calcium 580 mg, Mg 200 mg, vitamins C 100 mg, folic acid 0.4 mg, A 5000 IU, D 400 IU, B_1 3 mg, B_2 3 mg, B_6 5 mg, B_{12} 9 mcg, niacinamide 30 mg, pantothenic acid 5 mg, tocopherols (mixed) 10 mg, Fe 20 mg, Cu 1 mg, Mn 2 mg, K 10 mg, Zn 25 mg, I 0.1 mg/2 Tabs. Bot. 100s. *otc.*
Use: Mineral, vitamin supplement.

Chenix. (Solvay Pharmaceuticals) Chenodil.
Use: Anticholelithogenic. [Orphan Drug]

chenodeoxycholic acid.
Use: Urolithic.
See: Chenodiol.

•**chenodiol.** (KEEN-oh-DIE-ahl) USAN.
Formerly chenic acid.
Use: Anticholelithogenic. [Orphan Drug]

Cheracol. (Roberts Pharmaceuticals) Codeine phosphate 10 mg, guaifenesin 100 mg/5 ml, alcohol 4.75%. Bot. 2 oz, 4 oz, pt. *c-v.*
Use: Antitussive, expectorant.

Cheracol D. (Roberts Pharmaceuticals) Dextromethorphan HBr 10 mg, guaifenesin 100 mg/5 ml, alcohol 4.75%. Bot. 2 oz, 4 oz, 6 oz. *otc.*
Use: Antitussive, expectorant.

Cheracol Nasal. (Roberts Pharmaceuticals) Oxymetazoline HCl 0.05%, phenylmercuric acetate 0.02 mg/ml, benzalkonium chloride, glycine, sorbitol. Spray Bot. 30 ml. *otc.*
Use: Decongestant.

Cheracol Plus. (Roberts Pharmaceuticals) Phenylpropanolamine HCl 8.3 mg, dextromethorphan HBr 6.7 mg, chlorpheniramine maleate 1.3 mg/5 ml. Bot. 4 oz. *otc.*
Use: Antihistamine, antitussive, decongestant.

Cheracol Sore Throat. (Roberts Pharmaceuticals) Phenol 1.4%, saccharin, sorbitol, alcohol 12.5%. Spray Bot. 180 ml. *otc.*
Use: Mouth and throat product.

Cheratussin Cough Syrup. (Towne) Dextromethorphan HBr 45 mg, ammonium Cl 575 mg, citrate sodium 280 mg/fl oz. Bot. 4 oz. *otc.*
Use: Antitussive, expectorant.

Chero-Trisulfa-V. (Vita Elixir) Sulfadiazine 0.166 g, sulfacetamide 0.166 g, sulfamerazine 0.166 g, sodium citrate 0.5 g/5 ml. Susp. Bot. Pt.
Use: Anti-infective, sulfonamide.

cherry juice. N.F. 18.
Use: Flavoring.

cherry syrup.
Use: Pharmaceutic aid (vehicle).

Chestamine. (Leeds) Chlorpheniramine maleate 8 mg, 12 mg/Cap. Bot. 50s. *Rx.*
Use: Antihistamine.

Chest Throat Lozenges. (Lane) Eucalyptol, anise, horehound, tolu balsam, benzoin tincture, sugar, corn syrup. Pkg. 30s. *otc.*
Use: Antiseptic.

Chewable C. (Health for Life Brands, Inc.) Vitamin C 100 mg, 250 mg, 300 mg, 500 mg/Tab. Bot. 100s. *otc.*
Use: Vitamin supplement.

Chewable Multivitamins w/Fluoride. (H.L. Moore Drug Exchange Inc.) Fluo-

ride 1 mg, vitamins A 2500 IU, D 400 IU, E 15 IU, B_1 1.05 mg, B_2 1.2 mg, B_3 13.5 mg, B_6 1.05 mg, B_{12} 4.5 mcg, C 60 mg, folic acid 0.3 mg, sucrose/Tab. Bot. 100s. *Rx.*
Use: Mineral, vitamin supplement; dental caries agent.

Chew-Vims. (Barth's) Vitamins A 5000 IU, D 400 IU, B_1 3 mg, B_2 6 mg, niacin 1.71 mg, C 100 mg, B_{12} 5 mcg, E 5 IU/Tab. Bot. 30s, 90s, 180s, 360s. *otc.*
Use: Vitamin supplement.

Chew-Vi-Tab. (Halsey Drug Co.) Vitamins A 2500 IU, D 400 IU, E 15 IU, C 60 mg, folic acid 0.3 mg, B_1 1.05 mg, B_2 1.2 mg, niacin 13.5 mg, B_6 1.05 mg, B_{12} 4.5 mcg/Tab. Bot. 100s. *otc.*
Use: Vitamin supplement.

Chew-Vi-Tab with Iron. (Halsey Drug Co.) Vitamins A 5000 IU, C 60 mg, E 15 IU, folic acid 0.4 mg, B_1 1.5 mg, B_2 1.7 mg, niacin 20 mg, B_6 2 mg, B_{12} 6 mcg, D 400 IU, iron 18 mg/Tab. Bot. 100s. *otc.*
Use: Mineral, vitamin supplement.

Chibroxin. (Merck & Co.) Norfloxacin 3 mg/ml. Soln. Drop. Bot. 5 ml Ocumeters. *Rx.*
Use: Anti-infective, ophthalmic.

chicken pox vaccine.
See: Varivax (Merck & Co.).

Chiggerex. (Scherer Laboratories, Inc.) Benzocaine 0.02%, camphor, menthol, peppermint oil, olive oil, clove oil, pegosperse, methylparaben. Oint. Jar 50 g. *otc.*
Use: Anesthetic, counterirritant.

Chigger-Tox. (Scherer Laboratories, Inc.) Benzocaine 2.1%, benzyl benzoate 21.4%, soft soap, isopropyl alcohol. Liq. Bot. 30 ml. *otc.*
Use: Anesthetic, topical.

Children's Advil. (Wyeth-Ayerst Laboratories) Ibuprofen 100 mg/5 ml. Susp. Bot. 119 ml, 473 ml. *Rx.*
Use: Analgesic, NSAID.

Children's Allerest. (Novartis Pharmaceutical Corp.) Phenylpropanolamine HCl 9.4 mg, chlorpheniramine maleate 1 mg. Chew. Tab. Bot. 24s. *otc.*
Use: Antihistamine, decongestant.

Children's Cepacol. (J.B. Williams Co. Inc.) Acetaminophen 160 mg/5 ml, pseudophedrine HCl 15 mg/5 ml, benzoic acid, sorbitol, glycerin, grape, cherry flavors. Liq. Bot. 118 ml. *otc.*
Use: Decongestant.

Children's Dramamine. (Pharmacia & Upjohn) Dimenhydrinate 12.5 mg/5 ml, alcohol 5%, sucrose. Liq. Bot. 120 ml. *otc.*
Use: Antiemetic, antivertigo.

Children's Dynafed Jr. (BDI Pharmaceuticals, Inc.) Acetaminophen 80 mg, fruit flavor. Chew. Tab. Bot. 36s. *otc.*
Use: Analgesic.

Children's Feverall. (Upsher-Smith Labs, Inc.) Acetaminophen 120 mg or 325 mg/Supp. Pkg. 6s. *otc.*
Use: Analgesic.

Children's Formula Cough Syrup. (Pharmakon Laboratories, Inc.) Guaifenesin 50 mg, dextromethorphan HBr 5 mg/5 ml, sucrose, corn syrup. Alcohol free. Grape flavor. Syr. Bot. 118 ml, 236 ml. *otc.*
Use: Antitussive, expectorant.

Children's Hold 4-Hour Cough Suppressant & Decongestant. (Beecham Products) Dextromethorphan HBr 3.75 mg, phenylpropanolamine HCl 6.25 mg/Loz. Pkg. 10s. *otc.*
Use: Antitussive, decongestant.

Children's Kaopectate. (Pharmacia & Upjohn) Attapulgite 600 mg/5 ml. Liq. Bot. 180 ml. *otc.*
Use: Antidiarrheal.

Children's Mapap. (Major Pharmaceuticals) Acetaminophen 160 mg/5 ml, alcohol free. Elix. Bot. 120 ml. *otc.*
Use: Analgesic.

Children's Motrin. (Ortho McNeil Pharmaceutical) Ibuprofen 100 mg/5 ml, alcohol free. Susp. Bot. 120 ml, 480 ml. *Rx-otc.*
Use: Analgesic, NSAID.

Children's No Aspirin Elixir. (Walgreen Co.) Acetaminophen 80 mg/2.5 ml. Non-alcoholic. Bot. 4 oz. *otc.*
Use: Analgesic.

Children's No-Aspirin Tablets. (Walgreen Co.) Acetaminophen 80 mg/Tab. Bot. 30s. *otc.*
Use: Analgesic.

Children's Nyquil. (Procter & Gamble Pharm.) Pseudoephedrine HCl 10 mg, chlorpheniramine maleate 0.6 mg, dextromethorphan HBr 5 mg/5 ml. Bot. 120 ml, 240 ml. *otc.*
Use: Antihistamine, antitussive, decongestant.

Children's Nyquil Nighttime Head Cold, Allergy Formula. (Procter & Gamble Pharm.) Pseudoephedrine HCl 10 mg, chlorpheniramine maleate 0.67 mg/5 ml. Alcohol free. Sorbitol, sucrose. Grape flavor. Liq. Bot. 120 ml. *otc.*
Use: Antihistamine, decongestant.

Children's Silapap. (Silarx Pharmaceuticals, Inc.) Acetaminophen 80 mg/2.5 ml, sugar free, alcohol free. Liq. Bot.

237 ml. *otc.*
Use: Analgesic.

Children's Silfedrine. (Silarx Pharmaceuticals, Inc.) Pseudoephedrine HCl 30 mg/5 ml. Liq. Bot. 118 ml. *otc.*
Use: Decongestant, nasal.

Children's Sunkist Multivitamins Complete. (Novartis Pharmaceutical Corp.) Iron 18 mg, vitamin A 5000 IU, D_3 400 IU, E 30 IU, B_1 1.5 mg, B_2 1.7 mg, B_3 20 mg, B_5 10 mg, B_6 2 mg, B_{12} 6 mcg, C 60 mg, folic acid 0.4 mg, Ca, Cu, I, K, Mg, Mn, P, Zn 10 mg, biotin 40 mcg, vitamin K, sorbitol, aspartame, phenylalanine, tartrazine/Chew. Tab. Bot. 60s. *otc.*
Use: Mineral, vitamin supplement.

Children's Sunkist Multivitamins + Extra C. (Novartis Pharmaceutical Corp.) Vitamin A 2500 IU, E 15 IU, D_3 400 IU, B_1 1.05 mg, B_2 1.2 mg, B_3 13.5 mg, B_6 1.05 mg, B_{12} 4.5 mcg, C 250 mg, folic acid 0.3 mg, vitamin K_1 5 mcg, sorbitol, aspartame, phenylalanine, tartrazine. Chew. Tab. Bot. 60s. *otc.*
Use: Mineral, vitamin supplement.

Children's Sunkist Multivitamins + Iron. (Novartis Pharmaceutical Corp.) Iron 15 mg, vitamin A 2500 IU, E 15 IU, D_3 400 IU, B_1 1.05 mg, B_2 1.2 mg, B_3 13.5 mg, B_6 1.05 mg, B_{12} 4.5 mcg, C 60 mg, folic acid 0.3 mg, vitamin K_1 5 mcg, sorbitol, aspartame, phenylalanine, tartrazine. Chew. Tab. Bot. 60s. *otc.*
Use: Mineral, vitamin supplement.

Children's Tylenol Cold Liquid. (McNeil Consumer Products Co.) Pseudoephedrine HCl 15 mg, chlorpheniramine maleate 1 mg, acetaminophen 160 mg/5 ml, sorbitol, sucrose. Alcohol free. Grape flavor. Liq. Bot. 120 ml. *otc.*
Use: Analgesic, antihistamine, decongestant.

Children's Tylenol Cold Multi Symptom Plus Cough. (McNeil Consumer Products Co.) Acetaminophen 160 mg, dextromethorphan HBr 5 mg, chlorpheniramine maleate 1 mg, pseudoephedrine HCl 15 mg/5 ml. Liq. Bot. 120 ml. *otc.*
Use: Antihistamine, antitussive, decongestant.

Children's Tylenol Cold Plus Cough. (Ortho McNeil Pharmaceutical) Acetaminophen 80 mg, pseudoephedrine HCl 7.5 mg, dextromethorphan HBr 2.5 mg, chlorpheniramine maleate 0.5 mg/ Chew. Tab. Pkg. 24s. *otc.*
Use: Analgesic, antihistamine, antitussive, decongestant.

Children's Tylenol Cold Tablets. (McNeil Consumer Products Co.) Pseudoephedrine HCl 7.5 mg, chlorpheniramine maleate 0.5 mg, acetaminophen 80 mg, aspartame, sucrose, phenylalanine 4 mg. Grape flavor. Chew. Tab. Bot. 24s. *otc.*
Use: Analgesic, antihistamine, decongestant.

Children's Tylenol Elixir. (McNeil Consumer Products Co.) Acetaminophen 160 mg/5 ml. Elix. Bot. 60 ml, 120 ml. *otc.*
Use: Analgesic.

Children's Ty-Tabs. (Major Pharmaceuticals) Acetaminophen 80 mg. Tab. Bot. 100s, 1000s. *otc.*
Use: Analgesic.

chimeric A2 (human-murine) IgG monoclonal anti-TNF antibody (CA2). (Centocor, Inc.)
Use: Crohn's disease. [Orphan Drug]

chimeric M-t412 (human-murine) igg monoclonal anti-CD4.
Use: Multiple sclerosis. [Orphan Drug]

chimeric (murine variable, human constant) Mab (C2B8) to CD20. (IDEC Pharmaceuticals)
Use: Treatment of non-Hodgkin's B-cell lymphoma. [Orphan Drug]

chinese gelatin.
See: Agar.

chinese isinglass.
Use: Amebicide.

chiniofon.
Use: Amebicide.

Chinositol. (Vernon) 8-Hydroxyquinoline sulfate 7.5 gr/Tab. Vial 6s. Trit. Tab. (3/5 gr) Bot. 50s. Vial 110s. Pow. 1 oz.
Use: Antiseptic.

chlamydia trachomatis test.
Use: Diagnostic aid.
See: MicroTrak (Syva Co.).

Chlamydiazyme. (Abbott Diagnostics) Enzyme immunoassay for detection of *Chlamydia trachomatis* from urethral or urogenital swabs. Test Kit 100s.
Use: Diagnostic aid.

Chlo-Amine. (Bayer Corp. (Consumer Div.)) Chlorpheniramine maleate 2 mg/ Chew. Tab. Box 24 × 4 mg Tab. Pkg. *otc.*
Use: Antihistamine.

chlophedianol. (KLOE-fee-DIE-ah-nole) F.D.A.

•**chlophedianol hydrochloride.** (KLOE-fee-DIE-ah-nole) USAN.
Use: Antitussive.

Chloracol 0.5%. (Horizon Pharmaceutical Corp.) Chloramphenicol 5 mg/

ml with chlorobutanol, hydroxypropyl methylcellulose. Dropper bot. 7.5 ml. *Rx.*
Use: Anti-infective, ophthalmic.

Chlorafed. (Roberts Pharmaceuticals) Chlorpheniramine maleate 2 mg, pseudoephedrine HCl 30 mg/5 ml, alcohol, dye, sugar, and corn free. Liq. Bot. 120 ml, 480 ml. *otc.*
Use: Antihistamine, decongestant.

Chlorafed H.S. Timecelles. (Roberts Pharmaceuticals) Chlorpheniramine maleate 4 mg, pseudoephedrine HCl 60 mg/SR Cap. Bot. 100s. *Rx.*
Use: Antihistamine, decongestant.

Chlorafed Timecelles. (Roberts Pharmaceuticals) Chlorpheniramine maleate 8 mg, pseudoephedrine HCl 120 mg/SA Timecelles. Bot. 100s. *Rx.*
Use: Antihistamine, decongestant.

Chlorahist. (Evron) Chlorpheniramine maleate. **4 mg/Tab.:** Bot. 100s, 1000s. **8 mg, 12 mg/Cap.:** Bot. 250s, 1000s. **Syr. 2 mg/4 ml.:** Bot. qt. *Rx-otc.*
Use: Antihistamine.

•**chloral betaine.** (KLOR-uhl BEE-tah-een) USAN. N.F. XIV.
Use: Hypnotic, sedative.

•**chloral hydrate.** (KLOR-uhl HIGH-drate) U.S.P. 23.
Use: Sedative, hypnotic.
See: Aquachloral Supprettes, Supp. (PolyMedica Pharmaceuticals).
Generic Products:
Quality Generics (7.5 gr) Bot. 100s.
Parke, Davis-Cap (500 mg) Bot 100s, UD 100s.

chloral hydrate betaine (1:1) compound. Chloral Betaine.

chloralpyrine dichloralpyrine.
See: Dichloralantipyrine.

chloralurethane. Name used for Carbochloral.

Chloraman. (Rasman) Chlorpheniramine maleate 12 mg/Tab. Bot. 100s, 500s, 1000s. *Rx.*
Use: Antihistamine.

•**chlorambucil.** (klor-AM-byoo-sill) U.S.P. 23.
Use: Antineoplastic.
See: Leukeran, Tab. (GlaxoWellcome).

Chloramine-T. Sodium paratoluenesulfan chloramide, chloramine, chlorozone. **Lilly-Tab.:** (0.3 g), Bot. 100s, 1000s. **Robinson:** Pow., 1 oz.
Use: Antiseptic, deodorant.
See: Chlorazene (Badger).

chloramphenicol. (KLOR-am-FEN-ih-kahl) (Various Mfr.) **Soln.:** 5 mg/ml Bot. 7.5 ml, 15 ml; **Oint.:** 10 mg/g Tube 3.5 g; **Cap.:** 250 mg Bot. 100s.
Use: Anti-infective, antirickettsial.

•**chloramphenicol.** (KLOR-am-FEN-ih-kole) U.S.P. 23.
Use: Anti-infective, antirickettsial.
See: AK-Chlor, Preps. (Akorn, Inc.).
Chloromycetin, Preps. (Parke-Davis).
Chloroptic, Ophth. Oint. (Allergan, Inc.).
Chloroptic S.O.P., Ophth. Oint. (Allergan, Inc.).
Econochlor, Soln., Oint. (Alcon Laboratories, Inc.).
Mychel, Cap. (Houba).
Ophthochlor, Soln. (Parke-Davis).

•**chloramphenicol.** (KLOR-am-FEN-ih-kole) U.S.P. 23.
Use: Treatment of superficial ocular infections involving the conjunctiva and/or cornea caused by susceptible organisms.
See: Chloromyxin, Ophthalmic Oint. (Parke-Davis).

chloramphenicol and hydrocortisone acetate for ophthalmic suspension.
Use: Anti-infective, anti-inflammatory.
See: Chloromycetin, Prods. (Parke-Davis)

chloramphenicol and polymyxin b sulfate ophthalmic ointment.
Use: Anti-infective.

chloramphenicol, hydrocortisone acetate, and polymyxin b sulfate ophthalmic ointment.
Use: Anti-infective, anti-inflammatory.
See: Chloromycetin, Prods. (Parke-Davis).

•**chloramphenicol palmitate.** U.S.P. 23.
Use: Anti-infective, antirickettsial.
See: Chloromycetin Palmitate, Oral Susp. (Parke-Davis).

•**chloramphenicol pantothenate complex.** (KLOR-am-FEN-ih-kahl PAN-toe-THEH-nate) USAN.
Use: Anti-infective, antirickettsial.

chloramphenicol and prednisolone ophthalmic ointment.
Use: Anti-infective, steroid combination.
See: Chloromycetin, Prods. (Parke-Davis).

•**chloramphenicol sodium succinate.** U.S.P. 23.
Use: Anti-infective, antirickettsial.
See: Chloromycetin Succinate, Inj. (Parke-Davis).
Mychel-S, IV (Houba).

chloramphenicol sodium succinate. (Various Mfr.) 100 mg/ml. Inj. Vial. 1 g in 15 ml.
Use: Anti-infective, antirickettsial.

Chloraseptic Children's Lozenges.

(Procter & Gamble Pharm.) Benzocaine 5 mg/Loz. Pkg. 18s. *otc.*
Use: Anesthetic, local.

Chloraseptic Liquid. (Procter & Gamble Pharm.) Total phenol 1.4% as phenol and sodium phenolate, saccharin. Menthol and cherry flavors. Bot. 180 ml, 360 ml (mouthwash/gargle); 45 ml, 240 ml, 360 ml (throat spray). *otc.*
Use: Anesthetic, antiseptic, local.

Chloraseptic Lozenge. (Procter & Gamble Pharm.) Total phenol 32.5 mg/lozenge as phenol and sodium phenolate. Menthol and cherry flavors. Pkg. 18s, 36s. *otc.*
Use: Anesthetic, antiseptic.

Chlorazene. (Badger) Chloramine-T, sodium p-toluene-sulfonchloramide.
Pow.: UD Pkg. 20 g, 38 g, 50 g, 88 g, 200 g, 240 g, 320 g, Bot. 1 lb, 5 lb.
Aromatic Pow. (5%): Bot. 1 lb, 5 lb.
Tab. (0.3 g): Bot. 20s, 100s, 1000s, 5000s. *otc.*
Use: Antiseptic, deodorant.

chlorazepate dipotassium.
Use: Anxiolytic anticonvulsant.
See: Clorazepate dipotassium.

chlorazepate monopotassium.
See: Clorazepate monopotassium.

Chlorazine. (Major Pharmaceuticals) Prochlorperazine 5 mg, 10 mg/Tab. Bot. 100s.
Use: Antiemetic, antipsychotic, antivertigo.

chlorozone.
See: Chloramine-T.

Chlor Benzo Mor, A and D Ointment. (Wade) Vitamins A and D fortified, chlorobutanol 3%, benzocaine 2%, benzyl alcohol 3%, actamer 1%, in lanolin and petrolatum base. Tube 1 oz, Jar 1 oz, lb. *otc.*
Use: Anesthetic, antiseptic, local.

Chlor Benzo Mor Spray. (Wade) Vitamin A and D fortified, chlorobutanol 3%, benzocaine 2%, benzyl alcohol 3%, actamer 1%, in lanolin and mineral oil base. Bot. 2 oz, 11 oz. *otc.*
Use: Antiseptic, anesthetic, local.

chlorbutanol.
See: Chlorobutanol, N.F. 18.

chlorbutol.
See: Chlorobutanol, N.F. 18.

•**chlorcyclizine hydrochloride.** N.F. 18.
Use: Antihistamine.

•**chlordantoin.** (CLOR-dan-toe-in) USAN.
Use: Antifungal.

•**chlordiazepoxide.** (klor-DIE-aze-ee-POX-side) U.S.P. 23.
Use: Anxiolytic.
See: Brigen-G, Tab. (Grafton).
Libritabs, Tab. (Roche Laboratories).
W/Amitriptyline.
See: Limbitrol, Tab. (Roche Laboratories).

chlordiazepoxide and amitriptyline HCl tablets. (klor-DIE-aze-ee-POX-ide and am-ee-TRIP-tih-leen)
Use: Anxiolytic.
See: Limbitrol, Tab. (Roche Laboratories).

•**chlordiazepoxide hydrochloride.** (klor-DIE-aze-ee-POX-ide) U.S.P. 23.
Use: Hypnotic, sedative.
See: Chlordiazachel, Cap. (Houba).
Librium, Cap., Inj. (Roche Laboratories).
Screen, Cap. (Foy Laboratories).
Zetran, Cap. (Roberts Pharmaceuticals).
W/Clidinium bromide.
See: Librax, Cap. (Roche Laboratories).

chlordiazepoxide w/clindinium bromide. (Various Mfr.) Clindinium 2.5 mg, chlordiazepoxide HCl 5 mg/Cap. Bot. 30s, 100s, 500s, 1000s, UD 100s. *c-IV.*
Use: Gastrointestinal, anticholinergic.

chlordiazepoxide and clindinium bromide. (Chelsea Laboratories, Inc.) Clindinium bromide 2.5 mg, chlordiazepoxide HCl 5 mg/Cap. Bot. 100s, 500s, 1000s. *Formerly Clindex* (Rugby Labs, Inc.). *Rx.*
Use: Anticholinergic, antispasmodic.

Chlordrine S.R. (Rugby Labs, Inc.) Pseudoephedrine HCl 120 mg, chlorpheniramine maleate 8 mg/SR Cap. Bot. 100s. *Rx.*
Use: Antihistamine, decongestant.

Chloren 4. (Wren) Chlorpheniramine maleate 4 mg/Tab. Bot. 100s, 1000s. *otc.*
Use: Antihistamine.

Chloren 8 T.D. (Wren) Chlorpheniramine maleate 8 mg/Tab. Bot. 100s, 1000s. *otc.*
Use: Antihistamine.

Chloren 12 T.D. (Wren) Chlorpheniramine maleate 12 mg/Tab. Bot. 100s, 1000s. *Rx-otc.*
Use: Antihistamine.

Chloresium. (Rystan, Inc.) **Oint.:** Chlorophyllin copper complex 0.5% in hydrophilic base. Tube 1 oz, 4 oz, Jar lb.
Soln.: Chlorophyllin copper complex 0.2% in isotonic saline soln. Bot. 60 ml, 240 ml, qt. *otc.*
Use: Deodorant, healing agent.

Chloresium Tablets. (Rystan, Inc.) Chlorophyllin copper complex 14 mg/Tab. Bot. 100s, 1000s. *otc.*

Use: Deodorant, oral.

Chloresium Tooth Paste. (Rystan, Inc.) Chlorophyllin copper complex. Tube 3.25 oz. *otc.*
Use: Deodorant, oral.

chlorethyl.
See: Ethyl Chloride.

chlorguanide hydrochloride.
See: Chloroguanide HCl (Various Mfr.).

chlorhexidine. (klor-HEX-ih-deen) F.D.A. *otc.*
Use: Antiseptic.
See: Bacto Shield, Foam, Soln. (Steris Laboratories, Inc.).
Bacto Shield 2, Soln. (Steris Laboratories, Inc.).
Hibiclens (Zeneca Pharmaceuticals).

•**chlorhexidine gluconate.** (klor-HEX-ih-deen GLUE-koe-nate) USAN.
Use: Antimicrobial.
See: Bacto Shield, Foam, Soln. (Steris Laboratories, Inc.).
Bacto Shield 2, Soln. (Steris Laboratories, Inc.).
Hibiclens, Liq. (Zeneca Pharmaceuticals).
Hibistat, Liq. (Zeneca Pharmaceuticals).
Peridex (Procter & Gamble Pharm.).
PerioChip (Astra USA).
PerioGard (Colgate).

chlorhexidine gluconate mouthrinse.
Use: Amelioration of oral mucositis associated with cytoreductive therapy for conditioning patients for bone marrow transplantation. [Orphan Drug]
See: Peridex (Procter & Gamble Pharm.).
PerioGard, Oral Rinse (Colgate Oral Pharmaceuticals).

•**chlorhexidine hydrochloride.** (klor-HEX-ih-deen) USAN.
Use: Anti-infective, topical.

•**chlorhexidine phosphanilate.** (klor-HEX-ih-deen FOSS-fah-nih-LATE) USAN.
Use: Anti-infective.

chlorinated and iodized peanut oil. Chloriodized Oil.

•**chlorindanol.** (klor-IN-dah-nahl) USAN.
Use: Antiseptic, spermaticide.

chlorine compound, antiseptic. Antiseptics, Chlorine.

chloriodized oil. Chlorinated and iodized peanut oil.

•**chlormadinone acetate.** (klor-MAD-ih-nohn) USAN. N.F. XIII.
Use: Hormone, progestin.

Chlor Mal w/Sal + APAP S.C. (Global Source) Chlorpheniramine maleate 2 mg, acetaminophen 150 mg, salicylamide 175 mg/Tab. Bot. 1000s. *otc.*
Use: Analgesic, antihistamine.

chlormerodrin. Mercloran. *Rx.*
Use: Diuretic.

•**chlormerodrin hg 197.** USAN. U.S.P. XX.
Use: Diagnostic aid (renal function determination), radiopharmaceutical.

•**chlormerodrin hg 203.** USAN. U.S.P. XX.
Use: Diagnostic aid (renal function determination), radiopharmaceutical.

chlormezanone. Chlormethazanone. *Rx.*
Use: Anxiolytic.
See: Trancopal, Cap. (Sanofi Winthrop Pharmaceuticals).

Chlor-Niramine Allergy Tabs. (Whiteworth Towne) Chlorpheniramine maleate 4 mg/Tab. Bot. 24s, 100s. *otc.*
Use: Antihistamine.

•**chlorobutanol.** (Klor-oh-BYOO-tah-nole) N.F. 18.
Use: Anesthetic, antiseptic, hypnotic; pharmaceutic aid (antimicrobial).
See: Cerumenex, Drops (Purdue Frederick Co.).
Pre-Sert (Allergan, Inc.).

W/Atropine sulfate, chlorpheniramine maleate, phenylpropanolamine HCl.
See: Decongestant, Inj. (Century Pharmaceuticals, Inc.).

W/Calcium glycerophosphate, calcium levulinate.
See: Cal San, Inj. (Burgin-Arden).

W/Cetyltrimethylammonium Br, methapyrilene HCl, phenylephrine HCl, hydrocortisone.
See: T-Spray, Liq. (Saron).

W/Diphenhydramine HCl.
See: Ardeben, Inj. (Burgin-Arden).

W/Ephedrine HCl, sodium Cl.
See: Efedron HCl, Nasal Jelly (Hart).

W/Estradiol cypionate, testosterone cypionate.
See: Depo-Testadiol, Vial (Pharmacia & Upjohn).
Depotestogen, Vial (Hyrex Pharmaceuticals).

W/Glycerin, anhydrous.
See: Ophthalgan, Liq. (Wyeth-Ayerst Laboratories).

W/Liquifilm.
See: Liquifilm Tears (Allergan, Inc.).

W/Methylcellulose.
See: Lacril (Allergan, Inc.).

W/Myristyl-gamma-picolinium Cl.
See: Wet Tone, Soln. (3M Pharmaceuticals).

W/Nonionic lanolin derivative.

See: Lacri-Lube, Ophthalmic Oint. (Allergan, Inc.).
W/Polyethylene glycol, polyoxyl 40 stearate.
See: Ocean, Liq. (Fleming & Co.).
•**chlorocresol.** (KLOR-oh-KREE-sole) N.F. 18.
Use: Antiseptic, disinfectant.
chloroethane.
See: Ethyl Chloride. Anticholinergic, antispasmodic.
Chlorofair. (Bausch & Lomb Pharmaceuticals) **Soln.:** Chloramphenicol 5 mg/ml. Bot. 7.5 ml. **Oint.:** Chloramphenicol 10 mg/g in white petrolatum base with mineral oil, polysorbate 60. Tube 3.5 g. *Rx.*
Use: Anti-infective, ophthalmic.
chloroguanide hydrochloride. (Various Mfr.) Proguanil HCl. *Rx.*
Use: Antimalarial.
Chlorohist-LA. (Roberts Pharmaceuticals) Xylometazoline HCl 0.1%. Soln. Spray 15 ml. *otc.*
Use: Decongestant.
chloro-iodohydroxyquinoline.
See: Clioquinol, U.S.P. 23.
chloromethapyrilene citrate.
See: Chlorothen Citrate.
Chloromycetin. (Monarch Pharmaceuticals) Chloramphenicol. **Ophth. Oint.:** (1%) in base of petrolatum, polyethylene. Tube 3.5 g. **Inj.:** 100 mg/ml (as sodium succinate) when reconstituted. 1 g Vial. 15 ml. **Ophth. Soln.:** (25 mg) Bot. w/dropper 15 ml (dry). Soln. Plastic dropper Bot. 15 ml. **Oral:** 150 mg/5 ml (palmitate), alcohol, sucrose, sodium benzoate 0.5%. Custard flavor. Bot. 60 ml. **Otic Drops:** (0.5%) 5 mg/ml w/propylene glycol. Bot. 15 ml. *Rx.*
Use: Anti-infective.
Chloromycetin/Hydrocortisone. (Parke-Davis) Hydrocortisone acetate 0.5% (2.5% as powder), chloramphenicol 0.25% (1.25% as powder). Pow. Bot. with dropper 5 ml. *Rx.*
Use: Anti-infective, ophthalmic.
Chloromycetin Sodium Succinate I.V. (Monarch Pharmaceuticals) Chloramphenicol sodium succinate dried powder which when reconstituted contains chloromycetin 100 mg/ml. Steri-vial 1 g, 10s. *Rx.*
Use: Anti-infective.
chlorophenothane.
Use: Pediculicide.
chlorophyll. (Freeda Vitamins, Inc.) Chlorophyll 20 mg, sugar free/Tab. Bot. 100s, 250s, 500s. *otc.*
Use: Deodorant, oral.
Chlorophyll "A" Ointment.
See: Chloresium Oint. (Rystan, Inc.).
Chlorophyll "A" Solution. (Chlorophyllin).
See: Chloresium Soln. (Rystan, Inc.).
chlorophyll derivatives, systemic.
See: Chlorophyll (Freeda Vitamins, Inc.).
Derifil (Rystan, Inc.).
Chloresium (Rystan, Inc).
chlorophyll derivatives, topical.
See: Chloresium (Rystan, Inc.).
chlorophyll tablets. *otc.*
See: Derifil, Tab. (Rystan, Inc.).
chlorophyll, water-soluble. (Various Mfr.) Chlorophyllin.
See: Chloresium Prep. (Rystan, Inc.).
Derifil, Pow. (Rystan, Inc.).
chlorophyllin. (KLOR-oh-FILL-in)
Use: Deodorant, healing agent.
•**chlorophyllin copper complex.** (KLOR-oh-FILL-in KAHP-uhr) USAN.
Use: Deodorant.
See: PALS, Tab. (Palisades Pharmaceuticals, Inc.).
•**chlorophyllin copper complex sodium.** U.S.P. 23.
Use: Deodorant.
•**chloroprocaine hydrochloride.** (Klor-oh-PRO-cane) U.S.P. 23.
Use: Anesthetic, local.
See: Nesacaine, Inj. (Astra Pharmaceuticals, L.P.).
Nesacaine-MPF, Inj. (Astra Pharmaceuticals, L.P.).
Chloroptic. (Allergan, Inc.) Chloramphenicol 0.5%. **Soln.:** Dropper bot. 2.5 ml, 7.5 ml. *Rx.*
Use: Anti-infective, ophthalmic.
Chloroptic S.O.P. (Allergan, Inc.) Chloramphenicol 10 mg/g. Oint. Tube 3.5 g. *Rx.*
Use: Anti-infective, ophthalmic.
•**chloroquine.** (KLOR-oh-kwin) U.S.P. 23.
Use: Antiamebic, antimalarial.
See: Aralen HCl Prods. (Sanofi Winthrop Pharmaceuticals).
•**chloroquine hydrochloride injection.** U.S.P. 23.
Use: Antiamebic, antimalarial.
See: Aralen HCl (Sanofi Winthrop Pharmaceuticals).
•**chloroquine phosphate.** U.S.P. 23.
Use: Antiamebic, antimalarial, lupus erythematosus agent.
See: Aralen Phosphate, Tab. (Sanofi Winthrop Pharmaceuticals).
chloroquine phosphate. (KLOR-oh-kwin) (Various Mfr.) Cloroquine phosphate 250 mg (equiv. to 150 mg base).

Tab. Bot. 20s, 22s, 30s, 100s, 1000s, UD 100s. *Rx.*
Use: Amebicide.

chlorothen.
Use: Antihistamine.

chlorothen citrate. (Whittier) Tab., Bot. 100s.
Use: Antihistamine.
W/Pyrilamine, thenylpyramine.
See: Derma-Pax, Liq. (Recsei Laboratories).

chlorothenylpyramine. Chlorothen, Prep.

Chlorotheophyllinate w/Benadryl.
See: Dramamine, Prep. (Searle).

•**chlorothiazide.** U.S.P. 23.
Use: Diuretic.
See: Diuril, Tab., Susp. (Merck & Co.).
W/Methyldopa.
See: Aldoclor, Tab. (Merck & Co.).

•**chlorothiazide sodium for injection.** U.S.P. 23.
Use: Antihypertensive, diuretic.
See: Sodium Diuril, Vial (Merck & Co.).

chlorothymol.
Use: Anti-infective.

•**chlorotrianisene.** (klor-oh-try-AN-ih-seen) U.S.P. 23.
Use: Estrogen.
See: Placidyl, Cap. (Abbott Laboratories).

•**chloroxine.** (KLOR-ox-een) USAN.
Use: Antiseborrheic.

•**chloroxylenol.** (KLOR-oh-ZIE-len-ole) U.S.P. 23.
Use: Antibacterial.
W/Benzocaine, menthol, lanolin.
See: Unburn, Spray, Cream, Lot. (Leeming-Pacquin).
W/Hexachlorophene.
See: Desitin, Preps. (Leeming-Pacquin).
W/Hydrocortisone, pramoxine.
See: Cortic (Everett Lab.).
Otomar-HC, Otic Soln. (Marnel Pharmaceuticals, Inc.).
W/Methyl salicylate, menthol, camphor, thymol, eucalyptus oil, isopropyl alcohol.
See: Gordobalm, Balm (Gordon Laboratories).
W/Pramoxine HCl, hydrocortisone.
See: Oti-Med, Drops (Hyrex Pharmaceuticals).
Tri-Otic, Drops (Pharmics, Inc.).
Zoto-HC, Otic Drops (Horizon Pharmaceutical Corp.).

Chlorpazine. (Major Pharmaceuticals) Prochlorperazine maleate 5 mg, 10 mg, 25 mg/Tab. Bot. 100s, UD 100s (5 mg, 10 mg only). *Rx.*
Use: Antipsychotic.

Chlorphed Injection. (Roberts Pharmaceuticals) Brompheniramine maleate 10 mg/ml. Vial 10 ml. *Rx.*
Use: Antihistamine.

Chlorphed-LA. (Roberts Pharmaceuticals) Oxymetazoline 0.05%. Soln. Spray 15 ml. *otc.*
Use: Decongestant.

Chlorphedrine SR. (Zenith Goldline Pharmaceuticals) Chlorpheniramine maleate 8 mg, pseudoephedrine HCl 120 mg/Cap. Bot. 100s. *Rx.*
Use: Antihistamine, decongestant.

•**chlorphenesin carbamate.** (KLOR-fen-ee-sin CAR-bah-mate) USAN.
Use: Muscle relaxant.
See: Maolate, Tab. (Pharmacia & Upjohn).

•**chlorpheniramine maleate.** (klor-fen-IHR-ah-meen) U.S.P. 23.
Use: Antihistamine.
See: Aller-Chlor, Syr., Tab. (Rugby Labs, Inc.).
Allergy, Tab. (Major Pharmaceuticals).
Chestamine, Cap. (Leeds).
Chlo-Amine, Tab. (Bayer Corp. (Consumer Div.)).
Chloraman, Tab. (Rasman).
Chloren, Preps. (Wren).
Chloren 4, Tab. (Mills).
Chlor-Niramine, Tab. (Whiteworth Towne).
Chlorophen, Vial (Medical Chem.).
Chlor-Span, Cap. (Burlington).
Chlor-Trimeton (Schering-Plough Corp.).
Efidac 24 Chlorpheniramine, ER Tab. (Novartis Pharmaceutical Corp.).
Histacon, Tab., Syr. (Marsh Labs).
Nasahist (Keene Pharmaceuticals, Inc.).
Polaramine, Tab., Syr. (Schering-Plough Corp.).
Pedia Care Allergy Formula, Liq. (Ortho McNeil Pharmaceutical).
Teldrin, Spansule (SmithKline Beecham Pharmaceuticals).

chlorpheniramine maleate. (Various Mfr.) **Tab.:** Chlorpheniramine maleate 4 mg. Bot. 100s, 1000s. *otc.*
Use: Antihistamine.

chlorpheniramine maleate. (Various Mfr.) **Inj.:** 10 mg/ml, benzyl alcohol 1.5%. Multidose vial. *Rx.*
Use: Antihistamine.

chlorpheniramine maleate w/combinations.
See: Al-Ay, Preps. (Jones Medical Industries, Inc.).

Alka-Seltzer Plus, Tab. (Bayer Corp. (Consumer Div.)).
Allerdec, Cap. (Towne).
Allerest, Prods. (Novartis Pharmaceutical Corp.).
Alumadrine, Tab. (Fleming & Co.).
A.R.M., Tab. (SmithKline Beecham Pharmaceuticals).
Atuss DM, Syr. (Atley Pharmaceuticals, Inc.).
B.M.E., Liq. (Brothers).
Bobid, Cap. (Boyd).
Breacol Cough Medication, Liq. (Bayer Corp. (Consumer Div.)).
Brolade, Cap. (Brothers).
Bur-Tuss Expectorant (Burlington).
Children's Tylenol Cold Plus Cough, Chew. Tab. (Ortho McNeil Pharmaceuticals).
Chlor-Trimeton, Preps. (Schering-Plough Corp.).
Codimal, Tab. (Schwarz Pharma, Inc.).
Comtrex, Tab., Cap., Liq. (Bristol-Myers Squibb).
Contac, Cap. (SmithKline Beecham Pharmaceuticals).
Cophene No. 2, Cap. (Dunhall Pharmaceuticals, Inc.).
Cophene-S, Syr. (Dunhall Pharmaceuticals, Inc.).
Coricidin, Preps. (Schering-Plough Corp.).
Corilin, Liq. (Schering-Plough Corp.).
Cotylenol, Preps. (Ortho McNeil Pharmaceutical).
D.A. II, Tab. (Dura).
Dallergy, Tab., Cap., Syr. (Laser, Inc.).
Deconamine, Tab., Cap., Syr. (Berlex Laboratories, Inc.).
Deconhist L.A., SR Tab. (Zenith Goldline).
Demazin, Tab., Syr. (Schering-Plough Corp.).
Derma-Pax, Lot. (Recsei Laboratories).
Dezest, Cap. (Geneva Pharmaceuticals).
Donatussin, Liq., Syr. (Laser, Inc.).
Dristan, Preps. (Whitehall Robins Laboratories).
Drucon, Elix. (Standard Drug Co.).
Ex-Histine, Syr. (WE Pharm.).
Extendryl, Tab., Cap., Syr. (Fleming & Co.).
F.C.A.H., Cap. (Scherer Laboratories, Inc.).
Fedahist, Prods. (Donner).
Fitacol (Standex).
Histacon, Tab., Syr. (Marsh Labs).
Histapco, Tab. (Apco).
Hista-Vadrin, Tab., Cap., Syr. (Scherer Laboratories, Inc.).
Histine Prods. (Freeport).
Histine PV, Syr. (Ethex Corp.).
Hycomine Compound, Tab. (Du Pont Merck Pharmaceutical Co.).
Hyphed, Syr. (Cypress).
Iodal HD, Liq. (Iomed).
Iotussin HC, Syr. (Iomed).
Kronofed-A, Cap. (Ferndale Laboratories, Inc.).
Mapap CF, Tab. (Major Pharmaceuticals).
Marhist (Marlop Pharmaceuticals, Inc.).
Mescolor, Tab. (Horizon).
Nolamine , Tab. (Carnrick Laboratories Inc.).
Novahistine, Preps. (Hoechst Marion Roussel).
Pancof-HC, Liq. (Pan Am Labs).
Pannaz, Tab. (Pan Am Labs).
Partuss, Liq. (Parmed Pharmaceuticals Inc.).
Partuss T.D., Tab. (Parmed Pharmaceuticals Inc.).
Phenahist, Preps. (T.E. Williams Pharmaceuticals).
Phenchlor, Prods. (Freeport)
Polytuss-DM, Liq. (Rhode).
Pyma, Cap., Vial (Forest Pharmaceutical Inc.).
Pyristan, Cap., Elix. (Arcum).
Quelidrine, Syr. (Abbott Laboratories).
Ryna, Liq. (Wallace Laboratories).
Scotcof, Liq. (Scott/Cord).
Scotnord (Scott/Cord).
Shertus, Liq. (Sheryl)
Sinarest, Tab. (Novartis Pharmaceutical Corp.).
Sine-Off, Prods. (SmithKline Beecham Pharmaceuticals).
Sinucol, Cap., Vial (Tennessee Pharmaceutic).
Sinulin, Tab. (Carnrick Laboratories, Inc.).
Sinutab Extra Strength, Cap. (Warner Lambert).
Statomin Maleate CC, Tab. (Jones Medical Industries, Inc.).
Sudafed Plus, Tab., Syr. (Glaxo-Wellcome).
Triactin, Syr. (ProMetic Pharma).
Triaminic, Prods. (Novartis Pharmaceutical Corp.).
Triaminic Chewables (Novartis Pharmaceutical Corp.).
Turbilixir, Liq. (Burlington).
Turbispan, Leisurecaps, Cap. (Burlington).
Tusquelin, Syr. (Circle Pharmaceuticals, Inc.).

Tussar, Prods. (Rhone-Poulenc Rorer Pharmaceuticals, Inc.).
Unituss HC, Syr. (United Research Laboratories).

d-chlorpheniramine maleate.
See: Polaramine Expectorant, Tab., Syr. (Schering-Plough Corp.).

chlorpheniramine maleate w/pseudoephedrine hydrochloride. (Eon Labs Manufacturing, Inc.) Pseudoephedrine HCl 120 mg, chlorpheniramine maleate 8 mg/Cap. Bot. 100s, 250s, 1000s. *otc.*
Use: Antihistamine, decongestant.

•**chlorpheniramine polistirex.** (klor-fen-IHR-ah-meen pahl-ee-STIE-rex) USAN.
Use: Antihistamine.

chlorpheniramine tannate.
W/Carbetapentane tannate, ephedrine tannate, phenylephrine tannate.
See: Rynatuss Tab., Susp. (Wallace Laboratories).
W/Phenylephrine tannate, pyrilamine tannate.
See: Rynatan, Tab., Susp. (Wallace Laboratories).
W/Pseudoephedrine tannate.
See: Tanafed, Susp. (Horizon Pharmaceutical Corp.).

•**chlorphentermine hydrochloride.** (klor-FEN-ter-meen) USAN.
Use: Anorexic.

chlorphthalidone.
See: Chlorthalidone.

Chlor-Pro 10. (Schein Pharmaceutical, Inc.) Chlorpheniramine maleate 10 mg/ml, benzyl alcohol. Inj. Vial 30 ml. *Rx.*
Use: Antihistamine.

•**chlorpromazine.** (klor-PRO-muh-zeen) U.S.P. 23.
Use: Antiemetic, antipsychotic.

•**chlorpromazine hydrochloride.** U.S.P. 23.
Use: Antiemetic, antipsychotic.
See: Promachlor, Tab. (Geneva Pharmaceuticals).
Promaz, Inj. (Keene Pharmaceuticals, Inc.).
Thorazine, Tab., Cap., Liq., Syr., Supp., Amp. (SmithKline Beecham Pharmaceuticals).

chlorpromazine HCl injection. (Various Mfr.) Chlorpromazine HCl 25 mg/ml. Inj. Amp. 1 ml, 2 ml. Vial 10 ml. *Rx.*
Use: Antipsychotic.

chlorpromazine hydrochloride intensol oral solution. (Roxane Laboratories, Inc.) Chlorpromazine HCl concentrated oral soln. **30 mg/ml:** Bot. 120 ml. **100 mg/ml:** Bot. 60 ml, 240 ml. *Rx.*
Use: Antiemetic, antipsychotic.

chlorpromazine HCl tablets. (Various Mfr.) Chlorpromazine HCl 10 mg, 25 mg, 50 mg, 100 mg, 200 mg. Tab. Bot. 100s, 1000s, UD 100s. *Rx.*
Use: Antipsychotic.

•**chlorpropamide.** (klor-PRO-puh-mide) U.S.P. 23.
Use: Antidiabetic.
See: Diabinese, Tab. (Pfizer US Pharmaceutical Group).

chlorpropamide. (klor-PRO-puh-mide) (Various Mfr.) Chlorpropamide 100 mg, 250 mg. Tab. Bot. 100s, 250s (250 mg only), 500s, 1000s, UD 100s, 600s. *Rx.*
Use: Antidiabetic.

chlorprophenpyridamine maleate.
See: Chlorpheniramine Maleate, U.S.P. 23.

chlorquinol. Mixture of the chlorinated products of 8-hydroxyquinoline containing about 65% of 5,7-dichloro-8-hydroxyquinoline. Quixalin.

Chlor-Rest. (Rugby Labs, Inc.) Phenylpropanolamine HCl 18.7 mg, chlorpheniramine maleate 2 mg/Tab. Bot. 100s. *otc.*
Use: Decongestant, antihistamine.

Chlor-Span. (Burlington) Chlorpheniramine maleate 8 mg/SR Cap. Bot. 60s. *otc.*
Use: Antihistamine.

chlortetracycline and sulfamethazine bisulfates soluble powder.
Use: Anti-infective.

•**chlortetracycline bisulfate.** (klor-the-trah-SIGH-kleen) U.S.P. 23.
Use: Anti-infective; antiprotozoal.

•**chlortetracycline hydrochloride.** U.S.P. 23.
Use: Anti-infective; antiprotozoal.
See: Aureomycin, Oint. (Storz/Lederle Ophthalmic Pharmaceuticals).

•**chlorthalidone.** (klor-THAL-ih-dohn) U.S.P. 23.
Use: Antihypertensive, diuretic.
See: Hygroton, Tab. (Rhone-Poulenc Rorer Pharmaceuticals, Inc.).
Thalitone, Tab. (Horus Therapeutics, Inc.).
W/Reserpine.
See: Demi-Regroton, Tab. (Rhone-Poulenc Rorer Pharmaceuticals, Inc.).
Regroton, Tab. (Rhone-Poulenc Rorer Pharmaceuticals, Inc).

chlorthalidone. (Various Mfr.) 25 mg, 50 mg, 100 mg. Tab. Bot. 100s (25 mg); 100s, 250s, 1000s (50 mg); 100s, 500s, 1000s (100 mg). *Rx.*
Use: Diuretic, antihypertensive.

Chlor-Trimeton Allergy. (Schering-

Plough Corp.) Chlorpheniramine maleate 4 mg, lactose. Tab. Pkg. 24s. *otc.*
Use: Antihistamine.

Chlor-Trimeton Allergy 4 Hour. (Schering-Plough Corp.) **Tab.:** Chlorpheniramine maleate 4 mg, lactose. Bot. 48s. **Syr.:** Chlorpheniramine maleate 2 mg/5 ml, parabens, cherry flavor. Bot. 118 ml. *otc.*
Use: Antihistamine.

Chlor-Trimeton Allergy 8 Hour. (Schering-Plough Corp.) Chlorpheniramine maleate 8 mg, parabens, lactose, sugar. TR Tab. Bot. 24s. *otc.*
Use: Antihistamine.

Chlor-Trimeton Allergy 12 Hour. (Schering-Plough Corp.) Chlorpheniramine maleate 12 mg, parabens, lactose, sugar. TR Tab. Pkg. 15s. *otc.*
Use: Antihistamine.

Chlor-Trimeton Allergy Sinus. (Schering-Plough Corp.) Phenylpropanolamine HCl 12.5 mg, chlorpheniramine maleate 2 mg, acetaminophen 500 mg/Capl. Box 24s. *otc.*
Use: Analgesic, antihistamine, decongestant.

Chlor-Trimeton w/Combinations. (Schering-Plough Corp.) Chlorpheniramine maleate.

W/Acetaminophen.
See: Coricidin, Tab. (Schering-Plough Corp.).

W/Acetaminophen, phenylpropanolamine.
See: Coricidin "D", Prods. (Schering-Plough Corp.).

W/Phenylephrine HCl.
See: Demazin, Prods. (Schering-Plough Corp.).

W/Pseudoephedrine sulfate.
See: Chlor-Trimeton Decongestant, Tab. (Schering-Plough Corp.).
Chlor-Trimeton 12 Hour Allergy (Schering-Plough Corp.).

W/Salicylamide, phenacetin, caffeine, vitamin C.
See: Coriforte, Cap. (Schering-Plough Corp.).

W/Sodium salicylate, amino acetic acid.
See: Corilin, Liq. (Schering-Plough Corp.).

Chlor-Trimeton 4 Hour Relief Tablets. (Schering-Plough Corp.) Chlorpheniramine maleate 4 mg, pseudoephedrine sulfate 60 mg/Tab. Box 24s, 48s. *otc.*
Use: Antihistamine, decongestant.

Chlor-Trimeton 12 Hour Allergy. (Schering-Plough Corp.) Chlorpheniramine maleate 8 mg, pseudoephedrine sulfate 120 mg/SR Tab. Box 24s, 48s. UD 96s. *otc.*
Use: Antihistamine, decongestant.

Chlor-Trimeton 12 Hour Relief Tablets. (Schering-Plough Corp.) Chlorpheniramine 8 mg, pseudoephedrine sulfate 120 mg/Tab. Box 12s. Bot. 36s. *otc.*
Use: Antihistamine, decongestant.

Chlorzide. (Foy Laboratories) Hydrochlorothiazide 50 mg/Tab. Bot. 1000s. *Rx.*
Use: Diuretic.

•**chlorzoxazone.** (klor-ZOX-uh-zone) U.S.P. 23.
Use: Muscle relaxant.
See: Paraflex, Tab. (Ortho McNeil Pharmaceutical).
Parafon Forte DSC, Capl. (Ortho McNeil Pharmaceutical).
Remular-S (Inter. Ethical).

chlorzoxazone. (Various Mfr.) 250 mg, 500 mg/Tab. Bot. 100s, 500s (500 mg only), 1000s.
Use: Muscle relaxant.

chlorzoxazone and acetaminophen capsules.
Use: Analgesic, muscle relaxant.

chlorzoxazone and acetaminophen tablets.
Use: Analgesic, muscle relaxant.

Choice 10. (Whiteworth Towne) Potassium Cl 10% soln., unflavored. Bot. Gal. *Rx.*
Use: Electrolyte supplement.

Choice 20. (Whiteworth Towne) Potassium Cl 20% soln., unflavored. Bot. gal. *Rx.*
Use: Electrolyte supplement.

Choice dm. (Mead Johnson Nutritionals) Protein 10.6 g, fat 12 g, carbohydrate 25 g, vitamins A, D, E, K, C, FA, B_1, B_2, B_3, B_5, B_6, B_{12}, biotin, Ca, P, I, Fe, Mg, Cu, Zn, Mn, Cl, Na, Se, Cr, Mo, sucrose, 250 calories/240 ml. Lactose free/Liq. Ready-to-use can 240 ml. *otc.*
Use: Nutritional supplement, enteral.

Cholac. (Alra Laboratories, Inc.) Lactulose 10 g/15 ml. Bot. 240 ml, pt, UD 30 ml. *Rx.*
Use: Laxative.

cholacrylamine resin. Anion exchange resin consisting of a water-soluble polymer having a molecular weight equivalent between 350 and 360 in which aliphatic quaternary amine groups are attached to an acrylic backbone by ester linkages.

cholalic acid.
See: Cholic Acid.

Cholan-DH. (Medeva Pharmaceuticals, Inc.) Dehydrocholic acid 250 mg/Tab. Bot. 100s.

Use: Laxative.

cholanic acid. Dehydrodesoxycholic acid.

Cholebrine. (Mallinckrodt) Iocetamic acid (62% iodine) 750 mg/Tab. Bot. 100s, 150s.
Use: Radiopaque agent.

•**cholecalciferol.** (kole-eh-kal-SIH-fer-ole) U.S.P. 23. *Formerly 7-Dehydrocholesterol, activated.*
Use: Vitamin D_3 (antirachitic).
See: Decavitamin Cap., Tab.
Delta-D, Tab. (Freeda Vitamins, Inc.).

cholecystography agents.
See: Bilopaque, Cap. (Sanofi Winthrop Pharmaceuticals).
Iodized Oil (Various Mfr.).
Iophendylate Inj.
Pantopaque, Amp. (Lafayette Pharmaceuticals, Inc.).
Telepaque, Tab. (Sanofi Winthrop Pharmaceuticals).

Choledyl SA. (Parke-Davis) Oxtriphylline 400 mg, 600 mg/Tab. Bot. 100s, UD 100s. *Rx.*
Use: Bronchodilator.

•**cholera vaccine.** U.S.P. 23.
Use: Immunization.

cholera vaccine. (Wyeth-Ayerst Laboratories) 8 units each of Ogawa and Inaba strains/ml. Vial 1.5 ml, 20 ml.
Use: Immunization.

choleretic. Bile salts.
See: Bile Preps. and Forms.
Dehydrocholic Acid.
Tocamphyl, Tab. (Various Mfr.).

cholesterin.
See: Cholesterol.

•**cholesterol.** N.F. 18.
Use: Pharmaceutic aid (emulsifying agent).

cholesterol reagent strips. (Bayer Corp. (Consumer Div.)) A quantitative strip test for cholesterol in serum. Seralyzer reagent strips. Bot. 25s.
Use: Diagnostic aid.

cholestyramine. (koe-less-TIE-ruh-meen) An antihyperlipidemic agent used to lower cholesterol. Consists of anhydrous cholestyramine 4 g/dose.
Use: Ion-exchange resin (bile salts), antihyperlipoproteinemic.
See: Questran, Pow. (Bristol Labs.).
Questran Light, Pow. (Bristol Labs.).

cholestyramine powder. (Zenith Goldline Pharmaceuticals) 4 g (as anhydrous resin), phenylalanine 14.1 mg/5.5 g powder, aspartame/Pow. Single-dose 5.5 g Pkt. 42s, 60s. *Rx.*
Use: Bile acid sequestrant.

•**cholestyramine resin.** (koe-less-TEER-uh-meen) U.S.P. 23.
Use: Antihyperlipidemic, ion-exchange resin (bile salts).
See: LoCHOLEST (Warner Chilcott).
Questran, Pow. (Bristol-Myers Squibb).

Cholidase. (Freeda Vitamins, Inc.) Choline 450 mg, inositol 150 mg, vitamins B_6 2.5 mg, B_{12} 5 mcg, E 7.5 mg/Tab. Bot. 100s, 250s, 500s. *otc.*
Use: Lipid, vitamin supplement.

choline. (Various Mfr.) Choline. Tab.: **250 mg:** Bot. 100s, 250s, 500s, 1000s. **500 mg:** Bot. 100s. **650 mg:** Bot. 90s, 100s, 250s, 500s. *otc.*
Use: Lipotropic.

choline bitartrate.
W/Bile extract, pancreatic substance, dl-methionine.
See: Ilopan-Choline, Tab. (Pharmacia & Upjohn).

choline chloride. (Various Mfr.).
Use: Liver supplement. [Orphan Drug]
W/Inositol, methionine, vitamin B_{12}.
See: W/Methionine, vitamins, niacinamide, panthenol.

choline chloride, carbamate. Carbachol, U.S.P. 23.

choline chloride succinate.
See: Succinylcholine Chloride, U.S.P. 23.

choline dihydrogen citrate. 2-Hydroxyethyl trimethylammonium citrate US vitamin 0.5 g. Bot. 100s, 500s.
Use: Lipotropic.

choline magnesium trisalicylate. (Sidmak Laboratories, Inc.) 500 mg, 750 mg or 1000 mg. Tab. Bot. 100s, 500s. *Rx.*
Use: Analgesic.
See: Trilisate, Tab. (Purdue Frederick Co.).

cholinergic agents. Parasympathomimetic Agents.
See: Mecholyl Cl, Inj. (Baker Norton Pharmaceuticals, Inc.).
Mestinon, Tab., Syr., Amp. (Roche Laboratories).
Mytelase, Cap. (Sanofi Winthrop Pharmaceuticals).
Pilocarpine Nitrate (Various Mfr.).
Tensilon, Inj. (Roche Laboratories).
Urecholine, Inj, Tab. (Merck & Co.).

cholinergic blocking agents.
See: Parasympatholytic agents.

•**choline salicylate.** USAN.
Use: Analgesic.

cholinesterase inhibitors. Agents that inhibit the enzyme cholinesterase and enhance the effects of endogenous acetylcholine.

Use: Glaucoma therapy.
See: Eserine Sulfate, Oint. (Various Mfr.).
Isopto Eserine, Soln. (Alcon Laboratories, Inc.).
Eserine Salicylate, Soln. (Alcon Laboratories, Inc.).

cholinesterase inhibitors. Agents that inhibit the enzyme cholinesterase and enhance the effects of endogenous acetylcholine.
Use: Muscle stimulants.
See: Neostigmine Methylsulfate, Inj. (Various Mfr.).

choline theophyllinate.
See: Oxtriphylline.

Cholinoid. (Zenith Goldline Pharmaceuticals) Choline 111 mg, inositol 111 mg, vitamins B_1 0.33 mg, B_2 0.33 mg, B_3 3.33 mg, B_5 1.7 mg, B_6 0.33 mg, B_{12} 1.7 mcg, C 100 mg, lemon bioflavonoid complex 100 mg/Cap. Bot. 100s. *otc.*
Use: Lipid, vitamin supplement.

Chol Meth in B. (Esco) Choline bitartrate 235 mg, inositol 112 mg, methionine 70 mg, betaine anhydrous 50 mg, vitamins B_{12} 6 mcg, B_1 6 mg, B_6 3 mg, niacin 10 mg/Cap. Bot. 500s, 1000s. *otc.*
Use: Vitamin supplement.

Cholografin Meglumine. (Bracco Diagnostics) Iodipamide meglumine. 520 mg, iodine 257 mg/ml, EDTA. Vial 20 ml. *Rx.*
Use: Radiopaque agent.

Choloxin. (Knoll Pharmaceuticals) Sodium dextrothyroxine 1 mg/Tab. Bot. 100s. *Rx.*
Use: Antihyperlipidemic.

cholylglycine.
See: CG RIA, Kit (Abbott Laboratories).

chondodendron tomentosum.
See: Curare.

Chondroitinase. (Storz Ophthalmics)
Use: Surgical aid, ophthalmic. [Orphan Drug]

chondrotin sulfate and sodium hyaluronate. Surgical aid in anterior segment procedures including cataract extraction and intraocular lens implantation. *Rx.*
See: Viscoat, Soln. (Cilco).

chondrus. Irish Moss.
W/Petrolatum, Liq.
See: Kondremul, Liq. (Medeva Pharmaceuticals, Inc.).

Chooz. (Schering-Plough Corp.) Calcium carbonate 500 mg/Gum Tab. Pkg. 16s. *otc.*
Use: Antacid.

Chorex 5. (Hyrex Pharmaceuticals) Chorionic gonadotropin 5000 units, mannitol, benzyl alcohol 0.9%/Vial 10 ml. *Rx.*
Use: Hormone, chorionic gonadotropin.

Chorex 10. (Hyrex Pharmaceuticals) Chorionic gonadotropin 10,000 units. Mannitol, benzyl alcohol 0.9%/Vial 10 ml. *Rx.*
Use: Hormone, chorionic gonadotropin.

chorionic gonadotropin. 5000 units/Vial w/diluent 10 ml, 10,000 units/Vial w/ diluent 10 ml, 20,000 units/Vial w/diluent 10 ml (Various Mfr.) mannitol, benzyl alcohol 0.9%. Vial 10 ml.
Use: Prepubertal cryptorchidism or induction of ovulation and pregnancy in anovulatory women.
See: A.P.L., Inj. (Wyeth-Ayerst Laboratories).
Chorex 5, Vial (Hyrex Pharmaceuticals).
Chorex 10, Vial (Hyrex Pharmaceuticals).
Choron 10, Vial (Forest Pharmaceutical, Inc.).
Gonic, Vial (Roberts Pharmaceuticals).
Pregnyl, Vial (Organon).
Profasi, Vial (Serono Laboratories, Inc.).

Choron 10. (Forest Pharmaceutical, Inc.) Chorionic gonadotropin 10,000 units/ vial with diluent 10 ml, mannitol, benzyl alcohol 0.9%. Inj. Vial 10 ml. *Rx.*
Use: Hormone, chorionic gonadotropin.

Chromagen. (Savage Laboratories)
Cap.: Ferrous fumarate 66 mg, vitamins C 250 mg, B_{12} activity 10 mcg, desiccated stomach substances 100 mg/soft gelatin cap. Bot. 100s, 500s. *Rx.*
Use: Mineral, vitamin supplement.

Chromagen FA. (Savage Laboratories) Fe 66 mg, vitamin C 250 mg, folic acid 1 mg, B_{12} 10 mcg. Cap. UD 100s. *Rx.*
Use: Mineral, vitamin supplement.

Chromagen Forte. (Savage Laboratories) Fe 151 mg, vitamin C 60 mg, folic acid 1 mg, B_{12} 10 mcg. Cap. UD 100s. *Rx.*
Use: Mineral, vitamin supplement.

Chroma-Pak. (SoloPak Pharmaceuticals, Inc.) Chromium. **4 mcg/ml:** Vial 10 ml, 30 ml. **20 mcg/ml:** Vial 5 ml. *Rx.*
Use: Nutritional supplement, parenteral.

chromargyre.
See: Merbromin (Various Mfr.).

chromated. Solution (Cr^{51}).
See: Chromitope sodium (Bristol-Myers Squibb).

Chromelin Complexion Blender. (Summers Laboratories, Inc.) Dihydroxyac-

etone 5%, alcohol 50%. Bot. Oz. *otc.*
Use: Hyperpigmenting.

chromic acid, disodium salt. Sodium Chromate Cr^{51} Inj., U.S.P. 23.

•**chromic chloride.** U.S.P. 23.
Use: Supplement (trace mineral).

•**chromic chloride Cr^{51}.** USAN.
Use: Radiopharmaceutical.
See: Chromitope Cl (Bristol-Myers Squibb).

•**chromic phosphate Cr^{51}.** USAN.
Use: Radiopharmaceutical.

•**chromic phosphate P^{32} suspension.** U.S.P. 23.
Use: Radiopharmaceutical.

Chromitope Sodium. (Bristol-Myers Squibb) Chromate Cr^{51}, Sodium for Inj. 0.25 mCi.
Use: Radiopharmaceutical.

chromium. A trace metal used in IV nutritional therapy that helps maintain normal glucose metabolism and peripheral nerve function.
See: Chromium, Inj. (Various Mfr.).
Chromic Chloride, Inj. (Various Mfr.).
Chromium Chloride, Inj. (Various Mfr.).
Chroma-Pak, Inj. (Solopak Pharmaceuticals, Inc.).
Chromium Trace Metal Additive, Inj. (I.M.S, Ltd.).
Concentrated Chromic Chloride, Inj. (American Regent).

•**chromonar hydrochloride.** (KROE-moe-nahr) USAN.
Use: Coronary vasodilator.

Chronulac. (Hoechst Marion Roussel) Lactulose 10 g/15 ml (< 2.2 g galactose, 1.2 g lactose, 1.2 g other sugars). Bot. 473 ml, 1890 ml, UD 15 ml, 30 ml. Box 100s. *Rx.*
Use: Laxative.

Chur-Hist. (Churchill) Chlorpheniramine 4 mg/Kaptab. Bot. 100s.
Use: Antihistamine.

Chymex. (Pharmacia & Upjohn) Bentiromide 500 mg/7.5 ml w/propylene glycol 40%. Screening test for pancreatic exocrine insufficiency.
Use: Diagnostic aid.

Chymodiactin. (Smith & Nephew United) 4 nKat units, 1.4 mg sodium L-cysteinate HCl with diluent. Pow. for Inj. Vial 2 ml. *Rx.*
Use: Proteolytic enzyme.

•**chymopapain.** (KIE-moe-pap-ANE) USAN.
Use: Proteolytic enzyme.

Cibacalcin. (Novartis Pharmaceutical Corp.) Calcitonin-human for injection.
Use: Paget's disease. [Orphan Drug]

CI Basic Violet 3. Gentian Violet U.S.P. 23.

Ciba Vision Cleaner. (Ciba Vision) Cocoamphocarboxyglycinate, sodium lauryl sulfate, sorbic acid 0.1%, hexylene glycol, EDTA 0.2%. Soln. 5 ml or 15 ml. *otc.*
Use: Contact lens care.

Ciba Vision Saline. (Ciba Vision) Buffered, isotonic with NaCl, boric acid. Soln. Bot. 90 ml, 240 ml, 360 ml. *otc.*
Use: Contact lens care, rinsing, storage.

cibenzoline. (SIGH-BEN-zoe-leen)
See: Cifenline Succinate. USAN.

•**ciclafrine hydrochloride.** (SICK-lah-freen) USAN.
Use: Antihypotensive.

•**ciclazindol.** (sigh-CLAY-zin-dole) USAN.
Use: Antidepressant.

•**cicletanine.** (sick-LET-ah-neen) USAN.
Use: Antihypertensive.

•**ciclopirox.** (sigh-kloe-PEER-ox) USAN.
Use: Antifungal.

•**ciclopirox olamine.** (sigh-kloe-PEER-ox OLE-ah-meen) U.S.P. 23.
Use: Antifungal.
See: Loprox, Cream (Hoechst Marion Roussel).

•**cicloprofen.** (SICK-low-pro-fen) USAN.
Use: Anti-inflammatory.

•**cicloprolol hydrochloride.** (SIGH-kloe-PRO-lahl) USAN.
Use: Antiadrenergic (β-receptor).

Cidex. (Johnson & Johnson) Activated dialdehyde soln. Bot. Qt, gal, 2.5 gal.
Use: Disinfectant, sterlizing.

Cidex-7. (Johnson & Johnson) Glutaraldehyde 2% and vial of activator with aqueous potassium salt as buffer and sodium nitrite as a corrosive inhibitor. Soln. Bot. Qt, gal, 5 gal.
Use: Disinfectant, sterilizing.

Cidex Plus. (Johnson & Johnson) 3.2% glutaraldehyde. Soln. Gal.
Use: Disinfectant, sterilizing.

C.I. Direct Blue 53 Tetrasodium Salt. Evans Blue, U.S.P. 23. *Rx.*

•**cidofovir.** (sigh-DAH-fah-vihr) USAN.
Use: Antiviral.
See: Vistide (Gilead Sciences, Inc.).

•**cidoxepin hydrochloride.** (sih-DOX-eh-PIN) USAN.
Use: Antidepressant.

•**cifenline.** (sigh-FEN-leen) USAN. *Formerly cibenzoline.*
Use: Cardiovascular (antiarrhythmic).

•**cifenline succinate.** (sigh-FEN-leen) USAN.

Use: Cardiovascular agent (antiarrhythmic).

•**ciglitazone.** (sigh-GLIE-tah-ZONE) USAN.
Use: Antidiabetic.

cignolin.
See: Anthralin (Various Mfr.).

•**ciladopa hydrochloride.** (SIGH-lah-doe-pah) USAN.
Use: Antiparkinsonian, dopaminergic.

cilastatin-imipenem. A formulation of imipenem, a thienamycin antibiotic, and cilastatin sodium, the inhibitor of the renal dipeptidase, dehydropeptidase-1.
Use: Anti-infective.
See: Primaxin I.V., Pow. (Merck & Co.). Primaxin I.M., Pow. (Merck & Co.).

•**cilastatin sodium.** (SIGH-lah-STAT-in) U.S.P. 23.
Use: Enzyme inhibitor.
W/Imipenem.
See: Primaxin, Inj. (Merck & Co.).

•**cilazapril.** (sile-AZE-ah-PRILL) USAN.
Use: Antihypertensive.

•**cilexetil.** (sigh-LEX-eh-till) USAN.
Use: Anti-infective.

Cilfomide. (Sanofi Winthrop Pharmaceuticals) Inositol hexanicotinate. Tab. *Rx.*
Use: Hypolipidimic, peripheral vasodilator.

ciliary neutrotrophic factor (recombinant human). (Regeneron Pharmaceuticals, Inc.)
Use: Treatment of motor neuron disease. [Orphan Drug]

Cillium. (Whiteworth Towne) Psyllium seed husk. 4.94 g, 14 calories/rounded tsp. Pow. Bot. 420 g, 630 g. *otc.*
Use: Laxative.

•**cilmostim.** (SILL-moe-stim) USAN. *Formerly rhM-CSF, M-CSF, CSF-1.*
Use: Hematopoietic (macrophage colony-stimulating factor).

•**cilobamine mesylate.** (SIGH-low-BAM-een) USAN. *Formerly clobamine mesylate.*
Use: Antidepressant.

•**cilofungin.** (SIGH-low-FUN-jin) USAN.
Use: Antifungal.

•**cilostazol.** (sill-OH-stah-zole) USAN.
Use: Antithrombotic, platelet inhibitor, vasodilator.
See: Pletal, Tab. (Otsuka America Pharmaceuticals).

Ciloxan. (Alcon Laboratories, Inc.) Ciprofloxacin HCl 3.5 mg (equivalent to 3 mg base)/ml. Soln., Drop-Tainer dispensers. 2.5 ml, 5 ml. *Rx.*
Use: Anti-infective.

•**cimaterol.** (sigh-MAH-teh-role) USAN.
Use: Repartitioning agent.

•**cimetidine.** (sigh-MET-ih-deen) U.S.P. 23.
Use: Histamine H_2 antagonist.
See: Tagamet, Tab., Inj. (SmithKline Beecham Pharmaceuticals).

cimetidine. (Endo Laboratories) Cimetidine 150 mg, phenol 5 mg/ml. Inj. Vial 2 ml. Multidose vial 8 ml. *Rx.*
Use: Histamine H_2 receptor antagonist.

cimetidine. (Various Mfr.) Cimetidine 200 mg, 300 mg, 400 mg, 800 mg. Tab. Bot. 30s, 50s, 100s, 500s, 1000s. *Rx.*
Use: Histamine H_2 receptor antagonist.

•**cimetidine hydrochloride.** (sigh-MET-ih-deen) USAN.
Use: Histamine H_2 receptor antagonist.

cimetidine hydrochloride. (sigh-MET-ih-deen) (Endo Laboratories) Cimetidine HCl 150 mg, phenol 5 mg/ml. Inj. Vial 2 ml, Multi-dose vial 8 ml. *Rx.*
Use: Histamine H_2 antagonist.

cimetidine oral solution. (sigh-MET-ih-deen) (Alpharma USPD Inc.) 300 mg (as HCl)/5 ml. Bot. 240 ml, 470 ml. *Rx.*
Use: Histamine H_2 antagonist.

Cinacort Span. (Foy Laboratories) Triamcinolone acetonide 40 mg/ml. Vial 5 ml. *Rx.*
Use: Corticosteroid.

•**cinalukast.** (sin-ah-LOO-kast) USAN.
Use: Antiasthmatic (leukotriene antagonist).

•**cinanserin hydrochloride.** (sin-AN-ser-in) USAN.
Use: Serotonin inhibitor.

cinchona bark. (Various Mfr.).
Use: Antimalarial, tonic.
W/Anhydrous quinine, cinchonidine, cinchonine, quinidine, quinine.
See: Totaquine, Pow. (Various Mfr.).

cinchonine salts. (Various Mfr.).
Use: Quinine dihydrochloride.

cinchophen.
Use: Analgesic.

•**cinepazet maleate.** (SIN-eh-PAZZ-ett) USAN.
Use: Antianginal.

•**cinflumide.** (SIN-flew-mide) USAN.
Use: Muscle relaxant.

•**cingestol.** (sin-JESS-tole) USAN.
Use: Hormone, progestin.

•**cinnamedrine.** (sin-am-ED-reen) USAN.
Use: Muscle relaxant.
See: Midol, Tab. (Bayer Corp. (Consumer Div.)).

cinnamic aldehyde. Name previously used for Cinnamaldehyde.

cinnamon.

Use: Flavoring.

cinnamon oil. (Various Mfr.).
Use: Pharmaceutic aid.

•**cinnarizine.** (sin-NAHR-ih-zeen) USAN.
Use: Antihistamine.

cinnopentazone. INN for Cintazone.

Cinobac. (Oclassen Pharmaceuticals, Inc.) Cinoxacin **250 mg/Cap.:** Bot. 40s. **500 mg/Cap.:** Bot. 50s. *Rx.*
Use: Anti-infective, urinary.

•**cinoxate.** (sin-OX-ate) U.S.P. 23.
Use: Ultraviolet screen.

•**cinperene.** (SIN-peh-reen) USAN.
Use: Antipsychotic.

Cin-Quin. (Solvay Pharmaceuticals) Quinidine sulfate. (Contains 83% anhydrous quinidine alkaloid.) **Tab.:** 100 mg, 200 mg or 300 mg. Bot. 100s, 1000s, UD 100s. **Cap.:** 200 mg. Bot. 100s. 300 mg. Bot. 100s, 1000s, UD 100s. *Rx.*
Use: Antiarrhythmic.

•**cinromide.** (SIN-row-mide) USAN.
Use: Anticonvulsant.

•**cintazone.** (SIN-tah-zone) USAN.
Use: Anti-inflammatory.

•**cintriamide.** (sin-TRY-ah-mid) USAN.
Use: Antipsychotic.

•**cioteronel.** (SIGH-oh-TEH-row-nell) USAN.
Use: Dermatologic, acne; androgenic alopecia and keloid (antiandrogen).

•**cipamfylline.** (sigh-PAM-fih-lin) USAN.
Use: Antiviral.

Cipralan. (Roche Laboratories) Cifenline succinate, formerly cibenzoline. *Rx.*
Use: Antiarrhythmic.

•**ciprefadol succinate.** (sih-PREH-fah-dahl) USAN.
Use: Analgesic.

Cipro. (Bayer Corp. (Consumer Div.)) Ciprofloxacin HCl 100 mg, 250 mg, 500 mg, 750 mg/Tab. Bot. 50s (750 mg only), 100s (except 750 mg), UD 100s, 100 mg in *Cipro Cystitis Packs* 6s. *Rx.*
Use: Anti-infective, fluoroquinolone.

Cipro HC Otic. (Bayer Corp. (Allergy Div.)) Ciprofloxacin 2 mg, hydrocortisone 10 mg/ml, benzyl alcohol. Susp. Bot. 10 ml. *Rx.*
Use: Otic preparation.

Cipro I.V. (Bayer Corp. (Consumer Div.)) Ciprofloxacin 200 mg, 400 mg (with lactic acid). **Inj. Vial:** 20 ml (1%), 40 ml (1%). **Flex Bot:** 100 ml (in 5% dextrose) and 200 ml (in 5% dextrose). *Rx.*
Use: Anti-infective, fluoroquinolone.

•**ciprocinonide.** (sih-PRO-SIN-oh-nide) USAN.
Use: Adrenocortical steroid.

•**ciprofibrate.** (sip-ROW-FIE-brate) USAN.
Use: Antihyperlipoproteinemic.

•**ciprofloxacin.** (sip-ROW-FLOX-ah-sin) U.S.P. 23.
Use: Anti-infective.

•**ciprofloxacin hydrochloride.** (sip-ROW-FLOX-ah-sin) U.S.P. 23.
Use: Anti-infective.
See: Ciloxan, Soln. (Alcon Laboratories, Inc.).
Cipro Preps. (Bayer Corp. (Consumer Div.)).

•**ciprostene calcium.** (sigh-PRAHS-teen) USAN.
Use: Platelet aggregation inhibitor.

•**ciramadol.** (sihr-AM-ah-dole) USAN.
Use: Analgesic.

•**ciramadol hydrochloride.** (sihr-AM-ah-dole) USAN.
Use: Analgesic.

Cirbed. (Boyd) Papaverine HCl 150 mg/Cap. Bot. 100s. *Rx.*
Use: Antispasmodic.

Circavite-T. (Circle Pharmaceuticals, Inc.) Iron 12 mg, vitamins A 10,000 IU, D 400 IU, E 15 mg, B_1 10.3 mg, B_2 10 mg, B_3 100 mg, B_5 18.4 mg, B_6 4.1 mg, B_{12} 5 mcg, C 200 mg, Cu, I, Mg, Mn, Zn 1.5 mg. Bot. 100s. *otc.*
Use: Mineral, vitamin supplement.

•**cirolemycin.** (sih-ROW-leh-MY-sin) USAN.
Use: Anti-infective, antineoplastic.

•**cisapride.** (SIS-uh-PRIDE) USAN.
Use: Gastrointestinal, stimulant (peristaltic).
See: Propulsid, Tab. (Janssen Pharmaceutical, Inc.).

•**cisatracurium besylate.** (sis-ah-trah-CURE-ee-uhm BESS-ih-late) USAN.
Use: Nondepolarizing neuromuscular blocking agent; muscle relaxant.
See: Nimbex, Inj. (GlaxoWellcome).

•**cisconazole.** (SIS-KOE-nah-zahl) USAN.
Use: Antifungal.

•**cisplatin.** (SIS-plat-in) U.S.P. 23. *Formerly cis-Platinum II.*
Use: Antineoplastic.
See: Platinol, Inj. (Bristol-Myers Squibb).

cis-retinoic acid. (13-cis-Retinoic Acid). *Rx.*
Use: Antiacne.
See: Isotretinoin.
Accutane (Roche Laboratories).

9-cis retinoic acid. (Allergan, Inc.)
Use: Promyelocytic leukemia treatment; prevention of retinal detachment due to proliferative vitreoretinopathy.

[Orphan Drug]

citalopram hydrobromide.
Use: Antidepressant.
See: Celexa, Tab. (Forest Pharmaceuticals).

citanest hydrochloride. (Astra Pharmaceuticals, L.P.) **Plain:** Prilocaine HCl 4%/1.8 ml dental cartridge. *Rx.*
Use: Anesthetic, local.

Citanest Hydrochloride Forte. (Astra Pharmaceuticals, L.P.) Prilocaine HCl 4% with epinephrine 1:200,000. Contains sodium metabisulfite. Dental cartridge 1.8 ml. Inj. *Rx.*
Use: Anesthetic, local.

•**citenamide.** (sigh-TEN-ah-MIDE) USAN.
Use: Anticonvulsant.

Cithal Capsules. (Table Rock) Watermelon seed extract 2 gr, theobromine 4 gr, phenobarbital 0.25 gr/Cap. Bot. 100s, 500s. *Rx.*
Use: Antihypertensive.

•**citicoline sodium.** (SIGH-tih-koe-leen) USAN.
Use: Post-stroke and post-head trauma treatment.

Citracal. (Mission Pharmacal Co.) Calcium citrate 950 mg/Tab. Bot. 100s. *otc.*
Use: Calcium supplement.

Citracal 1500 + D. (Mission Pharmacal Co.) Calcium citrate 1500 mg, vitamin D 200 IU/Tab. Bot. 60s. *otc.*
Use: Mineral, vitamin supplement.

Citracal Liquitab. (Mission Pharmacal Co.) Calcium citrate 2376 mg/Effervescent tab. Box. 30s. *otc.*
Use: Mineral supplement.

Citra Forte. (Boyle and Co. Pharm.) Hydrocodone bitartrate 5 mg, ascorbic acid 30 mg, pheniramine maleate 2.5 mg, pyrilamine maleate 3.33 mg, potassium citrate 150 mg/5 ml. Bot. Pt, gal. *c-III.*
Use: Antihistamine, antitussive, vitamin supplement.

Citramin-500. (Thurston) Vitamin C 500 mg, rose hips, acerola with mixed bioflavonoids/Loz. Bot. 100s, 250s, 1000s. *otc.*
Use: Mineral, vitamin supplement.

Citranox. (Alconox)
Use: Liquid acid detergent for manual and ultrasonic washers.

Citra pH. (ValMed, Inc.) Sodium citrate dihydrate 450 mg/30 ml. Soln. 30 ml. *otc.*
Use: Antacid.

Citrasan B. (Sandia) Lemon bioflavonoid complex 300 mg, vitamins C 300 mg, B_1 30 mg, B_2 10 mg, B_6 5 mg, B_{12} 4 mcg, calcium pantothenate 10 mg, niacinamide 50 mg/Tab. Bot. 100s, 1000s. *otc.*
Use: Mineral, vitamin supplement.

Citrasan K-250. (Sandia) Vitamins C 250 mg, K 1 mg, lemon bioflavonoid 250 mg/Tab. Bot. 100s, 1000s. *otc.*
Use: Vitamin supplement.

Citrasan K Liquid. (Sandia) Vitamins C 125 mg, K 0.66 mg, lemon bioflavonoid complex 125 mg/5 ml. Bot. Pt, gal. *otc.*
Use: Vitamin supplement.

citrate acid.
See: Bicitra Soln. (Baker Norton Pharmaceuticals, Inc.).

citrate and citric acid solution.
Use: Alkalinizer.
See: Polycitra (Baker Norton Pharmaceuticals, Inc.).
Polycitra LC (Baker Norton Pharmaceuticals, Inc.).
Polycitra K (Baker Norton Pharmaceuticals, Inc.).
Oracit (Carolina Medical Products).
Bicitra (Baker Norton Pharmaceuticals, Inc.).

Citrate of Magnesia. (Various Mfr.) Magnesium citrate. Soln. Bot. 300 ml. *otc.*
Use: Laxative.

citrated normal human plasma.
See: Plasma, Normal Human.

Citresco-K. (Esco) Vitamins C 100 mg, K 0.7 mg, citrus bioflavonoid complex 100 mg/Cap. Bot. 100s, 500s, 1000s. *otc.*
Use: Vitamin supplement.

•**citric acid.** U.S.P. 23.
Use: Component of anticoagulant solutions and drug products.

citric acid and d-gluconic acid irrigant.
Use: Irrigant, genitourinary. [Orphan Drug]
See: Renacidin (Guardian Laboratories).

citric acid, glucono-delta-lactone and magnesium carbonate.
Use: Renal and bladder calculi of the apatite or struvite variety. [Orphan Drug]

citric acid, magnesium oxide, and sodium carbonate irrigation.
Use: Irrigant, ophthalmic.

citrin.
See: Vitamin P.

Citrin Capsules. (Table Rock) Watermelon seed extract 4 gr/Cap. Bot. 100s, 500s. *Rx.*
Use: Antihypertensive.

Citrocarbonate. (Pharmacia & Upjohn) Sodium bicarbonate 0.78 g, sodium

citrate anhydrous 1.82 g/3.9 g. Bot. 4 oz, 8 oz. *otc.*
Use: Antacid.

Citrocarbonate Effervescent Granules. (Roberts Pharmaceuticals) Sodium bicarbonate 780 mg, sodium citrate anhydrous 1820 mg, sodium 700.6 mg/5 mg. Bot. 150 g. *otc.*
Use: Analgesic, antacid.

Citro Cee, Super. (Marlyn Nutraceuticals, Inc.) Bioflavonoids 500 mg, rutin 50 mg, vitamin C 500 mg, rose hips powder 500 mg/Tab. Bot. 50s, 100s. *otc.*
Use: Vitamin supplement.

Citro-Flav 200. (Zenith Goldline Pharmaceuticals) Citrus bioflavonoid compound 200 mg/Cap. Bot. 100s, 1000s. *otc.*
Use: Vitamin supplement.

Citroleum Sunburn Creme. (Citroleum) Bot. 4 oz.

Citrolith. (Beach Pharmaceuticals) Potassium citrate 50 mg, sodium citrate 950 mg/Tab. Bot. 100s, 500s. *Rx.*
Use: Alkalinizer, urinary.

Citroma. (Century Pharmaceuticals, Inc.) Magnesium citrate. Oral Soln. Bot. 10 oz. *otc.*
Use: Laxative.

Citroma Low Sodium. (National Magnesia) Magnesium citrate. Oral soln w/lemon or cherry flavor in sugar-free vehicle. Bot. 10 oz. *otc.*
Use: Laxative.

Citrotein. (Novartis Pharmaceutical Corp.) Sucrose, pasteurized egg white solids, amino acids, maltodextrin, citric acid, natural and artificial flavors, mono- and diglycerides, partially hydrogenated soybean oil, 0.66 cal/ml, protein 40.7 g, carbohydrate 120.7 g, fat 1.55 g, Na 698 mg, K 698 mg/L. Tartrazine (orange flavor only). Pow. 1.57 oz/packet, Can 14.16 oz. Orange, grape, and punch flavors. *otc.*
Use: Nutritional supplement, enteral.

citrovorum factor. U.S.P. 23. Leucovorin Calcium.
See: Leucovorin Calcium (ESI Lederle Generics).

Citrucel. (SmithKline Beecham Pharmaceuticals) Methylcellulose 2 g/heaping tbsp. dose w/citric acid. Bot. 16 oz, 30 oz. *otc.*
Use: Laxative.

Citrucel Sugar Free. (SmithKline Beecham Pharmaceuticals) Methylcellulose 2 g, aspartame, phenylalanine 52 mg. Pow. Can. 479 g. *otc.*
Use: Laxative.

citrus bioflavonoid compound.
See: Bioflavonoid Compounds (Various Mfr.).
C.V.P., Syr. (Rhone-Poulenc Rorer Pharmaceuticals, Inc.).
Vitamin P.

Citrus-flav C 500. (Fibertone) Citrus bioflavonoids complex 200 mg, vitamin C 200 mg, hesperidin complex 40 mg, acerola 50 mg, rutin 10 mg, in citrus base of orange and lemon powder, grapefruit concentrate powder and citrus pectin. Tabs. Bot. 100s, 250s. *otc.*
Use: Nutritional supplement.

C-Ject. (Lincoln Diagnostics) Ascorbic acid 2000 mg, sodium bisulfite 0.1%, disodium sequestrene 0.01%/10 ml. Amp. 10 ml, "Score-Break" Box 25s. *Rx.*
Use: Nutritional supplement.

C-Ject with B. (Lincoln Diagnostics) When mixed with 10 ml of diluent, each vial contains: Vitamins C 2000 mg, B_1 50 mg, B_2 5 mg, B_6 10 mg, nicotinamide 100 mg, methylparaben 0.89 mg, propylparaben 0.22 mg, sodium bisulfite 10 mg, disodium sequestrene 1 mg. Box of 6 lyophilized plugs and 6 10 ml vials of Sterile Diluent. *Rx.*
Use: Nutritional supplement.

CKA Canker Aid. (Pannett Prod.) Benzocaine, aluminum hydrate, magnesium trisilicate, sodium acid carbonate. Pow. *otc.*
Use: Cancer, cold sores.

CK (CPK) Reagent Strips. (Bayer Corp. (Consumer Div.)) Seralyzer reagent strips for creatinine phosphokinase in serum or plasma. Bot. 25s.
Use: Diagnostic aid.

•**cladribine.** (KLAD-rih-BEAN) USAN.
Use: Antineoplastic. [Orphan Drug]
See: Leustatin (Ortho Biotech, Inc.).

Claforan. (Hoechst Marion Roussel) Cefotaxime sodium. **Pow. for Inj.:** 500 mg/Vial Pkg. 10s. 1 g, 2 g Vial. Pkg. 10s, 25s, 50s. Infusion bot. 10s, *ADD-Vantage* system Vial 25s. 10g. Bot. **Inj.:** 1 g, 2 g. Premixed, frozen. 50 ml Pkg. 12s. *Rx.*
Use: Anti-infective, cephalosporin.

•**clamoxyquin hydrochloride.** (KLAM-OX-ee-kwin) USAN.
Use: Amebicide.

•**clarithromycin.** (kluh-RITH-row-MY-sin) U.S.P. 23.
Use: Anti-infective.
See: Biaxin, Tab; Gran. for Oral Susp. (Abbott Laboratories).

clarithromycin. A semi-synthetic macrolide antibiotic. *Rx.*
Use: Anti-infective, antiulcerative, erythromycin.

See: Biaxin Tabs., Gran. for Oral Susp. (Abbott Laboratories).

Claritin. (Schering-Plough Corp.) Loratadine. **Tab.:** 10 mg, lactose. Bot. 100s, 500s, unit-of-use 14s, 30s, UD 100s. **Syr.:** 1 mg/ml. Bot. 16 oz. **Reditabs:** 10 mg, mannitol. Unit-of-use 30s. *Rx.*
Use: Antihistamine.

Claritin-D. (Schering-Plough Corp.) Loratadine 5 mg, pseudoephedrine sulfate 120 mg. Tab, SR Tab. Bot. 30s (except Tab.), 100s, unit-of-use 10s, 30s (except SR Tab.), UD 100s. *Rx.*
Use: Antihistamine, decongestant.

Claritin-D 24-Hour. (Schering-Plough Corp.) Loratadine 10 mg, pseudoephedrine sulfate 240 mg/ER Tab. Bot. 100s, UD 100s. *Rx.*
Use: Antihistamine, decongestant.

Claritin-12.
See: Vitamin B_{12}.

•**clavulanate potassium.** (CLAV-you-lah-nate) U.S.P. 23.
Use: Inhibitor (β-lactamase).

clavulanate potassium and ticarcillin.
Use: Anti-infective, pencillin.
See: Timentin (SmithKline Beecham Pharmaceuticals).

clavulanic acid/amoxicillin.
Use: Anti-infective, penicillin.
See: Augmentin, Tab. (SmithKline Beecham Pharmaceuticals).

clavulanic acid/ticarcillin.
Use: Anti-infective, penicillin.
See: Timentin Pow. for Inj. (SmithKline Beecham Pharmaceuticals).

•**clazolam.** (CLAY-zoe-lam) USAN.
Use: Anxiolytic.

•**clazolimine.** (clay-ZOLE-ih-meen) USAN.
Use: Diuretic.

Clean-N-Soak. (Allergan, Inc.) Cleaning agent with phenylmercuric nitrate 0.004%. Bot. 120 ml. *otc.*
Use: Contact lens care.

Clearasil 10%. (Procter & Gamble Pharm.) Benzoyl peroxide 10%. Bot. oz. *otc.*
Use: Dermatologic, acne.

Clearasil Adult Care Cream. (Procter & Gamble Pharm.) Sulfur, resorcinol, alcohol 10%, parabens. Cream Tube. 17 g. *otc.*
Use: Dermatologic, acne.

Clearasil Adult Care Medicated Blemish Stick. (Procter & Gamble Pharm.) Sulfur 8%, resorcinol 1%, bentonite 4%, laureth-4, titanium dioxide. Stick ⅛ oz. *otc.*
Use: Dermatologic, acne.

Clearasil Antibacterial Soap. (Procter & Gamble Pharm.) Triclosan 0.75%. Bar 92 g. *otc.*
Use: Dermatologic, acne.

Clearasil Clearstick, Maximum Strength. (Procter & Gamble Pharm.) Salicylic acid 2%, alcohol 39%, menthol, EDTA. Liq. 35 ml. *otc.*
Use: Dermatologic, acne.

Clearasil Clearstick, Regular Strength. (Procter & Gamble Pharm.) Salicylic acid 1.25%, alcohol 39%, aloe vera gel, menthol, EDTA. Liq. 35 ml. *otc.*
Use: Dermatologic, acne.

Clearasil Clearstick for Sensitive Skin, Maximum Strength. (Procter & Gamble Pharm.) Salicylic acid 2%, alcohol 39%, aloe vera gel, menthol, EDTA. Liq. 35 ml. *otc.*
Use: Dermatologic, acne.

Clearasil Daily Face Wash. (Procter & Gamble Pharm.) Triclosan 0.3%, glycerin, aloe vera gel, EDTA. Liq. Bot. 135 ml. *otc.*
Use: Dermatologic, acne.

Clearasil Double Clear. (Procter & Gamble Pharm.) **Pads, maximum strength:** Salicylic acid 2%, alcohol 40%, witch hazel distillate, menthol, Jar 32s. **Pads, regular strength:** Salicylic acid 1.25%, alcohol 40%, witch hazel distillate, menthol. Jar 32s. *otc.*
Use: Dermatologic, acne.

Clearasil Double Textured Pads. (Procter & Gamble Pharm.) **Pads, regular strength:** Salicylic acid 2%, alcohol 40%, glycerin, aloe vera gel, EDTA. Pkg. 32s, 40s. **Pads, maximum strength:** Salicylic acid 2%, alcohol 40%, menthol, aloe vera gel, EDTA. Pkg. 32s, 40s. *otc.*
Use: Dermatologic, acne.

Clearasil Maximum Strength Cream. (Procter & Gamble Pharm.) Benzoyl peroxide 10%, parabens in tinted or vanishing base. Tube 18 g, 28 g. *otc.*
Use: Dermatologic, acne.

Clearasil Maximum Strength Lotion. (Procter & Gamble Pharm.) Benzoyl peroxide 10%, cetyl alcohol, parabens in vanishing base. Bot. 29 ml. *otc.*
Use: Dermatologic, acne.

Clearasil Medicated Deep Cleanser. (Procter & Gamble Pharm.) Salicylic acid 0.5%, alcohol 42%, menthol, EDTA, aloe vera gel, hydrogenated castor oil. Liq. Bot. 229 ml. *otc.*
Use: Dermatologic, acne.

Clear Away. (Schering-Plough Corp.) Salicylic acid 40%. Disc Pck. 18s. *otc.*
Use: Dermatologic, acne.

Clear Away Plantar. (Schering-Plough Corp.) Salicylic acid 40%. Disc (for feet) Pck. 24s. *otc.*
Use: Dermatologic, acne.

Clear Blue Easy. (Unipath Diagnostics) Dipstick for in-home pregnancy test. Kit 1s, 2s.
Use: Diagnostic aid.

Clearblue Pregnancy Test. (VLI) Dip stick for pregnancy test. Kit 2s.
Use: Diagnostic aid.

Clearex Acne Cream. (Health for Life Brands, Inc.) Allantoin, sulfur, resorcinol, d-panthenol, isopropanol. Tube 1.5 oz. *otc.*
Use: Dermatologic, acne.

Clear Eyes ACR Eye Drops. (Ross Laboratories) Naphazoline HCl 0.012%. Bot. 15 ml, 30 ml. *otc.*
Use: Mydriatic, vasoconstrictor.

Clear Eyes Eye Drops. (Ross Laboratories) Naphazoline HCl 0.012%. Bot. 15 ml, 30 ml. *otc.*
Use: Mydriatic vasoconstrictor.

Clearly Cala-Gel. (Tec Laboratories, Inc.) Diphenhydramine HCl, zinc acetate, menthol, EDTA. Gel 180 g. *otc.*
Use: Antipruritic, topical.

Clearplan. (VLI) Ovulation prediction test. Box 10s.
Use: Diagnostic aid.

Clear Total Lice Elimination System. (Care Technologies, Inc.) **Shampoo:** Pyrethrum extract 0.3%, piperonyl butoxide 4%. 2 ml, 4 ml. **Lice egg remover:** Enzymes including oxidoreductase, tranferase, lyase, hydrolase, isomerase, ligase, hydroxyethyl cellulose, sodium benzoate. *otc.*
Use: Pediculicide.

Clear Tussin 30. (Zenith Goldline Pharmaceuticals) Dextromethorphan 15 mg, guaifenesin 100 mg/5 ml, alcohol, dye, sugar free. Liq. Bot. 118 ml. *otc.*
Use: Decongestant, expectorant.

•**clebopride.** (KLEH-boe-PRIDE) USAN.
Use: Antiemetic.

•**clemastine.** (KLEM-ass-teen) USAN.
Use: Antihistamine.
See: Tavist, Tab., Syr. (Novartis Pharmaceutical Corp.).

•**clemastine fumarate.** (KLEM-ass-teen) U.S.P. 23.
Use: Antihistamine.
See: Tavist, Tab., Syr. (Novartis Pharmaceutical Corp.).

clemastine fumarate. (Various Mfr.) Clemastine fumarate 0.5 mg/5 ml Syr. Bot. 118 ml, 480 ml. *Rx.*
Use: Antihistamine.

clemastine fumarate w/combinations.
See: Antihist-D, Tab. (Zenith Goldline Pharmaceuticals).

Clens. (Alcon Laboratories, Inc.) Cleansing agent with benzalkonium Cl 0.02%, EDTA 0.1%. Soln. Bot. 60 ml. *otc.*
Use: Contact lens care.

•**clentiazem maleate.** (klen-TIE-ah-zem) USAN.
Use: Antianginal, antihypertensive, antagonist (calcium channel).

Cleocin. (Pharmacia & Upjohn) Clindamycin HCl 75 mg, 150 mg, or 300 mg/Cap. Tartrazine, lactose. Bot. 100s (75 mg); 16s, 100s, UD 100s (150 mg, 300 mg). *Rx.*
Use: Anti-infective.

Cleocin Pediatric. (Pharmacia & Upjohn) Clindamycin palmitate 75 mg/5 ml. Gran. for Oral Soln. Bot. 100 ml. *Rx.*
Use: Anti-infective.

Cleocin Phosphate. (Pharmacia & Upjohn) Clindamycin phosphate 150 mg/ml. Vial 2 ml, 4 ml, 6 ml; *ADD-Vantage* Vial 4 ml, 6 ml; *Galaxy* Plastic Cont. 50 ml; Bulk pkg. 60 ml. *Rx.*
Use: Anti-infective.

Cleocin T. (Pharmacia & Upjohn) Clindamycin phosphate 10 mg/ml. Topical soln., gel, lot. Bot. 30 ml, 60 ml, pt. (topical soln.). Bot. 7.5 ml, 30 ml (gel). Lot. Bot. 60 ml (lotion). *Rx.*
Use: Anti-infective.

Cleocin Vaginal. (Pharmacia & Upjohn) Clindamycin phosphate 2%, mineral oil, benzyl alcohol, propylene glycol, polysorbate 60, sorbitan, monostearate. Cream. Tube with 7 disposable applicators 40 g. *Rx.*
Use: Anti-infective, vaginal.

Clerz Drops for Hard Lenses. (Ciba Vision) Hypertonic solution with hydroxyethylcellulose, sorbic acid, poloxamer 407, EDTA 0.1%, thimerosal 0.001%. Soln. Bot. 25 ml. *otc.*
Use: Contact lens care.

Clerz Drops for Soft Lenses. (Ciba Vision) Hypertonic solution with hydroxyethylcellulose, sodium borate, poloxamer 407, sorbic acid, thimerosal 0.001%, EDTA 0.1%. Soln. Bot. 25 ml. *otc.*
Use: Contact lens care.

Clerz 2 for Hard Lenses. (Ciba Vision) Isotonic solution with hydroxyethylcellulose, poloxamer 407, sodium Cl, potassium Cl, sodium borate, boric acid, sorbic acid, EDTA. Soln. Bot. 5 ml, 15 ml, 30 ml. *otc.*
Use: Contact lens care.

Clerz 2 for Soft Lenses. (Ciba Vision)

Isotonic solution with sodium Cl, potassium Cl, hydroxyethylcellulose, poloxamer 407, sodium borate, boric acid, sorbic acid, EDTA. Soln. Bot. 5 ml (2s), 15 ml, 30. *otc.*
Use: Contact lens care.

•**clidinium bromide.** (KLIH-dih-nee-uhm BROE-mide) U.S.P. 23.
Use: Anticholinergic.
See: Quarzan, Cap. (Roche Laboratories).
W/Chlordiazepoxide.
See: Librax, Cap. (Roche Laboratories).

Climara. (Berlex Laboratories, Inc.) Estradiol 3.9 mg, 5.85 mg, 7.8 mg/ Transdermal Patch. Box 4s. *Rx.*
Use: Estrogen.

•**clinafloxacin hydrochloride.** (klin-ah-FLOX-ah-sin) USAN.
Use: Anti-infective.

Clinda-Derm. (Paddock Laboratories) Clindamycin phosphate 10 mg/ml, isopropyl alcohol 51.5%, propylene glycol. Soln. Bot. 60 ml. *Rx.*
Use: Dermatologic, acne.

•**clindamycin.** (KLIN-dah-MY-sin) USAN.
Use: Anti-infective, dermatologic, acne. Oral as antibiotic. Vaginal as anti-infective. AIDS-associated pneumonia. [Orphan Drug]
See: Cleocin T (Pharmacia & Upjohn).
Cleocin (Pharmacia & Upjohn).
Cleocin Vaginal Cream (Pharmacia & Upjohn).
Clindets, Pledgets (Stiefel Laboratories, Inc.).

•**clindamycin hydrochloride.** (KLIN-dah-MY-sin) U.S.P. 23.
Use: Anti-infective.
See: Cleocin HCl A.D.T., Cap. (Pharmacia and Upjohn).

clindamycin hydrochloride. (KLIN-dah-MY-sin) (Various Mfr.) Clindamycin HCl 75 mg, 150 mg, Cap. Bot. 100s. *Rx.*
Use: Lincosamide.

•**clindamycin palmitate hydrochloride.** (KLIN-dah-MY-sin PAL-mih-tate) U.S.P. 23.
Use: Anti-infective.
See: Cleocin Pediatric (Pharmacia & Upjohn).
Cleocin T, Liq. (Pharmacia & Upjohn).

•**clindamycin phosphate.** (KLIN-dah-MY-sin) U.S.P. 23.
Use: Anti-infective.
See: Cleocin phosphate, Inj. (Pharmacia & Upjohn).
Clinda-Derm, Soln. (Paddock Laboratories).

clindamycin phosphate. (KLIN-dah-MY-sin) (Various Mfr.) **Inj.:** 150 mg/ml. Vial 2 ml, 4 ml, 6 ml, 60 ml, 100 ml. **Top. Soln., Gel, Lot.:** Clindamycin phosphate 10 mg/ml. Bot. 30 ml, 60 ml (Topical Soln.). Tube 30 ml (gel). Bot. 60 ml (lot.). *Rx.*
Use: Lincosamide; dermatologic, acne.

Clindets. (Stiefel Laboratories, Inc.) Clindamycin 1% (10 mg/ml). Pledgets. Pkg. 60s. *Rx.*
Use: Anti-infective.

Clindex. (Rugby Labs, Inc.)
See: Chlordiazepoxide and clindinium bromide (Chelsea Laboratories, Inc.).

Clinistix Reagent Strips. (Bayer Corp. (Consumer Div.)) Glucose oxidase, peroxidase and orthotolidine. Diagnostic test for glucose in urine. Bot. 50s.
Use: Diagnostic aid.

Clinitest. (Bayer Corp. (Consumer Div.)) 2-drop and 5-drop combination packages w/color charts for both 2-drop and 5-drop use. Reagent tablets containing copper sulfate, sodium hydroxide, heat-producing agents. Patient's plastic set; Tab. refills. **Box:** 100s, 500s, sealed in foil. **Child-resistant bot.:** 36s, 100s.
Use: Diagnostic aid.

clinocaine hydrochloride.
See: Procaine HCl.

Clinoril. (Merck & Co.) Sulindac 150 mg or 200 mg/Tab. Bot. 100s, UD 100s. Unit-of-use 60s, 100s. *Rx.*
Use: Analgesic, NSAID.

Clinoxide. (Geneva Pharmaceuticals) Clidinium 2.5 mg, chlordiazepoxide HCl, 5 mg. Cap. Bot. 100s, 500s. *c-IV.*
Use: Gastrointestinal, anticholinergic.

•**clioquinol.** (Klye-oh-KWIN-ole) U.S.P. 23. *Formerly Iodochlorhydroxyquin.*
Use: Antiamebic, anti-infective, topical.
See: HCV Cream (Saron).
Quin III, Cream (Teva Pharmaceuticals USA).
Quinoform, Oint., Cream, Lot. (C & M Pharmacal, Inc.).
Vioform, Prep. (Novartis Pharmaceutical Corp.).
W/Aluminum acetate solution, hydrocortisone.
See: Hysone, Cream (Roberts Pharmaceuticals).
W/Hydrocortisone acetate, lidocaine.
See: Lidaform-HC, Creme, Lot. (Bayer Corp. (Consumer Div.)).
W/Hydrocortisone, lidocaine.
See: HIL-20, Lot. (Solvay Pharmaceuticals).
W/Hydrocortisone, chlorobutanol.
See: HC-Form, Jelly (Recsei Laboratories).

W/Hydrocortisone, coal tar extract.
See: Sherform-HC, Oint. (Sheryl).
Enterex, Tab. (Person and Covey, Inc.).

clioquinol and hydrocortisone cream.
Use: Antifungal.
See: Caquin, Cream (Forest Pharmaceutical, Inc.).
Hysone, Cream (Roberts Pharmaceuticals).
Iohydro, Cream (Freeport).

clioquinol and hydrocortisone ointment.
Use: Antifungal.
See: Hysone, Cream (Roberts Pharmaceuticals).

•**clioxanide.** (klie-OX-ah-nide) USAN.
Use: Anthelmintic.

Clipoxide. (Schein Pharmaceutical, Inc.) Clidinium bromide 2.5 mg, chlordiazepoxide HCl 5 mg/Cap. Bot. 100s, 500s. *c-v.*
Use: Anticholinergic, antispasmodic.

•**cliprofen.** (klih-PRO-fen) USAN.
Use: Anti-inflammatory.

clobamine mesylate. (KLOE-bah-meen) Name previously used. See cilobamine mesylate.
Use: Antidepressant.

•**clobazam.** (KLOE-bazz-am) USAN.
Use: Anxiolytic.

•**clobetasol propionate.** (kloe-BEE-tah-sahl PRO-ee-oh-nate) U.S.P. 23.
Use: Anti-inflammatory.
See: Cormax, Oint. (Oclassen Pharmaceuticals, Inc.).
Temovate (GlaxoWellcome Dermatology).

clobetasol propionate. (Various Mfr.) **Cream:** 0.05%. Tube 15 g, 30 g, 45 g. **Ointment:** 0.05%, white petrolatum. 15 g, 30 g, 45 g.
Use: Corticosteroid, topical.

•**clobetasone butyrate.** (kloe-BEE-tih-sone BYOO-tah-rate) USAN.
Use: Corticosteroid, anti-inflammatory.

•**clocortolone acetate.** (kloe-CORE-toe-lone) USAN.
Use: Corticosteroid, topical.

•**clocortolone pivalate.** (kloe-CORE-toe-lone PIH-vah-late) U.S.P. 23.
Use: Corticosteroid, topical.

Clocream. (Pharmacia & Upjohn) Vitamins A and D in vanishing base. Tube oz. *otc.*
Use: Emollient.

•**clodanolene.** (Kloe-DAN-oh-leen) USAN.
Use: Muscle relaxant.

•**clodazon hydrochloride.** (KLOE-dah-zone) USAN.
Use: Antidepressant.

Cloderm. (Hermal Pharmaceutical Labs) Clocortolone pivalate cream 0.1%. Tube 15 g, 45 g. *Rx.*
Use: Corticosteroid, topical.

•**clodronic acid.** (kloe-DRAHN-ik acid) USAN.
Use: Calcium regulator.

•**clofazimine.** (kloe-FAZZ-ih-meen) U.S.P. 23.
Use: Anti-infective (tuberculostatic, leprostatic). [Orphan Drug]
See: Lamprene, Cap. (Novartis Pharmaceutical Corp.).

•**clofibrate.** (kloe-FIH-brate) U.S.P. 23.
Use: Antihyperlipidemic.
See: Atromid S, Cap. (Wyeth-Ayerst Laboratories).

•**clofilium phosphate.** (KLOE-FILL-ee-uhm) USAN.
Use: Cardiovascular agent (antiarrhythmic).

•**cloflucarban.** (KLOE-flew-CAR-ban) USAN.
Use: Antiseptic, disinfectant.

•**clogestone acetate.** (kloe-JESS-tone ASS-eh-tate) USAN. Under study.
Use: Hormone, progestin.

•**clomacran phosphate.** (KLOE-mah-KRAN) USAN. Under study.
Use: Antipsychotic.

•**clomegestone acetate.** (KLOE-meh-JESS-tone) USAN. Under study.
Use: Hormone, progestin.

•**clometherone.** (kloe-METH-ehr-OHN) USAN.
Use: Antiestrogen.

Clomid. (Hoechst Marion Roussel) Clomiphene citrate 50 mg/Tab. Ctn. 30s. *Rx.*
Use: Ovulation inducer.

•**clominorex.** (kloe-MEE-no-rex) USAN.
Use: Anorexic.

•**clomiphene citrate.** (KLOE-mih-feen SIH-trate) U.S.P. 23.
Use: Antiestrogen.
See: Clomid, Tab. (Hoechst Marion Roussel).
Serophene, Tab. (Serono Laboratories, Inc.).

clomiphene citrate. (Various Mfr.) 50 mg/Tab. Pkg. 10s, 30s. *Rx.*
Use: Ovulation inducer.

•**clomipramine hydrochloride.** (kloe-MIH-pruh-meen) USAN.
Use: Antidepressant.
See: Anafranil (Novartis Pharmaceutical Corp.).

clomipramine hydrochloride. (kloe-MIH-pruh-meen) (Apothecon, Inc.) Clomipramine HCl 25 mg, 50 mg, 75 mg. Cap. Bot. 100s. *Rx.*
Use: Antidepressant.

Clomycin. (Roberts Pharmaceuticals) Bacitracin 500 U, neomycin sulfate equivalent to 3.5 mg neomycin base, polymyxin B sulfate 5000 U, lidocaine 40 mg, yellow petrolatum, anhydrous, lanolin, light mineral oil/g. Oint. Tube 30 g. *otc.*
Use: Anti-infective, topical.

•**clonazepam.** (kloe-NAY-ze-pam) U.S.P. 23.
Use: Anticonvulsant.
See: Klonopin, Tab. (Roche Laboratories).

clonazepam. (Variuos Mfr.) 0.5 mg, 1 mg, 2 mg/Tab. Bot. 100s. *c-IV.*
Use: Anticonvulsant.

•**clonidine.** (KLOE-nih-DEEN) USAN.
Use: Antihypertensive.
See: Catapres (Boehringer Ingelheim, Inc.).

•**clonidine hydrochloride.** (KLOE-nih-DEEN) U.S.P. 23.
Use: Antihypertensive. Epidural use for pain in cancer patients. [Orphan Drug]
See: Catapres, Tab. (Boehringer Ingelheim, Inc.).
Duraclon, Inj. (Fujisawa USA, Inc.).

clonidine hydrochloride and chlorthalidone tablets. (Various Mfr.) Clonidine HCl 0.1 mg, 0.2 mg, 0.3 mg, chlorthalidone 15 mg/Tab. Bot. 100s, 500s, 1000s.
Use: Antihypertensive, diuretic.
See: Combipres, Tab. (Boehringer Ingelheim, Inc.).

•**clonitrate.** (KLOE-nye-trate) USAN.
Use: Coronary vasodilator.

•**clonixeril.** (kloe-NIX-ehr-ill) USAN.
Use: Analgesic.

•**clonixin.** (kloe-NIX-in) USAN.
Use: Analgesic.

•**clopamide.** (kloe-PAM-id) USAN.
Use: Antihypertensive, diuretic.

•**clopenthixol.** (KLOE-pen-THIX-ole) USAN.
Use: Antipsychotic.

•**cloperidone hydrochloride.** (KLOE-per-ih-dohn) USAN.
Use: Hypnotic, sedative.

clophenoxate hydrochloride.
Use: Cerebral stimulant.

•**clopidogrel bisulfate.** (kloe-PIH-doe-grell bye-SULL-fate) USAN.
Use: Platelet inhibitor.
See: Plavix, Tab. (Sanofi Winthrop Pharmaceuticals).

•**clopimozide.** (KLOE-PIM-oh-zide) USAN.
Use: Antipsychotic.

•**clopipazan mesylate.** (KLOE-pip-ah-ZAN) USAN.
Use: Antipsychotic.

•**clopirac.** (KLOE-pih-rack) USAN.
Use: Anti-inflammatory.

•**cloprednol.** (kloe-PRED-nahl) USAN.
Use: Corticosteroid, topical.

•**cloprostenol sodium.** (kloe-PROSTE-een-ole) USAN.
Use: Prostaglandin.

•**clorazepate dipotassium.** (klor-AZE-eh-PATE DIE-poe-TASS-ee-uhm) U.S.P. 23.
Use: Anxiolytic, anticonvulsant.
See: Tranxene, Prods. (Abbott Laboratories).

clorazepate dipotassium. (Various Mfr.) 3.75 mg, 7.5 mg, 15 mg/Tab. Bot. 30s, 100s, 500s. *c-IV.*
Use: Anxiolytic, anticonvulsant.

•**clorazepate monopotassium.** (clor-AZE-eh-PATE MAHN-oh-poe-TASS-ee-uhm) USAN.
Use: Anxiolytic.

•**clorethate.** (klahr-ETH-ate) USAN.
Use: Hypnotic, sedative.

•**clorexolone.** (KLOR-ex-oh-LONE) USAN.
Use: Diuretic.

Clorfed II. (Stewart-Jackson Pharmacal, Inc.) Chlorpheniramine 4 mg, pseudoephedrine 60 mg/Tab. Bot. 100s. *otc.*
Use: Antihistamine, decongestant.

Clorfed Capsules. (Stewart-Jackson Pharmacal, Inc.) Chlorpheniramine 8 mg, pseudoephedrine 120 mg/Cap. Bot. 100s. *Rx-otc.*
Use: Antihistamine, decongestant.

Clorfed Expectorant. (Stewart-Jackson Pharmacal, Inc.) Pseudoephedrine 30 mg, guaifenesin 100 mg, codeine 10 mg/5 ml. Bot. Pt. *c-v.*
Use: Antitussive, decongestant, expectorant.

•**cloroperone hydrochloride.** (KLOR-oh-PURR-ohn) USAN.
Use: Antipsychotic.

•**clorophene.** (KLOR-oh-feen) USAN.
Use: Disinfectant.

Clorpactin WCS-90. (Guardian Laboratories) Sodium oxychlorosene 2 g. Bot. 5s.
Use: Antiseptic.

•**clorprenaline hydrochloride.** (klor-PREN-ah-leen) USAN.
Use: Bronchodilator.

•**clorsulon.** (KLOR-sull-ahn) U.S.P. 23.
Use: Antiparasitic, fasciolicide.

•**clortermine hydrochloride.** (klor-TER-meen) USAN.
Use: Anorexic.

•**closantel.** (KLOSE-an-tell) USAN.
Use: Anthelmintic.

•**closiramine aceturate.** (kloe-SIH-rah-meen ah-SEE-tur-ate) USAN.
Use: Antihistamine.

clostridial collagenase.
Use: Dupuytren's disease. [Orphan Drug]

•**clothiapine.** (KLOE-THIGH-ah-peen) USAN.
Use: Antipsychotic.

•**clothixamide maleate.** (kloe-THIX-ah-mid) USAN.
Use: Antipsychotic.

•**cloticasone propionate.** (kloe-TICK-ah-SONE PRO-pee-oh-nate) USAN.
Use: Anti-inflammatory.

•**clotrimazole.** (kloe-TRIM-uh-zole) U.S.P. 23.
Use: Antifungal.
See: Fungoid, Cream, Soln. (Pedinol Pharmacal, Inc.).
Gyne-Lotrimin (Schering-Plough Corp.).
Lotrimin, Cream, Soln. (Schering-Plough Corp.).
Mycelex, Cream, Soln., Tab. (Bayer Corp. (Consumer Div.)).
Mycelex-7, Vaginal Cream, Tab. (Bayer Corp. (Consumer Div.)).
Mycelex-7 Combination Pack (Bayer Corp. (Consumer Div.)).
Mycelex-G, Vaginal Supp. (Bayer Corp. (Consumer Div.)).

clotrimazole. (Various Mfr.) **Vaginal Tab.:** 100 mg, in 7s with applicator. **Vaginal cream:** 1% Tube 45 g with applicator.
Use: Antifungal, *Candida* infections.

clotrimazole. (NMC Laboratories) Clotrimazole 1%, benzyl alcohol. Vaginal cream. In 45 g with 7 disposable applicators. *otc.*
Use: Antifungal, vaginal.

clotrimazole. (Taro Pharmaceuticals USA, Inc.) Clotrimazole 1% in a vanishing cream base, benzyl alcohol 1%, cetostearyl alcohol. Cream. Tube 15 g, 30 g, 45 g, 2 × 45 g. *otc.*
Use: Antifungal, topical.

clotrimazole and betamethasone dipropionate cream.
Use: Antifungal, anti-inflammatory.

clotrimidazole. (Fujisawa USA, Inc.)
Use: Sickle cell disease. [Orphan Drug]

clove oil.
Use: Pharmaceutic aid (flavor).

Cloverine. (Medtech Laboratories, Inc.) White salve. Tin Oz. *otc.*
Use: Dermatologic, counterirritant.

Clovocain. (Vita Elixir) Benzocaine, oil of cloves. *otc.*
Use: Anesthetic, local.

•**cloxacillin benzathine.** (KLOX-ah-SILL-in BENZ-ah-theen) U.S.P. 23.
Use: Anti-infective.

•**cloxacillin sodium.** (KLOX-ah-SILL-in) U.S.P. 23.
Use: Anti-infective, penicillin.
See: Cloxapen, Cap. (SmithKline Beecham Pharmaceuticals).

cloxacillin sodium. (KLOX-ah-SILL-in SO-dee-uhm) (Various Mfr.) **Cap.:** 250 mg, 500 mg. Bot. 100s, UD 100s (250 mg only). **Pow. for Oral Soln.:** 125 mg/5 ml when reconstituted. Bot. 100 ml, 200 ml. *Rx.*
Use: Anti-infective, penicillin.

Cloxapen. (SmithKline Beecham Pharmaceuticals) Cloxacillin sodium 250 mg or 500 mg/Cap. Bot. 30s (500 mg only), 100s, UD 100s (500 mg only). *Rx.*
Use: Anti-infective, penicillin.

•**cloxyquin.** (KLOX-ee-kwin) USAN.
Use: Anti-infective.

•**clozapine.** (KLOE-zuh-PEEN) USAN.
Use: Antipsychotic.
See: Clozaril (Novartis Pharmaceutical Corp.).

clozapine. (KLOE-zuh-PEEN) (Zenith Goldline) Clozapine 25 mg, 100 mg. Tab. Bot. 100s, 500s, 1000s, 4000s, 5000s. *Rx.*
Use: Antipsychotic.

Clozaril. (Novartis Pharmaceutical Corp.) Clozapine 25 mg, 100 mg/Tab. UD 100s, total daily dose packages of 150 mg, 200 mg, 250 mg, 300 mg, 400 mg, 500 mg, 600 mg/day. *Rx.*
Use: Antipsychotic.

Clysodrast. (Rhone-Poulenc Rorer Pharmaceuticals, Inc.) Tannic acid, 2.5 g, bisacodyl 1.5 mg/Pkt. Pow. Box 25s, 50s. *Rx.*
Use: Laxative.

C-Max. (Bio-Technology General Corporation) Vitamin C 1000 mg, Mg 40 mg, Zn 5 mg, K 10 mg, Mn 1 mg, pectin 10 mg in a base of rose hips. Tab. Bot. 100s. *otc.*
Use: Mineral, vitamin supplement.

C.M.C. Cellulose Gum.
See: Carboxymethylcellulose Sodium, Preps.

CMV. (Wampole Laboratories) Cyto-

megalovirus antibody test system for the qualitative and semi-quantitative detection of CMV antibody in human serum. Test 100s.
Use: Diagnostic aid.

CMV-IGIV.
Use: Immunization.
See: Cytogam, Vial (MedImmune, Inc.).
Cytomegalovirus Immune Globulin Intravenous (Human).

Coadvil. (Whitehall Robins Laboratories) Ibuprofen 200 mg, pseudoephedrine HCl 30 mg/Tab. Bot. 100s. *otc.*
Use: Analgesic, decongestant.

coagulation factor ix.
Use: Antihemophilic. [Orphan Drug]
See: Mononine (Centeon).

coagulation factor ix (human).
Use: Antihemophilic. [Orphan Drug]
See: AlphaNine (Alpha Therapeutic Corp.).

coagulation factor ix (recombinant).
Use: Antihemophilic. [Orphan Drug]
See: BeneFix (Genetics Institute).

coagulation factor VIIa (recombinant).
Use: Antihemophilic.
See: NovoSeven, Pow. for Inj. (Novo Nordisk).

coagulants.
See: Hemostatics.

•**coal tar.** U.S.P. 23.
Use: Topical antieczematic; antipsoriatic.
See: Balnetar, Liq. (Westwood Squibb Pharmaceuticals).
Creamy Tar, Shampoo (C & M Pharmacal).
Estar, Gel (Westwood Squibb Pharmaceuticals).
L.C.D. Compound, Oint., Soln. (Almay, Inc.).
Polytar Bath, Liq. (Stiefel Laboratories, Inc.).
Protar Protein, Shampoo (Dermol Pharmaceuticals, Inc.).
Tarbonis, Cream (Schwarz Pharma, Inc.).
Zetar, Preps. (Dermik Laboratories, Inc.).
W/Allantoin, hydrocortisone.
See: Alphosyl-HC, Lot., Cream (Schwarz Pharma, Inc.).
W/Hydrocortisone.
See: Doak Oil Forte, Liq. (Doak Dermatologics).
Ze Tar-Quin, Cream (Dermik Laboratories, Inc.).
W/Iodoquinol, hydrocortisone.
See: Tarcotin, Cream (Schwarz Pharma, Inc.).
W/Zinc oxide.
See: Tarpaste, Paste (Doak Dermatologics).

coal tar, distillate.
Use: Dermatologic, topical.
See: Lavatar, Liq. (Doak Dermatologics).
Syntar, Cream (Zeneca Pharmaceuticals).
W/Sulfur, salicylic acid.
See: Pragatar, Oint. (Menley & James).

coal tar extract.
Use: Dermatologic, topical.
See: Pentrax Gold, Shampoo (Gen Derm).
W/Allantoin, hexachlorophene.
See: Sebical Cream (Schwarz Pharma, Inc.).
W/Allantoin, hexachlorophene, glycerin, lanolin.
See: Pso-Rite, Cream (DePree).
W/Allantoin, salicylic acid, perhydrosqualene.
See: Skaylos, Cream (Ambix Laboratories, Inc.).
Skaylos, Lot. (Ambix Laboratories, Inc.).
W/Salicylic acid.
See: Neutrogena T/Sal, Shampoo (Neutrogena).

coal tar paste.
Use: Dermatologic, topical.
W/Zinc paste.
See: Tarpaste, Paste (Doak Dermatologics).

coal tar topical solution. Liquor Carbonis Detergens. L.C.D.
Use: Antieczematic, topical.
See: Advanced Formula Tegrin, Shampoo (Block Drug Co., Inc.).
Balnetar, Liq. (Westwood Squibb Pharmaceuticals).
Creamy Tar, Shampoo (C & M Pharmacal).
Estar, Gel (Westwood Squibb Pharmaceuticals).
High Potency Tar (C & M Pharmacal).
L.C.D. Compound Oint., Soln. (Almay, Inc.).
MG217 Medicated, Shampoo, Cond. (Triton Consumer Products, Inc.).
Psorigel, Gel (Galderma Laboratories, Inc.).
PsoriNail, Liq. (Summers Laboratories, Inc.).
Wright's, Soln. (E. Fougera and Co.).
Zetar, Emulsion, Shampoo (Dermik Laboratories, Inc.).
W/Allantoin, psorilan, myristate.
See: Iocon, Shampoo (Galderma Laboratories, Inc.).

Psorelief, Cream (Quality Formulations, Inc.).
W/Hydrocortisone, iodoquinol.
See: Cor-Tar-Quin, Cream, Lot. (Bayer Corp.).
W/Hydrocortisone alcohol, clioquinololine, diperodon HCl, vitamins A, D.
See: Pentarcort, Cream (Dalin).
W/Robane (perhydrosqualene).
See: Skaylos, Shampoo (Ambix Laboratories).
W/Salicylic acid.
See: Ionil T, Shampoo (Galderma Laboratories, Inc.).
W/Salicylic acid, sulfur, protein.
See: Vanseb-T Tar, Shampoo (Allergan).

Co-Apap. (Various Mfr.) Pseudoephedrine HCl 30 mg, chlorpheniramine maleate 2 mg, dextromethorphan HBr 15 mg, acetaminophen 325 mg/Tab. Bot. 24s, 50s, 1000s. *otc.*
Use: Analgesic, antihistamine, antitussive, decongestant.

cobalamine concentrate. U.S.P. 23.
Use: Hematopoietic vitamin.
See: Vitamin B_{12} (Various Mfr.).

cobalt chloride.
W/Ferrous gluconate, vitamin B_{12}, duodenum whole desiccated.
See: Bitrinsic-E, Cap. (Zeneca).

cobalt gluconate.
W/Ferrous gluconate, vitamin B_{12} activity, desiccated stomach substance, folic acid.
See: Chromagen, Cap., Inj. (Savage Laboratories).

cobalt-labeled vitamin B_{12}.
See: Rubratope-57 (Bristol-Myers Squibb).

cobalt standards for vitamin B_{12}.
See: Cobatope-57, and Cobatope-60 (Bristol-Myers Squibb).

•**cobaltous chloride Co 57.** (koe-BALL-tuss) USAN.
Use: Radiopharmaceutical.

•**cobaltous chloride Co 60.** USAN.
Use: Radiopharmaceutical.

cobatope-57. (Bristol-Myers Squibb) Cobaltous Cl Co 57.

cobex 1000. (Standex) Vitamin B_{12} 1000 mcg/10 ml. Vial 30 ml. *Rx.*
Use: Vitamin supplement.

Co-Bile. (Western Research) Hog bile 64.8 mg, pancreas substance 64.8 mg, papain-pepsin complex 97.2 mg, diatase malt 16.2 mg, papain 48.6 mg, pepsin 48.6 mg/Tab. Bot. 1000s. *Rx-otc.*
Use: Digestive enzyme.

•**cocaine.** (koe-CANE) U.S.P. 23.
Use: Anesthetic, local.

•**cocaine hydrochloride.** U.S.P. 23.
Use: Anesthetic, local.

cocaine HCl. Top. Soln.: Cocaine HCl 4%, 10%/Bot. 10 ml, UD 4 ml. (Various Mfr.). **Pow.:** 5 g, 25 g. (Mallinckrodt). *c-II.*
Use: Mucosal anesthetic.

cocaine viscous. (Various Mfr.) Cocaine viscous 4%, 10%/Soln. Top. Bot. 10 ml, UD 4 ml. *c-II.*
Use: Anesthetic, local.

•**coccidioidin.** (cox-id-ee-OY-din) U.S.P. 23.
Use: Diagnostic aid (dermal reactive indicator).
See: Spherulin (ALK Laboratories, Inc.).

cocculin.
See: Picrotoxin, Inj. (Various Mfr.).

Cocilan Syrup. (Health for Life Brands, Inc.) Euphorbia, wild lettuce, cocillana, squill, senega, cascarin (bitterless). Bot. Gal. Available w/codeine. Bot. Gal.

cocoa.
Use: Pharmaceutic aid (flavor; flavored vehicle).

•**cocoa butter.** N.F. 18.
Use: Pharmaceutic aid (suppository base).

Codamine Pediatric Syrup. (Alpharma USPD Inc.) Hydrocodone bitartrate 2.5 mg, phenylpropanolamine HCl 12.5 mg/5 ml. Bot. Pt. *c-III.*
Use: Antitussive, decongestant.

Codamine Syrup. (Zenith Goldline Pharmaceuticals) Hydrocodone bitartrate 5 mg, phenylpropanolamine HCl 25 mg/5 ml. Bot. Pt, gal. *c-III.*
Use: Antitussive, decongestant.

Codanol. (A.P.C.) Vitamins A, D, hexachlorophene, zinc oxide. Oint. Tube 1.5 oz, 4 oz, Jar lb. *otc.*
Use: Dermatologic, counterirritant.

Codap. (Solvay Pharmaceuticals) Codeine phosphate 32 mg, acetaminophen 325 mg/Tab. Bot. 250s. *c-III.*
Use: Analgesic combination.

Codegest Expectorant. (Great Southern Laboratories) Guaifenesin 100 mg, phenylpropanolamine HCl 12.5 mg, codeine phosphate 10 mg/5 ml. Alcohol, dye free. Liq. Bot. Pt, gal. *c-V.*
Use: Antitussive, decongestant, expectorant.

Codehist DH Elixir. (Geneva Pharmaceuticals) Pseudoephedrine 30 mg, chlorpheniramine maleate 2 mg, codeine phosphate 10 mg/5 ml, alcohol 5.7%. Bot. 120 ml, 480 ml. *c-V.*
Use: Antihistamine, antitussive, decongestant.

•**codeine.** (KOE-deen) U.S.P. 23.
Use: Analgesic, narcotic; antitussive.

codeine combinations.
See: Actifed, Expectorant, Syr. (GlaxoWellcome).
Anexsia w/Codeine, Tab. (SmithKline Beecham Pharmaceuticals).
APAP w/Codeine, Tab. (Schwarz Pharma, Inc.).
A.P.C. w/Codeine, Tab. (Various Mfr.).
Ascriptin W/Codeine No. 2, Tab. (Rhone-Poulenc Rorer Pharmaceuticals, Inc.).
Ascriptin W/Codeine No. 3, Tab. (Rhone-Poulenc Rorer Pharmaceuticals, Inc.).
Brontex (Procter & Gamble).
Calcidrine Syr. (Abbott Laboratories).
Capital w/Codeine, Susp. (Carnrick Laboratories, Inc.).
Cheracol, Syr. (Pharmacia & Upjohn).
Chlor-Trimeton Expectorant (Schering-Plough Corp.).
Cycofed Pediatric, Syr. (Cypress).
Deconsal Pediatric, Syr. (Medeva Pharmaceuticals, Inc.).
Drucon w/Codeine, Liq. (Standard Drug Co.).
Empirin No. 1, No. 2, No. 3, No. 4, Tab. (GlaxoWellcome).
Fiorinal w/Codeine, Cap. (Novartis Pharmaceutical Corp.).
Golacol, Syr. (Arcum).
Guaifenesin DAC, Liq. (Cypress).
Novahistine, Expectorant (Hoechst Marion Roussel).
Nucofed, Liq. (SmithKline Beecham).
Partuss AC (Parmed Pharmaceuticals, Inc.).
Pediacof, Syr. (Sanofi Winthrop Pharmaceuticals).
Phenaphen #2, #3, #4, Cap. (Wyeth-Ayerst Laboratories).
Phenergan Expectorant w/Codeine, Troches (Wyeth-Ayerst Laboratories).
Proval No. 3, Tab. (Solvay Pharmaceuticals).
Robitussin A-C, DAC (Wyeth-Ayerst Laboratories).
Tolu-Sed, Elix. (Scherer Laboratories, Inc).
Tussar-2, Syr. (Rhone-Poulenc Rorer Pharmaceuticals, Inc.).
Tussar SF, Liq. (Rhone-Poulenc Rorer Pharmaceuticals, Inc.).
Tussi-Organidin, Prods. (Wallace Laboratories).
Tylenol w/Codeine No. 1, No. 2, No. 3, No. 4 Tab. (Ortho McNeil Pharmaceutical).
Tylenol w/Codeine, Elix. (Ortho McNeil Pharmaceutical).
Vasotus, Liq. (Sheryl).

codeine methylbromide. Eucodin.
Use: Antitussive.

•**codeine phosphate.** (KOE-deen FOSS-fate) U.S.P. 23.
Use: Analgesic, narcotic; antitussive.

codeine phosphate. (KOE-deen FOSS-fate) (Roxane) **Oral Soln.:** 15 mg/5 ml. Bot. 500 ml, UD 5 ml. *c-II.*
Use: Analgesic, narcotic.

codeine phosphate. (Various Mfr.) **Inj.:** 30 mg, 60 mg. Vial 1 ml (30 mg only), *Tubex* 1 ml. *c-II.*
Use: Analgesic, narcotic; antitussive.

codeine phosphate and guaifenesin. (Zenith Goldline Pharmaceuticals) Codeine phosphate 10 mg, guaifenesin 300 mg/Tab. Bot. 100s. *c-III.*
Use: Expectorant, narcotic antitussive.

•**codeine polistirex.** (KOE-deen pahl-ee-STIE-rex) USAN.
Use: Antitussive.

codeine resin complex combinations.
See: Omni-Tuss, Liq. (Medeva Pharmaceuticals, Inc.).

•**codeine sulfate.** (KOE-deen) U.S.P. 23.
Use: Analgesic, antitussive, narcotic.

codeine sulfate. (KOE-deen) (Various Mfr.) Codeine sulfate 15 mg, 30 mg, 60 mg. Tab. Bot. 100s, UD 100s. *c-II.*
Use: Analgesic, narcotic.

codelcortone.
See: Prednisolone.

Codiclear DH. (Schwarz Pharma, Inc.) Hydrocodone bitartrate 5 mg, guaifenesin 100 mg/5 ml. Syr. Bot. 4 oz, pt. *c-III.*
Use: Antitussive, expectorant.

Codimal. (Schwarz Pharma, Inc.) Chlorpheniramine maleate 2 mg, pseudoephedrine HCl 30 mg, acetaminophen 325 mg/Cap. or Tab. Bot. 24s, 100s, 1000s. *otc.*
Use: Analgesic, antihistamine, decongestant.

Codimal DH Syrup. (Schwarz Pharma, Inc.) Hydrocodone bitartrate 1.66 mg, phenylephrine HCl 5 mg, pyrilamine maleate 8.33 mg/5 ml. Bot. 4 oz, pt, gal. *c-III.*
Use: Antihistamine, antitussive, decongestant.

Codimal DM. (Schwarz Pharma, Inc.) Dextromethorphan HBr 10 mg, phenylephrine HCl 5 mg, pyrilamine maleate 8.33 mg/5 ml, alcohol 4%, saccharin, sorbitol. Sugar free. Syr. Bot. 4 oz, pt, gal. *otc.*

Use: Antitussive, antihistamine, decongestant.

Codimal-L.A. (Schwarz Pharma, Inc.) Chlorpheniramine maleate 8 mg, pseudoephedrine HCl 120 mg/SR Cap. Bot. 100s, 1000s. *Rx.*
Use: Antihistamine, decongestant.

Codimal-L.A. Half Capsules. (Schwarz Pharma, Inc.) Pseudoephedrine HCl 60 mg, chlorpheniramine maleate 4 mg, sucrose. Cap. Bot. 100s. *Rx.*
Use: Antihistamine, decongestant.

Codimal PH Syrup. (Schwarz Pharma, Inc.) Codeine phosphate 10 mg, phenylephrine HCl 5 mg, pyrilamine maleate 8.33 mg/5 ml. Bot. 4 oz, pt, gal. *c-v.*
Use: Antihistamine, antitussive, decongestant.

Codimal Tablets. (Schwarz Pharma, Inc.) Chlorpheniramine maleate 2 mg, pseudoephedrine HCl 30 mg, acetaminophen 325 mg/Tab. Bot. 24s, 100s, 1000s.
Use: Analgesic, antihistamine, decongestant.

•**cod liver oil.** U.S.P. 23. Emulsion.
Use: Vitamin A and D therapy.
See: Cod Liver Oil Concentrate, Cap. (Schering-Plough Corp.).
W/Anesthesin, zinc oxide, hydroxyquinoline.
See: Medicone Dressing. (Medicore).
W/Benzocaine.
See: Morusan, Oint. (SmithKline Beecham Pharmaceuticals).
W/Creosote.
See: Cod liver oil 9 min, creosote 1 min/ Cap. Bot. 100s (Bryant).
W/Malt extract.
See: Vitamins A, D (GlaxoWellcome).
W/Methylbenzethonium Cl.
See: Benephen, Prods. (Halsted).
W/Viosterol.
See: Vitamins A, D (Abbott Laboratories).
Vitamins A, D (Bristol-Myers Squibb).
W/Zinc oxide.
See: Desitin, Preps. (Pfizer US Pharmaceutical Group).

cod liver oil concentrate. (Schering-Plough Corp.) Concentrate of cod liver oil with vitamins A and D added. **Cap.:** Bot. 40s, 100s. **Tab.:** Bot. 100s, 240s. Also W/Vitamin C. Bot. 100s. *otc.*
Use: Vitamin supplement.

cod liver oil ointment. *otc.*

codorphone hydrochloride. (KOE-dahr-fone) Name previously used for Conorphone HCl.
Use: Analgesic.
See: Conorphone HCl.

•**codoxime.** (CODE-ox-eem) USAN.
Use: Antitussive.

codoxy. (Halsey Drug Co.) Oxycodone HCl 4.5 mg, oxycodone terephthalate 0.38 mg, aspirin 325 mg/Tab. Bot. 100s.
Use: Analgesic combination.

Cogentin. (Merck & Co.) Benztropine mesylate. **Tab.:** 0.5 mg Bot. 100s; 1 mg Bot. 100s, UD 100s; 2 mg Bot. 100s, 1000s, UD 100s. **Inj.:** Benztropine mesylate 1 mg/ml w/sodium Cl 9 mg and water for injection q.s. to 1 ml Amp. 2 ml, Box 6s. *Rx.*
Use: Antiparkinsonian.

Co-Gesic. (Schwarz Pharma, Inc.) Hydrocodone bitartrate 5 mg, acetaminophen 500 mg/Tab. Bot. 100s, 500s. *c-III.*
Use: Analgesic combination.

Cognex. (Parke-Davis) Tacrine HCl 10 mg, 20 mg, 30 mg, 40 mg/Cap. Bot. 120s, UD 100s. *Rx.*
Use: Psychotherapeutic.

Co-Hep-Tral. (Davis & Sly) Folic acid 10 mg, vitamin B_{12} 100 mcg, liver injection q.s./ml. Vial 10 ml. *Rx.*
Use: Mineral, vitamin supplement.

Co-Hist. (Roberts Pharmaceuticals) Pseudoephedrine HCl 30 mg, chlorpheniramine 2 mg, acetaminophen 325 mg/Tab. Bot. 500s, 1000s. *otc.*
Use: Analgesic, antihistamine, decongestant.

Colabid. (Major Pharmaceuticals) Probenecid 500 mg, colchicine 0.5 mg/ Tab. Bot. 100s, 1000s. *Rx.*
Use: Antigout.

Colace. (Bristol-Myers Squibb) Docusate sodium. **Syr.:** 60 mg/15 ml with alcohol < 1%. Bot. 240 ml, 480 ml. **Liq.:** 150 mg/15 ml. Bot. 30 ml, 480 ml with calibrated droppers. *otc.*
Use: Laxative.

Colagyn. (Smith & Nephew United) Zinc sulfocarbolate, potassium, oxyquinoline sulfate, lactic acid, boric acid. Jelly. Tube w/applicator and refill 6 oz. Douche Pow. 3 oz, 7 oz, 14 oz. *otc.*

Colana Syrup. (Hance) Euphorbia pilulifera tincture 8 ml, wild lettuce syrup 8 ml, cocillana tincture 2.5 ml, squill compound syrup 1.5 ml, cascara 0.25 g, menthol 4.8 mg/fl oz. Bot. 4 fl oz, gal. Also w/Dionin 15 mg/fl oz. Bot. gal.

Co-Lav. (Copley Pharmaceutical, Inc.) Polyethylene glycol 3350 60 g, sodium chloride 1.46 g, potassium chloride 0.745 g, sodium bicarbonate 1.68 g, sodium sulfate 5.68 g per L/Pow. for Soln. Jug 4 L. *Rx.*

Use: Bowel evacuant.

Colax. (Rugby Labs, Inc.) Docusate sodium 100 mg, phenolphthalein 65 mg/Tab. Bot. 30s. *otc.*
Use: Laxative.

•**colchicine.** (KOHL-chih-seen) U.S.P. 23.
Use: Gout suppressant. Treat multiple sclerosis [Orphan Drug]
W/Benemid.
See: Benn-C, Tab. (Scrip).
Col-Probenecid, Tab. (Various Mfr.).
W/Sodium salicylate, calcium carbonate, dried aluminum hydroxide gel, phenobarbital.
See: Apcogesic, Tabs. (Apco).

colchicine. (Various Mfr.) Colchicine 0.5 mg, 0.6 mg. Tab. Bot. 100s. *Rx.*
Use: Gout suppressant. Treat multiple sclerosis [Orphan Drug]

colchicine salicylate.
W/Phenobarbital, sodium p-aminobenzoate, vitamin B_1, aspirin.
See: Doloral, Tab. (Alamed).

Cold & Allergy. (Zenith Goldline Pharmaceuticals) Phenylpropanolamine HCl 12.5 mg, brompheniramine maleate 2 mg/5 ml. Elix. Bot. 118 ml, 237 ml, 473 ml, gal. *otc.*
Use: Antihistamine, decongestant.

cold cream. U.S.P. 23.
Use: Emollient; water in oil emulsion ointment base.

Cold-Gest Cold. (Major Pharmaceuticals) Chlorpheniramine maleate 8 mg, pseudoephedrine HCl 75 mg/Cap. Pkg. 10s, 20s. *otc.*
Use: Antihistamine, decongestant.

Coldloc. (Fleming & Co.) Phenylpropanolamine HCl 20 mg, phenylephrine 5 mg, guaifenesin 100 mg/5 ml, sorbitol. Alcohol, sugar, dye free. Elix. Bot. Pt. *Rx.*
Use: Decongestant, expectorant.

Coldloc-LA. (Fleming & Co.) Phenylpropanolamine HCl 75 mg, guaifenesin 600 mg/SR Cap. Bot. 50s, 100s. *Rx.*
Use: Decongestant, expectorant.

Coldonyl. (Dover Pharmaceuticals) Acetaminophen, phenylephrine HCl/Tab. Sugar, lactose, salt free. UD 500s. *otc.*
Use: Analgesic, decongestant.

Coldran. (Halsey Drug Co.) Phenylephrine HCl 5 mg, chlorpheniramine maleate 2 mg, salicylamide 1.5 gr, acetaminophen 0.5 gr, caffeine/Tab. Bot. 30s. *otc.*
Use: Analgesic, antihistamine, decongestant.

Cold Relief. (Rugby Labs, Inc.) Phenylpropanolamine HCl 12.5 mg, chlorpheniramine maleate 2 mg, dextromethorphan HBr 10 mg, acetaminophen 325 mg/Tab. Bot. 50s. *otc.*
Use: Analgesic, antihistamine, antitussive, decongestant.

Coldrine. (Roberts Pharmaceuticals) Acetaminophen 325 mg, pseudoephedrine HCl 30 mg, sodium metabisulfite/Tab. Bot. 1000s, 500s (packets), 4-dose boxes. *otc.*
Use: Analgesic, decongestant.

Cold Sore Lotion. (Purepac Pharmaceutical Co.) Camphor, benzoin, aluminum Cl. Bot. 0.5 oz.
Use: Cold sores, fever blisters.

Cold Symptoms Relief. (Major Pharmaceuticals) Pseudoephedrine HCl 30 mg, chlorpheniramine maleate 2 mg, dextromethorphan HBr 10 mg, acetaminophen 325 mg/Tab. Bot. 50s. *otc.*
Use: Analgesic, antihistamine, antitussive, decongestant.

Cold Tablets. (Walgreen Co.) Phenylephrine HCl 5 mg, chlorpheniramine maleate 2 mg, acetaminophen 325 mg/Tab. Bot. 50s. *otc.*
Use: Analgesic, antihistamine, decongestant.

Cold Tablets Multiple Symptom. (Walgreen Co.) Acetaminophen 500 mg, pseudoephedrine HCl 30 mg, chlorpheniramine maleate 2 mg, dextromethorphan HBr 10 mg/Tab. Bot. 50s. *otc.*
Use: Analgesic, antihistamine, antitussive, decongestant.

•**colesevelam hydrochloride.** (koe-leh-SEH-veh-lam) USAN.
Use: Antihyperlipidemic.

Colestid. (Pharmacia & Upjohn) Colestipol HCl. **Unflavored Gran.:** Bot. 300 g, 500 g. Pkt. 5 g. **Flavored Gran.:** Bot. 450 g. Pkt. 7.5 g (5 g colestipol HCl). *Rx.*
Use: Antihyperlipidemic.

Colestid Tablets. (Pharmacia & Upjohn) Colestipol HCl 1 g/Tab. 120s, 250s. *Rx.*
Use: Antihyperlipidemic.

•**colestipol hydrochloride.** (koe-LESS-tih-pole) U.S.P. 23.
Use: Antihyperlipidemic.
See: Colestid (Pharmacia & Upjohn).

•**colestolone.** (koe-LESS-toe-LONE) USAN.
Use: Hypolipidemic.

Col-Evac. (Forest Pharmaceutical, Inc.) Potassium bitartrate, bicarbonate of soda and a blended base of polyethylene glycols. Supp. 2s, 12s.
Use: Laxative.

Colfed-A. (Parmed Pharmaceuticals, Inc.) Pseudoephedrine HCl 120 mg, chlorpheniramine maleate 8 mg. Cap. Bot 100s. *Rx.*
Use: Antihistamine, decongestant.

•**colforsin.** (kole-FAR-sin) USAN.
Use: Antiglaucoma agent.

•**colfosceril palmitate.** (kahl-FOSE-uhr-ILL PAL-mih-TATE) USAN.
Use: Pulmonary surfactant, antiatelectic; prevention/treatment of hyaline membrane disease. [Orphan Drug]
See: Exosurf (GlaxoWellcome).

colfosceril palmitate, cetyl alcohol, tyloxapol.
Use: Hyaline membrane disease; adult respiratory distress syndrome. [Orphan Drug]
See: Exosurf Neonatal for Intrathecal Suspension (GlaxoWellcome).

colimycin sodium methanesulfonate. (Parke-Davis)
See: Colistimethate Sodium.

colimycin sulfate.
See: Coly-Mycin, Preps. (Parke-Davis).

•**colistimethate sodium.** (koe-LISS-tih-METH-ate) U.S.P. 23.
Use: Anti-infective.
See: Coly-Mycin M Parenteral, Inj. (Parke-Davis).

colistin base.
W/Neomycin base, hydrocortisone acetate, thonzonium bromide, polysorbate 80, acetic acid, sodium acetate.
See: Coly-Mycin Otic W/Neomycin and Hydrocortisone, Liq. (Parke-Davis).
Cortisporin-TC, Otic Susp. (Monarch Pharmaceuticals).

colistin methanesulfonate.
See: Colistimethate Sodium.

colistin and neomycin sulfates and hydrocortisone acetate otic suspension.
Use: Anti-infective, anti-inflammatory.

Co-Liver. (Standex) Folic acid 1 mg, vitamin B_{12} 100 mcg, liver 10 mcg/ml. Inj. Vial 10 ml. *Rx.*
Use: Mineral, vitamin supplement.

Colladerm. (C & M Pharmacal, Inc.) Glycerin, soluble collagen, hydrolysed elastin, allantoin, ethylhydroxycellulose, sorbic, octoxynol-9. Bot. 2.3 oz. *otc.*
Use: Emollient.

collagenase.
See: Santyl (Knoll Pharmaceuticals).

collagenase abc ointment. (Advance Biofactures Corporation) Collagenase 250 units/g in white petrolatum. 25 g, 50 g. *otc.*
Use: Enzyme, topical.

collagen implant. (Lacrimedics, Inc.) 0.2 mm, 0.3 mm, 0.4 mm, 0.5 mm. 0.6 mm. Box 12s. *Rx.*
Use: Collagen implant, ophthalmic.

collagen implant.
See: Zyderm I (Collagen Corp.).
Zyderm II (Collagen Corp.).

collagenase (lyophilized) for injection.
Use: Peyronie's disease. [Orphan Drug]

•**collodion.** (kah-LOW-dee-uhm) U.S.P. 23.
Use: Topical protectant.

colloidal aluminum hydroxide.
See: Aluminum Hydroxide Gel, U.S.P. 23.

collodial oatmeal.
Use: Emollient.
See: Actibath, Effer. Tab. (The Andrew Jergens Co.).
Aveeno, Preps. (Rydelle Laboratories).

Colloral. (AutoImmune, Inc.) Purified type II collagen.
Use: Juvenile rheumatoid arthritis. [Orphan Drug]

Collyrium for Fresh Eyes. (Wyeth-Ayerst Laboratories) Boric acid, sodium borate, benzalkonium Cl. Bot. 120 ml. *otc.*
Use: Irrigant, ophthalmic.

Collyrium Fresh Eye Drops. (Wyeth-Ayerst Laboratories) Tetrahydrozoline HCl 0.05%. Drop. Bot. 15 ml. *otc.*
Use: Mydriatic, vasoconstrictor.

ColoCare. (Helena Laboratories) In-home fecal test. Kit. 3s.
Use: Diagnostic aid.

Coloctyl. (Eon Labs Manufacturing, Inc.) Docusate sodium 100 mg/Cap. Bot. 100s, 1000s, UD 1000s. *otc.*
Use: Laxative.

Cologel. (Eli Lilly and Co.) Methylcellulose 450 mg/5 ml, alcohol 5%, saccharin. Bot. 16 fl oz. *otc.*
Use: Laxative.

colony-stimulating factor.
Use: Adjunct during antineoplastic therapy.
See: Leukine (Immunex Corp.).
Neupogen (Amgen, Inc.).

color allergy screening test.
See: CAST (Biomerica, Inc.).

Color Ovulation Test. (Biomerica, Inc.) Monoclonal antibody-based enzyme immunoassay test for hLH in urine. Kit. 9-day test kit.
Use: Diagnostic aid, ovulation.

Coloscreen. (Helena Laboratories) Occult blood screening test. Kit 12s, 25s, 50s. 3 tests per kit.
Use: Diagnostic aid.

Coloscreen/VPI. (Helena Laboratories) Occult blood screening test. Box 100s, 1000s.
Use: Diagnostic aid.

Colovage. (Dyna Pharm, Inc.) Powder for reconstitution to produce 1 gal soln. Containing sodium Cl 5.53 g, potassium Cl 2.82 g, sodium bicarbonate 6.36 g, sodium sulfate anhydrous 21.5 g, polyethylene glycol 3350. Pkg. 1s. *Rx.*
Use: Laxative.

Col-Probenecid. (Various Mfr.) Probenecid 500 mg, colchicine 0.5 mg/Tab. Bot. 100s. *Rx.*
Use: Antigout.

Coltab Children's. (Roberts Pharmaceuticals) Phenylephrine HCl 2.5 mg, chlorpheniramine maleate 1 mg/Chew. Tab. Bot. 30s. *otc.*
Use: Antihistamine, decongestant.

•**colterol mesylate.** (KOLE-ter-ole) USAN.
Use: Bronchodilator.

Coly-Mycin M Parenteral. (Monarch Pharmaceuticals) Colistimethate sodium equivalent to 150 mg colistin base. Inj. Vial. *Rx.*
Use: Anti-infective.

Coly-Mycin S Otic Drops w/Neomycin and Hydrocortisone. (Parke-Davis) Colistin base as the sulfate 3 mg, neomycin base as the sulfate 3.3 mg, hydrocortisone acetate 10 mg, thonzonium bromide 0.5 mg/ml, polysorbate 80, acetic acid, sodium acetate, thimerosal. Dropper bot. 5 ml, 10 ml. *Rx.*
Use: Anti-infective.

CoLyte. (Schwarz Pharma, Inc.) **2L:** PEG (Polyethylene glycol-electrolyte solution) 3350 120 g, sodium sulfate 11.36 g, sodium bicarbonate 3.36 g, sodium Cl 2.92 g, potassium Cl 1.49 g. **1 gal:** PEG 3350 227.1 g, sodium sulfate 21.5 g, sodium bicarbonate 6.36 g, sodium Cl 5.53 g, potassium Cl 2.82 g. **6 L:** PEG 3350 360 g, sodium sulfate 34.08 g, sodium bicarbonate 10.08 g, sodium Cl 8.76 g, potassium Cl 4.47 g. Pack 5. Bot. 2 L, gal, 4 L, 6 L. *Rx.*
Use: Bowel evacuant.

Combichole. (Trout) Dehydrocholic acid 2 gr, desoxycholic acid 1 gr/Tab. Bot. 100s, 1000s. *Rx.*
Use: Hydrocholeretic.

CombiPatch. (Rhone-Poulenc Rorer) **Transdermal Patch 9 cm^2:** Estradiol 0.05 mg, norethindrone acetate 0.14 mg. **Transdermal Patch 16 cm^2:** Estradiol 0.05 mg, norethindrone acetate 0.25 mg. Box. 8s. *Rx.*
Use: Estrogen and progestin combination.

Combipres Tablets. (Boehringer Ingelheim, Inc.) **0.1 mg:** Clonidine HCl 0.1 mg, chlorthalidone 15 mg/Tab. Bot. 100s, 1000s. **0.2 mg:** Clonidine HCl 0.2 mg, chlorthalidone 15 mg/Tab. Bot. 100s, 1000s. **0.3 mg:** Clonidine HCl 0.3 mg, chlorthalidone 15 mg/Tab. Bot. 100s. *Rx.*
Use: Antihypertensive.

Combistix. (Bayer Corp. (Consumer Div.)) Urine test for glucose, protein and pH. In 100s.
Use: Diagnostic aid.

Combistix Reagent Strips. (Bayer Corp. (Consumer Div.)) Protein test area: tetrabromphenol blue, citrate buffer, protein-absorbing agent; glucose test area: glucose oxidase, orthotolidin and a catalyst; pH test area methyl red and bromthymol blue. Strip Box 100s.
Use: Diagnostic aid.

Combivent. (Boehringer Ingelheim, Inc.) Ipratropium bromide 18 mcg, albuterol sulfate 103 mcg/actuation. Aer. Metered dose inhaler 14.7 g (200 inhalations). *Rx.*
Use: Secondary treatment of chronic obstructive pulmonary disease (COPD).

Combivir. (GlaxoWellcome) Lamivudine 150 mg, zidovudine 300 mg. Tab. Bot. 60s. *Rx.*
Use: Antiviral.

ComfortCare GP Wetting & Soaking. (PBH Wesley Jessen) Buffered, isotonic. Chlorhexidine gluconate 0.005%, EDTA 0.02%, octylphenoxy (oxyethylene) ethanol, povidone, polyvinyl alcohol, propylene glycol, hydroxyethylcellulose, NaCl. Soln. Bot. 120 ml, 240 ml. *otc.*
Use: Contact lens care.

Comfort Drops. (PBH Wesley Jessen) Isotonic solution containing naphazoline 0.03%, benzalkonium Cl 0.005%, edetate disodium 0.02%. Bot. 15 ml. *otc.*
Use: Contact lens care.

Comfort Eye Drops. (PBH Wesley Jessen) Naphazoline HCl 0.03%. Bot. 15 ml. *otc.*
Use: Decongestant, ophthalmic.

Comfort Gel Liquid. (Walgreen Co.) Aluminum hydroxide compressed gel 200 mg, magnesium hydroxide 200 mg, simethicone 20 mg/5 ml. Bot. 12 oz. *otc.*
Use: Antacid, antiflatulent.

Comfort Gel Tablets. (Walgreen Co.) Magnesium hydroxide 85 mg, simethi-

cone 25 mg, aluminum hydroxide-magnesium carbonate co-dried gel 282 mg/Tab. Bot. 100s. *otc.*
Use: Antacid, antiflatulent.

Comfort Tears. (Allergan) Hydroxyethylcellulose, benzalkonium Cl 0.005%, edetate disodium 0.02%. Bot. 15 ml. *otc.*
Use: Artificial tear solution.

Comhist L.A. Capsules. (Roberts Pharmaceuticals) Phenylephrine HCl 20 mg, chlorpheniramine maleate 4 mg, phenyltoloxamine citrate 50 mg/Cap. Bot. 100s. *Rx.*
Use: Antihistamine, decongestant.

Comhist Tablets. (Roberts Pharmaceuticals) Phenylephrine HCl 10 mg, chlorpheniramine maleate 2 mg, phenyltoloxamine citrate 25 mg/Tab. Bot. 100s. *Rx.*
Use: Antihistamine, decongestant.

Compal. (Solvay Pharmaceuticals) Dihydrocodeine 16 mg, acetaminophen 356.4 mg, caffeine 30 mg/Cap. Bot. 100s. *c-III.*
Use: Analgesic combination.

Compat Nutrition Enteral Delivery System. (Novartis Pharmaceutical Corp.) Top fill feeding containers 600 ml, 1400 ml. Gravity delivery set. Pump delivery set. Compat enteral feeding pump.
Use: Nutritional supplement.

Compazine. (SmithKline Beecham Pharmaceuticals) Prochlorperazine as the maleate. **Tab.:** 5 mg, 10 mg Bot. 100s. **Inj.:** Edisylate salt 5 mg/ml. Amp. 2 ml, vial 10 ml, disposable syringe 2 ml. **SR Spansule:** Maleate salt 10 mg, 15 mg. Bot. 50s. **Supp.:** 2.5 mg, 5 mg, 25 mg. Box 12s. **Syr.:** Edisylate salt 5 mg/5 ml. Bot. 120 ml. *Rx.*
Use: Antiemetic, antipsychotic.

Compete. (Mission Pharmacal Co.) Iron 27 mg, vitamins A 5000 IU, D 400 IU, E 45 IU, B_1 2 mg, B_2 2.6 mg, B_3 30 mg, B_6 20.6 mg, B_{12} 9 mcg, C 90 mg, folic acid 0.4 mg, Zn 22.5 mg/Tab. Bot. 100s. *otc.*
Use: Mineral, vitamin supplement.

Compleat B Meat Base Formula. (Novartis Pharmaceutical Corp.) Beef, nonfat milk, hydrolyzed cereal solids, maltodextrin, pureed fruits and vegetables, corn oil, mono- and diglycerides. Bot. 250 ml, Can 250 ml. *otc.*
Use: Nutritional supplement, eternal.

Compleat Modified Formula Meat Base. (Novartis Pharmaceutical Corp.) Hydrolyzed cereal solids, calcium caseinate, pureed fruits and vegetables, corn oil, beef puree, mono- and diglycerides. Can 250 ml. *otc.*
Use: Enteral nutritional supplement.

Compleat Regular Formula. (Novartis Pharmaceutical Corp.) Deionized water, beef puree, hydrolyzed cereal solids, green bean puree, pea puree, nonfat milk, corn oil, maltodextrin, peach puree, orange juice, mono- and diglycerides, carrageenan, vitamins, minerals. Bot. 250 ml, Can 250 ml. *otc.*
Use: Nutritional supplement, eternal.

Complete All-In-One. (Allergan, Inc.) Buffered, isotonic. Sodium Cl, polyhexamethylene biguanide, EDTA. Soln. Bot. 60, 120, 360 ml. *otc.*
Use: Contact lens care.

Complete Solution. (Allergan, Inc.) Buffered, isotonic. Sodium Cl, polyhexamethylene biguanide 0.0001%, tromethamine, tyloxapol, EDTA. Soln. Bot. 15 ml. *otc.*
Use: Contact lens care.

Complete Vitamins. (Mission Pharmacal Co.) Vitamins A 5000 IU, D 400 IU, E 45 IU, C 90 mg, B_1 2.25 mg, folic acid 0.4 mg, B_2 2.6 mg, B_3 30 mg, B_6 25 mg, B_{12} 9 mcg, ferrous gluconate 233 mg, zinc 22.5 mg/Tab. Bot. 100s, 1000s. *otc.*
Use: Mineral, vitamin supplement.

Complete Weekly Enzymatic Cleaner. (Allergan, Inc.) Effervescing, buffering and tableting agents. Sublitisin A. Tab. Pkg. 8s. *otc.*
Use: Contact lens care.

Completone Elixir Fort. (Sanofi Winthrop Pharmaceuticals) Ferrous gluconate.
Use: Mineral supplement.

Complex 15 Cream. (Baker Cummins Dermatologicals, Inc.) Jar 4 oz. *otc.*
Use: Emollient.

Complex 15 Lotion. (Baker Cummins Dermatologicals, Inc.) Bot. 8 oz. *otc.*
Use: Emollient.

Complex Zinc Carbonates.
See: Zinc (Pharmaceutical Labs, Inc.).

Comply Liquid. (Sherwood Davis & Geck) Sodium caseinate, calcium caseinate, hydrolyzed cornstarch, sucrose, corn oil, soy lecithin, vitamins A, B_1, B_2, B_3, B_5, B_6, B_{12}, C, D, E, K, folic acid, biotin, choline, Ca, Cl, Cu, Fe, I, Mg, Mn, P, Zn. Can 250 ml, Bot. 200 ml. *otc.*
Use: Nutritional supplement, enteral.

compound 42.
See: Warfarin (Various Mfr.).

compound cb3025.
See: Alkeran, Tab. (GlaxoWellcome).

compound e.

See: Cortisone Acetate. (Various Mfr.).

compound f.
See: Hydrocortisone (Various Mfr.).

compound q.
Use: Antiviral.

compound s.
Use: Antiviral.
See: Retrovir (GlaxoWellcome). Zidovudine.

Compound W. (Whitehall Robins Laboratories) Salicylic acid 17% w/w in flexible collodion vehicle w/ether 63.5%. Bot. 0.31 oz. *otc.*
Use: Keratolytic.

Compoz. (Medtech Laboratories, Inc.) **Tab.:** Diphenhydramine HCl 50 mg. Pkg. 12s, 24s. **Cap.:** Diphenhydramine HCl 25 mg. Pkg. 16s. *otc.*
Use: Sleep aid.

comprecin.
See: Penetrex (Warner Lambert).

Comtrex. (Bristol-Myers Squibb) Acetaminophen 325 mg, pseudoephedrine HCl 30 mg, chlorpheniramine maleate 2 mg, dextromethorphan HBr 10 mg/Tab. Bot. 24s, 50s. *otc.*
Use: Analgesic, antihistamine, antitussive, decongestant.

Comtrex Allergy-Sinus. (Bristol-Myers Squibb) Pseudoephedrine HCl 30 mg, chlorpheniramine maleate 2 mg, acetaminophen 500 mg/Tab. or Capl. Bot. 24s, 50s. *otc.*
Use: Analgesic, antihistamine, decongestant.

Comtrex Caplets. (Bristol-Myers Squibb) Acetaminophen 325 mg, pseudoephedrine HCl 30 mg, chlorpheniramine maleate 2 mg, dextromethorphan HBr 10 mg/Capl. Bot. 24s, 50s. *otc.*
Use: Analgesic, antihistamine, antitussive, decongestant.

Comtrex Cough Formula. (Bristol-Myers Squibb) Pseudoephedrine HCl 15 mg, dextromethorphan 7.5 mg, guaifenesin 50 mg, acetaminophen 125 mg/5 ml, alcohol 20%. Bot. 120 ml, 240 ml. *otc.*
Use: Analgesic, antitussive, decongestant, expectorant.

Comtrex Day-Night. (Bristol-Myers Squibb) **Night:** Pseudoephedrine HCl 30 mg, chlorpheniramine maleate 2 mg, dextromethorphan HBr 10 mg, acetaminophen 325 mg/Tab. Pkg. 6s. **Day:** Pseudoephedrine HCl 30 mg, dextromethrophan HBr 10 mg, acetaminophen 500 mg/Tab. Pkg. 18s. *otc.*
Use: Antihistamine, antitussive, decongestant.

Comtrex Liquid. (Bristol-Myers Squibb) Pseudoephedrine HCl 10 mg, dextromethorphan HBr 3.3 mg, chlorpheniramine maleate 0.67 mg, acetaminophen 108.3 mg/5 ml, alcohol 20%, sucrose. Bot. 180 ml. *otc.*
Use: Antihistamine, antitussive, decongestant.

Comtrex Liquid Multi-Symptom Cold Reliever. (Bristol-Myers Squibb) Acetaminophen 650 mg, phenylpropanolamine HCl 25 mg, chlorpheniramine maleate 4 mg, dextromethorphan HBr 20 mg/30 ml, alcohol 20%. Bot. 6 oz, 10 oz. *otc.*
Use: Analgesic, antihistamine, antitussive, decongestant.

Comtrex Liqui-Gels. (Bristol-Myers Squibb) Acetaminophen 325 mg, phenylpropanolamine HCl 12.5 mg, chlorpheniramine maleate 2 mg, dextromethorphan HBr 10 mg/Tab. Blister pkg. 24s, 50s. *otc.*
Use: Analgesic, antihistamine, antitussive, decongestant.

Comtrex, Maximum Strength. (Bristol-Myers Squibb) Phenylpropanolamine HCl 12.5 mg, dextromethorphan HBr 15 mg, chlorpheniramine maleate 2 mg, acetaminophen 500 mg. Cap. 24s, 50s. *otc.*
Use: Antihistamine, antitussive, decongestant.

Comtrex Maximum Strength Multi-Symptom Cold & Flu Relief. (Bristol-Myers Squibb) Phenylpropanolamine HCl 12.5 mg, chlorpheniramine maleate 2 mg, dextromethorphan HBr 15 mg, acetaminophen 500 mg/Capl. or Tab. Pkg. 24s. *otc.*
Use: Analgesic, antihistamine, antitussive, decongestant.

Comtrex Maximum Strength Non-Drowsy. (Bristol-Myers Squibb) Pseudoephedrine HCl 30 mg, dextromethorphan HBr 15 mg, acetaminophen 500 mg/Capl. Pkg. 24s. *otc.*
Use: Analgesic, antitussive, decongestant.

Comvax. (Merck & Co.) *Haemophilus influenzae* type b and hepatitis b vaccines. Combined 7.5 mcg Hib polysaccharide, 5 mcg hepatitis B surface antigen/0.5 ml. Single-dose vial. *Rx.*
Use: Vaccine.

Conceive Ovulation Predictor. (Quidel Corp.) In vitro diagnostic test for luteinizing hormone in urine.
Use: Diagnostic aid, pregnancy.

Concentraid. (Ferring Pharmaceuticals, Inc.) Desmopressin acetate 0.1 mg/ml (0.1 mg equals 400 IU arginine vaso-

pressin). Soln. Disposable intranasal pipettes containing 20 mcg/2 ml. *Rx.*
Use: Hormone.

Concentrated Cleaner. (Bausch & Lomb Pharmaceuticals) Anionic sulfate surfactant with friction-enhancing agents and sodium chlorine. Soln. Bot. 30 ml. *otc.*
Use: Contact lens care.

Concentrated Milk of Magnesia-Cascara. (Roxane Laboratories, Inc.) Magnesium hydroxide 2.34 g, aromatic cascara fluid extract U.S.P. 5 ml, alcohol 7%/5 ml. Susp. UD 15 ml. *otc.*
Use: Laxative.

Concentrated Multiple Trace Element. (American Regent) Zinc (as sulfate) 5 mg, copper (as sulfate) 1 mg, manganese (as sulfate) 0.5 mg, chromium (as chloride) 10 mcg. Vial. 10 ml. *Rx.*
Use: Trace element supplement.

concentrated oleovitamin a & d.
See: Oleovitamin A & D, Concentrated, Cap. (Various Mfr.)

Concentrated Phillips' Milk of Magnesia. (Roxane Laboratories, Inc.) Magnesium hydroxide 800 mg/5 ml, sorbitol and sugar. Strawberry and orange vanilla creme flavors. Liq. 8 fl. oz. *otc.*
Use: Antacid, laxative.

Concentrin Caps. (Parke-Davis) Dextromethorphan HBr 15 mg, pseudoephedrine HCl 30 mg, guaifenesin 100 mg/Cap. Bot. 12s. *otc.*
Use: Antitussive, decongestant, expectorant.

Conceptrol Contraceptive Inserts. (Advanced Care Products) Nonoxynol-9 150 mg. Supp. 10s. *otc.*
Use: Contraceptive, spermicide.

Conceptrol Disposable Contraceptive. (Advanced Care Products) Nonoxynol-9 4%. Vaginal gel. Tube. 2.7 ml (6s, 10s). *otc.*
Use: Contraceptive, spermicide.

Condol Suspension. (Sanofi Winthrop Pharmaceuticals) Dipyrone, chlormezanone. *Rx.*
Use: Analgesic, muscle relaxant.

Condol Tablets. (Sanofi Winthrop Pharmaceuticals) Dipyrone, chlormezanone. *Rx.*
Use: Analgesic, muscle relaxant.

Condrin-LA. (Roberts Pharmaceuticals) Phenylpropanolamine HCl 75 mg, chlorpheniramine maleate 12 mg. Bot. 1000s. *otc.*
Use: Antihistamine, decongestant.

condylox. (Oclassen Pharmaceuticals, Inc.) Podofilox 0.5%, alcohol 95%. Soln. Bot. 3.5 ml. *Rx.*
Use: Keratolytic.

Conest. (Grafton) Conjugated estrogens 0.625 mg, 1.25 mg, 2.5 mg/Tab. Bot. 100s, 1000s. *Rx.*
Use: Estrogen.

Conex-DA. (Forest Pharmaceutical, Inc.) Phenylpropanolamine HCl 37.5 mg, chlorpheniramine maleate 4 mg/Tab. Bot. 100s, 1000s. *otc.*
Use: Antihistamine, decongestant.

Conex Plus. (Forest Pharmaceutical, Inc.) Phenylpropanolamine HCl 25 mg, chlorpheniramine maleate 4 mg, acetaminophen 325 mg/Tab. Bot. 1000s. *otc.*
Use: Analgesic, antihistamine, decongestant.

Confide. (Direct Access Diagnostics) Reagent kit for HIV blood tests. Kit contains materials to draw a blood sample, a test card, and a protective mailer for 1 test. *otc.*
Use: Diagnostic aid.

Confident. (Block Drug Co., Inc.) Carboxymethylcellulose gum, ethylene oxide polymer, petrolatum/mineral oil base. Tube 0.7 oz, 1.4 oz, 2.4 oz. *otc.*
Use: Denture adhesive.

Congess. (Fleming & Co.) **Sr.:** Guaifenesin 250 mg, pseudoephedrine HCl 120 mg/SR Cap. **Jr.:** Guaifenesin 125 mg, pseudoephedrine HCl 60 mg/TR Cap. Bot. 100s, 1000s. *Rx-otc.*
Use: Decongestant, expectorant.

Congess Jr. (Fleming & Co.) Pseudoephedrine HCl 60 mg, guaifenesin 125 mg/Cap. Bot. 100s, 1000s. *Rx.*
Use: Decongestant, expectorant.

Congess Sr. (Fleming & Co.) Pseudoephedrine HCl 120 mg, guaifenesin 250 mg/Cap. Bot. 100s, 1000s. *Rx.*
Use: Decongestant, expectorant.

Congestac. (Menley & James Labs, Inc.) Pseudoephedrine HCl 60 mg, guaifenesin 400 mg/Tab. Bot. 24s. *otc.*
Use: Decongestant, expectorant.

Congestant D. (Rugby Labs, Inc.) Phenylpropanolamine HCl 12.5 mg, chlorpheniramine maleate 2 mg, acetaminophen 325 mg, sucrose. Tab. Bot. 100s, 1000s. *otc.*
Use: Antihistamine, decongestant.

congo red. Injection.
Use: Hemostatic in hemorrhagic disorders.

conjugated estrogens.
Use: Estrogen.
See: Estrogens, Conjugated (Various Mfr.).

Conjunctamide. (Horizon Pharma-

ceutical Corp.) Prednisolone acetate 0.5%, sodium sulfacetamide 10%, hydroxypropyl methylcellulose, polysorbate 80, sodium thiosulfate, benzalkonium Cl 0.01%. Susp. Dropper bot. 5 ml, 15 ml. *Rx.*
Use: Anti-infective, corticosteroid, ophthalmic.

•**conorphone hydrochloride.** (KOE-nahr-fone) USAN. *Formerly Codorphone.*
Use: Analgesic.

Conray. (Mallinckrodt) Iothalamate meglumine 600 mg, iodine 282 mg/ml, EDTA. Inj. Vial 30 ml, 50 ml, 100 ml. Bot. 100 ml, 150 ml, 200 ml. Pre-filled Syringe. 50 ml, 125 ml. *Rx.*
Use: Radiopaque agent.

Conray 30. (Mallinckrodt) Iothalamate meglumine 300 mg, iodine 141 mg/ml, EDTA. Inj. Vial 50 ml. Bot. 150 ml, 300 ml. *Rx.*
Use: Radiopaque agent.

Conray 43. (Mallinckrodt) Iothalamate meglumine 430 mg, iodine 202 mg/ml, EDTA. Inj. Vial 50 ml, 100 ml. Bot. 150 ml, 200 ml, 250 ml. Pre-filled syr. 50 ml. *Rx.*
Use: Radiopaque agent.

Conray 325. (Mallinckrodt) Iothalamate sodium 54.3% (32.5% iodine), EDTA. Inj. Vial 30 ml, 50 ml. *Rx.*
Use: Radiopaque agent.

Conray 400. (Mallinckrodt) Iothalamate sodium 668 mg, iodine 400 mg/ml, EDTA. Inj. Vial 50 ml. Pre-filled Syringe. 50 ml. *Rx.*
Use: Radiopaque agent.

Consin Compound Salve. (Wisconsin Pharmacal Co.) Carbolic acid ointment. Jar 2 oz, lb. *otc.*
Use: Minor skin irritations.

Constilac. (Alra Laboratories, Inc.) Lactulose syrup 10 g/15 ml. Bot. 8 oz, 16 oz, UD 30 ml. *Rx.*
Use: Laxative.

Constonate 60. Docusate sodium 100 mg, 250 mg/Cap. Bot. 100s, 1000s. *otc.*
Use: Laxative.

Constulose. (Alpharma USPD Inc.) Lactulose 10 g, galactose < 2.2 g, lactose 1.2 g, other sugars ≤ 1.2 g/15 ml. Syr. Bot. 237 ml, 946 ml. *Rx.*
Use: Analgesic, laxative.

Contac-12 Hour Capsules. (SmithKline Beecham Pharmaceuticals) Phenylpropanolamine HCl 75 mg, chlorpheniramine maleate 8 mg/CA Cap. Pkg. 10s, 20s. *otc.*
Use: Antihistamine, decongestant.

Contac Cough & Chest Cold Liquid. (SmithKline Beecham Pharmaceuticals) Pseudoephedrine HCl 15 mg, dextromethorpan HBr 5 mg, guaifenesin 50 mg, acetaminophen 125 mg/5 ml, alcohol 10%, saccharin, sorbitol. Liq. Bot. 4 fl. oz. *otc.*
Use: Analgesic, antitussive, decongestant, expectorant.

Contac Cough and Sore Throat Formula. (SmithKline Beecham Pharmaceuticals) Dextromethorphan HBr 5 mg, acetaminophen 125 mg/5 ml, alcohol 10%. Bot. 120 ml. *otc.*
Use: Analgesic, antitussive.

Contac Day & Night Allergy/Sinus Caplets. (SmithKline Beecham Pharmaceuticals) **Day:** Pseudoephedrine HCl 60 mg, acetaminophen 650 mg/Capl. **Night:** Pseudoephedrine HCl 60 mg, diphenhydramine HCl 50 mg, acetaminophen 650 mg/Capl. Pkg. 20 (15 day; 5 night). *otc.*
Use: Analgesic, antihistamine, decongestant.

Contac Day & Night Cold & Flu Caplets. (SmithKline Beecham Pharmaceuticals) **Day:** Pseudoephedrine HCl 60 mg, dextromethorphan HRr 30 mg, acetaminophen 650 mg/Cap. Pkg. 15s. **Night:** Pseudoephedrine HCl 60 mg, diphenhydramine HCl 50 mg, acetaminophen 650 mg/Cap. Pkg. 5s. *otc.*
Use: Analgesic, antihistamine, antitussive, decongestant.

Contac Jr. (SmithKline Beecham Pharmaceuticals) Pseudoephedrine HCl 15 mg, acetaminophen 160 mg, dextromethorphan HBr 5 mg, saccharin, sorbitol/5 ml. Bot. 4 oz. *otc.*
Use: Analgesic, antitussive, decongestant.

Contac Maximum Strength 12-Hour Caplets. (SmithKline Beecham Pharmaceuticals) Phenylpropanolamine HCl 75 mg, chlorpheniramine maleate 12 mg/Capl. Pkg. 10s, 20s. *otc.*
Use: Antihistamine, decongestant.

Contac Nighttime Cold. (SmithKline Beecham Pharmaceuticals) Acetaminophen 167 mg, dextromethorphan HBr 5 mg, pseudoephedrine HCl 10 mg, doxylamine succinate 1.25 mg/5 ml, alcohol 25%. Bot. 177 ml. *otc.*
Use: Analgesic, antihistamine, antitussive, decongestant.

Contac Non-Drowsy Formula Sinus. (SmithKline Beecham Pharmaceuticals) Pseudoephedrine HCl 30 mg, acetaminophen 500 mg/Capl. or Tab. Pkg. 24s. *otc.*

Use: Analgesic, decongestant.

Contac Severe Cold Formula. (SmithKline Beecham Pharmaceuticals) Phenylpropanolamine HCl 12.5 mg, acetaminophen 500 mg, chlorpheniramine maleate 2 mg, dextromethorphan HBr 15 mg/Capl. Pkg. 10s, 20s. *otc.*
Use: Analgesic, antihistamine, antitussive, decongestant.

Contac Severe Cold & Flu Nighttime Liquid. (SmithKline Beecham Pharmaceuticals) Pseudoephedrine HCl 10 mg, chlorpheniramine maleate 0.67 mg, dextromethorphan HBr 5 mg, acetaminophen 167 mg, alcohol 18.5%, saccharin, sorbitol, glucose. Liq. Bot. 180 ml. *otc.*
Use: Antihistamine, antitussive, decongestant.

contact lens products, soft. *otc.*
Use: Contact lens care, rinsing, storage.
See: Allergan Hydrocare Preserved Saline (Allergan, Inc.).
Boil n Soak (Alcon Laboratories, Inc.).
Lensrins (Allergan, Inc.).
Opti-Soft (Alcon Laboratories, Inc.).
ReNu Saline (Bausch & Lomb Pharmaceuticals).
Saline Solution, Sterile Preserved (Bausch & Lomb Pharmaceuticals).
Murine Preserved All-Purpose Saline Solution (Ross Laboratories).
Sensitive Eyes Plus (Bausch & Lomb Pharmaceuticals).
Sensitive Eyes Saline (Bausch & Lomb Pharmaceuticals).
Soft Mate Saline for Sensitive Eyes (PBH Wesley Jessen).
Allergan Sorbi-Care Saline (Allergan, Inc.).
Sterile Saline (Bausch & Lomb Pharmaceuticals).
Blairex Sterile Saline (Blairex Labs, Inc.).
Hypo-Clear (Bausch & Lomb Pharmaceuticals).
Lens Plus Preservative Free (Allergan, Inc.).
Ciba Vision Saline (Ciba Vision).
Hypo-Clear (Bausch & Lomb Pharmaceuticals).
Unisol (PBH Wesley Jessen).
Unisol 4 (PBH Wesley Jessen).
Soft Mate Saline Preservative-Free (PBH Wesley Jessen).

contact lens products, soft, salt tablets for normal saline. *otc.*
Use: Salt tablets for normal saline.
See: Soft Rinse 135 (Professional Supplies).
Amcon 250 (Amcon Laboratories).
Easy Eyes (Eaton Medicals).
Marlin Salt System II (Marlin Industries).
Soft Rinse 250 (Professional Supplies).

contact lens products, surfactant cleaning solutions. *otc.*
See: Ciba Vision Cleaner (Ciba Vision).
Daily Cleaner (Bausch & Lomb Pharmaceuticals).
Preflex for Sensitive Eyes (Alcon Laboratories, Inc.).
DURAcare II (Blairex Labs, Inc.).
LC-65 (Allergan, Inc.).
Lens Clear (Allergan, Inc.).
Lens Plus Daily Cleaner (Allergan, Inc.).
Mira Flow Extra Strength (Ciba Vision).
Murine Contact Lens Cleaner (Ross Laboratories).
Opti-Clean II (Alcon Laboratories, Inc.).
Pliagel (PBH Wesley Jessen).
Sensitive Eyes Saline/Cleaning Solution (Bausch & Lomb Pharmaceuticals).
Sof/Pro-Clean (Sherman Pharmaceuticals, Inc.).
Soft Mate Hands Off Daily Cleaner (PBH Wesley Jessen).
Soft Mate Protein Remover (PBH Wesley Jessen).
Soft Mate Daily Cleaning for Sensitive Eyes (PBH Wesley Jessen).

contact lens products, enzymatic cleaners. *otc.*
See: Allergan Enzymatic (Allergan, Inc.).
Extenzyme Protein Cleaner (Allergan, Inc.).
Opti-zyme Enzymatic Cleaner (Alcon Laboratories).
ReNu Effervescent Enzymatic Cleaner (Bausch & Lomb Pharmaceuticals).
ReNu Thermal Enzymatic Cleaner (Bausch & Lomb Pharmaceuticals).
Ultrazyme Enzymatic Cleaner (Allergan, Inc.).

contact lens products, re-wetting solutions. *otc.*
See: Adapettes for Sensitive Eyes (Alcon Laboratories, Inc.).
Clerz Drops (PBH Wesley Jessen).
Clerz 2 (PBH Wesley Jessen).
Comfort Tears (PBH Wesley Jessen).
Lens Drops (Ciba Vision).
Lens Fresh (Allergan, Inc.).
Lens Lubricant (Bausch & Lomb Pharmaceuticals).

Lens Plus Rewetting Drops (Allergan, Inc.).
Lens-Wet (Allergan, Inc.).
Murine Sterile Lubricating and Rewetting Drops (Ross Laboratories).
Opti-Tears (Alcon Laboratories, Inc.).
Sensitive Eye Drops (Bausch & Lomb Pharmaceuticals).
Soft Mate Comfort Drops (PBH Wesley Jessen).
Soft Mate Lens Drops (PBH Wesley Jessen).
Sterile Lens Lubricant (Blairex Labs, Inc.).

contact lens products, disinfectant. *otc.*
See: Allergan Hydrocare Cleaning and Disinfecting (Allergan, Inc.).
Aosept (Ciba Vision).
Disinfecting Solution (Bausch & Lomb Pharmaceuticals).
Flex-Care (Alcon Laboratories, Inc.).
Lens Plus Oxysept System (Allergan, Inc.).
Lensept (Ciba Vision).
MiraSept System (PBH Wesley Jessen).
Opti-Free (Alcon Laboratories, Inc.).

ConTE-PAK-4. (SoloPak Pharmaceuticals, Inc.) Zn 5 mg, Cu 1 mg, Mn 0.5 mg, Cr 10 mcg/ml. Soln. Vial 1 ml, 10 ml. *Rx.*
Use: Nutritional supplement, parenteral.

contraceptives, intrauterine system.
See: Oral Contraceptives (Various Mfr.).
Progestasert (Alza Corp.).

contraceptives, miscellaneous.
See: Oral Contraceptives (Various Mfr.).
Norplant (Wyeth-Ayerst Laboratories).
VCF, Film (Apothecus, Inc.).

contraceptives, vaginal foams.
See: Oral Contraceptives (Various Mfr.).
Delfen, Vaginal Foam (Ortho McNeil Pharmaceutical).
Emko, Vaginal Foam (Schering-Plough Corp.).

contraceptives, vaginal jellies and creams.
See: Oral Contraceptives (Various Mfr.).
Colagyn, Jelly (Smith & Nephew United).
Colagyn, Jelly (Smith & Nephew United).
Conceptrol, Cream, Gel (Ortho McNeil Pharmaceutical).
Gynol II, Gel (Ortho McNeil Pharmaceutical).
Immolin, Cream-Jel (Durex).
Koromex-A, Jelly (Holland-Rantos).
Koromex, Cream or Jelly (Holland-Rantos).
Ortho-Gynol, Jelly (Ortho McNeil Pharmaceutical).

contraceptives, vaginal suppositories.
See: Oral Contraceptives (Various Mfr.).
Intercept, Inserts (Ortho McNeil).
Lorophyn, Supp., Jelly (Eaton Medical Corp.).

Contrin. (Geneva Pharmaceuticals) Iron (from ferrous fumarate) 110 mg, B_{12} 15 mcg, IFC (intrinisic factor as concentrate or from stomach preparations) 240 mg, C 75 mg, folic acid 0.5 mg/Cap. Bot. 100s. *Rx.*
Use: Mineral, vitamin supplement.

Control. (Thompson Medical Co.) Phenylpropanolamine HCl 75 mg/TR Cap. Bot. 14s, 28s, 56s. *otc.*
Use: Dietary aid.

Contuss Liquid. (Parmed Pharmaceuticals, Inc.) Phenylpropanolamine HCl 20 mg, phenylephrine HCl 5 mg, guaifenesin 100 mg/5 ml, alcohol 5%, saccharin, sorbitol, sucrose. Liq. Bot. 16 fl. oz. *Rx.*
Use: Decongestant, expectorant.

Converspaz. (B.F. Ascher and Co.) Cellulase 5 mg, protease 10 mg, amylase 30 mg, lipase 13 mg, l-hyoscamine sulfate 0.0625 mg/Cap. Bot. 100s. *Rx.*
Use: Decongestant, expectorant.

Cool-Mint Listerine. (Warner Lambert) Thymol, eucalyptol, methyl salicylate, menthol, alcohol 21.6%. Liq. Bot. 90 ml, 180 ml, 360 ml, 540 ml, 720 ml, 960 ml. *otc.*
Use: Mouthwash.

Coopervision Balanced Salt Solution. (Ciba Vision) Sterile intraocular irrigation soln. Bot. 15 ml, 500 ml.
Use: Irrigant, ophthalmic.

Copavin Pulvules. (Eli Lilly and Co.) Codeine sulfate 15 mg, papaverine HCl 15 mg/Cap. Bot. 100s. *c-v.*
Use: Antitussive.

Copaxone. (Teva Pharmaceuticals USA) Glatiramer acetate 20 mg, mannitol 40 mg. Inj. Vial, 2 ml. Diluent vial 1 ml. 32s. *Rx.*
Use: Multiple sclerosis agent.

COPE. (Mentholatum Co., Inc.) Aspirin 421 mg, magnesium hydroxide 50 mg, aluminum hydroxide 25 mg, caffeine 32 mg/Tab. Bot. 36s, 60s. *otc.*
Use: Analgesic, antacid.

Cophene #2. (Dunhall Pharmaceuticals, Inc.) Chlorpheniramine maleate 12 mg, pseudoephedrine HCl 120 mg/Time Cap. Bot. 100s, 500s. *Rx.*
Use: Antihistamine, decongestant.

Cophene Injectable. (Dunhall Pharmaceuticals, Inc.) Atropine sulfate 0.2 mg,

phenylpropanolamine HCl 12.5 mg, chlorpheniramine maleate 5 mg/ml. Pkg. 10 ml. *Rx.*
Use: Anticholinergic, antihistamine, antispasmodic, decongestant.

Cophene-PL. (Dunhall Pharmaceuticals, Inc.) Phenylephrine HCl 20 mg, phenylpropanolamine HCl 20 mg, chlorpheniramine maleate 5 mg/5 ml. Bot. 16 oz. *Rx-otc.*
Use: Antihistamine, decongestant.

Cophene-S. (Dunhall Pharmaceuticals, Inc.) Dihydrocodone bitartrate 3 mg, phenylephrine HCl 20 mg, phenylpropanolamine HCl 20 mg, chlorpheniramine maleate 5 mg/5 ml. Bot. Pt. *c-III.*
Use: Antihistamine, antitussive, decongestant.

Cophene-X. (Dunhall Pharmaceuticals, Inc.) Carbetapentane citrate 20 mg, phenylephrine HCl 10 mg, phenylpropanolamine HCl 10 mg, chlorpheniramine maleate 2.5 mg, potassium guaiacolsulfonate 45 mg/Cap. Bot. 100s. *Rx.*
Use: Antihistamine, antitussive, decongestant, expectorant.

Cophene-XP. (Dunhall Pharmaceuticals, Inc.) Carbetapentane citrate 20 mg, phenylephrine HCl 10 mg, phenylpropanolamine HCl 20 mg, chlorpheniramine maleate 2.5 mg, potassium guaiacolsulfonate 45 mg/5 ml. Syr. Bot. pt. *Rx.*
Use: Antihistamine, antitussive, decongestant, expectorant.

copolymer 1, (cop 1).
Use: Treat multiple sclerosis. [Orphan Drug]

copper. (Abbott Laboratories) Copper 0.4 mg/ml (as 0.85 mg cupric Cl.) Inj. Vial 10 ml, 30 ml. *Rx.*
Use: Nutritional supplement, parenteral.

•**copper gluconate.** U.S.P. 23.
Use: Supplement (trace mineral).

copperhead bite therapy.
See: Antivenin, (crotalidae) Polyvalent Inj. (Wyeth-Ayerst Laboratories).

Copperin. (Vernon) Iron ammonium citrate, copper (6 gr). "A" adult dose, "B" children dose. Bot. 30s, 100s, 500s.
Use: Mineral supplement.

Coppertone. (Schering-Plough Corp.) A series of sun-care products marketed under the Coppertone name including Waterproof Lotions SPF 4, 6, 8, 15, and 25. Bot. 4 fl oz, 8 fl oz. Oil SPF 2: Bot. 4 fl oz, 8 fl oz; Lite Formula Oil SPF 2: Bot. 4 fl oz; Lite Lotion SPF 4: Bot. 4 fl oz; Dark Tanning Body Mousse SPF 4: Tube 4 oz; Suntanning Gel SPF 4: Tube 3 oz; Noskote SPF 8: Tube 0.44 oz, Jar 1 oz; Noskote SPF-15: Jar 1 oz. Contain one or more of the following ingredients: Padimate O, oxybenzone, homosalate, ethylhexyl p-methocinnamate. *otc.*
Use: Sunscreen.

Coppertone Dark Tanning Spray. (Schering-Plough Corp.) Padimate O in spray base (SPF 2). Bot. 8 fl oz. *otc.*
Use: Sunscreen.

Coppertone Face. (Schering-Plough Corp.) A series of sunscreen lotions with SPF 2, 4, 6 and 15 in a non-greasy base with padimate O, oxybenzone (SPF 15 only). *otc.*
Use: Sunscreen.

Coppertone Kids Sunblock. (Schering-Plough Corp.) **SPF 15:** Ethylhexyl p-methoxycinnamate, oxybenzone, 2-ethylhexyl salicylate, homosalate. Lot. Bot. 120 ml, 240 ml. **SPF 30:** Octocrylene, ethylhexyl p-methoxycinnamate, oxybenzone, 2-ethylhexyl salicylate. Lot. Bot. 120 ml, 240 ml. *otc.*
Use: Sunscreen.

Coppertone Lipkote. (Schering-Plough Corp.) Ethylhexyl p-methoxycinnamate, oxybenzone. SPF 15. Stick 4.5 g. *otc.*
Use: Sunscreen.

Coppertone Moisturizing Sunblock. (Schering-Plough Corp.) **SPF 45:** Ethylhexyl p-methoxycinnamate, 2-ethylhexyl salicylate, octocrylene, oxybenzone. Lot. Bot. 120 ml, 300 ml. **SPF 25, 30:** Ethylhexyl p-methoxycinnamate, oxybenzone, 2-ethylhexyl salicylate, homosalate. Lot. Bot. SPF 30: 120 ml, 240 ml; SPF 25: 120 ml. **SPF 15:** Ethylhexyl p-methoxycinnamate, oxybenzone. Lot. Bot. 120 ml, 240 ml, 300 ml. *otc.*
Use: Sunscreen.

Coppertone Moisturizing Sunscreen. (Schering-Plough Corp.) Ethylhexyl p-methoxycinnamate, oxybenzone, benzyl alcohol, vitamin E, aloe. PABA free. SPF 6, 8. Waterproof. Lot. Bot. 120 ml, 240 ml. *otc.*
Use: Sunscreen.

Coppertone Moisturizing Suntan. (Schering-Plough Corp.) **SPF 2:** homosalate, vitamin E, aloe. PABA free. Waterproof. Oil. Bot. 120 ml. **SPF 4:** Ethylhexyl p-methoxycinnamate, oxybenzone, benzyl alcohol, vitamin E, aloe. PABA free. Waterproof. Lot. Bot. 120 ml, 240 ml. *otc.*
Use: Sunscreen.

Coppertone Noskote. (Schering-Plough Corp.) Homosalate 8%, oxybenzone 3%. (SPF 8) Oint. Jar 13.2 g, 30 g. *otc.*
Use: Sunscreen.

Coppertone SPF-25 Sunblock Lotion. (Schering-Plough Corp.) Ethylhexyl p-methoxycinnamate, oxybenzone, Padimate O in lotion base (SPF 25). Bot. 120 ml. *otc.*
Use: Sunscreen.

Coppertone Sport. (Schering-Plough Corp.) Ethylhexyl p-methoxycinnamate, oxybenzone. SPF 4, 8, 15, 30. Lot. Bot. 120 ml. *otc.*
Use: Sunscreen.

Coppertone Tan Magnifier Suntan. (Schering-Plough Corp.) **SPF 2:** Triethanolamine salicylate. Oil Bot. 120 ml. **SPF 4 Lotion:** Ethylhexyl p-methoxycinnamate. Bot. 120 ml. **Gel:** 2-phenylbenzimidazole-5-sulfonic acid. Tube 120 g. *otc.*
Use: Sunscreen.

Coppertone Water Babies. (Schering-Plough) SPF 30, SPF 45. Ethylhexyl p-methoxycinnamate, 2-ethylhexyl salicylate, oxybenzone, homosalate, alcohol, aloe, parabens. PABA free. Waterproof. Lot. Bot. 118 ml. *otc.*
Use: Sunscreen.

copper trace metal additive. (I.M.S., Ltd.) Copper 1 mg. Inj. Vial 10 ml. *Rx.*
Use: Copper supplement.

•**copper undecylenate.** USAN.
Use: Copper supplement.

Co-Pyronil 2. (Eli Lilly and Co.) Chlorpheniramine maleate 4 mg, pseudoephedrine HCl 60 mg/Pulvule. Bot. 100s. *otc.*
Use: Antihistamine, decongestant.

Corab. (Abbott Diagnostics) Radioimmunoassay for detection of antibody to hepatitis B core antigen. Test kit 100s.
Use: Diagnostic aid.

Corab-M. (Abbott Diagnostics) Radioimmunoassay for the qualitative determination of specific Ig antibody to hepatitis B virus core antigen (Anti-HBc Ig) in human serum or plasma and may be used as an aid in the diagnosis of acute or recent hepatitis B infection.
Use: Diagnostic aid.

Corace Injection. (Forest Pharmaceutical, Inc.) Cortisone acetate 50 mg/ml. Vial 10 ml. *Rx.*
Use: Corticosteroid, topical.

Coracin. (Roberts Pharmaceuticals) Hydrocortisone acetate 1%, neomycin sulfate 0.5%, bacitracin zinc 400 units, polymyxin B sulfate 10,000 units/g in white petrolatum and mineral oil base. Oint. Tube 3.5 g. *Rx.*
Use: Anti-infective, corticosteroid, ophthalmic.

Coral. (Young Dental) Fluoride ion 1.23%, 0.1 molar phosphate. Jar 250 g, Coral II: 180 disposable cup units/carton. *Rx.*
Use: Fluoride, dental.

Coral/Plus. (Young Dental) Free fluoride ion 2.2%, recrystallized kaolinite. Tube 250 g. *Rx.*

coral snake (North American Biologicals, Inc.) antivenin.
See: Antivenin (*Micrurus fulvius*). (Wyeth-Ayerst Laboratories).

Corane. (Forest Pharmaceutical, Inc.) Pyrilamine maleate 25 mg, pheniramine maleate 10 mg, phenylpropanolamine HCl 25 mg, phenylephrine HCl 10 mg/Cap. Bot. 100s, 500s, 1000s. *otc.*
Use: Antihistamine, decongestant.

Corbicin-125. (Arthrins) Vitamin C 125 mg/Cap. Bot. 100s. *otc.*
Use: Vitamin supplement.

Cordarone. (Wyeth-Ayerst Laboratories) **Tab.:** Amiodarone HCl 200 mg, lactose. Bot. 60s, UD 100s. **Inj.:** Amiodarone 50 mg/ml, benzyl alcohol 20.2 mg/ml. Amp. 3 ml. *Rx.*
Use: Antiarrhythmic.

Cordran. (Eli Lilly and Co.) Flurandrenolide 0.025%, 0.05% in emulsified petrolatum base/g. **0.025%:** Tube 30 g, 60 g, Jar 225 g. **0.05%:** Tube 15 g, 30 g, 60 g, Jar 225 g. *Rx.*
Use: Corticosteroid, topical.

Cordran Lotion. (Eli Lilly and Co.) Flurandrenolide 0.05%, cetyl alcohol, benzyl alcohol, stearic acid, glyceryl monostearate, polyoxyl 40 stearate, glycerin, mineral oil, menthol, purified water. Squeeze bot. 15 ml, 60 ml. *Rx.*
Use: Corticosteroid, topical.

Cordran-N Cream & Ointment. (Eli Lilly and Co.) Flurandrenolide 0.5 mg, neomycin sulfate 5 mg/g. Tube 15 g, 30 g, 60 g. *Rx.*
Use: Corticosteroid, topical.

Cordran SP. (Eli Lilly and Co.) Flurandrenolide 0.025%, 0.05% in emulsified base w/cetyl alcohol, stearic acid, polyoxyl 40 stearate, mineral oil, propylene glycol, sodium citrate, citric acid, purified water. **0.025%:** Tube 30 g, 60 g, Jar 225 g. **0.05%:** Tube 15 g, 30 g, 60 g, Jar 225 g. *Rx.*
Use: Corticosteroid, topical.

Cordran Tape. (Eli Lilly and Co.) Flurandrenolide 4 mcg/sq. cm. Roll 7.5 cm × 60 cm, 7.5 cm x 200 cm. *Rx.*
Use: Corticosteroid, topical.

Cordrol. (Vita Elixir) Prednisolone 5 mg, 10 mg, 20 mg/Tab. Bot. 100s. *Rx.*
Use: Corticosteroid.

Coreg. (SmithKline Beecham) Carvedilol

3.125 mg, 6.25 mg, 12.5 mg, 25 mg, lactose, sucrose. Tab. Bot. 100s. *Rx.*
Use: Antihypertensive.

Coreg Powder. (Block Drug Co., Inc.) Denture adhesive containing polyethylene oxide polymer w/peppermint oil, karaya gum. Pkg.: pocket 0.7 oz; medium 1.15 oz; economy 3.55 oz. *otc.*
Use: Denture adhesive.

Corgard. (Bristol-Myers Squibb) Nadolol 20 mg, 40 mg, 80 mg, 120 mg or 160 mg/Tab. Bot 100s, 1000s, UD 100s. *Rx.*
Use: Beta-adrenergic blocker.

coriander oil.
Use: Pharmaceutic aid (flavor).

Coricidin. (Schering-Plough Corp.) Chlorpheniramine maleate 2 mg, acetaminophen 325 mg/Tab. Bot. 100s. *otc.*
Use: Analgesic, antihistamine.

Coricidin "D" Tablets. (Schering-Plough Corp.) Chlorpheniramine maleate 2 mg, acetaminophen 325 mg, phenylpropanolamine HCl 12.5 mg/Tab. Bot. 12s, 24s, 48s, 100s. *otc.*
Use: Analgesic, antihistamine, decongestant.

Coricidin Demilets. (Schering-Plough Corp.) Phenylpropanolamine HCl 6.25 mg, chlorpheniramine maleate 1 mg, acetaminophen 80 mg, saccharin, lactose. Tab. Bot. 24s, 36s. *otc.*
Use: Analgesic, antihistamine, decongestant.

Coricidin Extra Strength Sinus Headache Tablets. (Schering-Plough Corp.) Acetaminophen 500 mg, phenylpropanolamine HCl 12.5 mg, chlorpheniramine maleate 2 mg/Tab. Box 24s. *otc.*
Use: Analgesic, antihistamine, decongestant.

Coricidin Maximum Strength Sinus Headache. (Schering-Plough Corp.) Phenylpropanolamine HCl 12.5 mg, chlorpheniramine maleate 2 mg, acetaminophen 500 mg/Tab. Box 24s. *otc.*
Use: Analgesic, antihistamine, decongestant.

Corilin Infant Liquid. (Schering-Plough Corp.) Chlorpheniramine maleate 0.75 mg, sodium salicylate 80 mg/ml, alcohol < 1%. Bot. 30 ml. *otc.*
Use: Analgesic, antihistamine.

Corlopam. (Neurex Corporation) Fenoldopam mesylate 10 mg/ml, sodium metabisulfite. Inj. Single-dose Amp. 5 ml. *Rx.*
Use: Antihypertensive.

Cormax. (Oclassen Pharmaceuticals, Inc.) Clobetasol propionate 0.05%, white petrolatum, sorbitan sesquioleate. Oint. Tube. 15 g, 45 g. *Rx.*
Use: Corticosteroid, topical.

•**cormethasone acetate.** (core-METH-ah-sone) USAN.
Use: Anti-inflammatory, topical.

Corn Huskers Lotion. (Warner Lambert) Glycerin 6.7%, SD alcohol, algin, TEA-oleoyl sarcosinate, guar gum, methylparaben, calcium sulfate, calcium Cl, TEA-fumarate, TEA-borate. Bot. 4 oz, 7 oz. *otc.*
Use: Emollient.

•**corn oil.** N.F. 18.
Use: Pharmaceutic aid (solvent, oleaginous vehicle).
See: G. B. Prep Emulsion (Gray Pharmaceutical Co.).

Corotrope. (Sanofi Winthrop Pharmaceuticals) Milrinone for IV use. *Rx.*
Use: Cardiovascular agent.

corpus luteum, extract (water soluble).
See: Progesterone, Preps. (Various Mfr.).

Corque. (Geneva Pharmaceuticals) Hydrocortisone 1%, iodochlorhydroxyquin 3%. Cream Tube 20 g. *Rx.*
Use: Corticosteroid, topical.

Correctol. (Schering-Plough Corp.) Bisacodyl 5 mg, talc, lactose, sugar. Tab. Bot. 60s. *otc.*
Use: Laxative.

Correctol Extra Gentle. (Schering-Plough Corp.) Docusate sodium 100 mg. Softgel Cap. Bot. 30s. *otc.*
Use: Laxative.

Cortaid Intensive Therapy. (Pharmacia & Upjohn) Hydrocortisone 1%, alcohols, parabens. Tube 56 g. *otc.*
Use: Corticosteroid, topical.

Cortaid, Maximum Strength. (Pharmacia & Upjohn) Hydrocortisone in parabens 1%, cetyl and stearyl alcohols, glycerin, white petrolatum. Cream Tube 15 g, 30 g. *otc.*
Use: Corticosteroids, topical.

Cortaid Maximum Strength Spray. (Pharmacia & Upjohn) Hydrocortisone 1%, alcohol 55%, glycerin, methylparaben. Liq. Pump spray 45 ml. *otc.*
Use: Corticosteroid, topical.

Cortan. (Halsey Drug Co.) Prednisone 5 mg/Tab. Bot. 1000s. *Rx.*
Use: Corticosteroid.

Cortane D.C. Expectorant. (Standex) Brompheniramine maleate 2 mg, guaifenesin 100 mg, phenylephrine HCl 5 mg, phenylpropanolamine HCl 5 mg, codeine phosphate 10 mg, alcohol 3.5%/5 ml. Bot. pt. *c-v.*
Use: Antihistamine, antitussive, decongestant, expectorant.

Cortane Expectorant. (Standex) Brompheniramine maleate 2 mg, guaifenesin 100 mg, phenylephrine 5 mg, phenylpropanolamine HCl 5 mg, alcohol 3.5%/5 ml. Bot. Pt. *otc.*
Use: Antihistamine, decongestant, expectorant.

Cortapp. (Standex) Brompheniramine maleate 5 mg, phenylephrine HCl 5 mg, phenylpropanolamine HCl 5 mg, alcohol 2.3%/5 ml. Elix. Bot. Pt. *otc.*
Use: Antihistamine, decongestant.

Cortatrigen Ear Suspension. (Zenith Goldline Pharmaceuticals) Hydrocortisone 1%, neomycin sulfate 5 mg, polymyxin B sulfate 10,000 units/ml. Bot. 10 ml. *Rx.*
Use: Anti-infective, corticosteroid, otic.

Cortatrigen Modified Ear Drops. (Zenith Goldline Pharmaceuticals) Hydrocortisone 1%, neomycin sulfate 5 mg/ml, polymyxin b 10,000 U/ml, propylene glycol, glycerin, potassium metabisulfite. Bot. 10 ml. *Rx.*
Use: Anti-infective; corticosteroid, otic.

Cort-Dome. (Bayer Corp. (Consumer Div.)) Hydrocortisone alcohol. **Cream:** 0.25%: 1 oz, 4 oz; 0.5%: 1 oz; 1%: 1 oz. **Lot.:** 0.25%: 4 oz; 0.5%: 4 oz; 1%: 1 oz. *Rx.*
Use: Corticosteroid, topical.

Cort-Dome High Potency. (Bayer Corp. (Consumer Div.)) Hydrocortisone acetate 25 mg in a monoglyceride base. *Rx.*
Use: Corticosteroid, topical.

Cortef Acetate Ointment. (Pharmacia & Upjohn) Hydrocortisone acetate 10 mg/g, lanolin (anhydrous), white petrolatum, mineral oil. Tube 20 g. *Rx.*
Use: Corticosteroid, topical.

Cortef Feminine Itch Cream. (Pharmacia & Upjohn) Hydrocortisone acetate equivalent to hydrocortisone 5 mg/g. Tube 0.5 oz. *Rx.*
Use: Corticosteroid, topical.

Cortef Oral Suspension. (Pharmacia & Upjohn) Hydrocortisone 10 mg/5 ml (as 13.4 mg hydrocortisone cypionate). Oral susp. Bot. 4 oz. *Rx.*
Use: Corticosteroid.

Cortef Tablets. (Pharmacia & Upjohn) Hydrocortisone. **5 mg/Tab.:** Bot. 50s. **10 mg or 20 mg/Tab.:** Bot. 100s. *Rx.*
Use: Corticosteroid.

Cortenema. (Solvay Pharmaceuticals) Hydrocortisone 100 mg in aqueous solution w/carboxypolymethylene, polysorbate 80, methylparaben 0.18%/60 ml. Bot. w/applicator. UD 1s. *Rx.*
Use: Corticosteroid, topical.

cortenil.
See: Desoxycorticosterone Acetate, Preps. (Various Mfr.).

cortical hormone products.
See: Adrenal Cortex Extract (Various Mfr.).
Aristocort, Preps. (ESI Lederle Generics).
Corticotropin, Preps. (Various Mfr.).
Hydrocortisone, Preps. (Various Mfr.).
Cortisone Acetate, Preps. (Various Mfr.).
Decadron LA, Inj. (Merck & Co.).
Decadron, Tab., Elix., Inj. (Merck & Co.).
Desoxycorticosterone Acetate, Preps. (Various Mfr.).
Dexamethasone, Tab. (Various Mfr.).
Fludrocortisone (Various Mfr.).
Hydeltrasol, Inj. (Merck & Co.).
Hydrocortone Acetate, Inj. (Merck & Co.).
Hydrocortone Phosphate, Inj. (Merck & Co.).
Medrol, Preps. (Pharmacia & Upjohn).
Methylprednisolone, Tab. (Various Mfr.).
Prednisolone, Tab. (Various Mfr.).
Prednisone, Tab. (Various Mfr.).
Triamcinolone, Tab. (Various Mfr.).

Cortic Ear Drops. (Everett Laboratories, Inc.) Hydrocortisone 10 mg, pramoxine HCl 10 mg, chloroxylenol 1 mg/ml. Drops. Vial 10 ml. *Rx.*
Use: Otic preparation.

•**corticorelin ovine triflutate.** (core-tih-kah-REH-lin OH-vine TRY-flew-TATE) USAN.
Use: Hormone (corticotropin-releasing); diagnostic aid (adrenocortical insufficiency, Cushing's syndrome). [Orphan Drug]
See: Acthrel (Ferring Pharmaceuticals, Inc.).

corticosteroid/mydriatic combo, ophthalmics. Prednisolone acetate 0.25%, atropine sulfate 1%. *Rx.*
Use: Treatment of anterior uveitis.

corticotropin highly purified.
See: H.P. Acthar Gel, Vial (Centeon).

•**corticotropin injection.** (core-tih-koe-TROE-pin) U.S.P. 23. ACTH, Adrenocorticotrophic hormone or adrenocorticotropin or corticotropin.
Use: Adrenocorticotrophic hormone; corticosteroid, topical; diagnostic aid (adrenocortical insufficiency).
See: ACTH.
Acthar (Centeon).

•**corticotropin, repository, injection.**

(core-tih-koe-TROE-pin) U.S.P. 23.
Use: Hormone (adrenocorticotrophic); corticosteroid, topical; diagnostic aid (adrenocortical insufficiency).
See: Acthar Gel, Vial (Centeon).
ACTH Gel Purified (Various Mfr.).
H.P. Acthar Gel, Vial (Centeon).

Cortifoam. (Schwarz Pharma, Inc.) Hydrocortisone acetate 10% in an aerosol foam w/propylene glycol, emulsifying wax, steareth 10, cetyl alcohol, methylparaben, propylparaben, trolamine, inert propellants. Container 20 g w/rectal applicator for 14 applicatorsful. *Rx.*
Use: Corticosteroid, topical.

cortisol.
Note: Cortisol was the official published name for hydrocortisone in U.S.P. 23. The name was changed back to Hydrocortisone, U.S.P. in Supplement 1 to the U.S.P. 23.
See: Hydrocortisone, U.S.P. 23.

cortisol cyclopentylpropionate.
See: Cortef Fluid, Susp., Tab. (Pharmacia & Upjohn).

•**cortisone acetate.** (CORE-tih-sone) U.S.P. 23.
Use: Corticosteroid, topical.
See: Cortistan (Standex).
Cortone Acetate, Inj. (Merck & Co.).

cortisone acetate. (Kendall Co. Health Care Pro.) 5 mg, 10 mg, 25 mg/Tab. Bot. 50s, 100s, 500s.
Use: Adrenocortical steroid (anti-inflammatory).

Cortisporin Cream. (GlaxoWellcome) Polymyxin B sulfate 10,000 units, neomycin sulfate 5 mg, hydrocortisone acetate 5 mg/g, methylparaben 0.25%. Tube 7.5 g. *Rx.*
Use: Anti-infective, corticosteroid, topical.

Cortisporin Ointment. (GlaxoWellcome) Polymyxin B sulfate 5000 units, bacitracin zinc 400 units, neomycin sulfate 5 mg, hydrocortisone (1%) 10 mg/g in petrolatum base. Tube 30 g. *Rx.*
Use: Anti-infective, corticosteroid, topical.

Cortisporin Ophthalmic Ointment. (GlaxoWellcome) Polymyxin B sulfate 10,000 units, bacitracin 400 units, neomycin sulfate 0.35%, hydrocortisone 0.1%. Tube 3.5 g. *Rx.*
Use: Anti-infective, corticosteroid, ophthalmic.

Cortisporin Ophthalmic Suspension. (GlaxoWellcome) Polymyxin B sulfate 10,000 units, neomycin sulfate 0.35%, hydrocortisone 1%. Dropper bot. 7.5 ml Sterile. *Rx.*
Use: Anti-infective, corticosteroid, ophthalmic.

Cortisporin Otic Solution Sterile. (GlaxoWellcome) Polymyxin B sulfate 10,000 units, neomycin sulfate 5 mg, hydrocortisone 10 mg/ml, glycerin, propylene glycol, vitamin K metabisulfite 0.1%. Dropper bot. 10 ml Sterile. *Rx.*
Use: Anti-infective, corticosteroid, otic.

Cortisporin Otic Suspension. (GlaxoWellcome) Polymyxin B sulfate 10,000 units, neomycin sulfate 5 mg, hydrocortisone free alcohol 10 mg/ml, cetyl alcohol, propylene glycol, polysorbate 80, thimerosal. Dropper bot. 10 ml Sterile. *Rx.*
Use: Anti-infective, corticosteroid, otic.

Cortisporin-TC. (Monarch Pharmaceuticals) Colistin sulfate 3 mg, neomycin sulfate 3.3 mg, hydrocortisone acetate 10 mg, thonzonium bromide 0.5 mg, polysorbate 80, acetic acid, sodium acetate. Otic Susp. Bot. 10 ml w/dropper. *Rx.*
Use: Otic preparation.

Cortistan. (Standex) Cortisone 25 mg/10 ml. *Rx.*
Use: Corticosteroid.

•**cortivazol.** (core-TIH-vah-zole) USAN.
Use: Corticosteroid, topical.

Cortizone-5. (Thompson Medical Co.) Hydrocortisone 0.5%, glycerin, mineral oil, white petrolatum. Tube 30 g. *otc.*
Use: Corticosteroid, topical.

Cortizone for Kids. (Pfizer) Hydrocortisone 0.5%, parabens, cetearyl alcohol, glycerin, white petrolatum. Cream Tube 14 g. *otc.*
Use: Corticosteroid, topical.

Cortizone-S, Maximum Strength. (Thompson Medical Co.) Hydrocortisone 0.5%. Tube. *otc.*
Use: Corticosteroid, topical.

•**cortodoxone.** (CORE-toe-dox-OHN) USAN.
Use: Anti-inflammatory.

Cortogen Acetate. Cortisone acetate.

Cortone Acetate. (Merck & Co.) Cortisone acetate 50 mg/ml. Inj. Vial 10 ml. *Rx.*
Use: Corticosteroid.

Cortril Topical Ointment 1%. (Pfizer US Pharmaceutical Group) Hydrocortisone 1%, cetyl and stearyl alcohol, propylene glycol, sodium lauryl sulfate, petrolatum, cholesterol, mineral oil, methyl- and propylparabens in ointment base. Tube 0.5 oz.
Use: Corticosteroid, topical.

Cortrosyn Injection. (Organon Teknika Corp.) Cosyntropin 0.25 mg, mannitol 10 mg, lyophilized powder/ml. Vial. Pkg. w/1 ml amp diluent. Box 10s. Vial. *Rx.*
Use: Corticosteroid.

Corubeen. (Spanner) Vitamin B_{12} crystalline 1000 mcg/ml. Vial 10 ml. *Rx.*
Use: Vitamin supplement.

Corvert. (Pharmacia & Upjohn) Ibutilide fumarate 0.1 mg/ml. Soln. Vial. 10 ml. *Rx.*
Use: Antiarrhythmic.

Coryza Brengle. (Roberts Pharmaceuticals) Pseudoephedrine HCl 30 mg, acetaminophen 200 mg/Cap. Bot. 1000s. *otc.*
Use: Analgesic, decongestant.

Corzide. (Bristol-Myers Squibb) Nadolol 40 mg, bendroflumethiazide 5 mg/Tab or nadolol 80 mg, bendroflumethiazide 5 mg/Tab. Bot. 100s. *Rx.*
Use: Antihypertensive.

Corzyme. (Abbott Diagnostics) Enzyme immunoassay for detection of antibody to hepatitis B core antigen in serum or plasma. Test kit 100s.
Use: Diagnostic aid.

Corzyme-M. (Abbott Diagnostics) Enzyme immunoassay for the detection of Ig antibody to hepatitis B core antigen. (Anti-HBc Ig) In human serum or plasma. Test kit 100s.
Use: Diagnostic aid.

Cosmegen. (Merck & Co.) Actinomycin D (dactinomycin) 0.5 mg (lyophilized powder)/3 ml. *Rx.*
Use: Antineoplastic.

Cosmoline.
See: Petrolatum.

Cosopt. (Merck) Dorzolamide 2%, timolol maleate 0.5%, benzalkonium chloride 0.0075%, mannitol. Ophth. Soln. Ocumeters 5 ml, 10 ml. *Rx.*
Use: Antiglaucoma agent.

Cosulid. (Novartis Pharmaceutical Corp.) Sulfachloropyridazine.

•**cosyntropin.** (koe-sin-TROE-pin) USAN.
Use: Hormone (adrenocorticotrophic).
See: Cortrosyn, Vial (Organon Teknika Corp.).

Cotaphylline. (Major Pharmaceuticals) Oxtriphylline 100 mg, 200 mg/Tab. Bot. 100s, 500s. *Rx.*
Use: Bronchodilator.

cotarnine chloride. Cotarnine hydrochloride.

cotarnine hydrochloride.
See: Cotarnine Chloride.

Cotazym. (Organon Teknika Corp.) Lipase 8000 units, protease 30,000 units, amylase 30,000 units, calcium carbonate 25 mg/Cap. Bot. 100s, 500s. *Rx.*
Use: Digestive enzymes.

Cotazym-S. (Organon Teknika Corp.) Pancrelipase spheres, lipase 5000 units, protease 20,000 units, amylase 20,000 units/Cap. Bot. 100s, 500s. *Rx.*
Use: Digestive enzyme.

•**cotinine fumarate.** (koe-TIH-neen) USAN.
Use: Antidepressant, psychomotor stimulant.

Cotolate Tabs. (Major Pharmaceuticals) Benztropine 1 mg, 2 mg/Tab. Bot. 100s, 1000s. *Rx.*
Use: Antiparkinsonian.

Cotrim. (Teva Pharmaceuticals USA) Sulfamethoxazole 400 mg, trimethoprim 80 mg/Tab. Bot. 100s, 500s. *Rx.*
Use: Anti-infective.

Cotrim D.S. (Teva Pharmaceuticals USA) Sulfamethoxazole 800 mg, trimethoprim 160 mg/Tab. Bot. 100s, 500s. *Rx.*
Use: Anti-infective.

Cotrim Pediatric. (Teva Pharmaceuticals USA) Sulfamethoxazole 200 mg, trimethoprim 40 mg/5 ml. Oral Susp. Bot. 473 ml. *Rx.*
Use: Anti-infective.

•**cotton, purified.** U.S.P. 23.
Use: Surgical aid.

•**cottonseed oil.** N.F. 18.
Use: Pharmaceutic aid, solvent, oleaginous vehicle.

Co-Tuss V Liquid. (Rugby Labs, Inc.) Hydrocodone bitartrate 5 mg, guaifenesin 100 mg. Bot. 480 ml. *c-III.*
Use: Antitussive, expectorant.

Cotylenol Chewable Cold Tablet. (McNeil Consumer Products Co.) Acetaminophen 80 mg, phenylpropanolamine HCl 3.125 mg, chlorpheniramine maleate 0.5 mg. Chew. Tab. Bot. 24s. *otc.*
Use: Analgesic, antihistamine, decongestant.

Cotylenol Children's Chewable Cold Tablet. (McNeil Consumer Products Co.) Acetaminophen 80 mg, chlorpheniramine maleate 0.5 mg, pseudoephedrine HCl 7.5 mg. Chew. Tab. Bot. 24s. *otc.*
Use: Analgesic, antihistamine, decongestant.

Cotylenol Children's Liquid Cold Formula. (McNeil Consumer Products Co.) Acetaminophen 160 mg, chlorpheniramine maleate 1 mg, pseudoephedrine HCl 15 mg, sorbitol/5 ml. Bot. 4 oz. *otc.*
Use: Analgesic, antihistamine, decongestant.

Cotylenol Cold Formula. (McNeil Consumer Products Co.) Chlorpheniramine maleate 2 mg, dextromethorphan HBr 15 mg, pseudoephedrine HCl 30 mg, acetaminophen 325 mg/Tab. or Capl. **Tab.:** Box 24s, Bot. 50s, 100s. **Capl.:** Bot. 24s, 50s. *otc.*
Use: Analgesic, antihistamine, antitussive, decongestant.

Cotylenol Liquid Cold Formula. (McNeil Consumer Products Co.) Acetaminophen 650 mg, chlorpheniramine maleate 4 mg, pseudoephedrine HCl 60 mg, dextromethorphan HCl 30 mg/30 ml, alcohol 7.5%, sorbitol. Bot. 5 oz. *otc.*
Use: Analgesic, antihistamine, antitussive, decongestant.

Cough Formula Comtrex. (Bristol-Myers Squibb) Pseudoephedrine HCl 15 mg, dextromethorphan HBr 7.5 mg/5 ml, guaifenesin, saccharin, sucrose. Liq. Bot. 120 ml, 240 ml. *otc.*
Use: Antitussive, expectorant.

Cough Syrup. (Zenith Goldline Pharmaceuticals) Phenylephrine HCl 5 mg, dextromethorphan HBr 10 mg, guaifenesin 100 mg, alcohol free. Bot. 120 ml. *otc.*
Use: Antitussive, decongestant, expectorant.

Cough-X. (B.F. Ascher and Co.) Dextromethorphan 5 mg, benzocaine 2 mg, dye free/Loz. Pkg. 9s. *otc.*
Use: Anesthetic, antitussive.

Coumadin. (Du Pont Pharma) Warfarin sodium crystalline. **Tab.:** 1 mg, 2 mg, 2.5 mg, 4 mg, 5 mg, 7.5 mg, 10 mg. Bot. 100s, 1000s, UD 100s. **Powd. for Inj., lyophilized:** Warfarin sodium 2 mg, sodium phosphate 4.98 mg, dibasic, heptahydrate, sodium phosphate 0.194 mg, NaCl 0.1 mg, mannitol 38 mg/ml when reconstituted. Vial. 5 mg. *Rx.*
Use: Anticoagulant.

coumarin.
Use: Anticoagulant; treat renal cell carcinoma. [Orphan Drug]

coumarin and indandione derivatives.
Use: Anticoagulant.
See: Coumadin, Tab. (Du Pont Merck Pharmaceutical Co.).
Warfarin Sodium, Tab. (Various Mfr.).
Miradon, Tab. (Schering-Plough Corp.).

•**coumermycin.** (KOO-mer-MY-sin) USAN.
Use: Anti-infective.

•**coumermycin sodium.** (KOO-mer-MY-sin) USAN.
Use: Anti-infective.

Counterpain Rub. (Bristol-Myers Squibb) Methyl salicylate, eugenol, menthol. Oint. Tube 1 oz. *otc.*
Use: Analgesic, topical.

Covangesic. (Wallace Laboratories) Phenylpropanolamine HCl 12.5 mg, phenylephrine HCl 7.5 mg, chlorpheniramine maleate 2 mg, pyrilamine maleate 12.5 mg, acetaminophen 275 mg, tartrazine/Tab. Bot. 24s. *otc.*
Use: Analgesic, antihistamine, decongestant.

Covera-HS. (Searle) Verapamil HCl 180 or 240 mg/ER Tab. Bot. 30s, 100s, UD 100s. *Rx.*
Use: Calcium channel blocker.

Covermark. (O'Leary) Neutral cream, hypoallergenic, opaque, greaseless. Jars 1 oz, 3 oz, available in eleven shades. *otc.*
Use: Conceals birthmarks and skin discolorations.

Covermark Stick. (O'Leary) For normal to oily skin, available in 7 shades. *otc.*
Use: Conceals birthmarks and skin discolorations.

Co-Xan Syrup. (Schwarz Pharma, Inc.) Theophylline anhydrous 150 mg, ephedrine HCl 25 mg, guaifenesin 100 mg, codeine phosphate 15 mg, alcohol 10%/15 ml. Bot. 1 pt. *Rx.*
Use: Antitussive, bronchodilator, decongestant, expectorant.

Cozaar. (Merck & Co.) Losartan potassium 25 mg, 50 mg, lactose. Tab. Bot. 30s (50 mg only), 90s, 100s, 1000s (50 mg only), UD 100s. *Rx.*
Use: Antihypertensive.

CPA TR. (Schein Pharmaceutical, Inc.) Phenylpropanolamine HCl 75 mg, chlorpheniramine maleate 12 mg/Cap. Bot. 100s, 1000s. *otc.*
Use: Antihistamine, decongestant.

Cplex. (Arcum) Vitamins B_1 10 mg, B_2 10 mg, B_6 5 mg, B_{12} 10 mcg, niacinamide 100 mg, calcium pantothenate 25 mg, C 150 mg, liver 50 mg, dried yeast 50 mg/Cap. Bot. 100s, 1000s. *otc.*
Use: Mineral, vitamin supplement.

C.P.M. Tablets. (Zenith Goldline Pharmaceuticals) Chlorpheniramine 4 mg/Tab. Bot. 1000s. *otc.*
Use: Antihistamine.

c-reactive protein test.
See: LA test-CRP kit. (Fischer Pharmaceuticals, Inc.).

Cream Camellia. (O'Leary) Jar 2 oz. *otc.*
Use: Emollient.

Creamy Tar. (C & M Pharmacal, Inc.) Coal tar topical solution 6.65%, crude coal tar 0.67%. Shampoo. Bot. 240 ml. *otc.*

Use: Antiseborrheic.

•**creatinine.** N.F. 18.
Use: Bulking agent for freeze drying.

creatinine reagent strips. (Bayer Corp. (Consumer Div.)) Seralyzer reagent strips. A quantitative strip test for creatinine in serum or plasma. Bot. 25s.
Use: Diagnostic aid.

Cremagol. (Cremagol) Emulsion of liquid petrolatum, agar agar, acacia, glycerin. Bot. 14 oz. W/cascara 11 gr/oz, Bot. 14 oz. W/phenolphthalein 2 gr/oz, Bot. 14 oz. *otc.*
Use: Laxative.

Creomulsion Cough Medicine. (Summit Industries, Inc.) Beechwood creosote, cascara, ipecac, menthol, white pine, wild cherry w/alcohol. For adults. Liq. Bot. 4 fl oz, 8 fl oz. *otc.*
Use: Cough preparation.

Creomulsion for Children. (Summit Industries, Inc.) Beechwood creosote, cascara, ipecac, menthol, white pine, wild cherry w/alcohol. For children. Liq. Bot. 4 fl oz, 8 fl oz. *otc.*
Use: Cough preparation.

Creon. (Solvay Pharmaceuticals) Lipase 8000 units, amylase 30,000 units, protease 13,000 units, pancreatin 300 mg/ Cap. Bot. 100s, 250s. *Rx.*
Use: Digestive enzyme.

Creon 10. (Solvay Pharmaceuticals) Lipase 10,000 USP units, amylase 33,200 USP units, protease 37,500 USP units. DR Cap. Bot. 100s, 250s. *Rx.*
Use: Digestive enzyme.

Creon 20. (Solvay Pharmaceuticals) Lipase 20,000 USP units, amylase 66,400 USP units, protease 75,000 USP units. DR Cap. Bot. 100s, 250s. *Rx.*
Use: Digestive enzyme.

Creon 25. (Solvay Pharmaceuticals) Lipase 25,000 units, amylase 74,700 units, protease 62,500 units, pancreatin 300 mg. Cap. Bot. 100s. *Rx.*
Use: Digestive enzyme.

creosote. Wood creosote, creosote, beechwood creosote.

Creo-Terpin. (Lee Pharmaceuticals) Dextromethorphan HBr 10 mg/15 ml, tartrazine, alcohol 25%, terpin hydrate, creosote, saccharin, corn syrup. Liq. Bot. 120 ml. *otc.*
Use: Antitussive.

Crescormon. (Pharmacia & Upjohn) Somatotropin 4 IU/Vial. IM administration. *Rx.*
Note: Crescormon will be available only for patients who qualify for treatment. Apply to Kabi Group Inc. for approval.
Use: Hormone, growth.

•**cresol.** (KREE-sole) N.F. 18.
Use: Antiseptic, disinfectant.

cresol preparations.
Use: Antiseptic, disinfectant.
See: Saponated Cresol Soln.

m-cresyl-acetate.
See: Cresylate, Liq. (Recsei Laboratories).

Cresylate. (Recsei Laboratories) M-cresyl-acetate 25%, isopropanol 25%, chlorobutanol 1%, benzyl alcohol 1%, castor oil 5%, propylene glycol/15 ml. Bot. 15 ml, pt. *Rx.*
Use: Otic.

cresylic acid. Same as Cresol.

•**crilvastatin.** (krill-vah-STAT-in) USAN.
Use: Antihyperlipidemic.

Crinone 8%. (Wyeth-Ayerst Laboratories) Progesterone 8% (90 mg). Mineral oil, glycerin. Gel. Single-use, one piece 1.125 g applicators. *Rx.*
Use: Assisted reproductive technology treatment.

•**crisnatol mesylate.** (KRISS-nah-tole) USAN.
Use: Antineoplastic.

Criticare HN. (Bristol-Myers Squibb) High nitrogen elemental diet. Protein 14%, fat 4.3%, carbohydrate 81.5%. Bot. 8 oz. *otc.*
Use: Nutritional supplement, enteral.

Crixivan. (Merck & Co.) Indinavir sulfate 200 mg, 400 mg, lactose/Cap. Bot. 270s, 360s (200 mg only), 180s (400 mg only). *Rx.*
Use: Antiviral.

Croferrin. (Forest Pharmaceutical, Inc.) Iron peptonate 50 mg, liver injection 2.5 mcg, vitamin B_{12} 12.5 mcg, lidocaine HCl 1%, phenol 0.5%, sodium citrate 0.125%, sodium bisulfite 0.009%/ml. Vial 10 ml, 30 ml. *Rx.*
Use: Mineral, vitamin supplement.

•**crofilcon A.** (kroe-FILL-kahn A) USAN.
Use: Contact lens material (hydrophilic).

Crolom. (Bausch & Lomb Pharmaceuticals) Cromolyn sodium 4%. Soln. Bot. 2.5 ml, 10 ml w/controlled drop tip. *Rx.*
Use: Antiallergic, ophthalmic.

Cro-Man-Zin. (Freeda Vitamins, Inc.) Cr 200 mcg, Mn 5 mg, Zn 25 mg, kosher, sugar free/Tab. Bot. 100s, 250s. *otc.*
Use: Electrolyte, mineral supplement.

•**cromitrile sodium.** (KROE-mih-TRILE) USAN.
Use: Antiasthmatic.

cromolyn sodium.

Use: Mastocytosis. [Orphan Drug]
See: Gastrocrom (Medeva Pharmaceuticals, Inc.).

•**cromolyn sodium.** (KROE-moe-lin) U.S.P. 23.
Use: Antiasthmatic, prophylactic.
See: Gastrocrom (Medeva Pharmaceuticals, Inc.).
Intal (Medeva Pharmaceuticals, Inc.).
Nasalcrom (Medeva Pharmaceuticals, Inc.).

cromolyn sodium. (Dey Laboratories, Inc.) **Inhalation:** 20 mg/2 ml. Vial 60 ml, 120 ml. **Soln. for Nebulization:** 20 mg/Vial. 2 ml. *Rx.*
Use: Antiasthmatic, prophylactic.

cromolyn sodium 4% ophthalmic solution.
Use: Antiallergic, ophthalmic. [Orphan Drug]
See: Crolom, Ophth. Soln. (Bausch & Lomb Pharmaceuticals).

Cronetal.
See: Disulfiram.

•**croscarmellose sodium.** (KRAHS-CAR-mell-ose) N.F. 18. *Formerly Cross-linked Carboxymethylcellulose Sodium and Modified Cellulose Gum.*
Use: Pharmaceutic aid (tablet disintegrant).

•**crospovidone.** N.F. 18.
Use: Pharmaceutic aid (tablet excipient).

Cross Aspirin. (Cross) Aspirin 325 mg/Tab. Sugar, salt and lactose free. Bot. 100s, 1000s. *otc.*
Use: Analgesic.

Crotab. (Therapeutic Antibodies, Inc.) *Rx.*
See: Antivenin, Polyvalent Crotalic (Ovine) Fab.

Crotalidae Antivenin Polyvalent. (Wyeth-Ayerst Laboratories) 1 vial of lyophilized serum, 1 vial of bacteriostatic water 10 ml, USP, 1 vial normal horse serum. Inj. Vial Combination Pkg. *Rx.*
Use: Antivenin.

crotaline antivenin, polyvalent. U.S.P. 23. Antivenin Crotalidae Polyvalent, North and South American antisnake-bite serum. *Rx.*
Use: Immunizing agent.

•**crotamiton.** (kroe-TAM-ih-tuhn) U.S.P. 23.
Use: Scabicide.
See: Eurax, Cream, Lot. (Novartis Pharmaceutical Corp.).

CRPA Latex Test. (Laboratory Diagnostics) Rapid latex agglutination test for the qualitative determination of C-reactive protein. CRPA, 1 ml CRP Positest Control, 0.5 ml CRPA Latex Test Kit.
Use: Diagnostic aid.

Cruex Cream. (Novartis Self-Medication) Total undecylenate 20% as undecylenic acid and zinc undecylenate. Tube 0.5 oz. *otc.*
Use: Antifungal, topical.

Cruex Spray Powder. (Novartis Pharmaceutical Corp.) Undecylenic acid 2% and zinc undecylenate 20%. Aerosol can 1.8 oz, 3.5 oz, 5.5 oz. *otc.*
Use: Antifungal, topical.

Cruex Squeeze Powder. (Novartis Pharmaceutical Corp.) Calcium undecylenate 10%. Plastic squeeze bot. 1.5 oz. *otc.*
Use: Antifungal, topical.

Cryptolin. (Hoechst Marion Roussel) Gonadorelin in nasal spray. *Rx.*
Use: Cryptorchism treatment.

cryptosporidium hyperimmune bovine colostrum IgG concentrate. (Immucell Corp.)
Use: Treat diarrhea in AIDS patients. [Orphan Drug]

cryptosporidium parvum bovine immunoglobulin concentrate.
Use: Treat infection of GI tract in immunocompromised patients. [Orphan Drug]

crystalline trypsin. Highly purified preparation of enzyme as derived from mammalian pancreas glands.

crystal violet.
See: Methylrosaniline Chloride, U.S.P. 23.

Crystamine. (Dunhall Pharmaceuticals, Inc.) Cyanocobalamin 100 mcg, 1000 mcg/ml, benzyl alcohol. Vial 10 ml, 30 ml. *Rx.*
Use: Vitamin supplement.

Crysti 1000. (Roberts Pharmaceuticals) Cyanocobalamin crystalline 1000 mcg/ml. Inj. Vial 10 ml, 30 ml. *Rx.*
Use: Vitamin B_{12}.

Crysti-Liver. (Roberts Pharmaceuticals) Liver injection (equivalent to B_{12} 10 mcg), crystalline B_{12} 100 mcg, folic acid 0.4 mg. Inj. Vial 10 ml. *Rx.*
Use: Mineral, vitamin supplement.

Crystodigin. (Eli Lilly and Co.) Digitoxin 0.05 mg, 0.1 mg/Tab. Bot. 100s. *Rx.*
Use: Cardiovascular agent.

C Speridin. (Marlyn Nutraceuticals, Inc.) Hesperidin 100 mg, lemon bioflavonoids 100 mg, vitamin C 500 mg/SR Tab. Bot. 100s. *otc.*
Use: Vitamin supplement.

CTab.
See: Cetyl Trimethyl Ammonium Bromide.

C/T/S. (Hoechst Marion Roussel) Clindamycin phosphate 10 mg/ml. Top. Soln. 30 ml, 60 ml. *Rx.*
Use: Dermatologic, acne.

C-Tussin. (Century Pharmaceuticals, Inc.) Codeine phosphate 10 mg, pseudoephedrine HCl 30 mg, guaifenesin 100 mg/5 ml, alcohol 7.5%. Bot. 120 ml, gal. *c-iv.*
Use: Antitussive, decongestant, expectorant.

Culminal. (Culminal) Benzocaine 3% in water-miscible cream base. Tube 1 oz. *otc.*
Use: Anesthetic, local.

Culturette 10 Minute Group A Step ID. (Hoechst Marion Roussel) Latex slide agglutination test for group A streptococcal antigen on throat swabs. Kit 55 determinations.
Use: Diagnostic aid.

•**cupric acetate Cu 64.** (koo-prik ASS-eh-tate) USAN.
Use: Radioactive agent.

•**cupric chloride.** U.S.P. 23.
Use: Supplement (trace mineral).

•**cupric sulfate.** U.S.P. 23.
Use: Antidote to phosphorus.

Cuprid. (Merck & Co.) Trientine HCl 250 mg/Cap. Bot. 100s. *Rx.*
Use: Chelating agent.

Cuprimine. (Merck & Co.) Penicillamine 125 mg, 250 mg/Cap. Bot. 100s. *Rx.*
Use: Chelating agent.

•**cuprimyxin.** (KUH-prih-mix-in) USAN.
Use: Antifungal.

Cupri-Pak. (SoloPak Pharmaceuticals, Inc.) Copper. **0.4 mg/ml:** Vial 10 ml, 30 ml. **2 mg/ml:** Vial 5 ml. *Rx.*
Use: Nutritional supplement, parenteral.

curare.
Use: Muscle relaxant.

curare antagonist.
See: Neostigine Methylsulfate, Inj. (Various Mfr.).
Tensilon, Amp. (Roche Laboratories).

Curel. (Bausch & Lomb Pharmaceuticals) Glycerin, petrolatum, dimethicone, parabens. Lot. 180, 300, 390 ml. Cream 90 g. *Rx-otc.*
Use: Emollient.

Curosurf. (Dey Laboratories, Inc.) Pulmonary Surfactant Replacement.
Use: Respiratory distress syndrome. [Orphan Drug]

curral.
See: Diallyl Barbituric Acid, Tab. (Various Mfr.).

Curretab. (Solvay Pharmaceuticals) Medroxyprogesterone acetate 10 mg/Tab. Bot. 50s. *Rx.*
Use: Hormone, progestin.

Cutar Bath Oil. (Summers Laboratories, Inc.) Liquor carbonis detergens 7.5% in liquid petrolatum, isopropyl myristate, acetylated lanolin, lanolin alcohols extract. Bot. 180 ml. *otc.*
Use: Emollient.

Cutemol Emollient Cream. (Summers Laboratories, Inc.) Allantoin 0.2%, liquid petrolatum, acetylated lanolin, lanolin alcohols extract, isopropyl myristate, water. Jar 2 oz. *otc.*
Use: Emollient.

Cuticura Medicated Shampoo. (DEP Corp.) Sodium lauryl sulfate, sodium stearate, salicylic acid, protein, sulfur. Tube 3 oz. *otc.*
Use: Antidandruff.

Cuticura Medicated Soap. (DEP Corp.) Triclocarban 1%, petrolatum, sodium tallowate, sodium cocoate, glycerin, mineral oil, sodium Cl, tetrasodium EDTA, sodium bicarbonate, magnesium silicate, iron oxides. Bar 3.5 oz, 5.5 oz. *otc.*
Use: Anti-infective, topical.

Cutivate. (GlaxoWellcome) Fluticasone propionate. **Cream:** 0.05%. Jar 15 g, 30 g, 60 g. **Oint.:** 0.005%. Jar 15 g, 30 g, 60 g. *Rx.*
Use: Corticosteroid, topical.

Cutter Insect Repellent. (Bayer Corp. (Consumer Div.)) N,N-Diethyl-meta-toluamide 28.5%, other isomers 1.5%. Vial 1 oz; Foam, Can 2 oz; Spray 7 oz, Aerosol can 14 oz; Assortment Pack; First Aid Kits, Trial Pack, 6s; Marine Pack 3s; Camp Pack 4s; Pocket Pack, Travel Pack.
Use: Insect repellent.

CY 1503. (Cytel Corp.)
Use: Antithromboembolic. [Orphan Drug]

CY 1899. (Cytel Corp.)
Use: Antiviral, hepatitis B. [Orphan Drug]

Cyanide Antidote Package. (Eli Lilly and Co.) 2 Amp. (300 mg/10 ml) sodium nitrite; 2 Amp. (12.5 g/50 ml), sodium thiosulfate; 12 aspirols amyl nitrite (0.3 ml), syringes, stomach tube, tourniquet/Pkg. Check exact dosage before administration. *Rx.*
Use: Antidote, cyanide poisoning.

Cyanocob. (Paddock Laboratories) Vitamin B_{12} 1000 mcg/ml. Bot. 1000 ml, Vial 10 ml. *Rx.*
Use: Vitamin supplement.

•**cyanocobalamin.** (sigh-an-oh-koe-BAL-uh-min) U.S.P. 23. *Formerly Vitamin* B_{12}.

Use: Vitamin, hematopoietic.
See: Nascobal, Intranasal Gel (Schwarz Pharma, Inc.).

•**cyanocobalamin Co 57.** (sigh-an-oh-koe-BAL-uh-min) U.S.P. 23.
Use: Diagnostic aid (pernicious anemia); radioactive agent.

•**cyanocobalamin Co 60.** (sigh-an-oh-koe-BAL-uh-min) USAN. U.S.P. XXII.
Use: Diagnostic aid (pernicious anemia), radioactive agent.

cyanocobalamin crystalline. *Rx-otc.*
Use: Vitamin B_{12} supplement.
See: Vitamin B_{12}, Inj., Tab. (Various Mfr.).
Cobex, Inj. (Taylor Pharmaceuticals).
Crystamine, Inj. (Dunhall Pharmaceuticals, Inc.).
Betalin 12, Inj. (Eli Lilly and Co.).
Crysti 1000, Inj. (Roberts Pharmaceuticals).
Cyanoject, Inj. (Merz Pharmaceuticals).
Cyomin, Inj. (Forest Pharmaceutical, Inc.).

Cyanoject. (Merz Pharmaceuticals) Vitamin B_{12} 1000 mcg/ml, benzyl alcohol. Vial 10 ml, 30 ml. *Rx.*
Use: Vitamin supplement.

Cyanover. (Research Supplies) Cyanocobalamin 100 mcg, liver injection 10 mcg, folic acid 10 mg/ml. Lyo-layer vial 10 ml with vial of diluent 10 ml. *Rx.*
Use: Mineral, vitamin supplement.

•**cyclacillin.** (SIGH-klah-SILL-in) U.S.P. 23.
Use: Anti-infective.

cyclamate sodium. Cyclohexanesulfamate dihydrate salt.

•**cyclamic acid.** (sigh-KLAM-ik) USAN.
Use: Sweetener (non-nutritive).

•**cyclazocine.** (SIGH-CLAY-zoe-seen) USAN. Under study.
Use: Analgesic.

•**cyclindole.** (sigh-KLIN-dole) USAN.
Use: Antidepressant.

Cyclinex-1. (Ross Laboratories) Protein 7.5 g (from carnitine, cystine, histidine, isoleucine, leucine, lysine, methionine, phenylalanine, taurine, threonine, tryptophan, tyrosine, valine), fat 27 g (from palm oil, hydrogenated coconut oil, soy oil), carbohydrate 52 g (from hydrolyzed corn starch), linoleic acid 2000 mg, Fe 10 mg, Na 215 mg, K 760 mg, Ca, vitamins A, B_1, B_2, B_3, B_5, B_6, B_{12}, C, D, E, K, biotin, choline, folic acid, inositol, Cl, Cu, I, Mg, Mn, P, Se, Zn and 515 Cal per 100 g. Nonessential amino acid free. Pow. Can 350 g. *otc.*
Use: Nutritional supplement.

Cyclinex-2. (Ross Laboratories) Protein 15 g (from carnitine, cystine, histidine, isoleucine, leucine, lysine, methionine, phenylalanine, taurine, threonine, tryptophan, tyrosine, valine), fat 20.7 g (from palm oil, hydrogenated coconut oil, soy oil), carbohydrate 40 g (from hydrolyzed cornstarch), Fe 17 mg, Na 1175 mg, K 1830 mg, Ca, vitamins A, B_1, B_2, B_3, B_5, B_6, B_{12}, C, D, E, K, biotin, choline, folic acid, inositol, Cl, Cu, I, Mg, Mn, P, Se, Zn and 480 Cal per 100 g. Nonessential amino acid free. Pow. Can 325 g. *otc.*
Use: Nutritional supplement.

•**cycliramine maleate.** (SIGH-klih-rah-meen) USAN.
Use: Antihistamine.

•**cyclizine.** (SIGH-klih-zeen) U.S.P. 23.
Use: Antihistamine.

•**cyclizine hydrochloride.** U.S.P. 23.
Use: Antiemetic.
See: Marezine HCl and lactate, Preps. (GlaxoWellcome).

•**cyclizine lactate injection.** U.S.P. 23.
Use: Antihistamine, antinauseant.

cyclobarbital.
Use: Central depressant.

cyclobarbital calcium.
Use: Hypnotic, sedative.

•**cyclobendazole.** (SIGH-kloe-BEN-dah-zole) USAN.
Use: Anthelmintic.

•**cyclobenzaprine hydrochloride.** (SIGH-kloe-BEN-zuh-preen) U.S.P. 23.
Use: Muscle relaxant.
See: Flexeril, Tab. (Merck & Co.).

cyclobenzaprine hydrochloride. (Various Mfr.) 10 mg/Tab. Bot. 30s, 100s, 1000s.
Use: Muscle relaxant.

Cyclocort Cream. (ESI Lederle Generics) Amcinonide 0.1% in Aquatain hydrophilic base. Tubes 15 g, 30 g, 60 g. *Rx.*
Use: Corticosteroid, topical.

Cyclocort Ointment. (ESI Lederle Generics) Amcinonide 0.1% in ointment base. Tube 15 g, 30 g, 60 g. *Rx.*
Use: Corticosteroid, topical.

cyclocumarol.
Use: Anticoagulant.

•**cyclofilcon a.** (SIGH-kloe-FILL-kahn A) USAN.
Use: Contact lens material (hydrophilic).

Cyclogen. (Schwarz Pharma, Inc.) Dicyclomine HCl 10 mg, sodium Cl 0.9%, chlorobutanol hydrate 0.5%. Vial 10 ml, Box 12s. *Rx.*

Use: Antispasmodic.

•**cycloguanil pamoate.** (SIGH-kloe-GWAHN-ill PAM-oh-ate) USAN.
Use: Antimalarial.

Cyclogyl. (Alcon Laboratories, Inc.) Cyclopentolate HCl Soln. 0.5%, 1%, or 2%. Droptainer 2 ml, 5 ml, 15 ml. *Rx.*
Use: Cycloplegic, mydriatic.

•**cycloheximide.** (sigh-KLOE-HEX-ih-mid) USAN.
Use: Antipsoriatic.

•**cyclomethicone.** (sigh-kloe-METH-ih-cone) N.F. 18.
Use: Pharmaceutic aid (wetting agent).

cyclomethycaine and methapyrilene.
Use: Anesthetic, local.

cyclomethycaine sulfate.
Use: Anesthetic, local.

Cyclomydril. (Alcon Laboratories, Inc.) Phenylephrine HCl 1%, cyclopentolate HCl 0.2%. Droptainer 2 ml, 5 ml. *Rx.*
Use: Mydriatic.

Cyclonil. (Seatrace Pharmaceuticals, Inc.) Dicyclomine HCl 10 mg/ml. Vial 10 ml. *Rx.*
Use: Anticholinergic, antispasmodic.

Cyclopar. (Parke-Davis) Tetracycline HCl 250 mg, 500 mg/Cap. **250 mg:** Bot. 100s, 1000s. **500 mg:** Bot. 100s, UD 100s. *Rx.*
Use: Anti-infective, tetracycline.

•**cyclopentamine hydrochloride.** U.S.P. 23.
Use: Adrenergic (vasoconstrictor).
See: Clopane Hydrochloride, Nasal Soln. (Eli Lilly and Co.).
W/Aludrine
See: Aerolone Compound, Soln. (Eli Lilly and Co.).

8 cyclopentyl 1,3-dipropylxanthine. (SciClone Pharmaceuticals, Inc.)
Use: Cystic fibrosis. [Orphan Drug]

•**cyclopenthiazide.** (SIGH-kloe-pen-THIGH-ah-zide) USAN.
Use: Antihypertensive, diuretic.
See: Navidrix.

•**cyclopentolate hydrochloride.** (sigh-kloe-PEN-toe-tate) U.S.P. 23.
Use: Anticholinergic (ophthalmic).
See: AK-Pentolate, Soln. (Akorn, Inc.).
Cyclogyl, Soln. (Alcon Laboratories, Inc.).
W/Phenylephrine HCl.
See: Cyclomydril, Soln. (Alcon Laboratories, Inc.).

cyclopentolate hydrochloride. (Various Mfr.) 1% Soln. Bot. 2 ml, 15 ml.
Use: Anticholinergic (ophthalmic).

cyclopentylpropionate.
See: Depo-Testosterone, Vial (Pharmacia & Upjohn).

•**cyclophenazine hydrochloride.** (SIGH-kloe-FEH-nazz-een) USAN.
Use: Antipsychotic.

•**cyclophosphamide.** (sigh-kloe-FOSS-fuh-mide) U.S.P. 23.
Use: Antineoplastic, immunosuppressant.
See: Cytoxan, Pow. for Inj. Tab., Vial (Mead Johnson Oncology).
Neosar, Pow. for Inj. (Pharmacia & Upjohn).

•**cyclopropane.** (sigh-kloe-PRO-pane) U.S.P. 23.
Use: Anesthetic, general.

•**cycloserine.** (sigh-kloe-SER-een) U.S.P. 23.
Use: Anti-infective (tuberculostatic).
See: Seromycin, Cap. (Eli Lilly and Co.).

l-cycloserine.
Use: Treat Gaucher's disease. [Orphan Drug]

cyclosporin a.
Use: Immunosuppressant.
See: Cyclosporine, U.S.P. 23.

•**cyclosporine.** (SIGH-kloe-spore-EEN) U.S.P. 23. *Formerly Cyclosporin A.*
Use: Immunosuppressant.
See: Neoral, Cap., Oral Soln. (Novartis Pharmaceutical Corp.).
Sandimmune, Preps. (Novartis Pharmaceutical Corp.).
SangCya, Oral Soln. (SangStat).

cyclosporine ophthalmic. (SIGH-kloe-spore-EEN)
Use: Severe keratoconjunctivitis sicca; graft rejection following keratoplasty. [Orphan Drug]

cyclosporine 2% ophthalmic ointment. (Allergan, Inc.)
Use: Treatment of graft rejection after keratoplasty and corneal melting syndromes. [Orphan Drug]

•**cyclothiazide.** (SIGH-kloe-thigh-AZZ-ide) USAN. U.S.P. XXII.
Use: Antihypertensive, diuretic.

Cycofed Pediatric. (Cypress) Codeine phosphate 10 mg, pseudoephedrine HCl 30 mg, guaifenesin 100 mg/5 ml, alcohol 6%. Syr. Bot. 480 ml. *c-v.*
Use: Antitussive, expectorant.

Cycrin. (ESI Lederle Generics) Medroxyprogesterone acetate 2.5 mg, 5 mg, 10 mg, lactose. Tab. Bot. 100s, 1000s. *Rx.*
Use: Hormone, progestin.

Cydonol Massage Lotion. (Gordon Laboratories) Isopropyl alcohol 14%, methyl salicylate, benzalkonium Cl. Bot. 4 oz, gal. *otc.*

Use: Counterirritant.
•**cyheptamide.** (sigh-HEP-tah-mid) USAN.
Use: Anticonvulsant.
Cyklokapron. (Pharmacia & Upjohn) **Tab.:** Tranexamic acid 500 mg. Bot. 100s. **Inj.:** 100 mg/ml. Amp. 10 ml. *Rx.*
Use: Hemostatic.
Cylert Chewable Tablets. (Abbott Laboratories) Pemoline 37.5 mg/Chew. Tab. Bot. 100s. *c-IV.*
Use: Psychotherapeutic.
Cylert Tablets. (Abbott Laboratories) Pemoline 18.75 mg, 37.5 mg, 75 mg/Tab. Bot. 100s. *c-IV.*
Use: Psychotherapeutic.
Cylex Sugar Free. (Pharmakon Laboratories, Inc.) Benzocaine 15 mg, cetylpyridinium Cl 5 mg, sorbitol. Loz. Pkg. 12s. *otc.*
Use: Antiseptic; analgesic, topical.
Cylex Throat. (Pharmakon Laboratories, Inc.) Benzocaine 15 mg, cetylpyridinium Cl 5 mg, sorbitol. Loz. Pkg. 12s. *otc.*
Use: Antiseptic; analgesic, topical.
Cynobal. (Arcum) Cyanocobalamin 100 mcg or 1000 mcg/ml. Inj. **100 mcg:** Vial 30 ml. **1000/mcg/ml.:** Vial 10 ml, 30 ml. *Rx.*
Use: Vitamin supplement.
Cyomin. (Forest Pharmaceutical, Inc.) Cyanocobalamin 1000 mcg/ml. Inj. Vial 10 ml, 30 ml. *Rx.*
Use: Vitamin B_{12} supplement.
•**cypenamine hydrochloride.** (sigh-PEN-ah-meen) USAN.
Use: Antidepressant.
•**cyprazepam.** (sigh-PRAY-zeh-pam) USAN.
Use: Hypnotic, sedative.
•**cyproheptadine hydrochloride.** (sip-row-HEP-tuh-deen) U.S.P. 23.
Use: Antihistamine, antipruritic.
See: Periactin, Tab., Syr. (Merck & Co.).
cyproheptadine hydrochloride. (sip-row-HEP-tuh-deen) (Various Mfr.) **Tab.:** Cyproheptadine HCl 4 mg. Bot. 100s, 250s, 500s, 1000s. **Syr.:** 2 mg/5 ml, alcohol. Bot. 118 ml, pt., gal. *Rx.*
Use: Antihistamine.
•**cyprolidol hydrochloride.** (sigh-PRO-lih-dahl) USAN.
Use: Antidepressant.
•**cyproterone acetate.** (sigh-PRO-ter-ohn) USAN.
Use: Antiandrogen.
•**cyproximide.** (sigh-PROX-ih-MIDE) USAN.
Use: Antidepressant, antipsychotic.
cyren a.
See: Diethylstilbestrol Prep. (Various Mfr.).
Cyronine. (Major Pharmaceuticals) Liothyronine sodium 25 mcg/Tab. Bot. 100s. *Rx.*
Use: Hormone, thyroid.
Cystadane. (Orphan Medical, Inc.) Betaine anhydrous 1 g/1.7 ml. Pow. for Inj. Bot. 180 g. *Rx.*
Use: Treatment of homocystinuria.
Cystagon. (Mylan Pharmaceuticals) Cysteamine bitartrate 50 mg, 150 mg/Cap. Bot. 100s, 500s. *Rx.*
Use: Urinary tract agent.
Cystamin.
See: Methenamine, Tab. (Various Mfr.).
Cystamine. (Tennessee Pharmaceutic) Methenamine 2 gr, phenyl salicylate 0.5 gr, phenazopyridine HCl 10 mg, benzoic acid 1/8 gr, hyoscyamine sulfate gr, atropine sulfate gr/SC Tab. Bot. 100s, 1000s. *Rx.*
Use: Anti-infective, urinary.
•**cysteamine.** (sis-TEE-ah-MEEN) USAN.
Use: Antiurolithic (cystine calculi), nephropathic cystinosis. [Orphan Drug]
•**cysteamine hydrochloride.** (sis-TEE-ah-MEEN) USAN.
Use: Antiurolithic (cystine calculi) treatment of nephropathic cystinosis.
See: Cystagon.
•**cysteine hydrochloride.** (SIS-teh-een) U.S.P. 23.
Use: Amino acid for replacement therapy, treatment of photosensitivity in erythropoietic protoporphyria. [Orphan Drug]
See: Cysteine HCl (Abbott Laboratories).
Cystex. (Numark Laboratories, Inc.) Methenamine 162 mg, sodium salicylate 162.5 mg, benzoic acid 32 mg/Tab. Bot. 40s, 100s. *otc.*
Use: Anti-infective, urinary.
cystic fibrosis gene therapy. (Genzyme Corp.)
Use: Cystic fibrosis. [Orphan Drug]
cystic fibrosis transmembrane conductance regulator gene. (Genetic Therapy, Inc., Genzyme)
Use: Cystic fibrosis. [Orphan Drug]
cystic fibrosis TR gene therapy (recombinant adenovirus). (Gerac)
Use: Cystic fibrosis. [Orphan Drug]
See: AdGVCFTR 10 (GenVec, Inc.).
•**cystine.** (SIS-TEEN) USAN.
Use: Amino acid replacement therapy, an additive for infants on TPN.
Cysto. (Freeport) Methenamine 40.8 mg, methylene blue 5.4 mg, phenyl salicy-

late 18.1 mg, atropine sulfate 0.03 mg, hyoscyamine 0.03 mg, benzoic acid 4.5 mg/Tab. Bot. 1000s. *Rx.*
Use: Anti-infective, urinary.

Cysto-Conray. (Mallinckrodt) Iothalamate meglumine 430 mg, iodine 202 mg/ml, EDTA. Inj. Vial 50 ml, 100 ml. Bot. 250 ml. *Rx.*
Use: Radiopaque agent.

Cysto-Conray II. (Mallinckrodt) Iothalamate meglumine 17.2% (iodine 8.1%) with EDTA. Soln. Bot. 250 ml, 500 ml.
Use: Radiopaque agent.

Cystografin. (Bracco Diagnostics) Diatrizoate meglumine 300 mg, iodine 141 mg/ml. Inj. Bot. 100 ml, 300 ml fill in 200 ml, 500 ml, EDTA 430 mg, iodine 202 mg/ml, EDTA. *Rx.*
Use: Radiopaque agent.

Cystografin Dilute. (Bracco Diagnostics) Diatrizoate meglumine 180 mg, iodine 85 mg/ml. Inj. Bot. 300 ml, 500 ml. *Rx.*
Use: Radiopaque agent.

Cystospaz. (PolyMedica Pharmaceuticals) l-hyoscyamine 0.15 mg/Tab. Bot. 100s. *Rx.*
Use: Anticholinergic, antispasmodic.

Cystospaz-M. (PolyMedica Pharmaceuticals) Hyoscyamine sulfate 375 mcg/Cap. Bot. 100s. *Rx.*
Use: Anticholinergic, antispasmodic.

Cytadren. (Novartis Pharmaceutical Corp.) Aminoglutethimide 250 mg/Tab. Bot. 100s. *Rx.*
Use: Adrenal steroid inhibitor; treatment of Cushing's syndrome.

•**cytarabine.** (SIGH-tar-ah-bean) U.S.P. 23.
Use: Antineoplastic, antiviral.
See: Cytosar, Inj. (Pharmacia & Upjohn).

cytarabine. (Various Mfr.) 100 mg, 500 mg/Pow. for Inj. Vials.
Use: Antineoplastic, antiviral.

cytarabine, depofoam encapsulated.
Use: Neoplastic meningitis. [Orphan Drug]

•**cytarabine hydrochloride.** (SITE-ah-rah-been HIGH-droe-KLOR-ide) USAN. *Formerly Cytosine Arabinoside Hydrochloride.*
Use: Antiviral management of acute leukemias.
See: Cytosar-U, Vial (Pharmacia & Upjohn).

CytoGam. (MedImmune, Inc.) Cytomegalovirus immune globulin IV (human) 2500 mg ± 500 mg/Inj. Solvent/detergent treated. Vial 2.5 g. *Formerly called cytomegalovirus immune globulin (human) IV. Rx.*
Use: Antiviral, cytomegalovirus.

cytomegalovirus immune globulin (human).
Use: Antiviral, cytomegalovirus. [Orphan Drug]
See: CytoGam, Vial (MedImmune, Inc.).

cytomegalovirus immune globulin (human) iv. Now named CytoGam (MedImmune, Inc.).
Use: CMV pneumonia in bone marrow transplants. [Orphan Drug]
See: CytoGam, Vial (MedImmune, Inc.).

cytomegalovirus immune globulin IV (human). (Bayer Corp. (Biological and Pharmaceutical Div.))
Use: With ganciclovir sodium for the treatment of CMV pneumonia in bone marrow transplant patients. [Orphan Drug]

Cytomel. (SmithKline Beecham Pharmaceuticals) Liothyronine sodium 5 mcg, 25 mcg, 50 mcg/Tab. Bot. 100s. 25 mcg: Bot. 100s. *Rx.*
Use: Hormone, thyroid.

Cytosar-U. (Pharmacia & Upjohn) Cytarabine 20 mg/ml in powder, 50 mg/ml reconstituted. Vial 100 mg, 500 mg. *Rx.*
Use: Antineoplastic.

cytosine arabinoside hydrochloride. Cytarabine HCl.
See: Cytosar-U (Pharmacia & Upjohn).

Cytosol. (Cytosol Laboratories, Inc.) Calcium chloride 48 mg, magnesium chloride 30 mg, potassium chloride 75 mg, sodium acetate 390 mg, sodium chloride 640 mg, sodium citrate 170 mg/100 ml. Soln. Bot. 200 ml, 500 ml. *Rx.*
Use: Irrigant.

Cytotec. (Searle) Misoprostol 200 mcg/Tab. Bot. 100s, UD 100s. *Rx.*
Use: Prostaglandins.

Cytovene. (Roche Laboratories) Ganciclovir (as sodium). **Cap.:** 250 mg, 500 mg. Tab. Bot. 180s. **Inj.:** 500 mg/Pow. Vial. 10 ml. *Rx.*
Use: Antiviral.

Cytox. (MPL) Cyanocobalamin 500 mcg, vitamins B_6 20 mg, B_1 100 mg, benzyl alcohol 2% in isotonic solution of sodium Cl/ml. Inj. Vial 10 ml. *Rx.*
Use: Vitamin supplement.

Cytoxan Lyophilized. (Mead Johnson Oncology) Cyclophosphamide. 100 mg, mannitol 75 mg. Pow. for Inj. Vial 100 mg, 200 mg, 500 mg, 1 g, 2 g. *Rx.*
Use: Antineoplastic.

Cytoxan Powder. (Bristol-Myers Oncology/Immunology) Cyclophosphamide powder 100 mg, 200 mg, 500 mg, 1 g,

or 2 g/Vial. *Rx.*
Use: Antineoplastic.

Cytoxan Tablets. (Mead Johnson Oncology) Cyclophosphamide 25 mg, 50 mg/ Tab. Bot. 100s, 1000s (50 mg only). *Rx.*
Use: Antineoplastic.

Cytra-2. (Cypress) Sodium citrate dihydrate 500 mg, citric acid monohydrate 334 mg/5 ml. Soln. Bot. 16 oz. *Rx.*
Use: Alkalinizer, systemic.

Cytra-3. (Cypress) Potassium citrate monohydrate 550 mg, sodium citrate dihydrate 500 mg, citric acid monohydrate 334 mg/5 ml. Syr. Bot. 480 ml. *Rx.*
Use: Alkalinizer, sysemic.

Cytra-K. (Cypress) Potassium citrate monohydrate 1100 mg, citric acid monohydrate 334 mg/5 ml. Soln. Bot. 473 ml. *Rx.*
Use: Alkalinizer, systemic.

Cytra-LC. (Cypress) Potassium citrate monohydrate 550 mg, sodium citrate dihydrate 500 mg, citric acid monohydrate 334 mg/5 ml. Soln. Bot. 473 ml. *Rx.*
Use: Alkalinizer, systemic.

D

D-2. D vitamin.
See: Ergocalciferol.

D-3. D vitamin.
See: Cholecalciferol.

daa.
See: Dihydroxy Aluminum Aminoacetate.

DAB_{389} IL-2. (Seragen)
Use: Cutaneous T-cell lymphoma. [Orphan Drug]

•**dacarbazine.** (da-CAR-buh-zeen) U.S.P. 23.
Use: Antineoplastic.
See: DTIC-Dome, Inj. (Bayer Corp. (Consumer Div.)).

D.A. Chew Tabs. (Dura Pharmaceuticals) Phenylephrine HCl 10 mg, chlorpheniramine 2 mg, methscopolamine nitrate 1.25 mg/Tab. Bot. 100s. *Rx.*
Use: Anticholinergic, antihistamine, decongestant.

D.A. II. (Dura Pharmaceuticals) Chlorpheniramine maleate 4 mg, phenylephrine HCl 10 mg, methscopolamine nitrate 1.25 mg/Tab. Bot. 100s. *Rx.*
Use: Anticholinergic, antihistamine, decongestant.

•**dacliximab.** (dak-LICK-sih-mab) USAN.
Use: Monoclonal antibody (immunosuppressant).
See: Zenapax, Inj. (Hoffmann-LaRoche).
Daclizumab.

Daclizumab. USAN.
Use: Immunosuppressant.
See: Zenapax (Roche Laboratories).

Dacodyl. (Major Pharmaceuticals) **Tab.:** Bisacodyl 5 mg/Tab. Bot. 100s, 250s, 1000s. UD 100s. **Supp.:** Bisacodyl 10 mg. Box 12s, 100s. *otc.*
Use: Laxative.

Dacriose. (Ciba Vision) Sodium Cl, potassium Cl, sodium hydroxide, sodium phosphate, benzalkonium Cl 0.01%, edetate disodium. Bot. 15 ml, 120 ml. *otc.*
Use: Irrigant, ophthalmic.

•**dactinomycin.** (DAK-tih-no-MY-sin) U.S.P. 23.
Use: Antineoplastic.
See: Cosmegen, Vial (Merck & Co.).

Daily Cleaner. (Bausch & Lomb Pharmaceuticals) Isotonic solution with sodium Cl, sodium phosphate, tyloxapol, hydroxyethylcellulose, polyvinyl alcohol with thimerosal 0.004%, EDTA 0.2%. Soln. Bot. 45 ml. *otc.*
Use: Contact lens care.

Daily Conditioning Treatment. (Blistex, Inc.) Padimate O 7.5%, oxybenzone 3.5%, petrolatum. Stick 11.4 g. SPF 15. *otc.*
Use: Lip protectant.

Daily Vitamins Liquid. (Rugby Labs, Inc.) Vitamins A 2500 IU, D 400 IU, E 15 IU, C 60 mg, B_1 1.2 mg, B_2 1.2 mg, B_6 1.05 mg, B_{12} 4.5 mcg, niacinamide 13.5 mg/5 ml. Bot. 273 ml, 473 ml. *otc.*
Use: Vitamin supplement.

Daily Vitamins Tablets. (Kirkman Sales Co., Inc.) Vitamins A 5000 IU, D 400 IU, C 50 mg, B_1 3 mg, B_2 2.5 mg, B_6 1 mg, B_{12} 1 mcg, niacinamide 20 mg, d-calcium pantothenate 1 mg/Tab. Bot. 100s. *otc.*
Use: Vitamin supplement.

Daily Vitamins w/Iron. (Kirkman Sales Co., Inc.) Vitamins A 5000 IU, D 400 IU, B_1 2 mg, B_2 2.5 mg, B_6 1 mg, B_{12} 1 mcg, niacinamide 20 mg, d-calcium pantothenate 1 mg, iron 18 mg/Tab. Bot. 100s. *otc.*
Use: Vitamin supplement.

Daily-Vite w/Iron & Minerals. (Rugby Labs, Inc.) Iron 18 mg, vitamins A 5000 IU, D 400 IU, E 30 mg, B_1 1.5 mg, B_2 1.7 mg, B_3 20 mg, B_5 10 mg, B_6 2 mg, B_{12} 6 mcg, C 60 mg, folic acid 0.4 mg, Ca, Cl, Cr, Cu, I, K, Mg, Mn, Mo, P, Se, zinc 15 mg, biotin, vitamin K/Tab. Bot. 100s. *otc.*
Use: Mineral, vitamin supplement.

Dairy Ease. (Sanofi Winthrop Pharmaceuticals) Lactase 3300 FCC units, mannitol. Tab. Bot. 60s. *otc.*
Use: Digestive enzyme.

Daisy 2 Pregnancy Test. (Advanced Care Products) Home pregnancy test. Test kit 2s.
Use: Diagnostic aid.

Dakin's Solution.
See: Sodium Hypochlorite Solution Diluted.

Dakin's Solution-Full Strength. (Century Pharmaceuticals, Inc.) Sodium hypochlorite 0.5%. Soln. Bot. Pt, gal. *otc.*
Use: Anti-infective, topical.

Dakin's Solution-Half Strength. (Century Pharmaceuticals, Inc.) Sodium hypochlorite 0.25%. Soln. Bot. Pt. *otc.*
Use: Anti-infective, topical.

Dalalone. (Forest Pharmaceutical, Inc.) Dexamethasone sodium phosphate 4 mg/ml, methyl- and propylparabens, sodium bisulfite. Vial 5 ml. *Rx.*
Use: Corticosteroid.

Dalalone D.P. (Forest Pharmaceutical, Inc.) Dexamethasone acetate 16 mg/

ml, polysorbate 80, carboxymethylcellulose, sodium bisulfite, EDTA, benzyl alcohol. Vial 1 ml, 5 ml. *Rx.*
Use: Corticosteroid.

Dalalone L.A. (Forest Pharmaceutical, Inc.) Dexamethasone 8 mg/ml, polysorbate 80, carboxymethylcellulose, sodium bisulfite, EDTA, benzyl alcohol. Vial 5 ml. *Rx.*
Use: Corticosteroid.

d-ala-peptide t.
Use: Antiviral.

•**daledalin tosylate.** (dah-LEH-dah-lin TAH-sill-ate) USAN.
Use: Antidepressant.

•**dalfopristin.** (dal-FOE-priss-tin) USAN.
Use: Anti-infective.

Dalgan. (Wyeth-Ayerst Laboratories) Dezocine 5 mg, 10 mg, or 15 mg/ml. **5 mg/ml:** Vial (SD) 1 ml. **10 mg/ml:** Vial (SD) 1 ml, Vial (MD) 10 ml, syringes (prefilled) 1 ml. **15 mg/ml:** Vial (SD) 1 ml, syringes (prefilled) 1 ml. *Rx.*
Use: Analgesic, narcotic.

Dallergy Caplets. (Laser, Inc.) Chlorpheniramine maleate 8 mg, phenylephrine HCl 20 mg, methscopolamine nitrate 2.5 mg/ER Capl. Bot. 100s. *Rx.*
Use: Anticholinergic, antihistamine, decongestant.

Dallergy-D Syrup. (Laser, Inc.) Chlorpheniramine maleate 2 mg, phenylephrine HCl 5 mg/5 ml. Bot. 118 ml. *otc.*
Use: Antihistamine, decongestant.

Dallergy-Jr. Capsules. (Laser, Inc.) Brompheniramine maleate 6 mg, pseudoephedrine HCl 60 mg/Cap. Bot. 100s. *Rx.*
Use: Antihistamine, decongestant.

Dallergy Syrup. (Laser, Inc.) Chlorpheniramine maleate 2 mg, phenylephrine HCl 10 mg, methscopolamine nitrate 0.625 mg/5 ml. Bot. 473 ml. *Rx.*
Use: Anticholinergic, antihistamine, antispasmodic, decongestant.

Dallergy Tablets. (Laser, Inc.) Chlorpheniramine maleate 4 mg, phenylephrine HCl 10 mg, methscopolamine nitrate 1.25 mg/Tab. Bot. 100s. *Rx.*
Use: Anticholinergic, antihistamine, antispasmodic, decongestant.

Dalmane. (Roche Laboratories) Flurazepam HCl 15 mg or 30 mg/Cap. Bot. 100s, 500s, Prescription Pak 300s. RNP (Reverse Numbered Packages) 4 rolls × 25 cap. or 4 cards × 25 cap. UD 100s. *c-IV.*
Use: Hypnotic, sedative.

•**dalteparin sodium.** (dal-TEH-puh-rin) USAN.
Use: Anticoagulant, antithrombotic.
See: Fragmin, Inj. (Pharmacia & Upjohn).

•**daltroban.** (DAL-troe-ban) USAN.
Use: Platelet aggregation inhibitor, immunosuppressant.

•**dalvastatin.** (DAL-vah-STAT-in) USAN.
Use: Antihyperlipidemic.

Damacet-P. (Mason Pharmaceuticals, Inc.) Hydrocodone bitartrate 5 mg, acetaminophen 500 mg/Tab. Bot. 100s, 500s. *c-III.*
Use: Analgesic combination, narcotic.

Damason-P. (Mason Pharmaceuticals, Inc.) Hydrocodone bitartrate 5 mg, aspirin 500 mg/Tab. Bot. 100s, 500s, 1000s. *c-III.*
Use: Analgesic combination, narcotic.

Dambose.
See: Inositol, Tabs.

•**danaparoid sodium.** (dan-AHP-ah-royd) USAN.
Use: Antithrombotic.
See: Orgaran, Inj. (Organon, Inc.).

Danatrol. (Sanofi Winthrop Pharmaceuticals) Danazol. Cap. *Rx.*
Use: Gonadotropin inhibitor.

•**danazol.** (DAN-uh-ZOLE) U.S.P. 23.
Use: Anterior pituitary suppressant.
See: Danocrine, Cap. (Sanofi Winthrop Pharmaceuticals).

danazol. (Various Mfr.) Danazol 200 mg/Cap. Bot. 50s, 60s, 100s, 500s. *Rx.*
Use: Anterior pituitary suppressant.

Dandruff Shampoo. (Walgreen) Zinc pyrithione 2 g/100 ml. Bot. 11 oz. Tube 7 oz. *otc.*
Use: Antiseborrheic.

•**daniplestim.** (dan-ih-PLEH-stim) USAN.
Use: Antineutroenic, hematopoietic stimulant, treatment of chemotherapy-induced bone marrow suppression.

Danocrine. (Sanofi Winthrop Pharmaceuticals) Danazol 50 mg, 100 mg, or 200 mg/Cap. Bot. 100s. *Rx.*
Use: Gonadotropin inhibitor.

Danogar Tablets. (Sanofi Winthrop Pharmaceuticals) Danazol. *Rx.*
Use: Gonadotropin inhibitor.

Danol Capsules. (Sanofi Winthrop Pharmaceuticals) Danazol. *Rx.*
Use: Gonadotropin inhibitor.

Dantrium. (Procter & Gamble Pharm.) Dantrolene sodium. **25 mg/Cap.:** Bot. 100s, 500s, UD 100s; **50 mg/Cap.:** Bot. 100s; **100 mg/Cap.:** Bot. 100s, UD 100s. *Rx.*
Use: Muscle relaxant.

Dantrium IV. (Procter & Gamble Pharm.)

Dantrolene sodium 20 mg. Vial. 70 ml. *Rx.*
Use: Muscle relaxant.

•**dantrolene.** (dan-troe-LEEN) USAN.
Use: Muscle relaxant.

•**dantrolene sodium.** (dan-troe-LEEN) USAN.
Use: Muscle relaxant.
See: Dantrium, Cap., I.V. (Procter & Gamble Pharm.).

Dapa Extra Strength Tablets. (Ferndale Laboratories, Inc.) Acetaminophen 500 mg. Bot. 50s, 100s, 1000s, UD 100s. *otc.*
Use: Analgesic.

Dapa Tablets. (Ferndale Laboratories, Inc.) Acetaminophen 324 mg/Tab. Bot. 100s, 1000s, UD 100s. *otc.*
Use: Analgesic.

Dapco. (Schlicksup) Salicylamide 300 mg, butabarbital 15 mg/Tab. Bot. 100s, 1000s. *c-III.*
Use: Analgesic, hypnotic, sedative.

•**dapiprazole hydrochloride.** (DAP-ih-PRAY-zole) USAN.
Use: Alpha-adrenergic blocker, antiglaucoma agent, neuroleptic, psychotherapeutic agent.
See: Rev-Eyes, Pow. (Storz/Lederle Ophthalmic Pharmaceuticals).

•**dapoxetine hydrochloride.** (dap-OX-eh-teen) USAN.
Use: Antidepressant.

•**dapsone.** (DAP-sone) U.S.P. 23. *Formerly Diaminodiphenylsulfone.*
Use: Anti-infective (leprostatic), dermatitis herpetiformis suppressant, prevention/treatment of *Pneumocystis carinii* pneumonia. [Orphan Drug]
See: Dapsone (Jacobus Pharmaceutical Co.).

dapsone. (Jacobus Pharmaceutical Co.) 25 mg or 100 mg/Tab. Bot. 100s. *Rx.*
Use: Anti-infective (leprostatic), dermitis herpetiformis suppressant, prevention/treatment of *Pneumocystis carinii* pneumonia. [Orphan Drug]

•**daptomycin.** (DAP-toe-MY-sin) USAN.
Use: Anti-infective.

Daragen. (Galderma Laboratories, Inc.) Collagen polypeptide, benzalkonium Cl in a mild amphoteric base. Shampoo. Bot. 8 oz. *otc.*
Use: Dermatologic.

Dara Soapless Shampoo. (Galderma Laboratories, Inc.) Purified water, potassium coco hydrolyzed protein, sulfated castor oil, pentasodium triphosphate, sodium benzoate, sodium lauryl sulfate, fragrance. Shampoo. Bot. 8 oz, 16 oz. *otc.*
Use: Dermatologic, scalp.

Daranide. (Merck & Co.) Dichlorphenamide 50 mg/Tab. Bot. 100s. *Rx.*
Use: Antiglaucoma agent.

Daraprim. (GlaxoWellcome) Pyrimethamine 25 mg/Tab. Bot. 100s. *Rx.*
Use: Antimalarial.

Darco G-60. (Zeneca Pharmaceuticals) Activated carbon from lignite.
Use: Purifier.

•**darglitazone sodium.** (dahr-GLIH-tah-zone) USAN.
Use: Oral hypoglycemic.

•**darodipine.** (DA-row-dih-PEEN) USAN.
Use: Antihypertensive, bronchodilator, vasodilator.

Darvocet-N 100. (Eli Lilly and Co.) Propoxyphene napsylate 100 mg, acetaminophen 650 mg/Tab. Bot. 100s (Rx Pak) 500s, UD 100s, 500s, RN 500s. *c-IV.*
Use: Analgesic combination, narcotic.

Darvon. (Eli Lilly and Co.) Propoxyphene HCl 65 mg/Pulv. Bot. 100s. Rx Pak 500s; Blister pkg. 10 × 10s; UD 20 rolls 25s. *c-IV.*
Use: Analgesic combination, narcotic.

Darvon Compound-65. (Eli Lilly and Co.) Propoxyphene HCl 65 mg, aspirin 389 mg, caffeine 32.4 mg/Pulv. Bot. 100s, Rx Pak 500s. *c-IV.*
Use: Analgesic combination, narcotic.

Darvon-N. (Eli Lilly and Co.) Propoxyphene napsylate 100 mg. Tab. Bot. 100s, 500s, UD 100s. *c-IV.*
Use: Analgesic, narcotic.

Darvon Pulvules. (Eli Lilly and Co.) Propoxyphene HCl 65 mg. Cap. Bot. 100s, 500s, UD 100s. *c-IV.*
Use: Analgesic, narcotic.

Da-Sed. (Sheryl) Butabarbital 0.5 gr/Tab. Bot. 100s. *c-III.*
Use: Hypnotic, sedative.

Dasin. (SmithKline Beecham Pharmaceuticals) Ipecac 3 mg, acetylsalicylic acid 130 mg, camphor 15 mg, caffeine 8 mg, atropine sulfate 0.13 mg/Cap. Bot. 100s, 500s. *Rx.*
Use: Analgesic, anticholinergic, antispasmodic.

Daturine Hydrobromide.
See: Hyoscyamine Salts (Various Mfr.).

•**daunorubicin hydrochloride.** (DAW-no-RUE-bih-sin) U.S.P. 23.
Use: Antineoplastic.
See: Cerubidine, Inj. (Bedford Laboratories)
DaunoXome (Nexstar Pharmaceutical).

daunorubicin citrate liposome. (DAW-no-RUE-bih-sin)
Use: Treatment of advanced HIV-associated Kaposi's sarcoma. [Orphan Drug]
See: DaunoXome (Nexstar Pharmaceutical).

DaunoXome. (Nexstar Pharmaceutical) Daunorubicin citrate liposomal 2 mg/ml (equivalent to 50 mg daunorubicin base). Inj. Vials. 1, 4, 10 unit packs. *Rx.*
Use: Treatment of advanced HIV-associated Kaposi's sarcoma.

Davitamon K.
See: Menadione Inj., Tab. (Various Mfr.).

Davosil. (Colgate Oral Pharmaceuticals) Silicon carbide in glycerin base. Jar 8 oz, 10 oz. *otc.*
Use: Agent for oral hygiene.

Dayalets. (Abbott Laboratories) Vitamins B_1 1.5 mg, B_2 1.7 mg, A 5000 IU, C 60 mg, D 400 IU, niacinamide 20 mg, B_6 2 mg, B_{12} 6 mcg, E 30 IU, folic acid 0.4 mg/Filmtab. Bot. 100s. *otc.*
Use: Vitamin supplement.

Dayalets + Iron. (Abbott Laboratories) Vitamins B_1 1.5 mg, B_2 1.7 mg, niacinamide 20 mg, B_6 2 mg, C 60 mg, A 5000 IU, D 400 IU, E 30 IU, B_{12} 6 mcg, iron 18 mg, folic acid 0.4 mg/Filmtab. Bot. 100s. *otc.*
Use: Mineral, vitamin supplement.

Daycare. (Procter & Gamble Pharm.) Pseudoephedrine HCl 10 mg, dextromethorphan HBr 3.3 mg, guaifenesin 33.3 mg, acetaminophen 108 mg, alcohol 10%, saccharin. Expectorant Liq. Bot. 180 ml, 300 ml. *otc.*
Use: Analgesic, antitussive, decongestant, expectorant.

Day-Night Comtrex. (Bristol-Myers Squibb) Pseudoephedrine HCl 30 mg, chlorpheniramine maleate 2 mg, dextromethorphan HBr 10 mg, acetaminophen 325 mg/Tab. Pkg. 6s. *otc.*
Use: Analgesic, antihistamine, antitussive, decongestant.

Daypro. (Searle) Oxaprozin 600 mg/Capl. Bot. 100s, 500s, UD 100s. *Rx.*
Use: Analgesic, NSAID.

Day Tab. (Towne) Vitamins A 5000 IU, D 400 IU, B_1 15 mg, B_2 10 mg, C 600 mg, niacinamide 20 mg, B_6 5 mg, folic acid 400 mcg, pantothenic acid 10 mg, zinc 15 mg, copper 2 mg, B_{12} 5 mcg/Tab. Bot. 100s, 200s. *otc.*
Use: Mineral, vitamin supplement.

Day Tab Essential. (Towne) Vitamins A 5000 IU, D 400 IU, E 15 IU, C 60 mg, folic acid 0.4 mg, B_1 1.5 mg, B_2 1.7 mg, niacin 20 mg, B_6 2 mg, B_{12} 6 mcg/Tab. Bot. 200s. *otc.*
Use: Vitamin supplement.

Day Tabs, New. (Towne) Vitamins A 5000 IU, E 15 IU, D 400 IU, C 60 mg, folic acid 0.4 mg, B_1 1.5 mg, B_2 1.7 mg, niacin 20 mg, B_6 20 mg, B_{12} 6 mcg/Tab. Bot. 100s, 250s. *otc.*
Use: Vitamin supplement.

Day Tab Plus Iron. (Towne) Iron 18 mg, vitamins A 5000 IU, D 400 IU, B_1 1.5 mg, B_2 1.7 mg, niacinamide 20 mg, C 60 mg, B_6 2 mg, pantothenic acid 10 mg, B_{12} 6 mcg, folic acid 0.1 mg/Tab. Bot. 100s. *otc.*
Use: Mineral, vitamin supplement.

Day Tabs Plus Iron, New. (Towne) Vitamins A 5000 IU, E 15 IU, D 400 IU, C 60 mg, folic acid 0.4 mg, B_1 1.5 mg, B_2 1.7 mg, niacin 20 mg, B_6 20 mg, B_{12} 6 mcg, iron 18 mcg/Tab. Bot. 250s. *otc.*
Use: Mineral, vitamin supplement.

Day Tab Stress Complex. (Towne) Vitamins A 5000 IU, C 600 mg, B_1 15 mg, B_2 10 mg, niacin 100 mg, D 400 IU, E 30 IU, B_6 5 mg, folic acid 400 mcg, B_{12} 6 mcg, pantothenic acid 20 mg, iron 18 mg, zinc 15 mg, copper 2 mg/Tab. Bot. 60s. *otc.*
Use: Mineral, vitamin supplement.

Day Tab with Iron. (Towne) Vitamins A 5000 IU, D 400 IU, E 15 IU, C 60 mg, folic acid 1.5 mg, B_1 15 mg, B_2 1.7 mg, niacin 20 mg, B_6 2 mg, B_{12} 6 mcg, iron 18 mg/Tab. Bot. 200s. *Rx.*
Use: Mineral, vitamin supplement.

Dayto-Anase. (Dayton Laboratories, Inc.) Bromelains 50,000 IU (protease activity). Tab. Bot. 60s. *otc.*
Use: Enzyme.

Dayto Himbin. (Dayton Laboratories, Inc.) Yohimbine 5.4 mg/Tab. Bot. 60s. *Rx.*
Use: Alpha-adrenergic blocker.

Dayto Sulf. (Dayton Laboratories, Inc.) Sulfathiazole 3.42%, sulfacetamide 2.86%, sulfabenzamide 3.7%, urea 0.64%. Cream. Tube 78 g with 8 disposable applicators. *Rx.*
Use: Anti-infective, vaginal.

•**dazadrol maleate.** (DAY-zah-drole) USAN.
Use: Antidepressant.

Dazamide Tabs. (Major Pharmaceuticals) Acetazolamide 250 mg/Tab. Bot. 100s, 250s, 1000s, UD 100s. *Rx.*
Use: Diuretic.

•**dazepinil hydrochloride.** (dahz-EH-pih-NILL) USAN.
Use: Antidepressant.

•**dazmegrel.** (DAZE-meh-grell) USAN.
Use: Inhibitor (thromboxane synthetase).

•**dazopride fumarate.** (DAY-zoe-PRIDE) USAN.
Use: Peristaltic stimulant.

•**dazoxiben hydrochloride.** (DAZE-OX-ih-ben) USAN.
Use: Antithrombotic.

DB Electrode Paste. (Day-Baldwin) Tube 5%.

Dbed. Dibenzylethylenediamine dipenicillin G.
Use: Anti-infective, penicillin.

DCA.
See: Desoxycorticosterone acetate preps. (Various Mfr.).

DCF. Pentostatin (2'-deoxycoformycin). *Rx.*
Use: Anti-infective.
See: Nipent, Pow. (Parke-Davis).

DCP. (Towne) Calcium 180 mg, phosphorus 105 mg, vitamins D 66.7 IU/Tab. Bot. 100s. *otc.*
Use: Mineral, vitamin supplement.

DC Softgels. (Zenith Goldline Pharmaceuticals) Docusate calcium 240 mg/Cap. Bot. 100s, 500s. *otc.*
Use: Laxative.

DC 240. (Zenith Goldline Pharmaceuticals) Docusate calcium 240 mg/Cap. Bot. 100s, 500s. *otc.*
Use: Laxative.

DDAVP Injection. (Rorer) Desmopressin acetate 15 mcg/ml, NaCl 9 mg/ml. Amp. 1 ml, 2 ml. *Rx.*
Use: Antidiuretic.

DDAVP Nasal. (Rhone-Poulenc Rorer Pharmaceuticals, Inc.) 0.1 mg/ml (0.1 mg equivalent to 400 IU arginine vasopressin). Soln. Sodium chloride 7.5 mg. Spray Pump. Bot. 5 ml w/ spray pump (50 doses of 10 mcg). *Rx.*
Use: Antidiuretic.

DDAVP Spray. (Rorer) Desmopressin acetate 0.1 mg, chlorobutanol 5 mg/ml. Bot. 5 ml. Vial 2.5 ml w/applicator tubes for nasal administration. *Rx.*
Use: Antidiuretic.

DDAVP Tablets. (Rhone-Poulenc Rorer Pharmaceuticals, Inc.) Desmopressin acetate 0.1 or 0.2 mg/Tab. Bot 100s. *Rx.*
Use: Antidiuretic.

ddC. Dideoxycytidine.
Use: Antiviral.
See: HIVID (Roche Laboratories).

ddI. Didanosine.
Use: Antiviral.

D-Diol. (Burgin-Arden) Testosterone cypionate 50 mg, estradiol cypionate 2 mg/ml. Vial 10 ml. *Rx.*
Use: Androgen, estrogen combination.

DDS.
See: Dapsone Tab., U.S.P. 23.

DDT.
See: Chlorophenothane.

Deacetyllanatoside C.
See: Deslanoside, U.S.P. 23.

deadly nightshade leaf.
See: Belladonna Leaf, U.S.P. 23.

1-deamino-8-d-arginine vasopressin. Desmopressin acetate.
Use: Hormone.
See: Concentraid, Soln. (Ferring Pharmaceuticals, Inc.).
DDAVP, Inj., Soln. (Rhone-Poulenc Rorer Pharmaceuticals, Inc.).

deba.
See: Barbital (Various Mfr.).

Debrisan. (Johnson & Johnson) Dextranomer. **Beads:** Spherical hydrophilic 0.1 to 0.3 mm diameter. Bot. 25 g, 60 g, 120 g. Pk. 7 × 4 g, 14 × 14 g. US distributor Johnson & Johnson Consumer Products. **Paste:** 10 g. Foil packets 6s. *otc.*
Use: Dermatologic, wound therapy.

•**debrisoquin sulfate.** (deb-RICE-oh-kwin) USAN.
Use: Antihypertensive.

Debrox. (Hoechst Marion Roussel) Carbamide peroxide 6.5% in anhydrous glycerol. Plastic squeeze bot. 0.5 oz, 1 oz. *otc.*
Use: Otic.

Decabid. (Eli Lilly and Co.) Indecainide HCl 50 mg, 75 mg, or 100 mg/SR tab. Bot. 100s, UD 100s. [Approved but not marketed].
Use: Antiarrhythmic.

Deca-Bon. (Barrows) Vitamins A 3000 IU, D 400 IU, C 60 mg, B_1 1 mg, B_2 1.2 mg, niacinamide 8 mg, B_6 1 mg, panthenol 3 mg, B_{12} 1 mcg, biotin 30 mcg/0.6 ml. Drops Bot. 50 ml. *otc.*
Use: Vitamin supplement.

Decaderm. (Merck & Co.) Dexamethasone 0.1% w/isopropyl myristate gel, wood alcohols, refined lanolin alcohol, microcrystalline wax, anhydrous citric acid, anhydrous sodium phosphate dibasic. Tube 30 g. *Rx.*
Use: Corticosteroid.

Decadron. (Paddock Laboratories) Dexamethasone sodium phosphate 4 mg/ml. Vial 5 ml. *Rx.*
Use: Corticosteroid.

Decadron. (Merck & Co.) Dexamethasone. **Tab.:** 0.5 mg: Bot. 100s, UD 100s; 0.75 mg: 100s, UD 100s; 4 mg: Bot. 50s, UD 100s. **Elix.:** 0.5 mg/5 ml,

benzoic acid 0.1%, alcohol 5% Bot. w/ dropper 100 ml, Bot. w/out dropper 237 ml. *Rx.*
Use: Corticosteroid.
W/Neomycin sulfate.
See: NeoDecadron, Ophth. Soln., Ophth. Oint., Topical, Cream (Merck & Co.).

Decadron Phosphate. (Merck & Co.) Dexamethasone sodium phosphate. **Ophth. Soln.:** 0.1%. Ocumeter dispenser 5 ml. **Ophth. Oint.:** 0.05%. Tube 3.5 g. *Rx.*
Use: Corticosteroid, ophthalmic.

Decadron Phosphate Injection. (Merck & Co.) Dexamethasone sodium phosphate 4 mg or 24 mg/ml, creatinine 8 mg, sodium citrate 10 mg, disodium edetate 0.5 mg (24 mg/ml only), sodium hydroxide to adjust pH, sodium bisulfite 1 mg, methylparaben 1.5 mg, propylparaben 0.2 mg/ml. **4 mg/ml:** Vial 1 ml, 5 ml, 25 ml. **24 mg/ml:** (for IV use only): Vial 5 ml, 10 ml. *Rx.*
Use: Corticosteroid.

Deca-Durabolin. (Organon, Inc.) Nandrolone decanoate injection w/benzyl alcohol 10%. **50 mg/ml:** Multidose vial 2 ml. **100 mg/ml:** Multidose vial 2 ml, syringe 1 ml. **200 mg/ml:** Multidose vial 1 ml, syringe 1 ml. *c-III.*
Use: Anabolic steroid.

Deca-Durabolin Rediject Syringes. (Organon, Inc.) Nandrolone decanoate 50 mg, 100 mg, or 200 mg/ml. Syringe 1 ml. Box 25s. *c-III.*
Use: Anabolic steroid.

Decagen. (Zenith Goldline Pharmaceuticals) Iron 18 mg, vitamins A 5000 IU, D 400 IU, E 30 IU, B_1 1.7 mg, B_2 2 mg, B_3 20 mg, B_5 10 mg, B_6 3 mg, B_{12} 6 mcg, C 60 mg, folic acid 0.4 mg, Ca, Cl, Cr, Cu, B, I, K, Mg, Mn, Mo, Ni, P, Se, Si, Sn, V, Zn 15 mg, vitamin K, biotin 30 mcg/Tab. Bot. 130s. *otc.*
Use: Mineral, vitamin supplement.

Decaject. (Merz Pharmaceutcials) Dexamethasone sodium phosphate 4 mg/ml. Vial 5 ml, 10 ml. *Rx.*
Use: Corticosteroid.

Decaject-L.A. (Merz Pharmaceutcials) Dexamethasone acetate 8 mg/ml suspension, polysorbate 80, carboxymethylcellulose, sodium bisulfite, EDTA, benzyl alcohol. Inj. Vial 5 ml. *Rx.*
Use: Corticosteroid.

Decalix. (Pharmed) Dexamethasone 0.5 mg/5 ml. Bot. 100 ml. *Rx.*
Use: Corticosteroid.

Decameth. (Foy Laboratories) Dexamethasone sodium phosphate injection 4 mg/5 ml vial. *Rx.*
Use: Corticosteroid.

Decameth L.A. (Foy Laboratories) Dexamethasone sodium phosphate injection 8 mg/ml. Vial/5 ml. *Rx.*
Use: Corticosteroid.

Decameth Tablets. (Foy Laboratories) Dexamethasone 0.75 mg/Tab. Bot. 1000s. *Rx.*
Use: Corticosteroid.

Decapryn. (Hoechst Marion Roussel) Doxylamine succinate 12.5 mg/Tab. Bot. 100s. *otc.*
Use: Antihistamine.

Decasone Injection. (Forest Pharmaceutical, Inc.) Dexamethasone sodium phosphate equivalent to dexamethasone phosphate 4 mg/ml. Vial 5 ml. *Rx.*
Use: Corticosteroid.

decavitamin. U.S.P. XXI. Vitamins A 4000 IU, D 400 IU, C 70 mg, calcium pantothenate 10 mg, B_{12} 5 mcg, folic acid 100 mcg, nicotinamide 20 mg, B_6 2 mg, B_2 2 mg, B_1 2 mg/Cap. or Tab. *otc.*
Use: Vitamin supplement.

Decholin. (Bayer Corp. (Consumer Div.)) Dehydrocholic acid 250 mg/Tab. Bot. 100s, 500s. *otc.*
Use: Hydrocholeretic.

Decicain. Tetracaine HCl.

•**decitabine.** (deh-SIGH-tah-BEAN) USAN.
Use: Antineoplastic.

declaben. (DEH-klah-BEN) *Formerly lodelaben.*
Use: Antiarthritic, emphysema therapy adjunct.

Declomycin Hydrochloride. (ESI Lederle Generics) Demeclocycline HCl. **Cap.:** 150 mg. Bot. 100s. **Tab.:** 150 mg. Bot. 100s; 300 mg. Bot. 48s. *Rx.*
Use: Anti-infective, tetracycline.

Decofed. (Various Mfr.) Pseudoephedrine HCl 30 mg/5 ml. Syr. Bot. 120 ml, 240 ml, pt, gal. *otc.*
Use: Decongestant.

Decohist. (Towne) Chlorphen-iramine maleate 1 mg, phenylpropanolamine HCl 12.5 mg, salicylamide 180 mg, caffeine 15 mg/Cap. Bot. 18s. *otc.*
Use: Analgesic, antihistamine, decongestant.

Decohistine. (Rosemont Pharmaceutical Corp.) Phenylephrine HCl 5 mg, chlorpheniramine maleate 2 mg, alcohol 5%. Elix. Bot. 120 ml, pt. and gal. *otc.*
Use: Antihistamine, decongestant.

Decohistine DH. (Morton Grove Pharmaceuticals, Inc.) Pseudoephedrine HCl 30 mg, chlorpheniramine maleate 2 mg,

codeine phosphate 10 mg, alcohol. Liq. Bot. 120 ml, pt and gal. *c-v.*
Use: Antihistamine, antitussive, decongestant.

Deconade. (H.L. Moore Drug Exchange, Inc.) Phenylpropanolamine HCl 75 mg, chlorpheniramine maleate 12 mg/Cap. Bot. 100s, 1000s. *otc.*
Use: Antihistamine, decongestant.

Deconamine CX Liquid. (Bradley Pharmaceutical) Hydrocodone bitartrate 5 mg, pseudoephedrine HCl 60 mg, guaifenesin 200 mg/5 ml. Bot. 480 ml. *Rx.*
Use: Antitussive, expectorant.

Deconamine CX Tablets. (Bradley Pharmaceutical) Hydrocodone bitartrate 5 mg, pseudoephedrine HCl 30 mg, guaifenesin 300 mg. Tab. Bot. 100s. *Rx.*
Use: Antitussive, expectorant.

Deconamine SR Capsules. (Bradley Pharmaceutical) Chlorpheniramine maleate 8 mg, d-pseudoephedrine HCl 120 mg/Cap. Bot. 100s, 500s. *Rx.*
Use: Antihistamine, decongestant.

Deconamine Syrup. (Bradley Pharmaceutical) Chlorpheniramine maleate 2 mg, d-pseudoephedrine HCl 30 mg/5 ml, sorbitol. Bot. 473 ml. *Rx.*
Use: Antihistamine, decongestant.

Deconamine Tablets. (Bradley Pharmaceutical) Chlorpheniramine maleate 4 mg, d-pseudoephedrine HCl 60 mg/Tab. Bot. 100s. *Rx.*
Use: Antihistamine, decongestant.

Decongestabs. (Various Mfr.) Phenylpropanolamine HCl 40 mg, phenylephrine HCl 10 mg, chlorpheniramine maleate 5 mg, phenyltoloxamine citrate 15 mg/Tab. Bot. 100s, 1000s. *Rx.*
Use: Antihistamine, decongestant.

Decongestant Expectorant Liquid. (Schein Pharmaceutical, Inc.) Pseudoephedrine HCl 30 mg, codeine phosphate 10 mg, guaifenesin 100 mg, alcohol 7.5%. Bot. 480 ml. *c-v.*
Use: Antitussive, decongestant, expectorant.

Decongestant Formula Mediquell. (Parke-Davis) Dextromethorphan HBr 30 mg, pseudoephedrine HCl 60 mg/Square.
Use: Antitussive, decongestant.

Decongestant Tablets, Extended Release. (Various Mfr.) Phenylpropanolamine HCl 40 mg, phenylephrine HCl 10 mg, chlorpheniramine maleate 5 mg, phenyltoloxamine citrate 15 mg/Tab. Bot. 50s, 100s, 1000s. *Rx.*
Use: Antihistamine, decongestant.

Deconhist L.A. (Zenith Goldline Pharmaceuticals) Phenylephrine HCl 25 mg, phenylpropanolamine HCl 50 mg, chlorpheniramine maleate 8 mg, hyoscyamine sulfate 0.19 mg, atropine sulfate 0.04 mg, scopolamine hydrobromide 0.01 mg/SR Tab. Bot. 100s, 250s, 500s, 1000s. *Rx.*
Use: Anticholinergic, antihistamine, decongestant.

Deconomed. (Iomed) Chlorpheniramine maleate 8 mg, pseudoephedrine HCl 120 mg/Cap. Bot. 100s, 500s. *Rx.*
Use: Antihistamine, decongestant.

Deconsal II Capsules. (Medeva Pharmaceuticals, Inc.) Pseudoephedrine 60 mg, guaifenesin 600 mg/Cap. Bot. 100s. *Rx.*
Use: Decongestant, expectorant.

•**dectaflur.** (DECK-tah-flure) USAN.
Use: Dental caries agent.

Decubitex. (I.C.P. Pharmaceuticals) **Oint.:** Biebrich scarlet red sulfonated 0.1%, balsam Peru, castor oil, zinc oxide, starch, sodium propionate, parabens. Jar 15 g, 60 g, 120 g, lb. **Pow.:** Biebrich scarlet red sulfonated 0.1%, starch, zinc oxide, sodium propionate, parabens. Bot. 30 g, UD 1 g. *otc.*
Use: Antipruritic; dermatologic, wound therapy; emollient.

Decylenes. (Rugby Labs, Inc.) Undecylenic acid, zinc undecylenate. Oint. Tube 30 g, lb. *otc.*
Use: Antifungal, topical.

Deep-Down Pain Relief Rub. (SmithKline Beecham Pharmaceuticals) Methyl salicylate 15%, menthol 5%, camphor 0.5%. Tube 1.25 oz, 3 oz. *otc.*
Use: Analgesic, topical.

Deep Strength Musterole. (Schering-Plough Corp.) Methyl salicylate 30%, menthol 3%, methyl nicotinate 0.5%. Tube 1.25 oz, 3 oz. *otc.*
Use: Analgesic, topical.

Defen-LA. (Horizon Pharmaceutical Corp.) Pseudoephedrine HCl 60 mg, guaifenesin 600 mg/SR Tab. Bot. 100s. *Rx.*
Use: Decongestant, expectorant.

•**deferoxamine.** (DEE-fer-OX-ah-meen) USAN.
Use: Chelating agent (iron).

•**deferoxamine hydrochloride.** (DEE-fer-OX-ah-meen) USAN.
Use: Chelating agent for iron.

•**deferoxamine mesylate.** (DEE-fer-OX-ah-meen) U.S.P. 23.
Use: Iron depleter, antidote to iron poisoning, chelating agent.
See: Desferal Mesylate, Pow. for Inj.

(Novartis Pharmaceutical Corp.).
defibrotide. (Crinos International)
Use: Thrombotic thrombocytopenic purpura. [Orphan Drug]
Deficol. (Vangard Labs, Inc.) Bisacodyl 5 mg/Tab. Bot. 100s, 1000s. *otc.*
Use: Laxative.
•**deflazacort.** (deh-FLAZE-ah-cart) USAN.
Use: Anti-inflammatory.
d4T.
Use: Antiviral.
See: Stavudine (Bristol-Myers Squibb).
Degas. (Invamed, Inc.) Simethicone 80 mg, sucrose, mannitol. Chew. Tab. Bot. 100s. *otc.*
Use: Antiflatulent.
Degest 2. (Akorn, Inc.) Naphazoline HCl 0.012%. Bot. 15 ml. *otc.*
Use: Decongestant, ophthalmic.
dehydrex. (Holles Laboratories, Inc.)
Use: Recurrent corneal erosion. [Orphan Drug]
dehydrocholate sodium inj.. U.S.P. XXI.
Use: Relief of liver congestion, diagnosis of cardiac failure.
See: Decholin Sodium, Inj. (Bayer Corp. (Consumer Div.)).
7-dehydrocholesterol, activated. (Various Mfr.) Vitamin D-3.
Use: Vitamin supplement.
•**dehydrocholic acid.** (dee-HIGH-droe-KOLE-ik) U.S.P. 23.
Use: Orally, hydrocholeretic and choleretic.
See: Atrocholin, Tab. (GlaxoWellcome).
Cholan-DH, Tab. (Medeva Pharmaceuticals, Inc.).
Decholin (Bayer Corp. (Consumer Div.)).
Dilabil (Sanofi Winthrop Pharmaceuticals).
Ketocholanic acid.
Neocholan, Tab. (Hoechst Marion Roussel).
Procholon (Bristol-Myers Squibb).
W/Amylolytic and proteolytic enzymes, desoxycholic acid.
See: Bilezyme, Tab. (Roberts Pharmaceuticals).
W/Bile, homatropine methylbromide, pepsin.
See: Biloric, Caps. (Arcum).
W/Bile, homatropine methylbromide, phenobarbital.
See: Bilamide, Tab. (Norgine).
W/Bile extract, pepsin, pancreatin.
See: Progestive, Tab. (NCP).
W/Desoxycholic acid.
See: Combichole, Tab. (F. Trout).
Ketosox, Tab. (B.F. Ascher and Co.).
W/Docusate sodium.
See: Dubbalax-B, Cap. (Redford).
Dubbalax-N, Cap. (Redford).
Neolax, Tab. (Schwarz Pharma, Inc.).
W/Docusate sodium, phenolphthalein.
See: Bolax, Cap. (Boyd).
Tripalax, Cap. (Redford).
W/Homatropine methylbromide.
See: Cholan V, Tab. (Medeva Pharmaceuticals, Inc.).
Homachol, Tab. (Teva Pharmaceuticals USA).
W/Methscopolamine, ox bile, amobarbital.
See: Hydrochol Plus, Tab. (Zeneca Pharmaceuticals).
W/Ox bile, homatropine methylbromide, phenobarbital.
See: Bilamide, Tab. (Norgine).
W/Pancreatin, pepsin, ox bile, belladonna extract.
See: Canz, Tab. (Cole).
W/Pepsin, pancreatin enzyme concentrate, cellulase.
See: Cholan-HMB, Tab. (Medeva Pharmaceuticals, Inc).
W/Phenobarbital, homatropine methylbromide, gerilase, geriprotase, desoxycholic acid.
See: Bilezyme Plus, Tabs. (Roberts Pharmaceuticals).
dehydrocholin.
Use: Hydrocholeretic.
See: Dehydrocholic acid.
dehydroepiandrosterone. (Genelabs Technologics, Inc.)
Use: Treatment of systemic lupus erythematosus (SLE). [Orphan Drug]
dehydroeiandrosterone sulfate sodium. (Pharmadigm, Inc.)
Use: Treat serious burns, accelerate reepithelialization of donor sites in autologous skin grafting. [Orphan Drug]
dehydrodesoxycholic acid.
See: Cholanic acid.
Dekasol. (Seatrace Pharmaceuticals, Inc.) Dexamethasone phosphate 4 mg/ml. Vial 5 ml, 10 ml. *Rx.*
Use: Corticosteroid.
Dekasol L.A. (Seatrace Pharmaceuticals, Inc.) Dexamethasone acetate 8 mg/ml. Vial 5 ml. *Rx.*
Use: Corticosteroid.
De-Koff. (Whiteworth Towne) Terpin hydrate w/dextromethorphan. Elix. Bot. 4 oz. *otc.*
Use: Antitussive, expectorant.
Delacort Lotion. (Mericon Industries, Inc.) Hydrocortisone 0.5%. Bot. 4 oz. *otc.*
Use: Corticosteroid, topical.

•**delapril hydrochloride.** (DELL-ah-prill) USAN.
Use: Antihypertensive, angiotensin-converting enzyme inhibitor.

Del Aqua-5. (Del-Ray Laboratory, Inc.) Benzoyl peroxide 5%. Tube 42.5 g. *Rx.*
Use: Dermatologic, acne.

Del Aqua-10. (Del-Ray Laboratory, Inc.) Benzoyl peroxide 10%. 42.5 g. *Rx.*
Use: Dermatologic, acne.

Delaquin Lotion. (Schlicksup) Hydrocortisone 0.5%, iodoquin 3%. Bot. 3 oz. *Rx.*
Use: Antifungal, corticosteroid.

Delatest. (Dunhall Pharmaceuticals, Inc.) Testosterone enanthate 100 mg/ml, chlorobutanol in sesame oil. Amp. 10 ml. *c-III.*
Use: Androgen.

Delatestadiol. (Dunhall Pharmaceuticals, Inc.) Testosterone enanthate 90 mg, estradiol valerate 4 mg/ml, chlorobutanol in sesame oil. Amp. 10 ml. *Rx.*
Use: Androgen, estrogen combination.

Delatestryl. (Bio-Technology General Corporation) Testosterone enanthate 200 mg/ml in sesame oil, chlorobutanol 0.5%. Vial 5 ml. *c-III.*
Use: Androgen.

•**delavirdine mesylate.** USAN.
Use: Antiviral.
See: Rescriptor, Tab. (Pharmacia & Upjohn).

Delcid. (SmithKline Beecham Pharmaceuticals) Aluminum hydroxide 600 mg, magnesium hydroxide 665 mg/5 ml, alcohol 0.3%, saccharin. Bot. 8 oz. *otc.*
Use: Antacid.

Del-Clens. (Del-Ray Laboratory, Inc.) Soapless cleanser. Bot. 8 oz. *otc.*
Use: Dermatologic, cleanser.

Delcort. (Lee Pharmaceuticals) Hydrocortisone 0.5% or 1%. Cream. Pack. 1 g, 20 g, 1 lb. (1% only). *otc.*
Use: Corticosteroid, topical.

Delco-Lax. (Delco) Bisacodyl 5 mg/Tab. Bot. 1000s. *otc.*
Use: Laxative.

Delcozine. (Delco) Phendimetrazine tartrate 70 mg/Tab. Bot. 1000s, 5000s. *c-III.*
Use: Anorexiant.

•**delequamine hydrochloride.** (deh-LEH-kwah-meen) USAN.
Use: Anti-impotence agent.

Delestrec. Estradiol 17-undecanoate. *Rx.*
Use: Estrogen.

Delestrogen. (Bristol-Myers Squibb) Estradiol valerate **10 mg/ml:** In sesame oil, chlorobutanol. Vial 5 ml. **20 mg/ml:** In castor oil, benzyl benzoate, benzyl alcohol. Vial 5 ml. **40 mg/ml:** In castor oil, benzyl benzoate, benzyl alcohol. Vial 5 ml. *Rx.*
Use: Estrogen.

Delfen Contraceptive Foam. (Advanced Care Products) Nonoxynol-9 12.5% in an oil-in-water emulsion at pH 4.5 to 5. Starter can with applicator 20 g. Refill 20 g, 42 g. *otc.*
Use: Contraceptive, spermicide.

delinal. Propenzolate HCl.

•**delmadinone acetate.** (del-MAD-ih-nohn ASS-eh-tate) USAN.
Use: Antiandrogen; antiestrogen; hormone, progestin.

Del-Mycin. (Del-Ray Laboratory, Inc.) Erythromycin 2%, ethyl alcohol 66%. Topical soln. Bot. 60 ml. *Rx.*
Use: Dermatologic, acne.

Del-Stat. (Del-Ray Laboratory, Inc.) Abradant cleaner. Jar 2 oz. *otc.*
Use: Dermatologic, acne.

Delsym Cough Suppressant. (McNeil Consumer Products Co.) Dextromethorphan HBr 30 mg/5 ml. Liq. Bot. 3 oz. *otc.*
Use: Antitussive.

delta-1-cortisone.
Use: Corticosteroid.
See: Deltasone, Tab. (Pharmacia & Upjohn).

delta-1-hydrocortisone.
Use: Corticosteroid.
See: Prednisolone (Various Mfr.).

Delta-Cortef. (Pharmacia & Upjohn) Prednisolone 5 mg/Tab. Bot. 100s, 500s. *Rx.*
Use: Corticosteroid.

Deltacortone. Prednisone.
Use: Corticosteroid.

Delta-Cortril. Prednisolone.
Use: Corticosteroid.

Delta-D. (Freeda Vitamins, Inc.) Vitamin D_3 400 IU/Tab. Bot. 250s, 500s. *otc.*
Use: Vitamin supplement.

•**deltafilcon a.** (DELL-tah-FILL-kahn A) USAN.
Use: Contact lens material, hydrophilic.

•**deltafilcon b.** (DELL-tah-FILL-kahn B) USAN.
Use: Contact lens material (hydrophilic).

Deltasone. (Pharmacia & Upjohn) Prednisone. **2.5 mg:** Tab. Bot. 100s. **5 mg:** Tab. Bot. 100s, 500s, UD 100s, Dosepak 21s. **10 mg, 20 mg:** Tab. Bot. 100s, 500s, UD 100s. **50 mg:** Tab. Bot. 100s, UD 100s. *Rx.*
Use: Corticosteroid.

Delta-Tritex. (Dermol Pharmaceuticals,

Inc.) Triamcinolone acetonide. **Cream:** 0.1% Tube 30 and 80 g. **Oint.:** 0.1% Tube 30 g. *Rx.*
Use: Corticosteroid, topical.

Del-Trac. (Del-Ray Laboratory, Inc.) Acne lotion. Bot. 2 oz. *otc.*
Use: Dermatologic, acne.

Deltastab.
Use: Corticosteroid.
See: Prednisolone (Various Mfr.).

•**deltibant.** (DELL-tih-bant) USAN.
Use: Antagonist (bradykinin).

Del-Vi-A. (Del-Ray Laboratory, Inc.) Vitamin A 50,000 IU/Cap. Bot. 100s. *Rx.*
Use: Vitamin supplement.

Delysid. Lysergic acid diethylamide.
Use: Potent psychotogenic.

Demadex. (Roche) **Tab.:** Torsemide 5 mg, 10 mg, 20 mg, 100 mg. Bot. UD 100s. **Inj.:** Torsemide 10 mg/ml. Amps. 2 ml or 5 ml. *Rx.*
Use: Diuretics.

Demazin. (Schering-Plough Corp.) **Syr.:** Chlorpheniramine maleate 2 mg, phenylpropanolamine HCl 12.5 mg/5 ml, alcohol 7.5%, menthol. Bot. 118 ml. **Tab.:** Chlorpheniramine maleate 4 mg, phenylpropanolamine HCl 25 mg. Box 24s. Bot. 100s. *otc.*
Use: Antihistamine, decongestant.

•**demecarium bromide.** (deh-meh-CARE-ee-uhm BROE-mide) U.S.P. 23.
Use: Cholinergic (ophthalmic).
See: Humorsol, Soln. (Merck & Co.).

•**demeclocycline.** (DEH-meh-kloe-SIGH-kleen) U.S.P. 23. *Formerly Demethylchlortetracycline.*
Use: Anti-infective.
See: Declomycin, Prods. (ESI Lederle Generics).

•**demeclocycline hydrochloride.** (DEH-meh-kloe-SIGH-kleen) U.S.P. 23.
Use: Anti-infective.
See: Declomycin HCl, Preps. (ESI Lederle Generics).

demeclocycline hydrochloride and nystatin tablets.
Use: Anti-infective.

•**demecycline.** (DEH-meh-SIGH-kleen) USAN.
Use: Anti-infective.

Demerol Hydrochloride. (Sanofi Winthrop Pharmaceuticals) Meperidine HCl. **Syr.:** 50 mg/5 ml, saccharin. Bot. 16 fl oz. **Tab.:** 50 mg or 100 mg. Bot. 100s, 500s, UD 25s (50 mg only). *c-II.*
Use: Analgesic, narcotic.

demethylchlortetracycline hydrochloride.
Use: Anti-infective, tetracycline.
See: Demeclocycline HCl

Demi-Regroton. (Rhone-Poulenc Rorer Pharmaceuticals, Inc.) Chlorthalidone 25 mg, reserpine 0.125 mg/Tab. Bot. 100s. *Rx.*
Use: Antihypertensive, diuretic.

•**demoxepam.** (dem-OX-eh-pam) USAN.
Use: Anxiolytic.

Demser. (Merck & Co.) Metyrosine 250 mg/Cap. Bot. 100s. *Rx.*
Use: Antihypertensive.

Demulen 1/35-21. (Searle) Ethynodiol diacetate 1 mg, ethinyl estradiol 35 mcg/Tab. Compack disp. 21s, 6 × 21, refill 21s. *Rx.*
Use: Contraceptive.

Demulen 1/35-28. (Searle) Ethynodiol diacetate 1 mg, ethinyl estradiol 35 mcg/Tab. Compack 28s: 21 active tabs, 7 placebo tabs. Compack 6 × 28, refill 28s. *Rx.*
Use: Contraceptive.

Demulen 1/50-21. (Searle) Ethynodiol diacetate 1 mg, ethinyl estradiol 50 mcg/Tab. Compack Disp. 21s, 6 × 21, refill 21s. *Rx.*
Use: Contraceptive.

Demulen 1/50-28. (Searle) Ethynodiol diacetate 1 mg, ethinyl estradiol 50 mcg/Tab. Compack 28s: 21 active tabs, 7 placebo tabs. Compack Disp. of 28, 6 × 28, refill 28s. *Rx.*
Use: Contraceptive.

Denalan Denture Cleanser. (Whitehall Robins Laboratories) Sodium percarbonate 30%. Bot. 7 oz., 13 oz. *otc.*
Use: Agent for oral hygiene.

•**denatonium benzoate.** (DEE-nah-TOE-nee-uhm BEN-zoh-ate) N.F. 18.
Use: Pharmaceutic aid (flavor, alcohol denaturant).

Denavir. (SmithKline Beecham) Penciclovir 10 mg/g Cream. Tube 2 g. *Rx.*
Use: Cold sores.

Dencorub. (Last) Methyl salicylate 20%, menthol 0.75%, camphor 1%, eucalyptus oil 0.5%. Tube 1.25 oz, 2.75 oz. *otc.*
Use: Analgesic, topical.

Dencorub Analgesic Liquid. (Last) Oleoresin capsicum suspension in aqueous vehicle. Bot. 6 oz. *otc.*
Use: Analgesic, topical.

•**denileukin diftitox.** (deh-nih-LOO-kin DIFF-tih-tox) USAN.
Use: Treatment of proliferative malignant diseases and autoimmune diseases expressing interleukin 2 receptors. Biological response modifier; antineoplastic.

See: Ontak (Ligand Pharm).

•**denofungin.** (DEE-no-FUN-jin) USAN.
Use: Antifungal, antibacterial.

Denorex. (Whitehall Robins Laboratories) Coal tar solution 9%, menthol 1.5%. Shampoo. Bot. 4 oz, 8 oz. *otc.*
Use: Antiseborrheic.

Denorex, Extra Strength. (Whitehall Robins Laboratories) Coal tar solution 12.5%, menthol 1.5%, alcohol 10.4%. Shampoo. Bot. 120, 240, 360 ml. *otc.*
Use: Antiseborrheic.

Denorex Mountain Fresh. (Whitehall Robins Laboratories) Coal tar solution 9%, menthol 1.5%. Bot. 4 oz, 8 oz. *otc.*
Use: Antiseborrheic.

Denorex with Conditioners. (Whitehall Robins Laboratories) Coal tar solution 9%, menthol 1.5%. Bot 4 oz, 8 oz. *otc.*
Use: Antiseborrheic.

Denquel. (Procter & Gamble Pharm.) Potassium nitrate 5%, calcium carbonate, glycerin, flavors. Tube 1.6 oz, 3 oz, 4.5 oz. *otc.*
Use: Dentrifice.

Dental Caries Preventive. (Colgate Oral Pharmaceuticals) Fluoride ion 1.2%, alumina abrasive. 2 g Box 200s, Jar 9 oz. *Rx.*
Use: Dental caries agent.

Dentipatch. (Noven) Lidocaine 23 mg or 46.1 mg^2 patch, aspartame/Patch. Box 50s, 100s. *Rx.*
Use: Anesthetic, local.

Dentrol. (Block Drug Co., Inc.) Carboxymethylcellulose, polyethylene oxide homopolymer, peppermint and spearmint in mineral oil base. Bot. 0.9 oz, 1.8 oz. *otc.*
Use: Denture adhesive.

Dent's Dental Poultice. (C. S. Dent & Co. Division) Glycerin, mineral oil, polyoxyethylene sorbitan monooleate. Bot. 0.125 oz, 0.25 oz. *otc.*
Use: Dental poultice.

Dent's Ear Wax Drops. (C. S. Dent & Co. Division) Glycerin, mineral oil, polyoxyethylene sorbitan monooleate. Bot. 0.125 oz, 0.25 oz. *otc.*
Use: Otic.

Dent's Extra Strength Toothache Gum. (C. S. Dent & Co. Division) Benzocaine. Box. 1 g. *otc.*
Use: Anesthetic, local.

Dent's Lotion-Jel. (C. S. Dent & Co. Division) Benzocaine in special base. Tube 2 oz. *otc.*
Use: Anesthetic, local.

Dent's Maximum Strength Toothache Drops. (C. S. Dent & Co. Division) Benzocaine, alcohol 74%, chlorobutanol anhydrous 0.09%. Liq. 3.7 ml. *otc.*
Use: Anesthetic, local.

Dent's Toothache Drops Treatment. (C. S. Dent & Co. Division) Alcohol 60%, chlorobutanol anhydrous (chloroform derivative) 0.09%, propylene glycol, eugenol. Bot. 3.75 ml. *otc.*
Use: Anesthetic, local.

Dent's Toothache Gum. (C. S. Dent & Co. Division) Benzocaine, eugenol, petrolatum in base of cotton and wax. Box 1.05 g. *otc.*
Use: Anesthetic, local.

Denture Orajel. (Del Pharmaceuticals, Inc.) Benzocaine 10%, saccharin. Gel. Tube. 9.45 g. *otc.*
Use: Anesthetic, local.

Dent-Zel-Ite. (Last) Oral Mucosal Analgesic: Benzocaine 5%, alcohol, glycerin. Bot. 1.875 g. **Temporary Dental Filling:** Sandarac gum, alcohol. Bot. 1 oz. **Toothache Drops:** Eugenol 85% in alcohol. Bot. 1 oz. *otc.*
Use: Anesthetic, local.

denyl sodium.
Use: Anticonvulsant.
See: Diphenylhydantoin Sodium, Cap. (Various Mfr.).

deodorizers, systemic. Chlorophyll derivatives (chlorophyllin). *otc.*
Use: Oral: Control of fecal and urinary odors in colostomy, ileostomy or incontinence. Topical: Reduce pain and inflammation (wounds, burns, surface ulcers, skin irritation).
See: Chloresium, Tab., Soln., Oint. (Rystan, Inc.).
Chlorophyll, Tab. (Freeda Vitamins, Inc.).
Derifil, Tab. (Rystan, Inc.).

deoxyadenosine, 2-chloro-2[1]. (St. Jude Children's Hospital)
Use: Antineoplastic. [Orphan Drug]

2'deoxycoformycin. Pentostatin.
Use: Antibiotic, antineoplastic.
See: Nipent, Pow. (Parke-Davis).

deoxycytidine (5-AZA-2'). (Pharmachemie USA, Inc.)
Use: Antineoplastic. [Orphan Drug]

deoxynojirmycin. (Searle) Butyl-DNJ. *Rx.*
Use: Antiviral.

Depacon. (Abbott Laboratories) Valproic acid 5 ml (as valproic sodium)/Inj. Vial 10s. *Rx.*
Use: Anticonvulsant.

Depade. (Mallinckrodt) Naltrexone HCl 50 mg/Tab. Bot. 50s. *Rx.*
Use: Antidote.

Depakene. (Abbott Laboratories) Valproic acid. **Cap.:** 250 mg. Bot. 100s, UD

100s. **Syr.:** 250 mg/5 ml, sorbitol. Bot. 480 ml. *Rx.*
Use: Anticonvulsant.

Depakote. (Abbott Laboratories) Divalproex sodium 125 mg, 250 mg or 500 mg/DR Tab and 125 mg/sprinkle cap. **DR Tab.:** Bot. 100s, 500s, UD 100s. **Sprinkle Cap.:** Bot. 100s, UD 100s. *Rx.*
Use: Anticonvulsant.

DepAndro 100. (Forest Pharmaceutical, Inc.) Testosterone cypionate in cottonseed oil 100 mg/ml, benzyl alcohol. Vial 10 ml. *c-III.*
Use: Androgen.

DepAndro 200. (Forest Pharmaceutical, Inc.) Testosterone cypionate in cottonseed oil 200 mg/ml, benzyl benzoate, benzyl alcohol. Vial 10 ml. *c-III.*
Use: Androgen.

DepAndrogyn. (Forest Pharmaceutical, Inc.) Testosterone cypionate 50 mg, estradiol cypionate 2 mg/ml. Vial 10 ml. *Rx.*
Use: Androgen, estrogen combination.

Depa-Syrup. (Alra Laboratories, Inc.) Valproic acid syrup 250 mg/5 ml. Bot. 4 oz, 16 oz. *Rx.*
Use: Anticonvulsant.

Depen. (Wallace Laboratories) Penicillamine 250 mg/Tab. Bot. 100s. *Rx.*
Use: Chelating agent.

depepsen. Amylosulfate sodium.
Use: Digestive aid.

depGynogen. (Forest Pharmaceutical, Inc.) Estradiol cypionate in cottonseed oil 5 mg/ml, cottonseed oil, chlorobutanol. Inj. Vial 10 ml. *Rx.*
Use: Estrogen.

depMedalone 40. (Forest Pharmaceutical, Inc.) Methylprednisolone acetate in aqueous suspension 40 mg/ml, polyethylene glycol, myristyl-gamma-picolinium Cl. Vial 5 ml. *Rx.*
Use: Corticosteroid.

depMedalone 80. (Forest Pharmaceutical, Inc.) Methylprednisolone acetate 80 mg/ml, polyethylene glycol, myristyl-gamma-picolinium Cl. Vial 5 ml. *Rx.*
Use: Corticosteroid.

Depoestra. (Tennessee Pharmaceutic) Estradiol cypionate 5 mg/ml. Vial 10 ml. *Rx.*
Use: Estrogen.

Depo-Estradiol Cypionate. (Pharmacia & Upjohn) Estradiol cypionate 5 mg/ml, chlorobutanol, cottonseed oil. Inj. Vial 5 ml. *Rx.*
Use: Estrogen.

Depofoam encapsulated cytarabine. (DepoTech Corp.)
Use: Neoplastic meningitis. [Orphan Drug]

DepoGen. (Hyrex Pharmaceuticals) Estradiol cypionate 5 mg/ml, cottonseed oil, chlorobutanol. Inj. Vial 10 ml. *Rx.*
Use: Estrogen.

Depoject. (Merz Pharmaceutcials) Methylprednisolone acetate 40 mg or 80 mg/ml suspension with polyethylene glycol and myristyl-gamma-picolinium Cl. Inj. Vial 5 ml. *Rx.*
Use: Corticosteroid.

Depo-Medrol. (Pharmacia & Upjohn) Methylprednisolone acetate, 20 mg/Inj. Vial. 5 ml, 10 ml. Methylprednisolone acetate, 40 mg/Inj. Vial. 5 ml, 10 ml. Methylprednisolone acetate 80 mg/Inj. Vial. 1 ml, 5 ml. *Rx.*
Use: Corticosteroid.

Deponit. (Schwarz Pharma, Inc.) Nitroglycerin transdermal delivery system containing 16 mg or 32 mg. Box 30s, 100s. *Rx.*
Use: Antianginal, vasodilator.

Depopred-40. (Hyrex Pharmaceuticals) Methylprednisolone acetate suspension 40 mg/ml, polyethylene glycol, myristyl-gamma-picolinium Cl. Vial 5 ml, 10 ml. *Rx.*
Use: Corticosteroid.

Depopred-80. (Hyrex Pharmaceuticals) Methylprednisolone acetate 80 mg/Inj. Vial. 5 ml. *Rx.*
Use: Corticosteroid.

Depo-Provera. (Pharmacia & Upjohn) Medroxyprogesterone acetate 400 mg/ml. Suspended in polyethylene glycol 3350 20.3 mg, sodium sulfate (anhydrous) 11 mg, myristyl-gamma-picolinium Cl 1.69 mg/ml. Vial 2.5 ml, 10 ml, 1 ml U-Ject. *Rx.*
Use: Hormone, progestin.

Depo-Provera Contraceptive Injection. (Pharmacia & Upjohn) Medroxyprogesterone acetate 150 mg/ml, with PEG-3350 28.9 mg, polysorbate 80 2.41 mg, sodium Cl 8.68 mg, methylparaben 1.37 mg, propylparaben 0.15 mg/Inj. Vial. 1 ml. *Rx.*
Use: Contraceptive.

Depotest. (Hyrex Pharmaceuticals) Testosterone cypionate. **100 mg:** With cottonseed oil, benzyl alcohol. **200 mg:** With cottonseed oil, benzyl benzoate, benzyl alcohol. Vial 10 ml. *c-III.*
Use: Androgen.

Depo-Testadiol. (Roberts Pharmaceuticals) Testosterone cypionate 50 mg, estradiol cypionate 2 mg/ml. Vial 10 ml. *Rx.*
Use: Androgen, estrogen combination.

Depotestogen. (Hyrex Pharmaceuticals) Testosterone cypionate 50 mg, estradiol cypionate 2 mg/ml. Vial 10 ml. *Rx.*
Use: Androgen, estrogen combination.

Depo-Testosterone. (Pharmacia & Upjohn) Testosterone cypionate. **100 mg/ml:** In benzyl alcohol 9.45 mg, cottonseed oil 736 mg/ml. Vial 1 ml, 10 ml. **200 mg/ml:** In benzyl benzoate 0.2 ml, benzyl alcohol 9.45 mg, cottonseed oil 560 mg/ml. Vial 1 ml, 10 ml. *c-III.*
Use: Androgen.

deprenyl. Selegiline HCl.
See: Eldepryl (Somerset Pharmaceuticals).

Deproist Expectorant/Codeine. (Geneva Pharmaceuticals) Pseudoephedrine HCl 30 mg, codeine phosphate 10 mg, guaifenesin 100 mg/5 ml. Bot. 120 ml, 480 ml. *c-v.*
Use: Antitussive, decongestant, expectorant.

•**deprostil.** (deh-PRAHST-ill) USAN.
Use: Antisecretory, gastric.

Dep-Test. (Sigma-Tau Pharmaceuticals, Inc.) Testosterone cypionate 100 mg/ml. Vial 10 ml. *c-III.*
Use: Androgen.

Dequasine. (Miller Pharmacal Group, Inc.) L-lysine 20 mg, l-cysteine 100 mg, dl-methionine 50 mg, vitamin C 200 mg, iron 5 mg, Cu, I, Mg, Mn, Zn. Tab. Bot. 100s. *otc.*
Use: Mineral, vitamin supplement.

Derifil. (Rystan, Inc.) Chlorophyllin copper complex 100 mg/Tab. Bot. 30s, 100s, 1000s. *otc.*
Use: Deodorant, oral.

Dermabase. (Paddock Laboratories) Mineral oil, petrolatum, cetostearyl alcohol, propylene glycol, sodium lauryl sulfate, isopropyl palmitate, imidazolidinyl urea, methyl- and propylparabens. Cream. Jar 1 lb. *otc.*
Use: Emollient.

Dermacoat Aerosol Spray. (Century Pharmaceuticals, Inc.) Benzocaine 4.5%. Bot. 7 oz. *otc.*
Use: Anesthetic, local.

Dermacort Cream. (Solvay Pharmaceuticals) Hydrocortisone 0.5% or 1% in a water soluble cream of stearyl alcohol, cetyl alcohol, isopropyl palmitate, citric acid, polyoxyethylene 40 stearate, sodium phosphate, propylene glycol, water, benzyl alcohol, buffered to pH 5. 0.5% in 30 g, 1% in 1 lb. *Rx.*
Use: Corticosteroid, topical.

Dermacort Lotion. (Solvay Pharmaceuticals) Hydrocortisone 1% in lotion base, buffered to pH 5. Paraben free. Bot. 120 ml. *Rx.*
Use: Corticosteroid, topical.

Derma-Cover. (Scrip) Sulfur, salicylic acid, hyamine 10x, isopropyl alcohol 22%, in powder film forming base. Bot. 2 oz. *otc.*
Use: Keratolytic.

DermaFlex. (Zila Pharmaceuticals, Inc.) Lidocaine 2.5%, alcohol 79%. Gel. Tube 15 g. *otc.*
Use: Anesthetic, local.

Derma-Guard. (Greer Laboratories, Inc.) Protective adhesive pow. Can w/sifter top, 4 oz. Spray Top Bot. 4 oz, pkg. 1 lb. Rings. Pkg. 5s, 10s. *otc.*
Use: Dermatologic, protectant.

Dermal-Rub Balm. (Roberts Pharmaceuticals) Menthol racemic 7%, camphor 1%, methyl salicylate 1%, cajuput oil 1%. Cream. Jar 1 oz, 1 lb. *otc.*
Use: Analgesic, topical.

Dermamycin. (Pfeiffer Co.) **Cream:** Diphenhydramine HCl 2% in a base of parabens, polyethylene glycol monostearate and propylene glycol. 28.35 g. **Spray:** Diphenhydramine HCl 2%, menthol 1%, alcohol, methylparaben. Bot. 60 ml. *otc.*
Use: Antihistamine, topical.

Dermaneed. (Hanlon) Zirconium oxide 4.5%, calamine 6%, zinc oxide 4%, actamer 0.1% in bland lotionized base. Bot. 4 oz. *otc.*
Use: Antipruritic, topical.

Derma-Pax. (Recsei Laboratories) Methapyrilene HCl 0.22%, chlorothenylpyramine maleate 0.06%, pyrilamine maleate 0.22%, benzyl alcohol 1%, chlorobutanol 1%, isopropyl alcohol 40%. Liq. 4 oz, pt. *otc.*
Use: Antihistamine, topical; antipruritic, topical.

Derma-Pax HC. (Recsei Laboratories) Hydrocortisone 0.5%, pyrilamine maleate 0.2%, pheniramine maleate 0.2%, chlorpheniramine 0.06%, benzyl alcohol 1%. Liq. Bot. 60 ml, 120 ml, 480 ml.
Use: Antihistamine, topical; corticosteroid, topical.

Dermarest. (Del Pharmaceuticals, Inc.) Diphenhydramine HCl 2%, resorcinol 2%, aloe vera gel, benzalkonium chloride, EDTA, menthol, methylparaben, propylene glycol. Gel Tube 29.25 g, 56.25 g. *otc.*
Use: Antihistamine, topical.

Dermarest Dricort. (Del Pharmaceuticals, Inc.) Hydrocortisone 1%, white petrolatum cream. Bot. 14 g. *otc.*
Use: Corticosteroid, topical.

Dermarest Plus. (Del Pharmaceuticals,

Inc.) **Gel:** Diphenhydramine HCl 2%, menthol 1%, aloe vera gel, benzalkonium chloride, isopropyl alcohol, methylparaben, propylene glycol. Tube 15 g, 30 g. **Spray:** Diphenhydramine HCl 2%, menthol 1%, aloe vera gel, benzalkonium chloride, methylparaben propylene glycol, SDA 40 alcohol, EDTA. Bot. 60 ml. *otc.*
Use: Antihistamine, topical.

Dermasept Antifungal. (Pharmakon Laboratories, Inc.) Tannic acid 6.098%, zinc Cl 5.081%, benzocaine 2.032%, methylbenzethonium HCl, tolnaftate 1.017%, undecylenic acid 5.081%, ethanol 38B 58.539%, phenol, benzyl alcohol, benzoic acid, coal tar, camphor, menthol. Liq. Bot. 30 ml. *otc.*
Use: Antifungal, topical.

Dermasil. (Chesebrough-Ponds USA, Inc.) Glycerin and dimethicone in a base containing cyclomethicone, sunflower oil, petrolatum, borage oil, lecithin, vitamin E acetate, vitamin A palmitate, vitamin D_3, corn oil, EDTA, methylparaben. Lot. Bot. 120 ml, 240 ml. *otc.*
Use: Emollient.

Derma-Smoothe/FS Oil. (Hill Dermaceuticals, Inc.) Fluocinolone acetonide 0.01%. Oil. Bot. 4 oz. *Rx.*
Use: Antipsoriatic; antiseborrheic, topical.

Derma-Smoothe Oil. (Hill Dermaceuticals, Inc.) Refined peanut oil, mineral oil in lipophilic base. *otc.*
Use: Antipruritic; dermatologic, protectant.

Derma Soap. (Ferndale Laboratories, Inc.) Dowicil 0.1%. 4 oz w/dispenser. *otc.*
Use: Antiseptic.

Derma-Soft. (Vogarell) Medicated cream. Salicylic acid, castor oil, triethanolamine. Tube ¾ oz. *otc.*
Use: Keratolytic.

Derma-Sone 1%. (Hill Dermaceuticals, Inc.) Hydrocortisone 1%, pramoxine HCl 1%, cetyl alcohol, glyceryl monostearate, isopropyl myristate, potassium sorbate, furcelleran. *Rx-otc.*
Use: Anesthetic; corticosteroid, local.

Dermasorcin. (Lamond) Resorcin 2%, sulfur 5%. Bot. 1 oz, 2 oz, 4 oz, 8 oz, pt, 32 oz, 0.5 gal. *otc.*
Use: Dermatologic, acne; antiseborrheic, topical.

Dermastringe. (Lamond) Bot. 4 oz, 6 oz, 8 oz, pt, 32 oz, gal. *otc.*
Use: Dermatologic, cleanser.

Dermasul. (Lamond) Sulfur 5%. Bot. 1 oz, 2 oz, 4 oz, 8 oz, pt, 32 oz, 0.5 gal, gal. *otc.*
Use: Dermatologic, acne; antiseborrheic, topical.

Dermathyn. (Davis & Sly) Benzyl alcohol 3%, benzocaine 3.5%, butyl-p-aminobenzoate 1%, phenylmercuric borate. Tube 1 oz. *otc.*
Use: Anesthetic, local.

Dermatic Base. (Whorton Pharmaceuticals, Inc.) Compounding cream base. Bot. 16 oz.
Use: Pharmaceutical aid, emollient base.

Dermatol.
See: Bismuth subgallate, Preps. (Various Mfr.).

Dermatop. (Hoechst Marion Roussel) Prednicarbate 0.1%, white petrolatum, lanolin alcohols, mineral oil, cetostearyl alcohol, EDTA, lactic acid. Cream 15 g, 60 g. *Rx.*
Use: Corticosteroid, topical.

Derma Viva. (Rugby Labs, Inc.) Mineral oil, glyceryl stearate, laureth-4, lanolin oil, PEG-100 stearate, PEG-40 stearate, PEG-4 dilaurate, trolamine, dioctyl sodium sulfosuccinate, parabens. Lot. Bot. 237 ml. *otc.*
Use: Emollient.

Dermed. (Holloway) Vitamins A and D with hydrogenated vegetable oil. Cream. Tube 60 g, 120 g. *otc.*
Use: Emollient.

Dermeze. (Premo) Thenylpyramine HCl 2%, benzocaine 2%, tyrothricin 0.25 mg/g. Massage Lot. Bot. 5¾ oz. *otc.*
Use: Anesthetic, antihistamine, anti-infective.

Dermolate Anti-Itch. (Schering-Plough Corp.) Hydrocortisone 0.5% petrolatum, mineral oil, chlorocresol. Cream Tube 15 g, 30 g. *otc.*
Use: Corticosteroid, topical.

Dermol HC. (Dermol Pharmaceuticals, Inc.) **Cream:** Hydrocortisone 1% or 2.5%. Tube 30 g. **Oint.:** Hydrocortisone 1%. Tube 30 g. *Rx.*
Use: Anorectal preparation.

Dermolin. (Roberts Pharmaceuticals) Menthol racemic, methyl salicylate, camphor, mustard oil, isopropyl alcohol 8%. Bot. 3 oz, pt, gal. *otc.*
Use: Liniment.

Dermoplast. (Whitehall Robins Laboratories) **Spray:** Benzocaine 20%, menthol, methylparaben, aloe, lanolin. Bot. 82.5 ml. **Lot.:** Benzocaine 8%, menthol, aloe, glycerin, parabens, lanolin. Bot. 90 ml. *otc.*
Use: Anesthetic, local.

Dermovan. (Galderma Laboratories, Inc.)

Glyceryl stearate, spermaceti, mineral oil, glycerin, cetyl alcohol, butylparaben, methylparaben, propylparaben, purified water. Vanishing-type base, Jar 1 lb. *otc.*
Use: Dermatologic, protectant.

Dermtex HC. (Pfeiffer Co.) Hydrocortisone 0.5% in a glycerin base. Tube 15 g. *otc.*
Use: Corticosteroid, topical.

Dermuspray. (Warner Chilcott Laboratories) Trypsin 0.1 mg, balsam Peru 72.5 mg, castor oil 650 mg/0.82 ml. Aer. Bot. 120 g. *Rx.*
Use: Enzyme, topical.

DES.
See: Diethylstilbestrol.

desacchromin. A nonprotein bacterial colloidal dispersion of polysaccharide.

•**desciclovir.** (DESS-sigh-kloe-veer) USAN.
Use: Antiviral.

•**descinolone acetonide.** (DESS-SIN-ole-ohn ah-SEE-toe-nide) USAN.
Use: Corticosteroid, topical.

Desenex. (Novartis Pharmaceutical Corp.) Total undecylenate (as undecylenic acid and zinc undecylenate). **Aer. Spray Pow.:** 25%, menthol, talc. Can 81 g. **Cream:** 25%, lanolin, parabens, white petrolatum. Tube 15 g. **Oint.:** 25%, parabens, white petrolatum, lanolin. Tube 14 g. **Pow.:** 25%, talc. Bot. 45 g. **Foam:** Total undecylenate (as undecylenic acid) 10%, isopropyl alcohol 29.2%. Can 45 g. *otc.*
Use: Antifungal, topical.

Desenex Antifungal, Maximum. (Novartis Pharmaceutical Corp.) Miconazole nitrate 2% Pow. Tube 14 g. *otc.*
Use: Antifungal, topical.

Desenex Foot & Sneaker Spray. (Novartis Pharmaceutical Corp.) Aluminum chlorhydrex w/alcohol 89.3%. Aerosol Can 2.7 oz. *otc.*
Use: Foot deodorant, antiperspirant.

Desenex Maximum Strength. (Medeva Pharmaceuticals, Inc.) Total undecylenate 25%, lanolin, parabens, white petrolatum. Oint. Tube 15 g. *otc.*
Use: Antifungal, topical.

De Serpa. (de Leon) Reserpine 0.25 mg or 0.5 mg/Tab. Bot. 100s, 500s, 1000s (0.25 mg only). *Rx.*
Use: Antihypertensive.

Desert Pure Calcium. (CalWhite Mineral Co.) Calcium (from mineral calcite) 500 mg, vitamin D 125 IU. Tab. Bot. 200s. *otc.*
Use: Mineral, vitamin supplement.

Desferal. (Novartis Pharmaceutical Corp.) Deferoxamine mesylate 500 mg/5 ml. Amp. 4s. *Rx.*
Use: Antidote.

•**desflurane.** (dess-FLEW-rane) U.S.P. 23.
Use: Anesthetic.
See: Suprane (Ohmeda Pharmaceuticals).

•**desipramine hydrochloride.** (dess-IPP-ruh-meen) U.S.P. 23.
Use: Antidepressant.
See: Norpramin, Tab. (Hoechst Marion Roussel).

•**desirudin.** (deh-SIHR-uh-din) USAN.
Use: Anticoagulant.

Desitin. (Pfizer US Pharmaceutical Group) **Pow.:** Talc. Can 3 oz, 7 oz, 10 oz. **Oint.:** Cod liver oil, zinc oxide 40%, talc, petrolatum, lanolin. Tube 1 oz, 2 oz, 4 oz, 8 oz, Jar 1 lb. *otc.*
Use: Astringent, skin protectant.

Desitin Creamy. (Pfizer US Pharmaceutical Group) Zinc oxide 10%, mineral oil, white petrolatum, parabens. Oint. Tube 57 g. *otc.*
Use: Antifungal, topical.

Desitin with Zinc Oxide. (Pfizer US Pharmaceutical Group) Cornstarch 88.2%, zinc oxide 10%. Pow. Bot. 28 g, 397 g. *otc.*
Use: Diaper rash preparation.

•**deslanoside.** (dess-LAN-oh-side) U.S.P. 23.
Use: Cardiovascular agent.

•**deslorelin.** (DESS-low-REH-lin) USAN.
Use: Gonadotropin inhibitor; LHRH agonist. [Orphan Drug]
See: Somagard [as acetate] (Roberts Pharmaceuticals).

Desma. (Tablicaps) Diethylstilbestrol 25 mg/Tab. Patient dispenser 10s. *Rx.*
Use: Estrogen.

•**desmopressin acetate.** (DESS-moe-PRESS-in) USAN.
Use: Treatment of diabetes insipidus, mild hemophilia A, and von Willebrand's disease, antidiuretic. [Orphan Drug]
See: DDAVP, Liq. (Rhone-Poulenc Rorer Pharmaceuticals, Inc.).
Stimate (Centeon).

desmopressin acetate. (Rhone-Poulenc Rorer Pharmaceuticals, Inc.)
Use: Treatment of mild hemophilia A and von Willebrand's disease. [Orphan Drug]

desmopressin acetate. (Various Mfr.) Desmopressin acetate 4 mcg/ml. Inj. 1 ml, 10 ml. *Rx.*
Use: Treatment of diabetes insipidus.

Desogen. (Organon, Inc.) Desogestrel

0.15 mg, ethinyl estradiol 0.03 mg/Tab. Pck. 28s. *Rx.*
Use: Contraceptive.

•**desogestrel.** (DESS-oh-JESS-trell) USAN.
Use: Hormone, progestin.
W/Ethinyl estradiol.
See: Desogen, Tab. (Organon, Inc.).
Mircette (Organon, Inc.).
Ortho-Cept, Tab. (Ortho McNeil Pharmaceutical).

•**desonide.** (DESS-oh-nide) USAN.
Use: Anti-inflammatory.
See: Tridesilon, Cream (Bayer Corp. (Consumer Div.)).

desonide. (Various Mfr.) Desonide 0.05%. Oint. Cream Tube 15 g, 60 g. *Rx.*
Use: Anti-inflammatory; corticosteroid, topical.

desonide cream. (Galderma Laboratories, Inc.) Desonide 0.05% in cream base. Tube 15 g, 60 g. *Rx.*
Use: Corticosteroid, topical.

DesOwen. (Galderma Laboratories, Inc.) Desonide 0.05%. Cream. Tube 15 g, 60 g. *Rx.*
Use: Corticosteroid, topical.

•**desoximetasone.** (dess-OX-ee-MET-ah-sone) U.S.P. 23.
Use: Anti-inflammatory; corticosteroid, topical.
See: Topicort (Hoechst Marion Roussel).

•**desoxycorticosterone acetate.** (dess-OX-ee-core-tih-koe-STURR-ohn ASS-eh-tate) U.S.P. 23.
Use: Adrenocortical steroid (salt-regulating).

•**desoxycorticosterone pivalate.** U.S.P. 23.
Use: Adrenocortical steroid (salt-regulating).

desoxycorticosterone pivalate injectable suspension.
Use: Adrenocortical steroid (salt-regulating).

desoxycorticosterone trimethylacetate. U.S.P. XVI.
Use: Adrenocortical steroid (salt-regulating).

desoxyephedrine hydrochloride. (Various Mfr.) *c-II.*
Use: CNS stimulant.
See: Methamphetamine HCl, Prep.

Desoxyn. (Abbott Laboratories) Methamphetamine HCl. **Tab.:** 5 mg. Bot. 100s. **Gradumets:** 5 mg. Bot. 100s; 10 mg. Bot. 100s; 15 mg. Bot. 100s. *c-II.*
Use: CNS stimulant.

desoxy norephedrine.
Use: CNS stimulant.
See: Amphetamine HCl, Preps. (Various Mfr.).

desoxyribonuclease.
Use: Enzyme, topical.
W/Fibrinolysin.
See: Elase, prep. (Parke-Davis).

Desquam-E 2, 5, & 10. (Westwood Squibb Pharmaceuticals) Benzoyl peroxide 5% or 10%. Gel. Tube 42.5 g. *Rx.*
Use: Dermatologic, acne.

Desquam-X 5% or 10% Gel. (Westwood Squibb Pharmaceuticals) Benzoyl peroxide 5% or 10%, water base with EDTA. Tube 42.5 ml; 85 g (5% only). *Rx.*
Use: Dermatologic, acne.

Desquam-X 5% or 10% Wash. (Westwood Squibb Pharmaceuticals) Benzoyl peroxide 5% or 10%, EDTA. Bot. 150 ml. *Rx.*
Use: Dermatologic, acne.

D-Est. (Burgin-Arden) Estradiol cypionate 5 mg/ml. Vial 10 ml. *Rx.*
Use: Estrogen.

de-Stat. (Sherman Pharmaceuticals, Inc.) Surfactant cleaner, benzalkonium Cl 0.01%, EDTA 0.25%. Soln. Bot. 118 ml. *otc.*
Use: Contact lens care.

de-Stat 3. (Sherman Pharmaceuticals, Inc.) Octylphenoxy polyethoxyethanol, benzyl alcohol 0.1%, EDTA 0.5%, lauryl sulfate salt of imidazoldinyl urea. Soln. Bot. 118 ml. *otc.*
Use: Contact lens care.

de-Stat 4. (Sherman Pharmaceuticals, Inc.) Benzyl alcohol 0.3%, EDTA 0.5%, lauryl sulfate, salt of imidazoldinyl urea, octylphenoxy polyethoxyethanol. Thimerasal free. Soln. Bot. 118 ml. *otc.*
Use: Contact lens care.

Desyrel. (Bristol-Myers Squibb) Trazodone HCl 50 mg or 100 mg. Bot. 100s, 1000s, UD 100s. *Rx.*
Use: Antidepressant.

Desyrel Dividose. (Bristol-Myers Squibb) Trazodone HCl 150 mg or 300 mg/Dividose Tab. Bot. 100s, 500s (150 mg). *Rx.*
Use: Antidepressant.

Detachol. (Ferndale Laboratories, Inc.) Bland, nonirritating liquid for removing adhesive tape. Pkg. 4 oz.
Use: Adhesive remover.

De Tal. (de Leon) Phenobarbital 0.25 gr, hyoscyamine sulfate 0.1037 mg, atropine sulfate 0.0194 mg, hyoscine HBr 0.0065 mg/Tab. or 5 ml. **Tab.:** Bot.

100s. **Elix.:** With alcohol 20%. Bot. pt. *Rx.*
Use: Anticholinergic, antispasmodic, hypnotic, sedative.

Detane. (Del Pharmaceuticals, Inc.) Benzocaine 7.5%. Tube 0.5 oz. *otc.*
Use: Anesthetic, local.

•**deterenol hydrochloride.** (dee-TEER-eh-nahl) USAN.
Use: Adrenergic, ophthalmic.

detergents. surface-active.
See: pHisoDerm, Liq. (Sanofi Winthrop Pharmaceuticals).
pHisoHex, Liq. (Sanofi Winthrop Pharmaceuticals).
Zephiran, Prods. (Sanofi Winthrop Pharmaceuticals).

detigon hydrochloride.
See: Chlophedianol HCl (Various Mfr.).

•**detirelix acetate.** (DEH-tih-RELL-ix) USAN.
Use: Antagonist (LHRH).

•**detomidine hydrochloride.** (deh-TOE-mih-deen HIGH-droe-KLOR-ide) USAN.
Use: Hypnotic, sedative.

Detrol. (Pharmacia & Upjohn) Tolerodine tartrate 1 mg, 2 mg /Tab. Bot. 60s, 500s. UD 140s. *Rx.*
Use: Urinary tract product.

Detussin Capsules. (Various Mfr.) Phenylpropanolamine HCl 75 mg, caramiphen edisylate 40 mg/TR Cap. Bot. 100s, 500s, 1000s. *otc.*
Use: Antitussive, decongestant.

Detussin Expectorant Liquid. (Various Mfr.) Pseudoephedrine HCl 60 mg, hydrocodone bitartrate 5 mg, guaifenesin 200 mg, alcohol. Liq. Bot. 480 ml. *c-III.*
Use: Antitussive, decongestant, expectorant.

Detussin Liquid. (Various Mfr.) Pseudoephedrine HCl 60 mg, hydrocodone bitartrate 5 mg. Liq. Bot. Pt, gal. *c-III.*
Use: Antitussive, decongestant.

•**deuterium oxide.** (doo-TEER-ee-uhm) USAN.
Use: Radiopharmaceutical.

•**devazepide.** (dev-AZE-eh-PIDE) USAN.
Use: Antagonist (cholecystokinin); antispasmodic, gastrointestinal.

Devrom. (Parthenon Co., Inc.) Bismuth subgallate 200 mg, lactose, sugar/ Chew. Tab. Bot. 100s.
Use: Deodorant, systemic.

Dex 4 Glucose. (Can-Am Care Corporation) Glucose. Tab. Bot. 10s, 50s. *otc.*
Use: Hyperglycemic.

Dexacidin Ointment. (Ciba Vision) Neomycin sulfate 0.35%, dexamethasone 0.1% polymyxin B sulfate 10,000 units. Tube 3.5 g. *Rx.*
Use: Anti-infective; corticosteroid, ophthalmic.

Dexacidin Ophthalmic Suspension. (Ciba Vision) Neomycin 0.35%, polymyxin B sulfate 10,000 units, dexamethasone 1%. Bot. 5 ml. *Rx.*
Use: Anti-infective; corticosteroid, ophthalmic.

Dexacort Phosphate Respihaler. (Medeva Pharmaceuticals, Inc.) Dexamethasone sodium phosphate equivalent to 0.1 mg dexamethasone phosphate (approximately 0.084 mg dexamethasone) w/fluorochlorohydrocarbons as propellants, alcohol 2%. Aerosol for oral inhalation, 170 sprays in 12.6 g pressurized container.
Use: Bronchodilator.

Dexacort Phosphate Turbinaire. (Medeva Pharmaceuticals, Inc.) Dexamethasone sodium phosphate 0.1 mg equivalent to dexamethasone 0.084 mg w/fluorochlorohydrocarbons as propellants and alcohol 2%. Aerosol w/nasal applicator. Container 170 sprays; refill package without nasal applicator.
Use: Nasal corticosteroid.

Dex-a-Diet Caffeine Free. (Columbia Laboratories, Inc.) Phenylpropanolamine HCl 75 mg/Cap. or Capl. Pkg. 3s, 6s, 20s, 40s.
Use: Dietary aid.

Dex-a-Diet Original Formula. (Columbia Laboratories, Inc.) Phenylpropanolamine HCl 75 mg, ascorbic acid 200 mg/Cap. Pkg. 3s, 6s, 10s, 24s, 48s.
Use: Dietary aid.

Dexafed. (Roberts Pharmaceuticals) Phenylephrine HCl 5 mg, dextromethorphan HBr 10 mg, guaifenesin 100 mg/5 ml. Syr. Bot. 120 ml. *otc.*
Use: Antitussive, decongestant, expectorant.

Dexameth. (Major Pharmaceuticals) **Tab.:** Dexamethasone 0.25 mg, 0.5 mg, 0.75 mg, 1.5 mg or 4 mg. Bot. 100s (0.25 mg, 0.5 mg, 1.5 mg); Bot. 100s, 1000s, Unipak 12s (0.75 mg); Bot. 50s, 100s (4 mg). **Elix.:** 0.5 mg/5 ml, alcohol 5%. Bot. 100 ml, 240 ml. *Rx.*
Use: Corticosteroid.

•**dexamethasone.** (DEX-uh-METH-uh-sone) U.S.P. 23.
Use: Adrenal corticosteroid (anti-inflammatory); corticosteroid, topical.
See: Aeroseb-Dex, Aerosol (Allergan, Inc.).
Decaderm in Estergel (Merck & Co.).

Decadron, Tab., Elix. (Merck & Co.).
Decameth, Inj. (Foy Laboratories).
Decameth L.A., Inj. (Foy Laboratories).
Dexaport, Tab. (Freeport).
Dexone TM, Tab. (Solvay Pharmaceuticals).
Hexadrol, Tab., Elix., Cream (Organon, Inc.).
Maxidex Ophth. Liq. (Alcon Laboratories, Inc.).

W/Neomycin sulfate.
See: NeoDecadron, Prep (Merck & Co.).

W/Neomycin sulfate, polymyxin B sulfate.
See: NeoDecaspray, Aerosol (Merck & Co.).
See: Maxitrol Ophth Susp, Oint. (Alcon Laboratories, Inc.).

dexamethasone. (Steris Laboratories, Inc.) 0.1%. Susp. Bot. 5 ml. *Rx.*
Use: Corticosteroid, ophthalmic.

•**dexamethasone acefurate.** (DEX-ah-METH-ah-sone ASS-eh-fer-ate) USAN.
Use: Anti-inflammatory, topical steroid.

•**dexamethasone acetate.** (DEX-ah-METH-ah-sone) U.S.P. 23.
Use: Adrenocortical steroid (anti-inflammatory).
See: Dalalone (Forest Pharmaceutical, Inc.).
Dexone LA, Ind. (Kay).

•**dexamethasone dipropionate.** (DEX-ah-METH-ah-sone die-PRO-pee-oh-nate) USAN.
Use: Anti-inflammatory, steroid.

Dexamethasone Intensol Oral Solution. (Roxane Laboratories, Inc.) Dexamethasone 1 mg/ml concentrated oral soln. Bot. 30 ml w/calibrated dropper. *Rx.*
Use: Corticosteroid.

dexamethasone ophthalmic. (Various Mfr.) Dexamethasone 0.1%. Susp. Bot. 5 ml. *Rx.*
Use: Corticosteroid.

•**dexamethasone sodium phosphate.** (DEX-ah-METH-ah-sone) U.S.P. 23.
Use: Adrenocortical steroid (anti-inflammatory); corticosteroid, topical.
See: AK-Dex, Soln., Oint. (Akorn, Inc.).
Dalalone (Forest Pharmaceutical, Inc.).
Decadron Phosphate, Preps. (Merck & Co.).
Decaject, Vial (Merz Pharmaceutcials).
Decameth, Inj. (Foy Laboratories).
Dexone, Inj. (Keene, Hauck).
Hexadrol Phosphate, Inj. (Organon, Inc.).
Maxidex, Oint. (Alcon Laboratories, Inc.).
Savacort D, Inj. (Savage Laboratories).
Solurex, Inj. (Hyrex Pharmaceuticals).

W/Neomycin sulfate.
See: NeoDecadron, Prods. (Merck & Co.).

W/Neomycin and polymyxin B sulfates.
See: Dexacidin, Prods. (Ciba Vision).

dexamethasone sodium phosphate. (Various Mfr.) **Soln.:** 0.1%. Bot. 5 ml; **Oint.:** 0.05%. Tube 3.5 g. *Rx.*
Use: Adrenocortical steroid (anti-inflammatory); corticosteroid, topical.

•**dexamisole.** (DEX-AM-ih-sole) USAN.
Use: Antidepressant.

dexamphetamine.
See: Dextroamphetamine (Various Mfr.).

Dexaphen-S.A. Tablets. (Major Pharmaceuticals) Pseudoephedrine sulfate 120 mg, dexbrompheniramine maleate 6 mg. Tab. Bot. 100s, 500s. *Rx.*
Use: Antihistamine, decongestant.

Dexaport. (Freeport) Dexamethasone 0.75 mg/Tab. Bot. 1000s. *Rx.*
Use: Corticosteroid.

Dexasone. (Various Mfr.) Dexamethasone sodium phosphate 4 mg/ml, methyl- and propylparabens, sodium bisulfite. Vial 5 ml, 10 ml, 30 ml. *Rx.*
Use: Corticosteroid.

Dexasone Injection. (Roberts Pharmaceuticals) Dexamethasone sodium phosphate 4 mg/ml. Vial 5 ml, 30 ml. *Rx.*
Use: Corticosteroid.

Dexasone L.A. Injection. (Roberts Pharmaceuticals) Dexamethasone acetate 8 mg/ml. Vial 5 ml. *Rx.*
Use: Corticosteroid.

Dexasporin Ointment. (Bausch & Lomb Pharmaceuticals) Dexamethasone 0.1%, neomycin sulfate equivalent to 0.35% neomycin base and 10,000 units polymyxin B sulfate. Ophth. Oint. Tube 3.5 g. *Rx.*
Use: Steroid; anti-infective, ophthalmic.

Dexasporin Suspension. (Various Mfr.) Dexamethasone 0.1%, neomycin sulfate equivalent to 0.35%, neomycin base and 10,000 units polymyxin B sulfate/ml, hydroxypropyl methylcellulose, polysorbate 20, benzalkonium chloride. Drops. Bot. 5 ml. *Rx.*
Use: Anti-infective; corticosteroid, ophthalmic.

Dexatrim-15. (Thompson Medical Co.)

Phenylpropanolamine HCl 75 mg/TR Cap. Bot. 20s, 40s. *otc.*
Use: Dietary aid.

Dexatrim-15 w/Vitamin C. (Thompson Medical Co.) Phenylpropanolamine HCl 75 mg, vitamin C 180 mg/TR Cap. Bot. 20s. *otc.*
Use: Dietary aid.

Dexatrim Maximum Strength. (Thompson Medical Co.) Phenylpropanolamine HCl 75 mg/Tab. ER Bot. 20s. *otc.*
Use: Dietary aid.

•**dexbrompheniramine maleate.** (dex-brome-fen-EER-ah-meen MAL-ee-ate) U.S.P. 23.
Use: Antihistamine.
W/Pseudoephedrine sulfate
See: Disophrol Chronotab, Tab. (Schering-Plough Corp.).
Drixomed (Iomed).
Drixoral S.A., Tab. (Schering-Plough Corp.).

•**dexchlorpheniramine maleate.** U.S.P. 23.
Use: Antihistamine.
See: Polaramine, Repetabs Tab., Tab., Syr. (Schering-Plough Corp.).
W/Pseudoephedrine sulfate, guaifenesin, alcohol.
See: Polaramine Expectorant (Schering-Plough Corp.).

dexchlorpheniramine maleate. (Various Mfr.) Dexchlorpheniramine maleate 4 mg, 6 mg/TR Tab. Bot. 100s. *Rx.*
Use: Antihistamine.

•**dexclamol hydrochloride.** (DEX-clay-mahl) USAN.
Use: Hypnotic, sedative.

Dexedrine. (SmithKline Beecham Pharmaceuticals) Dextroamphetamine sulfate. **Tab.:** 5 mg. Bot. 100s, 1000s. **Spansule:** 5 mg. Bot. 50s; 10 mg, 15 mg. Bot. 50s, 500s. *c-II.*
Use: CNS stimulant.

•**dexetimide.** (dex-ETT-ih-mid) USAN.
Use: Anticholinergic, antiparkinsonian.

DexFerrum. (American Regent) Elemental iron 50 mg/ml (as dextran)/Inj. Vial. 2 ml (single dose). *Rx.*
Use: Hematinic.

Dex4 Glucose. (Can-Am Care Corporation) Glucose, lemon, orange, raspberry, grape flavors. Chew. Tab. Bot. 10s, 50s. *otc.*
Use: Glucose-elevating agent.

•**dexibuprofen.** (dex-EYE-byoo-PRO-fen) USAN.
Use: Analgesic; anti-inflammatory.

•**dexibuprofen lysine.** (dex-EYE-byoo-PRO-fen LIE-seen) USAN.
Use: Analgesic (cyclooxygenase inhibitor), anti-inflammatory.

•**deximafen.** (dex-IH-mah-fen) USAN.
Use: Antidepressant.

•**dexivacaine.** (dex-IH-vah-CANE) USAN.
Use: Anesthetic.

•**dexmedetomidine.** (DEX-meh-dih-TOE-mih-deen) USAN.
Use: Anxiolytic.

Dexone. (Solvay Pharmaceuticals) Dexamethasone 0.5 mg, 0.75 mg, 1.5 mg, 4 mg/Tab. Bot. 100s, UD 100s. Box 1s, 10s, 150s. *Rx.*
Use: Corticosteroid.

Dexone. (Roberts Pharmaceuticals) Dexamethasone sodium phosphate 4 mg/ml. Amp. 5 ml. *Rx.*
Use: Corticosteroid.

Dexone. (Solvay Pharmaceuticals) Dexamethasone sodium phosphate 4 mg/ml, methyl- and propylparabens, sodium bisulfite. Vial 5 ml, 10 ml. *Rx.*
Use: Corticosteroid.

Dexone LA. (Keene Pharmaceuticals, Inc.) Dexamethasone acetate suspension equivalent to dexamethasone 8 mg, polysorbate 80, carboxymethylcellulose, sodium bisulfite, EDTA, benzyl alcohol. Vial 5 ml. *Rx.*
Use: Corticosteroid.

•**dexormaplatin.** (DEX-ore-mah-PLAT-in) USAN.
Use: Antineoplastic.

•**dexoxadrol hydrochloride.** (dex-OX-ah-drole) USAN.
Use: Antidepressant; stimulant (central); analgesic.

•**dexpanthenol.** (DEX-PAN-theh-nahl) U.S.P. 23.
Use: Treatment of paralytic ileus and postoperative distention, cholinergic.
See: Ilopan, Inj. (Pharmacia & Upjohn).
Panthoderm (Rhone-Poulenc Rorer Pharmaceuticals, Inc.).

dexpanthenol/choline bitartrate.
See: Ilopan-choline (Pharmacia & Upjohn).

•**dexpemedolac.** (dex-peh-MED-oh-lack) USAN.
Use: Analgesic.

•**dexpropanolol hydrochloride.** (DEX-pro-PRAN-oh-lole) USAN.
Use: Antiadrenergic (β-receptor); cardiovascular agent (antiarrhythmic).

•**dexrazoxane.** (dex-ray-ZOX-ane) USAN.
Use: Cardioprotectant. [Orphan Drug]
See: Zinecard, Pow. for Inj. (Pharmacia & Upjohn)

•**dexsotalol hydrochloride.** (DEX-ah-tah-lahl) USAN.

Use: Cardiovascular agent (antiarrhythmic).

dextran 1.
See: Promit (Pharmacia & Upjohn).

dextran 6%. (Abbott Laboratories) *Rx.*
See: Dextran 75, I.V. (Abbott Laboratories).

•**dextran 40.** (DEX-tran 40) USAN. Polysaccharide (m.w. 40,000) produced by the action of *Leuconostoc mesenteroides* on sucrose.
Use: Blood flow adjuvant, plasma volume extender.
See: Gentran 40 (Baxter Healthcare Corp.).
Rheomacrodex (Medisan).
10% LMD, Inj. (Abbott Laboratories).

dextran 40. (McGaw, Inc.) Dextran 40 10% with 0.9% sodium chloride or in 5% dextrose. Inj. 500 ml. *Rx.*
Use: Plasma expander.

dextran 45, 75. Polysaccharide (m.w. 45,000, 75,000) produced by the action of *Leuconostoc mesenteroides* on saccharose. Rheotran (45). *Rx.*
Use: Blood volume expander.

•**dextran 70.** (DEX-tran 70) USAN. Polysaccharide (m.w. 70,000) produced by the action of *Levconostoc mesenteroides* on sucrose.
Use: Plasma volume extender.
See: Aquasite (Ciba Vision).
Dextran 70, Inj. (McGaw, Inc.).
Gentran 70, Inj. (Baxter Pharmaceutical Products, Inc.).
Hyskon (Kabi Pharmacia & Upjohn).
Macrodex (Medisan).

dextran 70. (DEX-tran 70) (McGaw, Inc.) Dextran 70 6% in 0.9% sodium chloride. Inj. 500 ml. *Rx.*
Use: Plasma expander.

•**dextran 75.** (DEX-tran 75) USAN. Polysaccharide (m.w. 75,000) produced by the action of *Leuconostoc mesenteroides* on sucrose.
Use: Plasma volume extender.
See: Dextran 75, Inj. (Abbott Laboratories).
Macrodex, Inj. (Medisan).

dextran 75. (Abbott Laboratories) Dextran 75 6% in 0.9% sodium chloride or 5% dextrose. Inj. 500 ml. *Rx.*
Use: Plasma expander.

dextran adjunct. *Rx.*
Use: Plasma expander.
See: Promit, Inj. (Pharmacia & Upjohn).

dextran and deferoxamine.
Use: Acute iron poisoning. [Orphan Drug]
See: Bio-Rescue (Biomedical Frontiers, Inc.).

dextran sulfate, inhaled aerosolized.
Use: Antiviral. [Orphan Drug]
See: Uendex (Ueno Fine Chemicals Industry).

dextran sulfate sodium. (Ueno Fine Chemicals Industry)
Use: AIDS drug. [Orphan Drug]

•**dextrates.** (DEX-traytz) N.F. 18. Mixture of sugars (approximately 92% dextrose monohydrate and 8% higher saccharides; dextrose equivalent is 95% to 97%) resulting from the controlled enzymatic hydrolysis of starch.
Use: Pharmaceutic aid (tablet binder, diluent).

•**dextrin.** N.F. 18.
Use: Pharmaceutic aid (suspending, viscosity-increasing agent; tablet binder; tablet, capsule diluent).

•**dextroamphetamine.** (DEX-troe-am-FET-ah-meen) USAN.
Use: Stimulant (central).

dextroamphetamine phosphate. Monobasic d-a-methylphenethlyamine phosphate. (+)-α-Methylphenethylamine phosphate.
Use: CNS stimulant.

dextroamphetamine saccharate.
See: Adderall (Richwood Pahrmaceuticals).

•**dextroamphetamine sulfate.** (DEX-troe-am-FET-uh-meen) U.S.P. 23.
Use: CNS stimulant.
See: Adderall (Richwood Pharmaceuticals).
Dexampex, Cap., Tab. (Teva Pharmaceuticals USA).
Dexedrine, Preps. (SmithKline Beecham Pharmaceuticals).
Dextrostat, Tab. (Richwood Pharmaceuticals).
Tidex Tab. (Allison).

dextroamphetamine sulfate w/combinations.
Use: CNS stimulant.
See: Adderall. (Richwood Pharmaceuticals).

Dextro-Check Normal Control. (Bayer Corp. (Consumer Div.)) Clear liquid containing measured amount of glucose 0.1%
Use: Glucometer calibration aid

Dextro-Chek Calibrators. (Bayer Corp. (Consumer Div.)) Clear liquid soln. containing measured amounts of glucose. Low calibrator contains 0.05% w/v glucose. High calibrator contains 0.3% w/v glucose.
Use: Glucometer calibration aid.

Dextro-Chlorpheniramine Maleate.

Use: Antihistamine.
See: Polaramine, Repetab, Tab., Expect., Syr. (Schering-Plough Corp.).

•**dextromethorphan.** (DEX-troe-meth-OR-fan) U.S.P. 23.
Use: Cough suppressant, antitussive.

•**dextromethorphan hydrobromide.** (DEX-troe-meth-OR-fan HIGH-droe-BROE-mide) U.S.P. 23.
Use: Antitussive.
See: Benylin, Preps. (Parke-Davis).
Creo-Terpin, Liq. (Lee Pharmaceuticals).
Delsym, Liq. (Medeva Pharmaceuticals, Inc.).
Mediquell, Tab. (Warner Lambert).
Silphen DM, Syr. (Silarx Pharmaceuticals, Inc.).
St. Joseph Cough Syr. (Schering-Plough Corp.).
Sucrets 4-Hour Cough, Loz. (SmithKline Beecham).
Symptom 1, Liq. (Parke-Davis).
Tus-F, Liq. (Orbit).
W/Benzocaine, menthol, peppermint oil.
See: Vicks Formula 44 Cough Control Discs, Loz. (Procter & Gamble Pharm.).

dextromethorphan hydrobromide w/ benzocaine.
Use: Nonnarcotic antitussive.
See: Cough-X, Loz. (Archer).
Spec-T, Loz. (Apothecon, Inc.).
Vicks Cough Silencers, Loz. (Procter & Gamble Pharm.).
Vicks Formula 44 Cough Control Discs, Loz. (Procter & Gamble Pharm.).

dextromethorphan hydrobromide w/ combinations.
See: Ambenyl-D, Liq. (Hoechst Marion Roussel).
Anatuss DM, Syr., Tab. (Merz Pharmaceutcials).
Anti-Tuss D.M., Liq. (Century Pharmaceuticals, Inc.).
Anti-Tussive, Tab. (Canright).
Atuss DM, Syr. (Atley Pharmaceuticals, Inc.).
Bayer Prods. (Bayer Corp. (Consumer Div.)).
Benylin Multi-Symptom, Liq. (Glaxo-Wellcome).
Breacol Cough Medication, Liq. (Bayer Corp. (Consumer Div.)).
Bromadine-DM (Cypress).
Capahist-DMH, Cap. (Freeport).
Cerose, Liq. (Wyeth-Ayerst Laboratories).
Cheracol D, Cough Syr. (Pharmacia & Upjohn).
Cheratussin, Cough Syr. (Towne).
Children's Hold 4-Hour Cough Suppressant & Decongestant, Loz. (SmithKline Beecham Pharmaceuticals).
Children's Tylenol Cold Plus Cough (Ortho McNeil Pharmaceutical).
Clear Tussin 30 (Zenith Goldline).
Codimal DM, Liq. (Schwarz Pharma, Inc.).
Comtrex, Cap., Liq. Tab. (Bristol-Myers Squibb).
Contac Jr., Liq. (SmithKline Beecham Pharmaceuticals).
Coricidin Children's Cough Syrup (Schering-Plough Corp.).
Diabetic Tussin, Liq. (Roberts Pharmaceuticals).
Dimacol, Cap. (Wyeth-Ayerst Laboratories).
Donatussin, Syr. (Laser, Inc.).
Dorcol Ped. Cough Syr. (Sandoz Pharmaceutical).
Dristan Cough Formula, Syr. (Whitehall Robins Laboratories).
Fenesin DM, Tab. (Dura).
Formula 44 Prods. (Procter & Gamble Pharm.).
Hall's Mentho-Lyptus Decongestant Liquid, Liq. (Warner Lambert).
Histalet, DM, Syr. (Reid Provident).
Iobid DM, SR Tab. (Iomed).
Iohist DM, Syr. (Iomed).
Liqui-Histine DM, Syr. (Liquipharm).
Mapap CF, Tab. (Major Pharmaceuticals).
Maximum Strength Tylenol Flu, Tab. (McNeil-CPC).
Med-Rx DM (Iomed).
Monafed DM, TR Tab. (Monarch Pharmaceuticals).
Muco-Fen-DM, TR Tab. (Wakefield Pharmaceuticals, Inc.).
Multi-Symptom Tylenol Cough (Ortho McNeil Pharmaceutical).
Night Time Cold/Flu Relief (ProMetic Pharma.).
Nil Tuss, Syr. (Minn. Pharm.).
Nyquil, Liq. (Procter & Gamble Pharm.).
Orthoxicol, Syr. (Pharmacia & Upjohn).
Partuss, Liq. (Parmed Pharmaceuticals, Inc.).
Pediacon DX Preps. (Zenith Goldline Pharmaceuticals).
Phenadex, Preps. (Barre-National).
Phenergan, Pediatric, Liq. (Wyeth-Ayerst Laboratories).
Polytuss-DM, Liq. (Rhode).
Profen II DM, TR Tab. (Wakefield

Pharmaceuticals, Inc.).
Protuss DM (Horizon).
Respa-DM, SR Tab. (Respa Pharmaceuticals, Inc.).
Robitussin-DM, Syr., Loz. (Wyeth-Ayerst Laboratories).
Robitussin Cold & Cough, Preps. (Wyeth-Ayerst Laboratories).
Robitussin-CF (Wyeth-Ayerst Laboratories).
Rondec DM, Drops, Syr. (Ross Laboratories).
Scotcof, Liq. (Scott/Cord).
Scot-Tussin Senior Clear, Liq. (Scott-Tussin Pharm).
Shertus, Liq. (Sheryl).
Sildec-DM, Ped. Drops. (Silarx Pharmaceuticals, Inc.).
Siltapp with Dextromethorphan HBr Cold & Cough, Elix. (Silarx Pharmaceuticals, Inc.).
Siltussin Preps. (Silarx Pharmaceuticals, Inc.).
Sorbase Cough Syr. (Fort David).
Spec-T Sore Throat-Cough Suppressant, Loz. (Squibb).
Sudafed Cough, Syr. (Glaxo-Wellcome).
Synacol CF, Tab. (Roberts Pharmaceuticals).
Synatuss-One, Liq. (Freeport).
Thor, Cough Syr. (Towne).
Tolu-Sed DM, Liq. (Scherer Laboratories, Inc.).
Triaminic, Preps. (Sandoz Pharmaceutical).
Triaminicol, Liq. (Sandoz Consumer).
Tusibron-DM, Liq. (Kenwood Laboratories).
Tussi-Organidin DM NR, Liq. (Wallace Laboratories).
Tussi-Organidin DM-S NR, Liq. (Wallace Laboratories).
Tusquelin, Syr. (Circle Pharmaceuticals).
Tylenol, Preps. (McNeil).
Unproco, Cap. (Solvay Pharmaceuticals).
Vicks Cough Prods. (Procter & Gamble Pharm.).
Vicks Daycare, Liq. (Procter & Gamble Pharm.).
Vicks Formula 44 Prods. (Procter & Gamble Pharm.).
Vicks Nyquil, Liq. (Procter & Gamble Pharm.).
Wal-Tussin DM, Syr. (Walgreen Co.).

•**dextromethorphan polistirex.** (DEX-troe-meth-OR-fan pahl-ee-STIE-rex) USAN.
Use: Antitussive.

dextromoramide tartrate.
Use: Analgesic, narcotic.

dextro-pantothenyl alcohol.
See: Ilopan (Pharmacia & Upjohn).
Panthenol (Various Mfr.).

dextropropoxyphene hydrochloride.
c-iv.
Use: Analgesic.
See: Propoxyphene HCl, Cap. (Various Mfr.).

•**dextrorphan hydrochloride.** (DEX-trore-fan) USAN.
Use: Treatment of cerebral ischemia, vasospastic therapy adjunct.

•**dextrose.** (DEX-trose) U.S.P. 23.
Use: Fluid and nutrient replenisher.
W/Calcium ascorbate and benzyl alcohol injection.
See: Calscorbate, Amp. (Cole).
W/Psyllium mucilloid.
See: V-lax, Pow. (Century Pharmaceuticals, Inc.).

5% Dextrose and Electrolyte No. 48. (Baxter Pharmaceutical Products, Inc.) Dextrose 50 g, calories 180/L with Na^+ 25 mEq, K^+ 20 mEq, Mg^{++} 3 mEq, Cl^- 24 mEq, phosphate 3 mEq, acetate 23 mEq with osmolarity 348 mOsm/L. Soln. Bot. 250 ml, 500 ml, 1000 ml. *Rx.*
Use: Nutritional supplement, parenteral.

5% Dextrose and Electrolyte No. 75. (Baxter Pharmaceutical Products, Inc.) Dextrose 50 g, calories 180/L with Na^+ 40 mEq, K^+ 35 mEq, Cl^- 48 mEq, phosphate 15 mEq and lactate 20 mEq with osmolarity 402 mOsm/L. Soln. Bot. 250 ml, 500 ml, 1000 ml. *Rx.*
Use: Nutritional supplement, parenteral.

dextrose-alcohol injection. *Rx.*
Use: Nutritional supplement, parenteral.
See: 5% Alcohol and 5% Dextrose in Water (Abbott, Baxter, Kendall-McGaw Labs).

dextrose-electrolyte solution. *Rx.*
Use: Nutritional supplement, parenteral.
See: Dextrose 2.5% w/0.45% Sodium chloride (Various Mfr.) Soln. 250, 500, 1000 ml.
Dextrose 5% and Electrolyte #48 (Baxter Pharmaceutical Products, Inc.) Soln. 250, 500, 1000 ml.
Dextrose 5% and Electrolyte #75 (Baxter Pharmaceutical Products, Inc.) Soln. 250, 500, 1000 ml.
Dextrose 5% in Lactated Ringer's (Various Mfr.) Soln. 250, 500, 1000 ml.
Dextrose 5% in Ringer's (Various Mfr.) Soln. 500, 1000 ml.
Dextrose 5% w/0.11% Sodium chloride (Kendall McGaw) Soln. 500, 1000 ml.

Dextrose 5% w/0.2% Sodium chloride (Various Mfr.) Soln. 250, 500, 1000 ml.
Dextrose 5% w/0.33% Sodium chloride (Various Mfr.) Soln. 250, 500, 1000 ml.
Dextrose 5% w/0.45% Sodium chloride (Various Mfr.) Soln. 250, 500, 1000 ml.
Dextrose 5% w/0.9% Sodium chloride (Various Mfr.) Soln. 250, 500, 1000 ml.
Dextrose 10% and Electrolyte #48 injection (Baxter Pharmaceutical Products, Inc.). Soln 250 ml.
Dextrose 10% w/0.45% Sodium chloride (McGaw, Inc.) Soln. 1000 ml.
Dextrose 10% w/0.9% Sodium chloride (Various Mfr.) Soln. 500, 1000 ml.
Dextrose 10% with Electrolytes (Abbott Laboratories). Soln. 21 mEq gluconate Soln. 500 ml in 1000 ml partial fill container.
Dextrose 25% in Half-Strength Lactated Ringer's (Various Mfr.) Soln 250, 500, 1000 ml.
Ionosol B and 5% Dextrose (Abbott Laboratories). Soln. 500, 1000.
Ionosol MB and 5% Dextrose (Abbott Laboratories). Soln. 250, 500, 1000 ml.
Ionosol MB and 10% Dextrose (Abbott Laboratories). Soln. 500 ml.
Ionosol T and 5% Dextrose (Abbott Laboratories) Soln. 250, 500, 1000 ml.
Isolyte E with 5% Dextrose (McGaw, Inc.). 8 mEq citrate Soln. 1000 ml.
Isolyte G with 5% Dextrose (McGaw, Inc.) 70 mEq NH_4+. Soln. 1000 ml.
Isolyte G with 10% Dextrose (McGaw, Inc.) 70 mEq NH_4+. Soln. 1000 ml.
Isolyte H with 5% Dextrose (McGaw, Inc.). Soln. 1000 ml.
Isolyte M and 5% Dextrose (McGaw, Inc.) Soln. 1000 ml.
Isolyte P with 5% Dextrose (McGaw, Inc.). Soln. 250, 500, 1000.
Isolyte R with 5% Dextrose (McGaw, Inc.). Soln. 1000 ml.
Isolyte S with 5% Dextrose (McGaw, Inc.). 23 mEq gluconate Soln. 1000 ml.
Normosol-M and 5% Dextrose (Abbott Laboratories). Soln. 500, 1000.
Normosol-R and 5% Dextrose (Abbott Laboratories). 23 mEq gluconate Soln. 500, 1000 ml.
Plasma-Lyte 56 and 5% Dextrose (Baxter Pharmaceutical Products, Inc.). Soln. 500, 1000.
Plasma-Lyte 148 and 5% Dextrose (Baxter Pharmaceutical Products, Inc.). 23 mEq gluconate Soln. 500, 1000 ml.
Plasma-Lyte M and 5% Dextrose (Baxter Pharmaceutical Products, Inc.). Soln. 500, 1000 ml.
Plasma-Lyte R and 5% Dextrose (Baxter Pharmaceutical Products, Inc.). Soln. 1000 ml.
Potassium chloride 0.075% in 5% Dextrose and 0.2% Sodium chloride (Various Mfr.) Soln. 1000 ml.
Potassium chloride 0.075% in 5% Dextrose and 0.45% Sodium chloride (Various Mfr.) Soln. 1000 ml.
Potassium chloride 0.075% in D-5-W (Baxter Pharmaceutical Products, Inc.) Soln. 1000 ml.
Potassium chloride 0.15% in 5% Dextrose and 0.2% Sodium chloride (Various Mfr.) Soln. 250, 500, 1000 ml.
Potassium chloride 0.15% in 5% Dextrose and 0.33% Sodium chloride (Baxter Pharmaceutical Products, Inc.) Soln. 500, 1000 ml.
Potassium chloride 0.15% in 5% Dextrose and 0.45% Sodium chloride (Various Mfr.) Soln. 500, 1000 ml.
Potassium chloride 0.15% in 5% Dextrose and 0.9% Sodium chloride (Baxter Pharmaceutical Products, Inc.) Soln. 1000 ml.
Potassium chloride 0.15% in D-5-W (Various Mfr.) Soln. 1000 ml.
Potassium chloride 0.224% in 5% Dextrose and 0.2% Sodium chloride (Various Mfr.) Soln. 1000 ml.
Potassium chloride 0.224% in 5% Dextrose and 0.33% Sodium chloride (Baxter Pharmaceutical Products, Inc.) Soln. 1000 ml.
Potassium chloride 0.224% in 5% Dextrose and 0.45% Sodium chloride (Various Mfr.) Soln. 1000 ml.
Potassium chloride 0.224% in D-5-W (Various Mfr.) Soln. 1000 ml.
Potassium chloride 0.3% in 5% Dextrose and 0.2% Sodium chloride (Various Mfr.) Soln. 1000 ml.
Potassium chloride 0.3% in 5% Dextrose and 0.33% Sodium chloride (Various Mfr.) Soln. 1000 ml.
Potassium chloride 0.3% in 5% Dextrose and 0.45% Sodium chloride (Various Mfr.) Soln. 1000 ml.
Potassium chloride 0.3% in 5% Dextrose and 0.9% Sodium chloride (Baxter Pharmaceutical Products,

Inc.) Soln. 1000 ml.
Potassium chloride 0.3% in D-5-W (Various Mfr.) Soln. 500, 1000 ml.

•**dextrose excipient.** N.F. 18.
Use: Pharmaceutic aid (tablet excipient).

50% Dextrose/Electrolyte Pattern A. (McGaw, Inc.) Dextrose 500 g/L, calories 1700 cal/L, Na^+ 84 mEq, K^+ 40 mEq, Ca^{++}10 mEq, Mg^{++} 16 mEq, Cl^- 115 mEq, osmolarity 2800 mOsm/L, sulfate 16 mEq, gluconate 13 mEq. Soln. 500 ml in 1000 ml partial fill container. *Rx.*
Use: Nutritional supplement, parenteral.

50% Dextrose/Electrolyte Pattern B. (McGaw, Inc.) Dextrose 500 g/L, calories 1700 cal/L, Na^+ 32 mEq, Ca^{++} 9 mEq, Mg^{++} 16 mEq, Cl^- 32 mEq, osmolarity 2615 mOsm/L, sulfate 16 mEq, gluconate 4.2 mEq. Soln. 500 ml in 1000 ml partial fill container. *Rx.*
Use: Nutritional supplement, parenteral.

50% Dextrose/Electrolyte Pattern N. (McGaw, Inc.) Dextrose 500 g/L, calories 1700 cal/L, Na^+ 90 mEq, K^+ 80 mEq, Mg^{++} 16 mEq, Cl^- 150 mEq, phosphate 28 mEq, osmolarity 2875 mOsm/L, sulfate 16 mEq. 500 ml in 1000 ml partial fill container. *Rx.*
Use: Nutritional supplement, parenteral.

dextrose large volume parenterals. (Abbott Hospital Products) *Rx.*
Use: Nutritional supplement, parenteral.
See: Dextrose 2 0.5% in Water-1000 ml.
Dextrose 2 0.5% in 0.5 Sterile Lactated Ringer's or in 0.5 Sterile Saline. 1000 ml.
Dextrose 5% in Water-150 ml, 250 ml, 500 ml, 1000 ml in Abbo-Vac glass or LifeCare flexible plastic container; partial-fill glass: 50 in 200 ml, 50 in 300 ml, 100 in 300 ml, 400 in 500 ml; partial-fill plastic: 50 in 150 ml, 100 in 150 ml.
Dextrose 5% in Lactated Ringer's. 250 ml, 500 ml, 1000 ml glass; 500 ml, 1000 ml plastic container.
Dextrose 5% in Ringer's. 500 ml, 1000 ml.
Dextrose 5% in Saline 0.9% or in 0.25, 0.33, or 0.5 Sterile Saline. 250, 500, 1000 ml glass or plastic container.
Dextrose 10% in Water. 250 ml, 500 ml, 1000 ml containers.
Dextrose 20% in Water. 500 ml.
Dextrose 50% in Water. 500 ml. Dextrose 20%, 30%, 40%, 50%, 60%, 70% Injections, USP in partial-fill container, 500 ml in 1000 ml.
Dextrose 50% and Injection w/Electrolytes. Partial-Fill Container. 500 ml in 1000 ml
Dextrose Injection 50%. Bot. 1000 ml.
Dextrose Injection 70%. Bot. 1000 ml.

dextrose small volume parenterals. (Abbott Hospital Products) **Dextrose 5%:** 50 ml, 100 ml pressurized pintop vial. **Dextrose 10%:** 5 ml amp.; **Dextrose 25%:** 10 ml syringe. **Dextrose 50%:** 50 ml Abboject syringe (18 g × 1.5″), 50 ml Fliptop vial. **Dextrose 70%:** 70 ml pressurized pintop vial. *Rx.*
Use: Nutritional supplement, parenteral.

dextrose-sodium chloride injection. (Abbott Laboratories) 10% Dextrose and 0.225% Sodium Cl. Inj. Single-dose container. 500 ml.
Use: Nutritional supplement, parenteral.

Dextrostat. (Richwood Pharmaceuticals) Dextroamphetamine sulfate 5 mg, sucrose, lactose, tartrazine/Tab. Bot. 100s. *c-II.*
Use: CNS Stimulant.

Dextrostix. (Bayer Corp. (Consumer Div.)) A cellulose strip containing glucose oxidase and indicator system. Box 10s.
Use: Diagnostic aid, glucose.

•**dextrothyroxine sodium.** (dex-troe-thigh-ROX-een) USAN. U.S.P. XXI.
Use: Anticholesteremic, antihyperlipidemic.

Dexule. (Health for Life Brands, Inc.) Vitamins A 1333 IU, D 133 IU, B_1 0.33 mg, B_2 0.4 mg, C 10 mg, niacinamide 3.3 mg, iron 3.3 mg, calcium 29 mg, phosphorus 15 mg, methylcellulose 100 mg, benzocaine 3 mg/Cap. Bot. 21s, 90s. *otc.*
Use: Mineral, vitamin supplement.

Dexyl. (Pinex) Dextromethorphan HBr 15 mg, vitamin C 20 mg/Tab. Box 20s. *otc.*
Use: Antitussive, vitamin supplement.

•**dezaguanine.** (DEH-zah-GWAHN-een) USAN.
Use: Antineoplastic.

•**dezaguanine mesylate.** (DEE-zah-GWAHN-een MEH-sih-late) USAN.
Use: Antineoplastic.

Dezest. (Armenpharm Ltd.) Atropine sulfate, phenylpropanolamine HCl, chlorpheniramine maleate. Bot. 100s.
Use: Anticholinergic, antihistamine, antispasmodic, decongestant.

•**dezinamide.** (deh-ZIN-ah-mide) USAN.
Use: Anticonvulsant.

•**dezocine.** (DESS-oh-seen) USAN.
Use: Analgesic.
See: Dalgan (Wyeth-Ayerst Laboratories).

D-Film. (Ciba Vision) Poloxamer 407, EDTA 0.25%, benzalkonium Cl 0.025%. Gel Tube 25 g. *otc.*
Use: Contact lens care.

DFMO. Eflornithine HCl. *Rx.*
Use: Anti-infective.
See: Ornidyl, Inj. (Hoechst Marion Roussel).

DFP. Disopropyl fluorophosphate (Various Mfr.)

d-Glucose. Dextrose. *Rx.*
Use: Nutritional supplement, parenteral.
See: D-2½-W, Soln. (Various Mfr.). D-10-W, Soln. (Various Mfr.).

DHC Plus. (Purdue Frederick Co.) Dihydrocodeine bitartrate 16 mg, acetaminophen 356.4 mg, caffeine 30 mg. Cap. Bot. 100s. *c-III.*
Use: Analgesic combination, narcotic.

DHEA. (Athena Neurosciences, Inc.) EL10. *Rx.*
Use: Antiviral, immunomodulator.

D.H.E. 45. (Sandoz Pharmaceutical) Dihydroergotamine mesylate 1 mg/ml, methanesulfonic acid, alcohol 6.1%, glycerin 15%. Inj. Amp. 1 ml. *Rx.*
Use: Antimigraine.

DHPG. Ganciclovir sodium. *Rx.*
Use: Antiviral.
See: Cytovene, Pow. (Roche Laboratories).

DHS Conditioning Rinse. (Person and Covey, Inc.) Conditioning ingredients. Bot. 8 oz. *otc.*
Use: Dermatologic, hair.

DHS Shampoo. (Person and Covey, Inc.) Blend of cleansing surfactants and emulsifiers. Plastic bot. w/dispenser 8 oz, 16 oz. *otc.*
Use: Dermatologic, hair, and scalp.

DHS Tar Gel Shampoo. (Person and Covey, Inc.) Coal Tar, U.S.P. 0.5% Bot. 8 oz. *otc.*
Use: Antipsoriatic, antiseborrheic.

DHS Tar Shampoo. (Person and Covey, Inc.) Coal tar 0.5% in DHS shampoo. Bot. 4 oz, 8 oz, 16 oz. *otc.*
Use: Antipsoriatic, antiseborrheic.

DHS Zinc Shampoo. (Person and Covey, Inc.) Zinc pyrithione 2% in DHS shampoo. Bot. 6 oz, 12 oz. *otc.*
Use: Antiseborrheic.

DHT. (Roxane Laboratories, Inc.) Dihydrotachysterol. **Tab.:** 0.125 mg, 0.2 mg or 0.4 mg/Tab. Bot. 50s, 100s (0.2 mg only), UD 100s (except 0.4 mg). **Intensol Soln.:** 0.2 mg/ml, alcohol 20%. Bot. 30 ml w/dropper. *Rx.*
Use: Antihypocalcemic.

DiaBeta. (Hoechst Marion Roussel) Glyburide. **1.25 mg:** Bot. 50s. **2.5 mg:** Bot. 100s, 500s, UD 100s. **5 mg:** Bot. 100s, 500s, 1000s, UD 1000s. *Rx.*
Use: Antidiabetic.

Diabetes CF. (Scot-Tussin Pharmacal, Inc.) Sugar-free. Syr. Bot. 120 ml. *otc.*
Use: Antitussive, expectorant.

Diabetic Tussin. (Roberts Pharmaceuticals) Dextromethorphan HBr 10 mg, guaifenesin 100 mg, phenylephedrine 5 mg/5 ml. Liq. Bot. 120 ml. *otc.*
Use: Antitussive, decongestant, expectorant.

Diabetic Tussin DM. (Roberts Pharmaceuticals) Dextromethorphan HBr 10 mg, guaifenesin 100 mg, saccharin, methylparaben, menthol, alcohol & dye free. Liq. Bot. 118 ml. *otc.*
Use: Antitussive, expectorant.

Diabetic Tussin EX. (Health Care Products) Guaifenesin 100 mg/5 ml, saccharin, menthol, methylparaben. Liq. Bot. 118 ml. *otc.*
Use: Expectorant.

Diabinese. (Pfizer US Pharmaceutical Group) Chlorpropamide 100 mg, 250 mg. Tab. Bot. 100s, 250s (250 mg only), 500s (100 mg only), 1000s (250 mg only), UD 100s. *Rx.*
Use: Antidiabetic.

diacetic acid test.
See: Acetest, Tab. (Bayer Corp. (Consumer Div.)).

Diaceto w/Codeine. (Archer-Taylor) Codeine 0.25 gr, 0.5 gr/Tab. or Cap. Bot. 500s, 1000s. *c-II.*
Use: Analgesic, narcotic.

Diaceto w/Gelsemium. (Archer-Taylor) Phenobarbital 0.5 gr, gelsemium 3 min/Tab. Bot. 1000s. *c-IV.*
Use: Hypnotic, sedative.

•**diacetolol hydrochloride.** (DIE-ah-SEET-oh-lahl HIGH-droe-KLOR-ide) USAN.
Use: Antiadrenergic (β-receptor).

diacetrizoate, sodium.
See: Diatrizoate (Various Mfr.).

•**diacetylated monoglycerides.** N.F. 18.
Use: Pharmaceutic aid (plasticizer).

diacetylcholine chloride. Succinylcholine Cl.
See: Anectine Chloride, Inj., Pow. (Burroughs Wellcome Co.).

diacetyl-dihydroxydiphenylisatin.
See: Oxyphenisatin acetate (Various Mfr.).

diacetyldioxyphenylisatin.
See: Oxyphenisatin acetate (Various Mfr.).

diacetylmorphine salts. Heroin. Illegal in USA by federal statute because of its addiction potential.

Di-Ademil.
See: Hydroflumethiazide, Tab. (Various Mfr.).

diagniol.
See: Sodium Acetrizoate.

diagnostic agents.
See: Acholest, Kit (E. Fougera and Co.) (allergic extracts).
Aplisol (Parke-Davis).
Aplitest (Parke-Davis).
Candida Skin Test Antigen (Allermed, ALK).
Candin (Allermed, ALK).
Cardio-Green, Vial (Becton Dickinson & Co.).
Cardiografin, Vial (Squibb).
Cea-Roche, Kit (Roche Laboratories).
Cholografin, Prep. (Squibb).
Coccidioidin, Vial (ALK, Iatric).
Dextrostix, Strip (Bayer Corp. (Consumer Div.)).
Dey-Pak Sodium Chloride (Dey Laboratories, Inc.).
Evans Blue Dye, Inj. (New World Trading Corp.).
EZ Detect Strep-A Test (Biomerica, Inc.).
Fertility Tape (Weston Labs.).
First Choice (Polymer Technology Int.).
Fluorescein Sodium Ophth. Soln. (Various Mfr.).
Fluor-I-Strip (Wyeth-Ayerst Laboratories).
Fluor-I-Strip A.T. (Wyeth-Ayerst Laboratories).
Fluress, Ophth. Soln. (Pilkington Barnes Hind).
Hema-Combistix Strips (Bayer Corp. (Consumer Div.)).
Hemastix Strips (Bayer Corp. (Consumer Div.)).
Histalog, Amp (Eli Lilly and Co.).
Histolyn-CYL (ALK).
Histoplasmin, Vial (Parke-Davis).
Hymenoptera venoms.
Indigo Carmine (Various Mfr.).
HIVAB HIV-1/HIV-2 (rDNA) EIA (Abbot Laboratories).
Immunex CRP (Wampole).
Mannitol Soln, Inj. (Merck & Co.).
Mono-Latex (Wampole).
Mono-Plus (Wampole).
MSTA (Pasteur Merieux Connaught).
Multitest-CMI (Pasteur Merieux Connaught).
Mumps Skin Test Antigen (Pasteur Merieux Connaught).
Persantine IV (Du Pont Merck Pharmaceutical Co).
Pharmalgen (ALK).
Phentolamine Methanesulfonate, Inj. (Various Mfr.).
Prepen (Schwarz Pharma).
Regitine, Amp, Tab. (Novartis Pharmaceutical Corp.).
Rheumanosticon Slide Test (Organon, Inc.).
Rheumatex (Wampole).
Rheumaton (Wampole).
Spherulin (ALK).
SureCell Chlamydia Test (Kodak Dental).
SureCell Herpes (HSV) Test (Kodak Dental).
SureCell Strep A Test (Kodak Dental).
Sodium Dehydrochol, Inj. (Various Mfr.).
Tes-Tape (Eli Lilly and Co.).
Tine Test (Wyeth-Ayerst Laboratories).
True Test (GlaxoWellcome).
Tubersol (Pasteur Merieux Connaught).
Venomil (Bayer Corp.).
See: Cholecystography Agents.
Kidney Function Agents.
Liver Function Agents.
Urography Agents.

diagnostic agents for urine.
See: Acetest, Tab. (Bayer Corp. (Consumer Div.)).
Albustix, Strip (Bayer Corp. (Consumer Div.)).
Biotel Diabetes (Biotel Corp.).
Biotel Kidney (Biotel Corp.).
Biotel U.T.I. (Biotel Corp.).
Chemstrip Micral, Strips (Boehringer Mannheim Pharmaceuticals).
Clinistix, Strip (Bayer Corp. (Consumer Div.)).
Clinitest, Tab. (Bayer Corp. (Consumer Div.)).
Fortel Midstream (Biomerica, Inc.).
Fortel Plus (Biomerica, Inc.).
Hema-Combistix, Strip (Bayer Corp. (Consumer Div.)).
HCG-nostick (Organon Teknika Corp.).
Hemastix, Strip (Bayer Corp. (Consumer Div.)).
Hematest, Tab (Bayer Corp. (Consumer Div.)).
Ictotest, Tab (Bayer Corp. (Consumer Div.)).
Ketostix, Strip (Bayer Corp. (Consumer Div.)).
SureCell hCG-Urine Test (Kodak Dental).

Uristix, Strip (Bayer Corp. (Consumer Div.)).
Wampole One-Step hCG (Wampole).

diallylbarbituric acid. Allobarbital, Allobarbitone, Curral.

diallylamicol. Diallyl-diethylaminoethyl phenol di HCl.

dialminate. Mixture of magnesium carbonate and (aluminate) dihydroxyaluminum glycinate.
W/Aspirin.
See: Bufferin, Preps. (Bristol-Myers Squibb).

Dialose. (Merck & Co.) Docusate sodium 100 mg., lactose, sugar. Tab. Bot. 36s. *otc.*
Use: Laxative.

Dialose Plus. (Merck & Co.) **Cap.:** Docusate sodium 100 mg, yellow phenolphthalein 65 mg/Cap. Bot. 36s, 100s, 500s. **Tab.:** Docusate sodium 100 mg, yellow phenolphthalein 65 mg, sugar/Tab. Bot 100s. *otc.*
Use: Laxative.

Dialyte Pattern LM w/1.5% Dextrose. (Gambro, Inc.) Dextrose 15 g/L, Na^+ 131, Ca^{++} 3.5, Mg^{++} 0.5, Cl^- 94 and lactate 40 with osmolarity 345 mOsm/L. Soln. Bot. 1000 ml, 2000 ml, 4000 ml. *Rx.*
Use: Peritoneal dialysis solution.

Dialyte Pattern LM w/2.5% Dextrose. (Gambro, Inc.) Dextrose 25 g/L, Na^+ 131.5, Ca^{++} 3.5, Mg^{++} 0.5, Cl^- 94 and lactate 40 with osmolarity 395 mOsm/L. Soln. Bot. 1000 ml, 2000 ml, 4000 ml. *Rx.*
Use: Peritoneal dialysis solution.

Dialyte Pattern LM w/4.25%Dextrose. (Gambro, Inc.) Dextrose 42.5 g/L, Na^+ 131.5, Ca^{++} 3.5, Mg^{++} 0.5, Cl^- 94, and lactate 40 with osmolarity 485 mOsm/L. Soln. Bot. 1000 ml, 2000 ml, 4000 ml. *Rx.*
Use: Peritoneal dialysis solution.

diamethine.
See: Dimethyl tubocurarine (Various Mfr.).

di-amino acetate complex w/calcium aluminum carbonate. Cap. IU.
See: Ancid Tab., Susp. (Sheryl).

diaminodiphenylsulfone. Dapsone, U.S.P. 23.
Use: Antimalarial.

diaminopropyl tetramethylene.
See: Spermine.

3,4-diaminopyridine. (Jacobus Pharmaceutical Co.)
Use: Lambert-Eaton myasthenic syndrome. [Orphan Drug]

•**diamocaine cyclamate.** (die-AM-oh-CANE SIH-klah-mate) USAN.
Use: Anesthetic, local.

Diamox. (Wyeth-Ayerst) Acetazolamide. **Tab.:** 125 mg Bot. 100s. 250 mg Bot. 100s, 1000s, UD 10 × 10s. **Inj. Vial:** Sterile sodium salt 500 mg (sodium hydroxide to adjust pH). *Rx.*
Use: Anticonvulsant, diuretic.

Diamox Sequels. (Wyeth-Ayerst) Acetazolamide 500 mg/Cap. Bot. 30s, 100s. *Rx.*
Use: Anticonvulsant, diuretic.

diamthazole dihydrochloride. Asterol.

Dianeal w/1.5% Dextrose. (Baxter Pharmaceutical Products, Inc.) Dextrose 15 g/L, Na^+ 141, Ca^{++} 3.5, Mg^{++}1.5, Cl^- 101, lactate 45 with osmolarity 364 mOsm/L. Soln. Bot. 1000 ml, 2000 ml. *Rx.*
Use: Peritoneal dialysis solution.

Dianeal 137 w/1.5% Dextrose. (Baxter Pharmaceutical Products, Inc.) Dextrose 15 g/L, Na^+ 132, Ca^{++} 3.5, Mg^{++} 1.5, Cl^- 102, lactate 35 with osmolarity 347 mOsm/L. Soln. Bot. 2000 ml. *Rx.*
Use: Peritoneal dialysis solution.

Dianeal w/4.25% Dextrose. (Baxter Pharmaceutical Products, Inc.) Dextrose 42.5 g/L, Na^+ 141, Ca^{++} 3.5, Mg^{++} 1.5, Cl^- 101, lactate 45 with osmolarity 503 mOsm/L. Soln. Bot. 2000 ml. *Rx.*
Use: Peritoneal dialysis solution.

Dianeal 137 w/4.25% Dextrose. (Baxter Pharmaceutical Products, Inc.) Dextrose 42.5 g/L, Na^+ 132, Ca^{++} 3.5, Mg^{++} 1.5, Cl^- 102, lactate 35 with osmolarity 486 mOsm/L. Soln. Bot. 2000 ml. *Rx.*
Use: Peritoneal dialysis solution.

dianeal PD-2 peritoneal dialysis soln with 1.1% amino acid.
Use: Nutritional supplement for dialysis patients. [Orphan Drug]

•**diapamide.** (die-APP-am-ide) USAN.
Use: Antihypertensive, diuretic.

Diapantin. (Janssen Pharmaceutical, Inc.) Isopropamide bromide. *Rx.*
Use: Anticholinergic.

Diaparene. (Bayer Corp. (Consumer Div.)) Methylbenzethonium Cl. Pow. Bot. 4 oz, 9 oz, 12.5 oz, 14 oz.
Use: Disinfectant, surface active agent.

Diaparene Medicated. (Reckitt & Colman) Methylbenzethonium Cl with white petrolatum 0.1%, glycerin, mineral oil, stearyl alcohol. Cream. Tube 30, 60, 120 g. *otc.*
Use: Antimicrobial, topical.

Diaparene Ointment. (Bayer Corp. (Consumer Div.)) Methylbenzethonium Cl 0.1% w/petrolatum, glycerin. Tube 1 oz,

2 oz, 4 oz. *otc.*
Use: Antimicrobial, topical.

Diaparene Peri-Anal Cream. (Bayer Corp. (Consumer Div.)) Methylbenzethonium Cl 1:1000, zinc oxide, starch, cod liver oil, white petrolatum, lanolin, calcium caseinate. Cream Tube 1 oz, 2 oz, 4 oz. *otc.*
Use: Antimicrobial, astringent.

Diaper Guard. (Del Pharmaceuticals, Inc.) Dimethicone 1%, white petrolatum 66%, cocoa butter, parabens, vitamins A, D_3, E, zinc oxide. Oint. Tube 49.6 g, 99.2 g. *otc.*
Use: Diaper rash preparation.

Diaper Rash. (Various Mfr.) Zinc oxide, cod liver oil, lanolin, methylparaben, petrolatum, talc. Oint. Tube 113 g. *otc.*
Use: Diaper rash preparation.

diaphenylsulfone. Dapsone.
Use: Leprostatic.

Diapid. (Sandoz Pharmaceutical) Lypressin synthetic lysine-8-vasopressin. Equiv. to 50 U.S.P. units posterior pituitary/ml (0.185 mg/ml). Nasal spray. Bot. 8 ml. *Rx.*
Use: Pituitary hormone.

Di-Ap-Trol. (Foy Laboratories) Phendimetrazine tartrate 35 mg/Tab. Bot. 100s, 1000s. *c-III.*
Use: Anorexiant.

Diarrest. (Dover Pharmaceuticals) Calcium carbonate, pectin/Tab. Sugar, lactose, and salt free. UD box 500s. *otc.*
Use: Antidiarrheal.

diarrhea therapy.
See: Antidiarrheal.

Diaserp. (Major Pharmaceuticals) Chlorothiazide 250 mg or 500 mg/Tab. w/reserpine. Bot. 100s. *Rx.*
Use: Antihypertensive.

Diasorb. (Columbia Laboratories, Inc.) Activated nonfibrous attapulgite. **Liq.:** 750 mg per 5 ml. Bot. 120 ml. **Tab.:** 750 mg. Pkg. 24s. *otc.*
Use: Antidiarrheal.

Diasporal. (Doak Dermatologics) Formerly Sulfur Salicyl Diasporal. Sulfur 3%, salicylic acid 2%, isopropyl alcohol in diasporal base. Cream Jar 3¾ oz. *otc.*
Use: Antiseptic, topical.

Diastase.
See: Aspergillus oryzae enzyme.

Diastat. (Atheria) Diazapam. **Pediatric:** 2.5 mg, 5 mg, 10 mg. **Adult:** 10 mg, 15 mg, 20 mg. Rectal gel. Twin pack. Includes lubricating jelly, plastic applicator with flexible, molded tip in two lengths.
Use: Anticonvulsant.

Diastix Reagent Strips. (Bayer Corp. (Consumer Div.)) Broad range test for glucose in urine. Containing glucose oxidase, peroxidase, potassium iodide w/blue background dye. Tab. Pkg. 50s, 100s.
Use: Diagnostic aid.

•**diatrizoate meglumine.** (die-ah-TRIH-zoe-ate meh-GLUE-meen) U.S.P. 23.
Use: Diagnostic aid (radiopaque medium).
See: Angiovist 282, Inj. (Berlex Laboratories, Inc.).
Cardiografin, Vial (Squibb).
Cystografin, Inj. (Squibb).
Gastrografin, Liq. (Squibb).
Hypaque-Cysto, Liq. (Sanofi Winthrop Pharmaceuticals).
Hypaque Meglumine (Sanofi Winthrop Pharmaceuticals).
Hypaque-76 (Nycomed).
MD-Gastroview (Mallinckrodt).
MD-76 R (Mallinckrodt).
RenoCal-76 (Bracco Diagnostics).
Renografin 60, Inj. (Squibb).
Reno-DIP, Inj. (Squibb).
Reno-30, Inj. (Squibb).
Reno-60, Inj. (Squibb).
Urovist, Prods. (Berlex Laboratories, Inc.)
W/Iodipamide methylglucamine.
See: Sinografin, Vial (Squibb).
W/Sodium Diatrizoate.
See: Renovist, Inj (Squibb).

diatrizoate meglumine and diatrizoate sodium injection.
Use: Diagnostic aid (radiopaque medium).
See: Angiovist 292, Inj. (Berlex Laboratories, Inc.).
Angiovist 370, Inj. (Berlex Laboratories, Inc.).
Hypaque-M Prods (Sanofi Winthrop Pharmaceuticals).

diatrizoate meglumine and diatrizoate sodium solution.
Use: Diagnostic aid (radiopaque medium).
See: Gastrografin Soln. (Squibb).
Renografin-60, Soln. (Squibb).
Renografin-60, -76, Soln. (Squibb).
Renovist, Soln. (Squibb).

diatrizoate meglumine 52.7% and iodipamide meglumine 25.8% (38% iodine).
Use: Diagnostic aid (radiopaque agent).
See: Sinografin, Inj. (Bracco Diagnostics).

diatrizoate methylglucamine.
Use: Diagnostic aid (radiopaque medium).

See: Diatrizoate Meglumine, U.S.P. 23.

diatrizoate methylglucamine sodium.
Use: Diagnostic aid (radiopaque medium).

•**diatrizoate sodium.** U.S.P. 23.
Use: Diagnostic aid (radiopaque medium).
See: Hypaque Prods. (Sanofi Winthrop Pharmaceuticals).
Urovist Sodium, Inj. (Berlex Laboratories, Inc.).
W/Meglumine diatrizoate.
See: Gastrografin, Liq. (Squibb).
Renografin-60, -76, Vial (Squibb).
Renovist II, Vial (Squibb).
W/Methylglucamine diatrizoate, sodium citrate, disodium ethylenediamine tetraacetate dihydrate, methylparaben, propylparaben.
See: Renovist, Vial (Squibb).

diatrizoate sodium 41.66% (24.9% iodine).
Use: Diagnostic aid (radiopaque agent).
See: Hypaque sodium, Soln. (Sanofi Winthrop Pharmaceuticals).

diatrizoate sodium (59.87% iodine).
Use: Diagnostic aid (radiopaque agent).
See: Hypaque Sodium, Soln. (Sanofi Winthrop Pharmaceuticals).

•**diatrizoate sodium I-125.** USAN.
Use: Radiopharmaceutical.

•**diatrizoate sodium I-131.** USAN.
Use: Radiopharmaceutical.

•**diatrizoic acid.** (DIE-at-rih-ZOE-ik) U.S.P. 23.
Use: Diagnostic aid (radiopaque medium).
See: Hypaque sodium salt.

•**diaveridine.** (DIE-ah-ver-ih-deen) USAN.
Use: Anti-infective.

•**diazepam.** (DIE-aze-uh-pam) U.S.P. 23.
Use: Agent for control of emotional disturbances, anxiolytic, hypnotic, sedative.
See: Diastat, Rectal Gel. (Athena Neurosciences, Inc.).
Diazepam Intensol, Soln. (Roxane Laboratories, Inc.).
Dizac, Inj. (Ohmeda Pharmaceuticals).
Valium, Tab. (Roche Laboratories).

diazepam. (Various Mfr.) **Tab.:** 2 mg, 5 mg, 10 mg. Bot. 100s, 500s, 1000s; 5 mg or 10 mg. Bot. 100s, 500s, 1000s; **Inj.:** 5 mg/ml. Vial 1, 2, 10 ml; syringe 1 cartridge 1 ml. **Oral Soln.:** (Roxane Laboratories, Inc.) 1 mg/1 ml orange, spice, wintergreen flavor. 500 ml, UD 5 ml, 10 ml. **Concentrated Oral Soln.:** (Roxane Laboratories, Inc.) 5 mg/ml. 30 ml w/dropper. *c-IV.*
Use: Agent for control of emotional disturbances, anxiolytic, hypnotic, sedative.

Diazepam Intensol. (Roxane Laboratories, Inc.) Diazepam 5 mg/ml. Oral Soln. 30 ml with dropper. *c-IV.*
Use: Anxiolytic.

diazepam viscous rectal solution. (Athena Neurosciences, Inc.)
Use: To treat acute repetitive seizures. [Orphan Drug]

•**diaziquone.** (DIE-azz-ih-kwone) USAN.
Use: Antineoplastic.

diazomycins a, b, & c. Antibiotic obtained from *Streptomyces ambofaciens.* Under study.

•**diazoxide.** (DIE-aze-OX-ide) U.S.P. 23.
Use: Antihypertensive.
See: Proglycem, Cap. (Medical Market Specialists).
Proglycem, Susp. (Medical Market Specialists).

diazoxide, parenteral. (DIE-aze-OX-ide)
Use: Antihypertensive.
See: Diazoxide Injection USP, Inj. (Various Mfr.).
Hyperstat IV, Inj. (Schering-Plough Corp.).

dibasic calcium phosphate dihydrate.
Use: Replenisher (calcium); pharmaceutic aid (tablet base).
See: Diostate D, Tab. (Pharmacia & Upjohn).

Dibatrol. (Lexis Laboratories) Chlorpropamide 100 mg or 250 mg/Tab. Bot. 100s, 1000s. *Rx.*
Use: Antidiabetic.

Dibent. (Roberts Pharmaceuticals) Dicyclomine 10 mg/ml with chlorobutanol. Inj. Vial 10 ml. *Rx.*
Use: Gastrointestinal, anticholinergic.

•**dibenzepin hydrochloride.** (die-BEN-zeh-pin) USAN.
Use: Antidepressant.

•**dibenzothiophene.** (die-BEN-zoe-THIGH-oh-feen) USAN.
Use: Keratolytic.

Dibenzyline. (SmithKline Beecham Pharmaceuticals) Phenoxybenzamine HCl 10 mg/Cap. Bot. 100s. *Rx.*
Use: Antihypertensive.

dibromodulcitol. (Biopharmaceutics, Inc.)
Use: Antineoplastic. [Orphan Drug]

•**dibromsalan.** (die-BROME-sah-lan) USAN.
Use: Antimicrobial, disinfectant.

•**dibucaine.** (DIE-byoo-cane) U.S.P. 23.
Use: Local anesthetic.

See: D-Caine, Oint. (Century Pharmaceuticals, Inc.).
Nupercainal, Oint., Cream, Supp. (Novartis Pharmaceutical Corp.).
Nupercainal Heavy, Soln. (Novartis Pharmaceutical Corp.).
W/Dextrose.
See: Nupercaine Heavy Soln. (Novartis Pharmaceutical Corp.).
W/Sodium bisulfite.
See: Nupercainal, Cream, Oint. (Novartis Pharmaceutical Corp.).
W/Zinc oxide, bismuth subgallate, acetone sodium bisulfite.
See: Nupercainal, Oint., Supp. (Novartis Pharmaceutical Corp.).

•**dibucaine hydrochloride.** U.S.P. 23.
Use: Anesthetic, local.
See: Nupercaine HCl, Soln. (Novartis Pharmaceutical Corp.).
W/Antipyrine, hydrocortisone, polymyxin B sulfate, neomycin sulfate.
See: Otocort, Liq. (Teva Pharmaceuticals USA).
W/Colistin sodium methanesulfonate, citric acid, sodium citrate.
See: Coly-Mycin M, Injectable (Warner Chilcott Laboratories).

dibutoline sulfate. Ethyl (2-hydroxyethyl)-dimethylammonium sulfate (2:1) bis (dibutyl-carbam-ate).
Use: Anticholinergic, antispasmodic.

•**dibutyl sebacate.** N.F. 18.
Use: Pharmaceutic aid (plasticizer).

Dical. (Rugby Labs, Inc.) Calcium 116 mg, vitamin D 133 IU, phosphorus 90 mg. Captab. Bot. 1000s. *otc.*
Use: Mineral, vitamin supplement.

dicalcium phosphate. (Various Mfr.) Dibasic calcium phosphate, monocalcium phosphate. **Cap.:** 7.5 gr or 10 gr. **Tab.:** 7.5 gr, 10 gr, or 15 gr. **Wafer:** 15 gr. *otc.*
Use: Mineral supplement.
W/Calcium gluconate and Vitamin D. (Various Mfr.) Cap., Tab., Wafer
See: CalciCaps, Tab. (Nion Corp.).

Dical-D. (Abbott Laboratories) Calcium 117 mg, vitamin D 133 IU, phosphorus 90 mg. Tab. Bot. 100s, 500s. *otc.*
Use: Mineral, vitamin supplement.

Dical-D with Vitamin C. (Abbott Laboratories) Dibasic calcium phosphate containing calcium 116.7 mg, phosphorus 90 mg, vitamin D 133 IU, ascorbic acid 15 mg/Cap. Bot. 100s.
Use: Mineral, vitamin supplement.

Dical-Dee. (Alpharma USPD Inc.) Vitamin D 350 IU, dibasic calcium phosphate 4.5 gr, calcium gluconate 3 gr/Cap. Bot. 100s, 1000s. *otc.*
Use: Mineral, vitamin supplement.

Dicaldel. (Faraday) Dibasic calcium phosphate 300 mg, calcium gluconate 200 mg, vitamin D 33 IU/Cap. Bot. 100s, 250s, 500s, 1000s. *otc.*
Use: Mineral, vitamin supplement.

Dical-D Wafers. (Abbott Laboratories) Dibasic calcium phosphate containing calcium 232 mg, phosphorus 180 mg, vitamin D 200 IU/Wafer. Box 51s. *otc.*
Use: Mineral, vitamin supplement.

Dicaltabs. (Faraday) Dibasic calcium phosphate 108 mg, calcium gluconate 140 mg, vitamin D 35 IU/Tab. Bot. 100s, 250s, 1000s. *otc.*
Use: Mineral, vitamin supplement.

Dicarbosil. (BIRA Corp.) Calcium carbonate 500 mg/Chew. Tab. Roll 12s. *otc.*
Use: Antacid.

Di-Cet. (Sanford & Son) Methylbenzethonium Cl 24.4 g, sodium carbonate monohydrate 48.8 g, sodium nitrite 24.4 g, trisodium ethylenediamine tetra-acetate monohydrate 2.4 g. Pow. Pkg. 2.4 g. Box 24s.
Use: Disinfectant.

dichloralantipyrine. Dichloralphenazone. Chloralpyrine. A complex of 2 mol. chloral hydrate with 1 mol. antipyrine. Sominat.
W/Isometheptene mucate, acetaminophen.
See: Midrin, Cap. (Schwarz Pharma, Inc.).

•**dichloralphenazone.** (die-klor-al-FEN-ah-zone) U.S.P. 23.
Use: Hypnotic, sedative.

Dichloramine T. (Various Mfr.) (1% to 5% in chlorinated paraffin). P-Toluenesulfone-dichloramine.
Use: Antiseptic.

dichloren.
See: Mechlorethamine HCl, Sterile Inj. (Various Mfr.).

dichloroacetate sodium.
Use: Lactic acidosis; hypercholesterolemia. [Orphan Drug]

dichloroacetic acid. *Rx.*
Use: Cauterizing agent.

•**dichlorodifluoromethane.** (die-KLOR-oh-die-flure-oh-METH-ane) N.F. 18.
Use: Pharmaceutic aid (aerosol propellant).

dichlorodiphenyl trichloroethane.
See: Chlorophenothane (Various Mfr.).

dichlorophenarsine hydrochloride. (Chlorarsen, Clorarsen, Fontarsol, Halarsol).

dichlorophene. Related to hexachlorophene.
W/Undecylenic acid.
See: Onychomycetin, Liq. (Gordon Laboratories).

•**dichlorotetrafluoroethane.** (die-KLOR-oh-teh-trah-flur-oh-ETH-ane) N.F. 18.
Use: Pharmaceutic aid (aerosol propellant).

•**dichlorphenamide.** (die-klor-FEN-ah-mide) U.S.P. 23.
Use: Carbonic anhydrase inhibitor.

•**dichlorvos.** (DIE-klor-vahs) USAN.
Use: Anthelmintic.

•**dicirenone.** (die-sigh-REN-ohn) USAN.
Use: Hypotensive, aldosterone antagonist.

Dickey's Old Reliable Eye Wash. (Dickey Drug) Berberine sulfate, boric acid, propyl parabens, methyl parabens. Plastic dropper bot. 8 ml, 12 ml, 1 oz. *otc.*
Use: Counterirritant, ophthalmic.

•**diclofenac potassium.** (die-KLOE-fen-ak) USAN.
Use: Analgesic, NSAID.
See: Cataflam, Tab. (Norvartis Pharmaceutical Corp.).

diclofenac potassium. (Invamed) 50 mg, lactose. Tab. Bot. 100s, 500s. *Rx.*
Use: Analgesic, NSAID.

•**diclofenac sodium.** (die-KLOE-fen-ak) U.S.P. 23.
Use: Analgesic, NSAID.
See: Voltaren (Novartis Pharmaceutical Corp.).

diclofenac sodium. (Various Mfr.) 25 mg, 50 mg, or 75 mg/DR Tab. Bot. 60s, 100s, 1000s, UD 100s. *Rx.*
Use: Analgesic, NSAID.

diclofenac sodium and misoprostol.
Use: Arthritis treatment.
See: Arthrotec, Tab. (Searle).

diclofenac sodium ophthalmic solution 0.1%. Diclofenac sodium 0.1%, mannitol. Soln. Bot. 5 ml. *Rx.*
Use: Analgesic, NSAID, ophthalmic.

Dicloxacil. (Zenith Goldline Pharmaceuticals) Dicloxacillin sodium 250 mg, 500 mg. Cap. Bot. 100s. *Rx.*
Use: Anti-infective, penicillin.

•**dicloxacillin.** (DIE-klox-uh-SILL-in) USAN.
Use: Anti-infective.
See: Dynapen, Cap., Susp. (Bristol-Myers Squibb).
Pathocil, Cap., Susp. (Wyeth-Ayerst Laboratories).

•**dicloxacillin sodium.** (DIE-klox-uh-SILL-in) U.S.P. 23.
Use: Anti-infective.
See: Dycill, Cap. (SmithKline Beecham Pharmaceuticals).
Dynapen, Cap., Soln. (Bristol-Myers Squibb).
Pathocil (Wyeth-Ayerst).

dicloxacillin sodium. (DIE-klox-uh-SILL-in) (Various Mfr.) Dicloxacillin sodium 250 mg, 500 mg. Cap. Bot. 30s (500 mg only), 40s, 50s (500 mg only), 100s, 500s, UD 100s. *Rx.*
Use: Anti-infective

Dicole. (Halsey Drug Co.) Docusate sodium 100 mg/Cap. Bot. 100s. *otc.*
Use: Laxative.

dicophane.
Use: Pediculicide.
See: Chlorophenothane (Various Mfr.), DDT.

dicoumarin.
Use: Anticoagulant.
See: Dicumarol, Preps. (Various Mfr.).

dicoumarol.
Use: Anticoagulant.
See: Dicumarol, U.S.P. 23.

•**dicumarol.** (die-KUME-ah-rahl) USAN. U.S.P. XXII. *Formerly Bishydroxycoumarin.*
Use: Anticoagulant.

dicumarol. (Abbott Laboratories) 25 mg/Tab. Bot. 100s, 1000s.
Use: Anticoagulant.

•**dicyclomine hydrochloride.** (die-SIGH-kloe-meen) U.S.P. 23.
Use: Anticholinergic, antispasmodic.
See: Antispas, Inj. (Keene Pharmaceuticals, Inc.).
Bentyl, Amp. Syringe, Cap., Tab., Syr. (Hoechst Marion Roussel).
Dysaps, Tab., Liq., Inj. (Savage Laboratories).
Nospaz, Vial (Solvay Pharmaceuticals).
See: Triactin Liq., Tab. (Procter & Gamble Pharm.).
W/Phenobarbital.
See: Bentyl with Phenobarbital, Prods (Hoechst Marion Roussel)

Dicynene. (Baxter Pharmaceutical Products, Inc.) *Rx.*
Use: Hemostatic.
See: Ethamsylate.

dicysteine.
See: Cystine, Pow. (Various Mfr.).

•**didanosine.** (die-DAN-oh-SEEN) USAN.
Use: Antiviral.

didehydrodideoxythymidine.
Use: Antiviral.
See: Stavudine (Bristol-Myers Squibb).

Di-Delamine Gel. (Del Pharmaceuticals, Inc.) Tripelennamine HCl 0.5%, diphenhydramine HCl 1%, benzalkonium Cl 0.12% in clear gel. Tube 1.25 oz. *otc.*
Use: Antipruritic, topical.

Di-Delamine Spray. (Del Pharmaceuti-

cals, Inc.) Tripelennamine HCl 0.5%, diphenhydramine HCl 1%, benzalkonium Cl 0.12%. Spray pump 4 oz. *otc.*
Use: Antipruritic, topical.

dideoxycytidine. (Roche Laboratories) *Rx.*
Use: Antiviral.
See: HIVID.

2,3 dideoxycytidine. (Roche; NCI; Bristol-Myers) *Rx.*
Use: Antiviral (AIDS).

dideoxyinisine.
Use: Antiviral.

Didrex. (Pharmacia & Upjohn) Benzphetamine HCl. **25 mg/Tab.:** Bot. 100s; **50 mg/Tab.:** Bot. 100s, 500s. *c-III.*
Use: Anorexiant.

Didronel. (Procter & Gamble Pharm.) Etidronate disodium 200 mg or 400 mg/Tab. Bot. 60s. *Rx.*
Use: Antihypercalcemia.

Didronel IV. (MGI Pharma, Inc.) Etidronate disodium 300 mg/6 ml amp. Amp. 6 ml. *Rx.*
Use: Antihypercalcemia.

•**dienestrol.** (die-en-ESS-trole) U.S.P. 23.
Use: Estrogen therapy, atrophic vaginitis.
See: D V, Cream (Hoechst Marion Roussel).
D V, Supp. (Hoechst Marion Roussel).
Ortho Dienestrol, Cream (Ortho McNeil Pharmaceutical).

dienestrol. (Ortho McNeil Pharmaceutical) 0.01%. Tube 78 g w/applicator.
Use: Estrogen.

Diet-Aid, Maximum Strength. (Columbia Laboratories, Inc.) Phenylpropanolamine HCl 75 mg/Cap. Pkg. 20s. *otc.*
Use: Dietary aid.

Diet-Aid Plus Vitamin C, Maximum Strength. (Columbia Laboratories, Inc.) Phenylpropanolamine HCl 75 mg, vitamin C 180 mg/Cap. Pkg. 20s. *otc.*
Use: Dietary aid.

diet aids, nonprescription.
Use: Dietary aid.
See: Dex-A-Diet Plus Vitamin C, Cap. (Columbia Laboratories, Inc.).
Dieutrim T.D., Cap. (Legere Pharmaceuticals, Inc.).
Extra Strength Grapefruit Diet Plan w/ Diadax, Cap. (Columbia Laboratories, Inc.).
Maximum Strength Dexatrim Plus Vitamin C, Cap. (Thompson Medical Co).

•**diethanolamine.** N.F. 18.
Use: Pharmaceutic acid (alkalizing agent).

diethanolamine.
See: Diolamine.

diethazine hydrochloride.
Use: Antiparkinsonian.

diethoxin. Intracaine HCl.

•**diethyl phthalate.** N.F. 18.
Use: Pharmaceutic aid (plasticizer).

diethyldithiocarbamate.
Use: Trial drug for AIDS. [Orphan Drug]
See: Imuthiol (Pasteur Merieux Connaught).

diethylenediamine citrate. Piperazine Citrate, Piperazine Hexahydrate.

diethylmalonylurea.
See: Barbital, Tab. (Various Mfr.).

•**diethylcarbamazine citrate.** (die- ETH-ill-car-BAM-ah-zeen SIH-trate) U.S.P. 23.
Use: Anthelmintic.

diethylpropion. (Various Mfr.) **Tab.:** Diethylpropion 25 mg. Bot. 100s, 500s, 1000s. **SR Tab.:** Diethylpropion 75 mg. Bot. 100s, 250s, 500s, 1000s. *c-IV.*
Use: Anorexiant.

•**diethylpropion hydrochloride.** (die-ETH-uhl-PRO-pee-ahn) U.S.P. 23.
Use: Anorexic.
See: Tenuate, Tab. (Hoechst Marion Roussel).
Tepanil, Tab. (3M Pharm.).
Tepanil Ten-Tab, Tab. (3M Pharm.).

•**diethylstilbestrol diphosphate.** (die-ETH-uhl-still-BESS-trahl die-FOSS-fate) U.S.P. 23.
Use: Estrogen.
See: Stilphostrol, Inj., Tab. (Bayer Corp. (Consumer Div.)).

diethylstilbestrol dipropionate. (Various Mfr.) Amp. in oil, 0.5 mg, 1 mg, or 5 mg/ml. Tab. 0.5 mg, 1 mg, or 5 mg.
Use: Estrogen.

•**diethyltoluamide.** (die-ETH-ill-toe-LOO-ah-mide) U.S.P. 23.
Use: Repellent (arthropod).
See: RV Pellent, Oint. (Zeneca Pharmaceuticals).

n, n-diethylvanillamide.
See: Ethamivan, Inj. (Various Mfr.).

Diet-Tuss. (Health for Life Brands, Inc.) Dextromethorphan 30 mg, thenylpyramine HCl, pyrilamine maleate 80 mg, sodium salicylate 200 mg, sodium citrate 600 mg, ammonium Cl 100 mg/fl oz. Sugar free. Bot. 4 oz. *otc.*
Use: Analgesic, antihistamine, antitussive, expectorant.

Dieutrim T.D. (Legere Pharmaceuticals,

Inc.) Phenylpropanolamine 75 mg, benzocaine 9 mg, sodium carboxymethylcellulose 75 mg/SR Cap. Bot. 100s, 1000s. *otc.*
Use: Dietary aid.

•**difenoximide hydrochloride.** (DIE-fen-OX-ih-mid) USAN.
Use: Antiperistaltic.

•**difenoxin.** (DIE-fen-OX-in) USAN.
Use: Antidiarrheal, antiperistaltic.
W/Atropine sulfate.
See: Motofen (Schwarz Pharma, Inc.).

Differin. (Galderma Laboratories, Inc.) Adapalene 0.1%, propylene glycol, EDTA, methylparaben. Gel. Tube. 15 g, 45 g. *Rx.*
Use: Dermatologic, acne.

•**diflorasone diacetate.** (die-FLORE-ah-sone die-ASS-eh-tate) U.S.P. 23.
Use: Anti-inflammatory, topical; antipruritic.
See: Florone, Cream, Oint. (Pharmacia & Upjohn).
Maxiflor, Cream, Oint. (Allergan, Inc.).
Psorcon, Cream, Oint. (Dermik Laboratories, Inc.).

•**difloxacin hydrochloride.** (die-FLOX-ah-SIN) USAN.
Use: Anti-infective (DNA gyrase inhibitor).

•**difluanine hydrochloride.** (die-FLEW-an-EEN) USAN.
Use: CNS stimulant.

Diflucan. (Roerig) Fluconazole. **Tab.:** 50 mg. Bot. 30s, 100 mg, or 200 mg. Bot. 30s, UD 100s; 150 mg. 1s. **Inj.:** 2 mg/ml Vial with sodium chloride 9 mg/ml or *Viaflex Plus* 100 ml, 200 ml. **Pow. for Oral Susp.:** 10 mg/ml in 350 mg or 40 mg/ml in 1400 mg. *Rx.*
Use: Antifungal.

•**diflucortolone.** (die-flew-CORE-toe-lone) USAN.
Use: Corticosteroid, topical.

•**diflucortolone pivalate.** USAN.
Use: Corticosteroid, topical.

•**diflumidone sodium.** (die-FLEW-mih-DOHN) USAN.
Use: Anti-inflammatory.

•**diflunisal.** (die-FLOO-nih-sal) U.S.P. 23.
Use: Analgesic, NSAID.
See: Dolobid, Tab. (Merck & Co.).

diflunisal. (Various Mfr.) Diflunisal 250 mg or 500 mg/Tab. Bot. 100s, 500s, unit-of-use 60s. *Rx.*
Use: Analgesic, NSAID.

•**difluprednate.** (DIE-flew-PRED-nate) USAN.
Use: Anti-inflammatory.

•**diftalone.** (DIFF-tah-lone) USAN.
Use: Anti-inflammatory, analgesic.

•**digalloyl trioleate.** USAN.

Di-Gel, Advanced. (Schering-Plough Corp.) Magnesium hydroxide 128 mg, calcium carbonate 280 mg, simethicone 20 mg/Tab. Bot. 30s, 60s, 90s. *otc.*
Use: Antacid, antiflatulent.

Di-Gel Liquid. (Schering-Plough Corp.) Aluminum hydroxide (equivalent to dried gel) 200 mg, magnesium hydroxide 200 mg, simethicone 20 mg/5 ml, saccharin, sorbitol. Bot. 180 ml, 360 ml. *otc.*
Use: Antacid, antiflatulent.

Digepepsin. (Kenwood Laboratories) Pepsin 250 mg, pancreatin 300 mg, bile salts 150 mg/Tab. Bot. 60s. *Rx.*
Use: Digestive enzyme.

Digestamic. (Lexis Laboratories) Pancrelipase 300 mg, pepsin 100 mg/Tab. Bot. 50s. *Rx-otc.*
Use: Digestive aid.

Digestamic Liquid. (Lexis Laboratories) Belladonna leaf fluid extract 0.64 min/5 ml. Bot. 8 oz. *Rx-otc.*
Use: Anticholinergic, antispasmodic.

Digestant. (Canright) Pancreatin 5.25 gr, ox bile extract 2 gr, pepsin 5 gr, betaine HCl 1 gr/Tab. Bot. 100s, 1000s. *Rx-otc.*
Use: Digestive aid.

Digestive Compound. (Thurston) Betaine HCl 3.25 gr, pepsin 1 gr, papain 2 gr, mycozyme 2 gr, ox bile 2 gr/2 Tab. Bot. 100s, 500s. *Rx-otc.*
Use: Digestive aid.

digestive enzymes.
See: Cotazym, Cap. (Organon, Inc.).
Cotazym-S, Cap. (Organon, Inc.).
Creon, Cap. (Solvay Pharmaceuticals).
Festal II, Tab. (Hoechst Marion Roussel).
Hi-Vegi-Lip Tab. (Freeda Vitamins, Inc.).
Ilozyme, Tab. (Pharmacia & Upjohn).
Ku-Zyme HP, Cap. (Kremers Urban).
Pancrease, Cap. (McNeil Pharm).
Pancreatin Enseals, Tab. (Eli Lilly and Co.).
Pancreatin, Tab. (Eli Lilly and Co.).
Viokase, Pow., Tab. (Wyeth-Ayerst Laboratories).

digestive products, miscellaneous.
Use: Digestive enzyme supplement.
See: Ku-Zyme, Cap. (Kremers Urban).
Arco-Lase, Tabs. (Arco Pharmaceuticals, Inc.).
Digestozyme, Tab. (Various Mfr.).
Enzobile Improved (Roberts Pharmaceuticals).

Digestozyme Tabs. (Zenith Goldline Pharmaceuticals) Pancreatin, pepsin, bile salts. Bot. 1000s. *Rx.*
Use: Digestive aid.

Digibind. (GlaxoWellcome) Digoxin Immune Fab (ovine) fragments 38 mg, sorbitol 75 mg/Vial. Box 1s. *Rx.*
Use: Antidote.

Digidote. (Boehringer Mannheim Pharmaceuticals)
Use: Antidote. [Orphan Drug]

•**digitalis.** (dih-jih-TAL-iss) U.S.P. 23.
Use: Cardiovascular agent.
See: Crystodigin, Tab. Amp., Vial (Eli Lilly and Co.).
Deslanoside, Inj. (Various Mfr.).
Digitoxin, Preps. (Various Mfr.).
Digoxin, Preps. (Various Mfr.).
Lanoxin, Tab., Inj., Elix. (GlaxoWellcome).

digitalis leaf, powdered.
Use: Cardiovascular agent.

digitalis tincture.
Use: Cardiovascular agent.

•**digitoxin.** (dih-jih-TOX-in) U.S.P. 23.
Use: Cardiovascular agent.
See: Crystodigin, Tab. (Eli Lilly and Co.).

digitoxin. (Various Mfr.) **Amp.:** (0.2 mg/ml) 1 ml, **Cap. in oil:** 0.1 mg or 0.2 mg. **Tab.:** 0.1 mg, 0.2 mg.
Use: Cardiovascular agent.

digitoxin, acetyl.
Use: Cardiovascular agent.

α-digitoxin monoacetate.
Use: Cardiovascular agent.

•**digoxin.** (dih-JOX-in) U.S.P. 23.
Use: Cardiovascular agent.
See: Lanoxicaps (GlaxoWellcome).
Lanoxin, Preps. (GlaxoWellcome).

digoxin. (Roxane Laboratories, Inc.) Digoxin 0.05 mg/ml, alcohol 10%. Bot 60 ml, UD 2.5 ml, UD 5 ml. *Rx.*
Use: Cardiovascular agent.

digoxin antibody.
See: Digibind (GlaxoWellcome).

Digoxin Elixir. (Roxane Laboratories, Inc.) 0.05 mg/ml. Liq. Bot. 60 ml, UD 2.5 ml, 5 ml. *Rx.*
Use: Cardiovascular agent.

digoxin i-125 immunoassay. (Abbott Diagnostics) Digoxin diagnostic kit for the quantitative determination of serum digoxin. 100s, 300s.
Use: Diagnostic aid.

digoxin immune fab (ovine) fragments.
Use: Antidote. [Orphan Drug]
See: Digibind, Pow. for Inj. (GlaxoWellcome).
Digidote (Boehringer Mannheim Pharmaceuticals).

Digoxin Riabead. (Abbott Diagnostics) Solid-phase radioimmunoassay for quantitative measurement of serum digoxin. Test kit 100s, 300s.
Use: Diagnostic aid.

dihematoporphyrin ethers.
Use: Photodynamic therapy of transitional cell carcinoma in situ of urinary bladder or primary or recurrent obstructing esophageal carcinoma. [Orphan Drug]
See: Photofrin (QLT Phototherapeutics).

•**dihexyverine hydrochloride.** (die-HEX-ih-ver-een) USAN.
Use: Anticholinergic.

Dihistine DH. (Zenith Goldline Pharmaceuticals) Pseudoephedrine HCl 30 mg, chlorpheniramine maleate 2 mg, codeine phosphate 10 mg. Elix. Bot. 4 oz, pt, gal. *c-v.*
Use: Antihistamine, antitussive, decongestant.

Dihistine Elixir. (Various Mfr.) Phenylephrine HCl 5 mg, chlorpheniramine maleate 2 mg/5 ml. Bot. Pt, gal. *otc.*
Use: Antihistamine, decongestant.

Dihistine Expectorant. (Zenith Goldline Pharmaceuticals) Pseudoephedrine HCl 30 mg, codeine phosphate 10 mg, guaifenesin 100 mg, alcohol 7.5%. Bot. 4 oz, pt, gal. *c-v.*
Use: Antitussive, decongestant, expectorant.

dihydan soluble.
See: Phenytoin Sodium (Various Mfr.).

dihydrocodeine. Paracodin. Drocode.
Use: Analgesic, antitussive.

•**dihydrocodeine bitartrate.** (die-high-droe-KOE-deen bye-TAR-trate) U.S.P. 23.
Use: Analgesic.
See: Hydrocodone Bitartrate, U.S.P. 23.
W/Caffeine, phenacetin, aspirin.
See: Drocogesic #3, Tab. (Rand).
Duradyne DHC, Liq. (Forest Pharmaceutical, Inc.).
W/Caffeine, aspirin.
See: Synalgos-DC, Cap. (Wyeth-Ayerst Laboratories).
W/Caffeine, acetaminophen.
See: DHC Plus, Cap. (Purdue Frederick Co.).

dihydrocodeinone resin complex.
W/Phenyltoloxamine resin complex.
See: Tussionex, Preps. (Medeva Pharmaceuticals, Inc.).

dihydroergocornine. Ergot alkaline component of hydergine.

dihydroergocristine. Ergot alkaloid component of hydergine.

dihydroergocryptine. Ergot alkaloid component of hydergine.

dihydroergotamine. (D.H.E. 45) (Sandoz Pharmaceutical) Dihydroergotamine mesylate. Amp. *Rx.*
Use: Agent for migraine, antiadrenergic.

•**dihydroergotamine mesylate.** (DIE-high-droe-err-GOT-uh-meen) U.S.P. 23. Dihydroergotamine methanesulfonate.
Use: Antiadrenergic, antimigraine.
See: DHE 45, Amp. (Sandoz Pharmaceutical).
Migranal (Norvartis Pharmaceutical Corp.).

dihydroergotoxine. Ergoloid mesylate. *Rx.*
Use: Psychotherapeutic agent.
See: Gerimal, Tab. (Rugby Labs, Inc.).
Hydergine, Tab. (Sandoz Pharmaceutical).
Ergoloid Mesylates, Tab. (Various Mfr.).
Ergoloid Mesylates, Tab. (Various Mfr.).
Hydergine, Tab. (Sandoz Pharmaceutical).
Hydergine LC, Cap. (Sandoz Pharmaceutical).
Hydergine, Liq. (Sandoz Pharmaceutical).

5,6-dihydro-5-azacytidine. (Ilex Oncology Inc.)
Use: Antineoplastic. [Orphan Drug]

dihydrofollicular hormone.
See: Estradiol (Various Mfr.).

dihydrofolliculine.
See: Estradiol (Various Mfr.).

dihydrohydroxycodeinone. (Oxycodone. (Ducodal, Eukodal, Eucodal).) *c-II.*
Use: Analgesic, narcotic.

dihydrohydroxycodeinone hydrochloride or bitartrate. Oxycodone HCl or Bitartrate.
W/Combinations.
See: Cophene-S, Syr. (Dunhall Pharmaceuticals, Inc.).
Damason-P, Tab. (Mason Pharmaceuticals, Inc.).
Percodan, Tab. (Du Pont Merck Pharmaceutical Co).

dihydromorphinone hydrochloride.
See: Dilaudid, Preps. (Knoll Pharmaceuticals).

•**dihydrostreptomycin sulfate.** (die-HIGH-droe-strep-toe-MY-sin) U.S.P. 23.
Use: Anti-infective.

dihydrotachysterol. (die-HIGH-droe-tack-ISS-ter-ole) (Roxane Laboratories, Inc.) 0.2 mg/Tab. Bot. 100s, UD 100s.
Use: Antihypocalcemic.
See: DHT (Roxane).
Hytakerol, Cap. (Sanofi Winthrop Pharmaceuticals).

dihydrotachysterol. (Roxane Laboratories, Inc.) 0.2 mg/Tab. Bot. 100s, UD 100s.
Use: Antihypocalcemic.

dihydrotestosterone.
Use: AIDS. [Orphan Drug]
See: Androgel-DHT. (Unimed).

dihydrotheelin.
See: Estradiol (Various Mfr.).

dihydroxyacetone.
See: Chromelin, Liq. (Summers Laboratories, Inc.).
Sudden Tan, Liq. (Schering-Plough Corp.).

•**dihydroxyaluminum aminoacetate.** (die-high-DROX-ee-ah-LOO-min-uhm ah-MEE-no-ASS-eh-tate) U.S.P. 23.
Use: Antacid.
W/Methscopolamine bromide, sodium lauryl sulfate, magnesium hydroxide.
See: Alu-Scop, Cap., Susp. (Westerfield).

•**dihydroxyaluminum sodium carbonate.** U.S.P. 23.
Use: Antacid.
See: Rolaids (Parke-Davis).

dihydroxycholecalciferol.
See: Rocaltrol. (Roche Laboratories).

24,25 dihydroxycholecalciferol. (Lemmon Co.; Tag Pharmaceuticals)
Use: Uremic osteodystrophy. [Orphan Drug]

dihydroxyestrin.
See: Estradiol (Various Mfr.).

dihydroxyfluorane. Fluorescein.

dihydroxyphenylisatin.
See: Oxyphenisatin (Various Mfr.).

dihydroxyphenyloxindol.
See: Oxyphenisatin (Various Mfr.).

dihydroxypropyl theophylline. Dyphylline.
See: Neothylline, Tab., Elix., Inj. (Teva Pharmaceuticals USA)

dihydroxy (stearato) aluminum. Aluminum Monostearate, N.F. 18.

diiodohydroxyquin.
Use: Amebicide.
See: Iodoquinol, U.S.P. 23.

diiodohydroxyquinoline.
See: Iodoquinol, U.S.P. 23.

diisopromine hydrochloride. (Lab. for Pharmaceutical Development, Inc.)
See: Desquam-X (Westwood Squibb Pharmaceuticals).

diisopropyl phosphorofluoridate.
See: Floropryl, Oint. (Merck & Co.).

diisopropyl sebacate.

Use: Moisturizing agent.

Dilacor XR. (Rhone-Poulenc Rorer Pharmaceuticals, Inc.) Diltiazem HCl 120 mg, 180 mg, or 240 mg/SR Cap. 100s, UD 100s. *Rx.*
Use: Calcium channel blocker.

dilaminate. Mixture of magnesium carbide and dihydroxyaluminum glycinate. *otc.*
Use: Antacid.

Dilantin. (Parke-Davis) Phenytoin. **30 Susp.:** 30 mg/5 ml. Bot. 8 oz, UD 5 ml. **125 Susp:** 125 mg/5 ml. Bot. 8 oz, UD 5 ml. **Infatab:** 50 mg/Tab. Bot. 100s, UD 100s. *Rx.*
Use: Anticonvulsant.

Dilantin Sodium. (Parke-Davis) Extended phenytoin sodium. **Kapseal:** 30 mg, 100 mg. Bot. 100s, 1000s, UD 100s. **Amp.:** (w/propylene glycol 40%, alcohol 10%, sodium hydroxide) 100 mg/2 ml. UD 10s; 250 mg/5 ml. Amp. 10s, UD 10s. *Rx.*
Use: Anticonvulsant.

Dilantin Sodium w/Phenobarbital Kapseal. (Parke-Davis) Phenytoin sodium 100 mg, phenobarbital 16 mg or 32 mg/Cap. Bot. 100s, 1000s, UD 100s (32 mg only). *Rx.*
Use: Anticonvulsant, hypnotic, sedative.

Dilantin-30 Pediatric. (Parke-Davis) Phenytoin 30 mg/5 ml, alcohol 0.6%. Susp. Bot. 240 ml, 5 ml. *Rx.*
Use: Anticonvulsant.

Dilatrate-SR. (Schwarz Pharma, Inc.) Isosorbide dinitrate 40 mg/SR Cap. Bot. 60s, 100s. *Rx.*
Use: Antianginal.

Dilaudid. (Knoll Pharmaceuticals) Hydromorphone HCl. **Inj.:** 1 mg, 2 mg, 4 mg/ml. Amp. 1 ml. Vial 20 ml. Box 10s. 2 mg. Box 25s. **Liq.:** 5 mg/ml. Bot. Pt. **Multiple-Dose Vial:** 2 mg/ml. Bot. 20 ml. **Tab.:** 1 mg, 2 mg, 3 mg, 4 mg, 8 mg. Bot. 100s; 500s, UD 100s (2 mg, 4 mg only). **Pow:** Vial, 15 gr Multiple dose vial 10 ml, 20 ml. 2 mg/ml. **Rectal Supp.:** 3 mg. Box 6s. *c-II.*
Use: Analgesic, narcotic.
W/Guaifenesin.
See: Dilaudid Cough Syrup. (Knoll Pharmaceuticals).

Dilaudid Cough Syrup. (Knoll Pharmaceuticals) Hydromorphone HCl 1 mg, guaifenesin 100 mg/5 ml. Alcohol 5%. Bot. Pt. *c-II.*
Use: Analgesic, narcotic; expectorant.

Dilaudid-5. (Knoll Pharmaceuticals) Hydromorphone HCl 5 mg/5 ml. Liq. Bot. 480 ml. *c-II.*
Use: Analgesic, narcotic.

Dilaudid HP. (Knoll Pharmaceuticals) Hydromorphone. **Inj.:** 10 mg/ml. Vial 1 ml, 5 ml. **Pow. for Inj. (lyophilized):** 250 mg (10 mg/ml after reconstitution). Single-dose vial. *c-II.*
Use: Analgesic, narcotic.

•**dilevalol hydrochloride.** (DIE-LEV-ah-lole) USAN.
Use: Antihypertensive, antiadrenergic (β-receptor).

dilithium carbonate. Lithium Carbonate, U.S.P. 23.
Use: Antipsychotic.

Dilocaine. (Roberts Pharmaceuticals) Lidocaine HCl 1% or 2%. Bot. 50 ml. *Rx.*
Use: Anesthetic, local.

Dilor. (Savage Laboratories) Dyphylline. **Tab.:** 200 mg. Bot. 100s, 1000s, UD 100s. **Elix.:** 160 mg/15 ml. Bot. pt. *Rx.*
Use: Bronchodilator.

Dilor 400. (Savage Laboratories) Dyphylline 400 mg. Bot. 100s, 1000s, UD 100s. *Rx.*
Use: Bronchodilator.

Dilor G Liquid. (Savage Laboratories) Dyphylline 300 mg, guaifenesin 300 mg/15 ml. Bot. Pt, gal. *Rx.*
Use: Bronchodilator, expectorant.

Dilor G Tablets. (Savage Laboratories) Dyphylline 200 mg, guaifenesin 200 mg/Tab. Bot. 100s, 1000s, UD 100s. *Rx.*
Use: Bronchodilator, expectorant.

diloxaride furoate.
Use: Anti-infective.

•**diltiazem hydrochloride.** (dill-TIE-uh-zem) U.S.P. 23.
Use: Vasodilator (coronary).

diltiazem hydrochloride extended-release capsules. (Various Mfr.) Diltiazem HCl 60 mg, 90 mg, or 120 mg. Bot. 100s. *Rx.*
Use: Calcium channel blocker.
See: Tiazac, ER Cap. (Forest Pharmaceutical, Inc.).

diltiazem hydrochloride tablets. (Various Mfr.) Diltiazem HCl 30 mg, 60 mg, 90 mg, or 120 mg. Bot. 100s, 500s, 1000s and unit-of-issue 30s, 60s, 90s, 120s. *Rx.*
Use: Calcium channel blocker.

diltiazem injection. (Bedford Laboratories) Diltiazem 5 mg/ml, 71.4 mg/ml sorbitol solution. Vial 5 ml, 10 ml. *Rx.*
Use: Calcium channel blocker.

•**diltiazem maleate.** (dill-TIE-ah-zem MAL-ate) USAN.
Use: Calcium channel blocker, antihypertensive.

See: Tiamate (Hoechst Marion Roussel).

diltiazem maleate and enalapril maleate.
Use: Antihypertensive.
See: Teczem (Hoechst Marion Roussel).

Dimacol. (Wyeth-Ayerst Laboratories) Pseudoephedrine HCl 30 mg, dextromethorphan HBr 10 mg, guaifenesin 100 mg/Cap. or 5 ml. **Cap.:** Bot. 100s, 500s, Pre-Pack 12s, 24s. **Liq.:** (w/alcohol 4.75%) Bot. Pt. *otc.*
Use: Antitussive, decongestant, expectorant.

Dimaphen Elixir. (Major Pharmaceuticals) Phenylpropanolamine HCl 12.5 mg, brompheniramine maleate 2 mg. Bot. 237 ml. *otc.*
Use: Antihistamine, decongestant.

Dimaphen Release Tablets. (Major Pharmaceuticals) Phenylpropanolamine HCl 75 mg, brompheniramine maleate 12 mg/Tab. Bot. 12s. *otc.*
Use: Antihistamine, decongestant.

Dimaphen Tablets. (Major Pharmaceuticals) Phenylpropanolamine HCl 25 mg, brompheniramine maleate 4 mg. Tab. Bot. 24s. *otc.*
Use: Antihistamine, decongestant.

•**dimefadane.** (DIE-meh-fah-dane) USAN.
Use: Analgesic.

•**dimefilcon a.** (DIE-meh-FILL-kahn A) USAN.
Use: Contact lens material (hydrophilic).

•**dimefline hydrochloride.** (DIE-meh-fleen) USAN.
Use: Respiratory.

•**dimefocon a.** (DIE-meh-FOE-kahn A) USAN.
Use: Contact lens material (hydrophobic).

Dimenest. (Forest Pharmaceutical, Inc.) Dimenhydrinate 50 mg/ml. Vial 10 ml. *Rx.*
Use: Antiemetic, antivertigo.

•**dimenhydrinate.** (die-men-HIGH-drih-nate) U.S.P. 23.
Use: Antiemetic, antihistamine.
See: Dimenest, Inj. (Forest Pharmaceutical, Inc.).
Dimentabs, Tab. (Jones Medical Industries, Inc.).
Dramamine, Preps. (Pharmacia & Upjohn).
Dymenate, Inj. (Keene Pharmaceuticals, Inc.).
Hydrate, Vial (Hyrex Pharmaceuticals).
Signate, Inj. (Sigma-Tau Pharmaceuticals, Inc.).
Traveltabs, Tab. (Geneva Pharmaceuticals).
Vertab, Cap. (Forest Pharmaceutical, Inc.).

Dimentabs. (Jones Medical Industries, Inc.) Dimenhydrinate 50 mg/Tab. Bot. 100s. *otc.*
Use: Antiemetic, antivertigo.

•**dimepranol acedoben.** (DIE-MEH-prah-nahl ah-SEE-doe-BEN) USAN.
Use: Immunomodulator.

•**dimercaprol.** (die-mer-CAP-role) U.S.P. 23. *Formerly BAL.*
Use: Antidote to gold, arsenic, and mercury poisoning; metal complexing agent.
See: BAL in oil, Inj. (Becton Dickinson & Co.).

Dimetane-DC Cough Syrup. (Wyeth-Ayerst Laboratories) Brompheniramine maleate 2 mg, phenylpropanolamine HCl 12.5 mg, codeine phosphate 10 mg/5 ml w/alcohol 0.95%. Bot. pt, gal. *c-v.*
Use: Antihistamine, antitussive, decongestant.

Dimetane Decongestant Caplets. (Wyeth-Ayerst Laboratories) Brompheniramine maleate 4 mg, phenylephrine HCl 10 mg/Capl. Bot. 24s, 48s. *otc.*
Use: Antihistamine, decongestant.

Dimetane Decongestant Elixir. (Wyeth-Ayerst Laboratories) Brompheniramine maleate 2 mg, phenylephrine HCl 5 mg/5 ml, alcohol 2.3%. Bot. 120 ml. *otc.*
Use: Antihistamine, decongestant.

Dimetane-DX Cough Syrup. (Wyeth-Ayerst Laboratories) Pseudoephedrine HCl 30 mg, brompheniramine maleate 2 mg, dextromethorphan HBr 10 mg/5 ml, alcohol 0.95%, saccharin, sorbitol. Bot. Pt. *Rx.*
Use: Antihistamine, antitussive, decongestant.

Dimetapp Allergy. (Wyeth-Ayerst Laboratories) Brompheniramine maleate 4 mg, sorbitol. Liqui-gels. 24s. *otc.*
Use: Antihistamine.

Dimetapp Cold & Allergy. (Wyeth-Ayerst Laboratories) Brompheniramine maleate 1 mg, phenylpropanolamine HCl 6.25 mg, aspartame, phenylalanine 8 mg, sorbitol. Chew. Tab. Bot. 24s. *otc.*
Use: Antihistamine, decongestant.

Dimetapp Cold & Flu Caplet. (Wyeth-Ayerst Laboratories) Phenylpropanolamine HCl 12.5 mg, brompheniramine maleate 2 mg, acetaminophen 500 mg/Capl. Bot. 24s, 48s. *otc.*
Use: Analgesic, antihistamine, decongestant.

Dimetapp DM Elixir. (Wyeth-Ayerst Laboratories) Phenylpropanolamine HCl 12.5 mg, brompheniramine maleate 2 mg, dextromethorphan HBr 10 mg/5 ml, 2.3% alcohol, saccharin, sorbitol. Elix. Bot. 120 ml, 240 ml. *otc.*
Use: Antihistamine, antitussive, decongestant.

Dimetapp Elixir. (Wyeth-Ayerst Laboratories) Brompheniramine maleate 2 mg, phenylpropanolamine HCl 12.5 mg/5 ml. Bot. 120 ml, 240 ml, 360 ml, 473 ml, gal, UD 5 ml. *otc.*
Use: Antihistamine, decongestant.

Dimetapp Extentabs. (Wyeth-Ayerst Laboratories) Brompheniramine maleate 12 mg, phenylpropanolamine HCl 75 mg/Tab. Bot. 100s, 500s, UD 100s. Blister pack 12s, 24s, 48s. *otc.*
Use: Antihistamine, decongestant.

Dimetapp 4-Hour Liqui-Gels. (Wyeth-Ayerst Laboratories) Brompheniramine maleate 4 mg, phenylpropanolamine HCl 25 mg, sorbitol. Cap. Pck. 12s. *otc.*
Use: Antihistamine, decongestant.

Dimetapp Sinus. (Wyeth-Ayerst Laboratories) Pseudoephedrine HCl 30 mg, ibuprofen 200 mg/Cap. Bot. 20s, 40s. *otc.*
Use: Analgesic, decongestant.

Dimetapp Tablets. (Wyeth-Ayerst Laboratories) Brompheniramine maleate 4 mg, phenylpropanolamine HCl 25 mg/Tab. Blisterpak 24s. *otc.*
Use: Antihistamine, decongestant.

•**dimethadione.** (DIE-meth-ah-DIE-ohn) USAN.
Use: Anticonvulsant.

•**dimethicone.** (DIE-meth-ih-cone) N.F. 18.
Use: Prosthetic aid (soft tissue), component of barrier creams, lubricant and hydrophobic agent.
See: Silicone, Oint. (Various Mfr.).

•**dimethicone 350.** (DIE-meth-ih-cone 350) USAN.
Use: Prosthetic aid for soft tissue.

•**dimethindene maleate.** (DIE-METH-in-deen) USAN. U.S.P. XX.
Use: Antihistamine.

•**dimethisoquin hydrochloride.** (die-meh-THIGH-so-kwin) USAN.

•**dimethisterone.** (DIE-meth-ISS-ter-ohn) USAN. N.F. XIV.
Use: Hormone, progestin.

dimethoxyphenyl penicillin sodium.
Use: Anti-infective.
See: Methicillin sodium (Various Mfr.).

dimethpyridene maleate. Dimethindene Maleate, U.S.P. 23.
See: Dimethindene Maleate, U.S.P. XX.

dimethylaminophenazone.
See: Aminopyrine (Various Mfr.).

dimethylamino pyrazine sulfate.
See: Ampyzine Sulfate.

dimethylcarbamate. of 3-Hydroxy-1-Methylpyridinium Bromide.
See: Mestinon, Tab. (Roche Laboratories).

dimethylhexestrol dipropionate. Promethestrol Dipropionate.

dimethyl polysiloxane.
See: Dimethicone (Various Mfr.).

•**dimethyl sulfoxide.** (die-METH-uhl sull-FOX-ide) U.S.P. 23.
Use: Anti-inflammatory, topical.
See: Rimso-50 (Research Industries Corp.).

dimethyl sulfoxide. (Pharma 21)
Use: Increased intracranial pressure. [Orphan Drug]

dimethyl-tubocurarine iodide.
Use: Muscle relaxant.
See: Metocurine Iodide.

dimethylurethimine.
See: Meturedepa (Centeon).

•**dimoxamine hydrochloride.** (die-MOX-AH-meen) USAN.
Use: Memory adjuvant.

Dimycor. (Standard Drug Co.) Pentaerythritol tetranitrate 10 mg, phenobarbital 15 mg/Tab. Bot. 1000s. *Rx.*
Use: Antianginal, hypnotic, sedative.

Dinacrin. (Sanofi Winthrop Pharmaceuticals) Isonicotinic acid, hydrazide. *Rx.*
Use: Antituberculosal.

Dinate. (Blaine Co., Inc.) Dimenhydrinate 50 mg/ml. Vial 10 ml. *Rx.*
Use: Antiemetic, antivertigo.

•**dinoprost.** (DIE-no-proste) USAN.
Use: Oxytocic; prostaglandin.

•**dinoprost tromethamine.** (DIE-no-proste troe-METH-ah-meen) U.S.P. 23.
Use: Oxytocic, prostaglandin.

•**dinoprostone.** (DIE-no-PROSTE-ohn) USAN.
Use: Abortifacient, agent for cervical ripening, oxytocic, prostaglandin.
See: Cervidil, Insert (Forest Pharmaceutical, Inc.).
Prepidil, Gel (Pharmacia & Upjohn).
Prostin E_2, Supp. (Pharmacia & Upjohn).

Diocto. (Purepac Pharmaceutical Co.) Docusate sodium 100 mg or 200 mg/Cap. Bot. 100s. *otc.*
Use: Laxative.

Diocto C. (Various Mfr.) Docusate sodium 60 mg, casanthranol 30 mg/15 ml. Syr. Bot. 240 ml, pt, gal. *otc.*

Use: Laxative.

Diocto-K. (Rugby Labs, Inc.) Docusate potassium 100 mg/Cap. Bot. 100s, 1000s. *otc.*
Use: Laxative.

Diocto-K Plus. (Rugby Labs, Inc.) Docusate sodium 100 mg, casanthranol 30 mg. Cap. Bot. 100s, 1000s. *otc.*
Use: Laxative.

Dioctolose. (Zenith Goldline Pharmaceuticals) Docusate potassium 100 mg/Cap. Bot. 100s, 1000s.
Use: Laxative.

Dioctolose Plus Capsules. (Zenith Goldline Pharmaceuticals) Docusate 100 mg, casanthranol 30 mg/Cap. Bot. 100s, 1000s. *otc.*
Use: Laxative.

dioctyl calcium sulfosuccinate. (die-OCK-till SULL-foe-SUCK-sih-nate) Docusate Calcium.
Use: Laxative.

dioctyl sodium sulfosuccinate.
Use: Non-laxative fecal softener.
See: Docusate Sodium, U.S.P. 23

diodone injection.
See: Iodopyracet injection.

Dioeze. (Century Pharmaceuticals, Inc.) Dioctyl sodium sulfosuccinate 250 mg/Cap. Bot. 100s, 1000s. *otc.*
Use: Laxative.

•**diohippuric acid I 125.** USAN.
Use: Radiopharmaceutical.

•**diohippuric acid I 131.** USAN.
Use: Radiopharmaceutical.

Dio-Hist. (Health for Life Brands, Inc.) Dextromethorphan 30 mg, thenylpyramine HCl 80 mg, phenylephrine HCl 20 mg, potassium tartrate 1/24 gr/oz. Bot. 4 oz. *otc.*
Use: Antihistamine.

D-Diol. (Burgin-Arden) Testosterone cypionate 50 mg, estradiol cypionate 2 mg/ml. Vial 10 ml. *Rx.*
Use: Androgen, estrogen combination.

diolamine. Diethanolamine.

diolostene.
See: Methandriol.

Dionex. (Henry Schein, Inc.) Docusate sodium 100 mg or 250 mg/Cap. Bot. 100s, 250s, 1000s. *otc.*
Use: Laxative.

dionin. Ethylmorphine HCl.
Use: Orally; cough depressant, ocular lymphagogue.

Dionosil Oily. (GlaxoWellcome) Propyliodone 60% in peanut oil. Inj. Vial 20 ml.
Use: Radiopaque agent.

diophyllin.
See: Aminophylline, Preps. (Various Mfr.).

diopterin. Pteroylglutamic acid, PDGA, Pteroyl-alpha-glutamylglutamic acid.
Use: Antineoplastic.

Diorapin. (Standex) Estrogenic conjugate 0.625 mg, methyltestosterone 5 mg/Tab. Bot. 100s. Estrone 2 mg, testosterone 25 mg/ml. Inj. Vial 10 ml. *Rx.*
Use: Androgen, estrogen combination.

Diosate D. (Towne) Docusate sodium. Cap. 100 mg or 250 mg/Tab. Bot. 100s. *otc.*
Use: Laxative.

Diosmin. Buchu resin obtained from lvs. of barosma serratifolia and alliedrutaceae.

Dio-Soft. (Standex) Docusate sodium 100 mg, casanthranol 30 mg/Cap. Bot. 100s. *otc.*
Use: Laxative.

Diostate D. (Pharmacia & Upjohn) Vitamin D 400 IU, calcium 343 mg, phosphorus 265 mg/3 Tab. Bot. 100s. *otc.*
Use: Mineral, vitamin supplement.

•**diotyrosine I 125.** (die-oh-TIE-row-seen) USAN.
Use: Radiopharmaceutical.

•**diotyrosine I 131.** USAN.
Use: Radiopharmaceutical.

Diovan. (Novartis Pharmaceutical Corp.) Valsartan 80 mg, 160 mg/Cap. Bot. 100s, 4000s, UD blister 100s. *Rx.*
Use: Antihypertensive.

Diovan HCT. (Novartis Pharmaceutical Corp.) Valsartan 80 mg, hydrochlorothiazide 12.5 mg or valsartan 160 mg, hydrochlorothiazide 12.5 mg. Tab. Bot. 100s, 4000s, UD 100s. *Rx.*
Use: Antihypertensive.

Diovocylin. (Novartis Pharmaceutical Corp.)
See: Estradiol, Preps. (Various Mfr.).

•**dioxadrol hydrochloride.** (die-OX-ah-drole) USAN.
Use: Antidepressant.

dioxindol. Diacetylhydroxyphenylisatin.

dioxyanthranol.
See: Anthralin, N.F. (Various Mfr.).

•**dioxybenzone.** (die-ox-ee-BEN-zone) U.S.P. 23.
Use: Ultraviolet screen.
W/Oxybenzone, benzophene.
See: Solbar, Lot. (Person and Covey, Inc.).

dipalmitoylphosphatidylcholine. Colfosceril palmitate.
Use: Synthetic lung surfactant.
See: Exosurf Neonatal, Pow. (GlaxoWellcome).

dipalmitoylphosphatidylcholine/phosphatidylglycerol.

Use: Neonatal respiratory distress syndrome. [Orphan Drug]
See: ALEC (Forum Products, Inc.).
diparcol hydrochloride. Diethazine.
Dipegyl.
See: Nicotinamide, Preps. (Various Mfr.).
Dipentum. (Pharmacia & Upjohn) Osalazine sodium 250 mg/Cap. Bot. 100s, 500s. *Rx.*
Use: Gastrointestinal.
diperodon hydrochloride.
Use: Anesthetic.
See: Diothane, Oint. (Hoechst Marion Roussel).
Proctodon, Cream (Solvay Pharmaceuticals).
W/Bacitracin, neomycin sulfate, polymyxin.
See: Boro, Oint. (Scrip).
W/Furacin (nitrofurazone).
See: Furacin E Urethral Inserts (Eaton Medical Corp.).
Furacin H.C. Urethral Inserts (Eaton Medical Corp.).
W/Furacin (nitrofurazone) and Microfur (nituroxime).
See: Furacin Otic, Drops. (Eaton Medical Corp.).
W/Hydrocortisone, polymyxin B sulfate, neomycin.
See: My Cort Otic #1, Ear Drops (Scrip).
W/Hydroxyquinoline Benzoate.
See: Diothane, Oint. (Hoechst Marion Roussel).
W/Methapyrilene HCl, pyrilamine maleate, allantoin, benzocaine, menthol.
See: Antihistamine Cream (Towne).
diphenadione.
Use: Anticoagulant.
Diphen AF. (Morton Grove Pharmaceuticals, Inc.) Diphenhydramine HCl 6.25 mg/5 ml, saccharin, sugar, cherry flavor. Liq. Bot. 237 ml. *otc.*
Use: Antihistamine.
Diphenatol. (Rugby Labs, Inc.) Diphenoxylate HCl 2.5 mg, atropine sulfate 0.025 mg. Tab. Bot. 100s, 500s, 1000s.
Use: Antidiarrheal.
Diphen Cough. (Rosemont Pharmaceutical Corp.) Diphenhydramine HCl 12.5 mg/5 ml., alcohol 5.1%, menthol, sucrose, parabens. Syr. Bot. 118 ml. *otc.*
Use: Antitussive.
Diphendydramine 50. (H.L. Moore Drug Exchange Inc.) Diphenhydramine HCl 50 mg, lactose, bisulfites/Cap. Bot. 100s, 1000s. *otc.*
Use: Antihistamine.
Diphenhist. (Rugby Labs, Inc.) Diphenhydramine HCl. **Captabs, Cap. Softgels, Tab.:** 25 mg, lactose, parabens (soft gels) Bot. 100s. **Soln.:** 12.5 mg/5 ml, saccharin, sucrose. Bot. 118 ml. *otc.*
Use: Antihistamine.
•**diphenhydramine citrate.** (die-fen-HIGH-druh-meen SIH-trate) U.S.P. 23.
Use: Antihistamine.
diphenhydramine and pseudoephedrine capsules.
Use: Antihistamine, decongestant.
diphenhydramine citrate.
Use: Antihistamine.
diphenhydramine hydrochloride. (die-fen-HIGH-druh-meen) (Various Mfr.) Diphenhydramine HCl. **Cap. Softgels:** 25 mg. 30s, 100s, 1000s. **Cap.:** 50 mg. Bot. 100s. **Syrup:** 12.5 mg/5 ml, alcohol. Bot. 118 ml. **Inj.:** 50 mg/ml. Single-dose Amp. 1 ml, Multidose vial 10 ml. *Rx-otc.*
Use: Antihistamine.
•**diphenhydramine hydrochloride.** (die-fen-HIGH-druh-meen) U.S.P. 23.
Use: Antihistamine.
See: AllerMax, Preps. (Pfeiffer Co.).
Banophen (Major).
Bax, Cap., Elix., Expectorant (McKesson Drug Co.).
Benadryl Hydrochloride, Preps. (Parke-Davis).
Benahist, Preps. (Keene Pharmaceuticals, Inc.).
Benylin Cough Syrup (Warner Lambert).
Clearly Cala-gel (Tec Laboratories, Inc.).
Dermamycin (Pfeiffer).
Dermarest (Del).
Diphen, Preps. (Morton Grove Pharmaceuticals, Inc.).
Diphen-Ex, Syr. (Quality Generics).
Diphendrydramine 50, Cap. (H.L. Moore Drug Exchange Inc.).
Diphenhist, Preps. (Rugby Labs, Inc.).
Diphenhydramine HCl (Weeks & Leo).
Fenylhist, Cap. (Roberts Pharmaceuticals).
40 Winks, Cap. (Roberts Pharmaceuticals).
Genahist, Liq. (Zenith Goldline Pharmaceuticals).
Histine Prods. (Freeport).
Hyrexin, Inj. (Hyrex Pharmaceuticals).
Mouthkote P/R, Oint., Spray (Parnell Pharmaceuticals, Inc.).
Nighttime Sleep Aid, Tab. (Rugby Labs, Inc.).

Scot-Tussin Allergy (Scot-Tussin Pharmacal, Inc.).
Scot-Tussin Allergy DM, Liq. (Scot-Tussin Pharmacal, Inc.).
Siladryl, Elix. (Silarx Pharmaceuticals, Inc.).
Silphen Cough (Silarx Pharmaceuticals, Inc.).
Silphen DM, Syr. (Silarx Pharmaceuticals, Inc.).
Span-Lanin, Cap. (Scrip).
Snooze Fast, Tab. (BDI Pharmaceuticals, Inc.).
Tusstat, Expectorant (Century Pharmaceuticals, Inc.).
W/Acetaminophen.
See: Excedrin PM, Preps. (Bristol-Myers Squibb).
Legatrin PM, Capl. (Columbia Laboratories, Inc.).
Midol PM, Capl. (Bayer Corp. (Consumer Div.)).
W/Ammonium Cl, menthol.
See: Fenylex, Expectorant (Roberts Pharmaceuticals).
Tusstat Expectorant (Century Pharmaceuticals, Inc.).
W/Antihistamines.
See: Bendylate, Inj. (Solvay Pharmaceuticals).
W/Chlorobutanol.
See: Ardeben, Inj. (Burgin-Arden).

diphenhydramine w/combinations.
See: Banophen Decongestant (Major Pharmaceuticals).
Benadryl Itch, Preps. (Glaxo-Wellcome).
Dermaycin, Cream, Spray (Pfeiffer Co).
Dermarest, Gel (Del).
Dermarest Plus, Gel, Spray (Del).

•**diphenidol hydrochloride.** (die-FEN-ih-dahl) USAN.
Use: Antiemetic

•**diphenidol pamoate.** (die-FEN-ih-dahl) USAN.
Use: Antiemetic.

•**diphenoxylate hydrochloride.** (die-fen-OX-ih-late) U.S.P. 23.
Use: Antiperistaltic to treat diarrhea.
W/Atropine.
See: Lomotil, Tab., Liq. (Searle).

diphenoxylate hydrochloride and atropine sulfate. (die-fen-OX-ih-late and AT-troe-peen)
Use: Antiperistaltic.

diphenylhydroxycarbinol. Benzhydrol HCl.

diphenylhydantoin. Phenytoin.
Use: Anticonvulsant.

diphenylhydantoin sodium. Phenytoin Sodium.
Use: Anticonvulsant.

diphenylisatin.
See: Oxyphenisatin (Various Mfr.).

diphosphonic acid.
See: Etidronic acid.

diphosphopyridine (dpn).
Use: Antialcoholic. Under study.

diphosphothiamin. Cocarboxylase.

diphtheria, acellular pertussis, tetanus vaccine. (diff-THEER-ee-uh, ay-SELL-you-luhr per-TUSS-iss, TET-ah-nus)
Use: Immunization.
See: Acel-Imune (Wyeth Lederle).
Certiva (Ross Pediatrics).
Infanrix (SKB).
TriHIBit (Pasteur Merieux Connaught).
Tripedia (Pasteur Merieux Connaught).

•**diphtheria antitoxin.** (diff-THEER-ee-uh) U.S.P. 23.
Use: Passive immunizing agent.

diphtheria antitoxin. (Pasteur Merieux Connaught) 20,000 units, tricresol 4%/vial. (Biocine Sclavo) 20,000 units, m-cresol 0.3%/vial. (not < 500 units/ml).
Use: I.M. slow I.V. infusion; protection/treatment of diphtheria; immunization.

diphtheria equine antitoxin. *Rx.*
Use: Prophylaxis and treatment of diphtheria.

diphtheria & tetanus toxoids. (diff-THEER-ee-uh & TET-ah-nus)
Use: Immunization.

diphtheria & tetanus toxoids & acellular pertussis vaccine.
See: Acel-Imune, Vial (Wyeth Lederle).
Infanrix, Vial (SmithKline Beecham Pharmaceuticals).
Tripedia, Vial (Pasteur Merieux Connaught).

diphtheria & tetanus toxoids, aluminum phosphate adsorbed. (Wyeth Lederle) Tubex 0.5 ml. Vial 5 ml. Pkg. 10s. Available in pediatric and adult strengths. 10 Lf units diphtheria and 5 Lf units tetanus per 0.5 ml dose. 1.5 Lf units diphtheria, 5 Lf units tetanus per 0.5 ml dose. *Rx.*
Use: Immunization.

diphtheria & tetanus toxoids. Pediatric: (Pasteur Merieux Connaught) 6.6 Lf units diphtheria and 5 Lf units tetanus/0.5 ml dose. Vial 5 ml. (Wyeth Lederle) 12.5 Lf units diphtheria, 5 Lf units tetanus per 0.5 ml dose. Vial 5 ml. (Mass. Public Health Bio. Lab.) 7.5 Lf units diphtheria and 7.5 Lf units teta-

nus/0.5 ml dose. Vial, multidose. **Adult:** (Pasteur Merieux Connaught) 2 Lf units diphtheria and 5 Lf units tetanus/0.5 ml dose. Vial 5 ml, 30 ml. (Wyeth Lederle) 2 Lf units diphtheria and 5 Lf units tetanus per 0.5 ml dose. Vial 5 ml, disp. syringe 0.5 ml, vial 5 ml. (Mass Public Health Bio Lab) 2 Lf units diphtheria and 2 Lf units tetanus/0.5 ml dose Vial, multidose. *Rx.*
Use: Immunization

diphtheria & tetanus toxoids & whole-cell pertussis vaccine. (diff-THEER-ee-uh & TET-ah-nus & per-TUSS-iss) (Pasteur Merieux Connaught) 6.5 Lf units diphtheria, 5 Lf units tetanus, 4 Lf units pertussis/0.5 ml dose. Vial 2.5 ml, 5 ml, 7.5 ml. (Mass. Public Health Bio. Lab.) 10 Lf units diphtheria, 5.5 Lf units tetanus and 4 units pertussis/0.5 ml dose. Vial 5 ml.
Use: Prevention against diphtheria, tetanus and pertussis; immunization.
See: DTwP Michigan Department of Health; SmithKline Beecham Pharmaceuticals.
Tri-immunol, Vial (Wyeth Lederle).

diptheria & tetanus toxoids & acellular pertussis vaccine. (U-Line)
Use: Prevention against diphtheria, tetanus, and pertussis; immunizing agent.
See: Acel-Imune, Vial (Wyeth Lederle).
Infanrix, Vial (SKB).
TriHIBit, Kit (Pasteur Merieux Connaught).
Tripedia, Vial (Pasteur Merieux Connaught).

diphtheria & tetanus toxoids & pertussis vaccine adsorbed. (Wyeth Lederle) Vaccine Vial 7.5 ml. *Rx.*
Use: Immunization.

diphtheria & tetanus toxoids & pertussis vaccine combined, aluminum phosphate-adsorbed.
Use: Immunization.
See: Tri-Immunol, Vial (Wyeth Lederle).

•**diphtheria toxin for Schick Test.** (diff-THEER-ee-uh) U.S.P. 23. *Formerly Diphtheria Toxin, Diagnostic.*
Use: Diagnostic aid (dermal reactivity indicator).

•**diphtheria toxoid.** (diff-THEER-ee-uh) U.S.P. 23.
Use: Immunization (active).

•**diphtheria toxoid adsorbed.** (diff-THEER-ee-uh) U.S.P. 23.
Use: Immunization (active).

Dipimol. (Everett Laboratories, Inc.) Dipyridamole 25 mg, 50 mg, or 75 mg/Tab. Bot. 100s, 500s, 1000s.
Use: Antianginal.

dipivalyl epinephrine.
See: Propine (Allergan, Inc.).

•**dipivefrin.** (die-PIHV-eh-FRIN) USAN. *Formerly Dipivalyl Epinephrine.*
Use: Adrenergic, ophthalmic.

•**dipivefrin hydrochloride.** (die-PIHV-eh-FRIN) U.S.P. 23.
Use: Antiglaucoma agent.
See: AKPro (Akorn).
Propine, Soln. (Allergan, Inc.).

dipivefrin hydrochloride. (Various Mfr.) 0.1% Soln. 5 ml, 10 ml, 15 ml. *Rx.*
Use: Antiglaucoma agent.

Dipyridamole. (Foy Laboratories) Dipyridamole 25 mg/Tab. Bot. 1000s. *Rx.*
Use: Antianginal.

Diprivan. (Zeneca Pharmaceuticals) Propofol 10 mg/ml. Inj. Amp. 20 ml, 50 ml, 100 ml infusion vials. *Rx.*
Use: Anesthetic, general.

Diprolene AF Cream. (Schering-Plough Corp.) Betamethasone dipropionate cream equivalent to 0.05% betamethasone. 15 g, 45 g. *Rx.*
Use: Corticosteroid, topical.

Diprolene Cream 0.05%. (Schering-Plough Corp.) Betamethasone dipropionate 0.05% in cream base. Tube 15 g. *Rx.*
Use: Anti-inflammatory; antipruritic, topical.

Diprolene Ointment 0.05%. (Schering-Plough Corp.) Betamethasone dipropionate 0.05%, in ointment base. Tube 15 g, 45 g. *Rx.*
Use: Anti-inflammatory; antipruritic, topical.

dipropylacetic acid.
See: Valproic Acid.

Diprosone Aerosol 0.1%. (Schering-Plough Corp.) Betamethasone dipropionate 6.4 mg (equiv. to 5 mg betamethasone) in vehicle of mineral oil, caprylic-capric triglyceride w/isopropyl alcohol 10%, inert hydrocarbon propellants (propane and isobutane). Can. 85 g. *Rx.*
Use: Corticosteroid, topical.

Diprosone Cream 0.05%. (Schering-Plough Corp.) Betamethasone dipropionate 0.64 mg (equiv. to 0.5 mg betamethasone) w/mineral oil, white petrolatum, polyethylene glycol 1000 monocetyl ether, cetostearyl alcohol, phosphoric acid, monobasic sodium phosphate with 4-chloro-m-cresol as preservative. Tube 15 g, 45 g. *Rx.*
Use: Corticosteroid, topical.

Diprosone Lotion 0.05%. (Schering-Plough Corp.) Betamethasone di-

propionate 0.64 mg (equivalent to 0.5 mg betamethasone) w/isopropyl alcohol (46.8%). Bot. 20 ml, 60 ml. *Rx.*
Use: Corticosteroid, topical.

Diprosone Ointment 0.05%. (Schering-Plough Corp.) Betamethasone dipropionate 0.64 mg (equivalent to 0.5 mg betamethasone) in white petrolatum and mineral oil base. Tube 15 g, 45 g.
Use: Corticosteroid, topical.

•**dipyridamole.** (DIE-pih-RID-uh-mole) U.S.P. 23.
Use: Coronary vasodilator.
See: Persantine, Tab. (Boehringer Ingelheim, Inc.).
Persantine IV (Du Pont Merck Pharmaceutical Co.).

dipyridamole. (DIE-pih-RID-uh-mole) (Various Mfr.) **25 mg/Tab.:** Bot. 90s, 100s, 500s, 1000s, 5000s, UD 100s. **50 mg, 75 mg/Tab.:** Bot. 100s, 500s, 1000s, UD 100s.
Use: Coronary vasodilator.
See: Persantine (Boehringer Ingelheim, Inc.).

•**dipyrithione.** (DIE-pihr-ih-THIGH-ohn) USAN.
Use: Antifungal, anti-infective.

•**dipyrone.** (DIE-pie-rone) USAN. *Formerly Methampyrone.*
Use: Analgesic, antipyretic.

•**dirithromycin.** (die-RITH-row-MY-sin) USAN.
Use: Anti-infective.
See: Dynabac, Tab. (Sanofi Winthrop Pharmaceucticals).

disaccharide tripeptide glycerol dipalmitoyl.
Use: Antineoplastic. [Orphan Drug]
See: ImmTher (Immuno Therapy Co.).

Disalcid. (3M Pharm.) Salsalate. **Tab.:** 500 mg or 750 mg. Bot. 100s, 500s, UD 100s. **Cap.:** 500 mg. Bot. 100s. *Rx.*
Use: Analgesic.

Discase. (Omnis Surgical) Chymopapain 5 units/2 ml. Vial 5 ml. *Rx.*
Use: Intradiscal injection for herniated lumbar intervertebral discs.

Disinfecting Solution. (Bausch & Lomb Pharmaceuticals) Sodium Cl, sodium borate, boric acid, chlorhexidine 0.005%, EDTA 0.1%, thimerosal 0.001%. Bot. 355 ml. *otc.*
Use: Contact lens care.

•**disiquonium chloride.** (die-SIH-CONE-ee-uhm) USAN.
Use: Antiseptic.

Dismiss Douche. (Schering-Plough Corp.) Sodium Cl, sodium citrate, citric acid, cetearyl octoate, ceteareth-27, fragrance. Pow. for dilution. Pkg. 2s.
Use: Vaginal agent.

Disobrom. (Geneva Pharmaceuticals) Pseudoephedrine sulfate 120 mg, dexbrompheniramine maleate 6 mg Tab. Bot 100s, 1000s. *Rx.*
Use: Antihistamine, decongestant.

•**disobutamide.** (DIE-so-BYOO-tam-ide) USAN.
Use: Cardiovascular agent (antiarrhythmic).

disodium carbonate. Sodium Carbonate, N.F. 18.

disodium chromate. Sodium Chromate Cr 51 Injection, U.S.P. 23.

disodium chromoglycate.
See: Intal (Medeva Pharmaceuticals, Inc.).
Nasalcrom (Medeva Pharmaceuticals, Inc.).

disodium clodronate. (Discovery Experimental & Development, Inc.)
Use: Antihypercalcemic. [Orphan Drug]

disodium clodronate tetrahydrate.
Use: Increased bone resorption due to malignancy. [Orphan Drug]
See: Bonefos (Leiras Pharmaceuticals, Inc.).

disodium edathamil.
See: Edathamil Disodium (Various Mfr.).

disodium edetate. Disodium ethylenediaminetetra acetate.
See: Edetate Disodium, U.S.P. 23.

disodium phosphate.
See: Sodium Phosphate, U.S.P. 23.

disodium phosphate heptahydrate. Sodium Phosphate, U.S.P. 23.

disodium thiosulfate pentahydrate. Sodium Thiosulfate, U.S.P. 23.

di-sodium versenate.
See: Edathamil Disodium (Various Mfr.).

•**disofenin.** (DIE-so-FEN-in) USAN.
Use: Diagnostic aid (carrier agent).

Disophrol. (Schering-Plough Corp.) Pseudoephedrine sulfate 60 mg, dexbrompheniramine maleate 2 mg. Tab. Bot. 100s. *otc.*
Use: Antihistamine, decongestant.

Disophrol Chronotabs. (Schering-Plough Corp.) Dexbrompheniramine maleate 6 mg, pseudoephedrine sulfate 120 mg/SA Tab. Bot. 100s. *otc.*
Use: Antihistamine, decongestant.

•**disopyramide.** (DIE-so-PIR-uh-mide) USAN.
Use: Cardiovascular agent (antiarrhythmic).

•**disopyramide phosphate.** (DIE-so-PIHR-ah-mid) U.S.P. 23.
Use: Cardiovascular agent, antiarrhythmic.

See: Norpace (Searle).

disopyramide phosphate extended-release capsules. (DIE-so-PIHR-ah-mid)
Use: Cardiovascular agent, antiarrhythmic.

Disotate. (Steris Laboratories, Inc.) Edetate disodium 150 mg/ml. Inj. Vial 20 ml. *Rx.*
Use: Antihypercalcemic.

•**disoxaril.** (die-SOX-ar-ILL) USAN.
Use: Antiviral.

Di-Spaz. (Vortech Pharmaceuticals) Dicyclomine HCl. **Cap.:** 10 mg. Bot. 1000s. **Inj.:** 10 mg. Vial 10 ml. *Rx.*
Use: Gastrointestinal, anticholinergic.

Dispos-a-Med. (Parke-Davis) Isoetharine HCl 0.5% or 1%. Can of prefilled sterile tubes 0.5 ml, 50s. *Rx.*
Use: Bronchodilator.

distaquaine.
See: Penicillin V.

distigmine bromide. Hexamarium bromide.

•**disulfiram.** (die-SULL-fih-ram) U.S.P. 23.
Use: Alcohol deterrent.
See: Antabuse, Tab. (Wyeth-Ayerst Laboratories).

Dital. (Forest Pharmaceutical, Inc.) Phendimetrazine tartrate 105 mg/SR Cap. Bot. 100s. *c-III.*
Use: Anorexiant.

Ditate D.S. (Savage Laboratories) Testosterone enanthate 360 mg, estradiol valerate 16 mg, benzyl alcohol 2% in sesame oil. Syringe 2 ml. Box 10s. Vial 2 ml. *Rx.*
Use: Androgen, estrogen combination.

•**ditekiren.** (DIE-teh-KIE-ren) USAN.
Use: Antihypertensive.

dithranol.
See: Anthralin, U.S.P. 23. (Various Mfr.).

D.I.T.I. Creme. (Dunhall Pharmaceuticals, Inc.) Iodoquinol 100 mg, sulfanilamide 500 mg, diethylstilbestrol 0.1 mg/g Jar. 4 oz. *Rx.*
Use: Anti-infective, vaginal.

D.I.T.I.-2 Creme. (Dunhall Pharmaceuticals, Inc.) Sulfanilamide 15%, aminacrine HCl 0.2%, allantoin 2%. Tube 142 g. *Rx.*
Use: Anti-infective, vaginal.

Ditropan Syrup. (Alza Corp.) Oxybutynin Cl 5 mg/5 ml sorbitol, sucrose, methylparaben. Syr. Bot. 473 ml. *Rx.*
Use: Genitourinary.

Ditropan Tablets. (Alza Corp.) Oxybutynin Cl 5 mg, lactose/Tab. Bot. 100s, 1000s, UD 100s. *Rx.*
Use: Urinary tract agent.

Ditropan XL. (Alza Corp.) Oxybutynin chloride 5 mg, 10 mg, lactose. ER Tab. Bot. 100s *Rx.*
Use: Urinary tract agent.

Diucardin. (Wyeth-Ayerst Laboratories) Hydroflumethiazide 50 mg/Tab. Bot. 100s. *Rx.*
Use: Antihypertensive, diuretic.

Diulo. (Searle) Metolazone 2.5 mg, 5 mg or 10 mg/Tab. Bot. 100s. *Rx.*
Use: Antihypertensive, diuretic.

Diurese. (American Urologicals, Inc.) Trichlormethiazide 4 mg/Tab. Bot. 100s, 1000s. *Rx.*
Use: Diuretic.

diuretic combinations.
See: Moduretic, Tab. (Merck & Co.).
Spironolactone w/Hydrochlorothiazide, Tab. (Various Mfr.).
Alazide, Tab. (Major Pharmaceuticals).
Aldactazide, Tab. (Searle).
Dyazide, Cap. (SKB).
Maxzide, Tab. (ESI Lederle Generics).
Maxzide-25 MG, Tab. (ESI Lederle Generics).
Spironazide, Tab. (Schein Pharmaceutical, Inc.).
Spirozide, Tab. (Rugby Labs, Inc.).
Triamterene w/Hydrochlorothiazide, Cap. (Various Mfr.).
Triamterene w/Hydrochlorothiazide, Tab. (Various Mfr.).

diuretics, loop.
See: Bumex, Inj., Tab. (Roche Laboratories).
Edecrin, Tab. (Merck & Co.).
Edecrin Sodium, Inj. (Merck & Co.).
Furosemide, Inj., Tab. (Various Mfr.).
Furosemide, Oral Soln. (Roxane Laboratories, Inc.).
Lasix, Inj., Oral Soln., Tab. (Hoechst Marion Roussel).
Luramide, Tab. (Major Pharmaceuticals).

diuretics, osmotic.
See: Ismotic, Soln. (Alcon Laboratories, Inc.).
Mannitol, Inj. (Various Mfr.).
Osmitrol, Inj. (Baxter Pharmaceutical Products, Inc.).
Osmoglyn, Soln. (Alcon Laboratories, Inc).
Ureaphil, Inj. (Abbott Laboratories).

diuretics, potassium-sparing.
See: Alatone, Tab. (Major Pharmaceuticals).
Aldactone, Tab. (Searle).
Amiloride HCl, Tab. (Various Mfr.).
Dyrenium, Cap. (SmithKline Beecham Pharmaceuticals).

Midamor, Tab. (Merck & Co.).
Spironolactone, Tab. (Various Mfr.).

diuretics, thiazides.
See: Aquatensen, Tab. (Wallace Laboratories).
Chlorothiazide, Tab. (Various Mfr.).
Chlorthalidone, Tab. (Various Mfr.).
Diucardin, Tab. (Wyeth-Ayerst Laboratories).
Diulo, Tab. (Searle).
Diurese, Tab. (American Urologicals, Inc.).
Diurigen, Tab. (Zenith Goldline Pharmaceuticals).
Diuril, Oral Susp., Tab. (Merck & Co.).
Diuril Sodium, Inj. (Merck & Co.).
Enduron, Tab. (Abbott Laboratories).
Esidrix, Tab. (Novartis Pharmaceutical Corp.).
Ethon, Tab. (Major Pharmaceuticals).
Exna, Tab. (Wyeth-Ayerst Laboratories).
Hydrochlorothiazide, Tab. (Various Mfr.).
Hydrochlorothiazide, Oral Soln. (Roxane Laboratories, Inc.).
HydroDIURIL, Tab. (Merck & Co.).
Hydroflumethiazide, Tab. (Various Mfr.).
Hydromal, Tab. (Roberts Pharmaceuticals).
Hydromox, Tab. (ESI Lederle Generics).
Hydro-T, Tab. (Major Pharmaceuticals).
Hydro-Z-50, Tab. (Merz Pharmaceutcials).
Hygroton, Tab. (Rhone-Poulenc Rorer Pharmaceuticals, Inc.).
Hylidone, Tab. (Major Pharmaceuticals).
Lozol, Tab. (Rhone-Poulenc Rorer Pharmaceuticals, Inc.).
Metahydrin, Tab. (Hoechst Marion Roussel).
Methyclothiazide, Tab. (Various Mfr.).
Mictrin, Tab. (Econo Med Pharmaceuticals).
Mykrox (Medeva Pharmaceuticals, Inc.).
Naqua, Tab. (Schering-Plough Corp.).
Naturetin, Tab. (Bristol-Myers Squibb).
Niazide, Tab. (Major Pharmaceuticals).
Oretic, Tab. (Abbott Laboratories).
Renese, Tab. (Pfizer US Pharmaceutical Group).
Saluron, Tab. (Bristol-Myers Squibb).
Thalitone, Tab. (Boehringer Ingelheim, Inc.).
Trichlormethiazide, Tab. (Various Mfr.).
Zaroxolyn, Tab. (Medeva Pharmaceuticals, Inc.).

Diuretic Tablets. (Faraday) Buchu leaves 150 mg, uva ursi leaves 150 mg, juniper berries 120 mg, bone meal, parsley, asparagus/Tab. Bot. 100s. *Rx.*
Use: Diuretic.

Diurigen Tablets. (Zenith Goldline Pharmaceuticals) Chlorothiazide 500 mg. Tab Bot. 100s, 1000s. *Rx.*
Use: Diuretic.

Diurigen w/Reserpine 250 Tablets. (Zenith Goldline Pharmaceuticals) Chlorothiazide 250 mg, reserpine 0.125 mg. Tab. Bot. 100s, 1000s. *Rx.*
Use: Antihypertensive combination.

Diurigen w/Reserpine 500 Tablets. (Zenith Goldline Pharmaceuticals) Chlorothiazide 500 mg, reserpine 0.125 mg. Tab. Bot. 100s, 1000s. *Rx.*
Use: Antihypertensive combination.

Diuril. (Merck & Co.) Chlorothiazide, U.S.P. 23. **Tab.:** 250 mg Bot. 100s, 1000s; 500 mg Bot. 100s, 1000s, UD 100s. **Oral Susp.:** 250 mg/5 ml w/methylparaben 0.12%, propylparaben 0.02%, benzoic acid 0.1%, alcohol 0.5%. Bot. 237 ml. *Rx.*
Use: Antihypertensive, diuretic.
W/Methyldopa.
See: Aldoclor, Tab. (Merck & Co.).

Diuril Sodium Intravenous. (Merck & Co.) Chlorothiazide sodium equivalent to 0.5 g chlorothiazide w/mannitol 0.25 g sodium hydroxide, thimerosal 0.4 mg. Vial 20 ml. *Rx.*
Use: Antihypertensive, diuretic.

Diutensen-R. (Wallace Laboratories) Methyclothiazide 2.5 mg, reserpine 0.1 mg/Tab. Bot. 100s, 500s, 5000s. *Rx.*
Use: Antihypertensive combination.

•**divalproex sodium.** (die-VAL-pro-ex) USAN.
Use: Anticonvulsant.
See: Depakote (Abbott Laboratories).

divinyl oxide. Vinyl ether, divinyl ether.
Use: Inhalation anesthetic.

Dizac. (Ohmeda Pharmaceuticals) Diazepam 5 mg/ml, preservative free. Inj. Vial 3 ml. *c-iv.*
Use: Anxiolytic, anticonvulsant, muscle relaxant.

Dizmiss. (Jones Medical Industries, Inc.) Meclizine HCl 25 mg/Tab. Bot. 100s, 1000s. *otc.*
Use: Antiemetic, antivertigo.

•**dizocilpine maleate.** (die-ZOE-sill-PEEN) USAN.
Use: Neuroprotective.

dl-desoxyephedrine hydrochloride.
See: dl-Methamphetamine HCl.

dl-methamphetamine hydrochloride. dl-Desoxyephedrine HCl.
See: Oxydess, Tab. (Vortech Pharmaceuticals).
W/Pyrilamine maleate, phenyltoloxamine dihydrogen citrate, didesoxyephedrine HCl, codeine phosphate, ammonium Cl, potassium guaiacolsulfonate, chloroform, phenylpropanolamine tartar emetic.
See: Meditussin-X Liquid (Roberts Pharmaceuticals).

dl-norephedrine hydrochloride.
See: Phenylpropanolamine Hydrochloride (Various Mfr.).

DM Cough. (Rosemont Pharmaceutical Corp.) Dextromethorphan HBr 10 mg/5 ml, alcohol 5%. Syr. Bot. 120 ml, pt, gal. *otc.*
Use: Antitussive.

DMCT. (ESI Lederle Generics) Demethylchlortetracycline. *Rx.*
Use: Anti-infective, tetracycline.
See: Declomycin HCl, Preps. (ESI Lederle Generics).

d-methorphan hydrobromide.
See: Dextromethorphan HBr (Various Mfr.).

d-methylphenylamine sulfate.
See: Dextroamphetamine Sulfate, U.S.P. 23. (Various Mfr.).

DML Dermatological Moisturizing Lotion. (Person and Covey, Inc.) Purified water, petrolatum, glycerin, methyl glucose sesquisterate, dimethicone, methyl gluceth-20 sesquisterate, benzyl alcohol, volatile silicone, glyceryl stearate, stearic acid, palmitic acid, cetyl alcohol, xanthan gum, magnesium aluminum silicate carbomer 941, sodium hydroxide. Bot. 8 oz. *otc.*
Use: Emollient.

DML Facial Moisturizer. (Person and Covey, Inc.) Octyl methoxycinnamate 8%, oxybenzone 4%, benzyl alcohol, petrolatum, EDTA. SPF 15. Cream 45 g. *otc.*
Use: Sunscreen.

DML Forte. (Person and Covey, Inc.) Petrolatum, PPG-2 myristyl ether propionate, glyceryl stearate, glycerin, stearic acid, d-panthenol, DEA-cetyl phosphate, simethicone, PVP eicosene copolymer, benzyl alcohol, cetyl alcohol, silica, disodium EDTA, BHA, magnesium aluminum silicate, sodium carbomer 1342. Tube 113 g. *otc.*
Use: Emollient.

dmp 777. (Du Pont Merck Pharmaceutical Co.)
Use: Cystic fibrosis. [Orphan Drug]

DMSO.
See: Dimethyl sulfoxide.

Doak Tar Distillate. (Doak Dermatologics) Coal tar distillate 40%. Liq. Bot. 59 ml. *otc.*
Use: Antiseborrheic.

Doak Tar Lotion. (Doak Dermatologics) Tar distillate 5%. Bot. 118 ml. *otc.*
Use: Antiseborrheic.

Doak Tar Oil. (Doak Dermatologics) Tar distillate 2%. Liq. Bot. 237 ml. *otc.*
Use: Antiseborrheic.

Doak Tar Oil Forte. (Doak Dermatologics) Tar distillate 5%. Bot. 4 oz.
Use: Antiseborrheic.

Doak Tar Shampoo. (Doak Dermatologics) Tar distillate 3% in shampoo base. Bot. 237 ml. *otc.*
Use: Antiseborrheic.

Doak Tersaseptic. (Doak Dermatologics) Liquid cleanser, pH 6.8. Bot. 4 oz, pt, gal. *otc.*
Use: Detergent.

Doan's Backache Spray. (DEP Corp.) Methyl salicylate 15%, menthol 8.4%, methyl nicotinate 0.6%. Aerosol Can 4 oz. *otc.*
Use: Analgesic, topical.

Doan's PM, Extra Strength.
See: Extra Strength Doan's PM, Capl. (Ciba Vision).

Doan's Pills. (DEP Corp.) Magnesium salicylate 325 mg/Tab. Ctn. 24s, 48s. *otc.*
Use: Analgesic.

•**dobutamine for injection.** (doe-BYOOT-ah-meen) U.S.P. 23.
Use: Cardiovascular agent.

•**dobutamine hydrochloride.** (doe-BYOOT-ah-meen) U.S.P. 23.
Use: Cardiovascular agent.
See: Dobutrex, Inj. (Eli Lilly and Co.).

dobutamine hydrochloride. (Various Mfr.) 12.5 mg/ml. May contain sulfites. Inj. Vial 20 ml.
Use: Cardiovascular agent.

•**dobutamine lactobionate.** (doe-BYOOT-ah-meen) USAN.
Use: Cardiovascular agent.

•**dobutamine tartrate.** (doe-BYOOT-ah-meen) USAN.
Use: Cardiovascular agent.

Dobutrex Solution. (Eli Lilly and Co.) Dobutamine HCl 250 mg. Inj. Vial 20 ml. *Rx.*
Use: Cardiovascular agent.

•**docebenone.** (dah-SEH-beh-nohn) USAN.
Use: Inhibitor (5-lipoxygenase).

•**docetaxel.** (doe-seh-TAX-ehl) USAN.
Use: Antineoplastic.
See: Taxotere (Rhone-Poulenc Rorer Pharmaceuticals, Inc.).

•**doconazole.** (doe-KOE-nah-zole) USAN.
Use: Antifungal.

Doctar. (Savage Laboratories) Coal tar 0.5%, conditioner. Shampoo. Bot. 100 ml. *otc.*
Use: Antiseborrheic.

Doctase. (Purepac Pharmaceutical Co.) Docusate sodium 100 mg, casanthranol 30 mg/Cap. Bot. 100s. *otc.*
Use: Laxative.

Doctyl. (Health for Life Brands, Inc.) Docusate sodium 100 mg/Tab. Bot. 40s, 100s, 1000s. *otc.*
Use: Laxative.

Doctylax. (Health for Life Brands, Inc.) Docusate sodium 100 mg, acetophenolisatin 2 mg, prune conc. ¾ mg/Tab. Bot. 40s, 100s, 1000s. *otc.*
Use: Laxative.

Docucal-P Softgels. (Parmed Pharmaceuticals, Inc.) Docusate (as calcium) 60 mg, phenolphthalein 65 mg/Cap. Bot. 100s, 1000s. *otc.*
Use: Laxative.

•**docusate calcium.** (DOCK-you-sate) U.S.P. 23. *Formerly Dioctyl Calcium Sulfosuccinate.*
Use: Laxative, stool softener.
See: Surfak, Cap. (Hoechst Marion Roussel).
Doxidan, Cap. (Hoechst Marion Roussel).

docusate with casanthranol. (DOCK-you-sate) (Various Mfr.) Docusate (as sodium) 100 mg, casanthranol 30 mg/Cap. Bot. 100s, 1000s, UD 100s. *otc.*
Use: Laxative, stool softener.

•**docusate potassium.** U.S.P. 23.
Use: Laxative, stool softener.
See: Dialose, Cap. (Zeneca Pharmaceuticals).
Dialose Plus, Cap. (Zeneca Pharmaceuticals).
Kasof, Cap. (Zeneca Pharmaceuticals).

•**docusate sodium.** (DOCK-you-sate) U.S.P. 23. *Formerly Dioctyl Sodium Sulfosuccinate.*
Use: Pharmaceutical aid (surfactant), stool softener.
See: Colace, Cap., Liq., Syr. (Bristol-Myers Squibb).
Coloctyl, Cap. (Eon Labs Manufacturing, Inc.).
Comfolax, Cap. (Searle).
Correctol Extra Gentle, Cap. (Schering-Plough Corp.).
Dialose Preps. (Merck & Co.).
Diomedicone, Tab. (Medicore).
Diosate, Cap. (Towne).
Doss, Super Doss, Tab. (Ferndale Laboratories, Inc.).
Doxinate, Cap., Liq. (Hoechst Marion Roussel).
DSS (Parke-Davis).
Duosol, Cap. (Kirkman Sales Co., Inc.).
Dynoctol, Cap. (Solvay Pharmaceuticals).
Easy-Lax, Cap. (Walgreen).
Ex-Lax Stool Softener (Norvartis Pharmaceutical Corp.).
Konsto, Cap. (Freeport).
Laxatab, Tab. (Freeport).
Liqui-Doss, Liq. (Ferndale Laboratories, Inc.).
Modane Soft, Cap. (Pharmacia & Upjohn).
Peri-Doss, Cap. (Ferndale Laboratories, Inc.).
Phillips Laxative, Gelcaps (Bayer Corp. (Consumer Div.)).
Regul-Aid, Syr. (Quality Generics).
Silace, Syr. (Silarx Pharmaceuticals, Inc.).
Silace-C, Syr. (Silarx Pharmaceuticals, Inc.).
Stulex, Tab. (Jones Medical Industries, Inc.).
Surfak, Cap. (Hoechst Marion Roussel).

W/Ascorbic acid, ferrous fumarate.
See: Hemaspan, Cap. (Sanofi Winthrop Pharmaceucticals).

W/Betaine HCl, zinc, manganese, molybdenum.
See: Hemaferrin (Western Research).

W/Bisacodyl.
See: Laxadan, Supp. (Teva Pharmaceuticals USA).

W/Brewer's yeast.
See: Doss or Super Doss, Tab. (Ferndale Laboratories, Inc.).

W/Casanthranol.
See: Calotabs, Tab. (Calotabs).
Constiban (Quality Generics).
Diolax, Cap. (Century Pharmaceuticals, Inc.).
Dio-Soft (Standex).
Easy-Lax Plus, Cap. (Walgreen).
Genericace, Cap. (Forest Pharmaceutical, Inc.).
Neo-Vadrin D-D-S, Cap. (Scherer Laboratories, Inc.).
Nuvac, Cap. (LaCrosse).
Peri-Colace, Cap., Syr. (Bristol-Myers Squibb).

W/Casanthranol, sodium carboxymethylcellulose.
See: Dialose Plus, Cap. (Zeneca Pharmaceuticals).
Tri-Vac, Cap. (Rhode).
W/Dehydrocholic acid.
See: Dubbalax-B, Cap. (Redford).
Dubbalax-N, Cap. (Redford).
Neolax, Tab. (Schwarz Pharma, Inc.).
W/D-calcium pantothenate and acetaphenolisatin.
See: Peri-Pantyl, Tab. (McGregor Pharmaceuticals, Inc.).
W/Ferrous fumarate, Vitamin C.
See: Hemaspan, Cap. (Sanofi Winthrop Pharmaceucticals).
Recoup, Tab. (ESI Lederle Generics).
W/Ferrous fumarate, vitamins.
See: Bevitone, Tab. (Teva Pharmaceuticals USA).
W/Ferrous fumarate, betaine HCl, desiccated liver, vitamins, minerals.
See: Hemaferrin, Tab. (Western Research).
W/Glycerin.
See: Barc, Cream, Liq. (Del Pharmaceuticals, Inc.).
W/Petrolatum.
See: Milkinol, Liq, Emulsion (Kremers Urban).
W/Phenolphthalein.
See: Correctol, Tab. (Schering-Plough Corp).
Ex-Lax Prods. (Sandoz Pharmaceutical).
Feen-A-Mint, Pills (Schering-Plough Corp.).
W/Phenolphthalein, dehydrocholic acid.
See: Bolax, Cap. (Boyd).
Tripalax, Cap. (Redford).
W/Polyoxyethylene nonyl phenol, sodium edetate, 9-aminoacridine HCl.
See: Vagisec Plus Supp. (Durex).
W/Senna concentrate.
See: Gentlax S, Tab. (Blair Laboratories).
Senokap-DDS, Cap. (Purdue Frederick Co.).
Senokot S, Tab. (Purdue Frederick Co.).

•**dofetilide.** (doe-FEH-till-ide) USAN.
Use: Cardiovascular agent, antiarrhythmic.

Dofus. (Miller Pharmacal Group, Inc.) Freeze-dried *Lactobacillus acidophilus* minimum of 1 billion organisms/Cap. w/*Lactobacillus bifidus* organisms added. Bot. 60s. *otc.*
Use: Nutritional supplement, antidiarrheal.

DOK. (Major Pharmaceuticals) Docusate sodium. **Caps.:** 250 mg. Bot. 100s, 1000s. **Liq.:** 150 mg/15 ml. Bot. Pt. **Syrup:** 60 mg/15 ml. Bot. Pt, gal. *otc.*
Use: Laxative, stool softener.

DOK-250. (Major Pharmaceuticals) Docusate sodium 250 mg. Cap. Bot. 100s. *otc.*
Use: Laxative, stool softener.

Doktors Spray. (Scherer Laboratories, Inc.) Phenylephrine HCl 0.25%, chlorobutanol, sodium bisulfite, benzalkonium chloride. Soln. Bot. 30 ml. *otc.*
Use: Decongestant.

Dolacet. (Roberts Pharmaceuticals) Hydrocodone bitartrate 5 mg, acetaminophen 500 mg/Cap. Bot. 100s. *c-III.*
Use: Analgesic combination, narcotic.

Dolamide Tabs. (Major Pharmaceuticals) Chlorpropamide 100 mg, 250 mg/Tab. Bot. 100s, 500s, 1000s. *Rx.*
Use: Antidiabetic.

Dolamin. (Harvey) Ammonium sulfate 0.75% with sodium Cl, benzyl alcohol. Amp. 10 ml. In 12s, 25s, 100s. *Rx.*
Use: Antineuralgic.

dolantin.
See: Meperidine HCl, U.S.P. 23.

•**dolasetron mesylate.** (dahl-AH-set-rahn) USAN.
Use: Antiemetic, antimigraine.
See: Anzemet Tab., Inj. (Hoechst Marion Roussel).

Dolcin. (Dolcin) Aspirin 3.7 gr, calcium succinate 2.8 gr/Tab. Bot. 100s, 200s. *otc.*
Use: Analgesic.

Doldram. (Dram) Salicylamide 7.5 gr/Tab. Bot. 100s.
Use: Analgesic.

Dolene AP-65. (ESI Lederle Generics) Propoxyphene HCl 65 mg, acetaminophen 650 mg/Tab. Bot. 100s, 500s. *c-IV.*
Use: Analgesic combination, narcotic.

Dolene Compound-65. (ESI Lederle Generics) Propoxyphene HCl 65 mg, aspirin 389 mg, caffeine 32.4 mg/Cap. Bot. 100s, 500s. *c-IV.*
Use: Analgesic combination, narcotic.

Dolene Plain. (ESI Lederle Generics) Propoxyphene HCl 65 mg/Cap. Bot. 100s, 500s. *c-IV.*
Use: Analgesic, narcotic.

Dolobid. (Merck & Co.) Diflunisal 250 mg or 500 mg/Tab. Unit-of-use 60s, UD 100s. *Rx.*
Use: Analgesic.

Dolomite. (NBTY, Inc.) Magnesium 78 mg, calcium 130 mg/Tab. Bot. 100s, 250s. *otc.*
Use: Mineral supplement.

Dolomite. (Halsey Drug Co.) Calcium 426 mg, magnesium 246 mg/Tab. w/ guar and acacia gum. Bot. 250s. *otc.*
Use: Mineral supplement.

Dolomite Plus Capsules. (Barth's) Magnesium 37 mg, calcium 187 mg, phosphorus 50 mg, iodine 0.25 mg/Cap. Bot. 100s, 500s, 1000s. *otc.*
Use: Mineral supplement.

Dolomite Tablets. (Faraday) Calcium 150 mg, magnesium 90 mg/Tab. Bot. 250s. *otc.*
Use: Mineral supplement.

dolonil. (Parke-Davis)
See: Pyridium Plus, Tab. (Parke-Davis).

Dolophine Hydrochloride. (Eli Lilly and Co.) Methadone HCl. **Inj.:** 10 mg/ml, NaCl 0.9%. Vial 20 ml. **Tab.:** 5 mg, 10 mg. Bot. 100s. *c-II.*
Use: Analgesic, narcotic.

Dolopirona Tablets. (Sanofi Winthrop Pharmaceuticals) Dipyrone with chlormezanone. *Rx.*
Use: Analgesic, anxiolytic, muscle relaxant.

Dolorac. (GenDerm) Capsaicin 0.25%, benzyl alcohol, cetyl alcohol. Cream Tube 28 g. *otc.*
Use: Analgesic, topical.

Doloral. (Progressive Enterprises) Colchicine salicylate 0.1 mg, phenobarbital 8 mg, sodium para-aminobenzoate 15 mg, vitamins B_1 25 mg, aspirin 325 mg/Tab. Bot. 100s, 1000s. *Rx.*
Use: Antiarthritic, antigout.

dolosal.
See: Meperidine HCl.

Dolsed. (American Urologicals, Inc.) Methenamine 40.8 mg, phenylsalicylate 18.1 mg, atropine sulfate 0.03 mg, hyoscyamine 0.03 mg, benzoic acid 4.5 mg, methylene blue 5.4 mg. Tab. Bot. 100s, 1000s. *Rx.*
Use: Anti-infective, urinary.

dolvanol.
Use: Analgesic, narcotic.
See: Meperidine HCl.

•**domazoline fumarate.** (DOME-AZE-oh-leen) USAN.
Use: Anticholinergic.

Domeboro. (Bayer Corp. (Consumer Div.)) Aluminum sulfate and calcium acetate when added to water gives therapeutic effect of Burow's. One pkg. or Tab/pt. water approximately equivalent to 1:40 dilution. **Pkg.:** 2.2 g, 12s, 100s. **Effervescent Tab.:** Box 12s, 100s, 1000s. *otc.*
Use: Anti-inflammatory, topical.

Domeboro Otic. (Bayer Corp. (Consumer Div.)) Acetic acid 2% (in aluminum acetate solution). Soln. Bot. 60 ml with dropper. *Rx.*
Use: Otic.

Dome-Paste Bandage. (Bayer Corp. (Consumer Div.)) Zinc oxide, calamine and gelatin bandage. Pkg. 4″ × 10 yd. and 3″ × 10 yd. impregnated gauze bandage. *otc.*
Use: Dermatologic, wound therapy.

domestrol.
See: Diethylstilbestrol, Preps. (Various Mfr.).

D.O.M.F.
Use: Antimicrobial.
See: Merbromin (Mercurochrome) (City Chem.).

•**domiodol.** (dome-EYE-oh-DOLE) USAN.
Use: Mucolytic.

•**domiphen bromide.** (DOE-mih-fen) USAN.
Use: Antiseptic; anti-infective, topical.
See: Bradosol.

Domol Bath and Shower Oil. (Bayer Corp. (Consumer Div.)) D_1-isopropyl sebacate, isopropyl myristate with mineral oil. Bot. 240 ml. *otc.*
Use: Emollient.

•**domperidone.** (dome-PEH-rih-dohn) USAN.
Use: Antiemetic.
See: Motilium (Janssen Pharmaceutical, Inc.).

Donatussin DC Syrup. (Laser, Inc.) Hydrocodone bitartrate 2.5 mg, phenylephrine HCl 7.5 mg, guaifenesin 50 mg/5 ml. Bot. 120 ml, 480 ml. *c-III.*
Use: Antitussive, decongestant, expectorant.

Donatussin Pediatric Drops. (Laser, Inc.) Guaifenesin 20 mg, chlorpheniramine maleate 1 mg, phenylephrine HCl 2 mg/ml. Drop. Bot. 30 ml. *Rx.*
Use: Antihistamine, decongestant, expectorant.

Donatussin Syrup. (Laser, Inc.) Phenylephrine 10 mg, chlorpheniramine maleate 2 mg, dextromethorphan HBr 7.5 mg, guaifenesin 100 mg. Bot. Pt, gal. *Rx.*
Use: Antihistamine, antitussive, decongestant, expectorant.

Dondril. (Whitehall Robins Laboratories) Dextromethorphan HBr 10 mg, phenylephrine HCl 5 mg, chlorpheniramine maleate 1 mg/Tab. Bot. 24s. *otc.*
Use: Antihistamine, antitussive, decongestant.

donepezil HCl. (doe-NEPP-eh-zill HIGH-droe-KLOR-ide) (Eisai; Pfizer US Pharmaceutical Group)

Use: Treatment of mild to moderate dementia of the Alzheimer's type.
See: Aricept, Tab. (Eisai; Pfizer US Pharmaceutical Group).

•**donetidine.** (doe-NEH-tih-DEEN) USAN.
Use: Antiulcerative.

Donna. (Arcum) Menthol, thymol, eucalyptol, exsiccated alum, boric acid. 4 oz, 14 oz. *Rx.*
Use: Vaginal agent.

Donnagel. (Wyeth-Ayerst Laboratories) **Chew. Tab.:** Attapulgite 600 mg. Pkg. 18s. **Liq.:** Attapulgite 600 mg/5 ml. Bot. 120 ml, 240 ml. *otc.*
Use: Antidiarrheal.

Donnamar. (H.L. Moore Drug Exchange, Inc.) Atropine sulfate 0.0194 mg, scopolamine HBr 0.0065 mg, hyoscyamine HBr, or SO_4 0.1037 mg, phenobarbital 16.2 mg/5 ml, alcohol 23%. Elix. Bot. 120 ml, pt, gal. *Rx.*
Use: Anticholinergic, antispasmodic.

Donnamar. (Marnel Pharmaceuticals, Inc.) Hyoscyamine sulfate 0.125 mg. Tab. Bot. 100s. *Rx.*
Use: Anticholinergic, antispasmodic.

Donnaphen. (Health for Life Brands, Inc.) Phenobarbital 16.2 mg, hyoscyamine sulfate 0.1037 mg, atropine sulfate 0.0194 mg, hyoscine HBr 0.0065 mg/5 ml. Elix. Bot. Pt, gal. *Rx.*
Use: Anticholinergic, antispasmodic.

Donna-Sed Elixir. (Vortech Pharmaceuticals) Atropine sulfate 0.0194 mg, scopolamine HBr 0.0065, hyoscyamine HBr, or SO_4 0.1037 mg, phenobarbital 16.2 mg, alcohol 23%. Liq. Bot. 118 ml, gal. *Rx.*
Use: Gastrointestinal, anticholinergic.

Donnatal. (Wyeth-Ayerst Laboratories) Hyoscyamine sulfate 0.1037 mg, atropine sulfate 0.0194 mg, scopolamine HBr 0.0065 mg, phenobarbital 16.2 mg. Cap. or Tab. Bot. 100s, 1000s. *Rx.*
Use: Anticholinergic, antispasmodic, sedative.

Donnatal Dis-Co UD Pack. (Wyeth-Ayerst Laboratories) Hyoscyamine sulfate 0.1037 mg, atropine sulfate 0.0194 mg, hyoscine HBr 0.0065 mg, phenobarbital 16.2 mg (0.25 gr)/Tab. or 5 ml. **Tab.:** UD 100s. **Elix.:** UD (5 ml) 25s. *Rx.*
Use: Anticholinergic, antispasmodic, sedative.

Donnatal Elixir. (Wyeth-Ayerst Laboratories) Atropine sulfate 0.0194 mg, scopolamine HBr 0.0065 mg, hyoscyamine HBr or sulfate 0.1037 mg, phenobarbital 16.2 mg, alcohol 23%, glucose, saccharin/5 ml. Bot. 120 ml, pt., gal, Dis-Co pack 5 ml. *Rx.*
Use: Gastrointestinal, anticholinergic.

Donnatal Extentabs. (Wyeth-Ayerst Laboratories) Hyoscyamine sulfate 0.3111 mg, atropine sulfate 0.0582 mg, scopolamine HBr 0.0195 mg, phenobarbital 48.6 mg (3/4 gr)/Tab. Bot. 100s, 500s, Dis-Co pack 100s. *Rx.*
Use: Anticholinergic, antispasmodic, sedative.

Donnatal #2. (Wyeth-Ayerst Laboratories) Phenobarbital 32.4 mg (0.5 gr), hyoscyamine sulfate 0.1037 mg, atropine sulfate 0.0194 mg, scopolamine HBr 0.0065 mg/Tab. Bot. 100s, 1000s. *Rx.*
Use: Anticholinergic, antispasmodic, sedative.

Donnazyme. (Wyeth-Ayerst Laboratories) Hyoscyamine sulfate 0.0518 mg, atropine sulfate 0.0097 mg, scopolamine HBr 0.0033 mg, phenobarbital 8.1 mg (1/8 gr), pepsin 150 mg/Tab. in outer layer, pancreatin 300 mg, bile salts 150 mg/Tab. in core. Bot. 100s, 500s. *Rx.*
Use: Anticholinergic, antispasmodic, digestive aid.

Don't. (Del Pharmaceuticals, Inc.) Sucrose octa acetate 5%, isopropyl alcohol 54%. Bot. 0.45 oz. *otc.*
Use: Nail-biting deterrent.

•**dopamantine.** (DOE-pah-MAN-teen) USAN.
Use: Antiparkinsonian.

dopamine. (DOE-pah-meen) (Astra Pharmaceuticals, L.P.) Dopamine. **Amp.:** 200 mg/5 ml Amp. Box 10s; 400 mg/10 ml Amp. Box 5s. **Additive Syringe:** 200 mg/5 ml Syr. Box 1s; 400 mg/10 ml Syr. Box 1s. *Rx.*
Use: Inotropic agent.

•**dopamine hydrochloride.** (DOE-puh-meen) U.S.P. 23.
Use: Adrenergic.
See: Intropin, Amp. (Du Pont Merck Pharmaceutical Co.).

dopamine hydrochloride and dextrose injection. (DOE-pah-meen)
Use: Adrenergic, emergency treatment of low blood pressure.

Dopar. (Procter & Gamble Pharm.) Levodopa 100 mg or 250 mg/Cap. Bot. 100s. 500 mg/Cap. Bot. 100s, 1000s. *Rx.*
Use: Antiparkinsonian.

•**dopexamine.** (doe-PEX-ah-MEEN) USAN.
Use: Cardiovascular agent.

•**dopexamine hydrochloride.** (doe-PEX-ah-MEEN) USAN.

Use: Cardiovascular agent.

Dopram. (Wyeth-Ayerst Laboratories) Doxapram HCl 20 mg/ml, 0.9% benzyl alcohol. Vial 20 ml. *Rx.*
Use: Respiratory.

Doral. (Wallace Laboratories) Quazepam 7.5 mg or 15 mg/Tab. Bot. 100s, UD 100s. *c-IV.*
Use: Hypnotic, sedative.

•**dorastine hydrochloride.** (DAHR-ass-teen HIGH-droe-KLOR-ide) USAN.
Use: Antihistamine.

Dorcol Children's Cold Formula. (Sandoz Pharmaceutical) Pseudoephedrine HCl 15 mg, chlorpheniramine maleate 1 mg/5 ml. Bot. 120 ml. *otc.*
Use: Antihistamine, decongestant.

Dorcol Children's Cough Syrup. (Sandoz Pharmaceutical) Dextromethorphan HBr 5 mg, pseudoephedrine HCl 15 mg, guaifenesin 50 mg/5 ml. Bot. 120 ml, 240 ml. *otc.*
Use: Antitussive, decongestant, expectorant.

Dorcol Children's Decongestant Liquid. (Sandoz Pharmaceutical) Pseudoephedrine HCl 15 mg/5 ml. Bot. 4 oz. *otc.*
Use: Decongestant.

Dorcol Fever and Pain Reducer. (Sandoz Pharmaceutical) Acetaminophen 160 mg/5 ml. Bot. 4 oz. *otc.*
Use: Analgesic.

•**doretinel.** (DOE-REH-tin-ell) USAN.
Use: Antikeratinizing agent.

Doriglute Tabs DEA. (Major Pharmaceuticals) Glutethimide 0.5 g/Tab. Bot. 100s, 250s, 1000s. *c-II.*
Use: Hypnotic.

Dormeer. (Taylor Pharmaceuticals) Scopolamine aminoxide HBr 0.2 mg/Cap. Bot. 100s, 1000s. *Rx.*
Use: Hypnotic, sedative.

dormethan.
See: Dextromethorphan HBr (Various Mfr.).

Dormin Capsules. (Randob Laboratories, Ltd.) Diphenhydramine HCl 25 mg, lactose. Cap. Bot. 32s, 72s. *otc.*
Use: Sleep aid.

Dormin Sleeping Caplets. (Randob Laboratories, Ltd.) Diphenhydramine HCl 25 mg/Cap. Bot. 32s. *otc.*
Use: Sleep aid.

dormiral.
See: Phenobarbital, Preps. (Various Mfr.).

dormonal.
See: Barbital, Preps. (Various Mfr.).

Dormutol. (Health for Life Brands, Inc.) Scopolamine aminoxide HBr 0.2 mg/Cap. Bot. 24s, 60s. *Rx.*
Use: Hypnotic, sedative.

dornase alfa. (DOR-nace AL-fuh)
Use: Cystic fibrosis. [Orphan Drug]
See: Pulmozyme, Soln. (Genentech, Inc.).

Doryx Pellets. (Parke-Davis) Doxycycline hyclate 100 mg/Cap. Bot. 50s. *Rx.*
Use: Anti-infective, tetracycline.

•**dorzolamide hydrochloride.** (dore-ZOLE-lah-mide) USAN.
Use: Carbonic anhydrase inhibitor.
See: TruSopt, Soln. (Merck & Co.).

dorzolamide hydrochloride and timolol maleate.
Use: Antiglaucoma.
See: Cosopt, Ophth. Soln. (Merck & Co.).

Dosaflex. (Richwood Pharmaceuticals) Senna fruit extract, parabens, sucrose, alcohol 7%. Syr. Bot. 237 ml. *otc.*
Use: Laxative.

Dosalax. (Richwood Pharmaceuticals) Extract of senna fruit, parabens, sucrose, alcohol 7%. Syrup. Bot. 237 ml. *Rx.*
Use: Laxative.

DOS Caps. (Zenith Goldline Pharmaceuticals) Dioctyl sodium sulfosuccinate SG 100 mg or 250 mg/Cap. Bot. 100s, 1000s. *otc.*
Use: Laxative.

Doss Syrup. (Rosemont Pharmaceutical Corp.) Docusate sodium 20 mg/5 ml. Bot. Pt, gal. *otc.*
Use: Laxative, stool softener.

Dostinex. (Pharmacia & Upjohn) Cabergoline 0.5 mg/Tab. Bot. 8s. *Rx.*
Use: Antihyperprolactinemic.

•**dothiepin hydrochloride.** (DOE-THIGH-eh-pin) USAN.
Use: Antidepressant.

Dotirol. (Sanofi Winthrop Pharmaceuticals) Ampicillin trihydrate available in Cap, Susp., Inj. (IV, IM). *Rx.*
Use: Anti-infective, penicillin.

Double-Action Toothache Kit. (C. S. Dent & Co. Division) **Liquid:** Benzocaine, alcohol 74%, chlorobutanol anhydrous 0.09%. Bot. 3.7 ml. **Maronox Pain Relief Tablets:** Acetaminophen 325 mg/Tab. Box. 8s. *otc.*
Use: Analgesic, topical.

Double Sal. (Pal-Pak, Inc.) Sodium salicylate 648 mg/EC Tab. Bot. 1000s. *otc.*
Use: Analgesic.

Double Strength Gaviscon-2. (SmithKline Beecham Pharmaceuticals) Aluminum hydroxide 160 mg, magnesium trisilicate 40 mg, alginic acid, calcium stearate, sodium bicarbonate, sucrose.

Tab. Bot. 48s. *otc.*
Use: Antacid.

Dovacet Capsules. (Pal-Pak, Inc.) Dover's powder 24.3 mg, aspirin 324 mg, caffeine 32.4 mg. Bot. 1000s.
Use: Analgesic.

Dover's Powder. Ipecac 1 part, opium 1 part, lactose 8 parts.
Use: Analgesic, diaphoretic, sedative.
W/Acetophenetidin, atropine sulfate, aspirin, camphor, caffeine, sodium sulfate, dried.
See: Dovium, Cap. (Hance).
W/Acetophenetidin, camphor, aspirin, caffeine, atropine sulfate.
See: Analgestine, Cap. (Roberts Pharmaceuticals).
W/Acetophenetidin, sodium citrate, potassium guaiacolsulfonate.
See: Doverlyn, Cap., Tab. (Davis & Sly).
W/A.P.C. camphor monobromated.
See: Coldate, Tab. (Zeneca Pharmaceuticals).
W/Aspirin, phenacetin, camphor monobromated, caffeine.
See: Coldate, Tab. (Zeneca Pharmaceuticals).
W/Atropine sulfate, A.P.C., camphor.
See: Dasin, Cap. (SmithKline Beecham Pharmaceuticals).

Dovonex. (Westwood Squibb Pharmaceuticals) Calcipotreine 0.005% alcohols, EDTA, mineral oil. Oint. Tube 30, 60 or 100 g. Soln. Bot. 50 ml. Cream Tube 30, 60, 100 g. *Rx.*
Use: Dermatologic, antipsoriatic.

Dowicil 200.
See: Derma Soap (Ferndale Laboratories, Inc.).

Dow-Isoniazid. (Hoechst Marion Roussel) Isoniazid 300 mg/Tab. Bot. 30s. *Rx.*
Use: Antituberculousal.

•**doxacurium chloride.** (dox-ah-cure-ee-uhm) USAN.
Use: Neuromuscular blocker.
See: Nuromax (GlaxoWellcome).

Doxamin. (Forest Pharmaceutical, Inc.) Thiamine HCl 100 mg, vitamin B_6 100 mg/ml. Vial 10 ml. *Rx.*
Use: Vitamin supplement.

Doxapap-N. (Major Pharmaceuticals) Propoxyphene napsylate 100 mg, acetaminophen 650 mg. Tab. Bot. 100s, 500s. *c-IV.*
Use: Analgesic combination, narcotic.

Doxaphene Capsules. (Major Pharmaceuticals) Propoxyphene HCl 65 mg/Cap. Bot. 1000s. *c-IV.*
Use: Analgesic, narcotic.

Doxaphene Compound 65 Caps. (Major Pharmaceuticals) Propoxyphene HCl, acetaminophen. Cap. Bot. 1000s. *c-IV.*
Use: Analgesic combination, narcotic.

•**doxapram hydrochloride.** (DOX-uh-pram) U.S.P. 23.
Use: Respiratory and CNS stimulant.
See: Dopram, Vial (Wyeth-Ayerst Laboratories).

doxapram hydrochloride. (Various Mfr.) 20 mg/ml. Benzyl alcohol. Inj. Vial. 20 ml.
Use: Respiratory and CNS stimulant.

•**doxaprost.** (DOX-ah-proste) USAN.
Use: Bronchodilator.

Doxate. Docusate sodium. *otc.*
Use: Laxative.

•**doxazosin mesylate.** (DOX-uh-ZOE-sin) USAN.
Use: Antihypertensive.
See: Cardura, Tab. (Roerig).

•**doxepin hydrochloride.** (DOX-uh-pin) U.S.P. 23.
Use: Psychotherapeutic agent, antidepressant.
See: Sinequan, Cap. (Roerig).

doxepin hydrochloride. (Various Mfr.) Doxepin HCl 10 mg, 25 mg, 50 mg, 75 mg, 100 mg, 150 mg/Cap. Bot. 100s, 500s, 1000s, UD 100s; 10 mg/ml Oral Conc. Bot. 120 ml. *Rx.*
Use: Anxiolytic.

Doxidan. (Hoechst Marion Roussel) Yellow phenolphthalein 65 mg, docusate calcium 60 mg/Cap. Bot. 30s, 100s, 1000s, UD 100s, Display Pack 10s. *otc.*
Use: Laxative.

Doxil. (Sequus Pharmaceuticals, Inc.) Doxorubicin HCl 20 mg. Inj. Vial 10 ml. *Rx.*
Use: Antibiotic.

•**doxofylline.** (DOX-oh-fill-een) USAN.
Use: Bronchodilator.

•**doxorubicin.** (DOX-oh-ROO-bih-sin) USAN.
Use: Antineoplastic.

•**doxorubicin hydrochloride.** (DOX-oh-ROO-bih-sin) U.S.P. 23.
Use: Antineoplastic.
See: Adriamycin, Inj. (Pharmacia & Upjohn).
Rubex, Pow. for Inj. (Bristol-Myers Oncology/Immunology).

doxorubicin HCl. (Bedford Labs) Doxorubicin HCl. **Pow. for Inj.: 10 mg::** w/lactose 50 mg. **20 mg:** w/lactose 100 mg. **50 mg:** w/lactose 250 mg. Vial. **Inj., aqueous:** 2 mg/ml, sodium chloride 0.9%. Vial 5 ml, 10 ml, 25 ml. *Rx.*
Use: Antibiotic.

•**doxpicomine hydrochloride.** (DOX-PIH-koe-meen) USAN. *Formerly Doxpicodin hydrochloride.*
Use: Analgesic.

Doxy 100. (Fujisawa USA, Inc.) Doxycycline hyclate for injection. Pow. 100 mg/Vial. *Rx.*
Use: Anti-infective, tetracycline.

Doxy 200. (Fujisawa USA, Inc.) Doxycycline hyclate. Pow. 200 mg/Vial. *Rx.*
Use: Anti-infective, tetracycline.

Doxy Caps. (Edwards Pharmaceuticals, Inc.) Doxycycline hyclate 100 mg/Cap. Bot. 50s. *Rx.*
Use: Anti-infective, tetracycline.

Doxychel Capsules. (Houba Inc.) Doxycycline hyclate 50 mg or 100 mg/Cap. Bot. 50s, 500s, UD 100s. *Rx.*
Use: Anti-infective, tetracycline.

Doxychel Injectable. (Houba Inc.) Doxycycline hyclate 100 mg or 200 mg/Vial. *Rx.*
Use: Anti-infective, tetracycline.

Doxychel Tablets. (Houba Inc.) Doxycycline hyclate 50 mg or 100 mg/Tab. Bot. 50s, 500s. *Rx.*
Use: Anti-infective, tetracycline.

•**doxycycline.** (DOX-ee-SIGH-kleen) U.S.P. 23.
Use: Anti-infective.
See: Monodox (Oclassen).
Vibramycin for Oral Susp. (Pfizer US Pharmaceutical Group).
Vibramycin IV. (Roerig).

•**doxycycline calcium oral suspension.** (DOX-ee-SIGH-kleen) U.S.P. 23.
Use: Anti-infective, antiprotozoal.

•**doxycycline fosfatex.** (DOX-ee-SIGH-kleen foss-FAH-tex) USAN.
Use: Anti-infective.

•**doxycycline hyclate.** (DOX-ee-SIGH-kleen HIGH-klate) U.S.P. 23.
Use: Anti-infective.
See: Bio-Tab, Tab. (International Ethical Labs).
Doxy Caps, Cap. (Edwards Pharmaceuticals, Inc.).
Periostat (CollaGenex).
Vibra-Tabs, Tab. (Pfizer US Pharmaceutical Group).
Vibramycin, Cap., Tab., Vial (Pfizer US Pharmaceutical Group).

•**doxylamine succinate.** U.S.P. 23.
Use: Antihistamine.
See: Decapryn, Prep. (Hoechst Marion Roussel).
Unisom, Tab. (Pfizer US Pharmaceutical Group).
W/Acetominophen, ephedrine sulfate, dextromethorphan HBr, alcohol.
See: Nyquil, Liq. (Vicks).
W/Dextromethorphan HBr, alcohol.
See: Consotuss Antitussive, Syr. (Hoechst Marion Roussel).
W/Dextromethorphan HBr, sodium citrate, alcohol.
See: Vicks Formula 44 Cough Mixture, Syr. (Procter & Gamble Pharm.).

doxylamine succinate w/combinations.
See: Night Time Cold/Flu Relief (Pro-Metic Pharma.).
Vicks NyQuil Multi-Symptom Cold Flu Relief (Procter & Gamble).

Doxy-Lemmon Capsules. (Teva Pharmaceuticals USA) Doxycycline hyclate equivalent to 100 mg of doxycycline base/Cap. Bot. 50s, 500s, UD 100s. *Rx.*
Use: Anti-infective, tetracycline.

Doxy-Lemmon Tablets. (Teva Pharmaceuticals USA) Doxycycline hyclate equivalent to 100 mg doxycycline base/Tab. Bot. 50s, 500s, UD 100s. *Rx.*
Use: Anti-infective, tetracycline.

Doxy-Tabs. (Houba Inc.) Doxycycline hyclate 100 mg/FC Tab. Bot. 50s, 500s. *Rx.*
Use: Anti-infective, tetracycline.

Doxy-Tabs-50. (Houba Inc.) 50 mg/Tab. Bot. 50s. *Rx.*
Use: Anti-infective, tetracycline.

DPPC. Colfosceril palmitate. *Rx.*
Use: Lung surfactant.
See: Exosurf Neonatal (Glaxo-Wellcome).

•**draflazine.** (DRAFF-lah-ZEEN) USAN.
Use: Cardioprotectant.

Dramamine II. (Pharmacia & Upjohn) Meclizine HCl 25 mg, lactose/Tab. Pkg. 8s. *otc.*
Use: Antiemetic, antivertigo.

Dramamine, Children's. (Pharmacia & Upjohn) Dimenhydrinate 12.5 mg/5 ml, alcohol 5%, sucrose. Liq. Bot. 120 ml. *otc.*
Use: Antiemetic, antivertigo.

Dramamine Liquid. (Pharmacia & Upjohn) Dimenhydrinate 12.5 mg/4 ml Bot. 90 ml, pt. *otc.*
Use: Antiemetic, antivertigo.

Dramamine Tablets. (Pharmacia & Upjohn) Dimenhydrinate 50 mg/Tab. Bot. 36s, 100s, 1000s, Blister pkg. 12s, UD 100s. *otc.*
Use: Antiemetic, antivertigo.

Dramanate. (Taylor Pharmaceuticals) Dimenhydrinate 50 mg/ml. Inj. Vial 10 ml. *Rx.*
Use: Antiemetic, antivertigo.

dramarin.
See: Dramamine, Preps. (Searle).

dramyl.

See: Dramamine, Preps. (Searle).

Drawing Salve. (Whiteworth Towne) Tube oz. *otc.*
Use: Dermatologic, wound therapy.

Drawing Salve with Triquinodin. (Towne) Tube 2 oz. *otc.*
Use: Dermatologic, wound therapy.

Dr. Berry's Skin Toner. (Last) Hydroquinone 2%. Jar Oz. *Rx.*
Use: Dermatologic.

Dr. Brown's Home Drug Testing System. (Personal Health and Hygiene) 1 urine specimen collection kit for detecting drugs of abuse (marijuana, cocaine, amphetamine, methamphetamine, phencyclidine, codeine, morphine, heroin). Kit 1s. *otc.*
Use: Diagnostic aid.

Dr. Caldwell Senna Laxative. (Mentholatum Co., Inc.) Senna 7%, alcohol 4.5%. Bot. 130 ml, 360 ml. *otc.*
Use: Laxative.

DRC Peri-Anal Cream. (Xttrium Laboratories, Inc.) Lassar's paste 37.5%, anhydrous lanolin, U.S.P. 37.5%, cold cream 25%. Tube 5 oz. *otc.*
Use: Dermatologic protectant, perianal.

Dr. Dermi-Heal. (Quality Formulations, Inc.) Zinc oxide 25%, allantoin 1%, peruvian balsam, castor oil, white petrolatum. Oint. Tube 75 g. *otc.*
Use: Astringent.

Dr. Drake's Cough Medicine. (Last) Dextromethorphan HBr 10 mg/5 ml Bot. 2 oz. *otc.*
Use: Antitussive.

•**dribendazole.** (dry-BEN-dah-ZOLE) USAN.
Use: Anthelmintic.

Dri-A Caps. (Barth's) Vitamin A 10,000 IU/Cap. Bot. 100s, 500s. *otc.*
Use: Vitamin supplement.

Dri A & D Caps. (Barth's) Vitamins A 10,000 IU, D 400 IU/Cap. Bot. 100s, 500s. *otc.*
Use: Vitamin supplement.

Dri-E. (Barth's) Vitamin E. **100 IU/Cap.:** Bot. 100s, 500s, 1000s. **200 IU/Cap.:** Bot. 100s, 250s, 500s. **400 IU/Cap:** Bot. 100s, 250s. *otc.*
Use: Vitamin supplement.

Dri/Ear. (Pfeiffer Co.) Boric acid 2.75% in isopropyl alcohol. Soln. Dropper Bot. 30 ml. *otc.*
Use: Otic.

dried aluminum hydroxide gel.
Use: Antacid.
See: Aluminum Hydroxide Gel, dried.

dried yeast.
See: Yeast, dried.

Driminate Tabs. (Major Pharmaceuticals) Dimenhydrinate 50 mg/Tab. Bot. 100s, 1000s. *otc.*
Use: Antiemetic, antivertigo.

•**drinidene.** (DRIH-nih-deen) USAN.
Use: Analgesic.

Drisdol Drops. (Sanofi Winthrop Pharmaceuticals) Ergocalciferol (Vitamin D_2) 8000 IU/ml in propylene glycol. Bot. 60 ml. *otc.*
Use: Refractory rickets, hypophosphatemia, hypoparathyroidism.

Drisdol 50,000 Unit Capsules. (Sanofi Winthrop Pharmaceuticals) Vitamin D_2, 50,000 IU/Cap. Bot. 50s. *Rx.*
Use: Refractory rickets, hypophosphatemia, hypoparathyroidism.

Dristan 12 Hour. (Whitehall Robins Laboratories) Chlorpheniramine maleate 4 mg, phenylephrine HCl 20 mg/Cap. Bot. 6s, 10s, 15s. *otc.*
Use: Antihistamine, decongestant.

Dristan Allergy. (Whitehall Robins Laboratories) Pseudoephedrine HCl 60 mg, brompheniramine maleate 4 mg/Cap. Bot. 20s. *otc.*
Use: Antihistamine, decongestant.

Dristan Capsules. (Whitehall Robins Laboratories) Phenylephrine HCl 5 mg, chlorpheniramine maleate 2 mg, acetaminophen 325 mg/Cap. Bot. 16s, 36s, 75s. *otc.*
Use: Analgesic, antihistamine, decongestant.

Dristan Cold. (Whitehall Robins Laboratories) Pseudoephedrine HCl 30 mg, acetaminophen 500 mg/Capl. Bot. 20s, 40s. *otc.*
Use: Analgesic, decongestant.

Dristan Cold & Flu. (Whitehall Robins Laboratories) Acetaminophen 500 mg, pseudoephedrine HCl 60 mg, chlorpheniramine maleate 4 mg, dextromethorphan HBr 20 mg/Pow. Pkts. 6s. *otc.*
Use: Analgesic, antihistamine, antitussive, decongestant.

Dristan Cold Multi-Symptom Formula. (Whitehall Robins Laboratories) Phenylephrine HCl 5 mg, chlorpheniramine maleate 2 mg, acetaminophen 325 mg/Tab. Bot. 20s, 40s, 75s. *otc.*
Use: Analgesic, antihistamine, decongestant.

Dristan Juice Mix-In. (Whitehall Robins Laboratories) Acetaminophen 500 mg, pseudoephedrine HCl 60 mg, dextromethorphan 20 mg/Pow. Pkts. 5s. *otc.*
Use: Analgesic, antitussive, decongestant.

Dristan 12-Hr Nasal. (Whitehall Robins Laboratories) Oxymetazoline HCl

0.05%, benzalkonium Cl 1:5000, thimerosal 0.002%, hydroxypropylmethylcellulose. Spray. Bot. 15 ml, 30 ml. *otc.*
Use: Decongestant, nasal.

Dristan Maximum Strength. (Whitehall Robins Laboratories) Pseudoephedrine HCl 30 mg, acetaminophen 500 mg/Capl. Bot. 24s. *otc.*
Use: Analgesic, decongestant.

Dristan Menthol Nasal Mist. (Whitehall Robins Laboratories) Phenylephrine HCl 0.5%, pheniramine maleate 0.2%. Bot. 0.5 oz, 1 oz. *otc.*
Use: Antihistamine, decongestant.

Dristan Nasal Mist. (Whitehall Robins Laboratories) Phenylephrine HCl 0.5%, pheniramine maleate 0.2%. Bot. 15 ml, 30 ml. *otc.*
Use: Antihistamine, decongestant.

Dristan No Drowsiness Cold. (Whitehall Robins Laboratories) Pseudoephedrine HCl 30 mg, acetaminophen 500 mg/Cap. Bot. 20s. *otc.*
Use: Analgesic, decongestant.

Dristan Saline Spray. (Whitehall Robins Laboratories) Sodium chloride. Soln. Bot. 15 ml.
Use: Nasal product.

Dristan Sinus. (Whitehall Robins Laboratories) Pseudoephedrine HCl 30 mg, ibuprofen 200 mg/Cap. Pkg. 20s. Bot. 24s, 40s. *otc.*
Use: Analgesic, decongestant.

Dritho Creme. (Dermik Laboratories, Inc.) Anthralin 0.1%, 0.25%, 0.5%. Tube 50 g. *Rx.*
Use: Antipsoriatic.

Dritho Creme HP 1.0%. (Dermik Laboratories, Inc.) Anthralin 1%. Tube 50 g. *Rx.*
Use: Antipsoriatic.

Dritho-Scalp. (Dermik Laboratories, Inc.) Anthralin 0.25%, 0.5%. Tube 50 g. *Rx.*
Use: Antipsoriatic.

Drixomed. (Iomed) Dexbrompheniramine maleate 6 mg, pseudoephedrine sulfate 120 mg/SR Tab. Bot. 100s, 500s. *Rx.*
Use: Antihistamine, decongestant.

Drixoral. (Schering-Plough Corp.) Dexbrompheniramine maleate 6 mg, pseudoephedrine sulfate 120 mg. SA Tab. Box 10s, 20s, 40s. Bot. 48s, 100s. *otc.*
Use: Antihistamine, decongestant.

Drixoral. (Schering-Plough Corp.) Pseudoephedrine sulfate 30 mg, brompheniramine maleate 2 mg, sorbitol, sugar. Syrup. Bot. 118 ml. *otc.*
Use: Antihistamine, decongestant.

Drixoral Cold & Allergy. (Schering-Plough Corp.) Dexbrompheniramine maleate 6 mg, pseudoephedrine sulfate 120 mg/SR Tab. Pkg. 10s. *otc.*
Use: Antihistamine, decongestant.

Drixoral Cold & Flu. (Schering-Plough Corp.) Pseudoephedrine HCl 60 mg, dexbrompheniramine maleate 3 mg, acetaminophen 500 mg/Tab. Bot. 12s, 24s, 48s. *otc.*
Use: Analgesic, antihistamine, decongestant.

Drixoral Cough & Congestion Liquid Caps. (Schering-Plough Corp.) Pseudoephedrine HCl 60 mg, dextromethorphan HBr 30 mg/Cap. Pkg. 10s. *otc.*
Use: Antihistamine, decongestant.

Drixoral Cough & Sore Throat Liquid Caps. (Schering-Plough Corp.) Dextromethorphan HBr 15 mg, acetaminophen 325 mg, sorbitol. Cap. Pkg. 10s. *otc.*
Use: Analgesic, antitussive.

Drixoral Non-Drowsy Formula. (Schering-Plough Corp.) Pseudoephedrine sulfate 120 mg, sugar. Tab. Pkg. 10s, 20s. *otc.*
Use: Decongestant.

Drixoral Plus. (Schering-Plough Corp.) Pseudoephedrine sulfate 60 mg, dexbrompheniramine maleate 3 mg, acetaminophen 500 mg/TR Tab. Bot. 12s, 24s. *otc.*
Use: Analgesic, antihistamine, decongestant.

Drixoral Sustained-Action. (Schering-Plough Corp.) Pseudoephedrine sulfate 120 mg, dexbrompheniramine maleate 6 mg, sugar, lactose. Tab. Pkg. 10s. Bot. 20s, 40s. *otc.*
Use: Antihistamine, decongestant.

Drize. (Jones Medical Industries, Inc.) Phenylpropanolamine HCl 75 mg, chlorpheniramine maleate 12 mg/SR Cap. Bot. 100s. *Rx.*
Use: Antihistamine, decongestant.

•**drobuline.** (DROE-byoo-leen) USAN.
Use: Cardiovascular agent (antiarrhythmic).

•**drocinonide.** (droe-SIN-oh-nide) USAN.
Use: Anti-inflammatory.

drocode.
See: Dihydrocodeine.

•**droloxifene.** (drole-OX-ih-feen) USAN.
Use: Antineoplastic.

•**droloxifene citrate.** (drole-OX-ih-feen) USAN.
Use: Antineoplastic.

•**drometrizole.** (DROE-meh-TRY-zole) USAN.

Use: Ultraviolet screen.

•**dromostanolone propionate.** (DRAHM-oh-STAN-oh-lone) USAN. U.S.P. XX.
Use: Antineoplastic.

•**dronabinol.** (droe-NAB-ih-nahl) U.S.P. 23.
Use: Antiemetic. [Orphan Drug]
See: Marinol, Gel Cap. (Roxane Laboratories, Inc.).

drop chalk. (Various Mfr.) Calcium carbonate, prepared. Prepared chalk.

•**droperidol.** (dro-PER-i-dahl) U.S.P. 23.
Use: Antipsychotic; anxiolytic.
See: Inapsine, Inj. (Janssen Pharmaceutical, Inc.).
Innovar, Inj. (Janssen Pharmaceutical, Inc.).

•**droprenilamine.** (droe-preh-NILL-ah-meen) USAN.
Use: Vasodilator (coronary).

•**drospirenone.** (droe-SPYE-reh-nohn) USAN.
Use: Contraceptive, oral.

Drotic Sterile Otic Solution. (B.F. Ascher and Co.) Hydrocortisone 10 mg (1%), polymyxin B sulfate 10,000 units, neomycin 5 mg/ml, preservatives. Dropper bot. 10 ml. *Rx.*
Use: Otic.

•**droxacin sodium.** (DROX-ah-sin) USAN.
Use: Anti-infective.

•**droxifilcon a.** (DROX-ih-fill-kahn A) USAN.
Use: Contact lens material (hydrophilic).

•**droxinavir hydrochloride.** (drox-IN-ah-veer HIGH-droe-KLOR-ide) USAN.
Use: Antiviral.

Dr. Scholl's Advanced Pain Relief Corn Removers. (Schering-Plough Corp.) Salicylic acid 40% in a rubber-based vehicle. Disc. 6s. *otc.*
Use: Keratolytic.

Dr. Scholl's Athlete's Foot. (Schering-Plough Corp.) **Pow.:** Tolnaftate 1%. Talc. Bot. 63 g. **Spray Liq.:** Tolnaftate 1%, alcohol 36%. Bot. 113 ml. *otc.*
Use: Antifungal, topical.

Dr. Scholl's Athlete's Foot Cream. (Schering-Plough Corp.) Tolnaftate 1%. Tube 0.5 oz. *otc.*
Use: Antifungal, topical.

Dr. Scholl's Callus Removers. (Schering-Plough Corp.) Salicylic acid 40% in a rubber-based vehicle. 6 pads, 4 discs. Extra thick in 4 discs. *otc.*
Use: Keratolytic.

Dr. Scholl's Clear Away. (Schering-Plough Corp.) Salicylic acid 40% in a rubber-based vehicle. Disc 18s. *otc.*
Use: Keratolytic.

Dr. Scholl's Clear Away One Step. (Schering-Plough Corp.) Salicylic acid 40% in a rubber-based vehicle. Strip 14s. *otc.*
Use: Keratolytic.

Dr. Scholl's Clear Away Plantar. (Schering-Plough Corp.) Salicylic acid 40% in a rubber-based vehicle. Disc 24s. *otc.*
Use: Keratolytic.

Dr. Scholl's Corn/Callus Remover. (Schering-Plough Corp.) Salicylic acid 12.6% in a flexible collodion, alcohol 18%, ether 55%, hydrogenated vegetable oil. Liq. 10 ml with 3 cushions. *otc.*
Use: Keratolytic.

Dr. Scholl's Corn/Callus Salve. (Schering-Plough Corp.) Salicylic acid 15%. Tube 0.4 oz. *otc.*
Use: Keratolytic.

Dr. Scholl's Corn Remover. (Schering-Plough Corp.) Salicylic acid 40% in a rubber-based vehicle. Discs: 6s as wrap-arounds, 9s as ultra thin, small, waterproof, regular, soft, and extra-thick. *otc.*
Use: Keratolytic.

Dr. Scholl's Corn Salve. (Schering-Plough Corp.) Salicylic acid 15%. Jar 0.4 oz. *otc.*
Use: Keratolytic.

Dr. Scholl's Cracked Heel Relief. (Schering-Plough Corp.) Lidocaine 2%, benzalkonium Cl 0.13%. Cream 5.6 g. *otc.*
Use: Anesthetic, local.

Dr. Scholl's Ingrown Toenail Reliever. (Schering-Plough Corp.) Sodium sulfide 1%. Bot. 0.33 oz. *otc.*
Use: Foot preparation.

Dr. Scholl's Maximum Strength Tritan. (Schering-Plough Corp.) Tolnaftate 1%. **Pow.:** Talc, Bot. 56 g. **Spray Pow.:** SD alcohol 40 14%. Bot. 85 g. *otc.*
Use: Antifungal, topical.

Dr. Scholl's Moisturizing Corn Remover Kit. (Schering-Plough Corp.) Salicylic acid 40% in a rubber-based vehicle, moisturizing cream, pain relief cushions. Disc 6s. *otc.*
Use: Keratolytic.

Dr. Scholl's One Step Corn Removers. (Schering-Plough Corp.) Salicylic acid 40% in a rubber-based vehicle. Strips 6s. *otc.*
Use: Keratolytic.

Dr. Scholl's Pro Comfort Jock Itch Spray. (Schering-Plough Corp.) Tolnaftate 1%. Aerosol Can 3.5 oz. *otc.*
Use: Antifungal, topical.

Dr. Scholl's Wart Remover Kit. (Scher-

ing-Plough Corp.) Salicylic acid 17% in a flexible collodion, alcohol 17%, ether 52%. Liq. 10 ml with brush and 6 adhesive pads. *otc.*
Use: Keratolytic.

Dr. Scholl's Zino Pads/with Medicated Disks. (Schering-Plough Corp.) Salicylic acid 20% or 40%. Protective pads designed for use with and without salicylic acid-impregnated disks. *otc.*
Use: Keratolytic.

Drucon. (Standard Drug Co.) Phenylephrine HCl 5 mg, chlorpheniramine maleate 2 mg, menthol 1 mg, alcohol 5%/5 ml Elix. Bot. Pt, gal. *otc.*
Use: Antihistamine, decongestant.

Drucon C R. (Standard Drug Co.) Phenylephrine HCl 25 mg, chlorpheniramine maleate 4 mg/Tab. Bot. 100s. *otc.*
Use: Antihistamine, decongestant.

Drucon with Codeine. (Standard Drug Co.) Codeine phosphate 10 mg, phenylephrine HCl 10 mg, chlorpheniramine maleate 2 mg, menthol 1 mg, alcohol 5%/5 ml. Bot. Pt. *c-v.*
Use: Antihistamine, antitussive, decongestant.

Dry Eyes. (Bausch & Lomb Pharmaceuticals) White petrolatum, mineral oil, lanolin. Oint. Tube 3.5 g. *otc.*
Use: Lubricant, ophthalmic.

Dry Eyes Solution. (Bausch & Lomb Pharmaceuticals) Polyvinyl alcohol 1.4%, benzalkonium Cl 0.01%, sodium phosphate, EDTA, NaCl. Ophth. Soln. Bot. 15 ml. *otc.*
Use: Lubricant, ophthalmic.

Dry Eye Therapy. (Bausch & Lomb Pharmaceuticals) Glycerin 0.3%, potassium Cl, sodium Cl, sodium citrate, sodium phosphate, zinc Cl. Drop. Single-use Bot. 0.3 ml (UD 32s). *otc.*
Use: Ophthalmic.

Dryox 2.5, 10. (C & M Pharmacal, Inc.) Benzoyl peroxide 2.5%, 5%, 10%, 20%. Gel. Tube. 30 g, 60 g. *otc.*
Use: Dermatologic, acne.

Dryox 20S 5. (C & M Pharmacal, Inc.) Benzoyl peroxide 20%, sulfur 10%, methylparaben. Gel. Tube. 30 g, 60 g. *otc.*
Use: Dermatologic, acne.

Dry Skin Creme. (Gordon Laboratories) Cetyl alcohol, lubricating oils in a water-soluble base. Jar 2 oz, 1 lb, 5 lb. *otc.*
Use: Emollient.

Drysol. (Person and Covey, Inc.) Aluminum Cl hexahydrate 20% in 93% SD alcohol 40. Bot. 37.5 ml. *Rx.*
Use: Astringent.

Drysum Shampoo. (Summers Laboratories, Inc.) Alcohol 15%, acetone 6%. Plastic bot. 4 oz. *otc.*
Use: Dermatologic, hair.

Drytergent. (C & M Pharmacal, Inc.) TEA-dodecylbenzenesulfonate, boric acid, lauramide DEA, propylene glycol, tartrazine, purified water, color, fragrance. Liq. Bot. 240 ml, 480 ml. *otc.*
Use: Dermatologic, acne.

Drytex. (C & M Pharmacal, Inc.) Salicylic acid 2%, benzalkonium Cl 0.1%, acetone 10%, isopropyl alcohol 40%, tartrazine. Lot. Bot. 240 ml. *otc.*
Use: Dermatologic, acne.

DSMC Plus. (Geneva Pharmaceuticals) Docusate potassium 100 mg. Cap. Bot. 100s. *otc.*
Use: Laxative.

DSS. (Dioctyl sodium sulfosuccinate) Docusate sodium. *otc.*
Use: Laxative.
See: Colace, Cap. (Bristol-Myers Squibb).
Docusate Sodium, Cap. (Various Mfr.).
DOK, Cap. (Major Pharmaceuticals).
DOS, Softgel, Cap. (Zenith Goldline Pharmaceuticals).
D-S-S, Cap. (Warner Chilcott Laboratories).
Modane Soft, Cap. (Pharmacia & Upjohn).
Pro-Sof, Cap. (Vangard Labs, Inc).

D-S-S. (Warner Chilcott Laboratories) Docusate sodium 100 mg/Cap. Bot. 100s, 1000s and UD 100s. *otc.*
Use: Laxative, stool softener.

DST. Dihydrostreptomycin.
See: Dihydrostreptomycin, Preps. (Various Mfr.).

D-Test 100. (Burgin-Arden) Testosterone cypionate 100 mg/ml. Vial 10 ml. *c-III.*
Use: Androgen.

D-Test 200. (Burgin-Arden) Testosterone cypionate 200 mg/ml. Vial 10 ml. *c-III.*
Use: Androgen.

DTIC. Dacarbazine. *Rx.*
Use: Antineoplastic.
See: DTIC-Dome, Inj. (Bayer Corp. (Consumer Div.)).

DTIC-Dome. (Bayer Corp. (Consumer Div.)) Dacarbazine 10 mg/ml. Inj. Vial 10 ml, 20 ml. *Rx.*
Use: Antineoplastic.

DTP. Diphtheria and tetanus toxoids and pertussis vaccine, adsorbed. *Rx.*
Use: Immunization.
See: Acel-Imune, Vial (Wyeth Lederle).
Diphtheria and Tetanus Toxoids and whole-cell Pertussis Vaccine, Inj.

(Pasteur Merieux Connaught, Massachusetts Public Health Biologic Labs) Infanarix (SKB).
DTwP, Inj. (Michigan Dept of Public Health/SmithKline Beecham Pharmaceuticals).
Tri-Immunol, Vial, Inj. (Wyeth Lederle).
Tripedia, Vial (Pasteur Merieux Connaught).

DTwP. (Michigan Department of Health; SmithKline Beecham Pharmaceuticals) 10 Lf units diphtheria, 5.5 Lf units tetanus and 4 Lf units pertussis/0.5 ml. Vial 5 ml. *Rx*.
Use: Immunization.

Duadacin. (Kenwood Laboratories) Phenylpropanolamine HCl 12.5 mg, chlorpheniramine maleate 2 mg, acetaminophen 325 mg/Cap. Bot. 100s, 1000s. Dispense-A-Pak 1000s. *otc*.
Use: Analgesic, antihistamine, decongestant.

Dual-Wet. (Alcon, Vision Care) Polyvinyl alcohol, duasorb water-soluble polymetric system, benzalkonium Cl 0.01%, disodium edetate 0.05%. Bot. 2 oz. *otc*.
Use: Contact lens care.

•**duazomycin.** (doo-AZE-oh-MY-sin) USAN. Antibiotic isolated from broth filtrates of *Streptomyces ambofaciens*.
Use: Antineoplastic.

Duazomycin A. Name used for Duazomycin.
Use: Antineoplastic.

Duazomycin B. Name used for Azotomycin.
Use: Antineoplastic.

Duazomycin C. Name used for Ambomycin.
Use: Antineoplastic.

Dulcagen Suppositories. (Zenith Goldline Pharmaceuticals) Bisacodyl 10 mg/Supp. Box 12s, 100s. *otc*.
Use: Laxative.

Dulcagen Tablets. (Zenith Goldline Pharmaceuticals) Bisacodyl 5 mg/Tab. Bot. 100s. *otc*.
Use: Laxative.

Dulcolax. (Novartis Consumer Health) Bisacodyl. **EC Tab.:** 5 mg. Box 10s, 25s, 50s, 100s. Bot. 1000s, UD 100s. **Supp.:** 10 mg. Box 2s, 4s, 8s, 50s, 500s. **Bowel Prep Kit:** 4 tab., 1 supp./Kit. 5s/box. *otc*.
Use: Laxative.

Dull-C. (Freeda Vitamins, Inc.) Ascorbic acid 4 g/tsp. Pow. Bot. 100 g, 500 g, 1000 g. *otc*.
Use: Vitamin supplement.

•**duloxetine hydrochloride.** (doo-LOX-eh-teen) USAN.
Use: Antidepressant.

Dulphalac. (Solvay Pharmaceuticals) Lactulose 10 g/5 ml. Syr. Bot. 240 ml, 480 ml, 960 ml, UD 30 ml. *Rx*.
Use: Laxative.

Duo. (SmithKline Beecham Pharmaceuticals) Tube 0.5 oz.
Use: Adhesive.

Duocet. (Mason Pharmaceuticals, Inc.) Hydrocodone bitartrate 5 mg, acetaminophen 500 mg/Tab. Bot. 100s. *c-III*.
Use: Analgesic combination, narcotic.

Duo-Cyp. (Keene Pharmaceuticals, Inc.) Testosterone cypionate 50 mg, estradiol cypionate 2 mg/ml. Vial 10 ml. *Rx*.
Use: Androgen, estrogen combination.

DuoDerm. (ConvaTec) **Sterile dressing:** 10 cm × 10 cm. Pack 5s. 20 cm × 20 cm. Pack 3s. **Sterile gran:** Packet 4 g. Pack 5s. *otc*.
Use: Dermatologic, wound therapy.

Duoderm Extra Thin. (ConvaTec) Flexible hydroactive sterile dressings. 4″ × 4″, 6″ × 6″. Pck. 10s. *otc*.
Use: Dressing, topical.

DuoFilm. (Stiefel Laboratories, Inc.) Salicylic acid 16.7%, lactic acid 16.7% in flexible collodion. Bot. 15 ml w/applicator. *otc*.
Use: Keratolytic.

Duo-Flow. (Ciba Vision) Poloxamer 188, benzalkonium Cl 0.013%, EDTA 0.25%. Soln. Bot. 120 ml. *otc*.
Use: Contact lens care.

Duo-K. (Various Mfr.) Potassium 20 mEq, chloride 3.4 mEq/15 ml (from potassium gluconate and potassium Cl). Bot. Pt, gal. *Rx*.
Use: Mineral supplement.

Duolube. (Bausch & Lomb Pharmaceuticals) White petrolatum, mineral oil. Sterile, preservative and lanolin free. Oint. Tube 3.5 g. *otc*.
Use: Lubricant, ophthalmic.

duomycin.
See: Aureomycin, Preps. (ESI Lederle Generics).

•**duoperone fumarate.** (DOO-oh-per-OHN) USAN.
Use: Neuroleptic.

DuoPlant. (Stiefel Laboratories, Inc.) Salicylic acid 27%, alcohol 50%, flexible collodion, hydroxypropyl cellulose, lactic acid. Liq. Bot. 14 g. *otc*.
Use: Ketatolytic (wart removal).

Duosol. (Kirkman Sales Co., Inc.) Docusate sodium 100 mg or 250 mg/Cap. Bot. 100s, 1000s. *otc*.
Use: Laxative.

Duotal. (Health for Life Brands, Inc.) 1.5 gr: Secobarbital sodium ¾ gr, amobarbital gr/Cap. 3 gr: Secobarbital sodium 1.5 gr, amobarbital 1.5 gr/Cap. Bot. 100s, 500s, 1000s. *c-II.*
Use: Hypnotic, sedative.

duotal.
See: Guaiacol Carbonate (Various Mfr.).

Duo-Trach Kit. (Astra Pharmaceuticals, L.P.) Lidocaine HCl 4%. Inj. 5 ml disp. syringe with laryngotracheal cannula. *Rx.*
Use: Anesthetic, local.

Duotrate 30. (Jones Medical Industries, Inc.) Pentaerythritol tetranitrate 30 mg/SR Cap. Bot. 100s. *Rx.*
Use: Antianginal.

Duotrate 45. (Jones Medical Industries, Inc.) Pentaerythritol tetranitrate 45 mg/SR Cap. Bot. 100s. *Rx.*
Use: Antianginal.

Duovin-S. (Spanner) Estrone 2.5 mg, progesterone 25 mg/ml. Vial 10 ml. *Rx.*
Use: Estrogen, progestin combination.

Duo-WR, No. 1 & No. 2. (Whorton Pharmaceuticals, Inc.) **No. 1:** Salicylic acid, compound tincture benzoin. **No. 2:** Compound tincture benzoin, formaldehyde. Bot. 0.25 oz. *otc.*
Use: Keratolytic.

Duphalac. (Solvay Pharmaceuticals) Lactulose 10 g/15 ml (< 2.2 g galactose, 1.2 g lactose, 1.2 g or less of other sugars). Syr. Bot. 240 ml, pt, qt, UD 30 ml. *Rx.*
Use: Laxative.

Duplast. (Beiersdorf, Inc.) Adhesive coated elastic cloth. 8″ × 4″ Strip. Box 10s. 10″ × 5″; Strip. Box 8s, 10s.

Duplex. (C & M Pharmacal, Inc.) Sodium lauryl sulfate 15%, lauramide DEA. Shampoo. Bot. Pt. gal. *otc.*
Use: Dermatologic, cleanser.

Duplex Shampoo. (C & M Pharmacal, Inc.) Sodium lauryl sulfate 15%, lauramide DEA, purified water. Bot. Pt, gal. *otc.*
Use: Dermatologic.

Duplex T Shampoo. (C & M Pharmacal, Inc.) Sodium lauryl sulfate, purified water, lauramide DEA, solution of coal tar, alcohol 8.3%. Bot. Pt, gal. *otc.*
Use: Antiseborrheic.

duponol.
See: gardinol type detergents (Sodium Lauryl Sulfate) (Various Mfr.).

Durabolin. (Organon, Inc.) Nandrolone phenpropionate 25 mg/ml in sesame oil, benzyl alcohol 5%. Inj. Vial 5 ml. *c-III.*
Use: Anabolic steroid.
See: Deca-Durabolin, Inj. (Organon, Inc.).

Durabolin. (Organon, Inc.) Nandrolone phenpropionate 50 mg/ml in sterile sesame oil, benzyl alcohol 10%. Inj. Vial 2 ml. *c-III.*
Use: Anabolic steroid.

DURAcare. (Blairex Labs, Inc.) Buffered hypertonic salt solution, non-ionic detergents with thimerosal 0.004%, EDTA 0.1%. Soln. Bot. 30 ml. *otc.*
Use: Contact lens care.

DURAcare II. (Blairex Labs, Inc.) Buffered hypertonic, ethylene and propylene oxide, octylphenoxypolyethoxyethanol, lauryl sulfate salt of imidazoline, sodium bisulfite 0.1%, sorbic acid 0.1%, EDTA 0.25%. Soln. Bot. 30 ml. *otc.*
Use: Contact lens care.

Duraclon. (Fujisawa USA, Inc.) Clonidine HCl 100 mcg/ml. Inj. Vials. 10 ml. *Rx.*
Use: Analgesic.

Dura-Estrin. (Roberts Pharmaceuticals) Estradiol cypionate in oil 5 mg/ml. Inj. Vial 10 ml. *Rx.*
Use: Estrogen.

Duragen. (Roberts Pharmaceuticals) Estradiol valerate in oil 20 mg or 40 mg/ml. Inj. Vial 10 ml. *Rx.*
Use: Estrogen.

Duragesic. (Janssen Pharmaceutical, Inc.) Fentanyl 2.5 mg, 5 mg, 7.5 mg or 10 mg/transdermal patch. Carton 5s. *c-II.*
Use: Analgesic, narcotic.

Dura-Gest. (Dura Pharmaceuticals) Phenylpropanolamine HCl 45 mg, phenylephrine HCl 5 mg, guaifenesin 200 mg/Cap. Bot. 100s, 500s. *Rx.*
Use: Decongestant, expectorant.

Duralex. (American Urologicals, Inc.) Pseudoephedrine HCl 120 mg, chlorpheniramine maleate 8 mg/SR Cap. Bot. 100s, 1000s. *Rx.*
Use: Antihistamine, decongestant.

Duralone Injection. (Roberts Pharmaceuticals) Methylprednisolone acetate 40 mg or 80 mg/ml Susp. for Inj. **40 mg:** Vial 10 ml. **80 mg:** Vial 5 ml. *Rx.*
Use: Corticosteroid.

Duralutin Injection. (Roberts Pharmaceuticals) Hydroxyprogesterone caproate in oil 250 mg/ml. Vial 5 ml. *Rx.*
Use: Hormone, progesterone.

Dura-Meth. (Foy Laboratories) Methylprednisolone 40 mg/ml. Vial 5 ml, 10 ml. *Rx.*
Use: Corticosteroid.

Duramist Plus. (Pfeiffer Co.) Oxymeta-

zoline HCl 0.05%. Spray. 15 ml. *otc.*
Use: Decongestant.

Duramorph. (ESI Lederle Generics) Morphine sulfate 0.5 mg/ml or 1 mg/ml. Inj. Amp. 10 ml. Preservative free. *c-II.*
Use: Analgesic, narcotic.

Duranest. (Astra Pharmaceuticals, L.P.) Etidocaine HCl 1.5%, epinephrine 1:200,000, sodium metabisulfite. Dental cartridges 1.8 ml. *Rx.*
Use: Anesthetic, local.

Duranest-MPF. (Astra Pharmaceuticals, L.P.) Etidocaine. **1%:** w/epinephrine 1:200,000. Vial 30 ml. **1.5%:** w/epinephrine 1:200,000. Amp. 20 ml. *Rx.*
Use: Anesthetic, local.

Durapam. (Major Pharmaceuticals) Flurazepam HCl 15 mg, 30 mg/Cap. Bot. 100s, 500s. *c-IV.*
Use: Hypnotic, sedative.

•**durapatite.** (der-APP-ah-tite) USAN.
Use: Prosthetic aid.

Duraquin. (Parke-Davis) Quinidine gluconate 330 mg/SR Tab. Bot. 100s, UD 100s. *Rx.*
Use: Cardiovascular agent.

DuraScreen. (Schwarz Pharma, Inc.) SPF 30. Octyl methoxycinnamate, octyl salicylate, oxybenzone, 2-phenylbenzimidazole-sulfonic acid, titanium dioxide, cetearyl alcohol, diazolidinyl urea, parabens, shea butter. Lot. Bot. 105 ml. *otc.*
Use: Sunscreen.

DuraScreen SPF 15. (Schwarz Pharma, Inc.) SPF 15. Ethylhexyl p-methoxycinnamate, 2-ethylhexyl salicylate, oxybenzone, parabens, titanium dioxide. Lot. Bot. 105 ml. *otc.*
Use: Sunscreen.

Dura-Tap/PD. (Dura Pharmaceuticals) Pseudoephedrine HCl 60 mg, chlorpheniramine maleate 4 mg. Cap. Bot. 100s. *Rx.*
Use: Antihistamine, decongestant.

Duratears Naturale. (Alcon Laboratories, Inc.) White petroleum, anhydrous liquid lanolin, mineral oil. Oint. Tube 3.5 g. *otc.*
Use: Lubricant, ophthalmic.

Duratest-200/Duratest-100. (Roberts Pharmaceuticals) Testosterone cypionate in oil 100 mg or 200 mg/ml. Inj. Vial 10 ml. *c-III.*
Use: Androgen.

Duratestrin. (Roberts Pharmaceuticals) Estradiol cypionate 2 mg, testosterone cypionate 50 mg/ml. Vial 10 ml. *Rx.*
Use: Androgen, estrogen combination.

Durathate-200 Injection. (Roberts Pharmaceuticals) Testosterone enanthate in oil 200 mg/ml. Vial 10 ml. *c-III.*
Use: Androgen.

Duration Mentholated Vapor Spray. (Schering-Plough Corp.) Oxymetazoline HCl 0.05%, aromatics. Squeeze bot. 15 ml. *otc.*
Use: Decongestant.

Duration Mild Nasal Spray. (Schering-Plough Corp.) Phenylephrine HCl 0.5%. Bot. 15 ml. *otc.*
Use: Decongestant.

Duration Nasal Spray. (Schering-Plough Corp.) Oxymetazoline HCl 0.05%. Aqueous soln. Squeeze bot. 15 ml, 30 ml. *otc.*
Use: Nasal decongestant; androgen, estrogen combination.

Duratuss. (UCB Pharmaceuticals, Inc.) Pseudoephedrine HCl 120 mg, guaifenesin 600 mg. LA Tab. Bot. 100s. *Rx.*
Use: Decongestant, expectorant.

Duratuss-G. (UCB Pharmaceuticals, Inc.) Guaifenesin 1200 mg. Tab. Bot. 100s. *Rx.*
Use: Expectorant.

Duratuss HD. (UCB Pharmaceuticals, Inc.) Hydrocodone bitartrate 2.5 mg, pseudoephedrine HCl 30 mg, guaifenesin 100 mg, alcohol 5%. Elix. Bot. 473 ml. *c-III.*
Use: Antitussive, decongestant, expectorant.

Dura-Vent. (Dura Pharmaceuticals) Phenylpropanolamine HCl 75 mg, guaifenesin 600 mg. SR Tab. Bot. 100s. *Rx.*
Use: Decongestant, expectorant.

Dura-Vent/A. (Dura Pharmaceuticals) Phenylpropanolamine HCl 75 mg, chlorpheniramine maleate 10 mg. SR Cap. Bot. 100s. *Rx.*
Use: Antihistamine, decongestant.

Dura-Vent/DA. (Dura Pharmaceuticals) Phenylephrine HCl 20 mg, chlorpheniramine maleate 8 mg, methscopolamine nitrate 2.5 mg. SR Tab. Bot. 100s. *Rx.*
Use: Anticholinergic, antihistamine, decongestant.

Durazyme. (Blairex Labs, Inc.) Nonionic detergent preserved w/thimerosal 0.004%, EDTA 0.1% in sterile buffered hypertonic salt soln. Bot. 30 ml. *otc.*
Use: Contact lens care.

Duricef. (Mead Johnson Laboratories) Cefadroxil. **Tab.:** 1 g. Bot. 50s, 100s, UD 100s. **Cap.:** 500 mg. Bot. 50s, 100s, UD 100s. **Susp.:** 125 mg/5 ml, 250 mg/5 ml, or 500 mg/5 ml Bot. 50 ml, 75 ml (500 mg/5 ml), 100 ml. *Rx.*
Use: Anti-infective, cephalosporin.

Dusotal. (Harvey) Sodium amobarbital

¾ gr, sodium secobarbital gr/Cap. Bot. 1000s. (3 gr) Bot. 1000s. *c-II.*
Use: Hypnotic, sedative.

•**dusting powder, absorbable.** U.S.P. 23.
Use: Lubricant.

dusting powder, surgical.
See: B-F-I Powder (SmithKline Beecham Pharmaceuticals).

Dutch Drops. Oil of turpentine, sulfurated.

dutch oil. Oil of turpentine, sulfurated.

Duvoid. (Roberts Pharmaceuticals) Bethanechol Cl 10 mg, 25 mg, 50 mg/Tab. Bot. 100s, UD 100s. *Rx.*
Use: Genitourinary.

D V Cream. (Hoechst Marion Roussel) Dienestrol 0.01% w/lactose, propylene glycol, stearic acid, diglycol stearate, TEA, benzoic acid, butylated hydroxytoluene, disodium edetate, buffered w/lactic acid to an acid pH. Tube 3 oz, w/applicator. *Rx.*
Use: Estrogen.

D-Vaso-S. (Dunhall Pharmaceuticals, Inc.) Pentylenetetrazol 50 mg, niacin 50 mg, dimenhydrinate 25 mg, alcohol 18%, sherry wine vehicle. Bot. Pt. *Rx.*
Use: Respiratory.

D-10-W. (Various Mfr.) Dextrose in water injection 10% (amps 3 ml); vials 250 ml, 500 ml, 1000 ml; 17 ml fill in 20 ml, 500 ml fill in 1000 ml, 1000 ml fill in 2000 ml vials. *Rx.*
Use: Carbohydrate supplement.

Dwelle. (Dakryon Pharmaceuticals) EDTA 0.09%, sodium chloride, potassium chloride, boric acid, povidone, NPX 0.001%. Drop. Bot. 15 ml. *otc.*
Use: Artificial tears.

d-xylose.
See: Xylo-Pfan. (Pharmacia & Upjohn).

Dyantoin Caps. (Major Pharmaceuticals) Phenytoin sodium 100 mg/Cap. Bot. 100s, 1000s. *Rx.*
Use: Anticonvulsant.

DX 114 Foot Powder. (Amlab) Zinc undecylenate 1%, salicylic acid 1%, benzoic acid 1%, ammonium alum 5%, boric acid 10.5% w/zinc stearate, chlorophyll, talc, kaolin, starch, calcium silicate, oil of wormwood. Cont. 2 oz. *otc.*
Use: Antifungal, topical.

Dyazide. (SmithKline Beecham Pharmaceuticals) Triamterene 37.5 mg, hydrochlorothiazide 25 mg/Cap. Bot. 1000s, UD 100s, Patient Pack 100s. *Rx.*
Use: Antihypertensive, diuretic.

Dycill. (SmithKline Beecham Pharmaceuticals) Dicloxacillin sodium 250 mg, 500 mg/Cap. Bot. 100s. *Rx.*
Use: Anti-infective, penicillin.

Dyclone. (Astra Pharmaceuticals, L.P.) Dyclonine HCl 0.5%, 1%. Soln. Bot. 30 ml. *Rx.*
Use: Anesthetic, local.

•**dyclonine hydrochloride.** (DIE-kloe-neen) U.S.P. 23.
Use: Anesthetic, topical.
See: Dyclone, Soln. (Astra Pharmaceuticals, L.P.).
W/Benzethonium chloride.
See: Skin Shield, Liq. (Del Pharmaceuticals, Inc.).

Dycomene. (Hance) Hydrocodone bitartrate ⅙ gr, pyrilamine maleate 1 gr/fl. oz. Bot. 3 oz, gal. *c-III.*
Use: Antitussive, sleep aid.

•**dydrogesterone.** (DIE-droe-JESS-ter-ohn) U.S.P. 23.
Use: Hormone, progestin.

dyes.
See: Antiseptic, Dyes.

Dyflex-200 Tablets. (Econo Med Pharmaceuticals) Dyphylline 200 mg/Tab. Bot. 100s, 1000s. *Rx.*
Use: Bronchodilator.

Dyflex-G Tablets. (Econo Med Pharmaceuticals) Dyphylline 200 mg, guaifenesin 200 mg/Tab. Bot. 100s, 1000s. *Rx.*
Use: Bronchodilator, expectorant.

Dy-G Liquid. (Cypress Pharm) Dyphylline 100 mg, guaifenesin 100 mg/5 ml. Liq. Bot. Pt. *Rx.*
Use: Bronchodilator, expectorant.

dylate. Clonitrate.
Use: Coronary vasodilator.

Dyline-GG Liquid. (Seatrace Pharmaceuticals, Inc.) Dyphylline 300 mg, guaifenesin 300 mg/15 ml. Bot. Pt, gal. *Rx.*
Use: Bronchodilator, expectorant.

Dyline-GG Tablets. (Seatrace Pharmaceuticals, Inc.) Dyphylline 200 mg, guaifenesin 200 mg/Tab. Bot. 100s, 1000s. *Rx.*
Use: Bronchodilator, expectorant.

•**dymanthine hydrochloride.** (DIE-man-theen) USAN.
Use: Anthelmintic.

Dymelor. (Eli Lilly and Co.) Acetohexamide 250 mg or 500 mg/Tab. Bot. 50s (500 mg only), 200s. *Rx.*
Use: Antidiabetic.

Dymenate. (Keene Pharmaceuticals, Inc.) Dimenhydrinate 50 mg/ml. Vial 10 ml. *Rx.*
Use: Antiemetic, antivertigo.

Dynabac. (Sanofi Winthrop Pharmaceuticals) Dirithromycin 250 mg/Tab. Enteric coated. Bot. 60s. *Rx.*

Use: Anti-infective.

Dynacin. (Medicis Dermatologicals, Inc.) Minocycline HCl 50 mg, 100 mg. Cap. Bot. 100s (50 mg). 50s (100 mg). *Rx.*
Use: Anti-infective, tetracycline.

DynaCirc. (Norvartis Pharmaceutical Corp.) Isradipine. 2.5 mg, 5 mg/Cap. Bot. 60s, 100s, UD 100s. *Rx.*
Use: Calcium channel blocker.

DynaCirc CR. (Novartis Pharmaceutical Corp.) Isradipine 5 mg, 10 mg/CR Tab. Bot. 30s, 100s. *Rx.*
Use: Calcium channel blocker.

Dynafed Asthma Relief. (BDI Pharmaceuticals, Inc.) Ephedrine HCl 25 mg, guaifenesin 200 mg/Tab. Bot. 60s. *otc.*
Use: Decongestant, expectorant.

Dynafed Jr., Children's. (BDI Pharmaceuticals, Inc.)
See: Children's Dynafed Jr., Chew. Tab. (BDI Pharmaceuticals, Inc.).

Dynafed Ex, Extra Strength. (BDI Pharmaceuticals, Inc.)
See: Extra Strength Dynafed, Tab. (BDI Pharmaceuticals, Inc.).

Dynafed IB. (BDI Pharmaceuticals, Inc.) Ibuprofen 200 mg/Tab. Bot. 36s. *otc.*
Use: Analgesic.

Dynafed Plus, Maximum Strength. (BDI Pharmaceuticals, Inc.)
See: Maximum Strength Dynafed Plus, Tab. (BDI Pharmaceuticals, Inc.).

Dynafed Pseudo. (BDI Pharmaceuticals, Inc.) Pseudoephedrine HCl 60 mg/Tab. Bot. 60s. *otc.*
Use: Decongestant.

Dyna-Hex Skin Cleanser. (Western Medical) Chlorhexidine gluconate 4%, isopropyl alcohol 4%. Liq. Bot. 120 ml, 240 ml, 480 ml, 1 gal. *otc.*
Use: Antimicrobial, antiseptic.

Dyna-Hex 2 Skin Cleanser. (Western Medical) Chlorhexidine gluconate 2%, isopropyl alcohol 4%. Liq. Bot. 120 ml, 240 ml, 480 ml, 1 gal. *otc.*
Use: Antimicrobial, antiseptic.

dynamine. (Mayo Foundation)
Use: Antispasmodic, Lambert-Eaton myasthenic syndrome, hereditary motor and sensory neuropathy type I (Charcot-Marie-Tooth Disease). [Orphan Drug]

Dynapen. (Apothecon) Dicloxacillin sodium. **Cap.:** 125 mg, 250 mg, 500 mg. Bot. 24s (except 500 mg), 50s (500 mg only), 100s (except 500 mg). **Pow. for Oral Susp.:** 62.5 mg/5 ml. Bot. 100 ml, 200 ml. *Rx.*
Use: Anti-infective, penicillin.

Dynaplex. (Alton) Vitamin B complex. Bot. 100s, 1000s. *otc.*
Use: Vitamin supplement.

dynarsan.
See: Acetarsone, Tab.

Dy-O-Derm. (Galderma Laboratories, Inc.) Purified water, isopropyl alcohol, acetone, dihydroxyacetone, FD&C; yellow No. 6, FD&C; blue No. 1, FD&C; red No. 33. Bot. 4 oz.
Use: Dermatologic, vitiligo stain.

Dy-Phyl-Lin. (Foy Laboratories) Dyphylline 250 mg/ml with benzyl alcohol. Inj. Vial 10 ml. *Rx.*
Use: Bronchodilator.

•**dyphylline.** (DIE-fih-lin) U.S.P. 23.
Use: Vasodilator, bronchodilator.
See: Brophylline, Inj., Granucaps (Solvay Pharmaceuticals).
Dilor, Preps. (Savage Laboratories).
Emfabid TD, Tab. (Saron).
Lardet, Inj. (Standex).
Neothylline, Tab. (Teva Pharmaceuticals USA).
Prophyllin, Oint., Pow. (Rystan, Inc.).
W/Chlorpheniramine maleate, guaifenesin, dextromethorphan HBr, phenylephrine HCl.
See: Dilor G, Liq, Tab. (Savage Laboratories).
Neothylline GG, Liq. (Teva Pharmaceuticals USA).
W/Guaifenesin.
See: Dy-G Liquid (Cypress Pharm).

Dyphylline GG Elixir. (Various Mfr.) Dyphylline 100 mg, guaifenesin 100 mg/ 15 ml. Bot. 473 ml. *Rx.*
Use: Bronchodilator.

Dyprotex. (Blistex, Inc.) Micronized zinc oxide 40%, petrolatum 37.6%, dimethicone 2.5%, cod liver oil, aloe extract, zinc stearate. Pads. Pkgs. 3s (9 applications). *otc.*
Use: Astringent.

Dyrenium. (SmithKline Beecham Pharmaceuticals) Triamterene. **50 mg/Cap.:** Bot. 100s, UD 100s. **100 mg/Cap.:** Bot. 100s, 1000s, UD 100s. *Rx.*
Use: Diuretic.

Dyretic. (Keene Pharmaceuticals, Inc.) Furosemide 10 mg/ml. Vial 10 ml. *Rx.*
Use: Diuretic.

Dyrexan-OD. (Trimen Laboratories, Inc.) Phendimetrazine tartrate 105 mg/SR Cap. Bot. 100s. *c-III.*
Use: Anorexiant.

Dyspel. (Dover Pharmaceuticals) Acetaminophen, ephedrine sulfate, atropine sulfate. Sugar, lactose, and salt free. Tab. UD Box 500s. *Rx.*
Use: Analgesic.

E

Ease. (NeuroGenesis/Matrix Tech., Inc.) D, L-phenylalanine 500 mg, L-glutamine 15 mg, L-tyrosine 25 mg, L-carnitine 10 mg, L-arginine pyroglutamate 10 mg, L-ornithine/L-aspartate 10 mg, Cr 0.033 mg, Se 0.012 mg, B_1 0.33 mg, B_2 5 mg, B_3 3.3 mg, B_5 0.33 mg, B_6 0.33 mg, B_{12} 1 mcg, E 5 IU, biotin 0.05 mg, FA 0.066 mg, Fe 1 mg, Zn 2.5 mg, Ca 35 mg, I 0.25 mg, Cu 0.33 mg, Mg 25 mg/Cap. Bot. 42s. *otc.*
Use: Nutritional supplement.

EACA. (Lederle Standard Products) Epsilon aminocaproic acid. *Rx.*
Use: Antifibrinolytic.
See: Amicar (Lederle Standard Products).

Ear Drops. (Weeks & Leo) Carbamide peroxide 6.5% in an anhydrous glycerin base. Bot. oz. *otc.*
Use: Otic.

Ear-Dry. (Scherer Laboratories, Inc.) Isopropyl alcohol, boric acid 2.75%. Dropper bot. 30 ml. *otc.*
Use: Otic.

Earex Ear Drops. (Health for Life Brands, Inc.) Benzocaine 0.15 g, antipyrine 0.7 g/0.5 oz. Bot. 0.5 oz. *Rx.*
Use: Otic.

Ear-Eze. (Hyrex Pharmaceuticals) Hydrocortisone 1%, chloroxylenol 0.1%, pramoxine HCl 1%. Dropper bot. 15 ml. *Rx.*
Use: Anesthetic, local; anti-infective, corticosteroid.

Earocol Ear Drops. (Roberts Pharmaceuticals) Benzocaine 1.4%, antipyrine 5.4%, glycerin, oxyquinoline sulfate. Soln. Dropper bot. 15 ml. *Rx.*
Use: Otic.

earthnut oil. Peanut Oil.

Easprin. (Parke-Davis) Aspirin 15 gr/EC Tab. Bot. 100s. *Rx.*
Use: Analgesic.

East-A. (Eastwood) Therapeutic lotion. Bot. 16 oz. *otc.*
Use: Emollient.

Easy-Lax. (Walgreen Co.) Docusate sodium 100 mg/Cap. Bot. 60s. *otc.*
Use: Laxative, stool softener.

Easy-Lax Plus. (Walgreen Co.) Docusate sodium 100 mg, casanthranol 30 mg/Cap. Bot. 60s. *otc.*
Use: Laxative, stool softener.

Eazol. (Roberts Pharmaceuticals) Fructose, dextrose, orthophosphoric acid with controlled hydrogen ion concentration. Bot. 473 ml. *otc.*
Use: Antinauseant.

E-Base. (Barr Laboratories, Inc.) Erythromycin. **Cap.:** 333 mg. Bot. 100s, 500s, 1000s. **Tab.:** 333 mg, 500 mg. Bot. 100s, 500s. *Rx.*
Use: Anti-infective, erythromycin.

•**ebastine.** (EBB-ass-teen) USAN.
Use: Antihistamine.

EBV-VCA. (Wampole Laboratories) Epstein-Barr virus, viral capsid antigen antibody test. Qualitative and semiquantitative detection of EBV antibody in human serum. Test 100s.
Use: Diagnostic aid.

EBV-VCA Ig. (Wampole Laboratories) Epstein-Barr virus, viral capsid antigen Ig antibody. Qualitative and semiqualitative detection of EBV-VCA Ig antibody in human serum. Test 50s.
Use: Diagnostic aid.

•**ecadotril.** (ee-CAD-oh-trill) USAN.
Use: Antihypertensive.

•**ecamsule.** (eh-KAM-sool) USAN.
Use: Sunscreen.

Ecee Plus. (Edwards Pharmaceuticals, Inc.) Vitamin E 165 mg, ascorbic acid 100 mg, magnesium sulfate 70 mg, zinc sulfate 80 mg/Tab. Bot. 100s. *otc.*
Use: Mineral, vitamin supplement.

•**echothiophate iodide.** (eck-oh-THIGH-oh-fate EYE-oh-dide) U.S.P. 23.
Use: Antiglaucoma agent; cholinergic (ophthalmic).
See: Phospholine Iodide, Pow. (Wyeth-Ayerst Laboratories).

•**eclanamine maleate.** (eh-KLAN-ah-MEEN) USAN.
Use: Antidepressant.

•**eclazolast.** (eh-CLAY-zole-AST) USAN.
Use: Antiallergic, inhibitor (mediator release).

Eclipse After Sun. (Novartis Pharmaceutical Corp.) Petrolatum, glycerin, oleth-3 phosphate, carbomer-934, imidazolidinyl urea, benzyl alcohol, cetyl esters wax. Lot. Bot. 180 ml. *otc.*
Use: Emollient.

Eclipse Lip and Face Protectant. (Novartis Pharmaceutical Corp.) Padimate O, oxybenzone. Stick 4.5 g. *otc.*
Use: Lip protectant.

Eclipse Original Sunscreen. (Novartis Pharmaceutical Corp.) Padimate O, glyceryl PABA. Lot. Bot. 120 ml. *otc.*
Use: Sunscreen.

Eclipse Suntan, Partial. (Novartis Pharmaceutical Corp.) Padimate O. Lot. Bot. 120 ml. *otc.*
Use: Sunscreen.

EC-Naprosyn. (Roche Laboratories) Naproxen 375 mg or 500 mg/TR Tab. Bot.

100s. *Rx.*
Use: NSAID.

•**econazole.** (ee-CON-uh-zole) USAN.
Use: Antifungal.

•**econazole nitrate.** (ee-CON-uh-zole) U.S.P. 23.
Use: Antifungal.
See: Spectazole (Ortho McNeil Pharmaceutical).

Econo B & C. (Vangard Labs, Inc.) Vitamins B_1 15 mg, B_2 10.2 mg, B_3 50 mg, B_5 10 mg, B_6 5 mg, C 300 mg/Capl. Bot. 100s, UD 100s. *otc.*
Use: Vitamin supplement.

Econopred. (Alcon Laboratories, Inc.) Prednisolone acetate 0.125%. Susp. Drop-Tainer 5 ml, 10 ml. *Rx.*
Use: Corticosteroid, ophthalmic.

Econopred Plus. (Alcon Laboratories, Inc.) Prednisolone acetate 1%. Susp. Drop-Tainer 5 ml, 10 ml. *Rx.*
Use: Corticosteroid, ophthalmic.

Ecotrin Adult Low Strength. (SmithKline Beecham) Aspirin 81 mg, tartrazine/EC Tab. Bot. 36s. *otc.*
Use: Analgesic.

Ecotrin Maximum Strength. (SmithKline Beecham) Acetylsalicylic acid 500 mg. **Tab.:** Bot. 60s, 150s. **Cap.:** Bot. 60s. *otc.*
Use: Analgesic.

Ecotrin Regular Strength. (SmithKline Beecham) Aspirin 325 mg/EC Tab. Bot. 100s, 250s, 1000s. *otc.*
Use: Analgesic.

Ed A-Hist Liquid. (Edwards Pharmaceuticals, Inc.) Phenylephrine HCl 10 mg, chlorpheniramine maleate 4 mg/5 ml, alcohol 5%. Liq. Bot. 473 ml. *Rx.*
Use: Antihistamine, decongestant.

Ed A-Hist Tablets. (Edwards Pharmaceuticals, Inc.) Chlorpheniramine maleate 8 mg, phenylephrine HCl 20 mg/SR Tab. Bot. 100s. *Rx.*
Use: Antihistamine, decongestant.

edathamil. Edetate ethylenediamine tetraacetic acid.

edathamil calcium-disodium. Calcium disodium ethylenediamine tetraacetate.
See: Calcium Disodium Versenate, Amp. & Tab. (3M Pharm.).

edathamil disodium. Disodium salt of ethylene diamine tetraacetic acid.
See: Endrate, Amp. (Abbott Laboratories).

•**edatrexate.** (EE-dah-TREX-ate) USAN.
Use: Antineoplastic.

Edecrin. (Merck & Co.) Ethacrynic acid 25 mg or 50 mg/Tab. Bot. 100s. *Rx.*
Use: Diuretic.

Edecrin Sodium Intravenous. (Merck & Co.) Ethacrynate sodium equivalent to 50 mg ethacrynic acid w/mannitol 62.5 mg, thimerosal 0.1 mg/Vial. 50 ml for reconstitution. *Rx.*
Use: Diuretic.

•**edetate calcium disodium.** (EH-duh-tate) U.S.P. 23. *Formerly Edathamil.*
Use: Chelating agent (metal).
See: Calcium Disodium Versenate, Amp., Tab. (3M Pharm.).

•**edetate dipotassium.** (EH-deh-tate) USAN.
Use: Pharmaceutic aid (chelating agent).

•**edetate disodium.** (EH-duh-tate) U.S.P. 23.
Use: Chelating agent (metal); pharmaceutic aid (chelating agent).
See: Disotate, Inj. (Steris Laboratories, Inc.).
Endrate, Amp. (Abbott Laboratories).
W/Benzalkonium Cl, boric acid, potassium Cl, sodium carbonate anhydrous.
See: Swim-Eye Drops (Savage Laboratories).
W/Phenylephrine HCl, methapyrilene HCl, benzalkonium Cl, sodium bisulfite.
See: Allerest Nasal Spray (Novartis Pharmaceutical Corp.).
W/Phenylephrine HCl, benzalkonium Cl, sodium bisulfate.
See: Sinarest, Aerosol (Novartis Pharmaceutical Corp.).
W/Potassium Cl, benzalkonium Cl, isotonic boric acid.
See: Dacriose (Smith, Miller & Patch).
W/Prednisolone sodium phosphate, niacinamide, sodium bisulfite, phenol.
See: P.S.P. IV. Inj. (Solvay Pharmaceuticals).
W/Sodium thiosulfate, salicylic acid, isopropyl alcohol, propylene glycol, menthol, colloidal alumina.
See: Tinver Lotion (PBH Wesley Jessen).

edetate disodium. (Various Mfr.) Edetate disodium 150 mg/ml. Inj. Vial 20 ml. *Rx.*
Use: Antihypercalcemia, cadiovascular agent.

•**edetate sodium.** (EH-deh-tate) USAN.
Use: Chelating agent.
See: Disodium Versenate (3M Pharm.).
Vagisec, Liq. (Julius Schmid).

•**edetate trisodium.** (EH-deh-tate) USAN.
Use: Chelating agent.

•**edetic acid.** (ED-eh-tic) N.F. 18.
Use: Pharmaceutic aid (chelating agent).

•**edetol.** (eh-deh-TOLE) USAN.
Use: Pharmaceutic aid (alkalinizing agent).

Edex. (Schwarz Pharma, Inc.) Alprostadil 5 mcg, 10 mcg, 20 mcg, 40 mcg (after reconstitution), lactose. Inj. Single-dose Vial or Kit 5 mcg, 10 mcg, 20 mcg, 40 mcg. *Rx.*
Use: Treatment for impotence.

•**edifolone acetate.** (EH-DIH-fah-LONE) USAN.
Use: Cardiovascular agent (antiarrhythmic).

ED-IN-SOL. (Edwards) Ferrous sulfate 15 mg/0.6 ml, alcohol, sodium benzoate, sorbitol, sucrose. Drops. Bot. 50 ml. *otc.*
Use: Iron-containing product.

edithamil.
See: Edathamil.

•**edobacomab.** (eh-dah-BACK-ah-mab) USAN.
Use: Antiendotoxin monoclonal antibody.

•**edoxudine.** (ee-DOX-you-DEEN) USAN.
Use: Antiviral.

•**edrecolomab.** (edd-reh-KOE-lah-mab) USAN.
Use: Monoclonal antibody (antineoplastic adjuvant).

edrofuradene. Name used for Nifurdazil.

•**edrophonium chloride.** (eh-droe-FOE-nee-uhm) U.S.P. 23.
Use: Antidote to curare principles; diagnostic aid, myasthenia gravis.
See: Enlon, Inj. (Ohmeda Pharmaceuticals).
Reversol (Organon Teknika Corp.).
Tensilon Chloride, Vial (Roche Laboratories).

edrophonium chloride/atropine sulfate.
See: atropine sulfate/edrophonium chloride.

ED-SPAZ. (Edwards Pharmaceuticals, Inc.) Hyoscyamine sulfate 0.125 mg/Tab. Bot. 100s. *Rx.*
Use: Anticholinergic, antispasmodic.

EDTA.
See: Edathamil (Various Mfr.).

ED-TIC. (Edwards Pharmaceuticals, Inc.) Phenylephrine HCl 5 mg, chlorpheniramine maleate 2 mg, hydrocodone bitartrate 1.67 mg/5 ml. Liq. Bot. 473 ml. *c-III.*
Use: Antihistamine, antitussive, decongestant.

Ed Tuss HC. (Edwards Pharmaceuticals, Inc.) Phenylephrine HCl 10 mg, chlorpheniramine maleate 4 mg, hydrocodone bitartrate 2.5 mg, alcohol 5%/5 ml. Liq. Bot. 480 ml. *c-III.*
Use: Antihistamine, antitussive, decongestant.

E.E.S. 200. (Abbott Laboratories) Erythromycin ethylsuccinate 200 mg/5 ml. Bot. 100 ml, 480 ml. *Rx.*
Use: Anti-infective, erythromycin.

E.E.S. 400. (Abbott Laboratories) Erythromycin ethylsuccinate. **Tab.:** 400 mg. Bot. 100s, 500s, 1000s, UD 100s. **Susp.:** 400 mg/5 ml. Bot. 100 ml, 480 ml. *Rx.*
Use: Anti-infective, erythromycin.

E.E.S. Drops. (Abbott Laboratories) Erythromycin ethylsuccinate representing erythromycin activity 100 mg/2.5 ml when reconstituted w/water. Dropper Bot. 50 ml. *Rx.*
Use: Anti-infective, erythromycin.

E.E.S. Granules. (Abbott Laboratories) Erythromycin ethylsuccinate 200 mg/5 ml when reconstituted. Pow. for Oral Susp. Bot. 100 ml, 200 ml. *Rx.*
Use: Anti-infective, erythromycin.

efavirenz.
Use: Antiviral.
See: Sustiva (Du Pont Pharmaceuticals).

Efed-II. (Alto Pharmaceuticals, Inc.) Ephedrine sulfate 25 mg/Cap. Box 24s. *otc.*
Use: Decongestant.

Efedron Nasal. (Hyrex Pharmaceuticals) Ephedrine HCl 0.6%, chlorobutanol 0.5% w/sodium Cl, menthol, and cinnamon oil in a water-soluble jelly base. Tube 20 g. *otc.*
Use: Decongestant.

•**efegatran sulfate.** (EH-feh-GAT-ran) USAN.
Use: Antithrombotic.

E-Ferol Spray. (Forest Pharmaceutical, Inc.) Alpha tocopherol equivalent to 30 IU Vitamin E/ml. Can 6 oz. *otc.*
Use: Emollient.

E-Ferol Succinate. (Forest Pharmaceutical, Inc.) d-alpha tocopherol acid succinate, equivalent to Vitamin E. **100 or 400 IU/Cap.:** Bot. 100s, 500s, 1000s. **200 IU/Cap.:** Bot. 50s, 100s, 500s, 1000s. **50 IU/Tab.:** Bot. 100s, 500s, 1000s. *otc.*
Use: Vitamin supplement.

E-Ferol Vanishing Cream. (Forest Pharmaceutical, Inc.) Alpha tocopherol. Jar 2 oz. *otc.*
Use: Emollient.

Effectin Tablets. (Sanofi Winthrop Pharmaceuticals) Bitolterol mesylate. *Rx.*
Use: Bronchodilator.

Effective Strength Cough Formula. (Alpharma USPD Inc.) Chlorpheniramine maleate 2 mg, dextromethorphan HBr 15 mg, alcohol 10%. Liq. Bot. 240 ml. *otc.*
Use: Antihistamine, antitussive.

Effective Strength Cough w/Decongestant. (Alpharma USPD Inc.) Pseudoephedrine HCl 20 mg, dextromethorhan HBr 10 mg, alcohol 10%. Liq. Bot. 240 ml. *otc.*
Use: Antitussive, decongestant.

Effer-K. (Nomax, Inc.) Potassium 25 mEq (as bicarbonate and citrate), saccharin. Effervescent tab. Box foil 30s, 250s. *Rx.*
Use: Mineral supplement.

Effexor. (Wyeth-Ayerst Laboratories) Venlafaxine 25 mg, 37.5 mg, 50 mg, 75 mg, or 100 mg/Tab. Bot. 100s, Redipak 100s. *Rx.*
Use: Antidepressant.

Effexor XR. (Wyeth-Ayerst Laboratories) Venlafaxine 37.5 mg, 75 mg, 150 mg/ ER Cap. Bot. 100s, UD 100s. *Rx.*
Use: Antidepressant.

Efficol Cough Whip, Suppressant, Decongestant. (Block Drug Co., Inc.) Phenylpropanolamine HCl 6.25 mg, dextromethorphan HBr 2.5 mg/5 ml Bot. 8 oz. *otc.*
Use: Antitussive, decongestant.

Efficol Cough Whip, Suppressant, Decongestant, Antihistamine. (Block Drug Co., Inc.) Dextromethorphan HBr 2.5 mg, phenylpropanolamine HCl 6.25 mg, chlorpheniramine maleate 1 mg/5 ml Bot. 8 oz. *otc.*
Use: Antihistamine, antitussive, decongestant.

Efidac/24. (Novartis Pharmaceutical Corp.) Pseudoephedrine HCl 240 mg/ Tab. Pkg. 6s, 12s. *otc.*
Use: Decongestant.

Efidac 24 Chlorpheniramine. (Novartis Pharmaceutical Corp.) Chlorpheniramine maleate 16 mg/ER Tab. Pkg. 6s, 12s. *otc.*
Use: Antihistamine.

•**eflornithine hydrochloride.** (ee-FLAHR-nih-THEEN) USAN.
Use: Antineoplastic, antiprotozoal. [Orphan Drug]
See: Ornidyl (Hoechst Marion Roussel).

EfoDine Ointment. (E. Fougera and Co.) Povidone-iodine oint. Foilpac oz, Tube oz. Jar lb. *otc.*

Efudex. (Roche Laboratories) Fluorouracil. **Soln.:** Fluorouracil 2% or 5%, w/ propylene glycol, hydroxypropyl cellulose, parabens, disodium edetate. Drop Dispenser 10 ml. **Cream:** Fluorouracil 5%, in vanishing cream base w/white petrolatum, stearyl alcohol, propylene glycol, polysorbate 60, parabens. Tube 25 g. *Rx.*
Use: Antineoplastic.

egraine. A protein binder from oats.

•**egtazic acid.** (egg-TAY-zik) USAN.
Use: Pharmaceutic aid.

EHDP.
See: Etidronate Disodium.

EL 10. (Elan Pharma) *Rx.*
Use: Antiviral, immunomodulator.

•**elacridar hydrochloride.** (eh-LACK-rih-dahr) USAN.
Use: Potentiation of chemotherapy in cancer (multidrug resistance inhibitor in cancer); antineoplastic (adjunct).

•**elantrine.** (EL-an-treen) USAN.
Use: Anticholinergic.

•**elastofilcon a.** (ee-LASS-toe-FILL-kahn A) USAN.
Use: Contact lens material, hydrophilic.

Elavil. (Zeneca Pharmaceuticals) Amitriptyline HCl. **Tab.: 10 mg:** Bot. 100s, 1000s; 25 mg: Bot. 100s, 1000s. **50 mg:** Bot. 100s, 1000s. **75 mg, 100 mg:** Bot. 100s. **150 mg:** Bot. 30s, 100s. All strengths in UD 100s. **Inj.:** Vial 10 mg/ ml w/dextrose 44 mg, methylparaben 1.5 mg, propylparaben 0.2 mg/ml w/water for injection. q.s. Vial 1 ml, 10 ml. *Rx.*
Use: Antidepressant, tricyclic.

elcatonin. (Innapharma, Inc.)
Use: Intrathecal treatment of intractable pain. [Orphan Drug]

•**eldacimibe.** (ell-DASS-ih-mibe) USAN.
Use: Antiatherosclerotic, antihyperlipidemic.

Eldec Kapseals. (Parke-Davis) Elemental iron 3.3 mg, Vitamins A 1667 IU, E 10 mg, B_1 10 mg, B_2 0.9 mg, B_3 17 mg, B_5 10 mg, B_6 0.7 mg, B_{12} 2 mcg, C 67 mg, folic acid 0.3 mg, calcium iodine/ Cap. Bot. 100s. *otc.*
Use: Mineral, vitamin supplement.

Eldecort. (Zeneca Pharmaceuticals) Hydrocortisone 2.5%, light mineral oil, propylene glycol, allantoin. Cream Tube 15 g, 30 g. *Rx.*
Use: Corticosteroid, topical.

Eldepryl. (Somerset Pharmaceuticals) Selegiline HCl 5 mg, lactose. Cap. Bot. 60s, 300s. *Rx.*
Use: Antiparkinsonian.

Eldercaps. (Merz Pharmaceuticals) Vitamins A 4000 IU, D 400 IU, E 25 IU, B 10 mg, B_2 5 mg, B_3 25 mg, B_5 10 mg, B_6

2 mg, C 200 mg, folic acid 1 mg, Zn 15.8 mg, Mg, Mn/Cap. Bot. 100s. *Rx.*
Use: Mineral, vitamin supplement.

Elder's RVP. Red Vet. Petrolatum.
Use: Dermatoses.

Eldertonic. (Merz Pharmaceuticals) Vitamins B_1 0.17 mg, B_2 0.19 mg, B_3 2.22 mg, B_5 1.11 mg, B_6 0.22 mg, B_{12} 0.67 mcg, alcohol 13.5%, Mg, Mn, zinc 1.7 mg/5 ml. Bot. 473 ml. *otc.*
Use: Mineral, vitamin supplement.

Eldisine. (Eli Lilly and Co.)
See: Vindesine sulfate.

Eldo-B & C. (Canright) Vitamins C 250 mg, B_1 25 mg, B_2 10 mg, niacinamide 150 mg, B_6 5 mg, d-calcium pantothenate 20 mg/Tab. Bot. 100s, 1000s. *otc.*
Use: Mineral, vitamin supplement.

Eldofe. (Canright) Ferrous fumarate 225 mg/Chew. Tab. Bot. 100s, 1000s. *otc.*
Use: Mineral supplement.

Eldofe-C. (Canright) Ferrous fumarate 225 mg, ascorbic acid 50 mg/Tab. Bot. 100s. *otc.*
Use: Mineral, vitamin supplement.

Eldopaque. (ICN Pharmaceuticals, Inc.) Hydroquinone 2% in a tinted sunblocking cream base. Tube 15 g, 30 g. *otc.*
Use: Dermatologic.

Eldopaque-Forte. (ICN Pharmaceuticals, Inc.) Hydroquinone 4% in a tinted sunblocking cream base. Tube 15 g, 30 g. *Rx.*
Use: Dermatologic.

Eldoquin. (ICN Pharmaceuticals, Inc.) Hydroquinone 2% in a vanishing cream base. Tube 15 g, 30 g. *otc.*
Use: Dermatologic.

Eldoquin Forte. (ICN Pharmaceuticals, Inc.) Hydroquinone 4% in vanishing cream base. Tube 15 g, 30 g. *Rx.*
Use: Dermatologic.

Elecal. (Western Research) Calcium 250 mg, magnesium 15 mg/Tab. Bot. 1000s. *otc.*
Use: Mineral supplement.

Electrolyte #48 Injection. Pediatric maintenance electrolyte solution. Dextrose 5% in electrolyte #48 w/sodium 25 mEq, potassium 20 mEq, magnesium 3 mEq, chloride 22 mEq, lactate 23 mEq, phosphate 3 mEq/L. *Rx.*
Use: Water, caloric, electrolyte supplement.

Electrolyte #75 and 5% Dextrose.
See: 5% Dextrose and Electrolyte #75.

Elegen-G. (Grafton) Amitriptyline 10 mg, 25 mg or 50 mg/Tab. Bot. 100s, 1000s. *Rx.*
Use: Antidepressant, tricyclic.

Elevites. (Barth's) Vitamins A 6000 IU, D 400 IU, B_1 1.5 mg, B_2 3 mg, C 60 mg, B_{12} 10 mcg, niacin 1 mg, E 10 IU, malt diastase 15 mg, iron 15 mg, calcium 381 mg, phosphorus 0.172 mg, citrus bioflavonoid complex 15 mg, rutin 15 mg, nucleic acid 3 mg, red bone marrow 30 mg, peppermint leaves 10 mg, wheat germ 30 mg/Tab. or Cap. Bot. 100s, 500s, 1000s. *Rx.*
Use: Mineral, vitamin supplement.

Elimite. (Allergan, Inc.) Permethrin 5%. Cream. Tube 60 g. *Rx.*
Use: Scabicide, pediculicide.

Elixicon. (Berlex Laboratories, Inc.) Theophylline 100 mg/5 ml with methyl and propyl parabens. Susp. Bot. 237 ml. *Rx.*
Use: Bronchodilator.

Elixiral. (Vita Elixir) Phenobarbital 16.2 mg, hyoscyamine sulfate 0.1037 mg, atropine sulfate 0.194 mg, hyoscine HBr 0.0065 mg/5 ml. Liq. Pt, gal. *Rx.*
Use: Anticholinergic, antispasmodic, hypnotic, sedative.

Elixophyllin Capsules, Dye-Free. (Forest Pharmaceutical, Inc.) Anhydrous theophylline 100 mg or 200 mg/Cap. **100 mg:** Bot. 100s. **200 mg:** Bot. 100s, 500s, UD 100s. *Rx.*
Use: Bronchodilator.

Elixophyllin Elixir. (Forest Pharmaceutical, Inc.) Anhydrous theophylline 80 mg, alcohol 20%/15 ml. Bot. pt, qt, gal. *Rx.*
Use: Bronchodilator.

Elixophyllin GG Liquid. (Forest Pharmaceutical, Inc.) Theophylline 100 mg, guaifenesin 100 mg/15 ml. Alcohol free. Bot. 237, 480 ml. *Rx.*
Use: Antiasthmatic combination.

Elixophyllin-KI Elixir. (Forest Pharmaceutical, Inc.) Anhydrous theophylline 80 mg, potassium iodide 130 mg/15 ml. Bot. 237 ml. *Rx.*
Use: Antiasthmatic combination.

Ellesdine. (Janssen Pharmaceutical, Inc.) Pipenperone. *Rx.*
Use: Anxiolytic.

Elliot's B Solution. (Orphan Medical, Inc.)
Use: Acute lymphatic leukemias and acute lymphoblastic lymphomas. [Orphan Drug]

•**elm.** U.S.P. 23. Dried inner bark of *Ulmus rubra* Muhlenberg (*Ulmus fulva* Michaux).
Use: Pharmaceutic aid (suspending agent), demulcent.

Elmiron. (Baker Norton Pharmaceuticals, Inc.) Pentosan polysulfate 100 mg/

Cap. Bot. 100s. *Rx.*
Use: Relief of bladder pain associated with interstitial cystitis.

Elocon Cream. (Schering-Plough Corp.) Mometasone furoate 0.1%, hexylene glycol, phosphoric acid, propylene glycol stearate, stearyl alcohol, ceteareth-20, titanium dioxide, aluminum starch octenyl succinate, white wax, white petrolatum. 15 g, 45 g. *Rx.*
Use: Corticosteroid, topical.

Elocon Lotion. (Schering-Plough Corp.) Mometasone furoate 0.1%. Bot. 30 ml, 60 ml. *Rx.*
Use: Corticosteroid, topical.

Elocon Ointment. (Schering-Plough Corp.) Mometasone furoate 0.1%, hexylene glycol, propylene glycol stearate, white wax, white petrolatum. 15 g, 45 g. *Rx.*
Use: Corticosteroid, topical.

Elphemet. (Canright) Phendimetrazine tartrate 35 mg/Tab. Bot. 100s, 1000s. *c-III.*
Use: Anorexiant.

Elprecal. (Canright) Vitamins A 5000 IU, D 400 IU, B_1 3 mg, B_2 2 mg, B_6 0.1 mg, B_{12} 1 mcg, C 50 mg, E 2 IU, calcium pantothenate 2.5 mg, niacinamide 15 mg, inositol 5 mg, choline 5 mg, calcium lactate 500 mg, ferrous sulfate 50 mg, Cu 1 mg, Mn 1 mg, Mg 2 mg, K 2 mg, Zn 0.5 mg, sulfur 1 mg/Cap. Bot. 100s. *otc.*
Use: Mineral, vitamin supplement.

•**elsamitrucin.** (els-AM-ih-TRUE-sin) USAN.
Use: Antineoplastic.

Elserpine. (Canright) Reserpine 0.25 mg/Tab. Bot. 100s, 1000s. *Rx.*
Use: Antihypertensive.

Elspar. (Merck & Co.) Asparaginase 10,000 IU, mannitol 80 mg/Inj. Vial 10 ml. *Rx.*
Use: Antineoplastic.

•**elucaine.** (eh-LOO-cane) USAN.
Use: Anticholinergic, gastric.

Eltroxin. (Roberts Pharmaceuticals) Levothyroxine sodium 0.05 mg, 0.1 mg, 0.15 mg, 0.2 mg, 0.3 mg/Tab. Bot. 100s, 500s. *Rx.*
Use: Hormone, thyroid.

Elvanol. (Du Pont Merck Pharmaceutical Co.) Polyvinyl alcohol.
Use: Pharmaceutical aid.

Emadine. (Alcon Laboratories, Inc.) Emedastine difumarate 0.05% (0.5 mg/ml), benzalkonium chloride 0.01%. Ophth. Soln. Dispenser 5 ml. *Rx.*
Use: Antihistamine, ophthalmic.

embechine. Aliphatic chloroethylamine.
Use: Antineoplastic.

Emcodeine Tabs. (Major Pharmaceuticals) Aspirin with codeine as #2, #3, or #4. Bot. 100s, 500s. *c-III.*
Use: Analgesic combination, narcotic.

Emcyt. (Pharmacia & Upjohn) Estramustine phosphate sodium equivalent to 140 mg estramustine phosphate sodium 12.5 mg/Cap. Bot. 100s. *Rx.*
Use: Antineoplastic.

Emdol. (Health for Life Brands, Inc.) Salicylamide, para-aminobenzoic acid, sodium calcium succinate, vitamin D-1250. Bot. 100s, 1000s. *otc.*
Use: Analgesic combination.

•**emedastine difumarate.** (eh-meh-DASS-teen die-FEW-mah-rate) USAN.
Use: Management of allergic conjunctivitis, antiasthmatic, antiallergic, antihistamine (H_1-receptor).
See: Emadine, Ophth. Soln. (Alcon Laboratories, Inc.).

emergency kits.
See: Ana-Kit (Bayer Corp. (Consumer Div.)).
AtroPen Auto-Injector (Survival Technology, Inc.).
Cyanide Antidote Package (Eli Lilly and Co.).
Emergent-Ez Kit (Healthfirst Corp.).
EpiPen Auto-Injector (Center Labs).
EpiEZPen (Center Labs).
EpiEZPen Jr. (Center Labs).
EpiPen Jr. Auto-Injector (Center Labs).
LidoPen Auto-Injector (Survival Technology, Inc.).
Poison Antidote Kit (Jones Medical Industries, Inc.).

Emergent-Ez. (Healthfirst Corp.) Adrenalin 2 amp., aminophylline 1 amp., ammonia inhalants (3), amyl nitrite inhalants (2), atropine 2 amp., diazepam (2 amp), epinephrine (2 amp), Benadryl 2 amp., nitroglycerin 1 bottle, Solu-Cortef 1 mix-o-vial, Talwin 1 amp., Tigan 1 amp., Valium 2 amp., Wyamine 2 amp., plastic air way (1), disposable syringes, tracheotomy needle (1) and tourniquet (1)/kit. *Rx.*
Use: Emergency kit.

Emeroid. (Delta Pharmaceutical Group) Zinc oxide 5%, diperodon HCl 0.25%, bismuth subcarbonate 0.2%, pyrilamine maleate 0.1%, phenylephrine HCl 0.25%, in a petrolatum base containing cod liver oil. Tube 1.25 oz. *otc.*
Use: Anorectal preparation.

Emersal. (Medco Lab, Inc.) Ammoniated mercury 5%, salicylic acid 2.5%. Lot. Bot. 120 ml. *Rx.*

Use: Antipsoriatic.

Emerson 1% Sodium Fluoride Dental Gel. (Emerson Laboratories) Red and plain. Bot. 2 oz. *Rx.*
Use: Dental caries agent.

emetics.
See: Apomorphine HCl.
Cupric Sulfate.
Ipecac Syr.

•**emetine hydrochloride.** (EM-eh-teen) U.S.P. 23.
Use: Antiamebic.

Emetrol. (Pharmacia & Upjohn) Dextrose 1.87 g, fructose 1.87 g, phosphoric acid 21.5 mg, methylparaben, lemon, mint, or cherry flavor. Soln. Bot. 118 ml, 236 ml, 473 ml. *otc.*
Use: Antiemetic.

Emgel. (GlaxoWellcome) Erythromycin 2%. Gel. Tube 27 g. *Rx.*
Use: Dermatologic, acne.

EM-GG. (Econo Med Pharmaceuticals) Guaifenesin 100 mg/5 ml. Bot. Pt. *otc.*
Use: Expectorant.

•**emilium tosylate.** (EE-MILL-ee-uhm TAH-sill-ate) USAN.
Use: Cardiovascular agent (antiarrhythmic).

Eminase. (Roberts Pharmaceuticals) Anistreplase 30 units/Pow. for Inj. Vials. *Rx.*
Use: Thrombolytic enzyme.

Emitrip Tabs. (Major Pharmaceuticals) Amitriptyline. **10 mg or 25 mg/Tab.:** Bot. 100s, 250s, 1000s, UD 100s. **50 mg/Tab.:** Bot. 100s, 250s, 1000s, UD 100s. **75 mg/Tab.:** Bot. 100s, 250s, UD 100s. **100 mg/Tab.:** Bot. 100s, 250s, 1000s, UD 100s. **150 mg/Tab.:** Bot. 100s, 250s. *Rx.*
Use: Antidepressant, tricyclic.

Emko Because Contraceptor. (Schering-Plough Corp.) Nonoxynol 9 (8% concentration). Contraceptor container w/applicator. Tube 10 g. *otc.*
Use: Vaginal contraceptive.

EMLA. (Astra Pharmaceuticals, L.P.) Lidocaine 2.5%, prilocaine 2.5%/ Cream. Tube 5 g, 30 g. *Rx.*
Use: Anesthetic, local.

Emollia-Creme. (Gordon Laboratories) Cetyl alcohol, lubricating oils in water-soluble base. Jar 4 oz, 5 lb. *otc.*
Use: Emollient.

Emollia-Lotion. (Gordon Laboratories) Water-dispersable waxes, lubricating bland oils in a water-soluble lotion base Bot. 1 oz, 4 oz, gal.
Use: Emollient.

Empirin Aspirin. (GlaxoWellcome) Aspirin 325 mg/Tab. Bot. 50s, 100s, 250s. *otc.*
Use: Analgesic.

Empirin w/Codeine. (GlaxoWellcome) Aspirin 325 mg with codeine phosphate 15 mg, 30 mg or 60 mg/Tab. **No. 2:** Codeine phosphate 15 mg. Bot. 100s. **No. 3:** Codeine phosphate 30 mg. Bot. 100s, 500s, 1000s, Dispenserpak 25s. **No. 4:** Codeine phosphate 60 mg. Bot. 100s, 500s, Dispenserpak 25s. *c-III.*
Use: Analgesic combination, narcotic.

Emulave. (Rydelle Laboratories)
See: Aveenobar Oilated (Rydelle Laboratories).

Emul-O-Balm. (Medeva Pharmaceuticals, Inc.) Menthol, camphor, methyl salicylate. Bot. 2 oz, 8 oz, gal.
Use: Analgesic, topical.

Emulsoil. (Paddock Laboratories) Castor oil 95%. Bot. 60 ml. *otc.*
Use: Laxative.

E-Mycin. (Pharmacia & Upjohn) Erythromycin 250 mg, 333 mg/EC Tab. Bot. 40s (250 mg only), 100s, 500s, UD 100s. *Rx.*
Use: Anti-infective, erythromycin.

•**enadoline hydrochloride.** (en-AHD-ole-en) USAN.
Use: Analgesic; severe head injury. [Orphan Drug]

•**enalapril maleate.** (EH-NAL-uh-prill) U.S.P. 23.
Use: Antihypertensive.
See: Vasotec, Tab. (Merck & Co.).
W/Diltiazem maleate.
See: Teczem, ER Tab. (Hoechst Marion Roussel).
W/Felodipine.
See: Lexxel, ER Tab. (Astra Pharmaceuticals, L.P.).
W/Hydrochlorothiazide.
See: Vaseretic, Tab. (Merck & Co.).

•**enalaprilat.** (EH-NAL-uh-prill-at) U.S.P. 23.
Use: Antihypertensive.
See: Vasotec Inj. (Merck & Co.).

•**enalkiren.** (en-al-KIE-ren) USAN.
Use: Antihypertensive.

•**enazadrem phosphate.** (eh-NAZZ-ah-drem FOSS-fate) USAN.
Use: Antipsoriatic; inhibitor (5-lipoxygenase).

Enbrel. (Immunex) Etanercept 25 mg. Pow. for Inj. Single-use vial. *Rx.*
Use: Antiarthritic.

encapsulated porcine islet preparation.
Use: Type 1 diabetes. [Orphan Drug]
See: BetaRx (VivoRx, Inc.).

Encare. (Thompson Medical Co.) Nonoxynol 9 (2.27%). Supp. 12s. *otc.*
Use: Vaginal contraceptive.

•**enciprazine hydrochloride.** (en-SIH-PRAH-zeen) USAN.
Use: Anxiolytic.

•**enclomiphene.** (en-KLOE-mih-FEEN) USAN. *Formerly Ciscslomiphene.*

•**encyprate.** (en-SIGH-prate) USAN.
Use: Antidepressant.

Endafed. (Forest Pharmaceutical, Inc.) Pseudoephedrine HCl 120 mg, brompheniramine maleate 12 mg/SR Cap. Bot. 100s. *Rx.*
Use: Antihistamine, decongestant.

Endagen-HD. (Jones Medical Industries, Inc.) Phenylephrine HCl 5 mg, chlorpheniramine maleate 2 mg, hydrocodone bitartrate 1.67 mg. Bot. 473 ml. *c-III.*
Use: Antihistamine, antitussive, decongestant.

Endal. (Forest Pharmaceutical, Inc.) Phenylephrine HCl 20 mg, guaifenesin 300 mg/TR Tab. Dye free. Bot. 100s. *Rx.*
Use: Decongestant, expectorant.

Endal Expectorant. (Forest Pharmaceutical, Inc.) Codeine phosphate 10 mg, phenylpropanolamine HCl 12.5 mg, guaifenesin 100 mg/5 ml w/alcohol 5%. Bot. Pt. *c-IV.*
Use: Antitussive, decongestant, expectorant.

Endal-HD. (Forest Pharmaceutical, Inc.) Phenylephrine HCl 5 mg, chlorpheniramine maleate 2 mg, hydrocodone bitartrate 1.67 mg w/menthol, sucrose. Liq. Bot. 480 ml. *c-III.*
Use: Antihistamine, antitussive, decongestant.

Endal-HD Plus. (Forest Pharmaceutical, Inc.) Hydrocodone bitartrate 2 mg, phenylephrine HCl 5 mg, chlorpheniramine maleate 2 mg/5 ml. Liq. Bot. 473 ml. *c-III.*
Use: Antihistamine, antitussive, decongestant.

Endecon. (Du Pont Merck Pharmaceutical Co.) Phenylpropanolamine HCl 25 mg, acetaminophen 325 mg/Tab. Bot. 60s. *otc.*
Use: Analgesic, decongestant.

Endep. (Roche Laboratories) Amitriptyline HCl 10 mg, 25 mg, 50 mg, 75 mg, 100 mg or 150 mg/Tab. **10 mg:** Bot. 100s, Tel-E-Dose 100s. **25 mg:** Bot. 100s, 500s, Tel-E-Dose 100s. **50 mg:** Bot. 100s, 500s, Tel-E-Dose 100s. **75 mg:** Bot. 100s, Tel-E-Dose 100s. **100 mg:** Bot. 100s, Tel-E-Dose 100s. **150 mg:** Bot 100s. *Rx.*
Use: Antidepressant, tricyclic.

End Lice. (Thompson Medical Co.) Pyrethrins 0.3%, piperonyl butoxide technical 3%. Liq. Bot. 177 ml. *otc.*
Use: Pediculicide.

endobenziline bromide.
Use: Anticholinergic.

endocaine. Pyrrocaine.
Use: Anesthetic, local.

endojodin.
See: Entodon.

Endolor. (Keene Pharmaceuticals, Inc.) Butalbital 50 mg, caffeine 40 mg, acetaminophen 325 mg/Cap. Bot. 100s. *Rx.*
Use: Analgesic, hypnotic, sedative.

endomycin. A new antibiotic obtained from cultures of *Streptomyces endus.* **Under study.**

endophenolphthalein. (Roche Laboratories) Diacetyldioxyphenylisatin-isacenbisatin. *otc.*
Use: Laxative.

•**endralazine mesylate.** (en-DRAL-ah-zeen MEH-sih-late) USAN.
Use: Antihypertensive.

Endrate. (Abbott Hospital Products) Edetate disodium 150 mg/ml. Inj. Amp. 20 ml. *Rx.*
Use: Antihypercalcemic, cardiovascular agent.

•**endrysone.** (EN-drih-sone) USAN.
Use: Anti-inflammatory, topical; ophthalmic.

Enduron. (Abbott Laboratories) Methyclothiazide 5 mg/Tab. Bot. 100s, 1000s, UD 100s. *Rx.*
Use: Diuretic.

Enduronyl. (Abbott Laboratories) Methyclothiazide 5 mg, deserpidine 0.25 mg/Tab. Bot. 100s, 1000s, UD 100s. *Rx.*
Use: Antihypertensive, diuretic.

Enduronyl Forte. (Abbott Laboratories) Methyclothiazide 5 mg, deserpidine 0.5 mg/Tab. Bot. 100s, 1000s. *Rx.*
Use: Antihypertensive, diuretic.

Enebag 2. (Lafayette Pharmaceuticals, Inc.) Air contrast barium enema bag. Case 24s.
Use: Radiopaque agent.

Enebag XL. (Lafayette Pharmaceuticals, Inc.) Air contrast barium enema bag 3000 ml w/lumen tubing, enema tip, and side clamp. Case 24s.
Use: Radiopaque agent.

Enecat. (Lafayette Pharmaceuticals, Inc.) Barium sulfate 5%. Conc. Susp. Bot. 110 ml w/480 ml bot. for dilution w/flexible tubing, clamp, enema tip. *Rx.*

Use: Radiopaque agent.

Enemark. (Lafayette Pharmaceuticals, Inc.) Rectal marker. 85% w/v liquid barium. Case of 12 kits.
Use: Rectal marker during radiation therapy.

Enerjets. (Chilton Laboratories) Caffeine 65 mg/Loz. Pkg. 10s. *otc.*
Use: CNS stimulant.

Eneset 1. (Lafayette Pharmaceuticals, Inc.) Barium sulfate suspension 300 ml/air contrast examination kit. Unit-of-use kit. Case 12s.
Use: Radiopaque agent.

Eneset 2. (Lafayette Pharmaceuticals, Inc.) Barium sulfate suspension 450 ml/contrast examination kit. Unit-of-use kit. Case 12s.
Use: Radiopaque agent.

Eneset 600. (Lafayette Pharmaceuticals, Inc.) Barium sulfate suspension 600 ml/air contrast examination kit. Unit-of-use kit. Case 12s.
Use: Radiopaque agent.

Enfamil. (Bristol-Myers Squibb) Vitamins A 2000 IU, D 400 IU, E 20 IU, C 52 mg, B_1 0.5 mg, B_2 1 mg, B_6 0.4 mg, B_{12} 1.5 mcg, niacin 8 mg, Ca 440 mg, P 300 mg, folic acid 100 mcg, pantothenic acid 3 mg, inositol 30 mg, biotin 15 mcg, K-1 55 mcg, choline 100 mg, Fe 1.4 mg, K 650 mg, Cl 400 mg, Cu 0.6 mg, I 65 mcg, Na 175 mg, Mg 50 mg, Zn 5 mg, Mn 100 mg/Qt. Concentrated Liq. 13 fl oz, Instant Pow. lb. *otc.*
Use: Nutritional supplement.

Enfamil Human Milk Fortifier. (Bristol-Myers Squibb) Whey protein, casein, corn syrup solids, lactose, protein 0.7 g, carbohydrate 2.7 g, fat 0.04 g, calories 14. Pow. Packet 0.95 g, Box 100s. *otc.*
Use: Nutritional supplement.

Enfamil w/Iron. (Bristol-Myers Squibb) Iron 12 mg/Qt. Pkg. Con. Liq. 13 fl oz. 24s. Pow. 1 lb. 6s. *otc.*
Use: Nutritional supplement.

Enfamil with Iron Ready to Use. (Bristol-Myers Squibb) Ready-to-use Enfamil with Iron infant formula 20 kcal/fl oz. Can 8 fl oz, 6-can pack; 32 fl oz, 6 cans per case. *otc.*
Use: Nutritional supplement.

Enfamil LactoFree. (Mead Johnson Nutritionals) Protein 2.1 g, fat 5.3 g, carbohydrate 10.9 g, calories 100/serving, linoleic acid 860 mg, A 300 IU, D 60 IU, E 2 IU, K 8 mcg, B_1 80 mcg, B_2 140 mcg, B_6 60 mcg, B_{12} 0.3 mcg, B_3 1000 mcg, folic acid 16 mcg, B_5 500 mcg, biotin 3 mcg, C 12 mg, choline 12 mg, inositol (liquid only) 17 mg, inositol (powder only) 6 mg, Ca 82 mg, P 55 mg, Mg 8 mg, Fe 1.8 mg, Zn 1 mg, Mn 15 mcg, Cu 75 mcg, I 15 mcg, Se 2.8 mcg, Na 30 mg, K 110 mg, Cl 67 mg. Liq., Liq. Conc., Pow. Bot. 397 g (pow.), 384 ml (liq. conc.), 946 ml (liq.). *otc.*
Use: Nutritional therapy, enteral.

Enfamil Next Step. (Bristol-Myers Squibb) Protein 17.3 g, carbohydrates 74 g, fat 33.3 g/liter, with appropriate vitamins and minerals. **Liq.:** 390 ml concentrate, 1 qt ready-to-use. **Pow.:** 360 g, 720 g. *otc.*
Use: Nutritional supplement.

Enfamil Nursette. (Bristol-Myers Squibb) Ready-to-feed Enfamil 20 kcal/fl oz, 4 fl oz, 6 fl oz and 8 fl oz. 4 bottles/sealed carton. W/Iron. Ready to use. Bot. 6 fl oz 4s, 24s. *otc.*
Use: Nutritional supplement.

Enfamil Premature Formula. (Bristol-Myers Squibb) Nonfat milk, whey protein concentrate, corn syrup solids, lactose, coconut oil, corn oil, medium chain triglycerides, soy lecithin. Protein 2.8 g, carbohydrate 10.7 g, fat 4.9 g, calories 96. Pow. Nursettes 120 ml. *otc.*
Use: Nutritional supplement.

Enfamil Ready To Use. (Bristol-Myers Squibb) Ready-to-use Enfamil infant formula 20 kcal/fl oz. Can 8 fl oz, 6-can pack; 32 fl oz, 6 cans per case. *otc.*
Use: Nutritional supplement.

•**enflurane.** (EN-flew-rane) U.S.P. 23.
Use: Anesthetic, inhalation.
See: Ethrane (Ohmeda Pharmaceuticals).

enflurane. (Abbott Laboratories) Enflurane 125 ml and 250 ml/Inhalation. *Rx.*
Use: Anesthetic, inhalation.

Engerix-B. (SmithKline Beecham) Hepatitis B vaccine (recombinant). **Adult:** 20 mcg/ml hepatitis B surface antigen. Vial 1 ml single-dose; 10 ml multidose vial; 1 ml Disp. Single-Dose Syr. **Pediatric:** 10 mcg/0.5 ml hepatitis B surface antigen. Vial 0.5 ml single-dose; 0.5 ml Disp. Single-Dose Syr. *Rx.*
Use: Vaccine.

•**englitazone sodium.** (EN-GLIH-tah-zone) USAN.
Use: Antidiabetic.

Enhancer. (Lafayette Pharmaceuticals) Barium sulfate 98%. Susp. Bot. 312 g. *Rx.*
Use: Radiopaque agent.

•**enilconazole.** (EE-nill-KOE-nah-zole) USAN.

Use: Antifungal.

•**eniluracil.** (en-ill-YOUR-ah-sill) USAN.
Use: Potentiator of antineoplastic activity of fluorouracil (uracil reductase inhibitor); antineoplastic (adjunct).

•**enisoprost.** (en-EYE-so-prahst) USAN.
Use: Antiulcerative.

Enisyl. (Person and Covey, Inc.) L-Lysine monohydrochloride 334 mg or 500 mg/Tab. Bot. 100s, 250s. *otc.*
Use: Nutritional supplement.

•**enlimomab.** (en-LIE-moe-mab) USAN.
Use: Anti-inflammatory; monoclonal antibody.

Enlon Injection. (Ohmeda Pharmaceuticals) Edrophonium Cl 10 mg/ml, phenol 0.45%, sodium sulfite 0.2%. Vial 15 ml. *Rx.*
Use: Cholinergic muscle stimulant.

Enlon-Plus. (Ohmeda Pharmaceuticals) Edrophonium chloride 10 mg, atropine sulfate 0.14 mg. Inj. Amp. 5 ml, Multidose Vial 15 ml. *Rx.*
Use: Muscle stimulant.

•**enloplatin.** (en-LOW-PLAT-in) USAN.
Use: Antineoplastic.

Ennex Ointment. (Ennex) Aloe vera extract 37.5%. **Skin Oint.:** Zinc oxide 12.5%, coal tar 1.5%, alcohol 4.5%. Tube oz. **Hemorrhoidal Oint.:** Tube oz. *otc.*
Use: Anti-inflammatory, astringent, antipruritic.

•**enofelast.** (EE-no-fell-ast) USAN.
Use: Antiasthmatic.

•**enolicam sodium.** (ee-NO-lih-kam) USAN.
Use: Anti-inflammatory, antirheumatic.

Enomine. (Major Pharmaceuticals) Phenylpropanolamine 45 mg, phenylephrine 5 mg, guaifenesin 200 mg/Cap. Bot. 100s, 500s. *Rx.*
Use: Decongestant, expectorant.

Enovid-E 21. (Searle) Norethynodrel 2.5 mg, mestranol 0.1 mg/Tab. Compack disp. 21s, 6 × 21. Refill 21s, 12 × 21. *Rx.*
Use: Estrogen, progestin combination.

Enovil. (Roberts Pharmaceuticals) Amtriptyline HCl 10 mg/ml. Vial 10 ml. *Rx.*
Use: Antidepressant.

•**enoxacin.** (en-OX-ah-SIN) USAN.
Use: Anti-infective.
See: Penetrex (Rhone-Poulenc Rorer Pharmaceuticals, Inc.).

•**enoxaparin sodium.** (ee-NOX-ah-PAR-in) USAN.
Use: Antithrombotic.
See: Lovenox Inj. (Rhone-Poulenc Rorer Pharmaceuticals, Inc.).

•**enoximone.** (EN-ox-ih-MONE) USAN.
Use: Cardiovascular agent.

•**enpiroline phosphate.** (en-PIHR-oh-LEEN) USAN.
Use: Antimalarial.

•**enprofylline.** (en-PRO-fih-lin) USAN.
Use: Bronchodilator.

•**enpromate.** (EN-pro-mate) USAN.
Use: Antineoplastic.

•**enprostil.** (en-PRAHS-till) USAN.
Use: Antisecretory, antiulcerative.

Enrich. (Ross Laboratories) Liquid food with fiber providing complete, balanced nutrition as a full liquid diet, liquid supplement, or tube feeding. One serving provides 5 g dietary fiber. 1100 calories/L. 1530 calories provides 100% US RDA for vitamins and minerals. Can Ready-to-Use 8 fl oz (vanilla, chocolate). *otc.*
Use: Nutritional supplement, enteral.

Ensidon. (Novartis Pharmaceutical Corp.) Opipramol HCl. *Rx.*
Use: Antidepressant.

Ensure. (Ross Laboratories) Liquid food providing 1.06 calories/ml. Can be used as a full liquid diet, liquid supplement or tube feeding. Two quarts (2000 calories) provides 100% US RDA for vitamins and minerals for adults and children over 4 yrs. **Ready-to-Use:** Bot. 8 fl oz (vanilla). Can 8 fl oz (chocolate, black walnut, coffee, strawberry, eggnog, vanilla), 32 fl oz (vanilla, chocolate). **Pow.:** Can 14 oz (400 g) (vanilla). *otc.*
Use: Nutritional supplement.

Ensure HN. (Ross Laboratories) High nitrogen low residue liquid food providing complete, balanced nutrition as tube feeding or oral supplement with 1.06 calories/ml. Provides 100% US RDA for vitamins and minerals for adults and children over 4 yrs. 1400 calories (1321 ml). Ready-to-Use: Can 8 fl oz (vanilla). *otc.*
Use: Nutritional supplement.

Ensure High Protein. (Ross Laboratories) Protein 50.4 g, carbohydrate 129.4 g, fat 25.2 g, < 21 mg cholesterol, Na 1218 mg, K 2100 mg, vitamin A 5250 IU, D 420 IU, E 47.5 IU, K 84 mcg, C 125 mg, folic acid 420 mg, B_1 1.6 mg, B_2 1.8 mg, B_3 21 mg, B_5 10.5 mg, B_6 2.1 mg, B_{12} 6.3 mcg, biotin 315 mcg, Ca 1050 mg, Cl, P, Mg, I, Mn, Cu, Zn 24 mg, Fe 19 mg, Se, Cr, Mo, 945 calories/237 ml. Liq. Bot. 237 ml. *otc.*

Use: Nutritional supplement.

Ensure Osmolite. (Ross Laboratories) *See:* Osmolite (Ross Laboratories).

Ensure Plus. (Ross Laboratories) High-calorie liquid food w/caloric density of 1500 calories/L. Six servings (8 oz and 2130 calories each) provides 100% US RDA for vitamins and minerals for adults and children. Ready-to-Use: Bot. 8 fl oz (vanilla). Can 8 fl oz (chocolate, vanilla, eggnog, coffee, strawberry). *otc.*
Use: Nutritional supplement.

Ensure Plus HN. (Ross Laboratories) High-calorie, high-nitrogen liquid food providing 1.5 calories/ml; 1420 calories provides 100% US RDA for vitamins and minerals for adults and children. Calorie/nitrogen ratio is 150:1. Can 8 fl oz (vanilla). *otc.*
Use: Nutritional supplement.

Ensure Pudding. (Ross Laboratories) Protein 6.8 g (nonfat milk), carbohydrate 34 g (sucrose, modified food starch), fat 9.7 g (partially hydrogenated soybean oil), vitamin A 850 IU, D 68 IU, E 7.7 IU, K 12 mcg, C 15.4 mg, folic acid 68 mcg, B_1 0.25 mg, B_2 0.29 mg, B_6 0.34 mg, B_{12} 1.1 mcg, B_3 3.4 mg, choline, biotin, B_5 1.7 mg, Na 240 mg, K 330 mg, Cl 220 mg, Ca 200 mg, P, Mg, I, Mn, Cu, Zn 3.83 mg, Fe 3.06 mg, 250 calories/can. Pudding. 150 g. *otc.*
Use: Nutritional supplement.

Entab 650. (Merz Pharmaceuticals) Aspirin 650 mg/EC tab. Bot. 100s. *otc.*
Use: Analgesic.

•**entacapone.** (en-TACK-ah-pone) USAN.
Use: Antidyskinetic; antiparkinsonian.

Entero-Test. (HDC Corporation) Cap. to identify duodenal parasites; to diagnose and locate upper GI bleeding, pH disorders, achlorhydria and esophageal reflux. Bot. 10s, 25s.
Use: Diagnostic aid.

Entero-Test Pediatric. (HDC Corporation) To identify duodenal parasites; to diagnose and locate upper GI bleeding, pH disorders, achlorhydria and esophageal reflux. Cap. Bot. 10s, 25s.
Use: Diagnostic aid.

Enterotube. (Roche Laboratories) Culture-identification method for Enterobacteriaceae ACA. Test kit 25s.
Use: Diagnostic aid.

Entertainer's Secret Spray. (KLI Corp.) Sodium carboxymethylcellulose, potassium Cl, dibasic sodium phosphate, aloe vera gel, glycerin, parabens. Soln. 60 ml spray. *otc.*
Use: Saliva substitute.

Entex. (Procter & Gamble Pharm.) Phenylephrine HCl 5 mg, phenylpropanolamine HCl 45 mg, guaifenesin 200 mg/Cap. Bot. 100s, 500s. *Rx.*
Use: Decongestant, expectorant.

Entex LA. (Procter & Gamble Pharm.) Phenylpropanolamine HCl 75 mg, guaifenesin 400 mg/TR Tab. Bot. 100s, 500s. *Rx.*
Use: Decongestant, expectorant.

Entex Liquid. (Procter & Gamble Pharm.) Phenylephrine HCl 5 mg, phenylpropanolamine HCl 20 mg, guaifenesin 100 mg/5 ml, alcohol 5%. Elix. Bot. 480 ml. *Rx.*
Use: Decongestant, expectorant.

Entex PSE. (Procter & Gamble Pharm.) Pseudoephedrine 120 mg, guaifenesin 600 mg. Prolonged action. Tab. Bot. 100s. *Rx.*
Use: Decongestant, expectorant.

entoidoin.
See: Entodon.

Entolase HP. (Wyeth-Ayerst Laboratories) Lipase 8000 units, protease 50,000 units, amylase 40,000 units/Cap. (enteric coated microbeads). Bot. 100s, 250s. *Rx.*
Use: Digestive enzyme.

Entrition Half Strength. (Biosearch Medical Products) Calcium and sodium caseinates, maltodextrin, corn oil, soy lecithin, mono- and diglycerides, protein 17.5 g, carbohydrate 68 g, fat 17.5 g, Na 350 mg, K 600 mg, calories 0.5/ml, osmolarity 120 mOsm/kg, water, vitamins A, B_1, B_2, B_3, B_5, B_6, B_{12}, C, D, E, K, Ca, P, Mg, I, Fe, Zn, Mn, Cu, Cl, biotin, choline, folic acid. Pouch 1 liter. *otc.*
Use: Nutritional supplement.

Entrition HN Entri-Pak. (Biosearch Medical Products) Sodium and calcium caseinates, soy protein isolate, maltodextrin, corn oil, soy lecithin, mono- and diglycerides, vitamins A, B_1, B_2, B_3, B_5, B_6, B_{12}, C, D, E, K, folic acid, biotin, choline, Ca, Cl, Cu, Fe, I, Mg, Mn, P, Zn. Pouch 1 liter. *otc.*
Use: Nutritional supplement.

Entrobag Set. (Lafayette Pharmaceuticals, Inc.) Enteroclysis set. Case 6 sets.
Use: Enteroclysis of the small intestine.

Entrobar. (Lafayette Pharmaceuticals, Inc.) Barium sulfate 50%. Susp. Bot. 500 ml. *Rx.*
Use: Radiopaque agent.

Entrokit. (Lafayette Pharmaceuticals, Inc.) Barium sulfate susp. (Entrobar),

methylcellulose (Entrolcel). Case 4 kits.
Use: Radiopaque agent.

Entrolcel. (Lafayette Pharmaceuticals, Inc.) Methylcellulose 1.8% w/w concentrate for dilution at time of use. Bot. 500 ml, case 24 Bot.
Use: Diagnostic aid.

•**entsufon sodium.** (ENT-sue-fahn) USAN.
Use: Detergent.

E.N.T.. (Springbok) Brompheniramine maleate 4 mg, phenylephrine HCl 5 mg, phenylpropanolamine HCl 5 mg/5 ml. Syr. Bot. 16 oz. *Rx.*
Use: Antihistamine, decongestant.

Entuss. (Roberts Pharmaceuticals) **Tab.:** Hydrocodone bitartrate 5 mg, guaifenesin 300 mg/Tab. Bot. 100s. **Syr.:** 5 mg hydrocodone bitartate, 300 mg potassium guaiacolsulfonate/5 ml. Alcohol free. Bot. 120 ml, 480 ml. *c-III.*
Use: Antitussive, expectorant.

Entuss-D Junior. (Roberts Pharmaceuticals) Pseudoephedrine HCl 30 mg, hydrocodone bitartrate 2.5 mg, guaifenesin 100 mg w/alcohol 5%, saccharin, sorbitol, sucrose. Liq. Bot. 120 ml, Pt. *c-III.*
Use: Antitussive, expectorant combination.

Entuss-D Liquid. (Roberts Pharmaceuticals) Hydrocodone bitartrate 5 mg, pseudoephedrine 30 mg/5 ml. 473 ml. *c-III.*
Use: Antitussive, decongestant.

Entuss-D Tablets. (Roberts Pharmaceuticals) Pseudoephedrine 30 mg, hydrocodone bitartrate 5 mg, guaifenesin 300 mg/Tab. Bot. 100s. *c-III.*
Use: Antitussive, decongestant, expectorant.

Enuclene. (Alcon Laboratories, Inc.) Tyloxapol 0.25%. Soln. Drop-tainer 15 ml. *otc.*
Use: Artificial eye care.

Enulose. (Alpharma USPD Inc.) Lactulose 10 g, galactose 2.2 g, lactose 1.2 g, other sugars ≤ 1.2 g. Syr. Pt, 2 qt. *Rx.*
Use: Laxative.

•**enviradene.** (en-VIE-rah-DEEN) USAN.
Use: Antiviral.

Enviro-Stress. (Vitaline Corp.) Vitamins B_1 50 mg, B_2 50 mg, B_3 100 mg, B_5 50 mg, B_6 50 mg, B_{12} 25 mcg, C 600 mg, E 30 IU, folic acid 0.4 mg, zinc 30 mg, Mg, Se, PABA. SR Tab. Bot. 90s, 1000s. *otc.*
Use: Mineral, vitamin supplement.

•**enviroxime.** (en-VIE-rox-eem) USAN.
Use: Antiviral.

Envisan Treatment Multipack. (Hoechst Marion Roussel) Dextranomer with PEG 3000 and PEG 600. Paste 10 g packets with nylon net and semi-occlusive film. *otc.*
Use: Dermatologic, wound therapy.

Enzest. (Barth's) Seven natural enzymes, calcium carbonate 250 mg/Tab. Bot. 100s, 250s, 500s. *otc.*
Use: Digestive enzymes, antacid.

Enzobile Improved. (Roberts Pharmaceuticals) Pancreatic enzyme concentrate 100 mg, ox bile extract 100 mg, cellulase 10 mg in inner core and pepsin 150 mg in outer layer. EC tab. Bot. 100s. *Rx-otc.*
Use: Digestive enzymes.

Enzone. (Forest Pharmaceutical, Inc.) Hydrocortisone acetate 1%, pramoxine HCl 1% in hydrophilic base w/stearic acid, aquaphor, isopropyl palmitate, polyoxyl 40, stearate, triethanolamine lauryl sulfate. Cream. Tube 30 g w/rectal applicator. *Rx.*
Use: Corticosteroid combination.

Enzymatic Cleaner for Extended Wear. (Alcon Laboratories, Inc.) Highly purified pork pancreatin to dilute in saline solution. Tab. Pkg. 12s. *otc.*
Use: Contact lens care.

Enzyme Formula #E-2. (Barth's) Amylase 30 mg, lipase 25 mg, bile salts 1 gr, wilzyme 10 mg, pepsin 2 gr, pancreatin 0.5 gr, calcium carbonate 4 gr/Tab. Bot. 100s, 250s. *Rx-otc.*
Use: Digestive aid.

enzymes.
See: Alpha Chymar, Vial (Centeon).
Cholinesterase (Various Mfr.).
Chymotrypsin.
Cotazym, Cap. (Organon Teknika Corp.).
Creon (Solvay Pharmaceuticals).
Diastase (Various Mfr.).
Pancreatin (Various Mfr.).
Papain (Various Mfr.).
Pepsin (Various Mfr.).

EPA. (NBTY, Inc.) N-3 fat content (mg) EPA 180 mg, DHA 120 mg, vitamin E 1 IU/Cap. Bot. 50s, 100s. *otc.*
Use: Nutritional supplement.

•**eperezolid.** (eh-per-EH-zoe-lid) USAN.
Use: Anti-infective.

•**ephedrine.** (eh-FED-rin) U.S.P. 23.
Use: Adrenergic (bronchodilator).
See: Bofedrol Inhalant (Jones Medical Industries, Inc.).
Racephedrine HCl (Various Mfr.).
W/Procaine.
See: Ephedrine and Procaine, Rx A', Amp. (Eli Lilly and Co.).

•**ephedrine hydrochloride.** (eh-FED-rin) U.S.P. 23.
Use: Bronchodilator.

ephedrine hydrochloride. (Various Mfr.) Cryst. Box 0.25 oz, 4 oz.
Use: Bronchodilator.

ephedrine hydrochloride w/combinations.
See: Ceepa, Tab. (Geneva Pharmaceuticals).
Co-Xan, Elix. (Schwarz Pharma, Inc.).
Derma Medicone (Medicore).
Derma Medicone HC, Oint. (Medicore).
Dynafed Asthma Relief, Tab. (BDI Pharmaceuticals, Inc.).
Golacol, Syr. (Arcum).
Kie, Tab., Syr. (Laser, Inc.).
Lardet Expectorant, Tab. (Standex).
Lardet, Tab. (Standex).
Mini Thin Asthma Relief, Tab. (BDI Pharmaceuticals, Inc.).
Mudrane, Tab. (ECR Pharmaceuticals).
Mudrane GG, Tab. (ECR Pharmaceuticals).
Quelidrine, Syr. (Abbott Laboratories).
Quibron Plus (Bristol-Myers Squibb).

ephedrine hydrochloride nasal jelly.
See: Efedron Nasal (Hyrex Pharmaceuticals).

•**ephedrine sulfate.** (eh-FED-rin) U.S.P. 23.
Use: Adrenergic (bronchodilator, nasal decongestant).

ephedrine sulfate. (West-Ward) 25 mg. Cap. Bot. 100s, 1000s. *otc.*
Use: Adrenergic (bronchodilator, nasal decongestant).

ephedrine sulfate. (Various Mfr.) 50 mg/Amp. Inj. 1 ml. *Rx.*
Use: Adrenergic (bronchodilator, nasal decongestant).

ephedrine sulfate w/combinations.
See: B.M.E., Elix. (Brothers).
Bronkaid, Preps. (Sanofi Winthrop Pharmaceuticals).
Marax DF, Syr. (Roerig).
Marax, Tab., Syr. (Roerig).
Pazo, Oint, Supp. (Bristol-Myers Squibb).
Wyanoids, Preps. (Wyeth-Ayerst Laboratories).

ephedrine sulfate and phenobarbital capsules.
Use: Bronchodilator, hypnotic, sedative.

1-ephenamine penicillin g. Compenamine.

Ephenyllin. (CMC) Theophylline 130 mg, ephedrine HCl 24 mg, phenobarbital 8 mg/Tab. Bot. 100s, 500s, 1000s. *Rx.*
Use: Bronchodilator, decongestant, hypnotic, sedative.

Ephrine Nasal Spray. (Walgreen Co.) Phenylephrine HCl 0.5%. Bot. 20 ml. *otc.*
Use: Decongestant.

Epi-C. (Lafayette Pharmaceuticals, Inc.) Barium sulfate 150%. Susp. Bot. 450 ml. *Rx.*
Use: Diagnostic aid.

•**epicillin.** (EH-pih-SILL-in) USAN.
Use: Anti-infective.

epidermal growth factor (human). (Chiron Therapeutics)
Use: Accelerate corneal healing. [Orphan Drug]

Epi-Derm Balm. (Pedinol Pharmacal, Inc.) Methyl salicylate, menthol, propylene glycol, alcohol. Bot. Gal. *otc.*
Use: Analgesic, topical.

EpiEZPen Autoinjector. (Center Laboratories) Epinephrine injection 1:2000. Delivers single dose of 0.3 mg. *Rx.*
Use: Emergency kit, anaphylaxis.

EpiEZPen Jr. Autoinjector. (Center Laboratories) Epinephrine injection 1:2000. Delivers single dose of 0.15 mg. *Rx.*
Use: Emergency kit, anaphylaxis.

Epifoam. (Schwarz Pharma, Inc.) Hydrocortisone acetate 1%, pramoxine HCl 1% in base of propylene glycol, cetyl alcohol, PEG-100 stearate, glyceryl stearate, laureth-23, polyoxyl 40 stearate, methylparaben, propylparaben, trolamine, or hydrochloric acid to adjust pH, purified water, butane, propane inert propellant. Aerosol container 10 g. *Rx.*
Use: Corticosteroid, topical.

Epiform-HC. (Delta Pharmaceutical Group) Hydrocortisone 1%, iodohydroxyquin 3% in cream base. Tube 20 g. *Rx.*
Use: Antifungal; corticosteroid, topical.

Epifrin Sterile Ophthalmic Solution. (Allergan, Inc.) Epinephrine HCl 0.5%, 1%, 2%. Bot. w/dropper 15 ml. *Rx.*
Use: Antiglaucoma.

E-Pilo. (Ciba Vision) Pilocarpine HCl 1%, 2%, 3%, 4%, 6%, epinephrine bitartrate 1%. Soln. Bot. 10 ml w/dropper-tip plastic vial. *Rx.*
Use: Antiglaucoma.

Epilyt. (Stiefel Laboratories, Inc.) Propylene glycol, glycerin, oleic acid, quaternium-26, lactic acid, BHT. Lotion. Bot. 118 ml. *otc.*
Use: Emollient.

•**epimestrol.** (EH-pih-MESS-trole) USAN.
Use: Anterior pituitary activator.

Epinal. (Alcon Laboratories, Inc.) Epi-

nephrine borate 0.5%, 1%. Dropper Bot. 7.5 ml. *Rx.*
Use: Antiglaucoma.

epinephran.
See: Epinephrine, Preps. (Various Mfr.).

•**epinephrine.** (epp-ih-NEFF-rin) U.S.P. 23.
Use: Asthma, hayfever, acute allergic states, cardiac arrest, acute hypersensitivity reactions, adrenergic (vasoconstrictor).
See: Asthma Meter, Aerosol (Rexall Group).
Asmolin, Vial (Lincoln Diagnostics).
Emergency Ana-Kit (Bayer Corp. (Consumer Div.)).
W/Lidocaine HCl.
See: Ardecaine 1%, 2%, Inj. (Burgin-Arden).

epinephrine. (Abbott Laboratories) Epinephrine 0.01 mg/ml. Soln. (Pediatric Inj). Box. 5 ml single-dose Abboject Syringe. *Rx-otc.*
Use: Asthma, hayfever, acute allergic states, cardiac arrest, acute hypersensitivity reactions, adrenergic (vasoconstrictor).

•**epinephrine bitartrate.** (epp-ih-NEFF-rim) U.S.P. 23.
Use: Adrenergic, ophthalmic.

epinephrine borate.
Use: Adrenergic, ophthalmic.
See: Epinal Ophth. Soln. (Alcon Laboratories, Inc.).

epinephrine hydrochloride. (Ciba Vision) 0.1%. Soln. 1 ml Dropperettes (12s). *Rx.*
Use: Adrenergic, ophthalmic. Emergency kit, anaphylaxis.
See: Adrenalin Cl, Soln. (Parke-Davis).
Ana-Guard Epinephrine, Inj. (Burgin-Arden).
EpiEZPen (Center Labs).
EpiEZPen Jr. (Center Labs).
EpiPen (Center Labs).
EpiPen Jr. (Center Labs).
Epifrin, Ophth. Soln. (Allergan, Inc.).
Epinal, Ophth. Soln. (Alcon Laboratories, Inc.).
Sus-Phrine, Amp., Vial (Berlex Laboratories, Inc).
Vaponefrin Solution & Nebulizer, Vial (Medeva Pharmaceuticals, Inc.).
W/Benzalkonium Cl, sodium Cl, sodium metabisulfite.
See: Glaucon, Soln. (Alcon Laboratories, Inc.).

epinephrine hydrochloride. (Various Mfr.) 1 mg/ml (1:1000 solution). Inj. Amp 1 ml. 0.1 mg/ml (1:10,000 solution). Inj. Vial 10 ml. *Rx.*
Use: Bronchodilator.

epinephrine, racemic.
See: AsthmaNefrin Solution (SmithKline Beecham).

epinephrine-related compounds.
See: Sympathomimetic Agents.

•**epinephryl borate ophthalmic solution.** (EPP-ih-NEFF-rill) U.S.P. 23.
Use: Adrenergic.

epinephryl borate ophthalmic solution.
Use: Adrenergic, ophthalmic.
See: Epinal (Alcon Laboratories, Inc.).
Eppy (PBH Wesley Jessen).

EpiPen Auto-Injector. (Center Laboratories) Epinephrine injection 1:1000. Delivers dose of 0.3 mg. Pkg. 1s, 2s, 2 ml injectors. *Rx.*
Use: Emergency kit.

EpiPen Jr. Auto-Injector. (Center Laboratories) Epinephrine injection 1:2000. Delivers dose of 0.15 mg. Pkg. 1s, 2s, 2 ml injectors. *Rx.*
Use: Emergency kit.

•**epipropidine.** (EPP-ih-PRO-pih-deen) USAN.
Use: Antineoplastic.

epirenan.
See: Epinephrine (Various Mfr.).

•**epirizole.** (eh-PEER-IH-zole) USAN.
Use: Analgesic, anti-inflammatory.

•**epirubicin hydrochloride.** (EH-pih-ROO-bih-sin) USAN.
Use: Antineoplastic.

•**epitetracycline hydrochloride.** (epp-ih-TEH-trah-SIGH-kleen HIGH-droe-KLOR-ide) U.S.P. 23.
Use: Anti-infective.

•**epithiazide.** (EH-pih-THIGH-azz-ide) USAN.
Use: Antihypertensive, diuretic.

Epitol. (Teva Pharmaceuticals USA) Carbamazepine 200 mg/Tab. Bot. 100s. *Rx.*
Use: Anticonvulsant.

Epivir. (GlaxoWellcome) Lamivudine. **Tab.:** 150 mg. Bot. 60s. **Oral Soln.:** 5 mg, 10 mg/ml. Bot. 240 ml. *Rx.*
Use: Antiviral.

Epivir-HBV. (GlaxoWellcome) Lamivudine. **Tab.:** 100 mg. Bot. 60s. **Oral Soln.:** 5 mg/ml. Bot. 240 ml. *Rx.*
Use: Antiviral.

•**eplerenone.** (eh-PLER-en-ohn) USAN.
Use: Antihypertensive; aldosterone antagonist.

EPO.
See: Epogen (Amgen, Inc.).
Procrit (Ortho Biotech, Inc.).

•**epoetin alfa.** (eh-POE-eh-tin) USAN.
Use: Antianemic; hematinic, hematopoietic. [Orphan Drug]
See: Epogen (Amgen, Inc.).
Procrit (Ortho Biotech, Inc.).

•**epoetin beta.** (eh-POE-eh-tin) USAN.
Use: Hematopoietic, hematinic, antianemic. [Orphan Drug]

Epogen. (Amgen, Inc.) Epoetin alfa (Erythropoietin; EPO) 2000 units, 3000 units, 4000 units, 10,000 units. Preservative free w/ 2.5 mg albumin (human) per ml. Vial 1 ml and 10,000 units in 2 ml multidose vials (1% benzyl alcohol). *Rx.*
Use: Hematopoietic.

•**epoprostenol.** (EH-poe-PROSTE-eh-nole) USAN. *Formerly Prostacyclin, PGI_2, Prostagland in I_2, Prostaglandin X, PGX.*
Use: Inhibitor (platelet). Primary pulmonary hypertension.
See: Flolan (Orphan drug) (Glaxo-Wellcome).

•**epoprostenol sodium.** (EH-poe-PROSTE-eh-nole) USAN.
Use: Inhibitor (platelet).
See: Flolan (GlaxoWellcome).

•**epostane.** (EH-poe-stain) USAN.
Use: Interceptive.

epoxytropine tropate methylbromide.
See: Methscopolamine Bromide (Various Mfr.).

Eppy/N. (PBH Wesley Jessen) Epinephryl borate ophthalmic soln. 0.5%, 1%, 2%. Bot. 7.5 ml. *Rx.*
Use: Antiglaucoma.

•**epristeride.** (eh-PRISS-the-ride) USAN.
Use: Inhibitor (alpha reductase).

Epromate. (Major Pharmaceuticals) Aspirin 325 mg, meprobamate 200 mg Tab. Bot. 100s, 500s. *c-IV.*
Use: Analgesic, anxiolytic.

•**eprosartan.** (eh-pro-SAHR-tan) USAN.
Use: Antihypertensive.

•**eprosartan mesylate.** (eh-pro-SAHR-tan) USAN.
Use: Antihypertensive.

Epsal. (Press Chem. & Pharm Labs) Saturated soln. of epsom salts 80% in ointment form. Jar 0.5 oz, 2 oz. *otc.*
Use: Drawing ointment.

Epsivite 100. (Standex) Vitamin E 100 IU/Cap. Bot. 100s. *otc.*
Use: Vitamin supplement.

Epsivite 200. (Standex) Vitamin E 200 IU/Cap. Bot. 100s. *otc.*
Use: Vitamin supplement.

Epsivite 400. (Standex) Vitamin E 400 IU/Cap. Bot. 100s. *otc.*
Use: Vitamin supplement.

Epsivite Forte. (Standex) Vitamin E 1000 IU/Cap. Bot. 100s. *otc.*
Use: Vitamin supplement.

epsom salt.
See: Magnesium Sulfate.

e.p.t. Stick Test. (Parke-Davis) Reagent in-home kit for urine testing. Pregnancy test. Kit 1s. *otc.*
Use: Diagnostic aid.

eptifibatide.
Use: Acute coronary syndrome.
See: Integrilin, Inj. (COR Therapeutics, Inc.).

eptoin.
See: Phenytoin Sodium (Various Mfr.).

Epulor. (Vista Pharm) Fat 31 g, carbohydrate 5 g, protein 4 g, calories 315/serving, biotin 100 mcg, B 50 mcg, Ca 333 mg, chloride 12 mg, Cr 40 mcg, Cu 200 mcg, folic acid 133 mcg, I 50 mcg, Fe 6 mg, Mg 133 mg, Mn 667 mcg, Mo 25 mcg, B_3 7 mg, Ni 2 mcg, B_5 3 mg, P 333 mg, K 35 mg, Se 23 mcg, Si 667 mcg, Na 7 mg, Sn 3 mcg, V 3 mcg, vitamin A 1667 IU, B_1 500 mcg, B_{12} 2 mcg, B_2 567 mcg, B_6 667 mcg, C 20 mg, D 133 IU, E 58 IU, K 8 mcg, Zn 5 mg. Liq. Pkg. 24s.
Use: Nutritional therapy, enteral.

Equagesic. (Wyeth-Ayerst Laboratories) Meprobamate 200 mg, aspirin 325 mg/Tab. Bot. 100s, UD 100s. *c-IV.*
Use: Analgesic, anxiolytic.

Equal. (Nutrasweet) Aspartame. **Packet:** 0.035 oz. (1 g). Box 50s, 100s, 200s. **Tab.:** Bot. 100s. *otc.*
Use: Artificial sweetener.

Equalactin. (Numark Laboratories, Inc.) Polycarbophil 625 mg (as calcium polycarbophil) dextrose, citric acid flavor. Chew. Tab. Bot. 48s. *otc.*
Use: Antidiarrheal or laxative.

Equanil. (Wyeth-Ayerst Laboratories) Meprobamate 200 mg or 400 mg/Tab. **200 mg:** Bot. 100s. **400 mg:** Bot. 100s, 500s, Redipak 25s. *c-IV.*
Use: Anxiolytic.

Equazine M. (Rugby Labs, Inc.) Aspirin 325 mg, meprobamate 200 mg, tartrazine. Tab. Bot. 100s, 500s. *c-IV.*
Use: Analgesic, anxiolytic.

•**equilin.** U.S.P. 23.
Use: Estrogen.

Equipertine. (Sanofi Winthrop Pharmaceuticals) Oxypertine. Cap. *Rx.*
Use: Anxiolytic.

Eradacil. (Sanofi Winthrop Pharmaceuticals) Rosoxacin. Cap. *Rx.*
Use: Antigonococcal agent.

Eramycin. (Wesley Pharmacal Co., Inc.)

Erythromycin FC Tab. Bot. 100s, 500s. *Rx.*
Use: Anti-infective, erythromycin.

•**erbulozole.** (ehr-BYOO-low-zole) USAN.
Use: Radiosensitizer; antineoplastic (adjunct).

Ercaf. (Geneva Pharmaceuticals) Ergotamine tartrate 1 mg, caffeine 100 mg/Tab. Bot. 100s, 1000s. *Rx.*
Use: Antimigraine.

Ergamisol. (Janssen Pharmaceutical, Inc.) Levamisole (base) 50 mg/Tab. Blister pack 36s. *Rx.*
Use: Antineoplastic.

Ergo Caff. (Rugby Labs, Inc.) Ergotamine tartrate 1 mg, caffeine 100 mg/Tab. Bot. 100s. *Rx.*
Use: Antimigraine.

•**ergocalciferol.** (ehr-go-kal-SIFF-eh-role) U.S.P. 23. *Formerly Oleovitamin D, Synthetic; Calciferol.*
Use: Treatment of refractory ricket; familial hypophosphatemia; hypoparathyroidism, vitamin (antirachitic).
See: Calciferol, Preps. (Schwarz Pharma, Inc.).
Drisdol, Liq., Cap. (Sanofi Winthrop Pharmaceuticals).
Vitamin D, Preps. (Various Mfr.).

ergocornine. (Various Mfr.) Ergot alkaloid. *Rx.*
Use: Peripheral vascular disorders.

ergocristine. (Various Mfr.) Ergot alkaloid. *Rx.*
Use: Vascular disorders.

ergocryptine. (Various Mfr.) Ergot alkaloid. *Rx.*
Use: Peripheral vascular disorders.

•**ergoloid mesylates.** (err-GO-loyd) U.S.P. 23. *Formerly Dihydroergotoxine Mesylate; Dihydroergotoxine Methanesulfonate; Dihydrogenated Ergot Alkaloids, Hydrogenated Ergot Alkaloids.*
Use: Psychotherapeutic, cognition adjuvant.
See: Hydergine Prods. (Novartis Pharmaceutical Corp.).

ergoloid mesylates.
Use: Psychotherapeutic agent, cognition adjuvant.

Ergomar. (Lotus Biochemical) Ergotamine tartrate 2 mg, lactose, peppermint oil, saccharin/Sublingual Tab. Pkg. 20s. *Rx.*
Use: Antimigraine.

ergometrine maleate.
See: Ergonovine (Various Mfr.)

Ergonal. (Vita Elixir) Ergot powder 259.2 mg, aloin 8.1 mg, apiol fluid green 290 mg, oil pennyroyal 28 mg/Cap. Bot. 24s. *Rx.*
Use: Oxytocic.

ergonovine. (Various Mfr.) Ergobasine, ergometrine, ergostetrine, ergotocine. *Rx.*
Use: Oxytocic.
See: Ergonovine Maleate.

•**ergonovine maleate.** (ehr-go-NO-veen MAL-ee-ate) U.S.P. 23.
Use: Oxytocic.
See: Methergine, Inj., Tab. (Novartis Pharmaceutical Corp.).

ergosterol, activated or irradiated. U.S.P. 23.
See: Ergocalciferol.

ergostetrine.
See: Ergonovine (Various Mfr.).

Ergot Alkalside Dihydrogenated.
See: ergoloid mesylates.

•**ergotamine tartrate.** (ehr-GOT-ah-mean TAR-trate) U.S.P. 23.
Use: Analgesic (specific in migraine).
See: Ergomar, Tab. (Lotus Biochemical).
W/Belladonna alkaloids, pentobarbital.
See: Wigraine, Tab. (Organon Teknika Corp.).
W/Belladonna alkaloids, phenobarbital.
See: Cafergot P-B, Supp. (Novartis Pharmaceutical Corp.).
W/Caffeine.
See: Bellergal, Tab. (Novartis Pharmaceutical Corp.).
W/Caffeine, homatropine methylbromide.
See: Cafergot, Supp. (Novartis Pharmaceutical Corp.).
W/Cyclizine HCl, caffeine.
See: Ergotatropin, Tab. (Cole).

ergotamine tartrate and caffeine suppositories.
Use: Vascular headache; analgesic (specific in migraine).
See: Cafergot, Supp. (Novartis Pharmaceutical Corp.).

ergotamine tartrate and caffeine tablets.
Use: Vascular headache; analgesic (specific in migraine).

ergotamine tartrate w/combinations.
See: Folergot-DF, Tab. (Marnel).

ergot, fluid extract. (Various Mfr.) Ergot 1 g/ml Bot. 4 oz, Pt.

ergotidine.
See: Histamine (Various Mfr.).

ergotocine.
See: Ergonovine (Various Mfr.).

Ergotrate Maleate. (Bedford Laboratories) Ergonovine maleate 0.2 mg/ml. Inj. Vial 1 ml. *Rx.*
Use: Oxytocic.

ergot-related products.
See: Cafergot, Supp., Tab. (Novartis

Pharmaceutical Corp.).
Cafergot P-B, Tab., Supp. (Novartis Pharmaceutical Corp.).
D.H.E. 45, Amp. (Novartis Pharmaceutical Corp.).
Ergonovine (Various Mfr.).
Ergotamine (Various Mfr.).
Ergotrate (Various Mfr.).
Hydergine, Sub. Tab. (Novartis Pharmaceutical Corp.).
Hydro-Ergot, Tab. (Henry Schein, Inc.).
Methergine, Amp., Tab. (Novartis Pharmaceutical Corp.).
Wigraine, Supp., Tab. (Organon Teknika Corp.).

eriodictin.
See: Vitamin P & Rutin.

eriodictyon. Flext., Aromatic Syrup.
Use: Pharmaceutic aid (flavor).
See: Vitamin P & Rutin.

E-R-O. (Scherer Laboratories, Inc.) Propylene glycol, glycerol. Bot. w/dropper tip 15 ml. *otc.*
Use: Otic.

•**ersofermin.** (EER-so-FEER-min) USAN.
Use: Dermatologic, wound therapy.

Ertine. (Health for Life Brands, Inc.) Hexachlorophene, benzocaine, cod liver oil, allantoin, boric acid, lanolin. Tube 1.5 oz. *Rx.*
Use: Burn and first aid remedy.

Erwinase. (Porton Product Limited) Erwinia L-asparaginase.
Use: Acute lymphocytic leukemia. [Orphan Drug]

erwina L-asparaginase.
Use: Acute lymphocytic leukemia.
See: Erwinase (Porton Product Limited).

Eryc. (Warner Chilcott Laboratories) Erythromycin 250 mg/DR Cap. Bot. 100s. *Rx.*
Use: Anti-infective, erythromycin.

Erycette. (Ortho McNeil Pharmaceutical) Erythromycin 2%. Pkg. 60 pledgets. *Rx.*
Use: Dermatologic, acne.

EryDerm 2%. (Abbott Laboratories) Erythromycin 2%. Topical soln. Bot. 60 ml. *Rx.*
Use: Dermatologic, acne.

Erygel. (Allergan, Inc.) Erythromycin 2%. Gel Tube 30 g, 60 g, Erygel 6 in 5 g (6s). *Rx.*
Use: Anti-infective, topical.

Erymax. (Allergan, Inc.) Erythromycin 2% Soln. 59 ml, 118 ml. *Rx.*
Use: Dermatologic, acne.

Erypar. (Parke-Davis) Erythromycin stearate 250 mg or 500 mg/Filmseal. **250 mg:** Bot. 100s, 500s. **500 mg:** Bot. 100s. *Rx.*
Use: Anti-infective, erythromycin.

EryPed. (Abbott Laboratories) Erythromycin ethylsuccinate 200 mg. Chew. Tab. Bot. 40s. *Rx.*
Use: Anti-infective, erythromycin.

EryPed Drops. (Abbott Laboratories) Erythromycin ethylsuccinate 100 mg/2.5 ml. Susp. Bot. 50 ml. *Rx.*
Use: Anti-infective, erythromycin.

EryPed 200. (Abbott Laboratories) Erythromycin ethylsuccinate 200 mg/5 ml. Susp. Bot. 480 ml. *Rx.*
Use: Anti-infective, erythromycin.

EryPed 400. (Abbott Laboratories) Erythromycin ethylsuccinate 400 mg/5 ml. Susp. Bot. 60 ml, 100 ml, 200 ml, UD 5 ml (100s). *Rx.*
Use: Anti-infective, erythromycin.

Ery-Tab. (Abbott Laboratories) Erythromycin enteric coated 250 mg, 333 mg, or 500 mg/Tab. Bot. 100s, 500s (except 500 mg), UD 100s. *Rx.*
Use: Anti-infective, erythromycin.

Erythra-Derm. (Paddock Laboratories) Erythromycin 2%, alcohol 66%. Soln. Bot. 60 ml. *Rx.*
Use: Dermatologic, acne.

•**erythrityl tetranitrate, diluted.** (eh-RITH-rih-till TEH-trah-NYE-trate) U.S.P. 23. *Formerly Erythrol Tetranitrate.*
Use: Coronary vasodilator.
See: Cardilate (GlaxoWellcome).

erythrityl tetranitrate tablets. (eh-RITH-rih-till TEH-trah-NYE-trate) (Various Mfr.) Erythritol, erythrol tetranitrate, nitroerythrite, tetranitrin, tetranitrol.
Use: Coronary vasodilator.
See: Anginar, Tab. (Pasadena Research Labs).
W/Phenobarbital.
See: Cardilate, Tab. (GlaxoWellcome).

Erythrocin Lactobionate. (Abbott Hospital Products) Erythromycin lactobionate. Pow. for Inj. 500 mg, *ADD-Vantage* vial 1 g. *Rx.*
Use: Anti-infective, erythromycin.

•**erythromycin.** (eh-RITH-row-MY-sin) U.S.P. 23.
Use: Anti-infective.
See: AK-Mycin, Oint. (Akorn, Inc.).
A/T/S, Gel (Hoechst Marion Roussel).
Del-Mycin, Soln. (Del Ray).
E-Base (Barr).
Emgel, Gel (GlaxoWellcome).
E-Mycin, Tab. (Pharmacia & Upjohn).
Eryc (Warner Chilcott).
Erymax, Soln. (Allergan, Inc.).
EryDerm, Soln. (Abbott Laboratories).
Ery-Tab (Abbott Laboratories).
Erythrocin, Prep. (Abbott Laboratories).

Erythromycin, Pledgets (Glades Pharmaceuticals).
Erythromycin Base, Filmtab (Abbott Laboratories).
Ilotycin, Prep. (Eli Lilly and Co.).
PCE, Tab. (Abbott Laboratories).
Robimycin, Tab. (Wyeth-Ayerst Laboratories).
T-Stat, Pads (Westwood Squibb Pharmaceuticals).
Theramycin Z, Soln. (Medicis Dermatologicals, Inc.).

erythromycin. (Pharmacia & Upjohn) Tab. 100 mg. Bot. 100s; 250 mg. Bot. 25s, 100s. 5 mg/g Oint. Tube 3.5 g, 3.75 g, UD 1 g.
Use: Anti-infective.

erythromycin. (Glades Pharmaceuticals) Erythromycin 2%, alcohol 95%. Gel Tube 30 g, 60 g. *Rx.*
Use: Dermatologic, acne.

•**erythromycin acistrate.** (eh-RITH-row-MY-sin ass-IH-strate) USAN.
Use: Anti-infective.

erythromycin and benzoyl peroxide topical gel. (eh-RITH-row-MY-sin and BEN-zoyl per-OX-ide)
Use: Anti-infective.

erythromycin base. (Various Mfr.) 250 mg. DR Cap. Bot. 60s, 100s, 500s. *Rx.*
Use: Anti-infective.

•**erythromycin estolate.** (eh-RITh-row-MY-sin ESS-toe-late) U.S.P. 23. *Formerly Erythromycin Propionate Lauryl Sulfate.*
Use: Anti-infective, erythromycin.
See: Ilosone, Preps. (Eli Lilly and Co.).

erythromycin estolate. (Various Mfr.) **Cap.:** 250 mg. Bot. 100s. **Susp.:** 125 mg/5 ml, 250 mg/5 ml. Bot. 480 ml. *Rx.*
Use: Anti-infective.

•**erythromycin ethylsuccinate.** (eh-RITH-row-MY-sin ETH-il-SUX-i-nate) U.S.P. 23.
Use: Anti-infective, erythromycin.
See: E.E.S. Prods. (Abbott Laboratories).
EryPed (Abbott Laboratories).
Pediamycin Prods. (Ross Laboratories).
Pediazole, Liq. (Ross Laboratories).

erythromycin ethylsuccinate. (Various Mfr.) **Tab.:** 400 mg. Bot. 100s, 500s. **Susp.:** 200 mg/5 ml, 400 mg/5 ml. Bot. 480 ml. *Rx.*
Use: Anti-infective.

erythromycin ethylsuccinate and sulfisoxazole acetyl for oral suspension. (eh-RITH-row-MY-sin Eth-ill-SUCK-sih-nate and sull-fih-SOX-ah-zole ASS-eh-till)
Use: Anti-infective.
See: Pediazole, Susp. (Ross Laboratories).

erythromycin filmtab. (Abbott Laboratories) Erythromycin base 250 mg or 500 mg/Tab. Bot. 100s; 500s, UD 100s (except 500 mg). *Rx.*
Use: Anti-infective, erythromycin.

•**erythromycin gluceptate, sterile.** (eh-RITH-row-MY-sin glue-SEP-tate) U.S.P. 23.
Use: Anti-infective, erythromycin.
See: Ilotycin Gluceptate, Amp. (Eli Lilly and Co.).

erythromycin glucoheptonate. U.S.P. 23.
See: Erythromycin Gluceptate, Ilotycin Glucoheptonate, Amp. (Eli Lilly and Co.).

erythromycin lactobionate. (Various Mfr.) 500 mg, 1 g. Pow. for Inj. Vial, piggyback vial (500 mg only). *Rx.*
Use: Anti-infective.

•**erythromycin lactobionate for injection.** (eh-RITH-row-MY-sin lack-toe-BYE-oh-nate) U.S.P. 23.
Use: Anti-infective, erythromycin.
See: Erythrocin Lactobionate, Vial (Abbott Laboratories).

erythromycin 2-propionate dodecyl sulfate. U.S.P. 23. Erythromycin Estolate
Use: Anti-infective, erythromycin.

erythromycin pledgets. (eh-RITH-row-MY-sin)
Use: Anti-infective, erythromycin.

Erythromycin Pledgets. (Glades Pharmaceuticals) Erythromycin 2%, alcohol 68.5%. Pledgets. Bot. 60s. *Rx.*
Use: Anti-infective, erythromycin.

•**erythromycin propionate.** (eh-RITH-row-MY-sin PRO-pee-oh-nate) USAN.
Use: Anti-infective.

erythromycin propionate lauryl sulfate.
Use: Anti-infective, erythromycin.
See: Erythromycin Estolate. Ilosone, Preps. (Eli Lilly and Co.).

•**erythromycin salnacedin.** (eh-RITH-row-MY-sin sal-NAH-seh-din) USAN.
Use: Dermatologic, acne.

•**erythromycin stearate.** (eh-RITH-row-MY-sin STEE-ah-rate) U.S.P. 23.
Use: Anti-infective, erythromycin.

erythromycin stearate. (Abbott Laboratories) 250 mg, 500 mg. Film coated tab. Bot. 100s, 500s, 1000s, Abbo-Pac 100s. *Rx.*

Use: Anti-infective.

erythromycin stearate. (Various Mfr.) 250 mg, 500 mg. Film coated tab. Bot. 100s, 500s, 1000s (250 mg only), UD 100s (500 mg only). *Rx.*
Use: Anti-infective.

erythromycin sulfate.
Use: Anti-infective, erythromycin.

erythromycin topical. (Various Mfr.) 2% Gel. Tube 30 g, 60 g. 2% Soln. Bot. 60 ml. *Rx.*
Use: Dermatologic, acne.
See: Emgel (GlaxoWellcome).
Erygel (Allergan, Inc.).

erythropoietin (recombinant human). (Boeing)
Use: Antianemic. [Orphan Drug]

erythrosine sodium. U.S.P. 23.
Use: Diagnostic aid (dental disclosing agent).

Eryzole. (Alra Laboratories, Inc.) Erythromycin ethylsuccinate 200 mg, acetyl sulfisoxazole 600 mg/5 ml when reconstituted. Gran for Susp. 100 ml, 150 ml, 200 ml. *Rx.*
Use: Anti-infective.

esclabron. Guaithylline.
Use: Antiasthmatic.

Esclim. (Serono) Estradiol 5 mg (0.025 mg/day), 7.5 mg (0.0375 mg/day), 10 mg (0.05 mg/day), 15 mg (0.075 mg/day), 20 mg (0.1 mg/day). Patch. Pkg. 24s, Calendar packs 8 and 24 systems. *Rx.*
Use: Estrogen.

Eserdine Forte Tabs. (Major Pharmaceuticals) Methyclothiazide, reserpine 0.5 mg/Tab. Bot. 100s. *Rx.*
Use: Antihypertensive, diuretic.

Eserdine Tabs. (Major Pharmaceuticals) Methyclothiazide, reserpine 0.25 mg/Tab. Bot. 100s, 250s. *Rx.*
Use: Antihypertensive, diuretic.

Eserine. Physostigmine as alkaloid, salicylate or sulfate salt. *Rx.*
Use: Antiglaucoma.

Eserine Salicylate. (Alcon Laboratories, Inc.) Physostigmine 0.5%. Soln. 2 ml. *Rx.*
Use: Antiglaucoma.

Eserine Sulfate Sterile Ophthalmic Ointment. (Ciba Vision) Physostigmine sulfate 0.25%. Tube 3.5 g. *Rx.*
Use: Antiglaucoma.

Esgic Capsules. (Forest Pharmaceutical, Inc.) Butalbital 50 mg, caffeine 40 mg, acetaminophen 325 mg/Cap. Bot. 100s. *Rx.*
Use: Analgesic, hypnotic, sedative.

Esgic Tablets. (Forest Pharmaceutical, Inc.) Butalbital 50 mg, caffeine 40 mg, acetaminophen 325 mg/Tab. Bot. 100s, 500s. *Rx.*
Use: Analgesic, hypnotic, sedative.

Esgic-Plus. (Forest Pharmaceutical, Inc.) Acetaminophen 500 mg, butalbital 50 mg, caffeine 40 mg/Tab. Bot. 100s, 500s. *Rx.*
Use: Analgesic, hypnotic, sedative.

Esidrix. (Novartis Pharmaceutical Corp.) Hydrochlorothiazide 25 mg, 50 mg/Tab. **25 mg:** Bot. 100s, 1000s, UD 100s. **50 mg:** Bot. 100s, 360s, 720s, 1000s, UD 100s. *Rx.*
Use: Antihypertensive, diuretic.

W/Apresoline.
See: Apresoline-Esidrix, Tab. (Novartis Pharmaceutical Corp.).

Esimil. (Novartis Pharmaceutical Corp.) Hydrochlorothiazide 25 mg, guanethidine monosulfate 10 mg/Tab. Bot. 100s. *Rx.*
Use: Antihypertensive, diuretic.

Eskalith. (SmithKline Beecham) Lithium carbonate. **Cap.:** 300 mg. Bot. 100s, 500s; **Tab.:** 300 mg. Bot. 100s. *Rx.*
Use: Antipsychotic.

Eskalith CR. (SmithKline Beecham) Lithium carbonate 450 mg/CR Tab. Bot. 100s. *Rx.*
Use: Antipsychotic.

•**esmolol hydrochloride.** (ESS-moe-lahl) USAN.
Use: Short-acting beta-adrenergic blocker; antiadrenergic (β-receptor).
See: Brevibloc, Inj. (Ohmeda Pharmaceuticals).

•**esorubicin hydrochloride.** (ESS-oh-ROO-bih-sin) USAN.
Use: Antineoplastic.

Esoterica Dry Skin Treatment Lotion. (SmithKline Beecham) Bot. 13 fl oz. *otc.*
Use: Emollient.

Esoterica Facial. (SmithKline Beecham) Hydroquinone 2%, padimate O 3.3%, oxybenzone 2.5%, sodium bisulfites, parabens, EDTA. Cream Tube 85 g. *otc.*
Use: Dermatologic.

Esoterica Medicated Fade Cream. (SmithKline Beecham) Hydroquinone 2%, padimate O 3.3%, oxybenzone 2.5%. Cream. Jar 90 g. *otc.*
Use: Dermatologic.

Esoterica Medicated Fade Cream, Facial. (SmithKline Beecham) Hydroquinone 2%, padimate O 3.3%, oxybenzone 2.5% in cream base. Jar 90 g, scented or unscented. *otc.*
Use: Dermatologic.

Esoterica Medicated Fade Cream, Regular. (SmithKline Beecham) Hydro-

quinone 2%. Cream. Jar 90 g. *otc.*
Use: Dermatologic.

Esoterica Sensitive Skin Formula. (SmithKline Beecham) Hydroquinone 1.5% with mineral oil, sodium bisulfite, parabens, EDTA. Cream. Jar 85 g. *otc.*
Use: Dermatologic.

Espotabs. (Combe, Inc.) Yellow phenolphthalein 97.2 mg/Tab. Bot. 12s, 30s, 60s. *otc.*
Use: Laxative.

•**esproquin hydrochloride.** (ESS-pro-kwin) USAN.
Use: Adrenergic.

Essential-8. Liquid amino acid protein supplement.
Use: Protein supplement.
See: Vivonex Diets, Liq. (Procter & Gamble Pharm.).

Estar. (Westwood Squibb Pharmaceuticals) Tar equivalent to 5% coal tar, U.S.P. in a hydro-alcoholic gel w/alcohol 13.8%. Tube 3 oz. *otc.*
Use: Antipsoriatic, antipruritic.

•**estazolam.** (ess-TAZZ-OH-lam) USAN.
Use: Hypnotic, sedative.
See: ProSom (Abbott Laboratories).

estazolam. (Zenith Goldline Pharmaceuticals) Estazolam 1 mg, 2 mg Tab. Bot. 30s, 100s, 500s, 1000s. *Rx.*
Use: Hypnotic, sedative.

Ester-C Plus. (Solgar Co., Inc.) Vitamin C 500 mg, citrus bioflavonoid complex 25 mg, acerola 10 mg, rutin 5 mg, rose hips 10 mg, calcium 62 mg/Cap. Bot. 50s. *otc.*
Use: Mineral, vitamin supplement.

Ester-C Plus, Extra Potency. (Solgar Co., Inc.) Vitamin C 1000 mg, citrus bioflavonoid complex 200 mg, acerola 25 mg, rutin 25 mg, rose hips 25 mg, calcium 125 mg/Tab. Bot. 30s. *otc.*
Use: Mineral, vitamin supplement.

esterified estrogens.
See: estrogens, esterified.

•**esterifilcon a.** (ess-TER-ih-FILL-kahn A) USAN.
Use: Contact lens material (hydrophilic).

Estilben.
See: Diethylstilbestrol Dipropionate (Various Mfr.).

Estinyl. (Schering-Plough Corp.) Ethinyl estradiol. **0.02 mg, 0.05 mg/Tab., coated:** Bot. 100s, 250s; **0.5 mg/Tab.:** Bot. 100s. *Rx.*
Use: Estrogen.

estopen.
See: Benzylpenicillin 2-diethylaminoethyl ester HI.

Estrace. (Bristol-Myers Squibb) Estradiol micronized 0.5 mg, 1 mg or 2 mg/Tab. Bot. 100s, 500s (except 0.5 mg). *Rx.*
Use: Estrogen.

Estrace Vaginal Cream. (Bristol-Myers Squibb) Estradiol 0.1 mg/g in a nonliquefying base, EDTA, methylparaben. Tube w/ applicator 42.5 g. *Rx.*
Use: Estrogen.

Estracon. (Freeport) Conjugated estrogens 1.25 mg/Tab. Bot. 1000s. *Rx.*
Use: Estrogen.

Estraderm Transdermal. (Ciba) Estradiol 4 mg (0.05 mg/day), 8 mg (0.1 mg/day). Calendar packs of 8 and 24 systems. *Rx.*
Use: Estrogen.

•**estradiol.** (ESS-truh-DIE-ole) U.S.P. 23. The form now known to be physiologically active is the β form rather than the α.
Use: Estrogen.
See: Aquagen, Vial, Aq. (Remsen).
Estrace, Tab., Vaginal Creme (Bristol-Myers Squibb).
Estraderm, Transdermal (Novartis Pharmaceutical Corp.).
Estring, Vaginal ring (Pharmacia & Upjohn).
FemPatch, Transd. Sys. (Parke-Davis).
Femogen, Susp., Tab. (Fellows-Testagar).
Progynon, Pellets (Schering-Plough Corp.).
W/Estriol, estrone.
See: Hormonin No. 1 and 2, Tab. (Schwarz Pharma, Inc.).
W/Estrone, estriol.
See: Sanestro, Tab. (Sandia).
W/Estrone, potassium estrone sulfate.
See: Tri-Estrin, Inj. (Keene Pharmaceuticals, Inc.).
W/Progesterone, testosterone, procaine HCl, procaine base.
See: Horm-Triad, Vial (Bell).
W/Testosterone and chlorobutanol in cottonseed oil.
See: Depo-Testadiol, Vial (Pharmacia & Upjohn).
Estraderm, Patch (Novartis Pharmaceutical Corp.).
Climara, Patch (Berlex Laboratories, Inc.).

estradiol cyclopentylpropionate.
W/Testosterone cypionate.
See: Depo-Testadiol, Vial (Pharmacia & Upjohn).

•**estradiol cypionate.** (ESS-trah-DIE-ole SIP-ee-oh-nate) U.S.P. 23.
Use: Estrogen.
W/Estradiol cyclopentylpropionate.

See: depGynogen (Forest Pharmaceuticals).
Depo-Estradiol Cypionate, Inj. (Pharmacia & Upjohn).
DepoGen, Inj. (Hyrex Pharmaceuticals).
D-Est, Inj. (Burgin-Arden).
Estroject-L.A., Vial (Merz Pharmaceuticals).
Hormogen Depot, Inj. (Roberts Pharmaceuticals).
Span-F, Inj. (Scrip).
W/Testosterone cypionate.
See: D-Diol, Inj. (Burgin-Arden).
Dep-Testestro, Inj. (Zeneca Pharmaceuticals).
Duo-Cyp, Vial (Keene Pharmaceuticals, Inc.).
Menoject, L.A., Vial (Merz Pharmaceuticals).
W/Testosterone cypionate, chlorobutanol.
See: T.E. Ionate P.A., Inj. (Solvay Pharmaceuticals).
Depo-Testadiol (Pharmacia & Upjohn).
Span FM, Inj. (Scrip).
TE Ionate PA, Inj. (Solvay Pharmaceuticals).

estradiol cypionate. (Various Mfr.) Estradiol cypionate 5 mg/ml, cottonseed oil w/chlorobutanol. Inj. Vial. 10 ml. *Rx.*
Use: Estrogen.

estradiol dipropionate.
Use: Estrogen.

•**estradiol enanthate.** (ESS-trah-DIE-ole eh-NAN-thate) USAN.
Use: Estrogen.

estradiol, ethinyl.
See: Ethinyl Estradiol.

estradiol hemihydrate.
Use: Estrogen.
See: Vagifem (Novo Nordisk).

estradiol monobenzonate.
See: Estradiol Benzoate.

estradiol, oral. (Teva) Micronized estradiol 0.5 mg, 1 mg, 2 mg. Tab. Bot. 100s. *Rx.*
Use: Estrogen.

estradiol trensdermal system.
Use: Estrogen.
See: Alora (Procter & Gamble).
Climara (Berlex).
CombiPatch (Rhone-Poulenc Rorer).
Esclim (Serono).
Estraderm (Ciba).
FemPatch (Parke-Davis).
Vivelle (Ciba-Geigy).

•**estradiol undecylate.** (ESS-trah-DIE-ole UHN-DEH-sill-ate) USAN.
See: Delestrec.

estradiol vaginal cream. (ESS-trah-DIE-ole)
Use: Estrogen.

•**estradiol valerate.** (ESS-trah-DIE-ole VAL-eh-rate) U.S.P. 23.
Use: Estrogen.
See: Ardefem 10, 20, Inj. (Burgin-Arden).
Deladiol, Inj. (Steris Laboratories, Inc.).
Delestrogen, Vial (Bristol-Myers Squibb).
Depogen, Inj. (Sigma-Tau Pharmaceuticals, Inc.).
Dioval, Preps. (Keene Pharmaceuticals, Inc.).
Duragen, Inj. (Roberts Pharmaceuticals).
Duratrad, Inj. (B. F. Ascher and Co.).
Estate, Inj. (Savage Laboratories).
Estra-L, Inj. (Taylor Pharmaceuticals).
Gynogen L.A., Inj. (Forest Pharmaceutical, Inc.).
Span-Est, Inj. (Scrip).
Valergen, Inj. (Hyrex Pharmaceuticals).
W/Benzyl alcohol.
See: Estate, Vial (Savage Laboratories).
W/Hydroxyprogesterone caproate.
See: Depo-Testadiol, Inj. (Pharmacia & Upjohn).
W/Testosterone enanthate.
See: Ardiol 90/4, 180/8, Inj. (Burgin-Arden).
Deladumone, Vial (Bristol-Myers Squibb).
Delatestadiol, Vial (Dunhall Pharmaceuticals, Inc.).
Duoval-P.A, I.M. (Solvay Pharmaceuticals).
Estra-Testrin, Inj. (Taylor Pharmaceuticals).
Span-Est-Test 4, Inj. (Scrip).
Teev, Inj. (Keene Pharmaceuticals, Inc.).
Tesogen LA, Inj. (Sigma-Tau Pharmaceuticals, Inc.).
Valertest, Inj. (Hyrex Pharmaceuticals).

estradiol valerate. (Various Mfr.) Inj. 20 mg/ml, 40 mg/ml. Vial 10 ml. 40 mg/ml. Vial 10 ml. *Rx.*
Use: Estrogen.

Estra-L. (Taylor Pharmaceuticals) Estradiol valerate in oil. 40 mg/ml. Vial 10 ml. *Rx.*
Use: Estrogen.

Estralutin.

•**estramustine.** (ESS-truh-muss-TEEN) USAN.
Use: Antineoplastic.

•**estramustine phosphate sodium.** (Ess-truh-muss-TEEN) USAN.
Use: Antineoplastic.
See: Emcyt, Cap. (Pharmacia & Upjohn).
Estratab. (Solvay Pharmaceuticals) Esterified estrogens 0.3 mg, 0.625 mg, 2.5 mg/Tab. Bot. 100s, 1000s (0.625 mg only). *Rx.*
Use: Estrogen.
Estratest. (Solvay Pharmaceuticals) Esterified estrogens 1.25 mg, methyltestosterone 2.5 mg/Tab. Bot. 100s, 1000s. *Rx.*
Use: Estrogen, androgen combination.
Estratest H.S. (Solvay Pharmaceuticals) Esterified estrogens 0.625 mg, methyltestosterone 1.25 mg/Tab. Bot. 100s. *Rx.*
Use: Estrogen, androgen combination.
•**estrazinol hydrobromide.** (ESS-trazz-ih-nahl) USAN.
Use: Estrogen.
estrin.
See: Estrone.
Estrinex. (Pharmacia & Upjohn)
See: Toremifene.
Estring. (Pharmacia & Upjohn) Estradiol 2 mg/Vaginal ring. Single packs. *Rx.*
Use: Estrogen.
•**estriol.** (ESS-tree-ole) U.S.P. 23.
Use: Estrogen.
Estrobene DP.
See: Diethylstilbestrol Dipropionate (Various Mfr.).
Estrofem. (Taylor Pharmaceuticals) Estradiol cypionate 5 mg/ml in oil. Inj. Vial 10 ml.
Use: Estrogen.
•**estrofurate.** (ESS-troe-FYOOR-ate) USAN.
Use: Estrogen.
estrogen-androgen therapy.
See: Androgen-Estrogen Therapy.
estrogenic substances, conjugated. (Water-soluble) A mixture containing the sodium salts of the sulfate esters of the estrogenic substances, principally estrone and equilin that are of the type excreted by pregnant mares. *Rx.*
See: Aquagen, Inj. (Remsen).
Ces, Tab. (Zeneca Pharmaceuticals).
Estroject, I.V., Vial (Merz Pharmaceuticals).
Estroquin, Tab. (Sheryl).
Estrosan, Tab. (Recsei Laboratories).
Evestrone, Tab. (Delta Pharmaceutical Group).
Orapin, Tab. (Standex).
Prelestrin, Tab. (Taylor Pharmaceuticals).
Premarin, I.V. (Wyeth-Ayerst Laboratories).
Premarin, Tab. (Wyeth-Ayerst Laboratories).
Premarin Vaginal Cream (Wyeth-Ayerst Laboratories).
W/Ethinyl estradiol.
See: Demulen, Tab. (Searle).
W/Meprobamate.
See: Milprem, Tab. (Wallace Laboratories).
PMB 200, Tab. (Wyeth-Ayerst Laboratories).
PMB 400, Tab. (Wyeth-Ayerst Laboratories).
W/Methyltestosterone.
See: Estratest, Tab. (Solvay Pharmaceuticals).
Estratest HS, Tab. (Solvay Pharmaceuticals).
Premarin with Methyltestosterone, Tab. (Wyeth-Ayerst Laboratories).
estrogenic substances in aqueous suspension. (Wyeth-Ayerst Laboratories) Sterile estrone suspension 2 mg/ml. Vial 10 ml. *Rx.*
Use: Estrogen.
estrogenic substance aqueous. (Various Mfr.) Estrogenic substance or estrogens (mainly estrone) 2 mg/ml. Inj. Vial 10 or 30 ml. *Rx.*
Use: Estrogen.
estrogenic substances mixed. May be a crystalline or an amorphous mixture of the naturally occurring estrogens obtained from the urine of pregnant mares. **Aqueous Susp.:** *See:* Gravigen, Inj. (Bluco Inc./Med. Discnt. Outlet). **Cap.:** W/Androgen therapy, vitamins, iron, d-desoxyephedrine HCl.
See: Premarin w/methyltestosterone, Tab. (Wyeth-Ayerst Laboratories).
•**estrogens, conjugated.** (ESS-truh-janz KAHN-juh-gay-tuhd) U.S.P. 23.
Use: Estrogen.
See: Conest, Tab. (Century Pharmaceuticals, Inc.).
Ganeake, Tab. (Geneva Pharmaceuticals).
PMB, Tab. (Wyeth-Ayerst Laboratories).
Premarin, Tab., I.V. (Wyeth-Ayerst Laboratories).
Premarin Vaginal Cream (Wyeth-Ayerst Laboratories).
Premarin with Methyltestosterone, Tab. (Wyeth-Ayerst Laboratories).
estrogens equine.
See: Estrogen.
PMB, Tab. (Wyeth-Ayerst Laboratories).

Premarin, Tab., I.V. (Wyeth-Ayerst Laboratories).
Premarin Vaginal Cream (Wyeth-Ayerst Laboratories).
Premarin with Methyltestosterone, Tab. (Wyeth-Ayerst Laboratories).

•**estrogens, esterified.** (ESS-troe-jenz, ess-TER-ih-fide) U.S.P. 23.
Use: Estrogen.
See: Estratab (Solvay Pharmaceuticals).
Menest, Tab. (SmithKline Beecham).
Menogen, Tab. (Breckenridge Pharmaceuticals, Inc.).
Menogen HS, Tab. (Breckenridge Pharmaceuticals, Inc.).

estrogens, esterified & androgens.
Use: Estrogen, androgen supplement.
See: Estratest.
Estratab (Solvay Pharmaceuticals).
Menest (SmithKline Beecham).

estrogens, natural.
Use: Estrogen.
See: Depogen, Vial (Hyrex Pharmaceuticals).
Estradiol, Preps. (Various Mfr.).
Estrone, Preps. (Various Mfr.).
Estrogenic Substance (Various Mfr.).
PMB, Tab. (Wyeth-Ayerst Laboratories).
Premarin, Tab, I.V. (Wyeth-Ayerst Laboratories).
Premarin Vaginal Cream (Wyeth-Ayerst Laboratories).
Premarin with Methyltestosterone, Tab. (Wyeth-Ayerst Laboratories).

estrogens, synthetic.
See: Dienestrol, Preps. (Various Mfr.).
Diethylstilbestrol, Preps. (Various Mfr.).

Estrogestin A. (Harvey) Estrogenic substance 1 mg, progesterone 10 mg/ml in peanut oil. Vial 10 ml. *Rx.*
Use: Estrogen, progestin combination.

Estrogestin C. (Harvey) Estrogenic substance 1 mg, progesterone 12.5 mg/ml in peanut oil. Vial 10 ml. *Rx.*
Use: Estrogen, progestin combination.

•**estrone.** (ESS-trone) U.S.P. 23.
Use: Estrogen.
See: Bestrone Suspension, Inj. (Bluco Inc. Med. Discnt. Outlet).
Estrogenic Substances in Aqueous Susp. (Wyeth-Ayerst Laboratories).
Kestrone 5, Inj. (Hyrex Pharmaceuticals).
Foygen, Vial (Foy Laboratories).
Menagen, Cap. (Parke-Davis).
Menformon (A), Vial (Organon Teknika Corp.).
Par-Supp, Vag. Supp. (Parmed Pharmaceuticals, Inc.).
Propagon-S, Inj. (Spanner).
Theelin, Vial, Aqueous and Oil (Parke-Davis).
W/Hydrocortisone acetate.
See: Ovulin, Inj. (Sigma-Tau Pharmaceuticals, Inc.).
W/Estriol, estradiol.
See: Hormonin, Tab. (Schwarz Pharma, Inc.).
W/Estrogens.
See: Estrogenic Mixtures, Preps. (Various Mfr.).
Estrogenic Substances, Preps. (Various Mfr.).
W/Lactose.
See: Estrovag, Supp. (Fellows-Testagar).
W/Potassium estrone sulfate.
See: Mer-Estrone, Inj. (Keene Pharmaceuticals, Inc.).
Sodestrin, Inj. (Solvay Pharmaceuticals).
W/Progesterone.
See: Duovin-S, Inj. (Spanner).
W/Testosterone.
See: Andesterone, Vial (Lincoln Diagnostics).
Anestro, Inj. (Roberts Pharmaceuticals).
Di-Hormone, Susp. (Paddock Laboratories).
Di-Met, Susp. (Organon Teknika Corp.).
Diorapin (Standex).
Dl-Steroid, Vial (Kremers Urban).
Estratest, Tab. (Solvay Pharmaceuticals)
W/Testosterone, sodium carboxymethylcellulose, sodium Cl.
See: Android-G, Vial (ICN Pharmaceuticals, Inc.).
Geratic Forte, Inj. (Keene Pharmaceuticals, Inc.).
Geriamic, Tab. (Vortech Pharmaceuticals).
Geritag, Inj, Cap. (Solvay Pharmaceuticals).

estrone aqueous. (Various Mfr.) Estrone aqueous 5 mg/ml. Inj. Vial 10 ml. *Rx.*
Use: Estrogen.

estrone sulfate, piperazine.
See: Ogen, Tab., Vaginal Cream (Abbott Laboratories).

estrone sulfate, potassium.
See: Estrogen, Vial (Davol).

•**estropipate.** (ESS-troe-PIH-pate) U.S.P. 23. *Formerly Piperazine Estrone Sulfate.*
Use: Estrogen.
See: Ogen, Tab., Vaginal Cream (Abbott Laboratories).

Ortho-Est (Ortho Pharma).

estropipate. (Various Mfr.) Estropipate 0.625 mg, 1.25 mg, 2.5 mg, 5 mg/Tab. Bot. 30s, 100s, 500s. *Rx.*
Use: Estrogen.

Estroquin. (Sheryl) Purified conjugated estrogens 1.25 mg/Tab. Bot. 100s. *Rx.*
Use: Estrogen.

Estrostep Fe. (Parke-Davis) Norethindrone acetate 1 mg, ethinyl estradiol 20 mcg/Triangular Tab. Norethindrone acetate 1 mg, ethinyl estradiol 30 mcg/Square Tab. Norethindrone acetate 1 mg, ethinyl estradiol 35 mcg/Round Tab. Ferrous fumarate 75 mg, lactose. Box. 28s. *Rx.*
Use: Contraceptive.

Estrostep 21. (Parke-Davis) Norethindrone acetate 1 mg, ethinyl estradiol 20 mcg/Triangular Tab. Norethindrone acetate 1 mg, ethinyl estradiol 30 mcg/Square Tab. Norethindrone acetate 1 mg, ethinyl estradiol 35 mcg/Round Tab. Lactose. Box. 21s. *Rx.*
Use: Contraceptive.

•**etafedrine hydrochloride.** (EH-tah-FED-rin) USAN.
Use: Bronchodilator, adrenergic.
See: Nethamine (Hoechst Marion Roussel).

•**etafilcon a.** (EH-tah-FILL-kahn A) USAN.
Use: Contact lens material (hydrophilic).

Etalent. (Roger) Ethaverine HCl 100 mg/Cap. Bot. 50s, 500s. *Rx.*
Use: Vasodilator.

etanercept.
Use: Antiarthritic.
See: Enbrel (Immunex).

•**etanidazole.** (ETT-ah-NIDE-ah-zole) USAN.
Use: Antineoplastic (hypoxic cell radiosensitizer).

E-Tapp. (Edwards Pharmaceuticals, Inc.) Brompheniramine maleate 4 mg, phenylephrine HCl 5 mg, phenylpropanolamine HCl 5 mg/5 ml, alcohol 2.3%. Elix. Bot. gal. *otc.*
Use: Antihistamine, decongestant.

•**etarotene.** (ett-AHR-oh-teen) USAN.
Use: Keratolytic.

•**etazolate hydrochloride.** (eh-TAY-zoe-late) USAN.
Use: Antipsychotic.

Eterna 27. (Revlon) Pregnenolone acetate 0.5% in cream base. *otc.*
Use: Emollient.

•**eterobarb.** (ee-TEER-oh-barb) USAN.
Use: Anticonvulsant.

•**ethacrynate sodium for injection.** (ETH-ah-KRIN-ate) U.S.P. 23.
Use: Diuretic.
See: Edecrin Sodium I.V., Inj. (Merck & Co).

•**ethacrynic acid.** (eth-uh-KRIN-ik) U.S.P. 23.
Use: Diuretic.
See: Edecrin, Tab. (Merck & Co.).

•**ethambutol hydrochloride.** (eth-AM-byoo-tahl) U.S.P. 23.
Use: Anti-infective (tuberculostatic).
See: Myambutol HCl (Lederle Standard Products).

Ethamicort.
See: Hydrocortamate.

•**ethamivan.** (eth-AM-ih-van) USAN. U.S.P. XX.
Use: Stimulant (central and respiratory).

Ethamolin. (Schwarz Pharma, Inc.) Ethanolamine oleate 5%. Inj. Amp. 2 ml. *Rx.*
Use: Sclerosing agent.

•**ethamsylate.** (ETH-AM-sill-ate) USAN.
Use: Hemostatic.

ethanol. (Various Mfr.) Alcohol, anhydrous.

ethanolamine. Olamine.

•**ethanolamine oleate.** (ETH-ah-nahl-ah-MEEN OH-lee-ate) USAN.
Use: Sclerosing agent. [Orphan Drug]
See: Ethamolin (Schwarz Pharma, Inc.).

•**ethchlorvynol.** (eth-klor-VIH-nahl) U.S.P. 23.
Use: Hypnotic, sedative.
See: Placidyl, Cap. (Abbott Laboratories).

ethenol, homopolymer. U.S.P. 23. Polyvinyl Alcohol.

•**ether.** (EE-ther) U.S.P. 23.
Use: Anesthetic, general; inhalation.

•**ethinyl estradiol.** (ETH-in-ill ess-trah-DIE-ole) U.S.P. 23.
Use: Estrogen.
See: Estinyl, Tab. (Schering-Plough Corp.).
Feminone, Tab. (Pharmacia & Upjohn).
Menolyn, Tab. (Arcum).

ethinyl estradiol. (Bio-Technology General Corporation)
Use: Turner's syndrome. [Orphan Drug]

ethinyl estradiol w/combinations.
See: Alesse-21, Tab. (Wyeth-Ayerst Laboratories).
Alesse-28, Tab. (Wyeth-Ayerst Laboratories).
Brevicon, Tab. (Roche Laboratories).
Demulen, Tab. (Searle).
Desogen, Tab. (Organon Teknika Corp.).

GenCept, Tab. (Gencon).
Estrostep Fe, Tab. (Parke-Davis).
Estrostep 21, Tab. (Parke-Davis).
Jenest-28, Tab. (Organon Teknika Corp.).
Levlite 21 (Berlex Labs.).
Levlite 28 (Berlex Labs.).
Levora 0.15/30-21, Tab. (SCS).
Levora 0.15/30-28. Tab. (SCS).
Loestrin, Tab. (Parke-Davis).
Loestrin 1.5/30, Tab. (Parke-Davis).
Lo/Ovral, Tab. (Wyeth-Ayerst Laboratories).
Mircette (Organon).
Modicon 21 and 28, Tab. (Ortho McNeil Pharmaceutical).
Nelulen, Tab. (Watson Laboratories).
Nordette, Tab. (Wyeth-Ayerst Laboratories).
Norinyl, Prods. (Roche Laboratories).
Norlestrin, Tab. (Parke-Davis).
Norlestrin Fe, Tab. (Parke-Davis).
Ortho-Cept, Tab. (Ortho McNeil Pharmaceutical).
Ortho-Cyclen, Tab. (Ortho McNeil Pharmaceutical).
Ortho-Novum 1/35, 21, and 28 (Ortho McNeil Pharmaceutical).
Ortho Tri-Cyclen, Tab. (Ortho McNeil Pharmaceutical).
Ovcon-35, Tab. (Bristol-Myers Squibb).
Ovcon-50, Tab. (Bristol-Myers Squibb).
Ovlin, Vial (Zeneca Pharmaceuticals).
Ovral, Tab. (Wyeth-Ayerst Laboratories).
Preven (Gynetics).
Triphasil, Tab. (Wyeth-Ayerst Laboratories).
Zovia, Tab. (Watson Laboratories).

ethinyl estradiol and dimethisterone tablets.
Use: Estrogen, progestin combination.

ethinyl estrenol.
See: Lynestrenol (Organon Teknika Corp.).

•**ethiodized oil injection.** (eth-EYE-oh-dized) U.S.P. 23.
Use: Diagnostic aid (radiopaque medium).
See: Ethiodol, Inj. (Savage Laboratories).

•**ethiodized oil I 131.** (eth-EYE-oh-dized OIL I 131) USAN.
Use: Antineoplastic, radiopharmaceutical.

Ethiodol. (Savage Laboratories) Ethiodized oil. Poppy seed oil, iodine 475 mg/ml. Inj. Amp. 10 ml. *Rx.*
Use: Diagnostic aid.

Ethiofos. (eh-THIGH-oh-foss)
See: Amifostine.

•**ethionamide.** (eh-THIGH-ohn-ah-mide) U.S.P. 23.
Use: Anti-infective (tuberculostatic).
See: Trecator S.C., Tab. (Wyeth-Ayerst Laboratories).

ethisterone.
See: Anhydrohydroxyprogesterone (Various Mfr.).

Ethmozine. (Roberts Pharmaceuticals) Moricizine HCl 200 mg, 250 mg, or 300 mg/Tab. Bot. 21s, 100s, UD 100s. *Rx.*
Use: Antiarrhythmic.

Ethocaine.
See: Procaine HCl (Various Mfr.).

ethocylorvynol. U.S.P. 23.

ethodryl.
See: Diethylcarbamazine Citrate.

ethohexadiol. Used in Comp. Dimethyl Phthalate.
Use: Insect repellent.

•**ethonam nitrate.** (ETH-oh-nam NYE-trate) USAN.
Use: Antifungal.

•**ethosuximide.** (ETH-oh-SUX-ih-mide) U.S.P. 23.
Use: Anticonvulsant.
See: Zarontin, Cap., Syr. (Parke-Davis).

ethosuximide. (Copley Pharmaceutical, Inc.) Ethosuximide 250 mg/5 ml, saccharin, sucrose, raspberry flavor. Syr. Bot. 483 ml. *Rx.*
Use: Anticonvulsant.

•**ethotoin.** (ETH-oh-toyn) U.S.P. 23.
Use: Anticonvulsant.
See: Peganone (Abbott Laboratories).

ethovan. Ethyl Vanillin.

•**ethoxazene hydrochloride.** (eth-OX-ah-zeen) USAN.
Use: Analgesic.

ethoxzolamide.
Use: Carbonic anhydrase inhibitor.

Ethrane. (Ohmeda Pharmaceuticals) Enflurane. Volatile Liq. Bot. 125 ml, 250 ml. *Rx.*
Use: Anesthetic, general.

•**ethybenztropine.** (ETH-ih-BENZ-troe-peen) USAN.
Use: Anticholinergic.

•**ethyl acetate.** (ETH-ill ASS-eh-tate) N.F. 18.
Use: Pharmaceutic aid, flavoring; solvent.

ethyl aminobenzoate. Anesthesin, anesthrone, benzocaine, parathesin.
Use: Anesthetic, local.
See: Benzocaine (Various Mfr.).

ethyl bromide. (Various Mfr.) Bromoeth-

ane. *Rx.*
Use: Anesthetic, general.

ethyl carbamate.
See: Urethan (Various Mfr.).

•**ethylcellulose.** N.F. 18.
Use: Tablet binder, pharmaceutic aid.

ethylcellulose aqueous dispersion.
Use: Tablet binder, pharmaceutic aid.

ethyl chaulmoograte.
Use: Hansen's disease, sarcoidosis.

•**ethyl chloride.** (ETH-ill KLOR-ide) U.S.P. 23.
Use: Anesthetic, topical.

ethyl chloride. (Various Mfr.) Ethyl chloride 100 g chloroethane/Spray. Bot. 105 ml, 120 ml. *Rx.*
Use: Anesthetic, local.

•**ethyl dibunate.** (ETH-ill DIE-byoo-nate) USAN.
Use: Cough suppressant, antitussive.

ethyl diiodobrassidate. Iodobrassid. Lipoiodine.

ethyldimethylammonium bromide.
See: Ambutonium Bromide.

ethylene. (Various Mfr.) Ethene. *Rx.*
Use: Anesthetic, general.

•**ethylenediamine.** (eth-ih-leen-DIE-ah-meen) U.S.P. 23.
Use: Component of aminophylline injection.

ethylenediamine solution. (67% w/v).
Use: Solvent (Aminophylline Inj.).

ethylenediaminetetraacetic acid.
See: Edathamil, EDTA (Various Mfr.).

ethylenediamine tetraacetic acid disodium salt.
See: Endrate Disodium, Amp. (Abbott Laboratories).

•**ethylestrenol.** (ETH-ill-ESS-tree-nahl) USAN.
Use: Anabolic.

ethylhydrocupreine hydrochloride.
Use: Antiseptic.

ethylmorphine hydrochloride.
Use: Narcotic.

ethyl nitrite spirit. Ethyl nitrite. Sweet Spirit of Niter. Spirit of Nitrous Ether.

•**ethyl oleate.** (ETH-ill) N.F. 18.
Use: Pharmaceutic aid (vehicle).

ethyl oxide; ethyl ether.
Use: Solvent.

•**ethylparaben.** (eth-ill-PAR-ah-ben) N.F. 18.
Use: Pharmaceutic aid (antifungal preservative).

ethylstibamine. Astaril, neostibosan.
Use: Antimony therapy.

•**ethyl vanillin.** (ETH-ill) N.F. 18.
Use: Pharmaceutic aid (flavor).

•**ethynerone.** (eth-EYE-ner-ohn) USAN.
Use: Hormone, progestin.

•**ethynodiol diacetate.** (eh-THIN-oh-die-ole die-ASS-eh-tate) U.S.P. 23.
Use: Progesterone, progestin.
W/Ethinyl estradiol.
See: Ovulen, Tab. (Searle).
Demulen, Preps. (Searle).
Estrostep Fe, Tab. (Parke-Davis).
Estrostep 21, Tab. (Parke-Davis).
Nelulen, Tab. (Watson Laboratories).
Zovia, Tab. (Watson Laboratories).
W/Mestranol.
See: Ovulen, Tab. (Searle).

ethynodiol diacetate and ethinyl estradiol tablets.
Use: Contraceptive.

ethynodiol diacetate and mestranol tablets.
Use: Contraceptive.

ethynylestradiol.
See: Ethinyl Estradiol, U.S.P. (Various Mfr.).
Mestranol (Various Mfr.).

ethynylestradiol 3-methyl ether.
See: Enovid, Tab. (Searle).

Ethyol. (Alza/US Bioscience) Pow. for Inj. Lyophilized: 500 mg (anhydrous basis) 500 mg mannitol in 10 ml single-use vials. *Rx.*
Use: Cyto-protective agent.

•**etibendazole.** (eh-tie-BEN-dah-ZOLE) USAN.
Use: Anthelmintic.

Eticylol. (Novartis Pharmaceutical Corp.) Ethinyl estradiol. *Rx.*
Use: Estrogen.

•**etidocaine.** (eh-TIE-doe-cane) USAN.
Use: Anesthetic, local.
See: Duranest, Inj. (Astra Pharmaceuticals, L.P.).
Duranest-MPF, Inj. (Astra Pharmaceuticals, L.P.).

•**etidronate disodium.** (eh-TIH-DROE-nate) U.S.P. 23.
Use: Bone resorption inhibitor. Treatment of symptomatic Paget's disease of bone (osteitis deformans). Degenerative metabolic bone disease. [Orphan Drug]
See: Didronel, Tab. (Procter & Gamble Pharm.).

•**etidronic acid.** (eh-tih-DRAH-nik) USAN.
Use: Calcium regulator.

•**etifenin.** (EH-tih-FEN-in) USAN.
Use: Diagnostic aid.

•**etintidine hydrochloride.** (ett-IN-tih-DEEN) USAN.
Use: Antiulcerative.

etiocholanedoine. (SuperGen, Inc.)

Use: Aplastic anemia; Prader-Willi syndrome. [Orphan Drug]

•**etocrylene.** (EH-toe-KRIH-leen) USAN.
Use: Ultraviolet screen.

•**etodolac.** (EE-toe-DOE-lak) USAN.
Use: Analgesic, NSAID.
See: Lodine (Wyeth-Ayerst Laboratories).
Lodine XL, ER Tab. (Wyeth-Ayerst Laboratories).

etodolac. (Zenith Goldline Pharmaceuticals) Etodolac 400 mg, lactose, polyethylene glycol, povidone. Tab. Bot. 100s, 500s, 1000s. *Rx.*
Use: Analgesic.

•**etofenamate.** (EH-toe-FEN-am-ate) USAN.
Use: Analgesic, anti-inflammatory.

•**etoformin hydrochloride.** (EH-toe-FORE-min) USAN.
Use: Antidiabetic.

•**etomidate.** (eh-TAHM-ih-date) USAN.
Use: Hypnotic, sedative.
See: Amidate (Abbott Laboratories).

etomide hydrochloride. (ETT-oh-mide) Bandol. Carbiphene HCl.

•**etonogestrel.** (ETT-oh-no-JESS-trell) USAN.
Use: Hormone, progestin.

•**etoperidone hydrochloride.** (EH-toe-PURR-ih-dohn) USAN.
Use: Antidepressant.
See: Vepesid, Inj., Cap. (Bristol-Myers Squibb).

Etopophos. (Bristol-Myers Oncology/Immunology) Etoposide phosphate diethanolate 119.3 mg (100 mg etoposide), dextran 40 300 mg/Pow. for Inj. Vials. Single dose. *Rx.*
Use: Antineoplastic.

•**etoposide.** (EH-toe-POE-side) U.S.P. 23.
Use: Antineoplastic.
See: Etopophos, Pow. for Inj. (Bristol-Myers Oncology/Immunology).
Toposar, Inj. (Pharmacia & Upjohn).
Vepesid, Inj., Cap. (Bristol-Myers Squibb).

etoposide. (EH-toe-POE-side) (Various Mfr.) Etoposide 20 mg/ml, alcohol 30.5%, benzyl alcohol 30 mg, polysorbate 80 80 mg, PEG 300 650 mg, citric acid 2 mg/ml. Inj. Vial 5 ml, 12.5 ml, 25 ml. *Rx.*
Use: Antineoplastic.

•**etoposide phosphate.** (ee-toe-POE-side) USAN.
Use: Antineoplastic.
See: Etopophos, Pow. for Inj. (Bristol-Myers Oncology/Immunology).

•**etoprine.** (ETT-oh-preen) USAN.
Use: Antineoplastic.

etoquinol sodium. Name used for Actinoquinol sodium.

etoval.
See: Butethal, N.F. (Various Mfr.).

•**etoxadrol hydrochloride.** (eh-TOX-ah-drole) USAN.
Use: Anesthetic.

•**etozolin.** (EAT-oh-zoe-lin) USAN.
Use: Diuretic.

Etrafon (2-10). (Schering-Plough Corp.) Perphenazine 2 mg, amitriptyline HCl 10 mg/Tab. Bot. 100s, 500s, UD 100s. *Rx.*
Use: Psychotherapeutic combination.

Etrafon (2-25). (Schering-Plough Corp.) Perphenazine 2 mg, amitriptyline HCl 25 mg/Tab. Bot. 100s, 500s, UD 100s. *Rx.*
Use: Psychotherapeutic combination.

Etrafon-A (4-10). (Schering-Plough Corp.) Perphenazine 4 mg, amitriptyline HCl 10 mg/Tab. Bot. 100s, UD 100s. *Rx.*
Use: Psychotherapeutic combination.

Etrafon Forte (4-25). (Schering-Plough Corp.) Perphenazine 4 mg, amitriptyline HCl 25 mg/Tab. Bot. 100s, 500s, UD 100s. *Rx.*
Use: Psychotherapeutic combination.

•**etretinate.** (eh-TRETT-ih-nate) USAN.
Use: Antipsoriatic.

etrynit. Propatyl nitrate.
Use: Cardiovascular agent.

•**etryptamine acetate.** (ee-TRIP-tah-meen) USAN.
Use: Central stimulant.

E.T.S.-2%. (Paddock Laboratories) Erythromycin topical 2%. Soln. Bot. 60 ml. *Rx.*
Use: Dermatologic, acne.

ettriol trinitrate.
See: Propatyl nitrate.

etybenzatropine. Ethybenztropine.

etynodiol acetate. Ethynodiol Diacetate.

eubasin.
See: Sulfapyridine (Various Mfr.).

eucaine hydrochloride. (Novartis Pharmaceutical Corp.) Menthol 8%, eucalyptus oil, SD 3A alcohol. Gel. Tube 60 g. *otc.*
Use: Liniment.

Eucalyptamint. (Novartis Pharmaceutical Corp.) Menthol 8%, eucalyptus oil, SD 3A alcohol. Gel 60 g. *otc.*
Use: Liniment.

Eucalyptamint Maximum Strength. (Novartis Pharmaceutical Corp.) Menthol 16%, lanolin, eucalyptus oil. Oint.

Tube 60 ml. *otc.*
Use: Liniment.

•**eucalyptol.** USAN.
Use: Pharmaceutic aid (flavor); antitussive; decongestant, nasal.
See: Vicks Sinex, Nasal Spray (Procter & Gamble Pharm.).
Vicks Va-Tro-Nol, Nose Drops (Procter & Gamble Pharm.).
Vicks Prods. (Procter & Gamble Pharm.).

eucalyptus oil.
Use: Flavor; antitussive; decongestant, nasal; expectorant; analgesic, topical.
See: Vicks Prods. (Procter & Gamble Pharm.).
Victors Regular, Cherry Loz. (Procter & Gamble Pharm.).

•**eucatropine hydrochloride.** (you-CAT-troe-peen) U.S.P. 23.
Use: Pharmaceutical necessity for ophthalmic dosage form; anticholinergic, ophthalmic.

eucatropine hydrochloride. (Glogau) Crystal, Bot. g.
Use: Pharmaceutical necessity for ophthalmic dosage form; anticholinergic, ophthalmic.

Eucerin. (Beiersdorf, Inc.) Unscented moisturizing formula. **Creme:** Jar 120 g, lb. **Lot.:** Bot. 240 ml, 480 ml. *otc.*
Use: Emollient.

Eucerin Cleansing. (Beiersdorf, Inc.) Sodium laureth sulfate, cocoamphocarboxyglycinate, cocamidopropyl betaine, cocamide MEA, PEG-7 glyceryl cocoate, PEG-5 lanolate, PEG-120 methyl glucose dioleate, lanolin alcohol, imidazolidinyl urea. Soap free. Lot. Bot. 240 ml. *otc.*
Use: Dermatologic, cleanser.

Eucerin Dry Skin Care Daily Facial. (Beiersdorf, Inc.) Ethylhexyl p-methoxycinnamate, titanium dioxide, 2-phenylbenzimidazole-5-sulfonic acid, 2-ethylhexyl salicylate, mineral oil, cetearyl alcohol, castor oil, lanolin alcohol, EDTA. SPF 20. Lot. Bot. 120 ml. *otc.*
Use: Sunscreen.

Eucerin Plus. (Beiersdorf, Inc.) Mineral oil, hydrogenated castor oil, sodium lactate 5%, urea 5%, glycerin, lanolin alcohol. Lot. Bot. 177 ml. *otc.*
Use: Emollient.

eucodal.
See: Oxycodone.

eucupin dihydrochloride. Isoamylhydrocupreine dihydrochloride.

Eudal-SR. (Forest Pharmaceutical, Inc.) Pseudoephedrine 120 mg, guaifenesin 400 mg/SR Tab. Bot. 100s. *Rx.*
Use: Decongestant, expectorant.

euflavine.
See: Acriflavine (Various Mfr.).

•**eugenol.** (you-jeh-nole) U.S.P. 23.
Use: Dental analgesic, oral anesthetic.
See: Benzodent, Oint. (Procter & Gamble Pharm.).

eukadol.
See: Dihydrohydroxycodeinone, Preps. (No Manufacturer Available).

Eulcin. (Leeds) Methscopolamine bromide 2.5 mg, butabarbital sodium 10 mg, aluminum hydroxide gel, dried, 250 mg, magnesium trisilicate 250 mg/Tab. Bot. 100s. *Rx.*
Use: Antacid, anticholinergic, antispasmodic, hypnotic, sedative.

Eulexin. (Schering-Plough Corp.) Flutamide 125 mg/Cap. 100s, 500s, UD 100s. *Rx.*
Use: Antineoplastic.

Eumydrin Drops. (Sanofi Winthrop Pharmaceuticals) Atropine methonitrate. *Rx.*
Use: Anticholinergic, antispasmodic.

euneryl.
See: Phenobarbital (Various Mfr.).

Euphorbia Compound. (Sherwood Davis & Geck) Euphorbia pilulifera fluid extract 1.5 ml, lobelia tincture 2.2 ml, nitroglycerin spirit 0.29 ml, sodium iodide 1.04 g, sodium bromide 1.04 g, alcohol 24%/30 ml. Bot. Pt, gal. *Rx.*
Use: Expectorant, hypnotic, sedative.

euphorbia pilulifera.
W/Cocillana, squill, antimony potassium tartrate, senega.
See: Cylana, Syr. (Jones Medical Industries, Inc.).
W/Phenyl salicylate and various oils.
See: Rayderm, Oint. (Velvet Pharmacal).

Eupractone. (Baxter Pharmaceutical Products, Inc.) Dimethadione.

•**euprocin hydrochloride.** (YOU-pro-sin) USAN.
Use: Anesthetic, local.
See: Eucupin HCl.

euquinine. Quinine ethyl carbonate.
Use: Antimalarial, antipyretic.

Eurax. Albutoin.

Eurax Cream. (Westwood Squibb Pharmaceuticals) Crotamiton 10% in vanishing-cream base of glyceryl monostearate, anhydrous lanolin, PEG 6-32, glycerin, polysorbate 80, benzyl alcohol, mineral oil, white wax, quaternium-15, fragrance. Tube 60 g. *Rx.*
Use: Scabicide, pediculicide.

Eurax Lotion. (Westwood Squibb Phar-

maceuticals) Crotamiton 10% in emollient-lotion base of glyceryl monostearate, anhydrous lanolin, PEG 6-32, glycerin, polysorbate 80, benzyl alcohol, light mineral oil, carboxymethylcellulose, simethicone, quaternium-15, fragrance. Bot. 60 g, 454 g. *Rx.*
Use: Scabicide, pediculicide.

Evac-Q-Kit. (Pharmacia & Upjohn) Each kit contains: **Evac-Q-Mag:** Magnesium citrate 300 ml, citric acid, potassium citrate. **Evac-Q-Tabs:** 2 tab. phenolphthalein 130 mg/Tab. **Evac-Q-Sert:** Supp. containing potassium bitartrate, sodium bicarbonate/supp. in polyethylene glycol base. Patient instruction sheet. *otc.*
Use: Bowel evacuant.

Evac-Q-Kwik. (Pharmacia & Upjohn) Each kit contains: **Evac-Q-Mag:** Magnesium citrate 300 ml, citric acid, potassium citrate in cherry-flavored base. **Evac-Q-Tabs:** 2 tab. phenolphthalein 130 mg. **Evac-Q-Kwik Supp.:** Bisacodyl 10 mg. *otc.*
Use: Bowel evacuant.

Evac Suppositories. (Burgin-Arden) Sodium bicarbonate, sodium biphosphate, dioctyl sodium sulfosuccinate 50 mg/Supp. *otc.*
Use: Laxative.

Evac Tablets. (Burgin-Arden) Guar gum 300 mg, danthron 50 mg, sodium 100 mg/Tab. *otc.*
Use: Laxative.

Evactol. (Delta Pharmaceutical Group) Docusate sodium 100 mg, sodium carboxymethyl cellulose 200 mg/Cap. Pkg. 10s, Bot. 10s, 30s, 100s. *otc.*
Use: Laxative.

Evac-U-Gen. (Walker, Corp & Co., Inc.) Yellow phenolphthalein 97.2 mg w/corn syrup, lactose, saccharin/Chew. Tab. Bot. 35s, 100s. *otc.*
Use: Laxative.

Evac-U-Lax. (Roberts Pharmaceuticals) Yellow phenolphthalein 80 mg/Chew. Tab. Bot. 100s. *otc.*
Use: Laxative.

Evalose. (Copley Pharmaceutical, Inc.) Lactulose 10 g/15 ml, galactose < 1.6 g, lactose < 1.2 g, other sugars H 1.2 g/Syrup. Bot. 240 ml, 960 ml. *Rx.*
Use: Laxative.

evans blue. U.S.P. XXII.
Use: Diagnostic aid (blood volume determination).

Evans Blue Dye. (New World Trading Corp.) Evans blue dye 5 ml/Inj. *Rx.*
Use: Diagnostic aid.

Everone. (Hyrex Pharmaceuticals) Testosterone enanthate in oil 100 mg or 200 mg/ml. Vial 10 ml. *c-III.*
Use: Androgen.

Evicyl Tablets. (Sanofi Winthrop Pharmaceuticals) Inositol hexanicotinate. *Rx.*
Use: Hypolipidemic, peripheral vasodilator.

Eviron. (Delta Pharmaceutical Group) Ferrous fumarate 160 mg, copper 1 mg, ascorbic acid 75 mg/Tab. *otc.*
Use: Mineral, vitamin supplement.

Evista. (Eli Lilly and Co.) Raloxifene HCl, lactose/Tab. Bot. 30s, 100s, 2000s. *Rx.*
Use: Osteoporosis prevention.

E-Vital Creme. (Taylor Pharmaceuticals) Vitamins E 100 IU, A 250 IU, D 100 IU, d-panthenol 0.2%, allantoin 0.1%/g. Jar 2 oz, lb. *otc.*
Use: Emollient.

Ewin Ninos Tablets. (Sanofi Winthrop Pharmaceuticals) Aspirin. *otc.*
Use: Analgesic.

Exact. (Advanced Polymer Systems) Benzoyl peroxide 5%, cetyl and stearyl alcohol, parabens. Cream Jar 18 g. *otc.*
Use: Dermatologic, acne.

Exact Liquid. (Advanced Polymer Systems) Salicylic acid 2%, propylene glycol, aloe vera gel, disodium EDTA, menthol, parabens, glycerin, diazolidinyl urea. Liq. Bot. 118 ml. *otc.*
Use: Dermatologic, acne.

•**exametazime.** (EX-ah-MET-ah-zeen) USAN.
Use: Diagnostic aid (regional cerebral perfusion imaging).

•**exaprolol hydrochloride.** (EX-ah-PRO-lahl) USAN.
Use: Antiadrenergic (β-receptor).

Ex-Caloric Wafers. (Eastern Research) Carboxymethylcellulose 181 mg, methylcellulose 272 mg/Wafer. Bot. 100s, 500s, 5000s. *otc.*
Use: Dietary aid.

Excedrin Aspirin Free. (Bristol-Myers Squibb) Acetaminophen 500 mg, caffeine 65 mg/Cap. Bot. 24s, 50s, 100s. *otc.*
Use: Analgesic combination.

Excedrin Extra Strength. (Bristol-Myers Squibb) Acetaminophen 250 mg, aspirin 250 mg, caffeine 65 mg. **Capl.:** Bot. 24s, 50s, 80s. **Tab.:** Bot. 12s, 30s, 60s, 100s, 165s, 225s. *otc.*
Use: Analgesic combination.

Excedrin Extra Strength. (Bristol-Myers Squibb) Acetaminophen 500 mg, caffeine 65 mg, parabens, mineral oil. Geltab Bot. 40s. *otc.*

Use: Analgesic combination.

Excedrin P.M.. (Bristol-Myers Squibb) **Tab.:** Acetaminophen 500 mg, diphenhydramine citrate 38 mg, parabens, mineral oil. Bot. 50s. **Capl.:** Acetaminophen 500 mg, diphenhydramine citrate 38 mg. Bot. 30s, 50s. **Liquigels:** Acetaminophen 500 mg, diphenhydramine HCl 25 mg. Bot. 20s, 40s. **Liq.:** Acetaminophen 1000 mg, diphenhydramine HCl 50 mg/30 ml, alcohol 10%, sucrose. Bot. 180 ml. **Geltab:** Acetaminophen 500 mg, diphenhydramine citrate 38 mg, EDTA, parabens. Bot. 100s. *otc.*
Use: Analgesic, sleep aid.

Excedrin Sinus. (Bristol-Myers Squibb) Pseudoephedrine HCl 30 mg, acetaminophen 500 mg/Tab. Capl. Bot. 24s. *otc.*
Use: Analgesic, decongestant.

Excita Extra. (Durex) Nonoxynol-9 8% Ribbed Condom. Box 3s, 12s, 36s. *otc.*
Use: Condom with spermicide.

exemestane. (Pharmacia & Upjohn)
Use: Hormonal therapy of metastatic breast carcinoma. [Orphan Drug]

Exgest LA Tablets. (Schwarz Pharma, Inc.) Phenylpropanolamine HCl 75 mg, guaifenesin 400 mg. Bot. 100s or 500s. *Rx.*
Use: Decongestant, expectorant.

Ex-Histine. (WE Pharmaceuticals, Inc.) Phenylephrine 10 mg, chlorpheniramine 2 mg, methscopolamine 1.25 mg/5 ml, root beer flavor. Syr. Bot. 16 oz. *Rx.*
Use: Antihistamine, decongestant.

Exidine-2 Scrub. (Baxter Pharmaceutical Products, Inc.) Chlorhexidine gluconate 2%, isopropyl alcohol 4%. Soln. Bot. 120 ml. *otc.*
Use: Antiseptic, antimicrobial.

Exidine-4 Scrub. (Baxter Pharmaceutical Products, Inc.) Chlorhexidine gluconate 4%, isopropyl alcohol 4%. Soln. Bot. 120 ml, 240 ml, 480 ml, 887 ml, 1 gal. *otc.*
Use: Antiseptic, antimicrobial.

Exidine Skin Cleanser. (Xttrium Laboratories, Inc.) Chlorhexidine gluconate 4%, isopropyl alcohol 4%. Bot. 120 ml, 240 ml, 16 oz, 32 oz, gal. *otc.*
Use: Antiseptic, antimicrobial.

Ex-Lax. (Novartis Pharmaceutical Corp.) Yellow phenolphthalein 90 mg/chocolate Chew. Tab. or unflavored pill. Chocolate Tab. 6s, 18s, 48s, 72s. Unflavored pill 8s, 30s, 60s. *otc.*
Use: Laxative.

Ex-Lax Chocolated Regular Strength. (Novartis Pharmaceutical Corp.) Sennosides 15 mg. Pieces. Pkg. 18s. *otc.*
Use: Laxative.

Ex-Lax Maximum Relief. (Novartis Pharmaceutical Corp.) Yellow phenolphthalein 135 mg. Tab. Pkg. 24s. *otc.*
Use: Laxative.

Ex-Lax Maximum Strength. (Novartis Pharmaceutical Corp.) Sennosides 25 mg. Tab. Pkg. 24s. *otc.*
Use: Laxative.

Ex-Lax Regular Strength. (Novartis Pharmaceutical Corp.) Sennosides 15 mg. Tab. Bot. 30s. *otc.*
Use: Laxative.

Ex-Lax Stool Softner. (Novartis Pharmaceutical Corp.) Docusate sodium 100 mg. Capl. Bot. 40s. *otc.*
Use: Laxative.

Exna. (Wyeth-Ayerst Laboratories) Benzthiazide 50 mg/Tab. Bot. 100s. *Rx.*
Use: Diuretic, antihypertensive.

Exocaine Plus. (Del Pharmaceuticals, Inc.) Methyl salicylate 30%. Jar 4 oz, Tube 1.3 oz. *otc.*
Use: Analgesic, topical.

exol. Di-isobutyl ethoxy ethyl dimethyl benzyl ammonium Cl.

exonic ot. Dioctyl Sodium Sulphosuccinate.
Use: Laxative.

Exosurf Neonatal. (GlaxoWellcome) Colfosceril palmitate; dipalmitoyl phosphatidylcholine (DPPC). Lyophilized pow. Vial 10 ml. *Rx.*
Use: Synthetic lung surfactant.

Expectorant DM Cough Syrup. (Weeks & Leo) Dextromethorphan HBr 15 mg, guaifenesin 100 mg/5 ml, alcohol 7.125%. Bot. 6 oz. *otc.*
Use: Antitussive, expectorant.

Expendable Blood Collection Unit ACD. (Baxter Pharmaceutical Products, Inc.) Citric acid 540 mg, sodium citrate 1.49 g, dextrose 1.65 g/67.5 ml. *Rx.*
Use: Anticoagulant.

Exten Strone 10. (Schlicksup) Estradiol valerate 10 mg/ml. Vial 10 ml. *Rx.*
Use: Estrogen.

Extendryl Chewable Tablets. (Fleming & Co.) Chlorpheniramine maleate 2 mg, phenylephrine HCl 10 mg, methscopolamine nitrate 1.25 mg/Chew. Tab. Bot. 100s, 1000s. *Rx.*
Use: Anticholinergic, antihistamine, antispasmodic, decongestant.

Extendryl Junior. (Fleming & Co.) Chlorpheniramine maleate 4 mg, phenylephrine HCl 10 mg, methscopolamine

nitrate 1.25 mg/TD Cap. 100s, 1000s. *Rx.*
Use: Anticholinergic, antihistamine, antispasmodic, decongestant.

Extendryl S.R. (Fleming & Co.) Chlorpheniramine maleate 8 mg, phenylephrine HCl 20 mg, methscopolamine nitrate 2.5 mg/TD Cap. Bot. 100s, 1000s. *Rx.*
Use: Anticholinergic, antihistamine, antispasmodic, decongestant.

Extendryl Syrup. (Fleming & Co.) Chlorpheniramine maleate 2 mg, phenylephrine HCl 10 mg, methscopolamine nitrate 1.25 mg/5 ml. Bot. 473 ml, gal. *Rx.*
Use: Anticholinergic, antihistamine, antispasmodic, decongestant.

Extenzyme Soflens Protein Cleaner. (Allergan, Inc.) Papain, sodium Cl, sodium carbonate, sodium borate, edetate disodium. Vial w/Tab. 24s. Refill 36s. *otc.*
Use: Contact lens care.

Extra Action Cough. (Rugby Labs, Inc.) Dextromethorphan HBr 15 mg, guaifenesin 100 mg w/alcohol 1.4%, corn syrup, saccharin. Syr. Bot. 118 ml. *otc.*
Use: Antitussive, expectorant.

Extra Strength Adprin-B. (Pfeiffer Co.) Aspirin 500 mg, calcium carbonate, magnesium carbonate, magnesium oxide/Tab, coated. Bot. 130s. *otc.*
Use: Analgesic.

Extra Strength Alka-Seltzer Effervescent. (Bayer Corp. (Consumer Div.)) Sodium bicarbonate (heat-treated)1985 mg, aspirin 500 mg, citric acid 1000 mg, sodium 588 mg/Tab. Bot. 12s and 24s. *otc.*
Use: Antacid.

Extra Strength Alkets Antacid. (Roberts Pharmaceuticals) Calcium carbonate 750 mg/Chew. Tab. Bot. 96s. *otc.*
Use: Antacid.

Extra Strength Aspirin Capsules. (Walgreen Co.) Aspirin 500 mg/Cap. Bot. 80s. *otc.*
Use: Analgesic.

Extra Strength Bayer Enteric 500 Aspirin. (Bayer Corp. (Consumer Div.)) Aspirin 500 mg. Tab. Enteric coated. Bot. 60s. *otc.*
Use: Analgesic.

Extra Strength Bayer Plus. (Bayer Corp. (Consumer Div.)) Aspirin 500 mg buffered with calcium carbonate, magnesium carbonate, magnesium oxide. Capl. Bot. 30s, 60s. *otc.*
Use: Analgesic.

Extra Strength Doan's PM. (Novartis Pharmaceutical Corp.) Magnesium salicylate 500 mg, diphenhydramine HCl 25 mg/Capl. Pkg. 20s. *otc.*
Use: Sleep aid.

Extra Strength Dynafed EX. (BDI Pharmaceuticals, Inc.) Acetaminophen 500 mg, fruit favor. Tab. Bot. 36s. *otc.*
Use: Analgesic.

Extra Strength Excedrin Capsules and Tablets. (Bristol-Myers Squibb) Acetaminophen 250 mg, aspirin 250 mg, caffeine 65 mg. Cap. Bot. 24s, 50s, 80s. Tab. Bot. 30s, 60s, 100s, 165s, 225s, Pkg. 12s. *otc.*
Use: Analgesic combination.

Extra Strength 5 mg Biotin Forte. (Vitaline Corp.) Vitamins B_1 10 mg, B_2 10 mg, B_3 40 mg, B_5 10 mg, B_6 25 mg, B_{12} 10 mcg, C 100 mg, biotin 5 mg, FA 800 mcg/Tab. Bot. 60s, 1000s. *otc.*
Use: Mineral, vitamin supplement.

Extra Strength Gas-X. (Novartis Pharmaceutical Corp.) Simethicone 125 mg/Tab. Pkg. 18s. *otc.*
Use: Antiflatulent.

Extra Strength Tylenol PM. (McNeil Consumer Products Co.) Diphenhydramine 25 mg, acetaminophen 500 mg. **Tab.:** 24s, 50s. **Capl.:** 24s, 50s. **Gelcap:** 20s, 40s. *otc.*
Use: Sleep aid.

Extra Strength Vicks Cough Drops. (Procter & Gamble Pharm.) Menthol 8.4 mg (menthol flavor) or menthol 10 mg (cherry and honey lemon flavors), corn syrup, sucrose/Loz. Pkg. 9s, 30s. *otc.*
Use: Mouth and throat preparation.

Extreme Cold Formula. (Major Pharmaceuticals) Pseudoephedrine HCl 30 mg, chlorpheniramine maleate 1 mg, dextromethorphan HBr 15 mg, acetaminophen 500 mg/Cap. Bot. 10s. *otc.*
Use: Analgesic, antihistamine, antitussive, decongestant.

Eye Drops. (Bausch & Lomb Pharmaceuticals) Tetrahydrozoline HCl 0.05%. Drop. Bot. 15 ml. *otc.*
Use: Ophthalmic vasoconstrictor, mydriatic.

Eye Face and Body Wash Station. (Lavoptik Co., Inc.) Sodium Cl 0.49 g, sodium biphosphate 0.4 g, sodium phosphate 0.45 g/100 ml, benzalkonium Cl 0.005%. Bot. 32 oz.
Use: Emergency wash.

Eye Irrigating Solution. (Rugby Labs, Inc.) Sodium Cl, sodium phosphate mono- and dibasic, benzalkonium Cl, EDTA. Soln. Bot. 118 ml. *otc.*
Use: Irrigant, ophthalmic.

Eye Irrigating Wash. (Roberts Pharmaceuticals) Boric acid, potassium Cl, sodium carbonate anhydrous, EDTA 0.01%, benzalkonium Cl. Soln. Bot. 120 ml. *otc.*
Use: Irrigant, ophthalmic.

Eye-Lube-A. (Optopics Laboratories, Corp) Glycerin 0.25%, EDTA, NaCl, benzalkonium chloride. Soln. Bot. 15 ml. *otc.*
Use: Lubricant, ophthalmic.

Eye Mo. (Sanofi Winthrop Pharmaceuticals) Boric acid, benzalkonium Cl, phenylephrine HCl, zinc sulfate. *otc.*
Use: Astringent, ophthalmic.

Eye Scrub. (Ciba Vision) PEG-200 glyceryl monotallawate, disodium laureth sulfosuccinate, cocoamidopropylamineoxide, PEG-78 glyceryl monococoate, benzyl alcohol, EDTA/Soln. Bot. 240 ml. *otc.*
Use: Cleanser, ophthalmic.

Eye-Sed Ophthalmic Solution. (Scherer Laboratories, Inc.) Zinc sulfate 0.25%. Bot. 15 ml. *otc.*
Use: Astringent, ophthalmic.

Eyesine. (Akorn, Inc.) Tetrahydrozoline HCl 0.05%. Drops. Bot. 15 ml. *otc.*
Use: Mydriatic, vasoconstrictor.

Eye-Stream. (Alcon Laboratories, Inc.) Sodium Cl 0.64%, potassium Cl 0.075%, magnesium Cl hexahydrate 0.03%, calcium Cl dihydrate 0.048%, sodium acetate trihydrate 0.39%, sodium citrate dihydrate 0.17%, benzalkonium Cl 0.013%. Bot. 30 ml, 118 ml. *otc.*
Use: Irrigant, ophthalmic.

Eye Wash. (Bausch & Lomb Pharmaceuticals) Boric acid, potassium Cl, EDTA, sodium carbonate, benzalkonium Cl 0.01%. Soln. Bot. 118 ml. *otc.*
Use: Irrigant, ophthalmic.

Eye Wash. (Zenith Goldline Pharmaceuticals) Boric acid, potassium Cl, EDTA, anhydrous sodium carbonate, benzalkonium Cl 0.1%. Soln. Bot. 118 ml. *otc.*
Use: Irrigant, ophthalmic.

Eye Wash. (Lavoptik Co., Inc.) Sodium Cl 0.49%, sodium biphosphate 0.4%, sodium phosphate 0.45%, benzalkonium Cl 0.005%. Soln. Bot. 180 ml with eye cup. *otc.*
Use: Irrigant, ophthalmic.

EZ-Detect. (Biomerica, Inc.) Occult blood screening test. Kit 3s.
Use: Diagnostic aid.

EZ Detect Strep-A Test. (Biomerica, Inc.) Coated stick test for detection of group A streptococci taken directly from a throat swab.
Use: Diagnostic aid.

Eze Pain. (Halsey Drug Co.) Acetaminophen 2.5 gr, salicylamide, caffeine/Cap. Bot. 21s. *otc.*
Use: Analgesic combination.

Ezide. (Econo Med Pharmaceuticals) Hydrochlorothiazide 50 mg/Tab. Bot. 100s, 1000s. *Rx.*
Use: Diuretic.

Ezol. (Stewart-Jackson Pharmacal, Inc.) Butalbital 50 mg, caffeine 40 mg, acetaminophen 325 mg. Bot. 100s. *Rx.*
Use: Analgesic, hypnotic, sedative.

Ezol #3. (Stewart-Jackson Pharmacal, Inc.) Acetaminophen 650 mg, codeine 30 mg. Bot. 100s. *c-III.*
Use: Analgesic combination, narcotic.

F

Fabrase.
Use: Fabry's disease. [Orphan Drug]

Faces Only Moisturizing Sunblock by Coppertone. (Schering-Plough Corp.) Ethylhexyl p-methoxycinnamate, oxybenzone. SPF 15. Lot. Bot. 55.5 ml. *otc.*
Use: Sunscreen.

Fact Home Pregnancy Test. (Advanced Care Products) Accurate test for pregnancy in 45 minutes, for use as early as 3 days after a missed period. Test kit 1s.
Use: Diagnostic aid.

factor VIIa recombinant, DNA orgin. (Novo Nordisk Pharm., Inc.)
Use: Antihemophilic, von Willebrand's disease. [Orphan Drug]

factor VIII.
See: Antihemophilic factor.

•**factor IX complex.** (FAK-tuhr-[IX] KAHM-plex) U.S.P. 23.
Use: Hemostatic.
See: Alpha Nine SD (Alpha Therapeutic Corp.).
Konyne 80 (Bayer Corp. (Consumer Div.)).
Mononine (Centeon).
Profilnine SD (Alpha Therapeutic Corp.).
Proplex T (Baxter Pharmaceutical Products, Inc.).

factor IX, coagulation.
See: Coagulation factor ix.

factor XIII (plasma-derived).
Use: Congenital Factor XIII deficiency. [Orphan Drug]
See: Fibrogammin P (Behringwerke Aktiengesellschaft).

Fact Plus. (Advanced Care Products) Reagent in-home kit for urine testing. Pregnancy test. Kit 1s, 2s.
Use: Diagnostic aid.

Factrel. (Wyeth-Ayerst Laboratories) Gonadorelin HCl 100 mcg or 500 mcg/Vial w/Amp. of 2 ml sterile diluent. *Rx.*
Use: Diagnostic aid.

•**fadrozole hydrochloride.** (FAHD-rah-ZOLE) USAN.
Use: Antineoplastic.

Falgos. (Sanofi Winthrop Pharmaceuticals) Acetylsalicylic acid. Tab. *otc.*
Use: Analgesic.

•**famciclovir.** (fam-SIGH-kloe-veer) USAN.
Use: Antiviral.
See: Famvir, Tab. (SmithKline Beecham).

Falmonox. (Sanofi Winthrop Pharmaceuticals) Teclozan Susp., Tab. *Rx.*
Use: Amebicide.

•**famotidine.** (fah-MOE-tih-den) U.S.P. 23.
Use: Antiulcerative.
See: Pepcid (Merck & Co.).
Pepcid RPD, Tab. (Merck & Co.).

•**famotine hydrochloride.** (FAM-oh-teen) USAN.
Use: Antiviral.

•**fampridine.** (FAHM-prih-DEEN) USAN.
Use: Symptomatic treatment of multiple sclerosis.

Famvir. (SmithKline Beecham) Famciclovir 125 mg, lactose/Tab. Bot 30s, UD 100s. Famciclovir 250 mg, lactose/Tab. Bot. 30s. Famciclovir 500 mg, lactose/Tab. Bot. 30s, UD 50s. *Rx.*
Use: Management of acute herpes zoster (shingles).

•**fananserin.** (fan-AN-ser-in) USAN.
Use: Antipsychotic, antischizophrenic (dual dopamine D_4 and serotonin 5-HT_2 receptor antagonist).

•**fanetizole mesylate.** (fan-EH-tih-zole) USAN.
Use: Immunoregulator.

Fansidar. (Roberts Pharmaceuticals) Sulfadoxine 500 mg, pyrimethamine 25 mg/Tab. Box 25s. *Rx.*
Use: Antimalarial.

•**fantridone hydrochloride.** (FAN-trih-dohn) USAN.
Use: Antidepressant.

Faramals. (Faraday) Vitamins A 10,000 IU, D 2000 IU, B_1 6 mg, B_2 4 mg, B_6 0.5 mg, folic acid 0.1 mg, C 100 mg, calcium pantothenate 5 mg, niacinamide 30 mg, E 5 IU, B_{12} 3 mcg/Tab. Bot. 100s, 250s, 500s, 1000s. *otc.*
Use: Mineral, vitamin supplement.

Faramals-M. (Faraday) Faramals plus calcium 103 mg, cobalt 0.1 mg, Cu 1 mg, I 0.15 mg, Fe 10 mg, Mg 6 mg, Mo 0.2 mg, P 80 mg, K 5 mg, Zn 1.2 mg/Tab. Bot. 100s, 250s, 500s, 1000s. *otc.*
Use: Mineral, vitamin supplement.

Faramins. (Faraday) Vitamins B_1 20 mg, B_2 6 mg, C 40 mg, niacinamide 20 mg, calcium pantothenate 3 mg, B_6 0.5 mg, powdered whole dried liver 125 mg, dried debittered yeast 125 mg, choline dihydrogen citrate 20 mg, inositol 20 mg, dl-methionine 20 mg, folic acid 0.1 mg, B_{12} 10 mcg, ferrous gluconate 30 mg, dicalcium phosphate 250 mg, copper sulfate 5 mg, magnesium sulfate 10 mg, manganese sulfate 5 mg, cobalt sulfate 0.2 mg, potassium Cl 2 mg, potassium iodide 0.15 mg/Tab. Bot. 100s, 250s, 500s, 1000s. *otc.*

Use: Mineral, vitamin supplement.

Faratol. (Faraday) Vitamins A 12,500 IU, D 1000 IU, B_1 20 mg, B_2 6 mg, B_6 0.5 mg, B_{12} 15 mcg, folic acid 0.1 mg, niacinamide 10 mg, calcium pantothenate 3 mg, C 60 mg, E 5 IU, choline dihydrogen citrate 20 mg, inositol 20 mg, dl-methionine 20 mg, whole dried liver 100 mg, dried debittered yeast 100 mg, dicalcium phosphate 200 mg, ferrous gluconate 30 mg, potassium iodide 0.2 mg, magnesium sulfate 7.2 mg, copper sulfate 5 mg, manganese sulfate 3.4 mg, cobalt sulfate 0.2 mg, potassium Cl 1.3 mg, zinc sulfate 2 mg, molybdenum 0.2 mg in a base of alfalfa/Tab. Bot. 100s, 250s, 500s, 1000s. *otc.*
Use: Mineral, vitamin supplement.

Farbee with Vitamin C. (Major Pharmaceuticals) Vitamins B_1 15 mg, B_2 10.2 mg, B_3 50 mg, B_5 10 mg, B_5 5 mg, C 300 mg/Capl. Bot. 100s, 130s, 1000. *otc.*
Use: Vitamin supplement.

Farbital Compound. (Major Pharmaceuticals) Butalbital, caffeine, aspirin. Cap. Bot. 100s. *c-III.*
Use: Analgesic, hypnotic, sedative.

Farbital Compound with Codeine #3. (Major Pharmaceuticals) Butalbital, caffeine, aspirin, codeine 30 mg. Bot. 1000s. *c-III.*
Use: Analgesic, hypnotic, sedative.

Farbital. (Major Pharmaceuticals) Butalbital. Tab. Bot. 100s. *c-III.*
Use: Hypnotic, sedative.

Fareston. (Schering-Plough Corp.) Toremifene citrate 60 mg, lactose. Tab. Bot. 30s, 100s. *Rx.*
Use: Antiestrogen agent.

Fastin. (SmithKline Beecham) Phentermine HCl 30 mg/Cap. Bot. 100s, 450s. Pack 150s. (5 × 30s). *c-IV.*
Use: Anorexiant.

fat emulsion, intravenous.
See: Liposyn 10% (Abbott Laboratories).
Liposyn 20% (Abbott Laboratories).
Travamulsion 10% (Baxter Pharmaceutical Products, Inc.).
Travamulsion 20% (Baxter Pharmaceutical Products, Inc.).
Intralipid 10% (Pharmacia & Upjohn).
Intralipid 20% (Pharmacia & Upjohn).
Liposyn II 10% (Abbott Laboratories).
Liposyn II 20% (Abbott Laboratories).

•**fat, hard.** N.F. 18.
Use: Pharmaceutic aid (suppository base).

Father John's Medicine Plus. (Oakhurst Co.) Phenylephrine HCl 2.5 mg, chlorpheniramine maleate 1 mg, dextromethorphan HBr 7.5 mg, guaifenesin 30 mg, ammonium Cl 100 mg, sodium citrate/5 ml. Bot. 120 ml, 240 ml. *otc.*
Use: Antihistamine, antitussive, decongestant, expectorant.

Fattibase. (Paddock Laboratories) Preblended fatty acid suppository base composed of triglycerides of coconut oil and palm kernel oil. Jar 1 lb, 5 lb.
Use: Pharmaceutical aid, suppository base.

fazadinium bromide.
Use: Neuromuscular blocking agent.

•**fazarabine.** (fah-ZAY-rah-BEAN) USAN.
Use: Antineoplastic.

F.C.A.H.. (Scherer Laboratories, Inc.) Chlorpheniramine maleate 4 mg, acetaminophen 162 mg, salicylamide 162 mg/Cap. Bot. 100s, 500s. *otc.*
Use: Analgesic, antihistamine.

Fe_{50}. (UCB Pharmaceuticals, Inc.) Ferrous sulfate 160 mg (iron 50 mg), PEG. ER Capl. UD 100s. *otc.*
Use: Mineral supplement.

Fe_{50}. (UCB Pharmaceuticals, Inc.) Fe 160 mg (as dried ferrous sulfate equivalent to 50 mg elemental iron), PEG. Capl. Bot. 100s. *otc.*
Use: Mineral supplement.

Feberin. (Arcum) Ferrous gluconate 3 gr, vitamins C 25 mg, B_1 2 mg, B_6 1 mg, B_2 1 mg, niacinamide 5 mg/Tab. Bot. 100s, 1000s. *otc.*
Use: Mineral, vitamin supplement.

febrile antigens. (Laboratory Diagnostics) Group O antigens (somatic) are dyed blue and group ≤ antigens (flagellars) are dyed red for clear identification for detection of bacterial agglutinins, bacterial infections. Vial 5 ml.
Use: Diagnostic aid.

Febrinol. (Eon Labs Manufacturing, Inc.) Acetaminophen 325 mg/Tab. Bot. 100s, 1000s. *otc.*
Use: Analgesic.

Fe-Brone. (Forest Pharmaceutical, Inc.) Vitamins B_{12} 1 IU, folic acid 1 mg, ferrous sulfate exsiccated (powdered) 200 mg, ferrous sulfate exsiccated (timed) 200 mg, C acid 100 mg, B_6 0.5 mg, B_1 2 mg, B_2 1 mg, copper 0.9 mg, zinc 0.5 mg, manganese 0.3 mg/Cap. Bot. 30s, 100s, 1000s. *Rx.*
Use: Mineral, vitamin supplement.

Fedahist Expectorant. (Schwarz Pharma, Inc.) Guaifenesin 200 mg, pseudoephedrine HCl 20 mg/5 ml, sorbitol, alcohol free. *otc.*
Use: Antihistamine, decongestant.

Fedahist Gyrocaps. (Schwarz Pharma,

Inc.) Pseudoephedrine HCl 65 mg, chlorpheniramine maleate 10 mg/SR Cap. Bot. 100s. *Rx.*
Use: Antihistamine, decongestant.

Fedahist Timecaps. (Schwarz Pharma, Inc.) Pseudoephedrine HCl 120 mg, chlorpheniramine maleate 8 mg/SR Cap. Bot. 100s. *Rx.*
Use: Antihistamine, decongestant.

Fedahist Tablets. (Schwarz Pharma, Inc.) Pseudoephedrine HCl 60 mg, chlorpheniramine maleate 4 mg, sorbitol (alcohol and sugar free)/Tab. Bot. 100s. *Rx.*
Use: Antihistamine, decongestant.

Feen-a-Mint. (Schering-Plough Corp.) Bisacodyl 5 mg, talc, lactose, sugar. Tab. Pkg. 10s. *otc.*
Use: Laxative.

Feen-a-Mint Dual Formula. (Schering-Plough Corp.) Docusate sodium 100 mg, yellow phenolphthalein 65 mg/Tab. Box 15s, 30s, 60s. *otc.*
Use: Laxative.

Feen-a-Mint Gum. (Schering-Plough Corp.) Yellow phenolphthalein 97.2 mg/ Chewing gum Tab. Box 5s, 16s, 40s. *otc.*
Use: Laxative.

Feen-a-Mint Pills. (Schering-Plough Corp.) Docusate sodium 100 mg, yellow phenolphthalein 65 mg/Tab. Box 15s, 30s, 60s. *otc.*
Use: Laxative.

Feen-a-Mint Tablets. (Schering-Plough Corp.) Bisacodyl 5 mg, talc, lactose, sugar. Tab. 10s. *otc.*
Use: Laxative.

Feg-I. (Western Research) Ferrous gluconate 300 mg/Tab. Handicount 28s (36 bags of 28 tab.). *otc.*
Use: Mineral supplement.

Feiba VH Immuno. (Baxter Healthcare Corp.) Freeze-dried anti-inhibitor coagulant complex. Heparin free. Vapor heated. Inj. Vial with diluent and needle.
Use: Antihemophilic.

•**felbamate.** (FELL-buh-MATE) USAN.
Use: Antiepileptic; treatment of Lennox-Gastaut syndrome [Orphan Drug]
See: Felbatol (Wallace Laboratories).

Felbatol. (Wallace Laboratories) Felbamate 400 mg or 600 mg, lactose/Tab.; felbamate 600 mg/5 ml, sorbitol, parabens, saccharin/Susp. **Tab.:** Bot. 100s and UD 100s. **Susp.:** Bot. 240 ml and 960 ml. *Rx.*
Use: Antiepileptic. It has been recommended that use of this drug be discontinued if aplastic anemia or hepatic failure occurs unless, in the judgement of the physician, continued therapy is warranted. For further information contact Wallace Labs at 609-655-6000.
See: Lennox-Gastaut syndrome. [Orphan Drug]

•**felbinac.** (FELL-bih-nak) USAN.
Use: Anti-inflammatory.

Feldene. (Pfizer US Pharmaceutical Group) Piroxicam 10 mg or 20 mg/Cap. **10 mg:** Bot 100s. **20 mg:** Bot. 100s, 500s, UD 100s. *Rx.*
Use: Analgesic, NSAID.

Fellobolic Injection. (Forest Pharmaceutical, Inc.) Methandriol dipropionate 50 mg/ml. Vial 10 ml. *Rx.*

•**felodipine.** (feh-LOW-dih-peen) USAN.
Use: Vasodilator.
See: Plendil, Tab. (Merck & Co.).

feldopine and enalapril maleate.
Use: Antihypertensive.
See: Lexxel, ER Tab. (Astra Pharmaceuticals, L.P.).

•**felvizumab.** (fell-VYE-zoo-mab) USAN.
Use: Antiviral (systemic); monoclonal antibody.

•**felypressin.** (fell-ih-PRESS-in) USAN.
Use: Vasoconstrictor.

Femagene. (Tennessee Pharmaceutic) Boric acid, sodium borate, lactic acid, menthol, methylbenzethonium Cl, parachlorometaxylenol, lactose, surface-active agents. Pow. 6 oz. *otc.*
Use: Feminine hygiene.

Femara. (Novartis Pharmaceutical Corp.) Letrozole 2.5 mg, lactose/Tab. Bot. 30s. *Rx.*
Use: Breast cancer treatment.

Femazole Tabs. (Major Pharmaceuticals) Metronidazole 250 mg or 500 mg/Tab. **250 mg:** Bot. 100s, 250s, 500s. **500 mg:** Bot. 50s, 100s. *Rx.*
Use: Anti-infective.

Femcal. (Freeda Vitamins, Inc.) Calcium carbonate 250 mg, vitamin D_3 100 IU, B_1 100 mg, Mg, Mn, Si, kosher, sugar free/Tab. Bot. 100s and 250s. *otc.*
Use: Electrolyte, mineral supplement.

Femcaps. (Buffington) Acetaminophen, caffeine, ephedrine sulfate, atropine sulfate/Tab. Sugar, lactose, and salt free Dispens-a-Kit 500s, Aidpaks 100s. *Rx.*
Use: Analgesic, anticholinergic, antispasmodic, bronchodilator.

Femcet. (Russ Pharmaceuticals) Acetaminophen 325 mg, butalbital 50 mg, caffeine 40 mg/Cap. Bot. 100s. *Rx.*
Use: Analgesic, hypnotic, sedative.

femergin.

See: Ergotamine Tartrate (Various Mfr.).

Femidyn.
See: Estrone (Various Mfr.).

Femilax. (G & W Laboratories) Docusate sodium 100 mg, phenolphthalein 65 mg/Tab. Bot. 30s, 60s, 90s. *otc.*
Use: Laxative.

Feminique Disposable Douche. (Durex) Sodium benzoate, sorbic acid, lactic acid, octoxynol-9. Twin-pack Bot. 120 ml. *otc.*
Use: Douche.

Feminique Disposable Douche. (Durex) Vinegar and water. Soln. Twin-packs. Bot. 180 ml. *otc.*
Use: Douche.

Feminone. (Pharmacia & Upjohn) Ethinyl estradiol 0.05 mg/Tab. Bot. 100s. *Rx.*
Use: Estrogen.

Femiron. (Menley & James Labs, Inc.) Ferrous fumarate 63 mg (iron 20 mg)/Tab. Bot. 40s, 120s. *otc.*
Use: Mineral supplement.

Femiron Multi-Vitamins and Iron. (Menley & James Labs, Inc.) Iron 20 mg, vitamins A 5000 IU, D 400 IU, B_1 1.5 mg, riboflavin 1.7 mg, B_3 20 mg, C 60 mg, B_6 2 mg, B_{12} 6 mcg, B_5 10 mg, folic acid 0.4 mg, E 15 mg/Tab. Bot. 35s, 60s, 90s. *otc.*
Use: Mineral, vitamin supplement.

Femizol-M. (Lake Consumer Products) Miconazole nitrate 2%. Vaginal cream. Tube, with applicator. 45 g. *otc.*
Use: Antifungal, vaginal.

Fem-1. (BDI Pharmaceuticals, Inc.) Acetaminophen 500 mg, pamabrom 25 mg/Tab. Bot. 30s. *otc.*
Use: Analgesic.

Femotrone. (Bluco Inc./Med. Discnt. Outlet) Progesterone in oil 50 mg/ml. Vial 10 ml. *Rx.*
Use: Hormone, progestin.

FemPatch. (Parke-Davis) Estradiol 10.3 mg (0.025 mg/day)/Patch. Box. 4s. *Rx.*
Use: Estrogen.

Femstat 3. (Procter-Syntex) Butoconazole nitrate 2%, parabens, cetyl alcohol, mineral oil, stearyl alcohol. Cream. Three 5 g prefilled applicators and 20 g with applicators. *otc.*
Use: Antifungal, vaginal.

Femizol-M. (Lake Consumer Products) Miconazole nitrate 2%, mineral oil. Vag. Cream. Tube 45 g with applicator. *otc.*
Use: Vaginal preparation.

•**fenalamide.** (fen-AL-am-IDE) USAN.
Use: Muscle relaxant.

fenamisal. Phenyl aminosalicylate.

•**fenamole.** (FEN-ah-mole) USAN.
Use: Anti-inflammatory.

Fenaprin. (Sanofi Winthrop Pharmaceuticals) Aspirin, chlormezanone. Tab. *Rx.*
Use: Analgesic, anxiolytic.

Fenarol. (Sanofi Winthrop Pharmaceuticals) Chlormezanone 100 mg or 200 mg/Tab. Bot. 100s.
Use: Anxiolytic.

fenarsone.
See: Carbarsone (Various Mfr.).

•**fenbendazole.** (FEN-BEND-ah-zole) USAN.
Use: Anthelmintic.

•**fenbufen.** (FEN-byoo-fen) USAN.
Use: Anti-inflammatory.

•**fencibutirol.** (fen-sih-BYOO-tih-role) USAN.
Use: Choleretic.

•**fenclofenac.** (FEN-kloe-fen-ACK) USAN.
Use: Anti-inflammatory.

•**fenclonine.** (fen-KLOE-neen) USAN. Under study by Pfizer.
Use: Serotonin inhibitor.

•**fenclorac.** (FEN-kloe-rack) USAN.
Use: Anti-inflammatory.

Fend. (Mine Safety Appliances) **A-2:** Water-soluble cream which forms a physical barrier to water-insoluble irritants. Tube 3 oz, Jar lb. **E-2:** This cream combines the functions of the water-soluble Fend A-2 and water-insoluble Fend I-2 creams. Tube 3 oz, Jar lb. **I-2:** Water-insoluble cream which forms a physical barrier to water-soluble irritants. Tube 3 oz, Jar lb. **S-2:** A silicone cream which forms a barrier against a combination of water-soluble and water-insoluble irritants Tube 3 oz, Jar lb. **X:** Industrial cold cream which rubs well into the skin and serves as a skin conditioner. Tube 3 oz, Jar lb.
Use: Skin protectant.

Fendol. (Buffington) Salicylamide, caffeine, acetaminophen, phenylephrine HCl/Tab. Sugar, lactose and salt free. Dispens-A-Kit 500s. Bot., 100s. *otc.*
Use: Analgesic combination.

•**fendosal.** (FEN-doe-sal) USAN.
Use: Anti-inflammatory.

Fenesin. (Dura Pharmaceuticals) Guaifenesin 600 mg/SR Tab. Bot. 100s, 600s. *Rx.*
Use: Expectorant.

Fenesin DM. (Dura Pharmaceuticals) Dextromethorphan HBr 30 mg, guaifenesin 600 mg/Tab. Bot. 100s. *Rx.*
Use: Antitussive, expectorant.

•**fenestrel.** (feh-NESS-trell) USAN. Under study.

Use: Estrogen.

•**fenethylline hydrochloride.** (FEN-ETH-ill-in) USAN.
Use: Stimulant (central).

•**fengabine.** (FEN-GAH-bean) USAN.
Use: Mood regulator.

•**fenimide.** (FEN-ih-mid) USAN.
Use: Anxiolytic, antipsychotic.

•**fenisorex.** (fen-EYE-so-rex) USAN.
Use: Anorexigenic, anorexic.

•**fenmetozole hydrochloride.** (FEN-MET-oh-zole) USAN.
Use: Antidepressant, antagonist (to narcotics).

•**fenmetramide.** (fen-MEH-trah-mide) USAN.
Use: Antidepressant.

fennel oil.
Use: Pharmaceutic aid (flavor).

•**fenobam.** (FEN-oh-bam) USAN.
Use: Hypnotic, sedative.

•**fenoctimine sulfate.** (fen-OCK-tih-MEEN) USAN.
Use: Gastric antisecretory.

fenofibrate.
Use: Antihyperlipidemic.

•**fenoldopam mesylate.** (feh-NAHL-doe-pam) USAN.
Use: Antihypertensive, dopamine agonist.
See: Corlopam, Inj. (Neurex Corporation).

•**fenoprofen.** (FEN-oh-PRO-fen) USAN.
Use: Anti-inflammatory, analgesic.

•**fenoprofen calcium.** (FEN-oh-PRO-fen) U.S.P. 23.
Use: Anti-inflammatory, analgesic.
See: Nalfon, Cap., Tab. (Eli Lilly and Co.).

•**fenoterol.** (FEN-oh-TER-ahl) USAN.
Use: Bronchodilator.

•**fenpipalone.** (FEN-PIP-ah-lone) USAN.
Use: Anti-inflammatory.

•**fenprinast hydrochloride.** (fen-PRIH-nast) USAN.
Use: Bronchodilator (antiallergic).

•**fenprostalene.** (FEN-PRAHST-ah-leen) USAN.
Use: Luteolysin.

•**fenquizone.** (FEN-kwih-zone) USAN.
Use: Diuretic.

•**fenretinide.** (fen-RET-ih-nide) USAN.
Use: Antineoplastic.

•**fenspiride hydrochloride.** (fen-SPIH-rid) USAN.
Use: Bronchodilator, antiadrenergic (α-receptor).

fentanyl.
Use: Analgesic, narcotic.
See: Duragesic, Transdermal (Janssen Pharmaceutical, Inc.).

•**fentanyl citrate.** (FEN-tuh-nill) U.S.P. 23.
Use: Analgesic, narcotic.
See: Sublimaze, Inj. (Janssen Pharmaceutical, Inc.).

fentanyl citrate. (Various Mfr.) 0.05 mg/ml. Inj. Amp. 2 ml, 5 ml, 10 ml, 20 ml. Vial. 20 ml, 30 ml, 50 ml. Carpujects 2 ml, 5 ml. *c-II.*
Use: Analgesic, narcotic.

Fentanyl Citrate & Droperidol. (Astra Pharmaceuticals, L.P.) Fentanyl 0.05 mg, droperidol 2.5 mg/ml. Inj. Amp and Vial 2 ml, 5 ml. *c-II.*
Use: Anesthetic, general.
See: Innovar, Inj. (Janssen Pharmaceutical, Inc.).

Fentanyl Oralet. (Abbott Laboratories) Fentanyl 100 mcg, 200 mcg, 300 mcg, 400 mcg sucrose, liquid glucose. Loz. Box. 25s. *c-II.*
Use: Anesthetic, general.

fentanyl transdermal system. (FEN-tuh-nill)
Use: Analgesic, narcotic.
See: Duragesic-25 (Janssen Pharmaceutical, Inc.).
Duragesic-50 (Janssen Pharmaceutical, Inc.).
Duragesic-75 (Janssen Pharmaceutical, Inc.).
Duragesic-100 (Janssen Pharmaceutical, Inc.).

fentanyl transmucosal system.
Use: Analgesic, narcotic.
See: Fentanyl Oralet, Loz. (Abbott).
Actiq, Loz. (Abbott).

•**fentiazac.** (fen-TIE-azz-ACK) USAN.
Use: Anti-inflammatory.

•**fenticlor.** (FEN-tih-Klor) USAN.
Use: Antifungal; antiseptic, topical.

•**fenticonazole nitrate.** (FEN-tih-KOE-nah-zole) USAN.
Use: Antifungal.

Fenton Elixir. (Sanofi Winthrop Pharmaceuticals) Ferrous gluconate. *otc.*
Use: Mineral supplement.

Fenylhist. (Roberts Pharmaceuticals) Diphenhydramine HCl 25 mg or 50 mg/Cap. Bot. 1000s. *otc.*
Use: Antihistamine.

fenyramidol hydrochloride. Phenyramidol HCl.

•**fenyripol hydrochloride.** (FEH-nee-rih-pahl) USAN.
Use: Muscle relaxant.

Feocyte. (Dunhall Pharmaceuticals, Inc.) Iron 110 mg, vitamins C 100 mg, B_6 2 mg, B_{12} 50 mcg, copper sulfate, fo-

lic acid 0.8 mg, desiccated liver 15 mg/ Prolonged Action Tab. Bot. 100s. *Rx.*
Use: Mineral, vitamin supplement.

Feocyte Injectable. (Dunhall Pharmaceuticals, Inc.) Peptonized iron 15 mg, vitamin B_{12} 200 mcg, liver injection N.F. beef 10 units, sodium citrate 10 mg, benzyl alcohol 2%/ml. Vial 10 ml. *Rx.*
Use: Mineral, vitamin supplement.

Feosol Caplets. (SmithKline Beecham) Carbonyl iron 50 mg, lactose, sorbitol, PEG. Capl. Bot. 60s. *otc.*
Use: Mineral supplement.

Feosol Elixir. (SmithKline Beecham) Ferrous sulfate (44 mg iron) 220 mg/5 ml, alcohol 5%. Bot. 16 oz. *otc.*
Use: Mineral supplement.

Feosol Tablets. (SmithKline Beecham) Ferrous sulfate, exsiccated 200 mg (65 mg iron), glucose/Tab. Bot. 100s. *otc.*
Use: Mineral supplement.

Feostat. (Forest Pharmaceutical, Inc.) **Tab.:** Ferrous fumarate 100 mg (33 mg iron)/Chew. Tab. Bot. 100s, UD 100s. **Drops:** Ferrous fumarate 45 mg (15 mg iron)/0.6 ml, methylparaben 0.2%. Bot. 60 ml. **Susp.:** Ferrous fumarate 100 mg (iron 33 mg)/5 ml, methylparaben 0.2%. Bot. 240 ml. *otc.*
Use: Mineral supplement.

Feostat Suspension. (Forest Pharmaceutical, Inc.) Ferrous fumarate 100 mg (33 mg iron)/5 ml. Bot. 240 ml. *otc.*
Use: Mineral supplement.

FE-Plus Protein. (Miller Pharmacal Group, Inc.) Iron (as an iron-protein complex) 50 mg/Tab. Bot. 100s. *otc.*
Use: Mineral supplement.

Feratab. (Upsher-Smith Labs, Inc.) Ferrous sulfate 187 mg (60 mg iron)/Tab. Bot. UD 100s. *otc.*
Use: Mineral supplement.

Ferate-C. (Pal-Pak, Inc.) Ferrous fumarate 150 mg, ascorbic acid 200 mg, docusate sodium 25 mg/Tab. Bot. 100s, 1000s. *otc.*
Use: Mineral, vitamin supplement; stool softener.

Fer-gen-sol Drops. (Zenith Goldline Pharmaceuticals) Ferrous sulfate 75 mg/0.6 ml (iron 15 mg/0.6 ml), alcohol 0.2%, sodium bisulfite, sorbitol, sugar. Drops. Bot. 50 ml. *otc.*
Use: Mineral supplement.

Fergon. (Bayer Corp. (Allergy Div.)) Ferrous gluconate 240 mg (iron 27 mg), sucrose. Tab. Bot. 100s. *otc.*
Use: Mineral supplement.

Feridex I.V. (Berlex Laboratories, Inc.) Iron 11.2 mg, mannitol 61.3 mg/ml, dextran 5.6 to 9.1 mg/ml. Inj. Vial. 5 ml. *Rx.*
Use: Radiopaque agent.

Fer-In-Sol. (Bristol-Myers Squibb) **Drops:** Elemental iron 15 mg/0.6 ml, alcohol 0.02%, sodium bisulfite, sorbitol, sugar. Dropper Bot. 50 ml. **Syr.:** 18 mg/5 ml. Alcohol 5%. Bot. 480 ml. *otc.*
Use: Mineral supplement.

Fer-Iron. (Rugby Labs, Inc.) Ferrous sulfate 75 mg (iron 15 mg)/0.6 ml, alcohol 0.2%, sodium bisulfite, sorbitol, sugar. Dropper Bot. 50 ml. *otc.*
Use: Mineral supplement.

Ferocyl. (Arco Pharmaceuticals, Inc.) Ferrous fumarate 150 mg (iron 50 mg), docusate sodium 100 mg/TR Cap. Bot. 100s. *otc.*
Use: Mineral supplement, stool softener.

Fero-Folic 500. (Abbott Laboratories) Ferrous sulfate controlled-release (equivalent to 105 mg iron), vitamin C 500 mg, folic acid 0.8 mg/Filmtab. Bot. 100s, 500s. *Rx.*
Use: Mineral, vitamin supplement.

Fero-Grad 500. (Abbott Laboratories) Sodium ascorbate 500 mg, ferrous sulfate equivalent to 105 mg iron/TR Tab. Bot. 30s. *otc.*
Use: Mineral supplement.

Ferolix. (Century Pharmaceuticals, Inc.) Ferrous sulfate 5 gr, alcohol 5%/10 ml Elix. Bot. 8 oz, pt, gal. *otc.*
Use: Mineral supplement.

Ferosan Forte. (Sandia) Ferrous fumarate 300 mg, liver-stomach concentrate 150 mg, vitamin B_{12} w/intrinsic factor concentrate 7.5 mcg, intrinsic factor concentrate 150 mg, B_{12} 7.5 mcg, ascorbic acid 75 mg, folic acid 1 mg, sorbitol 50 mg/Tab. Bot. 100s. *Rx.*
Use: Mineral, vitamin supplement.

Ferosan Syrup. (Sandia) Ferrous fumarate 91.2 mg, B_1 10 mg, B_6 3 mg, B_{12} 25 mcg/5 ml 16 oz, gal. *otc.*
Use: Mineral, vitamin supplement.

Ferospace. (Hudson Corp.) Ferrous sulfate 250 mg (iron 50 mg)/TR Cap. Bot. 100s. *otc.*
Use: Mineral supplement.

Ferotrinsic. (Rugby Labs, Inc.) Iron 110 mg (from ferrous fumarate), vitamins B_{12} 15 mcg, C 75 mg, intrinsic factor (as concentrate or from stomach preparations) 240 mg, folic acid 0.5 mg/Cap. 100s, 500s, 1000s. *Rx.*
Use: Mineral, vitamin supplement.

Feroweet. (Barth's) Vitamins B_1 6 mg, B_2 12 mg, niacin 4 mg, iron 30 mg,

B_{12} 10 mcg, B_6 95 mcg, pantothenic acid 50 mcg/3 Cap. Bot. 100s, 500s, 1000s. *otc.*
Use: Mineral, vitamin supplement.

Ferracomp. (Roberts Pharmaceuticals) Liver 2 mcg, vitamins B_{12} 15 mcg, B_1 10 mg, B_2 5 mg, B_6 1 mg, calcium pantothenate 1 mg, niacinamide 10 mg, iron 31.3 mg/ml. Vial 30 ml. *otc.*
Use: Mineral, vitamin supplement.

Ferralet Plus. (Mission Pharmacal Co.) Ferrous gluconate equivalent to 46 mg iron, C 400 mg, folic acid 0.8 mg, vitamin B_{12} 25 mcg/Tab. Bot. 60s. *otc.*
Use: Mineral, vitamin supplement.

Ferrets. (Pharmics, Inc.) Ferrous fumarate 325 mg, iron 106 mg/Tab. Bot. 100s. *otc.*
Use: Mineral supplement.

ferric ammonium citrate. Ammonium iron (Fe^{+++}) citrate.
Use: Mineral supplement.

ferric ammonium sulfate. (Various Mfr.)
Use: Astringent.

ferric ammonium tartrate. (Various Mfr.)
Use: Mineral supplement.

ferric cacodylate. (Various Mfr.)
Use: Leukemias, hematinic.

ferric chloride. (Various Mfr.)
Use: Astringent.

•**ferric chloride Fe 59.** (FER-ik KLOR-ide) USAN.
Use: Radiopharmaceutical.

ferric citrochloride tincture. Iron (Fe^{+++}) chloride citrate.
Use: Hematinic.

•**ferric fructose.** (FER-ik FRUKE-tose) USAN.
Use: Hematinic.

ferric glycerophosphate. Glycerol phosphate iron (Fe^{+++}) salt.
Use: Pharmaceutic necessity.

ferric hypophosphate. Iron (Fe^{+++}) phosphinate.
Use: Pharmaceutic necessity.

•**ferriclate calcium sodium.** (fer-ih-KLATE) USAN.
Use: Hematinic.

•**ferric oxide.** (FER-ik) N.F. 18.
Use: Pharmaceutic aid (color).

ferric oxide, yellow.
Use: Pharmaceutic aid (color).

ferric "peptonate". (Various Mfr.)
See: Iron Peptonized.

ferric pyrophosphate, soluble. Iron (Fe^{+++}) citrate pyrophosphate.

ferric quinine citrate, "green". (Various Mfr.)
Use: Mineral supplement.

ferric subsulfate solution. (Various Mfr.)
Use: Local use on the skin.

•**ferristene.** (FER-ih-steen) USAN.
Use: Diagnostic aid (paramagnetic).

Ferrizyme. (Abbott Diagnostics) Enzyme immunoassay for qualitative determination of ferritin in human serum or plasma. Test kit 100s.
Use: Diagnostic aid, paramagnetic.

Ferrlecit. (Schein) Sodium ferric gluconate complex 62.5 mg/5 ml (12.5 mg/ml of elemental iron), benzyl alcohol 9 mg/ml, sucrose 20%. Inj. Amp. 5 ml. *Rx.*
Use: Iron-containing product.

ferrocholate.
See: Ferrocholinate.

ferrocholinate. Ferrocholate. Ferrocholine. A chelate prepared by reacting equimolar quantities of freshly precipitated ferric hydroxide with choline dihydrogen citrate.
Use: Mineral supplement.

ferrocholine.
See: Ferrocholinate.

Ferro-Cyte. (Spanner) Iron peptonate 20 mg, liver injection (20 mg/ml) 0.25 ml, vitamins B_1 22 mg, B_2 0.5 mg, B_6 2.5 mg, B_{12} 30 mcg, niacinamide 25 mg, panthenol 1 mg/ml. Inj. Multiple-dose vial 10 ml. *Rx.*
Use: Mineral, vitamin supplement.

Ferro-Docusate TR. (Parmed Pharmaceuticals, Inc.) Ferrous fumarate 150 mg (iron 50 mg), docusate sodium 100 mg/TR Cap. Bot. 100s. *otc.*
Use: Mineral supplement, stool softener.

Ferro-Dok TR. (Major Pharmaceuticals) Ferrous fumarate 150 mg (iron 50 mg), docusate sodium 100 mg/TR Cap. Bot. 100s. *otc.*
Use: Mineral supplement, stool softener.

Ferrodyl Chewable Tablets. (Arcum) Ferrous fumarate 320 mg, vitamin C 200 mg/Tab. Bot. 100s, 1000s. *otc.*
Use: Mineral, vitamin supplement.

Ferromar. (Marnel Pharmaceuticals, Inc.) Ferrous fumarate 201.5 mg (iron 65 mg), vitamin C 200 mg/SR Capl. Bot. 100s. *otc.*
Use: Mineral supplement.

Ferroneed. (Hanlon) Ferrous gluconate 300 mg, ascorbic acid 60 mg/Cap. Bot. 100s. *otc.*
Use: Mineral, vitamin supplement.

Ferroneed T-Caps. (Hanlon) Ferrous fumarate 250 mg, thiamine HCl 5 mg, ascorbic acid 50 mg/TD Cap. Bot. 100s. *otc.*
Use: Mineral, vitamin supplement.

Ferronex. (Taylor Pharmaceuticals) Iron from ferrous gluconate 2.9 mg, vitamins B_{12} equivalent 1 mcg, B_2 0.75 mg, B_3 50 mg, B_5 1.25 mg, B_{12} 15 mcg, procaine 2%/ml. Inj. Vial 30 ml. *Rx.*
Use: Mineral, vitamin supplement.

Ferro-Sequels. (Selfcare, Inc.) Ferrous fumarate equivalent to iron 50 mg, docusate sodium, lactose. TR Tab. Bot. 30s, 90s. *otc.*
Use: Mineral supplement.

Ferrospan. (Imperial Lab) Ferrous fumarate 200 mg, ascorbic acid 100 mg/ Tab. Bot. 100s, 1000s. *otc.*
Use: Mineral, vitamin supplement.

Ferrosyn Injection. (Standex) Cyanocobalamin 30 mcg, liver 2 mcg, ferrous gluconate 100 mg, riboflavin 1.5 mg, panthenol 2.5 mg, niacinamide 100 mg, procaine 2%. Vial 30 ml. *Rx.*
Use: Mineral, vitamin supplement.

Ferrosyn S.C. (Standex) Iron 60 mg, vitamin B_{12} 5 mcg, magnesium 0.6 mg, copper 0.3 mg, manganese 0.1 mg, potassium 0.5 mg, zinc 0.15 mg/Tab. Bot. 100s, 1000s. *otc.*
Use: Mineral, vitamin supplement.

Ferrosyn. (Standex) Fe 60 mg, vitamin B_{12} 5 mcg, Mg 0.6 mg, Cu 0.3 mg, Mn 0.1 mg, K 0.5 mg, Zn 0.15 mg/Tab. Bot. 100s. *otc.*
Use: Mineral, vitamin supplement.

Ferrosyn See. (Standex) Iron 34 mg, ascorbic acid 60 mg/Tab. Bot. 100s, 1000s. *otc.*
Use: Mineral, vitamin supplement.

ferrous bromide. (FER-uhs) (Various Mfr.)
Use: In chorea & tuberculous cervical adenitis.

ferrous carbonate mass. Vallet's mass. (Various Mfr.)
Use: Mineral supplement.

ferrous carbonate, saccharated. (Various Mfr.)
Use: Mineral supplement.

•**ferrous citrate Fe 59.** (FER-uhs SIH-trate) USAN.
Use: Radiopharmaceutical.

•**ferrous fumarate.** (FER-uhs FEW-mahrate) U.S.P. 23.
Use: Hematinic.
See: Childron, Susp. (Fleming & Co.).
Eldofe, Tab. (Canright).
El-Ped-Ron, Liq. (Zeneca Pharmaceuticals).
Farbegen, Cap. (Hickam).
Feco-T, Cap. (Blaine Co., Inc.).
Femiron, Tab. (Menley & James Labs, Inc.).
Feostat, Preps. (Forest Pharmaceutical, Inc.).
Ferretts, Tab. (Pharmics, Inc.).
Fumasorb, Tab. (Hoechst Marion Roussel).
Fumerin, Tab. (Laser, Inc.).
Hemocyte, Tab. (US Pharm.).
Ircon, Tab. (Key Pharmaceuticals).
Laud-Iron, Tab., Susp. (Amfre-Grant).
Maniron, Meltab. (Jones Medical Industries, Inc.).
Nephro-Fer, Tab. (R & D Labs).
W/Ascorbic Acid.
See: C-Ron, Preps. (Solvay Pharmaceuticals).
Cytoferin, Tab. (Wyeth-Ayerst Laboratories).
Eldofe-C, Tab. (Canright).
Ferancee, Tab. (J & J Merck Consumer Pharm.).
Ferancee-HP, Tab. (Zeneca Pharmaceuticals).
Ferrodyl Chewable Tab. (Arcum).
Ferromar, SR Cap. (Marnel Pharmaceuticals, Inc.).
Min-Hema Chewable, Tab. (Scrip).
W/Ascorbic acid and folic acid.
See: Fer-Regules, Cap. (Quality Formulations, Inc.).
Ferro-Docusate TR, Cap. (Parmed Pharmaceuticals, Inc.).
Ferro Dok TR, Cap. (Major Pharmaceuticals).
Ferro-DSS SR, Cap. (Geneva Pharmaceuticals).
Ferro-Sequels, Cap. (ESI Lederle Generics).
W/Norethindrone, mestranol.
See: Ortho Novum Fe-28, Fe-28, 1 mg Fe-28, Tab. (Ortho McNeil Pharmaceutical).
W/Vitamins and minerals.
See: Stuart Formula, Tab. (Zeneca Pharmaceuticals).
Stuart Prenatal, Tab. (Zeneca Pharmaceuticals).
Stuartnatal 1 + 1, Tab. (Zeneca Pharmaceuticals).

ferrous fumarate. (Mission Pharmacal Co.) Ferrous fumarate 200 mg (iron 66 mg), sugar/Tab. Bot. 100s. Ferrous fumarate 300 mg (iron 106 mg) Tab. Bot. 100s. *otc.*
Use: Mineral supplement.

ferrous fumarate and docusate sodium extended-release tablets.
Use: Mineral supplement.

•**ferrous gluconate.** ((FER-uhs)) U.S.P. 23.
Use: Hematinic.
See: Fergon Prods. (Sanofi Winthrop Pharmaceuticals).
W/Ascorbic acid, desiccated liver, vitamin B complex.

See: I.L.X. w/B_{12}, Tab. (Kenwood Laboratories).
Stuart Hematinic, Liq. (Zeneca Pharmaceuticals).
W/Polyoxyethylene glucitan monolaurate.
See: Simron, Cap. (Hoechst Marion Roussel).

ferrous gluconate. (Various Mfr.) Ferrous gluconate 325 mg (iron 36 mg). Tab. Bot. 100s, 1000s. *otc.*
Use: Mineral supplement.

ferrous iodide. (Various Mfr.)
Use: In chronic tuberculosis.

ferrous iodide syrup. (Various Mfr.)
Use: In chronic tuberculosis.

ferrous lactate. (Various Mfr.)
Use: Mineral supplement.

•**ferrous sulfate.** (FER-uhs SULL-fate) U.S.P. 23.
Use: Hematinic.
See: Feosol, Spansule, Tab., Elix. (SmithKline Beecham).
Fe^{50}, Capl. (UCB Pharmaceuticals, Inc.).
Fer-gen-sol, Drops (Zenith Goldline Pharmaceuticals).
Fer-Iron, Drops (Rugby Labs, Inc.).
Fer-In-Sol, Syr. Drops (Mead Johnson).
Fero-Gradumet, Tab. (Abbott Laboratories).
Ferolix, Elix. (Century Pharmaceuticals, Inc.).
Ferrous Sulfate Filmseals, Tab. (Parke-Davis).
Fesotyme SR, Cap. (Zeneca Pharmaceuticals).
Irospan, Cap., Tab. (Fielding Co.).
Mol-Iron, Prods. (Schering-Plough Corp.).
W/Ascorbic acid.
See: Fero-Grad-500, Tab. (Abbott Laboratories).
Mol-Iron W/Vitamin C, Chronosules (Schering-Plough Corp.).
W/Ascorbic acid, folic acid.
See: Fero-Folic-500, Tab. (Abbott Laboratories).
W/Cyanocobalamin, ascorbic acid, folic acid.
See: Intrin, Cap. (Merit).
W/Folic acid.
See: Folvron, Cap. (ESI Lederle Generics).

ferrous sulfate. (Various Mfr.) Ferrous sulfate. **Tab.:** 324 mg (iron 65 mg) UD 100s; 325 mg (iron 65 mg) Bot. 100s. **Elix.:** 220 mg/5 ml (iron 44 mg/5 ml) Bot. 473 ml. **Drops:** 75 mg/0.6 ml (iron 15 mg/0.6 ml) Bot. 50 ml. *otc.*
Use: Mineral supplement.

•**ferrous sulfate, dried.** (FER-uhs SULL-fate) U.S.P. 23.
Use: Antianemic.
See: Fer-In-Sol (Bristol-Myers Squibb).
Feosol (SmithKline Beecham).
Ferrous Sulfate (Various Mfr.).
Slow Fe (Novartis Pharmaceutical Corp.).

ferrous sulfate exsiccated.
Use: Mineral supplement.
See: Fe_{50}, ER Capl. (UCB Pharmaceuticals, Inc.).
Feosol, Tab. (SmithKline Beecham).
Feratab, Tab. (Upsher-Smith Labs, Inc.).
Slow FE, SR Tab. (Novartis Pharmaceutical Corp.).

•**ferrous sulfate Fe 59.** (FER-uhs SULL-fate) USAN.
Use: Radiopharmaceutical.

ferrous sulfate. (Zenith Goldline Pharmaceuticals) Ferrous sulfate 325 mg (elemental iron 65 mg)/Tab. Bot. 100s. *otc.*
Use: Mineral supplement.

Ferrous Sulfate Filmseals. (Parke-Davis) Ferrous sulfate 5 gr/DR Tab. Bot. 1000s, UD 100s. *otc.*
Use: Iron supplement.

Fertility Tape. (Weston Labs.) Regular, extrasensitive, less-sensitive. W/Fertility Testor, cervical glucose test. Pkg. test 60s.
Use: Diagnostic aid.

Fertinex. (Serono Laboratories, Inc.) Urofollitropin 75 IU/Pow. for Inj. Amp. 1, 10, 100 ml amps with diluent. Urofollitropin 150 IU/Pow. for Inj. Ampules. Single with diluent. Lactose 10 mg. *Rx.*
Use: Ovulation inducer.

•**ferucarbotran.** (fur-you-CAR-boe-tran) USAN.
Use: Diagnostic aid (paramagnetic).

•**ferumoxides.** (feh-roo-MOX-ides) USAN.
Use: Diagnostic aid (paramagnetic).

•**ferumoxsil.** (feh-roo-MOX-sill) USAN.
Use: Diagnostic aid (paramagnetic).
See: GastroMARK, Oral Susp. (Mallinckrodt).

ferumoxtran-10. (fur-you-MOX-tran 10)
Use: Diagnostic aid (paramagnetic).

Ferusal. (Eon Labs Manufacturing, Inc.) Ferrous sulfate 325 mg/Tab. *otc.*
Use: Mineral supplement.

Festalan. (Hoechst Marion Roussel) Lipase 6000 units, amylase 30,000 units, protease 20,000 units, atropine methylnitrate 1 mg/EC Tab. Bot. 100s, 1000s. *Rx.*
Use: Digestive enzyme.

Fetinic. (Roberts Pharmaceuticals) Iron 3.6 mg, vitamins B_{12} equivalent to 2 mcg, B_1 10 mg, B_2 0.5 mg, B_3 10 mg, B_5 1 mg, B_6 1 mg, B_{12}15 mcg, chlorobutanol 0.5%, benzyl alcohol 2%/ml. Vial 30 ml. *Rx.*
Use: Mineral, vitamin supplement.

Fetinic-MW. (Roberts Pharmaceuticals) Iron 66 mg (from ferrous fumarate), vitamins B_{12} 5 mcg, C 60 mg/SR Cap. Bot. 100s. *otc.*
Use: Mineral, vitamin supplement.

•**fetoxylate hydrochloride.** (fee-TOX-ih-LATE) USAN.
Use: Muscle relaxant.

Feverall Children's. (Upsher-Smith Labs, Inc.) Acetaminophen 120 mg/Supp. Pkg. 6s. *otc.*
Use: Analgesic.

Feverall, Infants'. (Upsher-Smith Labs, Inc.) Acetaminophen 80 mg. Supp. Pkg. 6s. *otc.*
Use: Analgesic.

Feverall, Junior Strength. (Upsher-Smith Labs, Inc.) Acetaminophen 325 mg/Supp. Pkg. 6s. *otc.*
Use: Analgesic.

Feverall Sprinkle. (Upsher-Smith Labs, Inc.) Acetaminophen 80 mg or 160 mg/Cap. Bot. 20s. *otc.*
Use: Analgesic.

•**fexofenadine hydrochloride.** (fex-oh-FEN-ah-deen) USAN.
Use: Antihistamine.
See: Allegra, Tab. (Hoechst Marion Roussel).
Allegra-D, ER Tab. (Hoechst Marion Roussel).

•**fezolamine fumarate.** (feh-ZOLE-ah-MEEN) USAN.
Use: Antidepressant.

fgn-1. Cell Pathways, Inc.
Use: Treatment of adenomatous polyposis coli. [Orphan Drug]

•**fiacitabine.** (fih-AH-sit-ah-BEEN) USAN.
Use: Antiviral.

•**fialuridine.** (fie-al-YOUR-ih-deen) USAN.
Use: Antiviral.

fiau. (Oclassen Pharmaceuticals, Inc.)
Use: Antiviral, hepatitis B. [Orphan Drug]

Fiberall. (Novartis Consumer Health) Calcium carbophil 1250 mg (equiv. to 1000 mg polycarbophil). Chew. Tab. Lemon flavor. Pkg. 18s. *otc.*
Use: Laxative.

Fiberall Natural Flavor. (Novartis Self-Medication) **Pow.:** Psyllium hydrophilic mucilloid 3.4 g, wheat bran, sodium < 10 mg, potassium 60 mg, calories 6/5.9 g, saccharin. Can 150 g, 300 g, 450 g. **Wafer:** Psyllium hydrophilic mucilloid 3.4 g, wheat bran, oats, sucrose. Box 14s. *otc.*
Use: Laxative.

Fiberall Orange Flavor. (Novartis Consumer Health) Psyllium hydrophilic mucilloid 3.4 g, wheat bran, sodium < 10 mg, potassium 60 mg, calories 6/5.9 g Pow. Can 150 g, 300 g, 450 g. *otc.*
Use: Laxative.

FiberCon. (ESI Lederle Generics) Calcium polycarbophil 500 mg/Tab. Bot. 36s, 60s. *otc.*
Use: Laxative.

Fiber Guard. (Wyeth-Ayerst Laboratories) All natural high-fiber supplement 530 mg/Tab. Bot. 100s, 200s. *otc.*
Use: Fiber supplement.

Fiberlan. (Elan Pharma) Protein 50 g, fat 40 g, carbohydrates 160 g, Na 920 mg, K 1.56 g, fiber 14 g/per L. With vitamins A, C, B, B_2, B_3, D, E, B_5, B_6, B_{12}, K, Ca, Fe, folic acid, P, I, Mg, Zn, Cu, biotin, Mn, choline, Cl, Se, Cr, Mo. Liq. Bot. 237 ml. *otc.*
Use: Nutritional supplement.

Fiber-Lax. (Rugby Labs, Inc.) Calcium polycarbophil 625 mg (equiv. to 500 mg polycarbophil)/Tab. Bot. 60s. *otc.*
Use: Laxative.

Fibermed High-Fiber Snacks. (Purdue Frederick Co.) One serving (15 snacks) contains 5 g dietary fiber. Box 8 oz. Packs of 24 × 1.3 oz. *otc.*
Use: Fiber supplement.

Fibermed High-Fiber Supplement. (Purdue Frederick Co.) Each supplement contains 5 g dietary fiber. Box 14s. Institutional pack, Box 144s of two supplements. *otc.*
Use: Fiber supplement.

FiberNorm. (G & W Laboratories) Calcium polycarbophil 625 mg/Tab. Bot. 60s. *otc.*
Use: Laxative.

Fiber Rich. (Columbia Laboratories, Inc.) Phenylpropanolamine HCl 75 mg/Tab. Bot. 24s. *otc.*
Use: Dietary aid.

Fibre Trim. (Schering-Plough Corp.) Grain and citrus fruit concentrated dietary fiber. Tab. Bot. 100s, 250s. *otc.*
Use: Dietary aid.

Fibre Trim w/Calcium. (Schering-Plough Corp.) Grain and citrus fruit concentrated dietary fiber w/calcium. Tab. Bot. 90s, 225s. *otc.*
Use: Dietary aid.

•**fibrinogen I 125.** (FIE-BRIN-oh-jen I 125) USAN.

Use: Diagnostic aid (vascular patency); radiopharmaceutical.

fibrinogen (human). (Alpha Therapeutic Corp.) Partially purified fibrinogen prepared by fractionation from normal human plasma.
Use: Coagulant (clotting factor). [Orphan Drug]

fibrinolysis inhibitor.
See: Amicar Syr., Tab., Vial (ESI Lederle Generics).

Fibrogammin P. (Behringwerke Aktiengesellschaft)
Use: Congenital Factor XIII deficiency. [Orphan Drug]

fibronectin (human plasma derived). (Melville Biologics)
Use: Treatment of nonhealing corneal ulcers or epithelial defects. [Orphan Drug]

•**filaminast.** (fih-LAM-in-ast) USAN.
Use: Antiasthmatic (selective phosphodiesterase IV inhibitor).

Filaxis. (Amlab) Vitamins A 25,000 IU, D 1250 IU, C 150 mg, E 5 IU, B_1 12 mg, B_2 5 mg, B_6 0.5 mg, B_{12} 5 mcg, calcium pantothenate 5 mg, niacinamide 100 mg, Fe 15 mg, I 0.15 mg, Mg 10 mg, K 5 mg, Ca 75 mg, P 60 mg/Tab. Bot. 30s, 100s. Available w/B_{12}. Bot. 30s, 60s, 100s. *otc.*
Use: Mineral, vitamin supplement.

•**filgrastim.** (fill-GRAH-stim) USAN.
Use: Biological response modifier, antineoplastic adjunct, antineutropenic, hematopoietic stimulant. [Orphan Drug]
See: Neupogen (Amgen, Inc.).

•**filipin.** (FIH-lih-pin) USAN.
Use: Antifungal.

Finac. (C & M Pharmacal, Inc.) Salicylic acid 2%, isopropyl alcohol 22.5%, propylene glycol, acetone in lotion base. Bot. 60 ml. *otc.*
Use: Dermatologic, acne.

•**finasteride.** (fih-NASS-teer-ide) USAN.
Use: Benign prostatic hypertrophy therapy, antineoplastic, antineutropenic, inhibitor (alpha-reductase).
See: Propecia, Tab. (Merck & Co.). Proscar, Tab. (Merck & Co.).

Fiogesic. (Novartis Pharmaceutical Corp.) Phenylpropanolamine HCl 25 mg, pyrilamine maleate 12.5 mg, pheniramine maleate 12.5 mg, calcium carbaspirin 382 mg (equiv. to 300 mg ASA)/Tab. Bot. 100s. *otc.*
Use: Analgesic, antihistamine, decongestant.

Fioricet. (Novartis Pharmaceutical Corp.) Acetaminophen 325 mg, butalbital 50 mg, caffeine 40 mg/Tab. Bot. 100s, 500s, UD 100s. *Rx.*
Use: Analgesic, hypnotic, sedative.

Fioricet Codeine. (Novartis Pharmaceutical Corp.) Codeine phosphate 30 mg, acetaminophen 325 mg, caffeine 40 mg, butalbital 50 mg/Cap. Bot. 100s, Control pak 25s. *c-III.*
Use: Analgesic combination, narcotic.

Fiorinal. (Novartis Pharmaceutical Corp.) Butalbital (Sandoptal) 50 mg, caffeine 40 mg, aspirin 325 mg/Tab. or Cap. **Tab.:** Lactose Bot. 100s, 1000s. UD 100s. **Cap.:** Benzyl alcohol, parabens. Bot. 100s, 500s, UD 25s. *c-III.*
Use: Analgesic, hypnotic, sedative.

Fiorinal w/Codeine No. 3. (Novartis Pharmaceutical Corp.) Butalbital 50 mg, caffeine 40 mg, aspirin 325 mg, codeine phosphate 30 mg/Cap. Bot. 100s. Control Pak 25s. *c-III.*
Use: Analgesic combination, hypnotic, sedative.

Fiorpap. (Geneva Pharmaceuticals) Butalbital 50 mg, acetaminophen 325 mg, caffeine 40 mg/Tab. Bot 100s, 500s. *Rx.*
Use: Analgesic.

Fiortal. (Geneva Pharmaceuticals) Aspirin 325 mg, caffeine 40 mg, butalbital 50 mg, benzyl alcohol, parabens. Cap. Bot. 100s. *c-III.*
Use: Analgesic.

fire ant venom, allergenic extract, imported.
Use: Dermatologic aid-skin test, immunotherapy. [Orphan Drug]

Firmdent. (Moyco Union Broach Division) Formerly Moy. Karaya gum 94.6%, sodium borate 5.36% Pkg. 3 oz. *otc.*
Use: Denture adhesive.

First Aid Cream. (Johnson & Johnson) Cetyl alcohol, glyceryl stearate, isopropyl palmitate, stearyl alcohol, synthetic beeswax. Tube 0.8 oz, 1.5 oz, 2.5 oz. *otc.*
Use: Antiseptic; dermatologic, protectant.

First Aid Cream. (Walgreen Co.) Benzocaine 3%, allantoin 0.2%, benzyl alcohol 4%, phenol 0.25%. Tube 1.5 oz. *otc.*
Use: Anesthetic, antiseptic.

First Choice. (Polymer Technology International) 50s.
Use: Diagnostic aid.

First Response Ovulation Predictor. (Tambrands, Inc.) Monoclonal antibody-based enzyme immunoassay test

for hLH in urine. Test kit 1s. *otc.*
Use: Diagnostic aid.

First Response Pregnancy Test. (Tambrands, Inc.) Reagent in-home kit for urine testing. Test kit 1s.
Use: Diagnostic aid.

fish oil concentrate, natural. Natural fish oil concentrate containing EPA (Eicosanoic acid) and DHA (Docosahexaenoic acid).
Use: Nutritional supplement.

Fitacol. (Standex) Atropine sulfate 0.2 mg, phenylpropanolamine 12.5 mg, chlorpheniramine maleate 0.5 mg, chlorobutanol 0.5 mg, water q.s./ml. Bot. pt. *Rx.*
Use: Anticholinergic, antihistamine, antispasmodic, decongestant.

Fitacol Stankaps. (Standex) Belladonna alkaloidal salts 0.16 mg (atropine sulfate 0.024 mg, scopolamine HBr 0.014 mg, hyoscyamine sulfate 0.122 mg), phenylpropanolamine HCl 50 mg, chlorpheniramine maleate 1 mg, pheniramine maleate 12.5 mg/Cap. Bot. 100s. *Rx.*
Use: Anticholinergic, antihistamine, antispasmodic, decongestant.

5-FC.
See: Flucytosine.

5-FU.
See: Fluorouracil.

523 Tablets. (Enzyme Process) Pancreatin 200 mg 4x/Tab. Tryspin, chymotrypsin, amylase, lipase enzymes from pancreatin, raw beef pancreas. Bot. 100s, 250s.
Use: Digestive enzyme.

Fixodent. (Procter & Gamble Pharm.) Calcium sodium poly (vinyl methyl ether-maleate), carboxymethylcellulose sodium in a petrolatum base. Tube 0.75 oz, 1.5 oz, 2.5 oz. *otc.*
Use: Denture adhesive.

FK506.
See: Prograf (Fujisawa USA, Inc.).

FK-565.
Use: Immunomodulator.

Flagyl ER. (Searle) Metronidazole 750 mg. ER Tab. Bot. 30s. *Rx.*
Use: Anti-infective.

Flagyl I.V. (Searle) Metronidazole HCl sterile lyophilized powder in single-dose vials equivalent to 500 mg metronidazole. Carton 10s. *Rx.*
Use: Anti-infective.

Flagyl I.V. RTU. (Searle) Metronidazole ready-to-use, premixed, 500 mg/100 ml Soln. Vial (glass), Box 6s; Container, (plastic), Box 24s. *Rx.*
Use: Anti-infective.

Flagyl Tablets. (Searle) Metronidazole 250 mg or 500 mg/Tab. **250 mg:** Bot. 50s, 100s, 250s, 1000s, 2500s, UD 100s. **500 mg:** Bot. 50s, 100s, 500s, UD 100s. *Rx.*
Use: Anti-infective.

Flagyl 375. (Searle) Metronidazole 375 mg/Cap. Bot. 50s, UD 100s. *Rx.*
Use: Anti-infective.

Flanders Buttocks Ointment. (Flanders, Inc.) Zinc oxide, castor oil, balsam peru, boric acid in an emollient base. 60 g. *otc.*
Use: Dermatologic, counterirritant.

Flarex. (Alcon Laboratories, Inc.) Fluorometholone acetate 0.1%. Susp. Bot. 2.5 ml, 5 ml, 10 ml Drop-Tainers. *Rx.*
Use: Corticosteroid, ophthalmic; anti-inflammatory.

Flatulence Tablets. (Pal-Pak, Inc.) Nux vomica 16.2 mg, cascara sagrada extract 64.8 mg, ginger 48.6 mg, capsicum 16.2 mg/Tab. w/asafetida. *otc.*
Use: Antiflatulent, laxative.

Flatulex. (Dayton Laboratories, Inc.) **Tab.:** Simethicone 80 mg, activated charcoal 250 mg/Tab. Bot. 100s. **Drops:** Simethicone 40 mg/0.6 ml. Bot. 30 ml with calibrated dropper. *otc.*
Use: Antiflatulent.

Flatus. (Foy Laboratories) Nux vomica extract 0.25 gr, cascara extract 1 gr, ginger ¾ gr, capsicum gr/Tab. w/asfetida qs. Bot. 1000s. *otc.*
Use: Antiflatulent, laxative.

Flav-A-D. (Kirkman Sales Co., Inc.) Vitamins A 5000 IU, D 1000 IU, C 100 mg/Tab. Bot. 100s, 1000s. Also w/fluoride. Bot. 100s, 1000s. *Rx-otc.*
Use: Vitamin supplement.

flavine.
See: Acriflavine Hydrochloride (Various Mfr.).

Flavinoid-C. (Barth's) **Tab.:** Vitamin C 150 mg, hesperidin complex 10 mg, citrus bioflavonoid 50 mg, rutin 20 mg/Tab. Bot. 100s, 500s, 1000s. **Liq.:** Vitamin C 100 mg, bioflavonoid complex 100 mg/5 ml. Bot. 4 oz. *otc.*
Use: Vitamin supplement.

•**flavodilol maleate.** (FLAY-voe-DILL-ole) USAN.
Use: Antihypertensive.

flavolutan.
See: Progesterone (Various Mfr.).

flavonoid compounds.
See: Bio-Flavonoid Compounds; Vitamin P.

Flavons-500. (Freeda Vitamins, Inc.) Citrus bioflavonoids complex 500 mg, hesperidin complex/Tab. Bot. 100s, 250s,

500s. *otc.*
Use: Vitamin supplement.

Flavorcee. (NBTY, Inc.) Ascorbic acid 100 mg or 250 mg/Chew. Tab. **100 mg:** Bot. 100s. **250 mg:** Bot. 250s. *otc.*
Use: Vitamin supplement.

flavored diluent. (Roxane Laboratories, Inc.) Flavored vehicle for the immediate administration of crushed tablet or capsule product. Bot. 500 ml, UD 15 ml × 100.
Use: Flavored vehicle.

•**flavoxate hydrochloride.** (flay-VOKES-ate) USAN.
Use: Antispasmodic, urinary; muscle relaxant.
See: Urispas, Tab. (SmithKline Beecham).

flavurol. Merbromin.
Use: Antiseptic.

•**flazalone.** (FLAY-zah-lone) USAN.
Use: Anti-inflammatory.

•**flecainide acetate.** (fleh-CANE-ide) U.S.P. 23.
Use: Cardiovascular agent.
See: Tambocor (3M Pharm.).

Fleet Babylax. (C. B. Fleet Co., Inc.) Glycerin 4 ml in disposable pre-lubricated rectal applicator. Liq. pkg. 6s. *otc.*
Use: Laxative.

Fleet Bagenema. (C. B. Fleet Co., Inc.) Castile soap or Fleets bisacodyl prep. *otc.*
Use: Laxative.

Fleet Bisacodyl Prep Packets. (C. B. Fleet Co., Inc.) Bisacodyl 10 mg/10 ml packet. 36 packets/box. *otc.*
Use: Laxative.

Fleet Enema. (C. B. Fleet Co., Inc.) Sodium biphosphate 19 g, sodium phosphate 7 g/118 ml. Bot. w/rectal tube 4.5 oz. Pediatric size 67.5 ml, 135 ml. *otc.*
Use: Laxative.

Fleet Flavored Castor Oil Emulsion. (C. B. Fleet Co., Inc.) 1 oz delivers 30 ml castor oil. Bot. 1.5 oz, 3 oz. *otc.*
Use: Laxative.

Fleet Glycerin Suppositories. (C. B. Fleet Co., Inc.) Adult: Jar 12s, 24s, 50s. Child Size: Jar 12s. *otc.*
Use: Laxative.

Fleet Laxative. (C. B. Fleet Co., Inc.) Bisacodyl. **EC Tab.:** 5 mg/Tab. Bot. 24s. **Supp.:** 10 mg. Box 4s. *otc.*
Use: Laxative.

Fleet Medicated Wipes. (C. B. Fleet Co., Inc.) Hamamelis water 50%, alcohol 7%, glycerin 10%, benzalkonium Cl, methylparaben. Rectal pads. 100s. *otc.*
Use: Perianal hygiene.

Fleet Mineral Oil Enema. (C. B. Fleet Co., Inc.) Mineral oil 4.5 fl oz in an unbreakable vinyl squeeze bottle. *otc.*
Use: Laxative.

Fleet Pain Relief. (C. B. Fleet Co., Inc.) Pramoxine HCl 1%, glycerin 12%. Pads. 100s. *otc.*
Use: Anorectal preparation.

Fleet Phospho-Soda. (C. B. Fleet Co., Inc.) Sodium phosphate 18 g, sodium biphosphate 48 g/100 ml (96.4 mEq sodium/20 ml). Bot. 45 ml, 90 ml, 240 ml. *otc.*
Use: Laxative.

Fleet Prep Kit #1. (C. B. Fleet Co., Inc.) Fleet Phospho-Soda 45 ml, Fleet Bisacodyl Tablets 45 mg, Fleet Bisacodyl Suppository 110 mg. *otc.*
Use: Laxative.

Fleet Prep Kit #2. (C. B. Fleet Co., Inc.) Fleet Phospho-Soda 45 ml, Fleet Bisacodyl Tablets 45 mg, 1 Fleet Bagenema set for large volume enema, including optional Castile Soap Packet. 20 ml. *otc.*
Use: Laxative.

Fleet Prep Kit #3. (C. B. Fleet Co., Inc.) Fleet Phospho-Soda 45 ml, Fleet Bisacodyl Tablets 45 mg, Fleet Bisacodyl Enema 130 ml. 10 mg. *otc.*
Use: Laxative.

Fleet Prep Kit #4. (C. B. Fleet Co., Inc.) Fleet Flavored Castor Oil Emulsion 45 ml, Fleet Bisacodyl Tablets 45 mg, Fleet Bisacodyl Suppository 110 mg. *otc.*
Use: Laxative.

Fleet Prep Kit #5. (C. B. Fleet Co., Inc.) Fleet Flavored Castor Oil Emulsion 45 ml, Fleet Bisacodyl Tablets 45 mg, 1 Fleet Bagenema set for large volume enema, including optional Castile Soap Packet 20 ml. *otc.*
Use: Laxative.

Fleet Prep Kit #6. (C.B. Fleet Co., Inc.) Fleet Flavored Castor Oil Emulsion 45 ml, Fleet Bisacodyl Tablets 45 mg, Fleet Bisacodyl Enema 130 ml 10 mg. *otc.*
Use: Laxative.

•**fleroxacin.** (fler-OX-ah-SIN) USAN.
Use: Anti-infective.

•**flestolol sulfate.** (FLESS-toe-lahl) USAN.
Use: Antiadrenergic (β-receptor).

•**fletazepam.** (FLET-AZE-eh-pam) USAN.
Use: Muscle relaxant.

Fletcher's Castoria for Children. (Mentholatum Co., Inc.) Senna 6.5%, alcohol 3.5%. Liq. Bot. 75 ml, 150 ml. *otc.*

Use: Laxative.

Flexall 454. (Chattem Consumer Products) Menthol 7%, alcohol, allantoin, aloe vera gel, boric acid, carbomer 940, diazolidinyl urea, eucalyptus oil, glycerin, iodine, parabens, methyl salicylate, peppermint oil, polysorbate 60, potassium iodide, propylene glycol, thyme oil, triethanolamine. Gel Tube. 240 g. *otc.*
Use: Analgesic, topical.

Flexall 454, Maximum Strength. (Chattem Consumer Products) Menthol 16%, aloe vera gel, eucalyptus oil, methylsalicylate, SD alcohol 38-B, thyme oil. Gel 90 mg. *otc.*
Use: Analgesic, topical.

Flex Anti-Dandruff Shampoo. (Revlon) Zinc pyrithione 1% in liquid shampoo. *otc.*
Use: Antiseborrheic.

Flex Anti-Dandruff Styling Mousse. (Revlon) Zinc pyrithione 0.1%. Aerosol foam. *otc.*
Use: Antiseborrheic.

Flexaphen. (Trimen Laboratories, Inc.) Chlorzoxazone 250 mg, acetaminophen 300 mg/Cap. Bot 100s. *Rx.*
Use: Muscle relaxant.

Flex-Care Especially for Sensitive Eyes. (Alcon Laboratories, Inc.) EDTA 0.1%, chlorhexidine gluconate 0.005%, sodium Cl, sodium borate, boric acid. Soln. Bot. 118 ml, 237 ml, 355 ml, 360 ml. *otc.*
Use: Contact lens care.

Flexeril. (Merck & Co.) Cyclobenzaprine HCl 10 mg/Tab. Bot. 100s, UD 100s. *Rx.*
Use: Muscle relaxant.

flexible hydroactive dressings/granules.
See: Intra Site (Smith & Nephew United).
Shur-Clens (SmithKline Beecham).
DuoDerm (ConvaTec).
Sorbsan (Dow Hickam, Inc.).

Flexoject. (Merz Pharmaceuticals) Orphenadrine citrate 30 mg/ml. Inj. Vial 10 ml, amps 2 ml. *Rx.*
Use: Muscle relaxant.

Flexon. (Keene Pharmaceuticals, Inc.) Orphenadrine citrate 30 mg/ml. Inj. Vial 10 ml. *Rx.*
Use: Muscle relaxant.

Flexsol. (Alcon, Vision Care) Sterile, buffered, isotonic aqueous soln. of sodium Cl, sodium borate, boric acid, adsorbobase. Bot. 6 oz. *otc.*
Use: Contact lens care.

Flextra-DS. (Poly Pharm) Acetaminophen 500 mg, phenyltoloxamine citrate. Tab. Bot. 100s. *otc.*
Use: Analgesic.

Flintstones Children's. (Bayer Corp. (Consumer Div.)) Vitamin A 2500 IU, E 15 mg, C 60 mg, folic acid 0.3 mg, B_1 1.05 mg, B_2 1.2 mg, B_3 13.5 mg, B_6 1.05 mg, B_{12} 4.5 mcg, D 400 IU/Chew. Tab. Bot. 60s, 100s. *otc.*
Use: Vitamin supplement.

Flintstones Complete. (Bayer Corp. (Consumer Div.)) Elemental iron 18 mg, vitamins A 5000 IU, D 400 IU, E 30 mg, B_1 1.5 mg, B_2 1.7 mg, B_3 20 mg, B_5 10 mg, B_6 2 mg, B_{12} 6 mcg, C 60 mg, folic acid 0.4 mg, biotin 40 mcg, Ca, Cu, I, Mg, P, zinc 15 mg/Chew. Tab. Bot. 60s, 120s. *otc.*
Use: Mineral, vitamin supplement.

Flintstones Plus Calcium. (Bayer Corp. (Consumer Div.)) Vitamin A 2500 IU, D IU 400, E 15 IU, C 60 mg, folic acid 0.3 mg, B_1 1.05 mg, B_2 1.2 mg, B_3 13.5 mg, B_6 1.05 mg, B_{12} 4.5 mcg, Ca 200 mg. Chew. Tab. Bot. 60s. *otc.*
Use: Mineral, vitamin supplement.

Flintstones Plus Extra C Children's. (Bayer Corp. (Consumer Div.)) Vitamins A 2500 IU, D 400 IU, E 15 mg, C 250 mg, folic acid 0.3 mg, B_1 1.05 mg, B_2 1.2 mg, niacin 13.5 mg, B_6 1.05 mg, B_{12} 4.5 mcg/Tab. Bot. 60s, 100s. *otc.*
Use: Vitamin supplement.

Flintstones Plus Iron Multivitamins. (Bayer Corp. (Consumer Div.)) Vitamins A 2500 IU, E 15 mg, C 60 mg, folic acid 0.3 mg, B_1 1.05 mg, B_2 1.2 mg, niacin 13.5 mg, B_6 1.05 mg, B_{12} 4.5 mcg, D 400 IU, iron 15 mg/Chew. Tab. Bot. 60s, 100s. *otc.*
Use: Mineral, vitamin supplement.

Flo-Coat. (Lafayette Pharmaceuticals, Inc.) Barium sulfate 100%. Susp. Bot. 1850 ml. *Rx.*
Use: Radiopaque agent.

•**floctafenine.** (FLOCK-tah-FEN-een) USAN.
Use: Analgesic.

Flolan. (GlaxoWellcome) Epoprostenol sodium 0.5 or 1.5 mg, mannitol, NaCl/Vial. Pow. for Inj. 17 ml. *Rx.*
Use: Antihypertensive.

Flomax. (Boehringer Ingelheim, Inc.) Tamsulosin HCl 0.4 mg/Cap. Bot. 100s, 1000s. *Rx.*
Use: Benign prostatic hyperplasia treatment.

Flonase. (GlaxoWellcome) Fluticasone propionate 50 mcg/actuation. Spray Bot. 16 g (120 actuations). *Rx.*
Use: Corticosteroid, nasal.

Flor-D Chewable Tab. (Derm Pharm.) Fluoride 1 mg, vitamins A 4000 IU, D 400 IU, C 75 mg, B_1 1.5 mg, B_2 1.8 mg, niacinamide 15 mg, B_6 1 mg, B_{12} 3 mcg, calcium pantothenate 10 mg/Tab. Bot. 100s. *Rx.*
Use: Mineral, vitamin supplement.

Flor-D Drops. (Derm Pharm.) Fluoride 0.5 mg, vitamins A 3000 IU, D 400 IU, C 60 mg, B_1 1 mg, B_2 1.2 mg, niacinamide 8 mg/0.6 ml. Bot. 60 ml. *Rx.*
Use: Mineral, vitamin supplement.

•**flordipine.** (FLORE-dih-peen) USAN.
Use: Antihypertensive.

Florical. (Mericon Industries, Inc.) Sodium fluoride 8.3 mg, calcium carbonate 364 mg (equivalent to 145.6 mg calcium)/Cap. Bot. 100s, 500s. *otc.*
Use: Mineral supplement.

Florida Foam. (Hill Dermaceuticals, Inc.) Benzalkonium Cl, aluminum subacetate, boric acid 2%. Bot. 8 oz. *otc.*
Use: Soap substitute, antiseborrheic, antifungal, dermatologic-acne.

Florida Sunburn Relief. (Pharmacel Laboratory, Inc.) Benzyl alcohol 3%, phenol 0.4%, camphor 0.2%, menthol 0.15%. Lot. Bot. 60 ml. *otc.*
Use: Sunburn relief.

Florinef Acetate. (Apothecon, Inc.) Fludrocortisone acetate, 0.1 mg/Tab. Bot. 100s. *Rx.*
Use: Corticosteroid.

Florone Cream. (Dermik Laboratories, Inc.) Diflorasone diacetate 0.5 mg/g (0.05%) w/stearic acid, sorbitan monooleate, polysorbate 60, sorbic acid, citric acid, propylene glycol, purified water. Tube 15 g, 30 g, 60 g. *Rx.*
Use: Corticosteroid, topical.

Florone E. (Dermik Laboratories, Inc.) Diflorasone diacetate 0.5 mg. Tube 15 g, 30 g, 60 g. *Rx.*
Use: Corticosteroid, topical.

Florone Ointment. (Dermik Laboratories, Inc.) Diflorasone diacetate 0.5 mg/g (0.05%) W/polyoxypropylene 15-stearyl ether, stearic acid, lanolin alcohol and white petrolatum. Tube 15 g, 30 g, 60 g. *Rx.*
Use: Corticosteroid, topical.

Floropryl. (Merck & Co.) Isoflurophate 0.025% in sterile ophthalmic ointment in polyethylene-mineral oil gel. Tube 3.5 g. *Rx.*
Use: Agent for glaucoma.

Florvite. (Everett Laboratories, Inc.) Vitamins, fluoride 0.5 mg/Chew. Tab. Bot 100s. *Rx.*
Use: Dental caries agent.

Florvite Half Strength. (Everett Laboratories, Inc.) Elemental fluoride 0.5 mg, vitamins A 2500 IU, D 400 IU, E 15 mg, B_1 1.05 mg, B_2 1.2 mg, B_3 13.5 mg, B_6 1.05 mg, B_{12} 4.5 mcg, C 60 mg, folic acid 0.3 mg/Chew. Tab. Bot. 100s. *Rx.*
Use: Mineral, vitamin supplement; dental caries agent.

Florvite + Iron Drops. (Everett Laboratories, Inc.) Elemental fluorine. **0.25 mg:** Vitamins A 1500 IU, D 400 IU, E 5 mg, B_1 0.5 mg, B_2 0.6 mg, B_3 8 mg, B_6 0.4 mg, C 35 mg, iron 10 mg/ml. **0.5 mg:** Vitamins A 1500 IU, D 400 IU, E 5 mg, B_1 0.5 mg, B_2 0.6 mg, B_3 8 mg, B_6 0.4 mg, C 35 mg, iron 10 mg/ml. Liq. Bot. 50 ml. *Rx.*
Use: Mineral, vitamin supplement; dental caries agent.

Florvite + Iron Chewable. (Everett Laboratories, Inc.) Fluoride 1 mg, iron 12 mg, vitamins A 2500 IU, D 400 IU, E 15 mg, B_1 1.05 mg, B_2 1.2 mg, B_3 13.5 mg, B_6 1.05 mg, B_{12} 4.5 mcg, C 60 mg, folic acid 0.3 mg, Cu, Zn 10 mg, sucrose/Chew. Tab. Bot. 100s. *Rx.*
Use: Mineral, vitamin supplement; dental caries agent.

Florvite Pediatric Drops. (Everett Laboratories, Inc.) Elemental fluorine. **0.25 mg/ml:** Vitamins A 1500 IU, D 400 IU, E 5 mg, B_1 0.5 mg, B_2 0.6 mg, B_3 8 mg, B_6 0.4 mg, B_{12} 2 mcg, C 35 mg/ml. **0.5 mg/ml:** Vitamins A 1500 IU, D 400 IU, E 5 mg, B_1 0.5 mg, B_2 0.6 mg, B_3 8 mg, B_6 0.4 mg, B_{12} 2 mcg, C 35 mg, iron 10 mg/ml Bot. 50 ml. *Rx.*
Use: Mineral, vitamin supplement; dental caries agent.

Florvite Tablets. (Everett Laboratories, Inc.) Fluoride 1 mg, vitamins A 2500 IU, D 400 IU, E 15 mg, B_1 1.05 mg, B_2 1.2 mg, B_3 13.5 mg, B_6 1.05 mg, B_{12} 4.5 mcg, C 60 mg, folic acid 0.3 mg/Chew. Tab. Bot. 100s, 1000s. *Rx.*
Use: Mineral, vitamin supplement; dental caries agent.

Florvite Drops. (Everett Laboratories, Inc.) Fluoride 0.25 mg or 0.5 mg, A 1500 IU, D 400 IU, E 5 IU, B_1 0.5 mg, B_2 0.6 mg, B_3 8 mg, B_6 0.4 mg, B_{12} 2 mcg, C 35 mg/Drop. Bot. 50 ml. *Rx.*
Use: Mineral, vitamin supplement; dental caries agent.

•**flosequinan.** (flow-SEH-kwih-NAHN) USAN.
Use: Antihypertensive (vasodilator).

Flovent. (GlaxoWellcome) Fluticasone propionate 44 mcg, 110 mcg, 220 mcg/Aerosol spray. Canister. 7.9 g (60 actuations) and 13 g (120 actuations). *Rx.*

Use: Corticosteroid.

Flovent Rotadisk. (GlaxoWellcome) Fluticasone propionate 50 mcg, 100 mcg, 250 mcg. Pow. Blisters 4 containing 15 Rotodisks w/inhalation device. *Rx.*
Use: Corticosteroid.

•**floxacillin.** (FLOX-ah-SILL-in) USAN.
Use: Anti-infective.

Floxin. (Ortho McNeil Pharmaceutical) **Tab.:** Ofloxacin, 200 mg, 300 mg, or 400 mg. Bot. 50s, 100s. **Inj.:** 200 mg flexible container; 400 mg Vial 10 ml, 20 ml; Bot. 100 ml; flexible container. *Rx.*
Use: Anti-infective, fluoroquinolone.

Floxin Otic Solution. (Daiichi Pharmaceutical) Ofloxacin 3 mg/ml, benzalkonium chloride, sodium chloride, sodium hydroxide. Otic Soln. Bot. 5 ml. *Rx.*
Use: Anti-infective, otic.

•**floxuridine.** (flox-YOUR-ih-deen) U.S.P. 23.
Use: Antiviral, antineoplastic.
See: FUDR, Vial (Roberts Pharmaceuticals).

•**fluazacort.** (flew-AZE-ah-kort) USAN.
Use: Anti-inflammatory.

•**flubanilate hydrochloride.** (flew-BAN-ill-ate) USAN.
Use: Antidepressant; CNS stimulant.

•**flubendazole.** (FLEW-BEN-dah-zole) USAN.
Use: Antiprotozoal.

flucarbril.
Use: Muscle relaxant, analgesic.

•**flucindole.** (flew-SIN-dole) USAN.
Use: Antipsychotic.

•**flucloronide.** (flew-KLOR-oh-nide) USAN.
Use: Corticosteroid, topical.

Flu, Cold & Cough Medicine. (Major Pharmaceuticals) Pseudoephedrine HCl 60 mg, chlorpheniramine 4 mg, dextromethorphan HBr 20 mg, acetaminophen 500 mg. Pow. Pck. 6s. *otc.*
Use: Analgesic, antihistamine, antitussive, decongestant.

•**fluconazole.** (flew-KOE-nuh-sole) USAN.
Use: Antifungal.
See: Diflucan (Roerig).

•**flucrylate.** (FLEW-krih-late) USAN.
Use: Surgical aid (tissue adhesive).

•**flucytosine.** (flew-SITE-oh-seen) U.S.P. 23.
Use: Antifungal.
See: Ancobon, Cap. (Roberts Pharmaceuticals).

•**fludalanine.** (flew-DAL-AH-neen) USAN.
Use: Anti-infective.

Fludara. (Berlex Laboratories, Inc.) Fludarabine 50 mg. Pow. for Recon. Vial. 6 ml. *Rx.*
Use: Antineoplastic.

•**fludarabine phosphate.** (flew-DAR-uh-BEAN) USAN.
Use: Antineoplastic. [Orphan Drug]
See: Fludara, Pow. (Berlex Laboratories, Inc.).

•**fludazonium chloride.** (FLEW-dazz-OH-nee-uhm) USAN.
Use: Anti-infective, topical.

•**fludeoxyglucose F 18 injection.** (FLEW-dee-OX-ee-GLUE-kose F 18) U.S.P. 23.
Use: Diagnostic aid (brain disorders, thyroid disorders, liver disorders, cardiac disease, and neoplastic disease); radiopharmaceutical.

•**fludorex.** (FLEW-doe-rex) USAN.
Use: Anorexic, antiemetic.

•**fludrocortisone acetate.** (flew-droe-CORE-tih-sone) U.S.P. 23.
Use: Adrenocortical steroid (salt-regulating).
See: Florinef Acetate, Tab. (Apothecon, Inc.).

•**flufenamic acid.** (FLEW-fen-AM-ik) USAN.
Use: Anti-inflammatory.

•**flufenisal.** (flew-FEN-ih-sal) USAN.
Use: Analgesic.

Fluidex. (Columbia Laboratories, Inc.) Natural botanical ingredients. Tab. Bot. 36s, 72s.
Use: Diuretic.

Flu-Imune. (Wyeth Lederle) Influenza virus vaccine. Vial 5 ml (10 doses). (Purified surface antigen). *Rx.*
Use: Immunization.

fluitran. Trichlormethiazide.

Flumadine. (Forest Pharmaceutical, Inc.) **Tab.:** Rimantadine HCl 100 mg. Bot. 20s, 100s, 500s, 1000s. **Syr.:** Rimantadine HCl 50 mg/5 ml. Bot. 60 ml, 240 ml, 480 ml. *Rx.*
Use: Antiviral.

•**flumazenil.** (flew-MAZ-ah-nil) USAN.
Use: Antagonist (to benzodiazepine).
See: Mazicon (Roberts Pharmaceuticals).
Romazicon, Inj. (Roberts Pharmaceuticals).

flumecinol.
Use: Hyperbilirubinemia in newborns. [Orphan Drug]
See: Zixoryn (Farmacon, Inc.).

•**flumequine.** (FLEW-meh-kwin) USAN.
Use: Anti-infective.

•**flumeridone.** (FLEW-MER-ih-dohn) USAN.
Use: Antiemetic.

•**flumethasone.** (FLEW-meth-ah-zone) USAN.
Use: Corticosteroid, topical.
See: Locorten [21-pivalate] (Novartis Pharmaceutical Corp.).

•**flumethasone pivalate.** (FLEW-meth-ah-zone PIH-vah-late) U.S.P. 23.
Use: Corticosteroid, topical.

flumethiazide.
Use: Diuretic.

•**flumetramide.** (flew-MEH-trah-mide) USAN.
Use: Muscle relaxant.

•**flumezapine.** (FLEW-MEZZ-ah-peen) USAN.
Use: Antipsychotic, neuroleptic.

•**fluminorex.** (flew-MEE-no-rex) USAN.
Use: Anorexic.

•**flumizole.** (FLEW-mih-zole) USAN.
Use: Anti-inflammatory.

•**flumoxonide.** (flew-MOX-OH-nide) USAN.
Use: Adrenocortical steroid.

flunarizine.
Use: Alternating hemiplegia. [Orphan Drug]
See: Sibelium (Janssen Pharmaceutical, Inc.).

•**flunarizine hydrochloride.** (flew-NAR-ih-zeen) USAN.
Use: Vasodilator.

•**flunidazole.** (FLEW-nih-dah-ZOLE) USAN.
Use: Antiprotozoal.

•**flunisolide.** (flew-NIH-sole-ide) U.S.P. 23.
Use: Corticosteroid, topical.
See: AeroBid, Aer. (Forest Pharmaceutical, Inc.).
AeroBid-M, Aer. (Forest Pharmaceutical, Inc.).
Nasalide, Sol. Spray (Dura Pharmaceuticals).
Nasarel, Sol. Spray (Dura Pharmaceuticals).

•**flunisolide acetate.** (flew-NIH-sole-ide) USAN.
Use: Anti-inflammatory.

•**flunitrazepam.** (flew-NYE-TRAY-zeh-pam) USAN.
Use: Hynoptic, sedative.

•**flunixin.** (flew-NIX-in) USAN.
Use: Analgesic, anti-inflammatory.

•**flunixin meglumine.** (flew-NIX-in meh-GLUE-meen) U.S.P. 23.
Use: Analgesic, anti-inflammatory.

Fluocet. (NMC Laboratories) Fluocinolone acetonide cream 0.025% or 0.01%. Tube 15 g, 60 g. *Rx.*
Use: Corticosteroid, topical.

fluocinolide. (flew-oh-SIN-oh-lide)
See: Fluocinonide.

•**fluocinolone acetonide.** (flew-oh-SIN-oh-lone ah-SEE-toe-nide) U.S.P. 23.
Use: Corticosteroid, topical.
See: Fluonid, Cream, Oint., Soln. (Allergan, Inc.).
Synalar, Cream, Oint., Soln. (Roche Laboratories).

•**fluocinonide.** (FLEW-oh-SIN-oh-nide) U.S.P. 23. *Formerly Fluocinolide.*
Use: Corticosteroid, topical.
See: Lidex, Cream, Oint., Soln. (Roche Laboratories).
Lidex-E, Cream (Roche Laboratories).

fluocinonide. (E. Fougera and Co.) 0.05%. Tube 15 g, 60 g.
Use: Corticosteroid, topical.

fluocinonide topical solution. (E. Fougera and Co.) 0.05%. Soln. Bot. 60 ml.
Use: Corticosteroid, topical.

•**fluocortin butyl.** (FLEW-oh-CORE-tin BYOO-tuhl) USAN.
Use: Anti-inflammatory.

•**fluocortolone.** (FLEW-oh-CORE-toe-lone) USAN.
Use: Corticosteroid, topical.

•**fluocortolone caproate.** (FLEW-oh-CORE-toe-lone) USAN.
Use: Corticosteroid, topical.

Fluogen. (Parke-Davis) Influenza virus vaccine, trivalent. Immunizing antigen, ether extracted. Vial 5 ml, UD syringe 0.5 ml. The 5 ml vial contains sufficient product to deliver ten 0.5 ml doses. *Rx.*
Use: Immunization.

Fluonex. (Zeneca Pharmaceuticals) Fluocinonide 0.05%. Cream. Tube. 15 g, 30 g. *Rx.*
Use: Corticosteroid, topical.

Fluonid. (Allergan, Inc.) Fluocinolone acetonide. **Soln.:** 0.01%. Bot. 20 ml, 60 ml. *Rx.*
Use: Corticosteroid, topical.

Fluoracaine. (Akorn, Inc.) Proparacaine HCl 0.5%, fluorescein sodium 0.25%. Dropper Bot. 5 ml. *Rx.*
Use: Anesthetic, local; ophthalmic.

•**fluorescein.** (FLURE-eh-seen) U.S.P. 23.
Use: Diagnostic aid (corneal trauma indicator).
See: Fluorescite (Alcon Laboratories, Inc.).

•**fluorescein sodium.** U.S.P. 23. *Formerly Fluorescein, soluble.*

Use: Diagnostic aid (corneal trauma indicator).
See: AK-Fluor, Amp., Vial (Akorn, Inc.).
Fluor-I-Strips (Wyeth-Ayerst Laboratories).
Fluorets, Strips (Akorn, Inc.).
Ful-Glo, Strips (PBH Wesley Jessen).
Funduscein, Amp. (Ciba Vision).

fluorescein sodium. (Various Mfr.) 2% Ophth. Soln. Bot. 1 ml, 2 ml, 15 ml.
Use: Diagnostic aid (corneal trauma indicator).

fluorescein sodium i.v.
See: Fluorescite, Amp. (Alcon Laboratories, Inc.).

fluorescein sodium 2%. (Ciba Vision) Sterile aqueous solution containing fluorescein sodium 2%. Dropperette 1 ml, Box 12s.
Use: Diagnostic aid, ophthalmic.

fluorescein sodium 2% solution. (Alcon Laboratories, Inc.) Drop-Tainer 15 ml, Steri-Unit 2 ml 12s.
Use: Diagnostic aid, ophthalmic.

fluorescein sodium w/combinations.
See: Flurate (Bausch & Lomb).

fluorescein sodium w/proparacaine hydrochloride. (Taylor Pharmaceuticals) Proparacaine HCl 0.5%, fluorescein sodium 0.25%. Ophthalmic soln. Bot. 5 ml. *Rx.*
Use: Anesthetic, local; diagnostic aid, ophthalmic.

fluorescein sodium/sodium hyaluronate.
See: Sodium Hyaluronate and Fluorescein Sodium Healon Yellow (Pharmacia & Upjohn).

Fluorescite. (Alcon Laboratories, Inc.) Fluorescein as sodium salt. Inj. Soln. **10%:** Amp. 5 ml with syringes. **25%:** Amp 2 ml. *Rx.*
Use: Diagnostic aid, ophthalmic.

Fluoresoft. (Various Mfr.) Fluorexon 0.35%. Soln. Pipette 0.5 ml, Box 12s. *otc.*
Use: Diagnostic aid, ophthalmic.

Fluorets. (Akorn, Inc.) Fluorescein sodium 1 mg. Strip. Box 100s. *otc.*
Use: Diagnostic aid, ophthalmic.

fluorexon.
See: Fluoresoft (Holles Laboratories, Inc.).

fluoride. (Kirkman Sales Co., Inc.) Fluoride 1 mg (sodium fluoride 2.21 mg). Tab. Bot. 1000s. *Rx.*
Use: Dental caries agent.

Fluoride Loz. (Kirkman Sales Co., Inc.) Fluoride 1 mg (sodium fluoride 2.21 mg). Loz. Bot. 1000s. *Rx.*
Use: Dental caries agent.

fluoride sodium.
See: Fluoride Loz. (Kirkman).
Fluoride, Tab. (Kirkman).
Karidium, Top. Soln., Tab. (Young Dental).
Karigel, Gel (Young Dental).
Luride, Drops, Gel (Colgate-Hoyt).
Luride Lozi-Tabs, Chew. Tab. (Colgate-Hoyt).

fluoride therapy.
See: Adeflor Preps. (Pharmacia & Upjohn).
Cari-Tab, Softab Tab. (Zeneca Pharmaceuticals).
Coral Prods. (Young Dental).
Fluorineed, Chew. Tab. (Hanlon).
Fluorinse, Liq. (Pacemaker).
Fluora, Loz. (Kirkman Sales Co., Inc.).
Luride Preps (Colgate Oral Pharmaceuticals).
Mulvidren-F, Softab Tab. (Zeneca Pharmaceuticals).
Point Two, Rinse (Colgate Oral Pharmaceuticals).
Poly-Vi-Flor, Drops, Tab. (Bristol-Myers Squibb).
Soluvite-F, Drops (Pharmics, Inc.).
Tri-Vi-Flor, Drops, Tab. (Bristol-Myers Squibb).

Fluorigard. (Colgate Oral Pharmaceuticals) Fluoride 0.02% (from sodium fluoride 0.05%), alcohol 6%, tartrazine. Bot. 180 ml, 300 ml, 480 ml. *Rx.*
Use: Dental caries agent.

Fluori-Methane Spray. (Gebauer Co.) Dichlorodifluoromethane 15%, trichloromonofluoromethane 85%. Bot. 4 oz. *Rx.*
Use: "Painful motion" syndromes.

Fluorineed. (Hanlon) Fluoride 1 mg/Chew. Tab. Bot. 100s, 1000s. *Rx.*
Use: Dental caries agent.

Fluorinse. (Oral-B Laboratories, Inc.) Fluoride 0.09% from sodium fluoride 0.2%. Bot. 480 ml. *Rx.*
Use: Dental caries agent.

Fluorinse. (Pacemaker) Fluoride mouthwash. Pack. Fluoride ion level 0.05% or 0.2%. UD Bot. 32 oz. Concentrate 1 oz, 4 oz, gal. *Rx.*
Use: Dental caries agent.

Fluor-I-Strip. (Wyeth-Ayerst Laboratories) Fluorescein sodium 9 mg/ophthalmic strip. Box. 300s. *Rx.*
Use: Diagnostic aid, ophthalmic.

Fluor-I-Strip-A.T. (Wyeth-Ayerst Laboratories) Fluorescein sodium 1 mg/ophthalmic strip. Box 300s. *Rx.*
Use: Diagnostic aid, ophthalmic.

Fluoritab. (Fluoritab Corp.) Sodium fluoride 2.2 mg equivalent to 1 mg of fluo-

rine (as fluoride ion) w/inert organic filler 75.8 mg/Tab. Bot. 100s; Liq. dropper bot. (fluorine 0.25 mg from 0.55 mg sodium fluoride/Drop) 19 ml. *Rx.*
Use: Dental caries agent.

5-fluorocytosine.
See: Ancobon, Cap. (Roberts Pharmaceuticals).

•**fluorodopa F 18 injection.** (FLEW-roe-DOE-pah) U.S.P. 23.
Use: Diagnostic aid (brain imaging), radiopharmaceutical.

fluorogestone acetate.
Use: Hormone, progestin.

fluorohydrocortisone acetate. 9-α-Fluorohydrocortisone.
See: Fludrocortisone Acetate (Various Mfr.).

•**fluorometholone.** (flure-oh-METH-oh-lone) U.S.P. 23.
Use: Corticosteroid, ophthalmic.
See: Fluor-Op, Susp. (Ciba Vision).
FML (Allergan, Inc.).

•**fluorometholone acetate.** (flure-oh-METH-oh-LONE) USAN.
Use: Corticosteroid, ophthalmic; anti-inflammatory.

fluorometholone ophthalmic suspension. (Various Mfr.) 0.1%, benzalkonium chloride 0.004%, EDTA, polysorbate 80, polyvinyl alcohol 1.4%. Ophth. Susp. Bot. 5 ml, 10 ml, 15 ml. *Rx.*
Use: Corticosteroid, ophthalmic; anti-inflammatory.

Fluor-Op. (Ciba Vision) Fluorometholone 0.1%, benzalkonium chloride 0.004%, EDTA, polysorbate 80, polyvinyl alcohol 1.4%. Susp. Bot. 3 ml, 5 ml, 10 ml, 15 ml. *Rx.*
Use: Corticosteroid, ophthalmic; anti-inflammatory.

fluorophene.
Use: Antiseptic.

Fluoroplex Topical. (Allergan, Inc.) **Soln.:** Fluorouracil 1% in a propylene glycol base. Plastic bot. w/dropper 30 ml. **Cream:** Fluorouracil 1% in emulsion base w/benzyl alcohol 0.5%, emulsifying wax, mineral oil, isopropyl myristate, sodium hydroxide, purified water. Tube 30 g. *Rx.*
Use: Topical treatment of multiple actinic (solar) keratoses.

fluoroquinolones.
Use: Anti-infective.
See: Ciloxan (Alcon Laboratories, Inc.).
Cipro (Bayer Corp. (Consumer Div.)).
Cipro I.V. (Bayer Corp. (Consumer Div.)).
Floxin (Ortho McNeil Pharmaceutical).
Maxaquin (Searle).
Noroxin (Merck & Co.).
Penetrex (Rhone-Poulenc Rorer Pharmaceuticals, Inc.).

•**fluorosalan.** (FLEW-oh-row-SAH-lan) USAN.
Use: Antiseptic, disinfectant.

fluorothyl.
See: Flurothyl.

•**fluorouracil.** (FLURE-oh-YOUR-uh-sill) U.S.P. 23.
Use: Antineoplastic. [Orphan Drug]
See: Adrucil, Inj. (Pharmacia & Upjohn).
Efudex, Soln., Cream (Roberts Pharmaceuticals).
Fluoroplex, Soln., Cream (Allergan, Inc.).

fluorouracil. (Roberts Pharmaceuticals) Amp. 10 ml, 500 mg. Box 10s.
Use: Antineoplastic. [Orphan Drug]

Fluothane. (Wyeth-Ayerst Laboratories) Halothane. Bot. 125 ml, 250 ml. *Rx.*
Use: Anesthetic, general.

•**fluotracen hydrochloride.** (FLEW-oh-TRAY-sen) USAN.
Use: Antipsychotic, antidepressant.

•**fluoxetine.** (flew-OX-eh-teen) USAN.
Use: Antidepressant.
See: Prozac, Pulv., Liq. (Eli Lilly and Co.).

•**fluoxetine hydrochloride.** (flew-OX-eh-teen) USAN.
Use: Antidepressant.
See: Prozac (Eli Lilly and Co.).

Flu-Oxinate. (Taylor Pharmaceuticals) Benoxinate HCl 0.4%, fluorescein sodium 0.25%. Ophthalmic Soln. Bot. 5 ml. *Rx.*
Use: Local anesthetic, diagnostic aid, ophthalmic.

•**fluoxymesterone.** (flew-ox-ee-MESS-teh-rone) U.S.P. 23.
Use: Androgen.
See: Android-F, Tab. (Zeneca Pharmaceuticals).
Halotestin, Tab. (Pharmacia & Upjohn).
Ora-Testryl, Tab. (Bristol-Myers Squibb).

fluoxymestrone. (Various Mfr.) 10 mg/Tab. Bot. 100s. *c-III.*
Use: Androgen.

•**fluparoxan hydrochloride.** (flew-pah-ROX-an) USAN.
Use: Antidepressant.

•**fluperamide.** (flew-purr-ah-mide) USAN.
Use: Antiperistaltic.

•**fluperolone acetate.** (FLEW-per-oh-lone) USAN.

Use: Corticosteroid, topical.

•**fluphenazine decanoate.** (flew-FEN-uh-zeen) U.S.P. 23.
Use: Antipsychotic.
See: Prolixin Decanoate Soln. (Apothecon, Inc.).

•**fluphenazine enanthate.** (flew-FEN-uh-zeen) U.S.P. 23.
Use: Antipsychotic, anxiolytic.
See: Prolixin Enanthate Prods. (Apothecon, Inc.).

•**fluphenazine hydrochloride.** (flew-FEN-uh-zeen) U.S.P. 23.
Use: Antipsychotic, anxiolytic.
See: Permitil, Preps. (Schering-Plough Corp.).
Prolixin, Preps. (Apothecon, Inc.).

fluphenazine HCl concentrate. (Copley Pharmaceutical, Inc.) Fluphenazine HCl 5 mg/ml. Conc. Bot. 120 ml. *Rx.*
Use: Antipsychotic.

fluphenazine HCl injection. (Quad Pharmaceuticals, Inc.) Fluphenazine HCl 2.5 mg/ml. Inj. Vial 10 ml. *Rx.*
Use: Antipsychotic.

fluphenazine HCl tablet. (Various Mfr.) Fluphenazine HCl 1 mg, 2.5 mg, 5 mg, 10 mg/Tab. Bot. 50s, 100s, 500s, 1000s, UD 100s. *Rx.*
Use: Antipsychotic.

•**flupirtine maleate.** (flew-PIHR-teen) USAN.
Use: Analgesic.

•**fluprednisolone.** (FLEW-pred-NIH-so-lone) USAN.
Use: Corticosteroid, topical.

•**fluprednisolone valerate.** (FLEW-pred-NIH-so-lone VAL-eh-rate) USAN.
Use: Corticosteroid, topical.

•**fluproquazone.** (FLEW-PRO-kwah-zone) USAN.
Use: Analgesic.

•**fluprostenol sodium.** (flew-PROSTE-een-ole) USAN.
Use: Prostaglandin.

•**fluquazone.** (FLEW-kwah-zone) USAN.
Use: Anti-inflammatory.

•**fluradoline hydrochloride.** (FLURE-ade-OLE-een) USAN.
Use: Analgesic.

Flura-Drops. (Kirkman Sales Co., Inc.) Fluoride. **Drops:** 0.25 mg (from 0.55 mg sodium fluoride). Bot. 30 ml. **Rinse:** 0.02% (from 0.05% sodium fluoride). Bot. 480 ml. *Rx.*
Use: Dental caries agent.

Flura-Loz. (Kirkman Sales Co., Inc.) Sodium fluoride 2.2 mg providing 1 mg fluoride/Loz. Bot. 100s, 1000s. *Rx.*
Use: Dental caries agent.

•**flurandrenolide.** (FLURE-an-DREEN-oh-lide) U.S.P. 23. *Formerly Flurandrenolone.*
Use: Corticosteroid, topical.
See: Cordran, Preps. (Eli Lilly and Co.).

flurandrenolone. (FLURE-an-DREE-nahl-ohn)
Use: Corticosteroid, topical.

Flura-Tablets. (Kirkman Sales Co., Inc.) Sodium fluoride 2.21 mg, equivalent to 1 mg fluoride ion/Tab. Bot. 100s, 1000s. *Rx.*
Use: Dental caries agent.

Flurate. (Bausch & Lomb Pharmaceuticals) Benoxinate HCl 0.4%, fluorescein sodium 0.25%, chlorobutanol 1%, povidone/Soln. Bot. 5 ml. *Rx.*
Use: Diagnostic aid, ophthalmic.

•**flurazepam hydrochloride.** (flure-AZE-uh-pam) U.S.P. 23.
Use: Anticonvulsant, hypnotic, muscle relaxant, sedative.
See: Dalmane, Cap. (Roberts Pharmaceuticals).

•**flurbiprofen.** (FLURE-bih-PRO-fen) U.S.P. 23.
Use: Analgesic, anti-inflammatory.
See: Ansaid (Pharmacia & Upjohn).

flurbiprofen. (FLURE-bih-PRO-fen) (Various Mfr.) Flurbiprofen 50 mg, 100 mg. Tab. 100s, 500s. *Rx.*
Use: Analgesic, NSAID.
See: Ansaid (Pharmacia & Upjohn).

•**flurbiprofen sodium.** (FLURE-bih-PRO-fen) U.S.P. 23.
Use: Analgesic, NSAID; prostaglandin synthesis inhibitor.
See: Ocufen, Drops (Allergan, Inc.).

flurbiprofen sodium ophthalmic. (FLURE-bih-PRO-fen) (Various Mfr.) Flurbiprofen sodium 0.03%, polyvinyl alcohol 1.4%, thimerosal 0.005%, EDTA. Soln. Bot. 2.5 ml. *Rx.*
Use: Analgesic, NSAID.

Fluress. (PBH Wesley Jessen) Fluorescein sodium 0.25%. Bot. 5 ml. *Rx.*
Use: Anesthetic, diagnostic aid.

•**fluretofen.** (flure-EH-TOE-fen) USAN.
Use: Anti-inflammatory, antithrombotic.

flurfamide. (FLURE-fah-MIDE)
Use: Enzyme inhibitor.

•**flurocitabine.** (FLEW-row-SIGH-tah-bean) USAN.
Use: Antineoplastic.

Fluro-Ethyl. (Gebauer Co.) Ethyl Cl 25%, dichlorotetrafluoroethane 75%. Spray. Can 270 g. *Rx.*
Use: Anesthetic, topical.

•**flurofamide.** (FLEW-row-fah-MIDE) USAN. *Formerly Flurfamide.*

Use: Enzyme inhibitor (urease).

•**flurogestone acetate.** (FLEW-row-JEST-ohn) USAN.
Use: Hormone, progestin.

Flurosyn. (Rugby Labs, Inc.) **Cream:** Fluocinolone acetonide 0.01%, 0.025%. Tube 15 g, 60 g, 425 g. **Oint.:** Fluocinolone acetonide 0.025% in a white petrolatum base. Tube 15 g, 60 g. *Rx.*
Use: Corticosteroid, topical.

•**flurothyl.** (FLURE-oh-thill) USAN.
Use: Stimulant (central).

•**fluroxene.** (flure-OX-een) USAN.
Use: General inhalation anesthetic.

FluShield. (Wyeth-Ayerst Laboratories) Influenza virus vaccine. Vial 5 ml. Tubex. 0.5 ml. *Rx.*
Use: Immunization.

•**fluspiperone.** (FLEW-spih-per-OHN) USAN.
Use: Antipsychotic.

•**fluspirilene.** (flew-SPIRE-ih-leen) USAN.
Use: Antipsychotic, anxiolytic.

•**flutamide.** (FLEW-tuh-mide) U.S.P. 23.
Use: Antiandrogen.
See: Eulexin, Cap. (Schering-Plough Corp.).

•**fluticasone propionate.** (flew-TICK-ah-SONE PRO-pee-oh-nate) USAN.
Use: Anti-inflammatory.
See: Cutivate (GlaxoWellcome).
Flonase, Spray (GlaxoWellcome).
Flovent, Aer. Spray (GlaxoWellcome).
Flovent Rotadisk (GlaxoWellcome).

Flutra. Trichlormethiazide.
Use: Diuretic.

•**flutroline.** (FLEW-troe-LEEN) USAN.
Use: Antipsychotic.

•**fluvastatin sodium.** (FLEW-vah-STAT-in) USAN.
Use: Antihyperlipidemic inhibitor (HMG-CoA reductase).
See: Lescol, Cap. (Novartis Pharmaceutical Corp.).

Fluvirin. (Medeva Pharmaceuticals, Inc.) Influenza virus vaccine. Vial 5 ml, 0.5 ml pre-filled syringes. *Rx.*
Use: Immunization.

•**fluvoxamine maleate.** (flew-VOX-ah-meen) USAN.
Use: Antidepressant; anti-obsessional agent.
See: Luvox, Tab. (Solvay Pharmaceuticals).

•**fluzinamide.** (flew-ZIN-ah-mide) USAN.
Use: Anticonvulsant.

Fluzone. (Pasteur Merieux Connaught) Influenza virus vaccine, thimerosal 0.01%. Vial 5 ml (whole virus). Vial 5 ml, Syr. 0.5 ml (split-virus). *Rx.*
Use: Immunization.

FML. (Allergan, Inc.) Fluorometholone 0.1%, benzalkonium chloride 0.004%, EDTA, polysorbate 80, polyvinyl alcohol. Ophth. Susp. Bot. 5 ml and 10 ml. *Rx.*
Use: Corticosteroid, ophthalmic; anti-inflammatory.

FML Forte. (Allergan, Inc.) Fluorometholone 0.25%, benzalkonium chloride 0.005%, EDTA, polysorbate 80, polyvinyl alcohol 1.4%. Ophth. Susp. Bot. 2 ml, 5 ml, 10 ml, 15 ml. *Rx.*
Use: Corticosteroid, ophthalmic; anti-inflammatory.

FML-S. (Allergan, Inc.) Fluorometholone 0.1%, sulfacetomide sodium 10%. Susp. Dropper Bot. 5 ml, 10 ml. *Rx.*
Use: Corticosteroid, ophthalmic.

FML S.O.P. (Allergan, Inc.) Fluorometholone 0.1%, phenylmercuric acetate 0.0008%, white petrolatum, mineral oil, lanolin alcohol. Oint. Tube 3.5 g. *Rx.*
Use: Corticosteroid, ophthalmic; anti-inflammatory.

Foamicon. (Invamed, Inc.) Aluminum hydroxide 80 mg, magnesium trisilicate 20 mg, alginic acid, calcium stearate, compressible sugar, sodium bicarbonate, sucrose. Chew. Tab. Bot. 100s. *otc.*
Use: Antacid.

•**focofilcon a.** (FOE-koe-FILL-kahn A) USAN.
Use: Contact lens material (hydrophilic).

Foille. (Blistex, Inc.) Benzocaine 2%, benzyl alcohol 4% in a bland vegetable oil base. Oint. Tube 30 g. *otc.*
Use: Anesthetic, local.

Foillecort. (Blistex, Inc.) Hydrocortisone acetate 0.5%. Cream. Tube 3.5 g. *otc.*
Use: Corticosteroid, topical.

Foille Medicated First Aid. (Blistex, Inc.) **Aerosol:** Benzocaine 5% with chloroxylenol 0.1% in a bland vegetable oil base with benzyl alcohol. Spray 92 g. **Oint.:** Benzocaine 5%, chloroxylenol 0.1% in a bland vegetable oil base. Tube 30 g. **Lot.:** Benzocaine 5%, chloroxylenol 0.1% in a bland vegetable oil base with benzyl alcohol 30 ml. **Oint.:** Benzocaine 5%, chloroxylenol, benzyl alcohol, EDTA, corn oil. 3.5 g, 28 g. **Spray:** Benzocaine 5%, chloroxylenol, benzyl alcohol, corn oil. 92 ml. *otc.*
Use: Anesthetic, local.

Foille Plus. (Blistex, Inc.) **Cream:** Benzocaine 5%, benzyl alcohol 4% in a non-staining washable base. Tube 3.5 g. **Soln.:** Benzocaine 5%, benzyl alcohol,

alcohol 77.8%. Aerosol spray 105 g.
Spray: Benzocaine 5%, chloroxylenol, alcohol. 105 ml. *otc.*
Use: Anesthetic, local.

Folabee. (Vortech Pharmaceuticals) Liver inj. B_{12} equivalent to 10 mcg, crystalline B_{12} 100 mcg, folic acid 0.4 mg. Inj. Vial 10 ml. *Rx.*
Use: Anemia.

folacin.
See: Folic acid.

folacine.
See: Folic acid. (Various Mfr.).

Folergot-DF. (Marnel Pharmaceuticals, Inc.) Phenobarbital 40 mg, ergotamine tartrate 0.6 mg, levorotatory alkaloids of belladonna 0.2 mg, dye-free. Tab. Bot. 100s. *Rx.*
Use: Anticholinergic, gastrointestinal.

Folex PFS Injection. (Pharmacia & Upjohn) Methotrexate sodium 25 mg/ml. Preservative free. Inj. Vial. 2 ml, 4 ml, 8 ml. *Rx.*
Use: Antineoplastic.

•**folic acid.** (FOLE-ik) U.S.P. 23.
Use: Anemia; vitamin (hematopoietic).

folic acid. (Various Mfr.) Tab. **0.4 mg:** Bot. 100s. **0.8 mg:** Bot. 100s. **1 mg:** Bot. 30s, 100s, 1000s, UD 100s. *Rx.*
Use: Vitamin supplement.

folic acid. (Fujisawa USA, Inc.) 5 mg/ml w/ benzyl alcohol 1.5%, EDTA. Inj. Vials 10 ml. *Rx.*
Use: Vitamin supplement.

folic acid antagonists.
See: Methotrexate Inj., Tab. (ESI Lederle Generics).

folinic acid. U.S.P. 23. (Various Mfr.) Leucovorin Calcium, U.S.P. 23.

Fol-Li-Bee. (Foy Laboratories) Liver inj. equivalent to cyanocobalamin 10 mcg, folic acid 1 mg, cyanocobalamin 100 mcg/ml, phenol 0.5% pH adjusted w/sodium hydroxide and/or HCl. Vial 10 ml multi-dose, Monovials. *Rx.*
Use: Anemia.

follicle-stimulating hormone, human. Menotropins, Pergonal.

follicormon.
See: Estradiol Benzoate. (Various Mfr.).

follicular hormones.
See: Estrone (Various Mfr.).

folliculin.
See: Estrone (Various Mfr.).

Follistim. (Organon, Inc.) FSH activity 75 IU (as follitropin beta), sucrose. Inj. Vial 1s, 5s with diluent. *Rx.*
Use: Ovulation inducer.

follitropin alpha.
See: Gonal-F, Inj. (Serono Laboratories, Inc.).

follitropin beta.
See: Follistim, Inj. (Organon, Inc.).

Foltrin. (Eon Labs Manufacturing, Inc.) Liver and stomach concentrate 240 mg, B_{12} 15 mcg, iron 110 mg, C 75 mg, folic acid 0.5 mg/Cap. Bot. 100s, 1000s. *Rx.*
Use: Mineral, vitamin supplement.

•**fomepizole.** (foe-MEH-pih-ZOLE) USAN.
Use: Antidote (alcohol dehydrogenase inhibitor).
See: Antizol (Orphan Medical, Inc.).

•**fomivirsen sodium.** (foe-MIH-vihr-sen) USAN.
Use: Antiviral (CMV retinitis).
See: Vitravene, Inj. (Isis).

fonatol.
See: Diethylstilbestrol (Various Mfr.).

•**fonazine mesylate.** (FAH-nazz-een) USAN.
Use: Serotonin inhibitor.

fontarsol.
See: Dichlorophenarsine Hydrochloride.

Foralicon Plus Elixir. (Forbes) Vitamins B_{12} 16.7 mcg, B_6 4 mg, iron 200 mg (equivalent to elemental iron 24 mg), niacinamide 40 mg, folic acid 0.8 mg, sorbitol soln. q.s./15 ml. Bot. 8 oz, 16 oz. *Rx.*
Use: Mineral, vitamin supplement.

Forane. (Ohmeda Pharmaceuticals) Isoflurane. Gas. Volume 100 ml. *Rx.*
Use: Anesthetic, general.

•**forasartan.** (far-ah-SAHR-tan) USAN.
Use: Antihypertensive.

Fordustin. (Sween) Cornstarch based powder with deodorizing action. Bot. 3 oz, 8 oz. *otc.*
Use: Powder, topical.

Formadon Solution. (Gordon Laboratories) Formalin solution 3.7% to 4% (10% of U.S.P. strength) in an aqueous perfumed base. Bot. 1 oz, 4 oz, 0.5 gal, gal.
Use: Bromhidrosis, hyperhidrosis agent.

•**formaldehyde solution.** (for-MAL-dehhide) U.S.P. 23.
Use: For poison ivy, fungus infections of the skin, hyperhidrosis and as an astringent, disinfectant.

formalin.
See: Formaldehyde Solution (Various Mfr.).

Formalyde-10. (Pedinol Pharmacal, Inc.) Formaldehyde 10%, FDA-40 alcohol. Spray Bot. 60 ml. *Rx.*
Use: Bromhidrosis, hyperhidrosis agent.

Forma-Ray Solution. (Gordon Laboratories) Formalin 7.4% to 8% (20% of USP

strength) in aqueous, scented, tinted solution. Bot. 1.5 oz, 4 oz. *otc.*
Use: Drying.

•**formocortal.** (FORE-moe-CORE-tal) USAN.
Use: Corticosteroid, topical.

•**formoterol fumarate.** (fore-MOE-ter-ole FEW-mah-rate) USAN.
Use: Bronchodilator.

Formula 44 Cough Control Discs. (Procter & Gamble Pharm.)
See: Vicks Formula 44 Cough Discs (Procter & Gamble Pharm.).

Formula 44 Cough Mixture. (Procter & Gamble Pharm.) Chlorpheniramine maleate 2 mg, dextromethorphan HBr 15 mg, alcohol 10%/5 ml. Liq. Bot. 120 ml, 240 ml. *otc.*
Use: Antihistamine, antitussive.

Formula 44D Decongestant Cough Mixture. (Procter & Gamble Pharm.) Pseudoephedrine HCl 20 mg, dextromethorphan HBr 10 mg, guaifenesin 67 mg, alcohol 10%/5 ml. Liq. Bot. 120 ml, 240 ml. *otc.*
Use: Antitussive, decongestant, expectorant.

Formula 44M Cough and Cold. (Procter & Gamble Pharm.) Pseudoephedrine HCl 15 mg, dextromethorphan HBr 7.5 mg, chlorpheniramine maleate 1 mg, acetaminophen 125 mg/5 ml, alcohol 20%, saccharin, sucrose. Liq. Bot. 120 ml, 240 ml. *otc.*
Use: Analgesic, antihistamine, antitussive, decongestant.

Formula No. 81. (Fellows) Liver (beef) for inj. 1 mcg, ferrous gluconate 100 mg, niacinamide 100 mg, B_2 1.5 mg, panthenol 2.5 mg, B_{12} 3 mcg, procaine HCl 25 mg/2 ml. Vial 30 ml. *otc.*
Use: Mineral, vitamin supplement.

Formula 405. (Doak Dermatologics) Sodium tallowate, sodium cocoate, Doak Additive A, PPF-20 methyl glucose ether, titanium dioxide, trochlorocarbanilide, pentasodium pentatate, EDTA. Bar 100 g. *otc.*
Use: Dermatologic, cleanser.

Formula 1207. (Thurston) Iodine, liver fraction No. 2, caseinates/Tab. Bot. 100s, 250s. *otc.*
Use: Mineral supplement.

Formula B. (Major Pharmaceuticals) Vitamins B_1 15 mg, B_2 15 mg, B_3 100 mg, B_5 18 mg, B_6 4 mg, B_{12} 5 mcg, C 500 mg, folic acid 0.5 mg/Tab. Bot 250 g. *Rx.*
Use: Vitamin supplement.

Formula B Plus. (Major Pharmaceuticals) Iron 27 mg, A 5000 IU, E 30 IU, B_1 20 mg, B_2 20 mg, B_3 100 mg, B_5 25 mg, B_6 25 mg, B_{12} 50 mcg, C 500 mg, folic acid 0.8 mg, biotin 0.15 mg, Cr, Cu, Mg, Mn, Zn/Tab. Bot 100s, 500s. *Rx.*
Use: Mineral, vitamin supplement.

Formula VM-2000 Tablets. (Solgar Co., Inc.) Iron 5 mg, A 12,500 IU, D 200 IU, E 100 IU, B_1 50 mg, B_2 50 mg, B_3 50 mg, B_5 50 mg, B_6 50 mg, B_{12} 50 mcg, C 150 mg, folic acid 0.2 mg, B, Ca, Cr, Cu, I, K, Mg, Mn, Mo, Se, Zn 7.5 mg, betaine, biotin 50 mcg, choline, bioflavonoids, amino acids, hesperidin, inositol, l-glutethione, PABA, rutin/Tab. Bot. 30s, 60s, 90s, 180s. *otc.*
Use: Mineral, vitamin supplement.

formyl tetrahydropteroylglutamic acid. U.S.P. 23. Leucovorin Calcium.

Forta Drink Powder. (Ross Laboratories) Whey protein concentrate, sucrose, vitamins A, B_1, B_2, B_3, B_5, B_6, B_{12}, C, D, E, folic acid, biotin, Ca, Cu, Fe, I, Mg, Mn, P, Zn. Can. 482 g. *otc.*
Use: Nutritional supplement.

Forta-Flora. (Barth's) Whey-lactose 90%, pectin. **Pow.:** Jar lb. **Wafer:** Bot. 100s.

Forta Instant Cereal. (Ross Laboratories) Lactose-free oat or bran cereal provides 6.25 g dietary fiber/serving. Can 1 lb 1 oz. *otc.*
Use: Nutritional supplement.

Forta Instant Pudding. (Ross Laboratories) Lactose-free in pudding base. Can 1 lb 12 oz. Vanilla, chocolate, butterscotch flavors. *otc.*
Use: Nutritional supplement.

Forta Pudding Mix. (Ross Laboratories) Milk protein isolate, sucrose, hydrolyzed cornstarch, modified tapioca starch, partially hydrogenated soybean oil, vitamins A, B_1, B_2, B_3, B_5, B_6, B_{12}, C, D, E, folic acid, biotin, Ca, Fe, P, I, Mg, Zn, Cu, Mn, tartrazine. Can 794 g. *otc.*
Use: Nutritional supplement.

Forta Shake Powder. (Ross Laboratories) Nonfat dry milk, sucrose, vitamins A, B_1, B_2, B_3, B_5, B_6, B_{12}, C, D, E, folic acid, biotin, Ca, Cu, Fe, I, Mg, Mn, P, Zn, tartrazine. Can lb, pkt. 1.4 oz. Can 1 lb 2.7 oz, pkt. 1.6 oz. *otc.*
Use: Nutritional supplement.

Forta Soup Mix. (Ross Laboratories) Milk protein isolate, sodium and calcium caseinate, hydrolyzed cornstarch, modified tapioca starch, powdered shortening (partially hydrogenated coconut oil), vitamins A, B_1, B_2, B_3, B_5, B_6, B_{12}, C, D, E, folic acid, biotin, Ca, Cu, Fe, I, Mg, Mn, P, Zn. Chicken flavor. Can. 454 g. *otc.*

Use: Nutritional supplement.

Fortaz. (GlaxoWellcome) Ceftazidime Pow. for Inj. **500 mg:** Vial. **1 g:** Vial, *ADD-Vantage* vial, Infusion Pack. **2 g:** Vial, *ADD-Vantage* vial, Infusion Pack. **6 g:** Bulk Pkg. **Inj.:** 1 g. Vial 50 ml, premixed, frozen. *Rx.*
Use: Anti-infective, cephalosporin.

Forte L.I.V. (Foy Laboratories) Cyanocobalamin 15 mcg liver injection equivalent to vitamin B_{12} activity 1 mcg, ferrous gluconate 50 mg, B_2 0.75 mg, panthenol 1.25 mg, niacinamide 50 mg, citric acid 8.2 mg, sodium citrate 118 mg/ml, procaine HCl 2%. Bot. 30 ml. *otc.*
Use: Mineral, vitamin supplement.

Fortel Midstream. (Biomerica, Inc.) Reagent in-home urine test for pregnancy. 1 test stick per kit.
Use: Diagnostic aid, pregnancy.

Fortel Ovulation. (Biomerica, Inc.) Monoclonal antibody-based home test to predict ovulation. Kit 1s.
Use: Diagnostic aid.

Fortel Plus. (Biomerica, Inc.) Reagent in-home urine pregnancy test. Kit contains urine collection cup, dropper, test device.
Use: Diagnostic aid, pregnancy.

Fortovase. (Roche Laboratories) Saquinavir 200 mg/Cap. Bot. 180s. *Rx.*
Use: Antiviral.

Fortral. (Sanofi Winthrop Pharmaceuticals) Pentazocine as solution and tablets. *c-IV.*
Use: Analgesic, narcotic.

Fortramin. (Thurston) Vitamins E 200 IU, A 6000 IU, D 600 IU, B_1 4.5 mg, B_2 4.5 mg, B_6 4.5 mg, B_{12} 5 mcg, C 2.75 mg, rutin 8 mg, hesperidin complex 10 mg, lemon bioflavonoids 15 mg, d-calcium pantothenate 50 mg, para-aminobenzoic acid 7.5 mg, biotin 10 mg, folic acid 24 mcg, niacinamide 20 mg, desiccated liver 25 mg, iron 3 mg, calcium 75 mg, phosphorus 34 mg, manganese 10 mg, copper 0.5 mg, zinc 0.5 mg, iodine 0.375 mg, potassium 500 mg, magnesium 5 mg/Tab. Bot. 100s, 250s. *otc.*
Use: Mineral, vitamin supplement.

40 Winks. (Roberts Pharmaceuticals) Diphenhydramine HCl 50 mg/Cap. Bot. 30s. *otc.*
Use: Sleep aid.

Fosamax. (Merck & Co.) Alendronate sodium 5 mg, 10 mg or 40 mg, lactose/Tab. Bot. 100s, UD 30s, UD 100s. *Rx.*
Use: Bone resorption inhibitor.

•**fosarilate.** (FOSS-ah-RILL-ate) USAN.
Use: Antiviral.

•**fosazepam.** (foss-AZZ-eh-pam) USAN.
Use: Hypnotic, sedative.

•**foscarnet sodium.** (foss-CAR-net) USAN.
Use: Antiviral.
See: Foscavir, Inj. (Astra Pharmaceuticals, L.P.).

Foscavir. (Astra Pharmaceuticals, L.P.) Foscarnet sodium 24 mg/ml. Inj. Bot. 250 ml, 500 ml. *Rx.*
Use: Anti-infective, antiviral.

•**fosfomycin.** (foss-foe-MY-sin) USAN.
Use: Anti-infective.
See: Monurol (Zambon Corp.).

•**fosfomycin tromethamine.** (foss-foe-MY-sin troe-METH-ah-meen) USAN.
Use: Anti-infective.
See: Monurol, Granules (Forest Pharmaceutical, Inc.).

•**fosfonet sodium.** (FOSS-foe-net) USAN.
Use: Antiviral.

Fosfree. (Mission Pharmacal Co.) Iron 14.5 mg, A 1500 IU, D_3 150 IU, B_1 4.5 mg, B_2 2 mg, B_3 10.5 mg, B_5 1 mg, B_6 2.5 mg, B_{12} 2 mcg, C 50 mg, Ca 175.5 mg, sugar/Tab. Bot. 120s. *otc.*
Use: Mineral, vitamin supplement.

fosinopril. (FAH-sen-oh-PRIL)
Use: Angiotensin-converting enzyme inhibitor, antihypertensive.
See: Monopril (Bristol-Myers Squibb).

•**fosinopril sodium.** (FAH-sen-oh-PRIL) USAN.
Use: Antihypertensive, enzyme inhibitor (angiotensin-converting).
See: Monopril, Tab. (Bristol-Myers Squibb).

•**fosinoprilat.** (fah-SIN-oh-prill-at) USAN.
Use: Antihypertensive.

•**fosphenytoin sodium.** (FOSS-FEN-ih-toe-in) USAN.
Use: Anticonvulsant.
See: Cerebyx, Inj. (Parke-Davis).

•**fosquidone.** (FOSS-kwih-dohn) USAN.
Use: Antineoplastic.

•**fostedil.** (FOSS-teh-dill) USAN.
Use: Vasodilator (calcium channel blocker).

Fostex. (Bristol-Myers Squibb) Benzoyl peroxide 10%, EDTA, urea. Bar. 106 g. *otc.*
Use: Dermatologic, acne.

Fostex Acne Cleansing Cream. (Westwood Squibb Pharmaceuticals) Salicylic acid 2%, EDTA, stearyl alcohol. Cream. 118 g. *otc.*
Use: Dermatologic, acne.

Fostex Acne Medication Cleansing

Bar. (Westwood Squibb Pharmaceuticals) Salicylic acid 2%, EDTA. Bar. 106 g. *otc.*
Use: Dermatologic, acne.

Fostex 10%BPO. (Westwood Squibb Pharmaceuticals) Benzoyl peroxide 10%, EDTA. Gel 42.5 g. *otc.*
Use: Dermatologic, acne.

Fostex 10% Wash. (Bristol-Myers Squibb) Benzoyl peroxide 10% with water base. Liq. Bot. 150 ml. *otc.*
Use: Dermatologic, acne.

•**fostriecin sodium.** (FOSS-try-eh-SIN) USAN.
Use: Antineoplastic.

Fostril. (Westwood Squibb Pharmaceuticals) Sulfur, zinc oxide, parabens, EDTA. Lot. Tube 28 ml. *otc.*
Use: Dermatologic, acne.

Fototar Cream. (Zeneca Pharmaceuticals) Coal tar 1.6% (from 2% coal tar extract) in emollient moisturizing cream base. Tube 90 g, 480 g. *otc.*
Use: Dermatologic.

4-Way Cold Tablets. (Bristol-Myers Squibb) Aspirin 324 mg, phenylpropanolamine HCl 12.5 mg, chlorpheniramine maleate 2 mg/Tab. Bot. 36s, 60s, Card 15s. *otc.*
Use: Analgesic, antihistamine, decongestant.

4 Hair Softgel. (Marlyn Nutraceuticals, Inc.) Iron 2.5 mg, A 1250 IU, E 10 IU, B_3 5 mg, B_5 2.5 mg, B_6 1.5 mg, B_{12} 44 mcg, C 25 mg, folic acid 33.3 mg, biotin 250 mcg, I, Mg, Cu, Zn 7.5 mg, choline bitartrate, inositol, Mn, methionine, PABA, B_1, L-cysteine, tyrosine, Si/Cap. Bot 60s. *otc.*
Use: Mineral, vitamin supplement.

4 Nails Softgel. (Marlyn Nutraceuticals, Inc.) Ca 167 mg, iron 3 mg, A 833 IU, D 67, E 10 mg, B_1 3.3 mg, B_2 1.7 mg, B_3 8.3 mg, B_5 8.3 mg, B_6 8.3 mg, B_{12} 8.3 mcg, C 10 mg, folic acid 33.3 mg, biotin 8.3 mcg, P, I, Mg, Cu, Zn 3.3 mg, Cr, Mn, methionine, inositol, choline bitartrate, Se, PABA, protein isolate, gelatin, lecithin, unsaturated fatty acid, predigested protein L-cysteine, B mucopolysaccharides, silicon amino acid chelate, Si/Cap. Bot. 60s. *otc.*
Use: Mineral, vitamin supplement.

4-Way Fast Acting Nasal Spray. (Bristol-Myers Squibb) Phenylephrine HCl 0.5%, naphazoline HCl 0.05%, pyrilamine maleate 0.2%, buffered isotonic aqueous soln., thimerosal. Atomizer 15 ml, 30 ml. *otc.*
Use: Antihistamine, decongestant.

4-Way Long Acting Nasal Spray. (Bristol-Myers Squibb) Oxymetazoline HCl 0.05% in isotonic buffered soln. Spray Bot. 15 ml. *otc.*
Use: Decongestant.

40 Winks. (Roberts Med) Diphenhydramine HCl 50 mg. Cap. Bot. 30s. *otc.*
Use: Nonprescription sleep aid.

Fowler's Solution. Potassium Arsenite Solution (Various Mfr.).

Foxalin. (Standex) Digitoxin 0.1 mg, sodium carboxymethylcellulose/Cap. Bot. 100s. *Rx.*
Use: Cardiovascular agent.

foxglove.
See: Digitalis (Various Mfr.).

Foygen Aqueous. (Foy Laboratories) Estrogenic substance or estrogens 2 mg/ml with sodium carboxymethylcellulose, povidone, benzyl alcohol, methyl and propyl parabens. Inj. Vial 10 ml. *Rx.*
Use: Estrogen.

Foyplex Injection. (Foy Laboratories) Sterile injectable soln. of nine water-soluble vitamins. Packaged as 2 separate solutions for extemporaneous combination. *Rx.*
Use: Nutritional supplement, parenteral.

Fragmin. (Pharmacia & Upjohn) Dalteparin sodium 2500 IU (16 mg/0.2 ml), 5000 IU (32 mg/0.2 ml), 10,000 IU (64 mg/ml). Inj. Single-dose prefilled Syr. (2500 IU and 5000 IU). Multi-dose vial 9.5 ml (10,000 IU). *Rx.*
Use: Anticoagulant.

FreAmine III. (McGaw, Inc.) Amino acid 8.5% or 10%. Bot. 500 ml, 1000 ml. *Rx.*
Use: Nutritional supplement, parenteral.

FreAmine III 3% w/Electrolytes. (McGaw, Inc.) Amino acid 3% with electrolytes. Bot. 1000 ml. *Rx.*
Use: Nutritional supplement, parenteral.

FreAmine III 8.5% w/Electrolytes. (McGaw, Inc.) Sodium 60 mEq/L, potassium 60 mEq/L, magnesium 10 mEq/L, Cl 60 mEq/L, phosphate 40 mEq/L, acetate 125 mEq/L. Soln. Bot. 500 ml, 1000 ml. *Rx.*
Use: Nutritional supplement, parenteral.

FreAmine HBC 6.9%. (American McGaw) High branched 6.9% amino acid formulation for hypercatabolic patients. Bot. 1000 ml. *Rx.*
Use: Nutritional supplement, parenteral.

Free & Clear. (Pharmaceutical Specialties, Inc.) Ammonium laureth sulfate, disodium cocamide MEA sulfosuccinate, cocamidopropyl hydroxysultaine, cocamide DEA, PEG-120 methyl glucose dioleate, EDTA, potassium sor-

bate, citric acid. Shampoo. Bot. 240 ml. *otc.*
Use: Dermatologic, cleanser.

Freedavite. (Freeda Vitamins, Inc.) Iron 10 mg (from ferrous fumarate), vitamins A 5000 IU, D 400 IU, E 3 IU, $B_1$5 mg, B_2 3 mg, B_3 25 mg, B_5 5 mg, B_6 2 mg, B_{12} 2 mcg, C 60 mg, choline, inositol, potassium iodide, Ca, Cu, K, Mg, Mn, Se, Zn 0.2 mg. Bot. 100s, 250s. *otc.*
Use: Mineral, vitamin supplement.

Freedox. (Pharmacia & Upjohn) Tirilazad.
Use: A 21 aminosteroid antioxidant.

•**frentizole.** (FREN-tih-zole) USAN.
Use: Immunoregulator.

FreshBurst Listerine. (Warner Lambert) Thymol 0.064%, eucalyptol 0.092%, methyl salicylate 0.06%, menthol 0.042%, alcohol 21.6%. Rinse. Bot. 250 ml. *otc.*
Use: Mouthwash.

Fresh n' Feminine. (Walgreen Co.) Benzethonium Cl 0.2% Bot. 8 oz. *otc.*
Use: Vaginal agent.

fructose. (Various Mfr.) Soln. 10%. Bot. 1000 ml.
Use: Nutritional supplement.
See: Frutabs, Tab. (Pfanstiehl).

•**fructose.** U.S.P. 23.
Use: Nutritional supplement.

fructose and sodium chloride injection.
Use: Electrolyte, fluid, nutrient replacement.

Fruity Chews. (Zenith Goldline Pharmaceuticals) Vitamins A 2500 IU, D 400 IU, E 15 mg, B_1 1.05 mg, B_2 1.2 mg, B_3 13.5 mg, B_6 1.05 mg, B_{12} 4.5 mcg, C (as sodium ascorbate and ascorbic acid) 60 mg, folic acid 0.3 mg/Chew. Tab. Bot. 100s. *otc.*
Use: Mineral, vitamin supplement.

Fruity Chews w/Iron. (Zenith Goldline Pharmaceuticals) Elemental iron 12 mg, vitamins A 2500 IU, D 400 IU, E 15 mg, B_1 1.05 mg, B_2 1.2 mg, B_3 13.5 mg, B_6 1.05 mg, B_{12} 4.5 mcg, C (as sodium ascorbate and ascorbic acid) 60 mg, folic acid 0.3 mg, zinc 8 mg/Chew. Tab. Bot. 100s. *otc.*
Use: Mineral, vitamin supplement.

frusemide.
See: Lasix.

Frutabs. (Pfanstiehl) Fructose 2 g. Tab. Bot. 100s.
Use: Carbohydrate supplement.

FTA-ABS. (Wampole Laboratories) Fluorescent treponemal antibody-absorbed test in vitro for confirming a positive reagent test for syphillis. Test 100s.
Use: Diagnostic aid.

AFT-ABS/DS. (Wampole Laboratories) Fluorescent treponemal antibody-absorbed test in vitro for confirming a positive reagent test for syphilis. Test 100s.
Use: Diagnostic aid.

•**fuchsin, basic.** (FYOO-sin) U.S.P. 23.
Use: Anti-infective, topical.

FUDR. (Roberts Pharmaceuticals) Floxuridine 500 mg sterile pow. for inj. Vial 5 ml. *Rx.*
Use: Antineoplastic.

Ful-Glo. (PBH Wesley Jessen) Fluorescein sodium 0.6 mg/Strip. Box 300s. *otc.*
Use: Diagnostic aid, ophthalmic.

Fuller. (Birchwood Laboratories, Inc.) Pkg. 1 shield.
Use: Anorectal preparation.

Fulvicin P/G. (Schering-Plough Corp.) Griseofulvin ultramicrosize 125 mg, 165 mg, 250 mg, or 330 mg/Tab. Bot. 100s. *Rx.*
Use: Antifungal.

Fulvicin U/F. (Schering-Plough Corp.) Griseofulvin microsize 250 mg or 500 mg/Tab. Bot. 60s, 250s. *Rx.*
Use: Antifungal.

•**fumaric acid.** (fyoo-MAR-ik) N.F. 18.
Use: Acidifier.

Fumatinic. (Laser, Inc.) Iron 90 mg (from ferrous fumarate), vitamins C 100 mg, B_{12} 15 mcg, folic acid 1 mg/SR Cap. Bot. 100s. *Rx.*
Use: Mineral, vitamin supplement.

Fumeron. (Eon Labs Manufacturing, Inc.) Ferrous fumarate 330 mg, vitamin B_1 5 mg/TR Cap. *otc.*
Use: Mineral, vitamin supplement.

•**fumoxicillin.** (fyoo-MOX-ih-SILL-in) USAN.
Use: Antibacterial.

Funduscein. (Ciba Vision) Fluorescein sodium. Inj. **10%:** Amp. 5 ml. **25%:** Amp. 3 ml. *Rx.*
Use: Diagnostic aid, ophthalmic.

Fungacetin Ointment. (Blair Laboratories) Triacetin (glyceryl triacetate) 25% in a water-miscible ointment base. Tube 30 g. *Rx.*
Use: Antifungal, topical.

Fungatin. (Major Pharmaceuticals) Tolnaftate 1%. Cream Tube 15 g. *otc.*
Use: Antifungal, topical.

fungicides.
See: Amphotericin B (Fujisawa USA, Inc.).
Ancobon (Roberts Pharmaceuticals).
Arcum, Preps. (Arcum).

Asterol.
Basic Fuchsin (Various Mfr.).
Desenex, Prods. (Novartis Pharmaceutical Corp.).
Dichlorophene.
Diflucan (Roerig).
Fungizone Intravenous (Bristol-Myers Squibb).
Fulvicin P/G (Schering-Plough Corp.).
Fulvicin U/F (Schering-Plough Corp.).
Grifulvin V (Advanced Care Products).
Grisactin, Prods. (Wyeth-Ayerst Laboratories).
Griseofulvin Ultramicrosize (Various Mfr.).
Gris-PEG (Allergan, Inc.).
Miconazole Nitrate (Various Mfr.).
Monistat IV (Janssen Pharmaceutical, Inc.).
Mycostatin (Apothecon, Inc.).
Nifuroxime (Various Mfr.).
Nilstat (ESI Lederle Generics).
Nizoral (Janssen Pharmaceutical, Inc.).
Nystatin (Various Mfr.).
Phenylmercuric Preps. (Various Mfr.).
Sporanox, Cap. (Janssen Pharmaceutical, Inc.).
Undecylenic Acid (Various Mfr.).

•**fungimycin.** (FUN-jih-MY-sin) USAN.
Use: Antifungal.

Fungi-Nail. (Kramer Laboratories, Inc.) Resorcinol 1%, salicylic acid 2%, parachlorometaxylenol 2%, benzocaine 0.5%, acetic acid 2.5%, propylene glycol, hydroxypropyl methylcellulose, alcohol 0.5%. Bot. 30 ml. *otc.*
Use: Antifungal, topical.

Fungizone. (Bristol-Myers Squibb) Amphotericin B 3%, thimerosal, titanium dioxide. **Lot.:** Plastic bot. 30 ml. **Cream, Oint.:** Tube 20 g. **Oral Susp.:** Amphotericin B 100 mg/ml, alcohol < 0.55%, parabens, sodium metabisulfite/ Bot. 24 ml w/dropper. *Rx.*
Use: Antifungal, topical.

Fungizone Intravenous. (Bristol-Myers Squibb) Amphotericin B 50 mg, as desoxycholate. Pow for Inj. Vial. *Rx.*
Use: Antifungal.

Fungizone for Laboratory Use in Tissue Culture. (Bristol-Myers Squibb) Amphotericin B 50 mg, sodium desoxycholate 41 mg/Vial 20 ml.
Use: Diagnostic aid.

Fungoid AF. (Pedinol Pharmacal, Inc.) Undecylenic acid 25%/Soln. Bot. 30 ml. *otc.*
Use: Antifungal, topical.

Fungoid Creme. (Pedinol Pharmacal, Inc.) Clotrimazole 1%, benzyl alcohol. Tube 45 g. *Rx.*
Use: Antifungal,topical.

Fungoid-HC Creme. (Pedinol Pharmacal, Inc.) Miconazole nitrate 2%, hydrocortisone 1%. In 56.7 g, 1 g dual packets. *Rx.*
Use: Antifungal, topical.

Fungoid Solution. (Pedinol Pharmacal, Inc.) Clotrimazole 10 mg in polyethylene glycol 400. Top. Soln. Bot. 30 ml. *Rx.*
Use: Anti-infective, topical.

Fungoid Tincture. (Pedinol Pharmacal, Inc.) Miconazole nitrate 2%, alcohol. Soln. Bot. with brush applicator 7.39 ml, 29.57 ml. *otc.*
Use: Antifungal, topical.

Furacin Soluble Dressing. (Roberts Pharmaceuticals) Nitrofurazone 0.2%, polyethylene glycol base. Oint. (soluble) Jar 454 g, Tube 28 g, 56 g. *Rx.*
Use: Burn therapy.

Furacin Topical Cream. (Roberts Pharmaceuticals) Nitrofurazone 0.2% in a water-miscible base, cetyl alcohol, mineral oil, parabens. Tube 28 g. *Rx.*
Use: Burn therapy.

Furacin Topical Solution. (Roberts Pharmaceuticals) Nitrofurazone 0.2%. Bot. 480 ml. *Rx.*
Use: Burn therapy.

Furadantin Oral Suspension. (Dura Pharmaceuticals) Nitrofurantoin 5 mg/ ml. Bot. 60 ml, 470 ml. *Rx.*
Use: Anti-infective, urinary.

furalazine hydrochloride.
Use: Antimicrobial compound.

Furanite Tabs. (Major Pharmaceuticals) Nitrofurantoin 50 mg or 100 mg/Tab. Bot. 100s. *Rx.*
Use: Anti-infective, urinary.

•**furaprofen.** (FYOOR-ah-PRO-fen) USAN. *Formerly Enprofen.*
Use: Anti-inflammatory.

•**furazolidone.** (fyoor-ah-ZOE-lih-dohn) U.S.P. 23.
Use: Anti-infective, topical; antiprotozoal (Trichomonas, topical).
See: Furoxone Tab., Susp. (Procter & Gamble Pharm.).

•**furazolium chloride.** (FYOOR-ah-zoe-lee-uhm) USAN.
Use: Anti-infective.

•**furazolium tartrate.** (FYOOR-ah-ZOE-lee-uhm) USAN.
Use: Anti-infective.

furazosin hydrochloride. (FYOOR-ah-zoe-sin) Under study.
Use: Antihypertensive.

•**furegrelate sodium.** (fyoor-eh-GRELL-ate) USAN.
Use: Inhibitor (thromboxane synthetase).

furethidine.

•**furobufen.** (FER-oh-BYOO-fen) USAN.
Use: Anti-inflammatory.

•**furodazole.** (fyoor-OH-dah-zole) USAN.
Use: Anthelmintic.

Furonatal FA. (Lexis Laboratories) Vitamins A 8000 IU, D 400 IU, E 30 IU, C 60 mg, folic acid 1 mg, B_1 2 mg, B_2 2.8 mg, B_6 2.5 mg, B_{12} 8 mcg, niacinamide 20 mg, iron 65 mg, calcium 125 mg/Tab. Bot. 100s, 1000s. *Rx.*
Use: Mineral, vitamin supplement.

•**furosemide.** (fyu-ROH-se-mide) U.S.P. 23.
Use: Diuretic.
See: Lasix, Tab., Inj., Soln. (Hoechst Marion Roussel).

furosemide. (Roxane Laboratories, Inc.) Furosemide. **10 mg/ml:** Soln. Dropper bot. 60 ml. **40 mg/5 ml:** Soln. Bot. 5 ml, 10 ml, 500 ml. *Rx.*
Use: Diuretic.

furosemide. (Various Mfr.) **Tab.: 20 mg or 80 mg:** Bot. 100s, 500s, 1000s, UD 100s. **40 mg:** Bot. 60s, 100s, 500s, 1000s, UD 100s. **Oral Soln.:** 10 mg/ml Bot. 60 ml, 120 ml. **Inj.:** 10 mg/ml Vial 10 ml; single-dose vial 2 ml, 10 ml; partial fill single-dose vial 4 ml. *Rx.*
Use: Diuretic.

Furoxone. (Procter & Gamble Pharm.) Furazolidone. **Tab.:** 100 mg. Bot. 20s, 100s. **Liq.:** 50 mg/15 ml. Bot. 60 ml, 473 ml. *Rx.*
Use: Anti-infective.

•**fursalan.** (FYOOR-sal-an) USAN. Under study.
Use: Disinfectant.

•**fusidate sodium.** (FEW-sih-DATE) USAN.
Use: Anti-infective.

•**fusidic acid.** (few-SIH-dik) USAN.
Use: Anti-infective.

G

G-4.
See: Dichlorophene.

G-11. (Givaudan) Hexachlorophene Pow. for mfg.
See: Hexachlorophene, U.S.P. 23.

•**gabapentin.** (GAB-uh-PEN-tin) USAN.
Use: Anticonvulsant; amyotrophic lateral sclerosis agent. [Orphan Drug]
See: Neurontin, Cap. (Warner Lambert).

gabbromicina. Aminosidine.
Use: Anti-infective. [Orphan Drug]

Gabitril. (Abbott Laboratories) Tiagabine HCl 4 mg, 12 mg, 16 mg, 20 mg lactose/Tab. Bot. 100s, 500s, Abbo-Pac 100s. *Rx.*
Use: Partial seizure treatment.

Gacid Tab. (Arcum) Magnesium trisilicate 500 mg, aluminum hydroxide 250 mg/Tab. Bot. 100s, 1000s. *otc.*
Use: Antacid.

•**gadobenate dimeglumine.** (gad-oh-BEN-ate die-meh-GLUE-meen) USAN.
Use: Diagnostic aid (paramagnetic), brain tumors, spine disorders.

•**gadodiamide.** (GAD-oh-DIE-ah-mide) USAN.
Use: Diagnostic aid (paramagnetic); brain and spine disorders.
See: Omniscan, Inj. (Nycomed).

gadodiamide/caldiamide.
Use: Radiopaque agent.
See: Omniscan Inj. (Sanofi Winthrop Pharmaceuticals).

•**gadopentetate dimeglumine injection.** (GAD-oh-PEN-teh-tate die-meh-GLUE-meen) U.S.P. 23.
Use: Radiopaque agent; diagnostic aid.
See: Magnevist (Berlex Laboratories, Inc.).

•**gadoteridol.** (GAD-oh-TER-ih-dahl) USAN.
Use: Diagnostic aid, paramagnetic.
See: ProHance, Inj. (Bracco Diagnostics).

•**gadoversetamide.** (gad-oh-ver-SET-ah-mide) USAN.
Use: Diagnostic aid (paramagnetic; brain and spine disorders).

•**gadoxanum.** (gad-oh-ZAN-uhm) USAN.
Use: Diagnostic aid.

•**gadozelite.** (gad-oh-ZEH-lite) USAN.
Use: Diagnostic aid.

Galardin. (Glycomed, Inc.) Matrix metalloproteinase inhibitor.
Use: Corneal ulcers. [Orphan Drug]

•**galdansetron hydrochloride.** (gahl-DAN-seh-trahn) USAN.
Use: Antiemetic.

•**gallamine triethiodide.** (GAL-ah-meen try-eth-EYE-oh-dide) U.S.P. 23.
Use: Neuromuscular blocker.

•**gallium citrate Ga 67 injection.** (GAL-ee-uhm SIH-trate) U.S.P. 23.
Use: Diagnostic aid (radiopaque medium); radiopharmaceutical.

•**gallium nitrate.** (GAL-ee-uhm NYE-trate) USAN.
Use: Calcium regulator; antihypercalcemic. [Orphan Drug]
See: Ganite, Inj. (Fujisawa USA, Inc.).

gallochrome.
See: Merbromin (Various Mfr.).

gallotannic acid.
See: Tannic Acid, Preps. (Various Mfr.).

gallstone solubilizing agents.
See: Actigall, Cap. (Novartis Pharmaceutical Corp.).
Chenix, Tab. (Solvay Pharmaceuticals).
Moctanin (Ethitek Pharmaceuticals).

Galzin. (Lemmon Co.) Zinc acetate.
Use: Wilson's disease. [Orphan Drug]

Gamazole Tabs. (Major Pharmaceuticals) Sulfamethoxazole 500 mg/Tab. Bot. 100s, 500s, 1000s. *Rx.*
Use: Anti-infective, sulfonamide.

•**gamfexine.** (gam-FEX-ine) USAN.
Use: Antidepressant.

Gamimune N 5%. (Bayer Corp. (Consumer Div.)) Immune globulin IV (human) 5%. Inj. in maltose 10% 500 mg, 2.5 g, 5 g, 10 g. *Rx.*
Use: Immunization.

Gamimune N 10%. (Bayer Corp. (Consumer Div.)) Immune globulin IV (human) 10%. Inj. 5 g, 10 g, 20 g. Vial 50 ml, 100 ml, 200 ml. *Rx.*
Use: Immunization.

Gammagard S/D. (Baxter Pharmaceutical Products, Inc.) Immune globulin IV (human) 2.5 g, 5 g or 10 g/Bot. Freeze-dried, solvent/detergent treated w/ sterile water for injection. 500 mg. *Rx.*
Use: Immunization.

gamma benzene hexachloride.
See: lindane.

gamma globulin.
See: Immune Globulin Intramuscular.
Immune Globulin Intravenous.

gamma-hydroxybutyrate. (Biocraft Laboratories, Inc., Orphan Medical, Inc.)
Use: Narcolepsy. [Orphan Drug]

gamma interferon. 1-b.
See: Actimmune (Genentech, Inc.).

gammalinolenic acid.

Use: Juvenile rheumatoid arthritis. [Orphan Drug]

Gammar-P I.V. (Centeon) Immune globulin (human). Sucrose 5%, albumin 3% (1 g or 5 g). In 1 g single-dose vial with 20 ml sterile water for inj.; 2.5 g single-dose vial with 50 ml sterile water for inj.; 5 g single-dose vial with 100 ml sterile water for inj.; 5 g pharmacy bulk pack, 10 g. *Rx.*
Use: Immunization.

Gamulin Rh. (Centeon) Rho (D) Immune globulin (Human). Vial, syringe 1 dose. *Rx.*
Use: Immunization, Rh.

ganaxolone. (Cocensys, Inc.)
Use: Infantile spasms. [Orphan Drug]

•**ganciclovir.** (gan-SIGH-kloe-VIHR) USAN.
Use: Antiviral.
See: Cytovene, Cap., Pow for Inj. (Roche Laboratories).

ganciclovir intravitreal free implant.
Use: Cytomegalovirus retinitis. [Orphan Drug]
See: Vitrasert, Implant (Chiron Vision).

•**ganciclovir sodium.** (gah-SIGH-kloe-VIHR) USAN.
Use: Antiviral.
See: Cytovene (Roche Laboratories).

Ganeake. (Geneva Pharmaceuticals) Conjugated Estrogens, 0.625 mg, 1.25 mg, or 2.5 mg/Tab. Bot. 100s, 1000s. *Rx.*
Use: Estrogen.

ganglionic blocking agents.
See: Dibenzyline HCl, Cap. (SmithKline Beecham Pharmaceuticals).
Hexamethonium Cl and Bromide (Various Mfr.).
Hydergine, Amp., Tab. (Novartis Pharmaceutical Corp.).
Priscoline HCl, Tab., Vial (Novartis Pharmaceutical Corp.).
Regitine, Amp, Tab. (Novartis Pharmaceutical Corp.).

gangliosides as sodium salts.
Use: Retinitis pigmentosa.

•**ganirelix acetate.** (gah-nih-RELL-ix ASS-eh-tate) USAN.
Use: Gonad-stimulating principle.

Ganite. (Fujisawa USA, Inc.) Gallium nitrate. 25 mg/ml. Vial. 20 ml. *Rx.*
Use: Antihypercalcemic.

Gantanol. (Roche Laboratories) Sulfamethoxazole. **Tab.:** 500mg/Tab. Bot. 100s, Tel-E-Dose 100s. *Rx.*
Use: Anti-infective, sulfonamide.

Gantanol DS. (Roche Laboratories) Sulfamethoxazole 1 g/Tab. Bot. 100s. *Rx.*
Use: Anti-infective, sulfonamide.

Garamycin. (Schering-Plough Corp.) **Cream:** Gentamicin sulfate 1.7 mg (equivalent to gentamicin base 1 mg). Methylparaben 1 mg, butylparaben 4 mg as preservatives, stearic acid, propylene glycol monostearate, isopropyl myristate, propylene glycol, polysorbate 40, sorbitol soln., water/g. Tube 15 g. **Oint.:** Gentamicin sulfate 1.7 mg (equivalent to gentamicin base 1 mg), methylparaben 0.5 mg, propylparaben 0.1 mg in petrolatum base/g. Tube 15 g. *Rx.*
Use: Anti-infective, topical.

Garamycin I.V. Piggyback. (Schering-Plough Corp.) Gentamicin sulfate equivalent to 1 mg gentamicin base, 8.9 mg sodium Cl, (no preservatives). Inj. Bot. 60 ml (60 mg), 80 ml (80 mg). *Rx.*
Use: Anti-infective, aminoglycoside.

Garamycin Ophthalmic Ointment-Sterile. (Schering-Plough Corp.) Gentamicin sulfate 3 mg/g. Tube 3.5 g. *Rx.*
Use: Anti-infective, ophthalmic.

Garamycin Ophthalmic Solution, Sterile. (Schering-Plough Corp.) Gentamicin sulfate 3 mg/ml. Dropper Bot. 5 ml. *Rx.*
Use: Anti-infective, ophthalmic.

gardenal.
See: Phenobarbital. (Various Mfr.).

gardinol type detergents. Aurinol, Cyclopon, Dreft, Drene, Duponol, Lissapol, Maprofix, Modinal, Orvus, Sandopan, Sadipan.
Use: Detergent.

gardol. Sodium Lauryl Sarcosinate.

Garfield. (Menley & James Labs, Inc.) Vitamin A 2500 IU, D 400 IU, E 15 IU, C 60 mg, folic acid 0.3 mg, B_1 1.05 mg, B_2 1.2 mg, B_3 13.5 mg, B_6 1.05 mg, B_{12} 4.5 mcg, sucrose, lactose. Chew. Tab. Bot. 60s. *otc.*
Use: Vitamin supplement.

Garfield Complete w/ Minerals. (Menley & James Labs, Inc.) Vitamin A 5000 IU, D 400 IU, E 30 IU, C 60 mg, folic acid 0.4 mg, B_1 1.5 mg, B_2 1.7 mg, B_3 20 mg, B_6 2 mg, B_{12} 6 mcg, biotin 40 mcg, B_5 10 mg, iron 18 mg, Ca, Cu, P, I, Mg, zinc 15 mg, aspartame, phenylalanine, sorbitol/Chew. Tab. Bot. 60s. *otc.*
Use: Mineral, vitamin supplement.

Garfield Plus Extra C. (Menley & James Labs, Inc.) Vitamin A 2500 IU, D 400 IU, E 15 IU, C 250 mg, folic acid 0.3 mg, B_1 1.05 mg, B_2 1.2 mg, B_3 13.5 mg, B_6

1.05 mg, B_{12} 4.5 mcg, sucrose, lactose/ Chew. Tab. Bot. 60s. *otc.*
Use: Vitamin supplement.

Garfield Plus Iron. (Menley & James Labs, Inc.) Vitamins A 2500 IU, D 400 IU, E 15 IU, C 60 mg, folic acid 0.3 mg, B_1 1.05 mg, B_2 1.2 mg, B_3 13.5 mg, B_6 1.05 mg, B_{12} 4.5 mcg, iron 15 mcg, sucrose, lactose. Chew. Tab. Bot. 60s. *otc.*
Use: Mineral, vitamin supplement.

Garfields Tea. (Last) Senna leaf powder 68.3%. Bot. 2 oz. *otc.*
Use: Laxative.

Garitabs. (Halsey Drug Co.) Iron 50 mg, vitamins B_1 5 mg, B_2 5 mg, C 75 mg, niacinamide 30 mg, B_5 2 mg, B_6 0.5 mg, B_{12} 3 mcg. Bot. 1000s. *otc.*
Use: Mineral, vitamin supplement.

Gari-Tonic Hematinic. (Halsey Drug Co.) Vitamins B_1 5 mg, niacinamide 100 mg, B_2 5 mg, pantothenic acid 4 mg, B_6 1 mg, B_{12} 6 mcg, choline bitartrate 100 mg, iron 100 mg/30 ml Bot. 16 oz. *otc.*
Use: Mineral, vitamin supplement.

garlic. Allium.
Use: Antispasmodic.

garlic capsules. (Miller Pharmacal Group, Inc.) Garlic 166 mg/Cap. Bot. 100s. *otc.*
Use: Antispasmodic.

garlic oil.
See: Natural Garlic Oil, Cap. (Spirt).

garlic oil capsules. (Kirkman Sales Co., Inc.) Bot. 100s. *otc.*

Gas Ban. (Roberts Pharmaceuticals) Calcium carbonate 300 mg, simethicone 40 mg/Tab. Bot. UD 8s, 1000s. *otc.*
Use: Antacid.

Gas Ban DS. (Roberts Pharmaceuticals) Aluminum hydroxide 400 mg, magnesium hydroxide 400 mg, simethicone 40 mg/5 ml. Liq. Bot. 150 ml. *otc.*
Use: Antacid.

Gas Permeable Daily Cleaner. (PBH Wesley Jessen) Potassium sorbate 0.13%, EDTA 2%, ethoxylated polyoxypropylene glycol, tris (hydroxymethyl) amino methane, hydroxymethylcellulose. Thimerosal free. Sol. Bot. 30 ml. *otc.*
Use: Contact lens care.

Gas Permeable Lens Starter System. (PBH Wesley Jessen) Daily cleanser, Bot. 3 ml, Wetting and soaking soln., Bot. 60 ml, Hydra-Mat II spin cleansing unit. Kit. *otc.*
Use: Contact lens care.

Gas Permeable Wetting & Soaking Solution. (PBH Wesley Jessen) Sterile aqueous, isotonic soln. of low viscosity, buffered to physiological pH. Bot. 60 ml, 120 ml. *otc.*
Use: Contact lens care.

gastric acidifiers.
See: Glutamic Acid HCl (Various Mfr.).

Gastroccult. (SmithKline Diagnostics) Occult blood screening test. In 40s.
Use: Diagnostic aid.

Gastrocrom. (Medeva Pharmaceuticals, Inc.) Cromolyn sodium 5 ml/100 mg Oral Conc. 8 UD Amps/foil pouch. *Rx.*
Use: Antiallergic.
See: Cromolyn Sodium.

Gastrografin. (Bristol-Myers Squibb) Diatrizoate meglumine 660 mg, sodium diatrizoate 100 mg, iodine 367 mg/ml. Soln. Bot. 120 ml. *Rx.*
Use: Radiopaque agent.

gastrointestinal tests.
See: Entero-Test, Cap. (HDC Corporation).
Entero-Test, Ped. Cap. (HDC Corporation).
Gastro-Test (HDC Corporation).

GastroMark. (Mallinckrodt) Ferumoxsil 175 mcg iron/ml, sorbitol, saccharin, parabens. Oral. Susp. Bot. 300 ml, 360 ml. *Rx.*
Use: Radiopaque agent.

Gastrosed. (Roberts Pharmaceuticals) Hyoscyamine sulfate. **Soln.:** 0.125 mg/ml. Dropper Bot. 5 ml. Alcohol free. **Tab.:** 0.125 mg. Bot. 100s. *Rx.*
Use: Anticholinergic, antispasmodic.

Gastro-Test. (HDC Corporation) To determine stomach pH and to diagnose and locate gastric bleeding. Test 25s.
Use: Diagnostic aid.

Gas-X. (Novartis Pharmaceutical Corp.) Simethicone 80 mg/Softgel cap. Pkg. 12s, 30s. *otc.*
Use: Antiflatulent.

Gas-X, Extra Strength. (Novartis Pharmaceutical Corp.) Simethicone 125 mg, sorbitol/Softgel Cap. Box 30s, 100s. *otc.*
Use: Antiflatulent.

•**gatifloxacin.** (gat-ih-FLOX-ah-sin) USAN.
Use: Antibacterial.

•**gauze, absorbent.** U.S.P. 23.
Use: Surgical aid.

•**gauze, petrolatum.** U.S.P. 23.
Use: Surgical aid.

Gaviscon. (SmithKline Beecham Pharmaceuticals) Aluminum hydroxide 80 mg, magnesium trisilicate 20 mg, alginic acid, sodium bicarbonate, sucrose, calcium stearate. Chew. Tab. Bot. 30s, 100s. *otc.*

Use: Antacid.

Gaviscon-2, Double Strength Tablets. (SmithKline Beecham Pharmaceuticals) Aluminum hydroxide 160 mg, magnesium trisilicate 40 mg, alginic acid, sodium bicarbonate, sucrose. Chew. Tab. Bot. 48s. *otc.*
Use: Antacid.

Gaviscon Extra Strength Relief Formula Liquid. (SmithKline Beecham Pharmaceuticals) Aluminum hydroxide 254 mg, magnesium carbonate 237.5 mg, parabens, EDTA, saccharin, sorbitol, simethicone, sodium alginate/5 ml. Bot. 355 ml. *otc.*
Use: Antacid.

Gaviscon Extra Strength Relief Formula Tablets. (SmithKline Beecham Pharmaceuticals) Aluminum hydroxide 160 mg, magnesium carbonate 105 mg, alginic acid, sodium bicarbonate, sucrose, calcium stearate. Chew. Tab. Bot. 30s, 100s. *otc.*
Use: Antacid.

Gaviscon Liquid. (SmithKline Beecham Pharmaceuticals) Aluminum hydroxide 31.7 mg, magnesium carbonate 119.3 mg/5 ml. Bot. 177 ml, 355 ml. *otc.*
Use: Antacid.

GBA.
See: Gamma hydroxybutyrate.

G.B.H. Lotion. (Century Pharmaceuticals, Inc.) Gamma benzene hexachloride 1%. Bot. 2 oz, pt, gal.
Use: Scabicide, pediculicide.

G.B.S. (Forest Pharmaceutical, Inc.) Dehydrocholic acid 125 mg, phenobarbital 8 mg, homatropine methylbromide 2.5 mg/Tab. 100s, 1000s. *Rx.*
Use: Hydrocholeretic.

G-CSF.
See: Neupogen (Amgen, Inc.).

Gebauer's 114. (Gebauer Co.) Dichlorotetrafluoroethane 100%. Can 8 oz.
Use: Anesthetic, local.

Gee-Gee. (Jones Medical Industries, Inc.) Guaifenesin 200 mg/Tab. Bot. 1000s. *otc.*
Use: Expectorant.

Geladine. (Barth's) Gelatin, protein, vitamin D/Cap. Bot. 100s, 500s. *otc.*

Gelamal. (Halsey Drug Co.) Magnesium-aluminum hydroxide gel. Bot. 12 oz. *otc.*
Use: Antacid.

•**gelatin.** N.F. 18.
Use: Pharmaceutic aid (encapsulating, suspending agent, tablet binder, tablet coating agent).

•**gelatin film, absorbable.** U.S.P. 23.
Use: Local hemostatic.
See: Gelfilm (Pharmacia & Upjohn).

gelatin film, sterile.
See: Neupogen (Amgen, Inc.).

gelatin powder, sterile.
See: Gelfoam Powder (Pharmacia & Upjohn).

gelatin sponge.
See: Gelfilm (Pharmacia & Upjohn).

•**gelatin sponge, absorbable.** U.S.P. 23.
Use: Hemostatic, local.
See: Gelfoam, Paks (Pharmacia & Upjohn).

gelatin, zinc.
See: Zinc gelatin. (Various Mfr.).

Gel-Clean. (PBH Wesley Jessen) Gel formulated with nonionic surfactant. Tube 30 g. *otc.*
Use: Contact lens care.

Gelfilm. (Pharmacia & Upjohn) Sterile, absorbable gelatin film. Envelope 1s. 100 mm × 125 mm. Also available as Ophth. Sterile 25 × 50 mm. Box 6s. *Rx.*
Use: Hemostatic, topical.

Gelfoam. (Pharmacia & Upjohn) Sterile Sponges. **Size 12 - 3 mm.:** 20 × 60 mm (12 sq. cm) × 3 mm. Box 4 sponges in individual envelopes. **Size 12 - 7 mm.:** 20 × 60 mm (12 sq. cm.) × 7 mm. Box 12 sponges in individual envelopes, jar 4 sponges. **Size 50 - 10 mm.:** 62.5 × 80 mm (50 sq. cm.) × 10 mm. Box 4 sponges in individual envelopes. **Size 100 - 10 mm.:** 80 × 125 mm (100 sq. cm.) × 10 mm. Box 6 sponges in individual envelopes. **Size 200 - 10 mm.:** 80 × 250 mm (200 sq. cm.) × 10 mm. Box 6 sponges in individual envelopes. **Compressed Size 100.:** Intended primarily for application in the dry state. 80 × 125 mm Boxes of 6 sponges in individual envelopes. **Packs:** Packs size 2 cm (Designed particularly for nasal packing) 2 × 40 cm Single jar (packing cavities). **Size 6 cm:** 6 × 40 cm Box 6 sponges in individual envelopes. *Rx.*
Use: Hemostatic, topical

Gelfoam Dental Pack. (Pharmacia & Upjohn) Size 4, 20 mm × 20 mm × 7 mm. Jar 15 sponges. *Rx.*
Use: Hemostatic, topical.

Gelfoam Powder. (Pharmacia & Upjohn) Sterile Jar 1 g. *Rx.*
Use: Hemostatic, topical.

Gelfoam Prostatectomy Cones. (Pharmacia & Upjohn) Prostatectomy cones (for use with Foley catheter). 13 cm, 18 cm in diameter. Box 6s. *Rx.*
Use: Hemostatic.

Gel Jet Gelatin Capsules. (Kirkman Sales Co., Inc.) Bot. 100s, 250s.

Gel Kam. (Scherer Laboratories, Inc.) Fluoride 0.1% (stannous fluoride 0.4%). Cinnamon flavor. Gel. Bot. w/applicator tip 69 g, 105 g, 129 g. *Rx.*
Use: Dental caries agent.

Gelocast. (Beiersdorf, Inc.) Unna's Boot medicated bandage: Semi-rigid cast impregnated with zinc oxide mixtures. Box 4 inches × 10 yd, 3 inches × 10 yd.
Use: Unna's cast dressing.

Gelpirin. Acetaminophen 125 mg, aspirin 240 mg, caffeine 32 mg. Tab. Bot. 100s, 1000s. *otc.*
Use: Analgesic combination.

Gelpirin-CCF. (Alra Laboratories, Inc.) Acetaminophen 325 mg, guaifenesin 25 mg, chlorpheniramine maleate 1 mg, phenylpropanolamine HCl 12.5 mg/Tab. Bot. 50s. *otc.*
Use: Analgesic, decongestant, expectorant.

gelsemium. (Various Mfr.) Pkg. oz.
Use: Neuralgia.
W/APC.
See: APC Combinations.

gelsemium w/combinations.
See: UB, Tab. (Scrip).
Urisan-P, Tab. (Sandia).

gelsolin, recombinant human. (Biogen)
Use: Cystic fibrosis. [Orphan Drug]

Gel-Tin. (Young Dental) Fluoride 0.1% (from stannous fluoride 0.4%) Gel Bot. 57 g, 623 g. *Rx.*
Use: Dental caries agent.

•**gemcadiol.** (JEM-kah-DIE-ole) USAN.
Use: Antihyperlipoproteinemic.

•**gemcitabine.** (JEM-sit-ah-BEAN) USAN.
Use: Antineoplastic.

•**gemcitabine hydrochloride.** (JEM-sit-ah-BEAN) USAN.
Use: Antineoplastic.
See: Gemzar (Eli Lilly and Co.).

•**gemeprost.** (JEH-meh-PRAHST) USAN.
Use: Prostaglandin.

•**gemfibrozil.** (gem-FIE-broe-ZILL) U.S.P. 23.
Use: Antihyperlipidemic.
See: Lopid, Cap. (Parke-Davis).

gemfibrozil. (Various Mfr.) 300 mg/Cap., Bot. 100s, 500s, 1000s. 600 mg/Tab., Bot. 60s, 100s, 500s, 1000s.
Use: Antihyperlipidemic.

Gemzar. (Eli Lilly and Co.) Gemcitabine HCl 20 mg/ml. Pow for Inj. Vials 10 and 50 ml. *Rx.*
Use: Antineoplastic.

Genac. (Zenith Goldline Pharmaceuticals) Triprolidine HCl 2.5 mg, pseudoephedrine HCl 60 mg/Tab. Bot. 24s, 100s. *otc.*
Use: Antihistamine, decongestant.

Genacol. (Zenith Goldline Pharmaceuticals) Pseudoephedrine HCl 30 mg, chlorpheniramine maleate 2 mg, dextromethorphan HBr 10 mg, acetaminophen 325 mg/Tab. Bot. 50s. *otc.*
Use: Analgesic, antihistamine, antitussive, decongestant.

Genagesic. (Zenith Goldline Pharmaceuticals) Propoxyphene HCl 165 mg, acetaminophen 650 mg/Tab. Bot. 100s, 500s. *c-IV.*
Use: Analgesic combination, narcotic.

Genahist. (Zenith Goldline Pharmaceuticals) Diphenhydramine HCl 12.5 mg/5 ml, alcohol 14%. Liq. Bot. 120 ml. *otc.*
Use: Antihistamine.

Genallerate. (Zenith Goldline Pharmaceuticals) Chlorpheniramine maleate 4 mg, lactose/Tab. Bot. 24s. *otc.*
Use: Antihistamine.

Genamin Cold Syrup. (Zenith Goldline Pharmaceuticals) Phenylpropanolamine HCl 6.25 mg, chlorpheniramine maleate 1 mg. Alcohol free. In 118 ml. *otc.*
Use: Antihistamine, decongestant.

Genamin Expectorant. (Zenith Goldline Pharmaceuticals) Phenylpropanolamine 12.5 mg, guaifenesin 100 mg, alcohol 5%. In 120 ml. *otc.*
Use: Decongestant, expectorant.

Genapap, Children's Chewable Tabs. (Zenith Goldline Pharmaceuticals) Acetaminophen 80 mg/Chew. Tab. Bot. 30s. *otc.*
Use: Analgesic.

Genapap, Children's Elixir. (Zenith Goldline Pharmaceuticals) Acetaminophen 160 mg/5 ml. Cherry flavor. Bot. 120 ml. *otc.*
Use: Analgesic.

Genapap, Infants' Drops. (Zenith Goldline Pharmaceuticals) Acetaminophen 100 mg/ml, alcohol 7%. Soln. Dropper bot. 15 ml. *otc.*
Use: Analgesic.

Genapap. (Zenith Goldline Pharmaceuticals) Acetaminophen 325 mg/Tab. Bot. 100s. *otc.*
Use: Analgesic.

Genapax. (Key Pharmaceuticals) Gentian violet 5 mg/tampon. Box 12s.
Use: Antifungal, vaginal.

Genaphed. (Zenith Goldline Pharmaceuticals) Pseudoephedrine HCl 30 mg/Tab. Bot. 24s, 100s. *otc.*
Use: Decongestant.

Genasal. (Zenith Goldline Pharmaceuticals) Oxymetazoline 0.05%. Soln. 15 ml, 30 ml. *otc.*

Use: Decongestant.

Genasoft. (Zenith Goldline Pharmaceuticals) Docusate sodium 100 mg/Cap. Bot. 60s. *otc.*
Use: Laxative, stool softener.

Genasoft Plus. (Zenith Goldline Pharmaceuticals) Docusate sodium 100 mg, casanthranol 30 mg/Cap. Bot. 60s. *otc.*
Use: Laxative, stool softener.

Genaspor Antifungal. (Zenith Goldline Pharmaceuticals) Tolnaftate 1%. Cream Bot. 15 g. *otc.*
Use: Antifungal, topical.

Genasyme. (Zenith Goldline Pharmaceuticals) Simethicone 80 mg/Tab. Bot. 100s. *otc.*
Use: Antiflatulent.

Genatap. (Zenith Goldline Pharmaceuticals) Brompheniramine maleate 2 mg, phenylpropanolamine HCl 12.5 mg/5 ml. Elix. Bot. 118 ml. *otc.*
Use: Antihistamine, decongestant.

Genaton. (Zenith Goldline Pharmaceuticals) Aluminum hydroxide 80 mg, magnesium trisilicate 20 mg, alginic acid, sodium bicarbonate, sodium 18.4 mg, sucrose, sugar. Chew. Tab. Bot. 100s. *otc.*
Use: Antacid.

Genaton, Extra Strength. (Zenith Goldline Pharmaceuticals) Aluminum hydroxide 160 mg, magnesium carbonate 105 mg, alginic acid, sodium bicarbonate, sodium 29.9 mg, sucrose, calcium stearate. Chew. Tab. Bot. 100s. *otc.*
Use: Antacid.

Genaton Liquid. (Zenith Goldline Pharmaceuticals) Aluminum hydroxide 31.7 mg, magnesium carbonate 137.3 mg, sodium alginate, sodium 13 mg, EDTA, saccharin, sorbitol/5 ml. Bot. 355 ml. *otc.*
Use: Antacid.

genatropine hydrochloride. (jen-AT-row-peen) Atropine-N-oxide HCl. Aminoxytropine Tropate HCl.
See: X-tro, Cap. (Xttrium Laboratories, Inc.).

Genatuss DM Syrup. (Zenith Goldline Pharmaceuticals) Dextromethorphan HBr 10 mg, guaifenesin 100 mg. Bot. 120 ml. *otc.*
Use: Antitussive, expectorant.

Genatuss Syrup. (Zenith Goldline Pharmaceuticals) Guaifenesin 100 mg/5 ml, alcohol 3.5%. Bot. 120 ml. *otc.*
Use: Expectorant.

Gen-bee with C. (Zenith Goldline Pharmaceuticals) Vitamins B_1 15 mg, B_2 10.2 mg, B_3 50 mg, B_5 10 mg, B_6 5 mg, C 300 mg/Cap. Bot. 130s, 1000s. *otc.*
Use: Vitamin supplement.

Gencalc 600. (Zenith Goldline Pharmaceuticals) Calcium 600 mg (from calcium carbonate 1.5 g)/Tab. Bot. 60s. *otc.*
Use: Mineral supplement.

Gencept. (Gencon) **0.5/35:** Norethindrone 0.5 mg, ethinyl estradiol, 35 mcg/Tab (with 7 inert tabs) Pkgs 21s and 28s. **1/35:** Norethindrone 1 mg, ethinyl estradiol 35 mcg/Tab (with 7 inert tabs) Pkgs 21s and 28s. **10/11:** Norethindrone 0.5 mg and 1 mg, ethinyl estradiol 35 mcg/Tab (with 7 inert tabs). Pkg 21s and 28s. *Rx.*
Use: Contraceptive.

Gencold. (Zenith Goldline Pharmaceuticals) Phenylpropanolamine HCl 75 mg, chlorpheniramine maleate 8 mg/SR Tab. Pkg. 10s. *otc.*
Use: Antihistamine, decongestant.

Gendecon. (Zenith Goldline Pharmaceuticals) Phenylephrine HCl 5 mg, chlorpheniramine maleate 2 mg, acetaminophen 325 mg/Tab. Bot. 50s. *otc.*
Use: Analgesic, antihistamine, decongestant.

Genebs Extra Strength. (Zenith Goldline Pharmaceuticals) Acetaminophen 500 mg/Cap. Bot. 100s, 1000s. *otc.*
Use: Analgesic.

Genebs Extra Strength Tablets. (Zenith Goldline Pharmaceuticals) Acetaminophen 500 mg/Tab. Bot. 100s, 1000s. *otc.*
Use: Analgesic.

Genebs Tablets. (Zenith Goldline Pharmaceuticals) Acetaminophen 325 mg/Tab. Bot. 100s, 1000s. *otc.*
Use: Analgesic.

Generet-500. (Zenith Goldline Pharmaceuticals) Iron 105 mg, Vitamins B_1 6 mg, B_2 6 mg, B_3 30 mg, B_5 10 mg, B_6 5 mg, B_{12} 25 mcg, C (as sodium ascorbate) 500 mg. TR Tab. Bot. 60s. *otc.*
Use: Mineral, vitamin supplement.

Generix-T. (Zenith Goldline Pharmaceuticals) Iron 15 mg, vitamins A 10,000 IU, D 400 IU, E 5.5 mg, B_1 15 mg, B_2 10 mg, B_3 100 mg, B_5 10 mg, B_6 2 mg, B_{12} 7.5 mcg, C 150 mg, Cu, I, Mg, Mn, zinc 1.5 mg/Tab. Bot. 100s. *otc.*
Use: Mineral, vitamin supplement.

GenESA. (Gensia Automedics) Arbutamine HCl 0.05 mg/ml. Inj. Syringe 20 mg (containing 1 mg arbutamine). *Rx.*
Use: Diagnostic aid.

Genex. (Zenith Goldline Pharmaceuticals) Phenylpropanolamine HCl 18 mg, acetaminophen 325 mg/Cap. Bot.

100s, 1000s. *otc.*
Use: Analgesic, decongestant.

Geneye. (Zenith Goldline Pharmaceuticals) Tetrahydrozoline HCl 0.05%. Drop. Bot. 15 ml. *otc.*
Use: Mydriatic, vasoconstrictor.

Geneye Extra. (Zenith Goldline Pharmaceuticals) Tetrahydrozoline HCl 0.05%, PEG 400 1%, benzalkonium Cl, EDTA/ Drops. Bot. 15 ml. *otc.*
Use: Ophthalmic vasoconstrictor.

genital herpes treatment.
See: Acyclovir.
Zovirax Cap., Oint. (GlaxoWellcome).

Genite. (Zenith Goldline Pharmaceuticals) Pseudoephedrine HCl 10 mg, doxylamine succinate 1.25 mg, dextromethorphan HBr 5 mg, acetaminophen 167 mg, alcohol 25%/5 ml. Bot. 177 ml. *otc.*
Use: Analgesic, antihistamine, antitussive, decongestant.

genitourinary irrigants.
See: Acetic acid for irrigation (Various Mfr.).
Glycine (Aminoacetic Acid) for Irrigation (Various Mfr.).
Neosporin G.U. Irrigant, Soln (GlaxoWellcome).
Renacidin, Pow., Soln. (Guardian Laboratories).
Resectisol, Soln. (McGaw, Inc.).
Sorbitol (Various Mfr.).
Sorbitol-Mannitol (Abbott Laboratories).
Sodium Chloride for Irrigation (Various Mfr.).
Sterile Water for Irrigation (Various Mfr.).
Suby's Solution G (Various Mfr.).

Gen-K Powder. (Zenith Goldline Pharmaceuticals) Potassium Cl. Pow. 20 mEq/ packet. Box 30s. *Rx.*
Use: Electrolyte supplement.

Gen-K Tabs. (Zenith Goldline Pharmaceuticals) Effervescent potassium. Bot. 30s. *Rx.*
Use: Electrolyte supplement.

Genna Tablets. (Zenith Goldline Pharmaceuticals) Senna concentrate 217 mg/ Tab. Bot. 100s, 1000s. *otc.*
Use: Laxative.

Gennin. (Zenith Goldline Pharmaceuticals) Buffered aspirin 5 gr. Tab. Bot. 100s. *otc.*
Use: Analgesic.

genophyllin.
See: Aminophylline (Various Mfr.).

Genoptic Liquifilm Sterile Ophthalmic Solution. (Allergan, Inc.) Gentamicin sulfate 3 mg/ml. Bot. 1 ml, 5 ml. *Rx.*
Use: Anti-infective, ophthalmic.

Genoptic S.O.P. Sterile Ophthalmic Ointment. (Allergan, Inc.) Gentamicin sulfate 3 mg/g. Oint. Tube 3.5 g. *Rx.*
Use: Anti-infective, ophthalmic.

Genora 0.5/35. (Rugby Labs, Inc.) Norethindrone 0.5 mg, ethinyl estradiol 0.035 mg/Tab. Pkg. 21s; 28s (7 inert tab.) *Rx.*
Use: Contraceptive.

Genora 1/35-21. (Rugby Labs, Inc.) Norethindrone 1 mg, ethinyl estradiol 0.035 mg/Tab. Pkg. 126s (6-pak). *Rx.*
Use: Contraceptive.

Genora 1/35-28. (Rugby Labs, Inc.) Norethindrone 1 mg, ethinyl estradiol 0.035 mg/Tab., 7 inert tab. Pkg. 168s (6-pak). *Rx.*
Use: Contraceptive.

Genora 1/50-21. (Rugby Labs, Inc.) Norethindrone 1 mg, mestranol 0.05 mg/ Tab. Pkg. 126s (6-pak). *Rx.*
Use: Contraceptive.

Genora 1/50-28. (Rugby Labs, Inc.) Norethindrone 1 mg, mestranol 0.05 mg/ Tab., 7 inert tab. Pkg. 168s (6-pak). *Rx.*
Use: Contraceptive.

Genotropin. (Pharmacia & Upjohn) Somatropin 1.5 mg (≈ F4 IU/ml), preservative free. In 1.5 mg Intra-Mix two-chamber cartridge with pressure-release needle. 5s. Somatropin 5.8 mg (≈ F15 IU/ml). In 5.8 Intra-Mix two-chamber cartridge with pressure-release needle. 1s, 5s. Pow. for Inj. *Rx.*
Use: Hormone.

Genprep Ointment. (Zenith Goldline Pharmaceuticals) Live yeast cell derivative supplying 2000 units skin respiratory factor/oz of ointment w/shark liver oil 3%, phenylmercuric nitrate 1:10,000. Tube 2 oz. *otc.*
Use: Anorectal preparation.

Genpril. (Zenith Goldline Pharmaceuticals) Ibuprofen 200 mg. Tab. 50s, 100s. *otc.*
Use: Analgesic, NSAID.

Genprin. (Zenith Goldline Pharmaceuticals) Aspirin 325 mg. Tab. 100s. *otc.*
Use: Analgesic.

gensalate sodium. Sodium gentisate. (Sodium salt of 2,5-dihydroxybenzoic acid).
Use: Analgesic.

Gensan. (Zenith Goldline Pharmaceuticals) Aspirin 400 mg, caffeine 32 mg/ Tab. Bot. 100s. *otc.*
Use: Analgesic combination.

Gentacidin Ophthalmic Ointment. (Ciba Vision) Gentamicin 3 mg/g. Oint. Tube 3.5 g. *Rx.*

Use: Anti-infective, ophthalmic.

Gentacidin Ophthalmic Solution. (Ciba Vision) Gentamicin sulfate 3 mg/ml. Soln. Bot. 5 ml. *Rx.*
Use: Anti-infective, ophthalmic.

Gentafair. (Bausch & Lomb Pharmaceuticals) **Oint.:** Gentamicin 3 mg/g with liquid lanolin, white petrolatum, mineral oil, parabens. Tube 3.75 g, 15 g. **Soln.:** Gentamicin 3 mg/ml, polyoxyl 40 stearate, polyethylene glycol. Dropper bot. 5 ml, 15 ml. *Rx.*
Use: Anti-infective, ophthalmic.

Gentak. (Akorn, Inc.) **Oint.:** Gentamicin 3 mg/g. Tube 3.5 g. **Soln.:** Gentamicin 3 mg/ml. Bot. 5 ml, 15 ml. *Rx.*
Use: Anti-infective, ophthalmic.

gentamicin impregnated PMMA beads on surgical wire.
Use: Chronic osteomyelitis. [Orphan Drug]

gentamicin liposome injection.
Use: Mycobacterium avium-intracellulare infection. [Orphan Drug]

•**gentamicin sulfate.** (JEN-tuh-MY-sin) U.S.P. 23.
Use: Anti-infective.
See: Genoptic, Inj. (Allergan, Inc.).
Gentacidin, Preps. (Ciba Vision).
Gentak, Preps. (Akorn, Inc.).

gentamicin sulfate. (Schering-Plough Corp.) Produced by *Micromonospora purpurea.* (Various Mfr.). **Ophthalmic Oint.:** 3 mg/g Tube 3.5 g. **Ophthalmic Soln.:** 3 mg/ml Bot. 5 ml, 15 ml. **Inj.:** 40 mg/ml. Vial 2 ml, 20 ml. Cartridge-needle units 1.5 ml, 2 ml. **Ped. Inj.:** 10 mg/ml. Vial 2 ml. *Rx.*
Use: Anti-infective.

gentamicin and prednisolone acetate ophthalmic suspension.
Use: Anti-infective, anti-inflammatory.

•**gentian violet.** (JEN-shun) U.S.P. 23.
Formerly Methylrosaniline Chloride.
Use: Anti-infective, topical.

gentian violet. (JEN-shun) (Various Mfr.) Gentian violet 1%, 2%. Soln. Bot. 30 ml. *otc.*
Use: Anti-infective, topical.

gentisate sodium.

•**gentisic acid ethanolamide.** N.F. 18.
Use: Pharmaceutic aid, complexing agent.

Gentlax. (Blair Laboratories) Standardized senna concentrate 326 mg, malt extract, sucrose/Gran. 180 g. *otc.*
Use: Laxative.

Gentlax S. (Blair Laboratories) Standardized senna concentrate 187 mg, docusate sodium 50 mg. Tab. Bot. 30s, 60s. *otc.*
Use: Laxative.

Gentle Nature Natural Vegetable Laxative. (Novartis Pharmaceutical Corp.) Sennosides A and B as calcium salts. 20 mg/Tab. Box 16s, 32s. *otc.*
Use: Laxative.

Gentle Shampoo. (Ulmer Pharmacal Co.) Bot. 4 oz, gal. *otc.*
Use: Dermatologic, hair.

Gentran 40. (Baxter Pharmaceutical Products, Inc.) Dextran 40 10% w/sodium Cl 0.9% or Dextran 40 10% w/dextrose 5%. Inj. Plastic Bot. 500 ml. *Rx.*
Use: Plasma expander.

Gentran 70. (Baxter Pharmaceutical Products, Inc.) Dextran 70 6% w/sodium Cl 0.9%. Inj. Plastic Bot. 500 ml. *Rx.*
Use: Plasma expander.

Gentran 75. (Baxter Pharmaceutical Products, Inc.) Dextran 75 6% in sodium Cl 0.9%. Inj. Bot. 500 ml. *Rx.*
Use: Plasma expander.

Gentrasul. (Bausch & Lomb Pharmaceuticals) Gentamicin 3 mg. **Oint.:** 3.5 g. **Soln.:** Dropper bot. 5 ml. *Rx.*
Use: Anti-infective, ophthalmic.

Gentz Rectal Wipes. (Roxane Laboratories, Inc.) Pramoxine HCl 1%, alcloxa 0.2%, witch hazel 50%, propylene glycol 10%. Box 100s, 120s (individually wrapped disposable wipes). *otc.*
Use: Anorectal preparation.

Genuine Bayer Aspirin. (Bayer Corp. (Consumer Div.)) Aspirin 325 mg/FC Tab. Bot. 12s, 24s, 50s, 200s, 300s. *otc.*
Use: Analgesic.

Gen-Xene. (Alra Laboratories, Inc.) Clorazepate dipotassium 3.75 mg, 7.5 mg, or 15 mg/Tab. Bot. 30s, 100s, 500s, UD 100s. *c-iv.*
Use: Anticonvulsant, anxiolytic.

Geocillin. (Roerig) Carbenicillin indanyl sodium 382 mg/Tab. Bot. 100s, UD 100s. *Rx.*
Use: Anti-infective, penicillin.

Geopen. (Roerig) Carbenicillin disodium. Inj. **Vial:** 1 g, 2 g, 5 g. Pkg. 10s. **Piggyback Vial:** 2 g, 5 g, 10 g. **Bulk Pharmacy Pack:** 30 g. *Rx.*
Use: Anti-infective, penicillin.

•**gepirone hydrochloride.** (jeh-PIE-rone) USAN.
Use: Anxiolytic.

Gera Plus. (Towne) Iron 50 mg, vitamins B_1 5 mg, B_2 5 mg, C 75 mg, niacinamide 30 mg, calcium pantothenate 2 mg, B_6 0.5 mg, B_{12} 3 mcg/Tab. Bot. 100s. *otc.*

Use: Mineral, vitamin supplement.

Geravim. (Major Pharmaceuticals) Vitamins B_1 0.83 mg, B_2 0.42 mg, B_3 8.3 mg, B_5 1.67 mg, B_6 0.17 mg, B_{12} 0.17 mg, I, Fe 2.5 mg, Zn 0.3 mg, choline, Mn, alcohol 18%. Liq. Bot. pt., gal. *otc.*
Use: Mineral, vitamin supplement.

Geravite. (Roberts Pharmaceuticals) Vitamins B_1 0.3 mg, B_2 0.4 mg, B_3 33.3 mg, B_{12} 3.3 mcg, L-lysine, alcohol 15%, parabens, sorbitol, sucrose. Elix. Bot. 480 ml. *otc.*
Use: Mineral, vitamin supplement.

Gerber Baby Formula Low Iron Formula. (Bristol-Myers Squibb) Protein (from non-fat milk) 14.7 g, carbohydrate (from lactose) 71.3 g, fat (from palm olein, soy, coconut and high oleic sunflower oils) 36 g, linoleic acid 5.9 g, vitamins A, D, E, K, C, B_1, B_2, B_3, B_5, B_6, B_{12}, folic acid, biotin, choline, inositol, Ca, P, Mg, Fe 3.4 mg, Zn, Mn, Cu, I, Na 220 mg, K 720 mg, Cl, taurine, calories per L 666.7. **Ready to use liq.:** Bot. 943 ml. **Concentrated liq.:** Bot. 433 ml. **Pow.:** Can 457 g and 914 g. *otc.*
Use: Nutritional supplement.

Gerber Baby Formula with Iron. (Bristol-Myers Squibb) Protein (from nonfat milk) 14.7 g, carbohydrate (from lactose) 71.3 g, fat (from palm olein, soy, coconut and high oleic sunflower oils) 36 g, with linoleic acid 5.9 g, vitamins A, D, E, K, C, B_1, B_2, B_6, B_{12}, B_3, folic acid, B_5, biotin, choline, inositol, Ca, P, Mg, Fe 12 mg, Zn, Mn, Cu, I, Na 220 mg, K 720 mg, Cl, taurine 666.7, calories/L. Conc. Liq. Bot. 943 ml. *otc.*
Use: Nutritional supplement.

Geref. (Serono Laboratories, Inc.) Sermorelin acetate 50 mcg (lyophilized). Pow. for Inj. Amp. 2 ml w/sodium Cl. 0.9%.
Use: Diagnostic aid.

Geri-All-D. (Barth's) Vitamins A 10,000 IU, D 400 IU, B_1 7 mg, B_2 14 mg, C 200 mg, niacin 4.17 mg, B_{12} 25 mcg, E 50 IU, B_6 0.35 mg, pantothenic acid 0.63 mg, trace minerals and other factors. 2 Cap. Bot. 1 mo., 3 mo. and 6 mo. supply of Geri-All regular and Geri-All-D. *otc.*
Use: Mineral, vitamin supplement.

geriatric supplements w/multivitamins/minerals.
See: Geravite, Elix. (Roberts Pharmaceuticals).
Gerimed, Tab. (Fielding Co.).
Hep-Forte, Cap. (Marlyn Nutraceuticals, Inc.).
Mega VM-80, Tab. (NBTY, Inc.).
Optivite P.M.T., Tab. (Optimox Corp.).
Strovite Plus, Tab. (Everett Laboratories, Inc.).
Ultra Freeda, Tab. (Freeda Vitamins, Inc.).
Ultra Freeda Iron Free, Tab. (Freeda Vitamins, Inc).
Vigortol, Liq. (Rugby Labs, Inc.).
Viminate, Elix. (Various Mfr.).
Vita-Plus G Softgels (Scot-Tussin Pharmacal, Inc.).

Geriatroplex. (Morton) Cyanocobalamin 30 mcg, liver inj. 0.1 ml vitamins B_{12} activity 2 mcg, ferrous gluconate 50 mg, B_2 1.5 mg, calcium pantothenate 2.5 mg, niacinamide 100 mg, citric acid 16.4 mg, sodium citrate 23.6 mg/2 ml. Vial 30 ml. *otc.*
Use: Mineral, vitamin supplement.

Geri-Derm. (Barth's) Vitamins A 400,000 IU, D 40,000 IU, E 200 IU, panthenol 800 mg/4 oz. Jar 4 oz. *otc.*
Use: Skin supplement.

Geridium Tablets. (Zenith Goldline Pharmaceuticals) Phenazopyridine HCl 100 mg or 200 mg/Tab. Bot. 100s, 1000s. *Rx.*
Use: Analgesic; anti-infective, urinary.

Gerifort Plus. (A.P.C.) Vitamins A 10,000 IU, B_1 5 mg, B_2 6 mg, B_6 2 mg, C 75 mg, D-2 1000 IU, niacinamide 60 mg, iron 10 mg, calcium 115 mg, phosphorus 83 mg, iodine 0.1 mg, calcium pantothenate 10 mg, d-alpha tocopheryl acid succinate 3 IU, cobalamin concentrate 3 mcg, choline bitartrate 70 mg, inositol 35 mg, biotin 15 mcg, Zn 0.2 mg, Mg 2 mg, Mn 0.5 mg, K 0.15 mg/Amcap. Bot. 100s. *otc.*
Use: Mineral, vitamin supplement.

Gerilets. (Abbott Laboratories) Vitamins A 5000 IU, D 400 IU, E 45 IU, C 90 mg (from sodium ascorbate), folic acid 0.4 mg, B_1 2.25 mg, B_2 2.6 mg, niacin 30 mg, B_6 3 mg, B_{12} 9 mcg, biotin 0.45 mg, pantothenic acid 15 mg, iron 27 mg (from ferrous sulfate)/Tab. Bot. 100s. *otc.*
Use: Mineral, vitamin supplement.

Gerimal. (Rugby Labs, Inc.) Ergoloid mesylates 0.5 mg or 1 mg. **Sublingual Tab.:** Bot. 100s, 500s, 1000s; 1 mg. **Oral Tab.:** Bot. 100s, 500s, 1000s. *Rx.*
Use: Psychotherapeutic agent.

Gerimed. (Fielding Co.) Vitamins A 5000 IU, D 400 IU, E 30 mg, B_1 3 mg, B_2 3 mg, B_3 25 mg, B_6 2 mg, B_{12} 6 mcg, C 120 mg, calcium 370 mg, zinc 15 mg, Mg, P/Tab. Bot. 60s. *otc.*
Use: Mineral, vitamin supplement.

Gerineed. (Hanlon) Vitamins A 5000 IU,

B_1 20 mg, B_2 5 mg, niacinamide 20 mg, B_6 0.5 mg, calcium pantothenate 5 mg, B_{12} 5 mcg, rutin 25 mg, C 50 mg, E 10 IU, choline 50 mg, inositol 50 mg, calcium lactate 1.64 mg, iron sulfate 10 mg, Cu 1 mg, iodine 0.5 mg, Mn 1 mg, magnesium sulfate 1 mg, potassium sulfate 5 mg, zinc sulfate 0.5 mg/Cap. Bot. 100s. *otc.*
Use: Mineral, vitamin supplement.

Geriot. (Zenith Goldline Pharmaceuticals) Iron 50 mg (from ferrous sulfate), A 6000 IU, D 400 IU, E 30 IU, B_1 1.5 mg, B_2 1.7 mg, B_3 20 mg, B_5 10 mg, B_6 2 mg, B_{12} 6 mcg, C 60 mg, folic acid 0.4 mg, biotin 45 mcg, Ca, Cl, Cr, Cu, I, K, Mg, Mn, Mo, Ni, P, Se, Si, Sn, V, Zn, vitamin K/Tab. Bot. 100s. *otc.*
Use: Mineral, vitamin supplement.

Geri-Plus Capsules. (Health for Life Brands, Inc.) Vitamins A 12,500 IU, D 1200 IU, B_1 15 mg, B_2 10 mg, C 75 mg, niacinamide 30 mg, calcium pantothenate 2 mg, B_6 0.5 mg, E 5 IU, Brewer's yeast 10 mg, B_{12} 15 mcg, iron 11.58 mg, desiccated liver 15 mg, choline bitartrate 30 mg, inositol 30 mg, Ca 59 mg, P 45 mg, Zn 0.68 mg, francium dicalcium phosphate 200 mg, Mn, enzymatic factors, amino acids/Cap. Bot. 50s, 100s, 1000s. *otc.*
Use: Mineral, vitamin supplement.

Geri-Plus Elixir. (Health for Life Brands, Inc.) Vitamins B_1 25 mg, B_2 10 mg, B_6 1 mg, niacinamide 100 mg, calcium pantothenate 5 mg, B_{12} 20 mcg, iron ammonium citrate 100 mg, choline 200 mg, inositol 100 mg, magnesium Cl 2 mg, manganese citrate 2 mg, zinc acetate 2 mg, amino acids/fl oz. Bot. pt. *otc.*
Use: Mineral, vitamin supplement.

Geritol Complete. (SmithKline Beecham Pharmaceuticals) Vitamins A 6000 IU, E 30 IU, C 60 mg, folic acid 400 mcg, B_1 1.5 mg, B_2 1.7 mg, B_3 20 mg, B_6 2 mg, B_{12} 6 mcg, D 400 IU, K, biotin 45 mcg, B_5 10 mg, iron 18 mg, Ca, Cl, Cr, Cu, I, K, Mg, Mn, Mo, Ni, P, Se, Si, Sn, V, Zn, vitamin K. Tab. Bot. 14s, 40s, 100s, 180s. *otc.*
Use: Mineral, vitamin supplement.

Geritol Extended. (SmithKline Beecham) Iron 10 mg, vitamins A 3333 IU, D 200 IU, E 15 IU, B_1 1.2 mg, B_2 1.4 mg, B_3 15 mg, B_6 2 mg, B_{12} 2 mg, C 60 mg, folic acid 0.2 mg, vitamin K, Ca, I, Mg, Se, Zn 15 mg. Capl. Bot. 40s, 100s. *otc.*
Use: Mineral, vitamin supplement.

Geritol Tonic Liquid. (SmithKline Beecham Pharmaceuticals) Iron 18 mg, vitamins B_1 2.5 mg, B_2 2.5 mg, B_3 50 mg, B_5 2 mg, B_6 0.5 mg, methionine 25 mg, choline bitartrate 50 mg/15 ml. Alcohol 12%. Bot. 120 ml, 360 ml. *otc.*
Use: Mineral, vitamin supplement.

Gerivite. (Zenith Goldline Pharmaceuticals) Vitamins B_1 0.8 mg, B_2 0.4 mg, B_3 8.3 mg, B_5 1.7 mg, B_6 0.2 mg, B_{12} 0.2 mcg, iron 0.3 mg, Zn 0.3 mg, choline, I Mg, Mn, alcohol 18%, methylparaben, sorbitol. Liq. Bot. 473 ml. *otc.*
Use: Mineral, vitamin supplement.

Gerivites. (Rugby Labs, Inc.) Iron (from ferrous sulfate) 50 mg, A 5000 IU, D 400 IU, E 30 IU, B_1 1.5 mg, B_2 1.7 mg, B_3 20 mg, B_5 10 mg, B_6 2 mg, B_{12} 300 mcg, C 60 mg, folic acid 400 mg, Ca, Cl, Cr, Cu, I, K, Mg, Mn, Mo, Ni, Se, Si, P, Zn 15 mg/Tab. 40s. *otc.*
Use: Mineral, vitamin supplement.

Gerix. (Abbott Laboratories) Vitamins B_1 6 mg, B_2 6 mg, niacin 100 mg, iron 15 mg, B_6 1.6 mg, cyanocobalamin 6 mcg, alcohol 20%/30 ml. Elix. Bot. 480 ml. *otc.*
Use: Mineral, vitamin supplement.

germanin. (CDC) *Rx.*
Use: Anti-infective.
See: Suramin sodium (Naphuride sodium).

Germicin. (CMC) Benzalkonium Cl 50%. Bot. Pt., gal. *otc.*
Use: Antiseptic, antimicrobial.

Ger-O-Foam. (Roberts Pharmaceuticals) Methyl salicylate 30%, benzocaine 3%, volatile oils. Aerosol Can 4 oz. *otc.*
Use: Analgesic, anesthetic.

Geroton Forte. (Kenwood Laboratories) Vitamin B_1 1.7 mg, B_2 1.9 mg, B_3 2.22 mg, B_5 1.11 mg, B_6 0.22 mg, B_{12} 0.67 mcg, Zn 1.7 mg, Mg, Mn, alcohol 13%. Liq. Bot. 473 ml. *otc.*
Use: Mineral, vitamin supplement.

Gerterol Depo. (Fellows) Medroxyprogesterone acetate 50 mg, 100 mg/ml. Vial 5 ml. *Rx.*
Use: Hormone, progestin.

Gesic. (Lexalabs) Aspirin 226.8 mg, caffeine 32.4 mg, codeine 32.4 mg/Tab. Bot. 100s. *c-III.*
Use: Analgesic combination, narcotic.

•**gestaclone.** (JEST-ah-klone) USAN.
Use: Hormone, progestin.

•**gestodene.** (JEST-oh-deen) USAN.
Use: Hormone, progestin.

Gestoneed. (Hanlon) Calcium lactate 1069 mg, vitamins C 100 mg, nicotinic acid 18 mg, B_2 2.4 mg, B_1 1.8 mg, B_6 9 mg, D 500 IU, A 6000 IU/Cap. Bot. 100s. *otc.*
Use: Mineral, vitamin supplement.

•**gestonorone caproate.** (jess-TOE-nore-ohn CAP-row-ate) USAN.
Use: Hormone, progestin.
•**gestrinone.** (JESS-trih-nohn) USAN.
Use: Hormone, progestin.
Get Better Bear Sore Throat Pops. (Whitehall) Pectin 19 mg, corn syrup, sucrose, parabens. Loz. on a stick. Pkg. 10s. *otc.*
Use: Mouth and throat product.
Gets-It. (Oakhurst Co.) Salicylic acid, zinc Cl, collodion in ether ≈ 35%, alcohol ≈ 28%. Liq. Bot. 12 ml. *otc.*
Use: Keratolytic.
•**gevotroline hydrochloride.** (jeh-VOE-troe-LEEN) USAN.
Use: Antipsychotic.
Gevrabon. (ESI Lederle Generics) Vitamins B_1 0.83 mg, B_2 0.42 mg, B_3 8.3 mg, B_5 1.67 mg, B_6 0.17 mg, B_{12} 0.17 mcg, Fe 2.5 mg, choline, I, Mg, Mn, Zn 0.3 mg, alcohol 18%. Liq. Bot. 480 ml. *otc.*
Use: Mineral, vitamin supplement.
Gevral. (ESI Lederle Generics) Vitamins A 5000 IU, B_1 1.5 mg, B_2 1.7 mg, B_6 2 mg, B_{12} 6 mcg, folic acid 0.4 mg, C 60 mg, E 30 mg, B_3 20 mg, Ca, P, iron 18 mg, Mg, I, lactose, parabens, sucrose/ Tab. Bot. 100s. *otc.*
Use: Mineral, vitamin supplement.
Gevral Protein. (ESI Lederle Generics) Calcium caseinate, sucrose, protein 15.6 g, carbohydrate 7.05 g, fat 0.52 g, Na 50 mg, K 13 mg, calories 95.3/26 g. Pow. Can. 8 oz, 5 lb. *otc.*
Use: Nutritional supplement.
GG-Cen. (Schwarz Pharma, Inc.) Guaifenesin 200 mg/Cap. Bot. 24s, 100s. *otc.*
Use: Expectorant.
GI stimulants.
See: Maxolon, Tab. (SmithKline Beecham Pharmaceuticals).
Metoclopramide, Tab. (Various Mfr.).
Metoclopramide HCl, Inj. (Quad Pharmaceuticals, Inc.).
Octamide, Tab. (Pharmacia & Upjohn).
Reclomide, Tab. (Major Pharmaceuticals).
Reglan, Inj., Syr., Tab. (Wyeth-Ayerst Laboratories).
GL-2 Skin Adherent. (Gordon Laboratories) Ready-to-use. Bot. Pt, qt, gal. *otc.*
GL-7 Skin Adherent. (Gordon Laboratories) Plastic material which may be used full strength or diluted with 3 to 10 parts 99% isopropyl alcohol, acetone or naphtha. Pkg. Pt, qt, gal. *otc.*
Glandosane. (Kenwood Laboratories) Sodium carboxymethylcellulose 0.51 g, sorbitol 1.52 g, sodium Cl 0.043 g, potassium Cl 0.061 g, calcium Cl 0.007 g, magnesium Cl 0.003 g, dipotassium hydrogen phosphate 0.017 g/50 ml. Soln. Spray Bot. 50 ml. *otc.*
Use: Saliva substitute.
glandubolin.
See: Estrone (Various Mfr.).
•**glatiramer acetate.** (glah-TEER-ah-mer ASS-eh-tate) USAN.
Use: Multiple sclerosis; immunomodulator.
See: Copaxone Inj. (Teva Pharamaceuticals USA).
glauber's salt.
See: Sodium Sulfate (Various Mfr.).
Glaucon Solution. (Alcon Laboratories, Inc.) Epinephrine HCl 1%, 2%. Drop-Tainers. 10 ml. *Rx.*
Use: Antiglaucoma.
GlaucTabs. (Akorn, Inc.) Methazolamide 25 mg, 50 mg. Tab. Bot. 100s. *Rx.*
Use: Diuretic.
•**glaze, pharmaceutical.** N.F. 18.
Use: Pharmaceutic aid (tablet coating agent).
•**glemanserin.** (gleh-MAN-ser-in) USAN.
Use: Anxiolytic.
Gliadel. (Rhone-Poulenc Rorer Pharmaceuticals, Inc.) Carmustine (BCNU) 7.7 mg. Wafer. Single-dose treatment box with 8 individually pouched wafers. *Rx.*
Use: Alkylating agent.
•**gliamilide.** (glie-AM-ih-lide) USAN.
Use: Antidiabetic.
glibenclamide.
See: Glyburide.
•**glibornuride.** (glie-BORN-you-ride) USAN.
Use: Oral hypoglycemic agent; antidiabetic.
•**glicetanile sodium.** (glie-SET-AH-nile) USAN. *Formerly Glydanile Sodium.*
Use: Antidiabetic.
•**gliflumide.** (GLIH-flew-mide) USAN.
Use: Antidiabetic.
glim.
See: Gardinol Type Detergents (Various Mfr.).
•**glimepiride.** (GLIE-meh-pie-ride) USAN.
Use: Hypoglycemic.
See: Amaryl, Tab. (Hoechst Marion Roussel).
•**glipizide.** (GLIP-ih-zide) U.S.P. 23.
Use: Antidiabetic.
See: Glucotrol (Pfizer).
glipizide. (GLIP-ih-zide) (Various Mfr.) 5 mg, 10 mg/Tab. 100s, 500s, 1000s, UD 100s. *Rx.*

Use: Antidiabetic.

globulin, cytomegalovirus immune.
See: CytoGam, Vial (MedImmune, Inc.).

globulin, gamma.
See: Immune Globulin Intramuscular.
Immune Globulin Intravenous.

globulin, hepatitis b immune.
See: BayHep B (Bayer Corp. (Consumer Div.)).
H-BIG, Vial (Abbott Laboratories).

•**globulin, immune.** (GLAH-byoo-lin) U.S.P. 23. *Formerly Globulin, Immune Human Serum.*
Use: IM, measles prophylactic and polio; immunization.

globulin, immune, IV.
Use: Immunodeficiency; immune thrombocytopenia purpura; Kawasaki syndrome.
See: Gamimune N (Bayer Corp. (Consumer Div.)).
Gammagard S/D (Hyland Therapeutics).
Gammar-P IV (Centeon).
Iveegam (Immuno Therapy Co.).
Polygam S/D (American Red Cross).
Sandoglobulin (Novartis Pharmaceutical Corp.).
Venoglobulin-I (Alpha Therapeutic Corp.).
Venoglobulin-S (Alpha Therapeutic Corp.).

globulin, rabies immune.
Use: Immunization.
See: Bayrab (Bayer Corp. (Consumer Div.)).
Imogam Rabies (Pasteur Merieux Connaught).

globulin, rho (d) immune.
Use: Prevention of Rh isoimmunization; immune thrombocytopenic purpura.
See: BayRho D (Centeon).
Gamulin Rh (Centeon).
MICRhoGAM (Ortho McNeil Pharmaceutical).
Mini-Gamulin Rh (Centeon).
RhoGAM (Ortho McNeil Pharmaceutical).
WinRho SD (Univax Biologics).

•**globulin serum, anti-human.** U.S.P. 23.
Use: Immunization.

globulin, tetanus immune.
Use: Immunization.
See: Baytet (Bayer Corp. (Consumer Div.)).

globulin, vaccinia immune.
Use: Immunization.

globulin, varicella-zoster immune.
Use: Immunization.
See: varicella-zoster immune globulin (VZIG) (Mass. Public Health Bio. Lab.).

•**gloximonam.** (GLOX-ih-MOE-nam) USAN.
Use: Anti-infective.

glubionate calcium.
See: Neo-Calglucon, Syrup (Novartis Pharmaceutical Corp.).

GlucaGen. (Novo Nordisk) **Diagnostic Kit:** 1 vial containing glucagon (rDNA origin) 1 mg (1 IU) for Inj.; 1 vial containing sterile water for reconstitution 1 ml. **Emergency kit:** 1 vial containing glucagon (rDNA origin) 1 mg (1 IU) for Inj.; 1 vial containing sterile water for reconstitution. Lactose. Disp. Syr. and needle. *Rx.*
Use: Glucose-elevating agent, diagnostic aid, and emergency kit.

•**glucagon.** (GLUE-kuh-gahn) U.S.P. 23.
Use: Emergency treatment of hypoglycemia; antidiabetic.
See: GlucaGen (Novo Nordisk).

glucagon. (Eli Lilly and Co.) 1 unit/ml w/ diluent. 10 units w/10 ml diluent. Glucagon HCl 1 mg, 10 mg w/diluent; soln. contains lactose, glycerin 1.6% w/phenol 0.2% as a preservative. Vial.
Use: Hypoglycemic shock; antidiabetic.

Glucagon Emergency Kit. (Eli Lilly and Co.) Glucagon 1 mg, 10 mg, lactose w/ diluent. Inj. 1 ml, 10 ml. *Rx.*

Glucamide. (Teva Pharmaceuticals USA) Chlorpropamide 100 mg, 250 mg/Tab. Bot. 100s, 250s, 500s, 1000s, UD 100s. *Rx.*
Use: Antidiabetic.

•**gluceptate sodium.** (GLUE-sep-tate) USAN.
Use: Pharmaceutic aid.

Glucerna. (Ross Laboratories) Protein 41 g (amino acids), carbohydrate 93 g (hydrolyzed cornstarch, fructose, soy fiber), fat 55 g (high oleic safflower oil, soy oil, soy lecithin), sodium 917 mg (40 mEq), potassium 1542 mg (40 mEq), vitamins A, B_1, B_2, B_3, B_5, B_6, B_{12}, C, D, E, K, folic acid, Cl, Ca, P, Mg, I, Mn, Cu, Zn, Fe, Se, Cr, Mo, biotin, choline. Liq. Can 240 ml, Cont. 1 L. Ready-to-use. *otc.*
Use: Nutritional supplement.

glucocerebrosidase-beta-glucosidase.
Use: Treatment of Gaucher's disease.
See: Ceredase, Inj. (Genzyme Corp.).

glucocerebrosidase (PEG).
See: PEG-glucocerebrosidase.

glucocerebrosidase, recombinant retroviral vector. (Genetic Therapy, Inc.)
Use: Treatment for Gaucher's disease. [Orphan Drug]

glucocorticoids.
See: Cortical Hormone Products.

Glucolet Automatic Lancing Device. (Bayer Corp. (Consumer Div.)) To obtain sample for blood glucose testing. Automatic spring-loaded lancing device.
Use: Diagnostic aid.

Glucolet Endcaps. (Bayer Corp. (Consumer Div.)) To obtain sample for blood glucose testing. Controls depth of lancet penetration. Regular or super puncture.
Use: Diagnostic aid.

Glucometer II Blood Glucose Meter. (Bayer Corp. (Consumer Div.)) Electronic meter for blood glucose testing. *otc.*
Use: Diagnostic aid.

d-gluconic acid, calcium salt. Calcium Gluconate.

gluconic acid salts.
See: Calcium Gluconate.
Ferrous Gluconate.
Magnesium Gluconate.
Potassium Gluconate.

•**gluconolactone.** (glue-koe-no-LACK-tone) U.S.P. 23.
Use: Chelating agent.

Glucophage. (Bristol-Myers Squibb) Metformin HCl 500 mg or 850 mg/Tab. Bot. 100s, 300s (850 mg only), 500s (500 mg only). *Rx.*
Use: Antidiabetic.

•**glucosamine.** (glue-KOSE-ah-meen) USAN.
Use: Pharmaceutic aid.
W/Tetracycline.
See: Tetracyn, Cap., Syr. (Roerig).
W/Oxytetracycline.
See: Terramycin, Prep. (Pfizer US Pharmaceutical Group).

glucose.
See: Glutose, Gel (Paddock Laboratories).
Insta-Glucose, Gel (ICN Pharmaceuticals, Inc.).

glucose-elevating agents.
See: B-D Glucose, Chew. Tab. (Becton Dickinson & Co.).
Insta-Glucose, Gel (ICN Pharmaceuticals, Inc.).
Glucagon, Pow. for Inj. (Eli Lilly and Co.).
Glutose, Gel (Paddock Laboratories).
Insta-Glucose, Gel (ICN Pharmaceuticals, Inc.).
Insulin Reaction, Gel (Sherwood Davis & Geck).
Proglycem, Cap, Oral Susp. (Medical Market).

glucose enzymatic test strip.
Use: Diagnostic aid (in vitro, reducing sugars in urine).

glucose (hk) reagent strips. Reagent strip test for detection of glucose in serum or plasma. Bot. 50s.
Use: Diagnostic aid.

Glucose & Ketone Urine Test. (Major Pharmaceuticals) Reagent test for glucose and ketones in urine. Bot. 100s.
Use: Diagnostic aid.

•**glucose, liquid.** (GLUE-kose) N.F. 18.
Use: As a 5% to 50% solution as nutrient; for acute hepatitis and dehydration; to increase blood volume; pharmaceutic aid (tablet binder, tablet coating agent).

d-glucose, monohydrate. Dextrose.

glucose oxidase.
W/peroxidase, potassium iodide.
See: Diastix, Vial, Tab. (Bayer Corp (Consumer Div.)).

glucose polymers.
See: Polycose, Pow., Liq. (Ross Laboratories).

Glucose Reagent Strips. (Bayer Corp. (Consumer Div.)) A quantitative strip test for glucose in serum or plasma. Seralyzer reagent strips. Bot. 50s.
Use: Diagnostic aid.

glucose test.
See: Combistix (Bayer Corp. (Consumer Div.)).
First Choice, Strips (Polymer Technology Inc.).
Glucose Reagent Strips (Bayer Corp. (Consumer Div.)).

Glucostix Reagent Strips. (Bayer Corp. (Consumer Div.)) Cellulose strip containing glucose oxidase and indicator system. Bot. 50s, 100s, UD 25s. *otc.*
Use: Diagnostic aid.

glucosulfone sodium, injection.
See: Sodium Glucosulfone Injection.

Gluco System Lancets. (Bayer Corp. (Consumer Div.)) Disposable lancets for use in Miles Diagnostic Autolet or Glucolet.
Use: Diagnostic aid.

Glucotrol. (Pfizer US Pharmaceutical Group) Glipizide 5 mg, 10 mg, lactose/Tab. Bot. 100s, 500s, UD 100s. *Rx.*
Use: Antidiabetic.

Glucotrol XL. (Pfizer US Pharmaceutical Group) Glipizide 5 mg, 10 mg. ER Tab. Bot. 100s, 500s. *Rx.*
Use: Antidiabetic.

Glucovite. (Pal-Pak, Inc.) Ferrous gluconate 260 mg, vitamins B_1 1 mg, B_2 0.5 mg, C 10 mg/Tab. Bot. 1000s, 5000s. *otc.*
Use: Mineral, vitamin supplement.

glucurolactone. Gamma lactone of glucofuranuronic acid.

Glu-K. (Western Research) Potassium gluconate 486 mg/Tab. Bot. 1000s. *otc.*
Use: Electrolyte supplement.

gluside.
See: Saccharin (Various Mfr.).

•**glutamic acid.** USAN.
Use: Nutritional supplement.
See: Glutamic Acid Tab. (Various Mfr.).
Glutamic Acid Pow. (J. R. Carlson Laboratories).

Glutamic Acid Tablets. (Various Mfr.) 500 mg. In 100s, 500s. *otc.*
Use: Nutritional supplement.

Glutamic Acid Powder. (J. R. Carlson Laboratories) Bot. 100 g. *otc.*
Use: Nutritional supplement.

glutamic acid hydrochloride. Acidogen, aciglumin, glutasin. *otc.*
Use: Gastric acidifier.

glutamic acid salts.
See: Calcium Glutamate (Various Mfr.).

glutamine. (Nutritional Restart)
Use: Treatment of short bowel syndrome. [Orphan Drug]

•**glutaral concentrate.** (GLUE-tah-ral) U.S.P. 23.
Use: Disinfectant.
See: Cidex (Surgikos).

glutaraldehyde.
Use: Sterilizing, disinfecting agent.
See: Cidex (J & J Medical).
Cidex-7 (J & J Medical).
Cidex Plus (J & J Medical).

Glutarex-1. (Ross Laboratories) Protein 15 g, fat 23.9 g, carbohydrates 46.3 g, linoleic acid 1800 mg, Fe 9 mg, Na 190 mg, K 675 mg, Ca, vitamins A, B_1, B_2, B_3, B_5, B_6, B_{12}, C, D, E, K, biotin, choline, folic acid, inositol, Cl, Cu, I, Mg, Mn, P, Se, Zn and 480 Cal per 100 g. Lysine and tryptophan free. Pow. Can 350 g. *otc.*
Use: Nutritional supplement.

Glutarex-2. (Ross Laboratories) Protein 30 g, fat 15.5 g, carbohydrates 30 g, Fe 13 mg, Na 880 mg, K 1370 mg, Ca, vitamins A, B_1, B_2, B_3, B_5, B_6, B_{12}, C, D, E, K, biotin, choline, folic acid, inositol, Cl, Cu, I, Mg, Mn, P, Se, Zn and 410 Cal per 100 g. Lysine and tryptophan free. Pow. Can 325 g. *otc.*
Use: Nutritional supplement.

l-glutathione.
Use: Treatment of AIDS-associated cachexia. [Orphan Drug]
See: Cachexon (Telluride Pharm. Corp.).

•**glutethimide.** (glue-TETH-ih-mide) U.S.P. 23.
Use: Hypnotic, sedative.

Glutofac. (Kenwood Laboratories) Vitamins A 500 IU, E 30 IU, B_1 15 mg, B_2 10 mg, B_3 50 mg, B_5 20 mg, B_6 50 mg, C 300 mg, Zn 5 mg, Ca, Cr, Cu, Fe, K, Mg, Mn, P, Se/Capl. Bot. 90s. *otc.*
Use: Mineral, vitamin supplement.

Glutol. (Paddock Laboratories) Dextrose 100 g/180 ml. Bot. 180 ml.
Use: Diagnostic aid.

Glutose. (Paddock Laboratories) Liquid glucose (40% dextrose). Concentrated glucose for insulin reactions. Gel. Bot. 60 g. *otc.*
Use: Hyperglycemic.

Glyate. (Geneva Pharmaceuticals) Guaifenesin 100 mg/5 ml, alcohol 3.5%. Syr. Bot. 118 ml, 480 ml. *otc.*
Use: Expectorant.

•**glyburide.** (glie-BYOO-ride) U.S.P. 23.
Use: Antidiabetic.
See: DiaBeta (Hoechst Marion Roussel).
Glynase, PresTab. (Pharmacia & Upjohn).
Micronase, Tab. (Pharmacia & Upjohn).

glyburide. (Various Mfr.) **1.25 mg:** Tab. Bot. 50s, 100s, 500s. **2.5 & 5 mg:** Tab. Bot. 90s, 100s, 500s, 1000s, UD 100s; Blister pack 25s, 100s, 600s. *Rx.*
Use: Antidiabetic.

glyburide, micronized. (Various Mfr.) Micronized glyburide 1.5 mg, 3 mg, 4.5 mg, 6 mg. Tab. Bot. 100s, 500s (except 4.5 mg), 1000s, UD 100s (1.5 mg and 3 mg only). *Rx.*
Use: Antidiabetic.

Glycate Chewables. (Forest Pharmaceutical, Inc.) Glycine 150 mg, calcium carbonate 300 mg/Chew. Tab. Bot. 1000s. *otc.*
Use: Antacid.

•**glycerin.** (GLIH-suh-rin) U.S.P. 23.
Use: Pharmaceutic aid (humectant, solvent).
See: Corn Huskers Lot. (Warner Lambert).
Ophthalgan Ophthalmic, Soln. (Wyeth-Ayerst Laboratories).
Osmoglyn (Alcon Laboratories, Inc.).
W/Dimethicone.
See: Dermasil, Lot. (Chesebrough-Ponds USA, Inc.).

glycerin. (Various Mfr.) Various concentrations from 10% to > 95% for use as sterile allergen-extract diluents.

glycerin suppositories. (Various Mfr.) Glycerin, sodium stearate. *otc.*
Use: Rectal evacuant, cathartic.

glycerol.
See: Glycerin.

•**glycerol, iodinated.** (GLIH-ser-ole EYE-oh-dih-nay-tehd) USAN.
Use: Expectorant.

•**glyceryl behenate.** N.F. 18.
Use: Pharmaceutic aid (tablet/capsule lubricant).

glyceryl guaiacolate.
Use: Expectorant.
See: Guaifenesin, U.S.P. 23.

glyceryl guaiacolate carbamate. Methocarbamol.
See: Robaxin, Tab., Inj. (Wyeth-Ayerst Laboratories).
Robaxin 750, Tab. (Wyeth-Ayerst Laboratories).

glyceryl guaiacolether.
See: Guaifenesin.

•**glyceryl monostearate.** N.F. 18.
Use: Pharmaceutic aid (emulsifying agent).

Glyceryl-T Capsules. (Rugby Labs, Inc.) Theophylline 150 mg, guaifenesin 90 mg/Cap. Bot. 100s. *Rx.*
Use: Bronchodilator, expectorant.

Glyceryl-T Liquid. (Rugby Labs, Inc.) Theophylline 150 mg, guaifenesin 90 mg/15 ml. Liq. Bot. 480 ml. *Rx.*
Use: Bronchodilator, expectorant.

glyceryl triacetate.
See: Triacetin.

glyceryl triacetin. (Various Mfr.) Triacetin.
See: Fungacetin, Oint., Liq. (Blair Labs.).

glyceryl trierucate.
Use: Adrenoleukodystrophy. [Orphan Drug]

glyceryl trinitrate ointment.
See: Nitrol, Oint. (Kremers Urban).

glyceryl trinitrate tablets.
See: Nitroglycerin, Tab. (Various Mfr.).
Nitroglyn, Tab. (Key Corp).

glyceryl trioleate.
Use: Adrenoleukodystrophy. [Orphan Drug]

Glycets-Antacid Tablets. (Weeks & Leo) Calcium carbonate 350 mg, simethicone 25 mg/Chew. Tab. Bot. 100s. *otc.*
Use: Antacid, antiflatulent.

glycinato dihydroxyaluminum hydrate.
See: Dihydroxyaluminum Aminoacetate, U.S.P. 23.

•**glycine.** (GLIE-seen) U.S.P. 23. *Formerly Aminoacetic Acid.*
Use: Myasthenia gravis treatment, irrigating solution.
W/Aluminum hydroxide-magnesium carbonate coprecipitated gel.
See: Glycogel, Tab., Susp. (Schwarz Pharma, Inc.).
W/Calcium Carbonate.
See: Antacid No. 6, Tab. (Jones Medical Industries, Inc.).
Glycate Chewables, Tab. (O'Neal).
Titralac, Liq., Tab. (3M Pharm.).
W/Calcium carbonate, amylolytic, proteolytic cellulolytic enzymes.
See: Co-gel, Tab. (Arco Pharmaceuticals, Inc.).
W/Chlor-Trimeton, sodium salicylate.
See: Corilin, Liq. (Schering-Plough Corp.).
W/Glutamic acid, alanine.
See: Prostall, Cap. (Metabolic Prods.).

glycine, aluminum salt.
See: Dihydroxyaluminum Aminoacetate, U.S.P. 23.

glycine hydrochloride. (Various Mfr.)
Use: Gastric acidifier.

glycobiarsol.
Use: Amebiasis, *Trichomonas vaginalis, Monilia albicans.*

glycocoll. Glycine.
See: Aminoacetic Acid (Various Mfr.).

glycocyamine. Guanidoacetic acid.

Glycofed. (Pal-Pak, Inc.) Pseudoephedrine 30 mg, guaifenesin 100 mg. Tab. Bot. 1000s. *otc.*
Use: Decongestant, expectorant.

•**glycol distearate.** (GLIE-kole dih-STEE-ah-rate) USAN.
Use: Pharmaceutic aid (thickening agent).

glycol monosalicylate.
W/Oil of mustard, camphor, menthol, methyl salicylate.
See: Musterole, Oint., Cream (Schering-Plough Corp.).

glycophenylate bromide.
See: Mepenzolate Methylbromide.

•**glycopyrrolate.** (glie-koe-PIE-row-late) U.S.P. 23.
Use: Anticholinergic.
See: Robinul, Tab., Inj. (Wyeth-Ayerst Laboratories).
Robinul Forte, Tab. (Wyeth-Ayerst Laboratories).

Glycotuss. (Pal-Pak, Inc.) Guaifenesin 100 mg/Tab. Bot. 100s, 1000s. *otc.*
Use: Expectorant.

Glycotuss-dM. (Pal-Pak, Inc.) Guaifenesin 100 mg, dextromethorphan HBr 10 mg/Tab. Bot. 100s, 1000s. *otc.*
Use: Antitussive, expectorant.

glycyrrhiza. Pure extract, Fluidextract. Licorice root.
Use: Flavoring agent.

glycyrrhiza extract, pure.
Use: Flavoring agent.

glycyrrhiza fluid extract.
Use: Flavoring agent.

glydanile sodium. (GLIE-dah-neel SO-dee-uhm)
Use: Antidiabetic.

•**glyhexamide.** (glie-HEX-ah-mid) USAN.
Use: Antidiabetic.

Glylorin. (Cellegy Pharmaceuticals, Inc.) Monolaurin.
Use: Congenital primary ichthyosis. [Orphan Drug]

•**glymidine sodium.** (GLIE-mih-deen) USAN.
Use: Oral hypoglycemic agent; antidiabetic.

glymol.
See: Petrolatum Liquid (Various Mfr.).

Glynase PresTab. (Pharmacia & Upjohn) Glyburide (micronized) **1.5 mg:** Tab. Bot. 100s, UD 100s. **3 mg:** Tab. Bot. 100s, 500s, 1000s, UD 100s. **6 mg:** Tab. Bot. 100s, 500s. *Rx.*
Use: Antidiabetic.

•**glyoctamide.** (glie-OCKT-am-id) USAN.
Use: Hypoglycemic agent; antidiabetic.

Gly-Oxide. (SmithKline Beecham Consumer Healthcare) Carbamide peroxide 10% in flavored anhydrous glycerol. Liq. Bot. 15 ml, 60 ml. *otc.*
Use: Mouth and throat preparation.

glyoxyldiureide.
See: Allantoin (Various Mfr.).

•**glyparamide.** (glie-PAR-am-ide) USAN.
Use: Oral hypoglycemic agent; antidiabetic.

Glypressin. (Ferring Pharmaceuticals, Inc.) Terlipressin.
Use: Bleeding esophageal varicies. [Orphan Drug]

Glyset. (Bayer Corp. (Consumer Div.)) Miglitol 25 mg, 50 mg, 100 mg/Tab. Bot. 100s, 1000s (except 25 mg), UD 100. *Rx.*
Use: Antidiabetic.

Glytuss. (Merz Pharmaceuticals) Guaifenesin 200 mg/Tab. Bot. 100s. *otc.*
Use: Expectorant.

GM-CSF. Granulocyte macrophage colony-stimulating factor.
See: Leukine (Immunex Corp.).

G-myticin Creme and Ointment. (Pedinol Pharmacal, Inc.) Gentamicin sulfate equivalent to gentamicin base 1 mg. Tube 15 g. *Rx.*
Use: Anti-infective, topical.

gododiamide.
Use: Diagnostic aid.

Go-Evac. (Copley Pharmaceutical, Inc.) Polyethylene glycol 3350 59 g, sodium sulfate 5.685 g, sodium bicarbonate 1.685 g, sodium chloride 1.465 g, potassium chloride 0.743 g/L. Pow. for soln. Jug 4 L. *Rx.*
Use: Bowel evacuants.

Golacol. (Arcum) Codeine sulfate 30 mg, papaverine HCl 30 mg, emetine HCl 2 mg, ephedrine HCl 15 mg, q.s./30 ml. Alcohol 6.25%. Syr. Bot. 4 oz, 16 oz, gal. Orange flavor. *c-III.*
Use: Antitussive, bronchodilator.

Gold Alka-Seltzer Effervescent. (Bayer Corp. (Consumer Div.)) Sodium bicarbonate (heat treated) 958 mg, citric acid 832 mg, potassium bicarbonate 312 mg/Tab. 20s, 36s. *otc.*
Use: Antacid.

•**gold Au^{198}.** USAN, U.S.P. XX.
Use: Antineoplastic, diagnostic aid (liver imaging), radiopharmaceutical.
See: Radio Gold (Au^{198}).

gold Au 198 injection.
Use: Antineoplastic; diagnostic for liver scanning.

gold compounds.
See: Gold Sodium Thiosulfate (Various Mfr.).
Ridaura, Cap. (SmithKline Beecham Pharmaceuticals).
Solganal, Vial (Schering-Plough Corp.).

Gold Seal Calcium 600. (Walgreen Co.) Calcium 1200 mg/Tab. Bot. 60s. *otc.*
Use: Mineral supplement.

Gold Seal Calcium 600 with Vitamin D. (Walgreen Co.) Calcium 1200 mg, vitamin D/Tab. Bot. 60s. *otc.*
Use: Mineral supplement.

Gold Seal Chewable Vitamin C. (Walgreen Co.) Ascorbic acid 250 mg, 500 mg/Tab. Bot. 100s. *otc.*
Use: Vitamin supplement.

Gold Seal Ferrous Gluconate. (Walgreen Co.) Iron 37 mg/Tab. Bot. 100s. *otc.*
Use: Mineral supplement.

Gold Seal Ferrous Sulfate. (Walgreen Co.) Ferrous sulfate 325 mg/Tab. Bot. 100s, 1000s. *otc.*
Use: Mineral supplement.

Gold Seal Time Release Ferrous Sulfate. (Walgreen Co.) Iron 50 mg/Tab. Bot. 100s. *otc.*
Use: Mineral supplement.

•**gold sodium thiomalate.** (gold SO-dee-uhm thigh-oh-MAL-ate) U.S.P. 23.
Use: Antirheumatic.
See: Aurolate, Inj. (Taylor Pharmaceuticals).

gold sodium thiosulfate. Sterile, Auricidine, Aurocidin, Aurolin, Auropin, Aurosan, Novacrysin, Solfocrisol, Thiochrysine.
Use: Antirheumatic.

gold thioglucose.
See: Aurothioglucose, U.S.P. 23.

Golden-West Compound. (Golden-West) Gentian root, licorice root, cascara sagrada, damiana leaves, senna leaves, psyllium seed, buchu leaves, crude pepsin. Box 1.5 oz. *otc.*
Use: Laxative.

Goldicide Concentrate. (Pedinol Pharmacal, Inc.) Bot. (Conc.) oz. Ctn. 10s.
Use: Distinfectant.

GoLYTELY. (Braintree Laboratories, Inc.) Pow. for oral soln. after reconstitution containing PEG-3350 236 g, sodium sulfate 22.74 g, sodium bicarbonate 6.74 g, sodium Cl 5.86 g, potassium Cl 2.97 g when made up to 4 L. Disposable container 4800 ml. *Rx.*
Use: Bowel evacuant.

gonacrine.
See: Acriflavine (Various Mfr.).

•**gonadorelin acetate.** (go-NAD-oh-RELL-in) USAN. *Formerly Luteinizing Hormone-releasing Factor Diacetate Tetrahydrate.*
Use: Gonad-stimulating principle. [Orphan Drug]
See: Cryptolin Prods. (Hoechst Marion Roussel).
Lutrepulse (Ferring Labs).

•**gonadorelin hydrochloride.** (go-NAD-oh-RELL-in) USAN. *Formerly Luteinizing Hormone-releasing Factor Dihydrochloride.*
Use: Gonad-stimulating principle.

gonadotropic substance.
See: Gonadotropin Chorionic.

gonadotropins.
See: Pergonal, Pow. for Inj. (Serono Laboratories, Inc.).

•**gonadotropin, chorionic.** (go-NAD-oh-TROE-pin, core-ee-AHN-ik) U.S.P. 23.
Use: Gonad-stimulating principle. In the female: Chronic cystic mastitis, functional sterility, dysmenorrhea, premenstrual tension, threatened abortion. In the male: Cryptorchidism, hypogenitalism, dwarfism, impotency, enuresis.
See: Android HCG, Inj. (Zeneca Pharmaceuticals).
Antuitrin "S", Vial (Parke-Davis).
A.P.L., Secules (Wyeth-Ayerst Laboratories).
Corgonject, Vial (Merz Pharmaceuticals).
Follutein Pow. (Bristol-Myers Squibb).
Libigen, Vial (Savage Laboratories).
Pregnyl, Amp. (Organon Teknika Corp.).

gonadotropin, pituitary ant. lobe. Extracted from anterior lobe of equine pituitaries (not pregnant mare urine) (rat unit = 1 Fevold-Hisaw unit).

gonadotropin-releasing hormone analog.
See: Lupron, Inj., Susp. (Tap Pharmaceuticals).
Zoladex, Implant (Zeneca Pharmaceuticals).

gonadotropin releasing hormones.
See: Lutrepulse, Pow. for Inj. (Ortho McNeil Pharmaceutical).
Supprelin, Inj. (Ortho McNeil Pharmaceutical).
Synarel, Soln. (Roche Laboratories).

gonadotropin serum. Pregnant mare's serum.

Gonak. (Akorn, Inc.) Hydroxypropyl methylcellulose 2.5%. Soln. Bot. 15 ml. *otc.*
Use: Ophthalmic.

Gonal-F. (Serono Laboratories, Inc.) Follitropin alfa 75 IU, 150 IU, sucrose 30 mg. Inj. Amp. 1s, 10s. 100s, with diluent. *Rx.*
Use: Ovulation induction.

Gonic. (Roberts Pharmaceuticals) Chorionic gonadotropin 10,000 units w/diluent/vial. Pow. for Inj. Vial 10 ml. *Rx.*
Use: Hormone, chorionic gonadotropin.

gonioscopic hydroxypropyl methylcellulose.
See: Goniosol Lacrivial, Soln. (Smith, Miller & Patch).

Gonioscopic Solution. (Alcon Laboratories, Inc.) Hydroxyethyl cellulose. Drop-Tainer 15 ml. *Rx.*
Use: Ophthalmic.

Goniosol. (Ciba Vision) Gonioscopic hydroxypropyl methylcellulose 2.5%. Bot. 15 ml. *otc.*
Use: Ophthalmic.

Gonodecten Test Kit. (United States Packaging) Tube test for urethral discharge from males, for detection of *Neisseria gonorrhoeae.* Test kit 10s, 25s.
Use: Diagnostic aid.

gonorrhea tests.
See: Biocult-GC (Orion Diagnostica).
Gonodecten Test Kit (United States Packaging).
Gonozyme Diagnostic Kit (Abbott Laboratories).
Isocult for *Neisseria gonorrhoeae* (SmithKline Diagnostics).
MicroTrak *Neisseria gonorrhoeae* Culture Test (Syva Co.).

Gonozyme. (Abbott Diagnostics) Enzyme immunoassay for detection of

Neisseria gonorrhoeae in urogenital swab specimens. Test kit 100s.
Use: Diagnostic aid.

Good Samaritan Ointment. (Good Samaritan) Tube 1.25 oz. *otc.*
Use: Counterirritant.

Goody's Headache Powders. (Goody's Manufacturing Corp.) Aspirin 520 mg, acetaminophen 260 mg, caffeine 32.5 mg/dose. Pow. Pkg. 2s, 6s, 24s, 50s. *otc.*
Use: Analgesic.

Gordobalm. (Gordon Laboratories) Chloroxylenol, methyl salicylate, menthol, camphor, thymol, eucalyptus oil, isopropyl alcohol 16%, fast-drying gum base. Bot. 4 oz, gal. *otc.*
Use: Analgesic, topical.

Gordochom. (Gordon Laboratories) Undecylenic acid 25%, chloroxylenol 3%, penetrating oil base. Liq. Bot. 15 ml, 30 ml w/applicator. *otc.*
Use: Antifungal, topical.

Gordofilm. (Gordon Laboratories) Salicylic acid 16.7%, lactic acid 16.7% in flexible colloidan. Bot. 15 ml. *otc.*
Use: Keratolytic.

Gordogesic Cream. (Gordon Laboratories) Methyl salicylate 10% in absorption base. Jar 2.5 oz, 1 lb. *otc.*
Use: Analgesic, topical.

Gordomatic Crystals. (Gordon Laboratories) Sodium borate, sodium bicarbonate, sodium Cl, thymol, menthol, eucalyptus oil. Jar 8 oz, 7 lb. *otc.*
Use: Counterirritant.

Gordomatic Lotion. (Gordon Laboratories) Menthol, camphor, propylene glycol, isopropyl alcohol. Bot. 1 oz, 4 oz, gal. *otc.*
Use: Counterirritant.

Gordomatic Powder. (Gordon Laboratories) Menthol, thymol camphor, eucalyptus oil, salicylic acid, alum bentonite, talc. Shaker can 3.5 oz. Can 1 lb, 5 lb. *otc.*
Use: Counterirritant.

Gordon's Urea. (Gordon Laboratories) Urea 40% in petrolatum base. Jar oz. *Rx.*
Use: Emollient.

Gordophene. (Gordon Laboratories) Neutral coconut oil soap 15%, glycerin with Septi-Chlor (trichlorohydroxy diphenyl ether) broad-spectrum antimicrobial and bacteriostatic agent. Bot. 4 oz, gal.
Use: Dermatologic, cleanser.

Gordo-Vite A Creme. (Gordon Laboratories) Vitamin A 100,000 IU/oz. in water-soluble base. Jar 0.5 oz, 2.5 oz, 4 oz, lb, 5 lb. *otc.*
Use: Emollient.

Gordo-Vite A Lotion. (Gordon Laboratories) Vitamin A 100,000 IU/oz. Plastic bot. 4 oz, gal. *otc.*
Use: Emollient.

Gordo-Vite E Creme. (Gordon Laboratories) Vitamin E 1500 IU/oz in water-soluble base. Jar 2.5 oz, lb. *otc.*
Use: Emollient.

Gormel Cream. (Gordon Laboratories) Urea 20% in emollient base. Jar 0.5 oz, 2.5 oz, 4 oz, 1 lb, 5 lb. *otc.*
Use: Emollient.

•**goserelin.** (GO-suh-REH-lin) USAN.
Use: LHRH agonist.
See: Zoladex, Implant (Zeneca Pharmaceuticals).

goserelin acetate. (GO-suh-REH-lin ASS-uh-TATE)
Use: Gonadotropin-releasing hormone analog.
See: Zoladex, Implant (Zeneca Pharmaceuticals).

gossypol.
Use: Antineoplastic. [Orphan Drug]

gotamine. (Vita Elixir) Ergotamine tartrate 1 mg, caffeine 100 mg/Tab. *Rx.*
Use: Antimigraine.

gout, agents for.
See: Allopurinol, Tab. (Various Mfr.).
Anturane, Tab., Cap. (Novartis Pharmaceutical Corp.).
Benemid, Tab. (Merck & Co.).
Colchicine, Inj. (Eli Lilly and Co.).
Colchicine, Tab. (Various Mfr.).
Col-Probenecid, Tab. (Various Mfr.).
Proben-C, Tab. (Various Mfr.).
Probenecid, Tab. (Various Mfr.).
Probenecid w/Colchicine, Tab. (Various Mfr.).
Sulfinpyrazone, Tab., Cap. (Various Mfr.).
Zyloprim, Tab. (GlaxoWellcome).

•**govafilcon a.** (GO-vaff-ILL-kahn A) USAN.
Use: Contact lens material (hydrophilic).

gp 100 adenoviral gene therapy. (Genzyme Corp.)
Use: Antineoplastic. [Orphan Drug]

GP-500. (Marnel Pharmaceuticals, Inc.) Pseudoephedrine HCl 120 mg, guaifenesin 500 mg. Tab. Bot. 100s. *Rx.*
Use: Decongestant, expectorant.

•**gramicidin.** (gram-ih-SIH-din) U.S.P. 23.
Use: Anti-infective.
W/Neomycin.
See: Spectrocin, Oint. (Bristol-Myers Squibb).
W/Neomycin sulfate, polymyxin B sulfate, thimerosal.

See: Neo-Polycin Ophthalmic Soln. (Hoechst Marion Roussel).
W/Neomycin sulfate, polymyxin B sulfate, benzocaine.
See: Mycolog Cream, Oint. (Bristol-Myers Squibb).
W/Polymyxin B sulfate, neomycin sulfate.
See: AK-Spore Ophth. Soln. (Akorn, Inc.).
Neosporin, Ophth. Soln. (GlaxoWellcome).
Neosporin-G, Cream (GlaxoWellcome).
Ocutricin, Ophth. Soln. (Bausch & Lomb Pharmaceuticals).
W/Polymyxin B sulfate, neomycin sulfate, hydrocortisone acetate.
See: Cortisporin, Cream (GlaxoWellcome).

•**granisetron.** (gran-IH-SEH-trahn) USAN.
Use: Antiemetic.
See: Kytril, Inj. (SmithKline Beecham Pharmaceuticals).

•**granisetron hydrochloride.** (gran-IH-SEH-trahn) USAN.
Use: Antiemetic.
See: Kytril Inj. (SmithKline Beecham Pharmaceuticals).

Granulderm. (Copley Pharmaceutical, Inc.) Trypsin 0.1 mg, balsam Peru 72.5 mg, castor oil 650 mg/0.82 ml. Aerosol Spray 113.4 g. *Rx.*
Use: Enzyme, topical.

Granulex. (Hickam) Trypsin 0.1 mg, balsam Peru 72.5 mg, castor oil 650 mg w/ emulsifier/0.82 ml. Spray Can 2 oz, 4 oz. *Rx.*
Use: Dermatologic, wound therapy.

granulocyte colony-stimulating factor.
See: Neupogen (Amgen, Inc.).

granulocyte macrophage colony-stimulating factor.
See: Leukine (Immunex Corp.).

gratus strophanthin. Ouabain.

Gravineed. (Hanlon) Vitamins C 100 mg, E 10 IU, B_1 3 mg, B_2 2 mg, B_6 10 mg, B_{12} 5 mcg, A 4000 IU, D 400 IU, niacin 10 mg, folic acid 0.1 mg, iron fumarate 40 mg, calcium 67 mg/Cap. Bot. 100s. *otc.*
Use: Mineral, vitamin supplement.

Green mint. (Block Drug Co., Inc.) Urea, glycine, polysorbate 60, sorbitol, alcohol 12.2%, peppermint oil, menthol, chlorophyllin-copper complex. Bot. 7 oz, 12 oz. *otc.*
Use: Mouth and throat preparation.

green soap.
Use: Detergent.

•**grepafloxacin hydrochloride.** (grep-ah-FLOX-ah-sin) USAN.
Use: Antibacterial.
See: Raxar, Tab. (GlaxoWellcome).

Grifulvin V. (Advanced Care Products) Griseofulvin microsize. **Tab:** 250 mg. Bot. 100s; 500 mg. Bot. 100s, 500s. **Susp:** 125 mg/5 ml. Bot. 120 ml. *Rx.*
Use: Antifungal.

Grisactin Ultra. (Wyeth-Ayerst Laboratories) Griseofulvin ultramicrosize 125 mg, 250 mg,or 330 mg/Tab. Bot. 100s. *Rx.*
Use: Antifungal.

•**griseofulvin.** (griss-ee-oh-FULL-vin) U.S.P. 23.
Use: Antifungal.
See: Fulvicin P/G, Tab. (Schering-Plough Corp.).
Fulvicin U/F, Tab. (Schering-Plough Corp.).
Grifulvin V, Tab., Susp. (Ortho McNeil Pharmaceutical).
Grisactin, Cap., Tab. (Wyeth-Ayerst Laboratories).
Grisactin Ultra, Tab. (Wyeth-Ayerst Laboratories).

griseofulvin. (Various Mfr.) 165 mg or 330 mg. Tab. Bot. 100s.
Use: Antifungal.

griseofulvin microcrystalline.
Use: Antifungal.
See: Fulvicin U/F, Tab. (Schering-Plough Corp.).
Grifulvin V, Tab., Susp. (Ortho McNeil Pharmaceutical).
Grisactin, Cap., Tab. (Wyeth-Ayerst Laboratories).

griseofulvin, ultramicrosize. (Various Mfr.) Griseofulvin ultramicrosize 165 mg and 330 mg/Tab. Bot. 100s.
Use: Antifungal.
See: Fulvicin P/G, Tab. (Schering-Plough Corp.).
Grisactin Ultra, Tab. (Wyeth-Ayerst Laboratories).
Gris-PEG, Tab. (Allergan, Inc.).

Gris-PEG. (Allergan, Inc.) Griseofulvin ultramicrosize 125 mg or 250 mg/Tab. Bot. 100s, 500s (250 mg only). *Rx.*
Use: Antifungal.

group b streptococcus immune globulin. (North American Biologicals, Inc.)
Use: Anti-infective. [Orphan Drug]

growth hormone. Extract of human pituitaries containing predominantly growth hormone.
See: Crescormon.

growth hormone releasing factor. (ICN Pharmaceuticals, Inc.)
Use: Long-term treatment of growth failure. [Orphan Drug]

g-strophanthin. Ouabain.

guaiacol carbonate. (Various Mfr.) Duotal.
Use: Expectorant.

guaiacol glyceryl ether.
See: Guaifenesin.

guaiacol potassium sulfonate. *Rx.*
See: Bronchial, Syr. (DePree).
W/Ammonium Cl, sodium citrate, benzyl alcohol, carbinoxamine maleate.
See: Clistin Expectorant, Syr. (Ortho McNeil Pharmaceutical).
W/Dextromethorphan HBr.
See: Bronchial DM, Syr. (DePree).
W/Pheniramine maleate, pyrilamine maleate, codeine phosphate.
See: Tritussin, Syr. (Towne).

guaianesin.
Use: Expectorant.
See: Guaifenesin.

•**guaiapate.** (GWIE-ah-pate) USAN.
Use: Antitussive.

Guaifed Capsules. (Muro Pharmaceutical, Inc.) Guaifenesin 250 mg, pseudoephedrine HCl 120 mg/TR Cap. Bot. 100s, 500s. *Rx.*
Use: Decongestant, expectorant.

Guaifed-PD Capsules. (Muro Pharmaceutical, Inc.) Pseudoephedrine HCl 60 mg, guaifenesin 300 mg/TR Cap. Bot. 100s, 500s. *Rx.*
Use: Decongestant, expectorant.

Guaifed Syrup. (Muro Pharmaceutical, Inc.) Pseudoephedrine HCl 30 mg, guaifenesin 200 mg/5 ml. Bot. 118 ml, 473 ml. *Rx.*
Use: Decongestant, expectorant.

•**guaifenesin.** (GWIE-fen-ah-sin) U.S.P. 23. *Formerly Glyceryl Guaiacolate.* Synonyms: Glyceryl guaiacolate, glyceryl guaiacol ether, guaianesin, guaifylline, guayanesin.
Use: Expectorant.
See: Anti-tuss, Liq. (Century Pharmaceuticals, Inc.).
Consin-GG, Syr. (Wisconsin Pharmacal Co.).
Diabetic Tussin EX, Liq. (Health Care Products).
Duratuss-G, Tab. (UCB Pharmaceuticals, Inc.).
2/G, Liq. (Hoechst Marion Roussel).
G-100, Syr. (Sanofi Winthrop Pharmaceuticals).
GG-Cen, Syr. (Schwarz Pharma, Inc.).
Glycotuss, Tab., Syr. (Pal-Pak, Inc.).
Glytuss, Tab. (Merz Pharmaceuticals).
G-Tussin, Syr. (Quality Formulations, Inc.).
Guaifenex LA, ER Tab. (Ethex Corp.).
Humibid L.A., Tab. (Medeva Pharmaceuticals, Inc.).
Hytuss, Tab., Cap. (Hyrex Pharmaceuticals).
Liquibid, SR Tab. (Ion).
Monafed, SR Tab. (Monarch Pharmaceuticals).
Muco-Fen-LA, TR Tab. (Wakefield Pharmaceuticals, Inc.).
Organidin NR, Tab., Liq. (Wallace Laboratories).
Pheunomist, SR Tab. (ECR Pharm).
Respa-GF, SR Tab. (Respa Pharmaceuticals, Inc.).
Siltussin, Syr. (Silarx Pharmaceuticals, Inc.).
Touro EX, SR Cap. (Dartmouth Pharmaceuticals).
Tusibron, Liq. (Kenwood Laboratories).
Robitussin, Syr. (Wyeth-Ayerst Laboratories).
Wal-Tussin, Syr. (Walgreen Co.).
W/Combinations.
See: Actifed C Expectorant, Liq. (GlaxoWellcome).
Airet G.G., Cap., Elix. (Baylor Labs).
Ambenyl-D, Liq. (Hoechst Marion Roussel).
Anatuss DM, Syr., Tab. (Merz Pharmaceuticals).
Anti-tuss D.M., Liq. (Century Pharmaceuticals, Inc.).
Antitussive Guaiacolate, Syr. (Davol).
Aspirin-Free Bayer Select Head & Chest Cold, Capl. (Bayer Corp. (Allergy Div.)).
Atuss EX, Syr. (Atley Pharmaceuticals, Inc.).
Atuss G, Syr. (Atley Pharmaceuticals, Inc.).
Benylin Multi-Symptom, Liq. (GlaxoWellcome).
Brexin, Cap., Liq. (Savage Laboratories).
Broncholate, Cap., Elix. (Sanofi Winthrop Pharmaceuticals).
Bronkaid Dual Action, Capl. (Bayer Corp. (Consumer Div.)).
Brontex, Tab. Liq. (Procter & Gamble Pharm.).
Bur-Tuss Expectorant (Burlington).
Cheracol D, Syr. (Pharmacia & Upjohn).
Chlor-Trimeton, Expectorant (Schering-Plough Corp.).
Clear Tussin 30, Liq. (Zenith Goldline Pharmaceuticals).
Codeine Phosphate and Guaifenesin, Tab. (Zenith Goldline Pharmaceuticals).

Coldloc, Elix. (Fleming & Co.).
Coldloc-LA, SR Capl. (Fleming & Co.).
Congestac, Tab. (SmithKline Beecham Pharmaceuticals).
Coricidin Children's Cough Syr. (Schering-Plough Corp.).
Cortane D.C., Exp. (Standex).
Cycofed Pediatric, Syr. (Cypress Pharmaceutical, Inc.).
Deconamine CX, Tab., Liq. (Bradley Pharmaceutical).
Deconsal Pediatric, Syr. (Medeva Pharmaceuticals, Inc.).
Defen-LA, SR Tab. (Horizon Pharmaceutical Corp.).
Diabetes CF, Syr. (Scot-Tissin).
Diabetic Tussin, Liq. (Roberts Pharmaceuticals).
Diabetic Tussin DM, Liq. (Roberts Pharmaceuticals).
Dilaudid, Syr. (Knoll Pharmaceuticals).
Dilor G, Tab., Liq. (Savage Laboratories).
Dimacol, Cap. (Wyeth-Ayerst Laboratories).
Dimetane Expectorant, Liq. (Wyeth-Ayerst Laboratories).
Dimetane Expectorant-DC, Liq. (Wyeth-Ayerst Laboratories).
DM Plus, Liq. (West-Ward).
Donatussin, Syr. (Laser, Inc.).
Dy-G, Liq. (Cypress).
Dynafed Asthma Relief, Tab. (BDI Pharmaceuticals, Inc.).
Entex, Cap., Liq. (Procter & Gamble Pharm.).
Fenesin DM, Tab. (Dura).
Formula 44D Decongestant Cough Mixture, Syr. (Procter & Gamble Pharm.).
Glycotuss-DM, Tab. (Pal-Pak, Inc.).
Guaifenesin DAC (Cypress).
Guaifenex, Liq. (Ethex Corp.).
Guaifenex, PPA 75, ER Tab. (Ethex Corp.).
Guaifenex PSE 60, ER Tab. (Ethex Corp.).
Guaifenex PSE 120, ER Tab. (Ethex Corp.).
Guaifenex Rx, DM Tab. (Ethex Corp.).
Guaifenex RX, ER Tab. (Ethex Corp.).
Guaitex, Cap. Liq. (Rugby Labs, Inc.).
Guiatex LA, Tab. (Rugby Labs, Inc.).
Guaitex PSE, Tab. (Rugby Labs, Inc.).
Guaivent (Ethex Corp.).
Guaivent PD, Cap. (Ethex Corp.).
Guai-Vent/PSE, SR Tab. (Dura).
Guiatussin w/Codeine, Liq. (Rugby Labs, Inc.).
Guistrey Fortis, Tab. (Jones Medical Industries, Inc.).
Hycotuss Expectorant, Liq. (Du Pont Merck Pharmaceutical Co.).
Hycoclear Tuss, Syr. (Ethex Corp.).
Hydrocodone GF, Syr. (Morton Grove Pharmaceuticals, Inc.).
Iobid DM, SR Tab. (Iomed).
Isoclor Expectorant (Du Pont Merck Pharmaceutical Co.).
Lardet Expectorant, Tab. (Standex).
Liquibid-D, SR Tab. (ION Laboratories, Inc.).
Med-Rx (Iomed)
Med-Rx, DM, CR Tab. (Iomed).
Med-Rx, CR Tab. (Iomed).
Mini Thin Asthma Relief Tab. (BDI Pharmaceuticals, Inc.).
Monafed DM, ER Tab. (Monarch Pharmaceuticals).
Muco-Fen-DM, TR Tab. (Wakefield Pharmaceuticals, Inc.).
Mudrane GG, Tab, Elix. (ECR Pharmaceuticals).
Nasabid (Jones Medical Industries, Inc.).
Nasabid, PA Cap. (Jones Medical Industries, Inc.).
Nasabid SR, LA Tab. (Jones Medical Industries, Inc.).
Nasatab LA, LA Tab. (ECR Pharmaceuticals).
Novahistine Cough Formula, Liq. (Hoechst Marion Roussel).
Novahistine DMX, Liq. (Hoechst Marion Roussel).
Novahistine, Expectorant (Hoechst Marion Roussel).
Norel, Cap. (US Pharmaceutical Corp.).
Panmist JR, LA Tab. (Pan American Labs).
Partuss AC (Parmed Pharmaceuticals, Inc.).
Pediacon DX Children's, Syr. (Zenith Goldline Pharmaceuticals).
Pediacon DX Pediatric, Drops (Zenith Goldline Pharmaceuticals).
Pediacon EX, Drops (Zenith Goldline Pharmaceuticals).
Phenylfenesin LA, EA Tab. (Zenith Goldline Pharmaceuticals).
PMP Expectorant, Syr. (Schlicksup).
Polaramine Expectorant (Schering-Plough Corp.).
Poly-Histine Expectorant (Sanofi Winthrop Pharmaceuticals).
Polytuss-DM, Liq. (Rhode).
Profen LA, TR Tab. (Wakefield Phar-

maceuticals, Inc.).
Profen II DM, TR Tab. (Wakefield Pharmaceuticals, Inc.).
Profen II, TR Tab. (Wakefield Pharmaceuticals, Inc.).
Protuss DM (Horizon).
Quibron, Cap., Liq. (Bristol-Myers Squibb).
Quibron-300, Cap. (Bristol-Myers Squibb).
Quibron Plus, Cap, Elix. (Bristol-Myers Squibb).
Respa-DM, SR Tab. (Respa Pharmaceuticals, Inc.).
Respa-1st, SR Tab. (Respa Pharmaceuticals, Inc.).
Robitussin AC, CF, DAC, DM, PE (Wyeth-Ayerst Laboratories).
Robitussin-DM Cough Calmers, Loz. (Wyeth-Ayerst Laboratories).
Robitussin Cold & Cough, Cap Liquigels (Wyeth-Ayerst Laboratories).
Robitussin Severe Congestion, Cap, LiquiGels (Wyeth-Ayerst Laboratories).
Rondec-DM, Syr. (Ross Laboratories).
Rymed, Prods. (Edwards Pharmaceuticals, Inc.).
Scotcof, Liq. (Scott/Cord).
Scot-Tussin Senior Clear, Liq. (Scot-Tussin Pharm).
Silaminic Expectorant, Liq. (Silarx Pharmaceuticals, Inc.).
Sildicon-E, Ped Drops (Silarx Pharmaceuticals, Inc.).
Sil-Tex, Liq. (Silarx Pharmaceuticals, Inc.).
Siltussin-CF, Liq. (Roberts Pharmaceuticals).
Siltussin DM, Syr. (Silarx Pharmaceuticals, Inc.).
Sinutab Non-Drying, Liquicaps (GlaxoWellcome).
Slo-Phyllin GG, Cap., Syr. (Dooner).
Sorbase Cough Syr. (Fort David).
Sorbase II Cough Syr. (Fort David).
Sudafed Cough Syr. (Glaxo-Wellcome).
Sudal 60/500, TR Tab. (Atley Pharmaceuticals, Inc.).
Sudal 120/600, SR Tab. (Atley Pharmaceuticals, Inc.).
Synacol CF, Tab. (Roberts Pharmaceuticals).
Syn-Rx, CR Tab. (Medeva Pharmaceuticals, Inc.).
Tolu-Sed, Liq. (Scherer Laboratories, Inc.).
Tolu-Sed DM, Liq. (Scherer Laboratories, Inc.).
Touro LA, LA Capl. (Dartmouth).
Triaminic Expectorant (Novartis Pharmaceutical Corp.).
Tri-Histin Expectorant (Recsei Laboratories).
Trind, Liq. (Bristol-Myers Squibb).
Tusibron-DM, Liq. (Kenwood Laboratories).
Tussafed, Expectorant (Calvital).
Tussar-2, Syr. (Rhone-Poulenc Rorer Pharmaceuticals, Inc.).
Tussar SF, Liq. (Rhone-Poulenc Rorer Pharmaceuticals, Inc.).
Tussend, Liq. (Hoechst Marion Roussel).
Tussi-Organidin DM NR, Liq. (Wallace Laboratories).
Tussi-Organidin DM-S, Liq. (Wallace Laboratories).
Tussi-Organidin NR, Liq. (Wallace Laboratories).
Vicks Cough Syr. (Procter & Gamble Pharm).
Vicks Formula 44D Decongestant Cough Mixture, Syr. (Procter & Gamble Pharm).
Vicks 44E, Liq. (Procter & Gamble Pharm).
Wal-Tussin DM, Syr. (Walgreen Co.).

guaifenesin and codeine phosphate syrup.
Use: Antitussive, expectorant.

Guaifenesin DAC. (Cypress Pharmaceutical, Inc.) Codeine phosphate 10 mg, pseudoephedrine HCl 30 mg, guaifenesin 100 mg/5 ml, alcohol 1.9%, saccharin, sorbitol. Liq. Bot. 480 ml. *otc.*
Use: Antitussive, decongestant, expectorant.

guaifenesin/phenylpropanolamine hydrochloride.
See: Phenylpropanolamine hydrochloride & guaifenesin tablets.

guaifenesin & pseudoephedrine hydrochloride & codeine phosphate syrup. (Schein Pharmaceutical, Inc.) Pseudoephedrine HCl 30 mg, codeine phosphate 10 mg, guaifenesin 100 mg, alcohol 1.4 %/5 ml. Bot. 473 ml. *c-v.*
Use: Antitussive, decongestant, expectorant.
See: Guaifenesin DAC, Liq. (Cypress Pharmaceutical, Inc.).

Guaifenex. (Ethex Corp.) Guaifenesin 100 mg, phenylpropanolamine HCl 20 mg, phenylephrine HCl 5 mg, parabens, sorbitol/5 ml. Liq. Bot. 118 ml, 473 ml. *Rx.*
Use: Decongestant, expectorant.

Guaifenex DM. (Ethex Corp.) Guaifenesin 600 mg, dextromethorphan HBr 30

mg/ER Tab. Bot. 100s, 500s, 1000s. *Rx.*
Use: Antitussive, expectorant.

Guaifenex LA. (Ethex Corp.) Guaifenesin 600 mg, lactose/ER Tab. Bot. 100s, 500s. *Rx.*
Use: Expectorant.

Guaifenex PPA 75. (Ethex Corp.) Guaifenesin 600 mg, phenylpropanolamine HCl 75 mg, lactose/ER Tab. Bot. 100s, 500s. *Rx.*
Use: Decongestant, expectorant.

Guaifenex PSE 120. (Ethex Corp.) Guaifenesin 600 mg, pseudoephedrine HCl 120 mg/ER Tab. Bot. 100s. *Rx.*
Use: Decongestant, expectorant.

Guaifenex PSE 60. (Ethex Corp.) Guaifenesin 600 mg, pseudoephedrine HCl 60 mg, lactose/ER Tab. Bot. 100s. *Rx.*
Use: Decongestant, expectorant.

Guaifenex Rx. (Ethex Corp.) **AM:** Guaifenesin 600 mg, pseudoephedrine HCl 60 mg. **PM:** Guaifenesin 600 mg. ER Tab. Pkg. 28s. *Rx.*
Use: Decongestant, expectorant.

Guaifenex Rx DM. (Ethex Corp.) Guaifenesin 600 mg, pseudoephedrine HCl 60 mg/Tab. Pkg. 28s. *Rx.*
Use: Decongestant, expectorant.

Guaimax-D. (Schwarz Pharma, Inc.) Pseudoephedrine HCl 120 mg, guaifenesin 600 mg. ER Tab. Bot. 100s. *Rx.*
Use: Decongestant, expectorant.

Guaipax. (Vitaline Corp.) Phenylpropanolamine HCl 75 mg, guaifenesin 400 mg/Tab. Bot. 100s, 500s, 1000s. *Rx.*
Use: Decongestant, expectorant.

Guaiphotol. (Foy Laboratories) Iodine 1/30 gr, calcium creosote 4 gr/Tab. Bot. 1000s. *Rx.*
Use: Expectorant.

Guaitab. (Muro Pharmaceutical, Inc.) Pseudoephedrine HCl 60 mg, guaifenesin 400 mg, lactose/Tab. Bot. 100s. *otc.*
Use: Decongestant, expectorant.

Guaitex. (Rugby) **Cap.:** Phenylephrine HCl 5 mg, phenylpropanolamine HCl 45 mg, guaifenesin 200 mg. Bot. 100s. **Liq.:** Phenylephrine HCl 5 mg, phenylpropanolamine HCl 20 mg, guaifenesin 100 mg/5 ml. Bot. pt. *Rx.*
Use: Decongestant, expectorant.

Guaitex LA. (Rugby) Phenylpropanolamine HCl 75 mg, guaifenesin 400 mg. Tab. Bot. 100s, 1000s. *Rx.*
Use: Decongestant, expectorant.

Guaitex PSE. (Rugby) Pseudoephedrine HCl 120 mg, guaifenesin 500 mg. Tab. Bot. 100s. *Rx.*
Use: Decongestant, expectorant.

•**guaithylline.** (GWIE-thill-in) USAN.
Use: Bronchodilator, expectorant.

Guaivent. (Ethex Corp.) Guaifenesin 250 mg, pseudoephedrine HCl 120 mg, parabens, EDTA, sucrose. Cap. Bot. 100s, 500s. *Rx.*
Use: Decongestant, expectorant.

Guaivent PD. (Ethex Corp.) Guaifenesin 600 mg, pseudoephedrine HCl 60 mg, parabens, EDTA, sucrose. Cap. Bot. 100s, 500s. *Rx.*
Use: Decongestant, expectorant.

Guai-Vent/PSE. (Dura Pharmaceuticals) Pseudoephedrine HCl 120 mg, guaifenesin 600 mg/SR Tab. Bot. 100s. *Rx.*
Use: Expectorant.

guamide.
See: Sulfaguanidine (Various Mfr.).

•**guanabenz.** (GWAHN-uh-benz) USAN.
Use: Antihypertensive.
See: Wytensin, Tab. (Wyeth-Ayerst Laboratories).

•**guanabenz acetate.** (GWAHN-uh-benz) U.S.P. 23.
Use: Antihypertensive.

guanabenz acetate. (Various Mfr.) 4 mg or 8 mg/Tab. Bot. 30s, 100s, 500s.
Use: Antihypertensive.

•**guanacline sulfate.** (GWAHN-ah-kleen) USAN.
Use: Antihypertensive.

•**guanadrel sulfate.** (GWAHN-uh-drell) U.S.P. 23.
Use: Antihypertensive.
See: Hylorel, Tab. (Medeva Pharmaceuticals, Inc.).

•**guancydine.** (GWAHN-sigh-deen) USAN.
Use: Antihypertensive.

•**guanethidine monosulfate.** (gwahn-ETH-ih-deen MAH-no-SULL-fate) U.S.P. 23.
Use: Antihypertensive. Reflex sympathetic dystrophy and causalgia. [Orphan Drug]
See: Ismelin (Novartis Pharmaceutical Corp.).

W/Hydrochlorothiazide.
See: Esimil, Tab. (Novartis Pharmaceutical Corp.).

•**guanethidine sulfate.** (gwahn-ETH-ih-deen) USAN, U.S.P. XXI.
Use: Antihypertensive.
See: Ismelin, Tab. (Novartis Pharmaceutical Corp.).

W/Hydrochlorothiazide.
See: Esimil, Tab. (Novartis Pharmaceutical Corp.).

•**guanfacine hydrochloride.** (GWAHN-fay-seen) U.S.P. 23.

Use: Antihypertensive.
See: Tenex, Tab. (Wyeth-Ayerst Laboratories).

guanidine hydrochloride. (Key Pharmaceuticals) Guanidine HCl 125 mg/Tab. Bot. 100s. *Rx.*
Use: Muscle stimulant.

guanisoquin. (GWAN-eye-so-KWIN)
Use: Antihypertensive.

•**guanisoquin sulfate.** (GWAHN-eye-so-kwin) USAN.
Use: Antihypertensive.

•**guanoclor sulfate.** (GWAHN-oh-klahr) USAN.
Use: Antihypertensive.

•**guanoctine hydrochloride.** (GWAHN-ock-teen) USAN.
Use: Antihypertensive.

•**guanoxabenz.** (gwahn-OX-ah-benz) USAN.
Use: Antihypertensive.

•**guanoxan sulfate.** (GWAHN-ox-an) USAN.
Use: Antihypertensive.

•**guanoxyfen sulfate.** (GWAHN-OX-eh-fen) USAN.
Use: Antihypertensive, antidepressant.

Guardal. (Morton) Vitamins A 10,000 IU, B_1 20 mg, B_2 8 mg, C 50 mg, niacinamide 10 mg, calcium d-pantothenate 5 mg, iron 10 mg, dried whole liver 100 mg, yeast 100 mg, choline bitartrate 30 mg, B_6 0.5 mg, B_{12}8 mcg, mixed tocopherols 5 mg, dicalcium phosphate anhydrous 150 mg, magnesium sulfate dried 7.2 mg, sodium 1 mg, potassium Cl 1.3 mg/Tab. Bot. 100s. *otc.*
Use: Mineral, vitamin supplement.

Guardex. (Archer-Taylor) Tube 4 oz, 1 lb, 4.5 lb. *otc.*
Use: Emollient.

•**guar gum.** N.F. 18.
Use: Pharmaceutic aid (tablet binder; tablet disintegrant).
W/Danthron, docusate sodium.
See: Guarsol, Tab. (Western Research).
W/Standardized senna concentrate.
See: Gentlax B, Gran., Tab. (Blair Laboratories).

guayanesin.
Use: Expectorant.
See: Guaifenesin (Various Mfr.).

GuiaCough CF Liquid. (Schein Pharmaceutical, Inc.) Phenylpropanolamine HCl 12.5 mg, dextromethorphan HBr 10 mg, guaifenesin 100 mg. Bot. 118 ml. *otc.*
Use: Antitussive, decongestant, expectorant.

GuiaCough PE Liquid. (Schein Pharmaceutical, Inc.) Pseudoephedrine HCl 30 mg, guaifenesin 100 mg, alcohol 1.4%. Bot. 118 ml. *otc.*
Use: Decongestant, expectorant.

Guiamid Expectorant. (Vangard Labs, Inc.) Guaifenesin 100 mg/5 ml, alcohol 3.5%. Bot. Pt, gal. *otc.*
Use: Expectorant.

Guiaphed. (Various Mfr.) Theophylline 45 mg, ephedrine sulfate 36 mg, guaifenesin 150 mg, phenobarbital 12 mg, alcohol 19%/15 ml. Elix. Bot. 480 ml. *Rx.*
Use: Antiasthmatic combination.

Guaitex. (Rugby Labs, Inc.) **Cap.:** Phenylephrine HCl 5 mg, phenylpropanolamine HCl, guaifenesin 200 mg. **Liq.:** Phenylephrine HCl 5 mg, phenylpropanolamine 20 mg, quaifenesin 100 mg. *Rx.*
Use: Antitussive, expectorant.

Guiatex PSE. (Rugby Labs, Inc.) Pseudoephedrine HCl, guaifenesin 500 mg/Tab. Bot. 100s. *Rx.*
Use: Decongestant, expectorant.

Guiatex LA. (Rugby Labs, Inc.) Phenylpropanolamine HCl 75 mg, guaifenesin 400 mg/Tab. Bot. 100s, 1000s. *Rx.*
Use: Antitussive, expectorant.

Guiatuss AC Syrup. (Various Mfr.) Codeine phosphate 10 mg, guaifenesin 100 mg, alcohol 3.5%/5 ml. Syr. Bot. 120 ml, Pt, gal. *c-v.*
Use: Antitussive, expectorant.

Guiatuss CF. (Alpharma USPD Inc.) Phenylpropanolamine HCl 12.5 mg, dextromethorphan HBr 10 mg, guaifenesin 100 mg/5 ml. Syr. Bot. 120 ml. *otc.*
Use: Antitussive, expectorant.

Guiatuss DAC Liquid. (Various Mfr.) Pseudoephedrine HCl 30 mg, codeine phosphate 10 mg, guaifenesin 100 mg, alcohol/5 ml. Liq. Bot. 120 ml, 480 ml. *c-v.*
Use: Antitussive, decongestant, expectorant.

Guiatuss-DM Liquid. (Various Mfr.) Dextromethorphan HBr 10 mg, guaifenesin 100 mg/5 ml. Bot. 120 ml, 240 ml, pt, gal. *otc.*
Use: Antitussive, expectorant.

Guiatuss PE. (Alpharma USPD Inc.) Pseudoephedrine HCl 30 mg, guaifenesin 100 mg, alcohol 1.4%/5 ml. Liq. Bot. In 120 ml. *otc.*
Use: Decongestant, expectorant.

Guiatuss Syrup. (Various Mfr.) Guaifenesin 100 mg/5 ml. Syr. Bot. 120 ml, 240 ml, pt, gal. *otc.*

Use: Expectorant.

Guiatussin/Codeine Expectorant. (Rugby Labs, Inc.) Codeine phosphate 10 mg, guaifenesin 100 mg/5 ml, alcohol 3.5%. Syr. Bot. 120 ml, pt, gal. *c-v.*
Use: Antitussive, expectorant.

Guiatussin/Dextromethorphan. (Rugby Labs, Inc.) Dextromethorphan HBr 15 mg, guaifenesin 100 mg, alcohol 1.4%/5 ml. Liq. Bot. 480 ml. *otc.*
Use: Antitussive, expectorant.

Guaivent. (Ethex Corp.) Guaifenesin 250 mg, pseudoephedrine HCl 120 mg. Cap. Bot. 100s, 500s. *Rx.*
Use: Expectorant.

Guaivent PD. (Ethex Corp.) Guaifenesin 300 mg, pseudoephedrine HCl 60 mg, parabens, sucrose. Cap. Bot. 100s, 500s. *Rx.*
Use: Expectorant.

Guistrey Fortis. (Jones Medical Industries, Inc.) Guaifenesin 100 mg, phenylephrine HCl 10 mg, chlorpheniramine maleate 1 mg/Tab. Bot. 1000s. *otc.*
Use: Antihistamine, decongestant, expectorant.

Gulfasin. (Major Pharmaceuticals) Sulfisoxazole 500 mg/Tab. Bot. 100s, 250s, 1000s.
Use: Anti-infective, sulfonamide.

guncotton, soluble. Pyroxylin.

gusperimus.
Use: Acute renal graft-rejection episodes.

•**gusperimus trihydrochloride.** (guss-PURR-ih-muss try-HIGH-droe-KLOR-ide) USAN.
Use: Immunosuppressant.

Gustalac. (Roberts Pharmaceuticals) Calcium carbonate 300 mg, defatted skim milk pow. 200 mg/Tab. Bot. 100s, 250s, 1000s. *otc.*
Use: Antacid, calcium supplement.

Gustase. (Roberts Pharmaceuticals) Amylase 30 mg, protease 6 mg, cellulase 2 mg. Tab. Bot. 42s, 100s, 500s. *otc.*
Use: Digestive aid.

Gustase Plus. (Roberts Pharmaceuticals) Phenobarbital 8 mg, homatropine methylbromide 2.5 mg, gerilase 30 mg, geriprotase 6 mg, gericellulase 2 mg/Tab. Bot. 42s, 100s, 500s. *Rx.*
Use: Anticholinergic, antispasmodic, digestive aid, hypnotic, sedative.

•**gutta percha.** U.S.P. 23.
Use: Dental restoration agent.

G-vitamin.
See: Riboflavin (Various Mfr.).

G-well Shampoo. (Zenith Goldline Pharmaceuticals) Lindane 1%. Bot. 2 oz, pt, gal. *Rx.*
Use: Pediculicide.

Gynecort 10, Extra Strength. (Combe, Inc.) Hydrocortisone acetate 1%, parabens, zinc pyrithione. Cream. Tube 15 g. *otc.*
Use: Corticosteroid, topical.

Gyne-Lotrimin 3. (Schering-Plough) **Comb. Pack:** Clotrimazole 1% (vaginal cream), clotrimazole 200 mg (inserts), benzyl alcohol. Pkg 3s w/applictor (inserts), Tube 7 g (cream). **Vag. Inserts:** Clotrimazole 200 mg. Pkg. 3s w/applicator. *otc.*
Use: Antifungal, vaginal.

Gyne-Lotrimin Combination Pack. (Schering-Plough Corp.) **Vaginal Tab.:** Clotrimazole 100 mg. Pkg. 7s. **Topical Cream:** Clotrimazole 1%. Tube 7 g. *otc.*
Use: Antifungal, vaginal.

Gyne-Lotrimin 7 Vaginal Cream 1%. (Schering-Plough Corp.) Clotrimazole ≈ 5 g/applicatorful. Tube 45 g, 45 g twin-packs w/applicator. *otc.*
Use: Antifungal, vaginal.

Gyne-Lotrimin 7 Vaginal Tablets. (Schering-Plough Corp.) Clotrimazole 100 mg/Tab. Box 7 Tab. w/applicator, Box 6s. *otc.*
Use: Antifungal, vaginal.

gynergon.
See: Estradiol (Various Mfr.).

Gyne-Sulf. (G & W Laboratories) Sulfathiazole 3.42%, sulfacetamide 2.86%, sulfabenzamide 3.7%, urea 0.64%. Cream. Tube with applicator 82.5 g. *Rx.*
Use: Anti-infective, vaginal.

Gynogen L.A. 10. (Forest Pharmaceutical, Inc.) Estradiol valerate in sesame oil 10 mg/ml. Vial 10 ml. *Rx.*
Use: Estrogen.

Gynogen L.A. 20. (Forest Pharmaceutical, Inc.) Estradiol valerate in castor oil 20 mg/ml. Inj. Multi-dose Vial 10 ml. *Rx.*
Use: Estrogen.

Gynogen L.A. 40. (Forest Pharmaceutical, Inc.) Estradiol valerate in castor oil 40 mg/ml. Inj. Vial 10 ml. *Rx.*
Use: Estrogen.

Gynol II Contraceptive. (Advanced Care Products) Nonoxynol-9 in 2% concentration. Starter 75 g tube w/applicator. Refill 75 g, 114 g/Tube. *otc.*
Use: Contraceptive.

Gynol II Extra Strength Contraceptive. (Advanced Care Products) Nonoxynol-9 3%. Jelly. 75 g, 114 g. *otc.*
Use: Contraceptive, spermicide.

Gyno-Petraryl. (Janssen Pharmaceutical, Inc.) Econazole nitrate. *Rx.*
Use: Antifungal, vaginal.

Gynovite Plus. (Optimox Corp.) Vitamins A 833 IU, D 67 IU, E 67 mg (as d-alpha tocopheryl acid succinate), B_1 1.7 mg, B_2 1.7 mg, B_3 3.3 mg, B_5 1.7 mg, B_6 3.3 mg, B_{12} 21 mcg, C 30 mg, calcium 83 mg, iron 3 mg, folic acid 0.07 mg, boron, betaine, biotin, Cr, Cu, hesperidin, I, inositol, Mg, Mn, PABA, pancreatin, rutin, Se, Zn 2.5 mg. Tab. Bot. 100s. *otc.*
Use: Mineral, vitamin supplement.

H

Habitrol. (Novartis Pharmaceutical Corp.) Nicotine transdermal system. Dose absorbed in 24 hours, 21 mg, 14 mg, 7; total nicotine content (respectively) 52.5 mg, 35 mg, 17.5. Patch. Box 30 systems. *Rx.*
Use: Smoking deterrent.

haemophilus b conjugate vaccine.
Use: Vaccine, bacterial.
See: ActHIB, Pow. for Inj. (Pasteur Merieux Connaught).
HibTITER, Inj. (Wyeth-Ayerst Laboratories).
OmniHIB, Pow. for Inj. (SmithKline Beecham Pharmaceuticals).
Pedvax HIB, Pow. (Merck & Co.).
ProHIBIT, Inj. (Pasteur Merieux Connaught).
W/DTP vaccine.
See: ActHIB/DTP, Set of DTwP vial plus Hib Pow for Inj. (Pasteur Merieux Connaught).
Tetramune, Vial (Wyeth-Ayerst Laboratories).

haemophilus influenzae type b and hepatitis vaccines, combined.
See: Comvax (Merck & Co.).

Hair Booster Vitamin. (NBTY, Inc.) Vitamin B_3 35 mg, B_5 100 mg, B_{12} 6 mcg, folic acid 0.4 mg, zinc 15 mg, Cu, iron 18 mg, I, Mn, choline bitartrate, inositol, PABA, protein/Tab. Bot. 60s. *otc.*
Use: Mineral, vitamin supplement.

•**halazepam.** (hal-AZE-uh-pam) USAN, U.S.P. XXII.
Use: Hypnotic, sedative.

•**halazone.** (HAL-ah-zone) U.S.P. 23.
Use: Disinfectant.

•**halcinonide.** (hal-SIN-oh-nide) U.S.P. 23.
Use: Corticosteroid, topical; anti-inflammatory.
See: Halog Cream, Oint., Soln. (Westwood Squibb Pharmaceuticals).

Halcion. (Pharmacia & Upjohn) Triazolam 0.125 mg or 0.25 mg/Tab. **0.125 mg:** Bot. 100s, Visipak 100s. (4 × 25s). **0.25 mg:** Bot. 100s, UD 100s, Visipak 100s. (4 × 25s). *c-iv.*
Use: Hypnotic, sedative.

Haldol. (Ortho McNeil Pharmaceutical) Haloperidol. **Tab.:** 0.5 mg, 1 mg, 2 mg, 5 mg, or 10 mg. 20 mg/Tab. Bot. 100s. **Conc. Soln.:** 2 mg/ml. Bot. 15 ml, 120 ml. **Inj.:** 5 mg/ml, parabens. Amp. 1 ml. Vial 10 ml. *Rx.*
Use: Antipsychotic.

Haldol Decanoate 50. (Ortho McNeil Pharmaceutical) Haloperidol 50 (70.5 mg decanoate), sesame oil, benzyl alcohol 1.2%. Amp. 1 ml. Vial 5 ml. *Rx.*
Use: Antipsychotic.

Haldol Decanoate 100. (Ortho McNeil Pharmaceutical) Haloperidol 100 mg/ml (141.04 mg decanoate), sesame oil, benzyl alcohol 1.2%. Amp. 1 ml. Vial 5 ml. *Rx.*
Use: Antipsychotic.

Haldrone. (Eli Lilly and Co.) Paramethasone acetate 1 mg or 2 mg/Tab. Bot. 100s. *Rx.*
Use: Corticosteroid.

Halenol Children's. (Halsey Drug Co.) Acetaminophen 160 mg/5 ml. Elix. Bot. 120 ml, 240 ml, pt, gal. *otc.*
Use: Analgesic.

Halercol. (Roberts Pharmaceuticals) Vitamins A 5000 IU, D 400 IU, E 1.36 mg, B_1 1.5 mg, B_2 2 mg, B_3 20 mg, B_5 1 mg, B_6 0.1 mg, B_{12} 1 mcg, C 37.5 mg/Cap. Bot. 100s. *otc.*
Use: Vitamin supplement.

Haley's M-O. (Bayer Corp. (Consumer Div.)) Mineral oil 25%, milk of magnesia in emulsion base. Flavored or regular. Bot. 240 ml, 480 ml, 960 ml. *otc.*
Use: Laxative.

Halfan. (SmithKline Beecham Pharmaceuticals) 250 mg/Tab. Bot. 60s. *Rx.*
Use: Antimalarial. [Orphan Drug]

Halfort-T. (Halsey Drug Co.) Vitamins C 300 mg, B_1 15 mg, B_2 10 mg, niacin 100 mg, B_6 5 mg, B_{12} 4 mcg, pantothenic acid 20 mg/Tab. Bot. 100s. *otc.*
Use: Vitamin supplement.

Halfprin 81. (Kramer Laboratories, Inc.) Aspirin 81 mg. EC Tab. Bot. 90s. *otc.*
Use: Analgesic.

Half Strength Entrition Entri-Pak. (Biosearch Medical Products) Protein 17.5 g (Na and Ca caseinates), carbohydrate 68 g (maltodextrin), fat 17.5 g (corn oil, soy lecithin, mono- and diglycerides), sodium 350 mg, potassium 600 mg, mOsm/120 kg H_2O, calories 0.5/ml, vitamins A, B_1, B_2, B_3, B_5, B_6, B_{12}, C, D, E, K, P, Ca, Mg, I, Fe, Zn, Mn, Cu, Cl, biotin, choline, folic acid. Liq. Pouch 1 liter. *otc.*
Use: Nutritional supplement.

Half Strength Florvite with Iron. (Everett Laboratories, Inc.) Fluoride 0.5 mg, Vitamins A 2500 IU, D 400 IU, E 15 IU, B_1 1.05 mg, B_2 1.2 mg, B_3 13.5 mg, B_6 1.05 mg, B_{12} 4.5 mcg, C 60 mg, folic acid 0.3 mg, Cu, iron 12 mg, Zn 10 mg, sucrose/Tab. Bot. 100s. *Rx.*
Use: Mineral, vitamin supplement; dental caries agent.

Half Strength Introlan. (Elan Pharma) Protein 22.5 g, fat 18 g, carbohydrates 70 g, Na 345 mg, K 585 mg/L. Vitamins A, C, B_1, B_2, B_3, D, E, B_6, B_{12}, B_5, K, Ca, Fe, folic acid, P, I, Mg, Zn, Cu, biotin, Mn, choline, Cl, Se, Cr, Mo. Liq. In 1000 ml New Pak closed systems with and without color check. *otc.*
Use: Nutritional supplement.

Hali-Best. (Barth's) Vitamins A 10,000 IU, D 400 IU/Cap. Bot. 100s, 500s. *otc.*
Use: Vitamin supplement.

halibut liver oil.
Use: Vitamin supplement.

haliver oil.
See: Halibut Liver Oil (Various Mfr.).

Hall's Mentho-Lyptus Decongestant Liquid. (Warner Lambert) Dextromethorphan HBr 15 mg, phenylpropanolamine HCl 37.5 mg, menthol 14 mg, eucalyptus oil 12.7 mg/10 ml, alcohol 22%. Bot. 90 ml. *otc.*
Use: Antitussive, decongestant.

Hall's Mentho-Lyptus Cough Lozenges. (Warner Lambert) Menthol and eucalyptus oil in varying amounts and flavors. Stick-Pack 9s. Bag 30s. *otc.*
Use: Mouth and throat preparation.

Hall's Mentho-Lyptus Sugar Free. (Warner Lambert) Menthol 5 mg or 6 mg, eucalyptus oil 2.8 mg/Tab. Pkg. 25s. *otc.*
Use: Mouth and throat preparation.

Hall's-Plus Maximum Strength. (Warner Lambert) Menthol 10 mg, corn syrup, sugar. Cherry, honey-lemon, and regular flavors. Tab. Pkg. 10s, 25s. *otc.*
Use: Mouth and throat preparation.

Hall's Zinc Defense. (Warner Lambert Consumer Healthcare) Zinc acetate 5 mg, sugar, cherry, or peppermint flavor. Loz. 24s. *otc.*
Use: Mineral supplement.

•**halobetasol propionate.** (hal-oh-BEH-tah-sahl PRO-pee-oh-nate) USAN.
Use: Anti-inflammatory; corticosteroid, topical.
See: Ultravate (Westwood Squibb Pharmaceuticals).

•**halofantrine hydrochloride.** (HAY-low-FAN-trin) USAN.
Use: Antimalarial. [Orphan Drug]
See: Halfan, Tab. (SmithKline Beecham Pharmaceuticals).

Halofed. (Halsey Drug Co.) **Tab.:** Pseudoephedrine HCl 30 mg or 60 mg. Bot. 100s, 1000s. **Syr.:** Pseudoephedrine HCl 30 mg/5 ml. Bot. 120 ml, 240 ml, pt, gal. *otc.*
Use: Decongestant.

•**halofenate.** (HAY-low-FEN-ate) USAN.
Use: Antihyperlipoproteinemic, uricosuric.

•**halofuginone hydrobromide.** (HAY-low-FOO-jin-ohn HIGH-droe-BROE-mide) USAN.
Use: Antiprotozoal.

Halog Cream. (Westwood Squibb Pharmaceuticals) Halcinonide 0.025% or 0.1%, in specially formulated cream base consisting of glyceryl monostearate, cetyl alcohol, myristyl stearate, isopropyl palmitate, polysorbate 60, propylene glycol, purified water. **0.1%:** Tube 15 g, 30 g, 60 g, Jar 240 g. **0.025%:** Tube 15 g, 60 g. *Rx.*
Use: Corticosteroid, topical.

Halog-E Cream. (Westwood Squibb Pharmaceuticals) Halcinonide 0.1% in hydrophilic vanishing cream base consisting of propylene glycol dimethicone 350, castor oil, cetearyl alcohol, ceteareth-20, propylene glycol stearate, white petrolatum, water. Tube 15 g, 30 g, 60 g. *Rx.*
Use: Corticosteroid, topical.

Halog Ointment. (Westwood Squibb Pharmaceuticals) Halcinonide 0.1%, in Plastibase (plasicized hydrocarbon gel), PEG 400, PEG 6000 distearate, PEG 300, PEG 1540, butylated hydroxy toluene. Tube 15 g, 30 g, 60 g, Jar 240 g. *Rx.*
Use: Corticosteroid, topical.

Halog Solution. (Westwood Squibb Pharmaceuticals) Halcinonide 0.1%, edetate disodium, PEG 300, purified water, butylated hydroxy toluene as preservative. Bot. 20 ml, 60 ml. *Rx.*
Use: Corticosteroid, topical.

•**halopemide.** (hay-LOW-PEH-mid) USAN.
Use: Antipsychotic.

•**haloperidol.** (HAY-low-PURR-ih-dahl) U.S.P. 23.
Use: Antipsychotic, tranquilizer; antidyskinetic (in Gilles de la Tourette's disease).
See: Haldol, Preps. (Ortho McNeil Pharmaceutical).

haloperidol. (Various Mfr.) Haloperidol. **Tab.:** 0.5 mg, 1 mg, 2 mg, 5 mg, 10 mg, 20 mg/Tab. Bot. 100s, 500s (except 20 mg), 1000s (except 20 mg), 1000s. **Conc.:** 2 mg/ml. Bot. 15 ml, 120 ml, UD 100s 5 ml, and 10 ml. **Inj.:** 5 mg/ml. Amp. 1 ml, Syr. 1 ml, Vial 1 ml, 2 ml, 2.5 ml, 10 ml. *Rx.*
Use: Antipsychotic.

•**haloperidol decanoate.** (HAY-low-

PURR-ih-dahl deh-KAN-oh-ate) USAN.
Use: Antipsychotic.

•**halopredone acetate.** (HAY-low-PREH-dohn) USAN.
Use: Anti-inflammatory, topical.

•**haloprogesterone.** (HAL-oh-pro-jeh-STEE-rone) USAN.
Use: Hormone, progestin.

•**haloprogin.** (hal-oh-PRO-jin) U.S.P. 23.
Use: Antimicrobial, topical; anti-infective.
See: Halotex, Cream, Soln. (Westwood Squibb Pharmaceuticals).

Halotestin. (Pharmacia & Upjohn) Fluoxymesterone 2 mg, 5 mg, or 10 mg. Tartrazine, lactose, sucrose. **2 mg:** Bot. 100s. **5 mg:** Bot. 100s. **10 mg:** Bot. 30s, 100s. *c-III.*
Use: Androgen.

Halotex Cream. (Westwood Squibb Pharmaceuticals) Haloprogin 1% in water-dispersible base composed of PEG-400, PEG-4000, diethyl sebacate, polyvinylpyrrolidone. Tube 15 g, 30 g. *Rx.*
Use: Antifungal, topical.

Halotex Solution. (Westwood Squibb Pharmaceuticals) Haloprogin 1% in a clear colorless vehicle of diethyl sebacate w/alcohol 75%. Bot. 10 ml, 30 ml. *Rx.*
Use: Antifungal, topical.

•**halothane.** (HAL-oh-thane) U.S.P. 23.
Use: General anesthetic, inhalation.
See: Fluothane, Liq. (Wyeth-Ayerst Laboratories).
Halothane, 250 ml Liq. (Abbott Laboratories).

Halotussin. (Halsey Drug Co.) Guaifenesin 100 mg/5 ml. Bot. 4 oz, 8 oz, pt, gal. *otc.*
Use: Expectorant.

Halotussin-DM. (Halsey Drug Co.) Dextromethorphan HBr 10 mg, guaifenesin 100 mg. In 120 ml, 240 ml, pt, gal. *otc.*
Use: Antitussive, expectorant.

Halotussin-DM Sugar-Free Liquid. (Halsey Drug Co.) Dextromethorphan HBr 10 mg, guaifenesin 100 mg. In 120 ml, 240 ml, 480 ml, gal. *otc.*
Use: Antitussive, expectorant.

•**halquinols.** (HAL-kwin-oles) USAN.
Use: Anti-infective, topical; antimicrobial.

Haltran. (Roberts Pharmaceuticals) Ibuprofen 200 mg/Tab. Bot. 30s, 50s. Blister pkg. 12s. *otc.*
Use: Analgesic, NSAID.

HAMA. Hydroxyaluminum magnesium aminoacetate.

hamamelis water.
See: Succus Cineraria Maritima, Soln. (Walker Pharmacal).
Witch hazel (Various Mfr.).
Tucks Preps. (GlaxoWellcome).

•**hamycin.** (HAY-MY-sin) USAN.
Use: Antifungal.

Hang-Over-Cure. (Silvers) Calcium carbonate, glycine, thiamine HCl, pyridoxine HCl, aspirin. Cont. Tab. 6 g. *otc.*
Use: Antacid, analgesic combination.

Haniform. (Hanlon) Vitamins A 25,000 IU, D 1000 IU, B_1 10 mg, B_2 5 mg, C 150 mg, niacinamide 150 mg/Cap. Bot. 100s. *otc.*
Use: Vitamin supplement.

Haniplex. (Hanlon) Vitamins B_1 20 mg, B_2 10 mg, B_6 1 mg, calcium pantothenate 10 mg, B_{12} 5 mcg, niacin 20 mg, liver concentrate 50 mg, C 150 mg/Cap. Bot. 100s. *otc.*
Use: Mineral, vitamin supplement.

Harbolin. (Arcum) Hydralazine HCl 25 mg, hydrochlorothiazide 15 mg, reserpine 0.1 mg/Tab. Bot. 100s, 1000s. *Rx.*
Use: Antihypertensive combination.

hard fat.
Use: Pharmaceutic necessity.

hartshorn. Ammonium carbonate.

Haugase. (Madland) Trypsin, chymotrypsin. Bot. 50s, 250s.
Use: Enzyme preparation.

Havab. (Abbott Diagnostics) Radioimmunoassay or enzyme immunoassay for detection of antibody to hepatitis A virus. Test kit 100s.
Use: Diagnostic aid.

Havab EIA. (Abbott Diagnostics) Enzyme immunoassay for the detection of antibody to hepatitis A virus.
Use: Diagnostic aid.

Havab-M. (Abbott Diagnostics) Radioimmunoassay for the detection of specific Ig antibody to hepatitis A virus. Test kit 100s.
Use: Diagnostic aid.

Havab-M EIA. (Abbott Diagnostics) Enzyme immunoassay for the detection of Ig antibody to hepatitis A virus.
Use: Diagnostic aid.

Havrix. (SmithKline Beecham Pharmaceuticals) Hepatitis A vaccine. **Adult:** 1440 ELU units/ml. Single-dose vial, prefilled syringe. **Pediatric:** 720 ELU/0.5 ml. Single-dose vial, prefilled syringe. *Rx.*
Use: Immunization.

Hawaiian Tropic Aloe Paba Sunscreen. (Tanning Research Labs, Inc.) Padimate O, oxybenzone. Cream Bot. 120

g. *otc.*
Use: Sunscreen.

Hawaiian Tropic Baby Faces. (Tanning Research Labs, Inc.) SPF 20. Octyl methoxycinnamate, octocrylene, benzophenone-3, menthyl anthranilate, PABA free, waterproof. Gel Tube 120 g. *otc.*
Use: Sunscreen.

Hawaiian Tropic Baby Faces Sunblock. (Tanning Research Labs, Inc.) Octyl methoxycinnamate, benzophenone-3, octyl salicylate, titanium dioxide, octocrylene, PABA free, waterproof. **SPF 35:** Lot. Bot. 60 ml, 120 ml, 300 ml. **SPF 50:** Lot. Bot. 120 ml. *otc.*
Use: Sunscreen.

Hawaiian Tropic Cool Aloe with I.C.E. (Tanning Research Labs, Inc.) Lidocaine, menthol, aloe, SD alcohol 40, diazolidinyl urea, EDTA, vitamins A and E, tartrazine. Gel. Jar 360 g. *otc.*
Use: Emollient.

Hawaiian Tropic Dark Tanning. (Tanning Research Labs, Inc.) **Gel:** Phenylbenzimidazole sulfonic acid. SPF 2. Bot. 240 ml. **Oil:** 2-ethylhexyl methoxycinnamate, octyl dimethyl PABA, waterproof. Bot. 240 ml. *otc.*
Use: Sunscreen.

Hawaiian Tropic Dark Tanning with Sunscreen. (Tanning Research Labs, Inc.) **Oil:** Ethylhexyl p-methoxycinnamate, octyl dimethyl PABA. Waterproof. SPF 4. Bot. 240 ml. **Gel:** Phenylbenzimidazole, sulfonic acid. PABA free. SPF 4. Tube 240 g. *otc.*
Use: Sunscreen.

Hawaiian Tropic Just for Kids Sunblock. (Tanning Research Labs, Inc.) **SPF 30:** Homosalate, octyl methoxycinnamate, benzophenone-3, menthyl anthranilate, octyl salicylate. PABA free. Waterproof. Lot. Bot. 88.7 ml. **SPF 45:** Octyl methoxycinnamate, benzophenone-3, octyl salicylate, octocrylene, titanium dioxide. PABA free. Waterproof. Lot. Bot. 88.7 ml. *otc.*
Use: Sunscreen.

Hawaiian Tropic Lip Balm Sunblock. (Tanning Research Labs, Inc.) Padimate O, oxybenzone. Stick 4 g. *otc.*
Use: Sunscreen.

Hawaiian Tropic 8 Plus. (Tanning Research Labs, Inc.) Octyl methoxycinnamate, benzophenone-3, menthyl anthranilate. PABA free. Waterproof. SPF 8+. Gel 120 g. *otc.*
Use: Sunscreen.

Hawaiian Tropic 10 Plus. (Tanning Research Labs, Inc.) Octyl methoxycinnamate, benzophenone-3, menthyl anthranilate. PABA free. Waterproof. SPF 10+. Gel 120 g. *otc.*
Use: Sunscreen.

Hawaiian Tropic 15 Plus. (Tanning Research Labs, Inc.) Octyl methoxycinnamate, octocrylene, benzophenone-3, menthyl anthranilate, PABA free, waterproof. Gel Tube 120 g. *otc.*
Use: Sunscreen.

Hawaiian Tropic 15 Plus Sunblock. (Tanning Research Labs, Inc.) Menthyl anthranilate, octyl methoxycinnamate, benzophenone-3. PABA free. Waterproof. Lot. Bot. 7.5 ml, 15 ml, 60 ml, 120 ml, 240 ml, 300 ml. *otc.*
Use: Sunscreen.

Hawaiian Tropic 15 Plus Sunblock Lip Balm. (Tanning Research Labs, Inc.) Padimate O, oxybenzone. SPF 15, waterproof. Stick 4.2 g. *otc.*
Use: Sunscreen.

Hawaiian Tropic 45 Plus Sunblock Lip Balm. (Tanning Research Labs, Inc.) Octyl methoxycinnamate, benzophenone-3, octyl salicylate, titanium dioxide, menthyl anthranilate. PABA free. Waterproof. SPF 45+. Lip balm 4.2 g. *otc.*
Use: Sunscreen.

Hawaiian Tropic Protective Tanning. (Tanning Research Labs, Inc.) Titanium dioxide. PABA free. Waterproof. SPF 6. Lot. Bot. 240 ml. *otc.*
Use: Sunscreen.

Hawaiian Tropic Protective Tanning Dry. (Tanning Research Labs, Inc.) SPF 6. **Oil:** 2-ethylhexyl p-methoxycinnamate, homosalate, menthyl anthranilate. Waterproof. Bot. 180 ml. **Gel:** Phenylbenzimidazole, sulfonic acid, benzophenone-4. Tube 180 g. *otc.*
Use: Sunscreen.

Hawaiian Tropic Self Tanning Sunblock. (Tanning Research Labs, Inc.) Octyl methoxycinnamate, benzophenone-3, aloe, cetyl alcohol, stearyl alcohol, cocoa butter, parabens, vitamin E. PABA free. SPF 15. Cream 93.75 ml. *otc.*
Use: Sunscreen.

Hawaiian Tropic Sport Sunblock. (Tanning Research Labs, Inc.) SPF 15, SPF 30. Methoxycinnamate, octocrylene, benzophenone-3, octyl salicylate, titanium dioxide. PABA free. Waterproof. Lot. Bot. 88.7 ml. *otc.*
Use: Sunscreen.

Hawaiian Tropic Sunblock. (Tanning Research Labs, Inc.) Titanium dioxide, octyl methoxycinnamate, benzophenone-3, octyl salicylate, octocrylene.

PABA free. Waterproof. **SPF 30+:** Lot. Bot. 120 ml. **SPF 45+:** Lot. Bot. 120 ml, 300 ml. *otc.*
Use: Sunscreen.

Hawaiian Tropic Swim n Sun. (Tanning Research Labs, Inc.) Padimate O, oxybenzone. Lot. Bot. 120 ml. *otc.*
Use: Sunscreen.

Hayfebrol Liquid. (Scot-Tussin Pharmacal, Inc.) Pseudoephedrine HCl 30 mg, chlorpheniramine 2 mg/Syr. Bot. 118 ml. *otc.*
Use: Antihistamine, decongestant.

Hazogel Body and Foot Rub. (Vortech Pharmaceuticals) Witch hazel 70%, isopropanol 20% in a neutralized resin vehicle. Bot. 4 oz. *otc.*
Use: Astringent, antipruritic.

H-BIG Hepatitis B Immune Globulin (Human). (North American Biologicals, Inc.) Hepatitis B immune globulin (human). Vial 1 ml, 5 ml. Syr. 0.5 ml. *Rx.*
Use: Immunization.

H-BIGIV. (Nabi) Hepatitis B immune globulin IV.
Use: Prophylaxis against hepatitis B virus reinfection in liver transplant patients. [Orphan Drug]

1% HC. (C & M Pharmacal, Inc.) Hydrocortisone 1%, petrolatum base. Oint. Tube 15, 20, 30, 60, 120, 240 g, lb. *otc.*
Use: Corticosteroid, topical.

HC Derma-Pax. (Recsei Laboratories) Hydrocortisone 0.5% in liquid base. Dropper Bot. 2 oz. *otc.*
Use: Corticosteroid, topical.

HCG.
See: Chorionic Gonadotropin.

HCG-Nostick. (Organon Teknika Corp.) Sol Particle Immunoassay (SPIA) for detection of hCG in urine. Stick 30s.
Use: Diagnostic aid, pregnancy.

HD 85. (Lafayette Pharmaceuticals, Inc.) Barium suspension 85%. Susp. Kit 150 ml, 450 ml. Bot. 1900 ml. *Rx.*
Use: Radiopaque agent.

HD 200 Plus. (Lafayette Pharmaceuticals, Inc.) Barium sulfate 98%. Pow. for Susp. Bot. 312 g. *Rx.*
Use: Radiopaque agent.

Head & Shoulders Conditioner. (Procter & Gamble Pharm.) Pyrithione zinc 0.3%. Bot. 4 oz, 11 oz. *otc.*
Use: Antiseborrheic.

Head & Shoulders Dry Scalp. (Procter & Gamble Pharm.) Pyrithione zinc 1%, regular and conditioning formulas. Shampoo. Bot. 210 ml, 330 ml, 450 ml. *otc.*
Use: Antiseborrehic.

Head & Shoulders Intensive Treatment Dandruff Shampoo. (Procter & Gamble Pharm.) Selenium sulfide 1%, regular and conditioning formulas. Shampoo. Bot. 120 ml, 210 ml, 330 ml. *otc.*
Use: Antiseborrehic.

Head & Shoulders Shampoo. (Procter & Gamble Pharm.) Pyrithione zinc 1%. **Cream:** Tube 51 g, 75 g, 120 g, 210 g. **Lot:** 120 ml, 210 ml, 330 ml, 450 ml. *otc.*
Use: Antiseborrheic.

Healon. (Pharmacia & Upjohn) Sodium hyaluronate 10 mg/ml Inj. Syringe 0.4 ml, 0.55 ml, 0.85 ml, 2 ml. *Rx.*
Use: Surgical aid, ophthalmic.

Healon GV. (Pharmacia & Upjohn) Sodium hyaluronate 14 mg/ml Inj. Syringe 0.55 ml, 0.85 ml. *Rx.*
Use: Surgical aid, ophthalmic.

Healon Yellow. (Pharmacia & Upjohn) Sodium hyaluronate 10 mg, fluorescein sodium 0.005 mg/ml Inj. Syringe 0.55 ml, 0.85 ml.
Use: Surgical and diagnostic aid, ophthalmic.

Healthbreak. (Lemar Labs) Silver acetate 6 mg. Chewing gum. Pack 24s. *otc.*
Use: Smoking deterrent.

Heartburn Antacid. (Walgreen Co.) Aluminum hydroxide dried gel 80 mg, magnesium trisilicate 60 mg/Tab. Bot. 100s. *otc.*
Use: Antacid.

Heartline. (BDI Pharmaceuticals, Inc.) Aspirin 81 mg/Tab. Enteric coated Bot. 36s. *otc.*
Use: Anti-inflammatory.

heavy metal poisoning, antidote.
See: BAL., Amp. (Becton Dickinson & Co.).
Calcium Disodium Versenate, Amp., Tab. (3M Pharmaceuticals).

Heet Liniment. (Whitehall Robins Laboratories) Methyl salicylate 15%, camphor 3.6%, oleoresin capsicum 0.025%, alcohol 70%. Bot. 2⅓ oz, 5 oz. *otc.*
Use: Analgesic-topical.

•**hefilcon a.** (heh-FILL-kahn A) USAN.
Use: Contact lens material (hydrophilic).

•**helfilcon b.** (heh-FILL-kahn B) USAN.
Use: Contact lens material (hydrophilic).

•**helfilcon c.** (heh-FILL-kahn C) USAN.
Use: Contact lens material (hydrophilic).

Helidac. (Procter & Gamble Pharm.) Bismuth subsalicylate 264.4 mg/Tab. Metronidazole 250 mg/Tab. Tetracycline

500 mg/Cap. Box. 4s, 8s (bismuth subsalicylate only). *Rx.*
Use: Antiulcerative.

Helistat. (Hoechst Marion Roussel) Absorbable collagen hemostatic sponge. 1" × 2" and 3" × 4" in 10s, 9" × 10" in 5s. *Rx.*
Use: Hemostatic.

•**helium.** (HEE-lee-uhm) U.S.P. 23.
Use: Diluent for gases.

Helixate. (Centeon) Concentrated recombitant hemophilic factor. After reconstitution, also contains glycine 10 to 30 mg, imidazole ≤ 500 mcg/1000 IU, polysorbate 80 H 600 mcg/1000 IU, Calcium Cl 2 to 5 mM, sodium 100 to 130 mEq/L, chloride 100 to 130 mEq/L, albumin (human) 4 to 10 mg/ml. IU 250, 500, 1000. *Rx.*
Use: Antihemophilic.

Hemabate. (Pharmacia & Upjohn) Carboprost tromethamine equivalent to 250 mcg carboprost, tromethamine 83 mcg/ml. Inj. Amp 1 ml. *Rx.*
Use: Abortifacient.

Hema-Chek Slides. (Bayer Corp. (Consumer Div.)) Fecal occult blood test containing slide tests, developer and applicators. Pkg. 100s, 300s, 1000s.
Use: Diagnostic aid.

Hema-Combistix Reagent Strips. (Bayer Corp. (Consumer Div.)) Fourway strip test for urinary pH, glucose, protein and occult blood. Strip. Bot. 100s.
Use: Diagnostic aid.

Hemaferrin. (Western Research) Ferrous fumarate 150 mg, desiccated liver 50 mg, docusate sodium 25 mg, betaine HCl 100 mg, folic acid 0.4 mg, vitamins C 50 mg, B_6 2 mg, Mn 2 mg, B_{12} 5 mcg, Cu 1 mg, Zn 2 mg, Mo 0.4 mg/Tab. 28 Pack 1000s. *otc.*
Use: Mineral, vitamin supplement; stool softener.

Hemafolate. (Canright) Ferrous gluconate 293 mg, liver fraction II 250 mg, gastric substance 100 mg, vitamins C 50 mg, B_{12} 10 mcg/Tab. Bot. 100s, 1000s. *otc.*
Use: Mineral, vitamin supplement.

Hemalive Liquid. (Barth's) Vitamins B_1 3.15 mg, B_2 3.33 mg, niacin 22.5 mg, B_6 0.81 mg, B_{12} 6 mcg, biotin 3.6 mcg, iron 60 mg, choline, inositol, liver fraction No. 1, pantothenic acid/15 ml. Bot. 8 oz, 24 oz. *otc.*
Use: Mineral, vitamin supplement.

Hemalive Tablets. (Barth's) Vitamins B_{12} 25 mcg, iron 75 mg, B_1 2.5 mg, B_2 5 mg, niacin 1.4 mg, C 30 mg, liver 240 mg, B_6, pantothenic acid, aminobenzoic acid, choline, inositol, biotin, Mg, Mn, Cu/3 Tab. Bot. 100s, 500s, 1000s. *otc.*
Use: Mineral, vitamin supplement.

Hemaneed. (Hanlon) Hematinic B_{12}, intrinsic factor, Fe/Cap. Bot. 100s. *otc.*
Use: Mineral, vitamin supplement.

Hemaspan Tablets. (Sanofi Winthrop Pharmaceucticals) Iron 110 mg (from ferrous fumarate), ascorbic acid 200 mg, docusate sodium 20 mg/Tab. Bot. 100s, 1000s. *otc.*
Use: Mineral, vitamin supplement; stool softener.

Hemastix Reagent Strips. (Bayer Corp. (Consumer Div.)) Cellulose strip, impregnated with a peroxide and orthotolidine for detection of hematuria and hemoglobinuria. Strip Bot. 50s.
Use: Diagnostic aid.

Hematest Reagent Tablets. (Bayer Corp. (Consumer Div.)) Reagent Tab. for blood in the feces. Bot. 100s.
Use: Diagnostic aid.

Hematinic. (Canright) Ferrous gluconate 180 mg, desiccated liver 200 mg, vitamins B_{12} 1 mcg, C 25 mg, B_1 3.3 mg, copper gluconate 0.3 mg/Tab. Bot. 100s, 1000s. *otc.*
Use: Mineral, vitamin supplement.

hematinics.
See: Iron Products.
Ferric Compounds.
Ferrous Compounds.
Liver Products.
Vitamin B_{12}.
Vitamin Products.

Hematrin. (Towne) Iron 50 mg, vitamins B_{12} 10 mcg, B_1 10 mg, B_2 10 mg, B_6 2 mg, C 150 mg, copper 2 mg, niacinamide 50 mg, calcium pantothenate 5 mg, desiccated liver 200 mg/Captab. Bot. 60s, 100s. *otc.*
Use: Mineral, vitamin supplement.

heme arginate.
Use: Acute porphyria; myelodysplastic syndromes. [Orphan Drug]

HemeSelect. (SmithKline Diagnostics) Occult blood screening test. Box 40 test kits.
Use: Diagnostic aid, fecal.

Hemex. Hemin and zinc mesoporphyrin.
Use: Acute porphyric syndromes. [Orphan Drug]

Hemiacidrin. Citric acid, glucono-delta-lactone, magnesium carbonate.
Use: Genitourinary irrigant.
See: Renacidin, Pow. (Guardian Laboratories).
Renacidin, Soln. (Guardian Laboratories).

Hemex. (Vogarell) Oint. Tube 1.25 oz. Supp. Box 12s.
Use: Anorectal preparation.

hemin.
Use: Acute intermittent porphyria. [Orphan Drug]
See: Panhematin, Inj. (Abbott Laboratories).

hemin and zinc mesoporphyrin.
Use: Acute porphyric syndromes. [Orphan Drug]
See: Hemex.

hemisine.
See: Epinephrine (Various Mfr.).

Hemoccult SENSA. (SmithKline Diagnostics) Occult blood screening tests.
Use: Diagnostic aid, fecal.

Hemoccult Slides. (SmithKline Diagnostics) Occult blood detection (fecal). In 100s, 1000s, and tape dispensers (test 100s).
Use: Diagnostic aid.

Hemoccult II. (SmithKline Diagnostics) Occult blood detection (fecal). In 102s, kit 100s.
Use: Diagnostic aid.

Hemocitrate. (Hemotec Medical Products, Inc.) Trisodium citrate concentrate.
Use: Leukapheresis procedures. [Orphan Drug]

Hemocyte. (US Pharmaceutical Corp.) Ferrous fumarate 324 mg (Fe 106 mg)/Tab. Bot. 100s. *otc.*
Use: Mineral supplement.

Hemocyte-F. (US Pharmaceutical Corp.) Iron 106 mg (from ferrous fumarate), folic acid 1 mg/Tab. 100s. *Rx.*
Use: Mineral supplement.

Hemocyte Plus. (US Pharmaceutical Corp.) Iron 106 mg (from ferrous fumarate), sodium ascorbate 200 mg, vitamins B_1 10 mg, B_2 6 mg, B_6 5 mg, B_{12} 15 mcg, folic acid 1 mg, B_3 30 mg, B_5 10 mg, zinc 18.2 mg, Mg, Mn sulfate, Cu/Tabule. Bot. 100s. *Rx.*
Use: Mineral, vitamin supplement.

Hemocyte Plus Elixir. (US Pharmaceutical Corp.) Polysaccharide iron complex 12 mg, vitamin B_3 13.3 mg, B_5 3.3 mg, B_6 1.3 mg, B_{12} 4 mcg, folic acid 0.33 mg, zinc 5 mg, Mn 1.3 mg/15 ml. Bot. 473 ml. *Rx.*
Use: Mineral, vitamin supplement.

Hemofil M. (Baxter Pharmaceutical Products, Inc.) Stable dried preparation of Antihemophilic Factor in concentrated form. Albumin (human) 12.5 mg/ml when reconstituted. Bot. 10 ml, 20 ml, 30 ml with diluent. *Rx.*
Use: Antihemophilic.

Hemofil T. (Baxter Pharmaceutical Products, Inc.) Antihemophilic Factor (Human), method four, dried, heat-treated 225-375 IU/10 ml; 450-650 IU/20 ml; 675-999 IU/30 ml; 1000-1600 IU/30 ml. *Rx.*
Use: Antihemophilic.

•**hemoglobin crosfumaril.** (HEE-moe-GLOBE-in CROSS-FEW-mah-ril) USAN.
Use: Red cell substitute; treatment of prefusion deficit disorders.

Hemoglobin Reagent Strips. (Bayer Corp. (Consumer Div.)) Seralyzer reagent strips. Bot. 50s. Quantitive strip test for hemoglobin in whole blood.
Use: Diagnostic aid.

Hemopad. (Astra Pharmaceuticals, L.P.) Fibrous absorbable collagen hemostat. 2.5 cm × 5 cm, 5 cm × 8 cm, 8 cm ×10 cm. *Rx.*
Use: Hemostatic.

hemorheologic agent. Pentoxifylline.
See: Trental, Tab. (Hoechst Marion Roussel).

Hemorid for Women. (Thompson Medical Co.) **Lotion:** Mineral oil, petrolatum, diazolidinyl urea, cetyl alcohol, glycerin, parabens. Bot. 118 ml. **Cream:** White petrolatum 30%, mineral oil 20%, pramoxine HCl 1%, phenylephrine HCl 0.25%, aloe vera gel, parabens, cetyl and stearyl alcohols. In 28.3 g. **Supp:** Zinc oxide 11%, phenylephrine HCl 0.25%, hard fat 88.25%, aloe vera. In 12s. *otc.*
Use: Perianal hygiene.

Hemorrhoidal HC. (Various Mfr.) Hydrocortisone acetate 25 mg/Supp. Bot. 12s, 24s, 50s, 100s, UD 12s. *Rx.*
Use: Anorectal preparation.

Hemorrhoidal Ointment. (Zenith Goldline Pharmaceuticals) Live yeast cell derivative supplying skin respiratory factor 2000 units/oz of ointment w/shark liver oil 3%, phenyl mercuric nitrate 1:10,000. *otc.*
Use: Anorectal preparation.

Hemorrhoidal Suppositories. (Zenith Goldline Pharmaceuticals) Bismuth subgallate 2.25%, bismuth resorcin compound 1.75%, benzyl benzoate 1.2%, balsam Peru 1.8%, zinc oxide 11%/Supp. Box 12s. *otc.*
Use: Anorectal preparation.

Hemorrhoidal Uniserts. (Upsher-Smith Labs, Inc.) Bismuth subgallate 2.25%, bismuth resorcin compound 1.75%, benzyl benzoate 1.2%, balsam Peru 1.8%, zinc oxide 11%/Supp. Carton 12s, 50s. *otc.*

Use: Anorectal preparation.
hemostatics, local.
See: Absorbable Gelatin Sponge (Pharmacia & Upjohn).
Gelfilm (Pharmacia & Upjohn).
Gelfoam, Preps. (Pharmacia & Upjohn).
Helistat (Hoechst Marion Roussel).
Hemotene (Astra Pharmaceuticals, L.P.).
Oxidized Cellulose.
Thrombin (Various Mfr.).
hemostatic topical. Thrombin.
See: Thrombinar, Pow. (Centeon).
Thrombostat, Pow. (Parke-Davis).
hemostatin.
See: Epinephrine (Various Mfr.).
Hemotene. (Astra Pharmaceuticals, L.P.) Absorbable collagen hemostat. 1 g. Pkg. 5s. *Rx.*
Use: Hemostatic, topical.
Hemozyme Elixir. (Barrows) Vitamins B_1 5 mg, B_2 5 mg, B_6 1 mg, panthenol 4 mg, niacinamide 100 mg, B_{12} 3 mcg, iron 100 mg, choline bitartrate 100 mg, dl-methionine 100 mg, yeast extract, alcohol 12%/fl oz. Bot. 12 oz. *otc.*
Use: Mineral, vitamin supplement.
Hem-Prep. (G & W Laboratories) Phenylephrine HCl 0.25%, zinc oxide 11%. Supp. Bot. 12s. *otc.*
Use: Anorectal preparation.
Hem-Prep Ointment. (G & W Laboratories) Phenylephrine HCl 0.025%, zinc oxide 11%, white petrolatum. Oint. 42.5 g. *otc.*
Use: Anorectal preparation.
Hemril-HC Uniserts. (Upsher-Smith Labs, Inc.) Hydrocortisone acetate 25 mg/Supp. 12s. *Rx.*
Use: Anorectal preparation.
Hemril Uniserts. (Upsher-Smith Labs, Inc.) Bismuth subgallate 2.25%, bismuth resorcin compound 1.75%, benzyl benzoate 1.2%, balsam Peru 1.8%, zinc oxide 11%/Supp. 12s, 50s. *otc.*
Use: Anorectal preparation.
henbane.
See: Hyoscyamus (Various Mfr.).
Henydin-M. (Arcum) Thyroid desiccated pow. 0.5 gr, vitamins B_1 1 mg, B_2 0.5 mg, B_6 0.5 mg, niacinamide 2.5 mg/Tab. Bot. 100s, 1000s. *Rx.*
Use: Vitamin supplement.
Henydin-R. (Arcum) Thyroid desiccated pow. 1 gr, vitamins B_1 2 mg, B_2 1 mg, B_6 1 mg, niacinamide 5 mg/Tab. Bot. 100s, 1000s. *Rx.*
Use: Vitamin supplement.
Hepandrin. (Bio-Technology General Corporation) Oxandrolone.
Use: Turner's syndrome; AIDS; growth delay; alcoholic hepatitis; malnutrition. [Orphan Drug]
heparin, 2-0-desulfated. (HEP-uh-rin)
Use: Cystic fibrosis. [Orphan Drug]
See: Aeropin.
heparin antagonist.
See: Protamine Sulfate (Various Mfr.).
heparin calcium. *Rx.*
Use: Anticoagulant.
•**heparin calcium.** (HEP-uh-rin KAL-see-uhm) U.S.P. 23.
Use: Anticoagulant.
heparin lock flush solution. (Sanofi Winthrop Pharmaceuticals) **10 USP units/1 ml:** Cartridge 2 ml HEP-PAK containing 1 cartridge heparin lock flush Soln. (1 ml) and 2 cartridges sodium Cl Inj. HEP-PAK-2 containing 1 cartridge heparin lock flush soln. (1 ml) and 1 cartridge sodium Cl Inj. **10 USP units/2 ml:** Cartridge 2 ml. **100 USP units/1 ml:** Cartridge 2 ml HEP-PAK containing 1 cartridge heparin lock flush soln (1 ml) and 2 cartridges sodium Cl Inj. HEP-PAK-2 containing 1 cartridge of heparin lock flush soln (1 ml) and 1 cartridge sodium Cl Inj. **100 USP units/2 ml:** Cartridge 2 ml. *Rx.*
Use: Catheter patency agent.
heparin lock flush solution. (Wyeth-Ayerst Laboratories) Heparin sodium 10 units or 100 units/1 ml vial. Pkg. 50 Tubex 1 ml, 2 ml. *Rx.*
Use: Infusion set patency agent.
•**heparin sodium.** (HEP-uh-rin SO-dee-uhm) U.S.P. 23.
Use: Anticoagulant. Note: Protamine sulfate is antidote.
See: Hepathrom, Amp., Vial (Fellows-Testagar).
Heprinar, Inj. (Centeon).
Lipo-Hepin, Amp., Vial (3M Pharmaceuticals).
Lipo-Hepin/BL, Amp., Vial (3M Pharmaceuticals).
Liquaemin, Vial (Organon Teknika Corp.)
heparin sodium. (Pharmacia & Upjohn) 1000 units/ml. Vial 10 ml, 30 ml 5000 units/ml. Vial 1 ml, 10 ml 10,000 units/ml. Vial 1 ml, 4 ml (Sanofi Winthrop Pharmaceuticals) 5000 USP units/1 ml. Carpuject 1 ml fill in 2 ml cartridge.
Use: Anticoagulant. Note: Protamine sulfate is antidote.
heparin sodium and 0.45% sodium chloride. (Abbott Laboratories) 12,500, 25,000 units in 250 ml Inj. *Rx.*
Use: Anticoagulant.
heparin sodium and 0.9%sodium

chloride. (Baxter Pharmaceutical Products, Inc.) Inj.: 1000 units in 500 ml Viaflex. 2000, 5000 units in 1000 ml Viaflex. *Rx.*
Use: Anticoagulant.

heparin sodium lock flush solution. *Rx.*
Use: Anticoagulant.
See: Heparin Lock Flush, Inj. (Various Mfr.).
Hep-Lock, Inj. (ESI Lederle Generics).
Hep-Lock U/P, Inj. (ESI Lederle Generics).

HepatAmine. (McGaw, Inc.) Amino acid 8%. Inj. Bot. 500 ml. *Rx.*
Use: Nutritional supplement, parenteral.

Hepatic-Aid II Instant Drink Powder. (McGaw, Inc.) Amino acids (high BCAA, low AAA), maltodextrin, sucrose, partially hydrogenated soybean oil, lecithin, mono- and diglycerides. In 3 oz packet of 12s. *otc.*
Use: Nutritional supplement.

hepatitis A vaccine, inactivated. (hep-uh-TIGHT-iss) *Rx.*
Use: Immunization.
See: Havrix, Inj. (SmithKline Beecham Pharmaceuticals).
Vaqta, Inj. (Merck & Co.).

hepatitis B and haemophilus type b vaccines, combined.
See: Comvax (Merck & Co.).

•**hepatitis B immune globulin.** (hep-uh-TIGHT-iss B ih-myoon GLAH-byoo-lin) U.S.P. 23.
Use: Immunization.
See: BayHep B, Vial, Syr. (Bayer Corp. (Consumer Div.)).
H-BIG, Vial, Syr. (North American Biologicals, Inc.).

hepatitis B immune globulin IV. (hep-uh-TIGHT-iss)
Use: Prophylaxis against hepatitis B virus reinfection in liver transplant patients. [Orphan Drug]
See: H-BIGIV (Nabi).

hepatitis B vaccine, recombinant. (hep-uh-TIGHT-iss) *Rx.*
Use: Immunization.
See: Engerix-B (SmithKline Beecham Pharmaceuticals).
Recombivax HB, Inj. (Merck & Co.).

•**hepatitis B virus vaccine inactivated.** (hep-uh-TIGHT-iss B vak-SEEN) U.S.P. 23.
Use: Immunization.

Hepfomin R Injection. (Keene Pharmaceuticals, Inc.) Liver inj. equivalent to cyanocobalamin 10 mcg, folic acid 0.4 mg, cyanocobalamin 100 mcg. Vial 10 ml. *Rx.*
Use: Nutritional supplement, parenteral.

Hep-Forte. (Marlyn Nutraceuticals, Inc.) Vitamins A 1200 IU, E 10 mg, B_1 1 mg, B_2 1 mg, B_3 10 mg, B_5 2 mg, B_6 0.5 mg, B_{12} 1 mcg, C 10 mg, folic acid 0.06 mg, zinc 0.5 mg, choline, inositol, biotin, dl-methionine, desiccated liver, liver concentrate, liver fraction No. 2/Cap. Bot. 100s, 300s, 500s. *otc.*
Use: Vitamin, liver supplement.

Hep-Lock. (ESI Lederle Generics) Sterile heparin sodium soln. in saline 10 units or 100 units/ml. Dosette 1 ml, 2 ml, multiple-dose vial 10 ml, 30 ml. *Rx.*
Use: Catheter patency agent.

Hep-Lock PF. (ESI Lederle Generics) Preservative-free heparin flush soln. 10 units/ml or 100 units/ml. Vial 1 ml. *Rx.*
Use: Catheter patency agent.

Heptalac. (Copley Pharmaceutical, Inc.) Lactulose 10 g/15 ml, galactose < 1.6 g, lactose < 1.2 g, other sugars H 1.2 g/Syrup. Bot. 473 ml, 1920 ml. *Rx.*
Use: Laxative.

Herbal Cellulex. (NBTY, Inc.) Vitamin C 83 mg, K 33 mg, iron 9 mg/Tab. Bot. 90s. *otc.*
Use: Vitamin supplement.

Herbal Laxative. (NBTY, Inc.) Senna concentrate 125 mg, cascara sagrada 20 mg, buckthorn bark PDR. Tab. Bot. 100s. *otc.*
Use: Laxative.

Herceptin. (Genentech) Trastuzumab 440 mg Lyophilized Pow. Vial. Preservative free. Diluent: 30 ml of Bacteriostatic Water for Inj. w/1.1% benzyl alcohol. *Rx.*
Use: Antineoplastic.

Hermal Bath Oil. (Hermal Pharmaceutical Labs) Soybean oil-based bath oil. Bot. 8 oz, 32 oz. *otc.*
Use: Emollient.

Herpecin-L. (Campbell Laboratories) Allantoin, octyl-p-(dimethylamino)-benzoate (Padimate O), titanium dioxide, pyridoxine HCl in a balanced, acidic lipid system. Lip balm. Tube 2.5 g. *otc.*
Use: Cold sores.

herpes simplex virus gene. (Genetic Therapy, Inc.)
Use: Antineoplastic. [Orphan Drug]

Herrick Lacrimal Plug. (Lacrimedics, Inc.) Silicone plug 0.3 mm or 0.5 mm Pkg. 2 plugs. *Rx.*
Use: Punctal plug.

HES. Hetastarch.
Use: Plasma expander.
See: Hespan, Inj. (Du Pont Merck Pharmaceutical Co.).

Hespan Injection. (Du Pont Merck Pharmaceutical Co.) Hetastarch 6 g, sodium Cl 0.9%/100 ml. Bot. 500 ml. *Rx.*
Use: Plasma volume expander.

hesperidin.
Use: Capillary fragility and permeability, hemorrhage.
See: Vitamin P; also Rutin.
W/Combinations.
See: A.C.N., Tab. (Person and Covey, Inc.).
Hesper Bitabs, Tab. (Hoechst Marion Roussel).
Nialex, Tab. (Roberts Pharmaceuticals).
Vita Cebus, Tab. (Cenci, H.R Labs, Inc).

Hesperidin w/C. (Various Mfr.).
Use: Vitamin supplement.

hesperidin methyl chalcone.
Use: Vitamin P supplement.

•**hetacillin.** (HET-ah-SILL-in) USAN, U.S.P. XXII.
Use: Anti-infective.

•**hetacillin potassium.** (HET-ah-SILL-in poe-TASS-ee-uhm) U.S.P. 23.
Use: Anti-infective.

•**hetaflur.** (HEH-tah-flure) USAN.
Use: Dental caries prophylactic.

•**hetastarch.** (HET-uh-starch) USAN.
Use: Plasma volume extender.
See: Hespan, Inj. (Du Pont Merck Pharmaceutical Co.).

•**heteronium bromide.** (HET-er-oh-nee-uhm) USAN.
Use: Anticholinergic.

Hexabamate #1. (Rugby Labs, Inc.) Tridihexethyl Cl 25 mg, meprobamate 200 mg/Tab. Bot. 100s, 500s. *Rx.*
Use: Anticholinergic combination.

Hexabamate #2. (Rugby Labs, Inc.) Tridihexethyl Cl 25 mg, meprobamate 400 mg/Tab. Bot. 100s, 500s. *Rx.*
Use: Anticholinergic combination.

Hexa-Betalin. (Eli Lilly and Co.) Pyridoxine HCl. Inj. Vial 100 mg/ml. Ctn. 10s, vial 10 ml. *Rx.*
Use: Vitamin supplement.

Hexabrix. (Mallinckrodt Chemical) Ioxaglate meglumine 393 mg, ioxaglate sodium 196 mg, iodine 320 mg/ml, EDTA. Vial 20 ml, 30 ml, 50 ml. Bot. 75 ml fill in 150 ml, 100 ml fill in 150 ml, 200 ml fill in 250 ml, 150 ml. Power Inj. Syr. 125 ml.
Use: Radiopaque agent.

•**hexachlorophene.** (hex-ah-KLOR-oh-feen) U.S.P. 23.
Use: Anti-infective, topical; antiseptic; detergent.
See: Derl.
Gamophen, Leaves, Bar (Arbrook).
pHisoHex Prods. (Sanofi Winthrop Pharmaceuticals).

hexachlorophene cleansing emulsion.
Use: Anti-infective, topical detergent.

hexachlorophene liquid soap, detergent liquid.
Use: Anti-infective, topical detergent.
See: pHisoHex Liq. Prods. (Sanofi Winthrop Pharmaceuticals).

hexacose. Mixture of C-6 alcohols derived from oxidation of tetracosane–$C_{24}H_{50}$.

hexadecadrol.
See: Dexamethasone.

hexadienol. Hexacose.

Hexadrol. (Organon Teknika Corp.) Dexamethasone. **Tab.:** 4 mg. Bot. 100s, UD 100s, Strip 10 x 10s. **Elix.:** 0.5 mg/5 ml, alcohol 5%. Bot. 120 ml. *Rx.*
Use: Corticosteroid.

Hexadrol Phosphate. (Organon Teknika Corp.) Dexamethasone sodium phosphate 4 mg/ml, 10 mg/ml or 20 mg/ml, benzyl alcohol. **4 mg/ml:** Vial 1 ml, 5 ml, disposable syringe 1 ml. **10 mg/ml:** Vial 10 ml, disposable syringe 1 ml. **20 mg/ml:** Vial 5 ml, disposable syringe 5 ml. *Rx.*
Use: Corticosteroid.

•**hexafluorenium bromide.** (HEK-sah-flure-EE-nee-uhm) USAN, U.S.P. XXI.
Use: Muscle relaxant, synergist (succinycholine).

hexafluorodiethyl ether. Name used for Flurothyl.

hexahydroxycyclohexane.
See: Inositol, Preps. (Various Mfr.).

hexakose. Mixture of tetracosanes and oxidation products.

Hexalen. (US Bioscience) Altretamine. *Rx.*
Use: Antineoplastic.

hexamethonium.

hexamethonium chloride. (Various Mfr.) Hexamethylene (bistrimethylammonium) Cl.

hexamethylamine.
See: Hexastat. Hypotensive.

hexamethylenamine.
See: Methenamine (Various Mfr.).

hexamethylenetetramine.
See: Methenamine, U.S.P. 23. Hexamethylenetetramine Mandelate.

hexamethylmelamine. Altretamine.
Use: Antineoplastic.
See: Hexalen.

hexamethylpararosaniline chloride.
See: Bismuth Violet, Soln. (Table Rock).

hexamethylrosaniline chloride.

See: Gentian Violet.

hexamine.
See: Methenamine (Various Mfr.).

hexapradol hydrochloride. a- (1-Aminohexyl) benzhydrol HCl.
Use: CNS stimulant.

Hexate. (Davis & Sly) Atropine sulfate 1/2000 gr, extract of hyoscyamus 0.25 gr, methylene blue gr, methanamine 0.5 gr, benzoic acid 0.5 gr, salol 0.5 gr./Tab. Bot. 1000s. *Rx.*
Use: Anti-infective, urinary.

Hexavitamin Tablets. (Various Mfr.) Vitamins A 5000 IU, B_1 2 mg, B_2 3 mg, C 75 mg, D 400 IU, B_3 20 mg/Tab. Bot. 100s, 1000s, UD 100s. *otc.*
Use: Vitamin supplement.

Hexavitamin SC. (Halsey Drug Co.)
Use: Vitamin supplement.

hexcarbacholine bromide.

•**hexedine.** (HEX-eh-deen) USAN.
Use: Anti-infective.

hexene-ol. Hexacose.

hexenol. Hexacose.

hexitol irrigants.
Use: Irrigant, genitourinary.
See: Resectisol, Soln. (McGaw, Inc.).
Sorbitol, Soln. (McGaw, Inc.).
Sorbitol, Soln. (Baxter Pharmaceutical Products, Inc.).
Sorbitol-Mannitol, Soln. (Abbott Laboratories).

hexobarbital. U.S.P. 23.

•**hexobendine.** (HEX-oh-BEN-deen) USAN.
Use: Vasodilator.

Hexopal. (Bayer Corp. (Consumer Div.)) Inositol hexanicotinate. *Rx.*
Use: Hypolipidemic, peripheral vasodilator.

•**hexoprenaline sulfate.** (hex-oh-PREN-ah-leen) USAN.
Use: Bronchodilator, tocolytic.

•**hexylene glycol.** N.F. 18.
Use: Pharmaceutic aid (humectant, solvent).

•**hexylresorcinol.** (hex-ill-reh-SORE-sih-nole) U.S.P. 23.
Use: Anthelmintic (intestinal roundworms and trematodes), throat preparation.
See: Sucrets Sore Throat Loz. (SmithKline Beecham Pharmaceuticals).

H-F Gel. (Paddock Laboratories) Calcium gluconate gel 2.5%.
Use: Emergency burn treatment. [Orphan Drug]

H.H.R. (Geneva Pharmaceuticals) Hydralazine HCl 25 mg, hydrochlorothiazide 15 mg, reserpine 0.1 mg/Tab. Bot. 100s, 1000s. *Rx.*
Use: Antihypertensive.

Hibiclens. (J & J Merck Consumer Pharm.) Chlorhexidine gluconate 4%, isopropyl alcohol 4%, in a non-alkaline base. Bot. 4 oz, 8 oz, 16 oz, 32 oz, gal. Packette 15 ml. *otc.*
Use: Antimicrobial, antiseptic.

Hibiclens Sponge Brush. (J & J Merck Consumer Pharm.) Chlorhexidine gluconate impregnated sponge brush. Unit-of-use 22 ml sponge brushes. *otc.*
Use: Antimicrobial, antiseptic.

Hibistat. (J & J Merck Consumer Pharm.) Chlorhexidine gluconate 0.5%. **Liq.:** Isopropyl alcohol 70%, emollients. Bot. 4 oz, 8 oz. **Towelettes:** Unit-of-use pocket-size towelette impregnated with 5 ml Hibistat. *otc.*
Use: Antimicrobial, antiseptic.

Hibplex. (Standex) Vitamins B_1 100 mg, B_2 2 mg, $B_3$100 mg, panthenol 2 mg/ml. Vial 30 ml. *Rx.*
Use: Vitamin supplement.

HibTITER Vaccine. (Wyeth-Ayerst Laboratories) Purified *Haemophilus b* saccharide 10 mcg, diphtheria CRM_{197} protein 25 mcg. Inj. 0.5 ml, 2.5 ml, 5 ml vials. *Rx.*
Use: Immunization.

Hi B with C. (Towne) Vitamin C 300 mg, B_1 15 mg, B_2 10.2 mg, niacin 50 mg, B_6 5 mg, pantothenic acid 10 mg/Cap. Bot. 100s. *Rx.*
Use: Vitamin supplement.

Hi-Cor 1.0. (C & M Pharmacal, Inc.) Hydrocortisone 1% in a nonionic, ester-free, salt-free, paraben-free washable base. Tube 30 g, Jar 60 g, lb. *Rx.*
Use: Corticosteroid, topical.

Hi-Cor 2.5. (C & M Pharmacal, Inc.) Hydrocortisone 2.5% in a nonionic, ester-free, salt-free, paraben-free washable base. Tube 30 g. Jar 60 g. *Rx.*
Use: Corticosteroid, topical.

hiestrone.
See: Estrone (Various Mfr.).

High B12. (Barth's) Vitamin B_{12}, desiccated liver. Cap. Bot. 100s, 500s. *otc.*
Use: Vitamin supplement.

High Potency Cold Cap. (Weeks & Leo) Salicylamide 325 mg, chlorpheniramine maleate 4 mg, dextromethorphan HBr 15 mg, caffeine 16.2 mg/Tab. Bot. 18s. *otc.*
Use: Analgesic, antihistamine, antitussive.

High Potency N-Vites. (Nion Corp.) Vitamins B_1 15 mg, B_2 10 mg, B_3 100 mg, B_5 20 mg, B_{12} 10 mcg, C 500 mg/Tab. Bot. 100s. *otc.*

Use: Vitamin supplement.

High Potency Pain Relievers. (Weeks & Leo) Acetaminophen 300 mg, salicylamide 300 mg/Cap. Bot. 20s, 40s. *otc.*
Use: Analgesic.

High Potency Tar. (C & M Pharmacal, Inc.) Coal tar topical solution 25%. Shampoo, gel. Bot. 240 ml. *otc.*
Use: Antiseborrheic.

High Potency Vitamins and Minerals. (Burgin-Arden) Vitamins A 25,000 IU, D 400 IU, B_1 10 mg, B_2 5 mg, C 150 mg, niacinamide 100 mg, calcium 103 mg, phosphorus 80 mg, iron 10 mg, B_6 1 mg, B_{12} 5 mcg, magnesium 5.5 mg, manganese 1 mg, potassium 5 mg, zinc 1.4 mg/Tab. Bot. 100s. *otc.*
Use: Mineral, vitamin supplement.

•**hilafilcon a.** (high-lah-FILL-kahn A) USAN.
Use: Contact lens material (hydrophilic).

Hill-Shade Lotion. (Hill Dermaceuticals, Inc.) Para-aminobenzoic acid, alcohol 65%. SPF 22. *otc.*
Use: Sunscreen.

Hi-Po-Vites Tablets. (Hudson Corp.) Iron 6 mg, vitamins A 10,000 IU, D 400 IU, E 13 mg, B_1 25 mg, B_2 25 mg, B_3 50 mg, B_5 12.5 mg, B_6 15 mg, B_{12} 50 mcg, C 150 mg, folic acid 0.4 mg, Ca, Cr, Cu, I, K, Mg, Mn, Mo, P, Se, Zn 5 mg, biotin 1 mg, bioflavonoids, bone meal, PABA, choline bitartrate, betaine, inositol, lecithin, desiccated liver, rutin/Tab. Bot. 100s. *otc.*
Use: Mineral, vitamin supplement.

•**hioxifilcon a.** (high-ock-sih-FILL-kahn A) USAN.
Use: Contact lens material (hydrophilic).

hippramine.
See: Methenamine hippurate.

hipputope. (Bristol-Myers Squibb) Radioiodinated sodium iodohippurate (^{131}I) Inj. Bot. 1 m Ci, 2 m Ci.
Use: Diagnostic aid.

Hipotest. (Marlop Pharmaceuticals, Inc.) Ca 53.5 mg, iron 50 mg, vitamins A 10,000 IU, D 400 IU, E 2.5 mg, B_1 25 mg, B_2 25 mg, B_3 50 mg, B_5 13 mg, B_6 15 mg, B_{12} 50 mcg, C 150 mg, choline, betaine, PABA, rutin, bioflavonoids, biotin 1 mg, desiccated liver, bone meal, Cu, Mg, Mn, Zn 2.2 mg, I, P, lecithin/Tab. Bot. 100s. *otc.*
Use: Mineral, vitamin supplement.

Hiprex. (Hoechst Marion Roussel) Methenamine hippurate 1 g/Tab. Bot. 100s. *Rx.*
Use: Anti-infective, urinary.

Histacon Tablets. (Marsh Labs) Chlorpheniramine maleate 12 mg, ephedrine HCl 15 mg/SR Tab. Bot. 100s, 1000s. *otc.*
Use: Antihistamine, decongestant.

Histacon Syrup. (Marsh Labs) Chlorpheniramine maleate 3 mg, ephedrine HCl 4 mg/5 ml, alcohol 5%. Bot. pt.
Use: Antihistamine, decongestant.

Histagesic D.M. (Jones Medical Industries, Inc.) Phenylpropanolamine HCl 25 mg, chlorpheniramine maleate 4 mg, dextromethorphan HBr 10 mg, acetaminophen 324 mg/Tab. Bot. 100s, 1000s. *otc.*
Use: Analgesic, antihistamine, antitussive, decongestant.

Histagesic Modified Tablets. (Jones Medical Industries, Inc.) Phenylephrine HCl 10 mg, chlorpheniramine maleate 4 mg, acetaminophen 324 mg/Tab. Bot. 1000s. *otc.*
Use: Analgesic, antihistamine, decongestant.

Histalet. (Solvay Pharmaceuticals) Pseudoephedrine HCl 45 mg, chlorpheniramine maleate 3 mg/5 ml. Syr. Bot. 473 ml. *Rx.*
Use: Antihistamine, decongestant.

Histalet Forte. (Major Pharmaceuticals) Phenylpropanolamine HCl 50 mg, phenylephrine HCl 10 mg, chlorpheniramine maleate 4 mg, pyrilamine maleate 25 mg, lactose, sugar. Tab. Bot. 100s, 250s. *Rx.*
Use: Antihistamine, decongestant.

Histalet X. (Solvay Pharmaceuticals) **Syr.:** Pseudoephedrine HCl 45 mg, guaifenesin 200 mg/5 ml, alcohol 15%. Bot. 480 ml. **Tab.:** Pseudoephedrine HCl 120 mg, guaifenesin 400 mg/Tab. Bot. 100s. *Rx.*
Use: Decongestant, expectorant.

Histamic Capsules. (Lexis Laboratories) Phenylpropanolamine HCl 50 mg, phenylephrine HCl 25 mg, phenyltoloxamine citrate 30 mg, chlorpheniramine maleate 12 mg/SR Cap. Bot. 100s, 1000s. *otc.*
Use: Antihistamine, decongestant.

Histamic Tablets. (Lexis Laboratories) Phenylpropanolamine HCl 40 mg, phenylephrine HCl 10 mg, phenyltoloxamine citrate 15 mg, chlorpheniramine maleate 5 mg/Tab. Bot. 100s, 1000s. *otc.*
Use: Antihistamine, decongestant.

Histamine.
Use: Diagnostic aid.

•**histamine dihydrochloride.** (HISS-tah-meen die-HIGH-droe-KLOR-ide) U.S.P. 23.

Use: Analgesic, topical.
histamine H_2antagonists.
See: Axid Pulvules, Cap. (Eli Lilly and Co.).
Cimetidine HCl, Inj. (Endo Laboratories).
Pepcid, Tab., Pow. (Merck & Co.).
Pepcid IV, Inj. (Merck & Co.).
Tagamet, Tab., Liq., Inj. (SmithKline Beecham Pharmaceuticals).
Zantac, Tab., Syr., Inj. (Glaxo-Wellcome; Roche Laboratories).
Histapco. (Apco) Chlorpheniramine maleate 4 mg, ipecac and opium pow. 0.25 gr (contains opium 0.025 gr), camphor monobromated ⅛ gr, salicylamide 2 gr, phenacetin 1.5 gr, caffeine alkaloid gr, atropine sulfate gr/Tab. *Rx.*
Use: Analgesic, anticholinergic, antihistamine combination.
Histatab Plus. (Century Pharmaceuticals, Inc.) Chlorpheniramine maleate 2 mg, phenylephrine HCl 5 mg/Tab. Bot. 100s. *otc.*
Use: Antihistamine, decongestant.
Histatime Forte. (Major Pharmaceuticals) Phenylpropanolamine HCl 50 mg, phenylephrine HCl 10 mg, chlorpheniramine maleate 4 mg, pyrilamine maleate 25 mg/Cap. Bot. 100s. *Rx.*
Use: Antihistamine, decongestant.
Histatrol. (Center Laboratories) 2.75 mg/ml histamine phosphate, equivalent to 1 ml/ml histamine base, in 50% glycerin w/v, 5 ml vial; available in a Multitest dosage form or dropper bottle; 0.275 mg/ml histamine phosphate, equivalent to 0.1 mg/ml histamine base, 5 ml vial.
Use: Diagnostic aid, skin test control.
Hista-Vadrin Syrup. (Scherer Laboratories, Inc.) Phenylpropanolamine HCl 20 mg, chlorpheniramine maleate 2 mg, phenylephrine HCl 2.5 mg, alcohol 2%/5 ml. Bot. pt. *Rx.*
Use: Antihistamine, decongestant.
Hista-Vadrin Tablets. (Scherer Laboratories, Inc.) Phenylpropanolamine HCl 40 mg, chlorpheniramine maleate 6 mg, phenylephrine HCl 5 mg/Tab. Bot. 100s. *Rx.*
Use: Antihistamine, decongestant.
Hista-Vadrin T.D. Capsules. (Scherer Laboratories, Inc.) Phenylpropanolamine HCl 50 mg, chlorpheniramine maleate 4 mg, belladonna alkaloids 0.2 mg/Cap. Bot. 50s, 250s. *otc.*
Use: Antihistamine, decongestant combination.
Histerone Injection. (Roberts Pharmaceuticals) Testosterone aqueous susp. 50 mg or 100 mg/ml. Vial 10 ml. *c-III.*
Use: Androgen.
•**histidine.** (HISS-tih-deen) U.S.P. 23.
Use: Amino acid.
histidine monohydrochloride.
Use: I.M., peptic and jejunal ulcers.
Histine-1. (Freeport) Diphenhydramine HCl 10 mg, alcohol 12% to 14%/4 ml. Bot. 4 oz. *otc.*
Use: Antihistamine with anticholinergic, antitussive, antiemetic, and sedative effects.
Histine-2. (Freeport) Diphenhydramine HCl 12.5 mg/5 ml w/alcohol 5%. Bot. 4 oz. *otc.*
Use: Antihistamine with anticholinergic, antitussive, antiemetic, and sedative effects.
Histine-4. (Freeport) Chlorpheniramine maleate 4 mg/Tab. Bot. 1000s. *otc.*
Use: Antihistamine.
Histine-8. (Freeport) Chlorpheniramine maleate 8 mg/TR Tab. Bot. 1000s. *otc.*
Use: Antihistamine.
Histine-12. (Freeport) Chlorpheniramine maleate 12 mg/TR Tab. Bot. 1000s. *otc.*
Use: Antihistamine.
Histine-25. (Freeport) Diphenhydramine HCl 25 mg/Cap. Bot. 1000s. *otc.*
Use: Antihistamine with anticholinergic, antitussive, antiemetic, and sedative effects.
Histine-50. (Freeport) Diphenhydramine HCl 50 mg/Cap. Bot. 1000s. *otc.*
Use: Antihistamine with anticholinergic, antitussive, antiemetic, and sedative effects.
Histine DM. (Ethex Corp.) Phenylpropanolamine HCl 12.5 mg, brompheniramine maleate 2 mg, dextromethorphan HBr 10 mg, parabens, saccharin. Syr. Bot. 120 ml, 480 ml. *Rx.*
Use: Antihistamine, antitussive, decongestant.
Histinex-D. (Ethex Corp.) Hydrocodone bitartrate 5 mg, pseudoephedrine HCl 60 mg/5 ml. Liq. Bot. 480 ml, 960 ml. *c-III.*
Use: Antitussive, decongestant.
Histinex HC. (Ethex Corp.) Hydrocodone bitartrate 2.5 mg, phenylephrine HCl 5 mg, chlorpheniramine maleate 2 mg/5 ml. Syr. Alcohol and sugar free. Bot. 473 ml. *c-III.*
Use: Antitussive, decongestant, antihistamine.
Histinex PV. (Ethex Corp.) Hydrocodone bitartrate 2.5 mg, pseudoephedrine HCl 30 mg, chlorpheniramine maleate 2 mg, parabens, saccharin, sorbitol/5 ml. Syrup. Alcohol and sugar free. Bot.

120 ml, 480 ml. *c-III.*
Use: Antihistamine, antitussive, decongestant.

Histolyn-CYL. (ALK Laboratories, Inc.) Histoplasmin sterile filtrate from yeast cells of *Histoplasma capsulatum.* Vial 1.3 ml. *Rx.*
Use: Diagnostic aid, skin test.

•**histoplasmin.** (hiss-toe-PLAZZ-min) U.S.P. 23. (Parke-Davis) An aqueous solution containing standardized sterile culture filtrate of *Histoplasma capsulatum* grown on liquid synthetic medium.
Use: Diagnostic aid (dermal reactivity indicator).
See: Histolyn-CYL, Inj. (ALK Laboratories, Inc.).
Histoplasmin, diluted (Parke-Davis).

histoplasmin, diluted. (Parke-Davis) 1:100 w/v. Standardized sterile filtrate from cultures of *Histoplasma capsulatum,* 0.5% phenol, polysorbate 80. 1 ml/Inj. *Rx.*
Use: Diagnostic aid.

Histosal. (Ferndale Laboratories, Inc.) Pyrilamine maleate 12.5 mg, phenylpropanolamine HCl 20 mg, acetaminophen 324 mg, caffeine 30 mg/Tab. Bot. 100s. *otc.*
Use: Analgesic, antihistamine, decongestant.

•**histrelin.** (hiss-TRELL-in) USAN.
Use: LHRH agonist. Treatment of porphyria [Orphan Drug]
See: Supprelin, Inj. (Ortho McNeil Pharmaceutical).

histrelin acetate.
Use: Central precocious puberty. [Orphan Drug]
See: Supprelin, Inj. (Roberts Pharmaceuticals).

Histussin D. (Sanofi Winthrop Pharmaceucticals) Hydrocodone bitartrate 5 mg, pseudoephedrine HCl 60 mg/5 ml. Liq. Bot. 480 ml. *c-III.*
Use: Antitussive, decongestant.

Histussin HC Syrup. (Sanofi Winthrop Pharmaceuticals) Phenylephrine HCl 5 mg, chlorpheniramine maleate 2 mg, hydrocodone bitartrate 2.5 mg. In 480 ml. *c-III.*
Use: Analgesic, antihistamine, decongestant, narcotic.

Hitone. (Lafayette Pharmaceuticals, Inc.) Barium sulfate suspension 125% w/v. Bot. 2000 ml. Case 4s.
Use: Radiopaque agent.

Hi-Tor. (Barth's) Vitamins B_{12} 15 mcg, niacin 1.5 mg, B_1 6 mg, B_2 12 mg, B_6 54 mcg, pantothenic acid 150 mcg, choline 3.75 mg, inositol 5.25 mg/Tab. Bot. 100s, 500s, 1000s. *otc.*
Use: Vitamin supplement.

Hi-Tor 900. (Barth's) Vitamins B_1 13.5 mg, B_2 5.2 mg, niacin 15 mg, B_6 0.6 mg, pantothenic acid 1.2 mg, biotin, B_{12} 2.5 mcg, iron 0.9 mg, protein 7.5 g, inositol 50 mg, choline 40 mg, aminobenzoic acid 0.15 to 2.4 mg/15 g. Bot. 1 lb, 3 lb. *otc.*
Use: Mineral, vitamin supplement.

HIVAB HIV-1/HIV-2 (rDNA) EIA. (Abbott Laboratories) Enzyme immunoassay for qualitative detection of antibodies to human immunodeficiency virus Type 1 or Type 2 in human serum or plasma. Test kits 100s, 1000s, 5000s.
Use: Diagnostic aid.

Hi-Vegi-Lip Tablets. (Freeda Vitamins, Inc.) Pancreatin 2400 mg, lipase 12,000 units, protease 60,000 units, amylase 60,000 units/Tab. Bot. 100s, 250s. *otc.*
Use: Digestive aid.

Hivid. (Roche Laboratories) Zalcitabine 0.375 mg or 0.75 mg/Tab. Bot. 100s. *Rx.*
Use: Antiviral (Phase II/III AIDS).

Hivig. (Nabi) Human immunodeficiency virus immune globulin.
Use: Antiviral, HIV. [Orphan Drug]

Hiwolfia. (Jones Medical Industries, Inc.) Rauwolfia 25 mg, 50 mg, or 100 mg/Tab. Bot. 100s, 1000s.
Use: Antihypertensive.

HMG-CoA Reductase Inhibitors. *Rx.*
Use: Antihyperlipidemic.
See: Lescol, Cap. (Novartis Pharmaceutical Corp.).
Mevacor, Tab. (Merck & Co.).
Pravachol, Tab. (Bristol-Myers Squibb).
Zocor, Tab. (Merck & Co.).

HMM.
See: Hexamethylmelamine.

HMS. (Allergan, Inc.) Medrysone 1%. Ophth. Susp. Bot. 5 ml, 10 ml. *Rx.*
Use: Anti-inflammatory, ophthalmic.

HN_2. Mechlorethamine HCl.
Use: Antineoplastic.
See: Mustargen, Pow. (Merck & Co.).

H_2 OEX. (Fellows) Benzthiazide 50 mg/Tab. Bot. 100s, 1000s. *Rx.*
Use: Diuretic.

Hold. (SmithKline Beecham Pharmaceuticals) Dextromethorphan HBr 5 mg/Loz. Plastic tube 10 Loz. *otc.*
Use: Antitussive.

Hold DM. (Menley & James Labs, Inc.) Dextromethorphan HBr 5 mg, corn syrup, sucrose. Loz. Pkg. 10s. *otc.*
Use: Antitussive.

Hold Lozenges (Children's Formula). (SmithKline Beecham Pharmaceuticals) Phenylpropanolamine HCl 6.25 mg, dextromethorphan HBr 3.75 mg/ Loz. Roll 10s. *otc.*
Use: Antitussive, decongestant.

holocaine hydrochloride. (Various Mfr.) Phenacaine HCl.
Use: Anesthetic, local.

homarylamine hydrochloride. N-Methyl-3,4-methylenedioxyphenethylamine HCl.

•**homatropine hydrobromide.** (hoe-MAT-troe-peen HIGH-droe-BROE-mide) U.S.P. 23.
Use: Anticholinergic, ophthalmic; mydriatic, cycloplegic.
See: Homatropine HBr, Soln. (Ciba Vision).
Isopto Homatropine, Soln. (Alcon Laboratories, Inc.).
Murocoll, Liq. (Muro Pharmaceutical, Inc.).

homatropine hydrobromide. (Various Mfr.) 5% Soln. Bot. 1 ml, 2 ml, 5 ml. *Rx.*
Use: Mydriatic, cycloplegic.

homatropine hydrochloride.
Use: Anticholinergic, topical; mydriatic, cycloplegic.

•**homatropine methylbromide.** U.S.P. 23.
Use: Anticholinergic.

homatropine methylbromide w/combinations.
Use: Anticholinergic.
See: Hycodan, Tab., Pow., Syr. (Du Pont Pharma.).
Panitol H.M.B., Tab. (Wesley Pharmacal Co., Inc.).
Spasmatol, Tab. (Pharmed).
Tapuline, Tab. (Wesley Pharmacal Co, Inc.).

homatropine methylbromide and phenobarbital combinations.
Use: Anticholinergic.
See: Gustase Plus, Tab. (Roberts Pharmaceuticals).

Hominex-1. (Ross Laboratories) Protein 15 g, fat 23.9 g, carbohydrate 46.3 g, linoleic acid 1800 mg, Fe 9 mg, Na 190 mg, K 675 mg, Ca, vitamins A, B_1, B_2, B_3, B_5, B_6, B_{12}, C, D, E, K, biotin, choline, folic acid, inositol, Cl, Cu, I, Mg, Mn, P, Se, Zn and 480 Cal per 100 g. Methionine free. Pow. Can 350 g. *otc.*
Use: Nutritional supplement.

Hominex-2. (Ross Laboratories) Protein 30 g, fat 15.5 g, carbohydrate 30 g, Fe 13 mg, Na 880 mg, K 1370 mg, Ca, vitamins A, B_1, B_2, B_3, B_5, B_6, B_{12}, C, D, E, K, biotin, choline, folic acid, inositol, Cl, Cu, I, Mg, Mn, P, Se, Zn and 410 Cal per 100 g. Methionine free. Pow. Can 325 g. *otc.*
Use: Nutritional supplement.

Homogene-S. (Spanner) Testosterone 25 mg, 50 mg or 100 mg/ml. Vial 10 ml. *c-III.*
Use: Androgen.

•**homosalate.** (hoe-moe-SAL-ate) USAN. *Formerly Homomenthyl Salicylate.*
Use: Ultraviolet screen.
W/Combinations.
See: Coppertone, Prods. (Schering-Plough Corp.).

honey bee venom.
See: Albay (Bayer Corp. (Consumer Div.)).
Pharmalgen (ALK Laboratories, Inc.).
Venomil (Bayer Corp. (Consumer Div)).

•**hoquizil hydrochloride.** (HOE-kwih-zill) USAN.
Use: Bronchodilator.

hormofollin.
See: Estrone (Various Mfr.).

hornet venom.
See: Albay (Bayer Corp. (Consumer Div.)).
Pharmalgen (ALK Laboratories, Inc.).
Venomil (Bayer Corp. (Consumer Div.)).

Hospital Foam Cleaner. (Health & Medical Techniques) 0-phenylphenol 0.1%, 4-chloro-2-cyclopentyl-phenol 0.08%, lauric diethanolamide 0.2%, triethanolamine dodecylbenzenesulfonate 0.3%. Aerosol spray 19 oz.
Use: Antimicrobial, disinfectant.

Hospital Lotion. (Paddock Laboratories) Diisobutylcresoxyethoxy-ethyl dimethyl benzyl ammonium Cl, menthol, lanolin, mineral and vegetable oils. Bot. 4 oz, 8 oz, gal. *otc.*
Use: Emollient.

12-Hour Antihistamine Nasal Decongestant. (United Research Laboratories) Pseudoephedrine sulfate 120 mg, dexbrompheniramine maleate 6 mg, sugar, sucrose. Tab. Pkg. 10s. *otc.*
Use: Antihistamine, decongestant.

12-Hour Cold. (Hudson Corp.) Phenylpropanolamine HCl 75 mg, chlorpheniramine maleate 4 mg/Cap. Pkg. 10s. *otc.*
Use: Antihistamine, decongestant.

HPA-23. (antimoniotungstate) An experimental compound developed at the Pasteur Institute in Paris to stop or slow the reproduction of the AIDS virus, at least temporarily.

H.P. Acthar Gel. (Centeon) Repository

corticotropin injection highly purified 40 U.S.P. units/1 ml. Vial 1 ml, 5 ml; 80 U.S.P. units/1 ml. Vial 1 ml, 5 ml. *Rx.*
Use: Corticosteroid.

H-R Lubricating Jelly. (Wallace Laboratories) Hydroxypropyl methycellulose, parabens. Jelly 150 g. *otc.*
Use: Lubricant.

HRC-Tylaprin. (Cenci, H.R. Labs, Inc.) Acetaminophen 120 mg, alcohol 7%/ 5 ml. Elix. Bot. 2 oz, 4 oz. *otc.*
Use: Analgesic.

H.S. Need. (Hanlon) Chloral hydrate 3¾ gr, 7.5 gr/Cap. Bot. 100s. *Rx.*
Use: Sedative.

HSV-1. (Wampole Laboratories) Herpes simplex virus type I test system. For the qualitative and semi-quantitative detection of HSV-1 antibody in human serum. Test 100s.
Use: Diagnostic aid.

HSV-2. (Wampole Laboratories) Herpes simplex virus type II antibody test. For the qualitative and semi-quantitative detection of HSV-2 antibody in human serum. Test 100s.
Use: Diagnostic aid.

H.T. Factorate. (Centeon) Antihemophilic factor (human) dried, heat treated for IV administration only. Single-dose vial w/diluent and needles. *Rx.*
Use: Antihemophilic.

H.T. Factorate Generation II. (Centeon) Antihemophilic factor (human) dried, heat treated for IV administration only. Single-dose vial w/diluent and needles. *Rx.*
Use: Antihemophilic.

HTSH EIA. (Abbott Diagnostics) Enzyme immunoassay for the quantitative determination of human thyroid-stimulating hormone (TSH) in human serum or plasma.
Use: Diagnostic aid.

HTSH RIAbead. (Abbott Diagnostics) Immunoradiometric assay for the quantitative measurement of human thyroid-stimulating hormone (TSH) in serum.
Use: Diagnostic aid.

H-Tuss-D. (Cypress Pharmaceutical, Inc.) Hydrocodone bitartrate 5 mg, pseudoephedrine HCl 60 mg/5 ml, Liq. Bot. 473 ml. *Rx.*
Use: Expectorant.

Hulk Hogan Multi-Vitamins Plus Extra C. (S.G. Labs, Inc.) Vitamins A 2500 IU, E 15 IU, D_3 400 IU, B_1 1.05 mg, B_2 1.2 mg, B_3 13.5 mg, B_6 1.05 mg, B_{12} 4.5 mcg, C 300 mg, folic acid 300 mcg, sucrose. Chew. Tab. Bot. 60s. *otc.*
Use: Mineral, vitamin supplement.

Humalog. (Eli Lilly and Co.) Insulin lispro 100 units/ml. Inj. Vial, 10 ml. Cartridge 1.5 ml. *Rx.*
Use: Antidiabetic.

human acid alphaglucosidase. (Pharmain BV)
Use: Glycogne storage disease type II. [Orphan Drug]

human albumin microspheres.
Use: Radiopaque agent.
See: Optison, Inj. Susp. (Mallinckrodt).

human antihemophilic factor.
See: Antihemophilic.

human growth hormone. (Nutritional Restart)
Use: With glutamine in the treatment of short bowel syndrome. [Orphan Drug]

human growth hormone function test.
See: R-Gene 10, Inj. (Pharmacia & Upjohn).

human immunodeficiency virus immune globulin.
Use: Antiviral-HIV. [Orphan Drug]

human insulin. U.S.P. 23. Insulin Human.
Use: Hypoglycemic.
See: Humulin Prods. (Eli Lilly and Co.).

humanized anti-tac.
Use: Immunosuppressant. [Orphan Drug]
See: Zenapax (Roche Laboratories).

human serum albumin.
See: Albumotope (Bristol-Myers Squibb).

human thyroid-stimulating hormone (THS).
Use: Diagnostic aid. [Orphan Drug]

human t-lymphotropic virus type III gp 160 antigens.
Use: AIDS. [Orphan Drug]
See: Vaxsyn HIV-1.

Humate-P. (Centeon) Pasteurized, purified lyophilized concentrate of antihemophilic factor (human). Inj. Single-dose vial. *Rx.*
Use: Antihemophilic.

Humatin Capsules. (Monarch Pharmaceuticals) Paromomycin sulfate 250 mg/Cap. Bot. 16s. *Rx.*
Use: Amebicide.

Humatrope. (Eli Lilly and Co.) Somatropin 5 mg ($\approx$ 15 IU/vial), sucrose, mannitol 25 mg, glycine 5 mg, m-cresol 0.3%, glycerin 1.7%, water for injection. Pow. for Inj. (lyophilized). *Rx.*
Use: Hormone, growth.

Humegon. (Organon Teknika Corp.) Follicle-stimulating hormone activity 75 IU or 150 IU, luteinizing hormone activity 75 IU or 150 IU. Pow. for Inj. Vial 2 ml NaCl. *Rx.*

Use: Gonadotropin.

Humibid DM. (Medeva Pharmaceuticals, Inc.) Dextromethorphan HBr 30 mg, guaifenesin 600 mg/Tab. Bot. 100s. *Rx.*
Use: Antitussive, expectorant.

Humibid L.A. (Medeva Pharmaceuticals, Inc.) Guaifenesin 600 mg/SR Tab. Bot. 100s. *Rx.*
Use: Expectorant.

Humibid Sprinkle. (Medeva Pharmaceuticals, Inc.) Dextromethorphan HBr 15 mg, guaifenesin 300 mg/SR Cap. Bot. 100s. *Rx.*
Use: Antitussive, expectorant.

HuMist. (Scherer Laboratories, Inc.) Sodium Cl 0.65%, chlorobutanol 0.35%. Soln. Bot. 45 ml. *Rx.*
Use: Decongestant combination.

Humorsol. (Merck & Co.) Demecarium bromide 0.125% or 0.25% ophthalmic soln. 5 ml Ocumeter. *Rx.*
Use: Antiglaucoma agent.

Humulin 50/50. (Eli Lilly and Co.) Isophane insulin suspension (50%) and insulin injection (50%), 100 units human insulin (rDNA)/ml Inj. Vial 10 ml. *otc.*
Use: Antidiabetic.

Humulin 70/30. (Eli Lilly and Co.) Isophane insulin suspension (70%) and insulin injection (30%), 100 units/ml human insulin (rDNA) Inj. Bot. 10 ml. *otc.*
Use: Antidiabetic.

Humulin L. (Eli Lilly and Co.) Lente human insulin (recombinant DNA origin) 100 units/ml. Inj. Bot. 10 ml. Cartridge 1.5 ml. *otc.*
Use: Antidiabetic.

Humulin N. (Eli Lilly and Co.) NPH human insulin (recombinant DNA origin) 100 units/ml. Bot. 10 ml. Cartridge 1.5 ml. *otc.*
Use: Antidiabetic.

Humulin U Ultralente. (Eli Lilly and Co.) Ultralente human insulin (recombinant DNA origin) 100 units/ml. Inj. Bot. 10 ml. *otc.*
Use: Antidiabetic.

Hurricaine. (Beutlich, Inc.) Benzocaine 20%. Liq.: 0.25 ml, 3.75 ml, 30 ml. Gel: 3.75 ml, 30 g. Spray: 60 ml. *otc.*
Use: Anesthetic, topical.

Hurricaine Topical Anesthetic Spray Kit. (Beutlich, Inc.) Benzocaine 20%. Kit: Aerosol 60 g plus 200 disposable extension tubes. *otc.*
Use: Anesthetic, topical.

HVS 1 & 2. (Chemi-Tech Laboratories) Benzalkonium Cl in a specially formulated base. Soln. Bot. 15 ml. *otc.*
Use: Cold sores, fever blisters, herpes virus.

Hyacide. (Niltig) Benzethonium Cl 0.1%, sodium nitrite 0.55%. Soln. Bot. oz. *otc.*
Use: Antiseptic.

Hyalex. (Miller Pharmacal Group, Inc.) Magnesium salicylate 260 mg, magnesium p-aminobenzoate 163 mg, vitamins A 1500 IU, C 30 mg, D 100 IU, E 3 IU, B_{12} 2 mcg, pantothenic acid 5 mg, zinc 0.7 mg/Tab. Bot. 100s. *otc.*
Use: Mineral, vitamin supplement.

Hyalgan. (Sanofi Winthrop Pharmaceuticals) Sodium hyaluronate 20 mg/2 ml. *Rx.*
Use: Antiarthritic.

hyalidase.
See: Hyaluronidase (Various Mfr.).

•**hyaluronidase injection.** (high-uhl-yur-AHN-ih-dase) U.S.P. 23. Hyalidase, Hydase Enzymes which depolymerize hyaluronic acid. Hyalase, Rondase.
Use: Hypodermoclyses, promotion of diffusion, spreading agent.
See: Wydase, Vial (Wyeth-Ayerst Laboratories).

hyamagnate. Hydroxy-Aluminum-Magnesium-Aminoacetate, Sodium-free.

Hybec Forte. (Amlab) Vitamins B_1 100 mg, B_2 20 mg, B_6 2.5 mg, niacinamide 25 mg, C 200 mg, B_{12} 10 mcg, calcium pantothenate 5 mg, iron 10 mg, choline bitartrate 24 mg, inositol 10 mg, biotin 5 mcg, liver 50 mg, yeast 100 mg/Tab. Bot. 30s, 100s. *otc.*
Use: Mineral, vitamin supplement.

Hybolin Decanoate. (Hyrex Pharmaceuticals) Nandrolone decanoate 50 mg or 100 mg/ml in oil. Vial 2 ml. *c-III.*
Use: Anabolic steroid.

Hybolin Improved. (Hyrex Pharmaceuticals) Nandrolone phenpropionate 25 mg or 50 mg/ml in oil. Vial 2 ml. *c-III.*
Use: Anabolic steroid.

Hycamtin. (SmithKline Beecham Pharmaceuticals) Topotecan HCl 4 mg (free base), mannitol 48 mg. Pow. for Inj. Vial. Single-dose. *Rx.*
Use: Antineoplastic.

•**hycanthone.** (HIGH-kan-thone) USAN.
Use: Antischistosomal.

Hyclorite. U.S.P. 23. Sodium Hypochlorite soln.

HycoClear Tuss. (Ethex Corp.) Hydrocodone bitartrate 5 mg, guaifenesin 100 mg/5 ml. Alcohol, dye, sugar free. Syrup. Bot. 118 ml, 473 ml. *c-III.*
Use: Antitussive, expectorant.

Hycodan. (Du Pont Merck Pharmaceutical Co.) Hydrocodone bitartrate 5 mg, homatropine methylbromide 1.5 mg/5 ml or Tab. **Syr.:** Bot. 473 ml. **Tab.:** Bot. 100s, 500s. *c-III.*

Use: Antitussive combination.

Hycomine Compound Tablets. (Du Pont Merck Pharmaceutical Co.) Hydrocodone bitartrate 5 mg, chlorpheniramine maleate 2 mg, phenylephrine HCl 10 mg, acetaminophen 250 mg, caffeine (anhydrous) 30 mg/Tab. Bot. 100s, 500s. *c-III.*
Use: Analgesic, antihistamine, antitussive, decongestant.

Hycomine Pediatric Syrup. (Du Pont Merck Pharmaceutical Co.) Hydrocodone bitartrate 2.5 mg, phenylpropanolamine HCl 12.5 mg/5 ml. Bot. 480 ml. *c-III.*
Use: Antitussive, decongestant.

Hycomine Syrup. (Du Pont Merck Pharmaceutical Co.) Hydrocodone bitartrate 5 mg, phenylpropanolamine HCl 25 mg/5 ml. Syr. Bot. pt, gal. *c-III.*
Use: Antitussive, decongestant.

Hycort Cream. (Everett Laboratories, Inc.) Hydrocortisone 1% in a cream base. Tube oz. *Rx.*
Use: Corticosteroid, topical.

Hycort Ointment. (Everett Laboratories, Inc.) Hydrocortisone 1% in ointment base. Tube oz. *Rx.*
Use: Corticosteroid, topical.

Hycortole. (Teva Pharmaceuticals USA) Hydrocortisone. **Cream:** 0.5%: 5 g, 20 g; 1%: 5 g, 20 g, 4 oz; 2.5%: Tube 5 g, 20 g. **Oint.:** 1% or 2.5%. Tube 5 g, 20 g.
Use: Corticosteroid, topical.

Hycotuss Expectorant. (Du Pont Merck Pharmaceutical Co.) Hydrocodone bitartrate 5 mg, guaifenesin 100 mg, alcohol 10% (v/v)/5 ml. Bot. 480 ml. *c-III.*
Use: Antitussive, expectorant.

hydantoin derivatives.
Use: Anticonvulsant.
See: Dilantin, Preps. (Parke-Davis).
Diphenylhydantoin Sodium, U.S.P. 23.
Ethotoin.
Mesantoin, Tab. (Novartis Pharmaceutical Corp.).
Phenantoin.

hydase.
Use: Hypodermoclyses, promotion of diffusion.
See: Hyaluronidase (Various Mfr.).

Hydeltrasol. (Merck & Co.) Prednisolone sodium phosphate 20 mg/ml w/niacinamide 25 mg, sodium hydroxide to adjust pH, disodium edetate 0.5 mg, sodium bisulfite 1 mg, phenol 5 mg, water for injection q.s. 1 ml. Inj. Vial 2 ml, 5 ml. *Rx.*
Use: Corticosteroid.

Hydergine LC Liquid Capsules. (Novartis Pharmaceutical Corp.) Ergoloid mesylates 1 mg/Cap. Bot. 100s, 500s. SandoPak 100s, 500s. *Rx.*
Use: Psychotherapeutic agent.

Hydergine Liquid. (Novartis Pharmaceutical Corp.) Equal parts of dihydroergocornine, dihydroergocristine, dihydroergocryptine. (Ergoloid Mesylates). 1 mg/ml. Bot. 100 ml w/dropper. *Rx.*
Use: Psychotherapeutic agent.

Hydergine, Oral. (Novartis Pharmaceutical Corp.) Equal parts of dihydroergocornine, dihydroergocristine, dihydroergocryptine (Ergoloid Mesylates). 1 mg/Tab. Bot. 100s, 500s. SandoPak (UD) 100s, 500s. *Rx.*
Use: Psychotherapeutic agent.

Hydergine, Sublingual. (Novartis Pharmaceutical Corp.) Equal parts of dihydroergocornine, dihydroergocristine, dihydroergocryptine (Ergoloid Mesylates). 0.5 mg or 1 mg/Tab. Bot. 100s, 1000s, SandoPak (UD) 100s. *Rx.*
Use: Psychotherapeutic agent.

Hydoril. (Cenci, H.R. Labs, Inc.) Hydrochlorothiazide 25 mg or 50 mg/Tab. Bot. 100s, 1000s. *Rx.*
Use: Diuretic.

hydrabamine phenoxymethyl penicillin.
See: Penicillin V Hydrabamine.

hydracrylic acid beta lactone.
See: Propiolactone.

hydralazine. (Solopak Pharmaceuticals, Inc.) Hydralazine HCl 20 mg/ml Inj. Vial 1 ml. *Rx.*
Use: Antihypertensive.

•**hydralazine hydrochloride.** (high-DRAL-uh-zeen) U.S.P. 23.
Use: Antihypertensive.
See: Apresoline, Amp., Tab. (Novartis Pharmaceutical Corp.).
W/Hydrochlorothiazide.
See: Apresazide, Cap. (Novartis Pharmaceutical Corp.).
Apresoline-Esidrix, Tab. (Novartis Pharmaceutical Corp.).
Hydralazide, Tab. (Zenith Goldline Pharmaceuticals).
Hydroserpine Plus, Tab. (Zenith Goldline Pharmaceuticals).
W/Reserpine.
See: Dralserp, Tab. (Teva Pharmaceuticals USA).
Serpasil-Apresoline, Tab. (Novartis Pharmaceutical Corp.).
W/Reserpine, hydrochlorothiazide (Esidrix).
See: Harbolin, Tab. (Arcum).
Ser-Ap-Es, Tab. (Novartis Pharmaceutical Corp.).

hydralazine hydrochloride. (Various Mfr.) **10 mg, 25 mg, 50 mg:** Tab. Bot. 100s, 1000s, UD 100s. **100 mg:** Tab. Bot. 100s, 1000s.
Use: Antihypertensive.

•**hydralazine polistirex.** (high-DRAL-ah-zeen pahl-ee-STIE-rex) USAN.
Use: Antihypertensive.

Hydra Mag Tablets. (Pal-Pak, Inc.) Aluminum hydroxide gel, dried, 195 mg, magnesium trisilicate 195 mg, kaolin 162 mg/Tab. Bot. 1000s. *otc.*
Use: Antacid.

Hydrap-ES. (Parmed Pharmaceuticals, Inc.) Hydrochlorothiazide 15 mg, reserpine 0.1 mg, hydralazine HCl 25 mg/Tab. Bot. 100s, 500s, 1000s. *Rx.*
Use: Antihypertensive.

Hydraserp. (Geneva Pharmaceuticals) Hydrochlorothiazide 25 mg or 50 mg, reserpine 0.1 mg/Tab. Bot. 100s, 1000s. *Rx.*
Use: Antihypertensive combination.

hydrastine hydrochloride. (Penick) Pow. Bot. oz.
Use: Hemostatic.

Hydrate. (Hyrex Pharmaceuticals) Dimenhydrinate 50 mg/ml w/propylene glycol 50%, benzyl alcohol 5%. Amp. 1 ml. Box 25s, 100s; Vial 10 ml. *Rx.*
Use: Antiemetic, antihistamine, antivertigo.

Hydrazide. (Zenith Goldline Pharmaceuticals) **25/25:** Hydrochlorothiazide 25 mg, hydralazine 25 mg/Cap. **50/50:** Hydrochlorothiazide 50 mg, hydralazine 50 mg/Cap. Bot. 100s. *Rx.*
Use: Antihypertensive.

Hydra-Zide. (Par Pharmaceuticals) Hydralazine HCl 50 mg, hydrochlorothiazide 50 mg/Cap. Bot. 100s, 500s, 1000s. *Rx.*
Use: Antihypertensive.

hydrazone.
Use: Pulmonary tuberculosis.
See: Rimactane, Cap. (Novartis Pharmaceutical Corp.).

Hydrea. (Bristol-Myers Squibb) Hydroxyurea. 500 mg, lactose/Cap. Bot. 100s. *Rx.*
Use: Antineoplastic.

hydriodic acid. (Various Mfr.).
Use: Expectorant.

hydriodic acid therapy.
See: Aminoacetic Acid HI.

Hydrisinol Creme and Lotion. (Pedinol Pharmacal, Inc.) Sulfonated hydrogenated castor oil. **Cream:** Spout Cap Jar 4 oz, lb. **Lot.:** Bot. 8 oz. *otc.*
Use: Emollient.

Hydro-12. (Table Rock) Crystalline hydroxocobalamin 1000 mcg/ml Pkg. 10 ml. *Rx.*
Use: Vitamin supplement.

Hydro-Ban. (Whiteworth Towne) Juniper oil 10 mg, uva ursi 50 mg, buchu extract 50 mg, parsley piert extract 50 mg, iron 6 mg/Cap. Bot. 42s. *otc.*
Use: Diuretic.

Hydrocare Cleaning and Disinfecting. (Allergan, Inc.) Tris (2-hydroxyethyl) tallow ammonium Cl, thimerosal 0.002%, bis (2-hydroxyethyl) tallow ammonium Cl, sodium bicarbonate, sodium phosphates, hydrochloric acid, propylene glycol, polysorbate 80, polyhema. Soln. Bot. 240 ml, 360 ml. *otc.*
Use: Contact lens care, disinfective.

Hydrocare Preserved Saline. (Allergan, Inc.) Isotonic, buffered, NaCl, sodium hexametaphosphate, boric acid, sodium borate, EDTA 0.01%, thimerosal 0.001%. Soln. Bot. 240 ml, 360 ml. *otc.*
Use: Contact lens care, rinsing/storage solution.

Hydrocet. (Carnrick Laboratories, Inc.) Hydrocodone bitartrate 5 mg, acetaminophen 500 mg/Cap. Bot. 100s. *c-III.*
Use: Narcotic analgesic combination.

hydrochlorate. Same as Hydrochloride.

•**hydrochloric acid.** N.F. 18.
Use: Well diluted, achlorhydria; pharmaceutic aid (acidifying agent).

hydrochloric acid. (Various Mfr.) Muriatic Acid, Absolute 38%. Diluted 10%.

hydrochloric acid therapy.
Use: Well diluted, achlorhydria; pharmaceutic aid (acidifying agent); gastric acidifier.
See: Betaine HCl (Various Mfr.).
Glutamic Acid HCl (Various Mfr.).
Glycine HCl (Various Mfr.).

Hydrochloroserpine. (Freeport) Hydralazine HCl 25 mg, hydrochlorothiazide 15 mg, reserpine 0.1 mg/Tab. Bot. 1000s.
Use: Antihypertensive combination.

•**hydrochlorothiazide.** (high-droe-klor-oh-THIGH-uh-zide) U.S.P. 23.
Use: Diuretic.
See: Chlorzide, Tab. (Foy Laboratories).
Delco-Retic, Tab. (Delco).
Diu-Scrip, Cap. (Scrip).
Esidrix, Tab. (Novartis Pharmaceutical Corp.).
Hydromal, Tab. (Roberts Pharmaceuticals).
HydroDiuril, Tab. (Merck & Co.).
Microzide, Cap. (Watson Laboratories).
Oretic, Tab. (Abbott Laboratories).
Zide, Tab. (Solvay Pharmaceuticals).

W/Deserpidine.
See: Oreticyl, Tab. (Abbott Laboratories).
W/Enalapril.
See: Vaseretic, Tab. (Merck & Co.).
W/Guanethidine monosulfate.
See: Esimil, Tab. (Novartis Pharmaceutical Corp.).
W/Hydralazine HCl.
See: Apresazide, Cap. (Novartis Pharmaceutical Corp.).
Apresoline-Esidrix, Tab. (Novartis Pharmaceutical Corp.).
Hydralazide, Tab. (Zenith Goldline Pharmaceuticals).
W/Lisinopril.
See: Prinzide, Tab. (Merck & Co.).
Zestoretic, Tab. (Zeneca Pharmaceuticals).
W/Losartan potassium.
See: Hyzaar (Merck).
W/Methyldopa.
See: Aldoril, Tab. (Merck & Co.).
W/Moexipril.
See: Uniretic, Tab. (Schwarz Pharma, Inc.).
W/Propranolol.
See: Inderide, Tab. (Wyeth-Ayerst Laboratories).
W/Reserpine.
See: Hydropres, Tab. (Merck & Co.).
Hydroserp, Tab. (Zenith Goldline Pharmaceuticals).
Hydroserpine, Tab. (Geneva Pharmaceuticals).
Hydrotensin-50, Tab. (Merz Pharmaceuticals).
Hyperserp, Tab. (Zeneca Pharmaceuticals).
Serpasil-Esidrix, Tab. (Novartis Pharmaceutical Corp.).
W/Reserpine, Hydralazine HCl.
See: Harbolin, Tab. (Arcum).
Hydroserpine Plus, Tab. (Zenith Goldline Pharmaceuticals).
Ser-Ap-Es, Tab. (Novartis Pharmaceutical Corp.).
See: Aldactazide, Tab. (Searle).
W/Timolol maleate.
See: Timolide, Tab. (Merck & Co.).
W/Triamterene.
See: Dyazide, Cap. (SmithKline Beecham Pharmaceuticals).

hydrochlorothiazide/amiloride.
See: Amiloride hydrochloride and hydrochlorothiazide tablets.

hydrochlorothiazide w/combinations.
See: Hyzaar, Tab. (Merck & Co.).

hydrochlorothiazide/hydralazine. (Various Mfr.) Hydrochlorothiazide 25 mg, hydralazine HCl 25 mg/Cap, or hydrochlorothiazide 50 mg, hydralazine HCl 50 mg/Cap. Bot. 100s, 500s, 1000s. *Rx.*
Use: Antihypertensive.

hydrochlorothiazide/reserpine. (Various Mfr.)
See: Reserpine and hydrochlorothiazide.

hydrocholeretics.
See: Bile Salts (Various Mfr.).
Dehydrocholic Acid (Various Mfr.).
Ox Bile Extract (Various Mfr.).

hydrocholeretic combinations.
See: G.B.S., Tab. (Forest Pharmaceutical, Inc.).

Hydrocil Instant. (Solvay Pharmaceuticals) Blond psyllium coating containing psyllium 3.5 g/3.7 g dose. Tan granular, instant mix, sugar-free, low sodium, low potassium powder. UD packets. 3.7 g in 30s, 500s, Jar 250 g. *otc.*
Use: Laxative.

Hydro Cobex. (Taylor Pharmaceuticals) Hydroxocobalamin 1000 mcg/Vial 30 ml. *Rx.*
Use: Vitamin B_{12} supplement.

hydrocodone w/acetaminophen. (HIGH-droe-KOE-dohn with ass-eet-ah-MEE-no-fen) (Pharmics, Inc.) Hydrocodone bitartrate 7.5 mg, acetaminophen 500 mg. Tab. Bot. 100s, 500s. *c-III.*
Use: Analgesic combination, narcotic.
See: Alor 5/500, Tab. (Atley Pharmaceuticals, Inc.).
Anexsia 10/660, Tab. (Mallinckrodt).
Lortab, Preps. (UCB Pharmaceuticals, Inc.).
Vicodin, Tab. (Knoll Pharmaceuticals).

•**hydrocodone bitartrate.** (HIGH-droe-KOE-dohn by-TAR-TRATE) U.S.P. 23. Dihydrocodeinone bitartrate.
Use: Antitussive; analgesic, narcotic.
W/Combinations.
See: Alor 5/500 (Atley).
Anexsia 10/660 (Mallinckrodt).
Atuss EX, Syr. (United Research Laboratories).
Atuss G, Syr. (Atley Pharmaceuticals, Inc.).
Atuss HD, Liq. (Atley Pharmaceuticals, Inc.).
Deconamine CX, Tab. (Bradley Pharmaceutical).
Histinex-D (Ethex Corp.).
Histinex HC, Syr. (Ethex Corp.).
Histinex PV, Syr. (Ethex Corp.).
Histussin D, Liq. (Sanofi Winthrop Pharmaceuticals).
H-Tuss-D, Liq. (Cypress Pharmaceutical, Inc.).

Hycoclear Tuss, Syr. (Ethex Corp.).
Hydrocet, Cap. (Carnrick Laboratories, Inc.).
Hydrocodone w/acetaminophen, Tab. (Pharmics, Inc.).
Hydrocodone CP, Liq. (Morton Grove Pharmaceuticals, Inc.).
Hydrocodone GF, Liq. (Morton Grove Pharmaceuticals, Inc.).
Hydrocodone HD, Liq. (Morton Grove Pharmaceuticals, Inc.).
Hydrocodone PA, Liq. (Morton Grove Pharmaceuticals, Inc.).
Hyphed (Cypress Pharm.).
Iodal HD, Liq. (Iomed Labs).
Iotussin HC (Iomed Labs).
Lortab (UCB Pharma).
Lortab 10/500 (UCB Pharma).
Norco (Watson Labs).
Panacet 5/500, Tab. (ECR Pharmaceuticals).
Panasal 5/500, Tab. (ECR Pharmaceuticals).
Pancof-HC, Liq. (Pan American Labs).
Protuss (Horizon Pharmaceutical Corp.).
Protuss-D, Liq. (Horizon Pharmaceutical Corp.).
Tussafed HC (Everett Laboratories).
Tussend, Syr. (Monarch Pharmaceuticals).
Tyrodone, Liq. (Major Pharmaceuticals).
Unituss HC, Syr. (United Research Laboratories).
Vetuss HC, Syr. (Cypress Pharmaceutical, Inc.).
Vicodin HP (Knoll).
Vicoprofen (Knoll).
Zydone (Endo).

hydrocodone bitartrate & acetaminophen capsules. (Various Mfr.) Hydrocodone bitartrate 5 mg, acetaminophen 500 mg/Cap. Bot. 100s, 500s. *c-III.*
Use: Analgesic combination.

hydrocodone bitartrate & acetaminophen caplets. (Various Mfr.) Hydrocodone bitartrate 7.5 mg, acetaminophen 650 mg. Capl. Bot. 100s, 500s. *c-III.*
Use: Analgesic combination, narcotic.

hydrocodone bitartrate & acetaminophen tablets. (Various Mfr.) Hydrocodone bitartrate 5 mg 7.5 mg, 10 mg, acetaminophen 500 mg, 650 mg/Tab. Hydrocodone bitartrate 7.5 mg, acetaminophen 650 mg. Tab. Bot. 100s, 500s. *c-III.*
Use: Analgesic combination, narcotic.

hydrocodone bitartrate and guaifenesin. (Halsey Drug Co., Inc.) Hydrocodone bitartrate 5 mg, guaifenesin 100 mg/5 ml. Syr. Bot. 473 ml. *c-III.*
Use: Antitussive, expectorant.

hydrocodone bitartrate, phenylephrine HCl, chlorpheniramine maleate. (Cypress) Hydrocodone bitartrate 1.67 mg, phenylephrine HCl 5 mg, chlorpheniramine maleate 2 mg/5 ml. Syr. Bot. Pt, gal. *c-III.*
Use: Decongestant, antihistamine, antitussive.

hydrocodone bitartrate & phenylpropanolamine hydrochloride pediatric syrup. (Rosemont Pharmaceutical Corp.) Phenylpropanolamine HCl 12.5 mg, hydrocodone bitartrate 2.5 mg/5 ml. Syr. Bot. 118 ml, pt, gal. *c-III.*
Use: Antitussive combination.

hydrocodone comp. syrup. (Various Mfr.) Hydrocodone bitartrate 5 mg, homatropine methylbromide 1.5 mg. Syr. Bot. 473 ml, gal. *c-III.*
Use: Antitussive.

Hydrocodone CP. (Morton Grove Pharmaceuticals, Inc.) Hydrocodone bitartrate 2.5 mg, phenylephrine 5 mg, chlorpheniramine maleate 2 mg/5 ml. Liq. Bot. 473 ml. *c-III.*
Use: Antitussive.

Hydrocodone GF. (Morton Grove Pharmaceuticals, Inc.) Hydrocodone bitartrate 5 mg, guaifenesin 100 mg/5 ml. Syr. Bot. 473 ml. *c-III.*
Use: Antitussive, expectorant.

Hydrocodone HD. (Morton Grove Pharmaceuticals, Inc.) Hydrocodone bitartrate 1.67 mg, phenylephrine HCl 5 mg, chlorpheniramine maleate 2 mg/5 ml. Liq. Bot. 473 ml. *c-III.*
Use: Antitussive, expectorant.

Hydrocodone PA Syrup. (Morton Grove Pharmaceuticals, Inc.) Hydrocodone bitartrate 5 mg, phenylpropanolamine HCl 25 mg/5 ml. Syr. Bot. 473 ml. *c-III.*
Use: Antitussive, decongestant.

Hydrocodone PA Pediatric Syrup. (Morton Grove Pharmaceuticals, Inc.) Hydrocodone bitartrate 2.5 mg, phenylpropanolamine HCl 12.5 mg/5 ml. Syr. Bot. 473 ml. *c-III.*
Use: Antitussive, decongestant.

•**hydrocodone polistirex.** (high-droe-KOE-dohn pahl-ee-STIE-rex) USAN.
Use: Antitussive.

hydrocodone resin complex.
Use: Antitussive.
W/Phenyltoloxamine resin complex.
See: Tussionex, Prods. (Medeva Pharmaceuticals, Inc.).

hydrocortamate hydrochloride. 17-Hydroxycorticosterone-21-diethylaminoacetate HCl.

Use: Anti-inflammatory, topical.
•**hydrocortisone.** (HIGH-droe-CORE-tih-sone) U.S.P. 23.
Use: Anti-inflammatory, topical; corticosteroid, topical.
See: Acticort Lotion 100. (Baker Norton Pharmaceuticals, Inc.).
Alphaderm, Cream (Procter & Gamble Pharm.).
Caldecort, Spray (Novartis Pharmaceutical Corp.).
Cetacort, Lot. (Galderma Laboratories, Inc.).
Cortaid Intensive Therapy, Cream (Pharmacia & Upjohn).
Cort-Dome, Cream, Lot., Supp. (Bayer Corp (Consumer Div.)).
Cortef, Tab., Cream, Oint. (Pharmacia & Upjohn).
Cortenema, Enema (Solvay Pharmaceuticals).
Cortizone for Kids (Pfizer).
Cortril, Oint. (Pfizer US Pharmaceutical Group).
Delacort, Lot. (Mericon Industries, Inc.).
Dermacort, Cream, Lot. (Solvay Pharmaceuticals).
Dermol HC, Cream, Oint. (Dermol Pharmaceuticals, Inc.).
Dermolate, Prods. (Schering-Plough Corp.).
Eldecort, Cream (Zeneca Pharmaceuticals).
HC Derma-Pax, Liq. (Recsei Laboratories).
Hi-Cor 1.0, Cream (C & M Pharmacal, Inc.).
Hi-Cor 2.5, Cream (C & M Pharmacal, Inc.).
Hycort, Cream, Oint. (Everett Laboratories, Inc.).
Hycortole, Cream, Oint. (Premo).
Hydrocortone, Tab. (Merck & Co.).
Hytone, Cream, Oint., Lot. (Dermik Laboratories, Inc.).
My Cort, Cream (Scrip).
Proctocort, Oint. (Solvay Pharmaceuticals).
Scalpicin, Liq. (Combe, Inc.).
Signef, Supp. (Forest Pharmaceutical, Inc.).
Synacort, Cream (Roche Laboratories).
T/Scalp, Liq. (Neutrogena).
Texacort 25, 50, Lot. (Rydelle Laboratories).

hydrocortisone. (Pharmacia & Upjohn) Micronized nonsterile powder for prescription compounding.
Use: Anti-inflammatory, topical; corticosteroid, topical.

hydrocortisone w/combinations.
See: Carmol HC, Cream (Ingram).
Cipro HC (Bayer Corp.).
Cortef, Preps. (Pharmacia & Upjohn).
Cortic (Everett Lab.).
Cortisporin, Prep. (GlaxoWellcome).
Cortisporin-TC (Monarch).
Doak Oil Forte, Liq. (Doak Dermatologics).
Drotic No. 2, Drops (B.F. Ascher and Co.).
Fostril HC, Lot. (Westwood Squibb Pharmaceuticals).
Hysone, Oint. (Roberts Pharmaceuticals).
Kleer, Spray (Scrip).
Neo-Cort Dome, Cream, Lot., Drops (Bayer Corp. (Consumer Div.)).
Neo Cort Top, Oint. (Standex).
Nutracort, Cream, Gel, Lot. (Galderma Laboratories, Inc.).
1 + 1 Creme, 1 + 1-F Creme (Dunhall Pharmaceuticals, Inc.).
Oti-Med (Hyrex Pharmaceuticals).
Oto, Drops (Solvay Pharmaceuticals).
Otobiotic, Soln. (Schering-Plough Corp.).
Otocalm-H Ear Drops (Parmed Pharmaceuticals, Inc.).
Otomar-HC (Marnell).
Pyocidin-Otic, Soln. (Berlex Laboratories, Inc.).
Rectal Medicone-HC (Medicore).
Sherform-HC, Creme (Sheryl).
Terra-Cortril, Preps. (Pfizer).
Tri-Otic (Pharmics).
Vanoxide-HC, Lot. (Dermik Laboratories, Inc.).
Vytone, Cream (Dermik Laboratories, Inc.).
Zoto-HC (Horizon).

•**hydrocortisone acetate.** U.S.P. 23.
Use: Glucocorticoid.
See: Anucort-HC, Supp. (G & W Laboratories).
Anuprep HC, Supp. (Great Southern Laboratories).
Anusol-HC, Supp. (Parke-Davis).
Caldecort, Cream (Novartis Pharmaceutical Corp.).
Caldecort Light, Cream (Novartis Pharmaceutical Corp.).
Cortef Acetate, Ophth. Oint., Inj. (Pharmacia & Upjohn).
Cortifoam, Aerosol (Schwarz Pharma, Inc.).
Cortril Acetate, Aqueous Susp., Oint. (Pfipharmecs).
Gynecort, Oint. (Combe, Inc.).
Hemril-HC Uniserts, Supp. (Upsher-Smith Labs, Inc.).

Hydrocort, Vial (Dunhall Pharmaceuticals, Inc.).
Hydrocortone Acetate, Inj. (Merck & Co.).
Hydrosone, Inj. (Sigma-Tau Pharmaceuticals, Inc.).
Maximum Strength Corticaine, Cream (UCB Pharmaceuticals, Inc.).
Maximum Strength Dermarest Dricort Creme (Del Pharmaceuticals, Inc.).
Pramosone Cream, Lot. (Ferndale Laboratories, Inc.).
Proctocort (Monarch Pharmaceuticals).

hydrocortisone acetate. (Pharmacia & Upjohn) Micronized non-sterile powder for prescription compounding.
Use: Anti-inflammatory, topical; corticosteroid, topical.

hydrocortisone acetate w/combinations.
See: Anusol-HC, Cream, Supp. (Parke-Davis).
Carmol HC, Cream (Ingram).
Coly-Mycin S Otic Drops w/Neomycin and Hydrocortisone, Soln. (Warner Chilcott Laboratories).
Cortaid, Cream, Lot., Oint. (Pharmacia & Upjohn).
Cortef Acetate, Inj., Oint., Susp. (Pharmacia & Upjohn).
Cortic (Everett Lab.).
Cortisporin-TC, Otic Susp. (Monarch Pharmaceuticals).
Derma Medicone-HC, Oint. (Medicore).
Epifoam, Aerosol (Schwarz Pharma, Inc.).
Furacin HC Urethral Inserts (Eaton Medical Corp.).
Lida-Mantle HC, Cream (Bayer Corp (Consumer Div)).
Neo-Cortef, Preps. (Pharmacia & Upjohn).
Otomar-HC, Otic Soln. (Marnel Pharmaceuticals, Inc.).
Proctofoam-HC, Aerosol (Schwarz Pharma, Inc.).
Rectal Medicone-HC, Supp. (Medicore).
Wyanoids HC, Supp. (Wyeth-Ayerst Laboratories).

hydrocortisone and acetic acid otic solution.
Use: Anti-inflammatory, otic.

•**hydrocortisone buteprate.** (HIGH-droe-CORE-tih-sone BYOO-teh-prate) USAN.
Use: Anti-inflammatory; corticosteroid, topical.
See: Pandel, Cream (Savage Laboratories).

•**hydrocortisone butyrate.** (HIGH-droe-CORE-tih-sone BYOO-tih-rate) U.S.P. 23.
Use: Corticosteroid, topical.
See: Locoid, Soln. (Ferndale Laboratories, Inc.).

hydrocortisone cypionate. U.S.P. XXII. Oral Susp., U.S.P. XXII. Hydrocortisone Cypionate.
Use: Corticosteroid, topical.

hydrocortisone diethylaminoacetate hcl.
See: Hydrocortamate.

hydrocortisone dypropionate.
See: Cortef, Fluid (Pharmacia & Upjohn).

•**hydrocortisone hemisuccinate.** (HIGH-droe-CORE-tih-sone hem-ih-SUCK-sih-nate) U.S.P. 23.
Use: Adrenocortical steroid.

hydrocortisone I.V.
See: A-Hydro Cort, Vial (Abbott Laboratories).
Solu-Cortef, Vial (Pharmacia & Upjohn).

hydrocortisone/iodochlorhydroxyquin. (Various Mfr.) **Cream:** Hydrocortisone 0.5% or 3%, iodochlorhydroxyquin 3%. 15 g, 30 g, 480 g. **Oint.:** Hydrocortisone 1%, iodochlorhydroxyquin 3%. 20 g, 30 g. *Rx-otc.*
Use: Corticosteroid, topical.

hydrocortisone-neomycin. (Various Mfr.) Hydrocortisone 1%, neomycin sulfate 0.5%. Oint. 20 g. *Rx-otc.*
Use: Corticosteroid, topical.

hydrocortisone phosphate.
See: Hydrocortone Phosphate, Inj. (Merck & Co.).

•**hydrocortisone sodium phosphate.** (HIGH-droe-CORE-tih-sone) U.S.P. 23.
Use: Adrenocortical steroid (anti-inflammatory); corticosteroid, topical.

•**hydrocortisone sodium succinate.** (HIGH-droe-CORE-tih-sone) U.S.P. 23.
Use: Adrenocortical steroid (anti-inflammatory); corticosteroid, topical.
See: A-hydroCort, Vial (Abbott Laboratories).
Solu-Cortef, Vial (Pharmacia & Upjohn).

•**hydrocortisone valerate.** (HIGH-droe-CORE-tih-sone VAL-eh-rate) U.S.P. 23.
Use: Corticosteroid, topical.
See: Westcort Cream, Oint. (Westwood Squibb Pharmaceuticals).

hydrocortisone valerate. (Copley) 0.2% in hydrophilic base, white petrolatum, alcohol. Cream Tube 15 g, 45 g, 60 g. *Rx.*

Use: Corticosteroid, topical.

hydrocortisone valerate. (Taro) 0.2% in hydrophilic base, white petrolatum, alcohol, mineral oil. Oint. Tube 15 g, 45 g, 60 g. *Rx.*
Use: Corticosteroid, topical.

Hydrocortone Acetate Saline Suspension. (Merck & Co.) Hydrocortisone acetate 25 mg or 50 mg/ml, sodium Cl 9 mg, polysorbate 80 4 mg, sodium carboxymethylcellulose 5 mg/ml, benzyl alcohol 9 mg q.s. water for injection to 1 ml. Vial 5 ml. *Rx.*
Use: Corticosteroid.

Hydrocortone Phosphate Injection. (Merck & Co.) Hydrocortisone sodium phosphate equivalent to hydrocortisone 50 mg/ml, creatinine 8 mg, sodium citrate 10 mg/ml, sodium hydroxide to adjust pH, sodium bisulfite 3.2 mg, methylparaben 1.5 mg, propylparaben 0.2 mg, water for injection q.s./ml. Vial 2 ml multiple dose, 10 ml multiple dose. Disposable syringe 2 ml single dose. *Rx.*
Use: Corticosteroid.

Hydrocortone Tablets. (Merck & Co.) Hydrocortisone 10 mg or 20 mg/Tab. Bot. 100s. *Rx.*
Use: Corticosteroid.

Hydrocream Base. (Paddock Laboratories) Petrolatum, mineral oil, woolwax alcohol, imidazolidinyl urea, methyl- and propylparabens. Cream Jar lb.
Use: Emollient.

Hydro-Crysti 12. (Roberts Pharmaceuticals) Hydroxocobalamin, crystalline (vitamin B_{12}) 1000 mcg/ml Inj. Vial 30 ml. *Rx.*
Use: Vitamin B_{12} supplement.

HydroDIURIL. (Merck & Co.) Hydrochlorothiazide **25 mg/Tab.:** Bot. 100s, 1000s, UD 100s. **50 mg/Tab.:** Bot. 100s, 1000s, UD 100s. *Rx.*
Use: Diuretic.

Hydro-D Tablets. (Halsey Drug Co.) Hydrochlorothiazide. 25 mg, 50 mg/Tab. Bot. 1000s. *Rx.*
Use: Diuretic.

Hydro-Ergot. (Henry Schein, Inc.) Hydrogenated ergot alkaloids 0.5 mg or 1 mg/Tab. Bot. 100s. *Rx.*
Use: Psychotherapeutic agent.

•**hydrofilcon a.** (HIGH-droe-FILL-kahn A) USAN.
Use: Contact lens material (hydrophilic).

•**hydroflumethiazide.** (HIGH-droe-flew-meth-EYE-ah-zide) U.S.P. 23.
Use: Antihypertensive, diuretic.
See: Diucardin, Tab. (Wyeth-Ayerst Laboratories).
Saluron, Tab. (Bristol-Myers Squibb).
W/Reserpine.
See: Salutensin, Tab. (Bristol-Myers Squibb).
Salutensin-Demi, Tab. (Bristol-Myers Squibb).

hydrogen dioxide.
See: Hydrogen Peroxide.

hydrogen iodide.
Use: Expectorant.
See: Hydriodic acid.

•**hydrogen peroxide concentrate.** (HIGH-droe-jen per-OX-ide) U.S.P. 23.
Use: Anti-infective, topical.

hydrogen peroxide solution 30%. Perhydrol, hydrogen peroxide. Bot. 0.25 lb, 0.5 lb, 1 lb.
Use: Dentistry, preparing the 3% solution.

hydrogen peroxide topical solution. (Various Mfr.) (3%). 4 oz, 8 oz, pt.
Use: Anti-infective, topical.

Hydrogesic. (Edwards Pharmaceuticals, Inc.) Hydrocodone bitartrate 5 mg, acetaminophen 500 mg/Cap. Bot. 100s. *c-III.*
Use: Analgesic combination, narcotic.

Hydroloid-G Sublingual. (Major Pharmaceuticals) Ergoloid mesylates. **0.5 mg/Tab.:** Bot. 100s, 250s, 500s, UD 100s. **1 mg/Tab.:** Bot. 100s, 250s, 1000s, UD 100s. *Rx.*
Use: Psychotherapeutic agent.

Hydroloid-G Tabs. (Major Pharmaceuticals) Ergoloid mesylates 1 mg/Tab. Bot. 100s, 250s, 1000s, UD 100s. *Rx.*
Use: Psychotherapeutic agent.

Hydromal. (Roberts Pharmaceuticals) Hydrochlorothiazide 50 mg/Tab. Bot. 1000s. *Rx.*
Use: Diuretic.

Hydromet. (Alpharma USPD Inc.) Hydrocodone bitartrate 5 mg, homatropine MBr 1.5 mg/Syr. Bot. 473 ml, gal. *c-III.*
Use: Antitussive.

hydromorphone. (HIGH-droe-MORE-phone) *c-II.*
Use: Analgesic, narcotic.

•**hydromorphone hydrochloride.** (HIGH-droe-MORE-phone) U.S.P. 23. *Formerly Dihydromorphinone Hydrochloride.*
Use: Analgesic, narcotic.
See: Dilaudid Prods. (Knoll Pharmaceuticals).
HydroStat IR (Richwood).

hydromorphone HCl. (Paddock) 3 mg. Supp. Box 6s. *c-II.*
Use: Analgesic, narcotic.

hydromorphone HCl. (Various Mfr.) **Tab.:** 2 mg, 4 mg, 8 mg. Bot. 100s, 500s (4 mg only), UD 100s (except 8 mg).

Liq.: 5 mg/5 ml. Bot. 120 ml, 250 ml, 500 ml; UD patient cups 4 ml, 8 ml. **Inj.:** 1 mg/ml, 2 mg/ml, 4 mg/ml. **Tubex:** 2 m w/1 ml fill; Vial 1 ml, 20 ml (2 mg/ml only). *c-II.*
Use: Analgesic, narcotic.

hydromorphone sulfate.
Use: Analgesic, narcotic.

Hydromox. (ESI Lederle Generics) Quinethazone 50 mg/Tab. Bot. 100s, 500s. *Rx.*
Use: Diuretic.

Hydromox-R. (ESI Lederle Generics) Quinethazone 50 mg, reserpine 0.125 mg/Tab. Bot. 100s, 500s. *Rx.*
Use: Antihypertensive combination.

Hydropane. (Halsey Drug Co.) Hydrocodone bitartrate 5 mg, homatropine methylbromide 1.5 mg. Pt, gal. *c-III.*
Use: Antitussive combination.

Hydropel. (C & M Pharmacal, Inc.) Silicone 30%, hydrophobic starch derivative 10%, petrolatum. Jar. 2 oz, lb. *otc.*
Use: Emollient.

Hydrophed. (Rugby Labs, Inc.) Theophylline 130 mg, ephedrine sulfate 25 mg, hydroxyzine HCl 10 mg/Tab. Bot. 100s, 1000s. *Rx.*
Use: Antiasthmatic combination.

Hydrophen Pediatric Syrup. (Rugby Labs, Inc.) Phenylpropanolamine HCl 12.5 mg, hydrocodone bitartrate 2.5 mg/5 ml. Bot. 480 ml. *c-III.*
Use: Antitussive, decongestant.

Hydrophen Syrup. (Rugby Labs, Inc.) Phenylpropanolamine HCl 25 mg, hydrocodone bitartrate 5 mg/5 ml. Bot. pt, gal. *c-III.*
Use: Antitussive, decongestant.

hydrophilic ointment. (E. Fougera and Co.) Stearyl alcohol, white petrolatum, propylene glycol, sodium lauryl sulfate, water. Jar lb.
Use: Pharmaceutic aid, ointment base.

hydrophilic ointment base. (Emerson Laboratories) Oil in water emulsion bases. 1 lb.
Use: Pharmaceutic aid, ointment base.
See: Aquaphilic Ointment (Medco Research, Inc.).
Cetaphil, Cream, Lot. (Texas Pharmacal).
Dermovan, Cream (Texas Pharmacal).
Lanaphilic Oint. (Medco Research, Inc.).
Polysorb, Oint. (Savage Laboratories).
Unibase, Oint. (Parke-Davis).

Hydropine. (Rugby Labs, Inc.) Hydroflumethiazide 25 mg, reserpine 0.125 mg/Tab. Bot. 100s. *Rx.*
Use: Antihypertensive combination.

Hydropine H.P. Tablets. (Rugby Labs, Inc.) Hydroflumethiazide 50 mg, reserpine 0.125 mg/Tab. Bot. 100s, 500s, 1000s. *Rx.*
Use: Antihypertensive combination.

Hydropres-50. (Merck & Co.) Hydrochlorothiazide 50 mg, reserpine 0.125 mg/Tab. Bot. 100s, 1000s. *Rx.*
Use: Antihypertensive combination.

•**hydroquinone.** (high-DROE-KWIN-ohn) U.S.P. 23.
Use: Depigmentor.
See: Artra Skin Tone, Cream (Schering-Plough Corp.).
Black and White Bleaching, Cream (Schering-Plough Corp.).
Eldopaque, Cream, Oint. (Zeneca Pharmaceuticals).
Eldopaque Forte, Cream, Oint. (Zeneca Pharmaceuticals).
Eldoquin, Cream, Lot. (Zeneca Pharmaceuticals).
Esoterica Medicated Cream Prods. (SmithKline Beecham Pharmaceuticals).
Melpaque HP, Cream (Stratus Pharmaceuticals, Inc.).
Melquin HP, Cream (Stratus Pharmaceuticals, Inc.).
Nuquin HP, Cream, Gel (Stratus Pharmaceuticals, Inc.).

hydroquinone. (Glades Pharmaceuticals) Hydroquinone 3%, SD Alcohol 45%, propylene glycol, isopropyl alcohol 4%/Soln. 30 ml with applicator. Hydroquinone 4%, padimate 0.5%, dioxybenzone 3%, EDTA, sodium metabisulfite, hydroalcoholic base.
Use: Depigmentor.

hydroquinone monobenzyl ether.
See: Benoquin, Oint., Lot. (Zeneca Pharmaceuticals).

Hydrosal. (Hydrosal Co.) Aluminum acetate 5%. **Susp.:** Bot. 16 oz, gal. **Oint.:** 54 g, 113.4 g, Jar 54 g, 454 g. *otc.*
Use: Astringent.

Hydro-Serp. (Zenith Goldline Pharmaceuticals) Hydrochlorothiazide 25 mg, 50 mg, reserpine 0.125 mg, 0.1 mg/Tab. Bot. 100s, 1000s. *Rx.*
Use: Antihypertensive combination.

Hydroserpine #1. (Various Mfr.) Hydrochlorothiazide 25 mg, reserpine. Bot. 100s, 1000s. *Rx.*
Use: Antihypertensive combination.

Hydroserpine #2. (Various Mfr.) Hydrochlorothiazide 50 mg, reserpine. Bot. 100s, 250s, 400s, 1000s. *Rx.*
Use: Antihypertensive combination.

Hydrosine 25. (Major Pharmaceuticals) Hydrochlorothiazide 25 mg, reserpine 0.125 mg/Tab. Bot. 100s. Tartrazine. *Rx.*
Use: Antihypertensive combination.

Hydrosine 50. (Major Pharmaceuticals) Hydrochlorothiazide 50 mg, reserpine 0.125 mg/Tab. Bot. 100s. *Rx.*
Use: Antihypertensive combination.

Hydrosone. (Sigma-Tau Pharmaceuticals, Inc.) Hydrocortisone acetate 25 mg or 50 mg, lactose/ml. Vial 5 ml. *Rx.*
Use: Corticosteroid.

HydroStat IR. (Richwood) Hydromorphone HCl 1 mg, 2 mg, 3 mg, 4 mg. Tab. Bot. 100s. *c-II.*
Use: Analgesic, narcotic.

Hydrotensin-50. (Merz Pharmaceuticals) Hydrochlorothiazide 50 mg, reserpine 0.125 mg/Tab. Bot. 100s, 1000s. *Rx.*
Use: Antihypertensive combination.

Hydro-T Tabs. (Major Pharmaceuticals) Hydrochlorothiazide. **25 mg/Tab:** Bot. 100s, 1000s, UD 100s. **50 mg/Tab:** Bot. 100s, 1000s, UD 100s. **100 mg/Tab:** Bot. 100s, 250s, 1000s, UD 100s. *Rx.*
Use: Diuretic.

•**hydroxocobalamin.** (high-DROX-oh-koe-BAL-ah-meen) U.S.P. 23.
Use: Treatment of megaloblastic anemia, vitamin (hematopoietic).

hydroxocobalamin, crystalline. (Various Mfr.) 1000 mcg/ml Inj. 30 ml. *Rx.*
Use: Vitamin supplement.
See: Hydroxocobalamin (Various Mfr.).
Hydro Cobex (Taylor Pharmaceuticals).
Hydro-Crysti (Roberts Pharmaceuticals).
LA-12 (Hyrex Pharmaceuticals).

hydroxocobalamin/sodium thiosulfate.
Use: Antidote, cyanide. [Orphan Drug]

•**hydroxyamphetamine hydrobromide.** (high-DROX-ee-am-FET-uh-meen HIGH-droe-BROE-mide) U.S.P. 23.
Use: Adrenergic (ophthalmic); mydriatic.
See: Paredrine (Pharmics, Inc.).

2-hydroxybenzamide.
See: Salicylamide.

hydroxy bis (acetato)aluminum. Aluminum Subacetate Topical Soln.

hydroxy bis (salicylato) aluminum diacetate.
See: Aluminum aspirin.

hydroxybutyrate, sodium/gamma.
See: Sodium gamma-hydroxybutyrate acid.

hydroxycholecalciferol. (D_3).
Use: Antihypocalcemia.
See: Calcifediol.

•**hydroxychloroquine sulfate.** (high-drox-ee-KLOR-oh-kwin) U.S.P. 23.
Use: Antimalarial, lupus erythematosus suppressant.

hydroxychloroquine sulfate. (Copley Pharmaceutical, Inc.) 200 mg/Tab. Bot. 100s, 500s.
Use: Antimalarial, lupus erythematosus suppressant.

•**hydroxyethyl cellulose.** (high-drox-ee-ETH-ill SELL-you-lohs) N.F. 18.
Use: Pharmaceutic aid (suspending, viscosity-increasing agent).
See: Gonioscopic, Soln. (Alcon Laboratories, Inc.).

hydroxyethyl starch. (HES).
Use: Plasma volume expander.
See: Hespan, Inj. (Du Pont Merck Pharmaceutical Co.).

hydroxyisoindolin. Under study.
Use: Antihypertensive.

hydroxymagnesium aluminate.
Use: Antacid.
See: Magaldrate.

hydroxymycin. An antibiotic substance obtained from cultures of *Streptomyces paucisporogenes.*

•**hydroxyphenamate.** (high-DROX-ee-FEN-ah-mate) USAN.
Use: Anxiolytic.

•**hydroxyprogesterone caproate.** (high-DROX-ee-pro-JESS-ter-ohn CAP-ROW-ate) U.S.P. 23.
Use: Hormone, progestin.
See: Delalutin, Vial (Bristol-Myers Squibb).
Duralutin, Inj. (Roberts Pharmaceuticals).
Gesterol L.A. 250, Inj. (Forest Pharmaceutical, Inc.).
Hy-Gestrone, Vial (Taylor Pharmaceuticals).
Hylutin, Inj. (Hyrex Pharmaceuticals).
Hyprogest 250, Inj. (Keene Pharmaceuticals, Inc.)

hydroxyprogesterone caproate. (Various Mfr.) **125 mg/ml:** Inj. Vial 10 ml. **250 mg/ml:** Inj. Vial 5 ml. *Rx.*
Use: Hormone, progestin.

•**hydroxypropyl cellulose.** (high-drox-ee-PRO-pill SELL-you-lohs) N.F. 18.
Use: Topical protectant; pharmaceutic aid, emulsifying tablet coating agent.

•**hydroxypropyl methylcellulose.** U.S.P. 23.
Use: Pharmaceutic aid (suspending, viscosity-increasing agent; tablet excipient).
See: Anestacon (Alcon Laboratories, Inc.).

Econopred, Susp. (Alcon Laboratories, Inc.).
Occucoat, Soln. (Storz Ophthalmics).
W/Benzalkonium Cl.
See: Gonak, Soln. (Akorn, Inc.).
Goniosol (Ciba Vision).
Isopto Tears (Alcon Laboratories, Inc).
Ultra Tears, Soln. (Alcon Laboratories, Inc.).

•**hydroxypropyl methylcellulose phthalate.** N. F. 18.
Use: Pharmaceutic aid (coating agent).
See: Hypromellose phthalate.

hydroxypropyl methylcellulose phthalate 200731.
Use: Pharmaceutic aid (coating agent).

hydroxypropyl methylcellulose phthalate 220824.
Use: Pharmaceutic aid (coating agent).

hydroxystearin sulfate. Sulfonate hydrogenated castor oil.

L-5 Hydroxytryptophan (L-5HTP). (Circa Pharmaceuticals, Inc.)
Use: Postanoxic intention myoclonus. [Orphan Drug]

•**hydroxyurea.** (high-DROX-ee-you-REE-uh) U.S.P. 23.
Use: Antineoplastic. Sickle cell disease. [Orphan Drug]
See: Hydrea, Cap. (Bristol-Myers Squibb).

hydroxyurea. (Roxane Laboratories, Inc.) Hydroxyurea 500 mg, lactose. Cap. Bot. 100s, UD 100s. *Rx.*
Use: Antineoplastic.

•**hydroxyzine hydrochloride.** (high-DROX-ih-zeen) U.S.P. 23.
Use: Anxiolytic, antihistamine.
See: Atarax, Syr., Tab. (Roerig).
Vistaril Isoject (Roerig).
Vistaril, Cap., Susp. (Pfizer US Pharmaceutical Group).
W/Ephedrine sulf., theophylline.
See: Marax DF, Syr. (Roerig).
Marax Tab. (Roerig).
Theo-Drox, Tab. (Quality Formulations, Inc.).

hydroxyzine hydrochloride. (Various Mfr.). **Tab.:** 10 mg, 25 mg. Bot. 20s, 30s, 50s, 100s, 250s, 500s, 1000s, UD 32s, 100s. 50 mg. Bot. 30s, 100s. **Syr.:** 10 mg/5 ml. Bot. 16 ml, 120 ml, 473 ml, UD 5 ml, 12.5 ml, 25 ml. **Inj.:** 25 mg/ml. Syr. 2 ml. Vial 1 ml, 10 ml; 50 mg/ml. Amp. 2 ml; Syr. 1 ml, 2 ml; Vial 1 ml, 2 ml, 10 ml. *Rx.*
Use: Antihistamine, anxiolytic.

•**hydroxyzine pamoate.** U.S.P. 23.
Use: Tranquilizer (minor), antihistamine.
See: Vistaril, Cap., Susp. (Pfizer US Pharmaceutical Group).

hydroxyzine pamoate. (Various Mfr.). Hydroxyzine pamoate 25 mg, 50 mg. Bot. 12s, 20s, 100s, 500s, 100s, UD 32s, 100s. 100 mg. Bot. 100s, 500s, 1000s, UD 100s. *Rx.*
Use: Antihistamine, anxiolytic.

Hydro-Z-50. (Merz Pharmaceuticals) Hydrochlorothiazide 50 mg/Tab. Bot. 100s, 1000s. *Rx.*
Use: Diuretic.

Hy-Flow Solution. (Ciba Vision) Polyvinyl alcohol with hydroxyethylcellulose, benzalkonium Cl, EDTA. Bot. 60 ml. *otc.*
Use: Contact lens care.

Hy-Gestrone. (Taylor Pharmaceuticals) Hydroxyprogesterone caproate. **125 mg/ml.:** Vial 10 ml. **250 mg/ml.:** Vial 5 ml. *Rx.*
Use: Hormone, progestin.

Hygienic Cleansing. (Rugby Labs, Inc.) Witch hazel 50%, glycerin, benzalkonium Cl, methylparaben. Pads. 100s. *otc.*
Use: Anorectal preparation.

Hygroton. (Rhone-Poulenc Rorer Pharmaceuticals, Inc.) Chlorthalidone 25 mg or 50 mg/Tab. Lactose (25, 50 mg). Bot. 100s. *Rx.*
Use: Diuretic.

Hylidone Tabs. (Major Pharmaceuticals) Chlorthalidone. **25 mg or 50 mg/Tab:** Bot. 100s, 250s, 1000s, UD 100s. **100 mg/Tab:** Bot. 100s, 250s, 500s, 1000s. *Rx.*
Use: Diuretic.

Hyliver Plus. (Hyrex Pharmaceuticals) Folic acid 0.4 mg, liver 10 mcg, vitamin B_{12} 100 mcg/ml. Vial 10 ml with phenol. *Rx.*
Use: Vitamin supplement.

Hylorel Tablets. (Medeva Pharmaceuticals, Inc.) Guanadrel sulfate 10 mg or 25 mg/Tab. Bot. 100s. *Rx.*
Use: Antihypertensive.

Hylutin Injectable. (Hyrex Pharmaceuticals) Hydroxyprogesterone caproate in oil 125 mg/ml, 250 mg/ml. Castor oil with benzyl benzoate and benzyl alcohol. Vial 5 ml (250 mg), 10 ml (125 mg). *Rx.*
Use: Hormone, progestin.

•**hymecromone.** (HIGH-meh-KROE-mone) USAN.
Use: Choleretic.

hymenoptera venom/venom protein. Purified venoms of honeybee, wasp, white faced hornet, yellow hornet, yellow jacket, and mixed vespids (both hornets and yellow jackets). *Rx.*
Use: Allergenic extract.

See: Albay (Bayer Corp. (Biological and Pharmaceutical Div.)).
Venomil (Bayer Corp. (Consumer Div.)).

HY-N.B.P. Ointment. (Jones Medical Industries, Inc.) Bacitracin zinc 400 units, neomycin sulfate 5 mg, polymixin B sulfate 10,000 units/g. Tube 1/8 oz. *Rx.*
Use: Anti-infective, topical.

hyoscine hydrobromide. U.S.P. 23.
Scopolamine HBr.
Use: Antispasmodic.

hyoscine-hyoscyamine-atropine.
Use: Anticholinergic.
See: Atropine w/hyoscyamine w/hyoscine.

•**hyoscyamine.** (high-oh-SIGH-ah-meen) U.S.P. 23.
Use: Anticholinergic.
See: Cystospaz, Tab. (PolyMedica Pharmaceuticals).

hyoscyamine-atropine-hyoscine.
Use: Anticholinergic.
See: Atropine w/hyoscyamine w/hyoscine.

•**hyoscyamine hydrobromide.** U.S.P. 23.
Use: Anticholinergic.

hyoscyamine hydrochloride. (Various Mfr.).

hyoscyamine salts.
Use: Anticholinergic.
W/Atropine salts
See: Atropine W/hyoscyamine.

•**hyoscyamine sulfate.** U.S.P. 23.
Use: Anticholinergic.
See: Anaspaz, Tab. (B.F. Ascher and Co.).
A-Spas SK, Tab. Subl. (Hyrex Pharmaceuticals).
A-Spas S/L (Hyrex Pharmaceuticals).
Cystospaz-M, Cap. (PolyMedica Pharmaceuticals).
Donnamar, Tab. (Marnel Pharmaceuticals, Inc.).
ED-SPAZ, Tab. (Edwards Pharmaceuticals, Inc.).
Gastrosed, Drops, Tab. (Roberts Pharmaceuticals).
Levbid, ER Tab. (Schwarz Pharma, Inc.).
Levsin/SL, Sublingual Tab. (Schwarz Pharma, Inc.).
W/Atropine sulfate, hyoscine HBr, phenobarbital.
See: DeTal, Elix., Tab. (DeLeon).
Donnatal, Prods. (Wyeth-Ayerst Laboratories).
Peece, Tab. (Scrip).
Sedamine, Tab. (Dunhall Pharmaceuticals, Inc.).
Spasaid, Cap. (Century Pharmaceuticals, Inc.).
See: Donnazyme, Tab. (Wyeth-Ayerst Laboratories).
W/Atropine sulfate, scopolamine HCl, phenobarbital.
See: Belladonna Prods.
W/Butabarbital.
See: Cystospaz-SR, Cap. (PolyMedica Pharmaceuticals).

hyoscyamine sulfate. (Ethex) **ER Tab.:** 0.375 mg. Bot. 100s. **Sublingual Tab.:** 0.125 mg. Bot. 100s. **Tab.:** 0.125 mg. Bot. 100s.
Use: Anticholinergic.

hyoscyamine sulfate. (Various Mfr.) 0.375 mg/ER Cap. 100s. *Rx.*
Use: Anticholinergic.

hyoscyamine sulfate. (Zenith Goldline Pharmaceuticals) 0.125 mg/ml, alcohol 5%/Soln. Bot. with dropper. 15 ml. *Rx.*
Use: Anticholinergic.

hyoscyamus extract.
W/A.P.C.
See: Valacet Junior, Tab. (Pal-Pak, Inc.).
W/A.P.C., gelsemium extract.
See: Valacet, Tab. (Pal-Pak, Inc.).

hyoscyamus products and phenobarbital combinations.
Use: Anticholinergic, sedative.
See: Anaspaz PB, Tab. (Taylor Pharmaceuticals).
Donnatal, Preps. (Wyeth-Ayerst Laboratories).
Elixiral, Elix. (Vita Elixir).

Hyosophen Elixir. (Rugby Labs, Inc.) Atropine sulfate 0.0194 mg, scopolamine HBr 0.0065 mg, hyoscyamine HBr or sulfate 0.1037 mg, phenobarbital 16.2 mg, alcohol 23%, sugar, sorbitol. 120 ml, pt, gal. *Rx.*
Use: Gastrointestinal, anticholinergic.

Hyosophen Tablets. (Rugby Labs, Inc.) Atropine sulfate 0.0194 mg, scopolamine HBr 0.0065 mg, hyoscyamine HBr or SO_4 0.1037 mg, phenobarbital 16.2 mg. In 1000s. *Rx.*
Use: Anticholinergic combination.

Hypaque 76. (Nycomed) Diatrizoate meglumine 660 mg, diatrizoate sodium 100 mg, iodine 370 mg/ml, EDTA. Bot. 50 ml, 200 ml. Dilution bot. 100 ml, 150 ml, 200 ml. *Rx.*
Use: Radiopaque agent.

Hypaque-Cysto. (Nycomed) Diatrizoate meglumine 300 mg, iodine 141 mg/ml, EDTA. Pediatric Bot.: 100 ml in 300 ml, 250 ml in 500 ml. *Rx.*
Use: Radiopaque agent.

Hypaque-M 75%. (Sanofi Winthrop Pharmaceuticals) Diatrizoate meglumine 50%, diatrizoate sodium 25%, iodine 38.5%, EDTA. Vial 20 ml, 50 ml.
Use: Radiopaque agent.

Hypaque-M 90%. (Sanofi Winthrop Pharmaceuticals) Diatrizoate meglumine 60%, diatrizoate sodium 30%, EDTA. Vial 50 ml.
Use: Radiopaque agent.

Hypaque Meglumine 30%. (Nycomed) Diatrizoate meglumine 300 mg, iodine 141 mg/ml. Bot. Vial 100 ml. Bot. 300 ml w/ and w/o I.V. infusion set. *Rx.*
Use: Radiopaque agent.

Hypaque Meglumine 60%. (Nycomed) Diatrizoate meglumine 600 mg, iodine 282 mg/ml, EDTA. Vial 50 ml, 100 ml. Bot. 150 fill ml in 200 bot., 200 ml fill in 250 ml bot. *Rx.*
Use: Radiopaque agent.

Hypaque Oral. (Sanofi Winthrop Pharmaceuticals) **Pow.:** Diatrizoate sodium oral pow. containing iodine 600 mg/g. Can 250 g, Bot. 10 g. **Liq.:** Soln. 41.66%. Bot. 120 ml.
Use: Radiopaque agent.

Hypaque Sodium. (Nycomed) **Soln.:** Diatrizoate sodium 416.7 mg, iodine 249 mg/ml. Soln. Bot. 120 ml. **Pow.:** Diatrizoate sodium (59.87% iodine), iodine 600 mg/ml. Bot. 10 g. Can 250 mg with measuring spoon. *Rx.*
Use: Radiopaque agent.

Hypaque Sodium 20%. (Nycomed) Diatrizoate sodium 200 mg, iodine 120 mg/ml, EDTA. Multi-dose Vial 100 ml. *Rx.*
Use: Radiopaque agent.

Hypaque Sodium 25%. (Nycomed) Diatrizoate sodium 250 mg, iodine 150 mg/ml. Bot. 300 ml. *Rx.*
Use: Radiopaque agent.

Hypaque Sodium 50%. (Nycomed) Diatrizoate sodium 500 mg, iodine 300 mg/ml. Vial. 50 ml.
Use: Radiopaque agent.

Hyperab.
See: Bayrab, Vial (Bayer Corp. (Consumer Div.)).

HyperHep.
See: BayHep B, Vial (Bayer Corp. (Consumer Div.)).

hypericin. (VIMRxyn Pharm/NIH) *Rx.*
Use: Antiviral.

hyperlipidemia, agents for.
See: Atromid-S (Wyeth-Ayerst Laboratories).
Choloxin (Knoll Pharmaceuticals).
Clofibrate (Various Mfr.).
Colestid (Pharmacia & Upjohn).
Lescol (Novartis Pharmaceutical Corp).
Lopid (Parke-Davis).
Lorelco (Hoechst Marion Roussel).
Mevacor (Merck & Co.).
Pravachol (Bristol-Myers Squibb).
Questran (Bristol-Myers Squibb).
Questran Light (Bristol-Myers Squibb).
Zocor (Merck & Co.).

Hyperlyte. (American McGaw) Sodium 25 mEq, potassium 40.5 mEq, calcium 5 mEq, magnesium 8 mEq, chloride 33.5 mEq, acetate 40.6 mEq, gluconate 5 mEq, 6050 mOsm/L. Inj. Vial 25 ml fill in 50 ml. *Rx.*
Use: Nutritional supplement, parenteral.

Hyperlyte CR. (American McGaw) Sodium 25 mEq, potassium 20 mEq, calcium 5 mEq, magnesium 5 mEq, chloride 30 mEq, acetate 30 mEq, 5500 mOsm/L. Inj. Super-vial 150 ml, 250 ml fill. *Rx.*
Use: Nutritional supplement, parenteral.

Hyperlyte R. (American McGaw) Sodium 25 mEq, potassium 20 mEq, calcium 5 mEq, magnesium 5 mEq, chloride 30 mEq, acetate 25 mEq, 4200 mOsm/L. Inj. Vial 25 ml fill in 50 ml. *Rx.*
Use: Nutritional supplement, parenteral.

Hypermune RSV. (MedImmune, Inc.) Respiratory syncytial virus immune globulin, human.
Use: Respiratory syncytial virus treatment. [Orphan Drug]

Hyperopto 5%. (Professional Pharmacal) Sodium Cl 5%. Oint. Tube 3.5 g. *otc.*
Use: Ophthalmic.

Hyperopto Ointment. (Professional Pharmacal) Sodium HCl 50 mg, D.I. water 150 mg, anhydrous lanolin 150 mg, liquid petrolatum 50 mg, white petrolatum 599 mg, methylparaben 7 mg, propylparaben 3 mg/g. Tube 3.5 g. *otc.*
Use: Ophthalmic.

hyperosmolar agents.
Use: Laxative.
See: Glycerin, USP (Various Mfr.).
Sani-Supp, Supp. (G & W Laboratories).
Fleet Babylax, Liq. (C. B. Fleet Co., Inc.).

Hyperstat IV Injection. (Schering-Plough Corp.) Diazoxide 15 mg/ml. Amp. 20 ml. *Rx.*
Use: Antihypertensive.

hypertension diagnosis.
See: Regitine, Amp., Tab. (Novartis Pharmaceutical Corp.).

hypertensive emergency drugs.
See: Diazoxide Injection (Quad Pharmaceuticals, Inc.).

Hyperstat IV, Inj. (Schering-Plough Corp.).
Nitropress, Inj. (Abbott Laboratories).

Hyper-Tet.
See: Baytet, Vial (Bayer Corp. (Consumer Div.)).

Hyphed. (Cypress Pharm.) Hydrocodone bitartrate 2.5 mg, pseudoephedrine HCl 30 mg, chlorpheniramine maleate 2 mg/5 ml, alcohol. Syr. Bot. 1 pt. *c-III.*
Use: Antitussive, decongestant.

Hy-Phen. (B.F. Ascher and Co.) Hydrocodone bitartrate 5 mg, acetaminophen 500 mg. Tab. Bot. 100s. *c-III.*
Use: Analgesic, antitussive.

Hyphylline. Dyphylline. *Rx.*
See: Neothylline, Elix., Amp., Tab. (Teva Pharmaceuticals USA).

hypnogene.
See: Barbital (Various Mfr.).

Hypnomidate. (Janssen Pharmaceutical, Inc.) Etomidate. *Rx.*
Use: Anesthetic, general.

hypnotics.
See: Sedative/hypnotic agents.

"hypo".
See: Sodium Thiosulfate (Various Mfr.).

Hypo-Bee. (Towne) Vitamins B_1 50 mg, B_2 20 mg, B_6 5 mg, B_{12} 15 mcg, niacinamide 25 mg, calcium pantothenate 5 mg, C 300 mg, E 200 IU, iron 10 mg/Tab. Bot. 30s, 100s. *otc.*
Use: Mineral, vitamin supplement.

hypochlorite preps.
See: Antiformin.
Dakin's Soln.
Hyclorite.

Hypoclear. (Bausch & Lomb Pharmaceuticals) Isotonic soln. with sodium Cl 0.9%. Aerosol soln. 240 ml, 300 ml. *otc.*
Use: Contact lens care.

hypoglycemic agents.
See: Chlorpropamide.
Diabeta, Tab. (Hoechst Marion Roussel).
Diabinese, Tab. (Pfizer US Pharmaceutical Group).
Dymelor, Tab. (Eli Lilly and Co.).
Glucotrol, Tab. (Roerig).
Glynase, Tab. (Pharmacia & Upjohn).
Micronase, Tab. (Pharmacia & Upjohn).
Orinase, Tab., Vial (Pharmacia & Upjohn).
Phenformin HCl.
Tolbutamide.
Tolinase, Tab. (Pharmacia & Upjohn).

α-hypophamine. Oxytocin.

•**hypophosphorous acid.** (high-poe-FOSS-for-uhs) N.F. 18.
Use: Pharmaceutic aid (antioxidant).

HypoTears Ophthalmic Liquid. (Ciba Vision) Polyvinyl alcohol 1%, PEG-400, dextrose 1%, benzalkonium Cl 0.01%, EDTA. Bot. 15 ml, 30 ml. *otc.*
Use: Lubricant, ophthalmic.

HypoTears Ophthalmic Ointment. (Ciba Vision) White petrolatum, light mineral oil. Tube 3.5 g. *otc.*
Use: Lubricant, ophthalmic.

HypoTears PF. (Ciba Vision) Polyvinyl alcohol 1%, PEG 400, dextrose and EDTA. Soln. In 0.6 ml. *otc.*
Use: Artificial tears.

hypotensive agents.
See: Antihypertensives.

HypRh$_O$-D.
See: BayRh$_O$ D, Vial (Bayer Corp. (Consumer Div.)).

HypRh$_O$-D Mini-Dose. (Bayer Corp. (Consumer Div.)) RH$_O$ (D) Immune Globulin Micro-Dose. Each package contains a single-dose syringe. *Rx.*
Use: Immunization.

•**hypromellose phthalate.** N.F. 18.
Use: Pharmaceutical aid (coating agent).

Hyrexin-50. (Hyrex Pharmaceuticals) Diphenhydramine HCl 50 mg/ml, benzethonium chloride. Vial 10 ml. Amp. 1 ml. *Rx.*
Use: Antihistamine.

Hyscorbic Plus Tablets. (Sanofi Winthrop Pharmaceuticals) Vitamins E 45 IU, C 600 mg, folic acid 400 mcg, B_1 20 mg, B_2 10 mg, niacinamide 100 mg, B_6 10 mg, B_{12} 25 mcg, pantothenic acid 25 mg, copper 3 mg, zinc 23.9 mg/Tab. Bot. 60s. *otc.*
Use: Mineral, vitamin supplement.

Hyserp. (Freeport) Reserpine alkaloid 0.25 mg/Tab. Bot. 1000s. *Rx.*
Use: Antihypertensive.

Hyskon. (Pharmacia & Upjohn) Dextran 70 32% in 10% w/v dextrose. Bot. 100 ml, 250 ml. *Rx.*
Use: Diagnostic aid. For distending the uterine cavity and irrigating and visualizing its surfaces.

Hysone. (Roberts Pharmaceuticals) Clioquinol 30 mg, hydrocortisone 10 mg/g. Cream. Tube. 20 g. *otc.*
Use: Antifungal; corticosteroid, topical.

hysteroscopy fluid.
Use: Diagnostic aid.
See: Hyskon (Pharmacia & Upjohn).

Hytakerol. (Sanofi Winthrop Pharmaceuticals) Dihydrotachysterol. 0.125 mg/Cap. Bot. 50s. *Rx.*
Use: Treatment of tetany and hypoparathyroidism.

Hytinic. (Hyrex Pharmaceuticals) Poly-

saccharide-iron complex. **Cap.:** 150 mg. Bot. 50s, 500s. **Elix.:** 100 mg/5 ml, alcohol 10%. Bot. 240 ml. *otc.*
Use: MIneral supplement.

Hytinic Injection. (Hyrex Pharmaceuticals) Ferrous gluconate 3 mg, liver equivalent to vitamins B_{12} 1 mcg, vitamins B_2 0.75 mg, B_3 50 mg, B_5 1.25 mg, B_{12} equivalent 15 mcg. Vial 30 ml. *Rx.*
Use: Mineral, vitamin supplement.

Hytone Cream. (Dermik Laboratories, Inc.) Hydrocortisone in cream base. **1%:** 1 oz. Jar 4 oz. **2.5%:** Tube 1 oz, 2 oz. *Rx-otc.*
Use: Corticosteroid, topical.

Hytone Lotion 1%. (Dermik Laboratories, Inc.) Hydrocortisone 1% (10 mg/ml). Bot. 120 ml. *Rx.*
Use: Corticosteroid, topical.

Hytone Lotion 2.5%. (Dermik Laboratories, Inc.) Hydrocortisone 2.5% (25 mg/ml) in lotion base. Bot. 60 ml. *Rx.*
Use: Corticosteroid, topical.

Hytone Ointment. (Dermik Laboratories, Inc.) Hydrocortisone in ointment base, mineral oil, white petrolatum. **1%:** Tube 28.3 g, 113.4 g. **2.5%:** Tube 28.3 g. *Rx.*
Use: Corticosteroid, topical.

Hytone Spray. (Dermik Laboratories, Inc.) Hydrocortisone 1%. 45 ml. *Rx.*
Use: Corticosteroid, topical.

Hytrin. (Abbott Laboratories) Terazosin HCl 1 mg, 2 mg, 5 mg, 10 mg, parabens. Cap. Bot. 100s, UD 100s. *Rx.*
Use: Antihypertensive.

Hytuss Tablets. (Hyrex Pharmaceuticals) Guaifenesin 100 mg/Tab. Bot. 100s, 1000s. *otc.*
Use: Expectorant.

Hytuss 2X. (Hyrex Pharmaceuticals) Guaifenesin 200 mg/Cap. Bot. 100s, 1000s. *otc.*
Use: Expectorant.

Hyzaar. (Merck & Co.) Losartan potassium 50 mg, hydrochlorothiazide 12.5 mg, potassium 4.24 mg, lactose/Tab. Bot. 30s, 90s, 100s, UD 100s. *Rx.*
Use: Antihypertensive.

Hyzine-50. (Hyrex Pharmaceuticals) Hydroxyzine HCl 50 mg as HCl/ml. Vial 10 ml. *Rx.*
Use: Anxiolytic.

I

•**ibafloxacin.** (ih-BAH-FLOX-ah-sin) USAN.
Use: Anti-infective.

•**ibandronate sodium.** (ih-BAN-droe-nate SO-dee-uhm) USAN.
Use: Bone resorption inhibitor; antihypercalcemic.

ibenzmethyzin. Name used for Procarbazine Hydrochloride.

Iberet. (Abbott Laboratories) Ferrous sulfate 105 mg, ascorbic acid 150 mg, vitamins B_{12} 25 mcg, B_1 6 mg, B_2 6 mg, niacinamide 30 mg, B_5 10 mg, B_6 5 mg/CR Filmtab. Bot. 60s. *Rx.*
Use: Mineral, vitamin supplement.

Iberet-500 Filmtab. (Abbott Laboratories) Ascorbic acid 500 mg, ferrous sulfate 105 mg, vitamins B_1 6 mg, B_2 6 mg, B_3 30 mg, B_5 10 mg, B_6 5 mg, B_{12} 25 mcg/CR Filmtab. Bot. 60s, 100s, Abbo-Pac 100s. *Rx.*
Use: Mineral, vitamin supplement.

Iberet-500 Liquid. (Abbott Laboratories) Ferrous sulfate 78.75 mg, vitamins B_1 4.5 mg, B_2 4.5 mg, B_3 22.5 mg, B_5 7.5 mg, B_6 3.75 mg, B_{12} 18.75 mcg, C 375 mg, sorbitol, parabens/5 ml. Bot. 240 ml. *Rx.*
Use: Mineral, vitamin supplement.

Iberet-Folic-500 Filmtab. (Abbott Laboratories) Ferrous sulfate 105 mg, vitamin C 500 mg, B_3 30 mg, B_5 10 mg, B_1 6 mg, B_2 6 mg, B_6 5 mg, B_{12} 25 mcg, folic acid 0.8 mg/CR Filmtab. Bot. 60s. *Rx.*
Use: Mineral, vitamin supplement.

Iberet Liquid. (Abbott Laboratories) Ferrous sulfate 78.75 mg, vitamins C 112.5 mg, B_{12} 18.75 mcg, B_1 4.5 mg, B_2 4.5 mg, B_3 22.5 mg, B_5 7.5 mg, B_6 3.75 mg/15 ml. Bot. 240 ml. *Rx.*
Use: Mineral, vitamin supplement.

•**ibopamine.** (EYE-BOE-pah-meen) USAN.
Use: Dopaminergic (peripheral).

IBU. (Knoll Pharmaceuticals) Ibuprofen 400, 600, or 800 mg/Tab. 100s, 500s. *Rx.*
Use: Analgesic, NSAID.

•**ibufenac.** (eye-BYOO-feh-nak) USAN.
Use: Antirheumatic (anti-inflammatory, analgesic, antipyretic).

Ibuprin. (Thompson Medical Co.) Ibuprofen 200 mg/Tab. Bot. 50s, 100s. *otc.*
Use: Analgesic, NSAID.

•**ibuprofen.** (eye-BYOO-pro-fen) U.S.P. 23.
Use: Anti-inflammatory, analgesic.
See: Advil, Tab. (Whitehall Robins Laboratories).
Children's Advil, Susp. (Whitehall Robins Laboratories).
Dynafed IB, Tab. (BDI Pharmaceuticals, Inc.).
Genpril, Tab. (Zenith Goldline Pharmaceuticals).
Haltran, Tab. (Pharmacia & Upjohn).
IBU, Tab. (Knoll Pharmaceuticals).
Ibuprin, Tab. (Thompson Med).
Junior Strength Advil, Tab. (Whitehall Robins Laboratories).
Junior Strength Motrin, Tab. (Ortho McNeil Pharmaceutical).
Menadol, Tab. (Rugby Labs, Inc.).
Midol IB, Tab. (Bayer Corp. (Consumer Div.)).
Motrin, Tab, Drops, Chew. Tab., Susp. (Pharmacia & Upjohn).
Motrin IB, Tab. (Pharmacia & Upjohn).
Nuprin, Tab. (Bristol-Myers Squibb).
Pediatric Advil Drops, Oral Susp. (Whitehall Robins Laboratories).
Saleto, Tab. (Roberts Pharmaceuticals).

ibuprofen. (Various Mfr.) 200, 300, 400, 600, 800 mg/Tab. 12s, 15s, 21s, 30s, 40s, 50s, 60s, 100s, 360s, 500s, UD 100s. *Rx-otc.*
Use: Analgesic, NSAID.

•**ibuprofen aluminum.** (eye-BYOO-pro-fen) USAN.
Use: Anti-inflammatory.

•**ibuprofen piconol.** (eye-BYOO-pro-fen PIK-oh-nahl) USAN.
Use: Topical anti-inflammatory.

ibuprofen suspension. (Various Mfr.) 100 mg/5 ml. UD 50s. *Rx.*
Use: Analgesic, NSAID.

•**ibutilide fumarate.** (ih-BYOO-tih-lide FEW-muh-rate) USAN.
Use: Cardiac depressant (antiarrhythmic).
See: Corvert, Soln. (Pharmacia & Upjohn).

ICAPS Plus. (Ciba Vision) Vitamin A 6000 IU, C 200 mg, E 60 IU, B_2 20 mg, Zn 14.25 mg, Cu, Se, Mn/Tab. Sugar free. Bot. 60s, 120s. *otc.*
Use: Mineral, vitamin supplement.

ICAPS Time Release. (Ciba Vision) Vitamin A 7000 IU, C 200 mg, E 100 IU, B_2 20 mg, Zn 14.25 mg, Cu, Se/Tab. Sugar free. Bot. 60s, 120s. *otc.*
Use: Mineral, vitamin supplement.

•**icatibant acetate.** (eye-CAT-ih-bant ASS-eh-tate) USAN.
Use: Bradykinin antagonist.

Ice Mint. (Westwood Squibb Pharmaceuticals) Stearic acid, synthetic cocoa butter, lanolin oil, camphor, menthol, beeswax, mineral oil, sodium borate, aromatic oils, emulsifiers. Jar 4 oz. *otc.*
Use: Emollient, counterirritant.

I-Chlor 0.5%. (Americal Pharmaceutical, Inc.) Chloramphenicol 5 mg/ml. Bot. 7.5 ml, 15 ml. *Rx.*
Use: Anti-infective, ophthalmic.

•**ichthammol.** (ICK-thah-mole) U.S.P. 23.
Use: Topical anti-infective.
W/Aluminum hydroxide, phenol, zinc oxide, camphor, eucalyptol.
See: Boil-Ease Anesthetic Drawing Salve (Del Pharmaceuticals, Inc.).
W/Hydrocortisone acetate, benzocaine, oxyquinoline sulfate, ephedrine HCl.
See: Derma Medicone-HC (Medicore).
W/Naftalan, calamine, amber pet.
See: Naftalan, Oint. (Paddock Laboratories).

ichthammol. (Eli Lilly and Co.) 10%, 20% Oint.

ichthammol. (NMC Laboratories) Ichthammol 10% or 20% in a lanolin-petrolatum base. Oint. Tube 28.4 g. *otc.*
Use: Antiseptic.

ichthynate.
See: Ichthammol.

•**icopezil maleate.** (eye-KOE-peh-zill MAL-ee-ate) USAN.
Use: Alzheimer's disease treatment (cognition enhancer), cognition adjuvant, acetylcholinesterase inhibitor.

•**icotidine.** (eye-KOE-tih-DEEN) USAN.
Use: Antagonist (to histamine H_2 and H_1 receptors).

•**ictasol.** (IK-tah-sahl) USAN.
Use: Disinfectant.

Ictotest Reagent Tablets. (Bayer Corp. (Consumer Div.)) Reagent Tab. for urinary bilirubin. Bot. 100s.
Use: Diagnostic aid.

Icy Hot Balm. (Procter & Gamble Pharm.) Methyl salicylate 29%, menthol 7.6%. Jar 3.5 oz, 7 oz. *otc.*
Use: Analgesic, topical.

Icy Hot Cream. (Procter & Gamble Pharm.) Methyl salicylate 30%, menthol 10%. Tube 0.25 oz, 1.25 oz, 3 oz. *otc.*
Use: Analgesic, topical.

Icy Hot, Extra Strength. (Procter & Gamble Pharm.) Methyl salicylate 30%, menthol 10%, ceresin, cyclomethicone, hydrogenated castor oil, PEG-150 distearate, propylene glycol, stearic acid, stearyl alcohol. Stick 52.5 g. *otc.*
Use: Liniment.

Icy Hot Stick. (Procter & Gamble Pharm.) Methyl salicylate 15%, menthol 8%. Stick 1.75 oz. *otc.*
Use: Analgesic, topical.

I.D.A. Capsules. (Zenith Goldline Pharmaceuticals) Isometheptene mucate 65 mg, dichloralphenazone 100 mg, acetaminophen 324 mg/Cap. Bot. 100s. *Rx.*
Use: Analgesic.

Idamycin. (Pharmacia & Upjohn) Idarubicin HCl. Lactose 50 mg/5 mg. Lactose 100 mg/10 mg. Lactose 200 mg/20 mg Pow. for Inj. *Rx.*
Use: Anti-infective.

Idamycin PFS. (Pharmacia & Upjohn) Idarubicin HCl 1 mg/ml. Inj. Vial 5 ml, 10 ml, 20 ml. *Rx.*
Use: Anti-infective (anthracycline).

•**idarubicin hydrochloride.** (eye-DUH-RUE-bih-sin) U.S.P. 23.
Use: Antineoplastic. [Orphan Drug]
See: Idamycin (Pharmacia & Upjohn).

•**idoxifene.** (ih-dox-ih-feen) USAN.
Use: Antineoplastic, hormone replacement therapy (estrogen receptor antagonist), osteoporosis treatment and prevention.

I-Drops. (Americal Pharmaceutical, Inc.) Tetrahydrozoline HCl 0.5%. Ophthalmic Soln. Bot. 0.5 oz. *Rx.*
Use: Mydriatic, vasoconstrictor.

IDU. Idoxuridine.
Use: Antiviral, ophthalmic.

Ifex. (Everett Laboratories, Inc.) Ibuprofen 400 mg, 600 mg/Tab. Bot. 100s, 500s. *Rx.*
Use: Analgesic.

•**ifetroban.** (ih-FEH-troe-ban) USAN.
Use: Antithrombotic.

•**ifetroban sodium.** (ih-FEH-troe-ban) USAN.
Use: Antithrombotic.

Ifex. (Bristol-Myers Squibb) Ifosfamide 1 g, 3 g. Pow. for Inj. Vial single dose. *Rx.*
Use: Antineoplastic.

•**ifosfamide.** (eye-FOSS-fuh-MIDE) U.S.P. 23.
Use: Antineoplastic.
See: Ifex, Pow. for Inj. (Mead Johnson Oncology).

I-Gent. (Americal Pharmaceutical, Inc.) Gentamicin sulfate 3 mg/ml. Ophthalmic soln. Bot. 5 ml. *Rx.*
Use: Anti-infective, ophthalmic.

Igepal Co-430. (General Aniline & Film) Nonoxynol-4. *otc.*
Use: Contraceptive, spermicide.

Igepal Co-730. (General Aniline & Film)

Nonoxynol-15. *otc.*
Use: Contraceptive, spermicide.

Igepal Co-880. (General Aniline & Film) Nonoxynol-30. *otc.*
Use: Contraceptive, spermicide.

igG monoclonal anti-CD4.
See: Chimeric m-t412 (human-murine) igG monoclonal anti-cd4.

IGIV. (Various Mfr.) Immune globulin IV. *Rx.*
Use: Immunomodulator (Phase II/III pediatric HIV), immunization.
See: Gamimune N, Inj. (Bayer Corp. (Consumer Div.)).
Gammagard S/D, Pow. (Baxter Pharmaceutical Products, Inc.).
Gammar-P IV, Pow. (Centeon).
Iveegam, Pow. (Immuno Therapy Co.).
Polygam S/D (American Red Cross).
Sandoglobulin, Pow. (Novartis Pharmaceutical Corp.).
Venoglobulin-I, Pow. (Alpha Therapeutic Corp.).
Venoglobulin-S (Alpha Therapeutic Corp.).

I-Homatrine 5%. (Americal Pharmaceutical, Inc.) Homatropine hydrobromide 5%. Ophth. Soln. Bot. 5 ml. *Rx.*
Use: Cycloplegic, mydriatic.

IL-2. (Various Mfr.) Interleukin-2. *Rx.*
Use: Immunomodulator.
See: Proleukin (Chiron).

•**ilepcimide.** (eye-LEPP-sih-mide) USAN. *Formerly antiepilepsirine.*
Use: Anticonvulsant.

Iletin I. (Eli Lilly and Co.) Regular and modified insulin products from beef and pork. **Regular:** 100 units/ml. Bot. 10 ml. **Lente:** 100 units/ml. Bot. 10 ml. **NPH:** 100 units/ml. Bot 10 ml. *otc.*
Use: Antidiabetic.

Iletin II. (Eli Lilly and Co.) Special insulin products prepared from purified beef or purified pork. **Regular:** 100 units/ml. Bot. 10 ml. **Lente:** 100 units/ml. Bot. 10 ml. **NPH:** 100 units/ml. Bot 10 ml. *otc.*
Use: Antidiabetic.

Iletin II Concentrated. (Eli Lilly and Co.) Purified pork regular insulin 500 units/ml. Vial 20 ml. *Rx.*
Use: Antidiabetic.

•**ilmofosine.** (ill-MOE-fose-een) USAN.
Use: Antineoplastic.

•**ilonidap.** (ile-OHN-ih-dap) USAN.
Use: Anti-inflammatory.

Ilopan. (Pharmacia & Upjohn) Dexpanthenol 250 mg/ml. Amp. 2 ml, Disp. syringe 2 ml. *Rx.*
Use: Gastrointestinal stimulant.

Ilopan-Choline. (Pharmacia & Upjohn) Ilopan 50 mg, choline bitartrate 25 mg/Tab. Bot. 100s, 500s. *Rx.*
Use: Gastrointestinal stimulant.

•**iloperidone.** (ill-oh-PURR-ih-dohn) USAN.
Use: Antipsychotic.

iloprost infusion solution. (Berlex Laboratories, Inc.) Raynaud's phenomenon secondary to systemic sclerosis. [Orphan Drug]

Ilosone. (Eli Lilly and Co.) Erythromycin estolate. **Tab.:** 500 mg, Bot. 50s. **Susp.:** 125 mg, 250 mg/5 ml. Bot. 100 ml (250 mg only), 480 ml. *Rx.*
Use: Anti-infective, erythromycin.

Ilosone Pulvules. (Eli Lilly and Co.) Erythromycin estolate 250 mg. Cap. Bot. 100s. *Rx.*
Use: Anti-infective, erythromycin.

Ilotycin Gluceptate. (Eli Lilly and Co.) Erythromycin gluceptate 1 g. Inj. Vial 30 ml. *Rx.*
Use: Anti-infective, erythromycin.

Ilotycin Ophthalmic Ointment. (Eli Lilly and Co.) Erythromycin 5 mg/g. Tube 3.5 g. *Rx.*
Use: Anti-infective, ophthalmic.

Ilozyme. (Pharmacia & Upjohn) Pancrelipase equivalent to lipase 11,000 units, protease 30,000 units, amylase 30,000 units/Tab. Bot. 250s. *Rx.*
Use: Digestive enzymes.

I-Lube. (Americal Pharmaceutical, Inc.) Petrolatum ophthalmic ointment. Tube 0.125 oz.
Use: Lubricant, ophthalmic.

I.L.X. B12 Elixir. (Kenwood Laboratories) Liver fraction 98 mg, iron 102 mg, vitamins B_1 5 mg, B_2 2 mg, B_3 10 mg, B_{12} 10 mcg/15 ml. Bot. 240 ml. *otc.*
Use: Mineral, vitamin supplement.

I.L.X. B12 Tablets and Caplets. (Kenwood Laboratories) Iron 37.5 mg, vitamins C 120 mg, B_{12} 12 mcg, desiccated liver 130 mg, B_1 2 mg, B_2 2 mg, B_3 20 mg/Tab. Bot. 100s. *otc.*
Use: Mineral, vitamin supplement.

I-L-X Elixir. (Kenwood Laboratories) Iron 70 mg, liver concentrate 98 mg, vitamins B_1 5 mg, B_2 2 mg, B_3 10 mg/15 ml. Bot. 240 ml. *otc.*
Use: Mineral, vitamin supplement.

•**imafen hydrochloride.** (IH-mah-fen) USAN.
Use: Antidepressant.

Imager ac. (Lafayette) Barium Sulfate 100%. Susp. Bot. 650 ml w/enema tip-tubing assemblies w/kit, 1900 ml bot. *Rx.*
Use: Radiopaque agent.

•**imazodan hydrochloride.** (ih-MAY-zoe-DAN) USAN.
Use: Cardiovascular agent.

•**imciromab pentetate.** (im-SIHR-ah-mab PEN-teh-tate) USAN.
Use: Monoclonal antibody (antimyosin). [Orphan Drug]
See: Myoscint (Centocor, Inc.).

Imdur. (Key Pharmaceuticals) Isosorbide mononitrate 30 mg, 60 mg, 120 mg. ER Tab. Bot. 30s, 100s, UD 100s. *Rx.*
Use: Antianginal.

Imenol. (Sigma-Tau Pharmaceuticals, Inc.) Guaiacol 0.1 g, eucalyptol 0.08 g, iodoform 0.02 g, camphor 0.05 g/ml. Vial 30 ml. *Rx.*
Use: Expectorant.

l-methorphinan levorphanol.
See: Levo-Dromoran, Amp., Tab., Vial (Roche Laboratories).

Imferon. (Medeva Pharmaceuticals, Inc.) An iron-dextran complex containing iron 50 mg/ml. Amp. 2 ml. Box 10s. Vial (w/ phenol 0.5%) 10 ml. Box 2s. *Rx.*
Use: Mineral supplement.

imexon. (Amplimed)
Use: Multiple myeloma. [Orphan Drug]

imidazole carboxamide. *Rx.*
Use: Antineoplastic.
See: Dacarbazine, Inj. (Various Mfr.).
DTIC-Dome, Inj. (Bayer Corp. (Consumer Div.)).

•**imidecyl iodine.** (IH-mih-DEH-sill EYE-uh-dine) USAN.
Use: Anti-infective, topical.

•**imidocarb hydrochloride.** (ih-MIH-doe-KARB) USAN.
Use: Antiprotozoal (Babesia).

•**imidoline hydrochloride.** (im-ID-oh-leen) USAN.
Use: Anxiolytic, antipsychotic.

•**imidurea.** (ih-mid-your-EE-ah) N.F. 18.
Use: Antimicrobial.

•**imiglucerase.** (ih-mih-GLUE-ser-ACE) USAN.
Use: Enzyme replenisher, treatment for Gaucher's disease (glucocerebrosidase). [Orphan Drug]
See: Cerezyme (Genzyme Corp.).

•**imiloxan hydrochloride.** (ih-mill-OX-ahn) USAN.
Use: Antidepressant.

imipemide. (ih-MIH-peh-MIDE)
Use: Anti-infective.
See: Imipenem, U.S.P. 23.

•**imipenem.** (ih-mih-PEN-em) U.S.P. 23.
Formerly imipemide.
Use: Anti-infective.
W/Cilastatin for Injection.
See: Primaxin, Inj. (Merck & Co.).

•**imipramine hydrochloride.** (im-IPP-ruh-meen) U.S.P. 23.
Use: Antidepressant.
See: Janimine, Tab. (Abbott Laboratories).
Tofranil, Tab., Amp. (Novartis Pharmaceutical Corp.).

imipramine pamoate.
Use: Antidepressant.
See: Tofranil-PM, Cap. (Novartis Pharmaceutical Corp.).

•**imiquimod.** (ih-mih-KWIH-mahd) USAN.
Use: Immunomodulator.
See: Aldara Cream (3M Pharm.).

Imitrex Injection. (GlaxoWellcome) Sumatriptan succinate 12 mg/ml, sodium chloride 7 mg/ml. Inj. Unit-of-use syringes: 0.5 ml in 2 ml; Single-dose vial: 6 mg; SELFdose system kit: 2 unit-of-use syringes, 1 SELFdose unit. *Rx.*
Use: Antimigraine.

Imitrex Nasal Spray. (GlaxoWellcome) Sumatriptan 5 mg, 20 mg. Nasal spray, unit-dose spray device 100 mcl. 6s. *Rx.*
Use: Antimigraine.

Imitrex Tablets. (GlaxoWellcome) Sumatriptan succinate 25 mg, 50 mg, lactose/ Tab. Pkg. 9s. *Rx.*
Use: Antimigraine.

ImmTher. (Immuno Therapy Co.) Disaccharide tripeptide glycerol dipalmitoyl.
Use: Antineoplastic. [Orphan Drug]

Immun-Aid. (McGaw, Inc.) A custard flavored liquid containing 18.5 g protein, 60 g carbohydrate, 11 g fat, sodium 290 mg, potassium 530 mg per liter. 1 calorie/ml. With appropriate vitamins and minerals. Pow. Packets 123 g. 24s. *otc.*
Use: Nutritional supplement, enteral.

immune globulin. (ih-MYOON GLAH-byoo-lin) Immune Serum Globulin Human. Gamma-globulin fraction of normal human plasma. Vial 10 ml. Tubex 1 ml, 2 ml w/thimerosal 1:10,000. *Rx.*
Use: Modification of active measles, prophylaxis of hepatitis A; treatment of immune deficiencies; prevention of infection associated with bone marrow transplantation (BMT); decrease frequency of certain pediatric HIV-related infections and conjunctive therapy for Kawasaki syndrome.
See: Gamimune N (Bayer Corp. (Consumer Div.)).
Gammagard S/D (Baxter Pharmaceutical Products, Inc.).
Gammar-P IV (Centeon).
Iveegam (Immuno Therapy Co.).
Polygam S/D (American Red Cross).
Sandoglobulin (Novartis Pharmaceutical Corp.).

Venoglobulin-I (Alpha Therapeutic Corp.).
Venoglobulin-S (Alpha Therapeutic Corp.).

immune globulin, cytomegalovirus.
See: CytoGam, Vial (MedImmune, Inc.).

immune globulin, hepatitis B.
See: BayHep B, Vial, Syr. (Bayer Corp. (Consumer Div.)).
H-BIG, Vial, Syr. (North American Biologicals, Inc.).

immune globulin IM.
Use: Immunization.

•**immune globulin intravenous pentetate.** (ih-MYOON GLAH-byoo-lin in-trah-VEE-nuhs PEN-teh-tate) USAN.
Use: Diagnostic aid.

immune globulin IV.
Use: Immunization. [Orphan Drug]
See: Gamimune N, Inj. (Bayer Corp. (Consumer Div.)).
Gammagard, Pow. (Baxter Pharmaceutical Products, Inc.).
Gammar-P IV, Pow. (Centeon).
Iveegam, Pow. (Immuno Therapy Co.).
Polygam S/D (American Red Cross).
Sandoglobulin, Pow. (American Red Cross, Novartis).
Venoglobulin-I, Pow. (Alpha Therapeutic Corp.).
Venoglobulin-S (Alpha Therapeutic Corp.).

immune globulin, rabies.
Use: Immunization.
See: Bayrab (Bayer Corp. (Consumer Div.)).
Imogam Rabies (Pasteur Merieux Connaught).

immune globulin, Rh_o(D).
See: Gamulin Rh (Centeon).
BayRho D (Bayer Corp. (Consumer Div.)).
MICRhoGAM (Ortho Diagnostic Systems, Inc.).
Mini-Gamulin Rh (Centeon).
RhoGAM (Ortho Diagnostic Systems, Inc).
WinRho SD (Univax Biologics).

immune globulin, tetanus.
Use: Immunization.
See: Bay Tet (Bayer Corp. (Consumer Div.)).

immune globulin, vaccinia.
Use: Immunization.

immune globulin, varicella-zoster.
Use: Immunization.

immune serums.
See: Cytomegalovirus Immune Globulin Intravenous (Human) (Mass. Public Health Bio. Lab.).
Hepatitis b immune globulin.
Immune globulin IM.
Immune globulin IV.
Immune Serum Globulin (Human).
Rabies immune globulin.
Rho (D) immune globulin.
Tetanus immune globulin.
Vaccinia immune globulin.
Varicella-zoster immune globulin.

immune serum (animal).
See: Botulism Antitoxin, Vial (Pasteur Merieux Connaught).
Diphtheria Antitoxin.

Immunex C-RP. (Wampole Laboratories) Two-minute latex agglutination slide test for the qualitative detection of C-Reactive protein in serum. Kit 100s.
Use: Diagnostic aid.

Immuno. Immune globulin IV (human).
Use: Immunosuppressant. [Orphan Drug]

Immuno-C. (Biomune Systems, Inc.) Bovine Whey Protein Concentrate.
Use: Cryptosporidiosis treatment. [Orphan Drug]

immunosuppressive drugs.
See: Atgam (Pharmacia & Upjohn).
Imuran (GlaxoWellcome).
Neoral (Novartis Pharmaceutical Corp.).
Orthoclone OKT3, Inj. (Ortho McNeil Pharmaceutical).
Prograf (Fujisawa USA, Inc.).
Sandimmune, Cap, Oral Soln. or IV Soln. (Novartis Pharmaceutical Corp.).
Zenapax (Roche Laboratories).

Immunorex. (Antigen Laboratories) Allergenic extracts, various. Vial. *Rx.*
Use: Allergen desensitization.

Immuraid. (Immunomedics) Technetium Tc-99M murine monoclonal antibody to hCG and human AFP.
Use: Diagnostic aid. [Orphan Drug]

Immurait. (Immunomedics) Iodine I^{131} murine monoclonal antibody IgG2a to B cell.
Use: Antineoplastic.

Imodium A-D Liquid. (Ortho McNeil Pharmaceutical) Loperamide 1 mg/5 ml, alcohol 5.25%. Bot. 60 ml, 90 ml, 120 ml. *otc.*
Use: Antidiarrheal.

Imodium Capsules. (Janssen Pharmaceutical, Inc.) Loperamide 2 mg/Cap. Bot. 100s, 500s, UD 100s. *Rx.*
Use: Antidiarrheal.

Imogam Rabies Immune Globulin. (Pasteur Merieux Connaught) Rabies immune globulin (human) 150 IU/ml. Vials 2 ml, 10 ml. *Rx.*

Use: Immunization, rabies.

Imovax Rabies I.D. (Pasteur Merieux Connaught) Rabies vaccine 0.25 IU/0.1 ml for intradermal administration for pre-exposure treatment only. Wistar rabies virus strain PM-1503-3M grown in human diploid cell culture. Pow. for Inj. in single-dose syringe w/1 vial diluent. *Rx.*
Use: Immunization, rabies.

Imovax Rabies Vaccine. (Pasteur Merieux Connaught) Merieux rabies vaccine, Wistar rabies virus strain PM-1503-3M grown in human diploid cell cultures. Rabies Vaccine G 2.5 IU/ml. Pow. for Inj. In single-dose vial with disposable needle and syringe containing diluent and disposable needle for administration. *Rx.*
Use: Immunization, rabies.

Impact. (Health for Life Brands, Inc.) Belladonna alkaloids 0.16 mg, phenylpropanolamine HCl 50 mg, chlorpheniramine maleate 1 mg, pheniramine maleate 12.5 mg/Cap. Pack 12s, 24s. Vial 15s, 30s, Bot. 1000s. *Rx.*
Use: Anticholinergic, antihistamine, antispasmodic, decongestant.

imported fire ant venom, allergenic extract. (ALK Laboratories, Inc.)
Use: Allergy testing. [Orphan Drug]

Impromen. (Janssen Pharmaceutical, Inc.) Bromperidol decanoate. *Rx.*
Use: Antipsychotic.

Impromen Decanoate. (Janssen Pharmaceutical, Inc.) Bromperidol decanoate. *Rx.*
Use: Antipsychotic.

•**impromidine hydrochloride.** (im-PRAH-mid-deen) USAN.
Use: Diagnostic aid (gastric secretion indicator).

Improved Congestant Tablets. (Rugby Labs, Inc.) Chlorpheniramine maleate 2 mg, acetaminophen 325 mg/Tab. Bot. 100s, 1000s. *otc.*
Use: Antihistamine, analgesic.

Imreg-1. (Imreg) *Rx.*
Use: Immunomodulator.

Imreg-2. (Imreg) *Rx.*
Use: Immunomodulator.

Imuran. (GlaxoWellcome) Azathioprine. **Tab.:** 50 mg/Tab. Bot. 100s, UD 100s. **Inj.:** 100 mg/20 ml. Vial. *Rx.*
Use: Immunosuppressant.

Imuthiol. (Pasteur Merieux Connaught) Diethyldithiocarbamate. *Rx.*
Use: Immunomodulator.

Imuvert. (Cell Technology) *Serratia marcescens* extract (polyribosomes).
Use: Primary brain malignancies. [Orphan Drug]

Inapsine. (Janssen Pharmaceutical, Inc.) Droperidol 2.5 mg/ml. Amp. 2 ml, 5 ml, 10 ml. Box 10s. Multi-dose Vial w/ methylparaben 1.8 mg, propylparaben 0.2 mg, lactic acid/10 ml. Box 10s. *Rx.*
Use: Anesthetic, general.
W/Fentanyl citrate.
See: Innovar, Inj. (Janssen Pharmaceutical, Inc.).

•**indacrinone.** (IN-dah-KRIH-nohn) USAN.
Use: Antihypertensive, diuretic.

indalone.
See: Butopyronoxyl (Various Mfr.).

indandione derivative.
Use: Anticoagulant.
See: Anisindione (Various Mfr.).

•**indapamide.** (IN-DAP-uh-mide) U.S.P. 23.
Use: Antihypertensive, diuretic.
See: Lozol, Tab. (Rhone-Poulenc Rorer Pharmaceuticals, Inc.).

indapamide. (IN-DAP-uh-mide) (Various Mfr.) Indapamide 2.5 mg, lactose/Tab. Bot. 100s, 1000s. *Rx.*
Use: Antihypertensive, diuretic.

•**indecainide hydrochloride.** (in-deh-CANE-ide) USAN.
Use: Cardiovascular agent.
See: Decabid (Eli Lilly and Co.).

•**indeloxazine hydrochloride.** (in-DELL-OX-ah-zeen) USAN.
Use: Antidepressant.

Inderal Injection. (Wyeth-Ayerst Laboratories) Propranolol HCl 1 mg/ml. Amp. 1 ml. Box 10s. *Rx.*
Use: Beta-adrenergic blocker.

Inderal LA. (Wyeth-Ayerst Laboratories) Propranolol HCl 60 mg, 80 mg, 120 mg, 160 mg/SR Cap. Bot. 100s, 1000s, UD 100s. *Rx.*
Use: Beta-adrenergic blocker.

Inderal Tablets. (Wyeth-Ayerst Laboratories) Propranolol HCl 10 mg, 20 mg, 40 mg, 60 mg, 80 mg/Tab. Bot. 100s, 1000s, UD 100s. *Rx.*
Use: Beta-adrenergic blocker.

Inderide. (Wyeth-Ayerst Laboratories) Propranolol HCl 40 mg, hydrochlorothiazide 25 mg/Tab. Bot. 100s, 1000s, UD 100s. Propranolol HCl 80 mg, hydrochlorothiazide 25 mg/Tab. Bot. 100s. *Rx.*
Use: Antihypertensive combination.

Inderide LA Capsules. (Wyeth-Ayerst Laboratories) Propranolol HCl/hydrochlorothiazide LA Caps: 80 mg/50 mg, 120 mg/50 mg, 160 mg/50 mg. Bot. 100s. *Rx.*

Use: Antihypertensive combination.

indian gum.
See: Karaya Gum.

indigo carmine. (Becton Dickinson & Co.) Sodium indigotindisulfonate 8 mg/ml. Amp. 5 ml. Box 10s, 100s.
Use: Diagnostic aid.
See: Sodium indigotindisulfonate.

indigo carmine solution. (Becton Dickinson & Co.) Indigotindisulfonate sodium (0.8% aqueous soln. sodium salt of indigotindisulfonic acid) 40 mg/5 ml. Inj. Amp. 5 ml, 10s.
Use: Diagnostic aid.

•**indigotindisulfonate sodium.** (IN-dih-go-tin-die SULL-foe-nate) U.S.P. 23. Indigo Carmine.
Use: Diagnostic aid (cystoscopy).
See: Sodium Indigotindisulfonate.

•**indinavir.** USAN.
Use: Antiviral (HIV-protease inhibitor).

•**indinavir sulfate.** (in-DIN-ah-veer) USAN.
Use: Antiviral.
See: Crixivan, Cap. (Merck & Co.).

•**indium chlorides In 113m.** (IN-dee-uhm) USAN. U.S.P. XX.
Use: Radiopharmaceutical.

•**indium In 111 chloride solution.** U.S.P. 23.
Use: Radiopharmaceutical.

indium In 111 murine monoclonal antibody fab to myosin.
Use: Diagnostic aid in myocarditis. [Orphan Drug]
See: Myoscint (Centocor, Inc.).

•**indium In 111 oxyquinoline solution.** (IN-dee-uhm OX-ee-KWIN-oh-lin) U.S.P. 23.
Use: Radiopharmaceutical, diagnostic aid.

•**indium In 111 pentetate injection.** (IN-dee-uhm In 111 PEN-teh-tate) U.S.P. 23.
Use: Diagnostic aid (radionuclide cisternography), radiopharmaceutical.

•**indium In 111 pentetreotide.** (IN-dee-uhm In 111 pen-teh-TREE-oh-tide) U.S.P. 23.
Use: Diagnostic aid, radiopharmaceutical.

•**indium In 111 satumomab pendetide.** (IN-dee-uhm sat-YOU-mah-mab PEN-deh-TIDE) USAN.
Use: Radiodiagnostic monoclonal antibody (ovarian and colorectal carcinoma), radiopharmaceutical.

Indochron E-R. (Inwood Laboratories, Inc.) Indomethacin 75 mg. SR Cap. Bot. 60s, 100s. *Rx.*
Use: Analgesic, NSAID.

Indocin. (Merck & Co.) Indomethacin. **Cap.:** 25 mg. Bot. 100s, 1000s, UD 100s. Unit-of-use 100s; 50 mg. Bot. 100s, UD 100s. **Supp.:** 50 mg. Pkg. 30s. **Oral Susp.:** 25 mg/5 ml, alcohol 1%, sorbitol 0.1%. Bot. 237 ml. *Rx.*
Use: Analgesic, NSAID.

Indocin I.V. (Merck & Co.) Indomethacin sodium trihydrate equivalent to 1 mg indomethacin/Vial. Vial single-dose. *Rx.*
Use: Arterial patency agent.

Indocin SR. (Merck & Co.) Indomethacin 75 mg/SR Cap. Unit-of-use 30s, 60s.
Use: Analgesic, NSAID.

•**indocyanine green.** (in-doe-SIGH-ah-neen green) U.S.P. 23.
Use: Diagnostic aid (cardiac output determination, hepatic function determination).
See: Cardio-Green, Inj. (Becton Dickinson and Co.).

Indogesic. (Century Pharmaceuticals, Inc.) Acetaminophen 32.5 mg, butalbital 50 mg/Tab. Bot. 100s, 1000s. *Rx.*
Use: Analgesic, hypnotic, sedative.

Indoklon. Hexafluorodiethyl ether. Flurothyl. Bis-(2,2,2-trifluorethyl) ether. *Rx.*
Use: Shock-inducing agent (convulsant).

•**indolapril hydrochloride.** (in-DAHL-ah-PRILL) USAN.
Use: Antihypertensive.

Indo-Lemmon. (Teva Pharmaceuticals USA) Indomethacin 25 mg, 50 mg/Cap. Bot. 100s, 500s, 1000s. *Rx.*
Use: Analgesic, NSAID.

•**indolidan.** (in-DOE-lih-DAN) USAN.
Use: Cardiovascular agent.

Indometh. (Major Pharmaceuticals) Indomethacin 25 mg or 50 mg. Cap. **25 mg:** Bot. 100s, 1000s. **50 mg:** Bot. 100s, 500s. *Rx.*
Use: Analgesic, NSAID.

•**indomethacin.** (in-doe-METH-ah-sin) U.S.P. 23.
Use: Anti-inflammatory, analgesic.
See: Indochron E-R, Cap. (Inwood Laboratories, Inc.).
Indocin, Cap., SR Cap., IV, Oral Susp., Supp. (Merck & Co.).
Indo-Lemmon, Cap. (Teva Pharmaceuticals USA).

indomethacin. (Various Mfr.) **Cap.: 25 mg:** 60s, 100s, 500s, 1000s, UD 100s. **50 mg:** 23s, 72s, 100s, 250s, 500s, UD 100s. **SR Cap.:** 75 mg. Bot. 60s, 100s. *Rx.*
Use: Anti-inflammatory.

indomethacin. (Roxane Laboratories,

Inc.) Indomethacin 25 mg/5 ml. Oral susp. Bot. 500 ml. *Rx.*
Use: Analgesic, NSAID.

•**indomethacin sodium.** (in-doe-METH-ah-sin) U.S.P. 23.
Use: Anti-inflammatory, analgesic.

indomethacin sodium trihydrate. *Rx.*
Use: Arterial patency agent.
See: Indocin IV, Pow. (Merck & Co.).

•**indoprofen.** (in-doe-PRO-fen) USAN.
Use: Analgesic, anti-inflammatory.

•**indoramin.** (in-DAHR-ah-min) USAN.
Use: Antihypertensive.

•**indoramin hydrochloride.** (in-DAHR-ah-min) USAN.
Use: Antihypertensive.

•**indorenate hydrochloride.** (in-DAHR-en-ATE) USAN.
Use: Antihypertensive.

•**indoxole.** (IN-dox-OLE) USAN.
Use: Antipyretic, anti-inflammatory.

•**indriline hydrochloride.** (IN-drih-leen) USAN.
Use: Stimulant, central.

I-Neocort. (American Pharmaceutical Co.) Neomycin sulfate 5 mg, hydrocortisone acetate 15 mg/5 ml. Ophth. Susp. Bot. 5 ml. *Rx.*
Use: Anti-infective, corticosteroid.

I-Neospor. (American Pharmaceutical Co.) Polymyxin B sulfate, gramicidin, neomycin sulfate. Ophth. Soln. Bot. 10 ml. *Rx.*
Use: Anti-infective, ophthalmic.

Infalyte Oral Solution. (Bristol-Myers Squibb) Electrolyte mixture with 30 g/L rice syrup solids containing 4.2 calories/fl. oz. In 1 liter. *otc.*
Use: Nutritional supplement.

Infanrix. (SmithKline Beecham Pharmaceuticals) Diphtheria toxoid 25 Lf units, tetanus toxoid 10 Lf units, acellular pertussis vaccine (pertussis toxin 25 mcg, filamentous hemagglutinin 25 mcg, pertactin 8 mcg)/0.5 ml. Vial 0.5 ml. *Rx.*
Use: Immunization.

infant foods.
Use: Nutritional supplement.
See: Enfamil (Bristol-Myers Squibb).
Enfamil Human Milk Fortifier (Bristol-Myers Squibb).
Enfamil Premature 20 Formula (Bristol-Myers Squibb).
RCF, Liq. (Ross Laboratories).
Similac (Ross Laboratories).
Similac PM 60/40, Liq. (Ross Laboratories).

infant foods, hypoallergenic.
Use: Nutritional supplement.
See: Isomil (Ross Laboratories).
Isomil SF (Ross Laboratories).
I-Soyalac (Mt. Vernon Foods, Inc.).
Nutramigen (Bristol-Myers Squibb).
Pregestimil, Pow. (Bristol-Myers Squibb).
ProSobee (Bristol-Myers Squibb).
Soyalac (Mt Vernon Foods, Inc.).

Infant's Feverall. (Upsher-Smith Labs, Inc.) Acetaminophen 80 mg/Supp. 6s. *otc.*
Use: Analgesic.

Infants' No-Aspirin Drops. (Walgreen Co.) Acetaminophen 80 mg/0.8 ml. Non-alcoholic. Bot. 15 ml. *otc.*
Use: Analgesic.

Infants' Silapap. (Silarx Pharmaceuticals, Inc.) Acetaminophen 80 mg/0.8 ml. Drops. Bot. 15 ml. Alcohol free. *otc.*
Use: Analgesic, antipyretic.

Infarub Cream. (Whitehall Robins Laboratories) Methyl salicylate 35%, menthol 10% in vanishing cream base. Tube 1.25 oz, 3.5 oz. *otc.*
Use: Analgesic, topical.

Infasurf. (Forest Pharmaceuticals) Phospholipids 35 mg/ml suspended in 0.9% sodium chloride solution, 0.65 mg proteins. Intratracheal Susp. Single-use vial 6 ml. *Rx.*
Use: Lung surfactant.

Infatuss. (Scott/Cord) Dextromethorphan HBr 7.2 mg, chlorpheniramine maleate 1.1 mg, phenylpropanolamine HCl 4.8 mg, ammonium Cl 50 mg/5 ml. Bot. 4 oz, pt, gal. *otc.*
Use: Antihistamine, antitussive, decongestant, expectorant.

Infectrol Ointment. (Bausch & Lomb Pharmaceuticals) Dexamethasone 0.1%, neomycin sulfate equivalent to 0.35% neomycin base, 10,000 units polymyxin B sulfate/g. White petrolatum, lanolin, mineral oil, parabens. Oint. Tube 3.5, 3.75 g. *Rx.*
Use: Anti-infective, corticosteroid, topical.

Infectrol Suspension. (Bausch & Lomb Pharmaceuticals) Dexamethasone 0.1%, neomycin sulfate equivalent to 0.35% neomycin base, 10,000 units polymyxin B sulfate/ml. Hydroxypropyl methylcellulose, polysorbate 20, benzalkonium chloride. Drop. Bot. 5 ml. *Rx.*
Use: Anti-infective, corticosteroid, ophthalmic.

InFeD. (Schein Pharmaceutical, Inc.) Iron 50/ml (as dextran), sodium chloride 0.9%. Inj. Vial 2 ml. *Rx.*
Use: Mineral supplement.

Infergen. (Amgen, Inc.) Interferon alfa-

con-1 9 mcg, 15 mcg, preservative free. Single-dose Vial 0.3 ml. Pack 6s. *Rx.*
Use: Antiviral.

Inflamase Forte. (Ciba Vision) Prednisolone sodium phosphate 1%. Bot. 5 ml, 10 ml, 15 ml. *Rx.*
Use: Corticosteroid, ophthalmic.

Inflamase Mild. (Ciba Vision) Prednisolone sodium phosphate 0.125%. Bot. 3 ml, 5 ml, 10 ml. *Rx.*
Use: Corticosteroid, ophthalmic.

infliximab.
Use: Crohn's disease.
See: Remicade (Centocor).

•**influenza virus vaccine.** (in-flew-EN-zuh) U.S.P. 23.
Use: Immunization.
See: FluShield, Inj. (Wyeth-Ayerst Laboratories).
Fluvirin, Inj. (Evans Medical).
Fluzone, Inj. (Pasteur Merieux Connaught).

InfraRUB. (Whitehall Robins Laboratories) Methyl salicylate 35%, menthol 10%. Cream. Jar 37.5, 90 g. *otc.*
Use: Analgesic, topical.

Infumorph 200 and 500. (ESI Lederle Generics) Morphine sulfate 10 mg, 25 mg /ml. Inj. Amp. 20 ml. Preservative free. *c-II.*
Use: Analgesic, narcotic.

Ingadine Tabs. (Major Pharmaceuticals) Guanethidine sulfate 10 mg, 25 mg/Tab. Bot. 100s, 1000s. *Rx.*
Use: Antihypertensive.

INH. (Novartis Pharmaceutical Corp.) Isoniazid 300 mg/Tab. *Rx.*
Use: Antituberculosal.

Inhal-Aid. (Key Pharmaceuticals)
Use: Respiratory drug delivery system.

Inhibace. (Roche Laboratories; Glaxo-Wellcome) Cilazapril. *Rx.*
Use: Antihypertensive.

Innerclean Herbal Laxative. (Last) Senna leaf powder, psyllium seed, buckthorne, anise seed, fennel seed. Bot. 1 oz, 2 oz. *otc.*
Use: Laxative.

Innertabs. (Last) Senna leaf powder and psyllium seed tablets. Bot. 80s, 200s. *otc.*
Use: Laxative.

InnoGel Plus. (Hogil Pharmaceutical Corp.) Pyrethrins 0.3%, piperonyl butoxide technical 3%. Gel. Kits contain 3 pre-dosed gel paks, 1 comb. *otc.*
Use: Pediculicide.

Innovar Injection. (Janssen Pharmaceutical, Inc.) Fentanyl citrate 0.05 mg, droperidol 2.5 mg/ml. Amp. 2 ml, 5 ml. Box of 10s. *c-II.*
Use: Analgesic, narcotic; anesthetic, general.

Inocor Lactate. (Sanofi Winthrop Pharmaceuticals) Amrinone lactate (base equivalent) 5 mg/ml, sodium metabisulfite 0.25 mg/Inj. Amp. 20 ml. Box 5s. *Rx.*
Use: Inotropic.

•**inocoterone acetate.** (ih-NO-koe-ter-ohn) USAN.
Use: Dermatologic, acne.

in-111 murine mab. (2B8-MX-DTPA).
Use: B-cell non-Hodgkin's lymphoma. [Orphan Drug]

inophylline.
See: Aminophylline (Various Mfr.).

inosine pranobex. Isoprinosine.
Use: Antiviral. [Orphan Drug]
See: Isoprinosine (Newport).

Inosiplex. (Newport Pharmaceuticals) Isoprinosine. *Rx.*
Use: Antiviral.

inosit.
See: Inositol (Various Mfr.).

inositol.
Use: Lipotropic.

•**inositol niacinate.** (in-OH-sih-tole NIE-ah-sin-ate) USAN.
Use: Vasodilator.

inositol nicotinate.
See: Inositol Niacinate.

Inotropin. (Faulding USA) Dopamine 40 mg/ml, sodium metabisulfite 1%. Inj. 5 ml. *Rx.*
Use: Vasoconstrictor.

Inspirease. (Key Pharmaceuticals) *Rx.*
Use: Respiratory drug delivery system.

Insta-Char. (Kerr Drug) **Regular:** Aqueous suspension activated charcoal 50 g/8 oz. **Pediatric:** Aqueous suspension activated charcoal 15 g/4 oz. *otc.*
Use: Antidote.

Insta-Glucose. (ICN Pharmaceuticals, Inc.) Undiluted USP glucose. UD tube containing liquid glucose 31 g. *otc.*
Use: Hyperglycemic.

Inst-E-Vite. (Barth's) Vitamin E 100 IU, 200 IU/Cap. **100 IU:** Bot 100s, 500s, 1000s. **200 IU:** Bot. 100s, 250s, 500s. *otc.*
Use: Vitamin supplement.

Insulatard NPH Human. (Novo/Nordisk Pharm, Inc.) Human insulin isophane suspension 100 IU/ml. *otc.*
Use: Antidiabetic.

•**insulin.** (IN-suh-lin) U.S.P. 23.
Use: Antidiabetic.
See: Humulin, Prods. (Eli Lilly and Co.).
Iletin, Prods. (Eli Lilly and Co.).
Insulin, Prods. (Bristol-Myers Squibb).

Novolin, Prods. (Novo/Nordisk Pharm, Inc.).
Velosulin Human BR, Inj. (Novo/Nordisk Pharm, Inc.).

insulin. (IN-suh-lin) (Novo/Nordisk Pharm, Inc.) Insulatard NPH Mixtard Velosulin. *otc.*
Use: Antidiabetic.

•**insulin, dalanated.** USAN.
Use: Antidiabetic.

•**insulin human.** (IN-suh-lin) U.S.P. 23.
Use: Antidiabetic.
See: Humulin (Eli Lilly and Co.).

•**insulin human, isophane, suspension.** U.S.P. 23.
Use: Antidiabetic.

•**insulin human zinc suspension.** (IN-suh-lin) U.S.P. 23.
Use: Antidiabetic.

•**insulin human zinc, extended, suspension.** (IN-suh-lin) U.S.P. 23.
Use: Antidiabetic.

•**insulin, isophane, suspension.** U.S.P. 23.
Use: Antidiabetic.
See: NPH (Novo/Nordisk Pharm, Inc.).

•**insulin I-125.** (IN-suh-lin) USAN.
Use: Radiopharmaceutical.

•**insulin I-131.** (IN-suh-lin) USAN.
Use: Radiopharmaceutical.

insulin-like growth factor-1.
Use: Amyotrophic lateral sclerosis. [Orphan Drug]

•**insulin lispro.** (IN-suh-lin LICE-pro) USAN.
Use: Antidiabetic.
See: Humalog, Tab. (Bayer Corp. (Consumer Div.)).

•**insulin, neutral.** (IN-suh-lin) USAN.
Use: Antidiabetic.

insulin Novo rapitard. Biphasic Insulin.

insulin, protamine zinc suspension. (IN-suh-lin PRO-tah-meen zingk) U.S.P. XXII. 40 units, 100 units/ml. Vials 10 ml.
Use: Antidiabetic.

insulin, regular.
Use: Antidiabetic.
See: Regular Iletin I (Beef and Pork), Inj. (Eli Lilly and Co.).
Regular Insulin (Pork), Inj. (Novo/Nordisk Pharm, Inc.).
Pork Regular Iletin II (Pork), Inj. (Eli Lilly and Co.).
Regular Purified Pork Insulin, Inj. (Novo/Nordisk Pharm, Inc.).
Velosulin (Pork), Inj. (Novo/Nordisk Pharm, Inc.).
Humulin R, Inj. (Eli Lilly and Co.).
Humulin BR, Inj. (Eli Lilly and Co.).
Novolin R, Inj. (Novo/Nordisk Pharm, Inc.).
Velosulin, Inj. (Novo/Nordisk Pharm, Inc.).
Novolin R PenFill, Cartridges (Novo/Nordisk Pharm, Inc.).

insulin, regular concentrate.
Use: Antidiabetic.

insulin suspension, isophane.
Use: Antidiabetic.
See: Humulin 50/50, Inj. (Eli Lilly and Co.).
Humulin 70/30, Inj. (Eli Lilly and Co.).
Novolin 70/30, Inj. (Novo/Nordisk Pharm, Inc.).
Novolin 70/30 PenFill, Cartridge (Novo/Nordisk Pharm, Inc.).

insulin suspension, lente.
Use: Antidiabetic.
See: Lente Insulin, Vial (Novo/Nordisk Pharm, Inc.).
Lente L, Vial (Novo/Nordisk Pharm, Inc.).
Novolin L, Vial (Novo/Nordisk Pharm, Inc.).
Lente Iletin I (Beef and Pork), Inj. (Eli Lilly and Co.).
Lente Insulin (Beef), Inj. (Novo/Nordisk Pharm, Inc.).
Lente Iletin II (Pork), Inj. (Eli Lilly and Co.).
Lente Iletin II (Beef), Inj. (Eli Lilly and Co.).
Lente Purified Pork Insulin, Inj. (Novo/Nordisk Pharm, Inc.).
Humulin L, Inj. (Eli Lilly and Co.).
Novolin L, Inj. (Novo/Nordisk Pharm, Inc.).

insulin suspension, NPH.
Use: Antidiabetic.
See: NPH Iletin I (Beef and Pork), Inj. (Eli Lilly and Co.).
NPH Insulin (Beef), Inj. (Novo/Nordisk Pharm, Inc.).
Beef NPH Iletin II, Inj. (Eli Lilly and Co.).
NPH-N Purified (Pork), Inj. (Novo/Nordisk Pharm, Inc.).
Pork NPH Iletin II, Inj. (Eli Lilly and Co.)
Insulatard NPH (Pork), Inj. (Novo/Nordisk Pharm, Inc.).
Humulin N, Inj. (Eli Lilly and Co.).
Insulatard NPH, Inj. (Novo/Nordisk Pharm, Inc.).
Novolin N, Inj. (Novo/Nordisk Pharm, Inc.).
Novolin N PenFill, Cartridge (Novo/Nordisk Pharm, Inc.).

insulin suspension, PZI. *otc.*
Use: Antidiabetic.

See: Humulin U Ultralente, Inj. (Eli Lilly and Co.).

insulin suspension semilente. *otc.*
Use: Antidiabetic.

insulin suspension, ultralente. *otc.*
Use: Antidiabetic.
See: Ultralente Insulin (Beef), Inj. (Novo/Nordisk Pharm, Inc.).
Humulin U Ultralente, Inj. (Eli Lilly and Co.).

•**insulin zinc suspension.** (IN-suh-lin) U.S.P. 23.
Use: Antidiabetic.
See: Humulin L, Bot. (Eli Lilly and Co.).
Lente Insulin, Vial (Eli Lilly and Co.).
Lente Insulin, Vial (Novo/Nordisk Pharm, Inc.).
Lente L, Vial (Novo/Nordisk Pharm, Inc.).
Novolin L, Vial (Novo/Nordisk Pharm, Inc.).

•**insulin zinc, suspension, extended.** (IN-suh-lin) U.S.P. 23.
Use: Antidiabetic.
See: Humulin U Ultralente, Bot. (Eli Lilly and Co.).
Ultralente U, Vial (Novo/Nordisk Pharm, Inc.).

•**insulin zinc, prompt, suspension.** (IN-suh-lin) U.S.P. 23.
Use: Antidiabetic.

Intal Inhaler. (Rhone-Poulenc Rorer) Cromolyn sodium inhalation aerosol 800 mcg/actuation. Canister 8.1 g, 14.2 g. *Rx.*
Use: Respiratory inhalant.

Intal Nebulizer Solution. (Rhone-Poulenc Rorer) Cromolyn sodium 20 mg. Amp. 2 ml. *Rx.*
Use: Respiratory inhalant.

Integrilin. (COR Therapeutics, Inc.) Eptifibatide 0.75 mg/ml, 2 mg/ml, sodium hydroxide. Vial 10 ml (2 mg/ml only), 100 ml (0.75 mg/ml only). *Rx.*
Use: Antiplatelet.

Integrin Caps. (Sanofi Winthrop Pharmaceuticals) Oxypertine. *Rx.*
Use: Anxiolytic.

Intensol. (Roxane Laboratories, Inc.) A system of concentrated solutions of drugs w/calibrated dropper: Chlorpromazine HCl 30 mg or 100 mg/ml; dexamethasone 1 mg/ml; dihydrotachysterol 0.2 mg/ml; hydrochlorothiazide 100 mg/ml; prednisone 5 mg/ml; thioridazine HCl 30 mg or 100 mg/ml.

interferon. (IN-ter-FEER-ahn) A family of naturally occurring, small protein molecules with molecular weights of approximately 15,000 to 21,000 daltons. They are formed by the interaction of animal cells with viruses capable of conferring on animal cells resistance to virus infection. Three major classes of interferons have been identified: alpha, beta, and gamma. Interferon was first derived from human white blood cells and originally used in Finland.
Use: Antineoplastic, antiviral; treatment of breast cancer lymphoma, multiple melanoma and malignant melanoma.
See: Actimmune (Genentech, Inc.).
Avonex (Biogen).
Betaseron (Berlex Laboratories, Inc.).
Intron A for Injection, Inj. (Schering-Plough Corp.).
Roferon-A (Roche Laboratories).

interferon alfacon-1.
See: Infergen (Amgen, Inc.).

•**interferon alfa-2a.** (IN-ter-FEER-ahn AL-fuh-2a) USAN.
Use: Antineoplastic, antiviral; biological response modifier. [Orphan Drug]
See: Roferon-A (Roche Laboratories).

•**interferon alfa-2b.** (IN-ter-FEER-ahn AL-fuh-2b) USAN.
Use: Antineoplastic, antiviral; biological response modifier. [Orphan Drug]
See: Intron A, Inj. (Schering-Plough Corp.).

interferon alfa-2b, recombinant and ribavirin.
Use: Antineoplastic.
See: Rebetron (Shering Corporation).

•**interferon alfa-n1.** (IN-ter-FEER-ahn AL-fuh-nl) USAN.
Use: Antineoplastic, antiviral, biological response modifier. [Orphan Drug]
See: Wellferon (GlaxoWellcome).

interferon, beta. (IN-ter-FEER-ahn BAY-tuh)
Use: Immunomodulator, treatment of multiple sclerosis.
See: Avonex (Biogen).
Betaseron (Berlex Laboratories, Inc.).

•**interferon beta-1a.** (in-ter-FEER-ohn BAY-tah-1a) USAN.
Use: Antineoplastic, biological response modifier, immunomodulator, antineoblast. [Orphan Drug]
See: Avonex (Berlex Laboratories, Inc.).

•**interferon beta-1b.** (IN-ter-FEER-ahn BAY-tah-1b) USAN.
Use: Immunomodulator.
See: Betaseron (Berlex Laboratories, Inc.).

interferon beta (recombinant).
Use: Immune therapy.
See: Antril [Orphan Drug] (Amgen, Inc.).
Avonex (Biogen).

r-IFN-beta (Serono Laboratories, Inc.).

•**interferon gamma-1b.** (IN-ter-FEER-ahn GAM-uh-1b) USAN.
Use: Antineoplastic, antiviral, immunoregulator, biological response modifier. [Orphan Drug]
See: Actimmune (Genentech, Inc.).

interleukin-1 receptor antagonist, human recombinant.
Use: Juvenile rheumatoid arthritis, graft-vs-host disease in transplant patients. [Orphan Drug]
See: Antril (Amgen, Inc.).

interleukin-2.
Use: Immunomodulator, antineoplastic. [Orphan Drug]
See: Proleukin (Chiron).
Teceleukin (Roche Laboratories).

interleukin-2, recombinant liposome encapsulated.
Use: Antineoplastic. [Orphan Drug]

interleukin-2 PEG. (Cetus) *Rx.*
Use: Immunomodulator.

interleukin-3, recombinant human. (Novartis Pharmaceutical Corp.) *Rx.*
Use: Immunomodulator. [Orphan Drug]

Intralipid 10% I.V. Fat Emulsion. (Pharmacia & Upjohn) IV fat emulsion containing soybean oil 10%, egg yolk phospholipids 1.2%, glycerin 2.25%, water for injection. I.V. Flask 50 ml, 100 ml, 250 ml, 500 ml. *Rx.*
Use: Nutritional supplement, parenteral.

Intralipid 20% I.V. Fat Emulsion. (Pharmacia & Upjohn) IV fat emulsion containing soybean oil 20%, egg yolk phospholipids 1.2%, glycerin 2.25%, water for injection. I.V. Flask 50 ml, 100 ml, 250 ml, 500 ml. *Rx.*
Use: Nutritional supplement, parenteral.

intranasal steroids.
See: Beconase AQ Nasal (Glaxo-Wellcome).
Beconase Inhalation (Glaxo-Wellcome).
Decadron Phosphate Turbinaire (Merck & Co.).
Flonase (GlaxoWellcome).
Nasalide (Roche Laboratories).
Nasacort (Rhone-Poulenc Rorer Pharmaceuticals, Inc.).
Vancenase Nasal Inhaler (Schering-Plough Corp.).
Rhinocort (Astra Pharmaceuticals, LP).
Vancenase AQ Nasal (Schering-Plough Corp.).

IntraSite. (Smith & Nephew United) Graft T starch copolymer 2%, water 8%, propylene glycol 20%. Sterile amorphous interactive hydrogel dressing. 25 g. *Rx.*
Use: Dermatologic, wound therapy.

intrauterine progesterone system. *Rx.*
Use: Contraceptive.
See: Progestasert (Alza Corp.).

intraval sodium.
See: Pentothal Sodium, Preps. (Abbott Laboratories).

•**intrazole.** (IN-trah-zole) USAN.
Use: Anti-inflammatory.

•**intriptyline hydrochloride.** (in-TRIP-tih-leen) USAN.
Use: Antidepressant.

Introlite. (Ross Laboratories) Protein 22.2 g, carbohydrate 70.5 g, fat 18.4 g, Na 930 mg, K 1570 mg/L with 200 mOsm/kg water, with appropriate vitamins and minerals, 0.53 Cal/ml. Liq. *otc.*
Use: Nutritional supplement.

Intron A for Injection. (Schering-Plough Corp.) Interferon alfa-2b (recombinant). **Pow. for Inj.:** 3 million IU/1 ml vial diluent; 5 million IU/1 ml vial diluent or syringe; 10 million IU/2 ml vial diluent, 10 million IU/1 ml syringe diluent; 18 million IU/3.8 ml vial diluent/multidose vial; 25 million IU/5 ml vial diluent/multidose vial; 50 million IU/1 ml vial diluent/multidose vial. **Soln:** 3 million IU/0.5 ml vial, pak-3 (6 vials, 6 syringes); 5 million IU/0.5 ml vial, pak-5 (6 vials, 6 syringes); 10 million IU/1 ml vial, pak-10 (6 vials, 6 syringes); 18 million IU/multidose vial (22.8 million IU/3.8 ml); 25 million IU/multidose vial (32 million IU/3.2 ml). *Rx.*
Use: Antineoplastic.

Intropaque Liquid. (Lafayette Pharmaceuticals, Inc.) Barium sulfate 60% w/v suspension. Bot. Gal. Case 4s.
Use: Radiopaque agent.

Intropaste. (Lafayette Pharmaceuticals, Inc.) Barium sulfate 70%. Paste Tube 454 g. *Rx.*
Use: Radiopaque agent.

Intropin 200 mg. (Du Pont Merck Pharmaceutical Co.) Dopamine HCl 40 mg/ml, sodium bisulfite 1% as an antioxidant. Vial 5 ml. Box 20s; Amp. 5 ml. Box 20s; Prefilled additive syringe 5 ml. Box 5s. *Rx.*
Use: Vasoconstrictor.

Intropin 400 mg. (Du Pont Merck Pharmaceutical Co.) Dopamine HCl 80 mg/ml, sodium bisulfite 1% as an antioxidant. Vial 5 ml. Box 20s; prefilled additive syringe 5 ml. Box 5s. *Rx.*
Use: Vasoconstrictor.

Intropin 800 mg. (Du Pont Merck Pharmaceutical Co.) Dopamine HCl 160 mg/ml, sodium bisulfite 1% as an antioxi-

dant. Vial 5 ml. Box 20s; prefilled additive syringe 5 ml. Box 5s. *Rx.*
Use: Vasoconstrictor.

inulin. (Du Pont Merck Pharmaceutical Co.) Purified inulin 5 g/50 ml sodium Cl 0.9%, sodium hydroxide to adjust pH. Amp. 50 ml.
Use: Diagnostic aid.

•**inulin.** (IN-you-lin) U.S.P. 23.
Use: Diagnostic aid (renal function determination).

invert sugar. (Abbott Laboratories) 10%. Soln. Bot. 1000 ml. *Rx-otc.*
Use: Nutritional supplement, parenteral.
See: Travert, Soln. (Baxter Pharmaceutical Products, Inc.).

invert sugar-electrolyte solutions. *Rx.*
Use: Nutritional supplement, parenteral.
See: Ionosol G and 10% Invert Sugar (Abbott Laboratories).
Multiple Electrolyte 2 w/5% Invert Sugar (McGaw, Inc.).
5% Travert and Electrolyte No. 2 (Baxter Pharmaceutical Products, Inc.).
Ionosol B and 10% Invert Sugar (Abbott Laboratories).
10% Travert and Electrolyte No 2 (Baxter Pharmaceutical Products, Inc.).
Multiple Electrolyte 2 w/10% Invert Sugar (McGaw, Inc.).
Ionosol D and 10% Invert Sugar (Abbott Laboratories).

invert sugar injection.
Use: Fluid, nutrient replacement.

Invirase. (Roche Laboratories) Saquinavir mesylate 200 mg, lactose/Cap. Bot. 270s. *Rx.*
Use: Antiviral.

•**iobenguane I 123 injection.** (EYE-oh-BEN-gwane) U.S.P. 23.
Use: Radiopharmaceutical.

•**iobenguane I 131.** (EYE-oh-BEN-gwane) USAN.
Use: Diagnostic aid, radiopharmaceutical.

•**iobenguane sulfate I 123.** (EYE-oh-BEN-gwane) USAN.
Use: Diagnostic aid, radioactive, adrenomedullary disorders and neuroendocrine tumors; radiopharmaceutical.

•**iobenguane sulfate I 131.** (EYE-oh-BEN-gwane) USAN.
Use: Diagnostic aid, radiopharmaceutical.

•**iobenzamic acid.** (EYE-oh-ben-ZAM-ik) USAN.
Use: Diagnostic aid (radiopaque medium, cholecystographic).

Iobid DM. (Iomed) Dextromethorphan HBr 30 mg, guaifenesin 600 mg/SR Tab. Bot. 100s, 500s. *Rx.*
Use: Antitussive, expectorant.

•**iocanlidic acid I 123.** (eye-oh-kan-LIH-dik) USAN.
Use: Diagnostic aid (radioactive, cardiac disease) for assessment of viable myocardium.

Iocare Balanced Salt Solution. (Ciba Vision) Sodium Cl 0.64%, potassium Cl 0.075%, magnesium Cl 0.03%, calcium Cl 0.048%, sodium acetate 0.39%, sodium citrate 0.17%, sodium hydroxide or hydrochloric acid. Soln. Bot. 15 ml. *Rx.*
Use: Irrigant, ophthalmic.

•**iocarmate meglumine.** (EYE-oh-CAR-mate meh-GLUE-meen) USAN.
Use: Diagnostic aid (radiopaque medium).

•**iocarmic acid.** (EYE-oh-CAR-mik) USAN.
Use: Diagnostic aid (radiopaque medium).

•**iocetamic acid.** (eye-oh-seh-TAM-ik) U.S.P. 23.
Use: Diagnostic aid (radiopaque medium).

i-octadecanol.
See: Stearyl Alcohol, N.F.

Iodal HD. (Iomed) Hydrocodone bitartrate 1.67 mg, phenylephrine HCl 5 mg, chlorpheniramine maleate 2 mg/5 ml. Liq. Bot. 473 ml. *c-III.*
Use: Antihistamine, antitussive, decongestant.

•**iodamide.** (EYE-oh-dah-mide) USAN.
Use: Diagnostic aid (radiopaque medium).

•**iodamide meglumine.** (EYE-oh-dah-MIDE meh-GLUE-meen) USAN.
Use: Diagnostic aid (radiopaque medium).
W/Combinations.
See: Renovue-65, Vial (Bristol-Myers Squibb).
Renovue-Dip, Vial (Bristol-Myers Squibb).

Iodex. (KM Lee) Iodine 4.7% in petrolatum ointment base. Jar 1 oz, 14 oz. *otc.*
Use: Antimicrobial, antiseptic.

Iodex w/Methyl Salicylate. (KM Lee) Iodine 4.7%, methyl salicylate 4.8% in petrolatum ointment base. *otc.*
Use: Antiseptic, analgesic, topical.

iodinated I-125 albumin injection.
Use: Diagnostic aid (blood volume de-

termination), radiopharmaceutical.
See: albumin, iodinated I-125.

iodinated I-131 albumin aggregated injection.
Use: Radiopharmaceutical.
See: albumin, aggregated iodinated I-131 serum.

iodinated I-131 albumin injection.
Use: Diagnostic aid (blood volume determination and intrathecal imaging), radiopharmaceutical.
See: albumin, iodinated I-131.

iodinated glycerol and codeine phosphate liquid. (Various Mfr.) Codeine phosphate 10 mg, iodinated glycerol 30 mg/Liq. Bot. Pt, gal. *c-v.*
Use: Antitussive, expectorant, narcotic.

iodinated glycerol/theophylline.
See: Iophylline (Various Mfr.).

iodinated human serum albumin.
See: Albumotope (Bristol-Myers Squibb).

•**iodine.** (EYE-uh-dine) U.S.P. 23.
Use: Anti-infective, topical; source of iodine.
See: Kelp, Tab. (Quality Formulations, Inc.).

iodine cacodylate, colloidal. Cacodyne Iodine.

iodine 131: capsules diagnostic - capsules therapeutic - solution therapeutic oral.
See: Iodotope (Bristol-Myers Squibb).

iodine combination.
See: Calcidrine, Syr. (Abbott Laboratories).

iodine I^{123} murine monoclonal antibody to alpha-fetoprotein. (Immunomedics)
Use: Diagnostic aid. [Orphan Drug]

iodine I^{123} murine monoclonal antibody to hCG. (Immunomedics)
Use: Diagnostic aid. [Orphan Drug]

iodine I^{131} 6b-iodomethyl-19-norcholesterol.
Use: Diagnostic aid. [Orphan Drug]

iodine I^{131} metaiodobenzylguanidine sulfate.
Use: Diagnostic aid. [Orphan Drug]

iodine I^{131} murine monoclonal antibody to alpha-fetoprotein. (Immunomedics)
Use: Antineoplastic. [Orphan Drug]

iodine I^{131} murine monoclonal antibody to hCG. (Immunomedics)
Use: Antineoplastic. [Orphan Drug]

iodine I^{131} murine monoclonal antibody IgG2a to B cell.
Use: Antineoplastic. [Orphan Drug]
See: Immurait (Immunomedics).

iodine-iodophor.
See: Betadine, Preps. (Purdue Frederick Co.).

iodine povidone.
See: Efodine, Oint. (E. Fougera and Co.).
Iodophor.
Mallisol, Liq. (Roberts Pharmaceuticals).

iodine products, anti-infective.
See: Anayodin.
Betadine, Preps. (Purdue Frederick Co.).
Chiniofon.
Diiodohydroxyquinoline (Various Mfr.).
Prepodyne, Soln., Scrub (West).
Quinoxyl.
Surgidine, Liq. (Continental Consumer Products).
Vioform, Preps. (Novartis Pharmaceutical Corp.).

iodine products, diagnostic.
See: Chloriodized Oil (Various Mfr.).
Ethyl Iodophenylundecylate (Various Mfr.).
Iodized Oil.
Iodoalphionic Acid (Various Mfr.).
Iodobrassid.
Iodohippurate Sodium (Various Mfr.).
Iodopanoic Acid (Various Mfr.).
Iodophthalein Sodium (Various Mfr.).
Iodopyracet, Preps. (Various Mfr.).
Optiray 350, Inj. (Mallinckrodt Medical, Inc.).
Methiodal Sodium (Various Mfr.).
Pantopaque, Amp. (Lafayette Pharmaceuticals, Inc.).
Sodium Acetrizoate (Various Mfr.).
Sodium Iodomethamate (Various Mfr.).
Telepaque, Tab. (Sanofi Winthrop Pharmaceuticals).

iodine products, nutritional.
See: Calcium Iodobehenate (Various Mfr.).
Entodon.
Hydriodic Acid (Various Mfr.).
Iodobrassid (Various Mfr.).
Potassium Iodide (Various Mfr.).

iodine ration. (Barth's) Iodine (from kelp) 0.15 mg, trace minerals/Tab. Bot. 90s, 180s, 360s. *otc.*
Use: Mineral supplement.

iodine ration. (Nion Corp.) Iodine (from kelp) 0.15 mg/3 Tab. Bot. 175s, 500s. *otc.*
Use: Mineral supplement.

iodide, sodium, I-123 capsules. (EYE-uh-dine SO-dee-uhm)
Use: Diagnostic aid (thyroid function determination).

iodide, sodium, I-123 tablets.

Use: Diagnostic aid (thyroid function determination).

iodide, sodium, I-125 capsules.
Use: Diagnostic aid (thyroid function determination), radiopharmaceutical.

iodide, sodium, I-125 solution.
Use: Diagnostic aid (thyroid function determination), radiopharmaceutical.

iodide, sodium, I-131 capsules.
Use: Antineoplastic, diagnostic aid (thyroid function determination), radiopharmaceutical.
See: Iodotope, Cap. (Bracco Diagnostics).

iodide, sodium, I-131 solution.
Use: Antineoplastic, diagnostic aid (thyroid function determination), radiopharmaceutical.
See: Iodotope, Oral Soln. (Bracco Diagnostics).

iodine surface active complex.
See: Ioprep, Soln. (Arbrook).

iodine tincture, strong.
Use: Anti-infective, topical.

•**iodipamide.** (eye-oh-DIH-pa-mide) U.S.P. 23.
Use: Pharmaceutic necessity for Iodipamide Meglumine Injection.

•**iodipamide meglumine injection.** U.S.P. 23.
Use: Diagnostic aid (radiopaque medium).
See: Cholografin Meglumine, Inj. (Bracco Diagnostics).

iodipamide methylglucamine. Also sodium salt inj.
W/Diatrizoate methylglucamine.
See: Sinografin, Vial (Bristol-Myers Squibb).

•**iodipamide sodium I-131.** USAN.
Use: Radiopharmaceutical.

iodipamide sodium injection.
See: Cholografin Sodium, Soln. (Various Mfr.).

•**iodixanol.** (EYE-oh-DIX-an-ole) USAN.
Use: Diagnostic aid (radiopaque medium).
See: Visipaque, Inj. (Nycomed Inc.).

iodized oil. A vegetable oil containing not less than 38% and not more than 42% of organically combined iodine.
Use: Diagnostic aid.

iodoalphionic acid. Biliselectan dikol, pheniodol.

•**iodoantipyrine I-131.** USAN.
Use: Radiopharmaceutical.

iodobehenate calcium. Calcium iododocosanoate.
Use: Antigoitrogenic.

iodobrassid. Ethyl Diiodobrassidate. Lipoiodine.

•**iodocetylic acid I-123.** (eye-OH-doe-SEE-till-ik) USAN.
Use: Diagnostic aid, radiopharmaceutical.

•**iodocholesterol I-131.** (EYE-oh-DOE-koe-LESS-teh-role) USAN.
Use: Radiopharmaceutical.

iodochlorhydroxyquin. Clioquinol, U.S.P. 23.

Iodo Cream. (Day-Baldwin) Clioquinol 3%. Tube 1 oz, Jar 1 lb. *otc.*
Use: Antifungal, topical.

Iodo H-C. (Day-Baldwin) Clioquinol 3%, hydrocortisone 1%. **Oint.:** Tube 20 g, Jar 1 lb. **Cream:** Tube 20 g, Jar 1 lb. *Rx.*
Use: Antifungal, corticosteroid.

•**iodohippurate sodium I-123 injection.** (EYE-oh-doe-HIP-you-rate) U.S.P. 23.
Use: Radiopharmaceutical, diagnostic aid (renal function determination).

•**iodohippurate sodium I-125.** (EYE-oh-doe-HIP-you-rate) USAN.
Use: Radiopharmaceutical.
See: Hipputope I-125 (Bristol-Myers Squibb).

•**iodohippurate, sodium I-131 injection.** (EYE-oh-doe-HIP-you-rate) U.S.P. 23.
Use: Diagnostic aid (renal function determination), radiopharmaceutical.
See: Hipputope (Bristol-Myers Squibb).

iodo-hippuric acid.
See: Hipputope (Bristol-Myers Squibb).

Iodo Ointment. (Day-Baldwin) Clioquinol 3%. Tube 1 oz, Jar 1 lb. *Rx.*
Use: Antifungal, topical.

Iodo-Pak. (SoloPak Pharmaceuticals, Inc.) Iodine 100 mcg/ml. Inj. Vial 10 ml. *Rx.*
Use: Nutritional supplement, parenteral.

iodopanoic acid.
Use: Diagnostic aid (radiopaque medium).

Iodopen. (Fujisawa USA, Inc.) Sodium iodide 118 mcg/ml. Vial 3 ml, 10 ml. *Rx.*
Use: Nutritional supplement, parenteral.

iodophene. Iodophthalein.

iodophene sodium.
See: Iodophthalein Sodium (Various Mfr.).

iodophor.
See: Betadine, Preps. (Purdue Frederick Co.).

iodophthalein sodium. Tetraiodophenolphthalein Sodium, Tetraiodophthalein Sodium, Tetiothalein Sodium (Antinosin, Cholepulvis, Cholumbrin, Foriod, Iodophene, Iodorayoral, Nosophene Sodium, Opacin, Photobiline, Piliophen, Radiotetrane).

Use: Radiopaque agent.

iodopropylidene glycerol.
See: Organidin, Elix., Tab., Soln. (Wampole Laboratories).

•**iodopyracet I 125.** USAN.
Use: Radiopharmaceutical.

•**iodopyracet I 131.** USAN.
Use: Radiopharmaceutical.

iodopyracet inj. Diatrast, Diodone, Iopyracil, Neo-Methiodal, NeoSkiodan.
Use: Radiopaque medium.

iodopyracet compound. Diodrast.

iodopyracet concentrated. Diodrast.

iodopyrine. Antipyrine iodide.
Use: Iodides, analgesic.

•**iodoquinol.** (EYE-oh-doe-KWIH-nole) U.S.P. 23. *Formerly Diiodohydroxyquin.*
Use: Antiamebic.
See: Floraquin (Searle).
Sebaquin, Shampoo (Summers Labs).
W/9-Aminoacridine HCl.
See: Vagitric, Cream (ICN Pharmaceuticals, Inc.).
Yodoxin, Tab., Pow. (Glenwood, Inc.).
W/Hydrocortisone alcohol.
See: Vytone, Cream (Dermik Laboratories, Inc.).
W/Hydrocortisone, coal tar solution.
See: Gynben, Vag. Insert, Cream (ICN Pharmaceuticals, Inc.).
Gynben Insufflate, Pow. (ICN Pharmaceuticals, Inc.).
W/Surfactants.
See: Lycinate, Supp. (Hoechst Marion Roussel).
W/Sulfanilamide, diethylstilbestrol.
See: Amide V/S, Vaginal Insert (Scrip).
D.I.TI Creme (Dunhall Pharmaceuticals, Inc.).

Iodotope (Diagnostic). (Bristol-Myers Squibb) Sodium iodide I-131 for oral use. 7, 14, 28, 70, 106 units Ci/Vial of 5, 10, 15, 20 Cap.
Use: Diagnostic aid.

Iodotope (Therapeutic Antibodies, Inc.). (Bracco Diagnostics) Sodium iodide I-131. 1 to 50 mCi Cap. Sodium iodide I-151 7.05 m Ci/ml. Vial 7, 14, 28, 70, 106 mCi, EDTA 1 mg/solution. *Rx.*
Use: Antithyroid agent.

•**iodoxamate meglumine.** (EYE-oh-DOX-ah-mate meh-GLUE-meen) USAN.
Use: Diagnostic aid (radiopaque medium).

•**iodoxamic acid.** (EYE-oh-dox-AM-ik) USAN.
Use: Diagnostic aid (radiopaque medium).

iodoxyl.
See: Sodium Iodomethamate (Various Mfr.).

Iofed. (Iomed) Brompheniramine maleate 12 mg, pseudoephedrine HCl 120 mg/ER Cap. Bot. 100s. *Rx.*
Use: Antihistamine, decongestant.

Iofed PD. (Iomed) Brompheniramine maleate 6 mg, pseudoephedrine HCl 60 mg/ER Cap. Bot. 100s. *Rx.*
Use: Antihistamine, decongestant.

•**iofetamine hydrochloride I 123.** (EYE-oh-FET-ah-meen) USAN.
Use: Diagnostic aid, radiopharmaceutical.

•**ioglicic acid.** (eye-oh-GLIH-sick) USAN.
Use: Diagnostic aid (radiopaque medium).

•**ioglucol.** (EYE-oh-GLUE-kahl) USAN.
Use: Diagnostic aid (radiopaque medium).

•**ioglucomide.** (EYE-oh-GLUE-koe-mide) USAN.
Use: Diagnostic aid (radiopaque medium).

•**ioglycamic acid.** (EYE-oh-glie-KAM-ik) USAN.
Use: Diagnostic aid (radiopaque medium, cholecystographic).

•**iogulamide.** (EYE-oh-GULL-ah-mide) USAN.
Use: Diagnostic aid (radiopaque medium).

•**iohexol.** (EYE-oh-HEX-ole) U.S.P. 23.
Use: Diagnostic aid (radiopaque medium).
See: Omnipaque (Nycomed).

Iohist D. (Iomed) Phenylpropanolamine HCl 25 mg, phenyltoloxamine citrate 4 mg, pyrilamine maleate 4 mg, pheniramine maleate 4 mg, alcohol 4 %/5 ml. Bot. Pt. *Rx.*
Use: Antihistamine, decongestant.

Iohist DM. (Iomed) Dextromethorphan HBr 10 mg, phenylpropanolamine HCl 12.5 mg, brompheniramine maleate 2 mg/5 ml. Syrup. Alcohol and sugar free. Bot. Pt. *Rx.*
Use: Antihistamine, antitussive, decongestant.

Iohydro Cream. (Freeport) Hydrocortisone 1%, clioquinol 3%, pramoxine HCl 0.5%/0.5 oz. Tube 0.5 oz.
Use: Anesthetic; antifungal; corticosteroid, topical.

•**iomeprol.** (EYE-oh-MEH-prole) USAN.
Use: Diagnostic aid (radiopaque medium).

•**iomethin I-125.** (EYE-oh-METH-in) USAN.
Use: Diagnostic aid (neoplasm); radiopharmaceutical.

•**iomethin I-131.** (EYE-o-METH-in) USAN.
Use: Diagnostic aid (neoplasm); radiopharmaceutical.

•**iometopane I-123.** (eye-oh-meh-TOE-pane) USAN.
Use: Diagnostic aid.

Ionamin. (Medeva Pharmaceuticals, Inc.) Phentermine resin 15 mg, 30 mg, lactose/Cap. Bot. 100s, 400s. *c-IV.*
Use: Anorexiant.

Ionax Astringent Cleanser. (Galderma Laboratories, Inc.) Isopropyl alcohol 48%, acetone, salicylic acid. Bot. 240 ml. *otc.*
Use: Dermatologic, acne.

Ionax Foam. (Galderma Laboratories, Inc.) Benzalkonium Cl, propylene glycol. Aerosol Can 150 ml. *otc.*
Use: Dermatologic, acne.

Ionax Scrub. (Galderma Laboratories, Inc.) SD alcohol 40, benzalkonium Cl. Tube 60 g, 120 g. *otc.*
Use: Dermatologic, acne.

I-131 radiolabeled b1 monoclonal antibody. (Coulter Corp.)
Use: Treatment for non-Hodgkin's B-cell lymphoma. [Orphan Drug]

ion-exchange resins.
See: Polyamine Methylene Resin. Resins, Sodium-Removing.

Ionil Plus Shampoo. (Galderma Laboratories, Inc.) Salicylic acid 2%, sodium laureth sulfate, lauramide DEA, quaternium-22, talloweth-60 myristyl glycol, laureth-23, TEA lauryl sulfate, glycol disterate, laureth-4, TEA-abietoyl hydrolyzed collagen, DMDM hydantoin, tetrasodium EDTA, sodium hydroxide, FD&C blue No. 1. Bot. 4 oz, 8 oz. *otc.*
Use: Antiseborrheic.

Ionil Rinse. (Galderma Laboratories, Inc.) Conditioners with benzalkonium Cl in water base. Bot. 16 oz. *otc.*
Use: Dermatologic, hair.

Ionil Shampoo. (Galderma Laboratories, Inc.) Salicylic acid, benzalkonium Cl, alcohol 12%, polyoxyethylene ethers. Plastic bot. w/dispenser cap 4 oz, 8 oz, 16 oz, 32 oz. *otc.*
Use: Antiseborrheic.

Ionil T. (Galderma Laboratories, Inc.) A nonionic/cationic foaming shampoo w/ coal tar, salicylic acid, benzalkonium Cl, alcohol 12%, polyoxyethylene ethers. Plastic bot. 4 oz, 8 oz, 16 oz, 32 oz. *otc.*
Use: Antiseborrheic.

Ionil-T Plus Shampoo. (Galderma Laboratories, Inc.) Owentar II (equivalent to 2% coal tar), sodium laureth sulfate, lauramide DEA, quaternium-22, laureth-23, talloweth-60 myristyl glycol, TEA lauryl sulfate, glycol distearate, laureth-4, TEA abietoyl hydrolyzed collagen, DMDM hydantoin, disodium EDTA, fragrance, FD&C blue No. 1, FD&C yellow No. 70. Bot. 4 oz, 8 oz. *otc.*
Use: Antiseborrheic.

Ionosol D-CM. (Abbott Hospital Products) Sodium Cl 516 mg, potassium Cl 89.4 mg, calcium Cl anhydrous 27.8 mg, magnesium Cl anhydrous 14.2 mg, sodium lactate 560 mg/100 ml. Bot. 1000 ml. *Rx.*
Use: Nutritional supplement, parenteral.

•**iopamidol.** (EYE-oh-PAM-ih-dahl) U.S.P. 23.
Use: Diagnostic aid (radiopaque medium).
See: Isovue (Bracco Diagnostics).

•**iopanoic acid.** (eye-oh-pan-OH-ik) U.S.P. 23.
Use: Diagnostic aid (radiopaque medium).
See: Telepaque, Tab. (Sanofi Winthrop Pharmaceuticals).

•**iopentol.** (EYE-oh-PEN-tole) USAN.
Use: Diagnostic aid (radiopaque medium).

Iophen-C. (Various Mfr.) Codeine phosphate 10 mg, iodinated glycerol 30 mg/5 ml. Liq. Bot. Pt., gal. *c-V.*
Use: Antitussive, expectorant.

Iophen-DM. (Various Mfr.) Dextromethorphan HBr, iodinated glycerol 30 mg/5 ml. Liq. Bot. 120 ml, pt., gal. *Rx.*
Use: Antitussive, expectorant.

•**iophendylate.** (eye-oh-FEN-dih-late) U.S.P. 23. Benzenedecanoic acid, iodo-t-methyl, ethyl ester.
Use: Diagnostic aid (radiopaque medium).

iophendylate injection. Ethiodan, Myodil. Ethyl Iodophenylundecylate.
Use: Diagnostic aid (radiopaque medium).
See: Pantopaque, Amp. (Lafayette Pharmaceuticals).

iophenoxic acid. (EYE-oh-pro-SEH-mik Acid) Tab.

Iophylline. (Various Mfr.) Theophylline 120 mg, iodinated glycerol 30 mg/15 ml. Elix. Bot. 480 ml. *Rx.*
Use: Antiasthmatic combination.

Iopidine. (Alcon Laboratories, Inc.) Apraclonidine 0.5%, 1%, benzalkonium Cl 0.01%. Dispenser Bot. 0.25 ml (1%), Drop-Tainer 5 ml (0.5%). *Rx.*
Use: Antiglaucoma agent.

iopodate sodium.
See: Ipodate Sodium.

Ioprep. (Johnson & Johnson) Nonyl-

phenoxypolyethylenoxy (4) ethanol and nonylphenoxypolyethyleneoxy (15) ethanol iodine complex 5.5%, nonylphenoxypolyethyleneoxy (30) ethanol 10%. Solution provides 1% available iodine. Plastic bot. Gal.
Use: Antiseptic.

•**ioprocemic acid.** (EYE-oh-pro-SEH-mik acid) USAN.
Use: Diagnostic aid (radiopaque medium).

•**iopromide.** (eye-oh-PRO-mide) USAN.
Use: Diagnostic aid (radiopaque medium).
See: Ultravist, Inj. (Berlex Laboratories, Inc.).

•**iopronic acid.** (eye-oh-PRO-nik acid) USAN.
Use: Diagnostic aid (radiopaque medium, cholecystographic).

•**iopydol.** (eye-oh-PIE-dahl) USAN.
Use: Diagnostic aid (radiopaque medium, bronchographic).

•**iopydone.** (eye-oh-PIE-dohn) USAN.
Use: Diagnostic aid (radiopaque medium, bronchographic).

Iosal II. (Iomed) Pseudoephedrine HCl 60 mg, guaifenesin 600 mg/ER Tab. 100s. Bot. *Rx.*
Use: Expectorant.

•**iosefamic acid.** (EYE-oh-seh-FAM-ik) USAN.
Use: Diagnostic aid; radiopaque medium.

•**ioseric acid.** (eye-oh-SEH-rik) USAN.
Use: Diagnostic aid (radiopaque medium).

Iosopan. (Zenith Goldline Pharmaceuticals) Magaldrate 540 mg/5 ml. Liq. Bot. 355 ml. *otc.*
Use: Antacid.

Iosopan Plus. (Zenith Goldline Pharmaceuticals) Magaldrate 540 mg, simethicone 40 mg/5 ml. Liq. Bot. 355 ml. *otc.*
Use: Antacid.

•**iosulamide meglumine.** (eye-oh-SULL-ah-mide meh-GLUE-meen) USAN.
Use: Diagnostic aid (radiopaque medium).

•**iosumetic acid.** (eye-oh-sue-MEH-tick) USAN.
Use: Diagnostic aid (radiopaque medium).

•**iotasul.** (EYE-oh-tah-sull) USAN.
Use: Diagnostic aid (radiopaque medium).

•**iotetric acid.** (eye-oh-TEH-trick) USAN.
Use: Diagnostic aid (radiopaque medium).

iothalamate meglumide and iothalmate sodium injection.
Use: Diagnostic aid (radiopaque medium).
See: Vascoray (Mallinckrodt).

•**iothalamate meglumine injection.** (eye-oh-THAL-am-ate meh-GLUE-meen) U.S.P. 23.
Use: Diagnostic aid (radiopaque medium).
See: Conray (Mallinckrodt).
Cysto-Conray (Mallinckrodt).

•**iothalamate sodium injection.** (eye-oh-THAL-am-ate) U.S.P. 23.
Use: Diagnostic aid (radiopaque medium).
See: Conray (Mallinckrodt).

•**iothalamate sodium I-125 injection.** (eye-oh-THAL-am-ate) U.S.P. 23.
Use: Radiopharmaceutical.

•**iothalamate sodium I-131.** (eye-oh-THAL-am-ate) USAN.
Use: Radiopharmaceutical.

•**iothalamic acid.** (eye-oh-THAL-am-ik) U.S.P. 23.
Use: Diagnostic aid (radiopaque medium).

iothiouracil sodium. Sodium salt of 5-iodo-2-thiouracil.

•**iotrolan.** (EYE-oh-TRAHL-an) USAN.
Formerly Iotrol.
Use: Diagnostic aid (radiopaque medium).

•**iotroxic acid.** (EYE-oh-TRAHK-sick) USAN.
Use: Diagnostic aid (radiopaque medium).

Iotussin HC. (Iomed) Hydrocodone bitartrate 2.5 mg, phenylephrine HCl 5 mg, chlorpheniramine maleate 2 mg/5 ml. Alcohol and sugar free. Syr. Bot. 473 ml. *c-III.*
Use: Antihistamine, antitussive, decongestant.

•**iotyrosine I-131.** USAN.
Use: Radiopharmaceutical.

•**ioversol.** (EYE-oh-ver-SAHL) U.S.P. 23.
Use: Diagnostic aid (radiopaque medium).
See: Optiray (Mallinckrodt Medical, Inc.).

•**ioxaglate meglumine.** (eye-ox-AGG-late meh-GLUE-meen) USAN.
Use: Diagnostic aid (radiopaque medium).
See: Hexabrix, Inj. (Wallace Laboratories).

ioxaglate meglumine/ioxaglate sodium.
Use: Radiopaque agent.

See: Hexabrix (Mallinckrodt).

•**ioxaglate sodium.** (eye-ox-AGG-late) USAN.
Use: Diagnostic aid (radiopaque medium).

•**ioxaglic acid.** (eye-ox-AGG-lick) U.S.P. 23.
Use: Diagnostic aid (radiopaque medium).

•**ioxilan.** (eye-OX-ee-lan) USAN.
Use: Diagnostic aid.

•**ioxotrizoic acid.** (eye-OX-oh-TRY-zoe-ik) USAN.
Use: Diagnostic aid (radiopaque medium).

•**ipazilide fumarate.** (ih-PAZZ-ih-LIDE) USAN.
Use: Cardiovascular agent.

•**ipecac.** (IPP-uh-kak) U.S.P. 23.
Use: Emetic.
W/Combinations.
See: Ipsatol, Syr. (Key Pharmaceuticals).
Mallergan, Liq. (Roberts Pharmaceuticals).

ipecac. (Various Mfr.) 1.5% to 1.75% alcohol, 2%. Syr. Bot. 15 ml, 30 ml. *otc.*
Use: Antidote.

•**ipexidine mesylate.** (eye-PEX-ih-DEEN) USAN.
Use: Dental caries agent.

I-Pilopine. (Akorn, Inc.) Pilocarpine HCl 1%. Ophthalmic soln. Bot. 15 ml. *Rx.*
Use: Antiglaucoma agent.

•**ipodate calcium.** (EYE-poe-date) U.S.P. 23.
Use: Diagnostic aid (radiopaque medium).
See: Oragrafin calcium, Granules (Bristol-Myers Squibb).

•**ipodate sodium.** U.S.P. 23.
Use: Diagnostic aid (radiopaque medium).
See: Oragrafin sodium, Cap. (Bracco Diagnostics).

IPOL. (Pasteur Merieux Connaught) Suspension of 3 types of poliovirus (Types 1, 2, and 3) grown in monkey kidney cell cultures. Inj. Single-dose syringe 0.5 ml. *Rx.*
Use: Immunization.

Ipran. (Major Pharmaceuticals) Propranolol HCl 10 mg, 20 mg, 40 mg, 60 mg, 80 mg, 90 mg/Tab. **10 mg, 20 mg, 40 mg:** Bot. 100s, 250s, 1000s, UD 100s. **60 mg:** Bot. 100s, 500s. **80 mg:** Bot. 100s, 500s, 1000s, UD 100s. **90 mg:** Bot. 100s, 500s. *Rx.*
Use: Beta-adrenergic blocker.

•**ipratropium bromide.** (IH-pruh-TROE-pee-uhm) USAN.
Use: Bronchodilator.
See: Atrovent, Aerosol (Boehringer Ingelheim, Inc.).

ipratropium bromide. (Dey Laboratories, Inc.) Ipratropium bromide 0.02% (500 mcg/vial) Soln. for Inh. Vial 2.5 ml each. 25, 30, 60 unit-dose. *Rx.*
Use: Anticholinergic.

ipratropium bromide/albuterol sulfate. (Boehringer Ingelheim, Inc.)
Use: Secondary treatment of chronic obstructive pulmonary disease (COPD).
See: Combivent, Inhalation aerosol (Boehringer Ingelheim, Inc.).

I-Pred. (Akorn, Inc.) Prednisolone sodium phosphate 0.5%, 1%. Ophth. Soln. Bot. 5 ml. *Rx.*
Use: Corticosteroid, ophthalmic.

I-Prednicet. (Akorn, Inc.) Prednisolone acetate 1%. Ophth. Soln. Bot. 5 ml, 10 ml. *Rx.*
Use: Corticosteroid, ophthalmic.

•**iprindole.** (IH-prin-dole) USAN.
Use: Antidepressant.

•**iprofenin.** (IH-pro-FEN-in) USAN.
Use: Diagnostic aid (hepatic funtion determination).

•**ipronidazole.** (ih-pro-NIH-dah-zole) USAN.
Use: Antiprotozoal *Histomonas.*

•**iproplatin.** (IH-pro-PLAT-in) USAN.
Use: Antineoplastic.

iproveratril. Name used for verapamil.

•**iproxamine hydrochloride.** (IH-PROX-ah-meen) USAN.
Use: Vasodilator.

•**ipsapirone hydrochloride.** (ipp-sah-PIE-rone) USAN.
Use: Anxiolytic.

Ipsatol Cough Formula Liquid for Children and Adults. (Kenwood Laboratories) Guaifenesin 100 mg, dextromethorphan HBr 10 mg, phenylpropanolamine HCl 9 mg/5 ml. Bot. 118 ml. *otc.*
Use: Antitussive, decongestant, expectorant.

IPV.
Use: Immunization.
See: IPOL (Pasteur Merieux Connaught).
Polio Virus Vaccine, Inactivated.

•**irbesartan.** (ihr-beh-SAHR-tan) USAN.
Use: Antihypertensive (angiotensin II receptor antagonist).
See: Avapro, Tab. (Sanofi Winthrop Pharmaceuticals).

Ircon. (Kenwood Laboratories) Ferrous

fumarate 200 mg/Tab. Bot. 100s. *otc.*
Use: Mineral supplement.

Ircon-FA. (Kenwood Laboratories) Ferrous fumarate 82 mg, folic acid 0.8 mg/Tab. Bot. 100s. *otc.*
Use: Mineral supplement.

Irgasan CF3. Cloflucarban.
Use: Antiseptic, topical.

•**iridium Ir 192.** (ih-RID-ee-uhm) USAN.
Use: Radioactive agent.

Irrigate Eye Wash. (Optopics Laboratories, Corp) Sodium Cl, sodium phosphate mono- and dibasic, benzalkonium Cl, EDTA. Soln. Bot. 118 ml. *otc.*
Use: Irrigant, ophthalmic.

•**irinotecan hydrochloride.** (eye-rih-no-TEE-can) USAN.
Use: Antineoplastic (DNA topoisomerase I inhibitor).
See: Camptosar, Inj. (Pharmacia & Upjohn).

irisin. A polysaccharide found in several species of iris.

irocaine.
See: Procaine HCl (Various Mfr.).

Irodex. (Keene Pharmaceuticals, Inc.) Iron dextran complex 50 mg/ml. Vial 10 ml. *Rx.*
Use: Mineral supplement.

Iromin-G. (Mission Pharmacal Co.) Ferrous gluconate 260 mg (iron 30 mg), vitamins B_{12} (crystalline on resin) 2 mcg, C 100 mg, A acetate 4000 IU, D 400 IU, B_1 5 mg, B_2 2 mg, B_6 20.6 mg, B_3 10 mg, B_5 1 mg, folic acid 0.8 mg, Ca. Tab. Bot. 100s. *otc.*
Use: Mineral, vitamin supplement.

iron (2+) fumarate. Ferrous Fumarate, U.S.P. 23.

iron (2+) gluconate.
See: Ferrous Gluconate, U.S.P. 23.

iron carbonate complex.
See: Polyferose.

•**iron dextran injection.** (iron DEX-tran) U.S.P. 23.
Use: Hematinic.
See: Dexferrum, Inj. (American Regent).
Imferon, Amp., Vial (Hoechst Marion Roussel).
InFeD, Inj. (Schein Pharmaceutical, Inc.).

Iron-Folic 500. (Major Pharmaceuticals) Ferrous sulfate 105 mg, B_1 6 mg, B_2 6 mg, B_3 30 mg, B_5 10 mg, B_{12} 25 mcg, C 500 mg, folic acid 0.8 mg/Tab. Bot. 100s, 500s. *otc.*
Use: Mineral, vitamin supplement.

iron/liver combinations, injection.
See: Hemocyte (US Pharmaceutical Corp.).
Hytinic (Hyrex Pharmaceuticals).
Liver-Iron B Complex w/Vitamin B_{12} (Akorn, Inc.).

iron/liver combination, oral.
See: Feocyte, Tab. (Dunhill).
I-L-X B_{12}, Tab. (Kenwood Laboratories).
Liquid Geritonic (Roberts Pharmaceuticals).
I-L-X B_{12}, Elix. (Kenwood Laboratories).
I-L-X, Elix. (Kenwood Laboratories).

iron oxide mixture with zinc oxide. Calamine, U.S.P. 23.

iron products, injection.
See: InFeD (Schein Pharmaceutical, Inc.).

•**iron sorbitex injection.** (SORE-bih-tex) U.S.P. 23.
Use: Hematinic.

iron with vitamin B_{12} and IFC.
See: Pronemia Hematinic Capsules (ESI Lederle Generics).
Contrin Capsules (Geneva Pharmaceuticals).
Ferotrinsic Capsules (Rugby Labs, Inc.).
Livitrinsic-f Capsules (Zenith Goldline Pharmaceuticals).
Trinsicon Capsules (UCB Pharmaceuticals, Inc.).
Fergon Plus Caplets (Sanofi Winthrop Pharmaceuticals).
TriHEMIC 600 Tablets (ESI Lederle Generics).
Chromagen Capsules (Savage Laboratories).

Ironco-B. (Pal-Pak, Inc.) Ferrous sulfate 120.4 mg, manganese sulfate 21.6 mg, dicalcium phosphate 129.6 mg, vitamins B_1 1 mg, B_2 1 mg, niacin 6 mg, D 100 IU/Tab. Bot. 100s, 1000s. *otc.*
Use: Mineral, vitamin supplement.

Irospan. (Fielding Co.) Ferrous sulfate 65 mg, vitamin C 150 mg. Cap.: Bot. 60s. Tab.: Bot. 100s. *otc.*
Use: Mineral, vitamin supplement.

irradiated ergosterol.
See: Calciferol.

Irrigate Eye Wash. (Optopics Laboratories Corp.) Sodium Cl, mono- and dibasic sodium phosphate, benzalkonium Cl, EDTA. Bot. 118 ml. *otc.*
Use: Irrigant, ophthalmic.

irrigating solutions, physiological.
Use: Irrigant.
See: Tis-U-Sol (Baxter Pharmaceutical Products, Inc.).
Lactated Ringer's Irrigation (Abbott Laboratories).
Physiolyte (American McGaw).

PhysioSol (Abbott Laboratories).
irrigating solutions, urinary.
Use: Irrigant.
See: Neosporin G.U. Irrigant (Glaxo-Wellcome).
Renacidin (Guardian Laboratories).
Resectisol (McGaw, Inc.).
Sorbitol-Mannitol (Abbott Laboratories).
Acetic Acid (Various Mfr.).
Glycine (Aminoacetic acid) (Various Mfr.).
Sodium Chloride (Various Mfr.).
Sterile Water (Various Mfr.).
•**irtemazole.** (ihr-TEH-mah-zole) USAN.
Use: Uricosuric.
isacen.
See: Oxyphenisatin, Preps. (Various Mfr.).
•**isamoxole.** (eye-SAH-MOX-ole) USAN.
Use: Antiasthmatic.
iscador. (Hiscia)
Use: Antiviral.
•**isepamicin.** (eye-SEP-ah-MY-sin) USAN.
Use: Antibacterial (aminoglycoside).
ISG. Immune globulin intramuscular. *Rx.*
Use: Immunization.
Ismelin. (Novartis Pharmaceutical Corp.) Guanethidine monosulfate 10 mg, 25 mg/Tab. Bot. 100s. *Rx.*
Use: Antihypertensive.
ISMO. (Wyeth-Ayerst Laboratories) Isosorbide mononitrate 20 mg/Tab. Bot. 100s, UD 100s. *Rx.*
Use: Antianginal.
Ismotic. (Alcon, Surgical Division) Isosorbide solution. W/sodium 4.6 mEq, potassium 0.9 mEq/220 ml, alcohol, saccharin, sorbitol. In 220 ml. *Rx.*
Use: Diuretic.
iso-alcoholic elixir.
Use: Vehicle.
isoamylhydrocupreine dihydrochloride.
See: Eucupin Dihydrochloride.
isoamyl nitrate.
See: Amyl Nitrite, U.S.P. 23.
isoamyne.
See: Amphetamine (Various Mfr.).
Iso-B. (Tyson & Associates, Inc.) Vitamins B_1 25 mg, B_2 25 mg, B_3 75 mg, B_5 125 mg, B_6 50 mg, B_{12} 100 mcg, FA 0.2 mg, pyridoxal 5 phosphate 2.5 mg, PABA 50 mg, inositol 50 mg, choline bitartrate 125 mg, biotin 100 mcg/Cap. Bot. 120s. *otc.*
Use: Mineral, vitamin supplement.
isobornyl thiocyanoacetate, technical.
Use: Pediculicide.
See: Barc, Liq. (Del Pharmaceuticals, Inc.).
W/Docusate sodium and related terpenes.
See: Barc, Cream (Del Pharmaceuticals, Inc.).
isobucaine hydrochloride. U.S.P. XXI.
Use: Anesthetic, local.
isobucaine hydrochloride & epinephrine injection. U.S.P. XXI.
Use: Anesthetic, local.
•**isobutamben.** (EYE-so-BYOO-tam-ben) USAN.
Use: Anesthetic, local.
•**isobutane.** (eye-so-BYOO-tane) N.F. 18.
Use: Aerosol propellant.
isobutylallylbarbituric acid.
W/Aspirin, phenacetin, caffeine.
See: Buff-A-Comp, Tab., Cap. (Merz Pharmaceuticals).
Fiorinal, Tab., Cap. (Novartis Pharmaceutical Corp.).
Palgesic, Tab., Cap. (Pan Amer.).
Tenstan, Tab. (Standex).
W/Codeine phosphate.
See: Fiorinal w/Codeine, Cap. (Novartis Pharmaceutical Corp.).
isobutyl p-aminobenzoate.
See: Isobutamben, USAN.
isobutyramide. (Vertex Pharmaceuticals, Inc.)
Use: Sickle cell disease, beta-thalassemia. [Orphan Drug]
isobutyramide oral solution. (Alpha Therapeutic Corp.)
Use: Sickle call disease, beta-thalassemia. [Orphan Drug]
isocaine. Isobutamben, U.S.P. 23.
Isocaine Hydrochloride. (Novocol Chemical Mfr. Co.) Mepivacaine HCl 3%: 1.8 ml (dental cartridge). 2%: w/levonordefrin 1:20,000, sodium bisulfite. 1.8 ml (dental cartridge). *Rx.*
Use: Anesthetic, local.
See: Isocaine HCl, Inj. (Novocol Chemical Mfr. Co.).
Isocal. (Bristol-Myers Squibb) Lactose-free isotonic liquid containing as a percentage of the calories protein 13% as caseinate and soy protein; fat 37% as soy oil and medium chain triglycerides; carbohydrate 50% as corn syrup solids w/vitamins and minerals for the tube-fed patient. Bot. 8 fl oz, 12 fl oz, 32 fl oz. *otc.*
Use: Nutritional supplement.
Isocal HCN. (Bristol-Myers Squibb) High calorie nitrogen nutritionally complete food. Protein 15%, fat 45%, carbohydrate 40%. Can 8 fl oz. *otc.*
Use: Nutritional supplement.
Isocal HN. (Bristol-Myers Squibb) $\approx$ 1 Kcal/ml with protein 44 g, fat 45 g, car-

bohydrates 124 g/L. In 237 ml. *otc.*
Use: Nutritional supplement.

•**isocarboxazid.** (eye-so-car-BOX-ah-zid) U.S.P. 23.
Use: Antidepressant.
See: Marplan (Hoffman LaRoche).

Isocet. (Rugby Labs, Inc.) Acetaminophen 325 mg, caffeine 40 mg, butalbital 50 mg/Tab. Bot. 100s. *Rx.*
Use: Analgesic combination.

Isoclor Expectorant. (Medeva Pharmaceuticals, Inc.) Codeine phosphate 10 mg, pseudoephedrine HCl 30 mg, guaifenesin 100 mg/5 ml, alcohol 5%. Bot. Pt. *c-v.*
Use: Antitussive, decongestant, expectorant.

isococaine. Pseudococaine.

Isocom. (Nutripharm Laboratories, Inc.) Isometheptene mucate 65 mg, dichloralphenazone 100 mg, acetaminophen 325 mg/Cap. Bot. 50s, 100s, 250s. *Rx.*
Use: Antimigraine.

•**isoconazole.** (EYE-so-CONE-ah-zole) USAN.
Use: Anti-infective, antifungal.

Isocult Test for Bacteriuria. (SmithKline Diagnostics)
Use: Diagnostic aid.

Isocult Test for Candida. (SmithKline Diagnostics)
Use: Diagnostic aid.

Isocult Test for Neisseria Gonorrhoeae. (SmithKline Diagnostics)
Use: Diagnostic aid.

Isocult Test for N. Gonorrhoeae and Candida. (SmithKline Diagnostics)
Use: Diagnostic aid.

Isocult Test for Pseudomonas Aeruginosa. (SmithKline Diagnostics)
Use: Diagnostic aid.

Isocult Test for Staphylococcus Aureus. (SmithKline Diagnostics)
Use: Diagnostic aid.

Isocult Test for Throat Streptococci. (SmithKline Diagnostics)
Use: Diagnostic aid.

Isocult Test for Trichomonas Vaginalis. (SmithKline Diagnostics)
Use: Diagnostic aid.

Isocult Test for T. Vaginalis/Candida. (SmithKline Diagnostics)
Use: Diagnostic aid.

Iso D. (Dunhall Pharmaceuticals, Inc.) Isosorbide dinitrate. **Cap.:** 40 mg. Bot. 100s, 1000s. **Tab.:** 5 mg (sublingual). Bot. 100s. *Rx.*
Use: Antianginal.

isoephedrine hydrochloride. d-Isoephedrine HCl.
See: Pseudoephedrine HCl.
W/Chlorpheniramine maleate.
See: Isoclor, Tab., Expectorant Timesule, Liq. (Arnar-Stone).
W/Chlorprophenpyridamine maleate.
See: Isoclor, Tab. (Arnar-Stone).

d-isoephedrine sulfate.
See: Pseudoephedrine sulfate.

•**isoetharine.** (EYE-so-ETH-uh-reen) USAN.
Use: Bronchodilator.

•**isoetharine hydrochloride.** (EYE-so-ETH-uh-reen) U.S.P. 23.
Use: Bronchodilator.

isoetharine hydrochloride. (Roxane) 1%. Soln. for Inh. Bot. 10 ml, 30 ml, w/ dropper. *Rx.*
Use: Bronchodilator.

•**isoetharine mesylate.** (EYE-so-ETH-uh-reen) U.S.P. 23.
Use: Bronchodilator.
See: Bronkometer, Aerosol (Sanofi Winthrop Pharmaceuticals).

•**isoflupredone acetate.** (eye-so-FLEW-PREH-dohn) USAN.
Use: Anti-inflammatory.

•**isoflurane.** (EYE-so-FLEW-rane) U.S.P. 23.
Use: Anesthetic, general.

•**isoflurophate.** (eye-so-FLURE-oh-fate) U.S.P. 23.
Use: Cholinergic, ophthalmic.
See: Floropryl, Oint. (Merck & Co.).

iso-iodeikon.
See: Phentetiothalein Sodium.

Isoject. (Roerig) A purified, sterile, disposable injection system.
Use: Injection system.
See: Permapen (benzathine pencillin G) aqueous soln. 1,200,000 units/2 ml. 10s.
Terramycin (oxytetracycline) Intramuscular Soln.

I-Sol Solution. (Dey Laboratories, Inc.) Sodium Cl 0.64%, potassium Cl 0.075%, calcium Cl 0.048%, magnesium Cl 0.03%, sodium acetate 0.39%, sodium citrate 0.17%, sodium hydroxide or hydrochloric acid. Soln. Bot. 20 ml, 200 ml. *otc.*
Use: Irrigant, ophthalmic.

Isolan. (Elan Pharma) Protein 40 g, fat 36 g, carbohydrates 144 g, Na 690 g, K 1.17 g/L, with appropriate vitamins and minerals. Lactose free. Liq. In 237 ml Tetra Pak containers and 1000 ml New Pak closed systems with and without Color Check. *otc.*
Use: Nutritional supplement.

Isolate Compound Elixir. (Various Mfr.)

Theophylline 45 mg, ephedrine sulfate 12 mg, isoproterenol HCl 2.5 mg, potassium iodide 150 mg, phenobarbital 6 mg/15 ml, alcohol 19%. Elix. Bot. Pt, gal. *Rx.*
Use: Antiasthmatic combination.

•**isoleucine.** (EYE-so-LOO-seen) U.S.P. 23.
Use: Amino acid.

isoleucine. (EYE-so-LOO-seen) (Pfaltz & Bauer) Pow. 10 g.
Use: Amino acid.

Isolyte G with Dextrose. (American McGaw) Sodium 65 mEq, potassium 17 mEq, chloride 150 mEq, NH_4 70 mEq, dextrose 50 g, 170 Cal, 555 mOsm/L. Bot. 1000 ml. *Rx.*
Use: Nutritional supplement, parenteral.

Isolyte H/5% Dextrose. (American McGaw) Sodium 70 mEq, potassium 13 mEq, magnesium 3 mEq, chloride 40 mEq, acetate 16 mEq, dextrose 50 g, 170 Cal, 370 mOsm/L. Inj. Soln. 1000 ml. *Rx.*
Use: Nutritional supplement, parenteral.

Isolyte M/5% Dextrose. (American McGaw) Sodium 38 mEq, potassium 35 mEq, chloride 44 mEq, phosphate 15 mEq, acetate 20 mEq, dextrose 50 g, 175 Cal, 405 mOsm/L. Inj. Soln. 1000 ml. *Rx.*
Use: Nutritional supplement, parenteral.

Isolyte P/5% Dextrose. (American McGaw) Sodium 25 mEq, potassium 19 mEq, magnesium 3 mEq, chloride 23 mEq, phosphate 3 mEq, acetate 23 mEq, dextrose 50 g, 175 Cal, 350 mOsm/L. Inj. Soln. 250 ml, 500 ml, 1000 ml. *Rx.*
Use: Nutritional supplement, parenteral.

Isolyte R/5% Dextrose. (American McGaw) Sodium 41 mEq, potassium 16 mEq, calcium 5 mEq, magnesium 3 mEq, chloride 40 mEq, acetate 24 mEq, dextrose 50 g, 175 Cal, 380 mOsm/L. Inj. Soln. 1000 ml. *Rx.*
Use: Nutritional supplement, parenteral.

Isolyte S ≤ 7.4. (American McGaw) Sodium 140 mEq, potassium 5 mEq, magnesium 3 mEq, chloride 98 mEq, acetate 27 mEq, gluconate 23 mEq, 295 mOsm/L. Inj. Soln. 500 ml, 1000 ml. *Rx.*
Use: Nutritional supplement, parenteral.

Isolyte S/5% Dextrose. (American McGaw) Sodium 140 mEq, potassium 5 mEq, magnesium 3 mEq, chloride 98 mEq, acetate 27 mEq, gluconate 23 mEq, dextrose 50 g, 185 Cal, 550 mOsm/L. Inj. Soln. 1000 ml. *Rx.*
Use: Nutritional supplement, parenteral.

•**isomazole hydrochloride.** (eye-SO-mah-ZOLE) USAN.
Use: Cardiovascular agent.

isomeprobamate.
See: Carisoprodol (Various Mfr.).

•**isomerol.** (EYE-so-MER-ole) USAN. *Formerly Parahydrecin.*
Use: Antiseptic.

isometheptene mucate/dichloralphenazone/acetaminophen. (eye-so-meth-EPP-teen MYOO-kate, die-klor-uhl-FEN-uh-zone and ASS-et-ah-MEE-noe-fen)

isometheptene/dichloralphenazone/acetaminophen.
Use: Antimigraine.
See: Isometheptene/Dichloralphenazone/Acetaminophen, Cap. (Various Mfr.).
Isocom, Cap. (Nutripharm Laboratories, Inc.).
Midchlor, Cap. (Schein Pharmaceutical, Inc.).
Midrin, Cap. (Carnrick Laboratories, Inc.).
Migratine, Cap. (Major Pharmaceuticals).

•**isometheptene mucate.** (eye-so-meth-EPP-teen MYOO-kate) U.S.P. 23.
See: Midrin, Cap. (Carnick Laboratories, Inc.).

Isomil. (Ross Laboratories) Soy protein isolate infant formula containing 20 calories/fl oz. **Pow.:** Can 14 oz. **Concentrated Liq.:** Can 13 fl oz. **Ready-to-feed:** Can 32 fl oz. **Nursing Bottles:** Hospital use. Bot. 8 fl oz. *otc.*
Use: Nutritional supplement.

Isomil DF. (Ross Laboratories) Protein 17.9 g, carbohydrates 67.3 g, fat 36.7 g, Fe 12 mg, Na 293 mg, K 720 mg, with appropriate vitamins and minerals. 676 cal/L. Lactose free. Liq. 960 ml prediluted, ready-to-use cans. *otc.*
Use: Nutritional supplement.

Isomil SF. (Ross Laboratories) Low osmolar sucrose-free soy protein isolate infant formula containing 20 calories/fl oz. **Concentrated Liq.:** Can 13 fl oz. **Ready-to-feed:** Can 32 fl oz. **Nursing Bottles:** Hospital use. Bot. 8 fl oz. *otc.*
Use: Nutritional supplement, enteral.

Isomune-CK. (Roche Laboratories) Rapid immunochemical separation method of the heart specific CK-MB isoenzyme for quantitation when used with an appropriate CK substrate reagent. Test kit 100s, 250s.
Use: Diagnostic aid.

Isomune-LD. (Roche Laboratories)

Rapid immunochemical separation method of the heart specific LD-1 isoenzyme for quantitation when used with an appropriate LD substrate reagent. Test kit 40s, 100s.
Use: Diagnostic aid.

•**isomylamine hydrochloride.** (EYE-so-MILL-ah-meen) USAN.
Use: Muscle relaxant.

isomyn.
See: Amphetamine (Various Mfr.).

Isonate Sublingual. (Major Pharmaceuticals) Isosorbide 2.5 mg, 5 mg/Sublingual Tab. Bot. 100s, 1000s, UD 100s. *Rx.*
Use: Antianginal.

Isonate Tablets. (Major Pharmaceuticals) Isosorbide 5 mg, 10 mg, 20 mg or 30 mg/Tab. **5 mg or 10 mg:** Bot. 100s, 1000s, UD 100s. **20 mg or 30 mg:** Bot. 100s, 1000s. *Rx.*
Use: Antianginal.

Isonate TD-Caps. (Major Pharmaceuticals) Isosorbide 40 mg/TD Cap. Bot. 100s, 1000s. *Rx.*
Use: Antianginal.

Isonate T.R. Tabs. (Major Pharmaceuticals) Isosorbide 40 mg/TR Tab. Bot. 100s, 1000s. *Rx.*
Use: Antianginal.

isoniazid. (eye-so-NYE-uh-zid) (Carolina Medical Products) Isoniazid 50 mg/5 ml. Syr. Bot. Pt. *Rx.*
Use: Antituberculosal.

•**isoniazid.** (eye-so-NYE-uh-zid) U.S.P. 23.
Use: Anti-infective (tuberculostatic).
See: Dow-Isoniazid, Tab. (Hoechst Marion Roussel).
INH, Tab. (Novartis Pharmaceutical Corp.).
Laniazid, Syr. (Lannett Co., Inc.).
Nydrazid, Inj. (Bristol-Myers Squibb).
Nydrazid, Tab. (Marsam Pharmaceuticals, Inc.).
Calpas-INH, Tab. (American Chem. & Drug).
W/Calcium p-aminosalicylate, vitamin B_6.
See: Calpas Isoxine, Tab. (American Chem. & Drug).
Calpas-INAH-6, Tab. (American Chem. & Drug).
W/Pyridoxine HCl (vitamin B_6).
See: Niadox, Tab. (PBH Wesley Jessen).
Teebaconin w/B_6 (Consolidated Midland Corp.).
Pasna, Tri-Pack 300, Gran. (PBH Wesley Jessen).
W/Rifampin.
See: Rifater, Tab. (Hoechst Marion Roussel).

isoniazid. (Various Mfr.) 50 mg/Tab. Bot. 100s, 500, 1000s.
Use: Anti-infective (tuberculostatic).

isonicotinic acid hydrazide.
See: Isoniazid, U.S.P. 23 (Various Mfr.).

isonicotinyl hydrazide.
See: Isoniazid, U.S.P. 23 (Various Mfr.).

isonipecaine hydrochloride.
See: Meperidine Hydrochloride, U.S.P. 23 (Various Mfr.).

isopentaquine.
Use: Antimalarial.

isophane insulin suspension.
Use: Hypoglycemic agent.
See: Humulin, Vial (Eli Lilly and Co.).
insulin, isophane.
Novolin, Vial (Novo/Nordisk Pharm, Inc.).
NPH Insulin, Vial (Novo/Nordisk Pharm, Inc.).
NPH Iletin, Vial (Eli Lilly and Co.).

isophane insulin suspension/insulin injection.
Use: Antidiabetic.
See: Humulin 50/50 (Eli Lilly and Co.).
Humulin 70/30 (Eli Lilly and Co.).
Novolin 70/30 (Novo/Nordisk Pharm, Inc.).
Novolin 70/30 Penfill (Novo/Nordisk Pharm, Inc.).

isopregnenone.
See: Dydrogesterone.

Isoprinosine. (Newport Pharmaceuticals) Inosine pranobex.
Use: Antiviral, immunomodulator.

isoprophenamine hydrochloride. Name used for Clorprenaline HCl.

isopropicillin potassium.
Use: Anti-infective.

•**isopropyl alcohol.** (eye-so-PRO-pill AL-koe-hahl) U.S.P. 23.
Use: Topical anti-infective; pharmaceutic aid (solvent).

isopropyl alcohol spray. (Morton) Isopropyl alcohol w/propellant. Aer. Can 6 oz. *otc.*
Use: Anti-infective.

isopropylarterenol hydrochloride.
Use: Asthma, vasoconstrictor and allergic states.

isopropylarterenol sulfate.
See: Isoproterenol Sulfate.

•**isopropyl myristate.** N.F. 18.
Use: Pharmaceutic aid (emollient).

iso-noradrenaline.
See: Isoproterenol.

isopropyl-noradrenaline hydrochloride.
See: Isoproterenol HCl, U.S.P. 23.

•**isopropyl palmitate.** N.F. 18.

Use: Pharmaceutic aid (oleaginous vehicle).

isopropyl phenazone. 4-Isopropyl antipyrine. Larodon.

isopropyl rubbing alcohol.
Use: Rubefacient, solvent.

isoproterenol. (eye-so-pro-TER-uh-nahl)
See: Norisodrine (Abbott Laboratories).
W/Butabarbital, theophylline, ephedrine HCl.
See: Medihaler-Iso, Vial (3M Pharm.).

•**isoproterenol hydrochloride.** (eye-so-pro-TER-uh-nahl) U.S.P. 23.
Use: Bronchodilator, vasoconstrictor.
See: Isuprel HCl, Prods. (Sanofi Winthrop Pharmaceuticals).
Medihaler-ISO (3M Pharm.).
Norisodrine, Aerotrol, Syr. (Abbott Laboratories).
W/Aminophylline, ephedrine sulfate, phenobarbital.
See: Asminorel, Tab. (Solvay Pharmaceuticals).
W/Clopane (clopentamine) HCl, propylene glycol, ascorbic acid.
See: Aerolone Compound, Soln. (Eli Lilly and Co.).

isoproterenol hydrochloride. (Various Mfr.) 0.2 mg/ml (1:5000 solution), 0.02 mg/ml (1:50,000 solution). Inj. Amp. 5 ml (0.2 mg only), 10 ml. *Rx.*
Use: Bronchodilator, sympathomimetic.

•**isoproterenol sulfate.** (eye-so-pro-TER-uh-nahl) U.S.P. 23.
Use: Bronchodilator.
See: Medihaler-Iso, Vial (3M Pharm.).
W/Calcium iodide (anhydrous), alcohol.
See: Norisodrine, Syr. (Abbott Laboratories).

Isoptin. (Knoll Pharmaceuticals) Verapamil HCl 5 mg/2 ml. Inj. 2 ml and 4 ml amps, vials and disp. syringes. *Rx.*
Use: Calcium channel blocker.

Isoptin SR. (Knoll Pharmaceuticals) Verapamil HCl 120 mg, 180 mg, 240 mg. Tab. Bot. 100s, 500s, UD 100s. *Rx.*
Use: Calcium channel blocker.

Isoptin Tablets. (Knoll Pharmaceuticals) Verapamil HCl 40 mg, 80 mg, 120 mg. Tab. Bot. 100s, 500s, 1000s, UD 100s. *Rx.*
Use: Calcium channel blocker.

Isopto Alkaline. (Alcon Laboratories, Inc.) Hydroxypropyl methylcellulose 1%, benzalkonium Cl 0.01%. Sterile ophthalmic soln. Dropper bot. 15 ml. *otc.*
Use: Artificial tears.

Isopto Atropine. (Alcon Laboratories, Inc.) Atropine sulfate 0.5%, 1%. **0.5%:** Drop-Tainer 5 ml. **1%:** Drop-Tainer 5 ml, 15 ml. *Rx.*
Use: Cycloplegic, mydriatic.

Isopto Carbachol. (Alcon Laboratories, Inc.) Carbachol U.S.P. 0.75%, 1.5%, 2.25%, 3%, in a sterile buffered solution of methylcellulose 1%. **2.25%:** Drop-Tainer 15 ml. **0.75%, 1.5%, or 3%:** Drop-Tainer 15 ml, 30 ml. *Rx.*
Use: Antiglaucoma agent.

Isopto Carpine. (Alcon Laboratories, Inc.) Pilocarpine HCl 0.5%, 1%, 2%, 4%, 5%, 6%, 8%. Soln. Bot. 15 ml, 30 ml (except 5%). *Rx.*
Use: Antiglaucoma agent.

Isopto Cetamide. (Alcon Laboratories, Inc.) Sodium sulfacetamide 15%. Soln. Drop-Tainer 5 ml, 15 ml. *Rx.*
Use: Anti-infective, ophthalmic.

Isopto Cetapred. (Alcon Laboratories, Inc.) Sulfacetamide sodium 10%, prednisolone 0.25%. Susp. Drop-Tainer 5 ml, 15 ml. *Rx.*
Use: Anti-infective, corticosteroid, ophthalmic.

Isopto Frin. (Alcon Laboratories, Inc.) Phenylephrine HCl 0.12% in a methylcellulose Soln. Drop-Tainer 15 ml. *Rx.*
Use: Mydriatic, vasoconstrictor.

Isopto Homatropine. (Alcon Laboratories, Inc.) Homatropine HBr 2%, 5%. Soln. Drop-Tainer 5 ml, 15 ml. *Rx.*
Use: Cycloplegic, mydriatic.

Isopto Hyoscine. (Alcon Laboratories, Inc.) Hyoscine HBr 0.25%. Soln. Drop-Tainer 5 ml, 15 ml. *Rx.*
Use: Cycloplegic, mydriatic.

Isopto Plain. (Alcon Laboratories, Inc.) Hydroxypropyl methylcellulose 2910 0.5%, benzalkonium Cl 0.01%, sodium Cl, sodium phosphate, sodium citrate. Drop-Tainer 15 ml. *otc.*
Use: Artificial tears.

Isopto Tears. (Alcon Laboratories, Inc.) Hydroxypropyl methylcellulose 0.5%, benzalkonium Cl 0.01%, sodium Cl, sodium phosphate, sodium citrate. Bot. Drop-Tainer 15 ml, 30 ml. *otc.*
Use: Artificial tears.

Isordil Sublingual. (Wyeth-Ayerst Laboratories) Isosorbide dinitrate 2.5 mg, 5 mg, 10 mg/Tab. **2.5 mg or 5 mg:** Bot. 100s, 500s, Redi-pak 100s. **10 mg:** Bot. 100s. *Rx.*
Use: Antianginal.

Isordil Tembids. (Wyeth-Ayerst Laboratories) Isosorbide dinitrate 40 mg/Tab. or Cap. **SR Tab.:** Bot. 100s, 500s, 1000s. **SR Cap.:** Bot. 100s, 500s. *Rx.*
Use: Antianginal.

Isordil Titradose Tablets. (Wyeth-Ayerst Laboratories) Isosorbide dinitrate 5 mg, 10 mg, 20 mg, 30 mg, 40 mg/Tab. **5**

mg, 10 mg: Bot. 100s, 500s, 1000s, Redi-pak 100s. **20 mg, 30 mg:** Bot. 100s, 500s, Redi-pak 100s. **40 mg:** Bot. 100s, Redi-pak 100s. *Rx.*
Use: Antianginal.

Isorgen-G. (Grafton) Isosorbide 5 mg, 10 mg/Tab. Bot. 1000s. *Rx.*
Use: Antianginal.

•**isosorbide concentrate.** (EYE-sos-ORE-bide) U.S.P. 23.
Use: Diuretic.

•**isosorbide dinitrate diluted.** (EYE-sos-ORE-bide die-NYE-trate) U.S.P. 23.
Use: Coronary vasodilator.
See: Dilatrate-SR, Cap. (Schwarz Pharma, Inc.).
Iso-Bid, Cap. (Roberts Pharmaceuticals)
Iso-D, Tab., Cap. (Dunhall Pharmaceuticals, Inc.).
Isordil, Tab. (Wyeth-Ayerst Laboratories).
Isordil Tembids Cap., Tab. (Wyeth-Ayerst Laboratories).
Nitromed, Tab. (U.S. Ethicals).
Onset, Tab. (Sanofi Winthrop Pharmaceuticals).
Sorbitrate, Tab. (Zeneca Pharmaceuticals).
W/Phenobarbital.
See: Sorbitrate w/Phenobarbital, Tab. (Zeneca Pharmaceuticals).

isosorbide dinitrate. (Various Mfr.) **Sublingual:** 2.5 mg, 5 mg, 10 mg. **2.5 mg:** Bot. 100s, 500s, 1000s, UD 100s. **5 mg:** Bot. 100s, 1000s, UD 100s. **10 mg:** Bot. 100s, 1000s. **Oral:** 5 mg, 10 mg, 20 mg, 30 mg/Tab. 40 mg/SR Tab. **5 mg:** Bot. 100s, 1000s, UD 100s. **10 mg:** Bot. 100s, 500s, 1000s, UD 100s. **20 mg:** Bot. 90s, 100s, 120s, 180s, 240s, 360s, 500s, 1000s, UD 100s. **30 mg:** Bot. 100s, 500s, 1000s, UD 100s. **40 mg:** Bot. 90s, 100s, 250s, 1000s, UD 100s. *Rx.*
Use: Coronary vasodilator.

•**isosorbide mononitrate.** (EYE-sos-ORE-bide MAH-no-NYE-trate) USAN.
Use: Coronary vasodilator.
See: Imdur, ER Tab. (Key Pharmaceuticals).
ISMO, Tab. (Wyeth-Ayerst Laboratories).
Isotrate ER (Apothecon).
Monoket, Tab. (Schwarz Pharma, Inc.).

isosorbide mononitrate. (Teva) 20 mg, lactose. Tab. Bot. 100s, 500s. *Rx.*
Use: Coronary vasodilator.

isosorbide mononitrate. (Kremers Urban) 60 mg, methylcellulose, lactose. ER Tab. Bot. 100s. *Rx.*
Use: Coronary vasodilator.

isosorbide oral solution.
Use: Diuretic.

Isosource. (Novartis Pharmaceutical Corp.) Protein (Ca and Na caseinate, soy protein isolate) 43.2 g, carbohydrate (maltodextrin) 1755 g, fat (MCT, canola oil, lecithin) 443.9 g, Na 760 mg, K 1182 mg, mOsm/kg H_2O 390, Cal/ml 1.2, vitamins A, B_1, B_2, B_3, B_5, B_6, B_{12}, C, D, E, K, FA, biotin, choline, Ca, Cl, Cu, Fe, I, Mg, Mn, P, Zn, Se, Cr, Mo. Liq. Bot. 250 ml, 1000 ml. *otc.*
Use: Nutritional supplement.

Isosource HN. (Novartis Pharmaceutical Corp.) Protein (Ca and Na caseinate, soy protein isolate) 56.1 g, carbohydrate (maltodextrin) 165 g, fat (MCT, canola oil, lecithin) 43.9 g, Na 760 mg, K 1772 mg, mOsm/kg H_2O 390, Cal/ml 1.2, vitamins A, B_1, B_2, B_3, B_5, B_6, B_{12}, C, D, E, K, FA, biotin, choline, Ca, P, I, Fe, Mg, Cu, Zn, Cl, Mn, Se, Cr, Mo. Liq. Bot. 250 ml, 1000 ml. *otc.*
Use: Nutritional supplement.

•**isostearyl alcohol.** (EYE-so-STEE-rill) USAN.
Use: Pharmaceutic aid (emollient, solvent).

•**isosulfan blue.** (EYE-so-SULL-fan) USAN.
Use: Diagnostic aid, lymphangiography.
See: Lymphazurin (United States Surgical Corp.).

Isotein HN. (Novartis Pharmaceutical Corp.) Vanilla Flavor. Maltodextrin, delactosed lactalbumin, partially hydrogenated soy oil with BHA, fructose, medium chain triglycerides, artificial flavor, sodium caseinate, mono- and diglycerides, sodium Cl, vitamins, minerals. Pow. Packet 2.75 oz. *otc.*
Use: Nutritional supplement.

•**isotiquimide.** (eye-so-TIH-kwih-MIDE) USAN.
Use: Antiulcerative.

Isotrate ER. (Apothecon) Isosoribide mononitrate 60 mg, lactose. ER Tab. Bot. 100s, 500s. *Rx.*
Use: Coronary vasodilator.

•**isotretinoin.** (EYE-so-TREH-tin-NO-in) U.S.P. 23.
Use: Keratolytic.
See: Accutane, Cap. (Roche Laboratories).

•**isotretinoin anisatil.** (eye-so-TRETT-ih-noyn ah-NIH-sah-till) USAN.
Use: Dermatologic, acne.

isovorin. (ESI Lederle Generics) L-leucovorin.
Use: Antineoplastic. [Orphan Drug]

Isovue-128. (Bracco Diagnostics) Iopamidol 261 mg, iodine 128 mg/ml. Inj. Vial 50 ml. *Rx.*
Use: Radiopaque agent.

Isovue-200. (Bracco Diagnostics) Iopamidol 408 mg, iodine 200 mg/ml. Inj. Vial 50 ml. Bot. 100 ml, 200 ml. *Rx.*
Use: Radiopaque agent.

Isovue-250. (Bracco Diagnostics) Iopamidol 510 mg, iodine 250 mg/ml. Inj. Vial 50 ml. Bot. 100 ml, 150 ml, 200 ml. Power Injector Syr. 150 ml. Bulk pkg. 200 ml. *Rx.*
Use: Radiopaque agent.

Isovue-300. (Bracco Diagnostics) Iopamidol 612 mg, iodine 300 mg/ml, tromethamine, edetate calcium disodium. Inj. Vial 30 ml, 50 ml. Bot. 75 ml, 100 ml, 150 ml w/wo infusion sets. Power Injector Syr. 150 ml, Bulk pkg. 200 ml, 500 ml. *Rx.*
Use: Radiopaque agent.

Isovue-370. (Bracco Diagnostics) Iopamidol 755 mg, iodine 370 mg/ml, tromethamine, edetate calcium disodium. Inj. Vial 20 ml, 30 ml, 50 ml. Bot. 50 ml, 75 ml, 100 ml, 125 ml, 150 ml, 175 ml, 200 ml. Power Injector Syr. 75 ml, 100 ml, Bulk pkg. 200 ml, 500 ml. *Rx.*
Use: Radiopaque agent.

Isovue-M 200. (Bracco Diagnostics) Iopamidol 408 mg, iodine 200 mg/ml, tromethamine, edetate calcium disodium. Vial 10 ml, 20 ml. *Rx.*
Use: Radiopaque agent.

Isovue-M 300. (Bracco Diagnostics) Iopamidol 612 mg, iodine 300 mg/ml. Inj. tromethamine, edetate calcium disodium. Vial 15 ml. *Rx.*
Use: Radiopaque agent.

•**isoxepac.** (EYE-SOX-eh-pack) USAN.
Use: Anti-inflammatory.

•**isoxicam.** (eye-SOX-ih-kam) USAN.
Use: Anti-inflammatory.

•**isoxsuprine hydrochloride.** (eye-SOX-you-preen) U.S.P. 23.
Use: Vasodilator.
See: Vasodilan, Tab. (Bristol-Myers Squibb).

I-Soyalac. (Mt. Vernon Foods, Inc.) P-soy protein isolate, l-methionine, CHO-sucrose, tapioca dextrin. F-soy oil, soy lecithin. Corn free. Protein 20.2 g, carbohydrate 63.4 g, fat 35.5 g, iron 12 mg, 640 Cal/serving (1 qt). Concentrate 390 ml, ready-to-use 1 qt. *otc.*
Use: Nutritional supplement.

•**isradipine.** (iss-RAHD-ih-peen) USAN.
Use: Calcium channel blocker; antagonist (calcium channel).
See: DynaCirc (Novartis Pharmaceutical Corp.).

I-Sulfacet. (American Pharmaceutical Co.) Sulfacetamide sodium 10%, 15%, 30% ophthalmic soln. Bot. 2 ml, 5 ml, 15 ml. *Rx.*
Use: Anti-infective, ophthalmic.

I-Sulfalone Suspension. (American Pharmaceutical Co.) Sulfacetamide sodium 100 mg, prednisolone acetate 5 mg. Ophthalmic susp. Bot. 5 ml, 15 ml. *Rx.*
Use: Anti-infective, ophthalmic.

Isuprel Inhalation Solution. (Sanofi Winthrop Pharmaceuticals) Isoproterenol HCl 0.5% (1:200), 1% (1:100). Soln. for Inh. Bot. 10 ml. *Rx.*
Use: Bronchodilator, sympathomimetic.

Isuprel Mistometer. (Sanofi Winthrop Pharmaceuticals) Isoproterenol HCl 103 mcg/dose. Aer. Bot. 15 ml. Refill 15 ml. *Rx.*
Use: Bronchodilator, sympathomimetic.

Isuprel Sterile Injection. (Sanofi Winthrop Pharmaceuticals) Isoproterenol HCl 0.2 mg/ml with sodium metabisulfite in 1:5000 solution. Inj. Amp. *Rx.*
Use: Bronchodilator, sympathomimetic.

isuprene.
See: Isoproterenol (Various Mfr.)

•**itasetron.** (eye-tah-SEH-trahn) USAN.
Use: Antidepressant; antiemetic; anxiolytic.

•**itazigrel.** (ih-TAY-zih-GRELL) USAN.
Use: Platelet aggregation inhibitor.

Itchaway. (Moyco Union Broach Division) Zinc undecylenate 20%, undecylenic acid 2%. Pow. Can 1.5 oz. *otc.*
Use: Antifungal, topical.

Itch-X. (B.F. Ascher and Co.) Pramoxine HCl 1%. **Gel:** Benzyl alcohol, aloe vera gel, diazolidinyl urea, SD alcohol 40, parabens. 35.4 g. **Spray:** Benzyl alcohol, aloe vera gel, SD alcohol 40. In 60 ml. *otc.*
Use: Anesthetic, local.

itobarbital.
W/Acetaminophen.
See: Panitol, Tab. (Wesley Pharmacal Co., Inc.).

•**itraconazole.** (ih-truh-KAHN-uh-zole) USAN.
Use: Antifungal.
See: Sporanox, Cap. (Janssen Pharmaceutical, Inc.).

I-Trol. (Akorn, Inc.) Neomycin sulfate-polymyxin B sulfate-dexamethasone

0.1%. Ophthalmic susp. Bot. 5 ml. *Rx.*
Use: Anti-infective, corticosteroid, ophthalmic.

I-Valex-1. (Ross Laboratories) Protein 15 g, fat 23.9 g, carbohydrates 46.3 g, linoleic acid 1800 mg, Fe 9 mg, Na 190 mg, K 675 mg, with appropriate vitamins and minerals. 480 Cal/100 g. Leucine free. Pow. Can 350 g. *otc.*
Use: Nutritional supplement.

I-Valex-2. (Ross Laboratories) Protein 30 g, fat 15.5 g, carbohyrates 30 g, Na 880 mg, K 1370 mg, with appropriate vitamins and minerals. 410 Cal/100 g. Leucine free. Pow. Can 325 g. *otc.*
Use: Nutritional supplement.

Ivarest. (Blistex, Inc.) Calamine 14%, benzocaine 5%. **Cream:** 60 g. **Lot.:** 120 ml. *otc.*
Use: Dermatologic, poison ivy.

Iveegam. (Immune Respone Corp.) Immune globulin 50 mg/ml IgG/Pow. for Inj. in 1000 mg with diluent, double-ended spike and filter needle; and 2500 and 5000 mg with diluent, double-ended spike and infusion set with filter. *Rx.*
Use: Immunization.

•**ivermectin.** (eye-VER-MEK-tin) USAN.
Use: Antiparasitic.

Ivocort. (Roberts Pharmaceuticals) Micronized hydrocortisone alcohol 0.5%, 1%. Bot. 4 oz. *otc.*
Use: Corticosteroid, topical.

Ivy-Chex. (Jones Medical Industries, Inc.) Polyvinyl pyrrolidone-vinyl acetate, benzalkonium Cl 1:1000 in alcohol acetone base. Aerosol Can 4 oz. *otc.*
Use: Dermatologic, poison ivy.

Ivy Dry. (Ivy Corporation) Tannic acid 10%, isopropyl alcohol 12.5% Liq. 4 oz. Cream 1 oz, 6 oz. *otc.*
Use: Poison ivy therapy, topical.

Ivy-Rid. (Roberts Pharmaceuticals) Polyvinyl pyrrolidone-vinyl acetate, benzalkonium Cl. Spray can 2.75 oz. *otc.*
Use: Poison ivy therapy, topical.

I-Wash. (Akorn, Inc.) Phosphate buffered saline soln. Bot. 4 oz, 8 oz. *otc.*
Use: Irrigant, ophthalmic.

I-White. (Akorn, Inc.) Phenylephrine 0.12%, polyvinyl alcohol, hydroxyethyl cellulose. Soln. Bot. 15 ml. *otc.*
Use: Mydriatic, vasoconstrictor.

Izonid. (Major Pharmaceuticals) Isoniazid 300 mg/Tab. Bot. 100s. *Rx.*
Use: Antituberculosal.

J

jalovis.
See: Hyaluronidase (Various Mfr.).

Janimine. (Abbott Laboratories) Imipramine HCl 10 mg, 25 mg or 50 mg/Tab. Bot. 100s, 1000s. *Rx.*
Use: Antidepressant.

japan agar.
See: Agar (Various Mfr.).

japan gelatin.
See: Agar (Various Mfr.).

japan isinglass.
See: Agar (Various Mfr.).

japanese encephalitis virus vaccine.
Use: Immunization.
See: JE-VAX.

JE-VAX. (Pasteur Merieux Connaught) Japanese encephalitis virus vaccine 2 to 3 mcg nitrogen content per ml. Pow. for Inj. single-dose vial with 1.3 ml diluent; 10-dose vial with 11 ml diluent. *Rx.*
Use: Immunization.

Jenest-28. (Organon Teknika Corp.) 7 white tablets norethindrone 0.5 mg, ethinyl estradiol 35 mcg; 14 peach tablets norethindrone 1 mg, ethinyl estradiol 35 mcg; 7 inert tablets. Cyclic dispenser of 28. *Rx.*
Use: Contraceptive.

Jeri-Bath. (Dermik Laboratories, Inc.) Concentrated moisturizing bath oil. Plastic Bot. 8 oz. *otc.*
Use: Dermatologic.

Jets. (Freeda Vitamins, Inc.) Lysine 300 mg, vitamins C 25 mg, B_{12} 25 mcg, B_6 5 mg, B_1 10 mg/Chew. Tab. Bot. 30s, 250s, 500s. *otc.*
Use: Vitamin supplement.

Jevity Liquid. (Ross Laboratories) Calcium and sodium caseinates, soy fiber, hydrolyzed cornstarch, MCT (fractionated coconut oil) soy oil, corn oil, soy lecithin, vitamins A, B_1, B_2, B_3, B_5, B_6, B_{12}, C, D, E, K, folic acid, biotin, choline, Ca, P, Mg, Fe, Mn, Cu, Zn, I, Cl. In 240 ml. *otc.*
Use: Nutritional supplement.

Jiffy. (Block Drug Co., Inc.) Benzocaine, menthol, eugenol in glycerin-water base with SD alcohol 38-B 76%. Bot. 0.125 oz. *otc.*
Use: Anesthetic, local.

J-Liberty. (J Pharmacal) Chlordiazepoxide HCl 5 mg, 10 mg or 25 mg/Cap. *C-IV.*
Use: Anxiolytic.

Johnson's Baby Cream. (Johnson & Johnson) Dimethicone 2%. Jar 4 oz, 6 oz, Tube 2 oz. *otc.*
Use: Dermatologic protectant.

Johnson's Baby Sunblock Cream. (Johnson & Johnson) Octyl methoxycinnamate, octyl salicylate, oxybenzone, titanium dioxide, benzyl alcohol, cetyl alcohol. PABA free. SPF 15. Waterproof. Cream. Bot. 60 g. *otc.*
Use: Sunscreen.

Johnson's Baby Sunblock Extra Protection. (Johnson & Johnson) Octyl methoxycinnamate, octyl salicylate, titanium dioxide, oxybenzone, C12-15 alcohols benzoate, cetyl alcohol, EDTA, vitamin E. Lot. Bot. 120 ml. *otc.*
Use: Sunscreen.

Johnson's Baby Sunblock Lotion. (Johnson & Johnson) **SPF 15:** Octyl methoxycinnamate, octyl salicylate, oxybenzone, titanium dioxide, benzyl alcohol, cetyl alcohol. PABA free. Waterproof. Bot. 60 g. **SPF 30:** Benzophenone-3, octyl methoxycinnamate, octyl salicylate, titanium dioxide. PABA free. Waterproof. Bot. 120 ml. *otc.*
Use: Sunscreen.

Johnson's Medicated Powder. (Johnson & Johnson) Bentonite, kaolin, talc, zinc oxide. Pow. Small, Medium, Large. *otc.*
Use: Diaper rash preparation.

•**josamycin.** (JOE-sah-MYsin) USAN.
Use: Anti-infective.

Junior Strength Advil. (Whitehall Robins Laboratories) Ibuprofen 100 mg, sucrose, parabens/Tab. Bot. 24s. *otc.*
Use: Analgesic, NSAID.

Junior-Strength Feverall. (Upsher-Smith Labs, Inc.) Acetaminophen 120 mg or 325 mg/Supp. Pkg 6s. *otc.*
Use: Analgesic.

Junior Strength Motrin. (Ortho McNeil Pharmaceutical) Ibuprofen 100 mg, phenylalanine 6 mg, aspartame/Chew. Tab. Bot. 24s. *otc.*
Use: Analgesic, NSAID.

Junior Strength Panadol. (Bayer Corp (Consumer Div.)) Acetaminophen 160 mg. Capl. 30s. *otc.*
Use: Analgesic.

•**juniper tar.** (JOO-nih-per tar) U.S.P. 23.
Use: Local antieczematic, pharmaceutic necessity.

Junyer-All. (Barth's) Vitamins A 6000 IU, D 400 IU, B_1 3 mg, B_2 6 mg, C 120 mg, niacin 1 mg, E 12 IU, B_{12} 10 mcg, calcium 217 mg, phosphorus 97.5 mg, red bone marrow 10 mg, organic iron 15 mg, iodine 0.1 mg, beef peptone 20 mg/2 Cap. Bot. 10 month, 3 month, 6 month supply. *otc.*
Use: Vitamin supplement.

Just Tears. (Blairex Labs, Inc.) Benzalkonium chloride, EDTA, NaCl, polyvinyl alcohol 1.4%. Soln. Bot. 15 ml. *otc.*
Use: Lubricant, ophthalmic.

juvocaine.
See: Procaine HCl (Various Mfr.).

K

K-1. Phytonadione.
Use: Vitamin K.
See: Mephyton, Tab. (Merck & Co.).
Aqua MEPHYTON, Inj. (Merck & Co.).

K-4. Menadiol sodium diphosphate.
Use: Vitamin K.

K+8. (Alra Laboratories, Inc.) Potassium chloride 8 mEq. ER Tab. Bot. 100s, 500s. *Rx.*
Use: Electrolyte supplement.

K+10. (Alra Laboratories, Inc.) Potassium Cl 10 mEq/Tab. Bot. 100s, 500s, 1000s. *Rx.*
Use: Electrolyte supplement.

K 34. Hexachlorophene.

K + Care. (Alra Laboratories, Inc.) Potassium chloride, saccharin. Soln. Pkt. 15, 20, 25 mEq, 30s, 100s. *Rx.*
Use: Electrolyte supplement.

Kabikinase. (Pharmacia & Upjohn) Streptokinase 250,000 IU, 600,000 IU, 750,000 IU or 1,500,000 IU/vial. Pow. for inj. Vial 5 ml, 10 ml. *Rx.*
Use: Thrombolytic.

Kadian. (Faulding) Morphine sulfate 20 mg, 50 mg, 100 mg, sucrose/SR Cap. Bot. 60s. *c-II.*
Use: Analgesic, narcotic.

Kaergona.
See: Menadione (Various Mfr.).

Kala. (Freeda Vitamins, Inc.) Soy-based acidophilus 2 million units/Tab. Bot. 100s, 250s, 500s. *otc.*
Use: Nutritional supplement.

•**kalafungin.** (kal-ah-FUN-jin) USAN.
Use: Antifungal.

Kalory-Plus. (Tyler) Thyroid 3 gr, amphetamine sulfate 15 mg, atropine sulfate 1/180 gr, aloin 0.25 gr, phenobarbital 0.25 gr/TR cap. Bot. 100s, 1000s.
Use: Anorexiant.

Kaltostat. (SmithKline Beecham Pharmaceuticals) Calcium-sodium alginate fiber, 3″ × 4¾″ sterile dressing. In 1s. *otc.*
Use: Dressing, hydroactive.

Kaltostat Forte. (SmithKline Beecham Pharmaceuticals) Calcium-sodium alginate fiber, 4″ × 4″ sterile dressing. In 1s. *otc.*
Use: Dressing, hydroactive.

Kamfolene. (Wade) Camphor, menthol, methyl salicylate, turpentine and eucalyptus oils, carbolic acid 2%, calamine, zinc oxide in lanolin base. Jar 2 oz, lb. *otc.*
Use: Antiseptic.

•**kanamycin sulfate.** (kan-uh-MY-sin) U.S.P. 23.
Use: Anti-infective.
See: Kantrex, Cap., Vial (Bristol-Myers Squibb).

Kank-A. (Blistex, Inc.) Benzocaine 5%, cetylpyridinium chloride, castor oil, benzoin compound. Liq. Bot. 3.75 ml. *otc.*
Use: Anesthetic, local.

Kantrex. (Bristol-Myers Squibb) Kanamycin sulfate. **Cap.:** 0.5 g. Bot. 20s, 100s. **Vial.:** 0.5 g/2 ml or 1 g/3 ml. **Pediatric Inj.:** 75 mg/2 ml. **Disposable Syringe:** 500 mg/2 ml. *Rx.*
Use: Anti-infective aminoglycoside.

Kaochlor 10% Liquid. (Pharmacia & Upjohn) Potassium and chloride 20 mEq/15 ml (potassium Cl 10%), alcohol 5%, saccharin, FD&C Yellow No. 5. Bot. pt. *Rx.*
Use: Electrolyte supplement.

Kaochlor-Eff. (Pharmacia & Upjohn) Elemental potassium 20 mEq, chloride 20 mEq/Tab. Supplied by: Potassium Cl 0.6 g, potassium citrate 0.22 g, potassium bicarbonate 1 g, betaine HCl 1.84 g, saccharin 20 mg, artificial fruit flavor, tartrazine (color)/Tab. Sugar free. Carton 60s. *Rx.*
Use: Electrolyte supplement.

Kaochlor S-F 10%. (Pharmacia & Upjohn) Potassium 20 mEq, chloride 20 mEq/15 ml, saccharin, flavoring, alcohol 5%. Sugar free. Liq. Bot. 4 oz, pt. *Rx.*
Use: Electrolyte supplement.

Kaodene Non-Narcotic. (Pfeiffer Co.) Kaolin 3.9 g, pectin 194.4 mg/30 ml, bismuth subsalicylate. Alcohol free. Liq. Bot. 120 ml.
Use: Antidiarrheal.

Kaodene with Codeine. (Pfeiffer Co.) Codeine phosphate 32.4 mg, kaolin 3.9 g, pectin 194.4 mg, sodium carboxymethylcellulose, bismuth subsalicylate/30 ml. Susp. Bot. 120 ml. *otc.*
Use: Antidiarrheal.

•**kaolin.** (KAY-oh-lin) U.S.P. 23.
Use: Adsorbent.
W/Belladonna, phenobarbital.
See: Bellkata, Tab. (Ferndale Laboratories, Inc.).
W/Bismuth compound.
See: Kaomine, Pow. (Eli Lilly and Co.).
W/Bismuth subgallate.
See: Diastop, Liq. (ICN Pharmaceuticals, Inc.).
W/Bismuth subgallate, pectin, zinc phenolsulfonate, opium powder.
See: Diastay, Tab. (ICN Pharmaceuticals, Inc.).

W/Cornstarch, camphor, zinc oxide, eucalyptus oil.
  See: Mexsana, Pow. (Schering-Plough Corp.).
W/Furazolidone, pectin.
  See: Furoxone, Liq. (Eaton Medical Corp.).
W/Hyoscyamine sulfate, sodium benzoate, atropine sulfate, hyoscine HBR, pectin.
  See: Donnagel, Susp. (Wyeth-Ayerst Laboratories).
W/Neomycin sulfate, pectin.
  See: Pecto-Kalin, Liq. (Harvey).
W/Pectin.
  See: Kaopectate, Liq. (Pharmacia & Upjohn).
  Kapectin, Liq. (Health for Life Brands, Inc.).
  Pecto-Kalin, Susp. (Teva Pharmaceuticals USA).
  B-K-P Mixture, Liq. (Sutliff & Case).
W/Pectin, bismuth subcarbonate, belladonna.
  See: Kay-Pec, Liq. (Case).
W/Pectin, bismuth subcarbonate, opium powder.
  See: Palsorb Improved, Liq. (Roberts Pharmaceuticals).
W/Pectin, pow. opium extract.
  See: Pecto-Kalin, Susp. (Teva Pharmaceuticals USA).
W/Pectin, opium pow., bismuth subgallate, zinc phenolsulfonate.
  See: Cholactabs, Tab. (Roxane Laboratories, Inc.).
  B.P.P., Tab. (Teva Pharmaceuticals USA).
W/Pectin, paregoric (equivalent).
  See: Duosorb, Liq. (Solvay Pharmaceuticals).
  Kaoparin, Liq. (McKesson Drug Co.).
  Kapectin, Liq. (Health for Life Brands, Inc.).
  Ka-Pek w/Paregoric, Liq. (APC).
W/Pectin, zinc phenolsulfonate.
  See: Pectocel, Susp. (Eli Lilly and Co.).
W/Phenobarbital, atropine sulfate, aluminum hydroxide gel.
  See: Kao-Lumin, Tab. (Roxane Laboratories, Inc.).

kaolin colloidal.
W/Bismuth subcarbonate.
  See: Bisilad, Susp. (Schwarz Pharma, Inc.).
W/Magnesium trisilicate, aluminum hydroxide dried gel.
  See: Kamadrox, Tab. (ICN Pharmaceuticals, Inc.).
  Kathmagel, Tab. (Mason Pharmaceuticals, Inc.).
W/Pectin, aromatics.
  See: Paocin, Susp. (SmithKline Beecham Pharmaceuticals).

kaolin w/pectin. (KAY-oh-lin with PECK-tin) (Various Mfr.) Kaolin 90 g, pectin 2 g/30 ml. Susp. Bot. 180 ml, pt, UD 30 ml. *otc.*
  Use: Antidiarrheal combination.

Kaon Cl. (Pharmacia & Upjohn) Potassium Cl 500 mg, FD&C Yellow No. 5. CR Tab. Bot. 100s, 250s, 1000s. *Rx.*
  Use: Electrolyte supplement.

Kaon Cl-10. (Pharmacia & Upjohn) Potassium Cl 750 mg/CR Tab. Bot. 100s, 500s, 1000s. Stat-Pak 100s. *Rx.*
  Use: Electrolyte supplement.

Kaon-Cl 20%. (Pharmacia & Upjohn) Potassium and chloride 40 mEq (to potassium Cl 3 g)/15 ml, saccharin, flavoring, alcohol 5%. Bot. Pt. *Rx.*
  Use: Electrolyte supplement.

Kaon Elixir. (Pharmacia & Upjohn) Elemental potassium 20 mEq (as potassium gluconate 4.68 g)/15 ml, aromatics, grape and lemon-lime flavors, alcohol 5%, saccharin. Unit pkg. Pt, gal. *Rx.*
  Use: Electrolyte supplement.

Kaon Tablets. (Pharmacia & Upjohn) Elemental potassium 5 mEq obtained from potassium gluconate 1.17 g/SC Tab. Bot. 100s, 500s. *Rx.*
  Use: Electrolyte supplement.

Kaopectate. (Pharmacia & Upjohn) Kaolin 5.85 g, pectin 130 mg/oz. Liq. Bot. 8 oz, 12 oz, 16 oz, 1 gal, UD pkg. 3 oz. *otc.*
  Use: Antidiarrheal.

Kaopectate, Advanced Formula. (Pharmacia & Upjohn) Attapulgite 750 mg/15 ml, sucrose, methylparaben, alcohol free. Regular and peppermint flavor. Liq. Bot. 354 ml. *otc.*
  Use: Antidiarrheal combination.

Kaopectate, Children's. (Pharmacia & Upjohn) Attapulgite 600 mg/15 ml. Liq. Bot. 180 ml. *otc.*
  Use: Antidiarrheal combination.

Kaopectate, Maximum Strength. (Pharmacia & Upjohn) Attapulgite 750 mg, Capl. Pkg. 12s, 20s.
  Use: Antidiarrheal combination.

Kaopectate Tablet Formula. (Pharmacia & Upjohn) Attapulgite 750 mg/Tab. Blister pak 12s, 20s. *otc.*
  Use: Antidiarrheal.

Kaophen Tablets. (Pal-Pak, Inc.) Phenobarbital 6.5 mg, belladonna extract 0.1 mg, kaolin 388.8 mg/Tab. Bot. 100s, 1000s. *otc.*
  Use: Antidiarrheal.

Kao-Spen. (Century Pharmaceuticals, Inc.) Kaolin 5.2 g, pectin 260 mg/30 ml. Susp. Bot. 120 ml, pt, gal. *otc.*
Use: Antidiarrheal.

Kao-Tin. (Major Pharmaceuticals) Kaolin 5.85 g, pectin 130 mg/30 ml. Susp. Bot. 120 ml, 240 ml, pt, gal. *otc.*
Use: Antidiarrheal.

Kapectin. (Health for Life Brands, Inc.) Kaolin 90 gr, pectin 2 gr/oz. Bot. Gal.
Use: Antidiarrheal.

Kapectolin. (Various Mfr.) Kaolin 90 g, pectin 2 g/30 ml. Susp. Bot. 360 ml. *otc.*
Use: Antidiarrheal.

Ka-Pek. (APC) Kaolin 90 gr, pectin 4.5 gr/fl oz. Bot. 6 oz, gal. *otc.*
Use: Antidiarrheal.

kapilin.
See: Menadione (Various Mfr.).

karaya gum. (Penick) Indian Gum. Sterculia gum.
See: Tri-Costivin (Prof. Lab.).
W/Psyllium seed, plantago ovata, brewers yeast.
See: Movicol (Norgine).
W/Refined psyllium mucilloid.
See: Hydrocil regular (Solvay Pharmaceuticals).

karaya powder. (Sween) Bot. 3 oz.
Use: Deodorant, ostomy.

Kareon.
See: Menadione (Various Mfr.).

Karidium. (Young Dental) **Tab.:** Sodium fluoride 2.21 mg, sodium Cl 94.49 mg, disintegrant 0.5 mg. Bot. 180s, 1000s. **Liq.:** Sodium fluoride 2.21 mg, sodium Cl 10 mg, purified water q.s./8 drops. Bot. 30 ml, 60 ml. *Rx.*
Use: Dental caries agent.

Karigel. (Young Dental) Fluoride ion 0.5%, pH 5.6. Gel. Bot. 30 ml, 130 ml, 250 ml. *Rx.*
Use: Dental caries agent.

Karigel-N. (Young Dental) Fluoride ion 0.5% in neutral pH gel. Bot. 24 ml, 125 ml. *Rx.*
Use: Dental caries agent.

kasal. (KAY-sal) USAN. Approximately $Na_8Al_2(OH)_2(PO_4)_4$ with about 30% of dibasic sodium phosphate; sodium aluminum phosphate, basic.
Use: Food additive.

Kasof. (J & J Merck Consumer Pharm.) Docusate potassium 240 mg/Cap. Bot. 30s, 60s. *otc.*
Use: Laxative.

kasugamycin. Under study.
Use: Anti-infective.

Kaviton.
See: Menadione, U.S.P. 23. (Various Mfr.).

Kay Ciel Elixir. (Forest Pharmaceutical, Inc.) Potassium Cl 1.5 g/15 ml. (20 mEq/15 ml), alcohol 4%. Bot. 120 ml, 473 ml, gal. *Rx.*
Use: Electrolyte supplement.

Kay Ciel Powder. (Forest Pharmaceutical, Inc.) Potassium chloride 1.5 g/Packette. (20 mEq/Packet), 4% alcohol. Box 30s, 100s, 500s. *Rx.*
Use: Electrolyte supplement.

Kayexalate. (Sanofi Winthrop Pharmaceuticals) Sodium polystyrene sulfonate sodium content ≈ 100 mg/g. Jar lb. *Rx.*
Use: Potassium-removing resin.

K-C. (Century Pharmaceuticals, Inc.) Kaolin 5.2 g, pectin 260 mg, bismuth subcarbonate 260 mg/30 ml. Susp. Bot. 120 ml, pt, gal. *otc.*
Use: Antidiarrheal.

K + Care ET. (Alra Laboratories, Inc.) Potassium bicarbonate 25 mEq/Effervescent Tab. Bot. 30s, 100s, 1000s. *Rx.*
Use: Electrolyte supplement.

K-C Liquid. (Century Pharmaceuticals, Inc.) Kaolin 5.2 g, pectin 260 mg, bismuth subcarbonate 260 mg/oz. Bot. 4 oz, pt, gal. *otc.*
Use: Antidiarrheal.

K-C Suspension. (Century Pharmaceuticals, Inc.) Kaolin 5.2 g, pectin 260 mg, bismuth subcarbonate 260 mg/30 ml. Bot. 120 ml, pt, gal. *otc.*
Use: Antidiarrheal.

KCl-20. (Western Research) Potassium Cl 1.5 g (potassium 20 mEq, chloride 20 mEq)/Packet. Box 30s. *Rx.*
Use: Electrolyte supplement.

K-Dur 10 & 20. (Key Pharmaceuticals) **10:** Potassium Cl 750 mg (10 mEq)/SR Tab. **20:** Potassium Cl 1500 mg (20 mEq)/SR Tab. Bot. 100s. *Rx.*
Use: Electrolyte supplement.

KE.
See: Cortisone Acetate (Various Mfr.).

Keelamin. (Mericon Industries, Inc.) Zinc 20 mg, manganese 5 mg, copper 3 mg/Tab. Bot. 100s. *otc.*
Use: Mineral supplement.

Keflex. (Eli Lilly and Co.) **Capl.:** Cephalexin 250 mg, 500 mg. Bot. 20s, 100s (250 mg only), UD 100s. **Pow. for Oral Susp.:** Cephalexin 125 mg/5 ml, 250 mg/5 ml. 100 ml, 200 ml, UD 100 ml (250 mg/5 ml only).
Use: Anti-infective, cephalosporin.

Keftab. (Eli Lilly and Co.) Cephalexin HCl monohydrate 500 mg/Tab. Bot. 100s. *Rx.*
Use: Anti-infective, cephalosporin.

Kefurox. (Eli Lilly and Co.) Cefuroxime

sodium 750 mg or 1.5 g/Vial. ADD-Vantage and Faspak. **750 mg:** Vial 10 ml, 100 ml. **1.5 g:** Vial 20 ml, 100 ml. **7.5 g:** Vial. Pharmacy bulk pkg. *Rx.*
Use: Anti-infective, cephalosporin.

Kefzol. (Eli Lilly and Co.) Cefazolin sodium. **Pow. for Inj. Vials:** 500 mg, 1 g. **100 ml Bulk Vials:** 10 g, 20 g. **Inj.:** 500 mg, 1g. In 10 ml Redi-vials, Faspacks, and ADD-Vantage vials. *Rx.*
Use: Cephalosporin.

Kell E. (Canright) dl-α Tocopheryl 100 IU, 200 IU, 400 IU. Bot. 100s. *otc.*
Use: Vitamin supplement.

Kellogg's Tasteless Castor Oil. (SmithKline Beecham Pharmaceuticals) Castor oil 100%. Bot. 2 oz. *otc.*
Use: Laxative.

Kelp. (Arcum) Tab. Bot. 100s, 1000s.

Kelp Plus. (Barth's) Iodine from kelp plus 16 trace minerals/Tab. Bot. 100s, 500s, 1000s.

Kelp Tablets. (Faraday) Iodine from kelp 0.15 mg/Tab. Bot. 100s.

Kemadrin. (GlaxoWellcome) Procyclidine HCl 5 mg/Tab. Bot. 100s. *Rx.*
Use: Antiparkinsonian.

Kenac Cream. (NMC Laboratories) Triamcinolone acetonide cream 0.025% or 0.1%. Tube 15 g, 60 g, 80 g, Jar 240 g. *Rx.*
Use: Corticosteroid, topical.

Kenac Ointment. (NMC Laboratories) Triamcinolone acetonide 0.1%. Tube 15 g, 80 g. *Rx.*
Use: Corticosteroid, topical.

Kenaject-40. (Merz Pharmaceuticals) Triamcinolone acetonide 40 mg/ml. Inj. Vial 5 ml. *Rx.*
Use: Corticosteroid.

Kenakion. (Harriett Lane Home of Johns Hopkins Hospital) Vitamin K-1 oxide. *Rx.*
Use: Vitamin K-induced kernicterus.

Kenalog. (Westwood Squibb Pharmaceuticals) Triamcinolone acetonide. **0.1% Cream:** Tube 15 g, 60 g, 80 g, Jar 240 g, in aqueous lotion base w/propylene glycol, cetyl and stearyl alcohols, glyceryl monostearate, sorbitan monopalmitate, polyoxyethylene sorbitan monolaurate, methylparaben, propylparaben, polyethylene glycol monostearate, simethicone, sorbic acid. **0.5% Cream:** Tube 20 g. **0.1% Oint.:** (w/base of polyethylene, mineral oil) Tube 15 g, 60 g, 80 g; Jar 240 g **0.5% Oint.:** Tube 20 g. **0.1% Lot.:** Bot. 15 ml, 60 ml. **Spray:** 6.6 mg/100 g, alcohol 10.3%. Can 23 g, 63 g. *Rx.*
Use: Corticosteroid, topical.

Kenalog 0.025%. (Westwood Squibb Pharmaceuticals) Triamcinolone acetonide. **Cream:** Tube 15 g, 80 g, Jar 240 g. **Lot.:** In aqueous lotion base w/propylene glycol, cetyl and stearyl alcohols, glyceryl monostearate, sorbitan monopalmitate, polyoxyethylene sorbitan monolaurate, methylparaben, propylparaben, polyethylene glycol monostearate, simethicone, sorbic acid, tinted in an isopropyl palmitate vehicle with alcohol (4.7%). Bot. 60 ml. **Oint.:** Plastibase (w/base of polyethylene and mineral oil gel). 15 g, 80 g, 240 g. *Rx.*
Use: Corticosteroid, topical.

Kenalog-H. (Westwood Squibb Pharmaceuticals) Triamcinolone acetonide cream USP 0.1%. Each g of cream provides 1 mg of triamcinolone acetonide in a specially formulated hydrophilic vanishing cream base containing propylene glycol, dimethicone 350, castor oil, cetearyl alcohol and ceteareth-20, propylene glycol stearate, white petrolatum, purified water. Tube 15 g, 60 g. *Rx.*
Use: Corticosteroid, topical.

Kenalog-10 Injection. (Bristol-Myers Squibb) Sterile triamcinolone acetonide suspension 10 mg/ml, sodium Cl for isotonicity, benzyl alcohol 0.9% (w/v) as a preservative, sodium carboxymethylcellulose 0.75%, polysorbate 80 0.04%. Sodium hydroxide or HCl acid may be present to adjust pH to 5 to 7.5. Nitrogen packed at the time of manufacture. Vial 5 ml. *Rx.*
Use: Corticosteroid.

Kenalog-40 Injection. (Bristol-Myers Squibb) Sterile triamcinolone acetonide suspension 40 mg/ml, sodium chloride for isotonicity, benzyl alcohol 0.9% (w/v) as a preservative, sodium carboxymethylcellulose 0.75%, polysorbate 80 0.04%. Sodium hydroxide or HCl acid may be present to adjust pH to 5 to 7.5. Nitrogen packed at the time of manufacture. Vial 1 ml, 5 ml, 10 ml. *Rx.*
Use: Corticosteroid.

Kenalog in Orabase. (Apothecon, Inc.) Triamcinolone acetonide 0.1% in Orabase. Triamcinolone acetonide 1 mg/g. Tube 5 g. *Rx.*
Use: Corticosteroid, topical.

Kendall's "Compound E".
See: Cortisone Acetate (Various Mfr.).

Kendall's "Desoxy Compound B".
See: Desoxycorticosterone Acetate (Various Mfr.).

Kenwood Therapeutic. (Kenwood Labo-

ratories) Vitamins A 3333 IU, D 133 IU, E 1.5 IU, C 50 mg, B_1 2 mg, B_2 1 mg, B_3 20 mg, B_5 2 mg, B_6 0.33 mg, Ca, K, Mg, Mn, P/5 ml. Liq. Bot. 240 ml. *otc.*
Use: Mineral, vitamin supplement.

keratolytics.
See: Condylox (Oclassen Pharmaceuticals, Inc.).

Keri Facial Soap. (Westwood Squibb Pharmaceuticals) Sodium tallowate, sodium cocoate, mineral oil, octyl hydroxystearate, fragrance, glycerin, titanium dioxide, PEG-75, lanolin oil, docusate sodium, PEG-4 dilaurate, propylparaben, PEG-40 stearate, glyceryl monostearate, PEG-100 stearate, sodium Cl, BHT, EDTA. Bar 3.25 oz. *otc.*
Use: Dermatologic cleanser.

Keri Light Lotion. (Westwood Squibb Pharmaceuticals) Stearyl alcohol, ceteareath-20, cetearyl octanoate, glycerin, stearyl heptanoate, stearyl alcohol, carbomer 934, sodium hydroxide, squalene, methylparaben, propylparaben, fragrance. Bot. 6.5 oz, 13 oz. *otc.*
Use: Emollient.

Keri Lotion. (Westwood Squibb Pharmaceuticals) Mineral oil, lanolin oil, water, propylene glycol, glyceryl stearate, PEG-100 stearate, PEG 40 stearate, PEG-4 dilaurate, laureth-4, parabens, docusate sodium, triethanolamine, quaternium 15, carbomer 934. Bot. 6.5 oz, 13 oz, 20 oz. *otc.*
Use: Emollient.

Kerlone. (Searle) Betaxolol HCl 10 mg or 25 mg/Tab. Bot. 100s, UD 100s. *Rx.*
Use: Beta-adrenergic blocker.

Kerocaine.
See: Procaine HCl (Various Mfr.).

Kerodex. (Wyeth-Ayerst Laboratories) **No. 51:** Water-miscible. Tube 4 oz, Jar lb. **No. 71:** Water-repellent Tube 4 oz, Jar lb. *otc.*
Use: Emollient.

kerohydric. A de-waxed, oil-soluble fraction of lanolin.
Use: Emollient, cleanser.
See: Alpha-Keri, Soap, Spray (Westwood Squibb Pharmaceuticals).
Keri, Cream, Lot. (Westwood Squibb Pharmaceuticals).

W/Docusate sodium, sodium alkyl polyether sulfonate, sodium sulfoacetate, sulfur, salicylic acid, hexachlorophene.
See: Sebulex, Cream, Liq. (Westwood Squibb Pharmaceuticals).

Kerr Insta-Char. (Kerr Drug) **Regular:** Aqueous suspension activated charcoal 50 g/8 oz. **Pediatric:** Aqueous suspension activated charcoal 15 g/4 oz. *otc.*
Use: Antidote.

Kerr Triple Dye. (Kerr Drug) Gentian violet, proflavine hemisulfate, brilliant green in water. Dispensing bot. 15 ml. Single Use Dispos-A-Swab 0.65 ml, Box 10s, Case 10 × 50 Box. *otc.*
Use: Antiseptic.

Kestrone 5. (Hyrex Pharmaceuticals) Estrone 5 mg/ml, sodium carboxymethylcellulose, povidone, benzyl alcohol, propylparabens/Inj. Multi-dose Vial 10 ml. *Rx.*
Use: Estrogen.

Ketalar. (Monarch Pharmaceuticals) Ketamine HCl, sodium Cl, benzethonium Cl. **10 mg/ml:** Vial 20 ml, 25 ml and 50 ml. Pkg. 10s; **50 mg/ml:** Vial 10 ml. **100 mg/ml:** Vial 5 ml. Pkg. 10s. *Rx.*
Use: Anesthetic, general.

•**ketamine hydrochloride.** (KEET-uh-MEEN) U.S.P. 23.
Use: Anesthetic.
See: Ketalar, Inj. (Parke-Davis).

•**ketanserin.** (KEET-AN-ser-in) USAN.
Use: Serotonin antagonist.

•**ketazocine.** (key-TAY-zoe-seen) USAN.
Use: Analgesic.

•**ketazolam.** (keet-AZE-oh-lam) USAN.
Use: Anxiolytic.

•**kethoxal.** (KEY-thox-al) USAN.
Use: Antiviral.

•**ketipramine fumarate.** (key-TIH-prah-MEEN) USAN.
Use: Antidepressant.

•**ketoconazole.** (KEY-toe-KOE-nuh-zole) U.S.P. 23.
Use: Antifungal.
See: Nizoral, Tab. (Janssen Pharmaceutical, Inc.).

Ketodestrin.
See: Estrone (Various Mfr.).

Keto-Diastix Reagent Strips. (Bayer Corp. (Consumer Div.)) Dip and read reagent strip test for glucose and ketones in urine. Two test areas: glucose levels from 30 mg to 5000 mg/dl; ketone test (acetoacetic acid) negative 5 mg, 40 mg, 80 mg, 160 mg/dl. Strip Bot. 50s, 100s.
Use: Diagnostic aid.

ketohexazine. (ESI Lederle Generics)
Use: Hypnotic.

ketohydroxyestratriene.
See: Estrone (Various Mfr.).

ketohydroxyestrin.
See: Estrone (Various Mfr.).

ketone tests.

Use: Diagnostic aid.
See: Acetest Reagent, Tab. (Bayer Corp. (Consumer Div.)).
Chemstrip K, Reagent paper (Boehringer Mannheim Pharmaceuticals).
Ketostix Strips, Reagent Strips (Bayer Corp. (Consumer Div)).

Ketonex-1. (Ross Laboratories) Protein 15 g, fat 23.9 g, carbohydrates 46.3 g, linoleic acid 1800 mg, Fe 9 mg, Na 190 mg, K 675 mg. With appropriate vitamins and minerals. 480 Cal/100 g. Isoleucine, leucine and valine free. Pow. Can 350 g. *otc.*
Use: Nutritional supplement.

Ketonex-2. (Ross Laboratories) Protein 30 g, fat 15.5 g, carbohydrates 30 g, Fe 13 mg, Na 880 mg, K 1370 mg. With appropriate vitamins and minerals. 410 Cal/100 g. Isoleucine, leucine and valine free. Pow. Can 325 g. *otc.*
Use: Nutritional supplement.

•**ketoprofen.** (KEY-to-pro-fen) U.S.P. 23.
Use: Anti-inflammatory.
See: Orudis, Cap. (Wyeth-Ayerst Laboratories).
Oruvail, Cap. (Wyeth-Ayerst Laboratories).

ketoprofen. (Various Mfr.) 25 mg, 50 mg, 75 mg. Cap. Bot. 100s, 500s.
Use: Anti-inflammatory.

ketoprofen. (Schein) 200 mg, sucrose. ER Cap. Bot. 100s, 500s, 1000s. *Rx.*
Use: Anti-inflammatory.

•**ketorfanol.** (key-TAR-fan-AHL) USAN.
Use: Analgesic.

•**ketorolac tromethamine.** (KEY-TOR-oh-lak tro-METH-uh-meen) U.S.P. 23.
Use: Analgesic, NSAID, ophthalmic.
See: Acular, Soln. (Allergan).

ketorolac tromethamine. (Various Mfr.) 10 mg/Tab. Bot. 100s, 500s, 1000s. *Rx.*
Use: Analgesic.

Ketostix Reagent Strips. (Bayer Corp. (Consumer Div.)) Sodium nitroprusside, sodium phosphate, glycine. Stick test for ketones in urine (measures acetoacetic acid). Bot. 50s, 100s, UD 20s.
Use: Diagnostic aid.

•**ketotifen fumarate.** (KEY-toe-TIE-fen) USAN.
Use: Antiasthmatic.

Key-Plex. (Hyrex Pharmaceuticals) Vitamins B_1 50 mg, B_2 5 mg, B_{12} 1000 mcg, pyridoxine HCl 5 mg, d-panthenol 6 mg, niacinamide 125 mg, ascorbic acid 50 mg/ml. Vial 10 ml. *Rx.*
Use: Nutritional supplement, parenteral.

Key-Pred. (Hyrex Pharmaceuticals) Prednisolone. **25 mg/ml:** Vial 10 ml, 30 ml; **50 mg/ml:** Vial 10 ml. *Rx.*
Use: Corticosteroid.

Key-Pred-SP. (Hyrex Pharmaceuticals) Prednisolone sodium phosphate 20 mg/ml. Inj. Vial 10 ml. *Rx.*
Use: Corticosteroid.

K-G Elixir. (Geneva Pharmaceuticals) Potassium (as potassium gluconate) 20 mEq/15 ml, alcohol 5%. Elix. Bot. Pt. *Rx.*
Use: Electrolyte supplement.

kharophen.
See: Acetarsone (Various Mfr.).

khellin.
Use: Coronary vasodilator.

Kiddie Powder. (Gordon Laboratories) Pure fine Italian talc. Can 3.5 oz. *otc.*
Use: Antifungal.

Kiddi-Vites, Improved. (Geneva Pharmaceuticals) Vitamins A 5000 IU, D 500 IU, B_1 1 mg, B_2 1.5 mg, B_{12} 2 mcg, C 50 mg, B_6 1 mg, pantothenate 2 mg, niacinamide 10 mg/Tab. Bot. 100s, 1000s. *otc.*
Use: Vitamin supplement.

kidney function agents.
See: Biotel Kidney (Biotel Corp.).
Indigo Carmine, Soln. (Various Mfr.).
Inulin, Amp. (Arnar-Stone).
Iodohippurate, Sodium. Mannitol Soln., Amp. (Merck & Co).
Methylene Blue (Various Mfr.).

KIE Syrup. (Laser, Inc.) Potassium iodide 150 mg, ephedrine HCl 8 mg/5 ml. Syr. Bot. Pt, gal. *Rx.*
Use: Decongestant, expectorant.

Kindercal. (Mead Johnson Nutritionals) Protein 13%, carbohydrate 50%, fat 37%, 30 cal/oz, sucrose, vanilla flavor, lactose free. 30 cal/oz. Liq. Can. 8 oz. *otc.*
Use: Nutritional supplement.

kinate. Hexahydrotetra hydroxybenzoate salt, quinic acid salt.

Kinevac. (Bristol-Myers Squibb) Sincalide 5 mcg/vial. For gallbladder, pancreatic secretion and cholecystography.
Use: Diagnostic aid.

Kin White. (Whiteworth Towne) Triamcinolone acetonide. **Cream:** 0.025% or 1%. Tube 15 g, 80 g. **Oint.:** 1%. Tube 15 g, 80 g.
Use: Corticosteroid, topical.

•**kitasamycin.** (kit-ah-sah-MY-sin) USAN. An antibiotic substance obtained from cultures of *Streptomyces kitasatoensis.* Under study.
Use: Anti-infective.

Klaron. (Dermik Laboratories, Inc.) Sodium sulfacetamide 10%, propylene

glycol, polyethylene glycol 400, methylparaben, EDTA/Lot. Bot. 59 ml. *Rx.*
Use: Dermatologic.

Klavikordal. (U.S. Ethicals) Nitroglycerin 2.6 mg/SR Tab. Bot. 100s, 1000s. *Rx.*
Use: Antianginal.

KLB6. (NBTY, Inc.) Vitamin B_6 mcg, soya lecithin 100 mg, kelp 25 mg, cider vinegar 80 mg/Softgels. Bot. 100s. *otc.*
Use: Vitamin supplement.

KLB6 Complete. (NBTY, Inc.) Vitamins A 833.3 IU, E 5 mg (as IU), B_3 3.3 mg, C 10 mg, soya lecithin 200 mg, kelp 25 mg, cider vinegar 40 mg, wheat bran 83.3 mg, D 66.7 IU, FA 0.067 mg, B_1 0.25 mg, B_2 0.28 mg, B_6 8.3 mg, B_{12} 1 mcg, biotin 0.05 mg/Tab. Bot. 100s. *otc.*
Use: Vitamin supplement.

K-Lease. (Pharmacia & Upjohn) Potassium chloride 10 mEq (750 mg). ER Cap. Bot. 100s, 500s, 1000s, 2500s, UD 100s. *Rx.*
Use: Electrolyte supplement.

Kleen-Handz. (American Medical Industries) Ethyl alcohol 62%, aloe vera. Soln. Bot. 60 ml. *otc.*
Use: Antiseptic.

Kleer Compound. (Scrip) Acetaminophen 300 mg, phenylpropanolamine HCl 35 mg, guaifenesin. Tab. Bot. 100s. *otc.*
Use: Analgesic, decongestant, expectorant.

Kleer Improved. (Scrip) Atropine sulfate 0.2 mg, chlorpheniramine maleate 5 mg/ml. *Rx.*
Use: Anticholinergic, antihistamine.

Klerist-D. (Nutripharm Laboratories, Inc.) **Cap. SR:** Pseudoephedrine HCl 120 mg, chlorpheniramine maleate 8 mg. Bot. 100s, 500s. **Tab.:** Pseudoephedrine HCl 60 mg, chlorpheniramine maleate 4 mg. Bot. 24s, 100s. *Rx.*
Use: Antihistamine, decongestant.

Kler-Ro Liquid. (Ulmer Pharmacal Co.) Surgical cleanser and laboratory detergent. Bot. Gal.
Use: Antiseptic.

Kler-Ro Powder. (Ulmer Pharmacal Co.) Surgical cleanser and laboratory detergent. Can 2 lb, Bot. 6 lb.
Use: Antiseptic.

KL4-Surfactant. (Acute Therapeutics)
Use: Treatment of acute respiratory distress syndrome. [Orphan Drug]

Klonopin. (Roche Laboratories) Clonazepam 0.5 mg, 1 mg, 2 mg, lactose/Tab. 100s. *c-IV.*
Use: Anticonvulsant.

K-Lor. (Abbott Laboratories) Potassium Cl equivalent to potassium 20 mEq and Cl 20 mEq/2.6 g for oral soln. w/saccharin. Pkg. 30s, 100s. 15 mEq/2 g Pkg. 100s. *Rx.*
Use: Electrolyte supplement.

Klor-Con 8. (Upsher-Smith Labs, Inc.) Potassium Cl 8 mEq/ER Tab. Bot. 100s, 500s. *Rx.*
Use: Electrolyte supplement.

Klor-Con 10. (Upsher-Smith Labs, Inc.) Potassium Cl 10 mEq/ER Tab. Bot. 100s, 500s. *Rx.*
Use: Electrolyte supplement.

Klor-Con/25 Powder. (Upsher-Smith Labs, Inc.) Potassium Cl for oral soln 25 mEq/Pkt. Ctn. 30s, 100s, 250s. *Rx.*
Use: Electrolyte supplement.

Klor-Con/EF. (Upsher-Smith Labs, Inc.) Potassium bicarbonate 25 mEq/Tab. Ctn. 30s, 100s. *Rx.*
Use: Electrolyte supplement.

Klor-Con Powder. (Upsher-Smith Labs, Inc.) Potassium Cl for oral soln. 20 mEq/Pkt. w/saccharin. Pkt. 1.5 g. Box 30s, 100s. *Rx.*
Use: Electrolyte supplement.

Klorvess Effervescent Granules. (Novartis Pharmaceutical Corp.) Potassium 20 mEq, Cl 20 mEq supplied by potassium Cl 1.125 g, potassium bicarbonate 0.5 g, L-lysine monohydrochloride 0.913 g/Pkt. w/saccharin. Box 30s. *Rx.*
Use: Electrolyte supplement.

Klorvess Effervescent Tablets. (Novartis Pharmaceutical Corp.) Potassium Cl 1.125 g, potassium bicarbonate 0.5 g, L-lysine HCl 0.913 g/Effervescent Tab. Sodium and sugar free, saccharin. Pkg. 60s, 1000s. *Rx.*
Use: Electrolyte supplement.

Klorvess Liquid. (Novartis Pharmaceutical Corp.) Potassium Cl 1.5 g (20 mEq)/15 ml, alcohol 0.75%. Bot. pt. *Rx.*
Use: Electrolyte supplement.

Klotrix. (Bristol-Myers Squibb) Potassium Cl 10 mEq/SR Tab. Bot. 100s, 1000s, UD 100s. *Rx.*
Use: Electrolyte supplement.

K-Lyte. (Bristol-Myers Squibb) Potassium bicarbonate and citrate 25 mEq, saccharin. Lime and orange flavors. Effervescent Tab. Pkg. 30s, 100s, 250s. *Rx.*
Use: Electrolyte supplement.

K-Lyte/Cl. (Bristol-Myers Squibb) Potassium Cl 25 mEq, saccharin. Citrus and fruit punch flavor. Effervescent Tab. Pkg. 30s, 100s, 250s. Bulk powder 225 g/Can. *Rx.*
Use: Electrolyte supplement.

K-Lyte/Cl 50. (Bristol-Myers Squibb) Potassium Cl 50 mEq, saccharin. Citrus and fruit punch flavors. Pkg. 30s, 100s. *Rx.*
Use: Electrolyte supplement.

K-Lyte DS. (Bristol-Myers Squibb) Potassium bicarbonate and citrate 50 mEq, saccharin. Lime and orange flavor. Effervescent Tab. Pkg. 30s, 100s. *Rx.*
Use: Electrolyte supplement.

K-Norm. (Medeva Pharmaceuticals, Inc.) Potassium Cl 10 mEq/CR Cap. Bot. 100s, 500s. *Rx.*
Use: Electrolyte supplement.

Koate HP. (Bayer Corp (Consumer Div.)) A stable dried concentrate of Anti-hemophilic Factor. When reconstituted, contains heparin ≤ 5 U/ml, PEG ≤ 1500 ppm, glycine ≤ 0.05 M glycine, polysorbate 80 ≤ 25 ppm, calcium chloride ≤ 3 mM, aluminum ≤ 1 ppm, histidine ≤ 0.06 M, albumin (human) ≤ 10 mg/ml. Includes Sterile Water for Injection, double-ended transfer needle, filter needle, and administration set. Pow. Bot. 250, 500, 1000, 1500 IU Factor VIII activity (approximate). *Rx.*
Use: Antihemophilic.

Kodonyl Expectorant. (Halsey Drug Co.) Bromodiphenhydramine HCl 3.75 mg, diphenhydramine HCl 8.75 mg, ammonium Cl 80 mg, potassium guaiacolsulfonate 80 mg, menthol 0.5 mg/5 ml. Bot. 16 oz. *otc.*
Use: Antihistamine, expectorant.

Kof-Eze. (Roberts Pharmaceuticals) Menthol 6 mg. Loz. Pkg. 4s, Bot. 500s. *otc.*
Use: Mouth and throat preparation.

KOGENATE. (Bayer Corp. (Consumer Div.)) Recombinant antihemophilic factor (Factor VIII). Pow. for inj. Bot. 250 IU, 500 IU, 1000 IU. *Rx.*
Use: Antihemophilic.

Kolephrin. (Pfeiffer Co.) Pseudoephedrine HCl 30 mg, chlorpheniramine maleate 2 mg, acetaminophen 325 mg/ Capl. Bot. 24s, 36s. *otc.*
Use: Analgesic, antihistamine, decongestant.

Kolephrin/DM. (Pfeiffer Co.) Pseudoephedrine HCl 30 mg, chlorpheniramine maleate 2 mg, dextromethorphan HBr 10 mg, acetaminophen 325 mg/Capl. Bot. 30s. *otc.*
Use: Analgesic, antihistamine, antitussive, decongestant.

Kolephrin GG/DM Expectorant. (Pfeiffer Co.) Dextromethorphan HBr 10 mg, guaifenesin 150 mg/5 ml. Alcohol free. Bot. 120 ml. *otc.*
Use: Antitussive, expectorant.

Kolephrin NN. (Pfeiffer Co.) Phenylpropanolamine HCl 12.5 mg, pyrilamine maleate 10 mg, dextromethorphan HBr 7.5 mg/5 ml. Alcohol free. Liq. Bot. 120 ml. *otc.*
Use: Antihistamine, antitussive, decongestant.

•**kolfocon a.** (KAHL-FOE-kahn A) USAN.
Use: Contact lens material (hydrophobic).

•**kolfocon b.** (KAHL-FOE-kahn B) USAN.
Use: Contact lens material (hydrophobic).

•**kolfocon c.** (KAHL-FOE-kahn C) USAN.
Use: Contact lens material (hydrophobic).

•**kolfocon d.** (KAHL-FOE-kahn D) USAN.
Use: Contact lens material (hydrophobic).

Kolyum. (Medeva Pharmaceuticals, Inc.) Potassium ion 20 mEq, chloride ion 3.4 mEq from potassium gluconate 3.9 g, potassium Cl 0.25 g/15 ml or 5 g/15 ml. w/saccharin, sorbitol. Liq. Bot. Pt, gal. *Rx.*
Use: Electrolyte supplement.

Kondon's Nasal Jelly. (Kondon) Tube 20 g w/ephedrine alkaloid. Tube 20 g. *otc.*
Use: Decongestant.

Kondremul. (Medeva Pharmaceuticals, Inc.) Mineral oil 55%, Irish moss. Emulsion Bot. Pt. **W/Phenolphthalein:** 2.2 gr/tbsp. Bot. Pt. **W/Cascara:** 0.66 g/15 ml. Bot. 14 oz. *otc.*
Use: Laxative.

Konsto. (Freeport) Docusate sodium 100 mg/Cap. Bot. 1000s. *otc.*
Use: Laxative.

Konsyl-D Powder. (Konsyl Pharmaceuticals) Psyllium hydrophilic mucilloid, dextrose. Canister 325 g, 500 g, Packet 6.5 g, Ctn. 25s. *otc.*
Use: Laxative.

Konsyl Fiber. (Konsyl Pharmaceuticals) Calcium polycarbophil 625 mg/Tab. Bot. 90s. *otc.*
Use: Laxative.

Konsyl-Orange. (Konsyl Pharmaceuticals) Psyllium fiber 3.4 g/tbsp., sucrose, orange flavor. Pow. Bot. 12 g, 538 g. *otc.*
Use: Laxative.

Konsyl Powder. (Konsyl Pharmaceuticals) Psyllium hydrophilic mucilloid. Canister 300 g, 450 g, Packet 6 g, Ctn. 25s. *otc.*
Use: Laxative.

Konyne 80. (Bayer Corp. (Consumer

Div.)) Dried plasma fraction of coagulation factors II, VII, IX and X. Heparin free. Heat treated. Vial. 10 ml and 20 ml. *Rx.*
Use: Antihemophilic.

Kophane Cough & Cold Formula. (Pfeiffer Co.) Phenylpropanolamine HCl 12.5 mg, chlorpheniramine maleate 2 mg, dextromethorphan HBr 10 mg/5 ml. Liq. Bot. 120 ml. *otc.*
Use: Antihistamine, antitussive, decongestant.

Koro-Flex. (Holland-Rantos) Improved contouring-spring, natural latex diaphragm 60 mm to 95 mm.
Use: Contraceptive.

Koromex Coil Spring Diaphragm. (Holland-Rantos) Diaphragm made of pure latex rubber, cadmium-plated coil spring. Koromex Jelly and Cream/kit. 50 mm to 95 mm at graduations of 5 mm.
Use: Contraceptive.

Koromex Combination. (Holland-Rantos) Diaphragm 50 mm to 95 mm, Koromex Jelly and Cream/Kit.
Use: Contraceptive.

Koromex Crystal Clear Gel. (Durex) Nonoxynol-9 2%. Tube 126 ml with or without applicator. *otc.*
Use: Contraceptive.

Koromex Jelly. (Durex) Nonoxynol-9 3%. Vaginal Jelly. 126 g. *otc.*
Use: Contraceptive, spermicide.

Korum. (Geneva Pharmaceuticals) Acetaminophen 5 gr/Tab. Bot. 1000s. *otc.*
Use: Analgesic.

Kotabarb. (Wesley Pharmacal Co., Inc.) Phenobarbital ¼ gr. Tab. Bot. 1000s. *Rx.*
Use: Hypnotic, sedative.

Kovitonic. (Freeda Vitamins, Inc.) Iron 42 mg, vitamins B_1 5 mg, B_6 10 mg, B_{12} 30 mcg, folic acid 0.1 mg, l-lysine 10 mg/15 ml. Liq. Bot. 120 ml, 240 ml. *otc.*
Use: Mineral, vitamin supplement.

K-Pek. (Rugby Labs, Inc.) Attapulgite 600 mg/15 ml. Susp. Bot. 237 ml, pt, gal. *otc.*
Use: Antidiarrheal.

K-Phos M.F. (Beach Pharmaceuticals) Potassium acid phosphate 155 mg, sodium acid phosphate 350 mg/Tab. Bot. 100s, 500s. *Rx.*
Use: Acidifier, urinary.

K-Phos Neutral. (Beach Pharmaceuticals) Dibasic sodium phosphate 852 mg, potassium acid phosphate 155 mg, sodium acid phosphate 130 mg/Tab. Bot. 100s, 500s. *Rx.*
Use: Mineral supplement.

K-Phos No. 2. (Beach Pharmaceuticals) Potassium acid phosphate 305 mg, sodium acid phosphate, anhydrous 700 mg/Tab. Bot. 100s, 500s. *Rx.*
Use: Acidifier, urinary.

K-Phos Original. (Beach Pharmaceuticals) Potassium acid phosphate 500 mg/Tab. Bot. 100s, 500s. *Rx.*
Use: Urinary acidifier, electrolyte supplement.

K.P.N. (Freeda Vitamins, Inc.) Vitamins C 333 mg, Fe 11 mg, A 2667 IU, D 133 IU, E 10 mg, B_1 2 mg, B_2 2 mg, B_3 10 mg, B_5 3.3 mg, B_6 0.83 mg, B_{12} 2 mcg, C 33 mg, FA 0.27 mg, I, Cu, Mn, K, Mg, Zn 6.7 mg, bioflavonoids/Tab. Bot. 100s, 250s, 500s. *otc.*
Use: Mineral, vitamin supplement.

K-P Suspension. (Century Pharmaceuticals, Inc.) Kaolin 5.2 g, pectin 260 mg/oz. Bot. Gal. *otc.*
Use: Antidiarrheal.

Kronofed-A. (Ferndale Laboratories, Inc.) Pseudoephedrine HCl 120 mg, chlorpheniramine maleate 8 mg/Cap. Bot. 100s, 500s. *Rx.*
Use: Antihistamine, decongestant.

Kronofed-A Jr. (Ferndale Laboratories, Inc.) Pseudoephedrine HCl 60 mg, chlorpheniramine maleate 4 mg/Cap. Bot. 100s, 500s. *Rx.*
Use: Antihistamine, decongestant.

Kronohist Kronocaps. (Ferndale Laboratories, Inc.) Chlorpheniramine maleate 4 mg, pyrilamine maleate 25 mg, phenylpropanolamine HCl 50 mg/Cap. Bot. 100s, 1000s. *otc.*
Use: Antihistamine, decongestant.

•**krypton clathrate Kr 85.** (KRIPP-tahn KLATH-rate) USAN.
Use: Radiopharmaceutical.

•**krypton Kr 81m.** (KRIP-tahn Kr 81 m) U.S.P. 23.
Use: Radiopharmaceutical.

K-Tab. (Abbott Laboratories) Potassium Cl (10 mEq) 750 mg/ER Tab. Bot. 100s, 1000s, UD 100s. *Rx.*
Use: Electrolyte supplement.

K.T.V. Tablets. (Knight) Vitamin B_{12}, minerals. Bot. 50s. *otc.*
Use: Mineral, vitamin supplement.

Kudrox Double Strength Suspension. (Schwarz Pharma, Inc.) Aluminum hydroxide 500 mg, magnesium hydroxide 450 mg, simethicone 40 mg/5 ml. Bot. 355 ml. *otc.*
Use: Antacid.

Kutapressin. (Kremers Urban) Liver derivative complex composed of peptides

and amino acids. Inj. Vial 20 ml. *Rx.*
Use: Nutritional supplement.

Kutrase. (Kremers Urban) Amylase 30 mg, protease 6 mg, lipase 25 mg, cellulase 2 mg, l-hyoscyamine sulfate 0.0625 mg, phenyltoloxamine citrate 15 mg/Cap. Bot. 100s, 500s. *Rx.*
Use: Digestive aid.

Ku-Zyme. (Kremers Urban) Amylase 30 mg, protease 6 mg, lipase 75 mg, cellulase 2 mg/Cap. Bot. 100s, 500s. *Rx.*
Use: Digestive aid.

Ku-Zyme HP. (Kremers Urban) Lipase 8000 units, protease 30,000 units, amylase 30,000 units/Cap. Bot. 100s. *Rx.*
Use: Digestive aid.

K-vescent Potassium Chloride. (Major Pharm.) Potassium and chloride 20 mEq from potassium chloride 1.5 g, saccharin. Pow. Pkt. 30s, 100s. *Rx.*
Use: Potassium replacement product.

Kwelcof. (B.F. Ascher and Co.) Hydrocodone bitartrate 5 mg, guaifenesin 100 mg/5 ml. Bot. Pt, UD 5 ml. Pkg. 10s, 100s. Alcohol, dye, sugar, and corn free. *c-III.*
Use: Antitussive, expectorant.

Kwikderm Cream. (NMC Laboratories) Tolnaftate 1%. Cream. Tube 15 g. *otc.*
Use: Antifungal, topical.

Kwikderm Solution. (NMC Laboratories) Tolnaftate 1%. Soln. Bot. 10 ml.
Use: Antifungal, topical.

Kwildane Shampoo. (Major Pharmaceuticals) Gamma benzene hexachloride 1%. Bot. 60 ml, pt, gal.
Use: Pediculicide.

K-Y. (Johnson & Johnson) Glycerin, methylparaben, hydroxyethylcellulose. Sterile or regular. Jelly Tube 12 g, 60 g, 120 g. *otc.*
Use: Lubricant.

Kyodex Reagent Strips. (Kyoto) A disposable plastic reagent strip for determination of glucose in whole blood. Vial 25s.
Use: Diagnostic aid.

Kyotest UG Reagent Strips. (Kyoto) Reagent strips for glucose and ketones in urine.
Use: Diagnostic aid.

Kyotest UGK Reagent Strip. (Kyoto) Disposable reagent strip for measurement of glucose and ketones in the urine. Vial 50s, 100s.
Use: Diagnostic aid.

Kyotest UK Reagent Strips. (Kyoto) Reagent strip for ketones in urine. Vial 50s.
Use: Diagnostic aid.

KY Plus. (Johnson & Johnson) Nonoxynol-9 2%, methylparaben. Nongreasy. 113 g. *otc.*
Use: Lubricant.

Kytril. (SmithKline Beecham Pharmaceuticals) Granisetron HCl. **Inj.:** 1.12 mg/ml. Inj. Single-use vial 1 ml, 4 ml multidose vial (w/benzyl alcohol). **Tab.:** 1.12 mg/Tab. Pkg. 20s, unit-of-use 2s. *Rx.*
Use: Antiemetic (cancer therapy).

L

LA-12. (Hyrex Pharmaceuticals) Hydroxocobalamin 1000 mcg/ml. Inj. Vial 30 ml. *Rx.*
Use: Vitamin supplement.

•**labetalol hydrochloride.** (la-BET-ul-lahl) U.S.P. 23.
Use: Antihypertensive, antiadrenergic, (α-receptor, β-receptor).
See: Normodyne, Inj., Tab. (Schering-Plough Corp.).
Trandate Inj., Tab. (GlaxoWellcome).
W/Hydrochlorothiazide.
See: Trandate HCT, Tab. (Glaxo-Wellcome).
Normodyne, Inj., Tab. (Schering-Plough Corp.).

labetalol hydrochloride. (Various Mfr.) 100 mg, 200 mg, 300 mg. Tab. Bot. 100s, 500s, 1000s. *Rx.*
Use: Antihypertensive.

Labstix Reagent Strips. (Bayer Corp. (Consumer Div.)) Urine screening test. Bot. 100s.
Use: Diagnostic aid.

Lac-Hydrin Lotion. (Westwood Squibb Pharmaceuticals) Lactic acid 12% neutralized w/ammonium hydroxide, light mineral oil, cetyl alcohol, parabens. Tube 150 ml, 360 ml. *Rx.*
Use: Emollient.

•**lacidipine.** (lah-SIH-dih-PEEN) USAN.
Use: Antihypertensive.

Laclede Cleaner. (Laclede) Container. 2 lb.
Use: Detergent.

Laclede Disclosing Swab. (Laclede) Swabs 6″. 100s, 500s, 1000s.
Use: Dentrifice.

Laclede Topi-Fluor A.P.F. Topical Cream. (Laclede) Fluoride ion 1.23% (from sodium fluoride) in orthophosphoric acid 0.98%. Jar 50 ml, 500 ml, 1000 ml, 2000 ml. *Rx.*
Use: Dental caries agent.

Lacotein. (Christina) Protein digest 5% w/preservatives. Vial 30 ml (w/iodochin), Vial 30 ml. *Rx.*
Use: Protein supplement.

Lacril. (Allergan, Inc.) Hydroxypropyl methylcellulose 0.5%, gelatin A 0.01%, chlorobutanol 0.5%, polysorbate 80, dextrose, magnesium Cl, sodium borate, sodium chloride. Soln. Dropper bot. 15 ml. *otc.*
Use: Lubricant, ophthalmic.

Lacri-Lube NP. (Allergan, Inc.) White petrolatum 55.5%, mineral oil 42.5%, petrolatum/lanolin alcohol 2%. Oint. 0.7 g. *otc.*
Use: Lubricant, ophthalmic.

Lacri-Lube S.O.P. (Allergan, Inc.) White petrolatum 56.8%, mineral oil 41.5%, lanolin alcohols, chlorobutanol. Tube 3.5 g, 7 g. *otc.*
Use: Lubricant, ophthalmic.

Lacrisert. (Merck & Co.) Hydroxypropyl cellulose 5 mg/insert. Pkg. 60s w/applicators. *Rx.*
Use: Artificial tears.

LactAid. (Ortho McNeil Pharmaceutical) **Liq.:** Beta-D-galactosidase derived from *Kluyveromyces lactis* yeast (1000 Neutral Lactase units/5 drop dosage) in carrier of glycerol 50%, water 30%, inert yeast dry matter 20%. Units of 4, 12, 30, 75 one-quart dosages at 5 drops/dose. **Tab.:** Beta-D-galactosidase from *Aspergillus oryzae* (3300 FCC lactase units/Tab.) In 12s, 100s. *otc.*
Use: Digestive aid.

lactalbumin hydrolysate.
See: Aminonat.

lactase enzyme.
Use: Digestive aid.
See: LactAid, Capl., Liq. (Ortho McNeil Pharmaceutical).
Lactrase, Cap. (Schwarz Pharma, Inc.).
Dairy Ease, Tabs. (Sanofi Winthrop Pharmaceuticals).
SureLac, Tab. (Caraco Pharmaceutical Labs, Ltd.).

lactated ringer's injection.
Use: Electrolyte, fluid replacement; alkalizer, systemic.

•**lactic acid.** (LACK-tick) U.S.P. 23.
Use: Pharmaceutic necessity for sodium lactate injection.
See: Penecare, Cream, Lot. (Reed & Carnrick).
W/Sodium pyrrolidone carboxylate.
See: LactiCare (Stiefel Laboratories, Inc.).
Lactinol, Lot., Creme (Pedinol Pharmacal, Inc.).

LactiCare Lotion. (Stiefel Laboratories, Inc.) Lactic acid 5%, sodium pyrrolidone carboxylate 2.5% in an emollient lotion base. Bot. 8 oz, 12 oz, w/pump dispenser. *otc.*
Use: Emollient.

LactiCare-HC Lotion. (Stiefel Laboratories, Inc.) Hydrocortisone lotion 1%, 2.5%. **1%:** Bot 4 oz. **2.5%:** Bot. 2 oz. *Rx.*
Use: Corticosteroid, topical.

Lactinex. (Becton Dickinson & Co.) *Lactobacillus acidophilus* & *Lactobacillus bulgaricus* mixed culture. Tab. 250 mg, Bot. 50s. Gran. 1 g pkt. Box 12s. *otc.*

Use: Antidiarrheal, nutritional supplement.

Lactinol. (Pedinol Pharmacal, Inc.) Lactic acid 10%. Lot. Bot. 237 ml. *Rx.*
Use: Emollient.

Lactinol-E Creme. (Pedinol Pharmacal, Inc.) Lactic acid 10%, vitamin E 3500 IU/30 g. Cream 56.7 g, 113.4 g. *Rx.*
Use: Emollient.

lactobacillus acidophilus. Preparation made from acid-producing bacterium.
Use: Antidiarrheal, nutritional supplement.
See: Bacid (Novartis Pharmaceutical Corp.).
DoFUS (Miller Pharmacal Group, Inc.).
More Dophilus (Freeda Vitamins, Inc.).
Pro-Bionate (Natren, Inc).
Superdophilus (Natren, Inc).

lactobacillus acidophilus & bulgaricus mixed culture.
See: Lactinex, Tab., Gran. (Becton Dickinson & Co.).

lactobacillus acidophilus, viable culture.
See: DoFus, Tab. (Miller Pharmacal Group, Inc.).
Lactinex Gran., Tab. (Becton Dickinson & Co.).

lactobin. (Roxane Laboratories, Inc.)
Use: AIDS-associated diarrhea. [Orphan Drug]

Lactocal-F. (Laser, Inc.) Vitamin A 4000 IU, D 400 IU, E 30 IU, C 100 mg, folic acid 1 mg, B_1 3 mg, B_2 3.4 mg, B_3 20 mg, B_6 5 mg, B_{12} 12 mcg, calcium 200 mg, I, Fe 65 mg, Mg, Cu, Zn 15 mg/Tab. Bot. 100s, 1000s. *Rx.*
Use: Mineral, vitamin supplement.

lactoflavin.
See: Riboflavin, U.S.P. 23. (Various Mfr.).

Lactofree. (Bristol-Myers Squibb) Protein 14.7 g, carbohydrates 69.3 g, fat 36.7 g, linoleic acid 6 g, Fe 12 mg, Na 200 mg, K 733.3 mg, with appropriate vitamins and minerals. Lactose free. 666.7 cal/L. Pow. Can 400 g. *otc.*
Use: Nutritional supplement, enteral.

lactose. Milk sugar.
Use: Pharmaceutic aid (tablet and capsule diluent).
See: Natur-Aid, Pow. (Scott/Cord).

•**lactose anhydrous.** (LACK-tohs an-HIGH-druss) N.F. 18.
Use: Pharmaceutic aid (tablet and capsule diluent).

•**lactose monohydrate.** N.F. 18.
Use: Pharmaceutic aid (tablet and capsule diluent).

Lactrase. (Rhone-Poulenc Rorer Pharmaceuticals, Inc.) Standardized enzyme lactase (β-D-galactosidase) 125 mg dispersed in maltodextrins. Cap. Bot. 100s. *otc.*
Use: Nutritional supplement.

Lactrodectus Mactans Antivenin. (Merck & Co.) Antivenin 6000 units per vial (with 1:10,000 thimerosal), supplied with a 2.5 ml vial of Sterile Water for Injection and a 1 mg vial (with 1:10,000 thimerosal) of normal horse serum (1:10 dilution) for sensitivity testing. *Rx.*
Use: Antivenin (Black Widow spider).
See: antivenin *Lactrodectus Mactans.*

•**lactulose concentrate.** (LAK-tyoo-lohs) U.S.P. 23.
Use: Laxative, treatment of hepatic coma and chronic constipation.
See: Cephulac, Syr. (Hoechst Marion Roussel).
Chronulac, Liq. (Hoechst Marion Roussel).
Evalose, Syr. (Copley Pharmaceutical, Inc.).
Heptalac, Syr. (Copley Pharmaceutical, Inc.).

ladakamycin.
Use: Refractory acute myelogenous leukemia (AML) agent.
See: Azacitidine.

Ladogal. (Sanofi Winthrop Pharmaceuticals) Danazol. *Rx.*
Use: Androgen.

Ladogar. (Sanofi Winthrop Pharmaceuticals) Danazol. *Rx.*
Use: Androgen.

Lady Esther. (Menley & James Labs, Inc.) Mineral oil. Cream. 120 g. *otc.*
Use: Emollient.

L.A.E. 20. (Seatrace Pharmaceuticals, Inc.) Estradiol valerate 20 mg/ml. Inj. Vial 10 ml. *Rx.*
Use: Estrogen.

L.A.E. 40. (Seatrace Pharmaceuticals, Inc.) Estradiol valerate 40 mg/ml. Inj. Vial 10 ml. *Rx.*
Use: Estrogen.

Lamictal. (GlaxoWellcome) Lamotrigine 25 mg, 100 mg, 150 mg, 200 mg/Tab. Bot. 25s (25 mg), 60s (150 mg, 200 mg), 100s (100 mg). *Rx.*
Use: Anticonvulsant.

Lamictal Chewable Dispersible Tablets. (GlaxoWellcome) Lamotrigine 5 mg, 25 mg. Chew. Tab. Bot. 100s. *Rx.*
Use: Anticonvulsant.

•**lamifiban.** (la-mih-FIE-ban) USAN.
Use: Antithrombotic, platelet aggregation inhibitor, fibrinogen receptor antagonist.

Lamisil. (Novartis Pharmaceutical Corp.) Terbinafine HCl 1%. Cream Tube 15 g, 30 g. 250 mg/Tab. Bot. 30s, 100s.
Use: Antifungal.

•**lamivudine.** (la-MIH-view-deen) USAN.
Use: Antiviral; treatment of HIV infection.
See: Epivir, Tab., Oral Soln. (GlaxoWellcome).
Epivir-HBV, Tab., Oral Soln. (GlaxoWellcome).

lamivudine and zidovudine.
Use: AIDS.
See: Combivir, Tab. (GlaxoWellcome).

•**lamotrigine.** (lah-MOE-trih-JEEN) USAN.
Use: Anticonvulsant; Lennox-Gestaut syndrome. [Orphan Drug]
See: Lamictal (GlaxoWellcome).

Lampit. (Bayer Corp. (Biological and Pharmaceutical Div.)) Nifurtimox.
Use: Anti-infective.

Lamprene. (Novartis Pharmaceutical Corp.) Clofazimine 50 mg/Cap. Bot. 100s. *Rx.*
Use: Leprostatic.

Lanabiotic. (Combe, Inc.) Polymyxin B sulfate 5000 units, neomycin (as sulfate) 3.5 mg, bacitracin 500 units, lidocaine 40 mg/g. Oint. 15 g, 30 g. *otc.*
Use: Anti-infective, anesthetic, local.

Lanacane. (Combe, Inc.) **Spray:** Benzocaine 20%, benzethonium Cl, ethanol, aloe extract. 113 ml. **Cream:** Benzocaine 6%, benzethonium Cl, aloe, parabens, castor oil, glycerin, isopropyl alcohol. 28 g, 56 g. *otc.*
Use: Anesthetic, local.

Lanacort 10. (Combe, Inc.) Hydrocortisone acetate 1% **Cream:** Tube 15, 30 g. **Oint.:** Tube 15 g. *otc.*
Use: Corticosteroid, topical.

Lanacort Cream. (Combe, Inc.) Hydrocortisone acetate 0.5%. Tube 0.5 oz, 1 oz. *otc.*
Use: Corticosteroid, topical.

Lanaphilic Ointment. (Medco Lab, Inc.) Sorbitol, isopropyl palmitate, stearyl alcohol, white petrolatum, lanolin oil, sodium lauryl sulfate, propylene glycol, methylparaben, propylparaben. Jar 16 oz. Also available w/urea 10% or 20%. *otc.*
Use: Emollient.

Lanaphilic w/Urea 10%. (Medco Lab, Inc.) Urea, stearyl alcohol, white petrolatum, isopropyl palmitate, propylene glycol, sorbitol, sodium lauryl sulfate, lactic acid, parabens. Oint. Jar lb. *otc.*
Use: Emollient.

•**lanolin.** (LAN-oh-lin) U.S.P. 23. *Formerly Anhydrous lanolin.*
Use: Pharmaceutic aid (ointment base, absorbent).
See: Kerohydric (Westwood Squibb Pharmaceuticals).
W/Coconut oil, pine oil, castor oil, cholesterols, lecithin, parachlorometaxylenol.
See: Sebacide, Liq. (Paddock Laboratories).
W/Diiosbutylcresoxyethoxyethyl, dimethyl benzyl ammonium Cl, menthol.
See: Hospital Lot. (Paddock Laboratories).

•**lanolin alcohols.** N.F. 18.
Use: Pharmaceutic aid (emulsifying agent).

•**lanolin, modified.** U.S.P. 23.
Use: Pharmaceutic aid (ointment base, absorbent).

Lanoline. (GlaxoWellcome) Perfumed emollient. Oint. Tube 1.75 oz. *otc.*
Use: Pharmaceutic aid, ointment base, absorbent, emollient.

Lano-Lo Bath Oil. (Whorton Pharmaceuticals, Inc.) 8 oz.

Lanolor. (Numark Laboratories, Inc.) Lanolin oil, glyceryl stearates, propylene glycol, sodium lauryl sulfate, simethicone, polyoxyl 40 stearate, cetyl esters wax, methylparaben. Cream Jar 60 g, 240 g. *otc.*
Use: Emollient.

Lanorinal. (Lannett Co., Inc.) Aspirin 325 mg, caffeine 40 mg, butalbital 50 mg. Cap., Tab. Bot. 100s (Cap. only), 1000s. *c-III.*

•**lanoteplase.** (lan-OH-teh-place) USAN.
Use: Thrombolytic, plasminogen activator.

Lanoxicaps. (GlaxoWellcome) Digoxin 0.05 mg, 0.1 mg, 0.2 mg. Soln. in cap. Bot. 100s. *Rx.*
Use: Cardiovascular agent.

Lanoxin. (GlaxoWellcome) Digoxin. **Tab.: 0.125 mg:** Bot. 100s, 1000s, Unit-of-use 30s, UD 100s. **0.25 mg:** Bot. 100s, 1000s, 5000s, UD 100s, Unit-of-use 30s. **Pediatric Elix.:** 0.05 mg/ml, alcohol 10%. Bot. 60 ml. **Inj.:** (w/propylene glycol 40%, alcohol 10%, sodium phosphate 0.3%, anhydrous citric acid 0.08%) Amp. 0.5 mg/2 ml. Amp. 10s, 50s. **Pediatric Inj.:** 0.1 mg/ml. Amp. 1 ml 10s. *Rx.*
Use: Cardiovascular agent.

•**lanreotide acetate.** (lan-REE-oh-tide) USAN.
Use: Antineoplastic.

•**lansoprazole.** (lan-SO-pruh-zole) USAN.

Use: Gastric acid pump inhibitor, antiulcerative, maintenance of healing of erosive esophagitis and gastric ulcers.
See: Prevacid, Cap. (Tap Pharmaceuticals).
W/Amoxicillin and clarithromycin.
See: Prevpac (TAP Pharmaceuticals).

Lanturil. (Sanofi Winthrop Pharmaceuticals) Oxypertine. *Rx.*
Use: Anxiolytic.

lanum. (Various Mfr.) Lanolin. *otc.*
Use: Pharmaceutic aid.

•**lapyrium chloride.** (LAH-pihr-ee-uhm KLOR-ide) USAN.
Use: Pharmaceutic aid (surfactant).

Lardet. (Standex) Phenobarbital 8 mg, theophylline 130 mg, ephedrine HCl 24 mg/Tab. Bot. 100s. *Rx.*
Use: Antiasthmatic combination.

Lardet Expectorant. (Standex) Phenobarbital 8 mg, theophylline 130 mg, ephedrine HCl 24 mg, guaifenesin 100 mg/Tab. Bot. 100s. *Rx.*
Use: Antiasthmatic combination.

Largon. (Wyeth-Ayerst Laboratories) Propiomazine HCl 20 mg/ml w/sodium formaldehyde sulfoxylate, sodium acetate buffer. Amp. 1 ml, 2 ml. Pkg. 25s, Tubex syringe 1 ml. *Rx.*
Use: Hypnotic, sedative.

Lariam. (Roche Laboratories) Mefloquine HCl 250 mg/Tab. UD 25s. *Rx.*
Use: Antimalarial.

Larodopa Capsules. (Roche Laboratories) Levodopa 100 mg, 250 mg, 500 mg/Cap. **100 mg:** Bot. 100s. **250 mg and 500 mg:** Bot. 100s, 500s. *Rx.*
Use: Antiparkinsonian.

Larodopa Tablets. (Roche Laboratories) Levodopa 100 mg, 250 mg, 500 mg. **100 mg:** Bot. 100s. **250 mg and 500 mg:** Bot. 100s, 500s. *Rx.*
Use: Antiparkinsonian.

Larotid. (SmithKline Beecham Pharmaceuticals) Amoxicillin. **Cap.: 250 mg:** Bot. 100s, 500s, UD 100s, unit-of-use 18s. **500 mg:** Bot. 50s, 500s. **Oral Susp.:** 125 mg, 250 mg (as trihydrate)/ 5 ml. Bot. 80 ml, 100 ml, 150 ml. **Pediatric drops:** 50 mg (as trihydrate)/ml. Bot. 15 ml. *Rx.*
Use: Anti-infective, penicillin.

Larynex. (Dover Pharmaceuticals) Benzocaine. Sugar, lactose and salt free. Loz. UD Box 500s. *otc.*
Use: Anesthetic, local.

Lasix. (Hoechst Marion Roussel) Furosemide. **Tab.:** 20 mg, 40 mg/Tab. Bot. 100s, 500s, 1000s, UD 100s; 80 mg/ Tab. Bot. 50s, 500s, UD 100s. **Inj.:** 10 mg/ml. 2 ml Amp. Box 5s, 50s, 4 ml Amp. Box 5s, 25s; 10 ml Amp. Box 5s, 25s; Syringe 2 ml, 4 ml, 10 ml. Box 5s. Single-use Vial 2 ml, 4 ml, 10 ml.
Use: Diuretic.

lassar's paste.
See: Zinc Oxide Paste, U.S.P. 23. (Various Mfr.).

•**latanoprost.** (lah-TAN-oh-prahst) USAN.
Use: Antiglaucoma agent.
See: Xalatan, Soln. (Pharmacia & Upjohn).

Latest-CRP Kit. (Fischer Pharmaceuticals, Inc.) Measures C-reactive protein in serum. Kit 1s.
Use: Diagnostic aid.

•**laureth 4.** (LAH-reth 4) USAN.
Use: Pharmaceutic aid (surfacant).

•**laureth 9.** (LAH-reth 9) USAN.
Use: Pharmaceutical aid (surfactant), emulsifier, spermaticide.

•**laureth 10.** (LAH-reth 10s) USAN.
Use: Spermaticide.

•**laurocapram.** (LAHR-oh-KAH-pram) USAN.
Use: Pharmaceutic aid (excipient).

lauromacrogol 400. Laureth 9.

•**lauryl isoquinolinium bromide.** (LAH-rill EYE-so-KWIN-oh-lih-nee-uhm) USAN.
Use: Anti-infective.

lauryl sulfoacetate.
See: Lowila, Cake, Liq., Oint. (Westwood Squibb Pharmaceuticals).

Lavacol. (Parke-Davis) Ethyl alcohol 70%. Bot. Pt.
Use: Anti-infective, topical.

Lavatar. (Doak Dermatologics) Coal tar distillate 25.5% in a bath oil base. Liq. Bot. 4 oz, pt.
Use: Antipsoriatic, antipruritic.

lavender oil.
Use: Perfume.

•**lavoltidine succinate.** (lahv-OLE-tih-DEEN) USAN. *Formerly Loxotidine.*
Use: Antiulcerative (histamine H_2-receptor blocker).

Lavoptik Emergency Wash. (Lavoptik Co., Inc.) Eye, face, body wash. 32 oz/Emergency station. *otc.*
Use: Emergency wash.

Lavoptik Eye Wash. (Lavoptik Co., Inc.) Sodium Cl 0.49%, sodium biphosphate 0.4%, sodium phosphate 0.45%/100 ml w/benzalkonium Cl 0.005%. Bot. 6 oz. *otc.*
Use: Irrigant, ophthalmic.

Lavoris. (Procter & Gamble Pharm.) Zinc Cl, glycerin, poloxamer 407, saccharin, polysorbate 80, flavors, clove oil, alcohol, citric acid, water. Bot. 6 oz, 12 oz,

18 oz, 24 oz. *otc.*
Use: Mouthwash.

Laxative Caps. (Weeks & Leo) Docusate sodium 100 mg, casanthranol 30 mg/Cap. Bot. 30s, 60s. *otc.*
Use: Laxative.

laxatives.
See: Aloe (Various Mfr.).
Aloin (Various Mfr.).
Bile Salts (Various Mfr.).
Bisacodyl, Tab., Supp. (Various Mfr.).
Bisacodyl Tannex (PBH Wesley Jessen).
Carboxymethylcellulose Sodium (Various Mfr.).
Casanthranol, Cap., Tab. (Various Mfr.).
Cascara Sagrada (Various Mfr.).
Cascara Sagrada Fluidextract, Liq. (Parke-Davis).
Cascara, Tab. (Various Mfr.).
Castor Oil (Various Mfr.).
Citrucel (SmithKline Beecham Pharmaceuticals).
Correctol, Tab. (Schering-Plough Corp.).
Docusate Sodium (Various Mfr.).
Ex-Lax, Tab., Pow. (Ex-Lax, Inc.).
Feen-a-Mint, Gum, Mints (Schering-Plough Corp.).
Karaya Gum (Penick).
Liquid Petrolatum, Liq. (Various Mfr.).
Magnesia Maga (Various Mfr.).
Maltsupex (Wallace Laboratories).
Methylcellulose (Various Mfr.).
Mucilloid of Psyllium Seed W/Dextrose (Searle).
Mylanta Natural Fiber Supplement (J & J-Merck).
Nature's Remedy (SmithKline Beecham Pharmaceuticals).
Oxyphenisatin Acetate (Various Mfr.).
Petrolatum, Liq. (Various Mfr.).
Petrolatum, Liq., Emulsion (Various Mfr.).
Phenolphthalein (Various Mfr.).
Plantago ovata, Coating (Various Mfr.).
Poloxalkol, Cap., Soln. (Various Mfr.).
Prune Concentrate, Tab, Cap. (Various Mfr.)
Prune Preps (Various Mfr.).
Psyllium Granules W/Dextrose (Davol).
Psyllium Husk, Pow. (Pharmacia & Upjohn).
Psyllium Hydrocolloid, Pow. (Zeneca Pharmaceuticals).
Psyllium Hydrophilic Mucilloid (Various Mfr.).
Psyllium Seed, Gel, Gran. (Various Mfr.).
Restore (Inagra).
Senna, Alexandrian, Liq, Tab. (Various Mfr.).
Senna, Cassia angustifolia, Tab. (Brayten).
Senna Conc, Standardized, Gran, Tab., Pow., Supp. (Various Mfr.).
Senna Fruit Extract, Liq. (Various Mfr.).
Sennosides A & B, Tab. (Novartis Pharmaceutical Corp.).
Sodium Biphosphate (Various Mfr.).
Sodium Phosphate (Various Mfr.).
Unifiber (Dow Hickam, Inc.).

W/Choline base, cephalin, lipositol.
See: Alcolec Cap., Gran. (American Lecithin Company).

W/Coconut oil, pine oil, castor oil, lanolin, cholesterols, parachlorometaxylenol.
See: Sebacide, Liq. (Paddock Laboratories).

W/Vitamins.
See: Lec-E-Plex, Cap. (Barth's).

Laxinate 100. (Roberts Pharmaceuticals) Dioctyl sodium sulfosuccinate 100 mg/Cap. Bot. 100s, 1000s.
Use: Laxative.

Lax Pills. (G & W Laboratories) Yellow phenolphthalein 90 mg/Tab. Bot. 30s, 60s. *otc.*
Use: Laxative.

layor carang.
See: Agar (Various Mfr.).

•**lazabemide.** (lazz-AH-bem-ide) USAN.
Use: Antiparkinsonian.

Lazer Creme. (Pedinol Pharmacal, Inc.) Vitamins E 3500 units, A 100,000 units/oz. Jar 2 oz. *otc.*
Use: Emollient.

Lazer Formalyde Solution. (Pedinol Pharmacal, Inc.) Formaldehyde 10%, polysorbate 20, hydroxyethyl cellulose. Bot. 3 oz. *Rx.*
Use: Drying agent.

LazerSporin-C Solution. (Pedinol Pharmacal, Inc.) Neomycin sulfate 3.5 mg, polymyxin B sulfate 10,000 units, hydrocortisone 1%/ml. Bot. 10 ml. *Rx.*
Use: Anti-infective combination, topical.

l-baclofen.
Use: Antispasmodic. [Orphan Drug]

l-bulgaricus. Antidiarrheal.
See: Bacid (Medeva Pharmaceuticals, Inc.).
Lactinex B (Becton Dickinson & Co.).
More Dophilus (Freeda Vitamins, Inc.).

LC-65 Daily Contact Lens Cleaner. (Allergan, Inc.) Daily cleaning solution for all hard, soft (hydrophilic), rigid gas

permeable contact lenses. Bot. 15 ml, 60 ml. *otc.*
Use: Contact lens care.

L-Caine E. (Century Pharmaceuticals, Inc.) Lidocaine HCl 1%, 2%, epinephrine 1:100,000/ml. Inj. 20 ml, 50 ml. *Rx.*
Use: Anesthetic, local.

L-Caine Viscous. (Century Pharmaceuticals, Inc.) Lidocaine HCl 2% with sodium carboxymethylcellulose. Soln. Bot. 100 ml. *Rx.*
Use: Anesthetic, local.

l-carnitine. Amino acid derivative 250 mg/Cap. Bot. 60s.
Use: Nutritional supplement.
See: Vitacarn.
Carnitor (Sigma-Tau Pharmaceuticals, Inc.).

L.C.D. (Almay, Inc.) Alcohol extractions of crude coal tar. Cream, soln. Bot. 4 oz, pt. *otc.*
Use: Antipsoriatic, antipruritic, topical.
See: Coal Tar Topical Soln., U.S.P. 23.

LCR. *Rx.*
Use: Antineoplastic.
See: Vincristine sulfate.

LCx Neisseria gonorrhoeae Assay. (Abbott Laboratories) Reagent kit for the detection of *Neisseria gonorrhoeae* in female endocervical, male urethral, and urine swab specimens. Kit. 96s. *Rx.*
Use: Diagnostic aid.

l-cycloserine.
Use: Gaucher's disease. [Orphan Drug]

l-cysteine. (Tyson & Associates, Inc.)
Use: Erythropoietic protoporphyria. [Orphan Drug]

l-deprenyl.
See: Selegiline HCl.

LDH Reagent Strip. (Bayer Corp. (Consumer Div.)) A quantitative strip test for LDH in serum or plasma. Seralyzer reagent strip. Bot. 25s. *Rx.*
Use: Diagnostic aid.

Leber Tabulae. (Paddock Laboratories) Aloe 0.09 g, extract of rhei 0.03 g, myrrh 0.01 g, frangula 5 mg, galbanum 2 mg, olibanum 3 mg/Tab. Bot. 100s, 500s, 1000s.

Lec-E-Plex. (Barth's) Vitamin E 100 IU, 200 IU, 400 IU/Cap. w/lecithin. Bot. 100s, 500s, 1000s. *otc.*
Use: Vitamin E supplement.

•**lecimibide.** (leh-SIM-ih-bide) USAN.
Use: Antihyperlipidemic.

lecithin. (Various Mfr.) Lecithin. **Cap.:** 520 mg. Bot. 100s, 250s, 1000s; 650 mg. Bot. 90s, 100s, 250s, 500s. **Pow.:** 120 g, kg, lb. *otc.*
Use: Nutritional supplement.

•**lecithin.** (LESS-ih-thin) N.F. 18.
Use: Pharmaceutic aid (emulsifying agent).

lecithin. (Arcum) 1200 mg. Cap. Bot. 100s, 1000s; Gran. Bot. 8 oz; Pow. Bot. 4 oz. (Barth's) 8 gr/Cap. Bot. 100s, 500s, 1000s; Gran. Can 8 oz, 16 oz; Pow. Can 10 oz. (Cavendish) Tab. (0.5 gr) Bot. 500s. (Quality Formulations, Inc.) 1200 mg, Cap. 100s. (De Pree) Cap Bot 100s. (Pfanstiehl) 25 g, 100 g, 500 g/Pkg.
Use: Pharmaceutic aid (emulsifying agent).

•**ledoxantrone trihydrochloride.** (led-OX-an-trone try-HIGH-droe-KLOR-ide) USAN.
Use: Antineoplastic.

leflunomide.
Use: Antiarthritic.
See: Arava, Tab. (Hoechst Marion Roussel).

Legatrin PM. (Columbia Laboratories, Inc.) Acetaminophen 500 mg, diphenhydramine HCl 50 mg/Capl. Bot. 30s, 50s. *otc.*
Use: Sleep aid.

lemon oil.
Use: Pharmaceutic aid (flavor).

•**lenercept.** (LEH-ner-sept) USAN.
Use: Treatment of septic shock, multiple sclerosis, inflammatory bowel disease, rheumatoid arthritis.

lenetran. Mephenoxalone.
Use: Anxiolytic.

lenicet.
See: Aluminum Acetate, Basic (Various Mfr.).

•**leniquinsin.** (LEN-ih-KWIN-sin) USAN. Under study.
Use: Antihypertensive.

Lenium Medicated Shampoo. (Sanofi Winthrop Pharmaceuticals) Selenium sulfide. *otc.*
Use: Antiseborrheic.

•**lenograstim.** (leh-no-GRAH-stim) USAN.
Use: Antineutropenic, hematopoietic stimulant, immunomodulator (granulocyte colony-stimulating factor).

•**lenperone.** (LEN-per-OHN) USAN.
Use: Antipsychotic.

Lens Clear. (Allergan, Inc.) Sterile, isotonic solution surfactant cleaner w/sorbic acid 0.1%, edetate disodium 0.2%. Bot. 15 ml. *otc.*
Use: Contact lens care.

Lens Drops. (Ciba Vision) Sodium chloride, borate buffer, carbamide, poloxamer 407, EDTA 0.2%, sorbic acid 0.15%. Soln. Bot. 15 ml. *otc.*

Use: Contact lens care, rewetting.

Lensept Disinfecting Solution. (Ciba Vision) Micro-filtered hydrogen peroxide with sodium stannate 3%, sodium nitrate, phosphate buffers. Soln. Bot. 237, 355 ml. *otc.*
Use: Disinfecting solution.

Lensept Rinse and Neutralizer. (Ciba Vision) Sodium chloride, sodium borate decahydrate, boric acid, bovine catalase, sorbic acid, EDTA. Soln. Bot. 237 ml. System includes lens cup and holder. *otc.*
Use: Contact lens care, rinsing, neutralizing.

Lens Fresh. (Allergan, Inc.) Sterile, buffered, isotonic aqueous soln. W/ hydroxyethyl cellulose, sodium Cl, boric acid, sodium borate, sorbic acid 0.1%, edetate disodium 0.2%. Bot. 0.5 oz. *otc.*
Use: Contact lens care.

Lensine Extra Strength. (Ciba Vision) Cleaning agent with benzalkonium Cl 0.01%, EDTA 0.1%. Soln. Bot. 45 ml. *otc.*
Use: Contact lens care.

Lens Lubricant. (Bausch & Lomb Pharmaceuticals) Povidone and polyoxyethylene with thimerosal 0.004%, EDTA 0.1% Soln. Bot. 15 ml. *otc.*
Use: Contact lens care, lubricant.

Lens Plus. (Allergan, Inc.) Isotonic soln. w/sodium Cl 0.9%. Aerosol 3 oz, 8 oz, 12 oz. Preservative free. *otc.*
Use: Contact lens care.

Lens Plus Daily Cleaner. (Allergan, Inc.) Buffered solution with cocoamphocarboxyglycinate, sodium lauryl sulfate, hexylene glycol, sodium chloride, sodium phosphate. Preservative free. Soln. Bot. 15 ml, 30 ml. *otc.*
Use: Contact lens care, cleanser.

Lens Plus Oxysept Disinfecting Solution. (Allergan, Inc.) Hydrogen peroxide with sodium stannate 3%, sodium nitrate, phosphate buffer. Soln. Bot. 240 ml. *otc.*
Use: Contact lens care.

Lens Plus Oxysept 2 Neutralizing. (Allergan, Inc.) Catalase with buffering agents used to neutralize the *Lens Plus Oxysept 1* disinfecting solution in a chemical lens care system. For soft contact lens. Tabs. Box 12s. Bot. 36s. *otc.*
Use: Contact lens care.

Lens Plus Oxysept Rinse and Neutralizer. (Allergan, Inc.) Isotonic with sodium chloride, mono- and dibasic sodium phosphates, catalytic neutralizing agent, EDTA. Soln. Bot. 15 ml. *otc.*
Use: Contact lens care.

Lens Plus Preservative Free. (Allergan, Inc.) Isotonic sodium chloride 9%. Soln. Bot. 90 ml, 240 ml, 360 ml. *otc.*
Use: Contact lens care.

Lens Plus Rewetting Drops. (Allergan, Inc.) Sterile, non-preserved isotonic solution w/sodium Cl, boric acid. 0.35 ml (30s). *otc.*
Use: Contact lens care.

Lens Plus Rewetting Drops. (Allergan, Inc.) Isotonic solution with sodium chloride and boric acid. Thimerosal and preservative free. Soln. Bot. 0.3 ml (30s). *otc.*
Use: Contact lens care.

Lens Plus Sterile Saline. (Allergan, Inc.) Sodium Cl, boric acid, nitrogen. Soln. Bot. 90 ml, 240 ml, 360 ml. Aerosol. *otc.*
Use: Contact lens care.

Lensrins. (Allergan, Inc.) Sterile preserved saline for heat disinfection, rinsing and storage of soft (hydrophilic) contact lenses; rinsing solution for chemical disinfection. Soln. Bot. 8 oz. *otc.*
Use: Contact lens care.

Lens-Wet. (Allergan, Inc.) Isotonic, buffered soln. of polyvinyl alcohol, thimerosal 0.002%, EDTA 0.01%. Bot. 0.5 fl oz. *otc.*
Use: Contact lens care.

Lente Iletin I. (Eli Lilly and Co.) Insulin zinc suspension 100 units/ml. Beef and pork. Inj. Vial. 10 ml. *otc.*
Use: Antidiabetic.

Lente Iletin II. (Eli Lilly and Co.) Insulin zinc suspension 100 units/ml. Purified pork. Inj. Bot. 10 ml.
Use: Antidiabetic.

lente insulin. Susp. of zinc insulin crystals. *otc.*
See: Iletin Lente, Vial (Eli Lilly and Co.).

lente insulin. (Novo/Nordisk Pharm, Inc.) Insulin zinc susp. 100 units/ml Beef. Inj. Vial 10 ml.
Use: Antidiabetic.

Lente L. (Novo/Nordisk Pharm, Inc.) Insulin zinc suspension 100 units/ml. Purified pork. Inj. Vial 10 ml. *otc.*
Use: Antidiabetic.

lentinan. (Lenti-Chemico Pharmaceuticals)
Use: Immunomodulator.

lepirudin.
Use: Heparin-associated thrombocytopenia Type II. [Orphan Drug]
See: Refludan (Behringwerke).

lepromin. (Louisiana State University) Lepromin, 30 to 40 million acid-fast bacilli/ml. Vial 5 ml, 10 ml, 20 ml, 50 ml.

leprostatics.
Use: Bactericidal.
See: Dapsone, Tab. (Jacobus Pharmaceutical Co.).
Lamprene, Cap. (Novartis Pharmaceutical Corp.).

•**lergotrile.** (LER-go-trill) USAN.
Use: Enzyme inhibitor (prolactin).

•**lergotrile mesylate.** (LER-go-trill) USAN.
Use: Enzyme inhibitor (prolactin).

Lerton Ovules. (Vita Elixir) Caffeine 250 mg/Cap. *otc.*
Use: CNS stimulant.

Lescol. (Novartis Pharmaceutical Corp.) Fluvastatin sodium 20 mg, 40 mg. Cap. Bot. 30s, 100s.
Use: Antihyperlipidemic.

Lesterol. (Dram) Nicotinic acid 500 mg/Tab. Bot. 250s. *otc.*
Use: Antihyperlipidemic.

•**letimide hydrochloride.** (LET-ih-mide) USAN.
Use: Analgesic.

•**letrozole.** (let-ROW-zahl) USAN.
Use: Antineoplastic.
See: Femara, Tab. (Novartis Pharmaceutical Corp.).

•**leucine.** (LOO-SEEN) U.S.P. 23.
Use: Amino acid.

leucomax. (Various Mfr.). Leucomax. Granulocyte-macrophage colony-stimulating factor (Recombinant). Molgramostin (Schering-Plough Corp. and Novartis Pharmaceutical Corp.).
Use: Immunomodulator.

l-leucovorin.
Use: Antineoplastic. [Orphan Drug]
See: Isovorin (Lederle).

•**leucovorin calcium.** (loo-koe-VORE-in) U.S.P. 23.
Use: Antianemic, folate-deficiency; antidote to folic acid antagonists.

leucovorin calcium. (loo-koe-VORE-in) (Various Mfr.) 5 mg. Tab. Bot. 30s, 100s, UD 50s.
Use: Antagonist of amithopterin, antianemic (folate-deficiency), antidote to folic acid antagonists, antineoplastic. [Orphan Drug]
See: Wellcovorin, Inj., Tab. (Glaxo-Wellcome).

leucovorin calcium. (Various Mfr.) **Tab.:** 15 mg, 25 mg as calcium. Pkg. 12s, 24s, 25s, UD 50s. **Inj.:** 3 mg/ml as calcium w/ benzyl alcohol 0.9%. Amps 1 ml. **Pow. for Inj.:** 50 mg/vial, 100 mg/vial, 350 mg/vial. *Rx.*
Use: Folic acid antagonist overdosage.

Leukeran. (GlaxoWellcome) Chlorambucil 2 mg/Tab. Bot. 50s. *Rx.*
Use: Antineoplastic.

Leukine. (Immunex Corp.) Sargramostim. **Pow. for Inj.:** 250 mcg, 500 mcg. Lyophilized. **Liq.:** 500 mcg/ml Vial. *Rx.*
Use: Bone marrow transplant adjunct.

leukocyte protease inhibitor, recombinant secretory.
Use: Alpha-1 antitrypsin deficiency; cystic fibrosis. [Orphan Drug]

leukocyte protease inhibitor, secretory.
Use: Bronchopulmonary dysplasia. [Orphan Drug]

•**leukocyte typing serum.** U.S.P. 23.
Use: Diagnostic aid (blood, in vitro).

leupeptin. (Neuromuscular Agents)
Use: Adjunct to nerve repair. [Orphan Drug]

•**leuprolide acetate.** (loo-PRO-lide) USAN.
Use: Antineoplastic, LHRH agonist, central precocious puberty. [Orphan Drug]
See: Lupron, Inj. (Tap Pharmaceuticals).
Lupron Depot, Microspheres for Inj. (Tap Pharmaceuticals).
Lupon Depot (Tap Pharmaceuticals).

leuprolide acetate. (Bedford) 5 mg/ml, benzyl alcohol, sodium chloride. Inj. Multi-dose Vial 2.8 ml. *Rx.*
Use: Antineoplastic.

leurocristine.
See: Vincristine Sulfate (Eli Lilly and Co.)

leurocristine sulfate (1:1) (salt). Vincristine Sulfate, U.S.P. 23.
Use: Antineoplastic.

Leustatin. (Ortho Biotech, Inc.) Cladribine. Soln. 1 mg/ml. Vial. 20 ml single-use. *Rx.*
Use: Antineoplastic.

leuteinizing hormone (recombinant) human.
Use: With recombinant human follicle-stimulating hormone for chronic anovulation due to hypogonadotropic hypogonadism. [Orphan Drug]

•**levalbuterol hydrochloride.** (lev-al-BYOO-ter-ole HIGH-droe-KLOR-ide) USAN.
Use: Bronchodilator; antiasthmatic.

•**levalbuterol sulfate.** (lev-al-BYOO-ter-ole SULL-fate) USAN.
Use: Bronchodilator; antiasthmatic.

levamfetamine. (LEV-am-FET-ah-meen) F.D.A.
Use: Anorexic.

•**levamfetamine succinate.** (LEV-am-

FET-ah-meen) USAN.
Use: Anorexic.

•**levamisole hydrochloride.** (lev-AM-ih-sole) U.S.P. 23.
Use: Biological response modifier; antineoplastic.
See: Ergamisol (Janssen Pharmaceutical, Inc.).

Levaquin. (Ortho McNeil Pharmaceutical) Levofloxacin 250 mg, 500 mg/Tab. Bot. 50s, UD 100s. Levofloxacin 500 mg/Inj. Vial. 20 ml. Levofloxacin 250 mg, 500 mg/Inj. (premix). 50 ml flexible containers with 5% Dextrose solution (250 mg). 100 ml flexible containers with 5% Dextrose Solution (500 mg). *Rx.*
Use: Fluoroquinolone.

levarterenol. *Rx.*
Use: Vasoconstrictor.
See: Levophed, Inj. (Sanofi Winthrop Pharmaceuticals).

levarterenol bitartrate.
See: Norepinephrine Bitartrate, U.S.P. 23.

Levatol. (Schwarz Pharma, Inc.) Penbutolol sulfate 20 mg. Tab. Bot. 100s. *Rx.*
Use: Beta-adrenergic blocker.

Levbid. (Schwarz Pharma, Inc.) Hyoscyamine sulfate 0.375 mg/ER Tab. Bot. 100s. *Rx.*
Use: Anticholinergic.

•**levcromakalim.** (lev-KROE-mah-KAY-lim) USAN.
Use: Antihypertensive; antiasthmatic.

•**levcycloserine.** (LEV-sigh-kloe-SER-een) USAN.
Use: Enzyme inhibitor (Gaucher's disease).

•**levdobutamine lactobionate.** (LEV-dah-BYOOT-ah-meen LACK-toe-BYE-oh-nate) USAN.
Use: Cardiovascular agent.

Leviron. (Health for Life Brands, Inc.) Desiccated liver 7 gr, iron and ammonium citrate 3 gr, vitamins B_1 1 mg, B_2 0.5 mg, B_6 0.5 mg, calcium pantothenate 0.3 mg, niacinamide 2.5 mg, B_{12} 1 mcg/Cap. Bot. 100s, 1000s. *otc.*
Use: Mineral, vitamin supplement.

Levlen 21 Tablets. (Berlex Laboratories, Inc.) Levonorgestrel 0.15 mg, ethinyl estradiol 0.03 mg/Tab. Slidecase 21s, Box 3s. *Rx.*
Use: Contraceptive.

Levlen 28 Tablets. (Berlex Laboratories, Inc.) Levonorgestrel 0.15 mg, ethinyl estradiol 0.03 mg/Tab. (21 active, 7 inert). Slidecase 28s, Box 3s. *Rx.*
Use: Contraceptive.

Levlite 21. (Berlex Labs) Levonorgestrel 0.1 mg, ethinyl estradiol 0.02, lactose, sucrose. Tab. Pkt. 21s *Rx.*
Use: Contraceptive.

Levlite 28. (Berlex Labs) Levonorgestrel 0.1 mg, ethinyl estradiol 0.02 mg, lactose, sucrose. Tab. Pkt. 28s. *Rx.*
Use: Contraceptive.

•**levoamphetamine.** (lee-voe-meth-am-FET-uh-meen) U.S.P. 23.
Use: Nasal decongestant.

levo-amphetamine. Alginate (l-isomer) alpha-2-phenylaminopropane succinate.

•**levobetaxolol hydrochloride.** (LEE-voe-beh-TAX-oh-lahl) USAN.
Use: Antiadrenergic (β-receptor).

•**levobunolol hydrochloride.** (LEE-voe-BYOO-no-lahl) U.S.P. 23.
Use: Antiadrenergic (β-receptor).
See: AKBeta, Ophth. Soln. (Akorn, Inc.).
Betagan, Ophth. Soln. (Allergan, Inc.).

levobunolol hydrochloride. (LEE-voe-BYOO-no-lahl) (Various Mfr.) 0.25%, 0.5% Ophth. Soln. Bot. 5 ml, 10 ml, 15 ml (0.5% only). *Rx.*
Use: Beta-adrenergic blocker.

•**levocabastine hydrochloride.** (LEE-voe-cab-ASS-teen) USAN.
Use: Antihistamine.
See: Livostin, Ophth. Susp. (Ciba Vision).

•**levocarnitine.** (LEE-voe-CAR-nih-teen) U.S.P. 23.
Use: Carnitine replenisher. [Orphan Drug]
See: Carnitor, Liq., Tab. (Sigma-Tau Pharmaceuticals, Inc.).
L-Carnitine, Cap. (R & D Laboratories, Inc.).
Vitacarn, Liq. (McGaw, Inc.).

•**levodopa.** (LEE-voe-DOE-puh) U.S.P. 23.
Use: Antiparkinsonian.
See: Bio Dopa, Cap. (Bio-Deriv.).
Dopar, Cap. (Procter & Gamble Pharm.).
Larodopa, Tab. or Cap. (Roche Laboratories).
Levora, Cap. (Zeneca Pharmaceuticals).

levodopa & carbidopa. (LEE-voe-DOE-puh and CAR-bih-doe-puh)
Use: Antiparkinsonian.
See: Carbidopa and Levodopa, Tab. (Lemmon Co.).
Sinemet 10/100, Tab. (DuPont Merck Pharmaceutical Co.).

Sinemet 25/100, Tab. (DuPont Merck Pharmaceutical Co.).
Sinemet 25/250, Tab. (DuPont Merck Pharmaceutical Co.).
Sinemet CR, SR Tab. (DuPont Merck Pharmaceutical Co.).

Levo-Dromoran. (ICN) Levorphanol tartrate. **Inj. (Amp.):** 2 mg/ml w/methyl- and propylparabens, sodium hydroxide. 1 ml. **Vial:** 2 mg/ml w/phenol. Multidose Vial 10 ml. **Tab.:** 2 mg. Bot. 100s. *c-II.*
Use: Analgesic, narcotic.

•**levofloxacin.** (lee-voe-FLOX-ah-sin) USAN.
Use: Anti-infective.
See: Levaquin, Tab. Inj. (Ortho McNeil Pharmaceutical).

•**levofuraltadone.** (LEE-voe-fer-AL-tah-dohn) USAN.
Use: Anti-infective, antiprotozoal.

•**levoleucovorin calcium.** (LEE-voe-loo-koe-VORE-in) USAN.
Use: Antidote to folic acid antagonist.
See: Isovorin (Immunex Corp.).

•**levomethadyl acetate.** (LEE-voe-METH-uh-dill) USAN.
Use: Analgesic, narcotic.

•**levomethadyl acetate hydrochloride.** (LEE-voe-METH-uh-dill) USAN.
Use: Analgesic, narcotic; treatment of heroin addicts.
See: ORLAAM (Roxane).

•**levonantradol hydrochloride.** (LEE-voe-NAN-trah-DAHL) USAN.
Use: Analgesic.

•**levonordefrin.** (lee-voe-nore-DEFF-rin) U.S.P. 23.
Use: Adrenergic (vasoconstrictor).

•**levonorgestrel.** (LEE-voe-nor-JESS-truhl) U.S.P. 23.
Use: Hormone, progestin.
See: Alesse, Tab. (Wyeth-Ayerst Laboratories).
Levora, Tab. (SCS).
Norplant (Wyeth-Ayerst Laboratories).

levonorgestrel and ethinyl estradiol tablets.
Use: Contraceptive.
See: Alesse (Wyeth-Ayerst Laboratories).
Levlite (Berlex Laboratories, Inc.).
Levoral (SCS Pharmaceuticals).
Nordette, Tab. (Wyeth-Ayerst Laboratories).
Preven (Gynetics).

Levophed. (Breon) Norepinephrine bitartrate 1 mg/ml. Amp. 4 ml. *Rx.*
Use: Vasoconstrictor.

Levophed Bitartrate. (Sanofi Winthrop Pharmaceuticals) Norepinephrine bitartrate w/sodium Cl, sodium metabisulfite 1 mg, 2 mg/ml. Amp. 4 ml. Box 10s. *Rx.*
Use: Vasoconstrictor.

Levoprome. (ESI Lederle Generics) Methotrimeprazine 20 mg/ml w/benzyl alcohol 0.9%, disodium edetate 0.065%, sodium metabisulfite 0.3%. Vial 10 ml. *Rx.*
Use: Analgesic.

•**levopropoxyphene napsylate.** (lee-voe-pro-POX-ee-feen NAP-sih-late) USAN. U.S.P. XXII.
Use: Antitussive.

•**levopropylcillin potassium.** (lee-voe-pro-pihl-SILL-in) USAN.
Use: Anti-infective.

Levora. (SCS Pharmaceuticals) Ethinyl estradiol 0.03 mg, levonorgestrel 0.15 mg. Tab. Pkt. 21s, 28s. *Rx.*
Use: Contraceptive.

levorenine.
See: Epinephrine, U.S.P. 23. (Various Mfr.).

Levoroxine. (Bariatric) Sodium levothyroxine 0.05 mg, 0.1 mg, 0.2 mg, 0.3 mg/Tab. Bot. 100s, 500s. *Rx.*
Use: Hormone, thyroid.

•**levorphanol tartrate.** (lee-VORE-fah-nole TAR-trate) U.S.P. 23.
Use: Analgesic, narcotic.
See: Levo-Dromoran (ICN).

Levo-T. (ESI Lederle Generics) Levothyroxine sodium 0.025, 0.05, 0.075, 0.1, 0.125, 0.15, 0.2, 0.3 mg. Tab. Bot. 100s (all strengths), 1000s (0.05, 0.1, 0.15, 0.2 mg only). *Rx.*
Use: Hormone, thyroid.

Levothroid. (Forest Pharmaceutical, Inc.) Levothyroxine sodium. **Tab.:** 25 mcg, 50 mcg, 75 mcg, 88 mcg, 100 mcg, 112 mcg, 125 mcg, 137 mcg, 150 mcg, 175 mcg, 200 mcg, 300 mcg/Tab. Bot. 100s (all strengths), UD 100s (50 mcg, 100 mcg, 150 mcg, 200 mcg, 300 mcg only). **Inj.:** 200 mcg, 500 mcg. Vial 6 ml. *Rx.*
Use: Hormone, thyroid.

•**levothyroxine sodium.** (lee-voe-thigh-ROX-een) U.S.P. 23.
Use: Hormone, thyroid.
See: Eltroxin, Tab. (Roberts Pharmaceuticals).
Levo-T, Tab. (ESI Lederle Generics).
Levothroid, Tab., Inj. (Forest Pharmaceutical, Inc.).
Levoxine, Inj. (Jones Medical Industries, Inc.).
Levoxyl, Tab. (Jones Medical Industries, Inc.).

Synthroid, Tab., Inj. (Boots).
W/Mannitol.
See: Levoxine, Inj. (Jones Medical Industries, Inc.).
Synthroid, Inj. (Knoll Pharmaceuticals).
W/Sodium liothyronine.
See: Thyrolar, Tab. (Rhone-Poulenc Rorer Pharmaceuticals, Inc.).

levothyroxine sodium. (Various Mfr.) **Pow. for Inj.:** Levothyroxine sodium 200 mcg, 500 mcg/Vial. Pow. for Inj. 6 ml, 10 ml. 0.1 mg, 0.15 mg, 0.2 mg, 0.3 mg. Bot. 100s, 1000s, UD 100s. *Rx.*
Use: Hormone, thyroid.

•**levoxadrol hydrochloride.** (lev-OX-ah-drole) USAN.
Use: Anesthetic, local; muscle relaxant.

Levoxyl. (Jones Medical Industries, Inc.) Levothyroxine sodium 0.025 mg, 0.05 mg, 0.75 mg, 0.088 mg, 0.1 mg, 0.112 mg, 0.125 mg, 0.137 mg, 0.15 mg, 0.175 mg, 0.2 mg, 0.3 mg/Tab. Bot. 100s, 1000s, UD 100s. *Rx.*
Use: Hormone, thyroid.

Levsin. (Schwarz Pharma, Inc.) L-hyoscyamine sulfate. **Tab.:** 0.125 mg. Bot. 100s, 500s. **Soln.:** 0.125 mg/ml, alcohol 5%. Bot. 15 ml. **Elix.:** 0.125 mg/5 ml, alcohol 20%. Bot. Pt. **Inj.:** 0.5 mg/ml. Vial 1 ml, 10 ml. *Rx.*
Use: Anticholinergic, antispasmodic.

Levsin-PB Drops. (Schwarz Pharma, Inc.) Hyoscyamine sulfate 0.125 mg, phenobarbital 15 mg/ml, alcohol 5%. Liq. Bot. 15 ml. *Rx.*
Use: Anticholinergic, antispasmodic, hypnotic, sedative.

Levsin/SL. (Schwarz Pharma, Inc.) Hyoscyamine sulfate 0.125 mg/Tab. Sublingual. Bot. 100s, 500s. *Rx.*
Use: Gastrointestinal, anticholinergic.

Levsinex Timecaps. (Schwarz Pharma, Inc.) L-hyoscyamine sulfate 0.375 mg/TR Cap. Bot. 100s, 500s. *Rx.*
Use: Anticholinergic, antispasmodic.

levulose. Fructose.

levulose-dextrose.
See: Invert Sugar.

•**lexipafant.** (lex-IH-pah-fant) USAN.
Use: Platelet-activating factor (PAP) antagonist.

•**lexithromycin.** (lex-ith-row-MY-sin) USAN.
Use: Anti-infective.

Lextron. (Eli Lilly and Co.) Liver-stomach concentrate 50 mg, iron 30 mg, vitamins B_{12} (activity equivalent) 2 mcg, B_1 1 mg, B_2 0.25 mg w/other factors of vitamin B complex present in the liver-stomach concentrate/Pulv. Bot. 84s. *otc.*
Use: Mineral, vitamin supplement.

Lexxel. (Astra Pharmaceuticals, L.P.) Enalapril maleate 5 mg, felodipine 2.5 mg, 5 mg/ER Tab. Bot. 30s, 100s, UD 100s. *Rx.*
Use: Antihypertensive combination.

L'Homme. (Armenpharm Ltd.) Vitamins A 4000 IU, D 400 IU, B_1 1 mg, B_2 1.2 mg, B_{12} 2 mcg, calcium pantothenate 5 mg, B_3 10 mg, C 30 mg, Ca 100 mg, P 76 mg, Fe 10 mg, Mn 1 mg, Mg 1 mg, Zn 1 mg. Bot. 100s. *otc.*
Use: Mineral, vitamin supplement.

L-5 hydroxytryptophan. (Circa Pharmaceuticals, Inc.)
Use: Postanoxic intention myoclonus. [Orphan Drug]

•**liarozole fumarate.** (lie-AHR-oh-zole) USAN.
Use: Antipsoriatic.

•**liarozole hydrochloride.** (lie-AHR-oh-zole) USAN.
Use: Antineoplastic.

Li Ban Spray. (Pfizer US Pharmaceutical Group) Synthetic pyrethroid 0.5%, related compounds 0.065%, aromatic petroleum hydrocarbons 0.664%. Bot. 5 oz, Box 6s. *otc.*
Use: Pediculicide, inanimate objects. (Not to be used on humans or animals).

•**libenzapril.** (lie-BENZ-ah-prill) USAN.
Use: ACE inhibitor.

Librax. (Roche Laboratories) Clidinium bromide (Quarzan) 2.5 mg, chlordiazepoxide HCl (Librium) 5 mg, parabens, lactose/Cap. Bot. 100s, 500s, Teledose 100s (10 strips of 10). *Rx.*
Use: Anticholinergic combination.

Libritabs. (Roche Laboratories) Chlordiazepoxide 10 mg, 25 mg/Tab. **10 mg:** Bot. 100s, 500s; **25 mg:** Bot. 100s. *c-iv.*
Use: Anxiolytic.

Librium. (Roche Laboratories) Chlordiazepoxide HCl 5 mg, 10 mg, 25 mg/Cap. Bot. 100s, 500s, Tel-E-Dose (10 strips of 10; 4 cards of 25) in RNP (Reverse Numbered Package). *c-iv.*
Use: Anxiolytic.

Librium Injectable. (Roche Laboratories) Chlordiazepoxide HCl 100 mg/dry filled amp. plus special IM diluent, 2 ml for IM administration/compound w/benzyl alcohol 1.5%, polysorbate 80 4%, propylene glycol 20%, w/maleic acid and sodium hydroxide to adjust pH to approx. 3. Amp. 5 ml w/2 ml diluent, Box

10s. *c-iv.*
Use: Anxiolytic.

Lice-Enz. (Copley Pharmaceutical, Inc.) Pyrethrins 0.3%, piperonyl butoxide 3%. Shampoo. Bot. 60 g. *otc.*
Use: Pediculicide.

•**licostinel.** USAN.
Use: Treatment of stroke (NMDA receptor antagonist, glycine site).

•**licryfilcon a.** (lih-krih-FILL-kahn) USAN.
Use: Contact lens material (hydrophilic).

•**licryfilcon b.** USAN.
Use: Contact lens material (hydrophilic).

Lida-Mantle-HC Creme. (Bayer Corp. (Consumer Div.)) Lidocaine 3%, hydrocortisone acetate 0.5% in cream base. Tube 1 oz. *Rx.*
Use: Corticosteroid, anesthetic, local.

•**lidamidine hydrochloride.** (LIE-DAM-ih-deen) USAN.
Use: Antiperistaltic.

Lidex Cream. (Roche Laboratories) Fluocinonide 0.05%. Cream 15 g, 30 g, 60 g, 120 g. *Rx.*
Use: Corticosteroid, topical.

Lidex-E. (Roche Laboratories) Fluocinonide 0.05% in aqueous emollient base. Tube 15 g, 30 g, 60 g, 120 g. *Rx.*
Use: Corticosteroid, topical.

Lidex Gel. (Roche Laboratories) Fluocinonide 0.05% in gel base. Tube 15 ml, 30 ml, 60 ml, 120 ml. *Rx.*
Use: Corticosteroid, topical.

Lidex Ointment. (Roche Laboratories) Fluocinonide 0.05% in ointment base. Tube 15 g, 30 g, 60 g, 120 g. *Rx.*
Use: Corticosteroid, topical.

Lidex Topical Solution. (Roche Laboratories) Fluocinonide 0.05%. Soln. Bot. 20 ml, 60 ml. *Rx.*
Use: Corticosteroid, topical.

•**lidocaine.** (LIE-doe-cane) U.S.P. 23.
Use: Anesthetic, local.
See: Dentipatch, Patch (Noven).
Dermaflex, Gel (Schering-Plough Corp.).
Solarcaine Aloe Extra Burn Relief, Cream, Gel, Spray (Schering-Plough Corp.).
Xylocaine, Oint. (Astra Pharmaceuticals, L.P.).
Zilactin-L, Liq. (Zila Pharmaceuticals, Inc.).

lidocaine and epinephrine injection.
Use: Local anesthetic.
See: L-Caine E, Vial (Century Pharmaceuticals, Inc.).
Xylocaine W/Epinephrine, Soln. (Astra Pharmaceuticals, L.P.).

•**lidocaine hydrochloride.** (LIE-doe-cane) U.S.P. 23.
Use: Cardiovascular agent; anesthetic, local.
See: Anestacon, Jelly (PolyMedica Pharmaceuticals).
Ardecaine 1%, 2%, Inj. (Burgin-Arden).
Dilocaine, Inj. (Roberts Pharmaceuticals).
Dolicaine, I.M. (Solvay Pharmaceuticals).
Duo-Track Kit, Inj. (Astra Pharmaceuticals, L.P.).
L-Caine, Inj., Liq. (Century Pharmaceuticals, Inc.).
Lidoject-1, Inj. (Merz Pharmaceuticals).
Lidoject-2, Inj. (Merz Pharmaceuticals).
Nervocaine, Inj. (Keene Pharmaceuticals, Inc.).
Norocaine, Inj. (Vortech Pharmaceuticals).
Octocaine HCl, Inj. (Novocol Chemical Mfr. Co.).
Xylocaine HCl, Oint., Liq., Soln., Jelly (Astra Pharmaceuticals, L.P.).
Xylocaine 10% Oral, Spray (Astra Pharmaceuticals, L.P.).
Xylocaine Viscous, Soln. (Astra Pharmaceuticals, L.P.).
W/Benzalkonium Cl.
See: Medi-Quik, Aer. (Reckitt & Colman).
W/Benzalkonium Cl, phenol, menthol, eugenol, thyme oil, eucalyptus oil.
See: Unguentine Spray (Procter & Gamble Pharm.).
W/Cetyltrimethylammonium bromide, hexachlorophene.
See: Hil-20, Lot. (Solvay Pharmaceuticals).
W/Methyl parasept.
See: L-Caine, Inj. (Century Pharmaceuticals, Inc.).
W/Methyl parasept, epinephrine.
See: L-Caine-E, Inj. (Century Pharmaceuticals, Inc.).
W/Orthohydroxyphenyl mercuric Cl, menthol, camphor, allantoin.
See: Unguentine Plus, Cream (Procter & Gamble Pharm.).
W/Combinations.
See: Clomycin (Roberts).
Neosporin Plus (GlaxoWellcome).

lidocaine hydrochloride. (Abbott Laboratories) **0.2%, 0.4%, 0.8%:** w/5% Dextrose. 250 ml single-dose container; **1%, 2%:** Abboject syringe 5 ml; Vial 1 g, 2 g. Premixed: 0.2%, 0.4% in 5%

dextrose. Inj. containers (flexible or glass) 500 ml. **1%:** 2 ml, 5 ml single-dose amp. **1.5%:** 20 ml single-dose amp. **2%:** 10 ml/20 ml vial (for dilution to prepare IV drip soln.) **5%:** w/ 7.5% Dextrose amp. 2 ml. (Maurry) 2%. Vial.
Use: Injection for infiltration block anesthesia and IV drip for cardiac arrhythmias.

Lidocaine HCl. (Abbott Laboratories) Lidocaine HCl. 1%: 2 ml, 5 ml, 20 ml, 30 ml, 50 ml. 1.5%: 20 ml. w/Epinephrine 1:200,000. 5 ml. 2%: 5 ml, 20 ml, 30 ml, 50 ml. *Rx.*
Use: Anesthetic, local.

lidocaine patch 5%.
Use: Post-herpetic neuralgia resulting from herpes zoster infection. [Orphan Drug]
See: Lidoderm Patch (Hind Health Care Inc.).

Lidocaine 2% Viscous. (Various Mfr.) Lidocaine HCl 2%. Soln. 100 ml, UD 20 ml. *Rx.*
Use: Anesthetic, local.

Lidoderm Patch. (Hind Health Care Inc.) Lidocaine 5%.
Use: Post-herpetic neuralgia resulting from herpes zoster infection. [Orphan Drug]

•**lidofenin.** (LIE-doe-FEN-in) USAN.
Use: Diagnostic aid (hepatic function determination).

•**lidofilcon a.** (lih-DAH-FILL-kahn A) USAN.
Use: Contact lens material (hydrophilic).

•**lidofilcon b.** (lih-DAH-FILL-kahn B) USAN.
Use: Contact lens material (hydrophilic).

•**lidoflazine.** (LIE-dah-FLAY-zeen) USAN.
Use: Coronary vasodilator.

Lidoject-1. (Merz Pharmaceuticals) Lidocaine HCl 1%. Vial 50 ml. *Rx.*
Use: Anesthetic, local.

Lidoject-2. (Merz Pharmaceuticals) Lidocaine HCl 2%. Vial 50 ml. *Rx.*
Use: Anesthetic, local.

Lidopen Auto-Injector. (Survival Technology, Inc.) Lidocaine HCl 10%. Auto-injection device. *Rx.*
Use: Antiarrhythmic.

Lidox Caps. (Major Pharmaceuticals) Chlordiazepoxide HCl 10 mg, clidinium bromide 2.5 mg. Cap. Bot. 100s, 500s, 1000s, UD 100s. *Rx.*
Use: Anticholinergic combination.

Lidoxide. (Henry Schein, Inc.) Chlordiazepoxide HCl 5 mg, clidinium bromide 2.5 mg/Tab. Bot. 100s, 500s. *Rx.*
Use: Anticholinergic combination.

lid scrubs.
Use: Cleanser, ophthalmic.
See: Lid Wipes-SPF, Soln. (Akorn, Inc.).
OCuSOFT, Soln. (Cynacon/OCuSOFT).

Lid Wipes-SPF. (Akorn, Inc.) PEG-200 glyceryl monotallowate, PEG-80 glyceryl monococoate, laureth-23, cocoamidopropylamine oxide, NaCl, glycerin, sodium phosphate, sodium hydroxide. Soln. Pads UD 30s. *otc.*
Use: Cleanser, ophthalmic.

•**lifarizine.** (lih-FAR-ih-ZEEN) USAN.
Use: Cerebral anti-ischemic; platelet aggregation inhibitor.

Lifer-B. (Burgin-Arden) Cyanocobalamin 30 mcg, liver inj. 0.1 ml, ferrous gluconate 100 mg, riboflavin 1.5 mg, panthenol 2.5 mg, niacinamide 100 mg, citric acid 16.4 mg, sodium citrate 23.6 mg/ml. Vial 30 ml. *Rx.*
Use: Mineral, vitamin supplement.

Life Saver Kit. (Whiteworth Towne) Ipecac syrup two 1 oz bottles, activated charcoal pow. 1 oz, poison treatment instruction booklet. *otc.*
Use: Antidote, poisons.

Life Spanner. (Spanner) Vitamins A 12,500 IU, D 400 IU, E 5 IU, B_1 10 mg, B_2 5 mg, B_6 2 mg, B_{12} 5 mcg, niacinamide 50 mg, calcium pantothenate 10 mg, biotin 10 mcg, C 100 mg, hesperidin complex 10 mg, rutin 20 mg, choline bitartrate 40 mg, inositol 30 mg, betaine anhydrous 15 mg, l-lysine monohydrochloride 25 mg, Fe 30 mg, Cu 1 mg, Mn 1 mg, K 5 mg, Ca 105 mg, P 82 mg, Mg 5.56 mg, Zn 1 mg/Cap. Bot. 100s. *otc.*
Use: Mineral, vitamin supplement.

•**lifibrate.** (lih-FIE-brate) USAN.
Use: Antihyperlipoproteinemic.

•**lifibrol.** (lie-FIB-rahl) USAN.
Use: Hypercholesterolemic.

Lifol-B. (Burgin-Arden) Liver inj. 10 mcg, folic acid 1 mg, cyanocobalamin 100 mcg, phenol 0.5%/ml. Inj. Vial 10 ml. *Rx.*
Use: Nutritional supplement.

Lifolex. (Taylor Pharmaceuticals) Liver 10 mcg, cyanocobalamin 100 mcg, folic acid 5 mg/ml. Inj. Vial 10 ml. *Rx.*
Use: Nutritional supplement.

Lilly Bulk Products. (Eli Lilly and Co.) The following products are supplied by Eli Lilly under the U.S.P., N.F., or chemical name as a service to the health professions:
See: Ammoniated Mercury Oint.
Amyl Nitrite.

Analgesic Balm.
Apomorphine HCl.
Aromatic Elix.
Aromatic Ammonia.
Atropine Sulfate.
Bacitracin, Oint.
Belladonna Tincture.
Benzoin.
Boric Acid.
Calcium Gluceptate.
Calcium Gluconate.
Calcium Gluconate with Vitamin D.
Calcium Hydroxide.
Calcium Lactate.
Carbarsone.
Cascara, Aromatic, fluid extract.
Cascara Sagrada, fluid extract.
Citrated Caffeine.
Cocaine HCl.
Codeine Phosphate.
Codeine Sulfate.
Colchicine.
Compound Benzoin.
Dibasic Calcium Phosphate.
Diethylstilbestrol.
Ephedrine Sulfate.
Ferrous Gluconate.
Ferrous Sulfate.
Folic Acid.
Glucagon for Inj.
Green Soap Tincture.
Heparin Sodium.
Histamine Phosphate.
Ipecac.
Isoniazid.
Isopropyl Alcohol, 91%.
Liver, Vial for Inj.
Magnesium Sulfate.
Mercuric Oxide, Yellow.
Methadone HCl.
Methenamine for Timed Burning.
Methyltestosterone.
Milk of Bismuth.
Morphine Sulfate.
Myrrh.
Neomycin Sulfate.
Niacin.
Niacinamide.
Nitroglycerin.
Opium (Deodorized).
Ox Bile Extract.
Pancreatin.
Papaverine HCl.
Paregoric.
Penicillin G Potassium.
Phenobarbital.
Phenobarbital Sodium.
Potassium Cl.
Potassium Iodide.
Powder Papers (Glassine).
Progesterone.
Propylthiouracil.
Protamine Sulfate.
Pyridoxine HCl.
Quinidine Gluconate.
Quinidine Sulfate.
Quinine Sulfate.
Riboflavin.
Silver Nitrate.
Sodium Bicarbonate.
Sodium Chloride.
Sodium Salicylate.
Streptomycin Sulfate.
Sulfadiazine.
Sulfapyridine.
Sulfur.
Terpin Hydrate.
Terpin Hydrate and Codeine.
Testosterone Propionate.
Thiamine HCl.
Thyroid.
Tubocurarine HCl.
Tylosterone.
Whitfield's Oint.
Wild Cherry Syrup.
Zinc Oxide.
Zinc Oxide, Paste.

limarsol.
See: Acetarsone (City Chemical Corp.).

Limbitrol. (Roche Laboratories) Chlordiazepoxide 5 mg, amitriptyline HCl 12.5 mg/Tab. Bot. 100s, 500s, Tel-E-Dose 100s, Prescription pak 50s. *c-IV.*
Use: Psychotherapeutic agent.

Limbitrol DS. (Roche Laboratories) Chlordiazepoxide 10 mg, amitriptyline HCl 25 mg/Tab. Bot. 100s, 500s, Tel-E-Dose 100s, Prescription pak 50s. *c-IV.*
Use: Psychotherapeutic agent.

•**lime.** U.S.P. 23.
Use: Pharmaceutical necessity.

lime solution, sulfurated. U.S.P. XXI.
Use: Scabicide.

lime sulfur solution. Calcium polysulfide, calcium thiosulfate.
Use: Wet dressing.

•**linarotene.** (lin-AHR-oh-teen) USAN.
Use: Antikeratolytic.

Lincocin. (Pharmacia & Upjohn) Lincomycin HCl. **Cap.:** 500 mg. Bot. 100s. **Soln.:** 300 mg/ml. Benzyl alcohol 9.45 mg/ml. Vial 2 ml, 10 ml. *Rx.*
Use: Anti-infective.

•**lincomycin.** (LIN-koe-MY-sin) USAN. Antibiotic produced by *Streptomyces lincolnensis* variant.
Use: Anti-infective; infections due to gram-positive organisms.

•**lincomycin hydrochloride.** (LIN-koe-MY-sin) U.S.P. 23.
Use: Anti-infective.

See: Lincocin (Pharmacia & Upjohn).
Lincorex (Hyrex).

lincomycin hydrochloride. (Steris) 300 mg/ml. Inj. Vial 10 ml. *Rx.*
Use: Anti-infective.

Lincorex. (Hyrex) Lincomycin HCl 300 mg/ml. Benzyl alcohol 9.45 mg/ml. Inj. Vial 10 ml. *Rx.*
Use: Anti-infective.

•**lindane.** (LIN-dane) U.S.P. 23. Gamma-benzene-hexachloride, hexachlorocyclohexane.
Use: Pediculicide, scabicide.

lindane. (Fidelity Lab) Pow. 50%, Pkg. 1 lb, 5 lb. (Imperial Lab) Pow. 50%, Pkg. 1 lb, 4 lb; 12%, Pkg. 1 lb, 4 lb.
Use: Pediculicide, scabicide.

Lindora. (Westwood Squibb Pharmaceuticals) Sodium laureth sulfate, cocamide DEA, sodium Cl, lactic acid, tetra sodium EDTA, benzophenone-4, FD&C Blue No. 1. Bot. 8 oz. *otc.*
Use: Dermatologic, cleanser.

•**linezolid.** (lin-EH-zoe-lid) USAN.
Use: Anti-infective.

Linodil Capsules. (Sanofi Winthrop Pharmaceuticals) Inositol hexanicotinate. *Rx.*
Use: Hyperlipidemic, peripheral vasodilator.

•**linogliride.** (lie-no-GLIE-ride) USAN.
Use: Antidiabetic.

•**linogliride fumarate.** (lih-no-GLIE-ride) USAN.
Use: Antidiabetic.

linomide. (Pharmacia & Upjohn) Roquinimex.
Use: Immunomodulator. [Orphan Drug]

•**linopirdine.** (lih-no-PIHR-deen) USAN.
Use: Treatment of Alzheimer's disease (cognition enhancer).

Lioresal. (Novartis Pharmaceutical Corp.) Baclofen 10 mg, 20 mg/Tab. Bot. 100s, UD 100s. *Rx.*
Use: Muscle relaxant.

•**liothyronine I 125.** (lie-oh-THIGH-row-neen) USAN.
Use: Radiopharmaceutical.

•**liothyronine I 131.** (lie-oh-THIGH-row-neen) USAN.
Use: Radiopharmaceutical.

•**liothyronine sodium.** (lie-oh-THIGH-row-neen) U.S.P. 23.
Use: Hormone, thyroid.
See: Cytomel, Tab. (SmithKline Beecham Pharmaceuticals).
Triostat, Inj. (SmithKline Beecham Pharmaceuticals).

liothyronine sodium. (Various Mfr.) 10 mg/ml. Tab. Bot. 100s.
Use: Hormone, thyroid.

liothyronine sodium injection.
Use: Myxedema coma/precoma. [Orphan Drug]

•**liotrix tablets.** (LIE-oh-trix) U.S.P. 23.
Use: Hormone, thyroid.
See: Thyrolar, Tab. (Rhone-Poulenc Rorer Pharmaceuticals, Inc.).

lipase. W/Amylase, Protease.
Use: Digestive enzyme.

W/Alpha-amylase W-100, proteinase W-300, cellase W-100, estrone, testosterone, vitamins, minerals.
See: Kutrase (Schwarz Pharma, Inc.).
Ku-Zyme (Schwarz Pharma, Inc.).

W/Amylase, bile salts, wilzyme, pepsin, pancreatin, calcium.
See: Enzyme, Tab. (Barth's).

W/Amylase, protease.
See: Creon, Prods. (Solvay).

W/Amylolytic, proteolytic, cellulolytic enzymes.
See: Arco-Lase, Tab. (Arco Pharmaceuticals, Inc.).

W/Amylolytic, proteolytic, cellulolytic enzymes, phenobarbital, hyoscyamine sulfate, atropine sulfate.
See: Arco-Lase Plus, Tab. (Arco Pharmaceuticals, Inc.).

W/Pancreatin, protease, amylase.
See: Dizymes, Cap. (Recsei Laboratories).

lipid/DNA human cystic fibrosis gene. (Genzyme Corp.)
Use: Cystic fibrosis. [Orphan Drug]

lipids.
Use: Intravenous nutritional therapy.
See: Intralipid 10%, Soln. (Clintec Nutrition).
Intralipid 20%, Soln. (Clintec Nutrition).
Liposyn II 10%, Soln. (Abbott Laboratories).
Liposyn II 20%, Soln. (Abbott Laboratories).
Liposyn III 10%, Soln. (Abbott Laboratories).
Liposyn III 20%, Soln. (Abbott Laboratories).

Lipisorb. (Bristol-Myers Squibb) Protein 35 g/L, fat 48 g/L, carbohydrates 115 g/L, Na 733.3 mg/L, K 1250 mg/L, H_2O 320 mOsm/kg. With appropriate vitamins and minerals. 1 calorie/ml. Vanilla flavored. Pow. Can 1 lb. *otc.*
Use: Nutritional supplement.

Lipitor. (Parke-Davis) Atorvastatin calcium 10 mg, 20 mg, 40 mg/Tab. Bot. 90s, 5000s (10 mg only), UD 100s (except 40 mg). *Rx.*
Use: Antihyperlipidemic.

Lipkote by Coppertone. (Schering-Plough Corp.) Padimate O, oxybenzone. SPF 15. Lip balm 4.2 g. *otc.*
Use: Sunscreen.

Lipkote SPF 15 Ultra Sunscreen Lipbalm. (Schering-Plough Corp.) Tube 0.15 oz. *otc.*
Use: Sunscreen.

Lip Medex. (Blistex, Inc.) Petrolatum, camphor 1%, phenol 0.54%, cocoa butter, lanolin. Oint. 210 g. *otc.*
Use: Fever blisters, lip protectant.

lipocholine.
See: Choline dihydrogen citrate. (Various Mfr.).

Lipoflavonoid Caplets. (Numark Laboratories, Inc.) Vitamins C 100 mg, B_1 0.33 mg, B_2 0.33 mg, B_3 3.33 mg, B_6 0.33 mg, B_{12} 1.66 mcg, B_5 1.66 mg, choline 111 mg, bioflavonoids 100 mg, inositol 111 mg. Bot. 100s, 500s. *otc.*
Use: Vitamin supplement.

Lipoflavonoid Capsules. (Numark Laboratories, Inc.) Choline 111 mg, inositol 111 mg, vitamins B_1 0.3 mg, B_2 0.3 mg, B_3 3.3 mg, B_5 1.7 mg, B_6 0.3 mg, B_{12} 1.7 mcg, C 100 mg, lemon bioflavonoid complex. Cap. Bot. 100s, 500s. *otc.*
Use: Vitamin supplement.

Lipogen Caplets. (Zenith Goldline Pharmaceuticals) Choline 111 mg, inositol 111 mg, vitamins B_1 0.33 mg, B_2 0.33 mg, B_3 3.33 mg, B_5 1.7 mg, B_6 0.33 mg, B_{12} 1.7 mcg, C 20 mg, A 1667 IU, E 10 IU, Zn 30 mg, Cu, Se. Bot. 60s. *otc.*
Use: Mineral, vitamin supplement.

Lipogen Capsules. (Various Mfr.) Choline 111 mg, inositol, vitamins B_1 0.33 mg, B_2 0.33 mg, B_3 3.33 mg, B_5 1.7 mg, B_6 0.33 mg, B_{12} 1.7 mcg, C 100 mg/Cap. Bot. 60s. *otc.*
Use: Vitamin supplement.

Lipomul. (Pharmacia & Upjohn) Corn oil 10 g/15 ml w/d-alpha tocopheryl acetate, butylated hydroxyanisole, polysorbate 80, glyceride phosphates, sodium saccharin, sodium benzoate 0.05%, benzoic acid 0.05%, sorbic acid 0.07%. Bot. Pt. *otc.*
Use: Nutritional supplement.

Lipo-Nicin/300 mg. (Zeneca Pharmaceuticals) Niacin 300 mg, vitamin C 150 mg, B_1 25 mg, B_2 2 mg, B_6 10 mg/TR Cap. 100s. *Rx.*
Use: Vasodilator.

Lipo-Nicin/100 mg. (Zeneca Pharmaceuticals) Nicotinic acid 100 mg, niacinamide 75 mg, vitamins C 150 mg, B_1 25 mg, B_2 2 mg, B_6 10 mg/Tab. Bot. 100s, 500s. *Rx.*
Use: Vasodilator combination.

Liponol Capsules. (Rugby Labs, Inc.) Choline, inositol 83 mg, methionine 110 mg, vitamins B_1 3 mg, B_2 3 mg, B_3 10 mg, B_5 2 mg, B_6 2 mg, B_{12} 2 mcg, desiccated liver 56 mg, liver concentrate 30 mg, sorbitol, lecithin/Cap. Bot. 60s. *otc.*
Use: Nutritional supplement.

liposomal amphotericin B.
Use: Antiviral. [Orphan Drug]

liposomal doxorubicin.
See: Doxorubicin hydrochloride.

liposomal prostaglandin E-1 injection. (Liposome Co.)
Use: Acute respiratory distress syndrome. [Orphan Drug]

liposome encapsulated recombinant interleukin-2. (Biomerica, Inc.)
Use: Antineoplastic. [Orphan Drug]

Liposyn. (Abbott Hospital Products) Intravenous fat emulsion containing safflower oil 10%, egg phosphatides 1.2%, glycerin 2.5% in water for inj. **10%:** Single-dose container 50 ml, 100 ml, 200 ml, 500 ml; Syringe Pump Unit 50 ml single-dose. **20%:** Single-dose container 200 ml, 500 ml Syringe Pump Unit 25 ml, 50 ml single-dose. *Rx.*
Use: Nutritional supplement, parenteral.

Liposyn II. (Abbott Hospital Products) Intravenous fat emulsion: **10%:** Safflower oil 5%, soybean oil 5%. Bot. 100 ml, 200 ml, 500 ml. **20%:** Safflower oil 10%, soybean oil 10% w/egg phosphatides 1.2%, glycerin 2.5%. 200 ml, 500 ml. Bot. Syringe pump unit 25 ml, 50 ml. *Rx.*
Use: Nutritional supplement, parenteral.

Liposyn III. (Abbott Laboratories) Oil, soybean, egg yolk phospholipids. **10%:** 100, 200, 500 ml. **20%:** 100, 500 ml. *Rx.*
Use: Nutritional supplement, parenteral.

Lipo-Tears. (Spectra Pharmaceuticals) Mineral oil, petrolatum. Preservative free. Drops. Bot. 1 ml. 30s. *otc.*
Use: Lubricant, ophthalmic.

Lipotriad. (Numark Laboratories, Inc.) Zn 30 mg, vitamin A 5000 IU, C 60 mg, E 30 IU, Cu, Se, B_3 20 mg, B_1 1.5 mg, B_2 1.7 mg, B_6 2 mg, B_{12} 6 mcg, B_5 10 mg, choline bitartrate, inositol. Capl. Bot. 60s. *otc.*
Use: Mineral, vitamin supplement.

lipotropics with vitamins.
Use: Nutritional supplement.
See: Lipotriad, Liq. (Numark Laboratories, Inc.).
Lipogen, Cap. (Various Mfr.).
Lipotriad, Cap. (Numark Laboratories, Inc.).

Lipoflavonoid, Cap. (Numark Laboratories, Inc.).
Cholinoid, Cap. (Zenith Goldline Pharmaceuticals).
Liponol, Cap. (Rugby Labs, Inc.).
Methatropic, Cap. (Zenith Goldline Pharmaceuticals).
Cholidase, Tab. (Freeda Vitamins, Inc.).

Lipoxide. (Major Pharmaceuticals) Chlordiazepoxide HCl 5 mg, 10 mg, 25 mg/Cap. Bot. 100s, 500s, 1000s. *c-IV.*
Use: Anxiolytic.

Liqua-Gel. (Paddock Laboratories) Boric acid, glycerine, propylene glycol, methylparaben, propylparaben, Irish moss extract, methylcellulose. Bot. 4 oz, 16 oz. *otc.*

Liquibid. (ION Laboratories, Inc.) Guaifenesin 600 mg, dye free. SR Tab. Bot. 100s. *Rx.*
Use: Expectorant.

Liquibid-D. (ION Laboratories, Inc.) Guaifenesin 600 mg, phenylephrine HCl 40 mg. SR Tab. Bot. 100s. *Rx.*
Use: Expectorant.

Liqui-Char. (Jones Medical Industries, Inc.) Activated charcoal. **Liq. Bot.:** 12.5 g/60 ml, 15 g/75 ml. **Squeeze container:** 25 g/120 ml, 50 g/240 ml, 30 g/120 ml.
Use: Antidote.

Liqui-Coat HD. (Lafayette Pharmaceuticals, Inc.) Barium sulfate 210%. Susp. Bot. 150 ml. *Rx.*
Use: Radiopaque agent.

Liqui-Doss. (Ferndale Laboratories, Inc.) Docusate sodium 60 mg, mineral oil. Bot. Pt. *otc.*
Use: Laxative.

Liquid Barosperse. (Lafayette Pharmaceuticals, Inc.) Barium sulfate 60%. Susp. Bot. 355 ml; 1900 ml. *Rx.*
Use: Radiopaque agents.

Liquid Geritonic. (Roberts Pharmaceuticals) Fe 105 mg, liver fraction 1 375 mg, B_1 3 mg, B_2 3 mg, B_3 30 mg, B_6 0.3 mg, B_{12} 9 mcg, inositol 60 mg, glycine 180 mg, yeast concentrate 375 mg, Ca, I, K, Mg, Mn, P, alcohol 20%. Liq. Bot. 240 ml, gal. *otc.*
Use: Nutritional supplement.

Liquid Lather. (Ulmer Pharmacal Co.) Gentle wash for hands, body, face, hair. Bot. 8 oz, gal. *otc.*
Use: Cleanser.

liquid petrolatum emulsion.
See: Mineral Oil Emulsion, U.S.P. 23.

Liquid Pred Syrup. (Muro Pharmaceutical, Inc.) Prednisone 5 mg/5 ml in syrup base. Alcohol 5%, saccharin, sorbitol. Bot. 120 ml, 240 ml. *Rx.*
Use: Corticosteroid.

Liquifilm Forte. (Allergan, Inc.) Polyvinyl alcohol 3%, thimerosal 0.002%, EDTA, sodium Cl. Soln. Bot. 15 ml, 30 ml. *otc.*
Use: Artificial tears.

Liquifilm Tears. (Allergan, Inc.) Polyvinyl alcohol 1.4%, chlorobutanol 0.5%, sodium Cl. Bot. 15 ml, 30 ml. *otc.*
Use: Artificial tears.

Liquifilm Wetting Solution. (Allergan, Inc.) Polyvinyl alcohol, hydroxypropyl methylcellulose, edetate disodium, sodium Cl, potassium Cl, benzalkonium Cl 0.004%. Bot. 60 ml. *otc.*
Use: Contact lens care.

Liqui-Histine-D Elixir. (Liquipharm) Phenylpropanolamine HCl 12.5 mg, pyrilamine maleate 4 mg, phenyltoloxamine citrate 4 mg, pheniramine maleate 4 mg/5 ml. Liq. Bot. 473 ml. *Rx.*
Use: Antihistamine, decongestant.

Liqui-Histine DM. (Liquipharm) Dextromethorphan HBr 10 mg, phenylpropanolamine HCl 12.5 mg, brompheniramine maleate 2 mg/5 ml. Alcohol free. Syr. Bot. 473 ml. *Rx.*
Use: Antihistamine, antitussive, decongestant.

Liquimat. (Galderma Laboratories, Inc.) Sulfur 5%, SD alcohol 40 22%, cetyl alcohol in drying makeup base. Plastic Bot. 45 ml. *otc.*
Use: Dermatologic, acne.

Liquipake. (Lafayette Pharmaceuticals, Inc.) Barium sulfate suspension 100% w/v for dilution. Bot. 1850 ml, Case 4s.
Use: Radiopaque agent.

Liquiprin. (Menley & James Labs, Inc.) Acetaminophen 80 mg/1.66 ml, saccharin. Soln. Bot. 35 ml w/dropper. *otc.*
Use: Analgesic.

liquor carbonis detergens.
See: Coal Tar Topical Soln., U.S.P. 23. (Various Mfr.).

•**lisadimate.** (liss-AD-ih-mate) USAN.
Use: Sunscreen.

•**lisinopril.** (lie-SIN-oh-pril) U.S.P. 23.
Use: Antihypertensive.
See: Prinivil, Tab. (Merck & Co.).
Zestril, Tab. (Zeneca Pharmaceuticals).
W/Hydrochlorothiazide.
See: Prinzide, Tab. (Merck & Co.).
Zestoretic, Tab. (Zeneca Pharmaceuticals).

•**lisofylline.** (lie-SO-fih-lin) USAN.
Use: Immunomodulator.

Listerine Antiseptic. (Warner Lambert

Consumer Healthcare) Thymol 0.06%, eucalyptol 0.09%, methyl salicylate 0.06%, menthol 0.04%. Alcohol 26.9% (regular flavor), 21.6% (cool mint flavor), sorbitol, saccharin. Bot. 90 ml, 180 ml, 360 ml, 540 ml, 720 ml, 960 ml, 1440 ml. *otc.*
Use: Mouthwash, antiseptic.

Listermint Arctic Mint Mouthwash. (Warner Lambert Consumer Healthcare) Glycerin, poloxamer 335, PEG 600, sodium lauryl sulfate, sodium benzoate, benzoic acid, zinc chloride, saccharin. Liq. 946 ml. *otc.*
Use: Antiseptic, mouthwash.

Lite Pred. (Horizon Pharmaceutical Corp.) Prednisolone sodium phosphate 0.125%. Soln. Bot. 5 ml. *Rx.*
Use: Corticosteroid, ophthalmic.

•**lithium carbonate.** (LITH-ee-uhm CAR-boe-nate) U.S.P. 23.
Use: Antipsychotic, manic-depressive state; antimanic; antidepressant.
See: Eskalith, Cap., Tab. (SmithKline Beecham Pharmaceuticals).
Lithonate, Cap. (Solvay Pharmaceuticals).
Lithotabs, Tab. (Solvay Pharmaceuticals).

lithium carbonate capsules and tablets. (Roxane Laboratories, Inc.) Lithium carbonate. **Tab.:** 300 mg. Bot. 100s, 1000s, UD 100s. **Cap.:** 150 mg, 300 mg, 600 mg. Bot. 100s, 1000s, UD 100s. *Rx.*
Use: Antipsychotic, manic-depressive state; antimanic; antidepressant.

•**lithium citrate.** (LITH-ee-uhm) U.S.P. 23.
Use: Antimanic.

lithium citrate. (Various Mfr.) Lithium citrate 8 mEq (equivalent to 300 mg lithium carbonate)/5 ml. Syr. Bot. 480 ml, 500 ml, UD 5 ml, 10 ml. *Rx.*
Use: Antipsychotic.

•**lithium hydroxide.** (LITH-ee-uhm high-DROX-ide) U.S.P. 23.
Use: Antipsychotic, manic-depressive state; antimanic; antidepressant.

Lithonate. (Solvay Pharmaceuticals) Lithium carbonate 300 mg/Cap. Bot. 100s, 1000s, UD 100s. *Rx.*
Use: Antipsychotic.

Lithostat. (Mission Pharmacal Co.) Acetohydroxamic acid 250 mg/Tab. Bot. 100s. *Rx.*
Use: Anti-infective, urinary.

Lithotabs. (Solvay Pharmaceuticals) Lithium carbonate 300 mg/Tab. Bot. 100s, 1000s, UD 100s. *Rx.*
Use: Antipsychotic.

Livec. (Enzyme Process) Vitamins A 5000 IU, B_1 1.5 mg, B_2 1.7 mg, niacin 20 mg, C 60 mg, B_6 2 mg, pantothenic acid 10 mg, E 30 IU, B_{12} 6 mcg, Ca 250 mg, Fe 5 mg, D 400 IU, folacin 0.075 mg/3 Tab. Bot. 100s, 300s. *otc.*
Use: Mineral, vitamin supplement.

Liverbex. (Spanner) Liver 2 mcg, vitamins B_1, B_2, B_6, B_{12}, niacinamide, pantothenate/ml. Vial 30 ml. *otc.*
Use: Nutritional supplement.

Liver Combo No. 5. (Rugby Labs, Inc.) Liver vitamin B_{12} equivalent 10 mcg, crystalline B_{12} 100 mcg, folic acid 0.4 mg/ml. Inj. Vial 10 ml. *Rx.*
Use: Nutritional supplement, parenteral.

liver derivative complex.
See: Kutapressin, Inj. (Schwarz Pharma, Inc.).

liver desiccated. Desiccated liver substance.

liver extract. Dry liver extract w/Vitamin B_{12}, folic acid.

liver function agents.
See: Iodophthalein (Various Mfr.).
Sulfobromophthalein Sodium, U.S.P. 23. (Gotham).

Livergran. (Rawl) Desiccated whole liver 9 g, vitamins B_1 18 mg, B_2 36 mg, niacinamide 90 mg, choline bitartrate 216 mg, B_6 3.6 mg, calcium pantothenate 3.6 mg, inositol 90 mg, biotin 6 mcg, vitamins B_{12} 5.4 mcg, methionine 198 mg, arginine 242 mg, cysteine 72 mg, glutamic acid 675 mg, histidine 99 mg, isoleucine 333 mg, leucine 495 mg, lysine 297 mg, phenylalanine 189 mg, threonine 333 mg, tryptophan 45 mg, tyrosine 180 mg, valine 306 mg/3 Tsp. Bot. 15 oz. *otc.*
Use: Nutritional supplement.

liver injection. (Various Mfr.) Liver extract for parenteral use. *Rx.*
Use: Parenteral liver supplement.

liver injection. (Arcum; Lederle Laboratories) Vitamin B_{12} 20 mcg/ml. Vial 10 ml. *Rx.*
Use: Nutritional supplement.

Liver Injection, Crude. (Eli Lilly and Co.) 2 mcg/ml. Vial 30 ml; (Medwick) 2 mcg/ml. Vial 30 ml. *Rx.*
Use: Liver supplement.

Liver Iron Vitamins Inj. (Arcum) Liver inj. (10 mcg B_{12} activity/ml) 0.1 ml, crude liver inj. (2 mcg B_{12} activity/ml) 0.125 ml, green ferric ammonium citrate 20 mg, niacinamide 50 mg, vitamin B_6 0.3 mg, B_2 0.3 mg, procaine HCl 0.5%, phenol 0.5%/2 ml. Vial 30 ml. *Rx.*
Use: Nutritional supplement.

Liver, Refined. (Medwick) 20 mcg/ml.

Vial 10 ml, 30 ml. *Rx.*
Use: Nutritional supplement.

liver vasoconstrictor.
See: Kutapressin, Vial, Amp. (Schwarz Pharma, Inc.).

Livifol. (Dunhall Pharmaceuticals, Inc.) Vitamin B_{12} activity from liver inj. equivalent to cyanocobalamin 10 mcg, folic acid 1 mg, cyanocobalamin 100 mcg/ml. Vial 10 ml. *Rx.*
Use: Vitamin supplement.

Livitrinsic-f. (Zenith Goldline Pharmaceuticals) Iron 110 mg, vitamins B_{12} 15 mcg, C 75 mg, intrinsic factor concentrate 240 mg, folic acid 0.5 mg/Cap. Bot. 100s, 1000s. *Rx.*
Use: Mineral, vitamin supplement.

Livostin. (Ciba Vision) Levocabastine HCl 0.05%. Susp. Dropper Bot. 2.5 ml, 5 ml, 10 ml. *otc.*
Use: Antiallergic, ophthalmic.

•**lixazinone sulfate.** (lix-AZE-ih-NOHN) USAN.
Use: Cardiotonic (phosphodiesterase inhibitor).

Lixoil. (Lixoil Labs.) Sulfonated fatty oils and one or more esters of higher fatty acids. Bot. 16 oz. *otc.*
Use: Dermatologic.

LKV-Drops. (Freeda Vitamins, Inc.) Vitamins A 5000 IU, D 400 IU, E 2 mg, B_1 1.5 mg, B_2 1.5 mg, B_3 10 mg, B_5 2 mg, B_6 2 mg, B_{12} 6 mcg, C 50 mg, biotin 50 mcg/0.6 ml. Bot. 60 ml. *otc.*
Use: Vitamin supplement.

LKV Infant Drops. (Freeda Vitamins, Inc.) Vitamins A 2500 IU, D 400 IU, E 5 IU, B_1 1 mg, B_2 1 mg, B_3 10 mg, B_5 3 mg, B_6 1 mg, B_{12} 4 mcg, C 50 mg, biotin 75 mcg/0.5 ml. Bot. 60 ml. *otc.*
Use: Vitamin supplement.

lld factor.
See: Vitamin B_{12}, Preps. (Various Mfr.).

l-leucovorin.
Use: Antineoplastic.
See: Isovorin.

lm-427. Ribabutin.
Use: CDC anti-infective agent.

LMD. (Abbott Laboratories) Dextran 40 10%. 500 ml. With 0.9% sodium chloride or in 5% dextrose. *Rx.*
Use: Plasma volume expander.

LMWD-Dextran 40. (Pharmachemie USA, Inc.) Normal saline 0.9%, dextrose 10%. *Rx.*
Use: Plasma volume expander.

Lobac. (Seatrace Pharmaceuticals, Inc.) Salicylamide 200 mg, phenyltoloxamine 20 mg, acetaminophen 300 mg/Cap. Bot. 100s. *Rx.*
Use: Analgesic, muscle relaxant.

Lobak. (Sanofi Winthrop Pharmaceuticals) Chlormezanone 250 mg, acetaminophen 300 mg/Tab. 40s, 100s, 1000s. *Rx.*
Use: Anxiolytic, analgesic.

Lobana Body. (Ulmer Pharmacal Co.) Mineral oil, triethanolamine stearate, stearic acid, lanolin, cetyl alcohol, potassium stearate, propylene glycol, parabens. Lot. Bot. 120, 240 ml, gal. *otc.*
Use: Emollient.

Lobana Body Shampoo. (Ulmer Pharmacal Co.) Chloroxylenol. Bot. 240 ml, gal. *otc.*
Use: Dermatologic, hair and skin.

Lobana Conditioning Shampoo. (Ulmer Pharmacal Co.) Bot. 8 oz, gal. *otc.*
Use: Dermatologic, hair and scalp.

Lobana Derm-Ade. (Ulmer Pharmacal Co.) Vitamin A, D, E. Cream Jar 2 oz, 8 oz. *otc.*
Use: Dermatologic, counterirritant.

Lobana Liquid Lather. (Ulmer Pharmacal Co.) Sodium laureth sulfate, sodium lauroyl sarcosinate, sodium myristyl sarcosonate, lauramide DEA, linoleamide DEA, octyl hydroxystearate, polyquaternium 7, tetrasodium EDTA, quaternium 15, sodium chloride, citric acid. Liq. Bot. 240 ml, gal. *otc.*
Use: Cleanser.

Lobana Peri-Gard. (Ulmer Pharmacal Co.) Water-resistant ointment containing vitamin A & D. Jar 2 oz, 8 oz. *otc.*
Use: Dermatologic, protectant.

Lobana Perineal Cleanser. (Ulmer Pharmacal Co.) Sprayer 4 oz, 8 oz. Bot. Gal. *otc.*
Use: Urine and fecal cleanser.

•**lobenzarit sodium.** (low-BENZ-ah-RIT) USAN.
Use: Antirheumatic.

Lobidram. (Dram) Lobeline sulfate 2 mg/Tab. Pkg. 15s, 30s. *otc.*
Use: Smoking cessation aid.

•**lobucavir.** (lah-BYOO-kah-vihr) USAN.
Use: Antiviral.

LoCHOLEST. (Warner Chilcott) Cholestyramine resin 4 g/9 g, fructose, sorbitol, sucrose. Pow. for Susp. Pouch 9 g, Can 378 g. *Rx.*
Use: Antihyperlipidemic.

LoCHOLEST Light. (Warner Chilcott) Cholestyramine resin 4 g/9 g, aspartame, fructose, mannitol, sorbitol, phenylalanine 3.93 mg/g. Pow. for Susp. Pouch 5.7 g, Can 239.4 g. *Rx.*
Use: Antihyperlipidemic.

Locoid. (Ferndale Laboratories, Inc.)
Cream: Hydrocortisone butyrate 0.1%.

Tube 15 g, 45 g. **Oint.:** Hydrocortisone butyrate 0.1%. Tube 15 g, 45 g. **Soln.:** Hydrocortisone butyrate 0.1%, isopropyl alcohol 50%, glycerin, povidone. Bot. 20 ml, 60 ml. *Rx.*
Use: Corticosteroid, topical.

•**lodelaben.** (low-DELL-ah-ben) USAN. *Formerly Declaben.*
Use: Antiarthritic; emphysema therapy adjunct.

•**lodenosine.** USAN.
Use: Antiviral (HIV reverse transcriptase inhibitor).

Lodine. (Wyeth-Ayerst Laboratories) **Cap.:** Etodolac 200, 300, 400 mg, lactose. Bot. 100s, UD 100s. **Tab.:** Etodolac 400 mg, lactose. Bot. 100s, UD 100s. *Rx.*
Use: Analgesic, NSAID.

Lodine XL. (Wyeth-Ayerst Laboratories) Etodolac 400 mg, 600 mg, lactose/ER Tab. Bot. 100s, UD 100s. *Rx.*
Use: Analgesic, NSAID.

Lodosyn. (Merck & Co.) Carbidopa 25 mg/Tab. Bot. 100s. *Rx.*
Use: Antiparkinsonian.

•**lodoxamide ethyl.** (low-DOX-ah-mide ETH-uhl) USAN.
Use: Antiasthmatic, antiallergic; bronchodilator.

•**lodoxamide tromethamine.** (low-DOX-ah-mide troe-METH-ah-meen) USAN.
Use: Antiasthmatic, antiallergic; bronchodilator; vernal keratoconjunctivitis.
See: Alomide, Soln. (Alcon Laboratories, Inc.).

Lodrane LD. (ECR Pharmaceuticals) Brompheniramine maleate 6 mg, pseudoephedrine HCl 60 mg/SR Cap. Bot. 100s. *Rx.*
Use: Antihistamine, decongestant.

Loestrin 21 1/20. (Parke-Davis) Norethindrone acetate 1 mg, ethinyl estradiol 20 mcg Tab. Petipac compact 21 Tab. Ctn. 5 compacts or Ctn. 5 refills. *Rx.*
Use: Contraceptive.

Loestrin 21 1.5/30. (Parke-Davis) Norethindrone acetate 1.5 mg, ethinyl estradiol 30 mcg/Tab. Petipac compact. Ctn. 5 compacts or Ctn. 5 refills. *Rx.*
Use: Contraceptive.

Loestrin Fe 1/20. (Parke-Davis) **White Tab.:** Norethindrone acetate 1 mg, ethinyl estradiol 20 mcg/Tab.; **Brown Tab.:** Ferrous fumarate 75 mg (7 tabs.) Carton 5 petipac compacts 28 Tab., carton of 5 refills 28 Tab. *Rx.*
Use: Contraceptive.

Loestrin Fe 1.5/30. (Parke-Davis) **Green Tab.:** Norethindrone acetate 1.5 mg, ethinyl estradiol 30 mcg. **Brown Tab.:** Ferrous fumarate 75 mg (7 tabs.). Carton 5 petipac compacts 28 Tab., carton of 5 refills 28 Tab. *Rx.*
Use: Oral contraceptive.

•**lofemizole hydrochloride.** (low-FEM-ih-ZOLE) USAN.
Use: Anti-inflammatory; analgesic; antipyretic.

Lofenalac. (Bristol-Myers Squibb) Corn syrup solids 49.2%, casein hydrolysate 18.7% (enzymic digest of casein containing amino acids and small peptides), corn oil 18%, modified tapioca starch 9.57%, protein equivalent 15%, fat 18%, carbohydrate 60%, minerals (ash) 3.6%, phenylalanine 75 mg/100 g pow., vitamins A 1600 IU, D 400 IU, E 10 IU, C 52 mg, folic acid 100 mcg, B_1 0.5 mg, B_2 0.6 mg, niacin 8 mg, B_6 0.4 mg, B_{12} 2 mcg, biotin 0.05 mg, pantothenic acid 3 mg, vitamin K-1 100 mcg, choline 85 mg, inositol 30 mg, Ca 600 mg, P 450 mg, I 45 mcg, Fe 12 mg, Mg 70 mg, Cu 0.6 mg, Zn 4 mg, Mn 1 mg, C 450 mg, K 650 mg, Na 300 mg/qt. at normal dilution of 20 k cal/fl oz, Can 2 1/2 lb. *otc.*
Use: Nutritional supplement.

•**lofentanil oxalate.** (low-FEN-tah-NILL OX-ah-late) USAN.
Use: Analgesic, narcotic.

•**lofepramine hydrochloride.** (low-FEH-prah-MEEN) USAN.
Use: Antidepressant.

•**lofexidine hydrochloride.** (low-FEX-ih-DEEN) USAN.
Use: Antihypertensive.

Logen Liquid. (Zenith Goldline Pharmaceuticals) Diphenoxylate HCl w/atropine sulfate. Bot. 2 oz. *c-v.*
Use: Antidiarrheal.

Logen Tablets. (Zenith Goldline Pharmaceuticals) Diphenoxylate HCl, atropine sulfate. Bot. 100s, 500s, 1000s. *c-v.*
Use: Antidiarrheal.

Lomanate. (Various Mfr.) Diphenoxylate HCl 2.5 mg, atropine sulfate 0.025 mg/5 ml. Bot. 60 ml. *c-v.*
Use: Antidiarrheal.

•**lomefloxacin.** (low-MEH-FLOX-ah-sin) USAN.
Use: Anti-infective.

•**lomefloxacin hydrochloride.** (low-MEH-FLOX-ah-sin) USAN.
Use: Anti-infective.
See: Maxaquin, Tab. (Searle).

•**lomefloxacin mesylate.** (low-MEH-FLOX-ah-sin) USAN.

Use: Anti-infective.

•**lometraline hydrochloride.** (low-MET-rah-LEEN) USAN.
Use: Antipsychotic, antiparkinsonian.

•**lometrexol sodium.** (LOW-meh-TREX-ole) USAN.
Use: Antineoplastic.

•**lomofungin.** (low-moe-FUN-jin) USAN.
Use: Antifungal.

Lomotil. (Searle) Diphenoxylate HCl 2.5 mg, atropine sulfate 0.025 mg/Tab. or 5 ml. **Tab.:** Bot. 100s, 500s, 1000s, 2500s, UD 100s. **Liq.:** Bot. w/dropper 2 oz. *c-v.*
Use: Antidiarrheal.

•**lomustine.** (LOW-muss-teen) USAN.
Use: Antineoplastic.
See: CeeNu, Cap. (Bristol-Myers Squibb).

Lonalac. (Bristol-Myers Squibb) Protein as casein 21%, fat as coconut oil 49%, carbohydrate as lactose 30%, vitamins A 1440 IU, B_1 0.6 mg, B_2 2.6 mg, niacin 1.2 mg, Ca 1.69 g, P 1.5 g, Cl 750 mg, K 1.88 g, Na 38 mg, Mg 135 mg/qt. Pow. Can 16 oz. *otc.*
Use: Nutritional supplement.

•**lonapalene.** (low-NAP-ah-LEEN) USAN.
Use: Antipsoriatic.

Long Acting Nasal Spray. (Weeks & Leo) Oxymetazoline HCl 0.05%. Soln. Bot. 0.75 oz. *otc.*
Use: Decongestant.

Long Acting Neo-Synephrine II Nose Drops and Nasal Spray. (Sanofi Winthrop Pharmaceuticals) Xylometazoline HCl 0.1% (adult strength) or 0.05% (child strength). Bot. 1 oz, Spray 0.5 oz (adult strength). *otc.*
Use: Decongestant.

Long Acting Neo-Synephrine II Vapor Spray. (Sanofi Winthrop Pharmaceuticals) Xylometazoline HCl 0.1%. Mentholated. Spray Bot. 0.5 fl oz. *otc.*
Use: Decongestant.

Loniten. (Pharmacia & Upjohn) Minoxidil 2.5 mg, 10 mg/Tab. **2.5 mg:** Unit-of-use Bot. 100s. **10 mg:** Bot. 500s, Unit-of-use Bot. 100s. *Rx.*
Use: Antihypertensive.

Lonox. (Geneva Pharmaceuticals) Diphenoxylate HCl 2.5 mg, atropine sulfate 0.025 mg/Tab. Bot. 100s, 500s, 1000s, UD 100s. *c-v.*
Use: Antidiarrheal.

Lo/Ovral. (Wyeth-Ayerst Laboratories) Norgestrel 0.3 mg, ethinyl estradiol 0.03 mg/Tab. Pilpak dispenser 6s, Tab. 21s. *Rx.*
Use: Contraceptive.

Lo/Ovral-28. (Wyeth-Ayerst Laboratories) Tab. 21s, each containing norgestrel 0.03 mg, ethinyl estradiol 0.03 mg, 7 pink inert. Tab. Pilpak dispenser 6s, Tab 28s. *Rx.*
Use: Contraceptive.

•**loperamide hydrochloride.** (low-PURR-ah-mide) U.S.P. 23.
Use: Antiperistaltic.
See: Imodium, Cap. (Ortho McNeil Pharmaceutical).
Neo-Diaral, Cap. (Roberts Pharmaceuticals).

Lopid. (Parke-Davis) Gemfibrozil 600 mg/Tab. Bot. 60s. *Rx.*
Use: Antihyperlipidemic.

Lopressor. (Novartis Pharmaceutical Corp.) Metoprolol tartrate. **Tab.:** 50 mg, 100 mg. Bot. 100s, 1000s, UD 100s, Gy-Pak 60s, 100s. **Amp.:** 5 mg/5 ml. *Rx.*
Use: Beta-adrenergic blocker.

Lopressor HCT. (Novartis Pharmaceutical Corp.) Metoprolol tartrate/hydrochlorothiazide. **Tab.:** 50/25 mg, 100/25 mg, or 100/50 mg. Bot. 100s. *Rx.*
Use: Antihypertensive combination.

Loprox. (Hoechst Marion Roussel) Ciclopirox olamine 1% in cream base. Tube 15 g, 30 g, 90 g. *Rx.*
Use: Antifungal, topical.

Lopurin. (Knoll Pharmaceuticals) Allopurinol 100 mg, 300 mg/Tab. Bot. 100s, 1000s, UD 100s. *Rx.*
Use: Antigout agent.

Lorabid. (Eli Lilly and Co.) Loracarbef. **Cap.:** 200 mg, 400 mg. Bot. 30s. **Pow. for Oral Susp.:** 100 mg/5 ml, 200 mg/5 ml, parabens, sucrose. Bot. 50 ml, 75 ml, 100 ml. *Rx.*
Use: Anti-infective, cephalosporin.

•**loracarbef.** (LOW-ra-CAR-beff) U.S.P. 23.
Use: Anti-infective.
See: Lorabid, Cap., Pow. (Eli Lilly and Co.).

•**lorajmine hydrochloride.** (lahr-AZH-meen) USAN.
Use: Cardiovascular agent.

•**loratadine.** (lore-AT-uh-DEEN) USAN.
Use: Antihistamine.
See: Claritin, Prods. (Schering-Plough Corp.).

•**lorazepam.** (lore-AZE-uh-pam) U.S.P. 23.
Use: Anxiolytic.
See: Alzapam, Tab. (Ultra).
Ativan, Tab., Inj. (Wyeth-Ayerst Laboratories).

lorazepam. (lore-AZE-uh-pam) (Purepac Pharmaceutical Co.) Lorazepam. **0.5 mg:** Tab. Bot. 100s, 500s. **1 mg, 2 mg:** Tab. Bot. 100s, 500s, 1000s. *c-iv.*
Use: Anxiolytic, hypnotic, sedative.

lorazepam. (lore-AZE-uh-pam) (Various Mfr.) Lorazepam, benzyl alcohol 2%. Inj. 2 mg/ml, 4 mg/ml. Vial 1 ml, 10 ml. *c-iv.*
Use: Anxiolytic, hypnotic, sedative.

Lorazepam Intensol. (Roxane Laboratories, Inc.) Lorazepam 2 mg/ml. Concentrated oral soln. Alcohol and dye free. Dropper Bot. 10 ml, 30 ml. *c-iv.*
Use: Anxiolytic, hypnotic, sedative.

•**lorbamate.** (lore-BAM-ate) USAN.
Use: Muscle relaxant.

•**lorcainide hydrochloride.** (lahr-CANE-ide) USAN.
Use: Cardiovascular agent; antiarrhythmic.

Lorcet-HD. (Forest Pharmaceutical, Inc.) Hydrocodone bitartrate 5 mg, acetaminophen 500 mg/Cap. Bot. 500s. *c-iii.*
Use: Analgesic combination, narcotic.

Lorcet Plus. (Forest Pharmaceutical, Inc.) Hydrocodone bitartrate 7.5 mg, acetaminophen 650 mg/Tab. Bot. 100s., 500s, UD 100s. *c-iii.*
Use: Analgesic combination, narcotic.

Lorcet 10/650. (Forest Pharmaceutical, Inc.) Hydrocodone bitartrate 10 mg, acetaminophen 650 mg/Tab. Bot. 20s, 100s, UD 100s. *c-iii.*
Use: Analgesic combination, narcotic.

•**lorcinadol.** (LORE-sin-ah-dole) USAN.
Use: Analgesic.

•**loreclezole.** (lahr-EH-kleh-zole) USAN.
Use: Antiepileptic.

Lorelco. (Hoechst Marion Roussel) Probucol 250 mg/Tab. Bot. 120s. *Rx.*
Use: Antihyperlipidemic.

•**lormetazepam.** (LORE-met-AZE-eh-pam) USAN.
Use: Hypnotic, sedative.

•**lornoxicam.** (lore-NOX-ih-kam) USAN.
Use: Anti-inflammatory; analgesic.

Loroxide. (Dermik Laboratories, Inc.) Benzoyl peroxide 5.5%, cetyl alcohol, parabens, EDTA, 1% silica, 64% calcium phosphate. Lot. Bot. 25 g. *otc.*
Use: Dermatologic, acne.

Lorprn. (UCB Pharmaceuticals, Inc.) Aspirin 325 mg, caffeine 40 mg, butalbital 50 mg/Cap. Bot. 100s. *c-iii.*
Use: Analgesic combination, narcotic.

Lortab 2.5/500. (UCB Pharmaceuticals, Inc.) Hydrocodone 2.5 mg, acetaminophen 500 mg/Tab. Bot. 100s, 500s. *c-iii.*
Use: Analgesic combination, narcotic.

Lortab 5/500. (UCB Pharmaceuticals, Inc.) Hydrocodone 5 mg, acetaminophen 500 mg/Tab. Bot. 100s, 500s, UD 100s. *c-iii.*
Use: Analgesic combination, narcotic.

Lortab 7/500. (UCB Pharmaceuticals, Inc.) Hydrocodone 7.5 mg, acetaminophen 500 mg/Tab. Bot. 100s, 500s, UD 100s. *c-iii.*
Use: Analgesic combination, narcotic.

Lortab 10/500. (UCB Pharmaceuticals, Inc.) Hydrocodone bitartrate 10 mg, acetaminophen 500 mg/Tab. Bot. 100s, 500s. *c-iii.*
Use: Analgesic combination, narcotic.

Lortab ASA. (UCB Pharmaceuticals, Inc.) Hydrocodone bitartrate 5 mg, aspirin 500 mg/Tab. Bot. 100s. *c-iii.*
Use: Analgesic combination, narcotic.

Lortab Elixir. (UCB Pharmaceuticals, Inc.) Hydrocodone bitartrate 2.5 mg, acetaminophen 167 mg/5 ml w/alcohol 7%, parabens, saccharin, sorbitol, sucrose. Bot. pt. *c-iii.*
Use: Analgesic combination, narcotic.

•**lortalamine.** (lahr-TAHL-ah-MEEN) USAN.
Use: Antidepressant.

•**lorzafone.** (LAHR-zah-FONE) USAN.
Use: Anxiolytic.

•**losartan potassium.** (low-SAHR-tan) USAN.
Use: Antihypertensive; treatment of CHF (angiotensin II receptor blocker).
See: Cozaar, Tab. (Merck & Co.).
W/Hydrochlorothiazide and potassium.
See: Hyzaar, Tab. (Merck & Co.).

Losec.
See: Prilosec.

Losopan Liquid. (Zenith Goldline Pharmaceuticals) Magaldrate 540 mg/5 ml. Bot. 12 oz. *otc.*
Use: Antacid.

Losopan Plus Liquid. (Zenith Goldline Pharmaceuticals) Magaldrate 540 mg, simethicone 20 mg/5 ml. Bot. 12 oz. *otc.*
Use: Antacid, antiflatulent.

Losotron Plus Liquid. (Various Mfr.) Magaldrate 540 mg, simethicone 20 mg/5 ml. Bot. 360 ml. *otc.*
Use: Antacid, antiflatulent.

•**losoxantrone hydrochloride.** (low-SOX-an-trone) USAN.
Use: Antineoplastic.

•**losulazine hydrochloride.** (low-SULL-ah-zeen) USAN.
Use: Antihypertensive.

Lotawin Capsules. (Sanofi Winthrop Pharmaceuticals) Oxypertine. *Rx.*

Use: Anxiolytic.

Lotemax. (Bausch & Lomb Pharmaceuticals) Loteprednol etabonate 0.5%, EDTA, benzalkonium chloride 0.01%. Ophth. Susp. Bot. 2.5 ml, 5 ml, 10 ml, 15 ml. *Rx.*
Use: Anti-inflammatory.

Lotensin. (Novartis Pharmaceutical Corp.) Benazepril HCl 5 mg, 10 mg, 20 mg, 40 mg, lactose/Tab. Bot. 100s, UD 100s. *Rx.*
Use: Antihypertensive.

•**loteprednol etabonate.** (low-TEH-PRED-nole ett-AB-ohn-ate) USAN.
Use: Anti-inflammatory, topical.
See: Alrex, Ophth. Susp. (Bausch & Lomb Pharmaceuticals).
Lotemax, Ophth. Susp. (Bausch & Lomb Pharmaceuticals).

lotio alba. White lotion. *otc.*
Use: Antiseborrheic; dermatologic, acne.

lotio alsulfa. (Doak Dermatologics) Colloidal sulfur 5%. Bot. 4 oz. *otc.*
Use: Antiseborrheic; dermatologic, acne.

Lotion-Jel. (C. S. Dent & Co. Division) Benzocaine in gel base. Tube 0.2 oz. *otc.*
Use: Anesthetic, local.

•**lotrafiban hydrochloride.** (low-TRAFF-ih-ban HIGH-droe-KLOR-ide) USAN.
Use: Antiplatelet.

Lotrel. (Novartis Pharmaceutical Corp.) Amlodipine 2.5 mg, 5 mg, benazepril HCl 10 mg/Cap., amlodipine 5 mg, benazepril HCl 20 mg/Cap. Bot. 100s. *Rx.*
Use: Antihypertensive combination.

Lotrimin. (Schering-Plough Corp.) Clotrimazole 1%. **Cream:** Tube 15 g, 30 g, 45 g, 90 g. **Lot.:** Bot. 30 ml. **Soln.:** 1%. Bot. 10 ml, 30 ml. *Rx.*
Use: Antifungal, topical.

Lotrimin AF. (Schering-Plough Corp.) Miconazole nitrate 2% **Pow.:** Talc. Bot. 90 g. **Spray Liq.:** SD alcohol 40 17%. Bot. 113 ml. **Spray Pow.:** SD alcohol 40 10%. Bot. 100 g. *otc.*
Use: Antifungal, topical.

Lotrisone. (Schering-Plough Corp.) Clotrimazole 1%, betamethasone dipropionate 0.05%/g. Tube 15 g, 45 g. *Rx.*
Use: Antifungal, topical.

Lo-Trop. (Vangard Labs, Inc.) Diphenoxylate HCl 2.5 mg, atropine sulfate 0.025 mg/Tab. Bot. 100s, 1000s. *c-v.*
Use: Antidiarrheal.

•**lovastatin.** (LOW-vuh-STAT-in) U.S.P. 23. *Formerly Mevinolin.*
Use: Antihypercholesterolemic; antihyperlipidemic; HMG-CoA reductase inhibitor.
See: Mevacor, Tab. (Merck & Co.).

Love Longer. (Durex) Benzocaine 7.5% in water-soluble lubricant base. Tube 0.5 oz. *otc.*
Use: Anesthetic, local.

Lovenox. (Rhone-Poulenc Rorer Pharmaceuticals, Inc.) Enoxaparin sodium. 30 mg/0.3 ml, 40 mg/0.4 ml, 60 mg/0.6 ml, 80 mg/0.8 ml, 100 mg/1 ml. Preservative free. Inj. Pk. 10 prefilled syringes w/26 guage x ½-inch needle. *Rx.*
Use: Anticoagulant.

•**loviride.** (LOW-vihr-ide) USAN.
Use: Antiviral for chronic oral treatment of HIV-seropositive patients (nonnucleoside reverse transcriptase inhibitor).

Lowila Cake. (Westwood Squibb Pharmaceuticals) Sodium lauryl sulfoacetate, dextrin, boric acid, urea, sorbitol, mineral oil, PEG 14 M, lactic acid, cellulose gum, docusate sodium. Cake 112.5 g. *otc.*
Use: Dermatologic, cleanser.

Low-Quel. (Halsey Drug Co.) Diphenoxylate HCl 2.5 mg, atropine sulfate 0.025 mg/Tab. Bot. 100s. *c-v.*
Use: Antidiarrheal.

Lowsium. (Rugby Labs, Inc.) Magaldrate 540 mg/5 ml. Susp. Bot. 360 ml. *otc.*
Use: Antacid.

Lowsium Plus. (Rugby Labs, Inc.) **Tab.:** Magaldrate 480 mg, simethicone 20 mg. Bot. 60s. **Susp.:** Magaldrate 540 mg, simethicone 40 mg/5 ml. Bot. 360 ml. *otc.*
Use: Antacid, antiflatulent.

•**loxapine.** (LOX-ah-peen) USAN.
Use: Anxiolyitc.

loxapine hydrochloride.
Use: Anxiolytic.
See: Loxitane-C Oral Concentrate (ESI Lederle Generics).
Loxitane, Inj. (ESI Lederle Generics).

•**loxapine succinate.** (LOX-ah-peen) U.S.P. 23.
Use: Anxiolytic.
See: Loxitane, Preps. (ESI Lederle Generics).

loxapine succinate. (Various Mfr.) 5 mg, 10 mg, 25 mg, 50 mg. Cap. Bot. 30s, 100s, 1000s. *Rx.*
Use: Antipsychotic.

Loxitane C. (ESI Lederle Generics) Loxapine HCl oral concentrate 25 mg/ml. Bot. 120 ml w/dropper. *Rx.*
Use: Antipsychotic.

Loxitane Capsules. (ESI Lederle Generics) Loxapine succinate. 10 mg, 50 mg/Cap.: Bot. 100s, 1000s, UD 100s. *Rx.*
Use: Antipsychotic.

Loxitane IM. (ESI Lederle Generics) Loxapine HCl (base equivalent) 50 mg/ml. Inj. Vial 10 ml. *Rx.*
Use: Antipsychotic.

•**loxoribine.** (LOX-ore-ih-BEAN) USAN.
Use: Immunostimulant; vaccine adjuvant.

L_2-oxothiazolidine$_4$-carboxylic acid.
Use: Treatment of adult respiratory distress syndrome. [Orphan Drug]
See: Procysteine (Transcend Therapeutics, Inc.).

Lozol. (Rhone-Poulenc Rorer Pharmaceuticals, Inc.) Indapamide 2.5 mg/Tab. Bot. 100s, 1000s, 2500s, Strip dispenser 100s. *Rx.*
Use: Diuretic, antihypertensive.

L-PAM.
See: Alkeran (GlaxoWellcome).

l-sarcolysin.
See: Alkeran, Tab. (GlaxoWellcome).

l-threonine.
Use: Antispasmodic.

l-triiodothyronine sod.
See: Cytomel, Tab. (SmithKline Beecham Pharmaceuticals).
Liothyronine Sod.

Lubafax. (GlaxoWellcome) Surgical lubricant, sterile; water-soluble, non-staining. Foil wrapper 2.7 g, 5 g. Box 144s.
Use: Lubricant.

Lubath. (Warner Lambert) Mineral oil, PPG-15, stearyl ether, oleth-2, nonoxynol 5, fragrance, FD&C Green No. 6. Bot. 4 oz, 8 oz, 16 oz. *otc.*
Use: Emollient.

•**lubeluzole.** (loo-BELL-you-zole) USAN.
Use: Stroke treatment.

Lubinol. (Purepac Pharmaceutical Co.) Light, heavy, and extra heavy mineral oil. Bot. Pt, qt, gal. (Extra heavy Bot.) 8 oz, pt, qt, gal. *otc.*
Use: Emollient.

Lubraseptic Jelly. (Guardian Laboratories) Water-soluble amyl phenyl phenol complex 0.12%, phenylmercuric nitrate, 0.007%. Bellows-type tube 10 g, 24s.
Use: Genitourinary aid.

LubraSOL Bath Oil. (Pharmaceutical Specialties, Inc.) Mineral oil, lanolin oil, PEG-200 dilaurate, oxybenzone. Bot. 240 ml, 480 ml, gal. *otc.*
Use: Emollient.

Lubricating Jelly. (Taro Pharmaceuticals USA, Inc.) Glycerin, propylene glycol. Jelly. 60 g, 125 g. *otc.*
Use: Vaginal agent.

Lubriderm Lotion. (Warner Lambert) Mineral oil, petrolatum, sorbitol, lanolin, lanolin alcohol, stearic acid, TEA, cetyl alcohol, fragrance (if scented), butylparaben, methylparaben, propylparaben, sodium Cl. Bot. (scented), 4 oz, 8 oz, 16 oz; (unscented) 8 oz, 16 oz. *otc.*
Use: Emollient.

Lubriderm Lubath Oil. (Warner Lambert) Mineral oil, PPG-15 stearyl ether, oleth-2, nonoxynol-5. Lanolin free. Bot. 240 ml, pt. *otc.*
Use: Emollient.

Lubrin. (Kenwood Laboratories) Glycerin, caprylic/capric triglyceride. Inserts. Pkg. 5s, 12s. *otc.*
Use: Lubricant.

LubriTears. (Bausch & Lomb Pharmaceuticals) White petrolatum, mineral oil, lanolin, chlorobutanol 0.5%. Oint. Tube 3.5 g. *otc.*
Use: Lubricant, ophthalmic.

LubriTears Solution. (Bausch & Lomb Pharmaceuticals) Hydroxypropyl methylcellulose 2906 0.3%, dextran 70 0.1%, EDTA, KCl, NaCl, benzalkonium chloride 0.01%. Bot. 15 ml. *otc.*
Use: Artificial tears.

•**lucanthone hydrochloride.** (LOO-kanthone) USAN.
Use: Antischistosomal.

Ludiomil. (Novartis Pharmaceutical Corp.) Maprotiline 25 mg, 50 mg, 75 mg/Tab. Bot. 100s, Accu-Pak 100s. *Rx.*
Use: Antidepressant.

•**lufironil.** (loo-FIHR-ah-nill) USAN.
Use: Collagen inhibitor.

Lufyllin. (Wallace Laboratories) Dyphylline. Inj. **Amp.:** (500 mg/2 ml) Box 25s. **Elix.:** 100 mg/15 ml; alcohol 20%. Bot. Pt, gal. **Tab.:** 200 mg. Bot. 100s, 1000s, UD 100s. *Rx.*
Use: Bronchodilator.

Lufyllin-400. (Wallace Laboratories) Dyphylline 400 mg/Tab. Bot. 100s, 1000s. *Rx.*
Use: Bronchodilator.

Lufyllin-EPG. (Wallace Laboratories) Ephedrine HCl 16 mg, dyphylline 100 mg, phenobarbital 16 mg, guaifenesin 200 mg/Tab. or 10 ml (Liq.). Tab. Bot. 100s. *Rx.*
Use: Antiasthmatic combination.

Lufyllin-EPG Elixir. (Wallace Laboratories) Dyphylline 150 mg, ephedrine HCl 24 mg, guaifenesin 300 mg, phenobarbital 24 mg, alcohol 5.5%/15 ml. Elix. Bot. 480 ml. *Rx.*
Use: Antiasthmatic combination.

Lufyllin-GG. (Wallace Laboratories) **Tab.:** Dyphylline 200 mg, guaifenesin 200 mg/Tab. Bot. 100s, 3000s, UD 100s. **Elix.:** Dyphylline 100 mg, guaifenesin 100 mg, alcohol 17%/15 ml. Elix. Bot. Pt, gal. *Rx.*
Use: Bronchodilator, expectorant.

Lugol's Solution. (Lyne Laboratories) Strong iodine soln, U.S.P. 23. Iodine 5 g, potassium iodide 10 g, in purified water to make 100 ml. Bot. 15 ml. (Wisconsin Pharmacal Co.) Bot. Pt. *Rx-otc.*
Use: Antithyroid, antiseptic, topical.

Luminal Injection. (Sanofi Winthrop Pharmaceuticals) Phenobarbital 130 mg/ml. Amp 1 ml. Box 100s.
Use: Hypnotic, sedative.

Lumopaque Capsules. (Sanofi Winthrop Pharmaceuticals) Tyropanoate sodium.
Use: Radiopaque agent.

lung surfactants.
Use: Surfactant replacement therapy in neonatal respiratory distress syndrome.
See: Exosurf (GlaxoWellcome).
Survanta (Ross Laboratories).

Lupron. (Tap Pharmaceuticals) Leuprolide acetate 5 mg/ml, benzyl alcohol 1.8 mg. Multiple-dose Vial 2.8 ml. *Rx.*
Use: Hormone.

Lupron Depot. (Tap Pharmaceuticals) Leuprolide acetate 3.75, 7.5 mg. Lyophilized microspheres for injection. Single-use kit. Preservative free. Microspheres for Inj. Kit. Single-dose vials. *Rx.*
Use: Hormone.

Lupron Depot-Ped. (Tap Pharmaceuticals) Leuprolide acetate 7.5 mg, 11.25 mg, 15 mg. Preservative free. Microspheres for Inj. Kit. *Rx.*
Use: Hormone.

Lupron Depot-3 Month. (Tap Pharmaceuticals) Leuprolide acetate 11.25 mg, 22.5 mg, 30 mg. Microspheres for injection. Single-use Kit. *Rx.*
Use: Hormone.

Lupron Depot-4 Month. (Tap Pharmaceuticals) Leuprolide acetate 11.25 mg, 30 mg, polylactic acid 264.8 mg, D-mannitol 51.9 mg. Inj. Single-use Kit. *Rx.*
Use: Antineoplastic.

Lupron Injection. (Tap Pharmaceuticals) Leuprolide acetate 1 mg/0.2 ml. Vial 2.8 ml. *Rx.*
Use: Antineoplastic.

Lupron for Pediatric Use. (Tap Pharmaceuticals) Leuprolide acetate 5 mg/ml, benzyl alcohol 1.8 mg. Multiple-dose Vial 2.8 ml. *Rx.*
Use: Hormone.

Luramide. (Major Pharmaceuticals) Furosemide 20 mg, 40 mg, 80 mg/Tab. Bot. 100s, 1000s. *Rx.*
Use: Diuretic.

Luride Drops. (Colgate Oral Pharmaceuticals) Sodium fluoride equivalent to 0.5 mg of fluoride/Drop. Plastic dropper bot. 50 ml. *Rx.*
Use: Dental caries agent.

Luride Gel. (Colgate Oral Pharmaceuticals) Fluoride (from sodium fluoride and hydrogen fluoride) 1.2%. Tube 7 g. *Rx.*
Use: Dental caries agent.

Luride Lozi-Tabs. (Colgate Oral Pharmaceuticals) Sodium fluoride 0.25 mg/ Chew. Tab. Sugar free. Bot. 120s. *Rx.*
Use: Dental caries agent.

Luride-F Lozi Tablets. (Colgate Oral Pharmaceuticals) Sodium fluoride in Lozi base tab. available as fluoride. **0.25 mg:** Bot. 120s; **0.5 mg:** Bot. 120s, 1200s; **1 mg:** Bot. 120s, 1000s, 5000s. *Rx.*
Use: Dental caries agent.

Luride Prophylaxis Paste. (Colgate Oral Pharmaceuticals) Acidulated phosphate sodium fluoride containing 0.4% fluoride ion w/silicon dioxide abrasive. UD 3 g, Jar 50 g. *otc.*
Use: Dentrifice.

Luride-SF Lozi Tablets. (Colgate Oral Pharmaceuticals) Sodium fluoride equivalent to 1 mg/Tab. Bot. 120s. *Rx.*
Use: Dental caries agent.

Luride Topical Gel. (Colgate Oral Pharmaceuticals) Fluoride 1.2%. Tube 7 g. *Rx.*
Use: Dental caries agent.

Luride Topical Solution. (Colgate Oral Pharmaceuticals) Acidulated phosphate sodium fluoride w/pH 3.2. Bot. 250 ml. *otc.*
Use: Dental caries agent.

Lurline PMS. (Fielding Co.) Acetaminophen 500 mg, pamabrom 25 mg, pyridoxine 50 mg/Tab. Bot. 24s, 50s. *otc.*
Use: Analgesic combination.

•**lurosetron mesylate.** (loo-ROW-set-rahn MEH-sih-late) USAN.
Use: Antiemetic.

Lurotin Caps. (BASF Wyandotte) Beta-carotene 25 mg/Cap. Bot. 100s. *otc.*
Use: Nutritional supplement.

•**lurtotecan dihyrdochloride.** (lure-toe-TEE-kan die-HIGH-droe-KLOR-ide) USAN.
Use: Antineoplastic (DNA topoisomerase I inhibitor).

luteogan.

See: Progesterone (Various Mfr.).

luteosan.
See: Progesterone (Various Mfr.).

lutocylol. (Novartis Pharmaceutical Corp.) Ethisterone.

Lutolin-F. (Spanner) Progesterone 25 mg, 50 mg/ml. Vial 10 ml. *Rx.*
Use: Hormone, progestin.

Lutolin-S. (Spanner) Progesterone 25 mg/ml. Vial 10 ml. *Rx.*
Use: Hormone, progestin.

•**lutrelin acetate.** (loo-TRELL-in ASS-eh-tate) USAN.
Use: LHRH agonist.

lutren.
See: Progesterone (Various Mfr.).

Lutrepulse. (Ortho McNeil Pharmaceutical) Gonadorelin acetate 0.8 mg, 3.2 mg/vial. Pow. for reconstitution (lyophilized). Vial 10 ml. *Rx.*
Use: Hormone, gonadotropin-releasing.

Luvox. (Solvay Pharmaceuticals) Fluvoxamine maleate 25 mg, 50 mg, 100 mg/Tab. Bot. 100s, 1000s (except 25 mg), UD 100s. *Rx.*
Use: Antidepressant.

•**lyapolate sodium.** (lie-APP-oh-late) USAN.
Use: Anticoagulant.
See: Peson (Hoechst Marion Roussel).

•**lycetamine.** (lie-SEET-ah-meen) USAN.
Use: Antimicrobial, topical.

lycine hydrochloride.
See: Betaine HCl (Various Mfr.).

Lydia E. Pinkham Herbal Compound. (Numark Laboratories, Inc.) Vitamin C, iron. Liq. Bot. 8 fl oz, 16 fl oz.

Lydia E. Pinkham Tablets. (Numark Laboratories, Inc.) Vitamin C, iron, calcium. Bot. 72s, 150s. *otc.*

•**lydimycin.** (lie-dih-MY-sin) USAN.
Use: Antifungal.

lyme disease vaccine.
Use: Vaccine.
See: LYMErix, Vac. (SmithKline Beecham).

LYMErix. (SmithKline Beecham) Lyme disease vaccine 30 mcg/0.5 ml. Single-dose vial 1s, 10s. Prefilled disp. *Tip-Lock* syringes w/1-inch 23-gauge needles. 5s *Rx.*
Use: Vaccine.

Lymphazurin 1%. (United States Surgical Corp.) Isosulfan blue 10 mg/ml. Vial 5 ml. *Rx.*
Use: Radiopaque agent.

lymphocyte immune globulin.
Use: Management of rejection in renal transplant.
See: Atgam, Inj. (Pharmacia & Upjohn).

LymphoScan. (Immunomedics) Technetium TC-99M murine monoclonal antibody (IgG2a) to B-cell.
Use: Diagnostic aid. [Orphan Drug]

•**lynestrenol.** (lin-ESS-tree-nahl) USAN.
Use: Hormone, progestin.

lynoestrenol. Lynestrenol.

lyophilized vitamin B complex and vitamin C with B_{12}. (McGuff Co., Inc.) B_1 50 mg, B_2 5 mg, B_3 125 mg, B_5 6 mg, B_6 5 mg, B_{12} 1000 mcg, C 50 mg/ml/Inj. Vial 10 ml. *Rx.*
Use: Vitamin supplement, parenteral.

Lyphocin P. (Fujisawa USA, Inc.) Vancomycin HCl 500 mg. Vial 10 ml. *Rx.*
Use: Anti-infective.

Lypholyte. (Fujisawa USA, Inc.) Multiple electrolye concentrate. Vial 20 ml, 40 ml, Maxivial 100 ml, 200 ml. *Rx.*
Use: Electrolyte supplement.

Lypholyte II. (Fujisawa USA, Inc.) Na^+ 35 mEq/L, K^+ 20 mEq/L, Ca^{++} 4.5 mEq/L, Mg^{++} 5 mEq/L, Cl 35 mEq/L, acetate 29.5 mEq/L. Single-dose flip-top vial 20 ml, 40 ml; flip-top vial 100 ml, 200 ml. *Rx.*
Use: Nutritional supplement, parenteral.

•**lypressin nasal solution.** (LIE-PRESS-in) U.S.P. 23.
Use: Antidiuretic; vasoconstrictor.
See: Diapid Nasal Spray (Novartis Pharmaceutical Corp.).

lysidin. Methyl glyoxalidin.

•**lysine.** (LIE-SEEN) USAN.
Use: Nutrient, rapid weight gain; amino acid.

l-lysine.
Use: Dietary supplement; amino acid.
See: Enisyl (Person and Covey, Inc.).
L-Lysine (Various Mfr.).

L-Lysine. (Various Mfr.) 312 mg, 500 mg/Tab. Bot. 100s. 1000 mg/Tab. Bot. 60s. 500 mg/Cap. Bot. 100s, 250s. *otc.*
Use: Dietary supplement; amino acid.

•**lysine acetate.** (LIE-SEEN) U.S.P. 23.
Use: Amino acid.

•**lysine hydrochloride.** (LIE-SEEN) U.S.P. 23.
Use: Amino acid.
See: Enisyl, Tab. (Person and Covey, Inc.).

Lysodase. (Enzon, Inc.) PEG-glucocerebrosidase.
Use: Gaucher's disease. [Orphan Drug]

Lysodren. (Bristol-Myers Oncology/Immunology) Mitotane 500 mg/Tab. Bot. 100s. *Rx.*
Use: Antineoplastic.

•**lysostaphin.** (LIE-so-STAFF-in) USAN. Enzyme produced by *Staphylococcus staphylolyticus.*

Use: Antibiotic; antibacterial enzyme.

Lytren. (Bristol-Myers Squibb) Dextrose, sodium citrate, citric acid, sodium Cl, potassium citrate. Ready-to-use Bot. 8 fl. oz. *otc.*
Use: Electrolyte, fluid replacement.

M

Maagel. (Health for Life Brands, Inc.) Aluminum and magnesium hydroxide. Bot. 12 oz, gal. *otc.*
Use: Antacid.

Maalox Antacid. (Rhone-Poulenc Rorer Pharmaceuticals, Inc.) Calcium carbonate 1000 mg, Na ≤ 0.4 mEq. Capl. Bot. 50s. *otc.*
Use: Antacid.

Maalox Anti-Diarrheal. (Rhone-Poulenc Rorer Pharmaceuticals, Inc.) Loperamide HCl 2 mg/Capl. Pkg. 12s. *otc.*
Use: Antidiarrheal.

Maalox Anti-Gas. (Rhone-Poulenc Rorer Pharmaceuticals, Inc.) Simethicone 80 mg, sucrose/Chew. Tab. Bot. 12s. *otc.*
Use: Antiflatulent.

Maalox Daily Fiber Therapy. (Rhone-Poulenc Rorer Pharmaceuticals, Inc.) Psyllium hydrophilic mucilloid fiber 3.4 g/dose, sucrose and 35 cal/12 g in regular; aspartame, 21 mg/tsp phenylalanine and 9 cal/5.8 g in sugar free. Pow. Can 283 g (sugar free), 369 g, 3 single-dose (12 g) packets. *otc.*
Use: Laxative.

Maalox Extra Strength Plus Suspension. (Rhone-Poulenc Rorer Pharmaceuticals, Inc.) Magnesium hydroxide 450 mg, aluminum hydroxide 500 mg, simethicone 40 mg/5 ml. Susp. Bot. 148 ml, 355 ml, 769 ml. *otc.*
Use: Antacid, antiflatulent.

Maalox Extra Strength Plus Tablets. (Rhone-Poulenc Rorer Pharmaceuticals, Inc.) Magnesium hydroxide 350 mg, aluminum hydroxide 350 mg, simethicone 30 mg. Chew. Tab. Bot. 38s, 75s. *otc.*
Use: Antacid, antiflatulent.

Maalox Extra Strength Suspension. (Rhone-Poulenc Rorer Pharmaceuticals, Inc.) Aluminum hydroxide 500 mg, magnesium hydroxide 450 mg, simethicone 40 mg, parabens, saccharin, sorbitol/5 ml. Susp. Bot. 148 ml, 355 ml, 769 ml. *otc.*
Use: Antacid, antiflatulent.

Maalox Extra Strength Tablets. (Rhone-Poulenc Rorer Pharmaceuticals, Inc.) Magnesium hydroxide 350 mg, dried aluminum hydroxide gel 350 mg/Tab. Bot. 38s, 75s. *otc.*
Use: Antacid.

Maalox Heartburn Relief. (Rhone-Poulenc Rorer Pharmaceuticals, Inc.) Aluminum hydroxide, magnesium carbonate 140 mg, magnesium carbonate 175 mg, tartrazine, saccharin, magnesium alginate, parabens, sorbitol/5 ml. Liq. Bot. 296 ml. *otc.*
Use: Antacid.

Maalox HRF. (Rhone-Poulenc Rorer Pharmaceuticals, Inc.) Aluminum hydroxide/magnesium carbonate codried gel 280 mg, magnesium carbonate 350 mg/10 ml, saccharin, tartrazine. Liq. Bot. 355 ml. *otc.*
Use: Antacid.

Maalox Plus. (Invamed, Inc.) Dried aluminum hydroxide 200 mg, magnesium hydroxide 200 mg, simethicone 25 mg, sugar/Chew. Tab. Bot. 100s. *otc.*
Use: Antacid.

Maalox Plus Tablets. (Rhone-Poulenc Rorer Pharmaceuticals, Inc.) Magnesium hydroxide 200 mg, dried aluminum hydroxide gel 200 mg, simethicone 25 mg/Tab. Bot. 50s, 100s, 144s. *otc.*
Use: Antacid, antiflatulent.

Maalox Suspension. (Rhone-Poulenc Rorer Pharmaceuticals, Inc.) Magnesium hydroxide 200 mg, aluminum hydroxide 225 mg/5 ml. Susp. Bot. 148 ml, 355 ml, 769 ml. *otc.*
Use: Antacid.

Maalox Tablets. (Rhone-Poulenc Rorer Pharmaceuticals, Inc.) Magnesium hydroxide 200 mg, dried aluminum hydroxide gel 200 mg/Tab. Bot. 100s. *otc.*
Use: Antacid.

Maalox Therapeutic Concentrate Suspension. (Rhone-Poulenc Rorer Pharmaceuticals, Inc.) Magnesium hydroxide 300 mg, aluminum hydroxide 600 mg/5 ml. Susp. Bot. 355 ml. *otc.*
Use: Antacid.

Maalox Therapeutic Concentrate Tablets. (Rhone-Poulenc Rorer Pharmaceuticals, Inc.) Magnesium hydroxide 300 mg, aluminum hydroxide 600 mg. Tab. Bot. 48s. *otc.*
Use: Antacid.

MacPac. (Procter & Gamble Pharm.) Nitrofurantoin macrocrystals 50 mg, 100 mg/Cap. UD 28s. *Rx.*
Use: Anti-infective, urinary.

macroaggregated albumin. (Bristol-Myers Squibb) Albumotope I-131.

Macrobid. (Procter & Gamble Pharm.) Nitrofurantoin 100 mg (as 25 mg nitrofurantoin macrocrystals and 75 mg nitrofurantoin monohydrate). Cap. Bot. 100s. *Rx.*
Use: Anti-infective, urinary.

Macrodantin. (Procter & Gamble Pharm.) Nitrofurantoin macrocrystals. **25 mg/Cap.:** Bot. 100s. **50 mg or 100 mg/Cap.:** Bot. 100s, 500s, 1000s, UD

100s. *Rx.*
Use: Anti-infective, urinary.

Macrodex. (Pharmacia & Upjohn) Dextran 6% w/v in normal saline, 6% w/v in dextrose 5% in water. Bot. 500 ml. *Rx.*
Use: Plasma volume expander.

macrogol stearate 2000. Polyoxyl 40 Stearate.

Macrotec. (Bristol-Myers Squibb) Technetium Tc 99m Medronate kit. Vial Kit 10s.
Use: Radiopaque agent.

•**maduramicin.** (mad-UHR-ah-MY-sin) USAN.
Use: Anticoccidal.

•**mafenide.** (MAY-feh-NIDE) USAN.
Use: Anti-infective.

•**mafenide acetate.** (MAY-feh-NIDE) U.S.P. 23.
Use: Anti-infective, topical.
See: Sulfamylon Cream (Bertek Pharmaceuticals).

mafenide acetate solution.
Use: Prevent graft loss on burn wounds. [Orphan Drug]

•**mafilcon a.** (MAY-fill-kahn A) USAN.
Use: Contact lens material (hydrophilic).

Mafylon Cream. (Sanofi Winthrop Pharmaceuticals) Mafenide acetate.
Use: Burn therapy.

•**magaldrate.** (MAG-al-drate) U.S.P. 23. (Wyeth-Ayerst Laboratories) Monalium Hydrate. Aluminum Magnesium Hydroxide.
Use: Antacid.
See: Iosopan (Zenith Goldline Pharmaceuticals).
Monalium Hydrate.
Riopan, Tab., Susp. (Wyeth-Ayerst Laboratories).

magaldrate and simethicone.
Use: Antacid, antiflatulent.
See: Lowsium (Rugby Labs, Inc.).
Lowsium Plus (Rugby Labs, Inc.).
Riopan Plus (Wyeth-Ayerst Laboratories).

magaldrate plus suspension. (Various Mfr.) Magaldrate 540 mg, simethicone 40 mg/5 ml. Susp. Bot. 360 ml. *otc.*
Use: Antacid, antiflatulent.

Magan. (Pharmacia & Upjohn) Magnesium salicylate (anhydrous) 545 mg/Tab. Bot. 100s, 500s. *Rx.*
Use: Analgesic.

Mag-Cal Tablets. (Fibertone) Calcium 416.7 mg (as carbonate), calcium 166.7 mg (as elemental), vitamin D 66.7 IU, Mg 83.3 mg, Cu 0.167 mg, Mn 0.83 mg, K 1.67 mg, Zn 0.167 mg/Tab. Bot. 90s, 180s. *otc.*
Use: Mineral, vitamin supplement.

Mag-Cal Mega. (Freeda Vitamins, Inc.) Mg 800 mg, Ca 400 mg, kosher, sugar free/Tab. Bot. 100s, 250s. *otc.*
Use: Mineral, vitamin supplement.

Magdrox. (Vita Elixir) Magnesium hydroxide, aluminum hydroxide. *otc.*
Use: Antacid.

Mag-G. (Cypress Pharmaceutical, Inc.) Magnesium gluconate dihydrate 500 mg (≈ 27 mg elemental Mg). Tab. Bot. 100s. *otc.*
Use: Mineral supplement.

Magmalin. (Pal-Pak, Inc.) Magnesium hydroxide 0.2 g, aluminum hydroxide gel, dried 0.2 g/Loz. Bot. 1000s. *otc.*
Use: Antacid.

Magnacal Liquid. (Biosearch Medical Products) Protein (from calcium, sodium caseinate), carbohydrate (from maltodextrin, sucrose), fat (partially hydrogenated from soy oil, lecithin, mono- and diglycerides). 1.5 Cal/ml, 590 mOsm/kg H_2O. Protein 70 g, CHO 250 g, fat 80 g, Na 1000 mg, K 1250 mg/L. Can 120 ml, 240 ml. *otc.*
Use: Nutritional supplement.

Magnalox Liquid. (Schein Pharmaceutical, Inc.) Aluminum hydroxide 225 mg, magnesium hydroxide 200 mg/5 ml. Liq. Bot. 360 ml. *otc.*
Use: Antacid.

Magnalum. (Global Source) Magnesium hydroxide 3.75 gr, aluminum hydroxide 2 gr/Tab. Bot. 1000s. *otc.*
Use: Antacid.

Magnaprin. (Rugby Labs, Inc.) Aspirin 325 mg, dried aluminum hydroxide gel 75 mg, magnesium hydroxide 75 mg/Tab. Bot. 100s, 500s. *otc.*
Use: Analgesic.

Magnaprin Arthritis Strength. (Rugby Labs, Inc.) Aspirin 325 mg, dried aluminum hydroxide gel 150 mg, magnesium hydroxide 150 mg/Tab. Bot. 100s, 500s. *otc.*
Use: Analgesic.

magnesia tablets.
Use: Antacid.

magnesia & alumina oral suspension. (Roxane Laboratories, Inc.) Oral Susp. 6 fl oz. 25s.
Use: Antacid.
See: Maalox, Liq. (Rhone-Poulenc Rorer Pharmaceuticals, Inc.).

magnesia & alumina tablets.
Use: Antacid.
See: Maalox, Tab. (Rhone-Poulenc Rorer Pharmaceuticals, Inc.).

magnesia magma. Milk of Magnesia.

Use: Antacid, cathartic, laxative.
See: Magnesium Hydroxide, Preps.

•**magnesia, milk of.** U.S.P. 23.
Use: Antacid, laxative.

magnesium acetylsalicylate. Apyron, Magnespirin, Magisal, Novacetyl.
Use: Analgesic.

magnesium aluminate hydrated.
Use: Antacid.
See: Riopan, Susp., Tab. (Wyeth-Ayerst Laboratories).

magnesium aluminum hydroxide.
Use: Antacid.
See: Maalox, Susp. (Rhone-Poulenc Rorer Pharmaceuticals, Inc.).
Malogel, Gel (Quality Formulations, Inc.).
Medalox, Gel (Davol).
W/APC.
See: Buffadyne, Tab. (Teva Pharmaceuticals USA).
W/Calcium carbonate.
See: Maalox Plus, Susp. (Rhone-Poulenc Rorer Pharmaceuticals, Inc).

•**magnesium aluminum silicate.** (mag-NEE-zee-uhm) N.F. 18.
Use: Pharmaceutic aid, suspending agent.

•**magnesium carbonate.** (mag-NEE-zee-uhm) U.S.P. 23.
Use: Antacid.

magnesium carbonate. (Baker, J.T.) Pow. 4 oz, 1 lb, 5 lb.
Use: Antacid.

magnesium carbonate and sodium bicarbonate for oral suspension.
Use: Antacid.

magnesium carbonate w/combinations.
Use: Antacid.
See: Alkets, Tab. (Pharmacia & Upjohn).
Antacid No. 2, Tab. (Jones Medical Industries, Inc.).
Bufferin, Tab. (Bristol-Myers Squibb).
Di-Gel, Tab., Liq. (Schering-Plough Corp.).
Marblen, Susp., Tab. (Fleming & Co.).

•**magnesium chloride.** U.S.P. 23.
Use: Electrolyte replacement, pharmaceutical necessity for hemodialysis and peritoneal dialysis.

•**magnesium citrate.** (mag-NEE-zee-uhm) U.S.P. 23.
Use: Cathartic; laxative.

•**magnesium gluconate.** U.S.P. 23.
Use: Vitamin supplement, replacement.
See: Almora, Tab. (Forest Pharmaceutical, Inc.).
Mag-G, Tab. (Cypress).

magnesium gluconate. (Western Research) Magnesium gluconate 500 mg/Tab. Bot. 1000s. *otc.*
Use: Vitamin supplement.

magnesium hydroxide. U.S.P. 23.
Use: Antacid, cathartic, laxative.
See: Magnesia Magma (Various Mfr.).
Milk of Magnesia (Various Mfr.).
Phillips' Milk of Magnesia (Bayer Corp. (Consumer Div.)).
Phillips' Chewable, Tab. (Bayer Corp. (Consumer Div.)).

magnesium hydroxide w/combinations.
See: Aludrox, Susp., Tab., Vial (Wyeth-Ayerst Laboratories).
Ascriptin, Tab. (Rhone-Poulenc Rorer Pharmaceuticals, Inc.).
Ascriptin A/D, Tab. (Rhone-Poulenc Rorer Pharmaceuticals, Inc.).
Ascriptin Extra Strength, Tab. (Rhone-Poulenc Rorer Pharmaceuticals, Inc.).
Ascriptin w/Codeine, Tab. (Rhone-Poulenc Rorer Pharmaceuticals, Inc.).
Banacid, Tab. (Buffington).
Delcid, Susp. (Hoechst Marion Roussel).
Gas Ban DS, Liq. (Roberts Pharmaceuticals).
Maalox, Susp., Tab. (Rhone-Poulenc Rorer Pharmaceuticals, Inc.).
Maalox Plus, Susp, Tab. (Rhone-Poulenc Rorer Pharmaceuticals, Inc.).
Mylanta, Mylanta II, Liq., Tab. (Zeneca Pharmaceuticals).

•**magnesium oxide.** (mag-NEE-zee-uhm OX-ide) U.S.P. 23.
Use: Pharmaceutic aid (sorbent).

magnesium oxide. (Manne) 420 mg/Tab. Bot. 250s, 1000s. (Stanlabs) 10 gr/Tab. Bot. 100s, 1000s. (Cypress) 400 mg. Tab. Bot. 120s. *otc.*
Use: Pharmaceutical aid (sorbant).
See: Mag-Ox, Tab. (Blaine Co., Inc.).
Mag-Ox 400, Tab. (Blaine Co., Inc.).
Niko-Mag, Cap. (Scruggs).
Par-Mag, Cap. (Parmed Pharmaceuticals, Inc.).
Uro-Mag, Cap. (Blaine Co., Inc.).
W/Calcium, Vitamin D.
See: Elekap, Cap. (Western Research).
W/Magnesium carbonate, calcium carbonate.
See: Alkets, Tab. (Pharmacia & Upjohn).
W/Ox bile (desiccated), hog bile (desiccated).
See: Hyper-Cholate, Tab. (Roberts Pharmaceuticals).

•**magnesium phosphate.** (mag-NEE-zee-uhm FOSS-fate) U.S.P. 23.
Use: Antacid.

•**magnesium salicylate.** U.S.P. 23.
Use: Analgesic, antipyretic, antirheumatic.
See: Analate, Tab. (Winston)
Backache Maximum Strength Relief, Capl. (Bristol-Myers Squibb).
Bayer Select Maximum Strength Backache, Capl. (Bayer Corp. (Consumer Div.)).
Efficin, Tab. (Pharmacia & Upjohn).
Magan, Tab. (Pharmacia & Upjohn).
Momentum Muscular Backache Formula, Capl. (Whitehall Robins Laboratories).
Nuprin Backache, Capl. (Bristol-Myers Squibb).
W/Diphenhydramine HCl.
See: Extra Strength Doan's PM, Capl. (Novartis Pharmaceutical Corp.).
W/Phenyltoloxamine citrate.
See: Mobigesic, Tab. (B.F. Ascher and Co.).
W/Combinations.
See: Maximum Strength Arthriten (Alva-Amco).

•**magnesium silicate.** N.F. 18.
Use: Pharmaceutic aid (tablet excipient).

•**magnesium stearate.** N.F. 18.
Use: Pharmaceutic aid (tablet and capsule lubricant).

•**magnesium sulfate.** (mag-NEE-zee-uhm SULL-fate) U.S.P. 23.
Use: Anticonvulsant, electrolyte replacement, laxative.

magnesium sulfate. (Various Mfr.) **10%:** (0.8 mEq/ml) Vial 20 ml, 50 ml. Amp. 20 ml. **12.5%:** (1 mEq/ml) Vial 20 ml. **50%:** (4 mEq/ml) Vial 2 ml, 5 ml, 10 ml, 20 ml, 50 ml. Syringe 5 ml, 10 ml. Amp. 2 ml, 10 ml. *Rx.*
Use: Anticonvulsant; electrolyte replacement; laxative.

•**magnesium trisilicate.** U.S.P. 23.
Use: Antacid.

magnesium trisilicate w/combinations.
See: Alsorb Gel C.T., Gel (Standex).
Arcodex, Tab. (Arcum).
Banacid, Tab. (Buffington).
Gacid, Tab. (Arcum).
Gaviscon, Tab. (Hoechst Marion Roussel).
Maracid 2, Tab. (Marlin Industries).

Magnevist. (Berlex Laboratories, Inc.) Gadopentetate dimeglumine 469.01 mg/ml. Inj. Vial 5 ml, 10 ml, 15 ml, 20 ml. Prefilled Disp. Syr. 10 ml, 15 ml, 20 ml. *Rx.*
Use: Radiopaque agent.

Magonate. (Fleming & Co.) Magnesium gluconate 500 mg/Tab. Bot. 100s, 1000s. *otc.*
Use: Vitamin supplement.

Mag-Ox 400. (Blaine Co., Inc.) Magnesium oxide 400 mg/Tab. Bot. 100s, 1000s. *otc.*
Use: Antacid, vitamin supplement.

Magsal. (US Pharmaceutical Corp.) Magnesium salicylate 600 mg, phenyltoloxamine citrate 25 mg/Tab. Bot. 100s. *Rx.*
Use: Analgesic combination.

Mag-Tab SR. (Niche Pharmaceuticals, Inc.) Magnesium (as lactate) 84 mg/SR Capl. Bot. 60s, 100s. *otc.*
Use: Vitamin supplement.

Maigret-50. (Ferndale Laboratories, Inc.) Phenylpropanolamine HCl 50 mg/Tab. Bot. 100s.
Use: Decongestant.

Maintenance Vitamin Formula w/Minerals. (Towne) Vitamins A palmitate 10,000 IU, D 400 IU, B_1 5 mg, B_2 2.5 mg, C 75 mg, niacinamide 40 mg, B_6 1 mg, calcium pantothenate 4 mg, B_{12} 2 mcg, E 2 IU, choline bitartrate 31.4 mg, inositol 15 mg, Ca 75 mg, P 58 mg, Fe 30 mg, Mg 3 mg, Mn 0.5 mg, K 2 mg, Zn 0.5 mg/Cap. Bot. 100s. *otc.*
Use: Mineral, vitamin supplement.

majeptil. Thioproperazine. Psychopharmacologic agent; pending release.

Major-gesic. (Major Pharmaceuticals) Phenyltoloxamine citrate 30 mg, acetaminophen 325 mg/Tab. Bot. 100s. *otc.*
Use: Antihistamine, analgesic.

malagride. Acetarsone.

Malaraquin. (Sanofi Winthrop Pharmaceuticals) Chloroquine phosphate. *Rx.*
Use: Antimalarial.

•**malathion.** (mal-ah-THIGH-ahn) U.S.P. 23.
Use: Pediculicide.

•**malethamer.** (mal-ETH-ah-mer) USAN.
Use: Antidiarrheal, antiperistaltic.

•**malic acid.** (MAL-ik) N.F. 18.
Use: Pharmaceutic aid (acidifying agent).

Mallamint. (Roberts Pharmaceuticals) Calcium carbonate 420 mg/Tab. Bot. 100s. *otc.*
Use: Antacid.

Mallazine Drops. (Roberts Pharmaceuticals) Tetrahydrozoline 0.05%. Soln. 15 ml. *otc.*
Use: Mydriatic, vasoconstrictor.

Mallergan-VC w/Codeine Syrup. (Rob-

erts Pharmaceuticals) Phenylephrine HCl 5 mg, promethazine HCl 6.25 mg, codeine phosphate 10 mg/5 ml, alcohol 7%. Syr. Bot. 120 ml. *c-v.*
Use: Antihistamine, antitussive, decongestant.

Mallisol. (Roberts Pharmaceuticals) Povidone-iodine. *otc.*
Use: Antimicrobial, antiseptic.

Malogen Injection Aqueous. (Forest Pharmaceutical, Inc.) Testosterone. **25 mg/ml:** 10 ml, 30 ml. **50 mg/ml:** 10 ml. **100 mg/ml:** 10 ml. *c-III.*
Use: Androgen.

Malogen 100 L.A. in Oil. (Forest Pharmaceutical, Inc.) Testosterone enanthate 100 mg/ml. Inj. 10 ml. *c-III.*
Use: Androgen.

Malogen 200 L.A. in Oil. (Forest Pharmaceutical, Inc.) Testosterone enanthate 200 mg/ml. Inj. 10 ml. *c-III.*
Use: Androgen.

Malogen Cyp. (Forest Pharmaceutical, Inc.) Testosterone cypionate in oil 100 mg, 200 mg/ml. Inj. Vial 10 ml. *c-III.*
Use: Androgen.

malonal. Barbital (Various Mfr.).

•**malotilate.** (mal-OH-tih-LATE) USAN.
Use: Liver disorder treatment.

•**maltitol solution.** (MAL-tih-tahl) N.F. 18.
Use: Sweetener.

Malotrone Aqueous Injection. (Bluco Inc./Med. Discnt. Outlet) Testosterone, USP 25 mg, 50 mg/ml in aqueous susp. Vial 10 ml. *c-III.*
Use: Androgen.

•**maltodextrin.** N.F. 18.
Use: Pharmaceutic aid (coating agent, tablet binder, tablet and capsule diluent, viscosity-increasing agent).

Maltsupex. (Wallace Laboratories) Laxative derived from natural barley malt extract for relief of constipation in children and adults. **Liq.:** Bot. 8 oz, pt. **Pow.:** Jar 8 oz, lb. **Tab.:** Malt soup extract 750 mg/Tab. Bot. 100s. *otc.*
Use: Laxative.
See: Syllamalt, Pow. (Wallace Laboratories).

Mammol Ointment. (Abbott Laboratories) Bismuth subnitrate 40%, castor oil 30%, anhydrous lanolin 22%, ceresin wax 7%, balsam Peru 1%. Tube ⅞ oz. Ctn. 12s. *otc.*
Use: Dermatologic, protectant, emollient.

mandameth. (Major Pharmaceuticals) Methenamine mandelate 0.5 g/EC Tab. Bot. 1000s. *Rx.*
Use: Anti-infective, urinary.

mandelic acid.
Use: Anti-infective, urinary.

mandelic acid salts. Calcium mandelate (Various Mfr.).

mandelyltropeine. Homatropine Salts (Various Mfr.).

Mandol. (Eli Lilly and Co.) Cefamandole nafate. 1 g/10 ml, 2 g/20 ml. Pow. for Inj. Vial. *Rx.*
Use: Anti-infective, cephalosporin.

Manganese.
Use: Dietary supplement.
See: Chelated manganese (Freeda Vitamins, Inc.).

•**manganese chloride.** (MANG-ah-neese) U.S.P. 23.
Use: Manganese deficiency treatment, trace mineral supplement.

•**manganese gluconate.** U.S.P. 23.
Use: Manganese deficiency, trace mineral supplement.

manganese glycerophosphate. Glycerol phosphate manganese salt.
Use: Pharmaceutical necessity.

manganese hypophosphite. Manganese^{++}phosphinate.
Use: Pharmaceutical necessity.

•**manganese sulfate.** U.S.P. 23.
Use: Trace mineral supplement.

Manga-Pak. (SoloPak Pharmaceuticals, Inc.) Manganese 0.1 mg/ml. Inj. Vial 10 ml, 30 ml. *Rx.*
Use: Nutritional supplement, parenteral.

mangofodopir trisodium.
Use: Diagnostic aid.
See: Teslascan, Inj. (Nycomed Inc.).

Maniron. (Jones Medical Industries, Inc.) Ferrous fumarate 3 mg/Tab. Bot. 100s, 1000s, 5000s. *otc.*
Use: Mineral supplement.

Mann Astringent Mouth Wash Concentrate. (Manne) Bot. 4 oz, qt, 0.5 gal, gal. Also mint flavored. Bot. 4 oz, qt, 0.5 gal, gal. *otc.*
Use: Mouthwash.

Mann Body Deodorant. (Manne) Bot. 4 oz, 8 oz, pt, qt. *otc.*

Mann Breath Deodorant. (Manne) Bot. 1 oz, 4 oz, 8 oz, pt, qt, 0.5 gal. *otc.*

Mann Emollient. (Manne) Jar. 100 g. *otc.*
Use: Emollient.

Mann Eugenol U.S.P. Extra. (Manne) 0.06 lb, 0.13 lb, 0.25 lb, 0.5 lb, 1 lb. *otc.*
Use: Dermatologic, protectant.

Mann Germicidal Solution. (Manne) **Regular:** Bot. Gal, 4 gal. **Conc.:** 12.8%. Bot. Pt, qt, 0.5 gal, gal. *otc.*
Use: Antimicrobial.

Mann Hand Lotion. (Manne) Twin pack,

gal. *otc.*
Use: Emollient.

Mann Hemostatic. (Manne) Bot. 1 oz, 4 oz, 8 oz, pt, qt. *otc.*
Use: Hemostatic.

Mann Liquid Soap. (Manne) Concentrated cococastile. Bot. Qt, 0.5 gal, gal. *otc.*
Use: Emollient.

Mann Lubricant and Cleanser. (Manne) Bot. Pt, qt. *otc.*
Use: Emollient.

Mann Superfatted Bar Soap. (Manne) Rich in lanolin. Cake. 12s. *otc.*
Use: Emollient.

Mann Talbot's Iodine. (Manne) Glycerin base. Bot. 1 oz, 4 oz, 8 oz, pt, qt. *otc.*
Use: Antiseptic.

Mann Topical Anesthetic. (Manne) Bot. 1 oz, 4 oz, 8 oz, pt. W/stain to indicate area treated. Bot. 1oz, 4 oz, 8 oz. *otc.*
Use: Anesthetic, local.

manna sugar. Mannitol (Various Mfr.).

Mannan. (Rugby Labs, Inc.) Purified glucomannan 500 mg/Cap. Bot. 90s. *otc.*
Use: Nutritional supplement.

Mannest. (Manne) Conjugated estrogens 0.625 mg, 1.25 mg, or 2.5 mg/Tab. Bot. 100s, 200s. *Rx.*
Use: Estrogen.

mannite.
See: Mannitol, U.S.P. 23.

•**mannitol.** (MAN-ih-tole) U.S.P. 23.
Use: Diagnostic aid.
See: Osmitrol (Baxter Pharmaceutical Products, Inc.).

mannitol hexanitrate.
Use: Coronary vasodilator.
See: Vascunitol, Tab. (Apco).

mannitol hexanitrate & phenobarbital tablets. (Jones Medical Industries, Inc.; Quality Generics) Mannitol hexanitrate 0.5 g, phenobarbital 0.25 g/Tab. Bot. 1000s. *c-IV.*
Use: Vasodilator.

mannitol hexanitrate with phenobarbital combinations.
See: Manotensin,Tab. (Dunhall Pharmaceuticals, Inc.).
Vascused, Tab. (Apco).

mannitol in sodium chloride injection.
Use: Diuretic.

mannitol injection. (Abbott Laboratories) 15%, 20%. Abbo-Vac single-dose container 500 ml.
Use: Diagnostic aid (renal function determination), diuretic.
See: Mannitol Solution, Amp. (Merck & Co.).

Manotensin. (Dunhall Pharmaceuticals, Inc.) Mannitol hexanitrate 32 mg, phenobarbital 16 mg/Tab. Bot. 100s, 1000s. *c-IV.*
Use: Vasodilator.

Mantoux Test.
Use: Tuberculin test.

manvene.
Use: Antineoplastic.

MAOI.
See: Monoamine Oxidase Inhibitors.

Maolate. (Pharmacia & Upjohn) Chlorphenesin carbamate 400 mg/Tab. Bot. 50s, 500s. *Rx.*
Use: Muscle relaxant, anxiolytic.

Maox 420. (Manne) Magnesium oxide 420 mg/Tab. Bot. 250s, 1000s. *otc.*
Use: Antacid.

Mapap Cold Formula. (Major Pharmaceuticals) Acetaminophen 325 mg, pseudoephedrine HCl 30 mg, dextromethorphan HBr 15 mg, chlorpheniramine maleate 2 mg. Tab. Pkg. 24s. *otc.*
Use: Antitussive combination.

Mapap Extra Strength. (Major Pharmaceuticals) Acetaminophen 500 mg/Tab. Bot. 30s, 60s, 100s, 200s, 1000s and UD 100s. *otc.*
Use: Analgesic.

Mapap Infant Drops. (Major Pharmaceuticals) Acetaminophen 100 mg/ml, alcohol free/Drops. Bot. 15 ml, 30 ml. *otc.*
Use: Analgesic.

Mapap Regular Strength. (Major Pharmaceuticals) Acetaminophen 325 mg/ Scored Tab. Bot. 100s, 1000s, UD 100s. *otc.*
Use: Analgesic.

Maprofix.
See: Gardinol Type Detergents (Various Mfr.).

•**maprotiline.** (map-ROW-tih-leen) USAN.
Use: Antidepressant.
See: Ludiomil, Tab. (Novartis Pharmaceutical Corp.).

•**maprotiline hydrochloride.** (map-ROW-tih-leen) U.S.P. 23.
Use: Antidepressant.

Maracid 2. (Marlin Industries) Magnesium trisilicate 150 mg, aluminum hydroxide dried gel 90 mg, aminoacetic acid 75 mg/Tab. Bot. *otc.*
Use: Antacid, adsorbent.

Maranox. (C.S. Dent & Co. Division) Acetaminophen 325 mg/Tab. Bot. 8s. *otc.*
Use: Analgesic.

Marax-DF Syrup. (Roerig) Hydroxyzine HCl 7.5 mg, ephedrine sulfate 18.75 mg, theophylline 97.5 mg/15 ml. Color free, dye free. Bot. Pt, gal. *Rx.*
Use: Antiasthmatic combination.

Marax Tab. (Roerig) Hydroxyzine HCl 10

mg, ephedrine sulfate 25 mg, theophylline 130 mg/Tab. Bot. 100s, 500s. *Rx.*
Use: Antiasthmatic combination.

Marbaxin 750. (Vortech Pharmaceuticals) Methocarbamol 750 mg/Tab. Bot. 500s. *Rx.*
Use: Muscle relaxant.

Marblen Liquid. (Fleming & Co.) Magnesium carbonate 400 mg, calcium carbonate 520 mg/5 ml. Bot. 473 ml. *otc.*
Use: Antacid.

Marblen Tablets. (Fleming & Co.) Calcium carbonate 520 mg, magnesium carbonate 400 mg. Tab. Bot. 100s, 1000s. *otc.*
Use: Antacid.

Marcaine. (Sanofi Winthrop Pharmaceuticals) Bupivacaine in sterile isotonic soln. containing sodium Cl pH adjusted 4 to 6.5 w/sodium hydroxide or hydrochloric acid. Multiple-dose vial also contains methylparaben 1 mg/ml as preservative. **0.25%:** Amp. 50 ml. Box 5s. Vial: Single-dose 10 ml, 30 ml. Box 10s; multiple-dose 50 ml. Box 1s. **0.5%:** Amp. 30 ml. Box 1s. Vial: Single-dose 10 ml, 30 ml. Box 10s; multiple-dose 50 ml. Box 1s. **0.75%:** Amp. 30 ml. Box 5s. Vial (single-dose) 10 ml, 30 ml. Box 10s. *Rx.*
Use: Anesthetic, local.

Marcaine with Epinephrine. (Sanofi Winthrop Pharmaceuticals) (1:200,000). **Bupivacaine 0.25%:** with epinephrine 1:200,000 in sterile isotonic soln. containing sodium Cl. Each 1 ml contains bupivacaine HCl 2.5 mg, epinephrine bitartrate 0.0091 mg, sodium metabisulfite 0.5 mg, monothioglycerol 0.001 ml, ascorbic acid 2 mg and edetate calcium disodium 0.1 mg. In multiple-dose vial, each 1 ml also contains methylparaben 1 mg as antiseptic preservative. pH adjusted to between 3.4 and 4.5 with sodium hydroxide or hydrochloric acid. Amp. 50 ml, 5s. Single-dose vial 10 ml, 30 ml. 10s. Multiple-dose vial 50 ml. 1s. **Bupivacaine 0.5%:** with epinephrine 1:200,000 in sterile isotonic soln. containing sodium Cl. Each 1 ml contains bupivacaine HCl 5 mg and epinephrine bitartrate 0.0091 mg, with sodium metabisulfite 0.5 mg, monothioglycerol 0.001 ml and ascorbic acid 2 mg, edetate calcium disodium 0.1 mg. In multiple-dose vial, each 1 ml also contains methylparaben 1 mg antiseptic preservative. pH adjusted to between 3.4 and 4.5 with sodium hydroxide or hydrochloric acid. Amp. 3 ml 10s, 30 ml. 5s. Single-dose vial 10 ml, 30 ml. 10s. Multiple-dose vial 50 ml. 1s. **Bupivacaine 0.75%:** with epinephrine 1:200,000 in sterile isotonic soln. containing sodium Cl. Each 1 ml contains bupivacaine HCl 7.5 mg, epinephrine bitartrate 0.0091 mg with sodium metabisulfite 0.5 mg, monothioglycerol 0.001 ml, ascorbic acid 2 mg as antioxidants, edetate calcium disodium 0.1 mg. pH adjusted to between 3.4 and 4.5 with sodium hydroxide or hydrochloric acid. Amp 30 ml. 5s. *otc.*
Use: Anesthetic, local.

Marcaine Spinal. (Sanofi Winthrop Pharmaceuticals) Bupivacaine HCl 15 mg/2 ml (0.75%) and dextrose 165 mg/2 ml (8.25%). Amp. 2 ml. *Rx.*
Use: Anesthetic, local.

Marcillin. (Marnel Pharmaceuticals, Inc.) Ampicillin trihydrate 500 mg. Cap. Bot. 100s. *Rx.*
Use: Anti-infective, penicillin.

Marcof Expectorant. (Marnel Pharmaceuticals, Inc.) Hydrocodone bitartrate 5 mg, potassium guaiacol sulfonate 300 mg/5 ml. Liq. Bot. 480 ml. *c-III.*
Use: Antitussive; expectorant, narcotic.

Mardon. (Armenpharm Ltd.) Propoxyphene HCl. **Cap.:** 32 mg Bot. 100s, 1000s. **65 mg:** Bot. 100s, 500s, 1000s. *c-IV.*
Use: Analgesic, narcotic.

Mardon Compound. (Armenpharm Ltd.) Propoxyphene compound 65 mg, aspirin 3.5 gr, phenacetin 2.5 gr, caffeine 0.5 gr/Cap. Bot. 100s, 500s, 1000s. *c-IV.*
Use: Analgesic combination, narcotic.

Marezine. (Himmel Pharmaceuticals, Inc.) Cyclizine HCl 50 mg/Tab. Bot. 100s. Box 12s. *otc.*
Use: Anticholinergic.

Margesic. (Marnel Pharmaceuticals, Inc.) Butalbital 50 mg, acetaminophen 325 mg, caffeine 40 mg/Cap. Bot. 100s. *Rx.*
Use: Analgesic, hypnotic, sedative.

Margesic H. (Marnel Pharmaceuticals, Inc.) Hydrocodone bitartrate 5 mg, acetaminophen 500 mg/Cap. Bot. 100s. *c-III.*
Use: Analgesic combination, narcotic.

Margesic No. 3. (Marnel Pharmaceuticals, Inc.) Codeine phosphate 30 mg, acetaminophen 300 mg/Tab. Bot. 100s. *c-III.*
Use: Analgesic combination, narcotic.

Marhist. (Marlop Pharmaceuticals, Inc.) Chlorpheniramine maleate 20 mg, phenylephrine HCl 2.5 mg, methscopolamine nitrate in special base/ Cap. Bot. 30s, 100s. Expectorant Bot.

4 oz, pt, gal. *Rx.*
Use: Anticholinergic, antihistamine, decongestant.

•**marimastat.** (mah-RIH-mah-stat) USAN.
Use: Antineoplastic (matrix metalloproteinase inhibitor).

Marine Lipid Concentrate. (Vitaline Corp.) Omega-3 1200 mg, EPA 360 mg, DHA 240 mg, E 5 IU/Cap., sodium free. Bot. 90s. *otc.*
Use: Nutritional supplement.

Marinol. (Roxane Laboratories, Inc.) Dronabinol 2.5 mg, 5 mg, 10 mg/Cap. Bot. 25s, 60s, 100s. *c-II.*
Use: Antiemetic.

Marlin Salt System. (Marlin Industries) Sodium Cl 250 mg/Tab. Bot. 200s with bot. 27.7 ml. *otc.*
Use: Contact lens care.

Marlyn Formula 50. (Marlyn Nutraceuticals, Inc.) Vitamin B_6 w/18 amino acids/ Cap. Bot. 100s, 250s, 1000s. *otc.*
Use: Nutritional supplement.

Marnatal-F. (Marnel Pharmaceuticals, Inc.) Ca 250 mg, Fe 60 mg, vitamins A 4000 IU, D 400 IU, E 30 mg, B_1 3 mg, B_2 3.4 mg, B_3 20 mg, B_6 5 mg, B_{12} 12 mcg, C 100 mg, folic acid 1 mg, Mg, Zn 25 mg, Cu, I/Tab. Bot. 30s, 100s. *Rx.*
Use: Mineral, vitamin supplement; dental caries agent.

Marplan. (Hoffman-LaRoche) Isocarboxazid 10 mg. Tab. Bot. 100s. *Rx.*
Use: Antidepressant.

Marthritic. (Marnel Pharmaceuticals, Inc.) Salsalate 750 mg. Tab. Bot. 100s. *Rx.*
Use: Analgesic.

•**masoprocol.** (mass-OH-prah-KOLE) USAN.
Use: Antineoplastic.
See: Actinex, Cream (Schwarz Pharma, Inc.).

Masse Breast Cream. (Advanced Care Products) Glyceryl monostearate, glycerin, cetyl alcohol, lanolin, peanut oil, Span-60, stearic acid, Tween-60, sodium benzoate, propylparaben, methylparaben, potassium hydroxide. Tube 2 oz. *otc.*
Use: Emollient.

Massengill Baking Soda Freshness. (SmithKline Beecham Pharmaceuticals) Sanitized water, sodium bicarbonate. Soln. Bot. 180 ml. *otc.*
Use: Vaginal agent.

Massengill Disposable Douche. (SmithKline Beecham Pharmaceuticals) Water, SD alcohol 40, lactic acid, sodium lactate, octoxynol-9, cetylpyridinium Cl, propylene glycol, diazolidinyl urea, EDTA, parabens, fragrance, color. Bot. 180 ml. *otc.*
Use: Vaginal agent.

Massengill Extra Cleansing w/Puraclean. (SmithKline Beecham Pharmaceuticals) Vinegar, water, cetylpyridinium chloride, diazolidinyl urea, EDTA. Soln. Bot. 180 ml. *otc.*
Use: Vaginal agent.

Massengill Feminine Cleansing Wash. (SmithKline Beecham Pharmaceuticals) Sodium laureth sulfate, magnesium oleth sulfate, sodium oleth sulfate, magnesium oleth sulfate, PEG-120 methyl glucose dioleate, parabens. Liq. Bot. 240 ml. *otc.*
Use: Vaginal agent.

Massengill Feminine Deodorant Spray. (SmithKline Beecham Pharmaceuticals) Aerosol Bot. 3 oz. *otc.*
Use: Vaginal agent.

Massengill Liquid. (SmithKline Beecham Pharmaceuticals) Lactic acid, SD alcohol 40, octoxynol-9, water, sodium bicarbonate. Bot. 120 ml. *otc.*
Use: Vaginal agent.

Massengill Medicated. (SmithKline Beecham Pharmaceuticals) Povidone-iodine 0.3% when added to sanitized fluid. Bot. 6 oz. *otc.*
Use: Vaginal agent.

Massengill Medicated Disposable Douche w/Cepticin. (SmithKline Beecham Pharmaceuticals) Povidone-iodine 10%. Liq. Vial 5 ml w/180 ml bot. of sanitized water. *otc.*
Use: Vaginal agent.

Massengill Medicated Douche w/Cepticin. (SmithKline Beecham Pharmaceuticals) Povidone-iodine 12%. Liq. concentrate. Bot. 120 ml, 240 ml. *otc.*
Use: Vaginal agent.

Massengill Powder. (SmithKline Beecham Pharmaceuticals) Ammonium alum, PEG-8, methyl salicylate, eucalyptus oil, menthol, thymol, phenol. Jar 120 g, 240 g, 480 g, 660 g. UD Packette 10s, 12s. *otc.*
Use: Vaginal agent.

Massengill Soft Cloth. (SmithKline Beecham Pharmaceuticals) Hydrocortisone 0.5%, diazolidinyl urea, DMDM hydantoin, isopropyl myristate, methylparaben, polysorbate 60, propylene glycol, propylparaben, sorbitan stearate, steareth-2, steareth-21. Towelettes 10s. *otc.*
Use: Vaginal agent.

Massengill Unscented. (SmithKline Beecham Pharmaceuticals) Water, SD alcohol 40, lactic acid, sodium lactate,

octoxynol-9, cetylpyridinium chloride, propylene glycol, diazolidinyl urea, parabens, EDTA. Soln. Bot. 180 ml. *otc.*
Use: Vaginal agent.

Massengill Vinegar-Water Disposable Douche. (SmithKline Beecham Pharmaceuticals) Water and vinegar solution. Bot. 180 ml. *otc.*
Use: Vaginal agent.

Massengill Vinegar & Water Extra Cleansing with Puraclean. (SmithKline Beecham Pharmaceuticals) Vinegar, water, cetylpyridinium chloride, diazolidinyl urea, EDTA. Soln. Bot. 180 ml. *otc.*
Use: Vaginal agent.

Massengill Vinegar & Water Extra Mild. (SmithKline Beecham Pharmaceuticals) Vinegar, water, preservative free. Soln. Bot. 180 ml. *otc.*
Use: Vaginal agent.

Master Formula. (Barth's) Vitamins A 10,000 IU, D 400 IU, C 180 mg, B_1 7 mg, B_2 14 mg, niacin 4.6 mg, B_6 292 mcg, pantothenic acid 210 mcg, B_{12} 25 mcg, biotin 2.9 mcg, E 50 IU, Ca 800 mg, P 387 mg, Fe 10 mg, I 0.1 mg, Cl 7.78 mg, inositol 11.6 mg, aminobenzoic acid 35 mcg, rutin 30 mg, citrus bioflavonoid complex 30 mg/4 Tab. Bot. 120s, 600s, 1200s. *otc.*
Use: Mineral, vitamin supplement.

Mastisol. (Ferndale Laboratories, Inc.) Nonirritating medical adhesive. Bot. 4 oz.
Use: Adhesive.

matrix metalloproteinase inhibitor.
Use: Corneal ulcers. [Orphan Drug]

Matulane. (Roche Laboratories) Procarbazine HCl 50 mg/Cap. Bot. 100s. *Rx.*
Use: Antineoplastic.

Mavik. (Knoll Pharmaceuticals) Trandolapril 1 mg, 2 mg, 4 mg, lactose/Tab. Bot. 100s, UD 100s. *Rx.*
Use: Antihypertensive.

Maxair Autohaler. (3M Pharmaceuticals) Pirbuterol acetate aerosol 0.2 mg/actuation. Metered dose inhaler 2.8 g (≥ 80 inhalations) and 14 g (≥ 400 inhalations). *Rx.*
Use: Sympathomimetic bronchodilator.

Maxair Inhaler. (3M Pharmaceuticals) Pirbuterol acetate aerosol 0.2 mg/actuation. Metered dose inhaler 25.6 g (≥ 300 inhalations). *Rx.*
Use: Sympathomimetic bronchodilator.

Maxalt. (Merck) Rizatriptan benzoate 5 mg, 10 mg, lactose. Tab. Bot. 500s, unit-of-use carrying case 6s. *Rx.*
Use: Antimigraine.

Maxalt-MLT. (Merck) Rizatriptan benzoate 5 mg, 10 mg. Orally disintegrating Tab. 2 unit-of-use carrying cases of 3 tabs (6 tabs total). *Rx.*
Use: Antimigraine.

Maxaquin. (Searle) Lomefloxacin HCl 400 mg/Tab. Bot. 20s, UD 100s. *Rx.*
Use: Anti-infective, fluoroquinolone.

Max EPA. (Various Mfr.) Omega-3 polyunsaturated fatty acids 1000 mg/Cap. containing EPA 180 mg, DHA 60 mg/Cap. Bot. 50s, 60s, 100s. *otc.*
Use: Nutritional supplement.

Maxidex. (Alcon Laboratories, Inc.) Dexamethasone 0.1%. Susp. Drop-Tainers 5 ml, 15 ml. *Rx.*
Use: Corticosteroid, ophthalmic.

Maxiflor Cream & Ointment. (Allergan, Inc.) Diflorasone diacetate 0.05%. Tubes 15 g, 30 g, 60 g. *Rx.*
Use: Corticosteroid, topical.

Maxilube. (Mission Pharmacal Co.) Water, silicone oil, glycerin, carbomer 934, triethanolamine, sodium lauryl sulfate, parabens. Jelly 90 g,150 g. *otc.*
Use: Vaginal agent.

Maximum Bayer Aspirin Tablets and Capsules. (Bayer Corp. (Consumer Div.)) Aspirin (Acetylsalicylic Acid; ASA) 500 mg. **Tab.:** 10s, 30s, 60s, 100s. **Capl.:** 60s. *otc.*
Use: Analgesic.

Maximum Blue Label. (Vitaline Corp.) Vitamins A 2500 IU, D 16.7 IU, E 66.7 mg, B_1 16.7 mg, B_2 8.3 mg, B_3 31.7 mg, B_5 66.7 mg, B_6 16.7 mg, B_{12} 16.7 mcg, C 200 mg, folic acid 0.13 mg, Zn 5 mg, Ca, Cr, Cu, I, K, Mg, Mn, Mo, Se, Si, V, biotin 50 mcg, SOD, l-lysine/Tab. Bot. 180s. *otc.*
Use: Mineral, vitamin supplement.

Maximum Green Label. (Vitaline Corp.) Vitamins A 2500 IU, D 16.7 IU, E 66.7 mg, B_1 16.7 mg, B_2 8.3 mg, B_3 31.7 mg, B_5 66.7 mg, B_6 16.7 mg, B_{12} 16.7 mcg, C 200 mg, folic acid 0.13 mg, Zn 5 mg, Ca, Cr, I, K, Mg, Mn, Mo, Se, Si, V, biotin 50 mcg, SOD, l-lysine/Tab. Bot. 180s. *otc.*
Use: Mineral, vitamin supplement.

Maximum Pain Relief Pamprin. (Chattem Consumer Products) Acetaminophen 250 mg, magnesium salicylate 250 mg, pamabrom 25 mg/Capl. Bot. 16s, 32s. *otc.*
Use: Analgesic combination.

Maximum Red Label. (Vitaline Corp.) Iron 3.3 mg, vitamins A 2500 IU, D 67 IU, E 66.7 mg, B_1 16.7 mg, B_2 8.3 mg, B_3 31.7 mg, B_5 66.7 mg, B_6 16.7 mg, B_{12} 16.7 mcg, C 200 mg, folic acid 0.13

mg, Zn 5 mg, Ca, Cr, Su,I, K, Mg, Mo, Se, Si, V, biotin 50 mcg, choline, inositol, bioflavonoids, l-lysine, PABA/Tab. Bot. 180s. *otc.*
Use: Mineral, vitamin supplement.

Maximum Strength Allergy Drops. (Bausch & Lomb Pharmaceuticals) Naphazoline HCl 0.03%.Soln. Bot. 15 ml. *otc.*
Use: Mydriatic, vasoconstrictor.

Maximum Strength Anbesol. (Whitehall Robins Laboratories) **Gel:** Benzocaine 20%, alcohol 60%, saccharin. Tube 7.2 g. **Liq.:** Benzocaine 20%, alcohol 60%, saccharin. Bot. 9 ml. *otc.*
Use: Anesthetic, local.

Maximum Strength Aqua-Ban. (Thompson Medical Co.) Pamabrom 50 mg, lactose/Tab. Bot. 30s. *otc.*
Use: Diuretic.

Maximum Strength Arthriten. (Alva/Amco Pharmacal Cos. Inc.) Acetaminophen 250 mg, magnesium salicylate 250 mg, caffeine anhydrous 32.5 mg, magnesium carbonate, magnesium oxide, calcium carbonate. Sugar free/Tab. Bot. 40s. *otc.*
Use: Analgesic.

Maximum Strength Benadryl. (Parke-Davis) **Cream:** Diphenhydramine HCl 2%, parabens in a greaseless base. Jar 15 g. **Spray, non-aerosol:** Diphenhydramine HCl 2%, alcohol 85%. Bot. 60 ml. *otc.*
Use: Antihistamine, topical.

Maximum Strength Benadryl Itch Relief. (Warner Lambert) Diphenhydramine HCl. **Cream:** 2%, zinc acetate 1%, parabens, aloe vera. 14.2 g. **Stick:** 2%, zinc acetate 1%. Alcohol 73.5%, aloe vera. 14 ml. *otc.*
Use: Antihistamine.

Maximum Strength Clearasil Clearstick.
See: Clearasil.

Maximum Strength Clearasil Clearstick for Sensitive Skin.
See: Clearasil.

Maximum Strength Comtrex.
See: Comtrex.

Maximum Strength Cortaid. (Pharmacia & Upjohn) Hydrocortisone 1% in parabens, mineral oil, white petrolatum. Oint. Tube 15 g, 30 g. *otc.*
Use: Corticosteroid, topical.

Maximum Strength Cortaid Faststick. (Pharmacia & Upjohn) Hydrocortisone 1%, alcohol 55%, methylparaben. Stick, roll-on. 14 g. *otc.*
Use: Corticosteroid, topical.

Maximum Strength Corticaine. (UCB Pharmaceuticals, Inc.) Hydrocortisone acetate 1%, glycerin, menthol, EDTA, parabens. Cream Tube 30 g. *otc.*
Use: Corticosteroid, topical.

Maximum Strength Dermarest Dricort Creme. (Del Pharmaceuticals, Inc.) Hydrocortisone (as acetate) 1%, white petrolatum. Cream Tube 14 g. *otc.*
Use: Corticosteroid, topical.

Maximum Strength Desenex Antifungal. (Novartis Pharmaceutical Corp.) Miconazole nitrate 2%, EDTA. Cream Tube 14 g. *otc.*
Use: Antifungal, topical.

Maximum Strength Dexatrim with Vitamin C. (Chattem Consumer Products) Phenylpropanolamine HCl, vitamin C 180 mg/Cap. Bot. 20s. *otc.*
Use: Dietary aid.

Maximum Strength Diet Aid Plus Vitamin C. (Columbia Laboratories, Inc.) Phenylpropanolamine HCl 75 mg, vitamin C 180 mg/Cap. Bot. 20s. *otc.*
Use: Dietary aid.

Maximum Strength Dristan. (Whitehall Robins Laboratories) Pseudoephedrine HCl 30 mg, acetaminophen 500 mg/Cap. Bot. 24s, 48s, 100s. *otc.*
Use: Analgesic, decongestant.

Maximum Strength Dristan Cold. (Whitehall Robins Laboratories) Pseudoephedrine HCl 30 mg, brompheniramine maleate 2 mg, acetaminophen 500 mg/Capl. Pkg. 16s, Bot. 36s. *otc.*
Use: Analgesic, antihistamine, decongestant.

Maximum Strength Dynafed Plus. (BDI Pharmaceuticals, Inc.) Acetaminophen 500 mg, pseudoephedrine 30 mg/Tab. Bot. 30s. *otc.*
Use: Analgesic, decongestant.

Maximum Strength Flexall 454. (Chattem Consumer Products) Menthol 16%, aloe vera gel, eucalyptus oil, methyl salicylate, SD alcohol 38-B, thyme oil. Gel Tube 90 g. *otc.*
Use: Liniment.

Maximum Strength Grapefruit Diet Plan w/Diadex. (Columbia Laboratories, Inc.) Phenylpropanolamine HCl 37.5 mg, grapefruit extract, sugar/Cap. Bot. 20s. *otc.*
Use: Dietary aid.

Maximum Strength Halls-Plus. (Warner Lambert) Menthol 10 mg, corn syrup, sucrose. Loz. Pkg. 10s, 20s. *otc.*
Use: Anesthetic.

Maximum Strength Kericort-10. (Bristol-Myers Squibb) Hydrocortisone 1%, parabens, cetyl alcohol, stearyl alcohol.

Cream Tube 56.7 g. *otc.*
Use: Corticosteroid, topical.

Maximum Strength Meted. (Medicis Dermatologicals, Inc.) Sulfur 5%, salicylic acid 3%. Shampoo. Bot. 118 ml. *otc.*
Use: Antiseborrheic combination.

Maximum Strength, Midol Multi-Symptom. (Bayer Corp. (Consumer Div.)) Acetaminophen 325 mg, pyrilamine maleate 12.5 mg/Tab. Bot. 30s. *otc.*
Use: Analgesic combination.

Maximum Strength Midol PMS. (Bayer Corp. (Consumer Div.)) Acetaminophen 500 mg, pamabrom 25 mg, pyrilamine maleate 15 mg/Capl. Pkg. 8s, 16s. Bot. 32s. Gelcaps. Pkg. 12s, 24s. *otc.*
Use: Analgesic combination.

Maximum Strength Nasal Decongestant. (Taro Pharmaceuticals USA, Inc.) Oxymetazoline HCl 0.05%, 0.002% phenylmercuric acetate, benzalkonium chloride. Spray Bot. 15 ml, 30 ml. *otc.*
Use: Decongestant.

Maximum Strength Neosporin. (GlaxoWellcome) Polymyxin B sulfate 10,000 units, neomycin 3.5 mg, bacitracin 500 units/g, white petrolatum. Oint. Tube 15 g. *otc.*
Use: Anti-infective, topical.

Maximum Strength No-Aspirin Sinus Medication. (Walgreen Co.) Acetaminophen 500 mg, pseudoephedrine HCl 30 mg/Tab. Bot. 50s. *otc.*
Use: Analgesic, decongestant.

Maximum Strength Nytol. (Block Drug Co., Inc.) Diphenhydramine HCl 50 mg/Tab., lactose. Pkg. 8s, 16s. *otc.*
Use: Sleep aid.

Maximum Strength Orajel Gel. (Del Pharmaceuticals, Inc.) Benzocaine 20%, saccharin. Tube 9.45 ml. *otc.*
Use: Anesthetic, local.

Maximum Strength Orajel Liquid. (Del Pharmaceuticals, Inc.) Benzocaine 20%, ethyl alcohol 44.2%, phenol, tartrazine, saccharin. Liq. Bot. 13.3 ml. *otc.*
Use: Anesthetic, local.

Maximum Strength Ornex. (Menley & James Labs, Inc.) Pseudoephedrine HCl 30 mg, acetaminophen 500 mg/Cap. Bot. 24s, 48s. *otc.*
Use: Analgesic, decongestant.

Maximum Strength Sine-Aid. (McNeil Consumer Products Co.) Pseudoephedrine HCl 30 mg, acetaminophen 500 mg/Cap., Tab., or Gelcap. **Cap. & Tab.:** Bot. 50s. **Gelcaps:** Bot. 40s. *otc.*
Use: Analgesic, decongestant.

Maximum Strength Sinutab Nighttime. (Warner Lambert Consumer Healthcare) Pseudoephedrine HCl 10 mg, diphenhydramine HCl 8.33 mg, acetaminophen 167 mg/5 ml. Liq. Alcohol free. 120 ml. *otc.*
Use: Analgesic, antihistamine, decongestant.

Maximum Strength Sinutab Without Drowsiness. (Warner Lambert) Pseudoephedrine HCl 30 mg, acetaminophen 500 mg/Tab. or Capl. Bot. 24s, 48s (tab. only). *otc.*
Use: Analgesic, decongestant.

Maximum Strength Sleepinal. (Thompson Medical Co.) **Cap.:** Diphenhydramine HCl 50 mg, lactose. Pkg. 16s. **Soft gel:** Diphenhydramine HCl 50 mg, sorbitol. Pkg. 16s. *otc.*
Use: Sleep aid.

Maximum Strength Sudafed Severe Cold Formula. (GlaxoWellcome) Dextromethorphan HBr 15 mg, pseudoephedrine HCl 30 mg, acetaminophen 500 mg/Tab. 10s. *otc.*
Use: Analgesic, antitussive, decongestant.

Maximum Strength Sudafed Sinus. (Warner Lambert) Pseudoephedrine HCl 30 mg, acetaminophen 500 mg/Tab. or Capl. Bot. 24s, 48s. *otc.*
Use: Analgesic, decongestant.

Maximum Strength Thera-Flu Non-Drowsy.
See: Thera-Flu.

Maximum Strength Tylenol Allergy Sinus. (McNeil Consumer Products Co.) Pseudoephedrine HCl 30 mg, chlorpheniramine maleate 2 mg, acetaminophen 500 mg/Tab. Bot. 24s, 60s. *otc.*
Use: Analgesic, antihistamine, decongestant.

Maximum Strength Tylenol Cough. (McNeil Consumer Products Co.) Dextromethorphan HBr 7.5 mg, acetaminophen 250 mg/5 ml, alcohol 10%. Liq. Bot. 120 ml. *otc.*
Use: Analgesic, antitussive.

Maximum Strength Tylenol Cough w/ Decongestant. (McNeil Consumer Products Co.) Pseudoephedrine HCl 15 mg, dextromethorphan HBr 7.5 mg, acetaminophen 250 mg/5 ml, alcohol 10%. Liq. Bot. 120 ml. *otc.*
Use: Analgesic, antitussive, decongestant.

Maximum Strength Tylenol Flu. (McNeil Consumer Products Co.) Acetaminophen 500 mg, pseudoephedrine HCl 30 mg, dextromethorphan HBR 15 mg. Gelcap. Pkg. 10s. *otc.*

Use: Analgesic, antitussive, decongestant.

Maximum Strength Tylenol Flu Night-Time Gelcaps. (McNeil Consumer Products Co.) Pseudoephedrine HCl 30 mg, chlorpheniramine maleate 2 mg, acetaminophen 500 mg/Gelcap. Pkg. 12s, 20s. *otc.*
Use: Analgesic, antihistamine, decongestant.

Maximum Strength Tylenol Flu Night-Time Powder. (McNeil Consumer Products Co.) Pseudoephedrine HCl 60 mg, diphenhydramine HCl 50 mg, acetaminophen 1000 mg. Powd. Pkt. 6s. *otc.*
Use: Analgesic, antihistamine, decongestant.

Maximum Strength Tylenol Select Allergy Sinus. (McNeil Consumer Products Co.) Pseudoephedrine HCl 30 mg, diphenhydramine HCl 25 mg, acetaminophen 500 mg. Cap. Bot. 24s. *otc.*
Use: Analgesic, antihistamine, decongestant.

Maximum Strength Tylenol Sinus. (McNeil Consumer Products Co.) Pseudoephedrine HCl 30 mg, acetaminophen 500 mg/Tab., Capl., or Gelcap. **Tab. and Capl.:** Bot. 24s, 50s. **Gelcap:** Bot. 24s, 60s. *otc.*
Use: Analgesic, decongestant.

Maximum Strength Unisom SleepGels. (Pfizer US Pharmaceutical Group) Diphendhydramine HCl 50 mg, sorbitol. Cap. Pkg. 8s. *otc.*
Use: Sleep aid.

Maximum Strength Wart Remover. (Stiefel Laboratories, Inc.) Salicylic acid 17%, alcohol 29%, castor oil, flexible collodion. Liq. 13.3 ml. *otc.*
Use: Keratolytic.

Maxipime. (Dura) Cefepime HCl 500 mg, 1 g, 2 g. Pow. for Inj. Vial 15 ml (500 mg, 1 g), 20 ml (2 g), *ADD-Vantage* Vial (1 g, 2 g), piggyback bottle 100 ml (1 g, 2 g). *Rx.*
Use: Antibiotic, cephalosporin.

maxiton.
See: Amphetamine (Various Mfr.).

Maxitrol Ointment. (Alcon Laboratories, Inc.) Dexamethasone 0.1%, neomycin 0.35%, polymyxin B sulfate 10,000 units/g. Tube 3.5 g. *Rx.*
Use: Anti-infective, ophthalmic.

Maxitrol Ophthalmic Suspension. (Alcon Laboratories, Inc.) Dexamethasone 0.1%, neomycin (as sulfate) 0.35%, polymyxin B sulfate 10,000 units/ml. Bot. 5 ml Drop-Tainer. *Rx.*
Use: Anti-infective, ophthalmic.

Maxivate. (Westwood Squibb Pharmaceuticals) Betamethasone dipropionate 0.05%. Cream, Oint. Tube 15 g, 45 g. *Rx.*
Use: Corticosteroid, topical.

Maxi-Vite. (Zenith Goldline Pharmaceuticals) Vitamins A 10,000 IU, D 400 IU, E 15 mg, B_1 10 mg, B_2 10 mg, B_3 100 mg, B_5 20 mg, B_6 5 mg, B_{12} 5 mcg, C 200 mg, Ca 53.5 mg, Fe 1.5 mg, folic acid 0.4 mg, biotin 1 mcg, I, P, Cu, Mg, Mn, Zn 1.5 mg, PABA, rutin, glutamic acid, inositol, choline bitartrate, bioflavonoids, l-lysine, betaine, lecithin/Tab. Bot. 60s. *otc.*
Use: Mineral, vitamin supplement.

Maxolon Tablets. (SmithKline Beecham Pharmaceuticals) Metoclopramide HCl 10 mg/Tab. Bot. 100s. *Rx.*
Use: Antiemetic, gastrointestinal stimulant.

Maxovite. (Tyson & Associates, Inc.) Vitamins A 2083 IU, D 16.7 IU, E 16.7 mg, B_1 5 mg, B_2 4.2 mg, B_3 4.2 mg, B_5 4.2 mg, B_6 54.2 mg, B_{12} 10.8 mcg, C 250 mg, folic acid 0.33 mg, Zn 5 mg, Ca, Cr, Cu, Fe, I, K, Mg, Mn, Se, biotin 11.7 mcg/Tab. Bot. 120s, 240s. *otc.*
Use: Mineral, vitamin supplement.

Maxzide. (ESI Lederle Generics) Hydrochlorothiazide 50 mg, triamterene 75 mg/Tab. Bot. 100s, 500s, UD 10 × 10s. *Rx.*
Use: Antihypertensive, diuretic.

Maxzide-25MG. (ESI Lederle Generics) Triamterene 37.5 mg, hydrochlorothiazide 25 mg/Tab. Bot. 100s, UD 100s. *Rx.*
Use: Diuretic combination.

Mayotic. (Merz Pharmaceuticals) Hydrocortisone 1%, neomycin sulfate 5 mg, polymyxin B sulfate 10,000 units/ml, thimerosal 0.01%. Susp. Bot. 10 ml w/ dropper. *Rx.*
Use: Otic.

•**maytansine.** (MAY-tan-SEEN) USAN.
Use: Antineoplastic.

May-Vita Elixir. (Merz Pharmaceuticals) Vitamins B_3 4.4 mg, B_5 1.1 mg, B_6 0.44 mg, B_{12} 1.33 mcg, FA 0.1 mg, Fe 4 mg, Mn, Zn 1.7 mg, alcohol 13%/Liq. Bot. 473 ml. *Rx.*
Use: Mineral, vitamin supplement.

Mazanor. (Wyeth-Ayerst Laboratories) Mazindol 1 mg/Tab. Bot. 30s. *c-IV.*
Use: Anorexiant.

•**mazapertine succinate.** (mazz-ah-PURR-teen) USAN.
Use: Antipsychotic.

Mazicon. (Roche Laboratories) Flumazenil 0.1 mg/ml. Inj. Vial 5 ml, 10 ml. *Rx.*

Use: Antidote.

•**mazindol.** (MAZE-in-dole) U.S.P. 23.
Use: Anorexic, appetite suppressant, Duchenne muscular dystrophy. [Orphan Drug]
See: Mazanor, Tab. (Wyeth-Ayerst Laboratories).
Sanorex, Tab. (Novartis Pharmaceutical Corp.).

M-Caps. (Mill-Mark) Methionine 200 mg/Cap. Bot. 50s, 1000s. *Rx.*
Use: Diaper rash preparation.

MCT Oil. (Bristol-Myers Squibb) Triglycerides of medium chain fatty acids. Lipid fraction of coconut oil; fatty acid shorter than C_8 < 6%, C_8 (octanoic) 67%, C_{10} (decanoic) 23%, longer than C_{10} 4%. Bot. Qt. *otc.*
Use: Nutritional supplement, enteral.

MD-Gastroview. (Mallinckrodt) Diatrizoate meglumine 660 mg, diatrizoate sodium 100 mg, iodine 367 mg/ml. Soln. Bot. 120 ml, 240 ml. *Rx.*
Use: Radiopaque agent.

MD-60. (Mallinckrodt) Diatrizoate meglumine 52%, diatrizoate sodium 8% (29.2% iodine). Inj. Vial 30 ml, 50 ml.
Use: Radiopaque agent.

MD-76R. (Mallinckrodt) Diatrizoate meglumine 660 mg, diatrizoate sodium 100 mg, iodine 370 mg/ml. Inj. Vial 50 ml. Bot. 100 ml, 150 ml, 200 ml. *Rx.*
Use: Radiopaque agent.

MDP-Squibb. (Bristol-Myers Squibb) Technetium Tc 99 medronate. Reaction vial pkg. 10s.
Use: Radiopaque agent.

meadinin. Mixture of Amoidin & Amidin alk. of Ammi Majus Linn.

measles prophylactic serum.
See: Immune Globulin (Intramuscular).

measles, mumps, and rubella virus vaccine live. (MEE-zuhls, mumps, and ru-BELL-uh vaccine)
Use: Immunization.
See: M-M-R II, Inj. (Merck & Co.).

measles and rubella virus vaccine live.
See: M-R-Vax II, Inj. (Merck & Co.).

•**measles virus vaccine, live.** (MEE-zuhls) U.S.P. 23. Modified live-virus measles vaccine.
Use: Immunization.
See: Attenuvax, Inj. (Merck & Co.).
W/Mumps virus vaccine, rubella virus vaccine.
See: M-M-R II (Merck & Co.).
W/Rubella virus vaccine.
See: M-R-Vax (Merck & Co.).

measles virus vaccine, live attenuated. Moratenline derived from Enders' attenuated Edmonston strain grown in cell cultures of chick embryos.
See: Attenuvax, Inj. (Merck & Co.).
W/Mumps virus vaccine, rubella virus vaccine.
See: M-M-R., Vial (Merck & Co.).
W/Rubella virus vaccine.
See: M-R-Vax, Inj. (Merck & Co.).

Mebaral. (Sanofi Winthrop Pharmaceuticals) Mephobarbital. Tab. **0.5 gr, 0.75 gr, or 1.5 gr:** Bot. 250s. *c-IV.*
Use: Anticonvulsant, sedative.

•**mebendazole.** (meh-BEND-uh-zole) U.S.P. 23.
Use: Anthelmintic.
See: Vermox, Tab. (Janssen Pharmaceutical, Inc.).

mebendazole. (Copley Pharmaceutical, Inc.) 100 mg/Chew. Tab. Pkg. 12s, 36s.
Use: Anthelmintic.

•**mebeverine hydrochloride.** (MEH-BEH-ver-een) USAN.
Use: Spasmolytic agent, muscle relaxant.

•**mebrofenin.** (MEH-broe-FEN-in) U.S.P. 23.
Use: Diagnostic aid (hepatobiliary function determination).

•**mebutamate.** (MEH-byoo-TAM-at) USAN.
Use: Antihypertensive.

•**mecamylamine hydrochloride.** (mek-ah-MILL-ah-meen) U.S.P. 23.
Use: Antihypertensive.

•**mecetronium ethylsulfate.** (MEH-seh-TROE-nee-uhm ETH-ill-SULL-fate) USAN.
Use: Antiseptic.

•**mechlorethamine hydrochloride.** (meh-klor-ETH-ah-meen) U.S.P. 23.
Use: Antineoplastic.
See: Mustargen, Pow. For Inj. (Merck & Co.).

mecholin hydrochloride.
See: Methacholine Cl, U.S.P. 23.

Mecholyl Ointment. (Gordon Laboratories) Methacholine Cl 0.25%, methyl salicylate 10% in ointment base. Jar 4 oz, 1 lb, 5 lb. *otc.*
Use: Analgesic, topical.

Meclan. (Advanced Care Products) Meclocycline sulfosalicylate 1%. Cream Tube 20 g, 45 g. *Rx.*
Use: Dermatologic, acne.

meclastine. Clemastine.

•**meclizine hydrochloride.** (MEK-lih-zeen) U.S.P. 23.
Use: Antinauseant, antiemetic.
See: Antivert, Chew. Tab. (Roerig).
Antrizine (Major Pharmaceuticals).

Bonine, Tab. (Roerig).
Dizmiss (Jones Medical Industries, Inc.).
Dramamine II, Tab. (Pharmacia & Upjohn).
Meclizine HCl (Various Mfr.).
Meni-D (Seatrace Pharmaceuticals, Inc.).
Vergon, Cap. (Marnel Pharmaceuticals, Inc.).

Meclizine HCl. (Various Mfr.). **Tab.: 12.5 mg:** Bot. 30s, 60s, 100s, 500s, 1000s, UD 100s. **25 mg:** In 12s, 20s, 30s, 60s, 100s, 500s, 1000s, UD 32s, 100s. **50 mg:** 100s. **Chew Tab.: 25 mg:** Bot. 20s, 30s, 60s, 100s, 1000s, UD 100s. *Rx-otc.*
Use: Antinauseant.

•**meclocycline.** (meh-kloe-SIGH-kleen) USAN.
Use: Anti-infective.

•**meclocycline sulfosalicylate.** (meh-kloe-SIGH-kleen SULL-foe-sah-LIH-sih-late) U.S.P. 23.
Use: Anti-infective.
See: Meclan, Cream (Ortho McNeil Pharmaceutical).

•**meclofenamate sodium.** (mek-loe-FEN-uh-mate) U.S.P. 23.
Use: Anti-inflammatory.

meclofenamate sodium. (Mylan Pharmaceuticals) Meclofenamate sodium 50 mg, 100 mg/Cap. Bot. 100s, 500s.
Use: Anti-inflammatory.

•**meclofenamic acid.** (MEH-kloe-fen-AM-ik Acid) USAN.
Use: Anti-inflammatory.

•**mecloqualone.** (MEH-kloe-KWAH-lone) USAN.
Use: Sedative, hypnotic.

•**meclorisone dibutyrate.** (MEH-KLAHR-ih-sone die-BYOO-tih-rate) USAN.
Use: Anti-inflammatory, topical.

•**mecobalamin.** (MEH-koe-BAHL-ah-min) USAN.
Use: Vitamin (hematopoietic).

mecodrin.
See: Amphetamine (Various Mfr.).

•**mecrylate.** (MEH-krih-late) USAN.
Use: Surgical aid (tissue adhesive).

mecysteine. Methyl Cysteine.

Meda Cap. (Circle Pharmaceuticals, Inc.) Acetaminophen 500 mg/Cap. Bot. 25s, 60s, 100s. *otc.*
Use: Analgesic.

Medacote. (Dal-Med Pharmaceuticals) Pyrilamine maleate 1%, dimethyl polysiloxane, zinc oxide, menthol, camphor in a greaseless base. Lot. Bot. 120 ml. *otc.*
Use: Antihistamine, topical.

Medadyne. (Dal-Med Pharmaceuticals) **Liq.:** Methyl benzethonium chloride, benzocaine, tannic acid, camphor, chlorothymol, menthol, benzyl alcohol, alcohol 61%. Bot. 15 ml, 30 ml. **Throat Spray:** Lidocaine, cetyl dimethyl ammonium chloride, ethyl alcohol. Bot. 30 ml. *otc.*
Use: Mouth and throat preparation.

Meda-Hist Expectorant. (Medwick) Bot. 4 oz, pt, gal.
Use: Decongestant, antitussive.

Medalox Gel. (Davol) Magnesium aluminum hydroxide gel. Bot. 12 oz, pt, gal. *otc.*
Use: Antacid.

Medamint. (Dal-Med Pharmaceuticals) Benzocaine 10 mg/Loz. Pkg. 12s, 24s. *otc.*
Use: Mouth and throat preparation.

Meda Tab. (Circle Pharmaceuticals, Inc) Acetaminophen 325 mg/Tab. Bot. 100s. *otc.*
Use: Analgesic.

Medatussin Pediatric. (Dal-Med Pharmaceuticals) Dextromethorphan HBr 5 mg, guaifenesin 50 mg, potassium citrate, citric acid, sorbitol, saccharin. Syr. Bot. 120 ml. *otc.*
Use: Antitussive, expectorant.

Medatussin Plus Cough. (Dal-Med Pharmaceuticals) Phenylpropanolamine HCl 25 mg, chlorpheniramine maleate 2 mg, phenyltoloxamine citrate 25 mg, dextromethorphan HBr 20 mg, guaifenesin 100 mg. Bot. Pt. gal. *otc.*
Use: Antihistamine, antitussive, decongestant, expectorant.

•**medazepam hydrochloride.** (med-AZE-eh-pam) USAN. Under study.
Use: Anxiolytic.

Medebar Plus. (Lafayette) Barium sulfate 100%. Susp. Bot. 1900 ml. Kit w/ enema tip-tubing assemblies 650 ml. *Rx.*
Use: Radiopaque agent.

Medent. (Stewart-Jackson Pharmacal, Inc.) Pseudoephedrine HCl 120 mg, guaifenesin 500 mg/Tab. Bot. 100s.
Use: Decongestant, expectorant.

Medescan. (Lafayette) Barium sulfate 2.3%. Susp. Bot. 250 ml, 450 ml, 1900 ml. *Rx.*
Use: Radiopaque agent.

Medicaine Cream. (Walgreen Co.) Benzocaine 3%, resorcinol 2%. Tube 1.25 oz. *otc.*
Use: Antipruritic.

Medicated Acne Cleanser. (C & M Pharmacal, Inc.) Sulfur 4%, resorcinol 2%,

SD alcohol 40 11.65%, methylparaben. Lot. Bot. 120 ml. *otc.*
Use: Dermatologic, acne.

Medicated Healer. (Walgreen Co.) Strong ammonia soln. 10%, camphor 2.6%. Bot. 6 oz. *otc.*
Use: Emollient.

Medicated Powder. (Johnson & Johnson) Zinc oxide, talc, fragrance, menthol. Plastic container 3 oz, 6 oz, 11 oz. *otc.*
Use: Antipruritic.

Medicone Derma. (Medicore) Benzocaine 2%, zinc oxide 13.73%, 8-hydroxyquinoline sulfate 1.05%, ichthammol 1%, menthol 0.48%, petrolatum-lanolin base 79.87%. Oint. Tube 42.5 g. *otc.*
Use: Anesthetic, local.

Medicone Dressing. (Medicore) Cod liver oil 125 mg, zinc oxide 125 mg, 8-hydroxyquinoline sulfate 0.5 mg, benzocaine 5 mg, menthol 1.8 mg/g w/ petrolatum, lanolin, talcum, paraffin, perfume. Tube 1 oz, 3 oz, Jar lb. *otc.*
Use: Anesthetic, local.

Medicone Ointment. (E. E. Dickinson Co.) Benzocaine 20%. Oint. 30 g. *otc.*
Use: Anorectal preparation.

Medicone Rectal. (Medicore) Benzocaine 130 mg, hydroxyquinoline sulfate 16 mg, zinc oxide 195 mg, menthol 9 mg, balsam Peru 65 mg. In a vegetable and petroleum oil base. Supp. 12s, 24s. *otc.*
Use: Anorectal preparation.

Medicone-HC Rectal. (Medicore) Hydrocortisone acetate 10 mg, benzocaine 2 gr, oxyquinoline sulfate 0.25 gr, zinc oxide 3 gr, menthol 1/7 gr, balsam Peru 1 gr, in a cocoa butter base/Supp. Box 12s. *Rx.*
Use: Anorectal preparation.

Medicone Suppositories. (E.E. Dickinson Co.) Phenylephrine HCl 0.25%, hard fat 88.7%, parabens. Pkg. 12s, 24s. *otc.*
Use: Anorectal preparation.

Medigesic. (US Pharmaceutical Corp.) Acetaminophen 325 mg, caffeine 40 mg, butalbital 50 mg/Cap. Bot. 100s. *Rx.*
Use: Analgesic, hypnotic, sedative.

Medihaler-Iso. (3M Pharmaceuticals) Isoproterenol sulfate 80 mcg/actuation. Aer. Inhaler 15 ml (≥ 300 doses) w/ adapter and 15 ml refill. *Rx.*
Use: Sympathomimetic bronchodilator.

Medi-Ject UD Vials. (Century Pharmaceuticals, Inc.) Tamper-proof rubber stoppered vial containing 1 ml sterile soln. Single-dose use. Atropine sulfate 0.4 mg/ml, 1.2 mg/ml. Scopolamine HBr 400 mcg/ml.

Medilax. (Mission Pharmacal Co.) Phenolphthalein 120 mg, aspartame, phenylalanine 1.5 mg/Chew. Tab. Bot. 24s. *otc.*
Use: Laxative.

Medipak. (Armenpharm Ltd.) First-aid kit.

Medi-Phite. (Davol) Vitamins B_1 and B_{12}. Syr. Bot. 4 oz, pt, gal. *otc.*
Use: Vitamin supplement.

Mediplast. (Beiersdorf, Inc.) Salicylic acid plaster 40%. Box 25s. *otc.*
Use: Keratolytic.

Mediplex Tabules. (US Pharmaceutical Corp.) Vitamins E 60 IU, B_1 25 mg, B_2 10 mg, B_3 100 mg, B_5 25 mg, B_6 10 mg, B_{12} 25 mcg, C 300 mg, Zn 4 mg, Cu, Mg, Mn/Tab. Bot. 100s. *otc.*
Use: Mineral, vitamin supplement.

Mediquell. (Parke-Davis) Dextromethorphan HBr 15 mg/Chewy Square. Pkg. 12s, 24s. *otc.*
Use: Antitussive.

Medi-Quik Aerosol. (Mentholatum Co., Inc.) Lidocaine 2.5%, benzalkonium Cl 0.1%, ethanol 38%. Aerosol 3 oz. *otc.*
Use: Antiseptic; anesthetic, local.

Medi-Quick Antibiotic Ointment. (Mentholatum Co., Inc.) Bacitracin neomycin, polymyxin B in ointment base. Tube 0.5 oz. *otc.*
Use: Anti-infective, topical.

Meditussin-X Liquid. (Roberts Pharmaceuticals) Codeine phosphate 50 mg, ammonium Cl 520 mg, potassium guaiacolsulfonate 520 mg, pyrilamine maleate 50 mg, phenylpropanolamine HCl 50 mg, dl-desoxyephedrine HCl 2 mg, tartar emetic 5 mg, phenyltoloxamine dihydrogen citrate 30 mg/30 ml. Bot. Pt, gal. *c-v.*
Use: Antihistamine, antitussive, expectorant.

•**medorinone.** (MEH-doe-RIH-nohn) USAN.
Use: Cardiovascular agent.

Medotar. (Medco Lab, Inc.) Coal tar 1%, polysorbate 80 0.5%, octoxynol-5, zinc oxide, starch, white petrolatum. Jar lb. *otc.*
Use: Antipsoriatic, antipruritic.

Medotopes. (Bristol-Myers Squibb) Radiopharmaceuticals.
See: A-C-D Solution Modified (Bristol-Myers Squibb).
Acid Citrate Dextrose Anticoagulant Solution Modified (Bristol-Myers Squibb).
Albumin, aggregated (Bristol-Myers Squibb).

Albumotope (Bristol-Myers Squibb).
Angiotensin Immutope Kit (Bristol-Myers Squibb).
Cobalt-Labeled Vitamin B_{12} (Bristol-Myers Squibb).
Cobalt Standards for Vitamin B_{12} (Bristol-Myers Squibb).
Cobatope (Bristol-Myers Squibb).
Digoxin (^{125}I) Immutope Kit (Bristol-Myers Squibb).
Hipputope (Bristol-Myers Squibb).
Human Serum Albumin (Bristol-Myers Squibb).
Iodinated Human Serum Albumin (Bristol-Myers Squibb).
Iodohippuric Acid (Bristol-Myers Squibb).
Macroaggregated Albumin (Bristol-Myers Squibb).
Macrotec (Bristol-Myers Squibb).
Minitec (Bristol-Myers Squibb).
Red Cell Tagging Solution (Bristol-Myers Squibb).
Rose Bengal (Bristol-Myers Squibb).
Selenomethionine (Bristol-Myers Squibb).
Sethotope (Bristol-Myers Squibb).
Technetium 99m (Bristol-Myers Squibb).
Technetium 99m-Iron-Ascorbate (DTPA) (Bristol-Myers Squibb).
Technetium 99m Sulfur Colloid Kit (Bristol-Myers Squibb).
Tesuloid (Bristol-Myers Squibb).

Medralone 40. (Keene Pharmaceuticals, Inc.) Methylprednisolone acetate 40 mg/ml. Vial 5 ml. *Rx.*
Use: Corticosteroid.

Medralone 80. (Keene Pharmaceuticals, Inc.) Methylprednisolone acetate 80 mg/ml. Vial 5 ml. *Rx.*
Use: Corticosteroid.

•**medrogestone.** (MEH-droe-JEST-ohn) USAN.
Use: Hormone, progestin.

Medrol. (Pharmacia & Upjohn) Methylprednisolone. **Tab.:** 2 mg. Bot. 100s; 4 mg Bot. 30s, 100s, 500s, UD 100s; 8 mg Bot. 25s; 16 mg Bot. 50s; 24 mg Bot. 25s; 32 mg Bot. 25s. **Dosepak:** 4 mg Pkg. 21s. **Alternate Daypak:** 16 mg Pkg. 14s. *Rx.*
Use: Corticosteroid.

•**medronate disodium.** (MEH-droe-nate die-SO-dee-uhm) USAN. *Formerly Disodium Methylene Diphosphonate; MDP.*
Use: Pharmaceutic aid.

•**medronic acid.** (meh-DRAH-nik acid) USAN.
Use: Pharmaceutic aid.

Medrosphol Hg-197. Merprane.

•**medroxalol.** (meh-DROX-ah-LAHL) USAN.
Use: Antihypertensive.

•**medroxalol hydrochloride.** (meh-DROX-ah-LAHL) USAN.
Use: Antihypertensive.

medroxyprogesterone acetate. (meh-DROX-ee-pro-JESS-tuh-rone) (ESI Lederle Generics) Medroxyprogesterone acetate 10 mg/Tab. Bot. 50s, 250s. *Rx.*
Use: Hormone, progestin.

•**medroxyprogesterone acetate.** (meh-DROX-ee-pro-JESS-tuh-rone) U.S.P. 23.
Use: Hormone, progestin.
See: Amen, Tab. (Carnrick Laboratories, Inc.).
Curretab, Tab. (Solvay Pharmaceuticals).
Cycrin, Tab. (ESI Lederle Generics).
Depo-Provera, Vial (Pharmacia & Upjohn).
Provera, Tab. (Pharmacia & Upjohn).

medroxyprogesterone acetate. (meh-DROX-ee-pro-JESS-tuh-rone) (CMC) 50 mg, 100 mg/ml. Vial 5 ml.
Use: Hormone, progestin.

medroxyprogesterone acetate. (Various Mfr.) Medroxyprogesterone acetate 2.5 mg, 5 mg, 10 mg/Tab. Bot. 30s, 40s (10 mg only), 50s, 90s (2.5 mg only), 100s, 250s, 500s, 1000s (2.5 and 5 mg only). *Rx.*
Use: Hormone, progestin.

MED-Rx. (Iomed) Pseudoephedrine HCl 60 mg, guaifenesin 600 mg/CR Tab. Box 28s. Guaifenesin 600 mg/CR Tab. Box 28s. *Rx.*
Use: Decongestant, expectorant.

MED-Rx DM. (Iomed) Pseudoephedrine 60 mg, guaifenesin 600 mg/CR Tab. Bot. 28s. Dextromethorphan hydrobromide 30 mg, guaifenesin 600 mg/CR Tab. Bot. 28s. *Rx.*
Use: Antitussive, expectorant.

•**medrysone.** (MEH-drih-sone) USAN. U.S.P. XXII.
Use: Corticosteroid, topical.
See: HMS, Ophth. Soln. (Allergan, Inc.).

•**mefenamic acid.** (MEH-fen-AM-ik) U.S.P. 23.
Use: Anti-inflammatory, analgesic.
See: Ponstel, Kapseal (Parke-Davis).

•**mefenidil.** (meh-FEN-ih-dill) USAN.
Use: Cerebral vasodilator.

•**mefenidil fumarate.** (meh-FEN-ih-dill) USAN.

Use: Cerebral vasodilator.

•**mefenorex hydrochloride.** (meh-FEN-oh-rex) USAN. Under study.
Use: Anorexic.

•**mefexamide.** (meh-FEX-am-IDE) USAN.
Use: Stimulant (central).

•**mefloquine.** (MEH-flow-kwin) USAN.
Use: Antimalarial.

•**mefloquine hydrochloride.** (MEH-flow-kwin) USAN.
Use: Antimalarial. [Orphan Drug]
See: Lariam (Roche Laboratories).

Mefoxin. (Merck & Co.) Sterile cefoxitin sodium. **Pow. for Inj.:** 1 g, 2 g, 10 g. Vial and Infusion Bot. (1 g, 2 g), Bulk Bot. (10 g). **Inj.:** 1 g, 2 g, dextrose. Premixed, frozen in 50 ml plastic containers. *Rx.*
Use: Anti-infective, cephalosporin.

Mefoxin in 5% Dextrose. (Merck & Co.) Cefoxitin sodium 1 g, 2 g in Dextrose in Water 5%. Inj. Containers 50 ml. *Rx.*
Use: Anti-infective, cephalosporin.

•**mefruside.** (MEFF-ruh-side) USAN.
Use: Diuretic.

Mega B. (Arco Pharmaceuticals, Inc.) Vitamins B_1 100 mg, B_2 100 mg, B_3 100 mg, B_5 100 mg, B_6 100 mg, B_{12} 100 mcg, folic acid 100 mcg, d-biotin 100 mcg, PABA 100 mg/Tab. Bot. 100s. *otc.*
Use: Vitamin supplement.

Megace. (Bristol-Myers Squibb) Megestrol acetate 20 mg, 40 mg/Tab. **20 mg/Tab.:** Bot. 100s. **40 mg/Tab.:** Bot. 100s, 250s, 500s. Megestrol acetate 40 mg/ml, alcohol $\leq$ 0.06%, sucrose. Susp. Bot. 236.6 ml. *Rx.*
Use: Antineoplastic; hormone, progestin.

•**megalomicin potassium phosphate.** (meh-GAL-OH-my-sin) USAN.
Use: Anti-infective.

Megaton. (Hyrex Pharmaceuticals) Vitamins B_3 4.4 mg, B_5 1.1 mg, B_6 0.44 mg, B_{12} 1.33 mcg, FA 0.1 mg, Fe 4 mg, Mn, Zn 1.7 mg, alcohol 13%/Liq. Bot. 473 ml. *Rx.*
Use: Mineral, vitamin supplement.

Mega VM-80. (NBTY, Inc.) Vitamins A 10,000 IU, D 1000 IU, E 100 mg, B_1 80 mg, B_2 80 mg, B_3 80 mg, B_5 80 mg, B_6 80 mg, B_{12} 80 mcg, C 250 mg, Fe 1.2 mg, folic acid 0.4 mg, Ca 4.5 mg, Zn 3.58 mg, choline, inositol, biotin 80 mcg, PABA, bioflavonoids, betaine, hesperidin, Cu, I, K, Mg, Mn. Tab. Bot. 60s, 100s. *otc.*
Use: Mineral, vitamin supplement.

•**megestrol acetate.** (meh-JESS-trole) U.S.P. 23.
Use: Antineoplastic; palliative treatment of advanced carcinoma of the breast or endometrium. AIDS-related weight loss. [Orphan Drug]
See: Megace, Susp. (Bristol-Myers Squibb).

•**meglumine.** (meh-GLUE-meen) U.S.P. 23.
Use: Diagnostic aid (radiopaque medium).

meglumine, diatrizoate inj.
Use: Diagnostic aid (radiopaque medium).
See: Cardiografin, Vial (Bristol-Myers Squibb).
Cystografin, Vial (Bristol-Myers Squibb).
Gastrografin, Soln. (Bristol-Myers Squibb).
Hypaque-76, Inj. (Sanofi Winthrop Pharmaceuticals).
Hypaque-M 75%, Inj. (Sanofi Winthrop Pharmaceuticals).
Hypaque-M 90%, Inj. (Sanofi Winthrop Pharmaceuticals).
Hypaque Meglumine, Vial (Sanofi Winthrop Pharmaceuticals).
Reno-M-30, -60, Vial (Bristol-Myers Squibb).
Reno-M-Dip, Vial (Bristol-Myers Squibb).
W/Meglumine iodipamide.
See: Sinografin, Soln. (Bristol-Myers Squibb).
W/Sodium diatrizoate.
See: Gastrografin, Soln. (Bristol-Myers Squibb).
Renografin-60, Inj. (Bristol-Myers Squibb).
Renografin-76, Inj. (Bristol-Myers Squibb).
Renovist II, Inj. (Bristol-Myers Squibb).

meglumine, iodipamide inj.
Use: Diagnostic aid; radiopaque medium.
See: Cholografin, Vial (Bristol-Myers Squibb).
W/Meglumine diatrizoate.
See: Sinografin, Soln. (Bristol-Myers Squibb).

meglumine, iothalamate inj.
Use: Diagnostic aid, radiopaque medium.

•**meglutol.** (MEH-glue-tahl) USAN.
Use: Antihyperlipoproteinemic.

•**melafocon a.** (MEH-lah-FOE-kahn A) USAN.
Use: Contact lens material (hydrophobic).

Melanex. (Neutrogena) Hydroquinone 3% in solution containing alcohol 47.3%. Bot. 1 oz w/Appliderm applicator and pinpoint rod applicator. *Rx.*
Use: Dermatologic.

melanoma vaccine.
Use: Stage III to IV melanoma. [Orphan Drug]

melanoma cell vaccine.
Use: Invasive melanoma. [Orphan Drug]

melarsoprol. (Mel B)
Use: Anti-infective.
See: Arsobal.

melatonin.
Use: Treatment of circadian rhythm sleep disorders in blind patients. [Orphan Drug]

Mel B.
See: Melarsoprol.

•**melengestrol acetate.** (meh-len-JESS-trole ASS-eh-tate) USAN.
Use: Antineoplastic; hormone, progestin.

Melhoral Child Tablet. (Sanofi Winthrop Pharmaceuticals) Acetylsalicylic acid. *otc.*
Use: Analgesic.

melitoxin.
See: Dicumarol (Various Mfr.).

•**melitracen hydrochloride.** (meh-lih-TRAY-sen) USAN.
Use: Antidepressant.

•**melizame.** (MEH-lih-zame) USAN.
Use: Sweetener.

Mellaril Concentrate. (Novartis Pharmaceutical Corp.) Thioridazine HCl 30 mg/ml, alcohol 3%. Soln. Bot. 118 ml. Concentrate 100 mg/ml, alcohol 4.2%. Pk. 4 oz. *Rx.*
Use: Antipsychotic.

Mellaril-S. (Novartis Pharmaceutical Corp.) Thioridazine 25 mg/5 ml, 100 mg/5 ml. Susp. Bot. Pt. *Rx.*
Use: Antipsychotic.

Mellaril Tablets. (Novartis Pharmaceutical Corp.) Thioridazine HCl 10 mg, 15 mg, 25 mg, 50 mg, 100 mg, 150 mg, 200 mg/Tab. Bot. 100s, 1000s, UD 100s (except 150 mg). *Rx.*
Use: Antipsychotic.

mellose. Methylcellulose.

Melonex. Metahexamide.
Use: Oral antidiabetic.

•**meloxicam.** (mell-OX-ih-kam) USAN.
Use: Anti-inflammatory.

Melpaque HP. (Stratus Pharmaceuticals, Inc.) Hydroquinone 4% in a sunblocking base of talc, EDTA, sodium metabisulfite. Cream. Tinted. Tube 14.2 g, 28.4 g. *Rx.*
Use: Dermatologic.

•**melphalan.** (MELL-fuh-lan) U.S.P. 23.
Use: Antineoplastic. [Orphan Drug]
See: Alkeran (GlaxoWellcome).

Melquin HP. (Stratus Pharmaceuticals, Inc.) Hydroquinone 4%, mineral oil, propylparaben, sodium metabisulfite. Vanishing base. Cream. Tube 14.2 g, 28.4 g. *Rx.*
Use: Dermatologic.

•**memotine hydrochloride.** (MEH-moe-teen) USAN.
Use: Antiviral.

•**menabitan hydrochloride.** (meh-NAB-ih-tan) USAN.
Use: Analgesic.

•**menadiol sodium diphosphate.** (men-ah-DIE-ole SO-dee-uhmdie-FOSS-fate) U.S.P. 23.
Use: Vitamin (prothrombogenic).

•**menadione.** (men-ah-DIE-ohn) U.S.P. 23.
Use: Oral & IM, Vitamin K therapy, vitamin (prothrombogenic).
W/Ascorbic acid, hesperidin.
See: Hescor-K, Tab. (Madland).

menadione diphosphate sodium.
See: Menadiol sodium diphosphate.

Menadol. (Rugby Labs, Inc.) Ibuprofen 200 mg/Tab. Bot. 50s, 100s. *otc.*
Use: Analgesic, NSAID.

menaphthene or menaphthone.
See: Menadione (Various Mfr.).

menaquinone.
See: Menadione (Various Mfr.).

Menest. (SmithKline Beecham Pharmaceuticals) Esterified estrogens. 0.3 mg, 0.625 mg, 1.25 mg, 2.5 mg. Tab. Bot. 50s. (2.5 mg only), 100s (except 2.5 mg). *Rx.*
Use: Estrogen combination.

Meni-D. (Seatrace Pharmaceuticals, Inc.) Meclizine 25 mg/Cap. Bot. 100s. *Rx.*
Use: Antiemetic, antivertigo.

meningococcal polysaccharide vaccine group A, C, Y, W-135. (Pasteur Merieux Connaught) Serogroup A, C, Y, and W-135 capsular polysaccharides 50 mcg/0.5 ml. Pow. for Inj.
Use: Immunization.
See: Menomune A/C/Y/W-135 (Pasteur Merieux Connaught).

•**meningococcal polysaccharide vaccine group A.** U.S.P. 23.
Use: Immunization.

•**meningococcal polysaccharide vaccine group C.** U.S.P. 23.
Use: Immunization.

•**menoctone.** (meh-NOCK-tone) USAN. Under study.
Use: Antimalarial.

•**menogaril.** (MEN-oh-gar-ILL) USAN.
Use: Antineoplastic.

Menogen. (Breckenridge Pharmaceuticals, Inc.) Esterified estrogen 1.25 mg, methyltestosterone 2.5 mg. Tab. Bot. 100s. *Rx.*
Use: Hormone.

Menogen H.S. (Breckenridge Pharmaceuticals, Inc.) Esterified estrogen 0.625 mg, methyltestosterone 1.25 mg. Tab. Bot. 100s. *Rx.*
Use: Hormone.

Menoject L.A. (Merz Pharmaceuticals) Testosterone cypionate, estradiol cypionate. Vial 10 ml. *Rx.*
Use: Androgen, estrogen combination.

Menolyn. (Arcum) Ethinyl estradiol 0.05 mg/Tab. Bot. 100s, 1000s. *Rx.*
Use: Estrogen.

Menomune-A/C/Y/W-135. (Pasteur Merieux Connaught) Serogroup A, C, Y, and W-135 capsular polysaccharides 50 mcg/0.5 ml. Pow. for Inj.
Use: Immunization.

Menoplex Tablets. (Fiske Industries) Acetaminophen 325 mg, phenyltoloxamine citrate 30 mg/ Tab. Bot. 20s. *otc.*
Use: Analgesic.

•**menotropins.** (MEN-oh-trope-inz) U.S.P. 23. *Formerly Human Follicle-Stimulating Hormone.*
Use: Hormone, gonadotropin; gonad-stimulating principle.
See: Humegon, Inj. (Organon Teknika Corp.).
Pergonal, Inj. (Serono Laboratories, Inc.).

Mentax. (Schering-Plough Corp.; Penederm, Inc.) Butenafine HCl 1%, benzyl and cetyl alcohol/Cream. Tube. 2 g, 15 g, 30 g. *Rx.*
Use: Antifungal.

Mentane. (Hoechst Marion Roussel) Velnacrine.
Use: Cholinesterase inhibitor for Alzheimer's disease.

•**menthol.** (MEN-thole) U.S.P. 23.
Use: Topical antipruritic, local analgesic, nasal decongestant, antitussive.
See: Blue Gel Muscular Pain Reliever (Rugby Labs, Inc.).
Robitussin Liquid Center Cough Drops, Loz. (Wyeth-Ayerst Laboratories).
Vicks Cough Silencers, Loz. (Procter & Gamble Pharm.).
Vicks Formula 44 Cough Control Discs, Loz. (Procter & Gamble Pharm.).
Vicks Inhaler (Procter & Gamble Pharm.).
Vicks Blue Mint, Lemon, Regular and Wild Cherry Medicated Cough Drops (Procter & Gamble Pharm.).
Vicks Medi-Trating Throat Loz. (Procter & Gamble Pharm.).
Vicks Oracin Regular and Cherry, Loz. (Procter & Gamble Pharm.).
Vicks Sinex, Nasal Spray (Procter & Gamble Pharm.).
Vicks Vaporub, Oint. (Procter & Gamble Pharm.).
Vicks Vaposteam, Liq. (Procter & Gamble Pharm.).
Vicks Va-Tro-Nol, Nose Drops (Procter & Gamble Pharm.).
Victors Regular and Cherry, Loz. (Procter & Gamble Pharm.).
W/Combinations.
See: Eucalyptamint, Gel (Novartis Pharmaceutical Corp.).
Eucalyptamint Maximum Strength, Oint. (Novartis Pharmaceutical Corp).
Hall's Mentho-Lyptus Sugar Free, Prods. (Warner Lambert).
Listerine Antiseptic, Liq. (Warner Lambert).

Mentholatum. (Mentholatum Co., Inc.) Menthol 1.35%, camphor 9%, titanium dioxide and fragrance in ointment base of petrolatum. Tube 0.4 oz, 1 oz. Jar 1 oz, 3 oz. *otc.*
Use: Analgesic, topical.

Mentholatum Deep Heating Lotion. (Mentholatum Co., Inc.) Menthol 6%, methyl salicylate 20%, lanolin derivative in lotion base. Bot. 2 oz, 4 oz. *otc.*
Use: Analgesic, topical.

Mentholatum Deep Heating Rub. (Mentholatum Co., Inc.) Menthol 5.8%, methyl salicylate 12.7%, eucalyptus oil, turpentine oil, anhydrous lanolin, vehicle and fragrance. Tube 1.25 oz, 3.33 oz, 5 oz. *otc.*
Use: Analgesic, topical.

Mentholin. (Apco) Methyl salicylate 30%, chloroform 20%, hard soap 3%, camphor gum 2.2%, menthol 0.8%, alcohol 35%. Bot. 2 oz. *otc.*
Use: Analgesic, topical.

menthyl valerate. Validol.
Use: Sedative.

•**meobentine sulfate.** (meh-OH-BEN-teen SULL-fate) USAN.
Use: Cardiovascular agent (antiarrhythmic).

mepacrine hydrochloride.

Use: Anthelmintic, antimalarial.
•**mepartricin.** (meh-PAR-trih-sin) USAN.
Use: Antifungal, antiprotozoal.
mepavlon. Meprobamate, U.S.P. 23.
•**mepenzolate bromide.** (meh-PEN-zoe-late BROE-mide) U.S.P. 23.
Use: Anticholinergic.
See: Cantil, Tab., Liq. (Hoechst Marion Roussel).
W/Phenobarbital.
See: Cantil w/phenobarbital (Hoechst Marion Roussel).
mepenzolate methyl bromide. Mepenzolate bromide.
Use: Anticholinergic.
Mepergan. (Wyeth-Ayerst Laboratories) Promethazine HCl 25 mg, meperidine HCl 25 mg/ml. Inj. Vial 10 ml, Tubex 2 ml. Box 10s. *c-II.*
Use: Analgesic combination, narcotic.
Mepergan Fortis. (Wyeth-Ayerst Laboratories) Meperidine HCl 50 mg, promethazine HCl 25 mg/Cap. Bot. 100s. *c-II.*
Use: Analgesic combination, narcotic.
meperidine hydrochloride. (meh-PEHR-ih-deen) U.S.P. 23.
Use: Analgesic, narcotic.
See: Demerol HCl, Prods. (Sanofi Winthrop Pharmaceuticals).
W/Acetaminophen.
See: Demerol APAP, Tab. (Sanofi Winthrop Pharmaceuticals).
W/Promethazine HCl.
See: Mepergan, Preps. (Wyeth-Ayerst Laboratories).
meperidine hydrochloride. (meh-PEHR-ih-deen) (Roxane) 50 mg/5 ml. Syr. Bot. 500 ml, UD 5 ml. *c-II.*
Use: Analgesic, narcotic.
meperidine hydrochloride. (meh-PEHR-ih-deen) (Various Mfr.) **Tab.:** 50 mg, 100 mg. Bot. 100s, UD 25s. **Inj.:** 10 mg/ml (single-dose vial 30 ml); 25 mg/ml (Amp., Syr. Vial 1 ml; 1 ml fill in 2 ml); 50 mg/ml (Vial 30 ml; Amp., Syr., Vial 1 ml; 1 ml fill in 2 ml); 75 mg/ml (Amp., Syr., Vial 1 ml; 1 ml fill in 2 ml); 100 mg/ml (Vial 20 ml; Amp., Syr., Vial 1 ml, 1 ml fill in 2 ml). *c-II.*
meperidine hydrochloride and atropine sulfate.
Use: Anesthetic, general.
See: Atropine and Demerol, Inj. (Sanofi Winthrop Pharmaceuticals).
mephenesin.
Use: Muscle relaxant.
See: Myanesin.
W/Acetaminophen, Vitamin C, butabarbital.
See: T-Caps, Cap. (Burlington).
W/Pentobarbital.
See: Nebralin, Tab. (Novartis Pharmaceutical Corp.).
W/Salicylamide, butabarbital sodium.
See: Metrogesic, Tab. (Lexis Laboratories).
mephenesin carbamate. Methoxydone.
•**mephentermine sulfate.** (meh-FEN-ter-meen) U.S.P. 23.
Use: Vasoconstrictor; decongestant, nasal. Also IV or IM; adrenergic (vasoconstrictor).
See: Wyamine Sulfate Inj. (Wyeth-Ayerst Laboratories).
•**mephenytoin.** (meh-FEN-ee-TOE-in) U.S.P. 23.
Use: Anticonvulsant.
See: Mesantoin, Tab. (Novartis Pharmaceutical Corp.).
•**mephobarbital.** (meh-foe-BAR-bih-tahl) U.S.P. 23.
Use: Anticonvulsant, hypnotic, sedative.
See: Mebaral, Tab. (Sanofi Winthrop Pharmaceuticals).
mephone. Mephentermine.
Mephyton. (Merck & Co.) Phytonadione (vitamin K_1) 5 mg/Tab. Bot. 100s. *Rx.*
Use: Anticoagulant.
Mepiben. (Schein Pharmaceutical, Inc.) Methylpiperidyl benzhydryl ether.
Use: Antihistamine.
mepiperphenidol bromide.
Use: Anticholinergic.
•**mepivacaine hydrochloride.** (meh-PIHV-ah-cane) U.S.P. 23.
Use: Anesthetic, local.
See: Carbocaine, Inj. (Sanofi Winthrop Pharmaceuticals).
Carbocaine Dental, Inj. (Cook-Waite Laboratories, Inc.).
Carbocaine with Neo-Cobefrin, Inj. (Cook-Waite Laboratories, Inc.).
Isocaine HCl, Inj. (Novocol Chemical Mfr. Co.).
Polocaine, Inj. (Astra Pharmaceuticals, L.P.).
Polocaine MPF, Inj. (Astra Pharmaceuticals, L.P.).
mepivacaine hydrochloride. (Zenith Goldline Pharmaceuticals) Mepivacaine HCl 1%, 2%, methylparaben. Inj. Vial 50 ml. *Rx.*
Use: Anesthetic, local.
mepivacaine hydrochloride and levonordefrin inj.
Use: Anesthetic, local.
See: Carbocaine, Cartridge, Vial (Cook-Waite Laboratories, Inc.).
•**meprednisone.** (meh-PRED-nih-sone)

U.S.P. 23.
Use: Corticosteroid, topical.

•**meprobamate.** (meh-pro-BAM-ate) U.S.P. 23.
Use: Anxiolytic, hypnotic, sedative.
See: Arcoban, Tab. (Arcum).
Bamate, Tab. (Century Pharmaceuticals, Inc.).
Equanil Tab., Cap. (Wyeth-Ayerst Laboratories).
Miltown, Tab. (Wallace Laboratories).
Tranmep, Tab. (Solvay Pharmaceuticals).
W/Acetylsalicylic acid.
See: Equagesic, Tab. (Wyeth-Ayerst Laboratories).
W/Benactyzine HCl.
See: Milprem, Tab. (Wallace Laboratories).
W/Pentaerythritol tetranitrate.
See: Miltrate, Tab. (Wallace Laboratories).
W/Premarin.
See: PMB 200, Tab. (Wyeth-Ayerst Laboratories).

meprobamate/aspirin. (Various Mfr.) Aspirin 325 mg, meprobamate 200 mg/Tab. Bot. 100s, 500s. *Rx.*
Use: Analgesic combination.

meprobamate/benactyzine.
Use: Miscellaneous psychotherapeutic agent.

meprobamate, n-isopropyl.
See: Carisoprodol.

Meprogesic Q. (Various Mfr.) Aspirin 325 mg, meprobamate 200 mg/Tab. Bot. 100s, 500s. *Rx.*
Use: Analgesic combination.

Meprolone Tabs. (Major Pharmaceuticals) Methylprednisolone 4 mg/Tab. Bot. 25s, 100s. *Rx.*
Use: Corticosteroid.

Mepron. (GlaxoWellcome) Atovaquone 750 mg/5 ml. Susp. Bot. 210 ml. *Rx.*
Use: Anti-infective.

meprylcaine hydrochloride. U.S.P. XXII.
Use: Anesthetic, local.

•**meptazinol hydrochloride.** (mep-TAZE-ih-nahl) USAN.
Use: Analgesic.

mepyrapone.
See: Metopirone, Tab., Amp. (Novartis Pharmaceutical Corp.).

•**mequidox.** (MEH-kwih-dox) USAN. Under study.
Use: Anti-infective.

mequinolate. (meh-KWIN-ole-ate) Name used for Proquinolate.

•**meralein sodium.** (MER-ah-leen) USAN.
Use: Anti-infective, topical.
See: Sodium Meralein.

merbromin. *otc.*
Use: Antiseptic, topical.

•**mercaptopurine.** (mer-cap-toe-PURE-een) U.S.P. 23.
Use: Antineoplastic.
See: Purinethol, Tab. (GlaxoWellcome).

mercazole.
See: Methimazole, U.S.P. 23.

mercufenol chloride. (MER-cue-FEEN-ole) USAN.
Use: Anti-infective, topical.

mercuranine.
See: Merbromin.

mercurial, antisyphilitics. Mercuric Oleate, Mercuric Salicylate.

mercuric oleate. Oleate of mercury.
Use: Parasitic and fungal skin diseases.

mercuric oxide ophthalmic ointment, yellow.
Use: Local anti-infective, ophthalmic.

mercuric salicylate. Mercury subsalicylate.
Use: Parasitic and fungal skin diseases.

mercuric succinimide. Bis-Succinimidato-mercury.

mercurocal.
See: Merbromin Soln. (Premo)

Mercurochrome. (Various Mfr.) Merbromin 2%. Soln. Bot. 15 ml, 30 ml. *otc.*
Use: Antiseptic, topical.

mercurome.
See: Merbromin Soln.

•**mercury, ammoniated.** U.S.P. 23.
Use: Anti-infective, topical.

mercury compounds.
See: Antiseptics, Mercurials.

mercury-197-203.
See: Chlormerodrin (Bristol-Myers Squibb).

mercury oleate. $Mercury^{++}$ oleate. Pharmaceutic aid.

Merdex. (Faraday) Docusate sodium 100 mg/Tab. Vial 60 ml. *Rx-otc.*
Use: Laxative.

Meridia. (Knoll Pharmaceuticals) Sibutramine 5 mg, 10 mg, 15 mg, lactose. Cap. 100s. *c-iv.*
Use: Anorexiant.

•**merisoprol acetate Hg 197.** (mer-EYE-so-prole) USAN.
Use: Radiopharmaceutical.

•**merisoprol acetate Hg 203.** (mer-EYE-so-prole) USAN.
Use: Radiopharmaceutical.

Meritene Powder. (Novartis Pharmaceutical Corp.) Vanilla flavor: Specially processed nonfat dry milk, corn syrup solids, sucrose, fructose, calcium caseinate, sodium Cl, natural and artificial

flavors, lecithin, vitamins and minerals. Can 1 lb, 4.5 lb, 25 lb. Packet 1.14 oz. Vanilla, chocolate, eggnog, milk chocolate, plain flavors. *otc.*
Use: Nutritional supplement.

merodicein. Sodium meralein.

•**meropenem.** (meh-row-PEN-em) USAN.
Use: Anti-infective.
See: Merrem IV. (Zeneca Pharmaceuticals).

meroxapol 105.
Use: Irrigating solution.
See: Saf-Clens, Spray (Calgon Vestal Laboratories).

merprane.
Use: Diagnostic aid.

Merrem IV. (Zeneca Pharmaceuticals) Meropenem 500 mg, 1 g. Pow. for Inj. Vial 20 ml (500 mg only), 30 ml (1 g only), 100 ml, *ADD-Vantage* Vial 15 ml. *Rx.*
Use: Anti-infective.

mersol. (Century Pharmaceuticals, Inc.) Thimerosal tincture, N.F. 1/1000. 1 oz, 4 oz, pt, gal. *otc.*
Use: Antiseptic.

Merthiolate. (Eli Lilly and Co.) Thimerosal. **Soln.:** 1:1000: 4 fl. oz, 16 fl oz, gal. **Tincture:** 1:1000: alcohol 50%, 0.75 oz, 4 fl oz, 16 fl oz, gal. *otc.*
Use: Antiseptic.

Meruvax II. (Merck & Co.) Lyophilized, live attenuated rubella virus of the Wistar Institute RA 27/3 strain. Each dose contains approximately 25 mcg of neomycin. Single-dose Vial w/diluent. Pkg. 1s, 10s.
Use: Immunization.
W/Attenuvax.
See: M-R-Vax II, Vial (Merck & Co.).
W/Attenuvax, Mumpsvax.
See: M-M-R II, Vial (Merck & Co.).
W/Mumpsvax.
See: Biavax II, Vial (Merck & Co.).

Mervan. (Continental Pharma, Belgium) Alclofenac.
Use: Anti-inflammatory.

•**mesalamine.** (me-SAL-uh-MEEN) USAN.
Use: Anti-inflammatory.
See: Asacol, DR Tab. (Procter & Gamble Pharm.).
Pentasa, CR Cap. (Hoechst Marion Roussel).
Rowasa, Enema, Supp. (Solvay Pharmaceuticals).

mesantoin. (Novartis Pharmaceutical Corp.) 100 mg/Tab. Bot. 100s. *Rx.*
Use: Anticonvulsant.

Mescolor. (Horizon Pharmaceutical Corp.) Chlorpheniramine maleate 8 mg, pseudoephedrine HCl 120 mg, methscopolamine nitrate 2.5 mg, dye free/ Tab. Bot. 100s.
Use: Anticholinergic, antihistamine, decongestant.

mescomine.
See: Methscopolamine bromide (Various Mfr.).

•**meseclazone.** (meh-SAK-lah-zone) USAN.
Use: Anti-inflammatory.

•**mesifilcon a.** (MEH-sih-FILL-kahn A) USAN.
Use: Contact lens material, hydrophilic.

•**mesna.** (MESS-nah) USAN.
Use: Hemorrhagic cystitis prophylactic; detoxifying agent. [Orphan Drug]
See: Mesnex, Inj. (Bristol-Myers Oncology/Immunology).

Mesnex. (Bristol-Myers Oncology/Immunology) Mesna 100 mg/ml, 0.25 mg/ml EDTA, benzyl alcohol 10.4 mg (10 ml)/ Inj. Vial 2 ml, 10 ml. *Rx.*
Use: Antidote.

•**mesoridazine.** (MESS-oh-RID-ah-zeen) USAN.
Use: Antipsychotic, anxiolytic.

•**mesoridazine besylate.** (MESS-oh-RID-ah-zeen BESS-ih-late) U.S.P. 23.
Use: Antipsychotic.
See: Serentil, Amp., Liq., Tab. (Boehringer Ingelheim, Inc.).

•**mespiperone c 11.** (meh-SPIH-peh-rone c 11) USAN.
Use: Radiopharmaceutical.

•**mesterolone.** (MESS-TER-oh-lone) USAN.
Use: Androgen.

mestibol. Monomestrol.

Mestinon. (Zeneca Pharmaceuticals) Pyridostigmine bromide 60 mg/Tab. Bot. 100s, 500s. Timespan 180 mg/Tab. Bot. 100s, 500s. *Rx.*
Use: Muscle stimulant.

Mestinon Injectable. (Zeneca Pharmaceuticals) Pyridostigmine bromide 5 mg/ml, w/methyl- and propylparabens 0.2%, sodium citrate 0.02%, pH adjusted to approximately 5 w/citric acid, sodium hydroxide. Amp. 2 ml. Box 10s. *Rx.*
Use: Muscle stimulant.

Mestinon Syrup. (Zeneca Pharmaceuticals) Pyridostigmine bromide 60 mg/5 ml, alcohol 5%. Bot. Pt. *Rx.*
Use: Muscle stimulant.

Mestinon Timespan. (Zeneca Pharmaceuticals) Pyridostigmine bromide 180 mg/Tab. Bot. 100s. *Rx.*
Use: Muscle stimulant.

•**mestranol.** (MESS-trah-nole) U.S.P. 23.
Use: Contraceptive, estrogen.
W/Ethynodiol Diacetate.
See: Ovulen, Tab. (Searle).
Ovulen-21, Tab. (Searle).
Ovulen-28, Tab. (Searle).
W/Norethindrone.
See: Norinyl, Tab. (Roche Laboratories).
Norinyl-1 Fe 28 (Roche Laboratories).
Ortho-Novum, Tab. (Ortho McNeil Pharmaceutical).
W/Norethindrone, ferrous fumarate.
See: Ortho Novum Fe-28, Fe-28, 1 mg Fe-28, Tab. (Ortho McNeil Pharmaceutical).
W/Norethynodrel.
See: Enovid, Tab. (Searle).
Enovid-E, Tab. (Searle).
Enovid-E 21, Tab. (Searle).

•**mesuprine hydrochloride.** (MEH-suh-PREEN) USAN.
Use: Vasodilator, muscle relaxant.

Metabolin. (Thurston) Vitamins A 833 IU, D 66 IU, B_1 833 mcg, B_2 500 mcg, B_6 0.083 mcg, calcium pantothenate 833 mcg, niacinamide 5 mg, folic acid 0.066 mcg, p-aminobenzoic acid 0.416 mcg, inositol 833 mcg, B_{12} 500 mcg, C 5 mg, Ca 33.1 mg, P 14.6 mg, Fe 2.5 mg, I 0.15 mg/Tab. Bot. 100s, 500s, 1000s. *otc.*
Use: Mineral, vitamin supplement.

•**metabromsalan.** (MET-ah-BROME-sah-lan) USAN.
Use: Antimicrobial, disinfectant.

metabutethamine hydrochloride.
Use: Anesthetic, local.

metabutoxycaine hydrochloride.
Use: Anesthetic, local.

metacaraphen hydrochloride. Netrin.

metacordralone.
See: Prednisolone (Various Mfr.).

metacortandracin.
See: Prednisone, Tab. (Various Mfr.).

metacortin.
See: Meticorten, Tab. (Schering-Plough Corp.).

•**metacresol.** (met-ah-KREE-sole) U.S.P. 23.
Use: Antiseptic, topical; antifungal.

meta-delphene. Diethyltoluamide U.S.P. 23.

metaglycodol.
Use: Central nervous system depressant.

Metahydrin. (Hoechst Marion Roussel) Trichlormethiazide 2 mg, 4 mg/Tab. Bot. 100s. *Rx.*
Use: Diuretic.

•**metalol hydrochloride.** (MEH-ta-lahl) USAN. Under study.
Use: Antiadrenergic β-receptor.

Metalone T.B.A. (Foy Laboratories) Prednisolone tertiary butylacetate 20 mg, sodium citrate 1 mg, polysorbate 80 1 mg, d-sorbitol 450 mg/ml, benzyl alcohol 0.9%, water for inj. Vial 10 ml. *Rx.*
Use: Corticosteroid.

Metamucil. (Procter & Gamble Pharm.) Psyllium hydrophilic mucilloid, sodium 1 mg, potassium 31 mg/Dose. **Regular Flavor:** w/ dextrose. Jar 7 oz, 14 oz, 21 oz. Packette 5.4 g. Box 100s. **Orange and Strawberry Flavors:** w/flavoring, sucrose and coloring. Jar 7 oz, 14 oz, 21 oz. *otc.*
Use: Laxative.

Metamucil Instant Mix. (Procter & Gamble Pharm.) Psyllium hydrophilic mucilloid with citric acid, sucrose, potassium bicarbonate, sodium bicarbonate. Powder when combined with water forms an effervescent, flavored liquid. **Lemon Lime Flavor:** w/calcium carbonate. Cartons of 16, 30, or 100 packets of 3.4 g. **Orange Flavor:** w/flavoring and coloring. Ctn. 16 or 30 packets of 3.4 g. *otc.*
Use: Laxative.

Metamucil, Sugar Free. (Procter & Gamble Pharm.) Psyllium hydrophilic mucilloidin sugar-free formula. **Regular Flavor:** Jar 3.7 oz, 7.4 oz, 11.1 oz. Packet 3.4 g. Box 100s. **Orange Flavor:** Jar 3.7 oz, 7.4 oz, 11.1 oz. *otc.*
Use: Laxative.

Metandren. (Novartis Pharmaceutical Corp.) Methyltestosterone. **Linguet:** 5 mg, 10 mg Bot. 100s. **Tab.:** 10 mg, 25 mg Bot. 100s. *Rx.*
Use: Androgen.

metaphenylbarbituric acid.
See: Mephobarbital.

metaphyllin.
See: Aminophylline (Various Mfr.).

Metaprel Syrup. (Novartis Pharmaceutical Corp.) Metaproterenol sulfate 10 mg/5 ml. Bot. Pt. *Rx.*
Use: Bronchodilator.

•**metaproterenol polistirex.** (MEH-tuh-pro-TEHR-uh-nahl pahl-ee-STIE-rex) USAN.
Use: Bronchodilator.

•**metaproterenol sulfate.** (MEH-tuh-pro-TEHR-uh-nahl) U.S.P. 23.
Use: Bronchodilator.
See: Alupent (Boehringer Ingelheim).

metaproterenol sulfate. (Various Mfr.) **Tab.:** 10 mg, 20 mg. Bot. 100s, 1000s. **Soln. for Inh.:** 0.4%, 0.6%. Vial 2.5

ml. 5%. Vial 10 ml, 30 ml. *Rx.*
Use: Bronchodilator.

•**metaraminol bitartrate.** (met-uh-RAM-in-ole by-TAR-trate) U.S.P. 23.
Use: Adrenergic.
See: Aramine, Amp., Vial (Merck & Co.).

Metastron. (Medi-Physics, Inc., Amersham Healthcare) Strontium-89 Cl 10.9 to 22.6 mg/ml. Preservative free. Inj. Vial 10 ml.
Use: Radiopharmaceutical.

Metatensin #2 & #4. (Hoechst Marion Roussel) Trichlormethiazide 2 mg, 4 mg, each containing reserpine 0.1 mg/Tab. Bot. 100s. *Rx.*
Use: Antihypertensive.

•**metaxalone.** (meh-TAX-ah-lone) USAN.
Use: Muscle relaxant.
See: Skelaxin (Carnrick Laboratories, Inc.).

Meted, Maximum Strength. (Medicis Dermatologicals, Inc.) Sulfur 5%, salicylic acid 3%. Shampoo. Bot. 118 ml. *otc.*
Use: Antiseborrheic combination.

•**meteneprost.** (meh-TEN-eh-PRAHST) USAN.
Use: Oxytocic, prostaglandin.

•**metesind glucuronate.** (MEH-teh-sind glue-CURE-oh-nate) USAN.
Use: Antineoplastic (specific thymidylate synthase inhibitor).

metethoheptazine.
Use: Analgesic.

•**metformin.** (MET-fore-min) USAN.
Use: Oral hypoglycemic, antidiabetic.
See: Glucophage, Tab. (Bristol-Myers Squibb).

•**metformin hydrochloride.** (MET-fore-min) USAN.
Use: Antidiabetic.

methacholine bromide. Mecholin bromide.
Use: Cholinergic.

•**methacholine chloride.** U.S.P. 23.
Use: Cholinergic.
See: Mecholyl Cl, Amp. (Mallinckrodt Baker, Inc.).
Provocholine, Amp. (Roche Laboratories).

methacholine chloride.
Use: Diagnostic aid.
See: Provocholine, Pow. for reconstitution (Roche Laboratories).

•**methacrylic acid copolymer.** (meth-ah-KRILL-ik ASS-id koe-PAHL-ih-mer) N.F. 18.
Use: Pharmaceutic aid (tablet coating agent).

•**methacycline.** (meth-ah-SIGH-kleen) USAN.
Use: Anti-infective.

methacycline hydrochloride. (meth-ah-SIGH-kleen) U.S.P. 23.
Use: Antibacterial.

•**methadone hydrochloride.** (METH-uh-dohn) U.S.P. 23.
Use: Analgesic, narcotic; narcotic abstinence syndrome suppressant.
See: Dolophine HCl (Eli Lilly and Co.).
Methadose (Mallinckrodt).

methadone hydrochloride. (Roxane) **Tab.:** 5 mg, 10 mg. Bot. 100s, UD 100s. **Oral Soln.:** 5 mg/5 ml, 10 mg/5 ml, alcohol 8%, sorbitol. Bot. 500 ml. *c-II.*
Use: Analgesic, narcotic.

methadone hydrochloride. (UDL) 10 mg/ml. Oral Conc. Bot. 1 qt. *c-II.*
Use: Analgesic, narcotic.

methadone hydrochloride diskets. (METH-uh-dohn) (Eli Lilly and Co.) Methadone HCl 40 mg/Dispersible Tab. Bot. 100s. *c-II.*
Use: Analgesic, narcotic.

methadone hydrochloride intensol. (METH-uh-dohn) (Roxane) Methadone HCl 10 mg/ml. Oral Conc. Bot. 30 mg. *c-II.*
Use: Analgesic, narcotic.

Methadose. (Mallinckrodt) Methadone. **Tab.:** 5 mg, 10 mg. Bot. 100s. **Disp. Tab.:** 40 mg. Bot. 100s. **Oral Conc.:** 10 mg/ml, Bot. 1 qt. **Pow.:** 50 g, 100 g, 500 g, 1 kg. *c-II.*
Use: Analgesic, narcotic.

•**methadyl acetate.** (METH-ah-dill ASS-eh-tate) USAN.
Use: Analgesic, narcotic.

•**methafilcon b.** (METH-ah-FILL-kahn B) USAN.
Use: Contact lens material (hydrophilic).

Methagual. (Gordon Laboratories) Guaiacol 2%, methyl salicylate 8% in petrolatum. Oint. 2 oz, lb. *otc.*
Use: Analgesic, topical.

methalamic acid. Name used for Iothalamic acid.

methalgen. (Alra Laboratories, Inc.) Camphor, menthol, mustard oil, methyl salicylate in non-greasy cream base. Bot. 2 oz, Jar 4 oz, lb.
Use: Analgesic, topical.

•**methalthiazide.** (METH-al-THIGH-ah-zide) USAN.
Use: Antihypertensive, diuretic.

methaminodiazepoxide.
See: Librium, Cap., Amp. (Roche Laboratories).

methamoctol.

Use: Adrenergic.
•**methamphetamine hydrochloride.** (meth-am-FET-uh-meen) U.S.P. 23.
Use: CNS stimulant.
See: Desoxyn, Gradumets, Tab. (Abbott Laboratories).
Methamphetamine HCl, Tab. (Various Mfr.).
W/Pamabrom, pyrilamine maleate, homatropine methylbromide, hyoscyamine-sulfate, scopolamine HBr.
See: Aridol, Tab. (MPL).
methamphetamine-dl hydrochloride.
See: dl-Methamphetamine HCl.
methampyrone.
See: Dipyrone.
methandriol. (Various Mfr.) Methylandrostenediol.
See: Anabol, Inj. (Keene Pharmaceuticals, Inc.).
methandriol dipropionate.
See: Arbolic, Inj. (Burgin-Arden).
methantheline bromide. U.S.P. XXII. Sterile, Tab.
Use: Parasympatholytic, anticholinergic.
See: Banthine, Vial, Tab. (Roberts Pharmaceuticals).
W/Phenobarbital.
See: Banthine w/Phenobarbital, Tab. (Roberts Pharmaceuticals).
Methaphor. (Borden) Protein hydrolysate (l-leucine, l-isoleucine, l-methionine, l-phenylalanine, l-tyrosine); methionine, camphor, benzethonium Cl, in Dermabase vehicle/Oint. Tube 1.5 oz. *otc.*
Use: Dermatologic, amino acid supplement.
•**methaqualone.** (METH-ah-kwan-lone) USAN.
Use: Hypnotic, sedative.
Methatropic Capsules. (Zenith Goldline Pharmaceuticals) Choline 115 mg, inositol 83 mg, methionine 110 mg, vitamins B_1 3 mg, B_2 3 mg, B_3 10 mg, B_5 2 mg, B_6 2 mg, B_{12} 2 mcg, desiccated liver 86 mg/Cap. Bot. 100s. *otc.*
Use: Vitamin supplement.
•**methazolamide.** (meth-ah-ZOLE-ah-mide) U.S.P. 23.
Use: Carbonic anhydrase inhibitor.
See: GlaucTabs, Tab. (Akorn, Inc.).
Neptazane, Tab. (ESI Lederle Generics).
methazolamide. (Various Mfr.) Methazolamide 25mg or 50 mg/Tab. Bot. 100s. *Rx.*
Use: Carbonic anhydrase inhibitor.
Methblue 65. (Manne) Methylene blue 65 mg/Tab. Bot. 100s, 1000s. *Rx.*
Use: Antidote, cyanide.
Meth-Choline. (Schein Pharmaceutical, Inc.) Choline 115 mg, inositol 83 mg, methionine 110 mg, vitamins B_1 3 mg, B_2 3 mg, B_3 10 mg, B_5 2 mg, B_6 2 mg, B_{12} 2 mcg, desiccated liver 56 mg, liver concentrate 30 mg/Cap. Bot. 100s, 250s, 1000s. *otc.*
Use: Vitamin supplement.
Meth-Dia-Mer Sulfa. Trisulfapyrimidines. Tab.
Use: Triple sulfonamide therapy.
See: Chemozine, Tab. (Tennessee Pharmaceutic).
Triple Sulfa, Tab. (Various Mfr.).
Meth-Dia-Mer Sulfonamides.
Use: Triple sulfonamide therapy.
W/Sulfacetamide.
See: Sulfa-Plex, Vaginal Cream (Solvay Pharmaceuticals).
Meth-Dia-Mer Sulfonamides Suspension. Trisulfapyrimidines Oral Suspension.
Use: Triple sulfonamide therapy.
See: Chemozine, Susp. (Tennessee Pharmaceutic).
Triple Sulfa, Susp. (CMC).
•**methdilazine.** U.S.P. 23.
Use: Antipruritic.
•**methenamine.** (meh-THEN-uh-meen) U.S.P. 23. *Formerly Hexamethylenamine.*
Use: Anti-infective, urinary.
methenamine w/combinations. (meh-THEN-uh-meen)
Use: Anti-infective, urinary.
See: Cystamine, Tab. (Tennessee Pharmaceutic).
Cystex, Tab. (Numark Laboratories, Inc.).
Cysto, Tab. (Freeport).
Prosed/DS, Tab. (Star Pharmaceuticals, Inc.).
Urimar-T, Tab. (Marnel Pharmaceuticals, Inc.).
Urisan-P, Tab. (Sandia).
Urised, Tab. (PolyMedica Pharmaceuticals).
Urogesic Blue, Tab. (Edwards Pharmaceuticals, Inc.).
Uro Phosphate, Tab. (ECR Pharmaceuticals).
U-Tran, Tab. (Scruggs).
methenamine and monobasic sodium phosphate tablets.
Use: Anti-infective, urinary.
methenamine anhydromethylene citrate. Formanol, Uropurgol, Urotropin.
•**methenamine hippurate.** (meth-EE-nah-meen HIP-you-rate) U.S.P. 23.

Use: Anti-infective, urinary.
See: Hiprex, Tab. (Hoechst Marion Roussel).
Urex, Tab. (3M Pharmaceuticals).

•**methenamine mandelate.** (meth-EE-nah-meen MAN-deh-late) U.S.P. 23.
Use: Anti-infective, urinary.

methenamine mandelate. (Various Mfr.) **Tab.:** 0.5 g, 1 g/Tab. 100s, 1000s. **Susp.:** 0.5 g/5 ml. Susp. Bot. 480 ml.
Use: Anti-infective, urinary.

methenamine mandelate w/combinations.
Use: Anti-infective, urinary.
See: Urisedamine, Tab. (PolyMedica Pharmaceuticals).

•**methenolone acetate.** (meth-EEN-oh-lone) USAN.
Use: Anabolic.

•**methenolone enanthate.** (meth-EEN-oh-lone eh-NAN-thate) USAN.
Use: Anabolic.

Metheponex. (Rawl) Choline 0.54 g, dl-methionine 1.80 g, inositol 0.27 g, whole desiccated liver 8.10 g, vitamins B_1 18 mg, B_2 36 mg, niacinamide 90 mg, B_6 3.6 mg, calcium pantothenate 3.6 mg, biotin 10.8 mcg, B_{12} 5.4 mcg and amino acid/daily therapeutic dose. Cap. Bot. 100s, 500s. *Rx.*
Use: Antidiabetic, nutritional supplement.

metheptazine.
Use: Analgesic.

Methergine. (Novartis Pharmaceutical Corp.) Methylergonovine maleate. **Amp.:** 0.2 mg/ml, tartaric acid 0.25 mg/ml, sodium Cl 3 mg/ml. **Tab.:** 0.2 mg. Bot. 100s, 1000s, SandoPak pkgs. 100s. *Rx.*
Use: Oxytocic.

methestrol.
See: Promethestrol (Various Mfr.).

methetharimide bemegride. USAN.
Use: Anticonvulsant.

•**methetoin.** (METH-eh-toe-in) USAN.
Use: Anticonvulsant.

Methibon. (Barrows) Choline dihydrogen citrate 278 mg, dl-methionine 111 mg, inositol 83.3 mg, vitamin B_{12} 2 mcg, liver concentrate, desiccated liver 86.6 mg/Cap. Bot. 100s. *Rx.*
Use: Antidiabetic, nutritional supplement.

methicillin sodium. (meth-ih-SILL-in) U.S.P. 23.
Use: Anti-infective.

•**methimazole.** (meth-IMM-uh-zole) U.S.P. 23.
Use: Thyroid inhibitor.
See: Tapazole, Tab. (Eli Lilly and Co.).

methiodal sodium. U.S.P. XXI. Sodium monoiodomethanesulfonate. Abrodil, Radiographol, Diagnorenol.
Use: Radiopaque medium.

Methiokaps. (Pal-Pak, Inc.) dl-methionine 200 mg/Cap. Bot. 1000s. *Rx.*
Use: Diaper rash product.

methiomeprazine hydrochloride. (SmithKline Beecham Pharmaceuticals)
Use: Antiemetic.

•**methionine C 11 injection.** (meh-THIGH-oh-NEEN) U.S.P. 23.
Use: Radiopharmaceutical.

•**methionine.** (meh-THIGH-oh-NEEN) U.S.P. 23.
Note: Also see Racemethionine, U.S.P. 23.
Use: Amino acid.

methionyl human stem cell factor (recombinant).
Use: Combination w/filgrastim to decrease the number of phereses required to collect blood progenitor cells following myelosuppressive/myeloblative therapy. [Orphan Drug]

methionyl neurotrophic (brain-derived, recombinant) factor.
Use: Amyotrophic lateral sclerosis agent. [Orphan Drug]

Methioplex. (Lincoln Diagnostics) Methionine 25 mg, vitamins B_1 50 mg, niacinamide 100 mg, B_2 2 mg, choline 50 mg, B_6 2 mg, panthenol 2 mg, benzyl alcohol 1%, distilled water q.s./ml. Vial 30 ml. *Rx.*
Use: Nutritional supplement.

•**methisazone.** (METH-eye-SAH-zone) USAN.
Use: Antiviral.

methitural sodium.
Use: Hypnotic, sedative.

•**methixene hydrochloride.** (meh-THIX-een) USAN.
Use: Muscle relaxant.

•**methocarbamol.** (meth-oh-CAR-buh-mahl) U.S.P. 23.
Use: Muscle relaxant.
See: Delaxin, Tab. (Ferndale Laboratories, Inc.).
Robaxin, Prods. (Wyeth-Ayerst Laboratories).
W/Aspirin.
See: Robaxisal, Tab. (Wyeth-Ayerst Laboratories).

methocarbamol. (Various Mfr.) **Tab.:** 500 mg, 750 mg. Bot. 60s (750 mg only), 100s, 500s, UD 100s. **Inj.:** 100 mg/ml Vial 10 ml.

Use: Muscle relaxant.

Methocarbamol/ASA. (Various Mfr.) Methocarbamol 400 mg, aspirin 325 mg/Tab. Bot. 15s, 30s, 40s, 100s, 500s, 1000.
Use: Muscle relaxant.

methocel. Methylcellulose.

•**methohexital.** (meth-oh-HEX-ih-tahl) U.S.P. 23.
Use: Pharmaceutic necessity for Methohexital Sodium for Injection.

•**methohexital sodium for injection.** U.S.P. 23.
Use: Anesthetic, general; anesthetic (intravenous).
See: Brevital, Amp., Pow. (Eli Lilly and Co.).

•**methopholine.** (METH-oh-foe-leen) USAN.
Use: Analgesic.
See: Versidyne.

Methopto 0.25%. (Professional Pharmacal) Methylcellulose pow. 2.5 mg (0.25% soln.), boric acid 12 mg, potassium Cl 7.3 mg, benzalkonium Cl 0.04 mg, glycerin 12 mg/ml w/sodium carbonate to adjust pH and purified water. Bot. 15 ml, 30 ml. *otc.*
Use: Artificial tears.

Methopto Forte 0.5%. (Professional Pharmacal) Methylcellulose pow. 5 mg (0.5% soln.), boric acid 12 mg, potassium Cl 7.3 mg, benzalkonium Cl 0.4 mg, glycerin 12 mg/ml w/sodium carbonate to adjust pH and purified water. Bot. 15 ml. *otc.*
Use: Artificial tears.

Methopto Forte 1%. (Professional Pharmacal) Methylcellulose pow. 10 mg (1% soln.), boric acid 12 mg, potassium Cl 7.3 mg, benzalkonium Cl 0.04 mg, glycerin 12 mg/ml w/sodium carbonate to adjust pH and purified water. Bot. 15 ml. *otc.*
Use: Artificial tears.

methopyraphone.
See: Metopirone, Tab., Amp. (Novartis Pharmaceutical Corp.).

methorate.
See: Dextromethorphan HBr.

Methorbate S.C. (Standex) Methenamine 40.8 mg, atropine sulfate 0.03 mg, hyoscyamine sulfate 0.03 mg, salol 18.1 mg, benzoic acid 4.5 mg, methylene blue 5.4 mg/Tab. Bot. 100s. *Rx.*
Use: Anti-infective, urinary.

d-methorphan hydrobromide.
See: Dextromethorphan HBr (Various Mfr.).

methorphinan. Racemorphan HBr. Dromoran.

•**methotrexate.** (meth-oh-TREK-sate) U.S.P. 23. *Formerly Amethopterin.*
Use: Leukemia in children, antineoplastic, antipsoriatic, juvenile rheumatoid arthritis. [Orphan Drug]

methotrexate. (Various Mfr.) Tab. 2.5 mg. Bot. 36s, 100s, UD 20s.
Use: Antineoplastic.

methotrexate. (Immunex Corp.) **Inj.:** 25 mg/ml as sodium, benzyl alcohol 0.9%, sodium Cl 0.26% and water for inj. Vials 2 ml, 10 ml. **Pow. for Inj.:** 20 mg or 1 g/vial as sodium. Single-use Vials. *Rx.*
Use: Antipsoriatic.

methotrexate sodium for injection. (ESI Lederle Generics) 2.5 mg/ml Vial 2 ml; 25 mg/ml. Vial 2 ml w/preservatives; 20 mg, 50 mg, 100 mg Vial cryodesiccated, preservative free; 50 mg, 100 mg, 200 mg Vial; 25 mg/ml solution preservative free.
Use: Leukemia therapy, psoriasis, osteogenic sarcoma. [Orphan Drug]
See: Folex, Inj. (Pharmacia & Upjohn).
Folex PFS. Inj. (Pharmacia & Upjohn).
Methotrexate, Inj., Pow. (ESI Lederle Generics)
Mexate, Inj. (Bristol-Myers Squibb)

methotrexate USP with laurocapram.
Use: Topical treatment of *Mycosis fungoides.* [Orphan Drug]

•**methotrimeprazine.** (METH-oh-trih-MEP-rah-zeen) U.S.P. 23.
Use: Analgesic, anxiolytic.
See: Levoprome, Amp., Vial (Immunex Corp.).

methoxamine hydrochloride. U.S.P. 23.
Use: Vasoconstrictor.
See: Vasoxyl (GlaxoWellcome).

•**methoxsalen.** (meth-OX-ah-len) U.S.P. 23.
Use: Pigmenting agent.
See: Oxsoralen, Cap., Lot. (Baxter Pharmaceutical Products, Inc.).
Oxsoralen Ultra, Cap. (Baxter Pharmaceutical Products, Inc.).
Uvadex, Soln. (Therakos).

8-methoxsalen.
Use: Treatment of diffuse systemic sclerosis, rejection of cardiac allografts. [Orphan Drug]
See: Uvadex.

methoxsalen topical solution.
Use: Pigmenting agent, topical.

methoxydone.
See: Mephenoxalone (Various Mfr.).

•**methoxyflurane.** (meth-OCK-sih-FLEW-rane) U.S.P. 23.

Use: Anesthetic, general.
See: Penthrane, Liq. (Abbott Laboratories).
methoxyphenamine hydrochloride. U.S.P. 23.
Use: Adrenergic (bronchodilator).
W/Chlorpheniramine maleate, acetophenetidin, acetylsalicylic acid, caffeine.
See: Pyrroxate, Cap., Tab. (Pharmacia & Upjohn).
W/Dextromethorphan HCl, orthoxine, sodium citrate.
See: Orthoxicol, Syr. (Pharmacia & Upjohn).
W/Dextromethorphan HBr, phenylephrine HCl, chlorpheniramine maleate.
See: Statuss, Syr., Cap. (Baxter Pharmaceutical Products, Inc.).
W/Medrol.
See: Medrol, Tab. (Pharmacia & Upjohn).
methoxypromazine maleate.
Use: CNS depressant.
methoxypsoralen, oral.
Use: Psoralen.
See: Oxsoralen (Baxter Pharmaceutical Products, Inc.).
Oxsoralen Ultra (Baxter Pharmaceutical Products, Inc.).
methscopolamine bromide. U.S.P. XXII. Tab.
Use: Anticholinergic.
See: Pamine, Tab., Vial (Pharmacia & Upjohn).
Scoline, Tab. (Westerfield).
W/Amobarbital.
See: Scoline-Amobarbital, Tab. (Westerfield).
W/Butabarbital sodium, dried aluminum hydroxide gel and magnesium trisilicate.
See: Eulcin, Tab. (Leeds Pharmacal).
W/Phenobarbital.
See: Pamine PB, Preps. (Pharmacia & Upjohn).
W/Phenylpropanolamine HCl, chlorpheniramine maleate.
See: Bobid, Cap. (Boyd).
methscopolamine nitrate. Scopolamine Methyl Nitrate, Preps. (Various Mfr.) Mescomine.
See: Dallergy, Cap., Tab., Syr. (Laser, Inc.).
Extendryl, Cap., Tab., Syr. (Fleming & Co.).
Sanhist T.D. 12, Tab. (Sandia).
Scotnord, Tab. (Scott/Cord).
W/Combinations.
See: D.A. II (Dura).
Ex-Histine (WE Pharm).
Mescolor (Horizon).

•**methsuximide.** (meth-SUCK-sih-mide) U.S.P. 23.
Use: Anticonvulsant.
See: Celontin Kapseal (Parke-Davis).
Methyclodine. (Rugby Labs, Inc.) Methyclothiazide 5 mg, deserpidine 0.25 mg/Tab. Bot. 100s. *Rx.*
Use: Antihypertensive, diuretic.
•**methyclothiazide.** (METH-ee-kloe-THIGH-ah-zide) U.S.P. 23.
Use: Antihypertensive, diuretic.
See: Enduron, Tab. (Abbott Laboratories).
Methyclodine, Tab. (Rugby Labs, Inc.).
W/Deserpidine.
See: Enduronyl, Tab. (Abbott Laboratories).
Enduronyl Forte, Tab. (Abbott Laboratories).
methylacetylcholine.
See: Methacholine.
•**methyl alcohol.** (METH-ill) N.F. 18.
Use: Pharmaceutic acid (solvent).
methylamphetamine hydrochloride & sulfate.
See: Desoxyephedrine HCl (Various Mfr.).
methylandrostenediol. Methandriol.
See: Hybolin, Vial (Hyrex Pharmaceuticals).
W/Adrenal cortex extract, Vitamin B_{12}.
See: Geri-Ace, Inj. (Baxter Pharmaceutical Products, Inc.).
W/Carboxymethylcellulose sodium, thimerosal.
See: Cenabolic, Vial (Century Pharmaceuticals, Inc.).
•**methylatropine nitrate.** (METH-ill-AT-row-peen) USAN.
Use: Anticholinergic.
•**methylbenzethonium chloride.** (meth-ill-benz-eth-OH-nee-uhm) U.S.P. 23.
Use: Bactericide, local anti-infective (topical).
See: Ammorid, Oint. (Kinney).
Benephen, Prods. (Halsted).
Cuticura Acne, Cream (Purex).
Cuticura Medicated First Aid, Cream (Purex).
Diaparene, Prods. (Bayer Corp. (Consumer Div.)).
Fordustin, Pow. (Sween).
Surgi-Kleen, Liq. (Sween).
W/Cod liver oil.
See: Benephen, Prods. (Halsted).
Sween, Cream (Sween).
W/Magnesium stearate.
See: Mennen Baby, Pow. (Mennen).
W/Phenol, acetanilid, zinc oxide, cala-

mine and eucalyptol.
See: Taloin, Oint. (Warren-Teed).
W/Phenylmercuric acetate, methylparaben.
See: Taloin, Tube (Warren-Teed).

methylbenztropine.
See: Ethybenztropine (Novartis Pharmaceutical Corp.).

methylbromtropin mandelate. Homatropine Methylbromide, U.S.P. 23.

•**methylcellulose.** (METH-ill-SELL-you-lohs) U.S.P. 23.
Use: Pharmaceutic aid (suspending agent).
See: Cellothyl, Tab. (International Drug).
Cologel, Soln. (Eli Lilly and Co.).
Isopto-Plain, Liq. (Alcon Laboratories, Inc.).
Melozets, Wafer (SmithKline Beecham Pharmaceuticals).
W/Boric acid, glycerin, propylene glycol, methylparaben, propylparaben, irish moss extract.
See: Canfield Lubricating Jelly (Paddock Laboratories).
W/Carboxymethylcellulose.
See: Ex-Caloric, Wafer (Eastern Research).
W/Dicyclomine HCl, magnesium trisilicate, aluminum hydroxide-magnesium carbonate, dried.
See: Triactin, Tab. (Procter & Gamble Pharm.).
W/Dicyclomine HCl, aluminum hydroxide, and magnesium hydroxide.
See: Triactin, Liq. (Procter & Gamble Pharm.).
W/Phenylephrine HCl, benzalkonium Cl.
See: Efricel (Professional Pharmacal).
W/Polysorbate 80, boric acid.
See: Lacril Artificial Tears (Allergan, Inc.).

methyl cysteine hydrochloride. Cysteine methyl ester hydrochloride.
Use: Mucolytic agent.

•**methyldopa.** (meth-ill-DOE-puh) U.S.P. 23. *Formerly Alpha-Methyldopa.*
Use: Antihypertensive.
See: Aldomet, Tab. (Merck & Co.).

methyldopa and chlorothiazide tablets.
Use: Antihypertensive.
See: Aldoclor, Tab. (Merck & Co.).

methyldopa/hydrochlorothiazide tablets.
Use: Antihypertensive.
See: Aldoril, Tab. (Merck & Co.).

methyldopa/hydrochlorothiazide. (Various Mfr.) Methyldopa 250 mg, hydrochlorothiazide 15 mg, 25 mg/Tab. Bot. 100s, 500s, 1000s, UD 100s. *Rx.*
Use: Antihypertensive combination.

methyldopa/hydrochlorothiazide. (Various Mfr.) Methyldopa 500 mg, hydrochlorothiazide 30 mg, 50 mg/Tab. Bot. 100s, 250s, 500s. *Rx.*
Use: Antihypertensive combination.

•**methyldopate hydrochloride.** (meth-ill-DOE-pate) U.S.P. 23.
Use: Antihypertensive.
See: Aldomet Ester HCl, Inj. (Merck & Co.).

methyldopate hydrochloride. (Fujisawa USA, Inc.) Methyldopate HCl 250 mg/5 ml. Inj. Vial. 6 ml. *Rx.*
Use: Antihypertensive.

•**methylene blue.** (METH-ih-leen blue) U.S.P. 23.
Use: Antidote, cyanide.
See: Methblue 65, Tab. (Manne).
Urolene Blue, Tab. (Star Pharmaceuticals, Inc.).

methylene blue. (Various Mfr.) 10 mg/ml. Inj. Vial 1 ml, 10 ml. *Rx.*
Use: GU antiseptic; antidote, cyanide.

methylene blue w/combinations.
See: Urised, Tab. (PolyMedica Pharmaceuticals).

•**methylene chloride.** N.F. 18.
Use: Pharmaceutic aid (solvent).

•**methylergonovine maleate.** (METH-ill-err-go-NO-veen MAL-ee-ate) U.S.P. 23.
Use: Oxytocic.
See: Methergine, Amp., Tab. (Novartis Pharmaceutical Corp.).

methylethylamino-phenylpropanol hydrochloride.
See: Nethamine HCl. (Various Mfr.).

methylglucamine diatrizoate, Inj. A water-soluble radiopaque iodine cpd. N-methylglucamine salt of Diatrizoate.
See: Diatrizoate Inj. (Various Mfr.).
Diatrizoate Meglumine Inj., U.S.P. 23.

methylglucamine iodipamide, inj.
See: Meglumine Iodipamide, Inj., U.S.P. 23. (Various Mfr.).
W/Diatrizoate methylglucamine.
See: Sinografin, Vial (Bristol-Myers Squibb).

methylglyoxal-bis-guanylhydrazone. Methyl GAG.

•**methyl isobutyl ketone.** (METH-ill eye-so-BYOO-till KEE-tone) N.F. 18.
Use: Pharmaceutic aid (alcohol denaturant).

methyliso-octenylamine.
See: Isometheptene HCl (Various Mfr.).

methylmercadone. Name used for Nifuratel.

•**methyl nicotinate.** USAN.
W/Histamine dihydrochloride, oleoresin capsicum, glycomonosalicylate.
See: Akes-N-Pain Rub, Oint. (H.L. Moore Drug Exchange Inc.).
W/Methyl salicylate, menthol.
See: Musterole Deep Strength Oint. (Schering-Plough Corp.).

Methylone. (Paddock Laboratories) Methylprednisolone acetate 40 mg/ml. Vial 5 ml. *Rx.*
Use: Corticosteroid.

•**methyl palmoxirate.** (METH-ill pal-MOX-ihr-ate) USAN.
Use: Antidiabetic.

•**methylparaben.** (meth-ill-PAR-ah-ben) N.F. 18.
Use: Pharmaceutic aid (antifungal agent).

•**methylparaben sodium.** (meth-ill-PAR-ah-ben) N.F. 18.
Use: Pharmaceutic aid (antimicrobial preservative).

methylphenethylamine.
See: Amphetamine HCl (Various Mfr.).

•**methylphenidate hydrochloride.** (meth-ill-FEN-ih-date) U.S.P. 23.
Use: CNS stimulant.
See: Ritalin HCl, Tab., Vial (Novartis Pharmaceutical Corp.).

methylphenidate hydrochloride. (Various Mfr.) **Tab.:** 5 mg, 10 mg, 20 mg. Bot. 100s, 1000s. **SR Tab.:** 20 mg. Bot. 100s.
Use: CNS stimulant.

methylphenidylacetate hydrochloride.
See: Methylphenidate HCl (Various Mfr.).

methylphenobarbital.
See: Mephobarbital.

d-methylphenylamine sulfate.
See: Dextroamphetamine Sulfate, (Various Mfr.).

methyl phenylethylhydantoin.
See: Mesantoin, Tab. (Novartis Pharmaceutical Corp.).

methylphenylsuccinimide.
See: Milontin, Kapseal, Susp. (Parke-Davis).

methylphytyl naphthoquinone.
Use: Vitamin supplement.
See: Phytonadione (Various Mfr.).

methyl polysiloxane.
See: Mylicon, Tab., Drops (Zeneca Pharmaceuticals).
Simethicone (Various Mfr.)

methylpred-40. (Seatrace Pharmaceuticals, Inc.) Methylprednisolone acetate 40 mg/ml. Vial 5 ml, 10 ml. *Rx.*
Use: Corticosteroid.

•**methylprednisolone.** (METH-ill-pred-NIH-suh-lone) U.S.P. 23.
Use: Corticosteroid, topical.
See: A-Methapred, Inj. (Abbott Laboratories).
Dura-Meth, Inj. (Foy Laboratories).
Medralone 40, Inj. (Keene Pharmaceuticals, Inc.).
Medralone 80, Inj. (Keene Pharmaceuticals, Inc.).
Medrol, Tab. (Pharmacia & Upjohn).
W/Neomycin sulfate
See: Solu-Medrol, Vial (Pharmacia & Upjohn).

•**methylprednisolone acetate.** (METH-ill-pred-NIH-suh-lone) U.S.P. 23.
Use: Corticosteroid.
See: Adlone, Inj. (Forest Pharmaceutical, Inc.).
Depo-Medrol, Inj., Rectal (Pharmacia & Upjohn).
Depopred-40, Vial (Hyrex Pharmaceuticals).

•**methylprednisolone hemisuccinate.** (METH-ill-pred-NIH-suh-lone hem-ih-SUCK-sih-nate) U.S.P. 23.
Use: Adrenocortical steroid.

•**methylprednisolone sodium phosphate.** (METH-ill-pred-NIH-suh-lone) USAN.
Use: Corticosteroid, topical.

•**methylprednisolone sodium succinate.** (METH-ill-pred-NIH-suh-lone) U.S.P. 23.
Use: Adrenocorticoid steroid; corticosteroid, topical.
See: Solu-Medrol, Mix-O-Vial (Pharmacia & Upjohn).

•**methylprednisolone suleptanate.** (METH-ill-pred-NIH-suh-lone sull-EPP-tah-NATE) USAN.
Use: Adrenocortical steroid, anti-inflammatory.

4-methylpyrazole.
Use: Methanol or ethylene glycol poisoning. [Orphan Drug]

methylpyrimal.
See: Sulfamerazine (Various Mfr.).

methylrosaniline chloride.
Use: Anthelmintic, anti-infective.
See: Gentian Violet (Various Mfr.).

•**methyl salicylate.** (METH-ill sal-ISS-ih-late) N.F. 18.
Use: Pharmaceutic aid (flavor).

methyl salicylate w/combinations.
Use: Rubefacient rub (topical).
See: Analbalm, Liq. (Schwarz Pharma, Inc.).
Analgesic Balm (Various Mfr.).
Banalg, Liniment (Forest Pharmaceutical, Inc.).

Cydonol, Lot. (Gordon Laboratories).
Emul-o-balm, Liq. (Medeva Pharmaceuticals, Inc.).
Gordobalm, Oint. (Gordon Laboratories).
Listerine Antiseptic, Liq. (Warner Lambert)
Musterole, Oint. (Schering-Plough Corp.).
Pain Bust-R II, Cream (Continental Consumer Products).
Sloan's Liniment, Liq. (Warner Lambert).
Ziks, Cream (Nnodum Corporation).

methyl sulfanil amidoisoxazole. Sulfamethoxazole.
See: Gantanol, Tab., Susp. (Roche Laboratories).

•**methyltestosterone.** (METH-ill-tess-TAHS-ter-ohn) U.S.P. 23.
Use: Androgen.
See: Android-10 or -25, Tab. (Zeneca Pharmaceuticals).
Arcosterone, Tab. (Arcum).
Metandren, Linguet, Tab. (Novartis Pharmaceutical Corp.).
Testred, Cap. (Zeneca Pharmaceuticals).
Virilon, Cap. (Star Pharmaceuticals, Inc.).

methyltestosterone. (Various Mfr.) 10 mg, 25 mg/Tab. Bot. 100s, 1000s. 10 mg/Tab., Buccal. Bot. 100s. *c-III.*
Use: Androgen.

methyltestosterone w/combinations.
Use: Androgen.
See: Android Tab. (Baxter Pharmaceutical Products, Inc.).
Menogen, Prods. (Breckenridge Pharmaceuticals, Inc.).
Premarin w/Methyltestosterone, Tab. (Wyeth-Ayerst Laboratories).
Virilon, Cap. (Star Pharmaceuticals, Inc.).

methylthionine chloride. Name used for Methylene Blue.

methylthionine hydrochloride. Name used for Methylene Blue.

methylthiouracil. U.S.P. XXI.
Use: Antithyroid agent.

methyl violet.
See: Gentian Violet, Crystal Violet, Methylrosaniline Cl.

methyndamine. Name used for Tetrydamine.

•**methynodiol diacetate.** (meh-THIN-oh-die-ole die-ASS-eh-tate) USAN.
Use: Hormone, progestin.

•**methysergide.** (METH-ih-SIR-jide) USAN.
Use: Antimigraine, vasoconstrictor.

•**methysergide maleate.** (METH-ih-SIR-jide) U.S.P. 23.
Use: Antimigraine, vasoconstrictor.
See: Sansert, Tab. (Novartis Pharmaceutical Corp.).

•**metiamide.** (meh-TIE-aim-id) USAN. Histamine H_2 antagonist.
Use: Treatment for peptic ulcer; antiulcerative.

•**metiapine.** (meh-TIE-ah-PEEN) USAN.
Use: Antipsychotic.

meticlopindol. Name used for Clopidol.

Meticorten. (Schering-Plough Corp.) Prednisone 1 mg/Tab. Bot. 100s. *Rx.*
Use: Corticosteroid.

Metimyd Ophthalmic Oint. Sterile. (Schering-Plough Corp.) Prednisolone acetate 0.5% (5 mg), sulfacetamide sodium 10%. Tube 3.5 g. *Rx.*
Use: Corticosteroid; sulfonamide, topical.

Metimyd Ophthalmic Susp. Sterile. (Schering-Plough Corp.) Prednisolone acetate 0.5%, sulfacetamide sodium 10%. Bot. dropper 5 ml. *Rx.*
Use: Corticosteroid; sulfonamide, topical.

•**metioprim.** (meh-TIE-oh-PRIM) USAN.
Use: Anti-infective.

•**metipranolol.** (meh-tih-PRAN-oh-lahl) USAN.
Use: Antihypertensive (β-blocker, ophthalmic).

metipranolol hydrochloride.
Use: Antihypertensive (β-blocker, ophthalmic).
See: OptiPranolol (Bausch & Lomb Pharmaceuticals).

metizoline. (meh-TIH-zoe-leen)
Use: Decongestant.

•**metizoline hydrochloride.** (meh-TIH-zoe-leen) USAN.
Use: Adrenergic vasoconstrictor.

•**metkephamid acetate.** (MET-KEFF-am-id) USAN.
Use: Analgesic.

•**metoclopramide hydrochloride.** (MET-oh-kloe-PRA-mide) U.S.P. 23.
Use: Antiemetic, gastrointestinal stimulant.
See: Reclomide, Tab. (Ultra).
Reglan, Amp. (Wyeth-Ayerst Laboratories).

metoclopramide intensol. (Roxane Laboratories, Inc.) Metoclopramide HCl 10 mg/ml, EDTA, sorbitol/Concentrated Soln. Dropper Bot. 10 ml, 30 ml. *Rx.*
Use: Antiemetic, gastrointestinal stimulant.

•**metocurine iodide.** (MEH-toe-CURE-een) U.S.P. 23. *Formerly Dimethyl Tubocurarine Iodide.*
Use: Neuromuscular blocker.
See: Metubine Iodide, Vial (Eli Lilly and Co.).

metofurone. (MET-oh-fyoor-OHN) Name used for Nifurmerone.

•**metogest.** (MET-oh-JEST) USAN.
Use: Hormone.

•**metolazone.** (meh-TOLE-uh-ZONE) U.S.P. 23.
Use: Antihypertensive, diuretic.
See: Mykrox, Tab. (Medeva Pharmaceuticals, Inc.).
Zaroxolyn, Tab. (Medeva Pharmaceuticals, Inc.).

•**metopimazine.** (meh-toe-PIH-mazz-EEN) USAN.
Use: Antiemetic.

Metopirone. (Novartis Pharmaceutical Corp.) Metyrapone 250 mg. Softgel Cap. Pkg. 18s. *Rx.*
Use: Diagnostic aid.

•**metoprine.** (MET-oh-preen) USAN.
Use: Antineoplastic.

•**metoprolol.** (meh-TOE-pro-lahl) USAN.
Use: Antiadrenergic β-receptor.

•**metoprolol fumarate.** (meh-TOE-pro-lahl) U.S.P. 23.
Use: Antihypertensive.

•**metoprolol succinate.** (meh-TOE-pro-lahl) USAN.
Use: Antihypertensive; antianginal; treatment of myocardial infarction.
See: Toprol XL, Extended-release Tab. (Astra Pharmaceuticals, L.P.).

•**metoprolol tartrate.** (meh-TOE-pro-lahl TAR-trate) U.S.P. 23.
Use: Antiadrenergic (β-receptor).
See: Lopressor, Tab. (Novartis Pharmaceutical Corp.).

metoprolol tartrate. (Various Mfr.) **Tab.:** 50 mg or 100 mg, lactose. Bot. 100s, 500s, 1000s, UD 100s. **Inj.:** 1 mg/ml. Amp. 5 ml.
Use: Antiadrenergic (β-receptor).

metoprolol tartrate and hydrochlorothiazide.
Use: Antihypertensive combination.
See: Lopressor HCT 100/50, Tab. (Novartis Pharmaceutical Corp.).
Lopressor HCT 100/25, Tab. (Novartis Pharmaceutical Corp.).
Lopressor HCT 50/25, Tab. (Novartis Pharmaceutical Corp.).

metoquine.
Use: Antimalarial.

•**metoquizine.** (MET-oh-kwih-zeen) USAN.
Use: Anticholinergic, antiulcerative.

Metreton Ophthalmic Solution. (Schering-Plough Corp.) Prednisolone sodium phosphate 5.5 mg/ml. Bot. 5 ml. *Rx.*
Use: Corticosteroid, ophthalmic.

Metric 21. (Fielding Co.) Metronidazole 250 mg/Tab. Bot. 100s. *Rx.*
Use: Anti-infective.

•**metrizamide.** (meh-TRIH-zam-ide) USAN.
Use: Myelography, diagnostic aid (radiopaque medium).
See: Amipaque, Inj. (Sanofi Winthrop Pharmaceuticals).

•**metrizoate sodium.** (meh-trih-ZOE-ate) USAN.
Use: Diagnostic aid (radiopaque medium).

MetroGel. (Galderma Laboratories, Inc.) Metronidazole 0.75%. Gel Tube 28.4 g. *Rx.*
Use: Dermatologic, acne.

MetroGel-Vaginal. (3M Pharmaceuticals) Metronidazole 0.75%, carbomer 934 P, EDTA, parabens, and propylene glycol. Gel Tube (with applicator) 70 g. *Rx.*
Use: Anti-infective, vaginal.

Metrogesic. (Lexis Laboratories) Salicylamide 325 mg, acetaminophen 162 mg, phenacetin 65 mg/Tab. Bot. 100s.
Use: Analgesic.

metrogestone. (MEH-troe-JEST-ohn)
Use: Hormone, progestin.

Metro I.V.. (McGaw, Inc.) Metronidazole 500 mg/100 ml. Inj. Vial 100 ml. Plastic containers 100 ml. *Rx.*
Use: Anti-infective.

MetroLotion. (Galderma) Metronidazole 0.75%, benzyl alcohol, stearyl alcohol, glycerin, mineral oil. Lot. Bot. 59 ml. *Rx.*
Use: Antiacne.

•**metronidazole.** (meh-troe-NID-uh-zole) U.S.P. 23.
Use: Antiprotozoal (trichomonas); antitrichomonal. [Orphan Drug]
See: Flagyl, Prods. (Searle).
MetroGel-Vaginal, Gel (3M Pharmaceuticals).
Metronid, Tab. (B.F. Ascher and Co.).
MetroLotion (Galderma).
Metryl, Tab, Vial (Teva Pharmaceuticals USA).
Noritate, Cream (Dermik Laboratories, Inc.).

•**metronidazole hydrochloride.** (meh-troe-NIH-dah-zole) USAN.
Use: Anti-infective.
See: Flagyl I.V. (Searle).

•**metronidazole phosphate.** (meh-troe-

NIH-dah-zole FOSS-fate) USAN.
Use: Antibacterial, anti-infective, antiprotozoal.

Metronidazole Redi-Infusion. (ESI Lederle Generics) Metronidazole 500 mg/100 ml Vial. *Rx.*
Use: Amebicide.

Metrozole. (Lexis Laboratories) Metronidazole 250 mg, 500 mg/Tab. **250 mg:** Bot. 100s, 250s. **500 mg:** Bot. 100s. *Rx.*
Use: Amebicide, anti-infective.

MET-RX. (Met-Rx USA) **Pow. for Drink:** Fat 2 g, Na 37 mg, K 900 mg, carbohydrate 22 g, protein, < 1 g dietary fiber, sugar, vitamins A, D, C, E, B_1, B_5, B_6, B_{12}, biotin, Mg, Zn, Ca, folate, P, Cu, Fe, riboflavin, iodine. Pow. For Drink. 72 g. **Food Bar:** Fat 4 g, Na 110 mg, K 700 mg, carbohydrate 50 g, protein 27 g, sugar, Ca, vitamins A, D, B_1, B_2, B_3, B_5, B_6, B_{12}, C, E, folate, biotin, P, Mg, Cu, Fe, I, Zn. Food Bar. 100 g. *otc.*
Use: Nutritional therapy.

Metryl. (Teva Pharmaceuticals USA) Metronidazole 250 mg/Tab. Bot. 100s, 250s, 500s, UD 100s. *Rx.*
Use: Amebicide, anti-infective.

Metryl 500. (Teva Pharmaceuticals USA) Metronidazole 500 mg/Tab. Bot. 100s, 500s. *Rx.*
Use: Amebicide, anti-infective.

Metubine Iodide. (Eli Lilly and Co.) Metocurine iodide 2 mg/ml. Vial 20 ml. *Rx.*
Use: Muscle relaxant.

•**meturedepa.** (meh-TOO-ree-DEH-pah) USAN.
Use: Antineoplastic.

Metussin. (Faraday) Dextromethorphan. Bot. 4 oz. *otc.*
Use: Antitussive.

Metussin Jr. (Faraday) Dextromethorphan. Bot. 4 oz. *otc.*
Use: Antitussive.

•**metyrapone.** (meh-TEER-ah-pone) U.S.P. 23.
Use: Diagnostic aid (pituitary function determination). Adrenocortical enzyme inhibitor.
See: Metopirone, Cap. (Novartis Pharmaceutical Corp.).

•**metyrapone tartrate.** (meh-TEER-ah-pone) USAN.
Use: Diagnostic aid (pituitary function determination).

metyrapone tartrate injection.
Use: Diagnostic aid.

•**metyrosine.** (meh-TIE-roe-seen) U.S.P. 23.
Use: Antihypertensive.
See: Demser (Merck & Co.)

Mevacor. (Merck & Co.) Lovastatin Tab. **10 mg:** Bot. 60. **20 mg:** Bot. 60s, 90s, 100s, 1000s, 10,000s, UD 100s. **40 mg:** Bot. 60s, 90s, 1000s, 10,000s. *Rx.*
Use: Antihyperlipidemic.

mevinolin.
See: Lovastatin.

Mexate-AQ. (Bristol-Myers Oncology/Immunology) Preservative-free liquid. Methotrexate 50 mg, 100 mg, 250 mg/Vial. *Rx.*
Use: Antineoplastic.

•**mexiletine hydrochloride.** (MEX-ih-leh-teen) U.S.P. 23.
Use: Cardiovascular agent (antiarrhythmic).
See: Mexitil, Cap. (Boehringer Ingelheim, Inc.).

mexiletine hydrochloride. (Various Mfr.) Mexiletine HCl 150 mg, 200 mg, 250 mg/Cap. Bot. 100s, UD 100s (except 250 mg). *Rx.*
Use: Cardiovascular agent (antiarrhythmic).

Mexitil. (Boehringer Ingelheim, Inc.) Mexiletine HCl 150 mg, 200 mg, 250 mg/Cap. Bot. 100s, UD 100s. *Rx.*
Use: Antiarrhythmic.

•**mexrenoate potassium.** (mex-REN-oh-ate poe-TASS-ee-uhm) USAN.
Use: Aldosterone antagonist.

Mexsana Medicated Powder. (Schering-Plough Corp.) Corn starch, kaolin, triclosan, zinc oxide. Can 3 oz, 6.25 oz, 11 oz. *otc.*
Use: Diaper rash preparation.

Meyenberg Goat Milk. (Jackson-Mitchell) Evaporated and powdered cans of goat milk. Foil pack 4 oz. (makes one quart). *otc.*
Use: Cows' milk allergies.

Mezlin. (Bayer Corp. (Consumer Div.)) Mezlocillin sodium 1 g, 2 g, 3 g, 4 g, 20 g. Pow. for Inj. Vial, infusion bot (except 1 g, 20 g), *ADD-Vantage* vial (only 3 g, 4 g), Bulk Pkg. (20 g only). *Rx.*
Use: Anti-infective, penicillin.

•**mezlocillin.** (MEZZ-low-SILL-in) USAN.
Use: Anti-infective.

•**mezlocillin sodium, sterile.** (MEZZ-low-SILL-in) U.S.P. 23.
Use: Anti-infective.
See: Mezlin, Pow. for Inj. (Bayer Corp. (Consumer Div.)).

MG Cold Sore Formula. (Outdoor Recreations) Menthol 1%, lidocaine, propylene glycol in alcohol base. Soln. Bot.

7.5 ml. *otc.*
Use: Cold sores, fever blisters.

MG-Oroate. (Miller Pharmacal Group, Inc.) Magnesium (as magnesium orotate) 33 mg/Tab. Bot. 100s. *otc.*
Use: Vitamin supplement.

MG217 Medicated. (Triton Consumer Products, Inc.) **Shampoo:** Coal tar solution 5%, salicylic acid 2%. Bot. 120 ml, 240 ml, 480 ml. **Conditioner:** Coal tar solution 2%. Bot. 120 ml. *otc.*
Use: Antiseborrheic.

MG217 Medicated Formula. (Triton Consumer Products, Inc.) Coal tar solution 5%, colloidal sulfur 1.5%, salicylic acid 2% in a special base of cleansers, wetting agents and lanolin. Shampoo 120 ml, 240 ml, 480 ml. *otc.*
Use: Antiseborrheic, antipruritic.

MG400. (Triton Consumer Products, Inc.) Colloidal sulfur in Guy-Base II 5%, salicylic acid 3%. Shampoo. Bot. 240 ml, pt. *otc.*
Use: Antiseborrheic.

MG-Plus Protein. (Miller Pharmacal Group, Inc.) Magnesium-protein complex made w/specially isolated soy protein 133 mg/Tab. Bot. 100s. *otc.*
Use: Vitamin supplement.

Miacalcin. (Novartis Pharmaceutical Corp.) Calcitonin-salmon 200 IU, acetic acid 2.25 mg, phenol 5 mg, sodium acetate trihydrate 2 mg, sodium chloride 7.5 mg/ml. Inj. Vial 2 ml. *Rx.*
Use: Hormone.

Miacalcin Nasal Spray. (Novartis Pharmaceutical Corp.) Calcitonin-salmon/activation (0.9 ml/dose) 200 IU, sodium chloride 8.5 mg/Spray. Bot. 2 ml. *Rx.*
Use: Antihypercalcemic.

Mi-Acid Gelcaps. (Major Pharmaceuticals) Calcium carbonate 311 mg, magnesium carbonate 232 mg, parabens, EDTA. Bot. 50s. *otc.*
Use: Antacid.

Mi-Acid Liquid. (Major Pharmaceuticals) Aluminum hydroxide 200 mg, magnesium hydroxide 200 mg, simethicone 20 mg/5 ml. Bot. 355 ml, 780 ml. *otc.*
Use: Antacid, antiflatulent.

Mi-Acid II Liquid. (Major Pharmaceuticals) Aluminum hydroxide 400 mg, magnesium hydroxide 400 mg, simethicone 40 mg/5 ml. Bot. 355 ml. *otc.*
Use: Antacid, antiflatulent.

miadone.
See: Methadone HCl. (Various Mfr.).

•**mianserin hydrochloride.** (my-AN-ser-in) USAN. Under study.
Use: Serotonin inhibitor, antihistamine.

•**mibolerone.** (my-BOLE-ehr-ohn) USAN.
Use: Anabolic, androgen.

Micanolol. (Bioglan Pharma) Anthralin 1%/Cream. Tube 50 g. *Rx.*
Use: Dermatologic.

Micardis. (Boehringer Ingelheim) Telmisartan 40 mg, 80 mg. Tab. Bot. 28s. *Rx.*
Use: Antihypertensive.

micasorb.
W/Red Veterinary Petrolatum.
See: RV Plus, Oint. (Baxter Pharmaceutical Products, Inc.).

Micatin. (Advanced Care Products) Miconazole nitrate 2%. **Cream:** Tube 0.5 oz, 1 oz. **Spray powder:** Aerosol 3 oz. **Spray Liquid Aerosol:** Bot. 3.5 oz. *otc.*
Use: Antifungal, topical.

Mi-Cebrin. (Eli Lilly and Co.) Vitamins B_1 10 mg, B_2 5 mg, B_6 1.7 mg, pantothenic acid 10 mg, niacinamide 30 mg, B_{12} (activity equiv.) 3 mcg, C 100 mg, E 5.5 IU, A 10,000 IU, D 400 IU, Fe 15 mg, Cu 1 mg, I 0.15 mg, Mn 1 mg, Mg 5 mg, Zn 1.5 mg/Tab. Pkg. 60s, 100s, 1000s, Blister pkg. 10 × 10s. *otc.*
Use: Mineral, vitamin supplement.

Mi-Cebrin T. (Eli Lilly and Co.) Vitamins B_1 15 mg, B_2 10 mg, B_6 2 mg, pantothenic acid 10 mg, niacinamide 100 mg, B_{12} 7.5 mcg, C 150 mg, E 5.5 IU, A 10,000 IU, D 400 IU, Fe 15 mg, Cu 1 mg, I 0.15 mg, Mn 1 mg, Mg 5 mg, Zn 1.5 mg/Tab. Bot. 30s, 100s, 1000s, Blister pkg. 10 × 10s. *otc.*
Use: Mineral, vitamin supplement.

micofur.
Use: Antifungal, anti-infective, topical.

Miconal. (Bioglan Pharma) Anthralin 1% Cream Tube 50 g. *Rx.*
Use: Antipsoriatic.

•**miconazole.** (my-KAHN-uh-zole) U.S.P. 23.
Use: Antifungal.
See: Monistat IV, Inj. (Janssen Pharmaceutical, Inc.).

•**miconazole nitrate.** (my-CONE-ah-zole NYE-trate) U.S.P. 23.
Use: Antifungal.
See: Breezee Mist Antifungal (Pedinol).
Femizol-M, Vag. Cream (Lake Consumer Products).
Fungoid Tincture, Soln. (Pedinol Pharmacal, Inc.).
Lotrimin AF, Pow., Spray Pow. (Schering-Plough Corp.).
Maximum Strength Desenex Antifungal, Cream (Novartis Pharmaceutical Corp.).
Monistat, Cream, Supp. (Ortho McNeil Pharmaceutical).

Monistat 3, Vaginal Supp. (Ortho McNeil Pharmaceutical).
Monistat 7, Vaginal cream, Supp. (Advanced Care Products).
Monistat-Derm, Prods. (Ortho McNeil Pharmaceutical).
M-Zole 7 Dual Pack (Alpharma).
Zeasorb-AF, Pow. (Stiefel Laboratories, Inc.).

miconazole nitrate. (Copley Pharmaceutical, Inc.) Miconazole nitrate 2%. Cream. Tube 45 g (100 mg/dose for 7 doses). *otc.*
Use: Antifungal, vaginal.

miconazole nitrate. (Taro Pharmaceuticals USA, Inc.) Miconazole nitrate 2%, benzoic acid, mineral oil, apricot kernel oil. Cream. Tube 15 g, 30 g. *otc.*
Use: Antifungal, topical.

micoren. (Novartis Pharmaceutical Corp.) A respiratory stimulant; pending release.

Micrainin. (Wallace Laboratories) Meprobamate 200 mg, aspirin 325 mg/Tab. Bot. 100s, UD 100s. *c-iv.*
Use: Analgesic combination.

MICRhoGAM. (Ortho Diagnostic Systems, Inc.) Rh_0 (D) immune globulin (human) micro-dose. Single-dose prefilled syringe. *Rx.*
Use: Agent to prevent immunization against Rh antigen.

microbubble contrast agent.
Use: Aid in ID of intracranial tumors. [Orphan Drug]

Microcult-GC Test. (Bayer Corp. (Consumer Div.)) Miniaturized culture test for the detection of *Neisseria Gonorrhoeae.* Test Kit 25s.
Use: Diagnostic aid.

microfibrillar collagen hemostat.
Use: Hemostatic, topical.
See: Avitene (Alcon Laboratories, Inc.).
Hemopad (Astra Pharmaceuticals, L.P.).
Hemotene (Astra Pharmaceuticals, L.P).

Micro-Guard. (Sween) Antimicrobial skin cream. Tube 0.5 oz, Jar 2 oz. *otc.*
Use: Antifungal, topical.

Micro-K Extencaps. (Wyeth-Ayerst Laboratories) Potassium Cl (8 mEq) 600 mg/Cap. Bot. 100s, 500s, Dis-Co pack 100s. *Rx.*
Use: Electrolyte supplement.

Micro-K 10 Extencaps. (Wyeth-Ayerst Laboratories) Potassium Cl 750 mg (10 mEq)/Cap. Bot. 100s, 500s, Dis-co UD 100s. *Rx.*
Use: Electrolyte supplement.

Micro-K LS. (Wyeth-Ayerst Laboratories) Potassium Cl 20 mEq (1500 mg). Extended release Susp. Packet 30s, 100s. *Rx.*
Use: Electrolyte supplement.

Microlipid. (Biosearch Medical Products) Fat emulsion 50%, safflower oil, polyglycerol esters of fatty acids, soy lecithin, xanthan gum, ascorbic acid. Cal 4500, fat 500 g/L, 80 mOsm/Kg. H_2O. 120 ml. *Rx.*
Use: Nutritional supplement.

Micronase. (Pharmacia & Upjohn) Glyburide 1.25, 2.5, 5 mg/Tab. **1.25 mg:** Bot. 100s. **2.5 mg:** Bot. 100s, 1000s, UD 100s. **5 mg:** Bot. 30s, 60s, 100s, 500s, 1000s, UD 100s. *Rx.*
Use: Antidiabetic.

microNefrin. (Bird Corp.) Racepinephrine HCl 2.25%, sodium bisulfite, potassium metabisulfite, chlorobutanol, benzoic acid, propylene glycol. Bot 15 ml, 30 ml. *otc.*
Use: Brochodilator, sympathomimetic.

Micronized Glyburide. (Copley Pharmaceutical, Inc.) 1.5 mg/Tab. Bot. 100s, UD 100s. 3 mg/Tab. Bot. 100s, 500s, 1000s, UD 100s. *Rx.*
Use: Antidiabetic.

Microsol. (Star Pharmaceuticals, Inc.) Sulfamethizole 0.5 g, 1 g/Tab. Bot. 100s, 1000s. *Rx.*
Use: Anti-infective, urinary.

Microsol-A. (Star Pharmaceuticals, Inc.) Phenazopyridine 50 mg, sulfamethizole 0.5 g/Tab. Bot. 100s, 1000s. *Rx.*
Use: Anti-infective, urinary.

Microstix Candida. (Bayer Corp. (Consumer Div.)) Test for *Candida* species in vaginal specimens. Box 25s.
Use: Diagnostic aid.

Microstix-3 Reagent Strips. (Bayer Corp. (Consumer Div.)) For recognition of nitrite in urine and for semi-quantitation of bacterial growth. Bot. 25s w/25 incubation pouches.
Use: Diagnostic aid.

MicroTrak Chlamydia Trachomatis Direct Specimen Test. (Syva Co.) To detect and identify chlamydia trachomatis. Slide test 60s.
Use: Diagnostic aid.

MicroTrak HSV 1/HSV 2 Culture Confirmation/Typing Test. (Syva Co.) For identification and typing of herpes simplex in tissue culture. Test kit 1s.
Use: Diagnostic aid.

MicroTrak Neisseria Gonorrhea Culture Test. (Syva Co.) For endocervical, urethral, rectal, and pharyngeal cultures. Test kit 85s.
Use: Diagnostic aid.

Microzide. (Watson Laboratories) Hydrochlorothiazide 12.5 mg, lactose. Cap. Bot. 100s. *Rx.*
Use: Diuretic.

micrurus fulvius antivenin. (Wyeth-Ayerst Laboratories) Inj. Combination package: One vial antivenin, one vial diluent (Bacteriostatic Water for Injection 10 ml.).
Use: Antivenin.

Mictrin Plus. (Johnson & Johnson) Water, SD alcohol 38-B, glycerin, poloxamer 407, flavor, sodium saccharin, glutamic acid buffer, cetylpyridinium Cl, FD & C Yellow #5, Blue #1. Bot. 12 oz, 24 oz. *otc.*
Use: Mouth preparation.

•**midaflur.** (MY-dah-flure) USAN.
Use: Hypnotic, sedative.

Midahist Expectorant. (Vangard Labs, Inc.) Codeine phosphate 10 mg, phenylpropanolamine HCl 18.75 mg, guaifenesin 100 mg/5 ml, alcohol 7.5%. Bot. Pt, gal. *c-v.*
Use: Antitussive, decongestant, expectorant.

midamaline hydrochloride.
Use: Anesthetic, local.

Midamor. (Merck & Co.) Amiloride 5 mg/Tab. Bot. 100s. *Rx.*
Use: Diuretic, antihypertensive.

Midaneed. (Hanlon) Vitamins A 5000 IU, D 500 IU, B_1 5 mg, B_2 3 mg, B_6 0.5 mcg, B_{12} 5 mcg, C 100 mg, niacinamide 10 mg, calcium pantothenate 5 mg/Cap. Bot. 100s. *otc.*
Use: Mineral, vitamin supplement.

Midatane DC Expectorant. (Vangard Labs, Inc.) Brompheniramine maleate 2 mg, guaifenesin 100 mg, phenylephrine HCl 5 mg, phenylpropanolamine HCl 5 mg, codeine phosphate 10 mg/5 ml, alcohol 3.5% Bot. Pt, gal. *c-v.*
Use: Antihistamine, antitussive, decongestant, expectorant.

Midatapp TR Tablets. (Vangard Labs, Inc.) Brompheniramine maleate 12 mg, phenylephrine HCl 15 mg, phenylpropanolamine HCl 15 mg/Tab. Bot. 100s, 500s, 1000s. *Rx.*
Use: Antihistamine, decongestant.

•**midazolam hydrochloride.** (meh-DAZE-oh-lam) USAN.
Use: Anesthetic (injectable).
See: Versed, Inj. (Roche Laboratories).

•**midazolam maleate.** (meh-DAZE-oh-lam) USAN.
Use: Anesthetic, intravenous.

Midchlor. (Schein Pharmaceutical, Inc.) Isometheptene mucate 65 mg, dichloralphenazone 100 mg, acetaminophen 325 mg/Cap. Bot. 100s. *Rx.*
Use: Antimigraine.

•**midodrine hydrochloride.** (MIH-doe-DREEN) USAN.
Use: Antihypotensive, vasoconstrictor.
See: ProAmatine, Tab. (Roberts Pharmaceuticals).

Midol for Cramps. (Bayer Corp. (Consumer Div.)) Aspirin 500 mg, caffeine 32.4 mg, cinnamedrine HCl 14.9 mg/Capl. In 8s, 16s, 32s. *otc.*
Use: Analgesic combination.

Midol IB. (Bayer Corp. (Consumer Div.)) Ibuprofen 200 mg. Tab. Bot. 50s. *otc.*
Use: Analgesic, NSAID.

Midol Maximum Strength. (Bayer Corp. (Consumer Div.)) Cinnamedrine HCl 14.9 mg, aspirin 500 mg, caffeine 32.4 mg/Tab. Bot. 12s, 30s, 60s. *otc.*
Use: Analgesic combination.

Midol Maximum Strength Multi-Symptom Menstrual. (Bayer Corp. (Consumer Div.)) Acetaminophen 500 mg, caffeine 60 mg, pyrilamine maleate 15 mg. Capl. Pkg. 8s, 16s, 32s. Gelcaps. Pkg. 12s, 24s. *otc.*
Use: Analgesic combination.

Midol Multi-Symptom, Maximum Strength. (Bayer Corp. (Consumer Div.)) Acetaminophen 500 mg, pyrilamine maleate 15 mg. Capl. Bot. 32s. *otc.*
Use: Analgesic combination.

Midol Multi-Symptom, Regular Strength. (Bayer Corp. (Consumer Div.)) Acetaminophen 325 mg, pyrilamine maleate 12.5 mg. Capl. Bot. 32s. *otc.*
Use: Analgesic combination.

Midol Original Formula. (Bayer Corp. (Consumer Div.)) Cinnamedrine HCl 14.9 mg, aspirin 454 mg, caffeine 32.4 mg/Tab. Bot. 30s, 60s. Strip pack 12s. *otc.*
Use: Analgesic combination.

Midol PM. (Bayer Corp. (Consumer Div.)) Acetaminophen 500 mg, diphenhydramine 25 mg. Capl. Pkg. 16s. *otc.*
Use: Analgesic combination.

Midol, Teen. (Bayer Corp. (Consumer Div.)) Acetaminophen 400 mg, pamabrom 25 mg/Cap. Pkg. 16s, 32s. *otc.*
Use: Analgesic combination.

Midrin. (Carnrick Laboratories, Inc.) Isometheptene mucate 65 mg, acetaminophen 325 mg, dichloralphenazone 100 mg/Cap. Bot. 50s, 100s. *Rx.*
Use: Antimigraine.

Midstream Pregnancy Test Kit. (Zenith

Goldline Pharmaceuticals) Stick for urine test. Kit 1s. *otc.*
Use: Pregnancy test.

•**mifobate.** (mih-FOE-bate) USAN.
Use: Antiatherosclerotic.

•**miglitol.** (mih-GLIH-tole) USAN.
Use: Antidiabetic.
See: Glyset, Tab. (Bayer Corp. (Consumer Div.)).

migraine agents.
See: Sansert, Tab. (Novartis Pharmaceutical Corp.).
Medihaler Ergotamine, Aerosol (3M Pharmaceuticals).
D.H.E. 45, Inj. (Novartis Pharmaceutical Corp.).
Imitrex (GlaxoWellcome).

migraine combinations.
See: Isometheptene/Dichloralphenazone/Acetaminophen. (Various Mfr.).
Isocom, Cap. (Nutripharm Laboratories, Inc.).
Midchlor, Cap. (Schein Pharmaceutical, Inc.).
Midrin, Cap. (Carnrick Laboratories, Inc).
Migratine, Cap. (Major Pharmaceuticals).

Migranal. (Novartis Pharmaceutical Corp.) Dihydroergotamine mesylate 4 mg/ml, caffeine, dextrose. Nasal spray. Bot. UD 4s. *Rx.*
Use: Antimigraine.

Migratine. (Major Pharmaceuticals) Isometheptene mucate 65 mg, dichloralphenazone 100 mg, acetaminophen 325 mg/Cap. Bot. 100s, 250s. *Rx.*
Use: Antimigraine.

MIH.
Use: Antineoplastic.
See: Matulane (Roche Laboratories).

•**milacemide hydrochloride.** (mill-ASS-eh-mide HIGH-droe-KLOR-ide) USAN.
Use: Anticonvulsant, antidepressant.

•**milameline hydrochloride.** (mill-AM-eh-leen) USAN.
Use: Antidementia (partial muscarinic agonist).

mild silver protein.
See: Silver Protein, Mild.

•**milenperone.** (mih-LEN-per-OHN) USAN.
Use: Antipsychotic.

Miles Nervine. (Bayer Corp. (Consumer Div.)) Diphenhydramine HCl 25 mg/Tab. Pkg. 12s, Bot. 30s.
Use: Nonprescription sleep aid.

•**milipertine.** (MIH-lih-PURR-teen) USAN.
Use: Antipsychotic.

Milkinol. (Schwarz Pharma, Inc.) Mineral oil in an emulsifying base. Bot. 240 ml. *otc.*
Use: Laxative.

milk of bismuth. (Various Mfr.) Bismuth hydroxide, bismuth subcarb.
Use: Orally, intestinal disturbances.

•**milk of magnesia.** (milk of mag-NEE-zhuh) U.S.P. 23. *Formerly Magnesia Magma.*
Use: Antacid, laxative.
See: Magnesium hydroxide (Various Mfr.).

milk of magnesia. (Various Mfr.). Magnesia (Magnesium hydroxide) 325 mg, 390 mg. **Tab.:** 250s, 1000s. **Liq.:** 120 ml, 360 ml, 720 ml, pt, qt, gal, UD 10 ml, 15 ml, 20 ml, 30 ml, 100 ml, 180 ml, 400 ml. **Susp.:** Pt, qt, gal, UD 15 and 30 ml.
Use: Antacid, laxative.

Milk of Magnesia-Concentrated. (Roxane Laboratories, Inc.) Magnesium hydroxide. Liq. Bot. 100 ml, 180 ml, 400 ml, UD 10 ml, 15 ml, 20 ml, 30 ml.
Use: Antacid.

Millazine. (Major Pharmaceuticals) Thioridazine. **10 mg, 15 mg/Tab.:** Bot. 100s. **25 mg/Tab.:** Bot. 100s, 1000s. **100 mg, 150 mg, 200 mg/Tab.:** Bot. 100s, 500s. *Rx.*
Use: Antipsychotic.

•**milodistim.** (my-low-DIH-stim) USAN.
Use: Immunomodulator (antineutropenic).

Milontin. (Parke-Davis) Phensuximide 0.5 g/Kapseal. Bot. 100s. *Rx.*
Use: Anticonvulsant.

Milpar. (Sanofi Winthrop Pharmaceuticals) Magnesium hydroxide, mineral oil. *otc.*
Use: Antacid, laxative.

•**milrinone.** (MILL-rih-nohn) USAN.
Use: Cardiovascular agent, congestive heart failure.
See: Primacor (Sanofi Winthrop Pharmaceuticals).

Milroy Artificial Tears. (Milton Roy) Bot. 22 ml.
Use: Artificial tears.

Miltown. (Wallace Laboratories) Meprobamate. **200 mg/Tab.:** Bot. 100s. **400 mg/Tab.:** Bot. 100s, 500s, 1000s. **600 mg/Tab.:** Bot. 100s. *c-IV.*
Use: Anxiolytic.

Miltown 600. (Wallace Laboratories) Meprobamate 600 mg/Tab. Bot. 100s. *c-IV.*
Use: Anxiolytic.

•**mimbane hydrochloride.** (MIM-bane) USAN.
Use: Analgesic.

•**minalrestat.** (min-AL-reh-stat) USAN.
Use: Aldose reductase inhibitor.

•**minaprine.** (MIN-ah-preen) USAN.
Use: Psychotherapeutic agent.

•**minaprine hydrochloride.** (MIN-ah-preen) USAN.
Use: Antidepressant.

•**minaxolone.** (min-AX-oh-lone) USAN.
Use: Anesthetic.

mincard.
Use: Diuretic.

Mineral Ice, Therapeutic. (Bristol-Myers Products) Menthol 2%, ammonium hydroxide, carbomer 934, cupric sulfate, isopropyl alcohol, magnesium sulfate, thymol. Gel Tube 105 g, 240 g, 480 g. *otc.*
Use: Liniment.

mineral-corticoids.
See: Desoxycorticosterone salts (Various Mfr.).

•**mineral oil.** U.S.P. 23.
Use: Laxative, pharmaceutic aid (solvent, oleaginous vehicle).
See: Petrolatum, Liq. (Various Mfr.).

mineral oil emulsion.
Use: Cathartic.

mineral oil enema.
Use: Cathartic.

•**mineral oil, light.** N.F. 18.
Use: Pharmaceutic aid (tablet and capsule lubricant, vehicle).

Minibex. (Faraday) Vitamins B_1 6 mg, B_2 3 mg, B_6 0.5 mg, C 50 mg, niacinamide 10 mg, calcium pantothenate 3 mg, B_{12} 2 mcg, folic acid 0.1 mg/Cap. Bot. 100s, 250s, 1000s. *otc.*
Use: Mineral, vitamin supplement.

Minidyne 10%. (Pedinol Pharmacal, Inc.) Povidone-iodine 10%, citric acid, sodium phosphate dibasic. Soln. Bot. 15 ml. *otc.*
Use: Antimicrobial, antiseptic.

Mini-Gamulin Rh. (Centeon) Rh_o (D) Immune Globulin (human). Single-dose Vial. *Rx.*
Use: Agent to prevent immunization against Rh antigen.

Minipress. (Pfizer US Pharmaceutical Group) Prazosin HCl 1 mg, 2 mg or 5 mg/Cap. **1 mg, 2 mg:** Bot. 250s, 1000s, UD 100s. **5 mg:** Bot. 250s, 500s, UD 100s. *Rx.*
Use: Antihypertensive.

Minitec. (Bristol-Myers Squibb) Sodium pertechnetate Tc 99 m generator.
Use: Radiopaque agent.

Minitec Generator (Complete with Components). (Bristol-Myers Squibb) Medotopes Kit.
Use: Diagnostic aid.

Mini Thin Asthma Relief. (BDI Pharmaceuticals, Inc.) Ephedrine HCl 25 mg, guaifenesin 100 mg, 200 mg/Tab. Bot. 60s (25/100 mg), 100s (25/200 mg). *otc.*
Use: Antiasthmatic.

Mini Thin Pseudo. (BDI Pharmaceuticals, Inc.) Pseudoephedrine HCl 60 mg/Tab. Bot. 60s. *otc.*
Use: Decongestant.

Minitran Transdermal Delivery System. (3M Pharmaceuticals) Nitroglycerin 9 mg, 18 mg, 36 mg, 54 mg. Patch 33s. *Rx.*
Use: Antianginal.

Minit-Rub. (Bristol-Myers Squibb) Methyl salicylate 15%, menthol 3.5%, camphor 2.3% in anhydrous base. Tube 1.5 oz, 3 oz. *otc.*
Use: Analgesic, topical.

Minizide. (Pfizer US Pharmaceutical Group) Prazosin HCl and polythiazide. **Minizide 1:** Prazosin 1 mg, polythiazide 0.5 mg/Cap. **Minizide 2:** Prazosin 2 mg, polythiazide 0.5 mg/Cap. **Minizide 5:** Prazosin 5 mg, polythiazide 0.5 mg/Cap. Bot. 100s. *Rx.*
Use: Antihypertensive.

Minocin. (ESI Lederle Generics) Minocycline HCl. **Cap., pellet-filled 50 mg:** Bot. 100s, 250s. **100 mg:** Bot. 50s, 250s. **IV:** 100 mg/Vial. **Oral Susp.:** 50 mg/5 ml, propylparaben 0.1%, butylparaben 0.06%, alcohol 5% v/v. Bot. 2 oz. *Rx.*
Use: Anti-infective, tetracycline.

•**minocromil.** (MIH-no-KROE-mill) USAN.
Use: Antiallergic (prophylactic).

•**minocycline.** (mihn-oh-SIGH-kleen) USAN.
Use: Anti-infective.

•**minocycline hydrochloride.** (mihn-oh-SIGH-kleen) U.S.P. 23.
Use: Anti-infective. [Orphan Drug]
See: Dynacin, Cap. (Medicis Dermatologicals, Inc.).
Minocin, Cap., Syr., Vial (ESI Lederle Generics).
Vectrin, Cap. (Warner Chilcott Laboratories).

minocycline hydrochloride. (Warner Chilcott Laboratories) Minocycline HCl 50 mg, 100 mg, Cap. Bot. 50s (100 mg only), 100s (50 mg only). *Rx.*
Use: Anti-infective.

•**minoxidil.** (min-OX-ih-dill) U.S.P. 23.

Use: Antihypertensive, vasodilator, hair growth stimulant (topical).
See: Loniten, Tab. (Pharmacia & Upjohn).

minoxidil. (min-OX-ih-dill) (Schein Pharmaceutical, Inc.) Minoxidil 2.5 mg/Tab. Bot. 100s, 500s, 1000s. *Rx.*
Use: Antihypertensive.

minoxidil. (min-OX-ih-dill) (Rugby Labs, Inc.) Minoxidil 10 mg/Tab. Bot. 500s. *Rx.*
Use: Antihypertensive.

Minoxidil for Men. (Lemmon Co.) Minoxidil 2%, alcohol 60%/Soln (topical). Pouches. 60 ml single and twin. *otc.*
Use: Male pattern baldness.

minoxidil, topical.
Use: Antialopecia agent.
See: Rogaine, Soln. (Pharmacia & Upjohn).

Mintezol. (Merck & Co.) Thiabendazole.
Susp.: 500 mg/5 ml. Bot. 120 ml.
Chew. Tab.: 500 mg. Pkg. 36s. *Rx.*
Use: Anthelmintic.

Minto-Chlor Syrup. (Pal-Pak, Inc.) Codeine sulfate 10 mg, potassium citrate 219 mg/5 ml, alcohol 2%. Gal. *c-v.*
Use: Antitussive, expectorant.

Mintox. (Major Pharmaceuticals) Aluminum hydroxide 200 mg, magnesium hydroxide 200 mg. Tab. Bot. 100s. *otc.*
Use: Antacid.

Mintox Plus Extra Strength Liquid. (Major Pharmaceuticals) Aluminum hydroxide 500 mg, magnesium hydroxide 450 mg, simethicone 40 mg/5 ml. Bot. 355 ml. *otc.*
Use: Antacid, antiflatulent.

Mintox Plus Tablets. (Major Pharmaceuticals) Aluminum hydroxide 200 mg, magnesium hydroxide 200 mg, simethicone 25 mg. Chew. Tab. 100s. *otc.*
Use: Antacid, antiflatulent.

Mintox Suspension. (Major Pharmaceuticals) Aluminum hydroxide 225 mg, magnesium hydroxide 200 mg, parabens, saccharin, sorbitol/5 ml. Susp. Bot. 355 ml, 780 ml. *otc.*
Use: Antacid, antiflatulent.

Mint Sensodyne. (Block Drug Co., Inc.) Potassium nitrate 5%, saccharin, sorbitol. Toothpaste. Tube 28.3 g. *otc.*
Use: Toothpaste for sensitive teeth.

Minute-Gel. (Oral-B Laboratories, Inc.) Acidulated phosphate fluoride 1.23% Gel. Bot. 16 oz. *Rx.*
Use: Dental caries agent.

Miochol-E. (Ciba Vision) Acetylcholine Cl 1:100, mannitol 2.8% when reconstituted. Soln. In 2 ml Univials. *Rx.*
Use: Antiglaucoma agent.

•**mioflazine hydrochloride.** (MY-ah-FLAY-zeen) USAN.
Use: Vasodilator (coronary).

Miostat Intraocular Solution. (Alcon, Surgical Division) Carbachol 0.01%. Vial 1.5 ml. Pkg. 12s.
Use: Antiglaucoma agent.

miotics, cholinesterase inhibitors.
Use: Antiglaucoma agents.
See: Humorsol, Soln. (Merck & Co.).
Eserine Sulfate, Oint. (Various Mfr.).
Isopto Eserine, Soln. (Alcon Laboratories, Inc.).
Eserine Salicylate, Soln. (Alcon Laboratories, Inc.).
Phospholine Iodide, Pow. (Wyeth-Ayerst Laboratories).
Floropryl, Oint. (Merck & Co.).

•**mipafilcon a.** (mih-paff-ILL-kahn A) USAN.
Use: Contact lens material (hydrophilic).

Miradon. (Schering-Plough Corp.) Anisindione 50 mg/Tab. Bot. 100s. *Rx.*
Use: Anticoagulant.

MiraFlow Extra Strength. (Ciba Vision) Isopropyl alcohol 15.7%, poloxamer 407, amphoteric 10. Thimerosal free. Soln. Bot. 12 ml. *otc.*
Use: Contact lens care.

Miral. (Armenpharm Ltd.) Dexamethasone 0.75 mg/Tab. Bot. 100s, 1000s.
Use: Corticosteroid.

Mirapex. (Pharmacia & Upjohn) Pramipexole 0.125 mg, 0.25 mg, 1 mg, 1.5 mg. Tab. Bot. 63s (0.125 mg only), 90s. *Rx.*
Use: Antiparkinson agent.

Mircette. (Organon) Desogestrel 0.15 mg, ethinyl estradiol 0.01 mg, 0.02 mg. Tab. Pkg. *Rx.*
Use: Contraceptive.

MiraSept. (Alcon Laboratories, Inc.) **Disinfecting Solution:** Hydrogen peroxide 3%, sodium stannate, sodium nitrate. Bot. 120 ml. **Rinse and neutralizer:** Boric acid, sodium borate, sodium Cl, sodium pyruvate, EDTA. Bot. 120 ml (2s). *otc.*
Use: Contact lens care.

MiraSept Step 2. (Alcon Laboratories, Inc.) Boric acid, sodium borate, sodium chloride, EDTA, sodium pyruvate. Soln. Bot. 120 ml. *otc.*
Use: Contact lens product.

•**mirfentanil hydrochloride.** (MIHR-FEN-tan-ill) USAN.
Use: Analgesic.

•**mirincamycin hydrochloride.** (mihr-IN-kah-MY-sin) USAN.
Use: Anti-infective, antimalarial.

•**mirisetron maleate.** (my-RIH-seh-trahn) USAN.
Use: Antianxiety.

•**mirtazapine.** (mihr-TAZZ-ah-PEEN) USAN.
Use: Antidepressant.
See: Remeron, Tab. (Organon Teknika Corp.).

•**misonidazole.** (MY-so-NIH-dah-zole) USAN.
Use: Antiprotozoal (trichomonas).

•**misoprostol.** (MY-so-PRAHST-ole) USAN.
Use: Antiulcerative.
See: Cytotec, Tab. (Searle).

misoprostol and diclofenac sodium.
Use: Arthritis; antiulcerative.
See: Arthrotec, Tab. (Searle).

Mission Prenatal. (Mission Pharmacal Co.) Ferrous gluconate 260 mg (iron 30 mg), vitamins C 100 mg, B_1 5 mg, B_6 3 mg, B_2 2 mg, B_3 10 mg, B_5 1 mg, B_{12} 2 mcg, A 4000 IU, D 400 IU, Ca, zinc 15 mg/Tab. Bot. 100s. *otc.*
Use: Mineral, vitamin supplement.

Mission Prenatal F.A. (Mission Pharmacal Co.) Ferrous gluconate 260 mg (iron 30 mg), vitamins C 100 mg, B_1 5 mg, B_6 10 mg, B_2 2 mg, B_3 10 mg, B_{12} 2 mcg, folic acid 0.8 mg, A acetate 4000 IU, D 400 IU, Ca, B_5 1 mg/Tab. Bot. 100s. *otc.*
Use: Mineral, vitamin supplement.

Mission Prenatal H.P. (Mission Pharmacal Co.) Ferrous gluconate 260 mg (iron 30 mg), vitamins C 100 mg, B_1 5 mg, B_6 25 mg, B_2 2 mg, B_3 10 mg, B_5 1 mg, B_{12} 2 mcg, folic acid 0.8 mg, A 4000 IU, D 400 IU, Ca/Tab. Bot. 100s. *otc.*
Use: Mineral, vitamin supplement.

Mission Prenatal Rx. (Mission Pharmacal Co.) Vitamins A 8000 IU, D 400 IU,C 240 mg, B_1 4 mg, B_2 2 mg, B_3 20 mg, B_5 10 mg, B_6 20 mg, B_{12} 8 mcg, folic acid 1 mg, Fe 60 mg, Ca 175 mg, I, Zn 15 mg, Cu/Tab. Bot. 100s. *Rx.*
Use: Mineral, vitamin supplement.

Mission Surgical Supplement. (Mission Pharmacal Co.) Vitamins C 500 mg, B_1 2.5 mg, B_2 2.6 mg, B_3 30 mg, B_5 16.3 mg, B_6 3.6 mg, B_{12} 9 mcg, A 5000 IU, D 400 IU, E 45 IU, Fe 27 mg, Zn 22.5 mg/Tab. Bot. 100s. *otc.*
Use: Mineral, vitamin supplement.

Mithracin. (Bayer Corp. (Consumer Div.)) Plicamycin 2500 mcg/Vial. Unit vial 10s. *Rx.*
Use: Antineoplastic, antihypercalcemic.

mithramycin. (MITH-rah-MY-sin)
Use: Antineoplastic.
See: Plicamycin.

•**mitindomide.** (my-TIN-doe-MIDE) USAN.
Use: Antineoplastic.

•**mitocarcin.** (MY-toe-CAR-sin) USAN. Antibiotic derived from *Streptomyces* species.
Use: Antineoplastic.

•**mitocromin.** (MY-toe-KROE-min) USAN. Produced by *Streptomyces virdochromogenes.*
Use: Antineoplastic.

•**mitogillin.** (MY-toe-GIH-lin) USAN. An antibiotic obtained from a "unique strain" of *Aspergillus restrictus.*
Use: Antitumorigenic antibiotic; antineoplastic.

mitoguazone. (CTRC Research Foundation)
Use: Treatment of diffuse non-Hodgkin's lymphoma. [Orphan Drug]

mitolactol.
Use: Adjuvant therapy in the treatment of primary brain tumors. [Orphan Drug]

•**mitomalcin.** (MY-toe-MAL-sin) USAN. Produced by *Streptomyces malayensis.* Under study.
Use: Antineoplastic.

•**mitomycin.** (MY-toe-MY-sin) U.S.P. 23. In literature as Mitomycin C. Antibiotic isolated from *Streptomyces caespitosis.*
Use: Anti-infective; antineoplastic.
See: Mutamycin, Inj. (Bristol-Myers Squibb).

•**mitosper.** (MY-toe-sper) USAN. Substance derived from *Aspergillus* of the glaucus group.
Use: Antineoplastic.

•**mitotane.** (MY-toe-TANE) U.S.P. 23. *Formerly o,p'-DDD.*
Use: Antineoplastic.
See: Lysodren, Tab. (Bristol-Myers Oncology/Immunology).

•**mitoxantrone hydrochloride.** (MY-toe-ZAN-trone) U.S.P. 23.
Use: Antineoplastic. [Orphan Drug]
See: Novantrone (ESI Lederle Generics).

Mitran. (Roberts Pharmaceuticals) Chlordiazepoxide HCl 10 mg/Cap. Bot. 100s. *c-IV.*
Use: Anxiolytic.

Mitrolan. (Wyeth-Ayerst Laboratories) Calcium polycarbophil equivalent to polycarbophil 500 mg/Tab. Blister Pak 36s, 100s. *otc.*
Use: Laxative.

•**mivacurium chloride.** (mih-vah-CURE-ee-uhm) USAN.

Use: Neuromuscular blocker.

•**mivobulin isethionate.** (mih-VOE-byoo-lin eye-seh-THIGH-oh-nate) USAN.
Use: Antineoplastic (microtubule inhibitor).

Mixed Respiratory Vaccine. Each ml contains *Staphylococcus aureus* 1,200 million organisms, *Streptococcus* (both *viridans* and non-hemolytic) 200 million organisms, *Streptococcus (Diplococcus) pneumoniae* 150 million organisms, *Moraxella (Branhamella, Neisseria) catarrhalis* 150 million organisms, *Klebsiella pneumoniae* 150 million organisms, and *Haemophilus influenzae* types a and b 150 million organisms. Vial. 20 ml.
Use: Bacterial vaccine.
See: MRV, Inj. (Bayer Corp. (Consumer Div.)).

mixed vespid Hymenoptera venom. *Rx.*
Use: Agent for immunization.
See: Albay (Bayer Corp. (Consumer Div.)).
Pharmalgen (ALK Laboratories, Inc.).
Venomil (Bayer Corp. (Consumer Div.)).

•**mixidine.** (MIX-ih-deen) USAN.
Use: Vasodilator (coronary).

mixture 612. Dimethyl Phthalate Solution, Compound.

M-M-R II. (Merck & Co.) Lyophilized preparation of live attenuated measles virus vaccine (Attenuvax), live attenuated mumps virus vaccine (Mumpsvax), live attenuated rubella virus vaccine (Meruvax II). See details under Attenuvax, Mumpsvax and Meruvax II. Single dose vial w/diluent. Pkg. 1s, 10s. *Rx.*
Use: Agent for immunization.

Moban. (Du Pont Merck Pharmaceutical Co.) Molindone HCl. **Liq.:** 20 mg/ml concentrate. Bot. 120 ml. **Tab.:** 5 mg, 10 mg, 25 mg, 50 mg, 100 mg, lactose. Tab. Bot. 100s. *Rx.*
Use: Antipsychotic.

mobenol. Tolbutamide, U.S.P. 23.

Mobidin. (B.F. Ascher and Co.) Magnesium salicylate, anhydrous 600 mg/Tab. Bot. 100s, 500s. *Rx.*
Use: Antiarthritic.

Mobigesic. (B.F. Ascher and Co.) Magnesium salicylate 325 mg, phenyltoloxamine citrate 30 mg. Tab. Bot. 50s, 100s, Pkg. 18s. *otc.*
Use: Analgesic combination.

Mobisyl Creme. (B.F. Ascher and Co.) Trolamine salicylate in vanishing creme base. Tube 100 g. *otc.*
Use: Analgesic, topical.

moccasin bite.
See: Antivenin (Crotalidae).

•**moclobemide.** (moe-KLOE-beh-mide) USAN.
Use: Antidepressant.

moctanin. (Ethitek Pharmaceuticals) Glyceryl-l-mono-octanoate (80% to 85%), glyceryl-l-mono-decanoate (10% to 15%), glyceryl-l-2-di-octanoate (10% to 15%), free glyceryl (2.5% maximum). Bot. 120 ml. *Rx.*
Use: Urolithic.

•**modafinil.** (moe-DAFF-ih-nill) USAN.
Use: Analeptic treatment of narcolepsy and hypersomnia.
See: Provigil, Tab. (Cephalon).

•**modaline sulfate.** (MODE-al-een) USAN.
Use: Antidepressant.

Modane. (Pharmacia & Upjohn) Phenolphthalein 130 mg/Tab. Pkg. 10s, 30s. Bot. 100s. *otc.*
Use: Laxative.

Modane Bulk. (Pharmacia & Upjohn) Powdered mixture of equal parts of psyllium and dextrose. Container 14 oz. *otc.*
Use: Laxative.

Modane Mild. (Pharmacia & Upjohn) Phenolphthalein 60 mg/Tab. Bot. 10s, 30s, 100s. *otc.*
Use: Laxative.

Modane Plus. (Pharmacia & Upjohn) Phenolphthalein 60 mg, docusate sodium 100 mg/Tab. Bot. 100s, Box 10s, 30s. *otc.*
Use: Laxative.

Modane Soft. (Pharmacia & Upjohn) Docusate sodium 100 mg/Cap. UD Pkg. 30s. *otc.*
Use: Laxative.

Modane Versabran. (Pharmacia & Upjohn) Psyllium hydrophilic mucilloid in wheat bran base. Dose 3.4 g, Bot. 10 oz. *otc.*
Use: Laxative.

•**modecainide.** (moe-deh-CANE-ide) USAN.
Use: Cardiovascular (antiarrhythmic).

Modicon 21. (Ortho McNeil Pharmaceutical) Norethindrone 0.5 mg, ethinyl estradiol 35 mcg/Tab. Dialpak 21s. *Rx.*
Use: Contraceptive.

Modicon 28. (Ortho McNeil Pharmaceutical) Norethindrone 0.5 mg, ethinyl estradiol 35 mcg/Tab., 7 inert Tab. Dialpak 28s. *Rx.*
Use: Contraceptive.

modinal.
See: Gardinol Type Detergents (Various Mfr.).

Moducal. (Bristol-Myers Squibb) Maltodextrin. Pow. Can 13 oz. *otc.*
Use: Nutritional supplement.

Moduretic. (Merck & Co.) Hydrochlorothiazide 50 mg, amiloride 5 mg/Tab. Bot. 100s, UD 100s. *Rx.*
Use: Antihypertensive, diuretic.

moenomycin. Phosphorus-containing glycolipide antibiotic. Active against gram-positive organisms. Under study.

•**moexipril hydrochloride.** (moe-EX-ah-prill) USAN.
Use: Antihypertensive, ACE inhibitor.
See: Univasc, Tab. (Schwarz Pharma, Inc.).

moexipril hydrochloride and hydrochlorothiazide.
Use: Antihypertensive.
See: Uniretic, Tab. (Schwarz Pharma, Inc.).

•**mofegiline hydrochloride.** (moe-FEH-jih-leen) USAN.
Use: Antiparkinsonian.

Moist Again. (Lake Consumer Products) Aloe vera, EDTA, methylparaben, glycerin. Gel. Tube 70.8 g. *otc.*
Use: Vaginal agent.

Moi-Stir. (Kingswood Laboratories, Inc.) Dibasic sodium phosphate, Mg, Ca, NaCl, KCl, sorbitol, sodium carboxymethylcellulose, parabens. Soln. 120 ml with pump spray. *otc.*
Use: Saliva substitute.

Moi-Stir Swabsticks. (Kingswood Laboratories, Inc.) Dibasic sodium phosphate, Mg, Ca, NaCl, KCl, sorbitol, sodium carboxymethylcellulose, parabens. Soln. Pkt. 3s. *otc.*
Use: Saliva substitute.

Moisture Drops. (Bausch & Lomb Pharmaceuticals) Hydroxypropyl methylcellulose 0.5%, povidone 0.1%, glycerin 0.2%, benzalkonium Cl 0.01%, EDTA, NaCl, boric acid, KCl, sodium borate. Soln. Bot. 0.5 oz, 1 oz. *otc.*
Use: Artificial tears.

molar phosphate.
W/Fluoride ion.
See: Coral Prods. (Young Dental).
Karigel, Gel. (Young Dental).

molecusol-carbamazepine.
See: PR-320.

•**molgramostim.** (mahl-GRAH-moe-STIM) USAN.
Use: Hematopoietic stimulant, antineutropenic.

•**molinazone.** (moe-LEEN-ah-zone) USAN.
Use: Analgesic.

•**molindone hydrochloride.** (moe-LIN-dohn) U.S.P. 23.
Use: Antipsychotic.
See: Moban, Tab. (Du Pont Merck Pharmaceutical Co.).

Mollifene Ear Drops. (Pfeiffer Co.) Glycerin, camphor, cajaput oil, eucalyptus oil, thyme oil. Soln. Bot. 24 ml. *otc.*
Use: Otic.

•**molsidomine.** (mole-SIH-doe-meen) USAN.
Use: Antianginal, vasodilator (coronary).

molybdenum solution. (American Quinine) Molybdenum 25 mcg/ml (as 46 mcg/ml ammonium molybdate tetrahydrate). Inj. Vial 10 ml. *Rx.*
Use: Nutritional supplement, parenteral.

Molycu. (Burns) Meprobamate 400 mg, copper 60 mg/ml. *Rx.*
Use: Antidote.

Moly-Pak. (SoloPak Pharmaceuticals, Inc.) Molybdenum 25 mcg. Inj. Vial 10 ml. *Rx.*
Use: Nutritional supplement, parenteral.

Molypen. (Fujisawa USA, Inc.) Ammonium molybdate tetrahydrate 46 mcg/ml. Vial 10 ml. *Rx.*
Use: Nutritional supplement, parenteral.

Momentum. (Whitehall Robins Laboratories) Aspirin 500 mg, phenyltoloxamine citrate 15 mg/Capl. Bot. 24s, 48s. *otc.*
Use: Analgesic.

Momentum Muscular Backache Formula. (Whitehall Robins Laboratories) Magnesium salicylate tetrahydrate 580 mg (equivalent to 467 mg magnesium salicylate anhydrous)/Capl. Box. 48s. *otc.*
Use: Analgesic compound.

•**mometasone furoate.** (moe-MET-uh-SONE FYU-roh-ate) U.S.P. 23.
Use: Topical steroid.
See: Elocon Cream, Oint., Lot. (Schering-Plough Corp.).
Nasonex, Nasal Spray (Schering-Plough Corp.).

monacetyl pyrogallol. Eugallol. Pyrogallol Monoacetate.
Use: Keratolytic.

Monafed. (Monarch Pharmaceuticals) Guaifenesin 600 mg, lactose/SR Tab. Bot. 100s. *Rx.*
Use: Expectorant.

Monafed DM. (Monarch Pharmaceuticals) Guaifenesin 600 mg, dextromethorphan HBr 30 mg/ER Tab. Bot. 100s. *Rx.*
Use: Antitussive, expectorant.

monalium hydrate. Hydrated magnesium aluminate. Magaldrate.
See: Riopan, Tab., Susp. (Wyeth-

Ayerst Laboratories).

•**monatepil maleate.** (moe-NAT-eh-pill) USAN.
Use: Antianginal; antihypertensive.

•**monensin.** (mah-NEN-sin) U.S.P. 23.
Use: Antifungal, anti-infective, antiprotozoal.

•**monensin sodium.** (mah-NEN-sin) U.S.P. 23.
Use: Antifungal, anti-infective, antiprotozoal.

Monistat Dual-Pak. (Ortho McNeil Pharmaceutical) Miconazole nitrate suppositories and cream. **200 mg/ Supp.:** Pkg. 3s w/applicator. **Cream 2%.:** Tube 15 g, 30 g, 90 g. *Rx.*
Use: Antifungal, vaginal.

Monistat 3 Vaginal Suppositories. (Ortho McNeil Pharmaceutical) Miconazole nitrate 200 mg/Supp. Pkg. 3s w/ applicator. *Rx.*
Use: Antifungal, vaginal.

Monistat 7 Vaginal Cream. (Advanced Care Products) Miconazole nitrate 2% in water-miscible cream. Tube 45 g w/ dose applicator. *otc.*
Use: Antifungal, vaginal.

Monistat 7 Vaginal Suppositories. (Advanced Care Products) Miconazole nitrate 100 mg/Supp. Pkg. 7s w/applicator. *otc.*
Use: Antifungal, vaginal.

Monistat 7 Combination Pack. (Advanced Care Products) **Vaginal Supp.:** Miconazole nitrate 100 mg. In 7s with applicator. **Topical Cream:** Miconazole nitrate 2%. Tube 9 g. *otc.*
Use: Antifungal, vaginal.

Monistat-Derm Cream. (Ortho McNeil Pharmaceutical) Miconazole nitrate 2%, pegoxol 7 stearate, peglicol 5 oleate, mineral oil, benzoic acid, butylated hydroxyanisole. Tube 15 g, 30 g, 90 g. *otc.*
Use: Antifungal, topical.

Monistat-Derm Lotion. (Advanced Care Products) Miconazole nitrate 2%, pegoxol 7 stearate, peglicol 5 oleate, mineral oil, benzoic acid, butylated hydroxyanisole. Squeeze bot. 30 ml, 60 ml. *Rx.*
Use: Antifungal, topical.

monoamine oxidase inhibitors.
Use: Antidepressant.
See: Parnate, Tab. (SmithKline Beecham Pharmaceuticals).
Nardil, Tab. (Parke-Davis).

•**mono and di-acetylated monoglycerides.** N.F. 18. A mixture of glycerin esterfied mono- and diesters of edible fatty acids followed by direct acetylation.
Use: Pharmaceutic aid (plasticizer).

•**mono- and diglycerides.** N.F. 18. A mixture of mono- and diesters of fatty acids from edible oils.
Use: Fatty acids, pharmaceutic aid (emulsifying agent).

•**monobenzone.** (mahn-oh-BEN-zone) U.S.P. 23.
Use: Depigmentor.
See: Benoquin, Oint., Lot. (Zeneca Pharmaceuticals).

monobenzyl ether of hydroquinone.
See: Benoquin, Oint., Lot. (Zeneca Pharmaceuticals).

Monocaps Tablets. (Freeda Vitamins, Inc.) Iron 14 mg, vitamins A 10,000 IU, D 400 IU, E 15 IU, B_1 15 mg, B_2 15 mg, B_3 41 mg, B_5 15 mg, B_6 15 mcg, B_{12} 15 mcg, C 125 mg, folic acid 0.1 mg, biotin 15 mg, PABA, L-lysine, Ca, Cu, I, K, Mg, Mn, Se, Zn 12 mg, lecithin/Tab. Bot. 100s, 250s, 500s. *otc.*
Use: Mineral, vitamin supplement.

Mono-Chlor. (Gordon Laboratories) Monochloroacetic acid 80%. Bot. 15 ml.
Use: Cauterizing agent.

monochloroacetic acid.
Use: Cauterizing agent.
See: Mono-Chlor, Soln. (Gordon Laboratories).

monchlorophenol-para.
See: Camphorated para-chlorophenol, Liq. (Novocol Chemical Mfr. Co.).

Monocid. (SmithKline Beecham Pharmaceuticals) Cefonicid sodium 500 mg, 1 g, 10 g/Vial and piggyback vial. Pharmacy Bulk Vial.
Use: Anti-infective, cephalosporin.

Monoclate. (Centeon) Monoclonal antibody derived stable lyophilized concentrate of Factor VIII: R heat-treated. With albumin (human) 1% to 2%, mannitol 0.8%, histadine 1.2 mM. Inj. Vial 1 ml single dose with diluent. *Rx.*
Use: Antihemophilic.

Monoclate-P. (Centeon) Stable concentrate of Factor VIII: C. $\approx$ 300 to 450 mmol sodium ions and $\approx$ 2 to 5 mmol calcium (as chloride) per L. With albumin (human) 1% to 2%, mannitol 0.8%, histadine 1.2 mmol, $\leq$ 50 ng/100 AHF activity units mouse protein. Pow. for Inj. *Rx.*
Use: Antihemophilic.

monoclonal antibodies (murine) anti-idiotype melanoma associated antigen.
Use: Invasive cutaneous melanoma. [Orphan Drug]

monoclonal antibodies (murine or hu-

man) B-cell lymphoma. (IDEC Pharmaceuticals)
Use: B-cell lymphoma. [Orphan Drug]

monoclonal antibodies PM-81.
Use: Adjunctive treatment for leukemia. [Orphan Drug]

monoclonal antibodies PM-81 and AML-2-23.
Use: Leukemic bone marrow transplantation. [Orphan Drug]

monoclonal antibody 17-1A.
Use: Pancreatic cancer. [Orphan Drug]

monoclonal antibody to CD4, 5a8. (Biogen)
Use: Postexposure prophylaxis for HIV. [Orphan Drug]

monoclonal antibody (human) against hepatitis B virus.
Use: Prophylaxis in hepatitis B reinfection in liver transplants. [Orphan Drug]

monoclonal antibody to lupus nephritis. (Medclone, Inc.)
Use: Immunization. [Orphan Drug]

•**monoctanoin.** (MAHN-ahk-tuh-NO-in) USAN.
Use: Anticholelithogenic (dissolution of gallstones). [Orphan Drug]
See: Moctanin, Inf. (Ethitek Pharmaceuticals).

monocycline hydrochloride.
See: Minocin I.V., Syr., Cap. (ESI Lederle Generics).

Mono-Diff Test. (Wampole Laboratories)
Use: Diagnostic aid, mononucleosis.

Monodox. (Oclassen Pharmaceuticals, Inc.) Doxycycline monohydrate equivalent to 50 mg, 100 mg doxycycline. Cap. Bot. 50s (100 mg only), 100s (50 mg only), 250s, (100 mg only) *Rx.*
Use: Anti-infective, tetracycline.

•**monoethanolamine.** (mahn-oh-eth-an-OLE-ah-meen) N.F. 18.
Use: Pharmaceutic aid (surfactant).

Mono-Gesic. (Schwarz Pharma, Inc.) Salsalate (salicylic acid) 750 mg/Tab. Bot. 100s, 500s. *Rx.*
Use: Analgesic.

monoiodomethanesulfonate sodium.
See: Methiodal Sodium, U.S.P. 23.

Monojel. (Sherwood Davis & Geck) Glucose 40%. UD 25 g. *otc.*
Use: Hyperglycemic.

Monoket. (Schwarz Pharma, Inc.) Isosorbide mononitrate 10 mg, 20 mg. Tab. Bot. 60s, 100s, 180s, UD 100s. *Rx.*
Use: Antianginal.

Mono-Latex. (Wampole Laboratories) Two-minute latex agglutination slide test for the qualitative or semiquantitative detection of infectious mononucleosis heterophile antibodies in serum or plasma. Test kit 20s, 50s, 1000s.
Use: Diagnostic aid.

monolaurin.
Use: Treatment of congenital primary ichthyosis. [Orphan Drug]
See: Glylorin.

monomercaptoundecahydrocloso-dodecaborate sodium.
Use: Treatment of glioblastoma multiforme. [Orphan Drug]

Mononine. (Centeon) Factor IX 100 IU/ml with nondetectable levelsof Factors II, VII and X with histidine ≈ 10 mM, mannitol ≈ 3%, mouse protein ≤ 50 ng/100 IU Factor IX activity units. Pow. for Inj. (lyophilized). Single-dose vials with diluent. *Rx.*
Use: Antihemophilic.

mononucleosis tests.
Use: Diagnostic aid.
See: Mono-Diff Test (Wampole Laboratories).
Mono-Latex (Wampole Laboratories).
Mono-Plus (Wampole Laboratories).
Monospot (Ortho Diagnostic Systems, Inc.).
Monosticon (Organon Teknika Corp.).
Monosticon Dri-Dot (Organon Teknika Corp.).
Mono-Sure Test (Wampole Laboratories).

Monopar. Stilbazium Iodide.
Use: Anthelmintic.

monophen.
Use: Orally, cholecystography.

Mono-Plus. (Wampole Laboratories) To diagnose infectious mononucleosis from serum, plasma, or fingertip blood. Test kits 24s.
Use: Diagnostic aid.

Monopril. (Bristol-Myers Squibb) Fosinopril sodium 10 mg, 20 mg, 40 mg, lactose. Tab. In 30s, 90s, 1000s. *Rx.*
Use: Antihypertensive; congestive heart failure.

•**monosodium glutamate.** (mahn-oh-SO-dee-uhm GLUE-tah-mate) N.F. 18.
Use: Pharmaceutic aid (flavor, perfume).

monosodium phosphate.
See: Sodium Biphosphate, U.S.P. 23.

Monospot. (Ortho Diagnostic Systems, Inc.) Diagnosis of infectious mononucleosis. Test kit 20s.
Use: Diagnostic aid.

monostearin. (Various Mfr.) Glyceryl monostearate.

Monosticon Dri-Dot. (Organon Teknika Corp.) Diagnosis of infectious mononucleosis.Test kit 40s, 100s.

Use: Diagnostic aid.

Mono-Sure Test. (Wampole Laboratories) One-minute hemagglutination slide test for the differential qualitative detection and quantitative determination of infectious mononucleosis heterophile antibodies in serum or plasma. Kit 20s.
Use: Diagnostic aid.

Monosyl. (Arcum) Secobarbital sodium 1 gr, butabarbital 0.5 gr/Tab.Bot. 100s, 1000s. *c-II.*
Use: Hypnotic, sedative.

Monotard Human Insulin. (Squibb/Novo) Human insulin zinc 100 units/ml. Susp. Vial 10 ml. *otc.*
Use: Antidiabetic.

•**monothioglycerol.** (mahn-oh-thigh-oh-GLIS-er-ole) N.F. 18.
Use: Pharmaceutic aid (preservative).

Mono-Vacc Test O.T. (Pasteur Merieux Connaught) 5 tuberculin units by the mantoux method. Multiple puncture disposable device. Box 25s (tamperproof). *Rx.*
Use: Diagnostic aid, tuberculosis.

monoxychlorosene. A stabilized, buffered, organichypochlorous acid derivative.
See: Oxychlorosene (Guardian Chem.).

Monsel Solution. (Wade) Bot. 2 oz, 4 oz.
Use: Styptic solution.

•**montelukast sodium.** (mahn-teh-LOO-kast) USAN.
Use: Antiasthmatic (leukotriene antagonist).
See: Singulair, Tab., Chew. Tab. (Merck & Co.).

Monurol. (Forest Pharmaceutical, Inc.) Fosfomycin tromethamine 3 g/Gran. Single-dose packet. *Rx.*
Use: Anti-infective, urinary.

•**morantel tartrate.** (moe-RAN-tell) USAN.
Use: Anthelmintic.

moranyl.
See: Suramin Sodium.

Morco. (Archer-Taylor) Cod liver oil ointment, zinc oxide, benzethonium Cl, benzocaine 1%. 1.5 oz, lb. *otc.*
Use: Antiseptic, antipruritic, topical.

More Dophilus. (Freeda Vitamins, Inc.) Acidophilus-carrot derivative 4 billion units/g. Pow. Bot. 120 g. *otc.*
Use: Antidiarrheal, nutritional supplement.

•**moricizine.** (MAHR-IH-sizz-een) USAN.
Use: Cardiovascular agent (antiarrhythmic).
See: Ethmozine (Du Pont Merck Pharmaceutical Co.).

•**morniflumate.** (MAR-nih-FLEW-mate) USAN.
Use: Anti-inflammatory.

Moroline. (Schering-Plough Corp.) Petrolatum. Jar 1.75 oz, 3.75 oz, 15 oz. *otc.*
Use: Dermatologic, lubricant, protectant.

Morpen. (Major Pharmaceuticals) Ibuprofen 400 mg, 600 mg/Tab. Bot. 500s. *Rx.*
Use: Analgesic, NSAID.

morphine and atropine sulfates tablets.
Use: Analgesic, parasympatholytic.

morphine hydrochloride. (Various Mfr.) Pow. Bot. 1 oz, 5 oz. *c-II.*
Use: Analgesic.

•**morphine sulfate.** (MORE-feen) U.S.P. 23.
Use: Analgesic, narcotic; sedative.
See: Astramorph PF, Inj. (Astra).
Duramorph, Inj. (ESI Lederle Generics).
Infumorph, Inj. (ESI Lederle Generics).
Kadian, SR Cap. (Zeneca Pharmaceuticals).
MS Contin (Purdue Frederick Co.).
MSIR (Purdue Frederick Co.).
OMS Concentrate, Soln. (Upsher-Smith Labs, Inc.).
Oramorph (Roxane Laboratories, Inc.).
RMS, Rec. Supp. (Upsher-Smith).
Roxanol, Soln. (Roxane Laboratories, Inc.).
Roxanol 100, Soln. (Roxane Laboratories, Inc.).
Roxanol Rescudose, Soln. (Roxane Laboratories, Inc.).
W/Tartar emetic, bloodroot, ipecac, squill, wild cherry.
See: Roxanol T, Soln. (Roxane Laboratories, Inc.).
Roxanol UD, Soln. (Roxane Laboratories, Inc.).

morphine sulfate. (Abbott) 0.5 mg/ml. Inj. Amps and vials 10 ml. *c-II.*
Use: Analgesic, narcotic.

morphine sulfate. (Eli Lilly) 10 mg, 15 mg, 30 mg, Soln. Tab. Bot. 100s. *c-II.*
Use: Analgesic, narcotic.

morphine sulfate. (Roxane) **Inj.:** 10 mg/5 ml, 20 mg/5 ml. Soln. Bot. 100 ml, 500 ml. UD 5 ml, 10 ml (10 mg/5 ml only). **Tab.:** 15 mg, 30 mg. Bot. 100s, UD 100s. *c-II.*
Use: Analgesic, narcotic.

morphine sulfate. (Various Mfr.) **Inj.:** 0.5 mg/ml (Amp. Vial 10 ml), 1 mg/ml (Vial 2 ml, 10 ml, 30 ml, 60 ml. Amp. 10 ml), 2 mg/ml (Vial 30 ml, Syr. and *Tu-*

bex 1 ml); 4 mg/ml (Disp. Syr. 1 ml, 2 ml. *Tubex* 1 ml), 5 mg/ml (Vial 1 ml, 30 ml), 8 mg/ml (Vial, Amp., Syr., 1 ml. 1 ml fill in 2 ml *Tubex*, Amp. Vial), 10 mg/ml (1 ml Syr., Vial, Amp.; Vial 10 ml, 30 ml; Syr. 30 ml; 1 ml fill in 2 ml *Tubex*, Amp., Vial), 15 mg/ml (Amp. and Vial 1 ml, 20 ml; 1 ml in fill in 2 ml *Tubex*, Amp. Vial), 25 mg/ml (Syr. 4 ml, 10 ml, 20 ml, 30 ml, 40 ml, 50 ml; Vial 10 ml, 20 ml, 40 ml); 50 mg/ml (Syr. 10 ml, 20 ml, 30 ml, 50 ml; Vial 20 ml, 40 ml, 50 ml). **Rec. Supp.:** 5 mg, 10 mg, 20 mg, 30 mg. Box 12s, 50s (30 mg only). *c-II.*
Use: Analgesic, narcotic.

•**morrhuate sodium injection.** (MORE-you-ate) U.S.P. 23.
Use: Sclerosing agent.

Morton Salt Substitute. (Morton Grove Pharmaceuticals, Inc.) Potassium Cl, fumaric acid, tricalcium phosphate, monocalcium phosphate. Na < 0.5 mg/5 g (0.02 mEq/5 g), K 2800 mg/5 g (72 mEq/5 g) 88.6 g. *otc.*
Use: Salt substitute.

Morton Seasoned Salt Substitute. (Morton Grove Pharmaceuticals, Inc.) Potassium chloride, spices, sugar, fumaric acid, triacalcium phosphate, monocalcium phosphate. Na < 1 mg/5 g (< 0.04 mEq/5 g), K 2165 mg/5 g (56 mEq/5 g). Bot. 85.1 g. *otc.*
Use: Salt substitute.

Mosco. (Medtech Laboratories, Inc.) 17.6% Salicylic acid. Jar 10 ml. *otc.*
Use: Keratolytic.

Motilium. (Janssen Pharmaceutical, Inc.) Domperidone maleate. *Rx.*
Use: Antiemetic.

Motion Aid. (Vangard Labs, Inc.) Dimenhydrinate 50 mg/Tab. Bot. 100s, 1000s, UD 10 × 10s.
Use: Antiemetic, antivertigo.

Motion Cure. (Wisconsin Pharmacal Co.) Meclizine 25 mg/Chew. Tab. 12s.
Use: Antiemetic, antivertigo.

motion sickness agents.
See: Antinauseants.
Bucladin, Softab Tab. (Zeneca Pharmaceuticals).
Dramamine, Preps. (Searle).
Emetrol, Liq. (Rhone-Poulenc Rorer Pharmaceuticals, Inc.).
Marezine, Tab, Amp. (Glaxo-Wellcome).
Scopolamine HBr (Various Mfr.).

Motofen. (Carnrick Laboratories, Inc.) Difenoxin HCl 1 mg, atropine sulfate 0.025 mg/Tab. Bot. 100s. *c-IV.*
Use: Antidiarrheal.

•**motretinide.** (MOE-TREH-tih-nide) USAN.
Use: Keratolytic.

Motrin. (Ortho McNeil Pharmaceutical) Ibuprofen. **Capl.: 100 mg:** Bot. 100s; **Tab: 50 mg or 100 mg:** Bot. 100s; **300 mg:** Bot. 500s, Unit-Of-Use 60s; **400 mg:** Bot. 500s, Unit-of-Use 100s, UD 100s; **600 mg:** Bot. 500s, Unit-of-Use 100s, UD 100s; **800 mg:** Bot. 500s, Unit-of-Use 100s, UD 100s. **Chew. Tab.: 50 mg:** 100s. **100 mg:** 100s. **Susp.:** 100 mg/5 ml, sucrose. 120, 480 ml. *Rx.*
Use: Analgesic, NSAID.

Motrin, Children's. (McNeil Consumer Products Co.) Ibuprofen 100 mg/5 ml, sucrose. Susp. Bot. 120 ml, 480 ml. *Rx-otc.*
Use: Analgesic, NSAID.

Motrin IB. (Pharmacia & Upjohn) Ibuprofen 200 mg. **Tab. or Capl.:** Bot. 24s, 50s, 100s, 165s. **Gelcaps:** Parabens. Bot. 24s, 50s. *otc.*
Use: Analgesic, NSAID.

Motrin IB Sinus. (Pharmacia & Upjohn) Pseudoephedrine HCl 30 mg, ibuprofen 200 mg. Capl. Pkg. 20s, Bot. 40s. *otc.*
Use: Decongestant, NSAID.

Motrin, Junior Strength. (Ortho McNeil Pharmaceutical) Ibuprofen 100 mg, aspartame, phenylalalanine 5 mg. Chew. Tab. Pkg. 24s. *otc.*
Use: Analgesic.

MouthKote. (Unimed) Xylitol, sorbitol, Mucoprotective Factor (MPF), yerba santa, saccharin. Alcohol free. Soln. Bot. 60, 240 ml, UD 5 ml. *otc.*
Use: Saliva substitute.

MouthKote O/R Rinse. (Unimed) Benzyl alcohol, menthol, sorbitol. Rinse. Sugar free. Bot. 240 ml. *otc.*
Use: Antiseptic.

MouthKote O/R Solution. (Unimed) Diphenhydramine HCl 1.25%, cetylpyridinium Cl, EDTA, saccharin. Soln. Bot. 40 ml. *otc.*
Use: Antiseptic.

MouthKote P/R. (Parnell Pharmaceuticals, Inc.) **Oint.:** Diphenhydramine HCl 25%. Tube 15 g. **Soln.:** Diphenhydramine HCl 1.25%, cetylpyridinium Cl, EDTA, saccharin. Bot. 40 ml.
Use: Mouth and throat preparation.

•**moxalactam disodium for injection.** (MOX-ah-LACK-tam die-SO-dee-uhm) U.S.P. 23.
Use: Anti-infective.
See: Moxam, Inj. (Eli Lilly and Co.)

Moxam. (Eli Lilly and Co.) Moxalactam di-

sodium. Vial 1 g/10 ml Traypak 10s; Vial 2 g/20 ml Traypak 10s; Vial 10 g/100 ml Traypak 6s. *Rx.*
Use: Anti-infective, cephalosporin.

•**moxazocine.** (MOX-AZE-oh-seen) USAN.
Use: Analgesic, antitussive.

•**moxilubant maleate.** USAN.
Use: Treatment of rheumatoid arthritis and psoriasis (leukotriene B_4 receptor antagonist).

•**moxnidazole.** (MOX-NIH-dazz-ole) USAN.
Use: Antiprotozoal (trichomonas).

Moxy Compound. (Major Pharmaceuticals) Theophylline 130 mg, ephedrine 25 mg, hydroxyzine HCl 10 mg/Tab. Bot. 100s. *Rx.*
Use: Antiasthmatic compound.

Moyco Fluoride Rinse. (Moyco Union Broach Division) Fluoride 2%. Flavor. Bot. 128 oz. with pump. *Rx-otc.*
Use: Dental caries agent.

6-MP.
Use: Antimetabolite.
See: Purinethol, Tab. (GlaxoWellcome).

M-Prednisol-40. (Taylor Pharmaceuticals) Methylprednisolone acetate 40 mg/ml. Inj. Susp. Vial 5 ml. *Rx.*
Use: Corticosteroid.

M-Prednisol-80. (Taylor Pharmaceuticals) Methylprednisolone acetate 80 mg/ml. Inj. Susp. Vial 5 ml.
Use: Corticosteroid.

MRV. (Bayer Corp. (Consumer Div.)) 2000 million organisms/ml from *Staphylococcus aureus* (1200 million), *Streptococcus*, viridans and non-hemolytic (200 million), *Streptococcus pneumoniae* (150 million), *Branhamella catarrhalis* (150 million), *Klebsiella pneumoniae* (150 million), *Haemophilus influenzae* (150 million). Inj. Vial 20 ml. *Rx.*
Use: Immunization.

M-R-VAX II. (Merck & Co.) Live attenuated measles virus vaccine (Attenuvax) and live attenuated rubella virus vaccine (Meruvax II). See details under Attenuvax and Meruvax II. Single-dose vial w/diluent. Pkg. 1s, 10s. *Rx.*
Use: Immunization.

MS Contin. (Purdue Frederick Co.) Morphine sulfate. **CR Tab.: 15 mg or 100 mg:** Bot. 100s, 500s, UD 25s. **30 mg:** Bot. 50s, 100s, 250s, 500s, UD 25s. **60 mg or 200 mg:** Bot. 100s, 500s, UD 25s. **200 mg:** Bot. 100s, UD 25s. *c-II.*
Use: Analgesic, narcotic.

MSIR. (Purdue Frederick Co.) Morphine sulfate. **Tab.:** 15 mg, 30 mg. Bot. 100s. **Cap.:** 15 mg, 30 mg. Bot. 100s. **Soln.:** 10 mg/5 ml, 20 mg/5 ml, 20 mg/ml. Bot. 30 ml. (20 mg/ml only), 120 ml. *c-II.*
Use: Analgesic, narcotic.

MSL-109. (Novartis Pharmaceutical Corp.) Monoclonal antibody.
Use: Antiviral. [Orphan Drug]

MS/L-Concentrate. (Richwood Pharmaceuticals) Morphine sulfate 100 mg/5 ml. Oral Soln. Bot. 120 ml w/calibrated dropper. *c-II.*
Use: Analgesic, narcotic.

MS/S. (Richwood Pharmaceuticals) Morphine sulfate 5 mg, 10 mg, 20 mg, 30 mg/Supp. 12s. *c-II.*
Use: Analgesic, narcotic.

MSTA. (Pasteur Merieux Connaught) Mumps skin test antigen 40 complement-fixing units/ml, Inj. Vial 1 ml. *Rx.*
Use: Diagnostic aid.

MTC. Mitomycin. *Rx.*
Use: Anti-infective.
See: Mutamycin, Pow. (Bristol-Myers Oncology/Immunology).

M.T.E.-4. (Fujisawa USA, Inc.) Zn 1 mg, Cu 0.4 mg, Cr 4 mcg, Mn 0.1 mg/ml. Inj. Vial 3 ml, 10 ml, MD Vial 30 ml. *Rx.*
Use: Mineral supplement.

M.T.E.-4 Concentrated. (Fujisawa USA, Inc.) Zn 5 mg, Cu 1 mg, Cr 10 mcg, Mn 0.5 mg/ml. Inj. Vial 1 ml, MD Vial 10 ml. *Rx.*
Use: Mineral supplement.

M.T.E.-5. (Fujisawa USA, Inc.) Zn 1 mg, Cu 0.4 mg, Cr 4 mcg, Mn 0.1 mg, Se 20 mcg/ml. Inj. Vial 10 ml. *Rx.*
Use: Mineral supplement.

M.T.E.-5 Concentrated. (Fujisawa USA, Inc.) Zn 5 mg, Cu 1 mg, Cr 10 mcg, Mn 0.5 mg, Se 60 mcg/ml. Inj. Vial 1 ml, MD vial 10 ml.
Use: Mineral supplement.

M.T.E.-6. (Fujisawa USA, Inc.) Zn 1 mg, Cu 0.4 mg, Cr 4 mcg, Mn 0.1 mg, Se 20 mcg, I 25 mcg/ml. Inj. Vial 10 ml. *Rx.*
Use: Mineral supplement.

M.T.E.-6 Concentrate. (Fujisawa USA, Inc.) Zn 5 mg, Cu 1 mg, Cr 10 mcg, Mn 0.5 mg, Se 60 mcg, I 75 mcg/ml. Inj. Vial 1 ml. MD vial 10 ml. *Rx.*
Use: Mineral supplement.

M.T.E.-7. (Fujisawa USA, Inc.) Zn 1 mg, Cu 0.4 mg, Mn 0.1 mg, Cr 4 mcg, Se 20 mcg, I 25 mcg, Mo 25 mcg/ml. Vial 10 ml. *Rx.*
Use: Mineral supplement.

MTP-PE. (Novartis Pharmaceutical Corp.) Muramyl-tripeptide.
Use: Immunomodulator.

MTX. *Rx.*

Use: Antineoplastic, antipsoriatic.
See: Methotrexate.

MUC 9 + 4 Pediatric. (Fujisawa USA, Inc.) Vitamin A 2300 IU, D 400 IU, E 7 mg, B_1 1.2 mg, B_2 1.4 mg, B_3 17 mg, B_5 5 mg, B_6 1 mg, B_{12} 1 mcg, C 80 mg, biotin 20 mcg, folic acid 0.14 mg, K 200 mcg/5ml, mannitol 375 mg. Pow. Vial. 10 ml. *Rx.*
Use: Nutritional supplement, parenteral.

mucilloid of psyllium seed.
W/Dextrose.
See: Metamucil, Liq. (Searle).

mucin.
See: Gastric Mucin (Wilson).

Muco-Fen-DM. (Wakefield Pharmaceuticals, Inc.) Guaifenesin 600 mg, dextromethorphan HBr 30 mg/TR Tab. Bot. 100s. *Rx.*
Use: Antitussive, expectorant.

Muco-Fen-LA. (Wakefield Pharmaceuticals, Inc.) Guaifenesin 600 mg, dye free/TR Tab. Bot. 100s. *Rx.*
Use: Expectorant.

mucolytics.
Use: Respiratory.
See: Mucomyst, Soln. (Bristol-Myers Squibb).

Mucomyst. (Bristol-Myers Squibb) A sterile 20% solution of acetylcysteine for nebulization or direct instillation into the lung as a mucolytic agent. Approved as antidote for acetaminophen overdose. Vial. **4 ml:** Ctn. 12s; **10 ml:** Ctn. 3s with dropper; **30 ml:** Ctn. 3s. *Rx.*
Use: Respiratory.

Mucomyst 10. (Bristol-Myers Squibb) A sterile 10% solution of acetylcysteine for nebulization or direct instillation into the lung as a mucolytic agent. Approved as antidote for acetaminophen overdose. Vial. **4 ml:** Ctn. 12s; **10 ml:** Ctn. 3s with dropper; **30 ml:** Ctn. 3s. *Rx.*
Use: Respiratory.

Mucosil-10 & -20 Solution. (Dey Laboratories, Inc.) Acetylcysteine sodium salt 10% or 20%. Soln. Vial 4 ml Box 12s. *Rx.*
Use: Respiratory.

Mudd. (Chattem Consumer Products) Natural hydrated magnesium aluminum silicate. Topical preparation. *otc.*
Use: Cleanser.

Mudrane. (ECR Pharmaceuticals) Aminophylline (anhydrous) 130 mg, phenobarbital 8 mg, ephedrine HCl 16 mg, potassium iodide 195 mg/Tab. Bot. 100s. *Rx.*
Use: Antiasthmatic combination.

Mudrane-2. (ECR Pharmaceuticals) Potassium iodide 195 mg, aminophylline (anhydrous) 130 mg/Tab. Bot. 100s. *Rx.*
Use: Antiasthmatic combination.

Mudrane GG. (ECR Pharmaceuticals) Aminophylline (anhydrous) 130 mg, ephedrine HCl 16 mg, guaifenesin 100 mg, phenobarbital 8 mg/Tab. Bot. 100s. *Rx.*
Use: Antiasthmatic combination.

Mudrane GG-2. (ECR Pharmaceuticals) Guaifenesin 100 mg, theophylline 111 mg/Tab. Bot. 100s. *Rx.*
Use: Antiasthmatic combination.

Mudrane GG Elixir. (ECR Pharmaceuticals) Theophylline 20 mg, ephedrine HCl 4 mg, guaifenesin 26 mg, phenobarbital 2.5 mg/5 ml, alcohol 20%. Bot. pt, 0.5 gal. *Rx.*
Use: Antiasthmatic combination.

Multa-Gen 12 + E. (Jones Medical Industries, Inc.) Vitamin A 5000 IU, D 400 IU, B_1 2 mg, B_2 2 mg, B_6 0.5 mg, B_{12} 3 mcg, C 37.5 mg, E 15 IU, folic acid 0.2 mg, nicotinamide 20 mg/Cap. Bot. 60s, 500s, 1000s. *otc.*
Use: Vitamin supplement.

MulTE-PAK-4. (SoloPak Pharmaceuticals, Inc.) Zn 1 mg, Cu 0.4 mg, Mn 0.1 mg, Cr 4 mg/ml. Inj. Vial 3 ml, 10 ml, 30 ml. *Rx.*
Use: Mineral supplement.

MulTE-PAK -5. (SoloPak Pharmaceuticals, Inc.) Zn 1 mg, Cu 0.4 mg, Mn 0.1 mg, Cr 4 mg, Se 20 mcg/ml. Inj. Vial 3 ml, 10 ml. *Rx.*
Use: Mineral supplement.

Multi-B-Plex. (Forest Pharmaceutical, Inc.) Vitamins B_1 100 mg, B_2 1 mg, nicotinamide 100 mg, pantothenic acid 10 mg, B_6 10 mg/ml. Inj. Vial 10 ml, 30 ml. *Rx.*
Use: Mineral, vitamin supplement.

Multi-B-Plex Capsules. (Forest Pharmaceutical, Inc.) Vitamins B_1 50 mg, B_2 5 mg, niacinamide 50 mg, calcium pantothenate 5.4 mg, B_6 0.2 mg, C 150 mg, B_{12} 1 mcg/Cap. Bot. 100s, 1000s. *otc.*
Use: Mineral, vitamin supplement.

Multi-Day. (NBTY, Inc.) Vitamins A 5000 IU, D 400 IU, E 30 mg, B_1 1.5 mg, B_2 1.7 mg, B_3 20 mg, B_5 10 mg, B_6 2 mg, B_{12} 6 mcg, C 60 mg, FA 0.4 ml/Tab. Bot. 100s. *otc.*
Use: Vitamin supplement.

Multi-Day Plus Iron. (NBTY, Inc.) Fe 18 mg, A 5000 IU, D 400 IU, E 15 mg, B_1 1.5 mg, B_2 1.7 mg, B_3 20 mg, B_6 2 mg, B_{12} 6 mcg, C 60 mg, FA 0.4 mg. Tab. Bot. 100s. *otc.*
Use: Vitamin supplement.

Multi-Day Plus Minerals. (NBTY, Inc.)

Fe 18 mg, A 6500 IU, D 400 IU, E 30 mg, B_1 1.5 mg, B_2 1.7 mg, B_3 20 mg, B_5 10 mg, B_6 2 mg, B_{12} 6 mcg, C 60 mg, FA 0.4 mg, Ca, Cl, Cr, Cu, I, K, Mg, Mn, Mo, P, Se, Zn 15 mg, biotin 30 mcg. Tab. Bot. 100s. *otc.*
Use: Vitamin supplement.

Multi-Day with Calcium and Extra Iron Tablets. (NBTY, Inc.) Fe 27 mg, A 5000 IU, D 400 IU, E 30 mg, B_1 1.5 mg, B_2 1.7 mg, B_3 20 mg, B_5 10 mg, B_6 2 mg, B_{12} 6 mcg, C 60 mg, FA 0.4 mg, Ca, Zn 15 mg, tartrazine/Tab. Bot. 100s. *otc.*
Use: Mineral, vitamin supplement.

Multi-Germ Oil. (Viobin) Corn, sunflower and wheat germ oils. Bot. 4 oz, 8 oz, pt, qt. *otc.*
Use: Nutritional supplement.

Multi-Jets. (Kirkman Sales Co., Inc.) Vitamins A 10,000 IU, D_2 400 IU, B_1 20 mg, B_2 8 mg, C 120 mg, niacinamide 10 mg, calcium pantothenate 5 mg, B_6 0.5 mg, E 50 IU, desiccated liver 100 mg, dried debittered yeast 100 mg, choline bitartrate 62 mg, inositol 30 mg, dl-methionine 30 mg, B_{12} 7 mcg, Fe 2.6 mg, Ca (dical phosphate) 58 mg, P (dical phosphate) 45 mg, I (potassium iodide) 0.114 mg, Mg sulfate 1 mg, Cu sulfate 1.99 mg, Mn sulfate 1.11 mg, KCl iodide 79 mg/Tab. Bot. 100s. *otc.*
Use: Mineral, vitamin supplement.

Multilex Tablets. (Rugby Labs, Inc.) Fe 15 mg, vitamins A 10,000 IU, D 400 IU, E 5.5 mg, B_1 10 mg, B_2 5 mg, B_3 30 mg, B_5 10 mg, B_6 1.7 mg, B_{12} 3 mcg, C 100 mg, Zn 1.5 mg, Cu, I, Mg, Mn/ Tab. Bot. 100s. *otc.*
Use: Mineral, vitamin supplement.

Multilex T & M Tablets. (Rugby Labs, Inc.) Fe 15 mg, vitamins A 10,000 IU, D 400 IU, E 5.5 mg, B_1 15 mg, B_2 10 mg, B_3 100 mg, B_5 10 mg, B_6 2 mg, B_{12} 7.5 mcg, C 150 mg, Cu, I, Mg, Mn, Zn 1.5 mg, sugar/Tab. Bot. 100s. *otc.*
Use: Mineral, vitamin supplement.

Multilyte. (Fujisawa USA, Inc.) Vitamins A 5000 IU, D 400 IU, E 15 mg, B_1 3 mg, B_2 3.4 mg, B_3 36 mg, B_5 14 mg, B_6 4.4 mg, B_{12} 6 mcg, C 120 mg, FA 0.4 mg, Zn 10.5 mg, biotin 100 mcg, Ca, K, Mg, Mn, phenylalanine. Tab. Pkg. 12s. *otc.*
Use: Mineral, vitamin supplement.

Multilyte-20. (Fujisawa USA, Inc.) Na 25 mEq/L, K 20 mEq/L, Ca 5 mEq/L, Mg 5 mEq/L, Cl 30 mEq/L, acetate 25 mEq/ L, gluconate 5 mEq/L. Vial 25 ml fill in 50 ml. *Rx.*
Use: Electrolyte, fluid replacement.

Multilyte-40. (Fujisawa USA, Inc.) Na 25 mEq/L, K 40.5 mEq/L, Ca 5 mEq/L, Mg 8 mEq/L, Cl 33.5 mEq/L, acetate 40.6 mEq/L, gluconate 5 mEq/L. Vial 25 ml fill in 50 ml. *Rx.*
Use: Electrolyte, fluid replacement.

Multi-Mineral Tablets. (NBTY, Inc.) Ca 166.7 mg, P 75.7 mg, I 25 mcg, Fe 3 mg, Mg 66.7 mg, Cu 0.33 mg, Zn 2.5 mg, K 12.5 mg, Mn 8.3 mg/Tab. Bot. 100s. *otc.*
Use: Mineral, vitamin supplement.

Multipals. (Faraday) Vitamins A 5000 IU, D 400 IU, C 50 mg, B_1 3 mg, B_6 0.5 mg, B_2 3 mg, calcium pantothenate 5 mg, niacinamide 20 mg, B_{12} 2 mcg/Tab. Bot. 100s, 250s, 1000s. *otc.*
Use: Mineral, vitamin supplement.

Multipals-M. (Faraday) Vitamins A 6000 IU, D 400 IU, B_1 3 mg, B_2 3 mg, B_6 0.5 mg, B_{12} 5 mcg, C 60 mg, E 2 IU, niacinamide 20 mg, calcium pantothenate 5 mg, Fe 10 mg, I 0.15 mg, Cu 1 mg, Mg 6 mg, Mn 1 mg, K 5 mg/Tab. Bot. 100s, 250s, 1000s. *otc.*
Use: Mineral, vitamin supplement.

Multiple Trace Element. (American Regent) Zinc sulfate 1 mg, copper sulfate 0.4 mg, manganese sulfate 0.1 mg, chromium Cl 4 mg/ml. Inj. Soln. Vial 10 ml. *Rx.*
Use: Mineral supplement.

Multiple Trace Element Concentrated. (American Regent) Zinc sulfate 5 mg, copper sulfate 1 mg, manganese sulfate 0.5 mg, chromium Cl 10 mcg/ml. Inj. Soln. Vial 10 ml. *Rx.*
Use: Mineral supplement.

Multiple Trace Element Neonatal. (American Regent) Zn 1.5 mg, Cu 0.1 mg, Mn 25 mcg, Cr 0.85 mcg/ml. Inj. Vial 2 ml single dose. *Rx.*
Use: Mineral supplement.

Multiple Trace Element Pediatric. (American Regent) Zinc sulfate 0.5 mg, copper sulfate 0.1 mg, manganese sulfate 0.03 mg, chromium Cl 1 mcg/ml. Inj. Soln. Vial 10 ml. *Rx.*
Use: Mineral supplement.

Multiple Vitamin Mineral Formula. (Kirkman Sales Co., Inc.) Vitamins A 5000 IU, D_2 400 IU, C 50 mg, B_1 2.5 mg, B_2 2.5 mg, B_6 0.5 mg, B_{12} 1 mcg, niacinamide 15 mg, calcium pantothenate 5 mg, E 0.1 IU, Ca 100 mg, Fe 7.5 mg, Mg 2.5 mg, K 2.5 mg, Zn 0.15 mg, Mn 0.5 mg, I 0.07 mg/Tab. Bot. 100s. *otc.*
Use: Mineral, vitamin supplement.

Multiple Vitamins Chewable. (Kirkman Sales Co., Inc.) Vitamins A 5000 IU, D 400 IU, C 50 mg, B_1 3 mg, B_2 2.5 mg,

B_6 1 mg, B_{12} 1 mcg, niacinamide 20 mg/Tab. Bot. 100s. *otc.*
Use: Vitamin supplement.

Multiple Vitamins w/Iron. (Kirkman Sales Co., Inc.) Vitamins A 5000 IU, D 400 IU, C 50 mg, B_1 3 mg, B_2 2.5 mg, B_6 1 mg, B_{12} 1 mcg, niacinamide 20 mg, Fe 10 mg/Tab. Bot. 100s. *otc.*
Use: Mineral, vitamin supplement.

Multi 75. (Fibertone) Vitamins A 25,000 IU, D 500 IU, E 150 IU, B_1 75 mg, B_2 75 mg, B_3 75 mg, B_5 75 mg, B_6 75 mg, B_{12} 75 mcg, C 250 mg, FA 0.4 mg, Ca 50 mg, Fe 10 mg, biotin, I, Mg, Zn 15 mg, Cu, PABA, K, Mn, Cr, Se, Mo, B, Si, choline bitartrate, inositol, rutin, lemon bioflavonoid complex, hesperidin, betaine, HCl/TR Tab. Bot. 60s, 90s. *otc.*
Use: Mineral, vitamin supplement.

Multistix 2 Reagent Strips. (Bayer Corp. (Consumer Div.)) Urinalysis reagent strip test for nitrite and leukocytes. Strip Bot. 100s.
Use: Diagnostic aid.

Multistix 7. (Bayer Corp. (Consumer Div.)) Urinalysis reagent strip test for glucose ketone, blood, pH, protein, nitrite, leukocytes. Strip Box 100s.
Use: Diagnostic aid.

Multistix 8. (Bayer Corp. (Consumer Div.)) Urinalysis reagent strip test for detecting glucose, ketone, blood, pH, protein, nitrite, bilirubin, leukocytes. Strip Box. 100s.
Use: Diagnostic aid.

Multistix 8 SG Reagent Strips. (Bayer Corp. (Consumer Div.)) Urinalysis reagent strip test for glucose, ketone, specific gravity, blood, pH, protein nitrite, leukocytes. Strip Box 100s.
Use: Diagnostic aid.

Multistix 9 Reagent Strips. (Bayer Corp. (Consumer Div.)) Urinalysis reagent strip test for glucose, bilirubin, ketone, blood, pH, protein, urobilinogen, nitrite, leukocytes. Strip Box 100s.
Use: Diagnostic aid.

Multistix 9 SG Reagent Strips. (Bayer Corp. (Consumer Div.)) Urinalysis reagent strip test for glucose, bilirubin, ketone, specific gravity, blood, pH, protein, nitrite, leukocytes. Strip Box 100s.
Use: Diagnostic aid.

Multistix 10 SG Reagent Strips. (Bayer Corp. (Consumer Div.)) Reagent strip test for glucose, bilirubin, ketone, specific gravity, blood, pH, protein, urobilinogen, nitrite, leukocytes in urine. Strip Box 100s.
Use: Diagnostic aid.

Multistix-N. (Bayer Corp. (Consumer Div.)) Glucose, protein, pH, blood, ketones, bilirubin, urobilinogen, nitrate, leukocytes. Kit. 100s.
Use: Diagnostic aid.

Multistix-N S.G. Reagent Strips. (Bayer Corp. (Consumer Div.)) Urinalysis reagent strip test for pH, protein, glucose, ketones, bilirubin, blood nitrite, urobilinogen, specific gravity. Strip Bot. 100s.
Use: Diagnostic aid.

Multistix Reagent Strips. (Bayer Corp. (Consumer Div.)) Urinalysis reagent strip test for pH, protein, glucose, ketone, bilirubin, blood. Strip Box 100s.
Use: Diagnostic aid.

Multistix S. G. Reagent Strips. (Bayer Corp. (Consumer Div.)) Urinalysis reagent strip test for pH, glucose, protein, ketones, bilirubin, blood, urobilinogen. Strip Box. 100s.
Use: Diagnostic aid.

Multi-Symptom Tylenol Cold. (McNeil Consumer Products Co.) Pseudoephedrine HCl 30 mg, chlorpheniramine maleate 2 mg, dextromethorphan HBr 15 mg, acetaminophen 325 mg/Capl. or Tab. Bot. 24s, 50s. *otc.*
Use: Analgesic, antihistamine, antitussive, decongestant.

Multi-Symptom Tylenol Cough. (Ortho McNeil Pharmaceutical) Dextromethorphan HBr 10 mg, acetaminophen 216.7 mg, alcohol 5%/5 ml. Liq. Bot. 120 ml. *otc.*
Use: Analgesic, antititussive.

Multi-Symptom Tylenol Cough with Decongestant. (Ortho McNeil Pharmaceutical) Dextromethorphan HBr 10 mg, acetaminophen 200 mg, pseudoephedrine HCl 20 mg, alcohol 5%, saccharin, sorbitol/5 ml. Liq. Bot. 120 ml. *otc.*
Use: Analgesic, antititussive, decongestant.

Multitest CMI. (Pasteur Merieux Connaught) One disposable applicator preloaded with 7 delayed hypersensitivity skin test antigens (tetanus toxoid, diphtheria toxoid, *Streptococcus*, old tuberculin, *Candida*, *Trichophyton*, *Proteus*) and glycerin-negative control. Single-use preloaded applicators. *Rx.*
Use: Diagnostic aid.

Multi-Thera Tablets. (NBTY, Inc.) Vitamins A 5500 IU, D 400 IU, E 30 mg, B_1 3 mg, B_2 3.4 mg, B_3 30 mg, B_5 10 mg, B_6 3 mg, B_{12} 9 mcg, C 120 mg, folic acid 0.4 mg, biotin 15 mcg/Tab. Bot. 100s. *otc.*
Use: Vitamin supplement.

Multi-Thera-M. (NBTY, Inc.) Iron 27 mg, vitamins A 5500 IU, D 400 IU, E 30 mg,

B_1 3 mg, B_2 3.4 mg, B_3 30 mg, B_5 10 mg, B_6 3 mg, B_{12} 9 mcg, C 120 mg, folic acid 0.4 mg, biotin 15 mcg, Zn 15 mg, Ca, Cl, Cr, Cu, I, K, Mg, Mn, Mo, Se/Tab. Bot. 130s. *otc.*
Use: Mineral, vitamin supplement.

Multitrace-5 Concentrate. (American Regent) Zinc sulfate 5 mg, copper sulfate 1 mg, manganese sulfate 0.5 mg, chromium Cl 10 mcg, selenium 60 mcg, benzyl alcohol 0.9%. Inj. Soln. Vial 1 ml, 10 ml. *Rx.*
Use: Mineral supplement.

Multi-Vit Drops. (Alpharma USPD Inc.) Vitamins A 500 IU, D 400 IU, E 5 mg, B_1 0.5 mg, B_2 0.6 mg, B_3 8 mg, B_6 0.4 mg, B_{12} 2 mcg, C 35 mg/ml. Bot. 50 ml. *otc.*
Use: Vitamin supplement.

Multi-Vit Drops w/Iron. (Alpharma USPD Inc.) Iron 10 mg, vitamins A 1500 IU, D 400 IU, E 5 IU, B_1 0.5 mg, B_2 0.6 mg, B_3 8 mg, B_6 0.4 mg, C 35 mg/ml. Methylparaben. Drop. Bot. 50 ml. *otc.*
Use: Mineral, vitamin supplement.

Multi-Vita. (Rosemont Pharmaceutical Corp.) Vitamins A 1500 IU, D 400 IU, E 5 mg, B_1 0.5 mg, B_2 0.6 mg, B_3 8 mg, B_6 0.4 mg, B_{12} 2 mcg, C 35 mg/ml. Alcohol free. Drop. Bot. 50 ml. *otc.*
Use: Vitamin supplement.

Multi-Vita Drops. (Rosemont Pharmaceutical Corp.) Vitamins A 1500 IU, D 400 IU, E 5 mg, B_1 0.5 mg, B_2 0.6 mg, B_3 8 mg, B_6 0.4 mg, B_{12} 2 mcg, C 35 mg/ml. Alcohol free. Drop. Bot. 50 ml. *otc.*
Use: Mineral, vitamin supplement.

Multi-Vita Drops w/Fluoride. (Rosemont Pharmaceutical Corp.) Fluoride 0.5 mg, vitamins A 1500 IU, D 400 IU, E 5 mg, B_1 0.5 mg, B_2 0.6 mg, B_3 8 mg, B_6 0.4 mg, B_{12} 2 mcg, C 35 mg/ml. Alcohol free. Drop. Bot. 50 ml. *Rx.*
Use: Vitamin supplement; dental caries agent.

Multi-Vita Drops w/Iron. (Rosemont Pharmaceutical Corp.) Iron 10 mg, vitamins A 1500 IU, D 400 IU, E 5 mg, B_1 0.5 mg, B_2 0.6 mg, B_3 8 mg, B_6 0.4 mg, C 35 mg/ml. Alcohol free. Drop. Bot. 50 ml. *otc.*
Use: Mineral, vitamin supplement.

Multivitamin with Fluoride Drops. (Major Pharmaceuticals) Fluoride 0.5 mg, vitamins A 1500 IU, D 400 IU, E 5 IU, B_1 0.5 mg, B_2 0.6 mg, B_3 8 mg, B_6 0.4 mg, B_{12} 2 mcg, C 35 mg, F 0.25 mg/Drop. Bot. 50 ml. *Rx.*
Use: Vitamin supplement; dental caries agent.

multivitamin concentrate injection. (Fujisawa USA, Inc.) Vitamins A 10,000 IU, D 1000 IU, E 5 IU, B_1 50 mg, B_2 10 mg, B_3 100 mg, B_5 25 mg, B_6 15 mg, C 500 mg/Inj. Vial 5 ml. *Rx.*
Use: Vitamin supplement.

multivitamin infusion (neonatal formula).
Use: Nutritional supplement for low birth weight infants. [Orphan Drug]

Multi-Vitamin Mineral w/Beta Carotene. (Mission Pharmacal Co.) Iron 27 mg, A 5000 IU, D 400 IU, E 30 IU, B_1 2.25 mg, B_2 2.6 mg, B_3 20 mg, B_5 10 mg, B_6 3 mg, B_{12} 9 mcg, C 90 mg, folic acid 0.4 mg, biotin, 0.45 mg, Ca, Cl, Cr, Cu, I, K, Mg, Mn, Mo, P, Se, Zn 15 mg, Vitamin K/Tab. Bot. 130s. *otc.*
Use: Mineral, vitamin supplement.

Multi-Vitamins Capsules. (Forest Pharmaceutical, Inc.) Vitamins A 5000 IU, D 400 IU, B_1 1.5 mg, B_2 2 mg, B_6 0.1 mg, C 37.5 mg, calcium pantothenate 1 mg, niacinamide 20 mg/Cap. Bot. 100s, 1000s, 5000s. *otc.*
Use: Mineral, vitamin supplement.

Multivitamins Capsules. (Solvay Pharmaceuticals) Vitamins A 5000 IU, D 400 IU, B_1 2.5 mg, B_2 2.5 mg, C 50 mg, B_3 20 mg, B_5 5 mg, B_6 0.5 mg, B_{12} 2 mcg, E 10 IU/Cap. Bot. 100s, UD 100s. *otc.*
Use: Mineral, vitamin supplement.

Multivitamin with Fluoride Drops. (Major Pharmaceuticals) Fluoride 0.5 mg, vitamins A 1500 IU, D 400 IU, E 4.1 IU, B_1 0.5 mg, B_2 0.6 mg, B_3 8 mg, B_6 0.4 mg, B_{12} 2 mg, C 35 mg/Drop. Bot. 50 ml. *otc.*
Use: Vitamin supplement; dental caries agent.

multizine.
See: Trisulfapyrimidines Tab., U.S.P. 23.

Multorex. (Health for Life Brands, Inc.) Vitamins A 6000 IU, D 1250 IU, C 50 mg, E 5 IU, B_1 3 mg, B_2 3 mg, B_6 0.5 mg, niacinamide 20 mg, calcium pantothenate 5 mg, B_{12} 5 mcg, Ca 59 mg, P 45 mg/Cap. Bot. 100s, 250s,1000s.
Use: Mineral, vitamin supplement.

Mulvidren-F Softabs. (Wyeth-Ayerst Laboratories) Fluoride 1 mg, vitamins A 4000 IU, D 400 IU, B_1 1.6 mg, B_2 2 mg, B_3 10 mg, B_5 2.8 mg, B_6 1 mg, B_{12} 3 mcg, C 75 mg, saccharin/Tab. Bot. 100s. *Rx.*
Use: Mineral, vitamin supplement; dental caries agent.

•**mumps skin test antigen.** U.S.P. 23.
Use: Diagnostic aid (dermal reactivity indicator).

See: MSTA, Inj. (Pasteur Merieux Connaught).
Mumpsvax. (Merck & Co.) Live mumps virus vaccine, Jeryl Lynn strain. Single-dose vial w/diluent Pkg. 1s, 10s. *Rx.*
Use: Agent for immunization.
W/Attenuvax, Meruvax II.
See: M-M-R II, Inj. (Merck & Co.).
W/Meruvax II.
See: Biavax II (Merck & Co.).
•**mumps virus vaccine live.** U.S.P. 23.
Use: Immunization.
See: Mumpsvax, Inj. (Merck & Co.).
mumps virus vaccine, live attenuated. Jeryl Lynn (B level) strain.
See: Mumpsvax (Merck & Co.).
W/Measles virus vaccine, rubella virus vaccine.
See: M-M-R, Inj. (Merck & Co.).
•**mupirocin.** (myoo-PIHR-oh-sin) U.S.P. 23.
Use: Anti-infective (topical and nasal).
See: Bactroban, Oint. (SmithKline Beecham Pharmaceuticals).
•**mupirocin calcium.** (myoo-PIHR-oh-sin KAL-see-uhm) USAN.
Use: Anti-infective, topical.
See: Bactroban, Cream (SmithKline Beecham).
•**muplestim.** (myoo-PLEH-stim) USAN.
Use: Hematopoietic stimulant; antineutropenic.
muriatic acid.
See: Hydrochloric Acid, N.F. 18.
Muri-Lube. (Fujisawa USA, Inc.) Mineral Oil "Light." Vial 2 ml, 10 ml. *Rx.*
Use: Lubricant.
Murine Ear Drops. (Ross Laboratories) Carbamide peroxide 6.5% in anhydrous glycerin. Bot. 0.5 oz. *otc.*
Use: Otic.
Murine Ear Wax Removal System. (Ross Laboratories) Carbamide peroxide 6.5% in anhydrous glycerin w/ear washing syringe. Bot. 0.5 oz. and ear washer 1 oz. *otc.*
Use: Otic.
Murine Eye Drops. (Ross Laboratories) Polyvinyl alcohol 0.5%, povidone 0.6%, benzalkonium chloride, dextrose, EDTA, NaCl, sodium bicarbonate, sodium phosphate. Soln. Bot. 15 ml, 30 ml. *otc.*
Use: Artificial tears.
Murine Plus Eye Drops. (Ross Laboratories) Tetrahydrozoline HCl 0.05%. Drop. Bot. 15 ml, 30 ml. *otc.*
Use: Vasoconstrictor, ophthalmic.
Murine Regular Formula. (Ross Laboratories) Sodium chloride, potassium chloride, sodium phosphate, glycerin, benzalkonium chloride 0.01%, EDTA 0.05%/Drop. Bot. 15, 30 ml. *otc.*
Use: Artificial tears.
Muro 128 Ointment. (Bausch & Lomb Pharmaceuticals) Sodium Cl 5% in sterile ointment base. Tube 3.5 g. *otc.*
Use: Hyperosmolar.
Muro 128 Solution. (Bausch & Lomb Pharmaceuticals) Sodium Cl 2%, 5%. Soln. Bot. 15 ml, 30 ml (5% only). *otc.*
Use: Hyperosmolar.
Murocel Solution. (Bausch & Lomb Pharmaceuticals) Methylcellulose 1%, propylene glycol, sodium Cl, methylparaben 0.046%, propylparaben 0.02%, boric acid, sodium borate. Soln. Bot. 15 ml. *otc.*
Use: Artificial tears.
Murocoll-2. (Bausch & Lomb Pharmaceuticals) Phenylephrine HCl 10%, scopolamine HBR 0.3% Bot. 5 ml. *Rx.*
Use: Cycloplegic, mydriatic.
•**muromonab-CD3.** (MYOO-row-MOE-nab cd 3) USAN.
Use: Monoclonal antibody (immunosuppressant).
See: Orthoclone OKT3, Inj. (Ortho McNeil Pharmaceutical).
Muroptic-5. (Optopics Laboratories, Corp) Sodium Cl, hypertonic 5%. Soln. Bot. 15 ml. *otc.*
Use: Hyperosmolar.
Muro's Opcon A Solution. (Bausch & Lomb Pharmaceuticals) Naphazoline HCl 0.025%, pheniramine maleate 0.3%. Bot. 15 ml. *otc.*
Use: Antihistamine (ophthalmic), decongestant.
Muro's Opcon Solution. (Bausch & Lomb Pharmaceuticals) Naphazoline HCl 0.1%. Bot. 15 ml. *otc.*
Use: Decongestant, ophthalmic.
Muro Tears Solution. (Bausch & Lomb Pharmaceuticals) Hydroxypropyl methylcellulose, dextran 40. Soln. Bot. 15 ml. *otc.*
Use: Artificial tears.
muscle adenylic acid. (Various Mfr.) Active form of adenosine 5-monophosphate.
See: Adenosine 5-monophosphate, Preps. (Various Mfr.).
muscle relaxants.
See: Arduan (Organon Teknika Corp.).
Curare (Various Mfr.).
Flexeril, Tab. (Merck & Co.).
Lioresal, Tab. (Novartis Pharmaceutical Corp.).
Mephenesin (Various Mfr.).
Meprobamate (Various Mfr.).

Metubine Iodine, Vial (Eli Lilly and Co.).
Neostig, Tab. (Freeport).
Norflex, Tab., Inj. (3M Pharmaceuticals).
Nuromax (GlaxoWellcome).
Parafon Forte, Tab. (Ortho McNeil Pharmaceutical).
Rela, Tab. (Schering-Plough Corp.).
Robaxin, Tab., Inj. (Wyeth-Ayerst Laboratories).
Soma, Tab, Cap. (Wallace Laboratories).
Succinylcholine Cl (Various Mfr.).

mustaral oil.
See: Allyl Isothiocyanate.

Mustargen. (Merck & Co.) Mechlorethamine HCl 10 mg Pow. For Inj. Vial. Treatment set vial 4s. *Rx.*
Use: Antineoplastic.

Musterole. (Schering-Plough Corp.) **Regular:** Camphor 4%, menthol 2%. Jar 0.9 oz. **Extra Strength:** Camphor 5%, menthol 3%. Jar 0.9 oz., Tube 1 oz, 2.25 oz. *otc.*
Use: Analgesic, topical.

Musterole Deep Strength. (Schering-Plough Corp.) Methyl salicylate 30%, menthol 3%, methyl nicotinate 0.5%. Jar 1.25 oz, Tube 3 oz. *otc.*
Use: Analgesic, topical.

Musterole Extra Strength. (Schering-Plough Corp.) Camphor 5%, menthol 3%, methyl salicylate, lanolin, oil of mustard, petrolatum. 27, 30, 67.5 g. *otc.*
Use: Liniment.

mustin.
See: Mechlorethamine HCl, Sterile.

mutalin. (Spanner) Protein and iodine. Vial 30 ml.

Mutamycin. (Bristol-Myers Oncology/Immunology) Mitomycin 5 mg, 20 mg, 40 mg/Vial. *Rx.*
Use: Antineoplastic.

•**muzolimine.** (MYOO-ZOLE-ih-meen) USAN.
Use: Antihypertensive, diuretic.

M.V.I.-12. (Astra Pharmaceuticals, L.P.) Vitamins A 3300 IU, D 200 IU, E 10 IU, B_1 3 mg, B_2 3.6 mg, B_3 40 mg, B_5 15 mg, B_6 4 mg, B_{12} 5 mcg, C 100 mg, biotin 60 mcg, FA 0.4 mg. Inj. Vials. 5 ml single-dose, 50 ml multiple-dose; Unit vial: 10 ml two-chambered vials. *Rx.*
Use: Nutritional supplement, parenteral.

M.V.I. Pediatric. (Astra Pharmaceuticals, L.P.) Vitamin A 2300 IU, D 400 IU, E 7 IU, B_1 1.2 mg, B_2 1.4 mg, B_3 17 mg, B_5 5 mg, B_6 1 mg, B_{12} 1 mcg, C 80 mg, biotin 20 mcg, FA 0.14 mg, vitamin K 200 mcg, mannitol 375 mg/Inj. Vial. *Rx.*
Use: Nutritional supplement, parenteral.

M.V.M. (Tyson & Associates, Inc.) Iron 3.6 mg, vitamins A 400 IU, E 60 IU, B_1 20 mg, B_2 10 mg, B_3 10 mg, B_5 100 mg, B_6 31 mg, B_{12} 160 mcg, C 50 mg, folic acid 0.08 mg, Ca, Cr, Cu, I, K, Mg, Mo, Zn 6 mg, biotin 160 mcg, PABA, Mn, Se, tryptophan/Cap. Bot 150s. *otc.*
Use: Mineral, vitamin supplement.

Myadec. (Parke-Davis) Iron 18 mg, A 5000 IU, D 400 IU, E 30 IU, B_1 1.7 mg, B_2 2 mg, B_3 20 mg, B_5 10 mg, B_6 3 mg, B_{12} 6 mcg, C 60 mg, folic acid 0.4 mg, biotin 30 mcg, vitamin K, Ca, P, I, Mg, Cu, Zn 15 mg, Mn, K, Cl, Cr, Mo, Se, Ni, Si, V, B, Sn/Tab. Bot. 130s. *otc.*
Use: Mineral, vitamin supplement.

myagen. Bolasterone.
Use: Anabolic agent.

Myambutol. (ESI Lederle Generics) Ethambutol HCl. Tab. **100 mg:** Bot. 100s. **400 mg:** Bot. 100s, 1000s, UD 10 × 10s. *Rx.*
Use: Antituberculous.

myanesin.
See: Mephenesin (Various Mfr.).

Myapap Drops. (Rosemont Pharmaceutical Corp.) Acetaminophen 80 mg/0.8 ml. Bot. 15 ml w/dropper. *otc.*
Use: Analgesic.

Myapap Elixir. (Rosemont Pharmaceutical Corp.) Acetaminophen 160 mg/5 ml. Bot. 4 oz, pt, gal. *otc.*
Use: Analgesic.

Myapap with Codeine Elixir. (Rosemont Pharmaceutical Corp.) Acetaminophen 120 mg, codeine phosphate 12 mg/5 ml. Bot. 4 oz, pt, gal. *c-v.*
Use: Analgesic, antitussive.

Mybanil. (Rosemont Pharmaceutical Corp.) Codeine phosphate 10 mg, bromodiphenhydramine HCl 12.5 mg/5 ml, alcohol 5%. Bot. 4 oz, pt, gal. *c-v.*
Use: Antihistamine, antitussive.

Mycadec DM Drops. (Rosemont Pharmaceutical Corp.) Pseudoephedrine 25 mg, carbinoxamine maleate 2 mg, dextromethorphan HBr 4 mg/ml. Bot. 30 ml. *Rx.*
Use: Antihistamine, antitussive, decongestant.

Mycadec DM Syrup. (Rosemont Pharmaceutical Corp.) Carbinoxamine maleate 4 mg, pseudoephedrine HCl 60 mg, dextromethorphan HBr 15 mg/5 ml, alcohol 0.6%. Bot. 4 oz, pt, gal. *Rx.*
Use: Antihistamine, antitussive, decongestant.

Mycadec Drops. (Rosemont Pharmaceutical Corp.) Pseudoephedrine HCl 25 mg, dextromethorphan HBr 4 mg, carbinoxamine maleate 2 mg/ml. Bot. 30 ml. *Rx.*
Use: Antihistamine, antitussive, decongestant.

Mycartal. (Sanofi Winthrop Pharmaceuticals) Pentaerythritol tetranitrate. *Rx.*
Use: Coronary vasodilator.

Mycelex. (Bayer Corp. (Consumer Div.)) Clotrimazole. **Cream:** 1%. Tube 15 g, 30 g, 90 g (2 × 45 g). **Topical Soln.:** 1%. Bot. 10 ml, 30 ml. *Rx-otc.*
Use: Antifungal, topical.

Mycelex-7. (Bayer Corp. (Consumer Div.)) **Vaginal Tab.:** Clotrimazole 100 mg. Pkg. 7s with applicator. **Vaginal Cream:** Clotrimazole 1%. Tube 45 g (7-day therapy) with applicator. *otc.*
Use: Antifungal, vaginal.

Mycelex-7 Combination Pack. (Bayer Corp. (Consumer Div.)) Clotrimazole. **Cream:** 1%. Tube 7 g. **Supp.:** 100 mg. Pkg. 7s w/applicator. *otc.*
Use: Antifungal, vaginal.

Mycelex-G. (Bayer Corp. (Consumer Div.)) Clotrimazole. **Vaginal Tab.:** 100 mg. Pkg. 7s w/applicator. **Cream:** 1%. Tube 45 g, 90 g. *Rx.*
Use: Antifungal, vaginal.

Mycelex-G 500. (Bayer Corp. (Consumer Div.)) Clotrimazole 500 mg/Vaginal Tab. w/applicator. *Rx.*
Use: Antifungal, vaginal.

Mycelex OTC. (Bayer Corp. (Consumer Div.)) Clotrimazole 1%, benzyl alcohol 1%. Cream Tube 15 g. *otc.*
Use: Anti-infective, topical.

Mycelex Troches. (Bayer Corp. (Consumer Div.)) Clotrimazole 10 mg/Troche 70s, 140s. *Rx.*
Use: Antifungal.

Mycelex Twin Pack. (Bayer Corp. (Consumer Div.)) Clotrimazole 500 mg/Vaginal Tab. w/applicator. Cream 1%. Tube 7 g. *Rx.*
Use: Antifungal, vaginal.

Mychel-S. (Rachelle) Sterile chloramphenicol sodium succinate. Vial 1 g/15 ml. Box 5s. *Rx.*
Use: Anti-infective.

Mycifradin. (Pharmacia & Upjohn) Neomycin sulfate 125 mg/5 ml (equivalent to 87.5 mg neomycin). Oral soln. Bot. Pt. *Rx.*
Use: Anti-infective.

Myciguent. (Pharmacia & Upjohn) Neomycin sulfate. **Cream:** 5 mg/g. Tube 0.5 oz. **Oint.:** 5 mg/g. Tube 0.5 oz, 1 oz, 4 oz. *otc.*
Use: Anti-infective, topical.

Mycinette. (Pfeiffer Co.) Benzocaine 15 mg, sorbitol, saccharin, menthol. Loz. 12s. *otc.*
Use: Anesthetic, local; antiseptic, expectorant.

Mycinette Sore Throat. (Pfeiffer Co.) Phenol 1.4%, alum 0.3%, alcohol free, sugar free. Spray 180 ml. *otc.*
Use: Mouth and throat preparation.

Myci-Spray. (Misemer Pharmaceuticals, Inc.) Phenylephrine HCl 0.25%, pyrilamine maleate 0.15%/ml. Bot. 20 ml. *otc.*
Use: Antihistamine, decongestant.

Mycitracin. (Pharmacia & Upjohn) Bacitracin 500 units, neomycin sulfate 5 mg, polymyxin B sulfate 5000 units/g. Oint. Tube 0.5 oz. Box 36s; 1 oz; UD 1/32 oz Box 144s. *otc.*
Use: Anti-infective, topical.

Mycitracin Plus. (Pharmacia & Upjohn) Polymyxin B sulfate 5000 units/g, neomycin 3.5 mg/g, bacitracin 500 units/g, lidocaine 40 mg, white petrolatum. Oint. Tube 15 g. *otc.*
Use: Anti-infective, topical.

Mycitracin Triple Antibiotic, Maximum Strength. (Pharmacia & Upjohn) Polymyxin B sulfate 5000 units/g, neomycin 3.5 mg/g, bacitracin 500 units/g, parabens, mineral oil, white petrolatum. Oint. Tube 30 g, UD 0.94 g. *otc.*
Use: Anti-infective, topical.

Mycobutin. (Pharmacia & Upjohn) Rifabutin. 150 mg/Cap. Bot. 100s. *Rx.*
Use: Antituberculosal.

Mycocide NS. (Woodward Laboratories, Inc.) Benzalkonium Cl, propylene glycol, methylparaben. Soln. Bot. 30 ml. *otc.*
Use: Antimicrobial, antiseptic.

Mycodone Syrup. (Rosemont Pharmaceutical Corp.) Hydrocodone bitartrate 5 mg, homatropine MBr 1.5 mg/5 ml. Bot. 4 oz, pt, gal. *c-III.*
Use: Antitussive.

Mycogen-II Cream. (Zenith Goldline Pharmaceuticals) Nystatin 100,000 units, triamcinolone acetonide 1 mg/g. Cream Tube 15 g, 30 g, 60 g, 120 g, lb. *Rx.*
Use: Antifungal, corticosteroid, topical.

Mycogen-II Ointment. (Zenith Goldline Pharmaceuticals) Nystatin 100,000 units, triamcinolone acetonide 1 mg/g. Oint. Tube 15 g, 30 g, 60 g. *Rx.*
Use: Antifungal, corticosteroid, topical.

Mycolog-II Cream and Ointment. (Bristol-Myers Squibb) Triamcinolone acetonide 1 mg, nystatin 100,000 units/g.

Ointment base w/Plastibase (polyethylene, mineral oil). Tube 15 g, 30 g, 60 g, Jar 120 g. *Rx.*
Use: Antifungal, corticosteroid, topical.

Mycomist. (Gordon Laboratories) Chlorophyll, formalin, benzalkonium Cl. Bot. 4 oz, plastic Bot. 1 oz. *otc.*
Use: Antifungal for clothing.

•**mycophenolate mofetil.** (my-koe-FEN-oh-LATE MOE-feh-till) USAN.
Use: Immunomodulator.
See: CellCept (Roche Laboratories).

•**mycophenolic acid.** (MY-koe-fen-AHL-ik acid) USAN.
Use: Antineoplastic.

Mycoplasma Pneumonia IFA IgM Test. (Wampole Laboratories) Indirect fluorescent assay for IgM antibodies to *Mycoplasma pneumoniae.* Box test 100s.
Use: Diagnostic aid.

Mycoplasma Pneumonia IFA Test. (Wampole Laboratories) Indirect fluorescent assay for antibodies to *Mycoplasma pneumoniae* Box test 100s.
Use: Diagnostic aid.

Mycostatin. (Apothecon, Inc.) Nystatin. **Tab.:** 500,000 units. Bot. 100s. **Cream:** 100,000 units/g in aqueous base. Tube 15 g, 30 g. **Oint.:** 100,000 units/g in Plastibase (polyethylene and mineral oil). Tube 15 g, 30 g. **Susp.:** 100,000 units/ml. In vehicle containing sucrose 50%, saccharin $< 1\%$ alcohol. Bot. 60 ml, 473 ml. **Troche:** 200,000 units. 30s. **Vaginal Tab:** 100,000 units, lactose 0.95 g, ethyl cellulose, stearic acid, starch. Pkg. 15s, 30s. **Pow.:** (topical) 100,000 units/g in talc. Shaker bot. 15 g. *Rx.*
Use: Antifungal.

Mycostatin Pastilles. (Bristol-Myers Oncology/Immunology) Nystatin, 200,000 units/Troche. 30s. *Rx.*
Use: Antifungal.

Myco-Triacet. (Various Mfr.) Triamcinolone acetonide 0.1%, neomycin sulfate 0.25%, gramicidin 0.25 mg, nystatin 100,000 units/g. **Cream:** 15 g, 30 g, 60 g, 480 g. **Oint.:** 15 g, 30 g, 60 g. *Rx.*
Use: Antifungal, corticosteroid, topical.

Myco-Triacet II Cream & Ointment. (Teva Pharmaceuticals USA) Nystatin 100,000 units, triamcinolone acetonide 1 mg/g. **Cream:** White petrolatum and mineral oil. Tube 15 g, 30 g, 60g. **Oint.:** Tube 15 g, 30 g, 60 g. *Rx.*
Use: Antifungal, corticosteroid, topical.

Mycotussin Expectorant. (Rosemont Pharmaceutical Corp.) Pseudoephedrine HCl 60 mg, hydrocodone bitartrate 5 mg, guaifenesin 200 mg/5 ml, alcohol 12.5%. Liq. Bot. 4 oz, pt, gal. *c-III.*
Use: Antitussive, decongestant, expectorant.

Mycotussin Liquid. (Rosemont Pharmaceutical Corp.) Pseudoephedrine HCl 60 mg, hydrocodone bitartrate 5 mg/5 ml, alcohol 5%. Bot. 4 oz, pt, gal. *c-III.*
Use: Antitussive, decongestant.

Mydacol. (Rosemont Pharmaceutical Corp.) Vitamins B_1 5 mg, B_2 2.5 mg, niacinamide 50 mg, B_6 1 mg, B_{12} 1 mcg, pantothenic acid 10 mg, I 100 mcg, Fe 15 mg, Mg 2 mg, Zn 2 mg, choline 100 mg, Mn 2 mg/30 ml. Liq. Bot. Pt, gal. *otc.*
Use: Mineral, vitamin supplement.

Mydfrin Ophthalmic 2.5%. (Alcon Laboratories, Inc.) Phenylephrine HCl 2.5%. Soln. Drop-Tainers. 3 ml, 5 ml. *Rx.*
Use: Mydriatic.

Mydriacyl. (Alcon Laboratories, Inc.) Tropicamide 0.5%, 1%. Soln. 3 ml (1% only), 15 ml Drop-Tainer. *Rx.*
Use: Cycloplegic, mydriatic.

mydriatics, parasympatholytic types.
See: Atropine Salts (Various Mfr.).
Homatropine Hydrobromide (Various Mfr.).
Scopolamine Salts (Various Mfr.).

mydriatics, sympathomimetic types.
See: Amphetamine Sulfate 3% (Various Mfr.).
Clopane HCl, Liq. (Eli Lilly and Co).
Ephedrine Sulfate (Various Mfr.).
Epinephrine HCl (Various Mfr.).
Neo-Synephrine HCl, Preps (Sanofi Winthrop Pharmaceuticals).
Phenylephrine HCl (Various Mfr.).

myelin.
Use: Multiple sclerosis. [Orphan Drug]

Myelo-Kit. (Sanofi Winthrop Pharmaceuticals) Omnipaque 180, 240 in various sizes and one sterile myelogram tray.
Use: Radiopaque agent.

Myfed. (Rosemont Pharmaceutical Corp.) Triprolidine HCl 1.25 mg, pseudoephedrine HCl 30 mg/5 ml. Syr. Bot. 4 oz, pt, gal. *otc.*
Use: Antihistamine, decongestant.

Myfedrine. (Rosemont Pharmaceutical Corp.) Pseudoephedrine 30 mg/5 ml. Liq. Bot. 473 ml. *otc.*
Use: Decongestant.

Myfedrine Plus. (Rosemont Pharmaceutical Corp.) Pseudoephedrine HCl 30 mg, chlorpheniramine maleate 2 mg/5 ml. Syr. Bot. 4 oz, pt, gal. *otc.*
Use: Antitussive, decongestant.

Mygel Liquid. (Geneva Pharmaceuticals) Aluminum hydroxide 200 mg, magnesium hydroxide 200 mg, simethi-

cone 20 mg, Na 1.38 mg/5 ml. Liq. Bot. 360 ml. *otc.*
Use: Antacid, antiflatulent.

Mygel Suspension. (Geneva Pharmaceuticals) Aluminum hydroxide 200 mg, magnesium hydroxide 200 mg, simethicone 20 mg/5 ml. Bot. 360 ml. *otc.*
Use: Antacid, antiflatulent.

Mygel II Suspension. (Geneva Pharmaceuticals) Aluminum hydroxide 400 mg, magnesium hydroxide 400 mg, simethicone 40 mg/5 ml. Bot. 360 ml. *otc.*
Use: Antacid, antiflatulent.

Myhistine DH. (Rosemont Pharmaceutical Corp.) Codeine phosphate 10 mg, chlorpheniramine maleate 2 mg, pseudoephedrine HCl 30 mg/5 ml. Liq. Bot. 4 oz, pt, gal. *c-v.*
Use: Antihistamine, antitussive, decongestant.

Myhistine Elixir. (Rosemont Pharmaceutical Corp.) Chlorpheniramine maleate 2 mg, phenylephrine HCl 5 mg/5 ml, alcohol 5%. Liq. Bot. 4 oz, pt, gal. *otc.*
Use: Antihistamine, decongestant.

Myhistine Expectorant. (Rosemont Pharmaceutical Corp.) Codeine phosphate 10 mg, guaifenesin 100 mg, pseudoephedrine HCl 30 mg/5 ml, alcohol 7.5%. Liq. Bot. 4 oz, pt, gal. *c-v.*
Use: Antitussive, decongestant, expectorant.

Myhydromine Pediatric. (Rosemont Pharmaceutical Corp.) Phenylpropanolamine HCl 12.5 mg, hydrocodone bitartrate 2.5 mg/5 ml. Bot. Pt, gal. *c-III.*
Use: Antitussive, decongestant.

Myhydromine Syrup. (Rosemont Pharmaceutical Corp.) Phenylpropanolamine HCl 25 mg, hydrocodone bitartrate 5 mg/5 ml. Syr. Bot. 4 oz, pt, gal. *c-III.*
Use: Antihistamine, antitussive, decongestive.

Myidone Tabs. (Major Pharmaceuticals) Primidone 250 mg/Tab. Bot. 100s, 1000s. *Rx.*
Use: Anticonvulsant.

Mykacet Cream. (NMC Laboratories) Nystatin 100,000 units, triamcinolone acetonide 0.1%/g. Tube 15 g, 30 g, 60 g. *Rx.*
Use: Antifungal, corticosteroid, topical.

My-K Elixir. (Rosemont Pharmaceutical Corp.) Potassium 20 mEq/15 ml, alcohol 5%, saccharin. Bot. Pt, gal. *Rx.*
Use: Electrolyte supplement.

My-K Formula 77D. (Rosemont Pharmaceutical Corp.) Phenylpropanolamine HCl 12.5 mg, dextromethorphan HBr 10 mg, guaifenesin 100 mg/5 ml, alcohol 10%. Liq. Bot. 180 ml. *otc.*
Use: Antitussive, decongestant, expectorant.

My-K Formula 77 Liquid. (Rosemont Pharmaceutical Corp.) Doxylamine succinate 3.75 mg, dextromethorphan HBr 7.5 mg/5 ml, alcohol 10%. Liq. Bot. 180 ml. *otc.*
Use: Antihistamine, antitussive.

Mykinac. (NMC Laboratories) Nystatin 100,000 units/g in cream base. Cream Tube 15 g, 30 g. *otc.*
Use: Antifungal, topical.

My-K Nasal Spray. (Rosemont Pharmaceutical Corp.) Oxymetazoline HCl 0.05%. Soln. Bot. 0.5 oz. *otc.*
Use: Decongestant.

Mykrox. (Medeva Pharmaceuticals, Inc.) Metolazone 0.5 mg/Tab. Bot. 100s. *otc.*
Use: Diuretic.

Mylagen Gelcaps. (Zenith Goldline Pharmaceuticals) Calcium carbonate 311 mg, magnesium carbonate 232 mg. Pkg. 24s. *otc.*
Use: Antacid.

Mylagen Liquid. (Zenith Goldline Pharmaceuticals) Magnesium hydroxide 200 mg, aluminum hydroxide 200 mg, simethicone 20 mg/5 ml. Bot. 355 ml. *otc.*
Use: Antacid, antiflatulent.

Mylagen II Liquid. (Zenith Goldline Pharmaceuticals) Aluminum hydroxide 400 mg, magnesium hydroxide 400 mg, simethicone 40 mg/5 ml. Bot. 355 ml. *otc.*
Use: Antacid, antiflatulent.

Mylanta. (J & J Merck Consumer Pharm.) Calcium carbonate 600 mg. Loz. 18s, 50s. *otc.*
Use: Antacid.

Mylanta Double Strength. (J & J Merck Consumer Pharm.) **Chew. Tab.:** Magnesium hydroxide 400 mg, aluminum hydroxide dried gel 400 mg, simethicone 40 mg, Bot. 24s, 60s. **Liq.:** Magnesium hydroxide 400 mg, aluminum hydroxide dried gel 400 mg, simethicone 40 mg, sorbitol/5 ml. Bot. 150 ml, 360 ml. **Susp.:** Magnesium hydroxide 400 mg, aluminum hydroxide dried gel 400 mg, simethicone 40 mg, Na 0.05 mEq/5 ml. Bot. 150 ml, 360 ml, 720 ml, UD 30, 150 ml. *otc.*
Use: Antacid.

Mylanta Gas. (J & J Merck Consumer Pharm.) Simethicone. **40 mg:** Chew. Tab. Bot. 100s, UD 100s. **80 mg:** Chew. Tab. Pkg. 12s, Bot. 48s, 100s, UD 100s. *otc.*

Use: Antiflatulent.

Mylanta Gas, Maximum Strength. (J & J Merck Consumer Pharm.) Simethicone 125 mg/Chew. Tab. Pkg. 12s, Bot. 60s. *otc.*
Use: Antiflatulent.

Mylanta Gelcaps. (J & J Merck Consumer Pharm.) Calcium carbonate 311 mg, magnesium carbonate 232 mg. Bot. 24s, 50s. *otc.*
Use: Antacid.

Mylanta Liquid. (J & J Merck Consumer Pharm.) Magnesium hydroxide 200 mg, aluminum hydroxide 200 mg, simethicone 20 mg, Na 0.68 mg/5 ml. Bot. 150 ml, 360 ml, 720 ml, UD 30 ml. *otc.*
Use: Antacid, antiflatulent.

Mylanta Natural Fiber Supplement. (J & J Merck Consumer Pharm.) Psyllium hydrophilic mucilloid fiber 3.4 g/dose, sucrose, orange flavor. Pow. Can 390 g. *otc.*
Use: Laxative.

Mylanta Soothing Antacids. (J & J Merck Consumer Pharm.) Calcium carbonate 600 mg, corn syrup, sucrose. Loz. Pkg. 18s. Bot. 50s. *otc.*
Use: Antacid.

Mylanta Tablets. (J & J Merck Consumer Pharm.) Magnesium hydroxide 200 mg, aluminum hydroxide 200 mg, simethicone 20 mg, Na 0.77 mg, sorbitol/Chew. Tab. Bot. 12s, 40s, 48s, 100s, 180s. *otc.*
Use: Antacid, antiflatulent.

Mylanta-II Liquid. (J & J Merck Consumer Pharm.) Magnesium hydroxide 400 mg, aluminum hydroxide 400 mg, simethicone 40 mg, Na 1.14 mg, sorbitol/5 ml. Bot. 0.5 oz, 12 oz, UD 30 ml, 100s. *otc.*
Use: Antacid, antiflatulent.

Mylanta-II Tablets. (J & J Merck Consumer Pharm.) Magnesium hydroxide 400 mg, aluminum hydroxide 400 mg, simethicone 40 mg, Na 1.3 mg/Chew. Tab. Box 24s, 60s. *otc.*
Use: Antacid, antiflatulent.

Mylase 100. Alpha-amylase.
See: Diastase.

Myleran. (GlaxoWellcome) Busulfan 2 mg/Tab. Bot. 25s. *Rx.*
Use: Alkylating agent.

Mylicon. (Zeneca Pharmaceuticals) Simethicone 40 mg. **Chew. Tab.:** Bot. 100s, 500s, UD 100s. **Drops:** 40 mg/0.6 ml. Bot. 30 ml. *otc.*
Use: Antiflatulent.

Mylicon-80. (Zeneca Pharmaceuticals) Simethicone 80 mg/Chew. Tab. Bot. 100s, Box 12s, 48s, UD 100s. *otc.*
Use: Antiflatulent.

Mylicon-125. (Zeneca Pharmaceuticals) Simethicone 125 mg/Chew. Tab. In 12s, 50s. *otc.*
Use: Antiflatulent.

Mylocaine 2% Viscous Solution. (Rosemont Pharmaceutical Corp.) Lidocaine HCl 2%. Bot. 100 ml. *Rx.*
Use: Anesthetic, local.

Mylocaine 4% Solution. (Rosemont Pharmaceutical Corp.) Lidocaine HCl 4%. Bot. 50 ml, 100 ml. *Rx.*
Use: Anesthetic, local.

Mymethasone. (Rosemont Pharmaceutical Corp.) Dexamethasone 0.5 mg/5 ml, alcohol 5%. Elix. Bot. 100 ml, 240 ml. *Rx.*
Use: Corticosteroid.

Myminic Expectorant. (Morton Grove Pharmaceuticals, Inc.) Phenylpropanolamine HCl 12.5 mg, guaifenesin 100 mg/5 ml, alcohol 5%. Bot. 4 oz, pt, gal. *otc.*
Use: Decongestant, expectorant.

Myminic Pediatric. (Rosemont Pharmaceutical Corp.) Phenylpropanolamine HCl 12.5 mg, guaifenesin 100 mg/5 ml, alcohol 5%. Liq. Bot. 4 oz, pt, gal. *otc.*
Use: Decongestant, expectorant.

Myminic Syrup. (Rosemont Pharmaceutical Corp.) Phenylpropanolamine HCl 12.5 mg, chlorpheniramine maleate 2 mg/5 ml. Alcohol free. Bot. 4 oz, pt, gal. *otc.*
Use: Antihistamine, decongestant.

Myminicol. (Morton Grove Pharmaceuticals, Inc.) Phenylpropanolamine HCl 12.5 mg, chlorpheniramine maleate 2 mg, dextromethorphan HBr 10 mg/5 ml. Liq. Bot. 4 oz, pt, gal. *otc.*
Use: Antihistamine, antitussive, decongestant.

Mynatal. (ME Pharmaceuticals, Inc.) Ca 300 mg, Fe 65 mg, vitamins A 5000 IU, D 400 IU, E 30 mg, B_1 3 mg, B_2 3.4 mg, B_3 20 mg, B_5 10 mg, B_6 10 mg, B_{12} 12 mcg, C 120 mg, folic acid 1 mg, biotin 30 mcg, Cr, Cu, I, Mg, Mn, Mo, Zn 25 mg/Cap. Bot. 100s, 500s. *Rx.*
Use: Mineral, vitamin supplement.

Mynatal FC. (ME Pharmaceuticals, Inc.) Ca 250 mg, Fe 60 mg, vitamin A 5000 IU, D 400 IU, E 30 IU, B_1 3 mg, B_2 3.4 mg, B_3 20 mg, B_5 10 mg, B_6 10 mg, B_{12} 12 mcg, C 100 mg, folic acid 1 mg, biotin 30 mcg, Zn 25 mg, I, Mg, Cr, Cu, Mo, Mn. Capl. Bot. 100s. *Rx.*
Use: Mineral, vitamin supplement.

Mynatal P.N. Captabs. (ME Pharmaceuticals, Inc.) Ca 125 mg, Fe 60 mg, vitamins A 4000 IU, D 400 IU, B_1 3 mg, B_2

3 mg, B_3 10 mg, B_6 2 mg, B_{12} 3 mcg, C 50 mg, folic acid 1 mg, Zn 18 mg/Tab. Bot. 100s. *Rx.*
Use: Mineral, vitamin supplement.

Mynatal P.N. Forte. (ME Pharmaceuticals, Inc.) Fe 60 mg, vitamin A 5000 IU, D 400 IU, E 30 IU, C 80 mg, B_1 3 mg, B_2 3.4 mg, B_3 20 mg, B_6 4 mg, B_{12} 12 mcg, folic acid 1 mg, Ca 250 mg, Zn 25 mg, I, Mg, Cu. Capl. Bot. 100s. *Rx.*
Use: Mineral, vitamin supplement.

Mynatal Rx. (ME Pharmaceuticals, Inc.) Ca 200 mg, Fe 60 mg, vitamin A 4000 IU, D 400 IU, E 15 mg, B_1 1.5 mg, B_2 1.6 mg, B_3 17 mg, B_5 7 mg, B_6 4 mg, B_{12} 2.5 mcg, C 80 mg, folic acid 1 mg, biotin 0.03 mg, Zn 25 mg, Mg, Cu. Capl. Bot. 100s. *Rx.*
Use: Mineral, vitamin supplement.

Mynate 90 Plus. (ME Pharmaceuticals, Inc.) Ca 250 mg, Fe 90 mg, vitamin A 4000 IU, D 400 IU, E 30 IU, B_1 3 mg, B_2 3.4 mg, B_3 20 mg, B_6 20 mg, B_{12} 12 mcg, C 120 mg, folic acid 1 mg, Zn 25 mg, DSS, I, Cu. Capl. Bot. 100s. *Rx.*
Use: Mineral, vitamin supplement.

Myo-B. (Sigma-Tau Pharmaceuticals, Inc.) Adenosine-5-monophosphoric acid, vitamin B_{12}. Inj. Vial 10 ml. *Rx.*

Myocide NS. (Woodward Laboratories, Inc.) Benzalkonium chloride, propylene glycol, methylparaben. Soln. 30 ml. *otc.*
Use: Antiseptic.

myodil.
See: Iophendylate Inj., U.S.P. 23.

Myoflex Creme. (Rhone-Poulenc Rorer Pharmaceuticals, Inc.) Trolamine salicylate 10% in a vanishing cream base. Tube 2 oz, 4 oz, Jar 8 oz, lb, Pump dispenser 3 oz. *otc.*
Use: Analgesic, topical.

Myolin. (Roberts Pharmaceuticals) Orphenadrine citrate 30 mg/ml. Inj. Vial 10 ml. *Rx.*
Use: Muscle relaxant.

Myorgal. (Mysuran.) Ambenonium Cl.
Use: Cholinergic.

Myotalis. (Vita Elixir) Digitalis 1.5 gr/EC Tab. *Rx.*
Use: Cardiovascular agent.

Myoscint. (Centocor, Inc.) Imciromab pentetate 0.5 mg for conjugation with indium-111. Kit. *Rx.*
Use: Radioimmunoscintigraphy agent.

Myotonachol. (Glenwood, Inc.) Bethanechol Cl 10 mg, 25 mg/Tab. Bot.100s. *Rx.*
Use: Urinary tract product.

Myotoxin. (Vita Elixir) **#1:** Digitoxin 0.1 mg/Tab. **#2:** Digitoxin 0.2 mg/Tab. *Rx.*
Use: Cardiovascular agent.

Myphentol Elixir. (Rosemont Pharmaceutical Corp.) Phenobarbital 16.2 mg, hyoscyamine SO_4 or HBr 0.1037 mg, atropine sulfate 0.0194 mg, scopolamine HBr 0.0065 mg/5 ml, alcohol 23%. Bot. 4 oz, pt, gal. *Rx.*
Use: Anticholinergic, antispasmodic, hypnotic, sedative.

Myphetane DC Cough. (Morton Grove Pharmaceuticals, Inc.) Codeine phosphate 10 mg, brompheniramine maleate 2 mg, phenylpropanolamine HCl 12.5 mg/5 ml, alcohol 1.2%. Syr. Bot. 4 oz, gal.
Use: Antihistamine, antitussive, decongestant.

Myphetane DX Cough. (Various Mfr.) Brompheniramine maleate 2 mg, pseudoephedrine HCl 30 mg, dextromethorphan HBr 10 mg/5 ml, alcohol 0.95%. Syr. Bot. 4 oz, pt, gal. *Rx.*
Use: Antihistamine, antitussive, decongestant.

Myphetane. (Rosemont Pharmaceutical Corp.) Brompheniramine maleate 2 mg/5 ml, alcohol. Elix. Bot. *otc.*
Use: Antihistamine.

Myphetapp. (Rosemont Pharmaceutical Corp.) Brompheniramine maleate 2 mg, phenylpropanolamine HCl 12.5 mg/5 ml, alcohol 2.3%. Elix. Bot. 4 oz, Pt. *otc.*
Use: Antihistamine, decongestant.

Myproic Acid. (Rosemont Pharmaceutical Corp.) Valproic acid 250 mg (as sodium valproate)/5 ml. Syr. Bot. Pt. *Rx.*
Use: Anticonvulsant.

Myriatin Drops. (Sanofi Winthrop Pharmaceuticals) Atropine methonitrate BP. *Rx.*
Use: Antispasmodic.

myristica oil.
Use: Flavor.

•**myristyl alcohol.** (mih-RIST-ill) N.F. 18.
Use: Pharmaceutic aid (stiffening agent).

myristyl-picolinium chloride.
See: Wet Tone, Soln. (3M Pharmaceuticals).

Myrj 45. (Zeneca Pharmaceuticals) Mixture of free polyoxyethylene glycol and its mono- and distearates. Polyoxyl 8 stearate.
Use: Surface active agent.

Myrj 52 and M2s. (Zeneca Pharmaceuticals) Polyoxyethylene 40 stearate. Mixture of free polyoxyethylene glycol and its mono- and distearates.

Use: Surface active agent.

Myrj 53. (Zeneca Pharmaceuticals) Polyoxyl 50 stearate.
Use: Surface active agent.

Mysoline. (Wyeth-Ayerst Laboratories) Primidone, lactose, saccharin. **Tab.:** 50 mg. Bot. 100s, 500s; 250 mg. Bot. 100s, 1000s, UD 100s. **Susp.:** 250 mg/5 ml. Bot. 240 ml. *Rx.*
Use: Anticonvulsant.

Mysuran. Ambenonium Cl.
Use: Muscle stimulant.
See: Mytelase Cl, Cap. (Sanofi Winthrop Pharmaceuticals).

Mytelase. (Sanofi Winthrop Pharmaceuticals) Ambenonium Cl 10 mg/Cap. Bot. 100s. *Rx.*
Use: Muscle stimulant.

Myticin G Creme and Ointment.
See: g-myticin creme and ointment.

Mytomycin-C. (IOP, Inc.)
Use: Antiglaucoma agent. [Orphan Drug]

Mytrex. (Savage Laboratories) Triamcinolone acetonide 0.1%, nystatin 100,000 units/g. Cream, Oint. 15 g, 30 g, 60 g, 120 g. *Rx.*
Use: Antifungal, topical; corticosteroid.

Mytussin. (Rosemont Pharmaceutical Corp.) Guaifenesin 100 mg/5 ml, alcohol 3.5%. Syr. Bot. 4 oz, pt, gal. *otc.*
Use: Expectorant.

Mytussin AC Cough. (Morton Grove Pharmaceuticals, Inc.) Guaifenesin 100 mg, codeine phosphate 10 mg/5 ml, alcohol 3.5%. Bot. 4 oz, pt, gal. *c-v.*
Use: Antitussive, expectorant.

Mytussin DAC. (Rosemont Pharmaceutical Corp.) Guaifenesin 100 mg, pseudoephedrine HCl 30 mg, codeine phosphate 10 mg/5 ml. Syr. Bot. 4 oz, pt, gal. *c-v.*
Use: Antitussive, decongestant, expectorant.

Mytussin DM Expectorant. (Morton Grove Pharmaceuticals, Inc.) Guaifenesin 100 mg, dextromethorphan HBr 10 mg/5 ml, alcohol 1.6%. Bot. 4 oz, pt, gal. *otc.*
Use: Antitussive, expectorant.

Myverol. (Eastman Kodak Co.) Glyceryl monostearate.

My-Vitalife. (ME Pharmaceuticals, Inc.) Ca 130 mg, Fe 27 mg, vitamins A 6500 IU, D 400 IU, E 30 mg, B_1 1.5 mg, B_2 1.7 mg, B_3 20 mg, B_5 10 mg, B_6 2 mg, B_{12} 6 mcg, C 60 mg, folic acid 0.4 mg, Cr, Cu, K, I, Mg, Mn, Mo, P, Se, Zn, 15 mg, vitamin K, biotin 30 mcg/Cap. Bot. 60s. *otc.*
Use: Mineral, vitamin supplement.

M-Zole 7 Dual Pack. (Alpharma USPD Inc.) Miconazole nitrate 100 mg. Vag. Supp. Miconazole nitrate 2%. Cream. *otc.*
Use: Vaginal preparation.

N

Na-Ana-Tal. (Churchill) Phenobarbital 0.25 g, phenacetin 2 g, aspirin 3 g, nicotinic acid 50 mg/Tab. Bot. 100s, Liq. Bot. 16 oz. *c-IV.*
Use: Analgesic, hypnotic, sedative.

•**nabazenil.** (nab-AZE-eh-nill) USAN.
Use: Anticonvulsant.

•**nabilone.** (NAB-ih-lone) USAN.
Use: Anxiolytic.

•**nabitan hydrochloride.** (NAB-ih-tan) USAN. *Formerly Nabutan Hydrochloride.*
Use: Analgesic.

•**naboctate hydrochloride.** (NAB-ock-tate) USAN.
Use: Antiglaucoma agent, antinauseant.

•**nabumetone.** (nab-YOU-meh-TONE) USAN.
Use: Anti-inflammatory.
See: Relafen (SmithKline Beecham Pharmaceuticals).

n-acetylcysteine.
See: Acetylcysteine.

n-acetyl-p-aminophenol. Acetaminophen, U.S.P. 23.

•**nadide.** (NAD-ide) USAN. *Formerly Diphosphopyridine Nucleotide, Nicotinamide Adenine Dinucleotide.*
Use: Antagonist to alcohol and narcotics.

Nadinola (Deluxe) for Oily Skin. (Strickland) Hydroquinone 2%. Bot. 1.25 oz, 2.25 oz. *Rx.*
Use: Dermatologic.

Nadinola for Dry Skin. (Strickland) Hydroquinone 2%. Bot. 1.25 oz, 2.25 oz. *Rx.*
Use: Dermatologic.

Nadinola (Ultra) for Normal Skin. (Strickland) Hydroquinone 2%. Bot. 1.25 oz, 3.75 oz, Tube 1.85 oz. *Rx.*
Use: Dermatologic.

•**nadolol.** (nay-DOE-lahl) U.S.P. 23.
Use: Antihypertensive, antianginal, beta-adrenergic blocker.
See: Corgard, Tab. (Bristol-Myers Squibb).

nadolol. (nay-DOE-lahl) (Various Mfr.) Tab.: **20 mg:** 100s, UD 100s. **40 mg, 80 mg:** 100s, 1000s, UD 100s. **120 mg:** 100s, 1000s. **160 mg:** 100s. *Rx.*
Use: Beta-adrenergic blocker.

nadolol and bendroflumethiazide.
Use: Antihypertensive, antianginal beta blocker.
See: Corzide (Bristol-Myers Squibb).

naepaine hydrochloride.
Use: Anesthetic, local.

•**nafamostat mesylate.** (naff-AM-oh-stat) USAN.
Use: Anticoagulant, antifibrinolytic.

•**nafarelin acetate.** (NAFF-uh-RELL-in) USAN.
Use: LHRH agonist; agonist, hormone. [Orphan Drug]
See: Synarel (Roche Laboratories).

Nafazair. (Bausch & Lomb Pharmaceuticals) Naphazoline HCl 0.1%. Soln. Bot. 15 ml. *Rx.*
Use: Mydriatic, vasoconstrictor.

Nafazair A. (Bausch & Lomb Pharmaceuticals) Naphazoline HCl 0.025%, pheniramine maleate 0.3%, benzalkonium chloride 0.01%, EDTA, boric acid, sodium borate. Bot. 15 ml. *Rx.*
Use: Decongestant combination, ophthalmic.

•**nafcillin, sodium.** (naff-SILL-in) U.S.P. 23.
Use: Anti-infective.
See: Unipen, Vial. (Wyeth-Ayerst Laboratories).
Nallpen, Pow. for Inj. (SmithKline Beecham Pharmaceuticals).

Na-Feen. (Pacemaker) Fluoride 1 mg/Dose. Tab. Bot. 100s, 500s, 1000s; Liq. 2 oz. *Rx.*
Use: Dental caries agent.

•**nafenopin.** (naff-EN-oh-pin) USAN.
Use: Antihyperlipoproteinemic.

•**nafimidone hydrochloride.** (naff-IH-mih-DOHN) USAN.
Use: Anticonvulsant.

•**naflocort.** (NAFF-lah-cort) USAN.
Use: Adrenocortical steroid (topical).

•**nafomine malate.** (NAFF-oh-meen) USAN.
Use: Muscle relaxant.

•**nafoxidine hydrochloride.** (naff-OX-ih-deen) USAN.
Use: Antiestrogen.

•**nafronyl oxalate.** (NAFF-row-NILL OX-ah-late) USAN.
Use: Vasodilator.

•**naftifine hydrochloride.** (NAFF-tih-FEEN) USAN.
Use: Antifungal.
See: Naftin, Cream (Allergan, Inc.).

Naftin. (Allergan, Inc.) Naftifine HCl 1%. Cream. 2 g, 15 g, 30 g. *Rx.*
Use: Antifungal, topical.

naganol.
See: Suramin Sodium. Naphuride Sodium.

•**nagrestipen.** USAN.
Use: Stem cell inhibitory protein.

Nailicure. (Purepac Pharmaceutical Co.) Denatonium benzoate in a clear nail polish base. Liq. Bot. 0.33 oz. *otc.*
Use: Nail-biting deterrent.

Nail Plus. (Faraday) Gelatin Cap. Bot. 100s, 200s.

•**nalbuphine hydrochloride.** (NAL-byoo-FEEN) USAN.
Use: Analgesic, narcotic.
See: Nubain, Vial (Du Pont Merck Pharmaceutical Co.).

Naldecon CX Adult Liquid. (Apothecon, Inc.) Phenylpropanolamine 12.5 mg, guaifenesin 200 mg, codeine phosphate 10 mg/10 ml. Alcohol free. Bot. 4 oz, pt. *c-v.*
Use: Antitussive, decongestant, expectorant.

Naldecon DX Adult Liquid. (Apothecon, Inc.) Phenylpropanolamine HCl 12.5 mg, guaifenesin 200 mg, dextromethorphan HBr 10 mg/10 ml, saccharin, sorbitol. Alcohol free. Bot. 4 oz, pt. *otc.*
Use: Antitussive, decongestant, expectorant.

Naldecon DX Children's Syrup. (Apothecon, Inc.) Phenylpropanolamine HCl 6.25 mg, dextromethorphan HBr 5 mg, guaifenesin 100 mg/5 ml. Bot. 4 oz, 16 oz. *otc.*
Use: Antitussive, decongestant, expectorant.

Naldecon DX Pediatric Drops. (Apothecon, Inc.) Phenylpropanolamine HCl 6.25 mg, guaifenesin 50 mg, dextromethorphan HBr 5 mg/ml, alcohol free, saccharin, sorbitol. Bot. 30 ml. *otc.*
Use: Antitussive, decongestant, expectorant.

Naldecon EX Children's Syrup. (Apothecon, Inc.) Phenylpropanolamine HCl 6.25 mg, guaifenesin 100 mg/5 ml, saccharin, sorbitol. Bot. 118 ml, 480 ml. *otc.*
Use: Decongestant, expectorant.

Naldecon EX Pediatric Drops. (Apothecon, Inc.) Phenylpropanolamine HCl 6.25 mg, guaifenesin 50 mg/ml. Bot. 30 ml. w/dropper. *otc.*
Use: Decongestant, expectorant.

Naldecon Pediatric Drops. (Apothecon, Inc.) Chlorpheniramine maleate 0.5 mg, phenyltoloxamine citrate 2 mg, phenylpropanolamine HCl 5 mg, phenylephrine HCl 1.25 mg/ml, sorbitol. Bot. 30 ml. *Rx.*
Use: Antihistamine, decongestant.

Naldecon Pediatric Syrup. (Apothecon, Inc.) Chlorpheniramine maleate 0.5 mg, phenyltoloxamine citrate 2 mg, phenylpropanolamine HCl 5 mg, phenylephrine HCl 1.25 mg/5 ml, sorbitol. Bot. 473 ml. *Rx.*
Use: Antihistamine, decongestant.

Naldecon Senior DX. (Apothecon, Inc.) Dextromethorphan HBr 10 mg, guaifenesin 200 mg/5 ml, saccharin, sorbitol, alcohol free. Liq. Bot. 118 ml. *otc.*
Use: Antitussive, expectorant.

Naldecon Senior EX. (Apothecon, Inc.) Guaifenesin 200 mg/5 ml, saccharin, sorbitol. Liq. Bot. 118 ml. *otc.*
Use: Expectorant.

Naldecon Syrup. (Apothecon, Inc.) Chlorpheniramine maleate 2.5 mg, phenyltoloxamine citrate 7.5 mg, phenylpropanolamine HCl 20 mg, phenylephrine HCl 5 mg/5 ml. Bot. 473 ml. *Rx.*
Use: Antihistamine, decongestant.

Naldecon Tablets. (Apothecon, Inc.) Phenylephrine HCl 10 mg, phenylpropanolamine HCl 40 mg, phenyltoloxamine citrate 15 mg, chlorpheniramine maleate 5 mg/SR Tab. Bot. 100s, 500s. *Rx.*
Use: Antihistamine, decongestant.

Naldegesic Tablets. (Bristol-Myers Squibb) Pseudoephedrine HCl 15 mg, acetaminophen 325 mg/Tab. Bot. 100s. *otc.*
Use: Analgesic, decongestant.

Naldelate DX Adult Liquid. (Alpharma USPD Inc.) Phenylpropanolamine HCl 12.5 mg, dextromethorphan HBr 10 mg, guaifenesin 200 mg. Bot. 120 ml, 480 ml. *otc.*
Use: Antitussive, decongestant, expectorant.

Naldelate Pediatric Syrup. (Various Mfr.) Phenylpropanolamine HCl 5 mg, phenylephrine HCl 1.25 mg, chlorpheniramine maleate 0.5 mg, phenyltoloxamine citrate 2 mg/5 ml. Bot. 120 ml, 473 ml, gal. *Rx.*
Use: Antihistamine, decongestant.

Naldelate Syrup. (Various Mfr.) Phenylpropanolamine HCl 20 mg, phenylephrine HCl 5 mg, chlorpheniramine maleate 2.5 mg, phenyltoloxamine citrate 7.5 mg/5 ml. Syr. Bot. 473 ml, gal. *Rx.*
Use: Antihistamine, decongestant.

Nalfon. (Eli Lilly and Co.) Fenoprofen calcium. **Cap.:** 200 mg. Rx Pak 100s. **300 mg.:** Rx Pak 100s, Bot. 500s. *Rx.*
Use: Analgesic, NSAID.

Nalgest. (Major Pharmaceuticals) Phenylpropanolamine HCl 40 mg, phenylephrine HCl 10 mg, chlorpheniramine maleate 5 mg, phenyltoloxamine citrate 15 mg/Tab. Bot. 100s, 500s,

1000s. *Rx.*
Use: Antihistamine, decongestant.
Nalgest Pediatric Drops. (Major Pharmaceuticals) Phenylpropanolamine HCl 5 mg, phenylephrine HCl 1.25 mg, chlorpheniramine maleate 0.5 mg, phenyltoloxamine citrate 2 mg, sorbitol/ml. Bot. 30 ml. *Rx.*
Use: Antihistamine, decongestant.
Nalgest Pediatric Syrup. (Major Pharmaceuticals) Phenylpropanolamine HCl 5 mg, phenylephrine HCl 1.25 mg, chlorpheniramine maleate 0.5 mg, phenyltoloxamine citrate 2 mg/5 ml. Syr. Bot. 473 ml, gal. *Rx.*
Use: Antihistamine, decongestant.
Nalgest Syrup. (Major Pharmaceuticals) Phenylpropanolamine HCl 20 mg, phenylephrine HCl 5 mg, chlorpheniramine maleate 2.5 mg, phenyltoloxamine citrate 7.5 mg/5 ml. Syr. Bot. 473 ml. *Rx.*
Use: Antihistamine, decongestant.
•**nalidixate sodium.** (nal-ih-DIK-sate) USAN. Under study.
Use: Anti-infective.
•**nalidixic acid.** (nal-ih-DIK-sik) U.S.P. 23.
Use: Anti-infective.
See: NegGram, Capl., Susp. (Sanofi Winthrop Pharmaceuticals).
Nallpen. (SmithKline Beecham Pharmaceuticals) Nafcillin sodium 500 mg, 1 g, 2 g, 10 g. Inj. Vial 500 mg, Piggyback 1 g, 2 g, Bulk 10 g. *Rx.*
Use: Anti-infective, penicillin.
•**nalmefene.** (NAL-meh-FEEN) USAN.
Formerly Naletrene.
Use: Antagonist to narcotics.
See: Revex, Inj. (Ohmeda Pharmaceuticals).
nalmetrene. (NAL-meh-treen)
Use: Antagonist to narcotics.
•**nalmexone hydrochloride.** (NAL-mex-ohn) USAN.
Use: Analgesic, narcotic.
•**nalorphine hydrochloride.** U.S.P. 23.
•**naloxone hydrochloride.** (NAL-ox-ohn) U.S.P. 23.
Use: Narcotic antagonist.
See: Narcan, Amp. (Du Pont Merck Pharmaceutical Co.).
naloxone hydrochloride. (Various Mfr.) **0.02 mg/ml:** Amp 2 ml. **0.4 mg/ml:** Amp 1 ml, syringe 1 ml, vial 1 ml, 2 ml, 10 ml. *Rx.*
Use: Narcotic antagonist.
Nalspan. (Rosemont Pharmaceutical Corp.) Phenylpropanolamine HCl 20 mg, phenylephrine HCl 5 mg, chlorpheniramine maleate 2.5 mg, phenyltoloxamine citrate 7.5 mg/ml, alcohol free. Syr. Bot. pt. *otc.*
Use: Antihistamine, decongestant.
•**naltrexone.** (nal-TREX-ohn) USAN.
Use: Antagonist to narcotics. [Orphan Drug]
See: Depade, Tab. (Mallinckrodt).
ReVia, Tab. (Du Pont Merck Pharmaceutical Co.).
namazene. Phenothiazine.
namol xenyrate. (NAY-mahl ZEH-neh-rate)
See: Namoxyrate.
•**namoxyrate.** (nam-OX-ee-rate) USAN.
Use: Analgesic.
See: Namol Xenyrate (Warner Chilcott Laboratories).
namuron.
See: Cyclobarbital Calcium (Various Mfr.).
•**nandrolone cyclotate.** (NAN-drole-ohn SIH-kloe-tate) USAN.
Use: Anabolic.
•**nandrolone decanoate.** (NAN-drole-ohn deh-KAN-oh-ate) U.S.P. 23.
Use: Androgen.
See: Anabolin LA-100, Vial (Alto Pharmaceuticals,Inc.).
Androlone-D, Inj. (Keene Pharmaceuticals, Inc.).
Androlone-D 50, Inj. (Keene Pharmaceuticals, Inc.).
Deca-Durabolin, Amp., Vial (Organon Teknika Corp).
Hybolin Decanoate, Inj. (Hyrex Pharmaceuticals).
•**nandrolone phenpropionate.** (NAN-droe-lone fen-PRO-pee-oh-nate) U.S.P. 23.
Use: Androgen.
See: Anabolin IM, Vial (Alto Pharmaceuticals, Inc.).
Androlone, Inj. (Keene Pharmaceuticals, Inc.).
Androlone 50, Inj. (Keene Pharmaceuticals, Inc.).
Durabolin Inj. (Organon Teknika Corp).
Hybolin Improved, Vial (Hyrex Pharmaceuticals).
nantradol hydrochloride. (NAN-trah-DAHL) USAN.
Use: Analgesic.
Naotin. (Drug Products) Sodium nicotinate. Amp. (equivalent to 10 mg nicotinic acid/ml)10 ml, Box 25s, 100s. *Rx.*
Use: Vitamin B_3 supplement.
NAPA. (Medco Research, Inc.; Parke-Davis) Acecainide hydrochloride.
Use: Cardiovascular agent.

•**napactadine hydrochloride.** (nap-ACK-tah-deen) USAN.
Use: Antidepressant.

•**napamezole hydrochloride.** (nap-am-EH-zole) USAN.
Use: Antidepressant.

NAPAmide Caps. (Major Pharmaceuticals) Disopyramide phosphate 100 mg or 150 mg/Cap. Bot. 100s, 500s, UD 100s. *Rx.*
Use: Antiarrhythmic.

•**naphazoline hydrochloride.** (naff-AZZ-oh-leen) U.S.P. 23.
Use: Adrenergic (vasoconstrictor).
See: AK-Con, Soln. (Akorn, Inc.).
Albalon, Soln. (Allergan America).
Allerest Eye Drops, Soln. (Novartis Pharmaceutical Corp.).
Comfort Eye Drops, Soln. (PBH Wesley Jessen).
Clear Eyes, Drops (Abbott Laboratories).
Degest 2, Soln. (PBH Wesley Jessen).
Maximum Strength Allergy Drops (Bausch & Lomb Pharmaceuticals).
Muro's Opcon, Soln. (Bausch & Lomb Pharmaceuticals).
Nafazair, Soln. (Bausch & Lomb Pharmaceuticals).
Naphcon, Drops (Alcon Laboratories, Inc.).
Privine HCl, Soln., Spray (Novartis Pharmaceutical Corp.).
VasoClear, Soln. (Ciba Vision).
Vasocon Regular, Liq. (Ciba Vision).
W/Antazoline phosphate, boric acid, phenylmercuric acetate, sodium Cl, sodium carbonate anhydrous.
See: Antazoline-V, Soln. (Rugby Labs, Inc.).
Vasocon-A Ophthalmic, Soln. (Ciba Vision).
W/Antazoline phosphate, polyvinyl alcohol.
See: AK-Con-A, Soln. (Akorn, Inc.).
Nafazair A, Soln. (Bausch & Lomb Pharmaceuticals).
Naphazole-A, Soln. (Major Pharmaceuticals).
Naphazoline Plus, Soln. (Parmed Pharmaceuticals, Inc.).
Naphcon A, Liq. (Alcon Laboratories, Inc).
Naphoptic-A, Soln. (Optopics Laboratories, Corp.).
W/PEG 300, benzalkonium Cl.
See: Allergy Drops (Bausch & Lomb Pharmaceuticals).
W/Phenylephrine HCl, pyrilamine maleate, phenylpropanolamine HCl.
See: 4-Way Nasal Spray (Bristol-Myers Squibb).
W/Polyvinyl alcohol.
See: Albalon, Ophth Soln. (Allergan, Inc.).
Albalon Liquifilm, Ophth. Soln. (Allergan, Inc.).

naphazoline hydrochloride. (Various Mfr.) 0.1% Soln. Bot. 15 ml. *Rx.*
Use: Adrenergic (vasoconstrictor).

naphazoline hydrochloride & antazoline phosphate. (Various Mfr.) Naphazoline HCl 0.05%, antazoline phosphate 0.5%. Soln. 5 ml, 15 ml. *otc.*
Use: Antihistamine, decongestant, ophthalmic.

naphazoline hydrochloride & pheniramine maleate. (Various Mfr.) Naphazoline HCl 0.025%, pheniramine maleate 0.3%. Soln. Bot. 15 ml. *otc.*
Use: Antihistamine, decongestant, ophthalmic.

naphazoline plus. (Parmed Pharmaceuticals, Inc.) Naphazoline HCl 0.025%, pheniramine maleate 0.3%. Bot. 15 ml. *otc.*
Use: Decongestant combination, ophthalmic.

Naphcon. (Alcon Laboratories, Inc.) Naphazoline HCl 0.012%. Soln. Bot. 15 ml. *otc.*
Use: Mydriatic, vasoconstrictor.

Naphcon-A. (Alcon Laboratories, Inc.) Naphazoline HCl 0.025%, pheniramine maleate 0.3%. Soln. Bot. 15 ml. *otc.*
Use: Decongestant combination, ophthalmic.

Naphcon Forte. (Alcon Laboratories, Inc.) Naphazoline HCl 0.1%/ml. Soln. Drop-Tainer Bot. 15 ml. *Rx.*
Use: Mydriatic, vasoconstrictor.

Napholine. (Horizon Pharmaceutical Corp.) Naphazoline HCl 0.1%. Soln. Bot. 15 ml. *Rx.*
Use: Mydriatic, vasoconstrictor.

Naphoptic-A. (Optopics Laboratories, Corp) Naphazoline HCl 0.025%, pheniramine maleate 0.3%. Soln. Bot. 15 ml. *Rx.*
Use: Decongestant combination, ophthalmic.

Naphthyl-B Salicylate. Betol, Naphthosalol, Salinaphthol.
Use: GI & GU, antiseptic.

naphuride sodium. Suramin Sodium.

•**napitane mesylate.** (NAP-ih-tane) USAN.
Use: Antidepressant.

Naprelan. (Wyeth-Ayerst Laboratories) Naproxen 375 mg, 500 mg/ER Tab. 100s (375 mg), 75s (500 mg). *Rx.*

Use: Analgesic.

•**napitane mesylate.** (NAP-ih-tane) USAN.
Use: Antidepressant.

Naprosyn. (Roche Laboratories) Naproxen. **Oral susp.:** 125 mg/5 ml, sorbitol. Bot. 480 ml. **250 mg/Tab.:** Bot. 100s, 500s, UD 100s; **375 mg/Tab.:** Bot. 100s, 500s, UD 100s; **500 mg/Tab.:** Bot. 100s, 500s, UD 100s. *Rx.*
Use: Analgesic, NSAID.

•**naproxen.** (nah-PROX-ehn) U.S.P. 23.
Use: Analgesic, anti-inflammatory, antipyretic.
See: Naprosyn, Susp., Tab. (Roche Laboratories).

naproxen. (Various Mfr.) 250, 375, 500 mg/Tab. 100s, 500s, 1000s, UD 100s. *Rx.*
Use: Analgesic, NSAID, antipyretic.

naproxen. (Roxane Laboratories, Inc.) 125 mg/5 ml, methylparaben, sorbitol, sucrose, pineapple-orange flavor. Oral Susp. 500 ml, UD 15 ml, 20 ml.
Use: Analgesic, NSAID.

•**naproxen sodium.** (nah-PROX-ehn) U.S.P. 23.
Use: Analgesic, anti-inflammatory, antipyretic.
See: Aleve, Tab. (Procter & Gamble Pharm.).
Anaprox, Tab. (Roche Laboratories).
Anaprox DS, Tab. (Roche Laboratories).
Naprosyn, Tab, Susp. (Roche Laboratories).

naproxen sodium. (Various Mfr.) 200 mg, 250 mg, 500 mg/Tab. 100s, 500s, 1000s, UD 100s. *Rx.*
Use: Analgesic, NSAID.

naproxen sodium. (Zenith Goldline Pharmaceuticals) Naproxen sodium 200 mg (220 mg naproxen sodium). Tab. Bot. 24s. *otc.*
Use: Anti-inflammatory.

•**naproxol.** (nay-PROX-ole) USAN.
Use: Analgesic, anti-inflammatory, antipyretic.

Naqua. (Schering-Plough Corp.) Trichlormethiazide 2 mg or 4 mg/Tab. Bot. 100s, 1000s. *Rx.*
Use: Diuretic.

•**napsagatran.** (nap-sah-GAT-ran) USAN.
Use: Antithrombotic.

•**naranol hydrochloride.** (NARE-ah-nahl) USAN.
Use: Antipsychotic.

•**naratriptan hydrochloride.** (NAHR-ah-trip-tan) USAN.
Use: Antimigraine.
See: Amerge, Tab. (GlaxoWellcome).

Narcan. (Du Pont Merck Pharmaceutical Co.) Naloxone HCl. **0.02 mg/ml:** Amp. 2 ml. **0.4 mg/ml:** Amp. 1 ml, Box 10s. Prefilled syringe 1 ml, Tray 10s; 1 ml, 2 ml, 10 ml Multiple-dose vials. **1 mg/ml:** Amp. 2 ml, Box 10s; Multiple-dose vial 10 ml. *Rx.*
Use: Narcotic antagonist.

Nardil. (Parke-Davis) Phenelzine sulfate 15 mg/Tab. Bot. 100s. *Rx.*
Use: Antidepressant.

Naropin. (Astra Pharmaceuticals, L.P.) Ropivacaine HCl 2, 5, 7.5, and 10 mg/ml concentrations/Inj. Single-dose amps, vials, and infusion bottles. *Rx.*
Use: Anesthetic, local.

Nasabid. (Jones Medical Industries, Inc.) Pseudoephedrine HCl 90 mg, guaifenesin 250 mg, sucrose. Cap., prolonged-action. Bot. 100s. *Rx.*
Use: Decongestant, expectorant.

Nasabid SR. (Jones Medical Industries, Inc.) Pseudoephedrine HCl 90 mg, guaifenesin 500 mg. LA Tab. Bot. 100s. *Rx.*
Use: Decongestant, expectorant.

Nasacort. (Rhone-Poulenc Rorer Pharmaceuticals, Inc.) Triamcinolone acetonide 55 mcg per actuation. Inhaler. Can. 10 g w/triamcinolone 15 mg ($\geq$ 100 sprays). *Rx.*
Use: Corticosteroid, nasal.

Nasacort AQ. (Rhone-Poulenc Rorer Pharmaceuticals, Inc.) Triamcinolone acetonide $\approx$ 55 mcg per actuation, benzalkonium chloride, dextrose, EDTA, carboxymethlycellulose sodium, polysorbate 80. Spray. Bot. 6.5 g and 16.5 g (30 and 120 actuations). *Rx.*
Use: Corticosteroid, nasal.

Nasadent. (Scherer Laboratories, Inc.) Sodium metaphosphate, glycerin, dicalcium phosphate dihydrate, sodium carboxymethylcellulose, oil of spearmint, sodium benzoate, saccharin. *otc.*
Use: Ingestible dentifrice.

Nasahist Capsules. (Keene Pharmaceuticals, Inc.) Phenylpropanolamine HCl 40 mg, phenylephrine HCl 10 mg, chlorpheniramine maleate 12 mg/Cap. Bot. 100s. *Rx.*
Use: Antihistamine, decongestant.

NaSal Saline Nasal. (Sanofi Winthrop Pharmaceuticals) Sodium Cl 0.65%. Drops, Spray. Bot. 15 ml. *otc.*
Use: Moisturizer, nasal.

Nasalcrom. (Ortho McNeil Pharmaceutical) Cromolyn sodium 40 mg/ml, benzalkonium Cl 0.01%, EDTA 0.01%. Nasal Soln. Metered dose spray. De-

livers 5.2 mg/spray. Metered spray device 13 ml or 26 ml. *otc.*
Use: Antiallergic, nasal.

Nasalide. (Dura) Flunisolide 0.025%. Spray Soln. Pump. Bot. 25 ml. *Rx.*
Use: Corticosteroid, nasal.

Nasal Jelly. (Kondon) Phenol, camphor, menthol, eucalyptus oil, lavender oil. Oint. Tube. 20 g. *otc.*
Use: Decongestant.

Nasal Saline. (Sanofi Winthrop Pharmaceuticals) Nasal spray and drops. Sodium Cl 0.65% buffered w/phosphates, preservatives. Bot. 15 ml. Spray Bot. 15 ml. *otc.*
Use: Moisturizer, nasal.

Nasarel. (Dura) Flunisolide 0.025%. Spray Soln. Bot. 25 ml. *Rx.*
Use: Anti-inflammatory.

Nasatab LA. (ECR Pharmaceuticals) Guaifenesin 500 mg, pseudoephedrine HCl 120 mg/LA Tab. Dye free. Bot. 100s. *Rx.*
Use: Decongestant, expectorant.

Nascobal. (Schwarz Pharma, Inc.) Cyanocobalamin 500 mcg/0.1 ml, benzalkonium chloride 500 mcg/actuation Intranasal Gel. Bot. 5 ml ($\approx$ 8 doses). *Rx.*
Use: Vitamin supplement.

Nasonex. (Schering-Plough Corp.) Mometasone furoate monohydrate 50 mcg, glycerin, phenylethyl alcohol. Nasal spray. Bot. 17 g. *Rx.*
Use: Corticosteroid.

Nasophen. (Premo) Phenylephrine HCl 0.25%, 1%. Bot. Pt. *otc.*
Use: Decongestant.

Natabec. (Parke-Davis) Vitamins A 4000 IU, D 400 IU, B_1 3 mg, B_2 2 mg, B_6 3 mg, C 50 mg, B_{12} 5 mcg, B_3 10 mg, elemental calcium 240 mg, elemental iron 30 mg/Kapseal. Bot. 100s. *otc.*
Use: Mineral, vitamin supplement.

Natabec-F.A. (Parke-Davis) Vitamins A 4000 IU, D 400 IU, B_1 3 mg, B_2 2 mg, B_6 3 mg, C 50 mg, B_{12} 5 mcg, B_3 10 mg, elemental calcium 240 mg, elemental iron 30 mg, folic acid 0.1 mg/Kapseal, magnesium, bisulfites. Bot. 100s. *otc.*
Use: Mineral, vitamin supplement.

Natabec with Fluoride. (Parke-Davis) Vitamins A 4000 IU, D 400 IU, B_1 3 mg, B_2 2 mg, B_6 3 mg, C 50 mg, B_{12} 5 mcg, B_3 10 mg, elemental calcium 240 mg, elemental iron 30 mg, elemental fluoride 1 mg/Kapseal. Bot. 100s. *Rx.*
Use: Vitamin supplement, dental caries agent.

Natacyn. (Alcon Laboratories, Inc.) Natamycin 5%. Bot. 15 ml. *Rx.*
Use: Antifungal agent, ophthalmic.

Natal Care Plus. (Ethex) Vitamin A 4000 IU, C 120 mg, calcium sulfate 200 mg, Fe 27 mg, D 400 IU, E 22 IU, B_1 1.84 mg, B_2 3 mg, niacinamide 20 mg, B_6 10 mg, folic acid 1 mg, B_{12} 12 mcg, Zn 25 mg, Cu 2 mg.Tab. Bot. 100s. *Rx.*
Use: Mineral, vitamin supplement.

Natalins. (Bristol-Myers Squibb) Ca 200 mg, Fe 30 mg, vitamins A 4000 IU, D 400 IU, E 15 IU, B_1 1.5 mg, B_2 1.6 mg, B_3 17 mg, B_6 2.6 mg, B_{12} 2.5 mcg, C 70 mg, folic acid 0.5 mg, Mg, Cu, Zn 15 mg/Tab. Bot. 100s. *otc.*
Use: Mineral, vitamin supplement.

•**natamycin.** (NAT-uh-MY-sin) U.S.P. 23.
Use: Anti-infective, ophthalmic.
See: Natacyn, Susp. (Alcon Laboratories, Inc.).

Natarex Prenatal. (Major Pharmaceuticals) Ca 200 mg, iron 60 mg, vitamins A 4000 IU, D 400 IU, E 15 mg, B_1 1.5 mg, B_2 1.6 mg, B_3 17 mg, B_5 7 mg, B_6 4 mg, B_{12} 2.5 mcg, C 80 mg, folic acid 1 mg, Cu, Mg, Zn 25 mg, biotin 30 mcg/ Tab. Bot 100s. *Rx.*
Use: Mineral, vitamin supplement.

Nata-San. (Sandia) Vitamins A 4000 IU, D 400 IU, B_1 5 mg, B_2 4 mg, B_6 10 mg, nicotinic acid 10 mg, C 100 mg, B_{12} activity 5 mcg, ferrous fumarate 200 mg (elemental iron 65 mg), calcium carbonate 500 mg (Ca 196 mg), Cu (sulfate) 0.5 mg, Mg (sulfate) 0.1 mg, Mn (sulfate) 0.1 mg, K (sulfate) 0.1 mg, Zn (sulfate) 0.5 mg/Tab. Bot. 100s, 1000s. *otc.*
Use: Mineral, vitamin supplement.

Nata-San F.A. (Sandia) Vitamins A 4000 IU, D 400 IU, B_1 5 mg, B_2 4 mg, B_6 10 mg, nicotinic acid 10 mg, C 100 mg, B_{12} activity 5 mcg, folic acid 1 mg, Fe 65 mg, Ca 200 mg, Cu (sulfate) 0.5 mg, Mg (sulfate) 0.1 mg, Mn (sulfate) 0.1 mg, K (sulfate) 0.1 mg, Zn (sulfate) 0.5 mg/Tab. Bot. 100s, 1000s. *Rx.*
Use: Mineral, vitamin supplement.

Natodine. (Faraday) Iodine in organic form as found in kelp 1 mg/Tab. Bot. 100s, 250s. *otc.*

Natrapel. (Tender) Citronella 10% in 15% Aloe vera base. *otc.*
Use: Insect repellent.

Natrico. (Drug Products) Potassium nitrate 2 g, sodium nitrite 1 g, nitroglycerin 0.25 g, cratageus oxycantha 0.25 gr/Pulvoid. Bot. 100s, 1000s. *Rx.*
Use: Antihypertensive.

Naturacil. (Bristol-Myers Squibb) Psyllium seed husks 3.4 g, carbohydrate 9.6 g, Na 11 mg, 54 cal/2 pieces. Ctn.

24s, 40s. *otc.*
Use: Laxative.

Natur-Aid. (Scott/Cord) Lactose, pectin, and Carob-lemon juice. Pow. 90%. Bot. 8 oz. *otc.*
Use: Increase in normal intestinal flora.

Natural Diuretic Water Tablet. (Amlab) Buchu leaves 1 g, uva ursi 1 g, trilicum 1 g, parsley 1 g, juniper berries 1 g, asparagus 1 g, alfalfa powder 1 gr/Tab. Bot. 100s. *otc.*
Use: Diuretic.

natural lung surfactant.
See: Survanta (Ross Laboratories).

natural vegetable powder. (Various Mfr.) Psyllium hydrophilic mucilloid 3.4 g, dextrose, sodium < 10 mg, 14 Cal/ Dose. Pow. 210 g, 420 g, 630 g. *otc.*
Use: Laxative.

natural vitamin a in oil.
See: Oleovitamin A, U.S.P. 23.

Naturalyte. (Unico Holdings) Na 45 mEq, K 20 mEq, Cl 35 mEq, citrate 48 mEq, dextrose 25 g/L. Soln. Bot. 240 ml, 1 liter. *otc.*
Use: Electrolyte, mineral supplement.

Naturalyte Oral Electrolyte Solution. (Unico Holdings) Dextrose 20 g, K 20 mEq, fructose 5 g, Cl 35 mEq, Na 45 mEq, citrate 30 mEq. Soln. Bot. 1 liter. *otc.*
Use: Mineral, electrolyte supplement.

Nature's Aid Laxative Tabs. (Walgreen Co.) Docusate sodium 100 mg, yellow phenolphthalein 65 mg/Tab. Bot. 60s. *otc.*
Use: Laxative.

Nature's Remedy Tablets. (SmithKline Beecham Pharmaceuticals) Aloe 100 mg, cascara sagrada 150 mg/FC Tab. Foil backed blister pkg. Box 12s, 30s, 60s. *otc.*
Use: Laxative.

Nature's Tears. (Rugby Labs, Inc.) Hydroxypropyl methylcellulose 2906 0.4%, KCl, NaCl, sodium phosphate, benzalkonium Cl 0.01%, EDTA. Soln. Bot. 15 ml. *otc.*
Use: Artificial tears.

Naturetin. (Bristol-Myers Squibb) Bendroflumethiazide. **5 mg/Tab.:** Bot. 100s, 1000s. **10 mg/Tab.:** Bot. 100s. *Rx.*
Use: Diuretic.

Natur-Lax Tablets. (Faraday) Rhubarb root, cape aloes, cascara sagrada extract, mandrake root, parsley, carrot. Protein coated tab. Bot. 100s. *otc.*
Use: Laxative.

Naus-A-Tories. (Table Rock) Pyrilamine maleate 25 mg, secobarbital 30 mg/ Supp. Box 12s. *c-II.*
Use: Antiemetic.

Nausea Relief. (Zenith Goldline Pharmaceuticals) Dextrose 1.87 g, fructose 1.87 g, phosphoric acid 21.5 mg, methylparaben. Soln. Bot. 118 ml. *otc.*
Use: Antiemetic.

Nausetrol. (Qualitest Products, Inc.) Fructose, dextrose, orthophosphoric acid with controlled hydrogen ion concentration. Soln. Bot. 118 ml, 473 ml, 3785 ml. *otc.*
Use: Antiemetic, antivertigo.

Navane. (Roerig) Thiothixene. **Cap.:** 1 mg, 2 mg, 5 mg, 10 mg or 20 mg. Bot. 100s, 500s, 1000s, UD 100s. **Liq.:** 5 mg/ml. Bot. 30 ml, 120 ml. *Rx.*
Use: Antipsychotic.

Navelbine. (GlaxoWellcome) Vinorelbine tartrate 10 mg/ml. Inj. Vial 1 ml, 5 ml. *Rx.*
Use: Antineoplastic.

Navidrix. Cyclopenthiazide. 3-Cyclopentylmethyl derivative of hydrochlorothiazide. *Rx.*
Use: Diuretic.

•**naxagolide hydrochloride.** (nax-AH-go-LIDE) USAN.
Use: Antiparkinsonian; dopamine agonist.

Nazafair. (Various Mfr.) Naphazoline HCl 0.1%. Soln. Bot. 15 ml. *Rx.*
Use: Mydriatic, vasoconstrictor.

N D Clear. (Seatrace Pharmaceuticals, Inc.) Chlorpheniramine maleate 8 mg, pseudoephedrine HCl 120 mg/TD Cap. Bot. 100s, 1000s. *Rx.*
Use: Antihistamine, decongestant.

n-diethyl meta-toluamide.
W/Red Veterinary Petrolatum.
See: RV Pellent, Oint. (ICN Pharmaceuticals, Inc.).

n-diethylvanillamide.
See: Ethamivan, Inj. (Various Mfr.).

ND-Gesic. (Hyrex Pharmaceuticals) Acetaminophen 300 mg, pyrilamine maleate 12.5 mg, chlorpheniramine maleate 2 mg, phenylephrine HCl 5 mg/Tab. Bot. 100s, 1000s. *otc.*
Use: Analgesic, antihistamine, decongestant.

NDNA. (Wampole Laboratories) Anti-native DNA test by IFA. Confirmatory test for active SLE. Test 48s.
Use: Diagnostic aid.

•**nebacumab.** (neh-BACK-you-mab) USAN. *Formerly Septomonab.*
Use: Monoclonal antibody (antiendotoxin).

Nebcin. (Eli Lilly and Co.) Tobramycin sulfate. **Inj.:** 10 mg/ml (Vial 6 ml, 8 ml),

40 mg/ml (*Hyporets* 1.5 ml, 2 ml). **Pow. for Inj.:** 1.2 g. Vial 1.2 g. **Pediatric Inj.:** 10 mg/ml Vial 2 ml. *Rx.*
Use: Anti-infective, aminoglycoside.

•**nebivolol.** (neh-BIV-oh-lole) USAN.
Use: Antihypertensive (beta blocker).

•**nebramycin.** (neh-brah-MY-sin) USAN. A complex of antibiotic substances produced by *Streptomyces tenebrarius.*
Use: Anti-infective.

NebuPent. (Fujisawa USA, Inc.) Pentamidine isethionate 300 mg. Aer. single-dose vial. *Rx.*
Use: Anti-infective.

Nebu-Prel. (Mahon) Isoproterenol sulfate 0.4%, phenylephrine HCl 2%, propylene glycol 10%. Liq. Vial 10 ml. *Rx.*
Use: Bronchodilator.

Nechlorin. (Henry Schein, Inc.) Chlorpheniramine 5 mg, phenylpropanolamine 40 mg, phenylephrine 20 mg, phenyltoloxamine 15 mg/Tab. Bot. 100s.
Use: Antihistamine, decongestant.

•**nedocromil.** (NEH-doe-KROE-mill) USAN.
Use: Antiallergic (prophylactic).

•**nedocromil calcium.** (NEH-doe-KROE-mill) USAN.
Use: Antiallergic (prophylactic).
See: Tilade Aer. (Medeva Pharmaceuticals, Inc.).

•**nedocromil sodium.** (NEH-doe-KROE-mill) USAN.
Use: Antiallergic (prophylactic).
See: Tilade, Aer. (Medeva Pharmaceuticals, Inc.).

N.E.E.. (Lexis Laboratories) Ethinyl estradiol 35 mcg, norethindrone 1 mg/Tab. 6 pcks. 21s, 28s. *Rx.*
Use: Contraceptive.

•**nefazodone hydrochloride.** (neff-AZE-oh-dohn) USAN.
Use: Antidepressant.
See: Serzone, Tab. (Bristol-Myers Squibb).

•**neflumozide hydrochloride.** (neh-FLEW-moe-ZIDE) USAN.
Use: Antipsychotic.

•**nefocon a.** (NEE-FOE-kahn A) USAN.
Use: Contact lens material (hydrophilic).

•**nefopam hydrochloride.** (NEFF-oh-pam) USAN.
Use: Muscle relaxant, analgesic.

Negacide. (Sanofi Winthrop Pharmaceuticals) Nalidixic acid. *Rx.*
Use: Anti-infective, urinary.

NegGram. (Sanofi Winthrop Pharmaceuticals) Nalidixic acid. Capl. **1 g:** UD 100s; **250 mg:** Bot. 56s. **500 mg:** Bot. 56s, 500s. *Rx.*
Use: Anti-infective, urinary.

•**nelezaprine maleate.** (neh-LEH-zah-PREEN) USAN.
Use: Muscle relaxant.

•**nelfilcon a.** (nell-FILL-kahn A) USAN.
Use: Contact lens material (hydrophilic).

•**nelfinavir mesylate.** (nell-FIN-ah-veer) USAN.
Use: Antiviral.
See: Viracept, Tab., Pow. (Agouron Pharmaceuticals, Inc.)

Nelova 0.5/35. (Warner Chilcott Laboratories) Ethinyl estradiol 35 mcg, norethindrone 0.5 mg/Tab. 6 Pcks. 21-day and 28-day w/ 7 inert tabs. *Rx.*
Use: Contraceptive.

Nelova 1/35E. (Warner Chilcott Laboratories) Norethindrone 1 mg, ethinyl estradiol 35 mcg/Tab. 21-day and 28-day (with 7 inert tabs). *Rx.*
Use: Contraceptive.

Nelova 1/50M. (Warner Chilcott Laboratories) Norethindrone 1 mg, mestranol 50 mcg/Tab. 21-day and 28-day (with 7 inert tabs). *Rx.*
Use: Contraceptive.

Nelova 10/11. (Warner Chilcott Laboratories) **Phase 1:** Norethindrone 0.5 mg, ethinyl estradiol 35 mcg/Tab., 10 tabs.; **Phase 2:** Norethindrone 1 mg, ethinyl estradiol 35 mcg/Tab., 11 tabs. 21-day and 28-day (with 7 inert tabs). *Rx.*
Use: Contraceptive.

Nelulen. (Watson Laboratories) **1/35 E:** Ethynodiol diacetate 1 mg, ethinyl estradiol 35 mcg. Tab. Pcks 21s, 28s. **1/50 E:** Ethynodiol diacetate 1 mg, ethinyl estradiol 50 mcg. Tab. Pcks. 21s, 28s. *Rx.*
Use: Contraceptive.

•**nelzarabine.** (nell-ZARE-ah-bean) USAN.
Use: Antineoplastic.

nemazine. Under study.
Use: Anti-inflammatory.

•**nemazoline hydrochloride.** (neh-MAZZ-oh-leen) USAN.
Use: Decongestant, nasal.

Nembutal Elixir. (Abbott Laboratories) Pentobarbital 20 mg/5 ml, alcohol 18%. Bot. Pt. *c-II.*
Use: Hypnotic, sedative.

Nembutal Sodium. (Abbott Laboratories) Pentobarbital sodium. **Inj.:** 50 mg/ml. Amp 2 ml; Vial 20 ml, 50 ml. Box 5s. **Cap.:** 50 mg. Bot. 100s; 100 mg. Bot. 100s, 500s. Display pack 100s. **Supp.:** 30 mg, 60 mg, 120 mg, 200 mg. Box 12s. *c-II.*

Use: Hypnotic, sedative.

Neo-Benz-All. (Xttrium Laboratories, Inc.) Benzalkonium Cl 20.1%. Packet 25 ml 15s. To make gal of 1:750 soln. Also Aqueous Neo-Benz-All 1:750 soln. Packet 20 ml, 50s. *otc.*
Use: Antiseptic, antimicrobial.

Neo Beserol. (Sanofi Winthrop Pharmaceuticals) Aspirin, methocarbamol. *Rx.*
Use: Analgesic, muscle relaxant.

Neocalamine. (Various Mfr.) Red ferric oxide 30 g, yellow ferric oxide 40 g, zinc oxide 930 g. *otc.*
Use: Astringent, antiseptic.

Neo-Calglucon. (Novartis Pharmaceutical Corp.) Glubionate calcium 1.8 g/5 ml. Syr. Bot. Pt. *Rx.*
Use: Mineral supplement.

Neocate One +. (Scientific Hospital Supplies, Inc.) Protein 2.5 g (amino acids 3 g), carbohydrates 14.6 g, fat 3.5 g, vitamins A, D, E, K, B_1, B_2, B_3, B_5, B_6, B_{12}, folic acid, biotin, C, choline, inositol, Ca, P, Mg, Fe, Zn, Mn, Cu, I, Mo, Cr, Se, Cl, Na 20 mg (0.9 mEq), K 93 mg (2.4 mEq) per 100 ml, 100 cal/ml. Liq. Bot. 237 ml. *otc.*
Use: Nutritional supplement, enteral.

Neo-Cholex. (Lafayette Pharmaceuticals, Inc.) Fat emulsion containing 40%/w/v pure vegetable oil. Bot. 60 ml.
Use: Cholecystokinetic.

Neocidin. (Major Pharmaceuticals) Polymyxin B sulfate 10,000 units, neomycin sulfate 1.75 mg, gramicidin 0.025 mg/ml. Soln. Bot. 10 ml. *Rx.*
Use: Anti-infective, ophthalmic.

neo-cobefrin.
Use: Vasoconstrictor.

Neo-Cultol. (Medeva Pharmaceuticals, Inc.) Refined mineral oil jelly. Chocolate flavored. Bot. 6 oz. *otc.*
Use: Laxative.

Neocurb. (Taylor Pharmaceuticals) Phendimetrazine tartrate 35 mg/Tab. Bot. 100s, 1000s. *c-III.*
Use: Anorexiant.

Neocylate. (Schwarz Pharma, Inc.) Potassium salicylate 280 mg, aminobenzoic acid 250 mg/Tab. Bot. 100s, 1000s. *otc.*
Use: Analgesic.

Neocyten. (Schwarz Pharma, Inc.) Orphenadrine citrate 30 mg/ml. Vial 10 ml. *Rx.*
Use: Muscle relaxant.

NeoDecadron Ophthalmic Solution. (Merck & Co.) Dexamethasone sodium phosphate equivalent to 0.1% dexamethasone phosphate, neomycin sulfate equivalent to 0.35% mg neomycin base. Ocumeter ophthalmic dispenser 5 ml. *Rx.*
Use: Anti-infective, corticosteroid, ophthalmic.

Neo-Dexair. (Bausch & Lomb Pharmaceuticals) Dexamethasone sodium phosphate 0.1%, neomycin sulfate 0.35%, polysorbate 80, EDTA, benzalkonium Cl 0.02%, sodium bisulfite 0.1%. Soln. Bot. 5 ml. *Rx.*
Use: Anti-infective, corticosteroid, ophthalmic.

Neo-Dexameth. (Major Pharmaceuticals) Dexamethasone sodium phosphate 0.1%, neomycin sulfate 0.35%. Soln. Bot. 5 ml. *Rx.*
Use: Anti-infective, corticosteroid, ophthalmic.

Neo-Diaral. (Roberts Pharmaceuticals) Loperamide 2 mg/Cap. Bot. UD 8s, 250s. *otc.*
Use: Antidiarrheal.

neodrenal.
See: Isoproterenol.

Neo-Durabolic. (Roberts Pharmaceuticals) Nandrolone decanoate injection. **50 mg/ml, 100 mg/ml:** Vial 2 ml. **200 mg/ml:** Vial 1 ml. *c-III.*
Use: Anabolic steroid.

Neo-fradin. (Pharma Tek, Inc.) Neomycin sulfate 125 mg/5 ml, parabens. Oral Soln. Bot. 480 ml. *Rx.*
Use: Amebicide.

Neogesic Tablets. (Pal-Pak, Inc.) Aspirin 194.4 mg, acetaminophen 129.6 mg, caffeine 32.4 mg/Tab. Bot. 1000s. *otc.*
Use: Analgesic combination.

Neoloid. (Kenwood Laboratories) Castor oil 36.4% (emulsified), sodium benzoate 0.1%, potassium sorbate 0.2%. Sugar free. Oil Bot. 118 ml. *otc.*
Use: Laxative.

Neo-Mist Nasal Spray. (A.P.C.) Phenylephrine HCl 0.5%, cetalkonium Cl 0.02%. Spray Bot. 20 ml. *otc.*
Use: Antiseptic, decongestant.

Neo-Mist Pediatric 0.25% Nasal Spray. (A.P.C.) Phenylephrine HCl 0.25%, cetalkonium Cl 0.02%. Squeeze Bot. 20 ml. *otc.*
Use: Antiseptic, decongestant.

Neomixin. (Roberts Pharmaceuticals) Bacitracin zinc 400 units, neomycin sulfate 3.5 mg, polymyxin B sulfate 5000 units in petrolatum base/g. Tube 15 g. *otc.*
Use: Anti-infective, topical.

neomycin base.
Use: Anti-infective.
W/Combinations.

See: Maxitrol, Oint., Susp. (Alcon Laboratories, Inc.).
Neosporin Plus (GlaxoWellcome).
Neotal, Oint. (Roberts Pharmaceuticals).

•**neomycin palmitate.** (NEE-oh-MY-sin PAL-mih-tate) USAN.
Use: Anti-infective.

neomycin and polymyxin B sulfates, bacitracin, and hydrocortisone acetate ointment.
Use: Anti-infective; antifungal; anti-inflammatory, topical.

neomycin and polymyxin B sulfates, bacitracin, and hydrocortisone acetate ophthalmic ointment.
Use: Anti-infective, antifungal, anti-inflammatory, topical.

neomycin and polymyxin B sulfates and bacitracin ointment.
Use: Anti-infective, topical.

neomycin and polymyxin B sulfates and bacitracin ophthalmic ointment.
Use: Anti-infective, topical.

neomycin and polymyxin B sulfates, bacitracin zinc, and hydrocortisone acetate ophthalmic ointment.
Use: Anti-infective, corticosteroid, topical.

neomycin and polymyxin B sulfates, bacitracin zinc, and hydrocortisone ointment.
Use: Anti-infective, corticosteroid, topical.

neomycin and polymyxin B sulfates, bacitracin zinc, and hydrocortisone ophthalmic ointment.
Use: Anti-infective, corticosteroid, topical.

neomycin and polymyxin B sulfates, bacitracin zinc, and lidocaine ointment.
Use: Anti-infective, topical.
See: Lanabiotic, Oint. (Combe, Inc.).

neomycin and polymyxin B sulfates and bacitracin zinc ointment.
Use: Anti-infective, topical.

neomycin and polymyxin B sulfates and bacitracin zinc ophthalmic ointment.
Use: Anti-infective, ophthalmic.

neomycin and polymyxin B sulfates and bacitracin zinc topical aerosol. U.S.P. XXI.
Use: Anti-infective, topical.

neomycin and polymyxin B sulfates and bacitracin zinc topical powder. U.S.P. XXI.
Use: Anti-infective, topical.

neomycin and polymyxin B sulfates cream.
Use: Anti-infective, topical.

neomycin and polymyxin B sulfates and dexamethasone ophthalmic ointment. (Various Mfr.) Dexamethasone 0.1%, neomycin sulfate 0.35%, polymyxin B sulfate 10,000 units. Tube 3.5 g.
Use: Anti-infective, corticosteroid, ophthalmic.

neomycin and polymyxin B sulfates and dexamethasone ophthalmic suspension. (Various Mfr.) Dexamethasone 0.1%, neomycin sulfate 0.35%, polymyxin B sulfate 10,000 units. Bot. 5 ml, 10 ml.
Use: Anti-infective, corticosteroid, ophthalmic.

neomycin and polymyxin B sulfates and gramicidin cream.
Use: Anti-infective, topical.

neomycin and polymyxin B sulfates, gramicidin, and hydrocortisone acetate cream.
Use: Anti-infective, corticosteroid, topical.

neomycin and polymyxin B sulfates and gramicidin ophthalmic solution.
Use: Anti-infective, ophthalmic.

neomycin and polymyxin B sulfates and hydrocortisone acetate cream.
Use: Anti-infective, corticosteroid, topical.

neomycin and polymyxin B sulfates and hydrocortisone acetate ophthalmic suspension.
Use: Anti-infective, corticosteroid, ophthalmic.

neomycin and polymyxin B sulfates and hydrocortisone ophthalmic suspension. (Various Mfr.) Hydrocortisone 1%, neomycin sulfate 0.35%, polymyxin B sulfate 10,000 units. Bot. 7.5 ml, 10 ml.
Use: Anti-infective, corticosteroid, ophthalmic.

neomycin and polymyxin B sulfates and hydrocortisone otic solution.
Use: Anti-infective, corticosteroid, otic.

neomycin and polymyxin B sulfates and hydrocortisone otic suspension. (Steris Laboratories, Inc.) Polymyxin B sulfate equiv. to 10,000 polymyxin B units, neomycin sulfate equiv. to 3.5 mg neomycin base/ml. Hydrocortisone 1%, thimerosal 0.01%, cetyl alcohol, propylene glycol, polysorbate 80. Susp. Bot. 10 ml.
Use: Anti-infective, corticosteroid, otic.

neomycin and polymyxin B sulfates ophthalmic ointment.
Use: Anti-infective, ophthalmic.

neomycin and polymyxin B sulfates and prednisolone acetate ophthalmic suspension.
Use: Anti-infective, corticosteroid, ophthalmic.

neomycin and polymyxin B sulfates solution for irrigation.
Use: Irrigant, ophthalmic, anti-infective, topical.
See: Neosporin G.U. Irrigant (GlaxoWellcome).

neomycin and polymyxin B sulfates ophthalmic solution.
Use: Anti-infective, ophthalmic.

•**neomycin sulfate.** (NEE-oh-MY-sin) U.S.P. 23.
Use: Anti-infective.
See: Mycifradin Sulfate, Tab., Soln. (Pharmacia & Upjohn).
Myciguent, Oint., Ophth. Oint., Cream (Pharmacia & Upjohn).
Neo-fradin, Soln. (Pharma Tek, Inc.).
Neo-Tabs (Pharma Tek, Inc.).
W/Combinations.
See: AK-Spore, Preps. (Akorn, Inc.).
Bacitracin Neomycin, Oint. (Various Mfr.).
Clomycin (Roberts).
Coracin, Oint. (Roberts Pharmaceuticals).
Cordran-N, Oint., Lot. (Eli Lilly and Co.).
Cortisporin, Preps. (GlaxoWellcome).
Maxitrol, Ophth., Oint., Susp. (Alcon Laboratories,Inc.).
Mycifradin Sulfate Sterile, Vial (Pharmacia & Upjohn).
Mycitracin, Oint., Ophth. Oint. (Pharmacia & Upjohn).
Neo-Cort Dome, Otic Soln. (Bayer Corp. (Consumer Div.)).
Neo-Cortef, Preps. (Pharmacia & Upjohn).
NeoDecadron Ophthalmic Solution (Merck & Co.).
Neosporin, Preps. (GlaxoWellcome).
Neotal, Ophth. Oint. (Roberts Pharmaceuticals).
Neo-Thrycex, Oint. (Del Pharmaceuticals, Inc.).
Ocutricin, Preps. (Bausch & Lomb Pharmaceuticals).
Spectrocin, Oint. (Bristol-Myers Squibb).
Tigo, Oint. (Burlington).
Tribiotic Plus (Thompson).
Trimixin, Oint. (Hance).

neomycin sulfate. (Pharmacia & Upjohn) (Pow. micronized for compounding. Bot. 100 g.)
Use: Anti-infective.

neomycin sulfate and bacitracin ointment.
Use: Anti-infective, topical.

neomycin sulfate and bacitracin zinc ointment.
Use: Anti-infective, topical.

neomycin sulfate and dexamethasone sodium phosphate cream.
Use: Anti-infective, corticosteroid, topical.

neomycin sulfate and dexamethasone sodium phosphate ophthalmic ointment.
Use: Anti-infective, corticosteroid, ophthalmic.

neomycin sulfate and dexamethasone sodium phosphate ophthalmic solution. (Various Mfr.) Dexamethasone sodium phosphate 0.1%, neomycin sulfate 0.35%. Bot. 5 ml.
Use: Anti-infective, corticosteroid, ophthalmic.

neomycin sulfate and fluocinolone acetonide cream.
Use: Anti-infective, corticosteroid, topical.

neomycin sulfate and fluorometholone ointment.
Use: Anti-infective, corticosteroid, topical.

neomycin sulfate and flurandrenolide.
Use: Anti-infective, corticosteroid, topical.
See: Cordran, Prods. (Eli Lilly and Co.).

neomycin sulfate and gramicidin ointment.
Use: Anti-infective, topical.

neomycin sulfate and hydrocortisone.
Use: Anti-infective, corticosteroid, topical.

neomycin sulfate and hydrocortisone acetate.
Use: Anti-infective, corticosteroid.

neomycin sulfate and methylprednisolone acetate cream.
Use: Anti-infective, corticosteroid, topical.

neomycin sulfate, polymyxin B sulfate, and gramicidin solution. (Various Mfr.) Polymyxin B sulfate 10,000 units/ml, neomycin sulfate 1.75 mg/ml, gramicidin 0.025 mg/ml. Bot. 2 ml, 10 ml. *Rx.*
Use: Anti-infective, ophthalmic.

neomycin sulfate, polymyxin B sulfate, and lidocaine.
Use: Anti-infective; anesthetic, local.
See: Clomycin, Oint. (Roberts Pharmaceuticals).
Neosporin Plus, Cream, Oint. (GlaxoWellcome).

Tribiotic Plus, Oint. (Thompson Medical Co.).

neomycin sulfate and prednisolone acetate ointment.
Use: Anti-infective, corticosteroid, topical.

neomycin sulfate and prednisolone acetate ophthalmic ointment.
Use: Anti-infective, corticosteroid, topical.

neomycin sulfate and prednisolone acetate ophthalmic suspension.
Use: Anti-infective, corticosteroid, topical.

neomycin sulfate and prednisolone sodium phosphate ophthalmic ointment.
Use: Anti-infective, corticosteroid, topical.

neomycin sulfate, sulfacetamide sodium, and prednisolone acetate ophthalmic ointment.
Use: Anti-infective, corticosteroid, topical.

neomycin sulfate and triamcinolone acetonide cream.
Use: Anti-infective, corticosteroid, topical.

neomycin sulfate and triamcinolone acetonide ophthalmic ointment.
Use: Anti-infective, corticosteroid, ophthalmic.

•**neomycin undecylenate.** (NEE-oh-MY-sin UHN-de-sih-LEN-ate) USAN.
Use: Anti-infective, antifungal.

Neopap. (PolyMedica Pharmaceuticals) Acetaminophen 125 mg/Supp. In 12s. *otc.*
Use: Analgesic.

Neopham 6.4%. (Pharmacia & Upjohn) Essential and non-essential amino acids 6.4%. Inj. 250 ml, 500 ml. *Rx.*
Use: Nutritional supplement, parenteral.

Neo Picatyl. (Sanofi Winthrop Pharmaceuticals) Glycobiarsoln. *Rx.*
Use: Amebicide.

Neo Quipenyl. (Sanofi Winthrop Pharmaceuticals) Primaquine phosphate. *Rx.*
Use: Antimalarial.

Neoral Capsules. (Novartis Pharmaceutical Corp.) Cyclosporine 25 mg, 100 mg/Soft gelatin Cap. 9.5% dehydrated alcohol. Bot. UD 30s. *Rx.*
Use: Immunosuppressant.

Neoral Oral Solution. (Novartis Pharmaceutical Corp.) Cyclosporine 100 mg/ml. Denatured alcohol 9.5% Bot. 50 ml. *Rx.*
Use: Immunosuppressant.

Neosar. (Pharmacia & Upjohn) Cyclophosphamide. 100 mg, sodium bicarbonate 82 mg. Pow. for Inj. Vial 100 mg, 200 mg, 500 mg, 1 g, 2 g. *Rx.*
Use: Antineoplastic.

neo-skiodan. Iodopyracet, Diodrast.

Neosporin Cream. (GlaxoWellcome) Polymyxin B sulfate, neomycin sulfate. Tube 0.5 oz, foil packet 1/32 oz. Ctn. 144s. *otc.*
Use: Anti-infective, topical.

Neosporin G.U. Irrigant. (GlaxoWellcome) Neomycin sulfate 40 mg, polymyxin B sulfate 200,000 units/ml. Amp. 1 ml. Box 10s, 50s, Multiple-dose vial 20 ml. *Rx.*
Use: Irrigant, genitourinary.

Neosporin Ointment. (GlaxoWellcome) Polymyxin B sulfate 5000 units, bacitracin zinc 400 units, neomycin sulfate 5 mg/g. Tube 0.5 oz, 1 oz. Foil packet 1/32 oz. Box 144s. *otc.*
Use: Anti-infective, topical.

Neosporin Maximum Strength. (GlaxoWellcome) Polymyxin B sulfate 10,000 units, neomycin 3.5 mg, bacitracin 500 units/g, white petrolatum. Oint. Tube 15 g. *otc.*
Use: Anti-infective, topical.

Neosporin Ophthalmic Ointment, Sterile. (GlaxoWellcome) Polymyxin B sulfate 10,000 units, bacitracin zinc 400 units, neomycin sulfate 3.5 mg/g. Tube 3.5 g. *Rx.*
Use: Anti-infective, ophthalmic.

Neosporin Ophthalmic Solution, Sterile. (GlaxoWellcome) Polymyxin B sulfate 10,000 units, neomycin sulfate 1.75 mg, gramicidin 0.025 mg/ml. Bot. 10 ml. Drop-dose. *Rx.*
Use: Anti-infective, ophthalmic.

Neosporin Plus. (GlaxoWellcome) **Cream:** Polymyxin B sulfate 10,000 units, neomycin 3.5 mg and lidocaine 40 mg/g, methylparaben 0.25%, mineral oil, white petrolatum. Tube 15 g. **Oint.:** Polymyxin B sulfate 10,000 units, bacitracin zinc 500 units, neomycin 3.5 mg, lidocaine 40 mg/g. White petrolatum base. Tube 15 g. *otc.*
Use: Anti-infective, topical.

neostibosan. Ethylstibamine.

neostigmine. (nee-oh-STIGG-meen)
Use: Cholinergic.
See: Neostigmine bromide (Lannett Co., Inc.).
Neostigmine Methylsulfate (Various Mfr.).
Prostigmin (Roche Laboratories).

neostigmine and atropine sulfate.
Use: Muscle stimulant.
See: Neostigmine Min-I-Mix (I.M.S., Ltd.).

•**neostigmine bromide.** (nee-oh-STIGG-meen BROE-mide) U.S.P. 23.
Use: Cholinergic.
See: Prostigmin Bromide, Tab. (Roche Laboratories).

neostigmine bromide. (Lannett Co., Inc.) 15 mg/Tab. 100s and 1000s.
Use: Cholinergic.

•**neostigmine methylsulfate.** (nee-oh-STIGG-meen METH-ill-SULL-fate) U.S.P. 23.
Use: Cholinergic.
See: Prostigmin methylsulfate, Vial (Roche Laboratories).

neostigmine methylsulfate. (Various Mfr.) 1:1000 Inj. In 10 ml vials. 1:2000 Inj. In 1 ml amps. and 10 ml vials. 1:4000 Inj. In 1 ml amps.
Use: Cholinergic.

Neostigmine Min-I-Mix. (I.M.S., Ltd.) Atropine sulfate 1.2 mg, neostigmine methylsulfate 2.5 mg. Inj. Vial. Use: Cholinergic muscle stimulant.
Use: Mydriatic, vasoconstrictor.

Neostrate AHA for Age Spots and Skin Lightening. (NeoStrata Company) Hydroquinone 2%, glycolic acid, propylene glycol, sodium bisulfite, sodium sulfite, EDTA/Gel. 48 ml. *otc.*
Use: Dermatologic.

neo-strepsan.
See: Sulfathiazole (Various Mfr.).

Neo-Synephrine. (Sanofi Winthrop Pharmaceuticals) Phenylephrine HCl 2.5% or 10%. Soln. Bot. 5 ml (10%), 15 ml (2.5%). *Rx.*
Use: Mydriatic, vasoconstrictor.

Neo-Synephrine Hydrochloride. (Sanofi Winthrop Pharmaceuticals) Phenylephrine HCl. **Spray:** 0.25% children and adult, 0.5% adult. **Regular:** Squeeze bot. 0.5 oz. **0.5% mentholated:** Squeeze bot. 0.5 oz. **Drops:** 0.125% infant; 0.25% children and adult; 0.5% adult; 1% adult extra strength. Bot. 1 oz; 0.25% and 1%, also bot. 16 oz. **Jelly:** 0.5%. Tube 18.75 g. *otc.*
Use: Decongestant.

Neo-Synephrine Hydrochloride. (Sanofi Winthrop Pharmaceuticals) Phenylephrine HCl. **Amp.:** 1%, Carpuject sterile cartridge-needle unit 10 mg/ml. (1 ml fill in 2 ml cartridge) w/22-gauge, 1.25 inch needle. Dispensing Bin 50s; Vial 1 ml. Box 25s. *Rx.*
Use: Vasoconstrictor.

Neo-Synephrine Viscous Ophthalmic. (Sanofi Winthrop Pharmaceuticals) Phenylephrine HCl 10%. Soln. Bot. 5 ml. *Rx.*
Use: Mydriatic, vasoconstrictor.

Neo-Tabs. (Pharma Tek, Inc.) Neomycin sulfate 500 mg (equivalent to 350 mg neomycin base)/Tab. Bot. 100s. *Rx.*
Use: Amebicide.

Neotal. (Roberts Pharmaceuticals) Zinc bacitracin 400 units, polymyxin B sulfate 5000 units, neomycin sulfate 5 mg, petrolatum and mineral oil base/g. Tube 3.5 g. *Rx.*
Use: Anti-infective, ophthalmic.

Neo-Thrycex Oint. (Del Pharmaceuticals, Inc.) Bacitracin, neomycin sulfate, polymyxin B sulfate. Tube 0.5 oz. *Rx.*
Use: Anti-infective, topical.

Neothylline. (Teva Pharmaceuticals USA) Dyphylline. **200 mg Tab.:** Bot. 100s, 1000s. **400 mg Tab.:** Bot. 100s, 500s. *Rx.*
Use: Bronchodilator.

Neothylline-GG. (Teva Pharmaceuticals USA) Dyphylline 200 mg, guaifenesin 200 mg/Tab. Bot. 100s, 1000s. *Rx.*
Use: Bronchodilator, expectorant.

Neotrace-4. (Fujisawa USA, Inc.) Zn 1.5 mg, Cu 0.1 mg, Cr 0.85 mcg, Mn 25 mcg/ml. Vial 2 ml. *Rx.*
Use: Mineral supplement.

Neotricin HC. (Bausch & Lomb Pharmaceuticals) Hydrocortisone acetate 1%, neomycin sulfate 0.35%, bacitracin zinc 400 units, polymyxin B sulfate 10,000 units. Oint. Tube 3.5 g. *Rx.*
Use: Anti-infective, corticosteroid, ophthalmic.

Neotricin Ophthalmic Ointment. (Bausch & Lomb Pharmaceuticals) Polymyxin B sulfate 10,000 units, neomycin sulfate 3.5 mg, bacitracin 400 units/g. In 3.5 g. *Rx.*
Use: Anti-infective, ophthalmic.

Neotricin Ophthalmic Solution. (Bausch & Lomb Pharmaceuticals) Polymyxin B sulfate 10,000 units, neomycin sulfate 1.75 mg, gramicidin 0.025 mg/ml. Dropper bot. 10 ml. *Rx.*
Use: Anti-infective, ophthalmic.

Neo-Trobex Injection. (Forest Pharmaceutical, Inc.) Vitamins B_1 150 mg, B_6 10 mg, riboflavin 5-phosphate sodium 2 mg, niacinamide 150 mg, panthenol 10 mg, choline Cl 20 mg, inositol 20 mg/ml. Vial 30 ml. *Rx.*
Use: Vitamin supplement.

Neotrol. (Horizon Pharmaceutical Corp.) Phenylephrine HCl 0.25%, pyrilamine maleate 0.2%, cetalkonium Cl 0.05%, tyrothricin 0.03%, phenylmercuric acetate 1:50,000. Soln. Squeeze Bot. 20 ml. *otc.*

Use: Antihistamine, decongestant.

Neo-Vadrin Stress Formula Vitamins Plus Zinc. (Scherer Laboratories, Inc.) Vitamins E 45 IU, C 600 mg, folic acid 400 mcg, B_1 20 mg, B_2 10 mg, B_{12} 25 mcg, biotin 45 mcg, pantothenic acid 25 mg, Cu 3 mg, Zn 23.9 mg/Tab. Bot. 60s. *otc.*
Use: Mineral, vitamin supplement.

Neo-Vadrin Time Release Vit. C. (Scherer Laboratories, Inc.) Vitamin C 500 mg/Cap. Bot. 50s, 100s. *otc.*
Use: Vitamin supplement.

Neo-Vadrin Vitamin B_6 TR. (Scherer Laboratories, Inc.) Vitamin B_6 100 mg/Cap. Bot. 100s. *otc.*
Use: Vitamin supplement.

Neoval. (Halsey Drug Co.) Vitamins A 10,000 IU, D 400 IU, B_1 10 mg, B_2 5 mg, B_6 2 mg, B_{12} 3 mcg, C 100 mg, E 5 mg, pantothenic acid 10 mg, niacinamide 30 mg, Fe 15 mg, Cu 1 mg, Mg 5 mg, Mn 1 mg, Zn 1.5 mg, I 0.15 mg/Tab. Bot. 100s. *otc.*
Use: Mineral, vitamin supplement.

Neoval T. (Halsey Drug Co.) Vitamins A 10,000 IU, D 400 IU, B_1 15 mg, B_2 10 mg, B_6 2 mg, C 150 mg, B_{12} 7.5 mcg, E 5 mg, pantothenic acid 10 mg, E 5 mg, niacinamide 100 mg, Fe 15 mg, Mg 5 mg, Mn 1 mg, Zn 1.5 mg, Cu 1 mg/Tab. Bot. 1000s. *otc.*
Use: Mineral, vitamin supplement.

Nephplex Rx. (Nephro-Tech, Inc.) B_1 1.5 mg, B_2 1.7 mg, B_3 20 mg, B_5 10 mg, B_6 10 mg, B_{12} 6 mcg, C 60 mg, folic acid 1 mg, d-biotin 300 mcg/Tab. Bot. 100s. *Rx.*
Use: Mineral, vitamin supplement.

5.4% NephrAmine. (McGaw, Inc.) Amino acid concentration 5.4%, nitrogen 0.65 g/100 ml. **Essential amino acids:** Isoleucine 560 mg, leucine 880 mg, lysine 640 mg, methionine 880 mg, phenylalanine 880 mg, threonine 400 mg, tryptophan 200 mg, valine 640 mg, histidine 250 mg/100 ml. **Nonessential amino acids:** Cysteine < 20 mg/100 ml, sodium 5 mEq, acetate 44 mEq, chloride 3 mEq/L, sodium bisulfite. Inj. 250 ml. *Rx.*
Use: Nutritional supplement, parenteral.

nephridine.
See: Epinephrine (Various Mfr.).

Nephro-Calci. (R & D Laboratories, Inc.) Calcium carbonate 1.5 g/Chew. Tab. (600 mg calcium). Bot. 100s, 200s, 500s, 1000s. *otc.*
Use: Mineral supplement.

Nephrocaps Capsules. (Fleming & Co.) Vitamins B_1 1.5 mg, B_2 1.7 mg, B_3 20 mg, B_5 5 mg, B_6 10 mg, B_{12} 6 mcg, C 100 mg, folic acid 1 mg, biotin 150 mcg/Cap. Bot. 100s. *Rx.*
Use: Vitamin supplement.

Nephro-Fer. (R & D Laboratories, Inc.) Ferrous fumarate 350 mg (Fe 115 mg)/Tab. Bot. 30s. *otc.*
Use: Mineral supplement.

Nephro-Fer RX. (R & D Laboratories, Inc.) Iron 106.9 mg, folic acid 1 mg. Tab. Bot. 120s. *Rx.*
Use: Mineral, vitamin supplement.

Nephron FA. (Nephro-Tech, Inc.) Fe 66.6 mg, C 40 mg, B_1 1.5 mg, B_2 1.7 mg, B_3 20 mg, B_5 10 mg, B_6 10 mg, B_{12} 6 mcg, biotin 300 mcg, FA 1 mg, docusate sodium 75 mg/Tab. Bot. 100s. *Rx.*
Use: Mineral, vitamin supplement.

Nephron Inhalant and Vaporizer. (Nephron Pharmaceuticals Corp.) Racepinephrine HCl 2.25% (epinephrine base 1.125%). Soln. for Inh. Bot. 15 ml. *otc.*
Use: Bronchodilator.

Nephro-Vite Rx. (R & D Laboratories, Inc.) Vitamins B_1 1.5 mg, B_2 1.7 mg, B_3 20 mg, B_5 10 mg, B_6 10 mg, B_{12} 6 mcg, C 60 mg, folic acid 1 mg, d-biotin 300 mcg/Tab. Bot. 100s. *Rx.*
Use: Mineral, vitamin supplement.

Nephro-Vite Rx + Fe. (R & D Laboratories, Inc.) Iron 100 mg, vitamins B_1 1.5 mg, B_2 1.7 mg, B_3 20 mg, B_5 10 mg, B_6 10 mg, B_{12} 6 mcg, C 60 mg, folic acid 1 mg, d-biotin 300 mcg, lactose/Tab. Bot. 120s. *Rx.*
Use: Mineral, vitamin supplement.

Nephro-Vite Vitamin B Complex & C Supplement. (R & D Laboratories, Inc.) Vitamins B_1 1.5 mg, B_2 1.7 mg, B_3 20 mg, B_5 10 mg, B_6 10 mg, B_{12} 6 mcg, C 60 mg, folic acid 800 mcg, biotin 300 mcg/Tab. Bot. 100s. *otc.*
Use: Mineral, vitamin supplement.

Nephrox. (Fleming & Co.) Aluminum hydroxide 320 mg, mineral oil 10%/5 ml. Bot. Pt. *otc.*
Use: Antacid.

Nepro. (Ross Laboratories) Protein 6.6 g (as Ca, Mg, and Na caseinates), fat 22.7 g (as 90% high-oleic safflower oil, 10% soy oil), carbohydrate 51.1 g (as-sucrose, hydrolyzed corn starch), vitamins A, D, E, K, C, B_1, B_2, B_5, B_6, B_{12}, biotin, FA, Na, K, Cl, Ca, P, Mg, I, Mn, Cu, Zn, Fe, Se/240 ml. 59.4 calories. Liq. Can. 240 ml. *otc.*
Use: Nutritional supplement, enteral.

Neptazane. (ESI Lederle Generics) Methazolamide 25 mg, 50 mg/Tab. Bot. 100s. *Rx.*

Use: Carbonic anhydrase inhibitor.

neraval.
Use: Anesthetic, general.

•**nerelimomab.** (neh-reh-LI-moe-mab) USAN.
Use: Monoclonal antibody.

Nervine Nighttime Sleep-Aid. (Bayer Corp. (Consumer Div.)) Diphenhydramine HCl 25 mg/Tab. Bot. 12s, 30s, 50s. *otc.*
Use: Sleep aid.

Nervocaine. (Keene Pharmaceuticals, Inc.) Lidocaine HCl 1%/Inj. Vial 50 ml. *Rx.*
Use: Anesthetic, local.

Nesacaine. (Astra Pharmaceuticals, L.P.) Chloroprocaine HCl 1%, 2%, methylparaben, EDTA. Inj. Vial 30 ml. *Rx.*
Use: Anesthetic, local.

Nesacaine-CE. (Astra Pharmaceuticals, L.P.) **Conc. 2%:** Chloroprocaine HCl 20 mg/ml in a sterile soln. containing sodium bisulfite, sodium Cl. Vial 30 ml. **Conc. 3%:** Chloroprocaine HCl 30 mg/ml in a sterile soln. containing sodium bisulfite, sodium Cl. Vial 30 ml. *Rx.*
Use: Anesthetic, local.

Nesacaine-MPF. (Astra Pharmaceuticals, L.P.) Chloroprocaine HCl 2% or 3%, EDTA, preservative-free. Inj. Vial 30 ml. *Rx.*
Use: Anesthetic, local.

Nesa Nine Cap. (Standex) Vitamins A 5000 IU, D 400 IU, C 37.5 mg, B_1 1.5 mg, B_2 2 mg, niacinamide 20 mg, B_6 0.1 mg, calcium pantothenate 1 mg, E 2 IU/Cap. Bot. 100s. *otc.*
Use: Mineral, vitamin supplement.

nesdonal sodium.
See: Pentothal Sodium, Prods. (Abbott Laboratories).
Thiopental Sodium, U.S.P. 23.

Nestabs. (Fielding Co.) Vitamins A 5000 IU, D 400 IU, E 30 mg, C 120 mg, B_1 3 mg, B_2 3 mg, B_3 20 mg, B_6 3 mg, B_{12} 8 mcg, Ca 200 mg, Fe 36 mg, folic acid 0.8 mg, Zn 15 mg, I/Tab. Bot. 100s. *otc.*
Use: Mineral, vitamin supplement.

Nestabs FA Tablets. (Fielding Co.) Vitamins A 5000 IU, D 400 IU, E 30 mg,C 120 mg, B_1 3 mg, B_2 3 mg, B_3 20 mg, B_6 3 mg, B_{12} 8 mcg, Ca 200 mg, Fe 36 mg, folic acid 1 mg, Zn 15 mg, I/Tab. Bot. 100s. *Rx.*
Use: Mineral, vitamin supplement.

Nestrex. (Fielding Co.) Pyridoxine 25 mg/Tab., dextrose. Bot. 100s. *otc.*
Use: Vitamin supplement.

Nethamine. W/Codeine phosphate, phenylephrine HCl, sodium citrate, doxylamine succinate.

•**netilmicin sulfate.** (neh-TILL-MY-sin SULL-fate) U.S.P. 23.
Use: Anti-infective.
See: Netromycin (Schering-Plough Corp.).

•**netrafilcon a.** (NET-rah-FILL-kahn A) USAN.
Use: Contact lens material (hydrophilic).

netrin. Under Study.
Use: Anticholinergic.
See: Metcaraphen HCl.

Netromycin. (Schering-Plough Corp.) Netilmicin 100 mg/ml. Inj. Vial 1.5 ml Box 10s, 25s. Multi-dose vial 15 ml Box 5s. Disp. Syringe 1.5 ml Box 10s. *Rx.*
Use: Anti-infective, aminoglycoside.

Neumega. (Genetics Institute) Oprelvekin 5 mg. Pow. for Inj. Box. Single-dose Vial with 5 ml diluent. *Rx.*
Use: Antithrombotic.

Neupogen. (Amgen, Inc.) Filgrastim (G-CSF) 300 mcg/ml. Vial 1 ml, 1.6 ml. *Rx.*
Use: Immunomodulator.

Neurodep-Caps. (Medical Products Panamericana) Vitamins B_1 125 mg, B_6 125 mg, B_{12} 1000 mcg/Cap. Bot. 50s. *otc.*
Use: Vitamin supplement.

Neurodep Injection. (Medical Products Panamericana) Vitamins B_1 50 mg, B_2 5 mg, B_3 125 mg, B_5 6 mg, B_6 5 mg, B_{12} 1000 mcg, C 50 mg/ml. Inj. Vial 10 ml. *Rx.*
Use: Vitamin supplement, parenteral.

Neurontin. (Parke-Davis) Gabapentin 100 mg, 300 mg, 400 mg; lactose. Cap. Bot. 100s, UD 50s. *Rx.*
Use: Anticonvulsant.

neurosin.
See: Calcium glycerophosphate (Various Mfr.).

Neut (sodium bicarbonate 4% additive solution). (Abbott Laboratories) Sodium bicarbonate 4%. Vial (2.4 mEq each of sodium and bicarbonate), disodium edetate anhydrous 0.05% as stabilizer. Pintop Vial 5 ml, 10 ml. Box 25s, 100s. *Rx.*
Use: Nutritional supplement, parenteral.

neutral acriflavine.
See: Acriflavine (Various Mfr.).

Neutralin. (Dover Pharmaceuticals) Calcium carbonate, magnesium oxide/Tab. Sugar, lactose and salt free. UD Box 500s. *otc.*
Use: Antacid.

neutral protamine hagedorn-insulin.
See: Insulin, N.P.H. Iletin (Eli Lilly and Co.).

•**neutramycin.** (NEW-trah-MY-sin) USAN. A neutral macrolide antibiotic produced by avariant strain of *Streptomyces rimosus*.
Use: Anti-infective.

Neutrexin. (US Bioscience) Trimetrexate glucuronate 25 mg. Pow. for Inj. (lyophilized). Vial 5 ml w/wo 50 mg leucovorin. *Rx.*
Use: Anti-infective.

neutroflavin.
See: Acriflavine (Various Mfr.).

Neutrogena Acne Mask. (Neutrogena) Benzoyl peroxide 5% in sebum absorbing facial mask vehicle, SD alcohol 40, glycerin, titanium dioxide. Tube 60 g. *otc.*
Use: Dermatologic, acne.

Neutrogena Antiseptic Cleanser for Acne-Prone Skin. (Neutrogena) Benzethonium Cl, butylene glycol, methylparaben, menthol, peppermint oil, eucalyptus, mint, rosemary oils, witch hazel extract, camphor. Liq. Bot. 135 ml. *otc.*
Use: Dermatologic, acne.

Neutrogena Baby Cleansing Formula Soap. (Neutrogena) Triethanolamine, glycerin, stearic acid, tallow, coconut oil, castor oil, sodium hydroxide, oleic acid, laneth-10 acetate, cocamide DEA, nonoxynol-14, PEG-4 octoate. Bar 105 g. *otc.*
Use: Dermatologic, cleanser.

Neutrogena Body Lotion. (Neutrogena) Glyceryl stearate, isopropyl myristate, PEG-100 stearate, butylene glycol, imidazolidinyl urea, carbomer 934, parabens, sodium lauryl sulfate, triethanolamine, cetyl alcohol. Lot. Bot. 240 ml. *otc.*
Use: Emollient.

Neutrogena Body Oil. (Neutrogena) Isopropyl myristate, sesame oil, PEG-40 sorbitan peroleate, parabens. Bot. 240 ml. *otc.*
Use: Emollient.

Neutrogena Chemical-Free Sunblocker. (Neutrogena) Titanium dioxide, parabens, diazolidinyl urea, shea butter. SPF 17. Lot. Bot. 120 ml. *otc.*
Use: Sunscreen.

Neutrogena Cleansing for Acne-Prone Skin. (Neutrogena) TEA-stearate, triethanolamine, glycerin, sodium tallowate, sodium cocoate, TEA-oleate, sodium ricinoleate, acetylated lanolin alcohol, cocamide DEA, TEA lauryl sulfate, tocopherol. Bar 105 g. *otc.*
Use: Dermatologic, cleanser.

Neutrogena Drying. (Neutrogena) Witch hazel, isopropyl alcohol, EDTA, parabens, tartrazine. Gel. Tube 22.5 ml. *otc.*
Use: Dermatologic, acne.

Neutrogena Dry Skin Soap. (Neutrogena) Triethanolamine, stearic acid, tallow, glycerin, coconut oil, castor oil, sodium hydroxide, oleic acid, laneth-10 acetate, cocamide DEA, nonoxynol-14, PEG-14 octoate, BHT, O-tolyl biguanide. Bar 105 g, 165 g. Scented or unscented. *otc.*
Use: Dermatologic, cleanser.

Neutrogena Glow Sunless Tanning. (Neutrogena) Octyl methoxycinnamate, cetyl alcohol, diazolidinyl urea, parabens, EDTA. SPF 8. Lot. Bot. 120 ml. *otc.*
Use: Sunscreen.

Neutrogena Intensified Day Moisture. (Neutrogena) Octyl methoxycinnamate, 2-phenylbenzimidazole sulfonic acid, titanium dioxide, cetyl alcohol, diazolidinyl urea, parabens, EDTA. SPF 15. Cream 67.5 g. *otc.*
Use: Dermatologic, moisturizer.

Neutrogena Lip Moisturizer. (Neutrogena) Octyl methoxycinnamate, benzophenone-3, corn oil, castor oil, mineral oil, lanolin oil, petrolatum, lanolin, stearyl alcohol. SPF 15. Lip balm 4.5 g. *otc.*
Use: Lip protectant.

Neutrogena Moisture SPF 5. (Neutrogena) Octyl methoxycinnamate, petrolatum, cetyl alcohol, parabens, diazolidinyl urea, EDTA, cetyl alcohol. Lot. Bot 60 ml,120 ml. *otc.*
Use: Dermatologic, moisturizer.

Neutrogena Moisture SPF 15. (Neutrogena) Octyl methoxycinnamate, benzophenone-3, glycerin, PEG-100 stearate, dimethicone, PEG-6000 monostearate, triethanolamine, parabens, imidazolidinyl urea, carbomer 954, PABA free. Lot. Bot. 120 ml. *otc.*
Use: Sunscreen.

Neutrogena Non-Drying Cleansing. (Neutrogena) Glycerin, caprylic/capric triglyceride, PEG-20 almond glycerides, cetyl ricinoleate, isohexadecane, TEA-cocoyl glutamate, PEG-20 methyl glucose sesquistearate, stearyl alcohol, cetyl alcohol, EDTA, dipotassium glycyrrhizate, stearyl glycyrrhetinate, bisabolol, parabens, acrylates/C 10-30 alkyl acrylate crosspolymer, triethanolamine, diazolidinyl urea. Lot. Bot. 165 ml. *otc.*
Use: Dermatologic, cleanser.

Neutrogena Norwegian Formula Emulsion. (Neutrogena) Glycerin base 2%.

Pump dispenser 5.25 oz. *otc.*
Use: Emollient.

Neutrogena Norwegian Formula Hand Cream. (Neutrogena) Glycerin base 41%. Tube 2 oz. *otc.*
Use: Emollient.

Neutrogena No-Stick Sunscreen. (Neutrogena) SPF 30. Homosalate 15%, octyl methoxycinnamate 7.5%, benzophenone-36%, octyl salicylate 5%, EDTA, parabens, diazolidinyl urea/ Cream. Waterproof 118 g. *otc.*
Use: Sunscreen.

Neutrogena Oil-Free Acne Wash. (Neutrogena) Salicylic acid 2%, EDTA, propylene glycol, tartrazine, aloe extract. Liq. Bot. 180 ml. *otc.*
Use: Dermatologic, acne.

Neutrogena Oily Skin Formula Soap. (Neutrogena) Triethanolamine, glycerin, fatty acids. Bar 3.5 oz. *otc.*
Use: Dermatologic, cleanser.

Neutrogena Original Formula Soap. (Neutrogena) Triethanolamine, glycerin, fatty acids. Bar 3.5 oz, 5.5 oz. *otc.*
Use: Dermatologic, cleanser.

Neutrogena Soap. (Neutrogena) TEA-stearate, triethanolamine, glycerin, sodium tallowate, sodium cocoate, sodium ricinoleate, TEA-oleate, cocamide DEA, tocopherol. Bar 105 g, 165 g. *otc.*
Use: Dermatologic, cleanser.

Neutrogena Sunblock. (Neutrogena) **SPF 8:** Octyl methoxycinnamate, menthyl anthranilate, titanium dioxide, mineral oil. Cream 67.5 g. **SPF 15:** Octyl methoxycinnamate, octyl salicylate, menthyl anthranilate, mineral oil, titanium dioxide, propylparaben. Cream 67.5 g. **SPF 25:** Octyl methoxycinnamate, benzophenone-3, octyl salicylate, castor oil, cetearyl alcohol, propylparaben, shea butter. Stick 12.6 g. **SPF 30:** Octocrylene, octyl methoxycinnamate, menthyl anthranilate, zinc oxide, mineral oil, vitamin E. Cream 67.5 g. *otc.*
Use: Sunscreen.

Neutrogena Sunscreen. (Neutrogena) Ethylhexyl p-methoxycinnamate 7%, oxybenzone 4%, titanium dioxide 2%. Tube 3 oz. *otc.*
Use: Sunscreen.

Neutrogena T/Gel. (Neutrogena) Coal tar extract 2%. Shampoo. Bot. 132 ml. *otc.*
Use: Antiseborrheic.

Neutrogena T/Sal. (Neutrogena) Salicylic acid 2%, solubilized coal tar extract 2%. Shampoo. Bot. 135 ml. *otc.*
Use: Antiseborrheic.

neutropin-1.
Use: Motor neuron disease/amyotrophic lateral sclerosis. [Orphan Drug]

•**nevirapine.** (neh-VIE-rah-peen) USAN.
Use: Antiviral.
See: Viramune, Tab. (Roxane Laboratories, Inc.).

New Decongest Pediatric Syrup. (Zenith Goldline Pharmaceuticals) Phenylpropanolamine HCl 5 mg, phenylephrine HCl 1.25 mg, chlorpheniramine maleate 0.5 mg, phenyltoloxamine citrate 2 mg/5 ml. Syr. Bot. Pt, gal. *Rx.*
Use: Antihistamine, decongestant.

New Decongestant. (Zenith Goldline Pharmaceuticals) Phenylpropanolamine HCl 40 mg, phenylephrine HCl 10 mg, chlorpheniramine maleate 5 mg/SR Tab. Bot. 100s, 1000s. *Rx-otc.*
Use: Antihistamine, decongestant.

•**nexeridine hydrochloride.** (NEX-eh-RIH-deen) USAN.
Use: Analgesic.

NG-29.
Use: Diagnostic aid. [Orphan Drug]

N.G.T. (Geneva Pharmaceuticals) Triamcinolone acetonide 0.1%, nystatin 100,000 units/g. Cream. Tube 15 g. *Rx.*
Use: Antifungal, corticosteroid, topical.

Nia-Bid. (Roberts Pharmaceuticals) Niacin 400 mg/TR Cap. Bot. 100s. *otc.*
Use: Vitamin supplement.

Niacal. (Jones Medical Industries, Inc.) Calcium lactate 324 mg, niacin 25 mg/ Tab. Peppermint flavor. Bot. 100s, 1000s. *otc.*
Use: Vasodilator, vitamin supplement.

•**niacin.** (NYE-uh-sin) U.S.P. 23.
Use: Antihyperlipidemic; vitamin (enzyme co-factor).
See: Niac, Cap. (Cole).
Niaspan, ER Tab. (Kos Pharmaceuticals).
Nico-400 (Hoechst Marion Roussel).
Ni Cord XL, Cap. (Scott/Cord).
Nicotinex, Elix. (Fleming & Co.).
Span Niacin 300, Tab. (Scrip).

niacin w/combinations.
See: Lipo-Nicin, Tab., Cap. (ICN Pharmaceuticals, Inc.).

•**niacinamide.** (nye-ah-SIN-ah-mide) U.S.P. 23.
Use: Vitamin (enzyme co-factor).
W/Pentylenetetrazol, thiamine HCl, cyanocobalamin, alcohol.
See: Cenalene, Tab., Elix. (Schwarz Pharma, Inc.).
W/Potassium iodide.
See: Riboflavin and Niacinamide, Amp.

(Eli Lilly and Co.).

Niacor. (Upsher-Smith Labs, Inc.) Niacin 500 mg/Tab. Bot. 100s. *Rx.*
Use: Vitamin supplement.

Nialexo-C. (Roberts Pharmaceuticals) Niacin 50 mg, vitamin C 30 mg/Tab. Bot. 100s. *otc.*
Use: Vitamin supplement.

Niarb Super. (Miller Pharmacal Group, Inc.) Magnesium 100 mg, vitamin C 200 mg, niacinamide 200 mg (as ascorbate)/Tab. Bot. 100s. *otc.*
Use: Mineral, vitamin supplement.

Niaspan. (Kos Pharmaceuticals) Niacin 375 mg, 500 mg, 750 mg, 1000 mg. ER Tab. Bot. 100s. Starter packs. *Rx.*
Use: Antihyperlipidemic.

Niazide. (Major Pharmaceuticals) Trichlormethiazide 4 mg/Tab. Bot. 100s, 1000s. *Rx.*
Use: Diuretic.

niazo. Neotropin.
Use: Antiseptic, urinary.

•**nibroxane.** (nye-BROX-ane) USAN.
Use: Antimicrobial, topical.

nicamindon.
See: Nicotinamide (Various Mfr.).

•**nicardipine hydrochloride.** (NYE-CAR-dih-peen) USAN.
Use: Vasodilator.
See: Cardene (Roche Laboratories).

nicardipine hydrochloride. (Mylan Pharmaceuticals) 20 mg, 30 mg/Cap. Bot. 90s, 500s. *Rx.*
Use: Vasodilator.

N'ice. (SmithKline Beecham Pharmaceuticals) Menthol 5 mg/Loz. in sugarless sorbitol base, saccharin. Pkg. 16s. *otc.*
Use: Anesthetic, local.

N'ice 'n Clear. (SmithKline Beecham Pharmaceuticals) Menthol 5 mg, sorbitol. Loz. Pkg. 16s. *otc.*
Use: Anesthetic, local.

N'ice Throat Spray. (SmithKline Beecham Pharmaceuticals) Menthol 0.12%, glycerin 25%, alcohol 23%, glucose, saccharin, sorbitol. Spray. 180 ml. *otc.*
Use: Mouth and throat preparation.

N'ice w/Vitamin C Drops. (SmithKline Beecham Consumer Healthcare) Ascorbic acid 60 mg, menthol, sorbitol, tartrazine/Loz. Pks. 16s. *otc.*
Use: Vitamin supplement, anesthetic, local.

•**nicergoline.** (nice-ERR-go-leen) USAN.
Use: Vasodilator.

Nichols Syphon Powder. (Last) Sodium bicarbonate, sodium Cl, sodium borate. Pouch 12.2 g (add to 32 oz. water to yield isotonic soln.).

•**niclosamide.** (nye-CLOSE-ah-mide) USAN.
Use: Antihelminthic.

Nico-400. (Jones Medical Industries, Inc.) Niacin 400 mg/Cap. Bot. 100s. *otc.*
Use: Vitamin supplement.

nicobion.
See: Nicotinamide (Various Mfr.).

Nicoderm. (Hoechst Marion Roussel) Total nicotine content 36 mg, 114 mg/patch. 14 systems/box. *Rx.*
Use: Smoking deterrent.

nicoduozide. A mixture of nicothazone and isoniazid.

•**nicorandil.** (NIH-CAR-an-dill) USAN.
Use: Coronary vasodilator.

Ni Cord XL Caps. (Scott/Cord) Nicotinic acid 400 mg/Cap. Bot. 100s, 500s. *otc.*
Use: Vitamin supplement.

Nicorette. (SmithKline Beecham Pharmaceuticals) Nicotine polacrilex 2 mg/Chew. Piece. Box 96s. *Rx.*
Use: Smoking deterrent.

nicotamide.
See: Nicotinamide (Various Mfr.).

nicothazone. Nicotinal dehydethiose micarbazone.

nicotilamide.
See: Nicotinamide (Various Mfr.).

nicotinamide. Niacinamide, U.S.P. 23. Vitamin B_3, Aminicotin, Dipegyl, Nicamindon, Nicotamide, Nicotilamide, Nicotinic Acid Amide.

nicotinamide adenine dinucleotide. Name used for Nadide.

•**nicotine.** (NIK-oh-TEEN) U.S.P. 23.
Use: Smoking cessation adjunct.
See: Nicotrol Inhaler (McNeil Consumer Products Co.).
Nicotrol NS, Spray (McNeil Consumer Products Co.).

nicotine transdermal systems.
Use: Smoking deterrent.
See: Habitrol (Novartis Pharmaceutical Corp.).
Nicoderm (Hoechst Marion Roussel).
Nicotrol (Parke-Davis).
Prostep (ESI Lederle Generics).

•**nicotine polacrilex.** (NIK-oh-TEEN PAHL-ah-KRILL-ex) U.S.P. 23.
Use: Smoking cessation adjunct.
See: Nicorette (Hoechst Marion Roussel).

nicotine resin complex.
See: Nicotine polacrilex.

Nicotinex Elixir. (Fleming & Co.) Niacin 50 mg/5 ml, alcohol 14%. Bot. Pt, gal.
Use: Vitamin B_3 supplement.

nicotinic acid. Niacin, U.S.P. 23.

nicotinic acid w/combinations.
See: Niacin w/Combinations (Various Mfr.).

nicotinic acid amide. Niacinamide, U.S.P. 23.
See: Niacinamide (Various Mfr.).

•**nicotinyl alcohol.** (NIK-oh-TIN-ill AL-koe-hahl) USAN.
Use: Vasodilator (peripheral).

nicotinyl tartrate. 3-Pyridinemethanol tartrate.

Nicotrol. (McNeil Consumer Products Co.) Nicotine 15 mg released gradually over 16 hours. Trans. system. Starter kit 7 patches, refill kit 7 patches. *otc.*
Use: Smoking deterrent.

Nicotrol Inhaler. (McNeil Consumer Products Co.) Nicotine 4 mg delivered (10 mg/cartridge). Inhaler Kit 1s. *Rx.*
Use: Smoking deterrent.

Nicotrol NS. (McNeil Consumer Products Co.) Nicotine 0.5 mg per actuation, methlyparaben, propylparaben, EDTA/Spray, pump. Bot. 10 ml. (200 sprays). *Rx.*
Use: Smoking deterrent.

nieraline.
See: Epinephrine (Various Mfr.).

•**nifedipine.** (nye-FED-ih-peen) U.S.P. 23.
Use: Coronary vasodilator, urinary tract agent. [Orphan Drug]
See: Adalat, Cap. (Bayer Corp. (Consumer Div.)).
Adalat CC, ER Tab. (Bayer Corp. (Consumer Div.)).
Procardia, Cap. (Pfizer US Pharmaceutical Group).

nifedipine. (Various Mfr.) Nifedipine 10 mg, 20 mg/Tab. In 100s, 300s, and UD 100s. *Rx.*
Use: Calcium channel blocker.

Niferex. (Schwarz Pharma, Inc.) **Elix.:** Iron 100 mg/5 ml polysaccharide-iron complex, alcohol 10%. Sugar and dye free. Bot. 236 ml. **Tab.:** Iron 50 mg. Bot. 100s. *otc.*
Use: Mineral supplement.

Niferex-150 Capsules. (Schwarz Pharma, Inc.) Polysaccharide iron complex equivalent to iron 150 mg/Cap. Bot. UD 100s. *otc.*
Use: Mineral supplement.

Niferex-150 Forte Capsules. (Schwarz Pharma, Inc.) Elemental iron as polysaccharide-iron complex 150 mg, folic acid 1 mg, vitamin B_{12} 25 mcg/Cap. Bot. 100s, 1000s. *Rx.*
Use: Mineral, vitamin supplement.

Niferex-PN Forte Tablets. (Schwarz Pharma, Inc.) Calcium 250 mg, iron 60 mg, vitamins A 5000 IU, D 400 IU, E 30 mg, B_1 3 mg, B_2 3.4 mg, B_3 20 mg, B_6 4 mg, B_{12} 12 mcg, C 80 mg, folic acid 1 mg, Cu, I, Mg, Zn 25 mg/Tab. Bot. 100s. *Rx.*
Use: Mineral, vitamin supplement.

Niferex-PN Tablets. (Schwarz Pharma, Inc.) Iron 60 mg, folic acid 1 mg, vitamins C 50 mg, B_{12} 3 mcg, A 4000 IU, D 400 IU, B_1 3 mg, B_2 3 mg, B_6 2 mg, B_3 10 mg, Zn 18 mg, Ca, sorbitol/Tab. Bot. 30s, 100s, 1000s. *Rx.*
Use: Mineral, vitamin supplement.

•**nifluridide.** (nye-FLURE-ih-DIDE) USAN.
Use: Ectoparasiticide.

•**nifungin.** (nih-FUN-jin) USAN. Substance derived from *Aspergillus giganteus.*

•**nifuradene.** (NYE-fyoor-ad-EEN) USAN.
Use: Anti-infective.

•**nifuraldezone.** (NYE-fer-AL-dee-zone) USAN. (Eaton Medical Corp.)
Use: Anti-infective.

•**nifuratel.** (NYE-fyoor-at-ell) USAN.
Use: Anti-infective, antifungal, antiprotozoal (trichomonas).

•**nifuratrone.** (nye-FYOOR-ah-trone) USAN.
Use: Anti-infective.

•**nifurdazil.** (NYE-fyoor-dazz-ill) USAN.
Use: Anti-infective.

nifurethazone.
Use: Anti-infective.

•**nifurimide.** (nye-FYOOR-ih-MIDE) USAN.
Use: Anti-infective.

•**nifurmerone.** (NYE-fyoor-MER-ohn) USAN.
Use: Antifungal.

nifuroxime.
Use: Antifungal, anti-infective, topical, antiprotozoal.
See: Micofur.

•**nifurpirinol.** (nye-fer-PIHR-ih-nole) USAN.
Use: Anti-infective.

•**nifurquinazol.** (NYE-fyoor-KWIN-azz-ole) USAN.
Use: Anti-infective.

•**nifurthiazole.** (NYE-fyoor-THIGH-ah-zole) USAN.
Use: Anti-infective.

nifurtimox.
Use: CDC anti-infective agent.
See: Lampit (Bayer Corp. (Diagnostic Div.)).

Night Time Cold/Flu Relief. (ProMetic Pharma) Doxylamine succinate 12.5 mg, dextromethorphan HBr 30 mg, acetaminophen 1000 mg, pseudo-

ephedrine HCl 60 mg/30 ml, alcohol 10%. Liq. Bot. 175 ml, 295 ml. *otc.*
Use: Antihistamine, antitussive, decongestant.

Night-Time Effervescent Cold Tablets. (Zenith Goldline Pharmaceuticals) Phenylpropanolamine HCl 15 mg, diphenhydramine citrate 38.33 mg, aspirin 325 mg/Tab. Pkg. 20s. *otc.*
Use: Analgesic, antihistamine, decongestant.

Nighttime Pamprin. (Chattem Consumer Products) Diphenhydramine HCl 50 mg, acetaminophen 650 mg. Pow. Pkg. 4s. *otc.*
Use: Sleep aid.

NightTime TheraFlu. (Novartis Pharmaceutical Corp.) Pseudoephedrine HCl 60 mg, chlorpheniramine maleate 4 mg, dextromethorphan HBr 30 mg, acetaminophen 1000 mg. Powd. 6s. *otc.*
Use: Analgesic, antihistamine, antitussive, decongestant.

nigrin. Streptonigrin.
Use: Antineoplastic.

Niko-Mag. (Scruggs) Magnesium oxide 500 mg/Cap. Bot. 100s, 1000s. *otc.*
Use: Antacid.

Nikotime TD Caps. (Major Pharmaceuticals) Niacin 125 mg, 250 mg/TD Cap. Bot. 100s, 1000s. *otc.*
Use: Vitamin supplement.

Nilandron. (Hoechst Marion Roussel) Nilutamide 50 mg/Tab. Bot. 90s. *Rx.*
Use: Antineoplastic.

Nilspasm. (Parmed Pharmaceuticals, Inc.) Phenobarbital 50 mg, hyoscyamine sulfate 0.31 mg, atropine sulfate 0.06 mg, scopolamine hydrobromide 0.0195 mg/Tab. Bot. 100s, 1000s. *Rx.*
Use: Anticholinergic, antispasmodic, hypnotic, sedative.

Nilstat Ointment & Cream. (ESI Lederle Generics) Nystatin 100,000 units/g. **Cream base:** w/Emulsifying wax, isopropyl myristate, glycerin, lactic acid, sodium hydroxide, sorbic acid 0.2%. Tube 15 g, Jar 240 g. **Oint. base:** w/light mineral oil, Plastibase 50 W. Tube 15 g. *Rx.*
Use: Antifungal, topical.

Nilstat Oral. (ESI Lederle Generics) Nystatin 500,000 units/FC Tab. Bot. 100s, UD 10 × 10s. *Rx.*
Use: Antifungal.

Nilstat Oral Suspension. (ESI Lederle Generics) Nystatin 100,000 units/ml, methylparaben 0.12%, propylparaben 0.03%, cherry flavor. Bot. 60 ml w/dropper, 16 fl oz. *Rx.*
Use: Antifungal.

Nilstat Powder. (ESI Lederle Generics) Nystatin pow. 150 million, 1 billion, 2 billion units/Bot. *Rx.*
Use: Antifungal.

Nil Tuss. (Minnesota Pharm) Dextromethorphan HBr 10 mg, chlorpheniramine maleate 1.25 mg, phenylephrine HCl 5 mg, ammonium Cl 83 mg/5 ml. Syr. Bot. Pt. *otc.*
Use: Antihistamine, antitussive, decongestant, expectorant.

•**nilutamide.** (nye-LOO-tah-mide) USAN.
Use: Antineoplastic.
See: Nilandron, Tab. (Hoechst Marion Roussel).

Nil Vaginal Cream. (Century Pharmaceuticals, Inc.) Sulfanilamide 15%, 9-aminoacridine HCl 0.2%, allantoin 1.5%. Bot. 4 oz. w/applicator. *otc.*
Use: Anti-infective, vaginal.

•**nilvadipine.** (NILL-vah-DIH-peen) USAN.
Use: Antagonist (calcium channel).

•**nimazone.** (nih-mah-ZONE) USAN.
Use: Anti-inflammatory.

Nimbex. (GlaxoWellcome) Cisatracurium besylate 2 mg/ml, Vial 5 ml, 10 ml; 10 mg/ml, Vial 20 ml. Inj. *Rx.*
Use: Nondepolarizing neuromuscular blocker; muscle relaxant.

Nimbus. (Biomerica, Inc.) Monoclonal antibody-based enzyme immunoassay. Screens for urinary chorionic gonadotropin. Pkg. 10s, 25s, 50s.
Use: Diagnostic aid.

•**nimodipine.** (NYE-MOE-dih-peen) USAN.
Use: Vasodilator.
See: Nimotop, Cap. (Bayer Corp. (Consumer Div.)).

Nimotop. (Bayer Corp. (Consumer Div.)) Nimodipine 30 mg Liq. Cap. Bot. UD 100s. *Rx.*
Use: Calcium channel blocker.

Nion B Plus C. (Nion Corp.) Vitamins B_1 15 mg, B_2 10.2 mg, B_3 50 mg, B_5 10 mg, C 300 mg/Capl. Bot 100s. *otc.*
Use: Vitamin supplement.

Niong. (U.S. Ethicals) Nitroglycerin 2.6 mg, 6.5 mg/CR Tab. Bot. 100s. *Rx.*
Use: Antianginal.

Nipent. (SuperGen, Inc.) Pentostatin 10 mg/Pow. Vial. Single-dose. *Rx.*
Use: Antineoplastic.

Niratron. (Progress) Chlorpheniramine maleate 4 mg/5 ml. Bot. pt.
Use: Antihistamine.

•**niridazole.** (nye-RIH-dah-ZOLE) USAN.
Use: Antischistosomal.

•**nisbuterol mesylate.** (NISS-BYOO-teh-role) USAN.

Use: Bronchodilator.

•**nisobamate.** (NYE-so-BAM-ate) USAN.
Use: Anxiolytic, hypnotic, sedative.

•**nisoldipine.** (nye-SOLE-idh-peen) USAN.
Use: Vasodilator (coronary).
See: Sular, ER Tab. (Zeneca Pharmaceuticals).

•**nisoxetine.** (NISS-OX-eh-teen) USAN.
Use: Antidepressant.

•**nisterime acetate.** (nye-STEER-eem) USAN.
Use: Androgen.

•**nitarsone.** (NITE-AHR-sone) USAN.
Use: Antiprotozoal (histomonas).

Nite Time Cold Formula. (Alpharma USPD Inc.) Pseudoephedrine HCl 10 mg, doxylamine succinate 1.25 mg, dextromethorphan HBr 5 mg, acetaminophen 167 mg, alcohol 25%. Liq. Bot. 180 ml, 300 ml. *otc.*
Use: Analgesic, antihistamine, antitussive, decongestant.

•**nitrafudam hydrochloride.** (NIGH-trah-FEW-dam) USAN.
Use: Antidepressant.

•**nitralamine hydrochloride.** (nye-TRAL-ah-meen) USAN.
Use: Antifungal.

•**nitramisole hydrochloride.** (nye-TRAM-ih-sole) USAN.
Use: Anthelmintic.

•**nitrazepam.** (nye-TRAY-zeh-pam) USAN.
Use: Anticonvulsant, hypnotic, sedative.

Nitrazine Paper. (Bristol-Myers Squibb) Determines pH of a solution, in pH 4.5 to 7.5 range. 15 ft. roll with dispenser and color chart.
Use: Diagnostic aid.

Nitrek. (Bertek Pharmaceuticals, Inc.) Nitroglycerin 22.4 mg/8 cm^2 (0.2 mg/hr), 44.8 mg/16 cm^2 (0.4 mg/hr), 67.2 mg/24 cm^2 (0.6 mg/hr). Patch. Box 30s. *Rx.*
Use: Antianginal.

•**nitrendipine.** (NIGH-TREN-dih-peen) USAN.
Use: Antihypertensive.

•**nitric acid.** (NYE-trick) N.F. 18.
Use: Pharmaceutic aid (acidifying agent).

nitric acid silver. Silver Nitrate, U.S.P. 23.

nitric oxide. (Ohmeda Pharmaceuticals)
Use: Primary pulmonary hypertension agent. [Orphan Drug]

Nitro-Bid IV. (Hoechst Marion Roussel) Nitroglycerin 5 mg/ml. Inj. Vial 1 ml box 10s; 5 ml Box 10s; 10 ml Box 5s. *Rx.*
Use: Antianginal.

Nitro-Bid Ointment. (Hoechst Marion Roussel) Nitroglycerin (glyceryl trinitrate) 2%, in lanolin and petrolatum base. Tube 20 g, 60 g, UD 1 g (100s). *Rx.*
Use: Antianginal.

Nitrocap. (Freeport) Nitroglycerin 2.5 mg/TR Cap. Bot. 100s. *Rx.*
Use: Antianginal.

•**nitrocycline.** (NYE-troe-SIGH-kleen) USAN.
Use: Anti-infective.

•**nitrodan.** (NYE-troe-dan) USAN.
Use: Anthelmintic.

Nitrodisc. (Roberts Pharmaceuticals) Nitroglycerin. Transcutaneous nitroglycerin discs releasing 16 mg, 24 mg, 32 mg/Patch. Ctn. 30s, 100s. *Rx.*
Use: Antianginal.

Nitro-Dur. (Key Pharmaceuticals) Nitroglycerin. Transdermal system releasing 20 mg, 40 mg, 60 mg, 80 mg, 120 mg, 160 mg/Patch. Ctn. 30s, 100s, UD 30s, 100s. *Rx.*
Use: Antianginal.

Nitrofan Caps. (Major Pharmaceuticals) Nitrofurantoin 50 mg, 100 mg/Cap. Bot. 100s, 500s. *Rx.*
Use: Anti-infective, urinary.

•**nitrofurantoin.** (nye-troe-FYOOR-an-toyn) U.S.P. 23.
Use: Anti-infective, urinary.
See: Furadantin, Soln. (Procter & Gamble Pharm.).

nitrofurantoin macrocrystals. (Various Mfr.) 50 mg, 100 mg/Cap. Bot. 100s, 500s, 1000s. *Rx.*
Use: Anti-infective, urinary.
See: Macrobid, Cap. (Procter & Gamble Pharm.).
Macrodantin, Cap. (Procter & Gamble Pharm.).

•**nitrofurazone.** U.S.P. 23.
Use: Anti-infective, topical.
See: Furacin, Preps. (Roberts Pharmaceuticals).

nitrofurazone. (Various Mfr.) **Top. Soln.:** 0.2%. Bot. Pt., gal. **Oint.:** 0.2%. Tube 480 g. *Rx.*
Use: Anti-infective, topical.

Nitrogard. (Parke-Davis) Transmucosal controlled-released nitroglycerin 1 mg, 2 mg, 3 mg/Tab. Bot. 100s. *Rx.*
Use: Antianginal.

•**nitrogen.** (NYE-troe-jen) N.F. 18.
Use: Pharmaceutic aid (air displacement).

nitrogen monoxide. Laughing Gas, Nitrous Oxide.
Use: Anesthetic, general; analgesic.

nitrogen mustard.
See: Mustargen, Vial (Merck & Co.).

nitrogen mustard derivatives.
See: Leukeran, Tab. (GlaxoWellcome).
Mustargen HCl, Vial (Merck & Co.).
Triethylene Melamine, Tab. (ESI Lederle Generics).

nitroglycerin. (nye-troe-GLIH-suh-rin) (Various Mfr.) 5 mg/ml. Inj. Vial 5 ml, 10 ml. *Rx.*
Use: Antianginal.

nitroglycerin. (Various Mfr.) Glyceryl Trinitrate, Glonoin, Nitroglycerol, Trinitrin, Trinitroglycerol Tab.
Use: Vasodilator.
See: Niglycon, Tab. (Consolidated Midland Corp.).
Niong, Tab. (U.S. Ethicals).
Nitrek (Bertek).
Nitro-Bid, Cap. (Hoechst Marion Roussel).
Nitrocels, Cap. (Winston).
Nitrodyl, Cap. (Sanofi Winthrop Pharmaceuticals).
Nitrogard (Parke-Davis).
Nitroglyn, Tab. (Key Pharmaceuticals).
Nitrol Oint. (Kremers Urban).
Nitro-Lyn, Cap. (Lynwood).
Nitrong, Tab. (Wharton).
NitroQuick (Ethex).
Nitrospan, Cap. (Rhone-Poulenc Rorer Pharmaceuticals, Inc.).
Nitro, TD Cap. (Fleming & Co.).
Nitro-Time, Cap. (Time-Cap Labs, Inc.).

•**nitroglycerin, diluted.** (nye-troe-GLIH-suh-rin) U.S.P. 23. *Formerly Glyceryl Trinitrate.*
Use: Vasodilator (coronary).

nitroglycerin in 5% dextrose. (Various Mfr.) **25 mg, 100 mg:** Inj. Soln. 250 ml. **50 mg:** Inj. Soln. 250, 500 ml. **200 mg:** Inj. Soln. 500 ml. *Rx.*
Use: Antianginal.

nitroglycerin injection. (Abbott Laboratories) 25 mg/ml. Vial 5 ml, 10 ml.
Use: Antianginal, vasodilator.
See: Tridil, Inj. (Du Pont Merck Pharmaceutical Co.).

nitroglycerin, intravenous.
Use: Vasodilator.
See: Nitro-Bid IV (Hoechst Marion Roussel).

nitroglycerin ointment. (Various Mfr.) 2% in lanolin-petrolatum base. Tube 30 g, 60 g. *Rx.*
Use: Vasodilator.

nitroglycerin patch.
Use: Antianginal.
See: Nitrek (Bertek Pharmaceuticals, Inc.).

nitroglycerin transdermal. (Various Mfr.) 16 mg to 62.5 mg, 32 mg to 125 mg, or 75 mg to 187.5 mg (some systems have different release rates). Box 30s.
Use: Vasodilator.
See: Deponit 5 and 10 (Wyeth-Ayerst Laboratories).
Nitrodisc (Searle).
NTS (Circa Pharmaceuticals, Inc.).
Transderm-Nitro (Novartis Pharmaceutical Corp.).

nitroglycerin transdermal system. (Hercon Lab) Nitroglycerin 37.3 mg, 74.6 mg, 111.9 mg. Patch Pkg. 30s. *Rx.*
Use: Vasodilator.

nitroglycerol.
See: Nitroglycerin (Various Mfr.).

Nitroglyn. (Key Pharmaceuticals) Nitroglycerin 2.5 mg, 6.5 mg, 9 mg/SRCap. Bot. 100s. *Rx.*
Use: Antianginal.

Nitrolan. (Elan Pharma) Protein 60 g, fat 40 g, carbohydrates 160 g, Na 690 mg, K 1.17 g/L, lactose free. With appropriate vitamins and minerals. Liq. In 237 ml Tetra Pak containers and 1000 ml New Pak closed systems with and without Color Check. *otc.*
Use: Nutritional supplement.

Nitrolin. (Schein Pharmaceutical, Inc.) Nitroglycerin 2.5 mg, 9 mg/SR Cap. **2.5 mg:** Bot. 100s. **9 mg:** Bot. 60s. *Rx.*
Use: Antianginal.

Nitrolingual Spray. (Rhone-Poulenc Rorer Pharmaceuticals, Inc.) Nitroglycerin lingual aerosol 0.4 mg/metered dose. Canister 13.8 g containing 200 metered doses. *Rx.*
Use: Antianginal.

Nitrol IV. (Rhone-Poulenc Rorer Pharmaceuticals, Inc.) Nitroglycerin 0.8 mg/ml. Amp.1 ml Box 25s; 10 ml Box 10s; 30 ml Box 5s. *Rx.*
Use: Antianginal.

Nitrol IV Concentrate. (Rhone-Poulenc Rorer Pharmaceuticals, Inc.) Nitroglycerin for infusion 50 mg/10 ml. Amp. Box 10s. *Rx.*
Use: Antianginal.

Nitrol Ointment. (Pharmacia & Upjohn) Nitroglycerin 2% in lanolin and petrolatum base. Tube 30 g, 60 g, Pack 6s. *Rx.*
Use: Antianginal.

Nitrol Ointment. (Savage Laboratories) Nitroglycerin 2% in a lanolin-petrola-

tum base. Tube 60 g, UD 3 g (50s). *Rx.*
Use: Antianginal agent.

Nitro-Lyn. (Lynwood) Nitroglycerin 2.5 mg/Cap. Bot. 100s. *Rx.*
Use: Antianginal.

nitromannite.
See: Mannitol Hexanitrate (Various Mfr.).

nitromannitol.
See: Mannitol Hexanitrate (Various Mfr.).

Nitromed. (U.S. Ethicals) Nitroglycerin 2.6 mg, 6.5 mg/CR Tab. Bot. 100s. *Rx.*
Use: Antianginal.

•**nitromersol.** (nye-troe-MER-sole) U.S.P. 23.
Use: Anti-infective, topical.

•**nitromide.** (NYE-troe-mid) USAN.
Use: Anti-infective.

•**nitromifene citrate.** (nye-TROE-mih-feen) USAN.
Use: Antiestrogen.

Nitronet. (U.S. Ethicals) Nitroglycerin 2.6 mg, 6.5 mg/CR Tab. Bot. 100s. *Rx.*
Use: Antianginal.

Nitrong Ointment. (Wharton) Nitroglycerin 2%. Oint. Tube 30 g, 60 g with dose applicator. *Rx.*
Use: Antianginal.

Nitrong Tablets. (Wharton) Nitroglycerin 2.6 mg, 6.5 mg, 9 mg/CR Tab. Bot. 30s, 60s (9 mg), 100s. *Rx.*
Use: Antianginal.

Nitropress. (Abbott Laboratories) Sodium nitroprusside 50 mg/2 ml. Vial. *Rx.*
Use: Antihypertensive.

nitroprusside sodium. (nye-troe-PRUSS-ide SO-dee-uhm)
Use: Antihypertensive.
See: Nitropress, Pow. for Inj. (Abbott Laboratories).
Sodium Nitroprusside, Pow. for Inj. (Various Mfr.).

NitroQuick. (Ethex) Nitroglycerin 0.3 mg (1/200 gr), 0.4 mg (1/150 gr), 0.6 mg (1/100 gr), lactose. Subling. Tab. Bot. 25s (0.4 mg only), 100s. *Rx.*
Use: Vasodilator.

nitrosoureas.
Use: Alkylating agent (antineoplastic).
See: CeeNu (Bristol-Myers Oncology/Immunology).
BiCNU (Bristol-Myers Oncology/Immunology).
Zanosar (Pharmacia & Upjohn).
Thiotepa (ESI Lederle Generics).

Nitrostat. (Parke-Davis) Nitroglycerin 0.3 mg, 0.4 mg, 0.6 mg/Tab. Bot. 25s, 100s, UD 100s. *Rx.*
Use: Antianginal.

Nitrostat IV. (Parke-Davis) Nitroglycerin for infusion. **0.8 mg/ml:** Amp. 10 ml. **5 mg/ml:** Amp. 10 ml, Vial 10 ml. **10 mg/ml:** Vial 10 ml. *Rx.*
Use: Antianginal.

Nitro-Time. (Time-Cap Labs, Inc.) Nitroglycerin 2.5 mg, 6.5 mg, 9 mg, lactose, sucrose/ER Cap. Bot. 60s, 90s, 100s. *Rx.*
Use: Antianginal.

nitrous acid, sodium salt. Sodium Nitrite, U.S.P. 23.

•**nitrous oxide.** U.S.P. 23. Laughing Gas. Nitrogen Monoxide.
Use: Anesthesia (inhalation).

•**nivazol.** (NIH-vah-ZOLE) USAN.
Use: Corticosteroid, topical.

Nivea Moisturizing. (Beiersdorf, Inc.) **Cream:** Mineral oil, petrolatum, lanolin alcohol, glycerin, microcrystalline wax, paraffin, magnesium sulfate, decyloleate, octyl dodecanol, aluminum stearate, citric acid, magnesium stearate. 120 g, 180 g, 300 g, 480 g. **Lot.:** Mineral oil, lanolin, isopropyl myristate, cetearyl alcohol, glyceryl stearate, acrylamide/sodium acrylate copolymer, simethicone, methychloroisothiazolinone, methylisothiazolinone. In 180 ml, 300 ml, 450 ml. *otc.*
Use: Emollient.

Nivea Moisturizing Creme Soap. (Beiersdorf, Inc.) Sodium tallowate, sodium cocoate, glycerin, petrolatum, titanium dioxide, NaCl, octyldodecanol, macadamia nut oil, aloe, sodium thiosulfate, lanolin alcohol, pentasodium pentetate, EDTA, BHT, beeswax. Bar 90 g, 150 g. *otc.*
Use: Dermatologic, cleanser.

Nivea Oil. (Beiersdorf, Inc.) Emulsion of neutral aliphatic hydrocarbons. **Liq.:** Bot. 2 oz, 4 fl oz, pt, qt. **Cream:** Tube 1 oz, 2⅓ oz, Jar 4 oz, 6 oz, 1 lb, 5 lb. tin. **Soap:** Bath or toilet size. *otc.*
Use: Emollient.
See: Basic, Soap (Beiersdorf, Inc.).

Nivea Sun. (Beiersdorf, Inc.) Octyl methoxycinnamate, octyl salicylate, benzophenone-3, 2-phenylbenzimidazole-5-sulfonic acid. Lot. Bot. 120 ml. *otc.*
Use: Sunscreen.

•**nivimedone sodium.** (nih-VIH-meh-dohn) USAN.
Use: Antiallergic.

Nix Creme Rinse. (GlaxoWellcome) Permethrin 1%. Bot. 2 oz. *otc.*
Use: Pediculicide.

•**nizatidine.** (nye-ZAT-ih-deen) U.S.P. 23.
Use: Antiulcerative.

See: Axid, Prods. (Eli Lilly and Co.).

Nizoral Cream. (Janssen Pharmaceutical, Inc.) Ketoconazole 2% cream. Tube 15 g, 30 g. *Rx.*
Use: Antifungal, topical.

Nizoral Tablets. (Janssen Pharmaceutical, Inc.) Ketoconazole 200 mg/Tab. Bot. 100s, UD 100s. *Rx.*
Use: Antifungal.

n-methylhydrazine.
Use: Antineoplastic.
See: Procarbazine.

n-methylisatin beta-thiosemicarbazone. Under study.
Use: Smallpox protection.

N-Multistix. (Bayer Corp. (Consumer Div.)) Glucose, protein, pH, blood, ketones, bilirubin, urobilinogen, nitrate, leukocytes. Kit 100s.
Use: Diagnostic aid.

N-Multistix S. G. Reagent Strips. (Bayer Corp. (Consumer Div.)) Urinalysis reagent strip test for pH, protein, glucose, ketones, bilirubin, blood, nitrite, urobilinogen and specific gravity. Bot. 100s.
Use: Diagnostic aid.

n, n-diethylvanillamide.
See: Ethamivan, Inj. (Various Mfr.).

No-Aspirin. (Walgreen Co.) Acetaminophen 325 mg/Tab. Bot. 100s. *otc.*
Use: Analgesic.

No-Aspirin Extra Strength. (Walgreen Co.) Acetaminophen 500 mg/Tab. **Tab.:** Bot. 60s, 100s. **Cap.:** Bot. 50s, 100s. *otc.*
Use: Analgesic.

•**noberastine.** (no-BER-ast-een) USAN.
Use: Antihistamine.

•**nocodazole.** (no-KOE-DAH-zole) USAN.
Use: Antineoplastic.

NoDoz. (Bristol-Myers Squibb) **Tab.:** Caffeine 200 mg, sucrose. Bot. 16s, 36s, 60s. **Chew. Tab.:** Caffeine 100 mg, aspartame, phenylalanine 15 mg, spearmint flavor. Pkg. 12s, 30s. *otc.*
Use: Analeptic.

No Drowsiness Allerest. (Novartis Pharmaceutical Corp.) Pseudoephedrine HCl 30 mg, acetaminophen 500 mg/Tab. Bot. 20s. *otc.*
Use: Analgesic, decongestant.

No Drowsiness Sinarest. (Medeva Pharmaceuticals, Inc.) Pseudoephedrine HCl 30 mg, acetaminophen 500 mg/Tab. Bot. 24s. *otc.*
Use: Analgesic, decongestant.

nofetumomab merpentan.
See: Verluma (Neorx Corp., Du Pont Merck Pharmaceuticals).

•**nogalamycin.** (no-GAL-ah-MY-sin) USAN.
Use: Antineoplastic.

No-Hist Capsules. (Dunhall Pharmaceuticals, Inc.) Phenylephrine HCl 5 mg, phenylpropanolamine HCl 40 mg, pseudoephedrine HCl 40 mg/Cap. Bot. 100s. *Rx.*
Use: Decongestant.

No-Hist-S Syrup. (Dunhall Pharmaceuticals, Inc.) Phenylephrine HCl 5 mg, phenylpropanolamine HCl 40 mg, pseudoephedrine HCl 40 mg/5 ml. Bot. pt. *Rx.*
Use: Decongestant.

Nokane. (Wren) Salicylamide 4 g, n-acetyl-p-aminophenol 4 g, caffeine 0.5 gr/Tab. Bot. 40s. *otc.*
Use: Analgesic combination.

Nolahist. (Carnrick Laboratories, Inc.) Phenindamine tartrate 25 mg/Tab. Bot. 100s. *otc.*
Use: Antihistamine.

Nolamine. (Carnrick Laboratories, Inc.) Chlorpheniramine maleate 4 mg, phenindamine tartrate 24 mg, phenylpropanolamine HCl 50 mg/Tab. Bot. 100s, 250s. *Rx.*
Use: Antihistamine, decongestant.

Nolex LA. (Carnrick Laboratories, Inc.) Phenylpropanolamine 75 mg, guaifenesin 400 mg/SR Tab. Bot. 100s. *Rx.*
Use: Decongestant, expectorant.

•**nolinium bromide.** (no-LIN-ee-uhm) USAN.
Use: Antisecretory, antiulcerative.

Nolvadex. (Zeneca Pharmaceuticals) Tamoxifen citrate 10 mg, 20 mg. Tab. Box 60s, 250s (10 mg only), 30s (20 mg only). *Rx.*
Use: Antineoplastic.

Nometic. Diphenidol.
Use: Antiemetic.

•**nomifensine maleate.** (NO-mih-FEN-seen) USAN.
Use: Antidepressant.

Nonamin. (Western Research) Ca 100 mg, Cl 90 mg, Mg 50 mg, Zn 3.75 mg, Fe 4.5 mg, Cu 0.5 mg, I 37.5 mcg, K 49 mg, P 100 mg/Tab. Bot. 1000s. *otc.*
Use: Mineral supplement.

Non-Drowsy Contac Sinus. (SmithKline Beecham Pharmaceuticals) Pseudoephedrine HCl 30 mg, acetaminophen 500 mg. Cap. Bot. 24s. *otc.*
Use: Analgesic, decongestant.

None. (Forest Pharmaceutical, Inc.) Heparin sodium 1000 units/ml. No preservatives. Amps 5 ml. Box 25s. *Rx.*
Use: Anticoagulant.

nonoxynol. (nahn-OCK-sih-nahl) (Ortho McNeil Pharmaceutical) *otc.*

Use: Contraceptive, spermicide.
See: Emko, Preps. (Schering-Plough Corp.).

•**nonoxynol-4.** (NAHN-ox-sih-nahl4) USAN.
Use: Pharmaceutic aid (surfactant).

•**nonoxynol-9.** (NAHN-ox-sih-nahl 9) U.S.P. 23.
Use: Spermaticide, pharmaceutic aid (wetting and solubilizing agent).
See: Conceptrol, Cream, Gel (Ortho McNeil Pharmaceutical).
Delfen, Foam (Ortho McNeil Pharmaceutical).
Encare, Insert (Eaton-Merz).
Gynol II, Jelly (Ortho McNeil Pharmaceutical).
Ortho-Gynol, Jelly (Ortho McNeil Pharmaceutical).

•**nonoxynol-10.** (nahn-OCK-sih-nahl 10) N.F. 18.
Use: Pharmaceutic aid (surfactant).

•**nonoxynol-15.** (NAHN-ox-sih-nahl15) USAN.
Use: Pharmaceutic aid (surfactant).

•**nonoxynol-30.** (NAHN-ox-sih-nahl 30) USAN. Under study.
Use: Pharmaceutic aid (surfactant).

nonspecific protein therapy.
See: Protein, Nonspecific Therapy.

nonsteroidal anti-inflammatory agents, ophthalmic.
See: Ocufen (Allergan, Inc.).
Profenal (Alcon Laboratories, Inc.).
Voltaren (Ciba Vision).

nonylphenoxypolyethoxy ethanol. Nonoxynol.
Use: Contraceptive, spermicide.
See: Delfen, Vaginal Foam (Ortho McNeil Pharmaceutical).

No Pain-HP. (Young Again Products) Capsaicin 0.075%. Roll-on. 60 ml. *otc.*
Use: Analgesic, topical.

•**noracymethadol hydrochloride.** (nahr-ASS-ih-METH-ah-dole) USAN.
Use: Analgesic.

•**norbolethone.** (nahr-BOLE-eth-ohn) USAN.
Use: Anabolic.

Norcet Tablets. (Holloway) Hydrocodone bitartrate 5 mg, acetaminophen 500 mg/Tab. Bot. 100s. *c-III.*
Use: Analgesic combination, narcotic.

Norco. (Watson Labs) Hydrocodone bitartrate 10 mg, acetaminophen 325 mg. Tab. Bot. 100s, 500s. *c-III.*
Use: Analgesic, narcotic.

Norcuron. (Organon Teknika Corp.) Vecuronium bromide 10 mg/5 ml. **With diluent:** Vial 5 ml lyophilized powder and 5 ml Amp. of sterile water for injection. Box 10s. **Without diluent:** Vial 5 ml lyophilized powder. Box 10s. **Prefilled syringe:** Vial 10 ml lyophilized powder and 10 ml syringe w/bacteriostatic water for injection. Box 10s. *Rx.*
Use: Muscle relaxant.

norcycline.
Use: Anti-infective.

Nordette. (Wyeth-Ayerst Laboratories) Levonorgestrel 0.15 mg, ethinyl estradiol 0.03 mg/Tab. 6 Pilpak dispensers, 21-day and 28-day w/ 7 inert tabs. *Rx.*
Use: Contraceptive.

Norditropin. (Novo/Nordisk Pharm, Inc.) Somatropin 4 mg (≈ to 12 IU), 8 mg (≈ to 24 IU), glycine 8.8 mg, mannitol 44 mg. Pow. for Inj. Benzyl alcohol 1.5%. Vials. *Rx.*
Use: Hormone, growth.

Norel. (US Pharmaceutical Corp.) Phenylephrine HCl 5 mg, phenylpropanolamine HCl 45 mg, guaifenesin 200 mg. Cap. Bot. 100s. *Rx.*
Use: Decongestant, expectorant.

Norel Plus Capsules. (US Pharmaceutical Corp.) Chlorpheniramine maleate 4 mg, phenyltoloxamine dihydrogen citrate 25 mg, phenylpropanolamine HCl 25 mg, acetaminophen 325 mg/Cap. Bot. 100s. *Rx.*
Use: Analgesic, antihistamine, decongestant.

•**norepinephrine bitartrate.** (NOR-eh-pih-NEFF-reen bye-TAR-trate) U.S.P. 23.
Formerly levarterenol bitartrate.
Use: Adrenergic (vasoconstrictor).
See: Levophed Bitartrate, Soln., Amp. (Sanofi Winthrop Pharmaceuticals).

Norethin 1/50M. (Roberts Pharmaceuticals) Norethindrone 1 mg, mestranol 50 mcg/Tab. 21-day and 28-day (with 7 inert tabs.). *Rx.*
Use: Contraceptive.

Norethin 1/35E. (Roberts Pharmaceuticals) Norethindrone 1 mg, ethinyl estradiol 35 mg/Tab. 21-day and 28-day (with 7 inert tabs.). *Rx.*
Use: Contraceptive.

•**norethindrone.** (nore-eth-IN-drone) U.S.P. 23.
Use: Progestin.
See: Norlutin, Tab. (Parke-Davis).
Nor-QD, Tab. (Roche Laboratories).
W/Ethinyl estradiol.
See: Brevicon 21 and 28, Tab. (Roche Laboratories).
GenCept, Tab. (Gencon).
Jenest-28, Tab. (Organon Teknika Corp.).
Modicon 21 and 28, Tab. (Ortho Mc-

Neil Pharmaceutical).
Ortho-Novum 21 and 28, Prods. (Ortho McNeil Pharmaceutical).
Ovcon-35, Tab. (Bristol-Myers Squibb).
Ovcon-50, Tab (Bristol-Myers Squibb).
W/Mestranol.
See: Norinyl, Prods. (Roche Laboratories).
Ortho-Novum, Prods. (Ortho McNeil Pharmaceutical).

•**norethindrone acetate.** U.S.P. 23.
Use: Hormone, progestin.
See: Aygestin, Tab. (Wyeth-Ayerst Laboratories).

norethindrone acetate and ethinyl estradiol.
Use: Contraceptive.
See: Brevicon, Tab. (Roche Laboratories).
CombiPatch (Rhone-Poulenc Rover).
Estrostep, Prods. (Parke-Davis).
Loestrin, Prods. (Parke-Davis).
Norinyl, Prods. (Roche Laboratories).
Norlestrin, Prods. (Parke-Davis).

norethindrone and ethinyl estradiol tablets.
Use: Contraceptive.

norethindrone and mestranol tablets.
Use: Contraceptive.

•**norethynodrel.** (nahr-eh-THIGH-no-drell) U.S.P. 23.
Use: Hormone, progestin.
See: Enovid, Prods. (Searle).

Norflex. (3M Pharm.) Orphenadrine citrate 100 mg/SR Tab. Bot. 100s, 500s. *Rx.*
Use: Muscle relaxant.

Norflex Injectable. (3M Pharm.) Orphenadrine citrate 30 mg, sodium bisulfite 2 mg, sodium Cl 5.8 mg, water for injection qs 2 ml. Amp. 2 ml 6s, 50s. *Rx.*
Use: Muscle relaxant.

•**norfloxacin.** (nor-FLOX-uh-SIN) U.S.P. 23.
Use: Anti-infective.
See: Chibroxin, Ophth. Soln. (Merck & Co.).
Noroxin, Tab. (Merck & Co.).

•**norflurane.** (nahr-FLEW-rane) USAN. Under study.
Use: Anesthetic, general.

Norgesic Forte Tablets. (3M Pharm.) Orphenadrine citrate 50 mg, aspirin 770 mg, caffeine 60 mg, lactose/Tab. Bot. 100s, 500s, UD 100s. *Rx.*
Use: Muscle relaxant, analgesic.

Norgesic Tablets. (3M Pharm.) Orphenadrine citrate 25 mg, aspirin 385 mg, caffeine 30 mg, lactose/Tab. Bot. 100s, 500s, UD 100s. *Rx.*
Use: Muscle relaxant, analgesic.

•**norgestimate.** (nore-JEST-ih-mate) USAN. *Formerly Dexnorgestrel Acetime.*
Use: Hormone, progestin.
W/Ethinyl estradiol.
See: Ortho-Cyclen, Tab. (Ortho McNeil Pharmaceutical).
Ortho Tri-Cyclen, Tab. (Ortho McNeil Pharmaceutical).

•**norgestomet.** (nore-JESS-toe-met) USAN.
Use: Hormone, progestin.

•**norgestrel.** (nahr-JESS-trell) U.S.P. 23.
Use: Contraceptive; hormone, progestin.
See: Ovrette, Tab. (Wyeth-Ayerst Laboratories).

norgestrel and ethinyl estradiol tablets.
Use: Contraceptive.
See: Lo/Ovral, Tab. (Wyeth-Ayerst Laboratories).

Norinyl 1 + 35. (Roche Laboratories) Norethindrone 1 mg, ethinyl estradiol 0.035 mg/Tab. Wallette 21- and 28-day (7 inert tabs). *Rx.*
Use: Contraceptive.

Norinyl 1 + 50. (Roche Laboratories) Norethindrone 1 mg, mestranol 0.05 mg/Tab. Wallette 21- and 28-day (7 inert tabs). *Rx.*
Use: Contraceptive.

Norinyl 2 mg. (Roche Laboratories) Norethindrone 2 mg, mestranol 0.1 mg/Tab. Memorette Disp. of 20s. Refill folders of 20s. *Rx.*
Use: Contraceptive.

Norisodrine Aerosol. (Abbott Laboratories) Norisodrine HCl (isoproterenol HCl) 0.25% (2.8 mg/ml) in inert chlorofluorohydrocarbon propellants, alcohol 33%, ascorbic acid 0.1% as preservative. Aerosol 15 ml. Box 12s. *Rx.*
Use: Bronchodilator.

Norisodrine/Calcium Iodide Syrup. (Abbott Laboratories) Isoproterenol sulfate 3 mg, calcium iodide, anhydrous 150 mg/5 ml, alcohol 6%. Bot. Pt. *Rx.*
Use: Bronchodilator.

Noritate. (Dermik Laboratories, Inc.) Metronidazole 1%. Cream Tube 30 g. *Rx.*
Use: Dermatologic, acne.

Norlestrin-21 1/50 Tablets. (Parke-Davis) Norethindrone acetate 1 mg, ethinyl estradiol 50 mcg/Tab. Compact

21s. Pkg. 5 compacts. Pkg. 5 refills; Ctn. 10 × 5 refills. *Rx.*
Use: Contraceptive.

Norlestrin-28 1/50 Tablet. (Parke-Davis) Norethindrone acetate 1 mg, ethinyl estradiol 50 mcg/Tab. Compact 21 yellow, 7 white (inert) tablets. Pkg. 5 compacts. Pkg. 5 refills; Ctn. 10 × 5 refills. *Rx.*
Use: Contraceptive.

Norlestrin-21 2.5/50 Tablets. (Parke-Davis) Norethindrone acetate 2.5 mg, ethinyl estradiol 50 mcg/Tab. Compact 21s. Pkg. 5 compacts. Pkg. 5 refills; Ctn. 10 × 5 refills. *Rx.*
Use: Contraceptive.

Norlestrin Fe 1/50 Tablets. (Parke-Davis) Norethindrone acetate 1 mg, ethinyl estradiol 50 mcg/Tab. Compact 21 yellow tab., 7 brown 75 mg ferrous fumarate tab. Pkg. 5 compacts. Pkg. 5 refills; Ctn. 10 × 5 refills. *Rx.*
Use: Contraceptive.

Norlestrin Fe 2.5/50 Tablets. (Parke-Davis) Norethindrone acetate 2.5 mg, ethinyl estradiol 50 mcg/Tab. Compact 21 Tab., 7 brown 75 mg ferrous fumarate Tab. Pkg. 5 compacts. Pkg. 5 refills; Ctn. 10 × 5 refills. *Rx.*
Use: Contraceptive.

Normaderm Cream & Lotion. (Doak Dermatologics) Buffered lactic acid in vanishing bases. **Cream:** Jar 3¾ oz, 16 oz. **Lot.:** Bot. 4 oz, 16 oz, 128 oz. *otc.*
Use: Dermatologic, emollient.

normal human serum albumin. Albumin Human, U.S.P. 23.

normal human serum albumin. (Baxter Healthcare Corp.) **5%/Inj.:** 50 ml, 250 ml, 500 ml **25%/Inj.:** 20 ml, 50 ml, 100 ml. *Rx.*
Use: Blood volume supporter.

normal saline.
See: 5% Sodium chloride (Various Mfr.).

Normaline Kit. (Apothecary Products, Inc.) Salt tablets for normal saline 250 mg/Tab. Preservative free. 200s with diluent Bot. 27.7 ml. *otc.*
Use: Ophthalmic.

Normiflo. (Wyeth-Ayerst Laboratories) Ardeparin sodium 5000 anti-factor Xa U in 0.5 ml, 10,000 anti-factor Xa U in 0.5 ml/Inj. Box. 10s w/25-gauge × ⅝ inch needle. *Rx.*
Use: Anticoagulant.

Normodyne. (Schering-Plough Corp.) Labetalol HCl. **Inj.:** 5 mg/ml. Amp. 20 ml. Vial 40 ml, 60 ml. **Tab.:** 100 mg, 200 mg, 300 mg. Bot. 100s, 500s, UD 100s. *Rx.*
Use: Antihypertensive.

Normol. (Alcon, Vision Care) Sterile, isotonic solution of thimerosal 0.004%, chlorhexidine gluconate 0.005%, edetate disodium 0.1%. Bot. 8 oz. *otc.*
Use: Contact lens care.

Normosol-M in D5W. (Abbott Hospital Products) Dextrose 5 g, sodium Cl 234 mg, potassium acetate 128 mg, magnesium acetate 21 mg, sodium bisulfite 30 mg/100 ml. Bot. 500 ml, 1000 ml in Abbo-Vac (glass) or Life Care (flexible) containers. *Rx.*
Use: Nutritional supplement, parenteral.

Normosol-R; Normosol-R pH 7.4; Normosol-R D5W. (Abbott Hospital Products) Sodium Cl 526 mg, sodium acetate 222 mg, sodium gluconate 502 mg, potassium Cl 37 mg, magnesium Cl 14 mg, pH of Normosol-R and Normosol R in D5W adjusted with HCl/100 ml. Bot. 500 ml, 1000 ml. in Life Care (flexible) containers. *Rx.*
Use: Nutritional supplement, parenteral.

Normotensin. (Marcen) IM soln. for inj. Mucopolysaccharide 20 mg, sodium nucleate 25 mg, epinephrine-neutralizing factor 25 units, sodium citrate 10 mg, inositol 5 mg, phenol 0.5%/ml. Multi-dose vial 10 ml, 30 ml.
Use: Antihypertensive.

Norolon. (Sanofi Winthrop Pharmaceuticals) Chloroquine phosphate. *Rx.*
Use: Antimalarial.

Noroxin. (Roberts Pharmaceuticals) Norfloxacin 400 mg/Tab. Bot. 100s, UD 20s, UD 100s. *Rx.*
Use: Urinary anti-infective.

Norpace. (Searle) Disopyramide phosphate 100 mg, 150 mg/Cap. Bot. 100s, 500s, 1000s, UD 100s. *Rx.*
Use: Antiarrhythmic.

Norpace CR. (Searle) Disopyramide phosphate 100 mg, 150 mg/CR Cap. Bot. 100s, 500s, UD 100s. *Rx.*
Use: Antiarrhythmic.

Norphyl. (Vita Elixir) Aminophylline 100 mg/Tab. *Rx.*
Use: Bronchodilator.

Norplant System. (Wyeth-Ayerst Laboratories) Levonorgestrel 36 mg. Implant kit 6s. *Rx.*
Use: Progestin contraceptive system.

Norpramin. (Hoechst Marion Roussel) Desipramine HCl 10 mg, 25 mg, 50 mg, 75 mg, 100 mg, 150 mg/Tab. **10 mg:** Bot. 100s; **25 mg:** Bot. 100s, 1000s, UD 100s; **50 mg:** Bot. 100s, 1000s, UD 100s; **75 mg:** Bot. 100s; **100 mg:** Bot. 100s. **150 mg:** Bot. 50s. *Rx.*
Use: Antidepressant.

nortriptyline. (nor-TRIP-tih-leen) (Schein

Pharmaceutical, Inc.) 10 mg, 25 mg, 50 mg, 75 mg. Cap. Bot. 100s; **25 mg:** Bot. 500s also. *Rx.*
Use: Antidepressant.

nortriptyline. (Various Mfr.) 10 mg, 25 mg, 50 mg, 75 mg/Cap. 100s, 500s. *Rx.*
Use: Antidepressant.

•**nortriptyline hydrochloride.** (nor-TRIP-tih-leen) U.S.P. 23.
Use: Antidepressant.
See: Aventyl HCl, Liq., Pulvule (Eli Lilly and Co.).
Pamelor, Cap., Liq. (Novartis Pharmaceutical Corp.).

Norval. Docusate sodium.
Use: Laxative.

Norvasc. (Pfizer US Pharmaceutical Group) Amlodipine **2.5 mg:** Bot. 100s; **5 mg:** Bot. 100s, UD 100s; **10 mg:** Bot. 100s, UD 100s. *Rx.*
Use: Calcium channel blocker.

Norvir. (Abbott Laboratories) Ritonavir 100 mg. Soln.: 80 mg/ml ritonavir, saccharin. *Rx.*
Use: Antiviral.

Norwich Extra Strength. (Procter & Gamble Pharm.) Aspirin 500 mg/Tab. Bot. 150s. *otc.*
Use: Analgesic.

Nosalt. (SmithKline Beecham Pharmaceuticals) Potassium Cl, potassium bitartrate, adipic acid, mineral oil, fumaric acid. Na < 10 mg/5 g (0.43 mEq/5 g), K 2502 mg/5 g (64 mEq/5 g). Pkg. 330 g. *otc.*
Use: Salt substitute.

Nosalt Seasoned. (SmithKline Beecham Pharmaceuticals) Potassium Cl, dextrose, onion, and garlic, spices, lactose, cream of tartar, paprika, silica, disodium inosinate, disodium guanylate, turmeric. Na < 5 mg/5 g (0.2 mEq/5 g), K 1328 mg/5 g (34 mEq/5 g). Pkg. 240 g. *otc.*
Use: Salt substitute.

•**noscapine.** (NAHS-kah-peen) U.S.P. 23.
Use: Antitussive.

noscapine hydrochloride. l-Narcotine-hydrochloride.
Use: Antitussive.
See: Noscaps, Cap. (Table Rock).

Noscaps. (Table Rock) Noscapine 7.5 mg, chlorpheniramine maleate 1 mg, phenylephrine HCl 5 mg, N-acetyl-p-aminophenol 150 mg, salicylamide 150 mg, vitamin C 20 mg/Cap. Bot. 100s, 500s. *otc.*
Use: Analgesic, antihistamine, decongestant, vitamin C.

Noskote. (Schering-Plough Corp.) Oxybenzone 3%, homosalate 8%. SPF 8. Cream 13.2 g, 30 g. *otc.*
Use: Sunscreen.

Noskote Sunblock. (Schering-Plough Corp.) Padimate O 8%, oxybenzone 3%, benzyl alcohol. SPF 15. Cream. Tube 30 g. *otc.*
Use: Sunscreen.

Nostril. (Boehringer Ingelheim, Inc.) Phenylephrine HCl 0.25%, 0.5%, benzalkonium Cl 0.004% in buffered aqueous soln. Bot. 15 ml, pump spray. *otc.*
Use: Decongestant.

Novacet. (Medicis Dermatologicals, Inc.) Sodium sulfacetamide 100 mg, sulfur 50 mg, benzyl alcohol, cetyl alcohol, sodium thiosulfate, EDTA. Lot. Bot. 30 ml. *Rx.*
Use: Dermatologic, acne.

Nova-Dec. (Rugby Labs, Inc.) Iron 18 mg, vitamins A 5000 IU, D 400 IU, E 30 IU, B_1 1.7 mg, B_2 2 mg, B_3 20 mg, B_5 10 mg, B_6 3 mg, B_{12} 6 mcg, C 60 mg, folic acid 0.4 mg, Ca, Cr, Cu, I, Mg, Mo, Mn, P, Se, K, Zn 15 mg, vitamin K, Cl, Ni, Sn, V, B, biotin 30 mcg/Tab. Bot. 130s. *otc.*
Use: Mineral, vitamin supplement.

Novadyne Expectorant. (Various Mfr.) Pseudoephedrine 30 mg, codeine phosphate 10 mg, guaifenesin 100 mg/5 ml, alcohol 7.5%. Bot. 120 ml, pt, gal. *c-III.*
Use: Antitussive, decongestant, expectorant.

Novagest Expectorant w/Codeine. (Major Pharmaceuticals) Pseudoephedrine HCl 30 mg, codeine phosphate 10 mg, guaifenesin 100 mg/5 ml, alcohol 8.2%. Liq. Bot. 118 ml. *c-v.*
Use: Antitussive, decongestant, expectorant.

novamidon.
See: Aminopyrine (Various Mfr.).

Novamine. (Clintec Nutrition) Amino acid concentration 11.4%, for infusion. Nitrogen 1.8 g/100 ml. Essential amino acids (mg/100 ml): Isoleucine 570, leucine 790, lysine 900, methionine 570, phenylalanine 790, threonine 570, tryptophan 190, valine 730. Nonessential amino acids (mg/100 ml): Alanine 1650, arginine 1120, histidine 680, proline 680, serine 450, tyrosine 30, glycine 790, glutamic acid 570, aspartic acid 330, acetate 114 mEq/L, sodium metabisulfite 30 mg/100 ml. In 250 ml, 500 ml, 1 liter. *Rx.*
Use: Parenteral nutritional supplement.

Novamine 15%. (Clintec Nutrition) Amino acids 15%: Lysine 1.18 g, leucine 1.04

g, phenylalanine 1.04 g, valine 960 mg, isoleucine 749 mg, methionine 749 mg, threonine 749 mg, tryptophan 250 mg, alanine 2.17 g, arginine 1.47 g, glycine 1.04 g, histidine 894 mg, proline 894 mg, glutamic acid 749 mg, serine 592 mg, aspartic acid 434 mg, tyrosine 39 mg, nitrogen 2.37 g/100 ml. Inj. 500 ml, 1000 ml. *Rx.*
Use: Nutritional supplement, parenteral.

Novamine Without Electrolytes. (Clintec Nutrition) Amino acid concentration 8.5%, for infusion. Nitrogen 1.35 g/100 ml. Essential amino acids (mg/100 ml): Isoleucine 420, leucine 590, lysine 673, methionine 420, phenylalanine 590, threonine 420, tryptophan 140, valine 550. Nonessential amino acids (mg/100 ml): Alanine 1240, arginine 840, histidine 500, proline 500, serine 340, tyrosine 20, glycine 590, glutamic acid 420, aspartic acid 250, acetate 88 mEq/L, sodium bisulfite 30 mg/100 ml. In 500 ml, 1 liter. *Rx.*
Use: Nutritional supplement, parenteral.

Novantrone. (Immunex Corp.) Mitoxantrone HCl 2 mg base/ml. Inj. Vial 10 ml, 12.5 ml, 15 ml. *Rx.*
Use: Antineoplastic.

novatropine.
See: Homatropine Methylbromide (Various Mfr.).

novobiocin calcium. U.S.P. XXII.
Use: Anti-infective.
See: Cathomycin Calcium.

novobiocin monosodium salt.
Use: Anti-infective.
See: Sodium Novobiocin.

•**novobiocin sodium.** U.S.P. 23.
Use: Anti-infective.
See: Albamycin, Cap. (Pharmacia & Upjohn).
Cathomycin Sodium.

Novocain. (Sanofi Winthrop Pharmaceuticals) Procaine HCl. **1%:** 2 ml, 6 ml, 30 ml. **2%:** 30 ml. **10%:** 2 ml/Inj. *Rx.*
Use: Anesthetic, local.

Novocain for Spinal Anesthesia. (Sanofi Winthrop Pharmaceuticals) Procaine HCl 10% soln. Amp. 2 ml. Box 25s. *Rx.*
Use: Anesthetic, spinal.

Novolin 70/30. (Novo/Nordisk Pharm, Inc.) Isophane susp. 70% (human), regular insulin 30% (human, semi-synthetic) 100 units/ml. Inj. Vial 10 ml. *otc.*
Use: Antidiabetic.

Novolin 70/30 PenFill. (Novo/Nordisk Pharm, Inc.) Isophane insulin suspension and insulin injection 100 U per ml human insulin. Cartridge 1.5 ml. *otc.*
Use: Antidiabetic.

Novolin 70/30 Prefilled. (Novo/Nordisk Pharm, Inc.) Isophane Insulin 100 units/ml human insulin (rDNA). Inj. Prefilled syringe 1.5 ml. *otc.*
Use: Antidiabetic.

Novolin L. (Novo/Nordisk Pharm, Inc.) Human insulin (semisynthetic) 100 units/ml. An insulin-zinc suspension (Lente). Inj. Vial 10 ml. *otc.*
Use: Antidiabetic.

Novolin N. (Novo/Nordisk Pharm, Inc.) Human insulin NPH (semisynthetic) 100 units/ml. Isophane insulin suspension (insulin w/protamine and zinc). Inj. Vial 10 ml. *otc.*
Use: Antidiabetic.

Novolin N PenFill. (Novo/Nordisk Pharm, Inc.) Isophane insulin suspension (NPH) 100 U per ml human insulin. Cartridge. 1.5 ml. *otc.*
Use: Antidiabetic.

Novolin N Prefilled. (Novo/Nordisk Pharm, Inc.) Isophane insulin suspension (NPH) 100 units/ml human insulin (rDNA). Inj. Prefilled syringe 1.5 ml. *otc.*
Use: Antidiabetic.

Novolin R. (Novo/Nordisk Pharm, Inc.) Human insulin, regular (semisynthetic) 100 units/ml. Inj. Vial 10 ml. *otc.*
Use: Antidiabetic.

Novolin R PenFill. (Novo/Nordisk Pharm, Inc.) Semisynthetic human regular insulin 100 units/ml. Inj. 1.5 ml cartridges. *otc.*
Use: Antidiabetic.

Novolin R Prefilled. (Novo/Nordisk Pharm, Inc.) Insulin 100 units/ml human insulin (rDNA). Inj. Prefilled syringe 1.5 ml. *otc.*
Use: Antidiabetic.

Novopaque. (LPI Diagnostics) Barium sulfate 60%. Susp. Bot. 355 ml, 1900 ml. *Rx.*
Use: Radiopaque agent.

NovoSeven. (Novo/Nordisk Pharm, Inc.) Human coagulation factor VIIa (recombinant) Vial 1.2 mg, 4.8 mg. *Rx.*
Use: Antihemophilic.

Noxzema Antiseptic Cleanser Sensitive Skin Formula. (Noxell Corp.) Benzalkonium Cl 0.13%. Bot. 4 oz, 8 oz. *otc.*
Use: Dermatologic, cleanser.

Noxzema Antiseptic Skin Cleanser. (Noxell Corp.) SD 40 alcohol 63%. Bot. 4 oz, 8 oz. *otc.*
Use: Dermatologic, cleanser.

Noxzema Antiseptic Skin Cleanser Extra Strength Formula. (Noxell Corp.)

SD 40 alcohol 36%, isopropyl alcohol 34%. Bot. 4 oz, 8 oz. *otc.*
Use: Dermatologic, cleanser.

Noxzema Clear Ups. (Noxell Corp.) Salicylic acid 0.5% on pads. Jar 50s. *otc.*
Use: Dermatologic, acne.

Noxzema Clear Ups Acne Medicine Maximum Strength Lotion. (Noxell Corp.) Benzoyl peroxide 10%. Bot. 1 oz. Vanishing formula. *otc.*
Use: Dermatologic, acne.

Noxzema Clear Ups Maximum Strength. (Noxell Corp.) Salicylic acid 2% on pads. Jar 50s. *otc.*
Use: Dermatologic, acne.

Noxzema Medicated Skin Cream. (Noxell Corp.) Menthol, camphor, clove oil, eucalyptus oil, phenol. Jar 2.5 oz, 4 oz, 6 oz, 10 oz. Tube 4.5 oz. Bot. 6 oz., 14 oz. Pump Bottle 10.5 oz. *otc.*
Use: Counterirritant.

Noxzema On-The-Spot. (Noxell Corp.) Benzoyl peroxide 10% in vanishing and tinted lotion. Bot. 0.25 oz. *otc.*
Use: Dermatologic, acne.

NPH Iletin I. (Eli Lilly and Co.) Insulin from beef and pork. 100 units/ml. Inj. Vial 10 ml. *otc.*
Use: Antidiabetic.

NPH-N. (Novo/Nordisk Pharm, Inc.) Purified pork insulin 100 units/ml in isophane insulin suspension (insulin w/ protamine and zinc). Inj. Vial 10 ml. *otc.*
Use: Antidiabetic.

NTBC.
Use: Tyrosinemia type 1. [Orphan Drug]

N-Trifluoroacetyladriamycin-14-valerate. (Anthra Pharmaceuticals, Inc.) *Rx.*
Use: Antineoplastic.

NTS Transdermal System. (Circa Pharmaceuticals, Inc.) Nitroglycerin transdermal system 5 mg/24 hours or 15 mg/24 hours. Box 30s. *Rx.*
Use: Antianginal.

NTZ Long-Acting. (Sanofi Winthrop Pharmaceuticals) Oxymetazoline HCl 0.05%, benzalkonium Cl, phenylmercuric acetate 0.002% as preservatives. Drops. Bot. 1 oz. Spray Bot. 1 oz. *otc.*
Use: Decongestant.

Nubain. (Du Pont Merck Pharmaceutical Co.) Nalbuphine HCl, sodium metabisulfite 0.1%. **10 mg/ml:** Amp 1 ml. Vial 10 ml. Box 1s. **20 mg/ml:** Amp 1 ml. Syringe 1 ml calibrated. Vial 10 ml. *Rx.*
Use: Analgesic, narcotic.

Nu-Bolic. (Seatrace Pharmaceuticals, Inc.) Nandrolone phenpropionate 25 mg/ml. Vial 5 ml. *c-III.*
Use: Anabolic steroid.

nucite.
See: Inositol (Various Mfr.).

Nucofed. (Roberts Pharmaceuticals) Codeine phosphate 20 mg, pseudoephedrine HCl 60 mg/5 ml or Cap. Syrup is alcohol-free. **Liq.:** Bot. Pt. **Cap.:** Bot. 60s. *c-III.*
Use: Antitussive, decongestant.

Nucofed Expectorant. (Roberts Pharmaceuticals) Codeine phosphate 20 mg, pseudoephedrine HCl 60 mg, guaifenesin 200 mg/5 ml, alcohol 12.5%, saccharin. Bot. 480 ml. *c-III.*
Use: Antitussive, decongestant, expectorant.

Nucofed Pediatric Expectorant. (Roberts Pharmaceuticals) Codeine phosphate 10 mg, pseudoephedrine HCl 30 mg, guaifenesin 100 mg/5 ml, alcohol 6%. Bot. Pt. *c-V.*
Use: Antitussive, decongestant, expectorant.

Nucotuss Expectorant. (Alpharma USPD Inc.) Pseudoephedrine HCl 60 mg, codeine phosphate 20 mg, guaifenesin 200 mg/5 ml, alcohol 12.5%, wintergreen flavor. Liq. Bot. 480 ml. *c-III.*
Use: Antitussive, decongestant, expectorant.

Nucotuss Pediatric Expectorant. (Alpharma USPD Inc.) Pseudoephedrine HCl 30 mg, codeine phosphate 10 mg, guaifenesin 100 mg/5 ml, strawberry flavor. Liq. Bot. 480 ml. *c-V.*
Use: Antitussive, decongestant, expectorant.

•**nufenoxole.** (NEW-fen-OX-ole) USAN.
Use: Antiperistaltic.

Nu-Iron 150. (Merz Pharmaceuticals) Polysaccharide-iron complex. 150 mg iron. Cap. Bot. 100s, 500s. *otc.*
Use: Mineral supplement.

Nu-Iron 150. (Merz Pharmaceuticals) Polysaccharide-Iron complex 100 mg/5 ml, alcohol 10%. Elix. 237 ml. *otc.*
Use: Mineral supplement.

Nu-Iron Plus Elixir. (Merz Pharmaceuticals) Polysaccharide iron complex 300 mg, folic acid 3 mg, vitamin B_{12} 75 mcg/15 ml. Bot. 237 ml. *Rx.*
Use: Mineral, vitamin supplement.

Nu-Iron-V. (Merz Pharmaceuticals) Polysaccharide iron 60 mg, folic acid 1 mg, vitamins A 4000 IU, C 50 mg, D 400 IU, $B_1$3 mg, B_2 3 mg, B_3 10 mg, B_6 2 mg, B_{12} 3 mcg, Ca/Tab. Bot. 100s. *Rx.*
Use: Mineral, vitamin supplement.

Nul-Tach. (Davis & Sly) Potassium 16 mg, magnesium 13 mg, ascorbic acid 250 mg/Tab. Bot. 100s. *Rx.*
Use: Antiarrythmic.

NuLytely. (Braintree Laboratories, Inc.) PEG 3350 420 g, sodium bicarbonate 5.72 g, sodium chloride 11.2 g, potassium chloride 1.48 g. Pow. Jugs. 4 L. *Rx.*
Use: Laxative.

Numorphan. (Endo Laboratories) Oxymorphone HCl. **1 mg/ml.:** Amp. 1 ml. **1.5 mg/ml.:** Multi-dose vial 10 ml. **Rectal Supp.:** 5 mg. Box 6s. *c-II.*
Use: Analgesic, narcotic.

Numotizine Cataplasm. (Hobart) Guaiacol 0.26 g, beechwood creosote 1.302 g, methyl salicylate 0.26 g/100 g. Jar 4 oz. *otc.*
Use: Analgesic, topical.

Numotizine Cough Syrup. (Hobart) Guaifenesin 5 g, ammonium Cl 5 g, sodium citrate 20 g, menthol 0.04 g/fl oz. Bot. 3 oz, pt, gal. *otc.*
Use: Expectorant.

Numzident. (Purepac Pharmaceutical Co.) Benzocaine 10%, PEG-400 NF 47.86%, PEG-3350 NF 10%, saccharin. Gel. 15 g. *otc.*
Use: Anesthetic, local.

Numzit. (Purepac Pharmaceutical Co.) Benzocaine, menthol, glycerin, methylparaben, alcohol 12%. Liq. Bot. 22.5 ml. *otc.*
Use: Anesthetic, local.

Numzit Gel. (Purepac Pharmaceutical Co.) Benzocaine, menthol. Tube 10 g. *otc.*
Use: Anesthetic, local.

Numzit Teething Gel. (Goody's Manufacturing Corp.) Benzocaine 7.5%, peppermint oil 0.018%, clove leaf oil 0.09%, PEG-400 66.2%, PEG-3350 26.1%, saccharin 0.036%. Tube. 14.1 g. *otc.*
Use: Anesthetic, local.

Numzit Teething Lotion. (Goody's Manufacturing Corp.) Benzocaine 0.2%, alcohol 12.1%, saccharin 0.02%, glycerin 2%, kelgin MU 0.5%, methylparaben. Lot. Bot. 15 ml. *otc.*
Use: Anesthetic, local.

nunol.
See: Phenobarbital (Various Mfr.).

Nupercainal. (Novartis Pharmaceutical Corp.) **Oint.:** Dibucaine 1%, acetone, sodium bisulfite, lanolin, mineral oil, white petrolatum. 30 g, 60 g. **Cream:** Dibucaine 0.5%, acetone, sodium bisulfite, glycerin. 42.5 g. **Supp.:** Cocoa butter, zinc oxide, sodium bisulfite. 12s, 24s. *otc.*
Use: Anesthetic, local (Oint., Cream); Anorectal preparation (Supp.).

Nuprin Backache. (Bristol-Myers Squibb) Magnesium salicylate tetrahydrate 580 mg (equivalent to 467 mg anhydrous magnesium salicylate). Capl. Bot. 50s. *otc.*
Use: Anti-inflammatory.

Nuprin Caplets. (Bristol-Myers Squibb) Ibuprofen 200 mg/Capl. Bot. 24s, 50s, 100s. *otc.*
Use: Analgesic, NSAID.

Nuprin Tablets. (Bristol-Myers Squibb) Ibuprofen 200 mg/Tab. Blister Pak 8s. Bot. 24s, 50s, 100s. *otc.*
Use: Analgesic, NSAID.

Nuquin HP. (Stratus Pharmaceuticals, Inc.) **Cream:** 4% hydroquinone, 30 mg dioxybenzone, 20 mg oxybenzone per g. Vanishing base. Stearyl alcohol, EDTA, sodium metabisulfite. Tube 14.2 g, 28.4 g, 56.7 g. **Gel:** 4% hydroquinone, 30 mg dioxybenzone per g. Alcohol, sodium metabisulfite, EDTA. Tube 14.2 g, 28.4 g. *Rx.*
Use: Dermatologic.

Nuromax. (GlaxoWellcome) Doxacurium chloride 1 mg/ml. Inj. Vial 5 ml. *Rx.*
Use: Neuromuscular blocker.

Nu-Salt. (Cumberland Packing Corp.) Potassium Cl, potassium bitartrate, calcium silicate, natural flavor derived from yeast. Sodium 0.85 mg/5 g (< 0.04 mEq/5 g), potassium 2640 mg/5 g (68 mEq/5 g). Pkg. 90 g. *otc.*
Use: Salt substitute.

Nu-Tears. (Optopics Laboratories, Corp) Polyvinyl alcohol 1.4%, EDTA, NaCl, benzalkonium chloride, potassium chloride. Soln. Bot. 15 ml. *otc.*
Use: Artificial tears.

Nu-Tears II. (Optopics Laboratories, Corp) Polyvinyl alcohol 1%, PEG-400 1%, EDTA, benzalkonium chloride. Soln. Bot. 15 ml. *otc.*
Use: Artificial tears.

Nu-Thera. (Kirkman Sales Co., Inc.) Vitamins A 10,000 IU, D 400 IU, B_1 10 mg, B_2 5 mg, niacinamide 100 mg, B_6 1 mg, B_{12} 5 mcg, C 150 mg, Ca 103 mg, P 80 mg, Fe 10 mg, Mg 5.5 mg, Mn 1 mg, K 5 mg, Zn 1.4 mg/Cap. Bot. 100s. *otc.*
Use: Mineral, vitamin supplement.

nutmeg oil.
Use: Pharmaceutic aid (flavor).

Nutracort. (Galderma Laboratories, Inc.) Hydrocortisone 1%. Cream Jar 4 oz. Tube 30 g, 60 g. *Rx.*
Use: Corticosteroid, topical.

Nutraderm. (Galderma Laboratories, Inc.) Oil-in-water emulsion. **Lot.:** Plastic bot. 8 oz, 16 oz. **Cream:** Tube 1.5 oz, 3 oz, Jar lb. *otc.*

Use: Emollient.

Nutraderm Bath Oil. (Galderma Laboratories, Inc.) Mineral oil, PEG-4 dilaurate, lanolin oil, butylparaben, benzophenone-3, fragrance, D & C Green No. 6. Bot. 8 oz. *otc.*
Use: Emollient.

Nutraloric. (Nutraloric) A chocolate, vanilla, or strawberry flavored liquid containing, when mixed with whole milk to make 1 L, 91.7 g protein, 175 g carbohydrates, 125 g fat, 875 mg Na, 3166.7 mg, K 2.2 calories/ml. Pow. Can 480 g. *otc.*
Use: Nutritional supplement.

Nutrament Drink Box. (Drackett) Protein 10 g, fat 7 g, carbohydrate 35 g, vitamins, minerals/240 calories/8 oz. Liq. Drink Box. *otc.*
Use: Nutritional supplement.

Nutrament Liquid. (Drackett) Protein 16 g, fat 10 g, carbohydrates 52 g, vitamins, minerals/360 calories/12 oz. Liq. Can. *otc.*
Use: Nutritional supplement.

Nutramigen. (Bristol-Myers Squibb) Hypoallergenic formula that supplies 640 calories/qt. Protein 18 g, fat 25 g, carbohydrates 86 g, vitamins A 2000 IU, D 400 IU, E 20 IU, C 52 mg, folic acid 100 mcg, B_1 0.5 mg, B_2 0.6 mg, niacin 8 mg, B_6 0.4 mg, B_{12} 2 mcg, biotin 50 mcg, pantothenic acid 3 mg, K-1 100 mcg, Cl 85 mg, inositol 30 mg, Ca 600 mg, P 400 mg, I 45 mcg, Fe 12 mg, Mg 70 mg, Cu 0.6 mg, Zn 5 mg, Mn 200 mcg, Cl 550 mg, K 700 mg, Na 300 mg/qt of formula (4.9 oz pow.). Liq. Can 16 oz, 390 ml concentrate, 1 qt ready-to-use. *otc.*
Use: Nutritional supplement.

Nutramin. (Thurston) Vitamins A 666 IU, D 66 IU, B_1 666 mcg, B_2 333 mcg, niacinamide 2 mg, folic acid 0.0444 mcg, Ca 16.6 mg, P 8.33 mg, Fe 1.33 mg, I 0.15 mg/Tab. Bot. 200s, 500s, 1000s. *otc.*
Use: Mineral, vitamin supplement.

Nutramin Granular. (Thurston) Vitamins A 333 IU, D 333 IU, B_1 3.3 mg, B_2 1.6 mg, niacinamide 10 mg, folic acid 0.133 mg, Ca 250 mg, P 115 mg, Fe 6.6 mg, I 0.15 mg/5 g. Bot. 10 oz, 32 oz. *otc.*
Use: Mineral, vitamin supplement.

Nutraplus. (Galderma Laboratories, Inc.) Urea 10% in emollient cream base or lotion base with preservatives. **Cream:** Tube 3 oz, Jar lb. **Lot.:** Bot. 8 oz, 16 oz. *otc.*
Use: Emollient.

Nutra-Soothe. (Pertussin) Colloidal oatmeal, light mineral oil. Emollient bath preparation. Pow. Pkts. 9s. *otc.*
Use: Dermatologic.

Nutravims. (Health for Life Brands, Inc.) Vitamins A 6000 IU, D 1250 IU, C 50 mg, E 5 IU, B_{12} 5 mcg, B_1 3 mg, B_2 3 mg, B_6 0.5 mg, niacinamide 20 mg, calcium pantothenate 5 mg, Zn 1.5 mg, Mn 1 mg, I 0.15 mg, K 5 mg, Mg 4 mg, Fe 15 mg, Ca 59 mg, P 45 mg/Cap. Bot. 100s, 250s, 1000s. *otc.*
Use: Mineral, vitamin supplement.

Nutren 1.0 Liquid. (Clintec Nutrition) Potassium and sodium caseinate, maltodextrin, sucrose, MCT, corn oil, lecithin, vitamins A, B_1, B_2, B_3, B_5, B_6, B_{12}, C, D, E, K, folic acid, biotin, choline, Ca, Cl, Cu, Fe, I, Mg, Mn, P, Zn. Can 250 ml. *otc.*
Use: Nutritional supplement.

Nutren 1.5 Liquid. (Clintec Nutrition) Casein, maltodextrin, corn syrup, sucrose, MCT, corn oil, vitamins A, B_1, B_2, B_3, B_5, B_6, B_{12}, C, D, E, K, folic acid, biotin, choline, Ca, Cl, Cu, Fe, I, Mg, Mn, P, Zn. 250 ml. *otc.*
Use: Nutritional supplement.

Nutren 2.0 Liquid. (Clintec Nutrition) Casein, maltodextrin, corn syrup, sucrose, MCT, corn oil, vitamins A, B_1, B_2, B_3, B_5, B_6, B_{12}, C, D, E, K, folic acid, biotin, choline, Ca, Cl, Cu, Fe, I, Mg, Mn, P, Zn. 250 ml. *otc.*
Use: Nutritional supplement.

Nutrex. (Holloway) Ca 162 mg, Fe 27 mg, vitamins A 5000 IU, D 400 IU, E 30 mg, B_1 2.25 mg, B_2 2.6 mg, B_3 20 mg, B_5 10 mg, B_6 3 mg, B_{12} 9 mcg, C 90 mg, folic acid 0.4 mg, Cu, I, K, Mg, Mn, P, Zn 22.5 mg, biotin 45 mcg/Tab. Bot. 100s. *otc.*
Use: Mineral, vitamin supplement.

Nutricon Tablets. (Taylor Pharmaceuticals) Ca 200 mg, Fe 20 mg, vitamins A 2500 IU, D 200 IU, E 15 mg, B_1 1.5 mg, B_2 1.5 mg, B_3 10 mg, B_5 5 mg, B_6 2 mg, B_{12} 5 mcg, C 50 mg, folic acid 0.4 mg, Cu, I, Mg, Zn 3.75 mg, biotin 150 mcg/Tab. Bot. 120s. *otc.*
Use: Mineral, vitamin supplement.

Nutri-E. (Nutri Lab.) Vitamin E. **Cream:** 200 IU/g. Jar 1 oz, 2 oz. **Oil:** 1 oz. **Oint.:** 200 IU/g. Tube 1 oz, 1.5 oz. **Cap.:** 200 IU. Bot. 80s; 400 IU. Bot. 60s, 100s; 800 IU. Bot. 55s. *otc.*
Use: Vitamin supplement.

Nutrilan. (Elan Pharma) A vanilla, chocolate, or strawberry flavored liquid containing 38 g protein, 37 g fat, 143 g carbohydrates, 632.5 mg Na, 1.073 g K/

L. With appropriate vitamins and minerals. In 237 ml Tetra Pak containers. *otc.*
Use: Nutritional supplement.

Nutrilipid. (McGaw, Inc.) Soybean oil intravenous fat emulsion. **10%:** Calories 1.1/ml. Bot. 250 ml, 500 ml. **20%:** Calories 2/ml. Bot. 250 ml, 500 ml. *Rx.*
Use: Nutritional supplement, parenteral.

Nutrilyte. (American Regent) Acetate 2.03 mEq, K 2.03 mEq, Cl 1.68 mEq, Na 1.25 mEq, Mg 0.4 mEq, Ca 0.25 mEq, gluconate 0.25 mEq/ml, ≈ 6212 mOsml/L. Concentrated Soln. Bot. 20 ml, 100 ml. *Rx.*
Use: Nutritional supplement, parenteral.

Nutrilyte II. (American Regent) Acetate 1.475 mEq, potassium 1 mEq, Cl 1.75 mEq, Na 1.75 mEq, Mg 0.25 mEq, Ca 0.225 mEq/ml, ≈ 6212 mOsml/L. Concentrated soln. Bot. 20 ml, 100 ml. *Rx.*
Use: Nutritional supplement, parenteral.

Nutri-Plex Tablets. (Faraday) Vitamins B_1 5 mg, B_2 5 mg, B_6 5 mg, pantothenic acid 25 mg, B_{12} 12.5 mcg, niacinamide 50 mg, iron gluconate 30 mg, choline bitartrate 50 mg, inositol 50 mg, PABA 15 mg, C 150 mg/2 Tab. Bot. 100s, 250s. *otc.*
Use: Mineral, vitamin supplement.

Nutrisource Modular System. (Novartis Pharmaceutical Corp.) Individual Nutrisource modules available: protein, amino acids, amino acids (high branched chain), carbohydrate, lipid (medium chain triglycerides), lipid (long branched chain triglycerides), vitamins, minerals. Cans of liquid. Packets of powder. *otc.*
Use: Nutritional supplement.

Nutri-Val. (Marcen) Vitamins A 5000 IU, D 500 IU, B_1 10 mg, B_2 5 mg, B_{12} activity 5 mcg, B_6 5 mcg, C 50 mg, hesperidin 5 mg, niacinamide 15 mg, folic acid 0.2 mg, calcium pantothenate 50 mg, choline bitartrate 50 mg, betaine HCl 25 mg, lipo-K 0.4 mg, duodenum substance 50 mg, pancreas substance 50 mg, inositol 25 mg, Cy-yeast hydrolysates 50 mg, rutin 5 mg, l-lysine HCl 5 mg, E 5 IU, Ossonate (glucuronic complex) 8 mg, glutamic acid 30 mg, lecithin 5 mg, Fe 20 mg, I 0.15 mg, Ca 50 mg, P 40 mg, B 0.1 mg, Cu 1 mg, Mn 1 mg, Mg 1 mg, K 5 mg, Zn 0.5 mg, biotin 0.02 mg/Cap. Bot. 100s, 500s, 1000s. *otc.*
Use: Mineral, vitamin supplement.

Nutri-Vite Natural Multiple Vitamin and Minerals. (Faraday) Vitamins A 15,000 IU, D 400 IU, B_1 1.5 mg, B_2 3 mg, B_{12} 15 mcg, niacin 500 mcg, B_6 20 mcg, choline 1.75 mg, folic acid 13 mcg, pantothenic acid 50 mcg, p-aminobenzoic acid 12 mcg, inositol 1.72 mg, C 60 mg, citrus bioflavonoids 15 mg, E 50 IU, iron gluconate 15 mg, Ca 192 mg, P 85 mg, I 0.15 mg, red bone marrow 30 mg/3 Tab. Protein coated Tab. Bot. 100s, 250s. *otc.*
Use: Mineral, vitamin supplement.

Nutrizyme. (Enzyme Process) Vitamins A 5000 IU, D 400 IU, C 60 mg, B_1 1.5 mg, B_2 1.7 mg, niacinamide 20 mg, B_6 2 mg, pantothenate 10 mg, B_{12} 6 mcg, E 30 IU, Fe 10 mg, Cu 1 mg, Zn 1 mg, Folac in 0.025 mg/Tab. Bot. 90s, 250s. *otc.*
Use: Mineral, vitamin supplement.

Nutropin. (Genentech, Inc.) Somatropin 5 mg (≈ 13 IU)/vial, 10 mg(≈ 26 IU)/vial. Pow. for Inj. (lyophilized). Vials with 10 ml diluent. *Rx.*
Use: Hormone, growth.

Nutropin AQ. (Genentech, Inc.) Somatropin 10 mg/Inj. (≈ 30 IU) Vial. *Rx.*
Use: Hormone, growth.

Nutrox Capsules. (Tyson & Associates, Inc.) Vitamins A 10,000 IU, E 150 IU, B_1 25 mg, B_2 25 mg, B_3 50 mg, B_5 22 mg, C 80 mg, l-cysteine, taurine, glutathione, zinc oxide 15 mg, Se/Cap. Bot. 90s. *otc.*
Use: Mineral, vitamin supplement.

Nuzine Ointment. (Hobart) Guaiacol 1.66 g, oxyquinoline sulfate 0.42 g, zinc oxide 2.5 g, glycerine 1.66 g, lanum (anhydrous) 43.76 g, petrolatum 50 g/100 g. Tube 1 oz. *otc.*
Use: Anorectal preparation.

Nycoff. (Dover Pharmaceuticals) Dextromethorphan HBr/Tab. UD Box 500s. Sugar, lactose and salt free. *otc.*
Use: Antitussive.

Nyco-White. (Whiteworth Towne) Nystatin, neomycin, gramicidin, triamcinolone. Cream. Tube 15 g, 30 g, 60 g. *Rx.*
Use: Anti-infective, topical.

Nyco-Worth. (Whiteworth Towne) Nystatin. Cream Tube 15 g. *Rx.*
Use: Antifungal, topical.

Nydrazid Injection. (Apothecon, Inc.) Isoniazid 100 mg/ml, chlorobutanol 0.25%, sodium hydroxide or hydrochloric acid to adjust pH. Vial 10 ml. *Rx.*
Use: Antituberculosal.

•**nylestriol.** (NYE-less-TRY-ole) USAN.
Use: Estrogen.

NyQuil Cough/Cold, Children's. (Procter & Gamble Pharm.) Pseudoephedrine HCl 10 mg, chlorpheniramine maleate 0.67 mg, dextromethorphan HBr

5 mg/5 ml, sucrose, alcohol free, cherry flavor. Liq. 120 ml. *otc.*
Use: Antihistamine, antitussive, decongestant.

NyQuil Hot Therapy. (Procter & Gamble Pharm.) Pseudoephedrine HCl 60 mg, doxylamine succinate 12.5 mg, dextromethorphan HBr 30 mg, acetaminophen 1000 mg/pkt. Powd. 6s. *otc.*
Use: Analgesic, antihistamine, antitussive, decongestant.

NyQuil Liqui-Caps. (Procter & Gamble Pharm.) Pseudoephedrine HCl 30 mg, diphenhydramine HCl 25 mg, dextromethorphan HBr 15 mg, acetaminophen 250 mg/Cap. Bot. 20s. *otc.*
Use: Analgesic, antihistamine, antitussive, decongestant.

NyQuil Nighttime Cold/Flu Medicine. (Procter & Gamble Pharm.) Pseudoephedrine HCl 10 mg, doxylamine succinate 2.1 mg, dextromethorphan HBr 5 mg, acetaminophen 167 mg/5 ml, alcohol 10%, sucrose, saccharin (cherry flavor), tartrazine (regular flavor). Liq. Bot. 295 ml. *otc.*
Use: Analgesic, antihistamine, antitussive, decongestant.

NyQuil Nighttime Cold Medicine Liquid. (Procter & Gamble Pharm.) Dextromethorphan HBr 30 mg, pseudoephedrine HCl 60 mg, doxylamine succinate 7.5 mg, acetaminophen 1000 mg/oz, alcohol 25%. Regular and cherry flavors. Regular flavor contains FDC Yellow #5 tartrazine. Bot. 6 oz, 10 oz, 14 oz. *otc.*
Use: Analgesic, antihistamine, antitussive, decongestant.

NyQuil Nighttime Head Cold Allergy Formula, Children's. (Procter & Gamble Pharm.) Pseudoephedrine HCl, chlorpheniramine maleate, 0.67 mg/5 ml, alcohol free, sorbitol, sucrose, grape flavor. Liq. Bot. 120 ml. *otc.*
Use: Antihistamine, decongestant.

Nyral. (Pal-Pak, Inc.) Cetylpyridinium Cl 0.5 mg, benzocaine 5 mg/Loz. w/parabens. Pkg. 100s, 1000s. *otc.*
Use: Antiseptic.

•**nystatin.** (nye-STAT-in) U.S.P. 23.
Use: Antifungal.
See: Mycostatin Preps. (Apothecon, Inc.).
Nilstat, Tab., Cream, Oint., Pow. (ESI Lederle Generics).
Nilstat, Oral Drops (ESI Lederle Generics).
Nilstat, Vaginal Tab. (ESI Lederle Generics).
Nystatin, Bulk Pow. (Paddock Laboratories).
Nystex, Cream, Oint., Susp. (Savage Laboratories).
O-V Statin, Tab. (Bristol-Myers Squibb).
Pedi-Dri, Pow. (Pedinol Pharmacal, Inc.).
W/Clioquinol.
See: Mycolog, Cream, Oint. (Bristol-Myers Squibb).
W/Tetracycline phosphate buffered.
See: Achrostatin-V, Cap. (ESI Lederle-Generics).

nystatin. (Various Mfr.) 100,000 units/ml.
Oral Susp.: Bot. 5 ml, 60 ml, 480 ml.
Vaginal Tab.: Pkg. 15s or 30s.
Use: Antifungal.

nystatin and triamcinolone acetonide cream.
Use: Antifungal, corticosteroid, topical.

nystatin and triamcinolone acetonide ointment.
Use: Antifungal, corticosteroid, topical.

nystatin, neomycin sulfate, gramicidin, and triamcinolone acetonide.
Use: Antifungal, anti-infective, corticosteroid, topical.
See: Mycolog, Prods. (Bristol-Myers Squibb).

Nystex Cream & Ointment. (Savage Laboratories) Nystatin 100,000 units/g. Tube 15 g, 30 g. *Rx.*
Use: Antifungal, topical.

Nystex Oral Suspension. (Savage Laboratories) Nystatin 100,000 units/ml in suspension. Bot. 60 ml. *Rx.*
Use: Antifungal, topical.

Nytcold Medicine. (Rugby Labs, Inc.) Pseudoephedrine HCl 10 mg, doxylamine succinate 1.25 mg, dextromethorphan HBr 5 mg, acetaminophen 167 mg, alcohol 25%, glucose, saccharin, sucrose, cherry flavor. Liq. Bot. 177 ml. *otc.*
Use: Analgesic, antihistamine, antitussive, decongestant.

Nytime Cold Medicine. (Rugby Labs, Inc.) Acetaminophen 1000 mg, doxylamine succinate 7.5 mg, pseudoephedrine HCl 60 mg, dextromethorphan HBr 30 mg/30 ml, alcohol 25%. Bot. 6 oz, 10 oz. *otc.*
Use: Analgesic, antihistamine, antitussive, decongestant.

Nytol. (Block Drug Co., Inc.) Diphenhydramine HCl 25 mg/Tab. Bot. 16s, 32s, 72s. *otc.*
Use: Sleep aid.

Nytol, Maximum Strength. (Block Drug Co., Inc.) Diphenhydramine HCl 50 mg, lactose. Tab. Bot. 8s. *otc.*
Use: Sleep aid.

O

O.A.D. (Sween) Ostomy. Bot. 1.25 oz, 4 oz, 8 oz. *otc.*
Use: Deodorant, ostomy.

Oasis. (Zitar) Artificial saliva. Bot. 6 oz. *otc.*
Use: Antixerostomia agent.

•**oatmeal, colloidal.** U.S.P. 23.
Use: Antipruritic, topical.

oatmeal, gum fraction.
See: Aveeno, Preps. (Rydelle Laboratories).

Obe-Nix 30. (Holloway) Phentermine HCl 30 mg/Cap. (equivalent to 24 mg base) Bot. 100s. *c-IV.*
Use: Anorexiant.

Obepar. (Tyler) Vitamins A 3000 IU, D 300 IU, B_1 3 mg, B_2 2 mg, nicotinamide 10 mg, B_6 3 mg, calcium pantothenate 2 mg, B_{12} 3 mcg, C 37.5 mg, Ca 150 mg, Fe 5 mg, Mg 1 mg, Mn 0.1 mg, K 1 mg, Zn 0.15 mg/Cap. Bot. 100s. *otc.*
Use: Mineral, vitamin supplement.

Obe-Tite. (Scott/Cord) Phendimetrazine tartrate 35 mg/Tab. Bot. 100s, 500s. *c-III.*
Use: Anorexiant.

Obezine. (Western Research) Phendimetrazine tartrate 35 mg/Tab. Handi count 28 (36 bags of 28s). *c-III.*
Use: Anorexiant.

•**obidoxime chloride.** (OH-bih-DOX-eem) USAN.
Use: Cholinesterase reactivator.

Obrical. (Canright) Calcium lactate 500 mg, vitamins D 400 IU, ferrous sulfate exsiccated 35 mg, B_1 1 mg, B_2 1 mg, C 10 mg/Tab. Bot. 100s, 1000s. *otc.*
Use: Mineral, vitamin supplement.

Obrical-F. (Canright) Ferrous sulfate 50 mg, calcium lactate 500 mg, vitamins D 400 IU, B_1 1 mg, B_2 1 mg, C 10 mg, folic acid 0.67 mg/Tab. Bot. 100s, 1000s. *otc.*
Use: Mineral, vitamin supplement.

Obrite. (Milton Roy) Contact lens and eye glass cleaner. Plastic spray Bot. 30 ml, 55 ml. *otc.*
Use: Contact lens and eye glass care.

OB-Tinic. (Roberts Pharmaceuticals) Fe 65 mg, vitamins A 6000 IU, D 400 IU, E 30 IU, B_1 1.1 mg, B_2 1.8 mg, B_3 15 mg, B_6 2.5 mg, B_{12} 5 mcg, C 60 mg, folic acid 1 mg, Ca/Tab. Bot. 100s. *Rx.*
Use: Mineral, vitamin supplement.

O-Cal f.a. (Pharmics, Inc.) **Tab.:** Ca 200 mg, Fe 66 mg, vitamins A 5000 IU, D 400 IU, E 30 mg, B_1 3 mg, B_2 3 mg, B_3 20 mg, B_6 4 mg, B_{12} 12 mcg, C 90 mg, folic acid 1 mg, fluoride 1.1 mg, Mg, I, Cu, Zn 15 mg. Bot. 100s. *Rx.*
Use: Mineral, vitamin supplement.

•**ocaperidone.** (oke-ah-PURR-ih-dohn) USAN.
Use: Antipsychotic.

Occlusal HP. (Medicis Dermatologicals, Inc.) Salicylic acid 17%. Soln. Bot. 10 ml. *otc.*
Use: Keratolytic.

Occucoat. (Storz Ophthalmics) Hydroxypropyl methylcellulose 2%. Soln. Syringe 1 ml with cannula. *Rx.*
Use: Ophthalmic.

Ocean. (Fleming & Co.) Sodium Cl 0.65%, benzyl alcohol. Soln. Bot. 45 ml, pt. *otc.*
Use: Moisturizer, nasal.

Ocean Plus. (Fleming & Co.) Caffeine 2.5%, benzyl alcohol. Soln. Bot. 15 ml. *otc.*
Use: Moisturizer, nasal.

•**ocfentanil hydrochloride.** (ock-FEN-tah-NILL) USAN.
Use: Analgesic, narcotic.

•**ocinaplon.** (oh-SIN-ah-plahn) USAN.
Use: Anxiolytic.

OCL Solution. (Abbott Hospital Products) Oral colonic lavage soln. Sodium Cl 146 mg, sodium bicarbonate 168 mg, sodium sulfate decahydrate 1.29 g, potassium Cl 75 mg, PEG-3350 6 g, polysorbate 80 30 ml/100 ml. 1.35 L 3-pack units. *Rx.*
Use: Laxative.

•**ocrylate.** (AH-krih-late) USAN.
Use: Surgical aid (tissue adhesive).

•**octabenzone.** (OCK-tah-BEN-zone) USAN.
Use: Ultraviolet screen.

octadecanoic acid.
See: Stearic Acid, N.F. 18

octadecanoic acid, sodium salt.
See: Sodium Stearate, N.F. 18.

octadecanoic acid, zinc salt.
See: Zinc Stearate, N.F. 18.

octadecanol-l.
See: Stearyl Alcohol, N.F. 18.

Octamide. (Pharmacia & Upjohn) Metoclopramide 10 mg/Tab. Bot. 100s, 500s. *Rx.*
Use: Gastrointestinal stimulant, antiemetic.

Octamide PFS. (Pharmacia & Upjohn) Metoclopramide HCl 5 mg/ml, preservative free. Vial. Single dose; 2, 10, 30 ml. *Rx.*
Use: Antiemetic, gastrointestinal stimulant.

•**octanoic acid.** (OCK-tah-NO-ik) USAN.

Use: Antifungal.

octapeptide sequence.
Use: Antiviral.
See: Flumadine (Roche Laboratories).

Octarex. (Health for Life Brands, Inc.) Vitamins A 5000 IU, D1000 IU, B_1 1.5 mg, B_2 2 mg, B_6 0.1 mg, calcium pantothenate 1 mg, niacinamide 20 mg, C 37.5 mg, E 1 IU, B_{12} 1 mcg/Cap. Bot. 100s, 1000s. *otc.*
Use: Mineral, vitamin supplement.

Octavims. (Health for Life Brands, Inc.) Vitamins A 6000 IU, D 1250 IU, C 50 mg, E 5 IU, B_1 3 mg, B_2 3 mg, B_6 0.5 mg, niacinamide 20 mg, calcium pantothenate 5 mg, B_{12} 5 mcg, Ca 59 mg, P 45 mg/Cap. Bot. 100s, 250s, 1000s. *otc.*
Use: Mineral, vitamin supplement.

•**octazamide.** (OCK-TAY-zah-mide) USAN.
Use: Analgesic.

•**octenidine hydrochloride.** (OCK-TEN-ih-deen) USAN.
Use: Anti-infective, topical.

•**octenidine saccharin.** (OCK-TEN-ih-deen SACK-ah-rin) USAN.
Use: Dental plaque inhibitor.

•**octicizer.** (OCK-tih-SIGH-zer) USAN. Santicizer 141.
Use: Pharmaceutic aid (plasticizer).

Octocaine HCl. (Novocol Chemical Mfr. Co.) Lidocaine HCl 2%, epinephrine 1:50,000 or 1:100,000. Inj. Dent. Cartridge 1.8 ml. *Rx.*
Use: Anesthetic, local.

•**octocrylene.** (OCK-toe-KRIH-leen) USAN.
Use: Ultraviolet screen.

•**octodrine.** (OCK-toe-DREEN) USAN. Under study.
Use: Adrenergic (vasoconstrictor); anesthetic, local.

•**octoxynol 9.** (ock-TOXE-ih-nahl 9) N.F. 18.
Use: Pharmaceutic aid (surfactant).

OctreoScan. (Mallinckrodt Chemical) Oxidronate sodium 2 mg, stannous chloride (anhydrous) 0.16 mg, gentisic acid 0.56 mg, NaCl 30 mg/vial. Pow. lyophilized. In kits containing 5 ml or 30 ml vials and additive-free sodium pertechnate Tc 99m (for reconstitution). *Rx.*
Use: Diagnostic aid, radiopaque agent.

•**octreotide.** (ock-TREE-oh-tide) USAN.
Use: Antisecretory (gastric).

•**octreotide acetate.** (ock-TREE-oh-tide) USAN.
Use: Antidiarrheal, gastrointestinal tumor; antihypotensive, carcinoid crisis; growth hormone suppressant, acromegaly, antisecretory (gastric).

•**octreotide pamoate.** (ock-TREE-oh-tide PAM-oh-ate) USAN.
Use: Antineoplastic.

•**octriptyline phosphate.** (ock-TRIP-tih-leen FOSS-fate) USAN.
Use: Antidepressant.

•**octrizole.** (OCK-TRY-zole) USAN.
Use: Ultraviolet screen.

•**octyldodecanol.** N.F. 18.
Use: Pharmaceutic aid (oleaginous vehicle).

octylphenoxy polyethoxyethanol. A mono-ether of a polyethylene glycol. Igepal CA 630 (Antara).

OcuClear. (Schering-Plough Corp.) Oxymetazoline HCl 0.025%. Soln. Bot. 30 ml. *otc.*
Use: Mydriatic, vasoconstrictor.

OcuCoat. (Storz Ophthalmics) Hydroxypropyl methylcellulose 2%. Soln. Syringe 1 ml. *Rx.*
Use: Lubricant, ophthalmic.

OcuCoat PF. (Storz Ophthalmics) Dextran 70 0.1%, hydroxypropyl methylcellulose, NaCl, KCl, dextrose, sodium phosphate. Preservative free. Drops. 0.5 ml single-dose containers. *otc.*
Use: Lubricant, ophthalmic.

Ocufen. (Allergan, Inc.) Flurbiprofen sodium 0.03%. Drops. Bot. 2.5 ml w/dropper. *Rx.*
Use: NSAID, ophthalmic.

•**ocufilcon a.** (OCK-you-FILL-kahn A) USAN.
Use: Contact lens material (hydrophilic).

•**ocufilcon b.** (OCK-you-FILL-kahn B) USAN.
Use: Contact lens material (hydrophilic).

•**ocufilcon c.** (OCK-you-FILL-kahn C) USAN.
Use: Contact lens material (hydrophilic).

•**ocufilcon d.** (OCK-you-FILL-kahn D) USAN.
Use: Contact lens material (hydrophilic).

•**ocufilcon e.** (OCK-you-FILL-kahn E) USAN.
Use: Contact lens material (hydrophilic).

Ocuflox. (Allergan, Inc.) Ofloxacin 3 mg/ml. Soln. Bot. 1 ml, 5 ml. *Rx.*
Use: Anti-infective, ophthalmic.

ocular lubricants.
Use: Ophthalmic.
See: Akwa Tears (Akorn, Inc.).
Artificial Tears (Rugby Labs, Inc.).
Dry Eyes (Bausch & Lomb Pharmaceuticals).
Duolube (Bausch & Lomb Pharmaceuticals).

Duratears Naturale (Alcon Laboratories, Inc.).
Hypotears (Novartis Vision).
Lacri-Lube NP (Allergan, Inc.).
Lacri-Lube S.O.P. (Allergan, Inc).
Lipo-Tears (Spectra Pharmaceuticals).
LubriTears (Bausch & Lomb Pharmaceuticals).
OcuCoat PF (Storz Ophthalmics).
Puralube (E. Fougera and Co.).
Refresh PM (Allergan, Inc.).
Tears Renewed (Akorn, Inc.).
Vit-A-Drops (Vision Pharmaceuticals, Inc.).

Ocu-Lube. (Bausch & Lomb Pharmaceuticals) Petrolatum sterile, preservative and lanolin free. Oint. Tube 3.5 g. *otc.*
Use: Lubricant, ophthalmic.

Ocumeter.
See: Decadron Phosphate, Preps. (Merck & Co.).
Humorsol, Ophth. Soln. (Merck & Co.).
NeoDecadron Ophthalmic Solution, Preps. (Merck & Co.).

Ocupress. (Otsuka America Pharmaceutical, Inc.) Carteolol HCl 1%. Soln. Bot. 5 ml, 10 ml, 15 ml w/dropper. *Rx.*
Use: Beta-adrenergic blocker, antiglaucoma agent.

Ocusert. (Alza Corp.) Pilocarpine ocular therapeutic system. **Pilo-20:** Releases 20 mcg pilocarpine/hour for one week. Pkg. 8s. **Pilo-40:** Releases 40 mcg pilocarpine/hour for one week. Pkg. 8s. *Rx.*
Use: Antiglaucoma agent.

OCuSOFT. (OCuSOFT) PEG-80 sorbitan laurate, sodium trideceth sulfate, PEG-150 distearate, cocoamido propyl hydroxysultaine, lauroamphocarboxyglycinate, sodium laureth-13 carboxylate, PEG-15 tallow polyamine, quaternium-15. Soln. Pads UD 30s, Bot. 30 ml, 120 ml, 240 ml, Compliance kit (120 ml and 100 pads). *otc.*
Use: Cleanser, ophthalmic.

OCuSOFT VMS. Vitamins A 5000 IU, E 30 IU, C 60 mg, Cu, Se, Zn 40 mg. Tab. Bot. 60s. *otc.*
Use: Mineral, vitamin supplement.

Ocusulf-10. (Optopics Laboratories, Corp) Sodium sulfacetamide 10%. Soln. Bot. 2 ml, 5 ml, 15 ml. *Rx.*
Use: Anti-infective, ophthalmic.

Ocutricin. (Bausch & Lomb Pharmaceuticals) Polymyxin B sulfate 10,000 units, bacitracin zinc 400 units, neomycin sulfate 3.5 mg. Oint. Tube 3.5 g. *Rx.*
Use: Antibiotic, ophthalmic.

Ocuvite. (Bausch & Lomb Pharmaceuticals) Formerly distributed by Storz. Vitamins A 5000 IU, E 30 IU, C 60 mg, Zn 40 mg, Cu, Se 40 mcg, lactose/Tab. Bot. 60s. *otc.*
Use: Mineral, vitamin supplement.

Ocuvite Extra. (Bausch & Lomb Pharmaceuticals) Vitamin A 6000 IU, C 200 mg, E 50 IU, Zn 40 mg, B_3 40 mg, B_2 3 mg, Cu, Se, Mn, l-glutathione. Tab. Bot. 50s. *otc.*
Use: Vitamin supplement.

Odara. (Young Dental) Alcohol 48%, carbolic acid less than 2%, zinc Cl, potassium iodide, glycerin, methyl salicylate, eucalyptus oil, myrrh tincture. Concentrated Liq. Bot. 8 oz. *otc.*
Use: Mouthwash.

oestergon.
See: Estradiol (Various Mfr.).

Oesto-Mins. (Tyson & Associates, Inc.) Ascorbic acid 500 mg, Ca 250 mg, Mg 250 mg, K 45 mg, vitamin D 100 IU/ 4.5 g. Pow. Bot. 200 g. *otc.*
Use: Vitamin supplement.

oestradiol.
See: Estradiol (Various Mfr.).

oestrasid.
See: Dienestrol (Various Mfr.).

oestrin.
See: Estrone (Various Mfr.).

oestroform.
See: Estrone (Various Mfr.).

oestromenin.
See: Diethylstilbestrol (Various Mfr.).

oestromon.
See: Diethylstilbestrol (Various Mfr.).

OFF-Ezy Corn & Callous Remover. (Del Pharmaceuticals, Inc.) Salicylic acid 17% in a collodion-like vehicle of 65% ether and 21% alcohol. Kit. 13.5 ml with callous smoother and 3 corn cushions. *otc.*
Use: Keratolytic.

OFF-Ezy Corn Remover. (Del Pharmaceuticals, Inc.) Salicylic acid 13.57% inflexible collodion base, ether 65%, alcohol 21%. Liq. Bot. 0.45 oz. *otc.*
Use: Keratolytic.

OFF-Ezy Wart Remover. (Del Pharmaceuticals, Inc.) Salicylic acid 17% in flexible collodion base, ether 65%, alcohol 21%. Liq. Bot. 13.5 ml. *otc.*
Use: Keratolytic.

•**ofloxacin.** (oh-FLOX-uh-SIN) U.S.P. 23.
Use: Anti-infective. [Orphan Drug]
See: Floxin (Daiichi Pharmaceutical).
Ocuflox, Ophth. Soln. (Allergan, Inc.).

•**ofornine.** (ah-FAR-neen) USAN.
Use: Antihypertensive.

Ogen. (Abbott Laboratories) Estropipate

0.75 mg, 1.5 mg, 3 mg/Tab. Bot. 100s. *Rx.*
Use: Estrogen.

Ogen Vaginal Cream. (Pharmacia & Upjohn) Estropipate 1.5 mg/g. Cream. Tube 42.5 g w/applicator. *Rx.*
Use: Estrogen.

Oilatum Soap. (Stiefel Laboratories, Inc.) Polyunsaturated vegetable oil 7.5%. Bar 120 g, 240 g. *otc.*
Use: Dermatologic, cleanser.

oil of camphor w/combinations.
See: Sloan's Liniment, Liq. (Warner Lambert).

oil of cloves w/alcohol.
See: Buckley "Z.O.", Liq. (Crosby).

Oil of Olay Daily UV Protectant. (Procter & Gamble Pharm.) SPF 15. **Cream:** Titanium dioxide, ethylhexyl p-methoxycinnamate, 2-phenylbenzimidazole-5-sulfonic acid, glycerin, triethanolamine, imidazolidinyl urea, parabens, carbomer, PEG-10, EDTA, castor oil, tartrazine. Scented and unscented. 51 g. **Lot.:** Ethylhexyl p-methoxycinnamate, 2-phenylbenzimidazole-5-sulfonic acid, titanium dioxide, cetyl alcohol, imidazolidinyl urea, parabens, EDTA, castor oil, tartrazine. Bot. 105 g, 157.7 g. *otc.*
Use: Sunscreen.

Oil of Olay Foaming Face Wash. (Procter & Gamble Pharm.) Potassium cocoyl hydrolyzed collagen, glycerin, EDTA. Liq. Bot. 90 ml, 210 ml. *otc.*
Use: Dermatologic, acne.

oil of pine w/combinations.
See: Sloan's Liniment, Liq. (Warner Lambert).

ointment base, washable.
See: Absorbent Base (Upsher-Smith Labs, Inc.).
Cetaphil, Cream, Lot. (Galderma Laboratories, Inc.).
Velvachol, Cream (Galderma Laboratories, Inc.).

•**ointment, bland lubricating ophthalmic.** U.S.P. 23.
Use: Lubricant, ophthalmic.

•**ointment, hydrophilic.** U.S.P. 23.
Use: Pharmaceutic aid (oil-in-water emulsion ointment base).

•**ointment, rose water.** U.S.P. 23.
Use: Pharmaceutic aid (emollient, ointment base).

•**ointment, white.** U.S.P. 23.
Use: Pharmaceutical aid (oleaginous ointment base).

•**ointment, yellow.** U.S.P. 23.
Use: Pharmaceutic aid (ointment base).

•**olaflur.** (OH-lah-flure) USAN.
Use: Dental caries agent.

olamine.
See: Ethanolamine.

•**olanzapine.** (oh-LAN-zah-PEEN) USAN.
Use: Antipsychotic.
See: Zyprexa, Tab. (Eli Lilly and Co.).

old tuberculin.
See: Mono-Vacc Test (OT), Box (Pasteur Merieux Connaught).
Tuberculin, Old, Tine Test, Jar (Wyeth-Ayerst Laboratories).

oleandomycin phosphate. Phosphate of an antibacterial substance produced by *Streptomyces antibioticus.*
Use: Anti-infective.

oleandomycin, triacetyl. Troleandomycin, U.S.P. XX.

•**oleic acid.** (oh-LAY-ik) N.F. 18.
Use: Pharmaceutic aid (emulsion adjunct).

•**oleic acid I 125.** USAN.
Use: Radiopharmaceutical.

•**oleic acid I 131.** USAN.
Use: Radiopharmaceutical.

oleovitamin a.
See: Vitamin A, U.S.P. 23

•**oleovitamin a & d.** U.S.P. 23.
Use: Vitamin supplement.
See: Super D, Perles, Liq. (Pharmacia & Upjohn)

oleovitamin d, synthetic.
Use: Vitamin supplement.
See: Viosterol in Oil.

•**oleyl alcohol.** (oh-LAY-il) N.F. 18.
Use: Pharmaceutic aid (emulsifying agent, emollient).
See: Patanol, Soln. (Alcon Laboratories, Inc.).

•**olive oil.** N.F. 18.
Use: Emollient, pharmaceutic aid (setting retardant for dental cements).

•**olopatadine hydrochloride.** (oh-low-pat-AD-een) USAN.
Use: Antiallergic (allergic rhinitis, urticria, allergic conjunctivitis, asthma).
See: Patanol, Soln. (Alcon Laboratories, Inc.).

•**olsalazine sodium.** (OLE-SAL-uh-zeen) USAN. *Formerly Sodium azodisalicylate, azodisal sodium.*
Use: Maintenance of remission of ulcerative colitis in patients intolerant of sulfasalazine; anti-inflammatory (gastrointestinal).
See: Dipentum (Pharmacia & Upjohn).

•**olvanil.** (OLE-van-ill) USAN.
Use: Analgesic.

OM 401.
Use: Sickle cell disease. [Orphan Drug]

omega-3 (n-3) polyunsaturated fatty acids. From cold water fish oils.
Use: Dietary supplement to reduce risk of coronary artery disease.
See: Cardi-Omega 3, Cap. (Thompson Medical Co.).
Marine 500, 1000, Cap. (Murdock).
Max EPA, Cap. (Various Mfr.).
Promega, Cap. (Parke-Davis).
Sea-Omega 50, Cap. (Rugby Labs, Inc.).

Omega Oil. (Block Drug Co., Inc.) Methyl nicotinate, methyl salicylate, capsicum oleoresin, histamine dihydrochloride, isopropyl alcohol 44%. Bot. 2.5 oz, 4.85 oz. *otc.*
Use: Analgesic, topical.

•**omeprazole.** (oh-MEH-pray-ZAHL) U.S.P. 23. (Astra Pharmaceuticals, L.P.)
Use: Depressant (gastric acid secretory); agent for gastroesophageal reflux disease.
See: Prilosec, Cap. (Merck & Co.).

•**omeprazole sodium.** (oh-MEH-pray-ZOLE) USAN.
Use: Antisecretory (gastric).

OmniCef. (Parke-Davis) **Cap.:** Cefdinir 300 mg. Bot. 60s. **Oral Susp.:** 125 mg/5 ml, sucrose. Bot. 60 ml, 100 ml. *Rx.*
Use: Anti-infective, cephalosporin.

Omnicol. (Delta Pharmaceutical Group) Dextromethorphan HBr 15 mg, chlorpheniramine maleate 4 mg, phenylephrine HCl 5 mg, phenindamine tartrate 4 mg, salicylamide 227 mg, acetaminophen 100 mg, caffeine alkaloid 10 mg, ascorbic acid 25 mg/Tab. Bot. 100s. *otc.*
Use: Antitussive, antihistamine, decongestant, analgesic.

Omnihemin. (Delta Pharmaceutical Group) Fe 110 mg, vitamins C 150 mg, B_{12} 7.5 mcg, folic acid 1 mg, Zn 1 mg, Cu 1 mg, Mn 1 mg, Mg 1 mg/Tab. or 5 ml. **Cap.:** Bot. 100s; **Soln.:** Bot. Pt. *Rx.*
Use: Mineral, vitamin supplement.

OmniHIB. (SmithKline Beecham Pharmaceuticals) Purified *Haemophilus influenza* type b capsular polysaccharide 10 mcg, tetanus toxoid 24 mcg/0.5 ml, sucrose 8.5%. Pow. for Inj. (lyophilized). Vial w/0.6 ml syringe of diluent. *Rx.*
Use: Immunization.

OMNIhist L.A. (WE Pharmaceuticals, Inc.) Phenylephrine 20 mg, chlorpheniramine maleate 8 mg, methscopolamine nitrate 2.5 mg/Tab. Bot. 100s. *Rx.*
Use: Anticholinergic, antihistamine, decongestant.

Omninatal. (Delta Pharmaceutical Group) Fe 60 mg, Cu 2 mg, Zn 15 mg, vitamins A 8000 IU, D 400 IU, C 90 mg, Ca 200 mg, folic acid 1.5 mg, B_1 2.5 mg, B_2 3 mg, niacinamide 20 mg, pyridoxine HCl 10 mg, pantothenic acid 15 mg, B_{12} 8 mcg/Tab. Bot. 100s. *Rx.*
Use: Mineral, vitamin supplement.

Omnipaque 140. (Nycomed) Iohexol 302 mg, iodine 140 mg/ml. Inj. Vial 50 ml, Bot. *Rx.*
Use: Radiopaque agent.

Omnipaque 180. (Nycomed) Iohexol 388 mg, iodine 180 mg/ml. Inj. Vial 10 ml, 20 ml; *Myelo-kit* 10 ml, 20 ml; *Redi-unit* 10 ml. *Rx.*
Use: Radiopaque agent.

Omnipaque 210. (Nycomed) Iohexol 453 mg, iodine 210 mg/ml. Inj. Vial 15 ml. *Rx.*
Use: Radiopaque agent.

Omnipaque 240. (Nycomed) Iohexol 518 mg, iodine 240 mg/ml. Inj. Vial 10 ml, 20 ml, 50 ml. Bot. 50 ml. Flex. Cont. 100 ml, 150 ml, 200 ml. Prefilled Syringe 50 ml. *Myelo-kit* 10 ml. 75 ml fill in 100 ml Bot. 100 ml fill in 100 ml Bot. 125 ml fill in 200 ml Bot. 150 ml fill in 200 ml Bot. 200 ml fill in 100 ml Bot. *Rx.*
Use: Radiopaque agent.

Omnipaque 300. (Nycomed) Iohexol 647 mg, iodine 300 mg/ml. Inj. Vial 10 ml, 30 ml, 50 ml. Bot. 50 ml. Flex. Cont. 100 ml, 150 ml. Prefilled Syringe 50 ml. 75 ml fill in 100 ml Bot. 100 ml fill in 100 ml Bot. 125 ml fill in 200 ml Bot. 150 ml fill in 200 ml Bot. 75 ml fill in 100 ml Flex. Cont., 125 ml fill in 150 ml Flex. Cont. Bulk Pack. *Rx.*
Use: Radiopaque agent.

Omnipaque 350. (Nycomed) Iohexol 755 mg, iodine 350 mg/ml. Inj. Vial 50 ml. Bot. 50 ml. Flex. Cont. 100 ml, 150 ml, 200 ml. Prefilled Syringe 50 ml. 75 ml fill in 100 ml bot, 100 ml fill in 100 ml bot, 125 ml fill in 200 ml bot, 150 ml fill in 200 ml bot, 175 ml fill in 200 ml bot, 200 ml fill in 200 ml bot., 250 ml fill in 300 ml bot, 75 ml fill in 100 ml Flex. Cont., 125 ml fill in 150 ml Flex. Cont. Bulk Pack. *Rx.*
Use: Radiopaque agent.

Omnipen. (Wyeth-Ayerst Laboratories) **Cap.:** Ampicillin anhydrous 250 mg, 500 mg. Bot. 100s, 500s. **Pow. for Oral Susp.:** Ampicillin trihydrate 125 mg, 250 mg/5 ml when reconstituted. Pow. for Oral Susp. Bot. 100 ml, 150 ml, 200 ml. *Rx.*
Use: Anti-infective, penicillin.

Omnipen-N. (Wyeth-Ayerst Laboratories)

Ampicillin sodium 125 mg, 250 mg, 500 mg, 1 g, 2 g, 10 g. Pow. for Inj. Vial, Piggyback and *ADD-Vantage* vials (only 500 mg, 1 g, 2 g), *Rx*.
Use: Anti-infective, penicillin.

Omniscan. (Nycomed) Gadodiamide 287 mg/ml. Inj. Vial 10 ml, 20 ml, 50 ml, 15 ml fill in 20 ml vials, 10 ml fill in 20 ml prefilled syringe, 15 ml fill in 20 ml prefilled syringe. Prefilled Syringe 20 ml. *Rx*.
Use: Radiopaque agent.

Omnitabs. (Halsey Drug Co.) Vitamins A 5000 IU, D 400 IU, C 50 mg, B_1 3 mg, B_2 2.5 mg, niacin 20 mg, B_6 1 mg, B_{12} 1 mcg, pantothenic acid 0.9 mg/Tab. Bot. 100s. *otc*.
Use: Vitamin supplement.

Omnitabs with Iron. (Halsey Drug Co.) Vitamins A 5000 IU, D 400 IU, B_1 3 mg, B_2 2.5 mg, B_6 1 mg, B_{12} 1 mcg, C 50 mg, niacinamide 20 mg, calcium pantothenate 1 mg, Fe 15 mg/Tab. Bot. 100s. *otc*.
Use: Mineral, vitamin supplement.

•**omoconazole nitrate.** (oh-moe-KAHN-ah-zole) USAN.
Use: Antifungal.

OMS Concentrate. (Upsher-Smith Labs, Inc.) Morphine sulfate 20 mg/ml. Soln. Bot. 30 ml, 120 ml w/dropper. *c-II*.
Use: Analgesic, narcotic.

Oncaspar. (Enzon, Inc.) Pegaspargase 750 IU/ml in a phosphate buffered saline solution. Inj. Single-use vials. *Rx*.
Use: Antineoplastic agent.

Oncet. (Wakefield Pharmaceuticals, Inc.) Hydrocodone bitartrate 5 mg, acetaminophen 500 mg/Cap. Bot. 100s. *c-III*.
Use: Analgesic, antitussive.

oncorad ov103.
Use: Antineoplastic. [Orphan Drug]

OncoScint CR/OV. (Cytogen) Satumomab pendetide labeled with indium-111, obtained separately. Kit with 1 mg/2 ml satumomab vial, vial of sodium acetate buffer, and filter.

Oncovin. (Eli Lilly and Co.) Vincristine sulfate for inj. 1 mg/ml, 2 mg/2 ml, or 5 mg/5 ml. Soln. Ctn. 10s. Hyporets 1 mg/Pkg 3s; 2 mg/Pkg 3s. *Rx*.
Use: Antineoplastic.

Oncovite. (Mission Pharmacal Co.) Vitamin A 10,000 IU, C 500 mg, D_3 400 IU, E 200 IU, B_1 0.37 mg, B_2 0.5 mg, B_6 25 mg, B_{12} 1.5 mcg, folate 0.4 mg, Zn 7.5 mg, sugar. Tab. Bot. 120s. *otc*.
Use: Vitamin supplement.

•**ondansetron hydrochloride.** (ahn-DAN-SEH-trahn) USAN.
Use: Anxiolytic, antiemetic, antischizophrenic.
See: Zofran, Preps. (GlaxoWellcome).

Ondrox. (Unimed) Ca 25 mg, iron 3 mg, vitamins A 2000 IU, D 100 IU, E 17 mg, B_1 0.25 mg, B_2 0.28 mg, B_3 3.33 mg, B_5 1.67 mg, B_6 0.33 mg, B_{12} 1 mcg, C 41.7 mg, folic acid 0.67, biotin 0.5 mcg, I, Mg, Cu, P, vitamin K, Cr, Mn, Mo, Se, V, B, Si, Zn 2.5 mg, inositol, bioflavonoids, N-acetylcysteine, l-glutathione, l-methionine, l-glutamine, taurine. Tab. Bot. 60s, 180s. *otc*.
Use: Mineral, vitamins supplements.

One-A-Day Essential. (Bayer Corp. (Consumer Div.)) Vitamins A 5000 IU, E 30 IU, C 60 mg, folic acid 0.4 mg, B_1 1.5 mg, B_2 1.7 mg, B_3 20 mg, B_6 2 mg, B_{12} 6 mcg, B_5 10 mg, D 400 IU/Tab. Sodium free. Bot. 75s, 130s. *otc*.
Use: Vitamin supplement.

One-A-Day Extras Antioxidant. (Bayer Corp. (Consumer Div.)) Vitamin E 200 IU, C 250 mg, A 5000 IU, Zn 7.5 mg, Cu, Se, Mn, tartrazine/Softgel Cap. Bot. 50s. *otc*.
Use: Vitamin Supplement.

One-A-Day Extras Vitamin C. (Bayer Corp. (Consumer Div.)) Vitamin C 500 mg/Tab. Bot. 100s. *otc*.
Use: Vitamin supplement.

One-A-Day Extras Vitamin E. (Bayer Corp. (Consumer Div.)) Vitamin E 400 IU/Softgel Cap. Bot. 60s. *otc*.
Use: Vitamin supplement.

One-A-Day Maximum Formula. (Bayer Corp. (Consumer Div.)) Fe 18 mg, vitamins A 5000 IU, D 400 IU, E 30 IU, B_1 1.5 mg, B_2 1.7 mg, B_3 20 mg, B_5 10 mg, B_6 2 mg, B_{12} 6 mcg, C 60 mg, folic acid 0.4 mg, Ca, Cl, Cr, Cu, I, K, Mg, Mn, Mo, P, Se, Zn 15 mg, biotin 30 mcg/Tab. Bot. 60s, 100s. *otc*.
Use: Mineral, vitamin supplement.

One-A-Day Men's Vitamins. (Bayer Corp. (Consumer Div.)) Vitamin A 5000 IU, C 200 mg, B_1 2.25 mg, B_2 2.55 mg, B_3 20 mg, D 400 IU, E 45 IU, B_6 3 mg, folic acid 0.4 mg, B_{12} 9 mcg, B_5 10 mg/Tab. Bot. 60s, 100s. *otc*.
Use: Mineral, vitamin supplement.

One-A-Day 55 Plus. (Bayer Corp. (Consumer Div.)) Vitamin A 6000 IU, C 120 mg, B_1 4.5 mg, B_2 3.4 mg, B_3 20 mg, D 400 IU, E 60 IU, B_6 6 mg, folic acid 0.4 mg, biotin 30 mcg, B_5 20 mg, K 25 mcg, Ca 220 mg, I, Mg, Cu, Zn 15 mg, Cr, Se, Mo, Mn, K, Cl/Tab. Bot. 50s, 80s. *otc*.
Use: Mineral, vitamin supplement.

One-A-Day Women's Formula. (Bayer Corp. (Consumer Div.)) **Tab.:** Ca 450 mg, Fe 27 mg, vitamins A 5000 IU, D

400 IU, E 30 mg, B_1 1.5 mg, B_2 1.7 mg, B_3 20 mg, B_5 10 mg, B_6 2 mg, B_{12} 6 mcg, C 60 mg, folic acid 0.4 mg, Zn 15 mg, tartrazine. Bot. 60s, 100s. *Rx.*
Use: Mineral, vitamin supplement.

One-Tablet-Daily. (Various Mfr.) Vitamins A 5000 IU, D 400 IU, E 30 mg, B_1 1.5 mg, B_2 1.7 mg, B_3 20 mg, B_5 10 mg, B_6 2 mg, B_{12} 6 mcg, C 60 mg, folic acid 0.4 mg. Tab. Bot. 30s, 100s, 250s, 365s, 1000s. *otc.*
Use: Vitamin supplement.

One-Tablet-Daily. (Various Mfr.) Vitamins A 5000 IU, D 400 IU, E 30 mg, B_1 1.5 mg, B_2 1.7 mg, B_3 20 mg, B_5 10 mg, B_6 2 mg, B_{12} 6 mcg, C 60 mg, folic acid 0.4 mg/Tab. Bot. 365s, 1000s. *otc.*
Use: Vitamin supplement.

One-Tablet-Daily Plus Iron. (Various Mfr.) Iron 18 mg, vitamins A 5000 IU, D 400 IU, E 15 mg, B_1 1.5 mg, B_2 1.7 mg, B_3 20 mg, B_6 2 mg, B_{12} 6 mcg, C 60 mg, folic acid 0.4 mg/Tab. Bot. 100s, 250s, 365s. *otc.*
Use: Mineral, vitamin supplement.

One-Tablet-Daily with Iron. (Zenith Goldline Pharmaceuticals) Fe 18 mg, A 5000 IU, D 400 IU, E 30 mg, B_1 1.5 mg, B_2 1.7 mg, B_3 20 mg, B_5 10 mg, B_6 2 mg, B_{12} 6 mcg, C 60 mg, folic acid 0.4 mg. Bot. 100s. *otc.*
Use: Mineral, viatmin supplement.

One-Tablet-Daily with Minerals. (Zenith Goldline Pharmaceuticals) Fe 18 mg, vitamins A 5000 IU, D 400 IU, E 30 IU, B_1 1.5 mg, B_2 1.7 mg, B_3 20 mg, B_5 10 mg, B_6 2 mg, B_{12} 6 mcg, C 60 mg, folic acid 0.4 mg, Ca, Cl, Cr, Cu, I, K, Mg, Mn, Mo, P, Se, Zn 15 mg, biotin 30 mcg/Tab. Bot. 100s, 1000s. *otc.*
Use: Mineral, vitamin supplement.

1000-BC, IM, or IV. (Solvay Pharmaceuticals) Vitamins B_1 25 mg, B_2 2.5 mg, B_6 5 mg, panthenol 5 mg, B_{12} 500 mcg, niacinamide 75 mg, C 100 mg/ml. Vial 10 ml. *Rx.*
Use: Vitamin supplement.

1+1-F Creme. (Dunhall Pharmaceuticals, Inc.) Hydrocortisone 1%, pramoxine HCl 1%, iodochlorhydroxyquin 3%. Tube 30 g. *Rx.*
Use: Corticosteroid; anesthetic, local; antifungal, topical.

1-2-3 Ointment No. 20. (Durel) Burow's solution, lanolin, zinc oxide (Lassar's paste). Jar oz, 1 lb, 6 lb. *otc.*
Use: Anti-inflammatory, topical.

1-2-3 Ointment No. 21. (Durel) Burow's solution 1 part, lanolin 2, zinc oxide (Lassar's paste) 1.5 oz, cold cream 1.5 oz. Jar oz, 1 lb, 6 lb. *otc.*
Use: Anti-inflammatory agent, topical.

Onoton Tablets. (Sanofi Winthrop Pharmaceuticals) Pancreatin, hemicellulose, ox bile extracts. *otc.*
Use: Digestive aid.

Ontak. (Ligand Pharm) Denileukin diftitox 150 mcg/ml. Soln. for Inj. Single-use Vial 2 ml. *Rx.*
Use: Antineoplastic.

•**ontazolast.** (ahn-TAH-zoe-last) USAN.
Use: Antiasthmatic (leukotriene antagonist).

ontosein.
See: Orgotein (Diagnostic Data).

Ony-Clear. (Pedinol Pharmacal, Inc.) Benzalkonium chloride. Soln. Bot. 1 oz w/applicator. *otc.*
Use: Antiseptic.

Opcon. (Bausch & Lomb Pharmaceuticals) Naphazoline HCl 0.1%. Soln. Bot. 15 ml. *otc.*
Use: Mydriatic, vasoconstrictor.

Opcon-A. (Bausch & Lomb Pharmaceuticals) 0.027% nephazoline HCl, 0.315% pheniramine maleate, 0.5% hydroxypropyl methylcellulose, 0.01% benzalkonium chloride, 0.1% EDTA, NaCl, boric acid, sodium buffers. Soln. Bot. 15 ml. *otc.*
Use: Mydriatic, vasoconstrictor, antihistamine.

o,p'-DDD.
Use: Miscellaneous antineoplastic.
See: Lysodren (Bristol-Myers Oncology/Immunology)

Operand. (Aplicare, Inc.) **Aerosal:** Iodine 0.5%. 90 ml. **Skin cleanser:** Iodine 1%. 90 ml. **Oint.:** Iodine 1%. 30 g, lb, packette 1.2 g, 2.7 g. **Perineal wash conc.:** Iodine 1%. 240 ml. **Prep soln.:** Iodine 1%. 60 ml, 120 ml, 240 ml, pt, qt. **Soln:** Prep pad 100s, swab stick 25s. **Surgical scrub:** Povidone-iodine 7.5%. 60 ml, 120 ml, 240 ml, pt, qt, gal, packette 22.5 ml. **Whirlpool conc.:** Iodine 1%. Gal. *otc.*
Use: Antiseptic, antimicrobial.

Operand Douche. (Aplicare, Inc.) Povidone-iodine. Soln. Bot. 60 ml, 240 ml, UD 15 ml. *otc.*
Use: Vaginal agent.

o-phenylphenol.
W/Amyl complex, phenylmercuric nitrate.
See: Lubraseptic Jelly (Gordon Laboratories).

Ophthacet. (Vortech Pharmaceuticals) Sodium sulfacetamide 10%. Soln. 15 ml. *Rx.*
Use: Anti-infective, ophthalmic.

Ophthalgan. (Wyeth-Ayerst Laborato-

ries) Glycerin ophthalmic soln. w/chlorobutanol 0.55% as preservative. Soln. Bot. 7.5 ml. *Rx.*
Use: Hyperosmolar.

Ophtha P/S. (Misemer Pharmaceuticals, Inc.) Prednisolone acetate 0.5%, sodium sulfacetamide 10%, hydroxyethyl cellulose, EDTA, polysorbate 80, sodium thiosulfate, benzalkonium chloride 0.025%. Susp. Bot. 5 ml. *Rx.*
Use: Corticosteroid; anti-infective, ophthalmic.

Ophtha P/S Ophthalmic Suspension. (Misemer Pharmaceuticals, Inc.) Sodium sulfacetamide 10%, prednisolone acetate 0.5%. Bot. 5 ml w/dropper. *Rx.*
Use: Corticosteroid; anti-infective, ophthalmic.

Ophthetic. (Allergan, Inc.) Proparacaine HCl 0.5%. Bot. 15 ml. *Rx.*
Use: Anesthetic, ophthalmic.

•**opipramol hydrochloride.** (oh-PIH-prah-mole) USAN.
Use: Antipsychotic, antidepressant, tranquilizer.

•**opium.** (OH-pee-uhm) U.S.P. 23.
Use: Pharmaceutic necessity for powdered opium.
See: Paregoric (Various Mfr.).

opium and belladonna. (Wyeth-Ayerst Laboratories) Powdered opium 60 mg, extract of belladonna 15 mg/Supp. Box 20s. *c-II.*
Use: Analgesic, narcotic; anticholinergic; antispasmodic.

•**opium powdered.** U.S.P. 23.
Use: Pharmaceutical necessity for Paregoric.
W/Albumin tannate, colloidal kaolin, pectin.
See: Ekrised, Tab. (Roberts Pharmaceuticals).
W/Belladonna extract.
See: B & O, Supp. (PolyMedica Pharmaceuticals).
W/Bismuth subgallate, kaolin, pectin, zinc phenolsulfonate.
See: Diastay, Tab. (ICN Pharmaceuticals, Inc.).

opium tincture.
W/Homatropine MBr, Pectin.
See: Dia-Quel, Liq. (I.P.C.).

opium tincture, camphorated.
Use: Antidiarrheal.
See: Paregoric, U.S.P. 23.

opium tincture, deodrized. (Eli Lilly and Co.) Opium 10%, alcohol 19%. Liq. Bot. 120 ml, pt. *c-II.*
Use: Analgesic, narcotic.

•**oprelvekin.** (oh-PRELL-veh-kin) USAN.
Use: Hematopoietic stimulant.
See: Neumega, Pow. for Inj. (Genetics Institute).

Opti-Bon Eye Drops. (Barrows) Phenylephrine HCl, berberine sulfate, boric acid, sodium Cl, sodium bisulfite, glycerin, camphor, water, peppermint water, thimerosal 0.004%. Bot. 1 oz. *otc.*
Use: Ophthalmic.

Opticaps. (Health for Life Brands, Inc.) Vitamins A 32,500 IU, D 3250 IU, B_1 15 mg, B_2 5 mg, B_6 0.5 mg, C 150 mg, E 5 IU, calcium pantothenate 3 mg, niacinamide 150 mg, B_{12} 20 mcg, Fe 11.26 mg, choline bitartrate 30 mg, inositol 30 mg, pepsin 32.5 mg, diastase 32.5 mg, Ca 30 mg, P 25 mg, Mg 0.7 mg, Fr. dicalcium phosphate 110 mg, Mn 1.3 mg, K 0.68 mg, Zn 0.45 mg, hesperidin compound 25 mg, biotin 20 mcg, brewer's yeast 50 mg, wheat germ oil 20 mg, hydrolyzed yeast 81.25 mg, protein digest. 47.04 mg, amino acids 34.21 mg/Cap. Bot. 30s, 60s, 90s, 1000s. *otc.*
Use: Mineral, vitamin supplement.

Opticare PMS. (Standard Drug Co.) Fe 2.5 mg, vitamins 2083 IU, D 17 IU, E 14 IU, B_1 4.2 mg, B_2 4.2 mg, B_3 4.2 mg, B_5 4.2 mg, B_6 50 mg, B_{12} 10.4 mcg, C 250 mg, folic acid 0.03 mg, Cr, Cu, I, K, Mg, Mn, Se, Zn 4.2 mg, biotin 10.4 mcg, choline bitartrate, bioflavonoids, inositol, PABA, rutin, Ca, amylase activity, protease activity, lipase activity, betaine, tartrazine. Bot. 150s. *otc.*
Use: Mineral, vitamin supplement.

Opti-Clean. (Alcon Laboratories, Inc.) Tween 21, polymeric cleaners, hydroxyethyl cellulose, thimerosal 0.004%, EDTA 0.1%. Bot 12 ml, 20 ml. *otc.*
Use: Contact lens care.

Opti-Clean II. (Alcon Laboratories, Inc.) Polymeric cleaning agent, Tween 21, EDTA 0.1%, polyquaternium 1 0.001%. Thimerosal free. Bot. 12 ml, 20 ml. *otc.*
Use: Contact lens care.

Opti-Clean II Especially For Sensitive Eyes. (Alcon Laboratories, Inc.) EDTA 0.1%, polyquaternium 1 0.001%, polymeric cleaners, Tween 21. Thimerosal free. Bot. 12 ml, 20 ml. *otc.*
Use: Contact lens care.

Opticyl. (Optopics Laboratories, Corp.) Tropicamide 0.5%, 1%. Soln. Bot. 2 ml, 15 ml. *Rx.*
Use: Cycloplegic, mydriatic.

Opti-Free Enzymatic Cleaner. (Alcon Laboratories, Inc.) Highly purified pork pancreatin. Tab. Pkg. 6s, 12s, 18s. *otc.*
Use: Contact lens care.

Opti-Free Non-Hydrogen Peroxide-Containing System. (Alcon Laboratories, Inc.) Citrate buffer, NaCl, EDTA 0.05%, polyquaternium 1 0.001%. Soln. 118 ml, 237 ml, 355 ml. *otc.*
Use: Ophthalmic.

Opti-Free Rewetting Solution. (Alcon Laboratories, Inc.) Citrate buffer, sodium Cl, EDTA 0.05%, polyquaternium 1 0.001%. Soln. Bot. 10 ml, 20 ml. *otc.*
Use: Contact lens care.

Opti-Free Surfactant Cleaning Solution. (Alcon Laboratories, Inc.) EDTA 0.01%, polyquaternium 1 0.001%, microclens polymeric cleaners, Tween 21. Thimerosal free. Soln. Bot. 12 ml, 20 ml. *otc.*
Use: Contact lens care.

Optigene. (Pfeiffer Co.) Sodium Cl, mono- and dibasic sodium phosphate, benzalkonium Cl, EDTA. Soln. Bot. 118 ml. *otc.*
Use: Irrigant, ophthalmic.

Optigene 3. (Pfeiffer Co.) Tetrahydrozoline HCl 0.05%. Soln. Bot. 15 ml. *otc.*
Use: Mydriatic, vasoconstrictor.

Optilets-500. (Abbott Laboratories) Vitamins B_1 15 mg, B_2 10 mg, B_3 100 mg, B_5 20 mg, B_6 5 mg, C 500 mg, A 10,000 IU, D 400 IU, E 30 IU, B_{12} 12 mcg/Filmtab. Bot. 120s. *otc.*
Use: Mineral, vitamin supplement.

Optilets-M-500. (Abbott Laboratories) Vitamins C 500 mg, B_3 100 mg, B_5 20 mg, $B_1$15 mg, A 5000 IU, B_2 10 mg, B_6 5 mg, D 400 IU, B_{12} 12 mcg, E 30 IU, Fe 20 mg, Mg, Zn 1.5 mg, Cu, Mn, I/ Filmtab. Bot. 120s. *otc.*
Use: Mineral, vitamin supplement.

Optimental. (Ross) Protein 12.2 g, fat 6.7 g, carbohydrate 32.9 g, vitamin A 1950 IU, D 67 IU, E 50 IU, K 20 mcg, C 50 mg, folic acid 135 mcg, B_1 0.5 mg, B_2 0.57 mg, B_6 0.67 mg, B_{12} 2 mcg, B_3 6.7 mg, choline 100 mg, biotin 100 mcg, B_5 3.4 mg, Na 250 mg, K 420 mg, chloride 320 mg, Ca 250 mg, P 250 mg, Mg 100 mg, I 38 mcg, Mn 0.84 mg, Cu 0.34 mg, Zn 3.8 mg, Fe 3 mg, Se 12 mcg, Cr 20 mcg, Mo 25 mcg, sucrose, canola oil, soy oil. Liq. Bot. 237 ml. *otc.*
Use: Nutritional therapy, enteral.

Optimine. (Schering-Plough Corp.) Azatadine maleate 1 mg/Tab. Bot. 100s. *Rx.*
Use: Antihistamine.

Optimoist. (Colgate Oral Pharmaceuticals) Xylitol, calcium phosphate monobasic, citric acid, sodium hydroxide, sodium benzoate, acesulfame potassium, hydroxyethyl cellulose, sodium monofluoro phosphate, 2 ppm fluoride. Soln. Bot. 60 ml, 330 ml. Spray. *otc.*
Use: Saliva substitute.

Optimox Prenatal. (Optimox Corp.) Ca 100 mg, iron 5 mg, vitamins A 833 IU, D 67 IU, E 2 mg, B_1 0.5 mg, B_2 0.6 mg, B_3 6.7 mg, B_5 3.3 mg, B_6 0.73 mg, B_{12} 0.87 mcg, C 30 mg, folic acid 0.13 mg, Cr, Cu, I, K, Mg, Mn, Se, Zn 3.17 mg. Tab. Bot. 360s. *otc.*
Use: Mineral, vitamin supplement.

Optimyd. (Schering-Plough Corp.) Prednisolone phosphate 0.5%, sodium sulfacetamide 10%, sodium thiosulfate. Sterile Soln. Drop Bot. 5 ml. *Rx.*
Use: Anti-infective, corticosteroid, ophthalmic.

Opti-One. (Alcon Laboratories, Inc.) EDTA 0.05%, polyquaternium 1 0.001%, NaCl, sodium citrate. Buffered, isotonic. Soln. 120 ml. *otc.*
Use: Contact lens care.

Opti-One Multi-Purpose. (Alcon Laboratories, Inc.) EDTA 0.05%, polyquaternium 0.001%, NaCl, mannitol. Buffered, isotonic. Soln. Bot. 118 ml, 237 ml, 355 ml, 473 ml. *otc.*
Use: Contact lens care.

Opti-One Rewetting. (Alcon Laboratories, Inc.) EDTA 0.05%, polyquaternium 1 0.001%, sodium chloride, citrate buffer, isotonic. Drops. Bot. 10 ml. *otc.*
Use: Contact lens care.

OptiPranolol. (Bausch & Lomb Pharmaceuticals) Metipranolol HCl 0.3%. Soln. Bot. 5 ml, 10 ml, 15 ml w/dropper. *Rx.*
Use: Antiglaucoma agent.

Optiray 160. (Mallinckrodt) Ioversol 339 mg, iodine 160 mg/ml. Inj. Vial 50 ml. 100 ml fill in 150 ml bot. *Rx.*
Use: Radiopaque agent.

Optiray 240. (Mallinckrodt) Ioversol 509 mg, iodine 240 mg/ml. Inj. Vial 50 ml. 100 ml fill in 150 ml Bot., 150 ml fill in 150 ml Bot., 200 ml fill in 250 ml Bot. Hand-held Syringe 50 ml. Power Injector Syringe 125 ml. *Rx.*
Use: Radiopaque agent.

Optiray 300. (Mallinckrodt) Ioversol 636 mg, iodine 300 mg/ml. Inj. 100 ml fill in 125 ml Power Injector Syringe. *Rx.*
Use: Radiopaque agent.

Optiray 320. (Mallinckrodt) Ioversol 678 mg, iodine 320 mg/ml. Inj. Vial 20 ml, 30 ml, 50 ml. Bot. 150 ml. 75 ml fill in 150 ml Bot. 100 ml fill in 150 ml Bot., 200 ml fill in 250 ml Bot. Hand-held Syringe 30 ml, 50 ml. 50 ml fill in 125 ml Power Injector Syringe. Power Injector Syringe 125 ml. *Rx.*

Use: Radiopaque agent.

Optiray 350. (Mallinckrodt) Ioversol 741 mg, iodine 350 mg/ml. Inj. Vial 30 ml, 50 ml. Bot. 150 ml. 75 ml fill in 150 ml Bot., 100 ml fill in 150 ml Bot., 200 ml fill in 250 ml Bot. Hand-held Syringe 30 ml, 50 ml. 50 ml fill in 125 ml Power Injector Syringe 125 ml. *Rx.*
Use: Radiopaque agent.

Opti-Soft. (Alcon Laboratories, Inc.) Isotonic soln of sodium Cl, borate buffer, EDTA 0.1%, polyquaternium 1 0.001%. Thimerosal free. Soln. Bot. 237 ml, 355 ml. *otc.*
Use: Contact lens care.

Opti-Soft Especially for Sensitive Eyes. (Alcon Laboratories, Inc.) Buffered, isotonic. EDTA 0.1%, polyquaternium 1 0.001%, NaCl, borate buffer. For lenses w/ $\leq$ 45% water content. Soln. Bot. 118 ml, 237 ml, 355 ml. *otc.*
Use: Contact lens care.

Optison. (Mallinckrodt) Human albumin microspheres 5 to 8 $\times$ 10^8, albumin human 10 mg, octafluoropropane 0.22 $\pm$ 0.11 mg/ml in aqueous sodium chloride 0.9%. Inj. Susp. 3 ml fill in single-use 3 ml vial. *Rx.*
Use: Radiopaque agent.

Opti-Tears. (Alcon Laboratories, Inc.) Isotonic solution with dextran, sodium Cl, potassium Cl, hydroxypropyl methylcellulose, EDTA 0.1%, polyquaternium 1 0.001%. Thimerosal and sorbic acid free. Soln. Bot. 15 ml. *otc.*
Use: Contact lens care.

Optivite for Women. (Optimox Corp.) Vitamins A 2083 IU, D 16.7 IU, E 14 mg, B_1 4.2 mg, B_2 4.2 mg, B_3 4.2 mg, B_5 4.2 mg, B_6 50 mg, B_{12} 10.4 mcg, C 250 mg, Fe 2.5 mg, folic acid 0.03 mg, Zn 4.2 mg, choline 52 mg, inositol 10 mg, Cr, Cu, I, K, Mg, Mn, Se, citrus bioflavonoids, PABA, rutin, pancreatin, biotin/Tab. Bot. 180s. *otc.*
Use: Mineral, vitamin supplement.

Optivite P.M.T. (Optimox Corp.) Vitamins A 2083 IU, D, E 16.7 mg, B_1 4.2 mg, B_2 4.2 mg, B_3 4.2 mg, B_5 4.2 mg, B_6 50 mg, B_{12} 10.4 mcg, C 250 mg, Fe 2.5 mg, FA 0.03 mg, Zn 4.2 mg, choline, Ca, Cr, Cu, I, K, Mg, Mn, Se, bioflavonoids, betaine, PABA, rutin, pancreatin, biotin, inositol/Tab. Bot. 180s. *otc.*
Use: Mineral, vitamin supplement.

Opti-Zyme Enzymatic Cleaner Especially For Sensitive Eyes. (Alcon Laboratories, Inc.) Pork pancreatin tablets. Pak 8s, 24s, 36s, 56s. *otc.*
Use: Contact lens care.

ORA5. (McHenry Laboratories, Inc.) Copper sulfate, iodine, potassium iodide, alcohol 1.5%. Liq. Bot. 3.75 ml, 30 ml. *otc.*
Use: Mouth preparation.

Orabase. (Colgate Oral Pharmaceuticals) Gelatin, pectin, sodium carboxymethylcellulose in hydrocarbon gel w/ polyethylene and mineral oil. 0.75 g Pkt. Box 100s. Tube 5 g, 15 g. *otc.*
Use: Mouth preparation.

Orabase-B. (Colgate Oral Pharmaceuticals) Benzocaine 20%, mineral oil. Paste. 5 g, 15 g. *otc.*
Use: Mouth and throat preparation.

Orabase Baby. (Colgate Oral Pharmaceuticals) Benzocaine 7.5%, alcohol free, fruit flavor. Gel. 7.2 ml. *otc.*
Use: Anesthetic, local.

Orabase Gel. (Colgate Oral Pharmceuticals) Benzocaine 15%, ethyl alcohol, tannic acid, salicylic acid, saccharin. Gel. 7 ml. *otc.*
Use: Anesthetic, local.

Orabase HCA. (Colgate Oral Pharmaceuticals) Hydrocortisone acetate 0.5%, polyethylene 5%, mineral oil. Gel Tube 5 ml. *Rx.*
Use: Corticosteroid, dental.

Orabase Lip. (Colgate Oral Pharmaceuticals) Benzocaine 5%, allantoin 1.5%, menthol 0.5%, petrolatum, lanolin, parabens, camphor, phenol/g. Cream. 10 g. *otc.*
Use: Anesthetic, local.

Orabase Plain. (Colgate Oral Pharmaceuticals) Gelatin, pectin & sodium carboxymethyl cellulose in polyethylene and mineral gel. Paste. 5, 15 g. *otc.*
Use: Mouth and throat preparation.

Orabase with Benzocaine. (Colgate Oral Pharmaceuticals) Benzocaine 20% in gelbase. Gel Pkt 0.75 g, Box 100s. Tube 5 ml, 15 ml. *otc.*
Use: Anesthetic, local.

Oracap. (Vangard Labs, Inc.) Phenylpropanolamine HCl 75 mg, chlorpheniramine maleate 12 mg/Cap. Bot. 100s, 1000s. *Rx.*
Use: Antihistamine, decongestant.

Oracit. (Carolina Medical Products) Sodium citrate 490 mg, citric acid 640 mg/5 ml, (sodium 1 mEq/ml equivalent to 1 mEq bicarbonate), alcohol 0.25%. Soln. Bot. Pt, UD 15 ml, 30 ml. *Rx.*
Use: Alkalinizer, systemic.

Oraderm Lip Balm. (Schattner) Sodium phenolate, sodium tetraborate, phenol, base containing an anionic emulsifier. ⅛ oz. *otc.*
Use: Anesthetic; antiseptic, local.

Orafix Medicated. (SmithKline Beecham Pharmaceuticals) Allantoin 0.2%, benzocaine 2%. Tube 0.75 oz. *otc.*
Use: Anesthetic, local; denture adhesive.

Orafix Original. (SmithKline Beecham Pharmaceuticals) Tube 1.5 oz, 2.5 oz, 4 oz. *otc.*
Use: Denture adhesive.

Orafix Special. (SmithKline Beecham Pharmaceuticals) Tube 1.4 oz, 2.4 oz. *otc.*
Use: Denture adhesive.

Oragrafin Calcium Granules. (Bristol-Myers Squibb) Ipodate calcium (61.7% iodine) 3 g/8 g Pkg. 25 × 1 dose pkg.
Use: Radiopaque agent.

Oragrafin Sodium Capsules. (Bristol-Myers Squibb) Ipodate sodium 500 mg, iodine 307 mg. Cap. Bot. 6s, UD 100s. *Rx.*
Use: Radiopaque agent.

Orahesive. (Colgate Oral Pharmaceuticals) Gelatin, pectin, sodium carboxymethylcellulose. Pow. Bot. 25 g. *otc.*
Use: Denture adhesive.

Orajel. (Del Pharmaceuticals, Inc.) Benzocaine 10% in a special base. Gel Tube 0.2 oz, 0.5 oz. *otc.*
Use: Anesthetic, local.

Orajel D. (Del Pharmaceuticals, Inc.) Benzocaine 10%, saccharin. Gel Tube 9.45 ml. *otc.*
Use: Anesthetic, local.

Orajel Mouth-Aid. (Del Pharmaceuticals, Inc.) Benzocaine 20%. **Liq.:** Cetylpyridinium 0.1%, ethyl alcohol 70%, tartrazine, saccharin, 13.5 ml. **Gel:** Benzalkonium Cl 0.02%, zinc Cl 0.1%, EDTA, saccharin. 5.6 g, 10 g. *otc.*
Use: Anesthetic, local

Orajel Perioseptic. (Del Pharmaceuticals, Inc.) Carbamide peroxide 15% in anhydrous glycerin, saccharin, methylparaben, EDTA. Liq. Bot. 13.3 ml. *otc.*
Use: Mouth preparation.

Oral-B Muppets Fluoride Toothpaste. (Oral-B Laboratories, Inc.) Fluoride 0.22%. Pump 4.3 oz. *otc.*
Use: Dental caries agent.

oralcid.
See: Acetarsone.

oral contraceptives.
See: Demulen, Tab. (Searle).
Desogen, Tab. (Organon Teknika Corp.).
Enovid-E, Tab. (Searle).
GenCept, Tab. (Gencon).
Jenest-28, Tab. (Organon Teknika Corp.).
Loestrin, Prods. (Parke-Davis).
Lo/Ovral, Prods. (Wyeth-Ayerst Laboratories).
Modicon, Prods. (Ortho McNeil Pharmaceutical).
Nelulen, Tab. (Watson Laboratories).
Norethin 1/35 E, Tab. (Roberts Pharmaceuticals).
Norethin 1/50 M, Tab. (Roberts Pharmaceuticals).
Nordette, Tab. (Wyeth-Ayerst Laboratories).
Norinyl, Prods. (Roche Laboratories).
Norlestrin, Prods. (Parke-Davis).
Ortho Cept, Tab. (Ortho McNeil Pharmaceutical).
Ortho-Cyclen, Tab. (Ortho McNeil Pharmaceutical).
Ortho Tri-Cyclen, Tab. (Ortho McNeil Pharmaceutical).
Ortho-Novum, Prods. (Ortho McNeil Pharmaceutical).
Ovcon-35, Tab. (Bristol-Myers Squibb).
Ovcon-50, Tab. (Bristol-Myers Squibb).
Ovral, Tab. (Wyeth-Ayerst Laboratories).
Ovrette, Tab. (Wyeth-Ayerst Laboratories).
Ovulen, Tab. (Searle)
Triphasil, Tab. (Wyeth-Ayerst Laboratories).

Oral Drops/Canker Sore Relief. (Weeks & Leo) Carbamide peroxide 10% in anhydrous glycerin base. Bot. 30 ml. *otc.*
Use: Mouth preparation.

Oralone Dental. (Thames Pharmacal Co., Inc.) Triamcinolone acetonide 0.1%. Paste 5 g. *Rx.*
Use: Corticosteroid, dental.

oral rehydration salts.
Use: Electrolyte combination.

Oramide. (Major Pharmaceuticals) Tolbutamide 0.5 g/Tab. Bot. 100s, 1000s. *Rx.*
Use: Antidiabetic.

Oraminic II. (Vortech Pharmaceuticals) Brompheniramine maleate 10 mg/ml. Inj. Vial. 10 ml multidose. *Rx.*
Use: Antihistamine.

Oramorph SR. (Roxane Laboratories, Inc.) Morphine sulfate 15 mg, 30 mg, 60 mg, 100 mg, lactose. SR Tab. Bot. 50s (30 mg only), 100s, 250s (30 mg only), 500s (15 mg only), UD 25s (60 mg and 100 mg only), 100s (15 mg and 30 mg only). *c-II.*
Use: Analgesic, narcotic.

orange flower oil. N.F. XVII.
Use: Flavor, perfume, vehicle.

orange flower water. N.F. XVI.
Use: Flavor, perfume.
orange oil. N.F. XVI.
Use: Flavor.
orange peel tincture, sweet. N.F.XVI.
Use: Flavor.
orange spirit, compound. N.F.XVI.
Use: Flavor.
orange syrup. N.F. XVI.
Use: Flavored vehicle.
Orap. (Ortho McNeil Pharmaceutical) Pimozide 2 mg/Tab. Bot. 100s. *Rx.*
Use: Antipsychotic.
Oraphen-PD. (Great Southern Laboratories) Acetaminophen 120 mg/5 ml, alcohol 5%, cherry flavor. Elix. 120 ml. *otc.*
Use: Analgesic.
orarsan.
See: Acetarsone.
Orasept. (Pharmakon Laboratories, Inc.) Tannic acid 12.16%, methyl benzethonium HCl 1.53%, ethyl alcohol 53.31%, camphor, menthol, benzyl alcohol, spearmint oil, cassia oil. Liq. Bot. 15 ml. *otc.*
Use: Mouth and throat preparation.
Orasept, Throat. (Pharmakon Laboratories, Inc.) Benzocaine 0.996%, methyl benzethonium Cl 1.037%, sorbitol 70%, menthol, peppermint, saccharin. Throat spray. 45 ml. *otc.*
Use: Mouth and throat preparation.
Orasol. (Zenith Goldline Pharmaceuticals) Benzocaine 6.3%, phenol 0.5%, alcohol 70%, povidone-iodine. Liq. Bot. 14.79 ml. *otc.*
Use: Anesthetic, local.
Orasone. (Solvay Pharmaceuticals) Prednisone **1 mg, 5 mg, 10 mg, 20 mg/Tab:** Bot. 100s, 1000s, UD 100s. **50 mg/Tab.:** Bot. 100s, UD 100s. *Rx.*
Use: Corticosteroid.
OraSure HIV-1. (Epitope Inc.) Collection kit: Cotton fiber on a stick with collection vial. Device for oral specimen collection. For professional use only.
Use: Diagnostic aid.
Oratuss TR. (Vangard Labs, Inc.) Caramiphen edisylate 20 mg, chlorpheniramine maleate 8 mg, phenylpropanolamine HCl 50 mg, isopropamide iodide 2.5 mg/TR Cap. Bot. 100s, 500s. *Rx.*
Use: Anticholinergic, antihistamine, antispasmodic, antitussive, decongestant.
Orazinc. (Mericon Industries, Inc.) Zinc sulfate 220 mg/Cap. Bot. 100s, 1000s. *otc.*
Use: Mineral supplement.
orbenin. Sodium cloxacillin.
Use: Anti-infective.
See: Cloxapen (SmithKline Beecham Pharmaceuticals).
Orbiferrous. (Orbit) Ferrous fumarate 300 mg, vitamins B_{12} 12 mcg, C 50 mg, B_1 3 mg, defatted desiccated liver 50 mg/Tab. Bot. 60s, 500s. *otc.*
Use: Mineral, vitamin supplement.
Orbit. (Spanner) Vitamins A 6250 IU, D 400 IU, B_1 3 mg, B_2 3 mg, B_6 2 mg, B_{12} 5 mcg, C 75 mg, niacinamide 20 mg, calcium pantothenate 10 mg, E 15 IU, biotin 15 mcg, Fe 20 mg/Tab. Bot. 100s. *otc.*
Use: Mineral, vitamin supplement.
•**orbofiban acetate.** (ore-boe-FIE-ban) USAN.
Use: Fibrinogen receptor antagonist; platelet aggregation inhibitor, antithrombotic.
•**orconazole nitrate.** (ahr-KOE-nah-zole NYE-trate) USAN.
Use: Antifungal.
Ordrine. (Eon Labs Manufacturing, Inc.) Chlorpheniramine maleate 12 mg, phenylpropanolamine HCl 75 mg/SR Cap. Bot. 100s, 1000s. *Rx.*
Use: Antihistamine, decongestant.
Ordrine AT Extended Release. (Eon Labs Manufacturing, Inc.) Phenylpropanolamine HCl 75 mg, caramiphen edisylate 40 mg/Cap. Bot. 50s, 100s, 500s. *Rx.*
Use: Cough preparation.
Oretic. (Abbott Laboratories) Hydrochlorothiazide 25 mg, 50 mg/Tab. Bot. 100s, 1000s, UD 100s. *Rx.*
Use: Diuretic.
Oreton Methyl. (Schering-Plough Corp.) Methyltestosterone. **Buccal Tab.:** 10 mg. Bot. 100s. **Tab.:** 10 mg, 25 mg. Bot. 100s. *c-III.*
Use: Androgen.
Orexin. (Roberts Pharmaceuticals) Vitamins B_1 8.1 mg, B_6 4.1 mg, B_{12} 25 mcg/Chew. Tab. Bot. 100s. *otc.*
Use: Vitamin supplement.
Organidin. (Wallace Laboratories) **Tab.:** 30 mg. Bot. 100s. **Elix.:** 60 mg/5 ml. 21.75% alcohol, glucose, saccharin. Bot. Pt., gal. **Soln.:** 50 mg/ml. Bot. 30 ml w/dropper.
Use: Expectorant.
Organidin NR. (Wallace Laboratories) **Tab:** Guaifenesin 200 mg/Tab. Bot. 100s. **Liq:** Guaifenesin 100 mg/5 ml. Bot. pt, gal. *Rx.*
Use: Expectorant.
Orgaran. (Organon Teknika Corp.) Danaparoid sodium 750 anti-Xa units/0.6 ml, sodium sulfite/Inj. Box. Single-dose

amps and pre-filled syringes. 10s. *Rx.*
Use: Anticoagulant.

Orglagen. (Zenith Goldline Pharmaceuticals) Orphenadrine citrate 100 mg/Tab. Bot. 100s, 1000s. *Rx.*
Use: Muscle relaxant.

•**orgotein.** (ORE-go-teen) USAN. A group of soluble metalloproteins isolated from liver, red blood cells, and other mammalian tissues.
Use: Anti-inflammatory, antirheumatic.

orgotein. (Diagnostic Data) Pure water-soluble protein with a compact conformation maintained by 4 g atoms of chelated divalent metals, produced from bovine liver as a Cu-Zn mixed chelate having superoxide dismutase activity. Ontosein, Palosein.

orgotein for injection.
Use: Familial amyotrophic lateral sclerosis. [Orphan Drug]

Original Alka-Seltzer Effervescent. (Bayer Corp. (ConsumerDiv.)) 1700 mg sodium bicarbonate, 325 mg aspirin, 1000 mg citric acid, 9 mg phenylalanine, 506 mg Na, aspartame. Tab. Pkg. 24s. *otc.*
Use: Antacid.

Original Eclipse Sunscreen. (Tri Tec Laboratories) Padimate O, glyceryl PABA, SPF 10. Lot. Bot. 120 ml. *otc.*
Use: Sunscreen.

Original Sensodyne. (Block Drug Co., Inc.) Strontium chloride hexahydrate 10%, saccharin, sorbitol. Toothpaste. Tube 59.5 g. *otc.*
Use: Mouth and throat preparation.

Orimune. (Wyeth-Ayerst Laboratories) Poliovirus vaccine. Live, Oral, Trivalent. Sabin strains Types 1, 2, and 3. Dose of 0.5 ml Dispette disposable pipette 1 dose. 10s, 50s. *Rx.*
Use: Immunization.

Orinase. (Pharmacia & Upjohn) Tolbutamide 500 mg/Tab. Bot. 200s, unit-of-use 100s. *Rx.*
Use: Antidiabetic.

Orinase Diagnostic. (Pharmacia & Upjohn) Tolbutamide sodium 1 g/Vial. Pow. for inj. Vial with 20 ml amp diluent.
Use: Diagnostic aid.

Orisul. (Novartis Pharmaceutical Corp.) Sulfaphenazole. A sulfonamide under study.

ORLAAM. (Roxane) Levomethadyl acetate HCl 10 mg, methylparaben, propylparaben. Soln. Bot. 500 ml. *c-II.*
Use: Analgesic, narcotic.

•**orlistat.** (ORE-lih-stat) USAN.
Use: Inhibitor (pancreatic lipase).
See: Xenical (Roche).

•**ormaplatin.** (ORE-mah-PLAT-in) USAN.
Use: Antineoplastic.

•**ormetoprim.** (ore-MEH-toe-PRIM) USAN.
Use: Anti-infective.

Ornade Spansules. (SmithKline Beecham Pharmaceuticals) Phenylpropanolamine HCl 75 mg, chlorpheniramine maleate 12 mg/Cap. Bot. 50s, 500s. *Rx.*
Use: Antihistamine, decongestant.

Ornex. (Menley & James Labs, Inc.) Acetaminophen 325 mg, phenylpropanolamine HCl 12.5 mg/Capl. Blister Pak 24s, 48s. Bot. 100s. Dispensary pak 792s. *otc.*
Use: Analgesic, decongestant.

Ornex Maximum Strength. (Menley & James Labs, Inc.) Pseudoephedrine HCl, acetaminophen 500 mg. Cap. Bot. 24s, 30s, 48s. *otc.*
Use: Analgesic, decongestant.

Ornex No Drowsiness. (Menley & James Labs, Inc.) Pseudoephedrine HCl 30 mg, acetaminophen 325 mg. Tab. Bot. 24s, 100s, 1000s. *otc.*
Use: Analgesic, decongestant.

•**ornidazole.** (ahr-NIH-DAH-zole) USAN.
Use: Anti-infective.

Ornidyl. (Hoechst Marion Roussel) Eflornithine HCl 200 mg/ml. Inj. Vial. 100 ml. *Rx.*
Use: Antiprotozoal.

•**orpanoxin.** (AHR-pan-OX-in) USAN.
Use: Anti-inflammatory.

Orpeneed VK. (Hanlon) Penicillin, buffered, 400,000 units/Tab. Bot. 100s. *Rx.*
Use: Anti-infective, penicillin.

•**orphenadrine citrate.** (ore-FEN-uh-dreen) U.S.P. 23.
Use: Antihistamine, muscle relaxant.
See: Banflex (Forest Pharmaceutical, Inc.).
Flexoject (Merz Pharmaceuticals).
Flexon, Inj. (Keene Pharmaceuticals, Inc.).
Myolin (Roberts Pharmaceuticals).
Norflex, Tab., Amp. (3M Pharmaceuticals).
Orphanate, Inj. (Hyrex Pharmaceuticals).
W/Aspirin, phenacetin, caffeine.
See: Norgesic, Tab. (3M Pharmaceuticals).
Norgesic Forte, Tab. (3M Pharmaceuticals).

orphenadrine citrate. (Various Mfr.) **Inj:** 30 mg/ml. Amps 2 ml, vial 10 ml. **Tab.:**

100 mg. Bot. 30s, 100s, 500s, 1000s.
Use: Antihistamine, muscle relaxant.

Orphengesic. (Various Mfr.) Orphenadrine citrate 25 mg, aspirin 385 mg, caffeine 30 mg/Tab. Bot. 100s, 500s, UD 100s. *Rx.*
Use: Analgesic, muscle relaxant.

Orphengesic Forte. (Various Mfr.) Orphenadrine citrate 50 mg, aspirin 770 mg, caffeine 60 mg/Tab. Bot. 100s, 500s. *Rx.*
Use: Analgesic, muscle relaxant.

Ortac-DM. (ION Laboratories, Inc.) Dextromethorphan 10 mg, phenylephrine HCl 5 mg, guaifenesin 100 mg/5 ml. Liq. Bot. 4 oz. *otc.*
Use: Antitussive, decongestant, expectorant.

ortal sodium. Sodium 5-ethyl-5-hexylbarbiturate. Hexethal sodium.

ortedrine.
See: Amphetamine (Various Mfr.).

orthesin.
See: Benzocaine.

Ortho All-Flex Diaphragm. (Ortho McNeil Pharmaceutical) Diaphragm kit (all flex arcing spring) in plastic compact, sizes 55, 60, 65, 70, 75, 80, 85, 90, 95 mm. *Rx.*
Use: Contraceptive.

orthocaine.
See: Orthoform.

Ortho-Cept. (Ortho McNeil Pharmaceutical) Desogestrel 0.15 mg, ethinyl estradiol 0.03 mg. Tab. Pkg. 28s w/7 inert Tab. and 21s. *Rx.*
Use: Contraceptive.

Orthoclone OKT3. (Ortho McNeil Pharmaceutical) Muromonab-CD3 5 mg/5 ml. Inj. Amps 5 ml. *Rx.*
Use: Immunosuppressant.

Ortho-Cyclen. (Ortho McNeil Pharmaceutical) Norgestimate 250 mcg, ethinyl estradiol 35 mcg. Tab. Pkg. 21s, 28s. *Rx.*
Use: Contraceptive.

Ortho Diaphragm. (Ortho McNeil Pharmaceutical) Diaphragm kit, coil spring sizes 50, 55, 60, 65, 70, 75, 80, 85, 90, 95, 100, 105 mm. *Rx.*
Use: Contraceptive.

Ortho Diaphragm-White. (Ortho McNeil Pharmaceutical) Diaphragm kit, flat spring sizes 55, 60, 65, 70, 75, 80, 85, 90, 95 mm. *Rx.*
Use: Contraceptive.

Ortho Dienestrol Vaginal Cream. (Ortho McNeil Pharmaceutical) Dienestrol 0.01% Cream Tube 78 g with or without applicator. *Rx.*
Use: Estrogen.

Ortho-Est. (Ortho McNeil Pharmaceutical) Estropipate 0.75 mg, 1.25 mg, lactose. Tab. Bot. 100s. *Rx.*
Use: Estrogen.

Orthoflavin. (Enzyme Process) Vitamins C 150 mg, E 25 mg/Tab. Bot. 100s, 250s. *otc.*
Use: Vitamin supplement.

Orthoform. (Columbus) Tyrothricin 0.5 mg, tetracaine HCl 0.5%, epinephrine 1/1000 Soln. 2%/g. Oint. Tube oz. *Rx.*
Use: Anti-infective, ophthalmic.

Ortho-Gynol Contraceptive. (Advanced Care Products) Oxtoxynol 9. Gel Tube. 75 g w/ applicator and 75 g, 114 g refills. *otc.*
Use: Contraceptive.

ortho-hydroxybenzoic acid. Salicylic Acid, U.S.P. 23.

orthohydroxyphenylmercuric chloride.
Use: Antiseptic.
W/Benzocaine, ephedrine HCl.
See: Myrimgacaine, Liq. (Pharmacia & Upjohn).
W/Benzocaine, parachlorometaxylenol, benzalkonium Cl, phenol.
See: Unguentine, Aer. (Procter & Gamble Pharm.).
W/Benzoic acid, salicylic acid.
See: NP-27, Liq. (Procter & Gamble Pharm.).

Ortho-Novum 1/35-21. (Ortho McNeil Pharmaceutical) Norethindrone 1 mg, ethinyl estradiol 0.035 mg/Tab. Dialpak 21s. *Rx.*
Use: Contraceptive.

Ortho-Novum 1/35-28. (Ortho McNeil Pharmaceutical) Norethindrone 1 mg, ethinyl estradiol 0.035 mg/Tab. w/7 inert Tab. Dialpak 28s. *Rx.*
Use: Contraceptive.

Ortho-Novum 1/50-21. (Ortho McNeil Pharmaceutical) Norethindrone 1 mg, mestranol 50 mcg/Tab. Dialpak 21s. *Rx.*
Use: Contraceptive.

Ortho-Novum 1/50-28. (Ortho McNeil Pharmaceutical) Norethindrone 1 mg, mestranol 50 mcg/Tab. w/7 inert Tab. Dialpak 28s. *Rx.*
Use: Contraceptive.

Ortho-Novum 7/7/7-21. (Ortho McNeil Pharmaceutical) Norethindrone 0.5 mg, ethinyl estradiol 0.035 mg/Tab.; norethindrone 0.75 mg, ethinyl estradiol 0.035 mg/Tab.; norethindrone 1 mg, ethinyl estradiol 0.035 mg/Tab. Dialpak 21s. *Rx.*
Use: Contraceptive.

Ortho-Novum 7/7/7-28. (Ortho McNeil Pharmaceutical) Same as Ortho-Novum 7/7/7/-21 w/7 inert Tab. Dialpak

28s. *Rx.*
Use: Contraceptive.
Ortho-Novum 10/11-21. (Ortho McNeil Pharmaceutical) Norethindrone 0.5 mg, ethinyl estradiol 0.035 mg/Tab; norethindrone 1 mg, ethinyl estradiol 0.035 mg/Tab. Dialpak 21s. *Rx.*
Use: Contraceptive.
Ortho-Novum 10/11-28. (Ortho McNeil Pharmaceutical) Norethindrone 0.5 mg, ethinyl estradiol 0.035 mg/Tab; norethindrone 1 mg, ethinyl estradiol 0.035 mg/Tab w/inert Tab. Dialpak 28s. *Rx.*
Use: Contraceptive.
Ortho Personal Lubricant. (Advanced Care Products) Greaseless, water-soluble, and non-staining aqueous hydrocolloid gel. Acid buffered to vaginal pH. Tube 2 oz, 4 oz. *otc.*
Use: Lubricant.
Ortho Tri-Cyclen. (Ortho McNeil Pharmaceutical) 7 white tablets containing norgestimate 0.18 mg, ethinyl estradiol 35 mcg; 7 light blue tablets containing norgestimate 0.215 mg, ethinyl estradiol 35 mcg; 7 blue tablets containing norgestimate 0.25 mg, ethinyl estradiol 35 mcg.Tab. Pkg. 21s, 28s. *Rx.*
Use: Contraceptive.
Orthoxicol Cough Syrup. (Roberts Pharmaceuticals) Phenylpropanolamine HCl 8.3 mg, chlorpheniramine maleate 1.3 mg, dextromethorphan HBr 6.7 mg/5 ml, alcohol 8%, sorbitol, parabens. Bot. 60 ml, 120 ml, 480 ml. *otc.*
Use: Antihistamine, antitussive, decongestant.
orthoxine. Methoxyphenamine.
orticalm.
Use: Hypotensive, tranquilizer.
See: Serpasil, Prod. (Bristol-Myers Squibb)
Orudis. (Wyeth-Ayerst Laboratories) Ketoprofen 25 mg, 50 mg, 75 mg/Cap. Bot. **25 mg, 50 mg:** 100s; **75 mg:** 100s, 500s, UD 100s. *Rx.*
Use: Analgesic, NSAID.
Orudis KT. (Whitehall Robins Laboratories) **Tab.:** 12.5 mg ketoprofen, tartrazine, sugar. In 50s. *otc.*
Use: Analgesic, NSAID.
Oruvail. (Wyeth-Ayerst Laboratories) **SR Tab.:** Ketoprofen 100 mg, 150 mg, 200 mg/SR Tab. Bot. 100s, Redipak 100s. **SR Cap.:** 100 mg, 150 mg. 100s, Redipak 100s. *Rx.*
Use: Analgesic, NSAID.
orvus.
See: Gardinol Type Detergents (Various Mfr.).
osarsal.
See: Acetarsone.
Os-Cal 250. (Hoechst Marion Roussel) Oyster shell powder as calcium 250 mg, vitamin D 125 IU, and trace minerals (Cu, Fe, Mg, Mn, Zn, silica)/Tab. Bot. 100s, 240s, 500s, 1000s. *otc.*
Use: Mineral, vitamin supplement.
Os-Cal 500. (SmithKline Beecham Pharmaceuticals) Calcium 500 mg/Tab. Bot. 60s, 120s. *otc.*
Use: Mineral supplement.
Os-Cal 250 + D. (SmithKline Beecham Pharmaceuticals) Calcium carbonate 625 mg, vitamin D 125 units/Tab. Bot. 100s. *otc.*
Use: Mineral, vitamin supplement.
Os-Cal 500 + D. (SmithKline Beecham Pharmaceuticals) Calcium carbonate 1250 mg, vitamin D 125 units/Tab. Bot. 60s. *otc.*
Use: Mineral, vitamin supplement.
Os-Cal 500 Chewable Tablets. (SmithKline Beecham Pharmaceuticals) Calcium 500 mg/Chew. Tab. Bot. 60s. *otc.*
Use: Mineral supplement.
Os-Cal Fortified. (SmithKline Beecham Pharmaceuticals) Ca 250 mg, Fe 5 mg, Mg, Mn, zinc 0.5 mg, vitamin A 1668 IU, D 125 IU, B_1 1.7 mg, B_2 1.7 mg, B_3 15 mg, B_6 2 mg, C 50 mg, E 0.8 IU, parabens/Tab. Bot. 100s. *otc.*
Use: Mineral, vitamin supplement.
Os-Cal Fortified Multivitamin & Minerals. (SmithKline Beecham Pharmaceuticals) 1668 IU vitamin A, 125 IU D, 0.8 IU E, 1.7 mg B_1, 1.7 mg B_2, 15 mg B_3, 2 mg B_6, 50 mg C, 5 mg Fe, 250 mg Ca, 0.5 mg Zn, Mn, Mg, EDTA, parabens. Tab. Bot. 100s. *otc.*
Use: Mineral, vitamin supplement.
Os-Cal Plus. (SmithKline Beecham Pharmaceuticals) Ca 250 mg, vitamins D 125 IU, A 1666 IU, C 33 mg, B_2 0.66 mg, B_1 0.5 mg, B_6 0.5 mg, niacinamide 3.33 mg, Zn 0.75 mg, Mn 0.75 mg, Fe 16.6 mg/Tab. Bot. 100s. *otc.*
Use: Mineral, vitamin supplement.
Osmitrol. (Baxter Pharmaceutical Products, Inc.) Mannitol in water. **5%:** 1000 ml; **10%:** 500 ml, 1000 ml; **15%:** 150 ml, 500 ml; **20%:** 250 ml, 500 ml. Mannitol in 0.3% Na. **5%:** 1000 ml. Mannitol in 0.45% Na. **20%:** 500 ml. *Rx.*
Use: Diuretic.
See: Mannitol.
Osmoglyn. (Alcon, Surgical Division) Glycerin 50% in flavored aqueous vehicle. Plastic Bot. 6 oz. *Rx.*
Use: Diuretic.
Osmolite. (Ross Laboratories) Isotonic

liquid food containing 1.06 calories/ml. Two quarts (2000 calories) provides 100% US RDA vitamins and minerals for adults and children. Osmolality: 300 mOsm/kg water. Ready-to-Use: Bot. Can 8 fl oz, 32 fl oz. *otc.*
Use: Nutritional supplement.

Osmolite HN. (Ross Laboratories) High nitrogen isotonic liquid food containing 1.06 calories/ml; 1400 calories provides 100% USRDA vitamins and minerals for adults and children. Osmolality: 300 mOsm/kg water. Ready-to-Use: Bot. 8 fl oz. Can 8 fl oz, 32 fl oz. *otc.*
Use: Nutritional supplement.

Osmotic Diuretics.
See: Mannitol (Various Mfr.).
Osmitrol (Baxter Pharmaceutical Products, Inc.).
Ureaphil (Abbott Laboratories).
Osmoglyn (Alcon Laboratories, Inc.).
Ismotic (Alcon Laboratories, Inc.).

ospolot.
Use: Anticonvulsant drug; pending release.

Ossonate. (Marcen) Cartilage mucopolysaccharide extract, chondroitin sulfate 50 mg/Cap. Bot. 100s, 500s, 1000s.

Ossonate-Plus. (Marcen) Ossonate-mucopolysaccharide extract 50 mg, acetaminophen 300 mg, salicylamide 200 mg/Cap. Bot. 100s, 500s, 1000s. *otc.*
Use: Antiarthritic.

Ossonate-Plus, Inj. (Marcen) Ossonate cartilage mucopolysaccharide extract 12.5 mg, case in hydrolysates 80 mg, sulfur 20 mg, sodium citrate 5 mg, benzyl alcohol 0.5%, phenol 0.5%/ml. Multidose 10 ml vial. *Rx.*
Use: Muscle relaxant, pain reliever.

Ossonate-75. (Marcen) Chondroitin sulfate 37.5 mg, benzyl alcohol 0.5%, phenol 0.5%, sodium citrate 5 mg/ml. Vial 10 ml. *Rx.*
Use: Infantile and atopic eczemas, drug allergies, dermatoses associated with intestinal toxemias.

Osteocalcin. (Arcola Laboratories) Calcitonin-salmon 200 IU, phenol 5 mg/ml. Inj. Vial 2 ml. *Rx.*
Use: Hormone.

Osteo-D. (Teva Pharmaceuticals USA)
See: Secalciferol.

Osteolate. (Fellows) Sodium thiosalicylate 50 mg, benzyl alcohol 2%/ml. Inj. Vial 30 ml. *Rx.*
Use: Analgesic.

Osteo-Mins. (Tyson & Associates, Inc.) **Powd.:** 500 mg vitamin C, 250 mg Ca, 250 mg Mg, 45 mg K, 100 IU D/4.5 g. Sugar free. 200 g. *otc.*
Use: Vitamin supplement.

Osteon/D. (Taylor Pharmaceuticals) Ca 600 mg, P 400 mg, Mg 240 mg, vitamin D 400 IU/6 Tab. Bot. 180s. *Rx.*
Use: Mineral, vitamin supplement.

Osti-Derm Lotion. (Pedinol Pharmacal, Inc.) Aluminum sulfate, zinc oxide. Bot. 42.5 g. *otc.*
Use: Antipruritic; astringent, topical.

Osti-Derm Roll-On. (Pedinol Pharmacal, Inc.) Aluminum chlorohydrate, camphor, alcohol, EDTA, diazolidinyl urea. Bot. 88.7 ml. *otc.*
Use: Antipruritic; astringent, topical.

Osto-K. (Parthenon Co., Inc.) Potassium 1 mEq (39 mg from gluconate, Cl, and citrate), vitamin C 25 mg, sodium 0.52 mg/Tab. Bot. 60s. *otc.*
Use: Mineral, vitamin supplement.

osvarsan.
See: Acetarsone.

Otic-Care. (Parmed Pharmaceuticals, Inc.) Hydrocortisone 1%, neomycin sulfate 5 mg, polymyxin B sulfate 10,000 units/ml, glycerin, hydrochloric acid, propylene glycol, potassium metabisulfite. Soln. Bot. *Rx.*
Use: Otic.

Otic Domeboro. (Bayer Corp. (Consumer Div.)) Acetic acid 2%, aluminum acetate solution. Plastic Dropper Bot. 2 oz. *Rx.*
Use: Otic.

Otic-HC. (Roberts Pharmaceuticals) Chloroxylenol 1 mg, pramoxine HCl 10 mg, hydrocortisone alcohol 10 mg, benzalkonium Cl 0.2 mg/ml. Bot. 12 ml. *Rx.*
Use: Otic.

Otic-Neo-Cort Dome.
See: Neo-Cort Dome Otic Soln. (Bayer Corp. (Consumer Div.))

Otic-Plain. (Roberts Pharmaceuticals) Chloroxylenol 1 mg, pramoxine HCl 10 mg, benzalkonium Cl 0.2 mg/ml. Bot. 12 ml. *Rx.*
Use: Otic.

Otic Solution No. 1. (Foy Laboratories) Hydrocortisone alcohol 10 mg, pramoxine HCl 10 mg, benzalkonium Cl 0.2 mg, acetic acid glacial 20 mg/ml w/ propylene glycol q.s. Bot. *Rx.*
Use: Otic.

Oti-Med. (Hyrex Pharmaceuticals) Chloroxylenol 1 mg, pramoxine HCl 10 mg, hydrocortisone 10 mg/ml, propylene glycol, benzalkonium chloride. Drops. Vial 10 ml. *Rx.*
Use: Otic.

Otobiotic Otic Solution. (Schering-

Plough Corp.) Polymyxin B, hydrocortisone in propylene glycol and glycerin vehicle w/edetate disodium, sodium bisulfite, anhydrous sodium sulfite, purified water. Bot. w/dropper 15 ml. *Rx.*
Use: Otic.

Otocain. (Holloway) Benzocaine 20%, benzethonium Cl 0.1%, glycerin 1%, polyethylene glycol. Soln. Bot. 15 ml. *Rx.*
Use: Otic.

Otocalm-H Ear Drops. (Parmed Pharmaceuticals, Inc.) Pramoxine HCl 10 mg, hydrocortisone alcohol 10%, p-chloro-m-xylenol 1 mg, benzalkonium Cl 0.2 mg, acetic acid glacial 20 mg, propylene glycol/ml. Bot. 10 ml. *Rx.*
Use: Otic.

Otocort Sterile Solution. (Teva Pharmaceuticals USA) Neomycin sulfate equivalent to 3.5 mg neomycin base, polymyxin B sulfate 10,000 units, hydrocortisone 10 mg/ml, propylene glycol, glycerin, potassium metabisulfite, HCl, purified water. Bot. 10 ml. *Rx.*
Use: Otic.

Otocort Sterile Suspension. (Teva Pharmaceuticals USA) Neomycin sulfate equivalent to 3.5 mg neomycin base, polymyxin B sulfate 10,000 units, hydrocortisone 10 mg/ml, cetyl alcohol, propylene glycol, polysorbate 80, thimerosal, water for injection. Bot. 10 ml. *Rx.*
Use: Otic.

Otogesic HC Solution. (Lexis Laboratories) Polymyxin B sulfate 10,000 IU, neomycin sulfate 3.5 mg, hydrocortisone 10 mg/ml, potassium metabisulfite 0.1%. Bot. 10 ml. *Rx.*
Use: Otic.

Otogesic HC Suspension. (Lexis Laboratories) Polymyxin B sulfate 10,000 units, neomycin sulfate 3.5 mg, hydrocortisone 10 mg/ml, benzalkonium Cl 0.01%. Bot. 10 ml. *Rx.*
Use: Otic.

Otomar-HC. (Marnel Pharmaceuticals, Inc.) Chloroxylenol 1 mg, hydrocortisone 10 mg, pramoxine HCl 10 mg/ml. Otic Soln. Plastic dropper vials 10 ml. *Rx.*
Use: Otic preparation.

Otomycin-HPN. (Misemer Pharmaceuticals, Inc.) Polymyxin B sulfate 10,000 units, neomycin sulfate 3.5 mg, hydrocortisone 10 mg/ml. Bot. w/dropper 10 ml. *Rx.*
Use: Otic.

Otrivin. (Novartis Pharmaceutical Corp.) Xylometazoline HCl. **Nasal Drops:** 0.1% w/sodium Cl, phenyl mercuric acetate 1:50,000. Dropper bot. 20 ml. **Nasal Spray:** 0.1% w/potassium phosphate monobasic, potassium Cl, sodium phosphate dibasic, sodium Cl, benzalkonium Cl 1:5000. Plastic squeeze spray 15 ml. **Ped. Nasal Soln. Drops:** 0.05%. Bot. 20 ml. *otc.*
Use: Decongestant.

ouabain octahydrate. Ouabain, U.S.P. XX

ovarian extract. Aqueous extract of whole ovaries of cattle.
Use: Estrogen.

ovarian substance. (Various Mfr.) Whole ovarian substance from cattle, sheep, or swine. *Rx.*
Use: Estrogen.

Ovastat. (Medac Gmbtt c/o Princeton Regulatory Assoc.)
See: Treosulfan.

Ovcon-35. (Bristol-Myers Squibb) Norethindrone 0.4 mg, ethinyl estradiol 0.035 mg/Tab. Ctn. 6 × 21s. *Rx.*
Use: Contraceptive.

Ovcon-35, 28 Day. (Bristol-Myers Squibb) Norethindrone 0.4 mg, ethinyl estradiol 0.035 mg, w/7 inert Tab/Ctn. 6 × 28s. *Rx.*
Use: Contraceptive.

Ovcon-50. (Bristol-Myers Squibb) Norethindrone 1 mg, ethinyl estradiol 0.05 mg/Tab. Ctn. 6 × 21s. *Rx.*
Use: Contraceptive.

Ovcon-50, 28 Day. (Bristol-Myers Squibb) Norethindrone 1 mg, ethinyl estradiol 0.05 mg, w/ 7 inert Tab/Ctn. 6 × 28s. *Rx.*
Use: Contraceptive.

Ovide. (Medicis Dermatologicals, Inc.) Malathion 0.5%. Lot. Bot. 59 ml. *Rx.*
Use: Pediculicide, scabicide.

ovifollin.
See: Estrone (Various Mfr.).

Ovlin. (Sigma-Tau Pharmaceuticals, Inc.) **Tab.:** Ethinyl estradiol 0.02 mg, conjugated estrogens 0.2 mg/Tab. Bot. 100s, 1000s. **Inj.:** Estrone 2 mg, ethinyl estradiol 0.05 mg, vitamin B_{12} 1000 mcg/ml. Vial 30 ml. *Rx.*
Use: Estrogen.

Ovocylin Dipropionate. (Novartis Pharmaceutical Corp.) Estradiol dipropionate. *Rx.*
Use: Estrogen.

Ovral. (Wyeth-Ayerst Laboratories) Norgestrel 0.5 mg, ethinyl estradiol 0.05 mg/Tab. 6 Pilpak dispensers, 21 Tab. Tripak 63s. *Rx.*
Use: Contraceptive.

Ovral-28. (Wyeth-Ayerst Laboratories)

Norgestrel 0.5 mg, ethinyl estradiol 0.05 mg/Tab. w/7 inert Tab. Pilpak dispenser 6s containing 21 Tab, 7 inert Tab. *Rx.*
Use: Contraceptive.

Ovrette. (Wyeth-Ayerst Laboratories) Norgestrel 0.075 mg/Tab. 6 Pilpak dispenser, Tab. 28s. *Rx.*
Use: Contraceptive.

OvuGen. (BioGenex Laboratories) In vitro diagnostic test for measurement of LH urine to determine ovulation. Kits. 6s, 10s.
Use: Diagnostic aid, ovulation.

OvuKIT Self-Test. (Monoclonal Antibodies) Monoclonal antibody-based enzyme immunoassay test for hLH in urine. Kit 6, 9 day.
Use: Diagnostic aid, ovulation.

ovulation stimulants.
See: Clomid (Hoechst Marion Roussel).
Serophene (Serono Laboratories, Inc.).

ovulation tests.
See: Answer Ovulation (Carter Wallace).
Clearplan Easy (Whitehall Robins Laboratories).
Color Ovulation Test (Biomerica, Inc.).
Conceive Ovulation Predictor (Quidel Corp.).
First Response Ovulation Predictor Test Kit (Carter Wallace).
Fortel Home Ovulation Test (Biomerica, Inc.).
OvuGen (BioGenex Laboratories).
OvuKIT Self-Test (Monoclonal Antibodies).

Ovulen-21. (Searle) Ethynodiol diacetate 1 mg, mestranol 0.1 mg/Tab. Compack Disp. 21s, 6 × 21, 24 × 21. Refill 21s, 12 × 21. *Rx.*
Use: Contraceptive.

Ovulen-28. (Searle) Ethynodiol diacetate 1 mg, mestranol 0.1 mg/Tab. w/ 7 inert Tab. Compack 28s: 21 active tab., 7 placebo tab. Compack dispenser 28s. Box 6 × 28. Refill 28s, Box 12 × 28. *Rx.*
Use: Contraceptive.

Ovustick Self-Test. (Monoclonal Antibodies) Home test for ovulation. Test kit 10s.
Use: Diagnostic aid.

Oxabid. (Jamieson-McKames) Magnesium oxide 140 mg or magnesium oxide heavy 400 mg/Cap. Bot. 100s. *otc.*
Use: Antacid.

•**oxacillin sodium.** (ox-uh-SILL-in) U.S.P. 23.
Use: Anti-infective.
See: Bactocill, Vial (SmithKline Beecham Pharmaceuticals).

oxacillin sodium. (Teva) 250 mg/5 ml when reconstituted. Pow. for Oral Soln. Bot. 100 ml. *Rx.*
Use: Anti-infective, penicillin.

oxacillin sodium. (Various Mfr.) **Cap.:** 250 mg, 500 mg, Bot. 100s (except 500 mg), UD 100s. **Pow. for Inj.:** 250 mg, 500 mg, 1 g, 2 g, 4 g, 10 g. Vial (except 10 g), piggyback vial (1 g, 2 g only), Bulk Vial (10 g only). *Rx.*
Use: Anti-infective, penicillin.

oxadimedine hydrochloride.
Use: Antiarrhythmic.

oxafuradene. (OX-ah-FYOOR-ah-deen) Name used for Nifuradene.
Use: Platelet aggregation agent.

•**oxagrelate.** (OX-ah-greh-LATE) USAN.
Use: Platelet aggregation inhibitor.

oxaliplatin. (Axion Pharmaceuticals)
Use: Antineoplastic. [Orphan Drug]

•**oxamarin hydrochloride.** (OX-ah-mah-rin) USAN.
Use: Hemostatic.

•**oxamisole hydrochloride.** (ox-AM-ih-sole) USAN.
Use: Immunoregulator.

•**oxamniquine.** (ox-AM-nih-kwin) U.S.P. 23.
Use: Antischistosomal, treatment of schistosomiasis.
See: Vansil, Cap. (Pfizer US Pharmaceutical Group).

oxanamide.
Use: Anxiolytic.

Oxandrin. (Bio-Technology General Corporation) 2.5 mg oxandrolone, lactose. Tab. Bot. 100s. *c-III.*
Use: Anabolic steroid.

•**oxandrolone.** (ox-AN-droe-lone) U.S.P. 23.
Use: Androgen, anabolic. [Orphan Drug]
See: Anavar, Tab. (Searle).

•**oxantel pamoate.** (OX-an-tell PAM-oh-ate) USAN.
Use: Anthelmintic.

•**oxaprotiline hydrochloride.** (OX-ah-PRO-tih-leen) USAN.
Use: Antidepressant.

•**oxaprozin.** (OX-ah-pro-zin) USAN.
Use: Anti-inflammatory.
See: Daypro, Capl. (Searle).

•**oxarbazole.** (ox-AHR-bah-zole) USAN.
Use: Antiasthmatic.

•**oxatomide.** (ox-AT-ah-mid) USAN.
Use: Antiallergic, antiasthmatic.

•**oxazepam.** (ox-AZE-uh-pam) U.S.P. 23.
Use: Anxiolytic, sedative.
See: Serax, Cap., Tab. (Wyeth-Ayerst Laboratories).

oxazolindinediones.
See: Tridione (Abbott Laboratories).

ox bile extract. Purified ox gall.
See: Bile Extract, Ox.

•**oxendolone.** (OX-en-doe-LONE) USAN.
Use: Antiandrogen (benign prostatic hypertrophy).

•**oxethazaine.** (OX-ETH-ah-zane) USAN.
Use: Anesthetic, local.

•**oxetorone fumarate.** (ox-EH-toe-rone) USAN.
Use: Antimigraine.

•**oxfendazole.** (ox-FEN-DAH-zole) USAN.
Use: Anthelmintic.

oxfenicine. (OX-FEN-ih-seen) USAN.
Use: Vasodilator.

ox gall.
See: Bile Extract, Ox.

•**oxibendazole.** (ox-ee-BEND-ah-zole) USAN.
Use: Anthelmintic.

•**oxiconazole nitrate.** (ox-ee-KAHN-ah-zole) USAN.
Use: Antifungal.
See: Oxistat Cream, Lot. (GlaxoWellcome).

oxidized bile acids.
See: Bile Acids, Oxidized.

oxidized cellulose. Absorbable cellulose. Cellulosic acid.
Use: Hemostatic.
See: Oxycel, Pad, Pledg., Strip. (Becton Dickinson & Co.).
Surgicel, Strip (Johnson & Johnson).

•**oxidopamine.** (OX-ih-DOE-pah-meen) USAN.
Use: Adrenergic (ophthalmic).

•**oxidronic acid.** (OX-ih-DRAHN-ik) USAN.
Use: Regulator (calcium).

Oxi-Freeda. (Freeda Vitamins, Inc.) Vitamin A 5000 IU, E 150 mg, B_3 40 mg, C 100 mg, B_1 20 mg, B_2 20 mg, B_5 20 mg, B_6 20 mg, B_{12} 10 mcg, Zn 15 mg, Se, glutathione, L-cysteine. Tab. Bot. 100s, 250s. *otc.*
Use: Mineral, vitamin supplement.

•**oxifungin hydrochloride.** (OX-ih-FUN-jin) USAN.
Use: Antifungal.

•**oxilorphan.** (ox-ih-LORE-fan) USAN.
Use: Narcotic antagonist.

•**oximonam.** (OX-ih-MOE-nam) USAN.
Use: Anti-infective.

•**oximonam sodium.** (OX-ih-MOE-nam) USAN.
Use: Anti-infective.

oxine.
See: Oxyquinoline sulfate (Various Mfr.).

•**oxiperomide.** (ox-ih-PURR-oh-mide) USAN.
Use: Antipsychotic.

Oxipor VHC Psoriasis Lotion. (Whitehall Robins Laboratories) Coal tar soln. 25%, alcohol 79%. Lot. Bot. 56 ml. *otc.*
Use: Antipsoriatic.

•**oxiramide.** (ox-EER-am-ide) USAN.
Use: Cardiovascular agent.

Oxistat. (GlaxoWellcome) Oxiconazole nitrate 1%. **Cream:** Tube 15 g, 30 g, 60 g; Lot. Bot. 30 ml. *Rx.*
Use: Antifungal, topical.

•**oxisuran.** (OX-ih-SUH-ran) USAN.
Use: Antineoplastic.

•**oxmetidine hydrochloride.** (ox-MEH-tih-DEEN) USAN.
Use: Antiulcerative.

•**oxmetidine mesylate.** (ox-MEH-tih-DEEN) USAN.
Use: Antiulcerative.

•**oxogestone phenpropionate.** (ox-oh-JESS-tone fen-PRO-pih-oh-nate) USAN.
Use: Hormone, progestin.

Oxolamine. (Arcum) Crystalline hydroxycobalamin 1000 mcg/ml. Vial 10 ml. *Rx.*
Use: Vitamin supplement.

•**oxolinic acid.** (ox-oh-LIH-nik acid) USAN.
Use: Anti-infective.

l-2-oxothiazolidine$_4$-carboxylicacid.
Use: Treatment of adult respiratory distress syndrome. [Orphan Drug]
See: Procysteine.

Oxothiazolidine Carboxylate. (Clintec Nutrition; Ben Venise Labs) Phase I restoration of glutathione depletion in HIV, ARC, AIDS; prevention of inflammation-induced HIV replication. *Rx.*
Use: Immunomodulator.

•**oxprenolol hydrochloride.** (ox-PREH-no-lole) U.S.P. 23. Under study.
Use: Beta-adrenergic receptor blocker, vasodilator (coronary).

Oxsoralen Lotion. (ICN Pharmaceuticals, Inc.) Methoxsalen 1% in an inert lotion vehicle of alcohol 71%, propylene glycol, acetone, water. Lot. Bot. oz. *Rx.*
Use: Dermatologic.

Oxsoralen Ultra. (ICN Pharmaceuticals, Inc.) 10 mg methoxsalen. Soft Cap. Bot. 50s, 100s. *Rx.*
Use: Dermatologic.

•**oxtriphylline.** (ox-TRY-fih-lin) U.S.P. 23.
Use: Bronchodilator.
See: Choledyl, Tab., Elix. (Parke-Davis).
W/Guaifenesin.

See: Brondecon, Tab., Elix. (Parke-Davis).

oxtriphylline and guaifenesin elixir. (Alpharma USPD Inc.) Oxtriphylline 300 mg, guaifenesin 150 mg, alcohol 20%/15 ml. Elix. Bot. Pt, gal. *Rx.*
Use: Bronchodilator, expectorant.

Oxy-5 Acne-Pimple Medication. (SmithKline Beecham Pharmaceuticals) Benzoyl peroxide 5% in lotion base. Lot. Bot. oz. *otc.*
Use: Dermatologic, acne.

Oxy 5 Tinted. (SmithKline Beecham Pharmaceuticals) Benzoyl peroxide 5%, titanium dioxide, sodium PCA, cetyl alcohol, silica, iron oxides, propylene glycol, citric acid, sodium lauryl sulfate, stearyl alcohol, parabens. Lot. Bot. 30 ml. *otc.*
Use: Dermatologic, acne.

Oxy 10 Maximum Strength Advanced Formula. (SmithKline Beecham Pharmaceuticals) Benzoyl peroxide 10%, EDTA. Gel. 30 ml. *otc.*
Use: Dermatologic, acne.

•**oxybenzone.** (ox-ee-BEN-zone) U.S.P. 23.
Use: Ultraviolet screen.
W/Dioxybenzone, benzophenone.
See: Solbar, Lot. (Person and Covey, Inc.).

oxybenzone with combinations.
See: Coppertone, Prods. (Schering-Plough Corp.).
Noskote, Cream (Schering-Plough Corp.).
Shade, Prods. (Schering-Plough Corp.).
Super Shade, Lot. (Schering-Plough Corp).

•**oxybutynin chloride.** (OX-ee-BYOO-tih-nin) U.S.P. 23.
Use: Anticholinergic.
See: Ditropan (Hoechst Marion Roussel).

oxybutynin chloride. (Various Mfr.) **Tab.:** 5 mg. Bot. 100s, 500s, 1000s, UD 100s. **Syr.:** 5 mg/5 ml, sorbitol, sucrose, methylparaben. Bot. 473 ml. *Rx.*
Use: Antispasmodic.

Oxycel. (Becton Dickinson & Co.) Cellulosic acid in absorbable hemostatic agent prepared from cellulose. Resembles ordinary surgical gauze or cotton. Pledget 2 × 1 × 1 inch. 10s. Pad 3 × 3 inch. 8 ply. 10s. Strip 5 × 0.5 inch. 4 ply. 18 × 2 inch. 4 ply. 10s. 36 × 0.5 inch. 4 ply. *Rx.*
Use: Hemostatic, topical.

Oxycet. (Halsey Drug Co.) Oxycodone HCl 5 mg, acetaminophen 325 mg/Tab. Bot. 100s, 500s, Hospital pack 250s. *c-II.*
Use: Narcotic analgesic combination.

Oxy-Chinol. (Ferndale Laboratories, Inc.) Potassium oxyquinoline sulfate 1 gr/Tab. Bot. 100s, 1000s. *otc.*
Use: Antimicrobial, deodorant.

•**oxychlorosene.** (OCK-sih-KLOR-ah-seen) USAN. Monoxychlorosene. Hydrocarbon derivative containing fourteen carbons and hypochlorous acid. The hydrocarbon chain also has a phenyl substituent which in turn holds a sulfonic acid group.
Use: Anti-infective, topical.
See: Clorpactin, Prod. (Scrip)

•**oxychlorosene sodium.** (OCK-sih-KLOR-ah-seen) USAN. Sodium salt of the complex derived from hypochlorous acid and tetradecylbenzene sulfonic acid. Action of active chlorine.
Use: Anti-infective, topical.

Oxy Clean Lathering Facial. (SmithKline Beecham Pharmaceuticals) Sodium tetraborate decahydrate dissolving particles in a base of surfactant cleaning agents. Soap free. Scrub 79.5 g. *otc.*
Use: Dermatologic, acne.

Oxy Clean Medicated Cleanser and Pads. (SmithKline Beecham Pharmaceuticals) **Cleanser and reg. strength pads:** Salicylic acid 0.5%, SD alcohol 40B 40%, citric acid, menthol, sodium lauryl sulfate. **Max. strength pads:** Salicylic acid 2%, SD alcohol 40B 50%, citric acid, menthol, sodium lauryl sulfate. Cleanser 120 ml. Pad. 50s. *otc.*
Use: Dermatologic, acne.

Oxy Clean Medicated Pads for Sensitive Skin. (SmithKline Beecham Pharmaceuticals) Salicylic acid 0.5%, SD alcohol 40B 16%. Jar 50s. *otc.*
Use: Dermatologic, acne.

Oxy Clean Scrub. (SmithKline Beecham Pharmaceuticals) Sodium tetraborate decahydrate dissolving particles in a base of surfactant cleaning agents. Soap Free. Lot. Bot. 79.5 g. *otc.*
Use: Dermatologic, acne.

Oxy Clean Soap. (SmithKline Beecham Pharmaceuticals) Salicylic acid 3.5%, sodium borate. Bar 97.5 g. *otc.*
Use: Dermatologic, acne.

•**oxycodone.** (OX-ee-KOE-dohn) USAN.
Use: Analgesic, narcotic.

oxycodone and aspirin. (Various Mfr.) Oxycodone HCl 4.5 mg, oxycodone terephthalate 0.38 mg, aspirin 325 mg/

Tab. Bot. 100s, 500s, 1000s, UD 25s. *c-II.*
Use: Analgesic combination, narcotic.

oxycodone and acetaminophen capsules. (OX-ee-KOE-dohn and ass-cet-ah-MEE-noe-fen) (Various Mfr.) Oxycodone HCl 5 mg, acetaminophen 500 mg/Cap. Bot. 100s, 500s, 1000s, UD 25s. *c-II.*
Use: Analgesic combination, narcotic.

oxycodone and acetaminophen tablets. (OX-ee-KOE-dohn and ass-cet-ah-MEE-noe-fen) (Various Mfr.) Oxycodone HCl 5 mg, acetaminophen 325 mg/Tab. Bot. 100s, 500s, 1000s, UD 25s. *c-II.*
Use: Analgesic combination, narcotic.

•**oxycodone hydrochloride.** (OX-ee-KOE-dohn) U.S.P. 23.
Use: Analgesic, narcotic.
See: Dihydrohydroxycodeinone HCl.
OxyContin, CR Tab. (Purdue Frederick).
OxyFAST (Purdue Frederick).
OxyIR, IR Cap. (Purdue Frederick).
Percolone (Endo Laboratories).
Roxicodone (Roxane).
W/Acetaminophen, oxycodone terephthalate.
See: Tylox, Cap. (Ortho McNeil Pharmaceutical).

•**oxycodone terephthalate.** (OX-ee-KOE-dohn teh-REFF-thah-late) U.S.P. 23.
Use: Analgesic, narcotic.

OxyContin. (Purdue Frederick) Oxycodone HCl 10 mg, 20 mg, 40 mg, 80 mg, lactose. CR Tab. Bot. 100s, UD 25s. *c-II.*
Use: Analgesic, narcotic.

Oxy Cover. (SmithKline Beecham Pharmaceuticals) Benzoyl peroxide 10%. Cream. 30 g. *otc.*
Use: Dermatologic, acne.

oxyethylene oxypropylene polymer.
See: Poloxalkol.
W/Danthron, vitamin B_1, carboxymethyl cellulose.
See: Evactol, Cap. (Delta Pharmaceutical Group).

OxyFAST. (Purdue Frederick) Oxycodone HCl 20 mg/ml. Conc. Soln. Dropper Bot. 30 ml. *c-II.*
Use: Analgesic, narcotic.

•**oxyfilcon a.** (OX-ee-FILL-kahn A) USAN.
Use: Contact lens material (hydrophilic).

•**oxygen.** U.S.P. 23.
Use: Gas, medicinal.

•**oxygen 93 percent.** U.S.P. 23.
Use: Gas, medicinal.

OxyIR. (Purdue Frederick) Oxycodone HCl 5 mg/IR Cap. Bot. 100s. *c-II.*
Use: Analgesic, narcotic.

Oxy Medicated Cleanser and Regular Strength Pads. (SmithKline Beecham Pharmaceuticals) Salicylic acid 0.5%, SD alcohol 28%, citric acid, menthol, propylene glycol. Cleanser. Bot. 120 ml. Pads 50s, 90s. *otc.*
Use: Dermatologic, acne.

Oxy Medicated Cleanser and Maximum Strength Pads. (SmithKline Beecham Pharmaceuticals) Salicylic acid 2%, SD alcohol 44%, citric acid, menthol, propylene glycol. Cleanser. Bot. 120 ml. Pads 50s, 90s. *otc.*
Use: Dermatologic, acne.

Oxy Medicated Cleanser and Sensitive Skin Pads. (SmithKline Beecham Pharmaceuticals) Salicylic acid 0.5%, alcohol 22%, disodium lauryl sulfosuccinate, menthol, trisodium EDTA. Cleanser. Bot. 120 ml. Pads 50s, 90s. *otc.*
Use: Dermatologic, acne.

Oxy Medicated Soap. (SmithKline Beecham Pharmaceuticals) Triclosan 1%, bentonite, cocoamphodipropionate, iron oxides, glycerin, magnesium silicate, sodium borohydride, sodium cocoate, sodium tallowate, talc, EDTA, titanium dioxide. Bar. 97.5 g. *otc.*
Use: Dermatologic, acne.

•**oxymetazoline hydrochloride.** (OX-ee-MET-azz-oh-leen) U.S.P. 23.
Use: Decongestant; adrenergic (vasoconstrictor); mydriatic.
See: Afrin, Nasal Spray, Soln. (Schering-Plough Corp.).
Cheracol Nasal, Spray (Roberts Pharmaceuticals).
Dristan 12-Hr Nasal, Spray (Whitehall Robins Laboratories).
Duration Nasal Spray (Schering-Plough Corp.).
Duration Nose Drops (Schering-Plough Corp.).
Duration Nose Drops for Children (Schering-Plough Corp.).
Ocuclear Soln. (Schering-Plough Corp.).
St Joseph Nasal Spray for Children (Schering-Plough Corp.).
St Joseph Nose Drops for Children (Schering-Plough Corp.).
Visine Soln. (Pfizer US Pharmaceutical Group).

•**oxymetholone.** (OCK-sih-METH-oh-lone) U.S.P. 23.
Use: Androgen.
See: Anadrol, Tab. (Roche Laboratories).

•**oxymorphone hydrochloride.** (ox-ee-MORE-fone) U.S.P. 23.
Use: Analgesic, narcotic. [Orphan Drug]
See: Numorphan Amp., Vial, Supp. (Du Pont Merck Pharmaceutical Co.).

Oxy Night Watch. (SmithKline Beecham Pharmaceuticals) Salicylic acid 1%, cetyl alcohol, silica, propylene glycol, stearyl alcohol, sodium laureth sulfate, parabens, EDTA. Lot. Bot. 60 ml. *otc.*
Use: Dermatologic, acne.

Oxy Night Watch Maximum Strength. (SmithKline Beecham Pharmaceuticals) Salicylic acid 2%, cetyl alcohol, EDTA, parabens, stearyl alcohol. Lot. Bot. 60 ml. *otc.*
Use: Dermatologic, acne.

Oxy Night Watch Sensitive Skin. (SmithKline Beecham Pharmaceuticals) Salicylic acid 1%, cetyl alcohol, EDTA, stearyl alcohol, parabens. Lot. Bot. 60 ml. *otc.*
Use: Dermatologic, acne.

•**oxypertine.** (OX-ee-PURR-teen) USAN. Integrin hydrochloride.
Use: Psychotherapeutic agent, antidepressant.

•**oxyphenbutazone.** (ox-ee-fen-BYOO-tah-zone) U.S.P. 23.
Use: Analgesic, antiarthritic, anti-inflammatory, antipyretic, antirheumatic.

•**oxyphenisatin acetate.** (OX-ee-fen-EYE-sah-tin) USAN.
Use: Laxative.
See: Endophenolphthalein (Roche Laboratories).
Isacen (No Manufacturer Available).
Prulet, Tab. (Mission Pharmacal Co.).
Prulet, Liquitab. (Mission Pharmacal Co).

•**oxypurinol.** (OX-ee-PYOO-ree-nahl) USAN.
Use: Xanthine oxidase inhibitor.

•**oxyquinoline.** (OX-ih-KWIN-oh-lin) USAN.
Use: Disinfectant.

oxyquinoline benzoate. (Merck&Co.) Pkg. lb.

W/Alkyl aryl sulfonate, disodium edetate, aminacrine HCl, copper sulfate, sodium sulfate.
See: NP-27 Cream (Procter & Gamble Pharm.).

•**oxyquinoline sulfate.** (OX-ih-KWIN-oh-lin) N.F. 18.
Use: Disinfectant, pharmaceutic aid (complexing agent).
See: Chinositol, Tab., Pow., Vial (Vernon).

oxyquinoline sulfate w/combinations.
See: Oxyzal Wet Dressing, Soln. (Gordon Laboratories).
Rectal Medicone, Oint. (Medicore).
Rectal Medicone-HC, Oint. (Medicore).
Rectal Medicone Unguent, Oint. (Medicore).

Oxy-Scrub. (SmithKline Beecham Pharmaceuticals) Abradant cleanser containing dissolving abradant particles of sodium tetraborate decahydrate. Tube 2.65 oz. *otc.*
Use: Dermatologic, acne.

Oxysept. (Allergan, Inc.) **Disinfecting Soln.:** Hydrogen peroxide 3%, sodium stannate, sodium nitrate, phosphate buffer. Bot. 240 ml, 360 ml. **Neutralizer Tab.:** Catalase, buffering agents. In 12s (w/Oxy-Tab cup), 36s. *otc.*
Use: Contact lens care.

Oxysept 1. (Allergan, Inc.) Microfiltered hydrogen peroxide 3% w/sodium tannate and sodium nitrate, preservative free, buffered. Soln. Bot. 355 ml. *otc.*
Use: Contact lens care.

Oxysept 2. (Allergan, Inc.) Catalytic neutralizing agent, EDTA, sodium Cl, mono- and dibasic sodium phosphates. Buffered, preservative free. Soln. In 15 ml single-use containers (25s). *otc.*
Use: Contact lens care.

•**oxytetracycline.** (ox-ee-teh-trah-SIGH-kleen) U.S.P. 23.
Use: Anti-infective.
See: Terramycin, Prods. (Pfizer US Pharmaceutical Group).

oxytetracycline and hydrocortisone acetate ophthalmic suspension.
Use: Anti-infective, anti-inflammatory.

oxytetracycline and nystatin capsules.
Use: Anti-infective, antifungal.

oxytetracycline and nystatin for oral suspension.
Use: Anti-infective, antifungal.

oxytetracycline and phenazopyridine hydrochlorides and sulfamethizole capsules.
Use: Analgesic; anti-infective; antispasmodic, urinary.

•**oxytetracycline calcium.** U.S.P. 23.
Use: Anti-infective.

•**oxytetracycline hydrochloride.** U.S.P. 23. An antibiotic from *Streptomyces rimosus.*
Use: Anti-infective, antirickettsial.
See: Terramycin HCl, Preps. (Pfizer Laboratories).
Urobiotic (Roerig).

oxytetracycline hydrochloride and hydrocortisone ointment.

Use: Anti-infective, anti-inflammatory.

oxytetracycline hydrochloride and polymyxin B sulfate.
Use: Anti-infective.

oxytetracycline hydrochloride and polymyxin B sulfate ophthalmic ointment.
Use: Anti-infective.

oxytetracycline hydrochloride and polymyxin B sulfate topical powder.
Use: Anti-infective.

oxytetracycline hydrochloride and polymyxin B sulfate vaginal tablets.
Use: Anti-infective.

oxytetracycline-polymyxin B. Mix of oxytetracycline HCl and polymyxin B sulfate.
Use: Anti-infective.
See: Terramycin HCl w/Polymyxin B.

oxytocics.
See: Ergotrate Maleate, Inj. (Bedford Laboratories).
Methergine, Inj. (Novartis Pharmaceutical Corp.).

•**oxytocin.** (ox-ih-TOE-sin) U.S.P. 23.
Use: Oxytocic.
See: Pitocin, Amp. (Parke-Davis).

oxytocin nasal solution. (ox-ih-TOE-sin)
Use: Oxytocic.

oxytocin, synthetic. (ox-ih-TOE-sin)
See: Pitocin, Amp. (Parke-Davis).

Oxy Wash. (SmithKline Beecham Pharmaceuticals) Benzoyl peroxide 10%. Liq. Bot. 120 ml. *otc.*
Use: Dermatologic, acne.

Oxyzal Wet Dressing. (Gordon Laboratories) Benzalkonium Cl 1:2000, oxyquinoline sulfate, distilled water. Dropper bot. 1 oz, 4 oz. *otc.*
Use: Dermatologic, counterirritant.

Oysco. (Rugby Labs, Inc.) Elemental calcium 500 mg/Tab. Bot. 60s. *otc.*
Use: Mineral supplement.

Oysco D. (Rugby Labs, Inc.) Ca 250 mg, D 125 IU. Tab. Bot. 100s, 250s, 1000s. *otc.*
Use: Mineral, vitamin supplement.

Oyst-Cal 500. (Zenith Goldline Pharmaceuticals) Calcium carbonate 1.25 g (calcium 500 mg)/Tab. Bot. 60s, 120s. *otc.*
Use: Mineral supplement.

Oyst-Cal-D. (Zenith Goldline Pharmaceuticals) Calcium 250 mg, vitamin D 125 IU/Tab. Bot. 100s, 1000s. *otc.*
Use: Mineral, vitamin supplement.

Oyster Calcium. (NBTY, Inc.) Ca 275 mg, D 200 IU, A 800 IU. Tab. Bot. 100s. *otc.*
Use: Mineral, vitamin supplement.

Oyster Shell Calcium-500. (Vangard Labs, Inc.) Calcium carbonate 1.25 g, (calcium 500 mg). Tab. Bot. 100s, UD 100s, 640s. *otc.*
Use: Mineral supplement.

oyster shells.
See: Os-Cal, Tab. (Hoechst Marion Roussel).

Oystercal 500. (NBTY, Inc.) Calcium carbonate 1.25 g (calcium 500 mg)/Tab. Bot. 100s. *otc.*
Use: Mineral supplement.

Oystercal-D. (NBTY, Inc.) Calcium 250 mg, vitamin D 125 IU/Tab. Bot. 100s, 250s. *otc.*
Use: Mineral, vitamin supplement.

•**ozolinone.** (oh-ZOE-lih-NOHN) USAN.
Use: Diuretic.

P

P_1E_1; P_2E_1; P_3E_1; P_4E_1; P_6E_1. (Alcon Laboratories, Inc.) Pilocarpine HCl 1%, 2%, 3%, 4%, 6%, respectively, with epinephrine bitartrate 1%. Plastic dropper vial 15 ml. *Rx.*
Use: Antigout agent.

P and S Liquid. (Baker Cummins Dermatologicals, Inc.) Bot. 4 oz, 8 oz. *otc.*
Use: Antiseborrheic.

P and S Shampoo. (Baker Cummins Dermatologicals, Inc.) Salicylic acid 2%, lactic acid 0.5%. Bot. 4 oz. *otc.*
Use: Antiseborrheic.

Pabalate. (Wyeth-Ayerst Laboratories) Sodium salicylate 300 mg, sodium aminobenzoate 300 mg/EC Tab. Bot. 100s, 500s. *otc.*
Use: Antirheumatic.

Pabalate-SF. (Wyeth-Ayerst Laboratories) Potassium salicylate 300 mg, potassium aminobenzoate 300 mg/Tab. Bot. 100s, 500s. *otc.*
Use: Antirheumatic.

PABA-Salicylate. (Various Mfr.) Sodium salicylate, p-aminobenzoate, vitamin C/ Tab. Bot. 100s, 500s. *otc.*
Use: Analgesic, vitamin combination.

PABA sodium. (Various Mfr.) Sodium p-aminobenzoate. *otc.*
Use: Vitamin supplement.

Pabasone. (Pinex) Sodium salicylate 5 gr, para-aminobenzoic acid 5 gr, ascorbic acid 20 mg/Tab. Bot. 100s. *otc.*
Use: Analgesic, vitamin supplement.

P-A-C. Preparations of phenacetin, aspirin, caffeine.
See: A.P.C. Preparations, Empirin Preparations.

p-acetylaminobenzaldehyde thiosemicarbazone.
Use: Antituberculous.
See: Amithiozone, Antib, Berculon A, Benzothiozon, Conteben, Myuizone, Neustab, Tebethion, Thiomicid, Thioparamizone, Thiacetazone.

P-A-C Revised Formula Analgesic. (Pharmacia & Upjohn) Aspirin 400 mg, caffeine 32 mg/Tab. Bot. 100s, 1000s. *otc.*
Use: Analgesic.

Pacemaker Prophylaxis Pastes with Fluoride. (Pacemaker) Silicone dioxide and diatomaceous earth, sodium fluoride 4.4%. Light abrasive, cinnamon/cherry. Medium abrasive, orange. Heavy abrasive, mint. Paste Bot. 8 oz.
Use: Dental caries agent.

Pacerone. (Upsher-Smith) Amiodarone HCl 200 mg. Tab. Bot. 60s, 500s, UD 100s. *Rx.*
Use: Antiarrhythmic.

Packer's Pine Tar Liquid Shampoo. (Rydelle Laboratories) Pine tar. Bot. 6 fl oz. *otc.*
Use: Antiseborrheic.

Packer's Pine Tar Soap. (Rydelle Laboratories) Bar 3.3 oz. *otc.*
Use: Dermatologic.

Paclin VK. (Armenpharm Ltd.) Penicillin phenoxymethyl 125 mg, 250 mg/Tab. Bot. 100s, 1000s. *Rx.*
Use: Anti-infective, penicillin.

•**paclitaxel.** (pak-lih-TAX-uhl) USAN.
Use: Antineoplastic.
See: Taxol, Inj. (Bristol-Myers Squibb).

•**padimate a.** (PAD-ih-mate A) USAN.
Use: Ultraviolet screen.

•**padimate o.** (PAD-ih-mate O) U.S.P. 23.
Use: Ultraviolet screen.
See: Coppertone, Prods. (Schering-Plough Corp.).
Eclipse, Prods. (Novartis Pharmaceutical Corp.).
Noskote, Prods. (Schering-Plough Corp.).
Shade, Prods. (Schering-Plough Corp.).
Super Shade, Prods. (Schering-Plough Corp.).
Tropical Blend Sunscreen, Lot. (Schering-Plough Corp.).

•**pagoclone.** (PAG-oh-klone) USAN.
Use: Anxiolytic.

PAH.
See: Sodium Aminohippurate Inj. (Various Mfr.).

Pain-a-Lay. (Glessner) Antiseptic, anesthetic soln. Bot. 4 oz w/sprayer, Bot. 4 oz, 8 oz, pt.
Use: Mouth and throat preparation.

Pain and Fever Capsules. (ESI Lederle Generics) Acetaminophen 500 mg/Cap. Bot. 50s, 100s. *otc.*
Use: Analgesic.

Pain and Fever Liquid. (ESI Lederle Generics) Acetaminophen 160 mg/5 ml (children's strength). Unit-of-use 4 oz, Bot. 16 oz. *otc.*
Use: Analgesic.

Pain and Fever Tablets. (ESI Lederle Generics) Acetaminophen 325 mg, 500 mg/Tab. **325 mg:** Bot. 100s, 1000s. **500 mg:** Bot. 50s, 100s. *otc.*
Use: Analgesic.

Pain Bust-R II. (Continental Consumer Products) Methyl salicylate 17%, menthol 12%. Cream Jar 90 g. *otc.*
Use: Liniment.

Pain Doctor. (E. Fougera and Co.) Cap-

saicin 0.025%, methyl salicylate 25%, menthol 10%, parabens, propylene glycol. Cream Tube. 60 g. *otc.*
Use: Anesthetic, local.

Pain Gel Plus. (Mentholatum Co., Inc.) Menthol 4%, aloe, vitamin E. Gel Tube 57 g. *otc.*
Use: Liniment.

Pain Relief, Aspirin Free. (Hudson Corp.) Acetaminophen 325 mg/Tab. Bot. 100s, 200s. *otc.*
Use: Analgesic, local.

Pain Relief Ointment. (Walgreen Co.) Methyl salicylate 15%, menthol 10%. Tube 1.5 oz, 3 oz. *otc.*
Use: Analgesic, topical.

Pain Reliever. (Rugby Labs, Inc.) Acetaminophen 250 mg, aspirin 250 mg, caffeine 65 mg/Tab. Bot. 100s, 1000s. *otc.*
Use: Analgesic combination.

Pain Relievers-Tension Headache Relievers. (Weeks & Leo) Acetaminophen 325 mg, phenyltoloxamine citrate 30 mg/Tab. Bot. 40s, 100s. *otc.*
Use: Analgesic combination.

Pain-X. (B.F. Ascher and Co.) Capsaicin 0.05%, menthol 5%, camphor 4%, alcohols, parabens. Gel Tube. 42.5 g. *otc.*
Use: Topical pain reliever.

Palbar No. 2. (Roberts Pharmaceuticals) Atropine sulfate 0.012 mg, scopolamine HBr 0.005 mg, hyoscyamine HBr 0.018 mg, phenobarbital 32.4 mg/Tab. Bot. 100s. *Rx.*
Use: Anticholinergic, antispasmodic, sedative, hypnotic.

•**paldimycin.** (pal-dih-MY-sin) USAN.
Use: Anti-infective.

palestrol.
See: Diethylstilbestrol (Various Mfr.).

•**palinavir.** (pal-LIH-nah-veer) USAN.
Use: Antiviral.

palinum.
Use: Hypnotic, sedative.
See: Cyclobarbital Calcium (Various Mfr.).

palivizumab.
Use: Antibody.
See: Synagis (MedImmune).

Palmitate-A 5000. Vitamin A 5000 IU. Tab. Bot. 100s. *otc.*
Use: Vitamin supplement.

•**palmoxirate sodium.** (pal-MOX-ihr-ate) USAN.
Use: Antidiabetic.

•**palonosetron hydrochloride.** (pal-oh-NO-seh-trahn) USAN.
Use: Antiemetic, antinauseant.

PALS. (Palisades Pharmaceuticals, Inc.) Chlorophyllin copper complex 100 mg. Tab. Bot. 30s, 100s, 1000s, UD 30s. *otc.*
Use: Deodorant, systemic.

PAM.
See: Melphalan.

•**pamabrom.** USAN.
See: Maximum Strength Aqua-Ban, Tab. (Thompson Medical Co.).
W/Acetaminophen.
See: Fem-1 (BDI).
Pamprin, Tab. (Chattem Consumer Products).
W/Acetaminophen, pyrilamine maleate.
See: Cardui, Tab. (Chattem Consumer Products).
Fem-1, Tab. (BDI Pharmaceuticals, Inc.).
Sunril, Cap. (Schering-Plough Corp.).
W/Pyrilamine maleate, homatropine methylbromide, hyoscyamine sulfate, scopolamine HBr, methamphetamine HCl.
See: Aridol, Tabs. (MPL).

•**pamaqueside.** (pam-ah-KWEH-side) USAN.
Use: Antiatherosclerotic, hypocholesterolemic.

•**pamatolol sulfate.** (PAM-ah-TOE-lole) USAN.
Use: Anti-adrenergic (β-receptor).

Pamelor. (Novartis Pharmaceutical Corp.) Nortriptyline HCl. Cap or Liq. **Cap.:** 10 mg, 25 mg, 50 mg, 75 mg base. **10 mg:** Bot. 100s, SandoPak 100s. **25 mg:** Bot. 100s, 500s, SandoPak 100s. **50 mg:** Bot. 100s, SandoPak 100s. **75 mg:** Bot. 100s. **Liq.:** Nortriptyline HCl equivalent to 10 mg base/5 ml. Bot. pt. *Rx.*
Use: Antidepressant.

•**pamidronate disodium.** (pam-IH-DROE-nate) USAN.
Use: Bone resorption inhibitor.
See: Aredia, Inj. (Novartis Pharmaceutical Corp.).

Pamine. (Kenwood Laboratories) Methscopolamine bromide 2.5 mg/Tab. Bot. 100s, 500s. *Rx.*
Use: Anticholinergic, antispasmodic.

p-aminobenzene-sulfonylacetylimide.
See: Sulfacetamide.

p-aminosalicylic acid salts.
See: Aminosalicylic acid salts.

Pamprin. (Chattem Consumer Products) Acetaminophen 400 mg, pamabrom 25 mg, pyrilamine maleate 15 mg/Tab. Bot. 24s, 48s. *otc.*
Use: Analgesic combination.

Pamprin Extra Strength Multi-Symp-

tom Relief Formula Tablets. (Chattem Consumer Products) Acetaminophen 400 mg, pamabrom 25 mg, pyrilamine maleate 15 mg/Tab. Bot. 12s, 24s, 48s. *otc.*
Use: Analgesic combination.

Pamprin Maximum Cramp Relief Formula Caplets. (Chattem Consumer Products) Acetaminophen 500 mg, pamabrom 25 mg, pyrilamine maleate 15 mg/Tab. Bot. 8s, 16s, 32s. *otc.*
Use: Analgesic combination.

Pamprin Multi-Symptom Caplets and Tablets. (Chattem Consumer Products) Acetaminophen 500 mg, pamabrom 25 mg, pyrilamine maleate 15 mg. Capl. Bot. 24s, 48s. Tab. Bot. 12s, 24s, 48s. *otc.*
Use: Analgesic combination.

Panacet 5/500. (ECR Pharmaceuticals) Hydrocodone bitartrate 5 mg, acetaminophen 500 mg. Tab. Bot. 100s. *c-III.*
Use: Analgesic combination, narcotic.

•**panadiplon.** (pan-ad-IH-plone) USAN.
Use: Anxiolytic.

Panadol. (Bayer Corp. (Consumer Div.)) Acetaminophen 500 mg/Tab. or Cap. **Tab.:** Bot. 2s, 30s, 60s, 100s. **Cap.:** Bot. 10s, 24s, 48s. *otc.*
Use: Analgesic.

Panadol, Children's. (Bayer Corp. (Consumer Div.)) Acetaminophen. **Tab.:** 80 mg. Bot. 30s. **Liq.:** 80 mg/0.8 ml. Bot. 2 oz, 4 oz. **Drops:** 80 mg/0.5 oz. Bot. 0.5 oz. *otc.*
Use: Analgesic.

Panadol, Infants' Drops. (Bayer Corp. (Consumer Div.)) Acetaminophen 100 mg/ml. Bot. 15 ml with 0.8 ml dropper. *otc.*
Use: Analgesic.

Panadol, Jr. (Bayer Corp. (Consumer Div.)) Acetaminophen 160 mg/Capl. Box. 30s. *otc.*
Use: Analgesic.

Panadyl. (Misemer Pharmaceuticals, Inc.) Pyrilamine maleate 25 mg, phenylpropanolamine HCl 50 mg, pheniramine maleate 25 mg/Tab. Bot. 100s, 1000s. *Rx.*
Use: Antihistamine, decongestant.

Panadyl Forte. (Misemer Pharmaceuticals, Inc.) Phenylpropanolamine HCl 50 mg, phenylephrine HCl 25 mg, chlorpheniramine maleate 8 mg/Tab. Bot. 100s. *Rx.*
Use: Antihistamine, decongestant.

Panafil. (Rystan, Inc.) Papain pow. 10%, urea 10%, chlorophyllin copper complex 0.5%, hydrophilic base. Oint. Tube oz, Jar lb. *Rx.*
Use: Enzyme, topical.

Panafil White Ointment. (Rystan, Inc.) Papain 10,000 units enzyme activity, hydrophilic base/g, urea 10%. Tube oz. *Rx.*
Use: Enzyme, topical.

Panalgesic Cream. (ECR Pharmaceuticals) Methyl salicylate 35%, menthol 4%. Jar 4 oz. *otc.*
Use: Analgesic, topical.

Panalgesic Liquid. (ECR Pharmaceuticals) Methyl salicylate 55.01%, menthol 1.25%, camphor 3.1%, in alcohol 22%, emollients, color. Bot. 4 oz, pt, 0.5 gal. *otc.*
Use: Analgesic, topical.

Panasal 5/500. (E.C. Robins) Hydrocodone bitartrate 5 mg, aspirin 500 mg. Tab. Bot. 100s. *c-III.*
Use: Analgesic combination, narcotic.

Panasol. (Seatrace Pharmaceuticals, Inc.) Prednisone 5 mg/Tab. Bot. 100s. *Rx.*
Use: Corticosteroid.

Panasol-S. (Seatrace Pharmaceuticals, Inc.) Prednisone 1 mg/Tab. Bot. 100s, 1000s. *Rx.*
Use: Corticosteroid.

Pan C-500. (Freeda Vitamins, Inc.) Hesperidin 100 mg, citrus bioflavonoids 100 mg, rutin 50 mg, vitamin C 500 mg/Tab. Bot. 100s, 250s, 500s. *otc.*
Use: Vitamin supplement.

Pancof-HC. (Pan American Labs) Hydrocodone bitartrate 2.5 mg, chlorpheniramine 2 mg, pseudoephedrine 15 mg/5 ml, dye and alcohol free. Liq. Bot. 25 ml, pt. *c-III.*
Use: Antihistamine, antitussive, decongestant.

•**pancopride.** (PAN-koe-pride) USAN.
Use: Antiemetic, anxiolytic, peristaltic stimulant.

Pancrease. (Ortho McNeil Pharmaceutical) Enteric coated pancrelipase capsules. **Regular:** Lipase 4500 units, amylase 20,000 units, protease 25,000 units/Cap. Sugar. Dye free. Bot. 100s, 250s. **MT4:** Lipase 4500 units, amylase 12,000 units, protease 12,000 units/Cap. Bot. 100s. **MT10:** Lipase 10,000 units, amylase 30,000 units, protease 30,000 units/Cap. Bot. 100s. **MT16:** Lipase 16,000 units, amylase 48,000 units, protease 48,000 units/Cap. Bot. 100s. **MT20:** Lipase 20,000 units, amylase 56,000 units, protease 44,000 units/Cap. Bot. 100s. **MT 25:** Lipase 25,000 units, amylase 70,000 units, protease 55,000 units. Cap. Bot. 100s. **MT 32:** Lipase 32,000 units, amylase

90,000 units, protease 70,000 units. Cap. Bot. 100s. *Rx.*
Use: Digestive enzyme.

pancreatic enzyme.
See: Pepsin, ox bile.

pancreatic substance. Substance from fresh pancreas of hog or ox, containing the enzymes amylopsin, trypsin, steapsin.
W/Bile extract, dl-methionine, choline bitartrate.
See: Pancobile, Tab. (Solvay Pharmaceuticals).
W/Lipase.
See: Cotazym, Cap., Pkt. (Organon Teknika Corp.).

•**pancreatin.** (PAN-kree-ah-tin) U.S.P. 23. Pancreatic enzymes obtained from hog or cattle pancreatic tissue.
Use: Enzyme (digestant adjunct).

•**pancrelipase.** (pan-KREE-lih-pace) U.S.P. 23. Preparation of hog pancreas with high content of steapsin and adequate amounts of pancreatic enzymes.
Use: Enzyme (digestant adjunct).
See: Cotazym, Cap., Pkt. (Organon Teknika Corp.).
W/Mixed conjugated bile salts, cellulase.
See: Viokase, Pow., Tab. (Wyeth-Ayerst Laboratories).

Pancretide. (Baxter Pharmaceutical Products, Inc.) Pancreatic polypeptide in normal saline.
Use: Fibrinolytic conditions.

pancuronium. (PAN-cue-ROW-nee-uhm)
See: Pancuronium Bromide (Organon Teknika Corp.).

•**pancuronium bromide.** (PAN-cue-ROW-nee-uhm) USAN.
Use: Neuromuscular blocker.
See: Pavulon, Inj. (Organon Teknika Corp.).

pancuronium bromide. (Various Mfr.) **1 mg/ml:** Vials 10 ml. **2 mg/ml:** Vials, amps, syringes. 2 ml, 5 ml.
Use: Neuromuscular blocker.

Pandel. (Savage Laboratories) Hydrocortisone buteprate 0.1%. Cream Tube 15 g, 45 g. *Rx.*
Use: Corticosteroid, topical.

Panex. (Roberts Pharmaceuticals) Acetaminophen 325 mg/Tab. Bot. 1000s. *otc.*
Use: Analgesic.

Panex 500. (Roberts Pharmaceuticals) Acetaminophen 500 mg/Tab. Bot. 1000s. *otc.*
Use: Analgesic.

Panhematin. (Abbott Laboratories) Hemin 301 mg/2 ml when reconstituted, 300 mg sorbitol. Inj. Vial 2 ml. *Rx.*
Use: Hematinic.

Panitol. (Wesley Pharmacal Co., Inc.) Allylisobutyl barbituric acid 15 mg, acetaminophen 300 mg/Tab. Bot. 100s, 1000s. *Rx.*
Use: Analgesic, hypnotic, sedative.

Panmist JR. (Pan American Labs) Pseudoephedrine 45 mg, guaifenesin 600 mg, dye free. LA Tab. Bot. 100s. *Rx.*
Use: Decongestant, expectorant.

Panmycin. (Pharmacia & Upjohn) Tetracycline HCl 250 mg/Cap. Bot. 100s, 1000s. *Rx.*
Use: Anti-infective, tetracycline.
See: Panmycin, Cap. (Pharmacia & Upjohn).

Pannaz. (Pan American Labs) Phenylpropanolamine 75 mg, chlorpheniramine 6 mg, methscopolamine 2.5 mg. Tab. Bot. 100s *Rx.*
Use: Anticholinergic, antihistamine, decongestant.

PanOxyl 5, 10 Acne Gel. (Stiefel Laboratories, Inc.) Benzoyl peroxide 5%, 10%, alcohol 20% in a hydroalcoholic gel base. Tube 56.7 g, 113.4 g. *Rx.*
Use: Dermatologic, acne.

PanOxyl AQ 2.5, 5, 10 Acne Gel. (Stiefel Laboratories, Inc.) Benzoyl peroxide 2.5%, 5%, 10%, methylparaben, EDTA in an aqueous gel base. Tube 56.7 g, 113.4 g. *Rx.*
Use: Dermatologic, acne.

PanOxyl Bar. (Stiefel Laboratories, Inc.) Benzoyl peroxide 5% cetostearyl alcohol, EDTA, glycerin, castor oil, mineral oil in a rich-lathering, mild surfactant cleansing base. Bar 113 g. *otc.*
Use: Dermatologic, acne.

PanOxyl-10 Bar. (Stiefel Laboratories, Inc.) Benzoyl peroxide 10% cetostearyl alcohol, castor oil, mineral oil, soap free in rich-lathering, mild surfactant cleansing base. Bar 113 g. *otc.*
Use: Dermatologic, acne.

panparnit hydrochloride. Caramiphen HCl.
Use: Antiparkinsonian.

Panretin. (Ligand Pharmaceuticals, Inc.) Alitretinoin 0.1%. Gel Tube 60 g. *Rx.*
Use: Endogenous retinoid.

Panscol. (Baker Cummins Dermatologicals, Inc.) Salicylic acid 3%, lactic acid 2%, phenol (< 1%). **Oint.:** Jar 3 oz. **Lot.:** Bot. 4 oz. *otc.*
Use: Emollient.

•**panthenol.** (PAN-theh-nahl) U.S.P. 23. Alcohol corresponding to pantothenic acid. Pantothenol. Pantothenylol.
Use: Treatment of paralytic ileus and

postoperative distention; vitamin.
See: Ilopan, Amp., Vial (Warren-Teed).
Panthoderm, Cream (Rhone-Poulenc Rorer Pharmaceuticals, Inc.).

panthenol w/combinations.
See: Lifer-B, Liq. (Burgin-Arden).

Panthoderm Cream. (Rhone-Poulenc Rorer Pharmaceuticals, Inc.) Dexpanthenol 2% in water-miscible cream. Tube 1 oz, Jar 2 oz, lb. *otc.*
Use: Emollient.

pantocaine.
See: Tetracaine HCl (Various Mfr.).

Pantocrin-F. (Spanner) Plurigland, ovarian, anterior and posterior pituitary, adrenal, thyroid extracts. Vial 30 ml. *Rx.*
Use: Hormone.

Pantopaque. (Alcon, Surgical Division) Iophendylate, ethyl iodophenylundecanoate. Amp. 3 ml 3s; 6 ml 6s; 1 ml 2s.
Use: Radiopaque agent.

•**pantoprazole.** (pahn-TOE-prazz-ole) USAN.
Use: Antiulcerative.

pantothenic acid. As calcium or sodium salt.
Use: Vitamin B_5 supplement.
See: Vitamin preparations.

pantothenic acid salts.
See: Calcium Pantothenate.
Sodium Pantothenate.

pantothenol.
See: Panthenol, Preps. (Various Mfr.).

pantothenyl alcohol.
See: Panthenol, Preps. (Various Mfr.).

pantothenylol.
See: Panthenol, Preps. (Various Mfr.).

Panvitex Geriatric. (Forest Pharmaceutical, Inc.) Safflower oil 340 mg, vitamins A 10,000 IU, D 400 IU, B_1 5 mg, B_6 1 mg, B_2 2.5 mg, B_{12} activity 2 mcg, C 75 mg, niacinamide 40 mg, calcium pantothenate 4 mg, E 2 IU, inositol 15 mg, choline bitartrate 31.4 mg, Ca 75 mg, P 58 mg, Fe 30 mg, Mn 0.5 mg, K 2 mg, Zn 0.5 mg, Mg 3 mg/Cap. Bot. 100s, 1000s. *otc.*
Use: Mineral, vitamin supplement.

Panvitex Plus Minerals. (Forest Pharmaceutical, Inc.) Vitamins A 5000 IU, D 400 IU, B_1 3 mg, B_2 2.5 mg, niacinamide 20 mg, B_6 1.5 mg, calcium pantothenate 5 mg, B_{12} 2.5 mcg, C 50 mg, E 3 IU, Ca 215 mg, P 166 mg, Fe 13.4 mg, Mg 7.5 mg, Mn 1.5 mg, K 5 mg, Zn 1.4 mg/Cap. Bot. 100s, 1000s. *otc.*
Use: Mineral, vitamin supplement.

Panvitex Prenatal. (Forest Pharmaceutical, Inc.) Ferrous fumarate 150 mg, cobalamin concentration 2 mcg, vitamins A 6000 IU, D 400 IU, B_1 1.5 mg, B_2 2.5 mg, niacinamide 15 mg, B_6 3 mg, C 100 mg, Ca 250 mg, calcium pantothenate 5 mg, folic acid 0.2 mg/Cap. Bot. 100s, 1000s. *otc.*
Use: Mineral, vitamin supplement.

Panvitex T-M. (Forest Pharmaceutical, Inc.) Vitamins A 10,000 IU, D 400 IU, B_1 10 mg, B_6 1 mg, B_2 5 mg, B_{12} 5 mcg, C 150 mg, niacinamide 100 mg, Ca 103 mg, P 80 mg, Fe 10 mg, Mn 1 mg, K 5 mg, Zn 1.4 mg, Mg 5.56 mg/Cap. Bot. 100s, 1000s. *otc.*
Use: Mineral, vitamin supplement.

PAP. (Abbott Diagnostics) Enzyme immunoassay for measurement of prostatic acid phosphatase. Test kit 100s.
Use: Diagnostic aid.

Papadeine #3. (Vangard Labs, Inc.) Codeine phosphate 30 mg, acetaminophen 300 mg/Tab. Bot. 100s, 1000s. *c-III.*
Use: Analgesic combination, narcotic.

•**papain.** (pap-ANE) U.S.P. 23. A proteolytic substance derived from *Carlica papaya.*
Use: Proteolytic enzyme.

papain w/combinations.
See: Accuzyme (Healthpoint Medical).
Panafil, Oint. (Rystan, Inc.).

Pap-a-Lix. (Freeport) n-acetyl-aminophenol 120 mg, alcohol 10%/5 ml. Bot. 4 oz, gal. *otc.*
Use: Analgesic.

•**papaverine hydrochloride.** (pap-PAV-uhr-een) U.S.P. 23.
Use: Muscle relaxant.
See: BP-Papaverine, Cap. (Burlington).
Cerespan, Cap. (Rhone-Poulenc Rorer Pharmaceuticals, Inc.).
Cirbed, Cap. (Boyd).
Delapav, Time Cap. (Dunhall Pharmaceuticals, Inc.).
Myobid, Cap. (Laser, Inc.).
P-200, Cap. (Knoll Pharmaceuticals).
Pavabid, Cap. (Hoechst Marion Roussel).
Pavacap, Unicells (Solvay Pharmaceuticals).
Pavacaps, Cap. (Freeport).
Pavacen Cenules, Cap. (Schwarz Pharma, Inc.).
Pavaclor, Cap. (Taylor Pharmaceuticals).
Pavadel, Cap. (Canright).
Pavadyl, Cap. (Sanofi Winthrop Pharmaceuticals).
Pavakey 300, Cap. (Key Pharmaceuticals).
Pavakey S.A., Cap. (Key Pharmaceuticals).

Pava-lyn, Cap. (Lynwood).
Pava Par, Cap. (Parmed Pharmaceuticals, Inc.).
Pavasule, Cap. (Jalco).
Pavatest T.D., Cap. (Fellows-Testagar).
Pavatym, Cap. (Everett Laboratories, Inc.).
Pavatran T.D., Cap. (Merz Pharmaceuticals).
Vasocap, Cap. (Keene Pharmaceuticals, Inc).

W/Codeine sulfate.
See: Vazosan, Tab. (Sandia).

W/Codeine sulfate, emetine HCl, ephedrine HCl.
See: Copavin Compound, Elix. (Eli Lilly and Co.).

W/Codeine sulfate, aloin, sodium salicylate.
See: Copavin, Pulvule, Tab. (Eli Lilly and Co.).

W/Phenobarbital.
See: Golacol, Syr. (Arcum).
See: Pavadel PB, Cap. (Canright).

Paplex Ultra. (Medicis Dermatologicals, Inc.) Salicylic acid 26% in flexible collodion. Bot. 15 ml. *otc.*
Use: Keratolytic.

para-aminobenzoic acid. (Various Mfr.). **Tab.:** 100 mg, 500 mg. Bot. 100s, 250s (100 mg only). **Pow.:** 120 g. *otc.*
Use: Sunscreen, agent for scleroderma.
See: Potaba, Tab., Cap., Powd., envules. (Glenwood, Inc.).

para-aminosalicylic acid. U.S.P. 23. Aminosalicylic Acid. *Rx.*
Use: Antituberculosis.

Parabaxin. (Parmed Pharmaceuticals, Inc.) Methocarbamol 500 mg, 750 mg/Tab. Bot. 100s. *Rx.*
Use: Muscle relaxant.

parabrom.
See: Pyrabrom.

parabromidylamine.
See: Brompheniramine, Dimetane, Preps. (Wyeth-Ayerst Laboratories).

paracain.
See: Procaine Hydrochloride (Various Mfr.).

paracarbinoxamine maleate. Carbinoxamine.

Paracet Forte. (Major Pharmaceuticals) Chlorzoxazone, acetaminophen. Tab. Bot. 100s, 1000s. *Rx.*
Use: Muscle relaxant.

paracetaldehyde. U.S.P. 23.
See: Paraldehyde.

parachloramine hydrochloride. U.S.P. 23. Meclizine HCl.
See: Bonine, Tab. (Pfizer US Pharmaceutical Group).

parachlorometaxylenol.
Use: Phenolic antiseptic.
See: D-Seb, Liq. (Rydelle Laboratories).
Nu-Flow, Liq. (Rydelle Laboratories).

W/9-aminoacridine HCl, methyl-dodecylbenzyl-trimethyl ammonium Cl, pramoxine HCl, hydrocortisone, acetic acid.
See: Drotic No. 2, Drops (B.F. Ascher and Co.).

W/Benzocaine.
See: TPO 20 (DePree).

W/Coconut oil, pine oil, castor oil, lanolin, cholesterols, lecithin.
See: Sebacide, Liq. (Paddock Laboratories).

W/Hydrocortisone, pramoxine HCl, benzalkonium Cl, acetic acid.
See: Oto Drops (Solvay Pharmaceuticals).

W/Lidocaine, phenol, zinc oxide.
See: Unguentine Plus, Cream (Procter & Gamble Pharm.).

W/Pramoxine HCl, hydrocortisone, benzalkonium Cl, acetic acid.
See: My Cort Otic #2, Drops (Scrip).
See: Rezamid, Lot. (Dermik Laboratories, Inc.).

•**parachlorophenol.** (par-ah-KLOR-oh-feh-nole) U.S.P. 23.
Use: Anti-infective, topical.

•**parachlorophenol, camphorated.** U.S.P. 23.
Use: Anti-infective, topical.

paracodin.
See: Dihydrocodeine.

Paraeusal Liquid. (Paraeusal) Liq. Bot. 2 oz, 6 oz, 12 oz.
Use: Minor skin irritations.

Paraeusal Solid. (Paraeusal) Oint. Jar 1 oz, 2 oz, 16 oz.
Use: Dermatologic, counterirritant.

•**paraffin.** (PAR-ah-fin) N.F. 18.
Use: Pharmaceutic aid (stiffening agent).

•**paraffin, synthetic.** N.F. 18.
Use: Pharmaceutic aid (stiffening agent).

Paraflex. (Ortho McNeil Pharmaceutical) Chlorzoxazone 250 mg/Tab. Bot. 100s. *Rx.*
Use: Muscle relaxant.

Parafon Forte DSC. (Ortho McNeil Pharmaceutical) Chlorzoxazone 500 mg/Capl. Bot. 100s, 500s, UD 100s. *Rx.*
Use: Muscle relaxant.

paraform. Paraformaldehyde (No Manufacturer Available).

paraformaldehyde.
Use: Essentially the same as formaldehyde.

See: Formaldehyde (Various Mfr.).
Trioxymethylene (an incorrect term for paraformaldehyde).

paraglycylarsanilic acid. N-carbamylmethyl-p-aminobenzenearsonic acid, the free acid of tryparsamide.

Parahist HD. (Pharmics, Inc.) Phenylephrine HCl 5 mg, chlorpheniramine maleate 2 mg, hydrocodone bitartrate 1.67 mg, alcohol free. Liq. Bot. 473 ml. *c-III.*
Use: Antihistamine, antitussive, decongestant.

Para-Jel. (Health for Life Brands, Inc.) Benzocaine 5%, cetyl dimethyl benzyl ammonium Cl. Tube 0.25 oz. *otc.*
Use: Anesthetic, local.

•**paraldehyde.** (par-AL-deh-hide) U.S.P. 23.
Use: Hypnotic, sedative.
See: Paral, Cap., Liq., Amp. (Forest Pharmaceutical, Inc.).

Paral Oral. (Forest Pharmaceutical, Inc.) Paraldehyde 30 ml. Bot. 12s, 25s. *c-IV.*
Use: Hypnotic, sedative.

paramephrin.
See: Epinephrine (Various Mfr.).

•**paramethasone acetate.** (PAR-ah-meth-ah-zone) U.S.P. 23.
Use: Corticosteriod, topical.
See: Haldrone, Tab. (Eli Lilly and Co.).

para-monochlorophenol.
See: Camphorated para-chlorophenol, Liq. (Novocol Chemical Mfr. Co.).

•**paranyline hydrochloride.** (PAR-ah-NYE-leen) USAN.
Use: Anti-inflammatory.

•**parapenzolate bromide.** (pa-rah-PEN-zoe-late BROE-mide) USAN.
Use: Anticholinergic.

Paraplatin. (Bristol-Myers Oncology/Immunology) Carboplatin 50 mg, 150 mg, 450 mg. Inj. Vial. *Rx.*
Use: Antineoplastic.

pararosaniline embonate. Pararosaniline pamoate.

•**pararosaniline pamoate.** (par-ah-row-ZAN-ih-lin PAM-oh-ate) USAN.
Use: Antischistosomal.

parasympatholytic agents. Cholinergic blocking agents.
See: Anticholinergic Agents.
Antispasmodics.
Mydriatics.
Parkinsonism Agents.

parasympathomimetic agents.
See: Cholinergic Agents.

Paratrol Liquid. (Walgreen Co.) Pyrethrins 0.2%, piperonyl butoxide technical 2%, deodorized kerosene 0.8%. Bot. 2 oz. *otc.*
Use: Pediculicide.

Parazone. (Henry Schein, Inc.) Chlorzoxazone 250 mg, acetaminophen 300 mg/Tab. Bot. 100s, 1000s. *Rx.*
Use: Muscle relaxant, analgesic.

•**parbendazole.** (par-BEN-dah-ZOLE) USAN. Under study.
Use: Anthelmintic.

Parcillin. (Parmed Pharmaceuticals, Inc.) Crystalline potassium penicillin G 240 mg, 400,000 units/Tab. Bot. 100s, 1000s. Pow. for Syr. 400,000 units/Tsp. 80 ml. *Rx.*
Use: Anti-infective, penicillin.

•**parconazole hydrochloride.** (par-KOE-nah-zole) USAN.
Use: Antifungal.

Par Decon. (Par Pharmaceuticals) Phenylpropanolamine HCl 40 mg, phenylephrine HCl 10 mg, chlorpheniramine maleate 5 mg, phenyltoloxamine citrate 15 mg/Tab. Bot. 100s, 500s, 1000s. *Rx.*
Use: Antihistamine, decongestant.

Paredrine. (Pharmics, Inc.) Hydroxyamphetamine HBr 1%. Bot. 15 ml. *Rx.*
Use: Mydriatic.

•**paregoric.** (par-eh-GORE-ik) U.S.P. 23.
Use: Antiperistaltic.

paregoric. (Various Mfr.) Morphine equivalent 2 mg/5 ml, alcohol 45%. Liq. Bot. Pt. gal. *c-III.*
Use: Antiperistaltic.

Paremyd. (Allergan, Inc.) Hydroxyamphetamine HBr 1%, tropicamide 0.25%. Soln. Bot. 5 ml, 15 ml. *Rx.*
Use: Cycloplegic, mydriatic.

parenabol. Boldenone undecylenate.

•**pareptide sulfate.** (PAR-epp-tide) USAN.
Use: Antiparkinsonian.

Par Estro. (Parmed Pharmaceuticals, Inc.) Conjugated estrogens 1.25 mg/Tab. Bot. 100s. *Rx.*
Use: Estrogen.

parethoxycaine hydrochloride.
W/Zirconium oxide, calamine.
See: Zotox, Spray, Cream (Del Pharmaceuticals).

Par-F. (Pharmics, Inc.) Fe 60 mg, Ca 250 mg, vitamins C 120 mg, A 5000 IU, D 400 IU, B_1 3 mg, B_2 3.4 mg, B_{12} 12 mcg, B_6 12 mg, B_3 20 mg, Cu, I, Mg, Zn 15 mg, E 30 IU, folic acid 1 mg/Tab. Bot. 100s. *Rx.*
Use: Mineral, vitamin supplement.

Par Glycerol. (Par Pharmaceuticals) Iodinated glycerol 60 mg/5 ml. Alcohol 21.75%, peppermint oil, corn syrup, saccharin. Caramel-mint flavor. Elix.

Bot. Pt. *Rx.*
Use: Expectorant.

•**pargyline hydrochloride.** (PAR-jih-leen) USAN. U.S.P. XXII
Use: Antihypertensive.

Parhist SR. (Parmed Pharmaceuticals, Inc.) Phenylpropanolamine HCl 75 mg, chlorpheniramine maleate 12 mg/Cap. Bot. 100s, 1000s. *Rx.*
Use: Antihistamine, decongestant.

paricalcitol.
Use: Vitamin supplement.
See: Zemplar, Inj. (Abbott).

Parkelp. (Phillip R. Park) Pacific sea kelp.
Tab.: Bot. 100s, 200s, 500s, 800s.
Gran.: Bot. 2 oz, 7 oz, 1 lb, 3 lb. *otc.*
Use: Nutritional supplement.

parkinsonism, agents for. Parasympatholytic agents.
See: Akineton, Tab., Inj. (Knoll Pharmaceuticals).
Artane, Elix., Tab., Sequels (ESI Lederle Generics).
Benztropine Mesylate, Tab. (Various Mfr.).
Caramiphen HCl.
Cogentin, Tab., Amp. (Merck & Co.).
Dopar, Cap. (Procter & Gamble Pharm.).
Eldepryl, Tab. (Somerset Pharmaceuticals).
Kemadrin, Tab. (GlaxoWellcome).
Larodopa, Tab. (Roche Laboratories).
Lodosyn, Tab. (Merck & Co.).
Parlodel, Tab., Cap. (Novartis Pharmaceutical Corp.).
Permax, Tab. (Eli Lilly and Co.).
Sinemet, Tab. (Du Pont Merck Pharmaceutical Co.).
Symmetrel, Cap, Syr. (Du Pont Merck Pharmaceutical Co.).
Trihexyphenidyl HCl (Various Mfr.).
Trihexy-2 (Geneva Pharmaceuticals).

Parlodel. (Novartis Pharmaceutical Corp.) Bromocriptine mesylate. Lactose. **Tab.:** 2.5 mg. Bot. 30s, 100s.
Cap.: 5 mg. Bot. 30s, 100s. *Rx.*
Use: Antiparkinsonian.

Parmeth. (Parmed Pharmaceuticals, Inc.) Promethazine HCl 50 mg/Cap. Bot. 100s, 1000s. *Rx.*
Use: Antiemetic, antihistamine, antivertigo.

parminyl. Salicylamide, phenacetin, caffeine, acetaminophen.

Par-Natal-FA. (Parmed Pharmaceuticals, Inc.) Vitamins A 4000 IU, D 400 IU, thiamine HCl 2 mg, riboflavin 2 mg, pyridoxine HCl 0.8 mg, ascorbic acid 50 mg, niacinamide 10 mg, I 0.15 mg, folic acid 0.1 mg, cobalamin concentrate 2 mcg, Fe 50 mg, Ca 240 mg/Cap. Bot. 100s, 1000s. *otc.*
Use: Mineral, vitamin supplement.

Par-Natal Plus 1 Improved. (Parmed Pharmaceuticals, Inc.) Elemental calcium 200 mg, elemental iron 65 mg, vitamins A 4000 IU, D 400 IU, E 11 mg, B_1 1.5 mg, B_2 3 mg, B_3 20 mg, B_6 10 mg, B_{12} 12 mcg, C 120 mg, folic acid 1 mg, Zn 25 mg, Cu/Tab. Bot. 500s. *Rx.*
Use: Mineral, vitamin supplement.

Parnate. (SmithKline Beecham Pharmaceuticals) Tranylcypromine sulfate 10 mg/Tab. Bot. 100s. *Rx.*
Use: Antidepressant.

parodyne.
See: Antipyrine (Various Mfr.).

paroleine.
See: Petrolatum Liquid (Various Mfr.).

•**paromomycin sulfate.** (par-oh-moe-MY-sin) U.S.P. 23. An antibiotic substance obtained from cultures of certain *Streptomyces* species, one of which is *Streptomyces rimosus.*
Use: Antiamebic.

parothyl. (Henry Schein, Inc.) Meprobamate 400 mg, tridihexethyl Cl 25 mg/Tab. Bot. 100s. *c-IV.*
Use: Anticholinergic, anxiolytic, antispasmodic.

•**paroxetine.** (puh-ROX-eh-teen) USAN.
Use: Antidepressant.

paroxetine hydrochloride.
Use: Antidepressant.
See: Paxil, Tab. (SmithKline Beecham Pharmaceuticals).

paroxyl.
See: Acetarsone (Various Mfr.).

parpanit.
See: Caramiphen HCl (Various Mfr.).

parsley concentrate. Garlic concentrate. *Rx.*

Par-Supp. (Parmed Pharmaceuticals, Inc.) Estrone 0.2 mg, lactose 50 mg/Vaginal Supp. Pkg. 12s.
Use: Estrogen.

Partapp TD. (Parmed Pharmaceuticals, Inc.) Phenylpropanolamine HCl 15 mg, phenylephrine HCl 15 mg, brompheniramine maleate 12 mg/TD Tab. Bot. 1000s.

Parten. (Parmed Pharmaceuticals, Inc.) Acetaminophen 10 gr/Tab. Bot. 100s, 1000s. *otc.*
Use: Analgesic.

•**partricin.** (PAR-trih-sin) USAN. Antibiotic produced by *Streptomyces aureofaciens.*
Use: Antifungal, antiprotozoal.

Partuss. (Parmed Pharmaceuticals, Inc.)

Dextromethorphan hydrobromide 60 mg, potassium guaiacolsulfonate 8 gr, chlorpheniramine maleate 6 mg, ammonium Cl 8 gr, tartar emetic 1/12 gr, chloroform 2 min/30 ml. Bot. 4 oz, pt, gal. *Rx.*
Use: Antihistamine, antitussive, expectorant.

Partuss A.C. (Parmed Pharmaceuticals, Inc.) Guaifenesin 100 mg, pheniramine maleate 7.5 mg, codeine phosphate 10 mg, alcohol 3.5%/5 ml. Bot. 4 oz. *c-v.*
Use: Antihistamine, antitussive, expectorant.

Partuss LA. (Parmed Pharmaceuticals, Inc.) Phenylpropanolamine HCl 75 mg, guaifenesin 400 mg/LA Tab. Bot. 100s, 500s. *Rx.*
Use: Decongestant, expectorant.

Parvlex. (Freeda Vitamins, Inc.) Iron 100 mg, vitamins B_1 20 mg, B_2 20 mg, B_3 20 mg, B_5 1 mg, B_6 10 mg, B_{12} 50 mcg, C 50 mg, folic acid 0.1 mg, Cu, Mn/ Tab. Bot. 100s, 250s. *otc.*
Use: Mineral, vitamin supplement.

Pas-C. (Hellwig) Pascorbic. p-aminosalicylic acid 0.5 g with vitamin C/Tab. Bot. 1000s. *Rx.*
Use: Antituberculosal.

Paser. (Jacobus Pharmaceutical Co.) Aminosalicylic acid 4 g/packet. Gran. Pkt. 30s. *Rx.*
Use: Adjunctive tuberculosis agent.

passiflora. Dried flowering and fruiting tops of *Passiflora incarnata*. Phenobarbital, valerian, hyoscyamus.

Patanol. (Alcon Laboratories, Inc.) Olopatadine HCl 0.1%/Soln. Drop-Tainer. 5 ml. *Rx.*
Use: Antihistamine, ophthalmic.

Path. (Parker) Buffered neutral formalin soln. 10%. Bot. 1 gal, 5 gal. Jar 4 oz.
Use: Tissue specimen fixative.

Pathilon. (ESI Lederle Generics) Tridihexethyl chloride 25 mg/Tab. Bot. 100s. *Rx.*
Use: Anticholinergic, antispasmodic.

Pathocil. (Wyeth-Ayerst Laboratories) Dicloxacillin sodium. **Cap.:** 250 mg, 500 mg. Bot. 50s (500 mg only), 100s (250 mg only). **Pow. for Oral Susp.:** 62.5 mg/5 ml. Bot. to make 100 ml. *Rx.*
Use: Anti-infective, penicillin.

•**paulomycin.** (PAW-low-MY-sin) USAN.
Use: Anti-infective.

Pavabid Plateau. (Hoechst Marion Roussel) Papaverine HCl 150 mg/TR Cap. Bot. 100s, 250s, 1000s, UD 100s. *Rx.*
Use: Vasodilator.

Pavacaps. (Freeport) Papaverine HCl 150 mg/TR Cap. Bot. 1000s. *Rx.*
Use: Vasodilator.

Pavacen Cenules. (Schwarz Pharma, Inc.) Papaverine HCl 150 mg/TR Cap. Bot. 100s. *Rx.*
Use: Vasodilator.

Pavadel. (Canright) Papaverine HCl 150 mg/Cap. Bot. 100s, 1000s. *Rx.*
Use: Vasodilator.

Pavadel PB. (Canright) Papaverine HCl 150 mg, phenobarbital 45 mg/Cap. Bot. 100s. *Rx.*
Use: Vasodilator.

Pavadyl. (Sanofi Winthrop Pharmaceuticals) Papaverine HCl 150 mg/Cap. Bot. 100s. *Rx.*
Use: Vasodilator.

Pavagen. (Rugby Labs, Inc.) Papaverine 150 mg/TR Cap. Bot. 500s, 1000s, UD 100s. *Rx.*
Use: Vasodilator.

Pava-Lyn. (Lynwood) Papaverine HCl 150 mg/Cap. Bot. 100s. *Rx.*
Use: Vasodilator.

Pavatine. (Major Pharmaceuticals) Papaverine 300 mg/Tab. Bot. 100s. *Rx.*
Use: Vasodilator.

Pavatine T.D. (Major Pharmaceuticals) Papaverine 150 mg/TD Cap. Bot. 100s, 1000s. *Rx.*
Use: Vasodilator.

Pavulon. (Organon Teknika Corp.) Pancuronium bromide. **1 mg/ml:** Vial 10 ml, Box 25s. **2 mg/ml:** Amp. 2 ml, 5 ml, Box 25s. *Rx.*
Use: Muscle relaxant, adjunct to anesthesia.

Paxarel. (Circle Pharmaceuticals, Inc.) Acetylcarbromal 250 mg/Tab. Bot. 100s. *Rx.*
Use: Hypnotic, sedative.

Paxil. (SmithKline Beecham Pharmaceuticals) Paroxetine. **Tab.:** 10 mg, 20 mg, 30 mg, 40 mg. Bot. 30s; 100s, SUP 100s (20 mg only). **Susp.:** 10 mg/5 ml. Bot. 250 ml. *Rx.*
Use: Antidepressant.

Paxil CR. (SmithKline Beecham Pharmaceuticals) Paroxetine HCl 12.5 mg, 25 mg. Tab. Bot. 30s, 100s, SUP 100s. *Rx.*
Use: Antidepressant.

•**pazinaclone.** (pah-ZIN-ah-klone) USAN.
Use: Anxiolytic.

Pazo Hemorrhoid Ointment. (Bristol-Myers Squibb) Zinc oxide 5%, ephedrine sulfate 0.2%, camphor 2% in lanolin-petrolatum base. Tube 28 g. *otc.*
Use: Anorectal preparation.

•**pazoxide.** (pay-ZOX-ide) USAN.
Use: Antihypertensive.

PB 100. (Schlicksup) Phenobarbital 1.5

gr/Tab. Bot. 1000s. *c-iv.*
Use: Hypnotic, sedative.

PBZ. (Novartis Pharmaceutical Corp.) Tripelennamine HCl 25 mg, 50 mg Tab. Bot. 100s. *Rx.*
Use: Antihistamine.

PBZ-SR. (Novartis Pharmaceutical Corp.) Tripelennamine HCl 100 mg/SR Tab. Bot. 100s. *Rx.*
Use: Antihistamine.

PCE Dispertab Tablets. (Abbott Laboratories) Erythromycin particles 333 mg, 500 mg. Tab. Bot. 60s (333 mg only), 100s (500 mg only). *Rx.*
Use: Anti-infective, erythromycin.

p-chlorometaxylenol. Benzocaine, benzyl alcohol, propylene glycol.
W/Hydrocortisone, pramoxine HCl.
See: 20-Caine Burn Relief (Alto Pharmaceuticals, Inc.).

p-chlorophenol.
See: Parachlorophenol.

PCMX.
See: Parachlorometaxylenol.

PDP Liquid Protein. (Wesley Pharmacal Co., Inc.) Protein 15 g (from protein hydrolysates), cal 60/30 ml. Bot. Pt, qt, gal. *otc.*
Use: Protein supplement.

P_1E_1. (Alcon) Pilocarpine HCl 1%, epinephrine bitartrate 1%. Soln. Drop-Tainers 15 ml. *Rx.*
Use: Antiglaucoma.

P_2E_1. (Alcon) Pilocarpine HCl 2%, epinephrine bitartrate 1%. Soln. Drop-Tainers 15 ml. *Rx.*
Use: Antiglaucoma.

P_4E_1. (Alcon) Pilocarpine HCl 4%, epinephrine bitartrate 1%. Soln. Drop-Tainers 15 ml. *Rx.*
Use: Antiglaucoma.

P_6E_1. (Alcon) Pilocarpine HCl 6%, epinephrine bitartrate 1%. Soln. Drop-Tainers 15 ml. *Rx.*
Use: Antiglaucoma.

Peacock's Bromides. (Natcon) **Liq.:** Potassium bromide 6 gr, sodium bromide 6 gr, ammonium bromide 3 gr/5 ml. Bot. 8 oz. **Tab.:** Potassium bromide 3 gr, sodium bromide 3 gr, ammonium bromide 1.5 gr. Bot. 100s. *Rx.*
Use: Hypnotic, sedative.

•**peanut oil.** N.F. 18.
Use: Pharmaceutic aid (solvent).

Pectamol. (British Drug House) Diethylaminoethoxyethyl-a,a-diethylphenylacetate citrate. Bot. 4 fl oz, 16 fl oz, 80 fl oz, 160 fl oz.
Use: Antitussive.

•**pectin.** (PECK-tin) U.S.P. 23.
Use: Protectant, pharmaceutic aid (suspending agent).

pectin w/combinations.
See: Donnagel Susp. (Wyeth-Ayerst Laboratories).
Furoxone, Liq., Tab. (Eaton Medical Corp.).
Kaopectate, Liq. (Pharmacia & Upjohn).

Pedameth. (Forest Pharmaceutical, Inc.) Racemethionine. **Cap.:** 200 mg. Bot. 50s, 500s. **Liq.:** 75 mg/5 ml. Bot. Pt. *Rx.*
Use: Diaper rash preparation.

Pedenex. (Health for Life Brands, Inc.) Caprylic acid, zinc undecylenate, sodium propionate. Tube 1.5 oz. Foot pow. spray 5 oz. *otc.*
Use: Antifungal, topical.

Pedia Care Allergy Formula. (McNeil Consumer Products Co.) Chlorpheniramine maleate 1 mg/5 ml, sorbitol, sucrose. Alcohol free. Grape flavor. Syr. Bot. 120 ml. *otc.*
Use: Antihistamine.

Pedia Care Cold Allergy Chewable Tablets. (McNeil Consumer Products Co.) Pseudoephedrine HCl 15 mg, chlorpheniramine maleate 1 mg, aspartame, phenylalanine 8 mg/Chew. Tab. Pkg. 18s. *otc.*
Use: Antihistamine, decongestant.

Pedia Care Cough-Cold. (McNeil Consumer Products Co.) **Chew. Tab.:** Pseudoephedrine HCl 15 mg, chlorpheniramine maleate 1 mg, dextromethorphan HBr 5 mg, aspartame (phenylalanine 6 mg), dextrose, sucrose. Fruit flavor. Pkg. 16s. **Liq.:** Pseudoephedrine HCl 15 mg, chlorpheniramine maleate 1 mg, dextromethorphan HBr 5 mg/5 ml, sorbitol, sucrose. Alcohol free. Cherry flavor. Syr. Bot. 120 ml. *otc.*
Use: Antihistamine, antitussive, decongestant.

Pedia Care Infants' Decongestant. (McNeil Consumer Products Co.) Pseudoephedrine HCl 7.5 mg/0.8 ml. Cherry flavor. Syr. Bot. 15 ml. *otc.*
Use: Decongestant.

Pedia Care NightRest. (McNeil Consumer Products Co.) Pseudoephedrine HCl 15 mg, chlorpheniramine maleate 1 mg, dextromethorphan HBr 7.5 mg/5 ml, sorbitol, sucrose. Alcohol free. Cherry flavor. Liq. Bot. 120 ml. *otc.*
Use: Antihistamine, antitussive, decongestant.

Pediacof. (Sanofi Winthrop Pharmaceuticals) Codeine phosphate 5 mg, phenylephrine HCl 2.5 mg, chlorpheniramine maleate 0.75 mg, potassium iodide 75 mg/5 ml, sodium benzoate 0.2%, al-

cohol 5%. Syr. Bot. 16 fl oz. *c-v.*
Use: Antihistamine, antitussive, decongestant, expectorant.

Pediacon DX Children's. (Zenith Goldline Pharmaceuticals) Phenylpropanolamine HCl 6.25 mg, guaifenesin 100 mg, dextromethorphan HBr 5 mg, alcohol 5%/5 ml. Syr. Bot. 118 ml. *otc.*
Use: Antitussive, decongestant, expectorant.

Pediacon DX Pediatric. (Zenith Goldline Pharmaceuticals) Phenylpropanolamine HCl 6.25 mg, guaifenesin 50 mg, dextromethorphan HBr 5 mg/ml. 5% alcohol. Sugar free. Drops. Bot. 30 ml. *otc.*
Use: Antitussive, decongestant, expectorant.

Pediacon EX. (Zenith Goldline Pharmaceuticals) Phenylpropanolamine 6.25 mg, guiafenesin 50 mg/ml. Sugar free. Drops. Bot. 30 ml. *otc.*
Use: Decongestant, expectorant.

Pediaflor Fluoride Drops. (Ross Laboratories) Fluoride 0.5 mg/ml as sodium fluoride 1.1 mg/ml. Bot. 50 ml. *Rx.*
Use: Dental caries agent.

Pedialyte. (Ross Laboratories) Na 45 mEq, K 20 mEq, chloride 35 mEq, citrate 30 mEq, dextrose 25 g/L. 100 calories/L. **Plastic Bot.:** 8 fl oz. (unflavored), 32 fl oz. (unflavored, fruit). **Nursing Bot.:** Hospital use. Bot. 8 fl oz. *otc.*
Use: Electrolytes, mineral supplement.

Pedialyte Electrolyte. (Zenith Goldline) Dextrose 25 g, K 20 mEq, Cl 35 mEq, Na 45 mEq, citrate 30 mEq, 100 cal/L. Oral Soln. Bot. 1 L. *otc.*
Use: Electrolyte, mineral supplement.

Pedialyte Freezer Pops. (Ross Laboratories) Na 45 mEq, K 20 mEq, Cl 35 mEq, citrate 30 mEq, dextrose 25 g/L, phenylalanine, aspartame/Liq. Ready-to-freeze pops. 2.1 fl oz. Box. 16s. *otc.*
Use: Electrolytes, mineral supplement.

Pediamycin Drops. (Ross Laboratories) Erythromycin ethylsuccinate for oral suspension 100 mg/2.5 ml. Bot. 50 ml (Dropper enclosed). *Rx.*
Use: Anti-infective, erythromycin.

Pediapred Oral Liquid. (Medeva Pharmaceuticals, Inc.) Prednisolone sodium phosphate 6.7 mg/5 ml. Bot. 4 oz. *Rx.*
Use: Corticosteroid.

PediaSure. (Ross Laboratories) Protein 30 g (Na caseinate, whey protein concentrate), carbohydrate 109.8 g (hydrolyzed cornstarch, sucrose), fat 49.8 g (hi-oleic safflower oil, soy oil, MCT [fractionated coconut oil], mono- and diglycerides, soy lecithin), Na 380 mg, K 1308 mg/L, vitamins A, B_1, B_2, B_3, B_5, B_6, B_{12}, C, D, E, K, inositol, Cl, Ca, P, Mg, I, Mn, Cu, Zn, Fe, biotin, choline, folic acid. < 310 mosm/kg H_2O, 1 cal/ml. Gluten free. Vanilla flavor. Ready-to-use can 240 ml. *otc.*
Use: Nutritional supplement.

Pediatric Advil Drops. (Whitehall Robins Laboratories) Ibuprofen 100 mg/2.5 ml, EDTA, glycerin, sorbitol, sucrose. Oral Susp. Bot. 15 ml. *otc.*
Use: Anti-inflammatory.

Pediatric Bear-E-Bag. (Lafayette) Barium 95%. Susp. Enema kit 170 g. *Rx.*
Use: Radiopaque agent.

Pediatric Cough Syrup. (Weeks & Leo) Ammonium Cl 300 mg, sodium citrate 600 mg/oz. Bot. 4 oz. *otc.*
Use: Expectorant.

Pediatric Electrolyte. (Zenith Goldline Pharmaceuticals) Dextrose 25 g, K 20 mEq, Cl 35 mEq, Na 45 mEq, citrate 48 mEq, calories 100/L. Soln. Bot. 1 L. *otc.*
Use: Nutritional supplement, enteral.

Pediatric Maintenance Solution. (Abbott Laboratories) IV solution w/dose calculated according to age, weight, clinical condition. Bot. 250 ml. *Rx.*
Use: Fluid, electrolyte, nutrient replacement.

Pediatric Multiple Trace Element. (American Regent) Zn (as sulfate) 0.5 mg, Cu (as sulfate) 0.1 mg, Mn (as sulfate) 0.03 mg, Cr (as chloride) 1 mcg/ml. Soln. Vial 10 ml. *Rx.*
Use: Nutritional supplement, parenteral.

Pediatric Triban. (Great Southern Laboratories) Trimethobenzamide HCl 100 mg, benzocaine 2%/Supp. Pkg. 10s. *Rx.*
Use: Antiemetic, antivertigo.

Pediatric Vicks 44d Dry Hacking Cough and Head Congestion. (Procter & Gamble Pharm.) Dextromethorphan HBr 15 mg/15 ml (1 mg/ml), sorbitol, sucrose, cherry flavor, alcohol free. Syr. Bot. 120 ml. *otc.*
Use: Antitussive.

Pediazole Suspension. (Ross Laboratories) Erythromycin ethylsuccinate 200 mg, sulfisoxazole acetyl 600 mg/5 ml. Bot. Granules reconstituted to 100 ml, 150 ml, 200 ml. *Rx.*
Use: Anti-infective, erythromycin.

Pedi-Boot Mist Kit. (Pedinol Pharmacal, Inc.) Cetylpyridinium Cl, triacetin, chloroxylenol. Bot. 2 oz. *otc.*
Use: Antifungal, antiseptic, deodorant.

Pedi-Boro Soak Paks. (Pedinol Pharmacal, Inc.) Astringent wet dressing w/ aluminum sulfate, calcium acetate, coloring agent. Box 12s, 100s. *otc.*
Use: Dermatologic, counterirritant.

Pedi-Cort V Creme. (Pedinol Pharmacal, Inc.) Clioquinol 3%, hydrocortisone 1%. Tube 20 g. *Rx.*
Use: Antifungal, corticosteroid, topical.

Pedicran with Iron. (Scherer Laboratories, Inc.) Vitamin B_{12} (crystallized) 25 mcg, ferric pyrophosphate, soluble (elemental iron 30 mg) 250 mg, thiamine mononitrate 10 mg, nicotinamide 10 mg, alcohol 1%/5 ml. Bot. 4 oz, pt. *otc.*
Use: Mineral, vitamin supplement.

pediculicides/scabicides.
See: Barc, Liq. (Del Pharmaceuticals, Inc.).
Blue, Gel (Various Mfr.).
Elimite, Cream (Allergan, Inc.).
Eurax, Preps. (Westwood Squibb Pharmaceuticals).
G-well, Preps. (Zenith Goldline Pharmaceuticals).
Lindane, Preps. (Various Mfr.).
Nix, Liq. (GlaxoWellcome).
Ovide, Lot. (Medicis Dermatologicals, Inc.).
Pronto Concentrate, Shampoo (Del Pharmaceuticals, Inc.).
Pyrinyl, Liq. (Various Mfr.).
R & C, Shampoo (Schwarz Pharma, Inc).
RID, Liq. (Pfizer US Pharmaceutical Group).
Step 2, Liq. (Medicis Dermatologicals, Inc.).
Tisit, Preps. (Pfeiffer Co.).
Tisit Blue, Gel (Pfeiffer Co.).
Triple X Kit, Liq. (Carter Wallace).

Pedi-Dri. (Pedinol Pharmacal, Inc.) Nystatin 100,000 U/g, corn starch, aluminum chlorhydroxide, menthol. Bot. 56.7 g. *Rx.*
Use: Antifungal, antiperspirant, deodorant, foot powder.

Pediotic. (GlaxoWellcome) Hydrocortisone 1%, neomycin 3.5 mg (as sulfate), polymyxin B sulfate 10,000 units/ml. Susp. Bot 7.5 ml with dropper. *Rx.*
Use: Otic.

Pedi-Pro Foot Powder. (Pedinol Pharmacal, Inc.) Aluminum chlorhydroxide, menthol, zinc undecylenate, chloroxylenol. Bot. 2 oz. *otc.*
Use: Antifungal, antiperspirant, deodorant.

Pedituss Cough. (Major Pharmaceuticals) Phenylephrine HCl 2.5 mg, chlorpheniramine maleate 0.75 mg, codeine phosphate 5 mg, potassium iodide 75 mg/5 ml, alcohol 5%, saccharin, sorbitol, sucrose. Syr. Bot. Pt., gal. *c-v.*
Use: Antihistamine, antitussive, decongestant, expectorant.

Pedolatum. (King Pharmaceuticals, Inc.) Salicylic acid, sodium salicylate. Oint. Pkg. 0.5 oz. *otc.*
Use: Analgesic, topical.

Pedric Senior. (Pal-Pak, Inc.) Acetaminophen 320 mg. *otc.*
Use: Analgesic.

PedTE-PAK-4. (SoloPak Pharmaceuticals, Inc.) Zn 1 mg, Cu 0.1 mg, Mn 0.025 mg, Cr 1 mcg. Vial 3 ml. *Rx.*
Use: Nutritional supplement, parenteral.

Pedtrace-4. (Fujisawa USA, Inc.) Zinc 0.5 mg, copper 0.1 mg, chromium 0.85 mcg, manganese 0.25 mg/ml. Vial 3 ml, 10 ml. *Rx.*
Use: Nutritional supplement, parenteral.

PedvaxHIB. (Merck & Co.) Purified capsular polysaccharide of *Haemophilus influenzae* type b, *Neisseria meningitidis* OMPC 250 mcg/dose when reconstituted, sodium chloride 0.9%, lactose 2 mg, thimerosal 1:20,000. Pow. for Inj. or Soln. Single-dose vial with vial of aluminum hydroxide diluent or single-dose vial. *Rx.*
Use: Immunization.

•**pefloxacin.** (PEH-FLOX-ah-sin) USAN.
Use: Anti-infective.

•**pefloxacin mesylate.** (PEH-FLOX-ah-sin) USAN.
Use: Anti-infective.

•**pegademase bovine.** (peg-AD-ah-MASE BOE-vine) USAN.
Use: Replacement therapy (adenosine deaminase deficiency); modified enzyme for use in ADA deficiency. [Orphan Drug]
See: Adagen (Enzon, Inc.).

Peganone. (Abbott Laboratories) Ethotoin 250 mg/Tab. or 500 mg/Cap. Bot. 100s. *Rx.*
Use: Anticonvulsant.

•**pegaspargase.** (peh-ASS-par-jase) USAN.
Use: Antineoplastic. [Orphan Drug]
See: Oncaspar, Inj. (Enzon, Inc.).

•**peglicol 5 oleate.** (PEG-lih-kahl 5 OH-lee-ate) USAN.
Use: Pharmaceutic aid (emulsifying agent).

PEG-glucocerebrosidase. (Enzon, Inc.)
Use: Treatment of Gaucher's disease. [Orphan Drug]

PEG-interleukin-2. (Cetus)
Use: Immunomodulator. [Orphan Drug]

PEG-L-asparaginase. (Enzon, Inc.) *Rx.*
Use: Antineoplastic.

PEG Ointment. (Medco Lab, Inc.) Polyethylene glycol. Jar 16 oz. *otc.*
Use: Pharmaceutical aid, ointment base.

•**pegorgotein.** (peg-AHR-gah-teen) USAN.
Use: Free oxygen radical scavenger.

•**pegoterate.** (PEG-oh-TEER-ate) USAN.
Use: Pharmaceutic aid (suspending agent).

•**pegoxol 7 stearate.** (peg-OX-ole 7 STEE-ah-rate) USAN.
Use: Pharmaceutic aid (emulsifying agent).

•**pelanserin hydrochloride.** (peh-LAN-ser-in) USAN.
Use: Antihypertensive; vasodilator (serotonin S_2 and α_1 adrenergic receptor blocker).

•**peldesine.** (PELL-deh-seen) USAN.
Use: Antineoplastic, antipsoratic.

pelentan. Ethyl Biscoumacetate. (No Manufacturer Available).

•**peliomycin.** (PEE-lee-oh-MY-sin) USAN. An antibiotic derived from *Streptomycin luteogriseus.*
Use: Antineoplastic.

•**pelretin.** (PELL-REH-tin) USAN.
Use: Antikeratinizer.

•**pelrinone hydrochloride.** (PELL-rih-nohn) USAN.
Use: Cardiovascular agent.

•**pemedolac.** (peh-MEH-doe-LACK) USAN.
Use: Analgesic.

•**pemerid nitrate.** (PEM-eh-rid) USAN.
Use: Antitussive.

•**pemetrexed disodium.** (pem-eh-TREX-ehd die-SO-dee-uhm) USAN.
Use: Antineoplastic.

•**pemirolast potassium.** (peh-mihr-OH-last) USAN.
Use: Antiallergic; inhibitor (mediator release).

•**pemoline.** (PEM-oh-leen) USAN.
Use: Stimulant (central); childhood attention-deficit syndrome (hyperkinetic syndrome).
See: Cylert, Prods. (Abbott Laboratories).

Penagen-VK. (Grafton) Penicillin V. **Tab.:** 250 mg. Bot. 100s. **Pow.:** 250 mg/100 ml. *Rx.*
Use: Anti-infective, penicillin.

•**penamecillin.** (PEN-ah-meh-SILL-in) USAN.
Use: Anti-infective.

•**penbutolol sulfate.** (pen-BYOO-toe-lole) U.S.P. 23.
Use: Beta-adrenergic blocking agent.
See: Levatol (Schwarz Pharma, Inc.).

•**penciclovir.** (pen-SIGH-kloe-VEER) USAN.
Use: Antiviral.
See: Denavir, Cream (SmithKline Beecham Pharmaceuticals).

Penecare. (Schwarz Pharma, Inc.) **Cream:** Lactic acid, mineral oil, imidurea. Tube. 120 g. **Lot.:** Lactic acid, imidurea. Bot. 240 ml. *otc.*
Use: Emollient.

Penecort Cream. (Allergan, Inc.) Hydrocortisone 1%, 2.5%, benzyl alcohol, petrolatum, stearyl alcohol, propylene glycol, isopropyl myristate, polyoxyl 40 stearate, carbomer 934, sodium lauryl sulfate, edetate disodium w/sodium hydroxide to adjust pH, purified water. **1%:** Tube 30 g, 60 g. **2.5%:** Tube 30 g. *Rx.*
Use: Corticosteroid, topical.

Penetrex. (Rhone-Poulenc Rorer Pharmaceuticals, Inc.) Enoxacin 200 mg, 400 mg/Tab. Bot. 50s. *Rx.*
Use: Anti-infective, fluoroquinolone.

•**penfluridol.** (pen-FLEW-rih-dahl) USAN.
Use: Antipsychotic.

•**penicillamine.** (PEN-ih-SILL-ah-meen) U.S.P. 23.
Use: Chelating agent; metal complexing agent, cystinuria, rheumatoid arthritis.
See: Cuprimine, Cap. (Merck & Co.).
Depen, Tab. (Wallace Laboratories).

penicillin. (pen-ih-SILL-in) Unless clarified, it means an antibiotic substance or substances produced by growth of the molds *Penicillium notatum* or *P. chrysogenum. Rx.*
Use: Anti-infective.

penicillin aluminum. *Rx.*
Use: Anti-infective, penicillin.

penicillin calcium. U.S.P. XIII. *Rx.*
Use: Anti-infective, penicillin.

penicillin, dimethoxy-phenyl. Methicillin Sodium.
Use: Anti-infective, penicillin.

•**penicillin g benzathine.** (pen-ih-SILL-in G BENZ-ah-theen) U.S.P. 23.
Use: Anti-infective.
See: Bicillin (Wyeth-Ayerst Laboratories).
Permapen, Aqueous Susp. (Pfizer US Pharmaceutical Group).

penicillin g benzathine & procaine combined. (pen-ih-SILL-in G BENZ-ah-theen and PRO-cane)

Use: Anti-infective, penicillin.
See: Bicillin C-R, Inj. (Wyeth-Ayerst Laboratories).
Bicillin C-R 900/300, Inj. (Wyeth-Ayerst Laboratories).

•**penicillin g potassium.** (pen-ih-SILL-in G peo-TASS-ee-uhm) U.S.P. 23.
Use: Anti-infective.
See: Pfizerpen, Syr. (Pfizer US Pharmaceutical Group).

penicillin g potassium. (Baxter) 1,000,000 units, 2,000,000 units, 3,000,000 units. Premixed frozen Inj. Galaxy cont. 50 ml. *Rx.*
Use: Anti-infective, penicillin.

penicillin g potassium. (Marsam) 1,000,000 units, 5,000,000 units, 10,000,000 units, 20,000,000 units/vial. Pow. for Inj. Vial. *Rx.*
Use: Anti-infective, penicillin.

•**penicillin g procaine.** (pen-ih-SILL-in G PRO-cane) U.S.P. 23.
Use: Anti-infective.

penicillin g procaine combinations.
See: Bicillin C-R, Tubex (Wyeth-Ayerst Laboratories).
Bicillin C-R 900/300, Inj. (Wyeth-Ayerst Laboratories).

penicillin g procaine and dihydrostreptomycin sulfate intramammary infusion.
Use: Anti-infective.

penicillin g procaine, dihydrostreptomycin sulfate, chlorpheniramine maleate and dexamethasone suspension, sterile. (pen-ih-SILL-in G PRO-cane, die-HIGH-droe-STREP-toe-MY-sin klor-fen-EAR-ah-meen MAL-ee-ate and DEX-ah-METH-ah-sone)
Use: Anti-infective, antihistamine, anti-inflammatory.

penicillin g procaine, dihydrostreptomycin sulfate, and prednisolone suspension, sterile.
Use: Anti-infective, anti-inflammatory.

penicillin g procaine and dihydrostreptomycin sulfate suspension, sterile.
Use: Anti-infective.

penicillin g procaine, neomycin and polymyxin B sulfates, and hydrocortisone acetate topical suspension.
Use: Anti-infective, anti-inflammatory.

penicillin g procaine and novobiocin sodium intramammary infusion.
Use: Anti-infective.

penicillin g procaine w/aluminum stearate suspension, sterile.
Use: Anti-infective.

penicillin g, procaine, sterile. Sterile Susp., Intramammary infusion, Procaine Penicillin.
Use: Anti-infective.
W/Parenteral, Aqueous Susp., (Procaine Penicillin, for Aqueous Inj.,) Procaine Penicillin and Buffered Penicillin for Aqueous, Inj.
See: Wycillin, Susp. (Wyeth-Ayerst Laboratories).
W/Parenteral, in oil w/aluminum monostearate.
See: Penicillin Procaine in Oil Inj.

•**penicillin g sodium for injection.** (pen-ih-SILL-in G so-dee-uhm) U.S.P. 23.
Use: Anti-infective.

penicillin g sodium. (Marsam) 5,000,000 units/Vial. Pow. for Inj. Vial. *Rx.*
Use: Anti-infective, penicillin.

penicillin hydrabamine phenoxymethyl.
Use: Anti-infective.

penicillin o chloroprocaine.
Use: Anti-infective, penicillin.

penicillin o, sodium. Allylmercaptomethyl penicillin.
Use: Anti-infective.

penicillin, phenoxyethyl.
Use: Anti-infective, penicillin.

penicillin phenoxymethyl benzathine.
Use: Anti-infective, penicillin.
See: Penicillin V Benzathine.

penicillin phenoxymethyl hydrabamine.
Use: Anti-infective, penicillin.
See: Penicillin V Hydrabamine.

penicillin s benzathine and penicillin g procaine suspension, sterile.
Use: Anti-infective.

•**penicillin v.** (pen-ih-SILL-in V) U.S.P. 23. *Formerly Penicillin Phenoxymethyl.* A biosynthetic penicillin formed by fermentation, with suitable precursors of *Penicillin notatum.*
Use: Anti-infective.
See: Penagen-VK, Tab., Pow. (Gafton).
V-Cillin, Preps. (Eli Lilly and Co.).

•**penicillin v benzathine.** (pen-ih-SILL-in V BEN-zah-theen) U.S.P. 23. *Formerly Penicillin Benzathine Phenoxymethyl.*
Use: Anti-infective.
See: Pen-Vee, Prods. (Wyeth-Ayerst Laboratories).

•**penicillin v hydrabamine.** (pen-ih-SILL-in V HIGH-drah-BAM-een) USAN. U.S.P. XX. *Formerly Penicillin Hydrabamine Phenoxymethyl.*
Use: Anti-infective.

penicillin vk. (Various Mfr.) **Tab.:** 250 mg, 500 mg. Bot. 20s, 30s, 40s, 80s (250 mg only), 100s, 500s, 1000s, UD 100s. **Pow. for Oral Soln.:** 125 mg/

5 ml, 250 mg/5 ml when reconstituted. Bot. 80 ml, 100 ml, 150 ml, 200 ml. *Rx.*
Use: Anti-infective, penicillin.

•**penicillin v potassium.** (pen-ih-SILL-in V poe-TASS-ee-uhm) U.S.P. 23. *Formerly Penicillin Potassium Phenoxymethyl.*
Use: Anti-infective.
See: Beepen VK, Tab., Syr. (SmithKline Beecham Pharmaceuticals).
Betapen VK., Soln., Tab. (Bristol-Myers Squibb).
Bopen, V-K, Tab. (Boyd).
Pen-Vee K, Soln., Tab. (Wyeth-Ayerst Laboratories).
Pfizerpen VK, Pow., Tab. (Pfizer US Pharmaceutical Group).
Suspen, Liq. (Circle Pharmaceuticals, Inc).
V-Cillin K, Tab., Oral Soln. (Eli Lilly and Co.).
Veetids, Soln., Tab. (Bristol-Myers Squibb).

penidural.
Use: Anti-infective.

Pen-Kera Creme with Keratin Binding Factor. (B.F. Ascher and Co.) Bot. 8 oz. *otc.*
Use: Emollient.

Penntuss. (Medeva Pharmaceuticals, Inc.) Codeine (as polistirex) 10 mg, chlorpheniramine maleate 4 mg/5 ml. Bot. Pt. *c-v.*
Use: Antitussive, antihistamine.

•**pentabamate.** (PEN-tah-BAM-ate) USAN.
Use: Anxiolytic.

Pentacarinat. (Armour) Pentamidine isethionate 300 mg. Inj. Single-dose vial. *Rx.*
Use: Anti-infective.

pentacosactride.
Use: Corticotrophic peptide.

•**pentaerythritol tetranitrate diluted.** (pen-tuh-eh-Rith-rih-tole teh-truh-NYE-trate) U.S.P. 23.
Use: Vasodilator.
See: Arcotrate Nos. 1 and 2, Tab. (Arcum).
Duotrate 45, Cap. (Hoechst Marion Roussel).
Pentetra, Tab. (Paddock Laboratories).
Peritrate, Tab. (Parke-Davis).
Petro-20 mg, Tab. (Foy Laboratories).
Tetratab, Tab. (Freeport).
Tetratab No. 1, Tab. (Freeport).
Vasolate, Cap. (Parmed Pharmaceuticals, Inc.).
Vasolate-80, Cap. (Parmed Pharmaceuticals, Inc.).

•**pentaerythritol tetranitrate, diluted.** U.S.P. 23.
Use: Vasodilator.

pentaerythritol tetranitrate w/combinations.
See: Arcotrate No. 3, Tab. (Arcum).
Bitrate, Tab. (Arco Pharmaceuticals, Inc.).
Dimycor, Tab. (Standard Drug Co.).
Pentetra w/Phenobarbital, Tab. (Paddock Laboratories).
Peritrate w/Nitroglycerin, Tab. (Parke-Davis).

•**pentafilcon a.** (PEN-tah-FILL-kahn A) USAN.
Use: Contact lens material (hydrophilic).

•**pentagastrin.** (PEN-tah-ASS-trin) USAN.
Use: Diagnostic aid (gastric secretion indicator).
See: Peptavlon, Amp. (Wyeth-Ayerst Laboratories).

•**pentalyte.** (PEN-tah-lite) USAN.
Use: Electrolyte combination.

Pentam 300. (Fujisawa USA, Inc.) Pentamidine isethionate 300 mg/Vial. *Rx.*
Use: Anti-infective.

pentamidine isethionate. (pen-TAM-ih-deen ice-uh-THIGH-uh-nate) (Abbott Laboratories) 300 mg. Pow. for Inj., lyophilized. Single-dose fliptop vials. *Rx.*
Use: Anti-infective. [Orphan Drug]
See: Pentam 300, Inj. (Fujisawa USA, Inc.).
Pentacarinat, Inj. (Armour).

pentamidine isethionate (inhalation).
Use: Anti-infective. [Orphan Drug]

•**pentamorphone.** (PEN-tah-MORE-fone) USAN.
Use: Analgesic (narcotic).

pentamoxane hydrochloride.
Use: Anxiolytic.

•**pentamustine.** (PEN-tah-MUSS-teen) USAN.
Use: Antineoplastic.

pentaphonate. Dodecyltriphenylphosphonium pentachlorophenolate.
Use: Anti-infective.

•**pentapiperium methylsulfate.** (PEN-tah-PIP-ehr-ee-uhm METH-ill-SULL-fate) USAN.
Use: Anticholinergic.

pentapyrrolidinium bitartrate.
See: Pentolinium Tartrate.

Pentasa. (Hoechst Marion Roussel) Mesalamine 250 mg. CR Cap. Bot. 240s, UD 80s. *Rx.*
Use: Anti-inflammatory.

pentasodium colistinmethanesulfonate. U.S.P. 23. Sterile Colistimethate Sodium.

•**pentastarch.** (PEN-tah-starch) USAN.
Use: Leukopheresis adjunct (red cell sedimenting agent). [Orphan Drug]

Penta-Stress. (Penta) Vitamins A 10,000 IU, D 500 IU, B_1 10 mg, B_2 10 mg, B_6 1 mg, calcium pantothenate 5 mg, niacinamide 50 mg, C 100 mg, E 2 IU, B_{12} 3.3 mcg/Cap. Bot. 90s, 1000s, Jar 250s. *otc.*
Use: Mineral, vitamin supplement.

Penta-Viron. (Penta) Calcium carbonate 500 mg, ferrous fumarate 100 mg, vitamins C 50 mg, D 167 IU, A 3.333 IU, B_1 3.3 mg, B_2 3.3 mg, B_6 2 mg, calcium pantothenate 1.6 mg, niacinamide 16.7 mg, E 2 IU/Cap. Bot. 100s, 1000s, Jar 250s. *otc.*
Use: Mineral, vitamin supplement.

Pentazine Inj. (Century Pharmaceuticals, Inc.) Promethazine 50 mg/ml. Inj. Vial 10 ml. *Rx.*
Use: Antihistamine.

Pentazine w/Codeine. (Century Pharmaceuticals, Inc.) Promethazine expectorant. Bot. 4 oz, 16 oz, gal.
Use: Antihistamine.

Pentazine VC w/Codeine Liquid. (Century Pharmaceuticals, Inc.) Promethazine HCl 6.25 mg, codeine phosphate 10 mg. Liq. Bot. 118 ml, pt, gal. *c-v.*
Use: Antihistamine, antitussive.

•**pentazocine.** (pen-TAZ-oh-seen) U.S.P. 23.
Use: Analgesic.

•**pentazocine hydrochloride.** (pen-TAZ-oh-seen) U.S.P. 23.
Use: Analgesic.
W/ Acetaminophen.
See: Talacen, Cap. (Sanofi Winthrop Pharmaceuticals).

pentazocine hydrochloride and aspirin tablets.
Use: Analgesic.
See: Talwin Compound, Tab. (Sanofi Winthrop Pharmaceuticals).

•**pentazocine lactate injection.** (pen-TAZ-oh-seen LACK-tate) U.S.P. 23.
Use: Analgesic.
See: Talwin Injection, Inj. (Sanofi Winthrop Pharmaceuticals).

pentazocine and naloxone hydrochloride tablets. (Royce Laboratories, Inc.) Pentazocine 50 mg, naloxone HCl 0.5 mg/Tab. Box. 100s, 500s, 1000s. *Rx.*
Use: Analgesic.
See: Talwin NX, Tab. (Sanofi Winthrop Pharmaceuticals).

•**pentetate calcium trisodium.** (PEN-teh-tate KAL-see-uhm try-SO-dee-uhm) USAN.
Use: Chelating agent (plutonium).

•**pentetate calcium trisodium Yb 169.** (PEN-teh-tate KAL-see-uhm TRY-SO-dee-uhm Yb 169) USAN.
Use: Radiopharmaceutical.

•**pentetate indium disodium In 111.** (PEN-teh-tate IN-dee-uhm) USAN.
Use: Diagnostic aid, radiopharmaceutical.

•**pentetic acid.** (PEN-teh-tick) U.S.P. 23.
Use: Diagnostic aid.

Pentetra-Paracote. (Paddock Laboratories) Pentaerythritol tetranitrate 30 mg, 80 mg/Cap. Bot. 100s, 500s, 1000s. *Rx.*
Use: Antianginal.

Penthrane. (Abbott Hospital Products) Methoxyflurane. Bot. 15 ml, 125 ml. *Rx.*
Use: Anesthetic, general.

•**pentiapine maleate.** (pen-TIE-ah-PEEN) USAN.
Use: Antipsychotic.

•**pentigetide.** (pent-EYE-jeh-TIDE) USAN.
Use: Antiallergic.

Pentina. (Freeport) *Rauwolfia serpentina*, 100 mg/Tab. Bot. 1000s. *Rx.*
Use: Antihypertensive.

•**pentisomicin.** (pent-IH-so-MY-sin) USAN.
Use: Anti-infective.

•**pentizidone sodium.** (pen-TIH-ZIH-dohn) USAN.
Use: Anti-infective.

•**pentobarbital.** (pen-toe-BAR-bih-tahl) U.S.P. 23.
Use: Hypnotic, sedative.
See: Nembutal, Elix., Gradumets (Abbott Laboratories).
Penta, Tab. (Dunhall Pharmaceuticals, Inc.).

pentobarbital combinations.
Use: Sedative/hypnotic.
See: Cafergot P-B, Supp., Tab. (Novartis Pharmaceutical Corp.).
Nembutal, Preps. (Abbott Laboratories).

•**pentobarbital, sodium.** (pen-toe-BAR-bih-tahl) U.S.P. 23.
Use: Hypnotic, sedative.
See: Maso-Pent, Tab. (Mason Pharmaceuticals, Inc.).
Nembutal Sodium, Preps. (Abbott Laboratories).
Night-Caps, Cap. (Jones Medical Industries, Inc.).
W/Adiphenine HCl, pharmasorb, aluminum hydroxide.
See: Ephedrine and Nembutal-25, Cap. (Abbott Laboratories).

W/Ergotamine tartrate, caffeine alkaloid, bellafoline.
See: Cafergot-P.B., Tab. (Novartis Pharmaceutical Corp.).
W/Homatropine methylbromide, dehydrocholic acid, ox bile extract.
See: Homachol, Tab. (Teva Pharmaceuticals USA).
W/Pyrilamine maleate.
See: A-N-R, Rectorette (Roberts Pharmaceuticals).
pentobarbital sodium. (Various Mfr.) 100 mg/Cap. Bot. 100s.
Use: Hypnotic, sedative.
pentobarbital sodium. (Wyeth-Ayerst Laboratories) 50 mg/ml. Inj. *Tubex* 2 ml. *c-II.*
Use: Hypnotic, sedative.
pentobarbital, soluble.
See: Pentobarbital Sodium, U.S.P. 23.
Pentol Tabs. (Major Pharmaceuticals) Pentaerythritol tetranitrate. **10 mg/Tab.:** Bot. 1000s. **20 mg/Tab.:** Bot. 100s, 1000s. **80 mg/SA Tab.:** Bot. 250s, 1000s. *Rx.*
Use: Antianginal.
Pentolair. (Bausch & Lomb Pharmaceuticals) Cyclopentolate HCl 1%. Soln. Squeeze Bot. 2 ml, 15 ml. *Rx.*
Use: Cycloplegic mydriatic.
pentolinium tartrate. Pentamethylene-1:5-bis (1'-methylpyrrolidinium bitartrate).
Use: Antihypertensive.
•**pentomone.** (PEN-toe-MONE) USAN.
Use: Prostate growth inhibitor.
•**pentopril.** (PEN-toe-prill) USAN.
Use: Enzyme inhibitor (angiotensin-converting).
•**pentosan polysulfate sodium.** (PEN-toe-san PAHL-in-SULL-fate SO-dee-uhm) USAN.
Use: Anti-inflammatory (interstitial cystitis).
pentosan sodium polysulfate.
Use: Treatment of interstitial cystitis. [Orphan Drug]
See: Elmiron, Cap. (Ivax).
•**pentostatin.** (PEN-toe-STAT-in) USAN.
Use: Potentiator; leukemia. [Orphan Drug]
Pentothal. (Abbott Laboratories) **Pow. for Inj.:** Thiopental sodium 20 mg/ml. In 1, 2.5, 5 g kits, 400 mg syringes; 25 mg/ml. In 1, 2.5, 5 g, 500 mg kits, 250, 400, 500 mg syringes. **Rectal Susp.:** Thiopental sodium 400 mg/g. In 2 g syringe. *Rx.*
Use: Anesthetic.
•**pentoxifylline.** (pen-TOX-IH-fill-in) USAN.
Use: Hemorrheologic, vasodilator.
See: Trental (Hoechst Marion Roussel).
pentoxifylline. (Copley Pharmaceutical, Inc.) Pentoxifylline 400 mg. Tab. Bot. 100s, 500s, 5000s. *Rx.*
Use: Hemorrheologic, vasodilator.
pentoxifyline extended release. (Purepac Pharmaceutical Co.) Pentoxifylline 400 mg. ER Tab. Bot. 100s, 500s, 1000s. *Rx.*
Use: Hemorrheologic, vasodilator.
Pentrax Gold. (Medicis Dermatologicals, Inc.) Solubilized coal tar extract 4%. Shampoo. Bot. 168 ml. *otc.*
Use: Antiseborrheic.
Pentrax Shampoo. (Rydelle Laboratories) Tar extract 8.75%, detergents, conditioning agents. Bot. 4 oz, 8 oz. *otc.*
Use: Antiseborrheic.
•**pentrinitrol.** (pen-TRY-nye-TROLE) USAN.
Use: Vasodilator (coronary).
Pent-T-80. (Mericon Industries, Inc.) Pentaerythritol tetranitrate 80 mg/T.D. Cap. Bot. 100s, 1000s. *Rx.*
Use: Antianginal.
Pen-V. (Zenith Forest Pharmaceutical) Penicillin 250 mg, 500 mg/Tab. Bot. 100s, 1000s. *Rx.*
Use: Anti-infective, penicillin.
Pen-Vee K. (Wyeth-Ayerst Laboratories) Penicillin V 250 mg, 500 mg Tab. Bot. 100s, 500s, UD 100s. *Rx.*
Use: Anti-infective, penicillin.
Pen-Vee K for Oral Solution. (Wyeth-Ayerst Laboratories) Penicillin V 125 mg/5 ml, 250 mg/5 ml. Bot. 100 ml, 150 ml (250 mg/5 ml only), 200 ml. *Rx.*
Use: Anti-infective, penicillin.
Pepcid. (Merck & Co.) Famotidine. **Tab.:** 20 mg, 40 mg. Bot. 30s, 90s, 100s, UD 100s. **Oral Susp.:** 40 mg/5 ml. Bot. 400 mg. **I.V. Inj. Premixed:** 20 mg/50 ml in 0.9% NaCl. 50 ml *Galaxy* container. *Rx.*
Use: Antiulcerative.
Pepcid AC. (J & J Merck Consumer Pharm.) Famotidine 10 mg, phenylalanine 1.4 mg, lactose, mannitol. Chew. Tab. Pkg. 6s, 18s, 30s, 50s. *otc.*
Use: Histamine H_2 agonist.
Pepcid AC Acid Controller. (J & J Merck Consumer Pharm.) Famotidine 10 mg/Tab. Pkg. 12s. *otc.*
Use: Antiulcerative.
Pepcid AC Chewable. (J & J Merck Consumer Pharm.) Famotidine 10 mg, aspartame, lactose, phenylalanine 1.4 mg. Chew. Tab. Pkg. 18s. *otc.*
Use: Histamine H_2 agonist.

Pepcid RPD. (Merck & Co.) Famotidine 20 mg, 40 mg, aspartame, mint flavor, gelatin, mannitol. Orally disintegrating Tab. UD 30s, 100s. *Rx.*
Use: Histamine H_2 agonist.

•**peplomycin sulfate.** (PEP-low-MY-sin) USAN.
Use: Antineoplastic.

•**peppermint.** N.F. 18.
Use: Pharmaceutic aid (flavor, perfume), antitussive, expectorant, nasal decongestant.
See: Vicks Prods. (Procter & Gamble Pharm.).

•**peppermint oil.** N.F. 18.
Use: Pharmaceutic aid (flavor).

•**peppermint spirit.** U.S.P. 23.
Use: Pharmaceutic aid (flavor, perfume).

•**peppermint water.** N.F. 18.
Use: Pharmaceutic aid (vehicle, flavored).

Pepsamar Comp. Tablets. (Sanofi Winthrop Pharmaceuticals) Aluminum hydroxide, magnesium hydroxide. *otc.*
Use: Antacid.

Pepsamar Esp Liquid. (Sanofi Winthrop Pharmaceuticals) Aluminum hydroxide, glycerin. *otc.*
Use: Antacid.

Pepsamar Esp Tablets. (Sanofi Winthrop Pharmaceuticals) Aluminum hydroxide, magnesium hydroxide, mannitol powder. *otc.*
Use: Antacid.

Pepsamar HM Tablets. (Sanofi Winthrop Pharmaceuticals) Aluminum hydroxide, starch. *otc.*
Use: Antacid.

Pepsamar Liquid. (Sanofi Winthrop Pharmaceuticals) Aluminum hydroxide. *otc.*
Use: Antacid.

Pepsamar Suspension. (Sanofi Winthrop Pharmaceuticals) Aluminum hydroxide, magnesium hydroxide, sorbitol. *otc.*
Use: Antacid.

Pepsamar Tablets. (Sanofi Winthrop Pharmaceuticals) Aluminum hydroxide. *otc.*
Use: Antacid.

Pepsicone Gel. (Sanofi Winthrop Pharmaceuticals) Aluminum hydroxide, magnesium hydroxide, simethicone. *otc.*
Use: Antacid, antiflatulent.

Pepsicone Tablet. (Sanofi Winthrop Pharmaceuticals) Aluminum hydroxide, magnesium hydroxide, simethicone. *otc.*
Use: Antacid, antiflatulent.

pepsin.
Use: Digestive aid.

pepsin w/combinations.
See: Biloric, Cap. (Arcum).
Donnazyme, Tab. (Wyeth-Ayerst Laboratories).
Enzobile, Tab. (Roberts Pharmaceuticals).
Leber Taurine, Liq. (Paddock Laboratories).

•**pepstatin.** (pep-STAT-in) USAN.
Use: Enzyme inhibitor (pepsin).

Peptamen Liquid. (Clintec Nutrition) Enzymatically hydrolyzed whey proteins, maltodextrin, starch, MCT, sunflower oil, lecithin, vitamins A, B_1, B_2, B_3, B_5, B_6, B_{12}, C, D, E, K, folic acid, biotin, choline, Ca, Cl, Cu, Fe, I, Mg, Mn, P, Zn. Can 500 ml. *otc.*
Use: Nutritional supplement.

Peptavlon. (Wyeth-Ayerst Laboratories) Pentagastrin 0.25 mg, NaCl/ml. For evaluation of gastric acid secretion. Amp. 2 ml, Ctn. 10s.
Use: Diagnostic aid.

Peptenzyme. (Schwarz Pharma, Inc.) Alcohol 16%. Pleasantly aromatic. Bot. Pt.
Use: Pharmaceutic aid.

Pepto-Bismol Caplets. (Procter & Gamble Pharm.) Bismuth subsalicylate 262 mg, < 2 mg sodium/Capl. Sugar free. Bot. 24s, 40s. *otc.*
Use: Antidiarrheal.

Pepto-Bismol Liquid. (Procter & Gamble Pharm.) Bismuth subsalicylate 262 mg/15 ml. Bot. 4 oz, 8 oz, 12 oz, 16 oz. *otc.*
Use: Antidiarrheal.

Pepto-Bismol Maximum Strength Liquid. (Procter & Gamble Pharm.) 524 mg/15 ml. Bot. 120 ml, 240 ml, 360 ml. *otc.*
Use: Antidiarrheal.

Pepto-Bismol Tablets. (Procter & Gamble Pharm.) Bismuth subsalicylate 262.5 mg/Chew. Tab. Pkg. 24s, 42s. *otc.*
Use: Antidiarrheal.

Perandren Phenylacetate. (Novartis Pharmaceutical Corp.) Testosterone phenylacetate. *c-III.*
Use: Androgen.

percaine.
Use: Local anesthetic.
See: Dibucaine HCl, U.S.P. 23.

Perchloracap. (Mallinckrodt) Potassium perchlorate 200 mg/Cap. Bot. 100s. *Rx.*

Use: Radiographic adjunct.
perchlorethylene. U.S.P. 23.
See: Tetrachlorethylene.
perchlorperazine.
See: Compazine, Preps. (SmithKline Beecham Pharmaceuticals).
Percocet. (Du Pont Merck Pharmaceutical Co.) Oxycodone HCl 5 mg, acetaminophen 325 mg/Tab. Bot. 100s, 500s, UD 100s. *c-II.*
Use: Analgesic combination, narcotic.
Percodan. (Du Pont Merck Pharmaceutical Co.) Oxycodone HCl 4.5 mg, oxycodone terephthalate 0.38 mg, aspirin 325 mg/Tab. Bot. 100s, 500s, 1000s, UD 250s. *c-II.*
Use: Analgesic combination, narcotic.
Percodan-Demi. (Du Pont Merck Pharmaceutical Co.) Oxycodone HCl 2.25 mg, oxycodone terephthalate 0.19 mg, aspirin 325 mg/Tab. Bot. 100s. *c-II.*
Use: Analgesic combination, narcotic.
Percogesic. (Procter & Gamble Pharm.) Acetaminophen 325 mg, phenyltoloxamine citrate 30 mg/Tab. Bot. 24s, 50s, 90s. *otc.*
Use: Analgesic, antihistamine.
Percolone. (Endo Laboratories) Oxycodone HCl 5 mg. Tab. Bot. 100s, UD 100s. *c-II.*
Use: Analgesic, narcotic.
Percomorph Liver Oil. May be blended with 50% other fish liver oils; each g contains vitamins A 60,000 IU & D 8500 IU.
Percy Medicine. (Merrick Medicine) Bismuth subnitrate 959 mg, calcium hydroxide 21.9 mg/10 ml, alcohol 5%. *otc.*
Use: Antidiarrheal.
Perdiem. (Rhone-Poulenc Rorer Pharmaceuticals, Inc.) Blend of psyllium 82%, senna 18% as active ingredients in granular form. Sodium content (0.08 mEq) 1.8 mg/rounded tsp. (6 g). Canister 100 g, 250 g, UD 6 g. *otc.*
Use: Laxative.
Perdiem Fiber. (Rhone-Poulenc Rorer Pharmaceuticals, Inc.) Psyllium 100% as active ingredient in granular form. Sodium content (0.08 mEq) 1.8 mg/ rounded tsp. (6 g). Canister 100 g, 250 g, UD 6 g. *otc.*
Use: Laxative.
Pere-Diosate. (Towne) Docusate sodium 100 mg, casanthranol 30 mg/Cap. Bot. 100s. *otc.*
Use: Laxative.
Perestan. (Henry Schein, Inc.) Docusate sodium 100 mg, casanthranol 30 mg/ Cap. Bot. 100s, 1000s. *otc.*
Use: Laxative.
•**perfilcon a.** (per-FILL-kahn A) USAN.
Use: Contact lens material (hydrophilic).
•**perflenapent.** (per-FLEN-ah-pent) USAN.
Use: Diagnostic aid (ultrasound contrast agent).
•**perflisopent.** USAN.
Use: Diagnostic aid (ultrasound contrast agent).
•**perflubron.** (per-FLEW-brahn) U.S.P. 23.
Use: Contrast agent; blood substitute.
•**perfosfamide.** (per-FOSS-fam-ide) USAN.
Use: Antineoplastic. [Orphan Drug]
pergalen.
See: Sodium Apolate.
•**pergolide mesylate.** (PURR-go-lide) USAN.
Use: Dopamine agonist.
See: Permax, Tab. (Athena Neurosciences, Inc.).
Pergonal (menotropins). (Serono Laboratories, Inc.) Follicle-stimulating hormone (FSH) and luteinizing hormone (LH) 75 IU, 150 IU. Inj. Amp 2 ml. *Rx.*
Use: Hormone, gonadotropin.
Pergrava. (Arcum) Vitamins A 2000 IU, D 300 IU, B_1 2 mg, B_2 2 mg, nicotinamide 10 mg, B_6 2 mg, B_{12} 5 mcg, C 60 mg, Ca 40 mg/Cap. Bot. 100s, 1000s. *otc.*
Use: Mineral, vitamin supplement.
Pergrava No. 2. (Arcum) Vitamins A 2000 IU, D 300 IU, B_1 2 mg, B_2 2 mg, nicotinamide 10 mg, B_6 2 mg, C 60 mg, calcium lactate monohydrate 200 mg, ferrous gluconate 31 mg, folic acid 0.1 mg/Cap. Bot. 100s, 1000s. *otc.*
Use: Mineral, vitamin supplement.
perhexiline. (per-HEX-ih-leen)
Use: Antianginal.
•**perhexiline maleate.** (per-HEX-ih-leen) USAN.
Use: Vasodilator (coronary).
perhydrol.
See: Hydrogen Peroxide 30% (Various Mfr.).
Peri Sofcap. (Alton) Docusate sodium with peristim. Bot. 100s, 1000s. *otc.*
Use: Laxative.
Periactin. (Merck & Co.) Cyproheptadine HCl 4 mg/Tab. Bot. 100s. *Rx.*
Use: Antihistamine.
Periactin Syrup. (Merck & Co.) Cyproheptadine HCl 2 mg/5 ml, alcohol 5%, sucrose, saccharin. Bot. 473 ml. *Rx.*
Use: Antihistamine.
Peri-Care. (Sween) Vitamins A and D in petroleum ointment base. Tube 0.5 oz,

1.75 oz. Jar 2 oz, 5 oz, 8 oz. *otc.*
Use: Emollient.

Peri-Colace. (Bristol-Myers Squibb) **Cap.:** Docusate sodium 100 mg, casanthranol 30 mg/Cap. Bot. 30s, 60s, 250s, 1000s, UD 100s. **Syr.:** Docusate sodium 60 mg, casanthranol 30 mg/15 ml, ethyl alcohol 10%. Bot. 8 oz, pt. *otc.*
Use: Laxative.

Peridex. (Procter & Gamble Pharm.) Chlorhexidine gluconate 0.12%, alcohol 11.6%, glycerin, PEG-40 sorbitan diisostearate, flavor, sodium saccharin, FD& C blue No. 1, water. Bot. 480 ml. *Rx.*
Use: Mouth preparation.

Peridin-C. (Beutlich, Inc.) Hesperidin methyl chalcone 50 mg, hesperidin complex 150 mg, ascorbic acid 200 mg/Tab. Bot. 100s, 500s. *otc.*
Use: Vitamin supplement.

Peri-Dos. (Zenith Forest Pharmaceutical) Docusate sodium 100 mg, casanthranol 30 mg/Cap. Bot. 30s, 60s, 100s, 1000s. *otc.*
Use: Laxative.

Peries. (Xttrium Laboratories, Inc.) Medicated pads w/witch hazel, glycerin. Jar pad 40s. *otc.*
Use: Hygienic wipe and local compress.

•**perindopril.** (per-IN-doe-prill) USAN.
Use: ACE inhibitor.

•**perindopril erbumine.** (per-IN-doe-prill ehr-BYOO-meen) USAN.
Use: Antihypertensive.
See: Aceon, Tab. (Ortho McNeil Pharmaceutical).

PerioChip. (Astra USA) Chlorhexidine gluconate 2.5 mg. Chip Blister pack 10s. *Rx.*
Use: Anesthetic.

Perio-Eze-20. (Moyco Union Broach Division) Oral paste.
Use: Analgesic, topical.

PerioGard. (Colgate Oral Pharmaceuticals) Chlorhexidine gluconate 0.12%, alcohol 11.6%, glycerin, PEG-40, sorbitol diisostearnate, saccharin. Rinse. Bot. 473 ml w/15 ml dose cup. *Rx.*
Use: Anesthetic.

Periostat. (CollaGenex) Doxycycline hyclate 20 mg. Cap. Bot. 100s. *Rx.*
Use: Anti-infective.

Peritinic. (ESI Lederle Generics) Elemental iron 100 mg, docusate sodium 100 mg, vitamins B_1 7.5 mg, B_2 7.5 mg, B_6 7.5 mg, B_{12} 50 mcg, C 200 mg, niacinamide 30 mg, folic acid 0.05 mg, pantothenic acid 15 mg/Tab. Bot. 60s. *otc.*
Use: Mineral, vitamin supplement; laxative.

Peritrate. (Parke-Davis) Pentaerythritol tetranitrate. **10 mg/Tab.:** Bot. 100s, 1000s. **20 mg/Tab.:** Bot. 100s, 1000s, UD 100s. **40 mg/Tab.:** Bot. 100s. *Rx.*
Use: Antianginal.

Peritrate S.A. (Parke-Davis) Pentaerythritol tetranitrate 80 mg (20 mg in immediate release layer, 60 mg in sustained release base)/Tab. Bot. 100s, 1000s, UD 100s. *Rx.*
Use: Antianginal.

Peri-Wash. (Sween) Bot. 4 oz, 8 oz, 1 gal., 5 gal., 30 gal., 55 gal.
Use: Anorectal preparation.

Peri-Wash II. (Sween) Bot. 4 oz, 8 oz, 1 gal., 5 gal., 30 gal., 55 gal.
Use: Anorectal preparation.

•**perlapine.** (PURR-lah-peen) USAN.
Use: Hypnotic, sedative.

perlatan.
See: Estrone (Various Mfr.).

permanganic acid, potassium salt. U.S.P. 23. Potassium permanganate.

Permapen. (Roerig) Penicillin benzathine G 1,200,000 units/dose. Inj. Isoject 2 ml. *Rx.*
Use: Anti-infective, penicillin.

Permax. (Athena Neurosciences, Inc.) Pergolide mesylate. 0.05 mg, 0.25 mg, 1 mg. Tab. Bot. 30s (0.05 mg only), 100s. *Rx.*
Use: Antiparkinsonian.

•**permethrin.** (per-METH-rin) USAN. Synthetic pyrethrin.
Use: Pediculicide for treatment of head lice, ectoparasiticide.
See: Acticin, Cream (Alpharma USPD Inc.).
Nix, Cream (GlaxoWellcome).

Permitil. (Schering-Plough Corp.) Fluphenazine HCl. **2.5 mg or 5 mg/Tab.:** Bot. 100s. **10 mg/Tab.:** Bot. 1000s. *Rx.*
Use: Antipsychotic.

Permitil Oral Concentrate. (Schering-Plough Corp.) Fluphenazine HCl 5 mg/ml, alcohol 1%, parabens. Dropper Bot. 118 ml. *Rx.*
Use: Antipsychotic.

Pernox Lathering Abradant Scrub. (Westwood Squibb Pharmaceuticals) Sulfur, salicylic acid. Lot. Bot. 141 g. *otc.*
Use: Dermatologic, acne.

Pernox Lotion. (Westwood Squibb Pharmaceuticals) Microfine granules of polyethylene 20%, sulfur 2%, salicylic acid 2% in a combination of soapless cleansers and wetting agents. Bot. 6

oz. *otc.*
Use: Dermatologic, acne.

Pernox Medicated Lathering Scrub Cleanser. (Westwood Squibb Pharmaceuticals) Polyethylene granules 26%, sulfur 2%, salicylic acid 1.5% w/soapless surface-active cleansers and wetting agents. Regular or lemon. Tube 2 oz, 4 oz. *otc.*
Use: Dermatologic, acne.

Pernox Scrub for Oily Skin. (Westwood Squibb Pharmaceuticals) Sulfur, salicylic acid, EDTA. Cleanser. 56 g, 113 g. *otc.*
Use: Dermatologic, acne.

Pernox Shampoo. (Westwood Squibb Pharmaceuticals) Sodium laureth sulfate, water, lauramide DEA, quaternium 22, PEG-75 lanolin/hydrolyzed animal protein, fragrance, sodium Cl, lactic acid, sorbic acid, disodium EDTA, FD&C yellow No. 6 and blue No. 1. Bot. 8 oz. *otc.*
Use: Cleanser, conditioner.

peroxidase.
W/Glucose oxidase, potassium, iodide.
See: Diastix Reagent Strips (Bayer Corp. (Consumer Div.)).

peroxide, dibenzoyl. Benzoyl Peroxide, Hydrous.

peroxides.
See: Hydrogen Peroxide (Various Mfr.).
Urea Peroxide.
Zinc Peroxide.

Peroxin A5. (Dermol Pharmaceuticals, Inc.) Benzoyl peroxide 5%. Gel Tube 45 ml. *Rx.*
Use: Dermatologic, acne.

Peroxin A10. (Dermol Pharmaceuticals, Inc.) Benzoyl peroxide 10%. Gel Tube 45 ml. *Rx.*
Use: Dermatologic, acne.

Peroxyl Dental Rinse. (Colgate Oral Pharmaceuticals) Hydrogen peroxide 1.5% in mint-flavored base, alcohol 6%. Bot. 240 ml, pt. *otc.*
Use: Mouth preparation.

Peroxyl Gel. (Colgate Oral Pharmaceuticals) Hydrogen peroxide 1.5% in a mint-flavored base. Gel Tube. 15 ml. *otc.*
Use: Mouth preparation.

•**perphenazine.** (per-FEN-uh-ZEEN) U.S.P. 23.
Use: Antiemetic, antipsychotic, anxiolytic.
See: Trilafon, Prods. (Schering-Plough Corp.).

perphenazine. (Various Mfr.) Perphenazine 2 mg, 4 mg, 8 mg, 16 mg. Tab. Bot. 100s, 250s (8 mg only), 500s. *Rx.*
Use: Antipsychotic.

perphenazine/amitriptyline tablets. (per-FEN-uh-zeen am-ee-TRIP-tih-leen) (Various Mfr.). Perphenazine (mg): 2, 2; Amitriptyline (mg): 10, 25. Bot. 21s, 100s, 500s, 1000s; Bot. 100s, 500s, 1000s.
Use: Miscellaneous psychotherapeutic.
See: Etrafon, Prods. (Schering-Plough Corp.).

Persa-Gel. (Advanced Care Products) Benzoyl peroxide 5%, 10%, acetone base. Tube 45 ml, 90 ml. *Rx.*
Use: Dermatologic, acne.

Persa-Gel W 5%, 10%. (Advanced Care Products) Benzoyl peroxide 5%, 10% in water base. Tube 45 ml, 90 ml. *Rx.*
Use: Dermatologic, acne.

Persangue. (Arcum) Ferrous gluconate 192 mg, vitamins C 150 mg, B_1 3 mg, B_2 3 mg, B_{12} 50 mcg/Cap. Bot. 100s, 500s. *otc.*
Use: Mineral, vitamin supplement.

Persantine. (Boehringer Ingelheim, Inc.) Dipyridamole 25 mg, 50 mg, 75 mg. Tab. **25 mg , 50 mg:** Bot. 100s, 1000s, UD 100s. **75 mg:** Bot. 100s, 500s, UD 100s. *Rx.*
Use: Antiplatelet.

Persantine IV. (Du Pont Merck Pharmaceutical Co.) Dipyridamole. Inj. For evaluation of coronary artery disease.
Use: Diagnostic aid.

persic oil. N.F. XVII.
Use: Vehicle.

pertechnetic acid, sodium salt. Sodium Pertechnetate Tc 99 m Solution.

Pertscan-99m. (Abbott Diagnostics) Radiodiagnostic. Inj. Tc-99m.
Use: Diagnostic aid.

Pertussin All-Night PM. (Pertussin Labs) Acetaminophen 167 mg, doxylamine succinate 1.25 mg, pseudoephedrine HCl 10 mg, dextromethorphan HBr 5 mg/5 ml, alcohol 25%. Liq. Bot. 240 ml. *otc.*
Use: Analgesic, antihistamine, antitussive, decongestant.

Pertussin CS. (Pertussin) Dextromethorphan HBr 3.5 mg, guaifenesin 25 mg/5 ml, 8.5% alcohol. Bot. 90 ml. *otc.*
Use: Antitussive, expectorant.

Pertussin ES. (Pertussin) Dextromethorphan HBr 15 mg/5 ml, alcohol 9.5%, sugar, sorbitol. Liq. Bot. 120 ml. *otc.*
Use: Antitussive.

Pertussin Syrup. (Pertussin) Dextromethorphan HBr 15 mg/5 ml, alcohol 9.5%. Bot. 3 oz, 6 oz. *otc.*
Use: Antitussive.

•**pertussis immune globulin.** (per-TUSS-iss) U.S.P. 23. *Formerly Pertussis Im-*

mune Human Globulin.
Use: Immunization.
•**pertussis vaccine.** U.S.P. 23.
Use: Immunization.
W/diphtheria and tetanus toxoids.
See: Acel-Imune, Vial (Wyeth-Ayerst Laboratories).
Certiva (Ross Pediatrics).
Infanrix (SKB).
Tri-Immunol, Vial (Wyeth-Ayerst Laboratories).
Tripedia, Vial (Pasteur Merieux Connaught).
pertussis vaccine. (Michigan Department of Health) Vial 5 ml.
Use: Immunization.
•**pertussis vaccine adsorbed.** U.S.P. 23.
Use: Immunization.
pertussis vaccine and diphtheria and tetanus toxoids, combined.
Use: Immunization.
See: Acel-Imune, Vial (Wyeth-Ayerst Laboratories).
Infanrix (SKB).
Tri-Immunol, Vial (Wyeth-Ayerst Laboratories).
Tripedia, Vial (Pasteur Merieux Connaught).
peruvian balsam.
Use: Local protectant, rubefacient.
W/Benzocaine, zinc oxide, bismuth subgallate, boric acid.
See: Hemorrhoidal Oint. (Towne).
W/Ephedrine sulfate, belladonna extract, zinc oxide, boric acid, bismuth oxyiodide, subcarbonate.
See: Wyanoids, Preps. (Wyeth-Ayerst Laboratories).
W/Lidocaine, bismuth subgallate, zinc oxide, aluminum subacetate.
See: Xylocaine, Supp. (Astra Pharmaceuticals, L.P.).
peson. Sodium Lyapolate. Polyethylene sulfonate sodium.
Use: Anticoagulant.
Peterson's Ointment. (Peterson) Carbolic acid, camphor, tannic acid, zinc oxide. Tube w/pipe 1 oz. Jar 16 oz. Can 1.4 oz, 3 oz. *otc.*
Use: Anorectal preparation.
Pethadol. (Halsey Drug Co.) Meperidine HCl 50 mg, 100 mg/Tab. Bot. 100s, 1000s. *c-II.*
Use: Analgesic, narcotic.
pethidine hydrochloride. U.S.P. 23.
See: Meperidine HCl.
PETN.
See: Pentaerythritol tetranitrate.
petrichloral. Pentaerythritol chloral.
Use: Sedative.
Petro-20. (Foy Laboratories) Pentaerythritol tetranitrate 20 mg/Tab. Bot. 100s, 1000s. *Rx.*
Use: Antianginal.
•**petrolatum.** (pen-troe-LAY-tum) U.S.P. 23.
Use: Pharmaceutic aid (ointment base).
See: Lipkote, Stick (Schering-Plough Corp.).
petrolatum gauze.
Use: Surgical aid.
•**petrolatum, hydrophilic.** U.S.P. 23.
Use: Pharmaceutic aid (absorbent, ointment base) topical protectant.
See: Lipkote (Schering-Plough Corp.).
petrolatum, liquid. U.S.P. 23. Mineral Oil, Light Mineral Oil, Adepsine Oil, Glymol, Liquid Paraffin, Parolein, White Mineral Oil, Heavy Liquid Petrolatum.
Use: Laxative.
See: Fleet Mineral Oil Enema (C.B. Fleet Co., Inc.).
Mineral Oil (Various Mfr.).
Saxol (Various Mfr.).
petrolatum, liquid, emulsion.
Use: Lubricant, laxative.
See: Milkinol, Liq. (Schwarz Pharma).
W/Agar-Gel.
See: Agoral Plain, Liq. (Parke-Davis).
Milkinol, Liq. (Schwarz Pharma).
W/Irish moss, casanthranol.
See: Haley's M. O., Liq. (Sanofi Winthrop Pharmaceuticals).
W/Phenolphthalein.
See: Agoral, Emulsion (Parke-Davis).
Phenolphthalein in liquid Petrolatum Emulsion.
petrolatum, red veterinarian. (Zeneca Pharmaceuticals) Also known as RVP.
W/Micasorb.
See: RV Plus, Oint. (ICN Pharmaceuticals, Inc.).
W/N-diethyl metatoluamide.
See: RV Pellent, Oint. (Zeneca Pharmaceuticals).
W/Zinc oxide, 2-ethoxyethyl p-methoxycinnamate.
See: RV Paque, Oint. (ICN Pharmaceuticals, Inc.).
•**petrolatum, white.** U.S.P. 23.
Use: Pharmaceutic aid (oleaginous ointment base) topical protectant.
See: Moroline, Oint. (Schering-Plough Corp.).
Petro-Phylic Soap. (Doak Dermatologics) Hydrophilic Petrolatum. Cake 4 oz.
Use: Emollient, anti-infective, topical.
PF4RIA. (Abbott Diagnostics) Platelet factor 4 radioimmunoassay for the quantitative measurement of total PF4 levels in plasma.

Use: Diagnostic aid.

Pfeiffer's Cold Sore. (Pfeiffer Co.) Gum benzoin 7%, camphor, menthol, thymol, eucalyptol, alcohol 85%. Lot. Bot. 15 ml. *otc.*
Use: Cold sores, fever blisters, moisturizer.

Pfizerpen. (Roering) Penicillin G potassium 1,000,000 units, 5,000,000 units, 20,000,000 units/vial. Pow. for Inj. Vial. *Rx.*
Use: Anti-infective, penicillin.

Pfizerpen VK. (Pfizer US Pharmaceutical Group) Penicillin V potassium 250 mg, 500 mg/Tab. **250 mg:** Bot. 1000s. **500 mg:** Bot. 100s. *Rx.*
Use: Anti-infective, penicillin.

PGA. U.S.P. 23.
See: Folic Acid.

PGE.
Use: Prostaglandin.
See: Alprostadil.

pHacid. (Baker Cummins Dermatologicals, Inc.) Bot. 8 oz.
Use: Dermatologic.

Phadiatop RIA Test. (Pharmacia & Upjohn) Determination of IgE antibodies specific to inhalant allergens in human serum. Kit 60s.
Use: Diagnostic aid.

Phanacol Cough. (Pharmakon Laboratories, Inc.) Phenylpropanolamine HCl 25 mg, dextromethorphan HBr 10 mg, guaifenesin 100 mg, acetaminophen 325 mg/5 ml. Syrup. Bot. 118 ml, 236 ml. *otc.*
Use: Antitussive, decongestant, expectorant.

Phanadex Cough Syrup. (Pharmakon Laboratories, Inc.) Phenylpropanolamine HCl 25 mg, pyrilamine maleate 40 mg, dextromethorphan HBr 15 mg, guaifenesin 100 mg/5 ml, sugar, potassium citrate, citric acid. Syr. Bot. 118 ml, 236 ml. *otc.*
Use: Antihistamine, antitussive, decongestant, expectorant.

Phanatuss Cough Syrup. (Pharmakon Laboratories, Inc.) Dextromethorphan HBr 10 mg, guaifenesin 85 mg, potassium citrate 75 mg, citric acid 35 mg/5 ml, sorbitol, menthol. Syr. Bot. 118 ml. *otc.*
Use: Antitussive, expectorant.

pH Antiseptic Skin Cleanser. (Walgreen Co.) Alcohol 63%. Bot. 16 oz. *otc.*
Use: Astringent, cleanser.

Pharazine. (Halsey Drug Co.) Bot. 4 oz, pt, gal.
Use: A series of cough and cold products.

Pharmadine. (Sherwood Davis & Geck) Povidone-iodine. **Oint.:** Pkt. 1 g, 1.5 g, 2 g, 30 g, 1 lb. **Perineal wash:** 240 ml. **Skin cleanser:** 240 ml. **Soln.:** 15 ml, 120 ml, 240 ml, pt, qt. **Soln., swabs:** 100s. **Soln., swabsticks:** 1 or 3/packet in 250s. **Spray:** 120 g. **Surgical scrub:** 30 ml, pt, qt, gal, foil-pack 15 ml. **Surgical scrub sponge/brush:** 25s. **Swabsticks, lemon glycerin:** 100s. **Whirlpool soln.:** Gal. *otc.*
Use: Antiseptic.

Pharmaflur. (Pharmics, Inc.) Sodium fluoride 2.21 mg. Tab. Bot. 1000s. *Rx.*
Use: Dental caries agent.

Pharmalgen Hymenoptera Venoms. (ALK Laboratories, Inc.) Freeze-dried venom or venom protein. Vials of 120 mcg, 1100 mcg for each of honey bee, white-faced hornet, yellow hornet, yellow jacket, or wasp. Vials of 360 mcg, 3300 mcg for mixed vespids (white-faced hornet, yellow hornet, yellow jacket). Diagnostic kit: 5 x 1 ml vial. Treatment kit: 6 x 1 ml vial or 1 x 1.1 mg multiple-dose vial. Starter Kit: 6 x 1 ml, pre-diluted 0.01 mcg to 100 mcg/ml.
Use: Antivenim.

Pharmalgen Standardized Allergenic Extracts. (ALK Laboratories, Inc.) 100,000 allergenic units/Vial. Box 5 x 1 ml.
Use: Diagnostic aid.

Phazyme. (Schwarz Pharma, Inc.) Simethicone 60 mg/Tab. Bot. 50s, 100s, 1000s. *otc.*
Use: Antiflatulent.

Phazyme 95. (Schwarz Pharma, Inc.) Simethicone 95 mg/Tab. Bot. 100s. *otc.*
Use: Antiflatulent.

Phazyme 125. (Schwarz Pharma, Inc.) Simethicone 125 ml. Cap. Bot. 50s. *otc.*
Use: Antiflatulent.

Phazyme Drops. (Schwarz Pharma, Inc.) Simethicone 40 mg/0.6 ml, saccharin. Bot. 30 ml w/dropper. *otc.*
Use: Antiflatulent.

•**phemfilcon a.** (FEM-fill-kahn A) USAN.
Use: Contact lens material (hydrophilic).

phenacaine hydrochloride. U.S.P. XXI.
Use: Anesthetic, local.

Phenacal. (NeuroGenesis/Matrix Tech., Inc.) D,l-phenylalanine 500 mg, l-glutamine 15 mg, l-tyrosine 25 mg, l-carnitine 10 mg, l-arginine pyroglutamate 10 mg, l-ornithine/l-aspartate 10 mg, Cr 0.033 mg, Se 0.012 mg, vitamin B_1 0.33 mg, B_2 5 mg, B_3 3.3 mg, B_5 0.33 mg, B_6 0.33 mg, B_{12} 1 mcg, E 5 IU,

biotin 0.05 mg, folic acid 0.066 mg, Fe 1 mg, Zn 2.5 mg, Ca 35 mg, I 0.25 mg, Cu 0.33 mg, Mg 25 mg/Cap. Bot. 42s, 180s. *otc.*
Use: Nutritional supplement.

phenacetin. Acetophenetidin. Ethoxy-acetanilide.
Note: This drug has been withdrawn from the market due to liver and kidney toxicity. This drug is no longer official in the U.S.P.
Use: Antipyretic, analgesic.

Phenadex Senior. (Alpharma USPD Inc.) Dextromethorphan HBr 10 mg, guaifenesin 200 mg/5 ml. Liq. Bot. 118 ml. *otc.*
Use: Antitussive, expectorant.

Phenahist Injectable. (T.E. Williams Pharmaceuticals) Atropine sulfate 0.2 mg, phenylpropanolamine HCl 12.5 mg, chlorpheniramine maleate 5 mg/ml. Vial 10 ml. *Rx.*
Use: Anticholinergic, antihistamine, antispasmodic, decongestant.

Phenahist-TR Tablets. (T.E. Williams Pharmaceuticals) Phenylephrine HCl 25 mg, phenylpropanolamine HCl 50 mg, chlorpheniramine maleate 8 mg, hyoscyamine sulfate 0.19 mg, atropine 0.04 mg, scopolamine HBr 0.01 mg. Tab. Bot. 100s. *Rx.*
Use: Anticholinergic, antihistamine, antispasmodic, decongestant.

phenamazoline hydrochloride.
Use: Vasoconstrictor.

Phenameth DM. (Major Pharmaceuticals) Promethazine HCl 6.25 mg, dextromethorphan HBr 15 mg/5 ml, alcohol. Syr. Bot. 120 ml. *Rx.*
Use: Antihistamine, antitussive.

Phenameth Tablets. (Major Pharmaceuticals) Promethazine 25 mg. Tab. Bot. 1000s. *Rx.*
Use: Antiemetic, antihistamine.

Phenameth VC w/Codeine. (Major Pharmaceuticals) Phenylephrine HCl 5 mg, promethazine HCl 6.25 mg, codeine phosphate 10 mg/5 ml, alcohol 7%. Syr. Bot. Pt, gal. *c-v.*
Use: Antihistamine, antitussive, decongestant.

Phenameth w/Codeine. (Major Pharmaceuticals) Promethazine HCl 6.25 mg, codeine phosphate 10 mg/5 ml, alcohol 7%. Syr. Bot. 4 oz, pt, gal. *c-v.*
Use: Antihistamine, antitussive.

phenantoin. Mephenytoin.
See: Mesantoin, Tab. (Novartis Pharmaceutical Corp.).

Phenapap Sinus Headache & Congestion. (Rugby Labs, Inc.) Pseudoephedrine HCl 30 mg, chlorpheniramine 2 mg, acetaminophen 325 mg. Tab. Bot. 30s, 100s, 1000s. *otc.*
Use: Analgesic, antihistamine, decongestant.

Phenaphen w/Codeine No. 3. (Wyeth-Ayerst Laboratories) Codeine phosphate 30 mg, acetaminophen 325 mg/Tab. *c-III.*
Use: Analgesic combination, narcotic.

phenaphthazine. Sodium dinitro phenylazonaphthol disulfonate.
See: Nitrazine Paper, Roll (Bristol-Myers Squibb).

phenarsone sulfoxylate. Methanesulfinic acid disodium salt.
Use: Antiamebic.

Phenaspirin Compound. (Davis & Sly) Phenobarbital 0.25 gr, aspirin 3.5 gr. Cap. Bot. 1000s. *Rx.*
Use: Analgesic, hypnotic, sedative.

Phenate. (Roberts Pharmaceuticals) Phenylpropanolamine HCl 40 mg, chlorpheniramine maleate 4 mg, acetaminophen 325 mg. CR Tab. Bot. 100s, 1000s. *Rx.*
Use: Analgesic, antihistamine, decongestant.

phenazocine hydrobromide.
Use: Analgesic.

phenazone.
See: Antipyrine (Various Mfr.).

•**phenazopyridine hydrochloride.** (fen-AZZ-oh-PIH-rih-deen) U.S.P. 23.
Use: Analgesic, urinary.
See: Azo-Standard, Tab. (PolyMedica Pharmaceuticals).
Pyridium, Tab. (Warner Chilcott Laboratories).

phenazopyridine hydrochloride w/ combinations.
See: Azo Gantanol, Tab. (Roche Laboratories).
Azo Gantrisin, Tab. (Roche Laboratories).
Azo-sulfisoxazole (Various Mfr.).
Triurisul, Tab. (Sheryl).
Uridium, Tab. (Ferndale; Pharmex).
Urisan-P, Tab. (Sandia).
Urobiotic, Cap. (Pfizer US Pharmaceutical Group).
Urogesic, Tab. (Edwards Pharmaceuticals, Inc.).

•**phenbutazone sodium glycerate.** (fen-BYOO-tah-zone so-dee-uhm GLIH-seh-rate) USAN.
Use: Anti-inflammatory.

•**phencarbamide.** (FEN-car-BAM-id) USAN.
Use: Anticholinergic, spasmolytic.

Phenchlor-Eight. (Freeport) Chlorpheniramine maleate 8 mg. TR Cap. Bot. 1000s. *Rx.*
Use: Antihistamine.

Phenchlor S.H.A. (Rugby Labs, Inc.) Phenylpropanolamine HCl 50 mg, phenylephrine HCl 25 mg, chlorpheniramine maleate 8 mg, hyoscyamine sulfate 0.19 mg, atropine sulfate 0.04 mg, scopolamine HBr 0.01mg/SR Tab. Bot. 100s, 500s. *Rx.*
Use: Anticholinergic, antihistamine, decongestant.

Phenchlor-Twelve. (Freeport) Chlorpheniramine maleate 12 mg. TR Cap. Bot. 1000s. *Rx.*
Use: Antihistamine.

•**phencyclidine hydrochloride.** (fen-SIGH-klih-deen) USAN.
Use: Anesthetic.

•**phendimetrazine tartrate.** (fen-die-MEH-trah-zeen TAR-trate) U.S.P. 23.
Use: Appetite suppressant (systemic).
See: Adipost, Cap. (B.F. Ascher and Co.).
Anorex, Cap., Tab. (Dunhall Pharmaceuticals, Inc.).
Bontril PDM, Tab. (Carnrick Laboratories, Inc.).
Bontril Slow Release, Cap. (Carnrick Laboratories, Inc.).
Delcozine, Tab. (Delco).
Di-Ap-Trol, Tab. (Foy Laboratories).
Elphemet, Tab. (Canright).
Obepar, Tab. (Parmed Pharmaceuticals, Inc.).
Obe-Tite, Tab. (Scott/Cord).
Phen-70, Tab. (Parmed Pharmaceuticals, Inc.).
Prelu-2, Cap. (Boehringer Ingelheim, Inc.).
Reducto, Tab. (Arcum).
Rexigen Forte, SR Cap. (ION Laboratories, Inc.).
Slim-Tabs, Tab. (Wesley Pharmacal Co, Inc.).

Phendry. (LuChem Pharmaceuticals, Inc.) Diphenhydramine HCl 12.5 mg/5 ml, alcohol 14%. Elix. Bot. Pt, gal. *otc.*
Use: Antihistamine.

Phendry Children's Allergy Medicine. (LuChem Pharmaceuticals, Inc.) Diphenhydramine HCl 12.5 mg/5 ml, alcohol 14%. Elix. Bot. 120 ml. *otc.*
Use: Antihistamine.

phenelzine dihydrogen sulfate.
See: Nardil, Tab. (Parke-Davis).

•**phenelzine sulfate.** (FEN-uhl-zeen) U.S.P. 23.
Use: Antidepressant.
See: Nardil, Tab. (Parke-Davis).

Phenerbel-S. (Rugby Labs, Inc.) Phenobarbital 40 mg, ergotamine tartrate 0.6 mg, l-alkaloids of belladonna 0.2 mg. Tab. Bot. 100s. *Rx.*
Use: Anticholinergic, hypnotic, sedative.

Phenergan-D. (Wyeth-Ayerst Laboratories) Promethazine HCl 6.25 mg, pseudoephedrine HCl 60 mg. Tab. Bot. 100s. *Rx.*
Use: Antihistamine, decongestant.

Phenergan Fortis. (Wyeth-Ayerst Laboratories) Promethazine HCl 25 mg/5 ml, alcohol 1.5%, saccharin. Bot. 473 ml. *Rx.*
Use: Antihistamine.

Phenergan Injection. (Wyeth-Ayerst Laboratories) Promethazine HCl 25 mg, 50 mg/ml, EDTA, phenol. Inj. Amp. 1 mg. *Rx.*
Use: Antihistamine.

Phenergan Plain. (Wyeth-Ayerst Laboratories) Promethazine HCl 6.25 mg/5 ml, alcohol 7%, saccharin. Syr. Bot. 118 ml, 473 ml. *Rx.*
Use: Antihistamine.

Phenergan Suppositories. (Wyeth-Ayerst Laboratories) Promethazine HCl 12.5 mg, 25 mg, 50 mg. Supp. Box. 12s. *Rx.*
Use: Antihistamine.

Phenergan Syrup Plain. (Wyeth-Ayerst Laboratories) Promethazine HCl 6.25 mg/5 ml. Bot. 4 oz, 6 oz, 8 oz, pt, gal. *Rx.*
Use: Antihistamine.

Phenergan Tablets. (Wyeth-Ayerst Laboratories) Promethazine HCl 12.5 mg, 25 mg, 50 mg. Tab. Bot. 100s. Redipak 100s. *Rx.*
Use: Antihistamine.

Phenergan VC. (Wyeth-Ayerst Laboratories) Promethazine HCl 6.25 mg, phenylephrine HCl 5 mg/5 ml. Syr. Bot. 118 ml, 473 ml. *Rx.*
Use: Antihistamine, decongestant.

Phenergan VC with Codeine. (Wyeth-Ayerst Laboratories) Promethazine HCl 6.25 mg, codeine phosphate 10 mg, phenylephrine HCl 5 mg/5 ml, alcohol 7%. Bot. 4 oz, 6 oz, 8 oz, pt, gal. *c-v.*
Use: Antihistamine, antitussive, decongestant.

Phenergan with Codeine. (Wyeth-Ayerst Laboratories) Promethazine HCl 6.25 mg, codeine phosphate 10 mg/5 ml. Bot. 4 oz, 6 oz, 8 oz, pt, gal. *c-v.*
Use: Antihistamine, antitussive.

Phenergan with Dextromethorphan. (Wyeth-Ayerst Laboratories) Pro-

methazine HCl 6.25 mg, dextromethorphan HBr 15 mg/5 ml, alcohol 7%. Bot. 4 oz, 6 oz, pt, gal. *Rx.*
Use: Antihistamine, antitussive.

pheneridine.
Use: Analgesic.

i-phenethylbiguanide monohydrochloride. Phenformin HCl.

Phenex-1. (Ross Laboratories) Protein 15 g, fat 23.9 g, carbohydrates 46.3 g, linoleic acid 1800 mg, Fe 9 mg, Na 190 mg, K 675 mg, Cal 480/100 g. With appropriate vitamins and minerals. Phenylalanine free. Pow. Can 350 g. *otc.*
Use: Nutritional supplement.

Phenex-2. (Ross Laboratories) Protein 30 g, fat 15.5 g, carbohydrates 30 g, Na 880 mg, K 1370 mg, Cal 410/ml. With appropriate vitamins and minerals. Phenylalanine free. Pow. Can 325 g. *otc.*
Use: Nutritional supplement.

phenformin hydrochloride. *Rx.*
Note: Withdrawn from market in 1978. Available under IND exemption.
Use: Hypoglycemic.

Phenhist DH w/Codeine. (Rugby Labs, Inc.) Pseudoephedrine HCl 30 mg, chlorpheniramine maleate 2 mg, codeine phosphate 10 mg/5 ml, alcohol 5%. Liq. Bot. 120 ml, 480 ml. *c-v.*
Use: Antihistamine, antitussive, decongestant.

Phenhist Expectorant. (Rugby Labs, Inc.) Pseudoephedrine HCl 30 mg, codeine phosphate 10 mg, guaifenesin 100 mg/5 ml, alcohol 7.5%. Liq. Bot. 118 ml, pt, gal. *c-v.*
Use: Antihistamine, antitussive, decongestant.

pheniform.
See: Phenformin HCl.

•**phenindamine tartrate.** USAN.
Use: Antihistamine.
See: Nolahist, Tab. (Carnrick Laboratories, Inc.).
W/Chlorpheniramine maleate, phenylpropanolamine HCl.
See: Nolamine, Tab. (Carnrick Laboratories, Inc.).
W/Phenylephrine HCl, aspirin, caffeine, aluminum hydroxide, magnesium carbonate.
See: Dristan, Tab. (Whitehall Robins Laboratories).
W/Phenylephrine HCl, caramiphen ethanedisulfonate.
See: Dondril, Tab. (Whitehall Robins Laboratories).
W/Phenylephrine HCl, chlorpheniramine maleate, drytane.
See: Comhist, Tab., Elix. (Baylor).
W/Phenylephrine HCl, chlorpheniramine maleate, belladonna alkaloids.
See: Comhist L.A., Cap. (Baylor Labs).
W/Phenylephrine HCl, pyrilamine maleate, chlorpheniramine maleate, dextromethorphan HBr.
See: Histalet, Histalet-DM, Histalet-Forte, Syr. (Solvay Pharmaceuticals).

pheniodol.
See: Iodoalphionic Acid (Various Mfr.).

pheniprazine hydrochloride.
Use: Antihypertensive.

•**pheniramine maleate.** USAN.
Use: Antihistamine.
See: Citra Forte, Cap., Syr. (Boyle and Co. Pharm).
Partuss AC (Parmed Pharmaceuticals, Inc.).
Poly-Histine Cap., Elix., Lipospan (Sanofi Winthrop Pharmaceuticals).
Thor, Cap. (Towne).
Tritussin, Syr. (Towne).
W/Combinations.
See: Iohist D (Iomed).
Statuss Green (Huckaby).
Tri-P Oral Infant Drops (Cypress).
Vetuss HC, Syr. (Cypress).

•**phenmetrazine hydrochloride.** (fen-MEH-trah-zeen) U.S.P. 23.
Use: Anorexic.

•**phenobarbital.** (fee-no-BAR-bih-tahl) U.S.P. 23.
Use: Anticonvulsant, hypnotic, sedative.
See: Solfoton, Tab., Cap. (ECR Pharmaceuticals).

phenobarbital. (Various Mfr.) **Tab.: 15 mg, 30 mg:** Bot. 100s, 1000s, 5000s, UD 100s. **60 mg:** Bot. 100s, 1000s, UD 100s. **100 mg:** 100s, 1000s. **Elix.:** 20 mg/5 ml. Bot. Pt, gal, UD 5 ml, UD 7.5 ml.
Use: Anticonvulsant, hypnotic, sedative.

phenobarbital. (Pharmaceutical Associates, Inc.) 15 mg/5 ml. Elix. Bot. Pt, UD 5 ml, 10 ml, 20 ml. *c-iv.*
Use: Anticonvulsant, hypnotic, sedative.

phenobarbital w/aminophylline.
See: Aminophylline (Various Mfr.).

phenobarbital w/atropine sulfate.
See: Atropine Sulfate (Various Mfr.).

phenobarbital w/belladonna.
See: Belladonna Products and Phenobarbital Combinations.

phenobarbital with central nervous system stimulants.
See: Arcotrate No. 3, Tab. (Arcum).

Sedamine, Tab. (Dunhall Pharmaceuticals, Inc.).
Spabelin, Elix., Tab. (Arcum).

phenobarbital combinations.
See: Aminophylline w/Phenobarbital, Combinations.
Aspirin-Barbiturate, Combinations.
Atropine-Hyoscine-Hyoscyamine Combinations.
Atropine Sulfate w/Phenobarbital.
Belladonna Extract Combinations.
Belladonna Products and Phenobarbital Combinations.
Bellatal, Tab. (Richwood Pahrmaceuticals).
Folergot-DF, Tab. (Marnel Pharmaceuticals, Inc.).
Homatropine Methylbromide and Phenobarbital Combinations.
Hyoscyamus Products and Phenobarbital Combinations.
Mannitol Hexanitrate w/Phenobarbital Combinations.
Mephenesin and Barbiturates Combinations.
Phenobarbital w/Central Nervous System Stimulants.
Secobarbital Combinations.
Sodium Nitrite Combinations.
Theobromine w/Phenobarbital Combinations.
Theophylline w/Phenobarbital Combinations.
Veratrum Viride w/Phenobarbital Combinations.

phenobarbital w/homatropine methylbromide.
See: Homatropine Methylbromide and Phenobarbital Combinations.

phenobarbital w/hyoscyamus.
See: Hyoscyamus Products and Phenobarbital Combinations.

phenobarbital w/mannitol hexanitrate.
Use: Anticonvulsant, sedative, hypnotic.
See: Mannitol Hexanitrate w/Phenobarbital Combinations.

•**phenobarbital sodium.** U.S.P. 23.
Use: Anticonvulsant, hypnotic, sedative.
See: Luminal Sodium, Inj. (Sanofi Winthrop Pharmaceuticals).

phenobarbital sodium. (Wyeth-Ayerst Laboratories) Inj. **30 mg/ml, 60 mg/ml:** *Tubex* 1 ml. **65 mg/ml:** Vial 1 ml. **130 mg/ml:** *Tubex* 1 ml, vial 1 ml. *c-IV.*
Use: Anticonvulsant, hypnotic, sedative.

phenobarbital sodium in propylene glycol. Vitarine. Amp. 0.13 g: 1 ml, Box 25s, 100s. *c-IV.*
Use: Anticonvulsant, hypnotic, sedative.

phenobarbital and theobromine combinations.
See: Theobromine w/Phenobarbital Combinations.

phenobarbital w/theophylline.
See: Theophylline w/Phenobarbital Combinations.

phenobarbital w/veratrum viride.
See: Veratrum Viride w/Phenobarbital Combinations.

Pheno-Bella. (Ferndale Laboratories, Inc.) Belladonna extract 10.8 mg, phenobarbital 16.2 mg/Tab. Bot. 100s, 1000s. *Rx.*
Use: Anticholinergic, antispasmodic, hypnotic, sedative.

•**phenol.** (FEE-nole) U.S.P. 23.
Use: Pharmaceutic aid (preservative), topical antipruritic.
W/Aluminum hydroxide, zinc oxide, camphor, eucalyptol, ichthammol, thyme oil.
See: Solarcaine Pump Spray (Schering-Plough Corp.).
W/Dextromethorphan.
See: Chloraseptic DM, Loz. (Eaton Medical Corp.).
W/Resorcinol.
See: Black & White, Oint. (Schering-Plough Corp.).
W/Resorcinol, boric acid, basic fuchsin, acetone.
See: Castellani's Paint, Liq. (Various Mfr.).

•**phenol, liquefied.** U.S.P. 23.
Use: Topical antipruritic.

•**phenolate sodium.** (FEEN-oh-late) USAN.
Use: Disinfectant.

Phenolax. (Pharmacia & Upjohn) Phenolphthalein 64.8 mg/Wafer. Bot. 100s. *otc.*
Use: Laxative.

•**phenolphthalein.** (fee-nahl-THAY-leen) U.S.P. 23.
Use: Laxative.
See: Espotabs, Tab. (Combe, Inc.).
Evac-U-Lax, Wafer (Roberts Pharmaceuticals).
Ex-Lax, Prods. (Novartis Pharmaceutical Corp.).
Feen-A-Mint, Tab., Gum (Schering-Plough Corp.).
Phenolax, Wafer (Pharmacia & Upjohn).
Veracolate, Tab. (Numark Laboratories, Inc.).

phenolphthalein. (Various Mfr.) Pkg. 1 oz, 0.25 lb, 1 lb.

Use: Laxative.

phenolphthalein w/combinations.
See: Correctol, Tab. (Schering-Plough Corp.).
Dialose Plus, Cap. Tab. (Merck & Co.).
Evac-Q-Kit, Tab., Supp. (Warren-Teed).
Dual Formula Feen-A-Mint Pills (Schering-Plough Corp.).
Feen-A-Mint, Gum, Mint, Pill (Schering-Plough Corp.).
4-Way Cold Tab. (Bristol-Myers Squibb).
Phillips' Laxative Gel-Cap (Bayer Corp. (Consumer Div.)).
Veracolate, Tab. (Numark Laboratories, Inc.).

phenolphthalein in liquid petrolatum emulsion. (Various Mfr.).
See: Petrolatum, Liq.

phenolphthalein. (Various Mfr.). Pkg. 1 oz, 0.25 lb., 1 lb.
Use: Laxative.

•**phenolphthalein yellow.** (fee-nahl-THAY-leen) U.S.P. 23.
Use: Laxative.

phenolsulfonates.
See: Sulfocarbolates.

phenolsulfonic acid. Sulfocarbolic acid.
Note: Used in Sulphodine, Tab. (Strasenburgh).

phenoltetrabromophthalein. Disulfonate Disodium.
See: Sulfobromophthalein Sodium, U.S.P. 23.

Pheno Nux Tablets. (Pal-Pak, Inc.) Phenobarbital 16.2 mg, nux vomica extract 8.1 mg, calcium carbonate 194.4 mg/Tab. Bot. 1000s. *c-IV.*
Use: Sedative, hypnotic, antacid.

Phenoptic. (Optopics Laboratories, Corp.) Phenylephrine HCl 2.5%. Soln. Bot. 2 ml, 5 ml, 15 ml. *Rx.*
Use: Mydriatic, vasoconstrictor.

phenothiazine. Thiodiphenylamine.

Phenoturic. (Truett) Phenobarbital 40 mg/5 ml. Elix. Bot. Pt, gal. *c-IV.*
Use: Hypnotic, sedative.

•**phenoxybenzamine hydrochloride.** (fen-ox-ee-BEN-zuh-meen) U.S.P. 23.
Use: Antihypertensive.
See: Dibenzyline, Cap. (SmithKline Beecham Pharmaceuticals).

phenoxymethyl penicillin.
See: Penicillin V.

phenoxymethyl penicillin potassium.
See: Penicillin V Potassium.

phenoxynate. Mixture of phenylphenols 17-18%, octyl and related alkylphenols 2-3%.

•**phenprocoumon.** (fen-PRO-koo-mahn) USAN.
Use: Anticoagulant.

Phen-70. (Parmed Pharmaceuticals, Inc.) Phendimetrazine tartrate 70 mg/Tab. Bot. 100s, 1000s. *c-III.*
Use: Anorexiant.

•**phensuximide.** (fen-SUCK-sih-mide) U.S.P. 23.
Use: Anticonvulsant.
See: Milontin, Preps. (Parke-Davis).

Phental. (Armenpharm Ltd.) Belladonna alkaloids, phenobarbital 0.25 gr/Tab. Bot. 1000s. *c-IV.*
Use: Anticholinergic, antispasmodic, hypnotic, sedative.

Phentamine. (Major Pharmaceuticals) Phentermine HCl 30 mg/Cap. (equivalent to 24 mg base). Bot. 100s. *c-IV.*
Use: Anorexiant.

•**phentermine.** (FEN-ter-meen) USAN.
Use: Anorexic.
See: Adipex, Tab. (Teva Pharmaceuticals USA).
Adipex-P, Cap. (Teva Pharmaceuticals USA).
Fastin, Cap. (SmithKline Beecham Pharmaceuticals).
Tora, Tab. (Solvay Pharmaceuticals).
Wilpowr, Cap. (Foy Laboratories).

phentermine as resin complex.
See: Ionamin, Cap. (Medeva Pharmaceuticals, Inc.).

•**phentermine hydrochloride.** (Fen-ter-meen) U.S.P. 23.
Use: Appetite suppressant (systemic).
See: Zantryl, Cap. (ION Laboratories, Inc.).

phentetiothalein sodium. Iso-Iodeikon.
Use: Radiopaque agent.

phentolamine hydrochloride. (fen-TOLE-uh-meen)
Use: Antihypertensive.
See: Regitine HCl, Tab. (Novartis Pharmaceutical Corp.).

•**phentolamine mesylate.** (fen-TOLE-uh-meen) U.S.P. 23. *Formerly Phentolamine Methanesulfonate.*
Use: Antiadrenergic.
See: Regitine, Inj. (Novartis Pharmaceutical Corp.).

phentolamine mesylate for injection. (Bedford) 5 mg, mannitol. Pow. for Inj. Vial 2 ml. *Rx.*
Use: Antiadrenergic.

phentolamine methanesulfonate. U.S.P. 23. Phentolamine mesylate.

Phentolox w/APAP. (Global Source) Phenyltoloxamine citrate 30 mg, acetaminophen 325 mg/Tab. Bot. 1000s. *Rx.*

Use: Antihistamine, analgesic.

Phentox Compound. (Rosemont Pharmaceutical Corp.) Phenylpropanolamine HCl 20 mg, phenylephrine HCl 5 mg, chlorpheniramine maleate 2.5 mg, phenyltoloxamine citrate 7.5 mg/5 ml. Bot. Pt, gal. *Rx.*
Use: Decongestant, antihistamine.

phentydrone.
Use: Systemic fungicide.

n-phenylacetamide.
See: Acetanilid (Various Mfr.).

phenylalanine ammonia-lyase.
Use: Hyperphenylalaninemia. [Orphan Drug]

•**phenyl aminosalicylate.** (FEN-ill ah-MEE-no-sah-LIH-sih-late) USAN.
Use: Anti-infective.

•**phenylalanine.** (fen-ill-AL-ah-NEEN) U.S.P. 23.
Use: Amino acid.
W/Combinations.
See: Alka-Seltzer Plus Cold & Sinus (Bayer Corp. (Alergy Div.)).
Pepcid AC (J & J Merck Consumer Pharm).

phenylalanine mustard.
See: Melphalan, U.S.P. 23, analgesic.

phenylazodiaminopyridine.
See: Phenazopyridine (Various Mfr.).

phenylazodiaminopyridine hcl or hbr.
See: Phenazopyridine HCl or HBr (Various Mfr.).

phenylazo sulfisoxazole. (A.P.C.) Sulfisoxazole 0.5 g, phenylazopyridine 50 mg/Tab. Bot. 1000s. *Rx.*
Use: Anti-infective, sulfonamide.

phenylazo tablets. (A.P.C.) Phenylazodiaminopyridine HCl 1.5 gr/Tab. Bot. 1000s. *Rx.*
Use: Analgesic, urinary.

•**phenylbutazone.** (fen-ill-BYOO-tahzone) U.S.P. 23.
Use: Antirheumatic.

phenylbutyrate sodium.
Use: Treatment of blood disorders. [Orphan Drug]

phenylcarbinol.
See: Benzyl Alcohol, N.F. 18.

phenylcinchoninic acid. Name used for cinchophen.

phenylephedrine w/combinations.
See: Diabetic Tussin (Roberts Med.).

•**phenylephrine hydrochloride.** (fen-ill-EFF-rin) U.S.P. 23.
Use: Adrenergic, mydriatic, sympathomimetic, vasoconstrictor.
See: AH-Chew D, Chew. Tab. (WE Pharmaceuticals, Inc.).
AK-Dilate (Akorn, Inc.).
AK-Nefrin (Akorn, Inc.).
Alcon-Efrin, Soln. (PolyMedica Pharmaceuticals).
Allerest Nasal Spray (Novartis Pharmaceutical Corp.).
Coricidin Decongestant Nasal Mist (Schering-Plough Corp.).
Ephrine, Spray (Walgreen Co.).
Isopto Frin (Alcon Laboratories, Inc.).
Mydfrin 2.5% (Alcon Laboratories, Inc.).
Neo-Synephrine HCl, Preps. (Sanofi Winthrop Pharmaceuticals).
Phenoptic (Optopics Laboratories, Corp.).
Prefrin Liquifilm Ophth. Soln. (Allergan, Inc.).
Relief (Allergan, Inc.).
Sinarest, Nasal Spray (Novartis Pharmaceutical Corp.).
Super-Anahist Nasal Spray (Warner Lambert).
W/Combinations.
See: Acotus, Liq. (Whorton Pharmaceuticals, Inc.).
Anodynos Forte, Tab. (Buffington).
Atuss DM, Syr. (Atley Pharmaceuticals, Inc.).
Atuss G, Syr. (Atley Pharmaceuticals, Inc.).
Atuss HD, Liq. (Atley Pharmaceuticals, Inc.).
Bur-Tuss Expectorant (Burlington).
Chlor-Trimeton Expectorant (Schering-Plough Corp.).
Chlor-Trimeton Expectorant w/Codeine (Schering-Plough Corp.).
Coldloc, Elix. (Flemming).
Coricidin Demilets (Schering-Plough Corp.).
D.A. II (Dura).
Dallergy, Syr., Cap., Tab., Inj. (Laser, Inc.).
Deconhist L.A. (Zenith Goldline).
Demazin, Syr. (Schering-Plough Corp.).
Diabetic Tussin, Liq. (Roberts Pharmaceuticals).
Dimetane Decongestant, Tab., Elix. (Wyeth-Ayerst Laboratories).
Dimetane Expectorant, Liq. (Wyeth-Ayerst Laboratories).
Dimetane Expectorant-DC, Liq. (Wyeth-Ayerst Laboratories).
Dimetapp, Elix., Extentabs (Wyeth-Ayerst Laboratories).
Doktors, Drops, Spray (Scherer Laboratories, Inc.).
Entex, Prods. (Procter & Gamble Pharm.).
Ex-Histine, Syr. (WE Pharmaceuticals, Inc.).

4 Way Tab., Spray (Bristol-Myers Squibb).
Furacin Nasal Soln. (Eaton Medical Corp.).
Guaifenex, Liq. (Ethex Corp.).
Guiatex, Preps. (Rugby Labs, Inc.).
Histinex HC, Syr. (Ethex Corp.).
Hydrocodone CP, Liq. (Morton Grove Pharmaceuticals, Inc.).
Hydrocodone HD, Liq. (Morton Grove Pharmaceuticals, Inc.).
Hydrocodone PA (Morton Grove Pharmaceuticals, Inc.).
Iodal HD, Liq. (Iomed).
Iotussin HC, Syr. (Iomed).
Liquibid-D, SR Tab. (ION Laboratories, Inc.).
Mydfrin Ophthalmic, Liq. (Alcon Laboratories, Inc.).
Nasahist, Cap. (Keene Pharmaceuticals, Inc.).
Norel, Cap. (US Pharmaceutical Corp.).
Pediacof, Syr. (Sanofi Winthrop Pharmaceuticals).
Phenoptic, Soln. (Muro Pharmaceutical, Inc.).
Phenylzin Drops, Ophth. Soln. (Ciba Vision).
Pyristan, Cap., Elix. (Arcum).
Rhinall, Liq. (Scherer Laboratories).
Rymed, Prods. (Edwards Pharmaceuticals, Inc.).
Sil-Tex, Liq. (Silarx Pharmaceuticals, Inc.).
Sinex, Nasal Spray (Procter & Gamble Pharm.).
Singlet, Tab. (Hoechst Marion Roussel).
Spec-T Sore Throat-Decongestant Loz. (Bristol-Myers Squibb).
Statuss Green (Huckaby).
Sucrets Cold Decongestant Loz. (SmithKline Beecham Pharmaceuticals).
Trind, Liq. (Bristol-Myers Squibb).
Turbilixir, Liq. (Burlington).
Turbispan Leisurecaps, Cap. (Burlington).
Tussafed HC, Syr. (Everett Laboratories).
Tympagesic, Liq. (Pharmacia & Upjohn).
Unituss HC, Syr. (United Research Laboratories).
Vasocidin, Ophth. Soln. (Ciba Vision).
Vasosulf, Ophth. Soln. (Novartis Pharmaceutical Corp.).
Vetuss HC, Syr. (Cypress).

phenylephrine hydrochloride. (Various Mfr.) **Ophth. Soln. 2.5%:** Bot. 15 ml. **10%:** Bot. 2 ml, 5 ml. **Inj. 1%:** Vial 5 ml. *Rx.*
Use: Adrenergic, mydriatic, sympathomimetic, vasoconstrictor.

phenylephrine tannate, chlorpheniramine tannate and pyrilamine tartrate. (Zenith Forest Pharmaceutical) Phenylephrine tannate 25 mg, chlorpheniramine tannate 8 mg, pyrilamine tannate 25 mg/Tab. Bot. 100s, 500s. *Rx.*
Use: Antihistamine, decongestant.

phenylephrine tannate w/combinations.
See: Tussi-12 (Wallace Labs).

•**phenylethyl alcohol.** (fen-ill-ETH-ill) U.S.P. 23.
Use: Pharmaceutic aid (antimicrobial).

phenyl-ethyl-hydrazine, beta. Phenelzine dihydrogen sulfate.
See: Nardil, Tab. (Parke-Davis).

phenylethylmalonylurea.
See: Phenobarbital (Various Mfr.).

Phenylfenesin L.A. (Zenith Goldline Pharmaceutical) Phenylpropanolamine HCl 75 mg, guaifenesin 400 mg/ER Tab. Bot. 100s, 500s. *Rx.*
Use: Decongestant, expectorant.

Phenylgesic. (Zenith Goldline Pharmaceutical) Phenyltoloxamine citrate 30 mg, acetaminophen 325 mg/Tab. Bot. 100s, 1000s. *otc.*
Use: Analgesic, antihistamine.

phenylic acid.
See: Phenol, U.S.P 23.

•**phenylmercuric acetate.** (fen-ill-mer-CURE-ik ASS-eh-tate) N.F. 18.
Use: Pharmaceutic aid (antimicrobial), preservative (bacteriostatic).
W/9-Aminoacridine HCl, tyrothricin, urea, lactose.
See: Trinalis, Vaginal Supp. (Poly-Medica Pharmaceuticals).
W/Benzocaine, chlorothymol, resorcin.
See: Lanacane Creme (Combe, Inc.).
W/Boric acid, polyoxyethylenenonylphenol or oxyquinoline benzoate.
See: Koromex, Preps. (Holland-Rantos).

phenylmercuric acetate. (Various Mfr.) Bot. 1 lb, 5 lb, 10 lb.
Use: Pharmaceutic aid (antimicrobial), preservative (Bacteriostatic).

phenylmercuric borate. (F. W. Berk) Pkg. Custom packed.
W/Benzyl alcohol, benzocaine, butyl p-aminobenzoate.
See: Dermathyn, Oint. (Davis & Sly).

phenylmercuric chloride. Chlorophenylmercury.

•**phenylmercuric nitrate.** N.F. 18.
Use: Pharmaceutic aid (antimicrobial); preservative (bacteriostatic).
See: Preparation H, Oint., Supp. (Whitehall Robins Laboratories).
W/Amyl, phenylphenol complex.
See: Lubraseptic Jelly (Guardian Laboratories).

phenylmercuric nitrate. (A.P.L.) **Oint. 1:1500:** 1 oz, 4 oz, lb. (Chicago Pharm) Loz. w/benzocaine. Bot. 100s, 1000s. **Ophth. Oint., 1:3000:** Tube 1/8 oz. **Soln. 1:20,000:** Bot. pt, gal. **Vaginal supp., 1:5000:** Box 12s.
Use: Pharmaceutic aid (antimicrobial), preservative (bacteriostatic).

phenylmercuric picrate.
Use: Antimicrobial.

phenylphenol-o.
W/Amyl complex, phenylmercuric nitrate.
See: Lubraseptic Jelly. (Guardian Laboratories).

•**phenylpropanolamine bitartrate.** (fen-ill-pro-pan-OLE-uh-meen bye-TAR-trate) U.S.P. 23.
Use: Adrenergic, vasoconstrictor.

•**phenylpropanolamine hydrochloride.** (fen-ill-pro-pan-OLE-uh-meen) U.S.P. 23.
Use: Adrenergic, vasoconstrictor.
See: Acu Trim Diet Gum (Heritage Consumer Products).
Maximum Strength Dexatrim, ER Tab. (Thompson Medical Co.).
Propagest, Tab. (Carnrick Laboratories, Inc.).
Spray-U-Thin (Caprice-Greystoke).

phenylpropanolamine hydrochloride w/combinations.
See: Allerest, Prods. (Novartis Pharmaceutical Corp.).
Alka-Seltzer Plus Cold & Sinus (Bayer Corp. (Allergy Div.)).
Alka-Seltzer Plus Sinus, Tab. (Bayer Corp. (Allergy Div.)).
Antihist-D, Tab. (Zenith-Goldline).
A.R.M., Tab. (SmithKline Beecham Pharmaceuticals).
Bayer, Prods. (Bayer Corp. (Consumer Div.)).
Breacol Cough Medication, Liq. (Bayer Corp. (Consumer Div.)).
Bur-Tuss Expectorant (Burlington).
Coldloc, Elix. (Fleming & Co.).
Coldloc-LA, SR Capl. (Fleming & Co.).
Comtrex, Cap., Liq., Tab. (Bristol-Myers Squibb).
Contac, Prods. (SmithKline Beecham Pharmaceuticals).
Cophene No. 2, Cap. (Dunhall Pharmaceuticals, Inc.).
Coricidin Cough Formula (Schering-Plough Corp.).
Coricidin "D" Decongestant, Tab. (Schering-Plough Corp.).
Coricidin Sinus Headache, Tab. (Schering-Plough Corp.).
Deconhist L.A. (Zenith Goldline Pharmaceuticals).
Dex-A-Diet, Prods. (Columbia Laboratories, Inc.).
Dezest, Cap. (Geneva Pharmaceuticals).
Dimetane Expectorant, Liq. (Wyeth-Ayerst Laboratories).
Dimetapp, Elix., Extentabs (Wyeth-Ayerst Laboratories).
Dynafed Asthma Relief, Tab. (BDI Pharmaceuticals, Inc.).
Entex, Cap., Liq. (Procter & Gamble Pharm.).
Entex LA, Tab. (Procter & Gamble Pharm.).
Guaifenex, Liq. (Ethex Corp.).
Guaifenex PPA 75, ER Tab. (Ethex Corp.).
Guiatex, Prods. (Rugby Labs, Inc.).
Hall's Mentho-Lyptus Cough Lozenges, Liq. (Warner Lambert).
Histalet Forte T. D., Tab. (Solvay Pharmaceuticals).
Hista-Vadrin, Syr., Tab., Cap. (Scherer Laboratories, Inc.).
Hydrocodone PA Pediatric, Syr. (Morton Grove Pharmaceuticals, Inc.).
Iohist DM, Syr. (Iomed).
Kleer Compound, Tab. (Scrip).
Liquibid-D, SR Tab. (ION Laboratories, Inc.).
Liqui-Histine DM, Syr. (Liquipharm).
Meditussin-X, Liq. (Roberts Pharmaceuticals).
Naldecon, Drop, Syr., Tab. (Bristol-Myers Squibb).
Nasahist, Cap., Inj. (Keene Pharmaceuticals, Inc.).
Nolamine, Tab. (Carnrick Laboratories, Inc.).
Norel, Cap. (US Pharmaceutical Corp.).
Ornade, Cap. (SmithKline Beecham Pharmaceuticals).
Ornex, Cap. (SmithKline Beecham Pharmaceuticals).
Panadyl, Tab., Cap. (Misemer Pharmaceuticals, Inc.).
Pannaz, Tab. (Pan A).
Partuss T.D. Tab. (Parmed Pharmaceuticals, Inc.).
Pediacon DX Children's, Syr. (Zenith Goldline Pharmaceuticals).

Pediacon EX, Drops (Zenith Goldline Pharmaceuticals).
Phenadex Children's Cough/Cold, Syr. (Alpharma USPD Inc.).
Phenadex Pediatric Cough/Cold, Drops (Alpharma USPD Inc.).
Phenylfenesin LA, EA Tab. (Zenith Goldline Pharmaceuticals).
Profen LA, TR Tab. (Wakefield Pharmaceuticals, Inc.).
Profen II (Wakefield Pharmaceuticals, Inc.).
Profen II DM, TR Tab. (Wakefield Pharmaceuticals, Inc.).
Pyristan, Cap., Elix. (Arcum).
Rymed, Prods. (Edwards Pharmaceuticals, Inc.).
Sanhist TD, Tab., Vial (Sandia).
Silaminic Expectorant, Liq. (Silarx Pharmaceuticals, Inc.).
Sildicon-E, Ped. Drops (Silarx Pharmaceuticals, Inc.).
Siltapp with Dextromethorphan HBr Cold & Cough, Elix. (Silarx Pharmaceuticals, Inc.).
Sil-Tex, Liq. (Silarx Pharmaceuticals, Inc.).
Siltussin-CF, Liq. (Silarx Pharmaceuticals, Inc.).
Sinarest, Tab. (Pharmcraft).
Sine-Off Tab. (Carnick Laboratories, Inc.).
Sinulin, Tab. (Carnick Laboratories, Inc.).
Spec-T Sore Throat-Decongestant, Loz. (Bristol-Myers Squibb).
St. Joseph Cold Tablets for Children (Schering-Plough Corp.).
Status Green (Huckaby).
Sucrets Cold Decongestant Loz. (SmithKline Beecham Pharmaceuticals).
Triactin (ProMetic Pharma).
Triminic, Preps. (Novartis Pharmaceutical Corp.).
Triminic, Chew. Tab. (Novartis Pharmaceutical Corp.).
Triaminicol, Syr. (Novartis Pharmaceutical Corp.).
Tri-P Oral Infant Drops (Cypress Pharm).
Vanex Forte-R (Schwarz Pharma, Inc).
Vetuss HC (Cypress Pharm).

phenylpropanolamine hydrochloride & chlorpheniramine maleate capsules. (Various Mfr.) Chlorpheniramine maleate 12 mg, pseudoephedrine HCl 75 mg/Cap. Bot. 50s, 100s, 1000s. *Rx-otc.*
Use: Antihistamine, decongestant.

phenylpropanolamine hydrochloride & guaifenesin tablets. (fen-ill-pro-pan-OLE-uh-meen HIGH-droe-KLOR-ide & GWIE-fen-ah-sin) (Various Mfr.) Phenylpropanolamine HCl 75 mg, guaifenesin 400 mg. Tab. Bot. 100s, 500s. *c-III.*
Use: Decongestant, expectorant.

phenylpropanolamine hydrochloride & hydrocodone syrup. (Rosemont Pharmaceutical Corp.) Phenylpropanolamine HCl 25 mg, hydrocodone bitartrate 5 mg. Bot. 480 ml.
Use: Antitussive, decongestant.

•**phenylpropanolamine polistirex.** (fen-ill-pro-pan-OLE-ah-meen pahl-ee-STIE-rex) USAN.
Use: Adrenergic, vasoconstrictor.

phenylpropylmethylamine hydrochloride. Vonedrine HCl.

phenyl salicylate. Salol.
W/Atropine sulfate, hyoscyamine, methenamine, methylene blue, gelsemium, benzoic acid.
See: Rayderm Oint. (Velvet Pharmacal).
W/Methenamine, methylene blue, benzoic acid, hyoscyamine alkaloid, atropine sulfate.
See: Urised, Tab. (PolyMedica Pharmaceuticals).

phenyl-tert-butylamine.
See: Phentermine.

phenylthilone.
Use: Anticonvulsant.

phenyltoloxamine citrate.
Use: Antihistamine.

phenyltoloxamine citrate w/combinations.
See: Flextra-DS (Poly Pharm).
Iohist D (Iomed).
Meditussin-X, Liq. (Roberts Pharmaceuticals).
Naldecon, Preps. (Bristol-Myers Squibb).
Poly-histine Prods. (Sanofi Winthrop Pharmaceuticals).

phenyltoloxamine resin w/combinations.
See: Tussionex, Cap., Liq., Tab. (Medeva Pharmaceuticals, Inc.).

Phenylzin. (Ciba Vision) Zinc sulfate 0.25%, phenylephrine HCl 0.12%. Bot. 15 ml. *Rx.*
Use: Decongestant, ophthalmic.

•**phenyramidol hydrochloride.** (FEN-ih-RAM-ih-dole) USAN.
Use: Analgesic; muscle relaxant.

•**phenytoin.** (FEN-ih-toe-in) U.S.P. 23.
Formerly Diphenylhydantoin.

Use: Anticonvulsant.
See: Dilantin Prods. (Parke-Davis).

phenytoin. (Alpharma USPD Inc.) Phenytoin 125 mg/5 ml. Oral Susp. Bot. 240 ml. *Rx.*
Use: Anticonvulsant.

•**phenytoin sodium.** (FEN-in-toe-in) U.S.P. 23. *Formerly Diphenylhydantoin Sodium.*
Use: Anticonvulsant, cardiac depressant (antiarrhythmic).
See: Dilantin Sodium, Preps. (Parke-Davis).

phenytoin sodium with phenobarbital.
Use: Anticonvulsant.
See: Dilantin with Phenobarbital Kapseals, Cap. (Parke-Davis).

pheochromocytoma, agents for.
See: Demser, Cap. (Merck & Co.).
Dibenzyline, Cap. (SmithKline Beecham Pharmaceuticals).
Regitine, Inj. (Novartis Pharmaceutical Corp.).

Pherazine DM. (Halsey Drug Co.) Promethazine 6.25 mg, dextromethorphan HBr 15 mg, alcohol 7%/5 ml. Bot. 4 oz, 6 oz, pt, gal. *Rx.*
Use: Antihistamine, antitussive.

Pherazine VC with Codeine Syrup. (Halsey Drug Co.) Phenylephrine HCl 5 mg, promethazine HCl 6.25 mg, codeine phosphate 10 mg, alcohol 7%/5 ml. Bot. Pt, gal. *c-v.*
Use: Antihistamine, antitussive, decongestant.

Pherazine VC Syrup. (Halsey Drug Co.) Phenylephrine HCl 5 mg, promethazine HCl 6.25 mg, alcohol 7%/5 ml. Bot. Pt, gal. *Rx.*
Use: Antihistamine, decongestant.

Pherazine w/Codeine. (Halsey Drug Co.) Promethazine HCl 6.25 mg, codeine phosphate 10 mg/5 ml, alcohol 7%, sorbitol, sucrose. Syr. Bot. 120 ml, pt, gal. *c-v.*
Use: Antihistamine, antitussive.

phethenylate. Also sodium salt.

Phicon. (T.E. Williams Pharmaceuticals) Pramoxine HCl 0.5%, vitamin A 7500 IU, E 2000 IU/30 g. Cream. Tube 60 g. *otc.*
Use: Anesthetic, local.

Phicon F. (T.E. Williams Pharmaceuticals) Undecylenic acid 8%, pramoxine HCl 0.05%. Cream. 60 g. *otc.*
Use: Anesthetic, local; antifungal.

Phillips' Chewable. (Bayer Corp. (Consumer Div.)) Magnesium hydroxide 311 mg. Tab. 100s, 200s.
Use: Laxative, antacid.

Phillips' Laxcaps. (Bayer Corp. (Consumer Div.)) Docusate sodium 83 mg, phenolphthalein 90 mg/Cap. Bot. 8s, 24s, 48s. *otc.*
Use: Laxative.

Phillips' Milk of Magnesia. (Bayer Corp. (Consumer Div.)) Magnesium hydroxide. Reg. and Mint. Bot. 4 oz, 12 oz, 26 oz; Tab. Bot. 30s, 100s, 200s. *otc.*
Use: Laxative, antacid.

Phillips'Milk of Magnesia Concentrated. (Bayer Corp. (Consumer Div.)) Magnesium hydroxide 800 mg/5 ml, sorbitol, sugar. Liq. Bot. 240 ml. *otc.*
Use: Antacid.

Phish Omega. (Pharmics, Inc.) Natural salmon oil concentrate containing EPA 120 mg, DHA 100 mg/Cap. Bot. 60s. *otc.*
Use: Vitamin supplement.

Phish Omega Plus. (Pharmics, Inc.) Natural fish oil concentrate containing EPA 300 mg, DHA 200 mg/Cap. Bot. 60s. *otc.*
Use: Vitamin supplement.

pHisoDerm. (Chattem Consumer Products) Sodium octoxynol-2 ethane sulfonate, white petrolatum, water, mineral oil (with lanolin alcohol and oleyl alcohol), sodium benzoate, octoxynol-3, tetrasodium EDTA, methylcellulose, cocamide MEA, imidazolidinyl urea.
Regular: 150 ml, 270 ml, 480 ml, gal.
Oily skin: 150 ml, 480. *otc.*
Use: Dermatologic, cleanser.

pHisoDerm for Baby. (Chattem Consumer Products) Sodium octoxynol-2 ethane sulfonate, petrolatum, octoxynol-3, mineral oil (with lanolin alcohol and oleyl alcohol), cocamide MEA, imidazolidinyl urea, sodium benzoate, tetrasodium EDTA, methylcellulose, hydrochloric acid. Liq. Bot. 150 ml, 270 ml. *otc.*
Use: Dermatologic, cleanser.

pHisoDerm Gentle Cleansing Bar. (Chattem Consumer Products) Sodium tallowate, sodium cocoate, petrolatum, glycerin, lanolin, sodium Cl, BHT, trisodium EDTA, titanium dioxide. Bar 99 g. *otc.*
Use: Dermatologic, cleanser.

pHisoHex. (Sanofi Winthrop Pharmaceuticals) Entsufon sodium, hexachlorophene 3%, petrolatum, lanolin cholesterols, methylcellulose, polyethylene glycol, polyethylene glycol monostearate, lauryl myristyl diethanolamide, sodium benzoate, water, pH adjusted with hydrochloric acid. Emulsion, Bot. 5 oz, pt, gal. Wall dispensers pt. Unit packets 0.25 oz. Box 50s, Pedal oper-

ated dispenser 30 oz. *otc.*
Use: Antimicrobial, antiseptic.

pHisoMed. (Sanofi Winthrop Pharmaceuticals) Hexachlorophene. *otc.*
Use: Antimicrobial, antiseptic.

pHisoPuff. (Sanofi Winthrop Pharmaceuticals) Nonmedicated cleansing sponge. Box sponge 1s. *otc.*
Use: Dermatologic, cleanser.

PhosChol. (American Lecithin Company) Phosphatidylcholine (highly purified lecithin). **Softgel:** 565 mg, 900 mg. Bot. 100s, 300s. **Liq. Conc.:** 3000 mg/5 ml. Bot. 240 ml, 480 ml. *otc.*
Use: Nutritional supplement.

phoscolic acid.
Use: Adjuvant.

Phos-Flur Oral Rinse Supplement. (Colgate Oral Pharmaceuticals) Acidulated phosphate sodium fluoride 0.05%, fluoride 1 ml/5 ml. Bot. 250 ml, 500 ml, gal. *Rx.*
Use: Dental caries preventative.

PhosLo. (Braintree Laboratories, Inc.) Calcium acetate 667 mg (calcium 169 mg)/Tab. Bot. 200s. *Rx.*
Use: Electrolytes, mineral supplement.

phosphate.
See: Potassium Phosphate, Inj. (Abbott Laboratories).
Sodium Phosphate, Inj. (Abbott Laboratories).

phosphentaside. Adenosine-5-monophosphate. Adenylic acid.
W/Vitamin B_{12}, niacin.
See: Denylex Gel, Vial (Westerfield).
W/Vitamin B_{12}, niacin, B_1.
See: Adenolin, Vial (Lincoln Diagnostics).

phosphocol P 32. (Mallinckrodt) Chromic phosphate P 32: 15 mCi with a concentration of up to 5 mCi/ml and specific activity of up to 5 mCi/mg at time of standardization. Susp. Vial 10 ml.
Use: Radiopharmaceutical.

phosphocysteamine.
Use: Cystinosis. [Orphan Drug]

Phospholine Iodide. (Wyeth-Ayerst Laboratories) Echothiophate Iodide for Ophthalmic Solution. 0.03%, 0.06%, 0.125%, 0.25% potencies/5 ml of sterile eye drops. Package: 1.5 mg for 0.03%; 3 mg for 0.06%; 6.25 mg for 0.125%;12.5 mg for 0.25% w/5 ml diluent. *Rx.*
Use: Antiglaucoma. [Orphan Drug]

phosphonoformic acid.
See: Foscarnet sodium.

phosphorated carbohydrate solution.
See: Emetrol, Liq. (Sanofi Winthrop Pharmaceuticals).
Nausea Relief, Soln. (Zenith Goldline Pharmaceuticals).
Nausetrol, Soln. (Various Mfr.).

•**phosphoric acid.** (foo-FORE-ik) N.F. 18.
Use: Pharmaceutic aid (solvent).

phosphoric acid, diluted.
Use: Pharmaceutic aid (solvent).

phosphorus.
Use: Phosphorus replacement.
See: Uro-KP-Neutral, Tab. (Star Pharmaceuticals, Inc.).
K-Phos Neutral, Tab. (Beach Pharmaceuticals).

Phospho-Soda. (C. B. Fleet Co., Inc.) Sodium biphosphate 48 g, sodium phosphate 18 g/100 ml. Bot. 1.5 oz, 3 oz, 8 oz. Flavored, unflavored. *otc.*
Use: Laxative.

Phosphotec. (Bristol-Myers Squibb) Technetium Tc 99m pyrophosphate kit. 10 vials/kit.
Use: Radiodiagnostic.

Photofrin. (QLT Phototherapeutics, Inc.) Porfimer sodium 75 mg. Freeze-dried cake or Pow. for Inj. Vial. *Rx.*
Use: Antineoplastic.

Photoplex Sunscreen. (Allergan, Inc.) Butyl methoxydibenzoylmethane 3%, padimate O 7%. Lot. 120 ml. *otc.*
Use: Sunscreen.

Phrenilin Forte Capsules. (Schwarz Pharma, Inc.) Acetaminophen 650 mg, butalbital 50 mg/Cap. Bot. 100s, 500s. *Rx.*
Use: Analgesic, hypnotic, sedative.

Phrenilin Tablets. (Schwarz Pharma, Inc.) Butalbital 50 mg, acetaminophen 325 mg/Tab. Bot. 100s. *Rx.*
Use: Analgesic, hypnotic, sedative.

Phrenilin with Codeine #3. (Schwarz Pharma, Inc.) Acetaminophen 325 mg, butalbital 50 mg, codeine phosphate 30 mg/Cap. Bot. 100s. *c-III.*
Use: Analgesic combination, hypnotic, sedative.

Phresh 3.5 Finnish Cleansing Liquid. (3M Pharm) Water, cocamidopropyl betaine, lactic acid, polyoxyethylene distearate, polyoxyethylene monostearate, hydroxyethyl cellulose, sodium phosphate, methylparaben. Bot. 6 oz. *otc.*
Use: Soapless cleansing agent.

pH-Stabil Cream. (Hermal Pharmaceutical Labs) Skin protection cream. Bot. 8 oz. Tube 2 oz. *otc.*
Use: Dermatologic.

Phthalamaquin. (Penick) Quinetolate.
Use: Antiasthmatic.

phthalazine, i-hydrazino-, monohydrochloride. U.S.P. 23. Hydralazine Hydrochloride.

phylcardin.
See: Aminophylline (Various Mfr.).
phyllindon.
See: Aminophylline (Various Mfr.).
Phyllocontin. (Purdue Frederick Co.) Aminophylline 225 mg/CR Tab. Bot. 100s. *Rx.*
Use: Bronchodilator.
phylloquinone. 2-Methyl-3-phytyl-1,4-naphthoquinine, vitamin K.
See: Phytonadione, U.S.P., Inj., Tab. (Various Mfr.).
Vitamin K-1 (Various Mfr.).
Phylorinol Liquid. (Schaffer Laboratories) Phenol 0.6%, boric acid, strong iodine solution, sorbitol 70% solution, sodium copper chlorophyll. 240 ml. *otc.*
Use: Mouth and throat preparation.
Phylorinol Mouthwash. (Schaffer Laboratories) Phenol 0.6%, methyl salicylate, sorbitol. Mouthwash. 240 ml. *otc.*
Use: Mouth and throat preparation.
physiological irrigating solution.
See: TIS-U-SOL, Soln. (Baxter Pharmaceutical Products, Inc.).
Physiosol, Soln. (Abbott Laboratories).
Physiolyte, Soln. (American McGaw).
Physiolyte. (American McGaw) Sodium Cl 530 mg, sodium acetate 370 mg, sodium gluconate 500 mg, potassium Cl 37 mg, magnesium Cl 30 mg/100 ml. Soln. Bot. 500 ml, 2 L, 4 L. *Rx.*
Use: Irrigant, ophthalmic.
PhysioSol Irrigation. (Abbott Hospital Products) Bot. 250 ml, 500 ml, 1000 ml glass or Aqualite (semi-rigid) containers. *Rx.*
Use: Irrigant, ophthalmic.
•**physostigmine salicylate.** (fie-zoe-STIG-meen) U.S.P. 23.
Use: Cholinergic (ophthalmic); parasympathomimetic agent, Friedreich's and other inherited ataxias. [Orphan Drug]
See: Antilirium, Amp. (Forest Pharmaceutical, Inc.).
Isopto-Eserine, Ophthalmic, Soln. (Alcon Laboratories, Inc.).
W/l-Hyoscyamine HBr.
See: Phyatromine-H, Amp., Vial (Schwarz Pharma).
W/Pilocarpine, methylcellulose.
See: Isopto P-ES, Soln. (Alcon Laboratories, Inc.).
physostigmine salicylate. (Forest Pharmaceutical, Inc.) Pow., Tube 1 gr, 5 gr, 15 gr.
Use: Cholinergic (ophthalmic).
•**physostigmine sulfate.** U.S.P. 23.
Use: Cholinergic (ophthalmic).
•**phytate persodium.** (FIE-tate per-SO-dee-uhm) USAN.
Use: Pharmaceutic aid.
•**phytate sodium.** (FIE-tate) USAN. Sodium salt of inositol hexaphosphoric acid.
Use: Chelating agent (calcium).
phytic acid. Inositol hexophosphoric acid.
•**phytonadione.** (fye-toe-nuh-DIE-ohn) U.S.P. 23.
Use: Vitamin (prothrombogenic).
See: Aquamephyton, Inj. (Merck & Co.).
Mephyton, Tab. (Merck & Co.).
phytonadione. (I.M.S., Ltd.) 2 mg/ml (Vitamin K_1). Inj. 0.5 ml, Min-I-ject prefilled syringes. *Rx.*
Use: Vitamin (prothrombogenic).
•**picenadol hydrochloride.** (pih-SEN-AID-ole) USAN.
Use: Analgesic.
•**piclamilast.** (pih-KLAM-ill-ast) USAN.
Use: Antiasthmatic (type IV phosphodiesterase inhibitor).
•**picotrin diolamine.** (PIH-koe-trin die-OH-lah-meen) USAN.
Use: Keratolytic.
picric acid, trinitrophenol.
See: Silver Salts (Various Mfr.).
picrotoxin. Cocculin.
Use: Respiratory.
•**picumeterol fumarate.** (PIKE-you-MEH-teh-role) USAN.
Use: Bronchodilator.
•**pifarnine.** (pih-FAR-neen) USAN.
Use: Antiulcerative (gastric).
Pilagan. (Allergan, Inc.) Pilocarpine nitrate 1%, 2%, or 4%. Soln. Bot. 15 ml. *Rx.*
Use: Antiglaucoma.
Pilocar. (Ciba Vision) Pilocarpine HCl 0.5%, 1%, 2%, 3%, 4%, or 6%. Bot. 15 ml; Twinpack 2 x 15 ml 0.5%, 1%, 2%, 3%, 4%, or 6%; 1 ml Dropperettes 1%, 2%, or 4%. *Rx.*
Use: Antiglaucoma.
•**pilocarpine.** (pie-low-CAR-peen) U.S.P. 23.
Use: Antiglaucoma, ophthalmic cholinergic, miotic.
See: Ocusert Pilo-20, Pilo-40 (Novartis Pharmaceutical Corp.).
•**pilocarpine hydrochloride.** (pie-low-CAR-peen) U.S.P. 23.
Use: Cholinergic (ophthalmic), topically as a miotic, xerostomia and keratoconjunctivitis sicca. [Orphan Drug]
See: Almocarpine (Wyeth-Ayerst Laboratories).
Isopto Carpine (Alcon).

Mi-Pilo, Soln. (PBH Wesley Jessen).
Pilocar, Soln. (Ciba Vision).
Pilomiotin, Soln. (Ciba Vision).
Piloptic, Soln. (Muro Pharmaceutical, Inc.).
Salagen, Tab. (MGI Pharma, Inc.).
W/Epinephrine HCl.
See: E-Carpine, Inj. (Alcon Laboratories, Inc.).
W/Physostigmine salicylate, methylcellulose.
See: E-Pilo, Soln. (Ciba Vision).
Isopto P-ES, Soln. (Alcon Laboratories, Inc.).

pilocarpine hydrochloride. (Various Mfr.) Pilocarpine HCl. **0.5%:** 15 ml, 30 ml. **1%:** 2 ml, 15 ml, 30 ml, UD 1 ml. **2% and 4%:** 2 ml, 15 ml, 30 ml. **6%:** 15 ml. **8%:** 2 ml.
Use: Cholinergic (ophthalmic), topically as a miotic, xerostomia and keratoconjunctivitis sicca. [Orphan Drug]

•**pilocarpine nitrate.** (pie-low-CAR-peen) U.S.P. 23.
Use: Cholinergic (ophthalmic).
See: P.V. Carpine (Allergan, Inc.).

Pilopine. (International Pharm) Pilocarpine HCl 1%, 2%, 4%. Soln. Bot. 15 ml. *Rx.*
Use: Antiglaucoma.

Pilopine HS Gel. (Alcon Laboratories, Inc.) Pilocarpine HCl 4%. Tube 3.5 g. *Rx.*
Use: Antiglaucoma.

Piloptic. (Optopics Laboratories, Corp) Pilocarpine HCl 0.5%, 1%, 2%, 3%, 4%, 6%. Soln. Bot. 15 ml. *Rx.*
Use: Antiglaucoma.

Pilostat. (Bausch & Lomb Pharmaceuticals) Pilocarpine HCl 0.5%, 1%, 2%, 3%, 4%, 6%. Soln. Bot. 15 ml, twin pack 2 x 15 ml. *Rx.*
Use: Antiglaucoma.

Pima Syrup. (Fleming & Co.) Potassium iodide 5 gr/5 ml. Bot. Pt, gal. *Rx.*
Use: Expectorant.

•**pimagedine hydrochloride.** (pih-MAH-jeh-deen) USAN.
Use: Inhibitor (advanced glycosylation end-product formation inhibitors).

•**pimetine hydrochloride.** (PIM-eh-teen) USAN.
Use: Antihyperlipoproteinemic.

piminodine esylate.
Use: Analgesic.

piminodine ethanesulfonate.
Use: Analgesic, narcotic.

•**pimobendan.** (pie-MOE-ben-dan) USAN.
Use: Cardiovascular agent.

•**pimozide.** (pih-moe-ZIDE) U.S.P. 23.
Use: Antipsychotic.
See: Orap, Tab. (Ortho McNeil Pharmaceutical).

•**pinacidil.** (pie-NASS-ih-DILL) USAN.
Use: Antihypertensive.

•**pinadoline.** (pih-nah-DOE-leen) USAN.
Use: Analgesic.

•**pindolol.** (PIN-doe-lahl) U.S.P. 23.
Use: Beta-adrenergic blocking agent, vasodilator.
See: Visken (Novartis Pharmaceutical Corp.).

pine needle oil. N.F. XVI.
Use: Perfume; flavor.

pine tar. U.S.P. XXI.
Use: Local antieczematic; rubefacient.

Pinex Concentrate Cough Syrup. (Last) Dextromethorphan HBr 7.5 mg/5 ml (after diluting 3 oz. concentrate to make 16 oz. solution). Bot. 3 oz. *otc.*
Use: Antitussive.

Pinex Cough Syrup. (Last) Dextromethorphan HBr 7.5 mg/5 ml. Bot. 3 oz, 6 oz. *otc.*
Use: Antitussive.

Pinex Regular. (Pinex) Potassium guaiacolsulfonate, oil of pine and eucalyptus, extract of grindelia, alcohol 3%/30 ml. Syr. Bot. 3 oz, 8 oz. Also cherry flavored 3 oz. Super and concentrated 3 oz. *otc.*
Use: Expectorant.

Pink Bismuth. (Zenith Forest Pharmaceutical) 130 mg/15 ml. Liq. Bot. 240 ml. *otc.*
Use: Antidiarrheal.

•**pinoxepin hydrochloride.** (pih-NOX-eh-PIN) USAN.
Use: Antipsychotic.

Pin-Rid. (Apothecary Products, Inc.) **Soft gelcap:** Pyrantel pamoate 180 mg (equivalent to 62.5 mg pyrantel base). Pkg. 24s. **Liq.:** Pyrantel pamoate 144 mg/ml (equivalent to 50 mg/ml pyrantel base), saccharin, sucrose. Bot. 30 ml. *otc.*
Use: Anthelmintic.

Pin-X. (Effcon Labs, Inc.) Pyrantel base (as pamoate) 50 mg/ml, sorbitol. Liq. Bot. 30 ml. *otc.*
Use: Anthelmintic.

•**pioglitazone hydrochloride.** (PIE-oh-GLIH-tah-zone) USAN.
Use: Antidiabetic.

•**pipamperone.** (pih-PAM-peer-OHN) USAN. *Formerly Floropipamide.*
Use: Antipsychotic.

•**pipazethate.** (pip-AZZ-eh-thate) USAN.
Use: Cough suppressant; antitussive.

pipazethate hydrochloride.

Use: Antitussive.

•**pipecuronium bromide.** (pih-peh-cure-OH-nee-uhm) USAN.
Use: Neuromuscular blocker.

•**piperacetazine.** (pih-PURR-ah-SET-ah-zeen) USAN.
Use: Antipsychotic.

•**piperacillin.** (PIH-per-uh-SILL-in) U.S.P. 23.
Use: Anti-infective.

•**piperacillin sodium.** (PIH-per-uh-SILL-in) U.S.P. 23.
Use: Anti-infective.
See: Pipracil (ESI Lederle Generics).
W/Tazobactam.
See: Zosyn, Inj. (ESI Lederle Generics).

•**piperamide maleate.** (PIH-per-ah-mid) USAN.
Use: Anthelmintic.

•**piperazine.** (pie-PEAR-ah-zeen) U.S.P. 23.
Use: Anthelmintic.

•**piperazine citrate.** (pie-PEAR-ah-zeen) U.S.P. 23. Piperazine Citrate Telra Hydrous Tripiperazine Dicitrate.
Use: Anthelmintic.
See: Bryrel, Syr. (Sanofi Winthrop Pharmaceuticals).
Ta-Verm, Syr., Tab. (Table Rock).

•**piperazine edetate calcium.** (pie-PEAR-ah-zeen EH-deh-tate) USAN.
Use: Anthelmintic.

piperazine estrone sulfate. (pie-PEAR-ah-zeen)
See: Estropipate.

piperazine hexahydrate. Tivazine.

piperazine phosphate.
Use: Anthelmintic.

piperidine phosphate.
Use: Psychiatric drug.

piperidolate hydrochloride.
Use: Anticholinergic.

•**piperoxan hydrochloride.** Fourneau 933. Benzodioxane. Diagnosis of hypertension.
Use: Diagnostic aid.

pipethanate hydrochloride.
Use: Anxiolytic.

•**piposulfan.** (PIP-oh-SULL-fan) USAN.
Use: Antineoplastic.

•**pipotiazine palmitate.** (PIP-oh-TIE-ah-zeen PAL-mih-tate) USAN.
Use: Antipsychotic.

•**pipoxolan hydrochloride.** (pih-POX-oh-lan) USAN.
Use: Muscle relaxant.

Pipracil. (ESI Lederle Generics) Piperacillin sodium 42.5 mg, 2 g, 3 g, 4 g, 40 g. Pow. for Inj. Vial, *ADD-Vantage* vial (except 40 g), Infusion Bot. (3 g, 4 g only), Bulk Vial (40 g only). *Rx.*
Use: Anti-infective, penicillin.

•**piprozolin.** (PIP-row-ZOE-lin) USAN.
Use: Choleretic.

•**piquindone hydrochloride.** (PIH-kwin-dohn) USAN.
Use: Antipsychotic.

•**piquizil hydrochloride.** (PIH-kwih-zill) USAN.
Use: Bronchodilator.

•**piracetam.** (PIHR-ASS-eh-tam) USAN.
Use: Cognition adjuvant, cerebral stimulant, myoclonus. [Orphan Drug]

•**pirandamine hydrochloride.** (pih-RAN-dah-meen) USAN.
Use: Antidepressant.

•**pirazmonam sodium.** (pihr-AZZ-moe-nam SO-dee-uhm) USAN.
Use: Antimicrobial.

•**pirazolac.** (PIHR-AZE-oh-lack) USAN.
Use: Antirheumatic.

•**pirbenicillin sodium.** (pihr-ben-IH-SILL-in) USAN.
Use: Anti-infective.

•**pirbuterol acetate.** (pihr-BYOO-tuh-role) USAN.
Use: Bronchodilator.
See: Maxair, Aerosol (3M Pharm.).

•**pirbuterol hydrochloride.** USAN.
Use: Bronchodilator.

•**pirenperone.** (PIHR-en-PURR-ohn) USAN.
Use: Anxiolytic.

•**pirenzepine hydrochloride.** (PIHR-en-zeh-PEEN) USAN.
Use: Antiulcerative.

•**piretanide.** (pihr-ETT-ah-nide) USAN.
Use: Diuretic.
See: Arlix, Prods. (Hoechst Marion Roussel).

•**pirfenidone.** (PEER-FEN-ih-dohn) USAN.
Use: Analgesic, anti-inflammatory, antipyretic.

piridazol.
See: Sulfapyridine, Tab. (Various Mfr.).

•**piridicillin sodium.** (pihr-RIH-dih-SILL-in) USAN.
Use: Anti-infective.

•**piridronate sodium.** (pihr-IH-DROE-nate) USAN.
Use: Regulator (calcium).

•**piriprost.** (PIHR-ih-prahst) USAN.
Use: Antiasthmatic.

•**piriprost potassium.** (PIHR-ih-prahst) USAN.
Use: Antiasthmatic.

piriton.
See: Chlorpheniramine (Various Mfr.).

•**piritrexim isethionate.** (pih-rih-TREX-im eye-seh-THIGH-oh-nate) USAN.
Use: Antiproliferative. [Orphan Drug]

•**pirlimycin hydrochloride.** (PIHR-lih-MY-sin) USAN.
Use: Anti-infective.

•**pirmagrel.** (PIHR-mah-GRELL) USAN.
Use: Inhibitor (thromboxane synthetase).

•**pirmenol hydrochloride.** (PIHR-MEH-nahl) USAN.
Use: Cardiovascular agent, antiarrhythmic.

•**pirnabine.** (PIHR-NAH-bean) USAN.
Use: Antiglaucoma agent.

•**piroctone.** (pihr-OCK-TONE) USAN.
Use: Antiseborrheic.

•**piroctone olamine.** (pihr-OCK-TONE OH-lah-meen) USAN.
Use: Antiseborrheic.

•**pirodavir.** (pih-ROW-dav-ihr) USAN.
Use: Antiviral.

•**piroglide tartrate.** (PIHR-oh-GLIE-ride) USAN.
Use: Antidiabetic.

•**pirolate.** (PIHR-oh-late) USAN.
Use: Antiasthmatic.

•**pirolazamide.** (PIHR-ole-aze-ah-mide) USAN.
Use: Cardiovascular agent, antiarrhythmic.

•**piroxantrone hydrochloride.** (PIH-row-ZAN-trone) USAN.
Use: Antineoplastic.

•**piroxicam.** (pihr-OX-ih-kam) U.S.P. 23.
Use: Anti-inflammatory.
See: Feldene, Cap. (Pfizer US Pharmaceutical Group).

piroxicam. (Various Mfr.) 10 mg, 20 mg. Cap. Bot. 100s, 500s, 1000s.
Use: Anti-inflammatory.

•**piroxicam betadex.** (pihr-OX-ih-kam BAY-tah-dex) USAN.
Use: Analgesic, anti-inflammatory, antirheumatic.

•**piroxicam cinnamate.** (pihr-OX-ih-kam SIN-ah-mate) USAN.
Use: Anti-inflammatory.

•**piroxicam olamine.** (pihr-OX-ih-kam OH-lah-meen) USAN.
Use: Anti-inflammatory, analgesic.

•**piroximone.** (PIHR-ox-ih-MONE) USAN.
Use: Cardiovascular agent.

•**pirprofen.** (pihr-PRO-fen) USAN.
Use: Anti-inflammatory.

•**pirquinozol.** (PIHR-KWIN-oh-zole) USAN.
Use: Antiallergic.

•**pirsidomine.** (pihr-SIH-doe-meen) USAN.
Use: Vasodilator.

Piso's. (Pinex) Ipecac, ammonium Cl, menthol in syrup base. Bot. 3 oz, 5 oz. *otc.*
Use: Expectorant.

pitayine.
See: Quinidine, Preps. (Various Mfr.).

Pitocin. (Monarch Pharmaceuticals) Oxytocin w/chlorobutanol 0.5%, acetic acid to adjust pH. Amp. 5 units/0.5 ml; 10 units/ml. Box 10s, Steri-dose syringe; 10 units/ml 10s. *Rx.*
Use: Oxytocic.

Pitressin Synthetic. (Parke-Davis) Vasopressin w/chlorobutanol 0.5%, pH adjusted with acetic acid. Amp. 0.5 ml, 1 ml (20 pressor units). Box 10s. *Rx.*
Use: Hormone.

Pitts Carminative. (Del Pharmaceuticals, Inc.) Bot. 2 oz.
Use: Antiflatulent.

pituitary, anterior. The anterior lobe of the pituitary gland supplies protein hormones classified under following headings.
See: Corticotropin, Preps. (Various Mfr.).
Gonadotropin, Preps. (Various Mfr.).
Growth Hormone.
Thyrotropic Principle.

Pituitary Function Test.
See: Metopirone, Tab. (Novartis Pharmaceutical Corp.).

pituitary, posterior, hormones.
W/ (a) Vasopressin. Pressor principle, β-hypophamine, postlobin-V.
See: Pitressin, Amp. (Parke-Davis).
W/ (b) Oxytocin. Oxytocic principle. α-hypophamine, postiobin-O.
See: Oxytocin, Inj. (Various Mfr.).
Pitocin, Amp. (Parke-Davis).

•**pituitary, posterior, injection.** U.S.P. 23.
Use: Hormone (antidiuretic).

•**pivampicillin hydrochloride.** (pihv-AM-pih-SILL-in) USAN.
Use: Anti-infective.

•**pivampicillin pamoate.** (pihv-AM-pih SILL-in PAM-oh-ate) USAN.
Use: Anti-infective.

•**pivampicillin probenate.** (pihv-AM-pih-SILL-in PRO-ben-ate) USAN.
Use: Anti-infective.

•**pivopril.** (PIH-voe-PRILL) USAN.
Use: Antihypertensive.

pix carbonis.
See: Coal Tar, Preps. (Various Mfr.).

pix juniperi.
Use: Sunscreen, moisturizer.
See: Juniper Tar, Comp. (Various Mfr.).

•**pizotyline.** (pih-ZOE-tih-leen) USAN.
Use: Anabolic, antidepressant, serotonin inhibitor (migraine).

placebo capsules. (Cowley) No. 3 orange red; No. 4 yellow. Bot. 1000s.
Use: Placebo.

placebo tablets. (Cowley) 1 gr white; 2 gr white; 3 gr white, red or yellow, pink, orange; 4 gr white; 5 gr white. Bot. 1000s.
Use: Placebo.

Placidyl. (Abbott Laboratories) Ethchlorvynol. **200 mg/Cap.:** Bot. 100s. **500 mg/Cap.:** Bot. 100s, 500s, UD 100s. **750 mg/Cap.:** Bot. 100s. *c-iv.*
Use: Hypnotic, sedative.

•**plague vaccine.** U.S.P. 23.
Use: Immunization.

plague vaccine. (Greer Laboratories, Inc.) 2000 million killed *Pasteurella pestis*/ml. Vial 20 ml.
Use: Immunization.

planocaine.
See: Procaine HCl, Preps. (Various Mfr.).

planochrome.
See: Merbromin, Soln. (Various Mfr.).

plantago, ovata coating.
See: Konsyl, Pow. (Burton, Parsons).
L.A. Formula, Pow. (Burton, Parsons).
Metamucil, Pow. (Searle).

•**plantago seed.** (PLAN-tah-go seed) U.S.P. 23.
Use: Laxative.

Plaquenil Sulfate. (Sanofi Winthrop Pharmaceuticals) Hydroxychloroquine sulfate 200 mg/Tab. (equivalent to base 155 mg). Bot. 100s. *Rx.*
Use: Antimalarial, antirheumatic.

Plaquenil Tablet. (Sanofi Winthrop Pharmaceuticals) Hydroxychloroquine sulfate. *Rx.*
Use: Antimalarial, antirheumatic.

Plasbumin-5. (Bayer Corp. (Consumer Div.)) Normal serum albumin (human) 5% U.S.P. fractionated from normal serum plasma, heat treated against hepatitis virus. Albumin 12.5 g/250 ml. Inj. Vial 50 ml. Bot. with IV set 250 ml, 500 ml. *Rx.*
Use: Plasma protein fraction.

Plasbumin-25. Bayer Corp. (Consumer Div.) Normal serum albumin (Human) 25% U.S.P. fractionated from normal serum plasma, heat treated against hepatitis virus. Albumin 12.5 g/50 ml. Inj. Vial 20 ml. Bot. with IV set 50 ml, 100 ml. *Rx.*
Use: Plasma protein fraction.

plasma.
See: Normal Human Plasma (Various Mfr.).

plasma expanders or substitutes.
See: Dextran 6% and LMD 10% (Abbott Laboratories).
Macrodex, Soln. (Pharmacia & Upjohn).

Plasma-Lyte A Injection. (Baxter Pharmaceutical Products, Inc.) Na 140 mEq, K 5 mEq, Mg 3 mEq, Cl 98 mEq, acetate 27 mEq, gluconate 23 mEq/L w/pH adjusted to 7.4. Plastic Bot. 500 ml, 1000 ml. *Rx.*
Use: Nutritional supplement, parenteral.

Plasma-Lyte 148 Injection. (Baxter Pharmaceutical Products, Inc.) Na 140 mEq, K 5 mEq, Mg 3 mEq, Cl 98 mEq, acetate 27 mEq, gluconate 23 mEq/L. Plastic Bot. 500 ml, 1000 ml. *Rx.*
Use: Nutritional supplement, parenteral.

Plasma-Lyte M and 5% Dextrose Injection. (Baxter Pharmaceutical Products, Inc.) Na 40 mEq, K 16 mEq, Ca 5 mEq, Mg 3 mEq, Cl 40 mEq, acetate 12 mEq, lactate 12 mEq/L. Plastic Bot. 500 ml, 1000 ml. *Rx.*
Use: Nutritional supplement, parenteral.

Plasma-Lyte R and 5% Dextrose Injection. (Baxter Pharmaceutical Products, Inc.) Na 140 mEq, K 10 mEq, Ca 5 mEq, Mg 3 mEq, Cl 103 mEq, acetate 47 mEq, lactate 8 mEq/L. Bot. 500 ml, 1000 ml. *Rx.*
Use: Nutritional supplement, parenteral.

Plasma-Lyte 56 and 5% Dextrose. (Baxter Pharmaceutical Products, Inc.) Na 40 mEq, K 13 mEq, Mg 3 mEq, Cl 40 mEq, acetate 16 mEq/L. Plastic Bot. 500 ml, 1000 ml. *Rx.*
Use: Nutritional supplement, parenteral.

Plasma-Lyte 148 and 5% Dextrose. (Baxter Pharmaceutical Products, Inc.) Dextrose 50 g, calories 190, Na 140 mEq, K 5 mEq, Mg 3 mEq, Cl 98 mEq, acetate 27 mEq, 547 mOsm, gluconate 23 mEq/L. Soln. Bot. 500 ml, 1000 ml. *Rx.*
Use: Nutritional supplement, parenteral.

Plasma-Lyte 56 in Water. (Baxter Pharmaceutical Products, Inc.) Na 40 mEq, K 13 mEq, Mg 3 mEq, Cl 40 mEq, acetate 16 mEq/L. Plastic Bot. 500 ml, 1000 ml. *Rx.*
Use: Nutritional supplement, parenteral.

Plasma-Lyte R Injection. (Baxter Pharmaceutical Products, Inc.) Na 140 mEq, K 10 mEq, Ca 5 mEq, Mg 3

mEq, Cl 103 mEq, acetate 47 mEq, lactate 8 mEq/L. Bot. 1000 ml. *Rx.*
Use: Nutritional supplement, parenteral.

Plasmanate. (Bayer Corp. (Consumer Div.)) Plasma protein fraction (human) 5%. U.S.P. Vial 50 ml. Bot. 250 ml, 500 ml with set. *Rx.*
Use: Plasma protein fraction.

Plasma-Plex. (Centeon) Plasma protein fraction 5%. Inj. Vial 250 ml, 500 ml. *Rx.*
Use: Plasma protein fraction.

•**plasma protein fraction.** U.S.P. 23. *Formerly Plasma Protein Fraction, Human.*
Use: Blood-volume supporter.
See: Plasmanate, Soln. (Bayer Corp. (Consumer Div.)).
Plasma-Plex, Soln. (Centeon).
Plasmatein, Soln. (Abbott Laboratories).
Protenate, Soln. (Baxter Pharmaceutical Products, Inc.).

plasma protein fraction. (Baxter Pharmaceutical Products, Inc.) For the plasma protein preparation obtained from human plasma using the Cohn fractionation technique. Bot. 250 ml.
Use: Blood volume supporter.

Plasmatein. (Alpha Therapeutic Corp.) Plasma protein fraction 5%. Inj. Vial w/injection set 250 ml, 500 ml. *Rx.*
Use: Plasma protein fraction.

plasmochin naphthoate. Pamaquine naphthoate.
Use: Antimalarial.

•**platelet concentrate.** U.S.P. 23.
Use: Platelet replenisher.

Platelet Factor 4. (Abbott Diagnostics) Radioimmunoassay for quantitative measurement of total PF4 levels in plasma. Test kit 100s.
Use: Diagnostic aid.

Platinol-AQ. (Bristol-Myers Oncology/Immunology) Cisplatin (CDDP) 1 mg/ml. Inj. Vial. 50 ml, 100 ml. *Rx.*
Use: Antineoplastic.

Plavix. (Sanofi Winthrop Pharmaceuticals) Clopidogrel 75 mg (as bisulfate), lactose. Tab. Bot. 100s, 500s, UD 100s. *Rx.*
Use: Antiplatelet.

•**pleconaril.** (pleh-KOE-nah-rill) USAN.
Use: Antiviral.

Plegisol. (Abbott Hospital Products) Calcium Cl dihydrate 17.6 mg, magnesium Cl hexahydrate 325.3 mg, potassium Cl 119.3 mg, sodium Cl 643 mg/100 ml. Approximately 260 mOsm/L. Single-Dose Container 1000 ml without sodium bicarbonate. *Rx.*
Use: Cardiovascular agent.

Plendil. (Astra Pharmaceuticals, L.P.) Felodipine 2.5 mg, 5 mg, 10 mg/ER Tab. Bot. 30s, 100s, UD 100s. *Rx.*
Use: Calcium channel blocker.

Pletal. (Otsuka America Pharmaceuticals) Cilostazol 50 mg, 100 mg. Tab. Bot. 60s, UD 100s. *Rx.*
Use: Antiplatelet.

Plewin Tablets. (Sanofi Winthrop Pharmaceuticals) Glycobiarsol, chloroquine phosphate. *Rx.*
Use: Amebicide.

Plexolan Cream. (Last) Zinc oxide, lanolin. Tube 1.25 oz, 3 oz. Jar 16 oz. *otc.*
Use: Dermatologic.

Plexon. (Sigma-Tau Pharmaceuticals, Inc.) Testosterone 10 mg, estrone 1 mg, liver 2 mcg, pyridoxine HCl 10 mg, panthenol 10 mg, inositol 20 mg, choline Cl 20 mg, vitamin B_2 2 mg, B_{12} 100 mcg, procaine HCl 1%, niacinamide 100 mg/ml. Vial 10 ml.
Use: Hormone, mineral, vitamin supplement.

Pliagel. (Alcon Laboratories, Inc.) NaCl, KCl, poloxamer 407, sorbic acid 0.25%, EDTA 0.5%. Soln. Bot. 25 ml. *otc.*
Use: Contact lens care.

•**plicamycin.** (PLY-kae-MY-sin) U.S.P. 23. Antibiotic derived from *Streptomyces agrillaceus* & *S. tanashiensis. Formerly Mithramycin.*
Use: Antineoplastic.
See: Mithracin, Pow. (Bayer Corp. (Consumer Div.)).

•**plomestane.** (PLOE-mess-TANE) USAN.
Use: Antineoplastic (aromatase inhibitor).

Plova. (Washington Ethical) Psyllium mucilloid. Pow. (flavored) 12 oz., (plain) 10 0.5 oz. *otc.*
Use: Laxative.

Pluravit Drops. (Sanofi Winthrop Pharmaceuticals) Multivitamin.
Use: Vitamin supplement.

PMB 200. (Wyeth-Ayerst Laboratories) Conjugated estrogens 0.45 mg, meprobamate 200 mg, lactose, sucrose/Tab. Bot. 60s. *Rx.*
Use: Anxiolytic, estrogen.

PMB 400. (Wyeth-Ayerst Laboratories) Conjugated estrogens 0.45 mg, meprobamate 400 mg, lactose, sucrose/Tab. Bot. 100s. *Rx.*
Use: Anxiolytic, estrogen.

P.M.P. Compound. (Mericon Industries, Inc.) Chlorpheniramine maleate 4 mg, phenylephrine HCl 15 mg, salicylamide 300 mg, scopolamine methylnitrate 0.8 mg/Tab. Bot. 100s, 1000s. *Rx.*

Use: Analgesic, antihistamine, decongestant.

PMP Expectorant. (Mericon Industries, Inc.) Codeine phosphate 10 mg, phenylephrine HCl 10 mg, guaifenesin 40 mg, chlorpheniramine maleate 2 mg/5 ml. Bot. Gal. *c-v.*
Use: Antihistamine, antitussive, decongestant, expectorant.

pneumococcal vaccine, polyvalent. (new-moe-KAH-kuhl) Purified capsular polysaccharides from 23 pneumococcal types. 25 mcg each of 23 polysaccharides per 0.5 ml.
Use: Immunization.

Pneumomist. (ECR Pharmaceuticals) Guaifenesin 600 mg. SR Tab. Bot. 100s. *Rx.*
Use: Expectorant.

Pneumotussin HC. (ECR Pharmaceuticals) Hydrocodone bitartrate 5 mg, guaifenesin 100 mg/5 ml. Syr. Bot. 120 ml, 480 ml. *c-III.*
Use: Antitussive, expectorant.

PNS Unna Boot. (Pedinol Pharmacal, Inc.) Non-sterile gauze bandage 10 yds x 3". Box 12s.
Use: Ambulatory procedure in treatment of leg ulcers and varicosities.

Pnu-Imune 23. (Wyeth-Ayerst Laboratories) Pneumococcal vaccine 0.5 ml dose. 5-dose vials. Lederject disposable syringe 5 x 1 dose. *Rx.*
Use: Immunization.

•**pobilukast edamine.** (poe-BIH-loo-kast EH-dah-meen) USAN.
Use: Antiasthmatic (leukotriene antagonist).

pochlorin. Prophyrinic and chlorophyllic compound.
Use: Antihypercholesteremic agent.

Pod-Ben-25. (C & M Pharmacal, Inc.) Podophyllin 25% in benzoin tincture. Bot. 1 oz. *Rx.*
Use: Keratolytic.

Podoben. (American Pharmaceutical Co.) Podophyllum resin extract 25%. Bot. 5 ml. *Rx.*
Use: Keratolytic.

Podocon-25. (Paddock Laboratories) Podophyllum resin 25% in benzoin tincture. Soln. 15 ml. *Rx.*
Use: Keratolytic.

•**podofilox.** (pah-dah-FILL-ox) USAN.
Use: Antimitotic.
See: Condylox (Oclassen Pharmaceuticals, Inc.).

podophyllin.
See: Podophyllum resin.

•**podophyllum.** (poe-doe-FILL-uhm) U.S.P. 23.
Use: Pharmaceutic necessity.

•**podophyllum resin.** U.S.P. 23.
Use: Caustic.
See: Podoben, Liq. (Maurry).

podophyllum resin. (Various Mfr.) Podophyllin. Pkg. 1 oz, 0.25 lb, 1 lb.
Use: Caustic.

Point-Two Mouthrinse. (Colgate Oral Pharmaceuticals) Sodium fluoride 0.2% in a flavored neutral liquid. Bot. 120 ml. *Rx.*
Use: Dental caries agent.

Poison Antidote Kit. (Jones Medical Industries, Inc.) Charcoal suspension. Bot. 60 ml, 4s. Ipecac syrup, Bot. 30 ml, 1/Kit. *otc.*
Use: Antidote.

•**poison ivy extract, alum precipitated.** (poly-zuhn EYE-vee EX-tract, AL-uhm pree-SIP-ih-tay-tehd) USAN.
Use: Ivy poisoning counteractant.

Poison Oak-N-Ivy Armor. (Tec Laboratories, Inc.) Trioctyl citrate, mineral oil, monostearyl citrate, beeswax. Lot. Bot. 59.1 ml. *otc.*
Use: Dermatologic, poison ivy.

•**polacrilin.** (pahl-ah-KRILL-in) USAN. Methacrylic acid with divinylbenzene. A synthetic ion-exchange resin, supplied in the hydrogen or free acid form. Amberlite IRP-64.
Use: Pharmaceutic aid.

•**polacrilin potassium.** N.F. 18. A synthetic ion-exchange resin, prepared through the polymerization of methacrylic acid and divinylbenzene, further neutralized with potassium hydroxide to form the potassium salt of methacrylic acid and divinylbenzene. Supplied as a pharmaceutical-grade ion-exchange resin in a particle size of 100- to 500-mesh.
Use: Pharmaceutic aid (tablet disintegrant).
See: Amberlite IRP-88 (Rohm and Haas).

Poladex Tabs. (Major Pharmaceuticals) Dexchlorpheniramine maleate. **4 mg/Tab.:** Bot. 100s, 250s, 1000s. **6 mg/Tab.:** Bot. 100s, 1000s. *Rx.*
Use: Antihistamine.

polamethene resin caprylate. The physiochemical complex of the acid-binding ion exchange resin, polyamine-methylene resin and caprylic acid.

Polaramine. (Schering-Plough Corp.) Dexchlorpheniramine maleate. **Tab.:** 2 mg, Bot. 100s. **Repetab.:** 4 mg, 6 mg/Tab. Bot. 100s. **Syr.:** 2 mg/5 ml alcohol

6%. Bot. 473 ml. *Rx.*
Use: Antihistamine.

Polaramine Expectorant. (Schering-Plough Corp.) Dexchlorpheniramine maleate 2 mg, pseudoephedrine sulfate 20 mg, guaifenesin 100 mg/5 ml, alcohol 7.2%. Bot. 16 oz. *Rx.*
Use: Antihistamine, decongestant, expectorant.

Poldeman AD Suspension. (Sanofi Winthrop Pharmaceuticals) Kaolin. *otc.*
Use: Antidiarrheal.

Poldeman Suspension. (Sanofi Winthrop Pharmaceuticals) Kaolin. *otc.*
Use: Antidiarrheal.

Poldemicina Suspension. (Sanofi Winthrop Pharmaceuticals) Kaolin. *otc.*
Use: Antidiarrheal.

•**poldine methylsulfate.** (POLE-deen METH-ill-SULL-fate) USAN. U.S.P. XX.
Use: Anticholinergic.

•**policapram.** (PAH-lee-CAP-ram) USAN.
Use: Pharmaceutic aid (tablet binder).

Polident Dentu-Grip. (Block Drug Co., Inc.) Carboxymethylcellulose gum, ethylene oxide polymer. Pkg. 0.675 oz, 1.75 oz, 3.55 oz. *otc.*
Use: Denture adhesive.

•**polifeprosan 20.** (pahl-ee-FEH-pro-SAHN 20) USAN.
Use: Pharmaceutic aid (biodegradable polymer for controlled drug delivery).

•**poligeenan.** (PAHL-ih-JEE-nan) USAN. Polysaccharide produced by extensive hydrolysis of carragheen from red algae.
Use: Pharmaceutic aid (dispersing agent).

•**poliglecaprone 25.** (poe-lih-GLEH-kah-prone 25) USAN.
Use: Surgical aid (surgical suture material, absorbable).

•**poliglecaprone 90.** (poe-lih-GLEH-kah-prone 90) USAN.
Use: Surgical aid (surgical suture coating, absorbable).

•**poliglusam.** (pahl-ee-GLUE-sam) USAN.
Use: Antihemorrhagic, hemostatic, dermatologic, wound therapy.

•**polignate sodium.** (poe-LIG-nate) USAN.
Use: Enzyme inhibitor (pepsin).

Poli-Grip. (Block Drug Co., Inc.) Karaya gum, magnesium oxide in petrolatum mineral oil base, peppermint and spearmint flavor. Tube 0.75 oz, 1.5 oz, 2.5 oz. *otc.*
Use: Denture adhesive.

poliomyelitis vaccine, inactivated. (Pasteur Merieux Connaught) (Purified, Salk Type IPV) Amp. 5 x 1 ml. Vial 10 dose. *Rx.*
Use: Immunization.
See: IPOL.
Poliovirus vaccine, inactivated

•**poliovirus vaccine, inactivated.** (POE-lee-oh-VYE-russ) U.S.P. 23. *Formerly Poliomyelitis Vaccine.*
Use: Immunization.
See: IPOL (Connaught).

poliovirus vaccine, inactivated. (Pasteur Merieux Connaught) Amp. 1 ml. Box 5s. Vial 10 dose. Subcutaneous administration.
Use: Agent for immunization (active).

•**poliovirus vaccine live oral.** (POE-lee-oh-VYE-russ) U.S.P. 23. Poliovirus vaccine, live, oral, type I, II, or III. Poliovirus vaccine, live, oral, trivalent.
Use: Immunization.
See: Orimune Trivalent I, II & III, Vial (Wyeth-Ayerst Laboratories).

poliovirus vaccine, live, oral, trivalent. Immunization against polio strains 1, 2, & 3. *Rx.*
Use: Immunization.
See: Orimune (Wyeth-Ayerst Laboratories).

•**polipropene 25.** (pahl-ee-PRO-peen 25) USAN.
Use: Pharmaceutic aid (tablet excipient).

•**polixetonium chloride.** (pahl-ix-eh-TOE-nee-uhm) USAN.
Use: Pharmaceutic aid (preservative).

Polocaine. (Astra Pharmaceuticals, L.P.) Mepivacaine. **1%, 2%:** Inj. Vial 50 ml. **3%:** Inj. Dental cartridge 1.8 ml. **2% w/ levonordefrin 1:20,000:** Sodium bisulfite. Inj. Dental cartridge 1.8 ml. *Rx.*
Use: Anesthetic, local.

Polocaine MPF. (Astra Pharmaceuticals, L.P.) Mepivacaine HCl. **1%, 1.5%:** Inj. Vial 30 ml. **2%:** Inj. Vial 20 ml. *Rx.*
Use: Anesthetic, local.

Poloris Poultices. (Block Drug Co., Inc.) Benzocaine 7.5 mg, capsicum 4.6 mg in poultice base. Pkg. 5 unit, 12 unit. *Rx.*
Use: Anesthetic, local.

•**poloxalene.** (PAHL-OX-ah-leen) USAN. Liquid nonionic surfactant polymer of polyoxypropylene polyoxyethylene type.
Use: Pharmaceutic aid (surfactant).

poloxalkol. Polyoxyethylene polyoxypropylene polymer.
See: Magcyl, Cap. (ICN Pharmaceuticals, Inc.).
W/Casanthrol.
See: Casakol, Cap. (Pharmacia & Upjohn).

•**poloxamer.** (pahl-OX-ah-mer) N.F. 18.
Use: Pharmaceutic aid (ointment and suppository base, surfactant, tablet binder and coating agent, emulsifying agent).

poloxamer 182 d. (pahl-OX-ah-mer 182D)
Use: Pharmaceutic aid (surfactant).

poloxamer 182 lf. (pahl-OX-ah-mer 182 LF)
Use: Food additive; pharmaceutic aid.

poloxamer 188. (pahl-OX-ah-mer 188)
Use: Cathartic; sickle cell crisis, severe burns. [Orphan Drug]

poloxamer 188 lf. (pahl-OX-ah-mer 188LF)
Use: Pharmaceutic aid (surfactant).

poloxamer 331. (pahl-OX-ah-mer 331)
Use: Food additive (surfactant); AIDS-related toxoplasmosis. [Orphan Drug]

poloxamer-iodine.
See: Prepodyne, Soln. (West).

polyamine resin.
See: Polyamine-Methylene Resin (Various Mfr.).

polyanhydroglucose. Polyanhydroglucuronic acid.
See: Dextran, Inj., Soln. (Various Mfr.).

Polybase. (Paddock Laboratories) Preblended polyethylene glycol suppository base for incorporation of medications where a water-soluble base is indicated. Jar 1 lb, 5 lb.
Use: Pharmaceutical aid, suppository base.

polybenzarsol. Benzocal.

Poly-Bon Drops. (Barrows) Vitamins A 3000 IU, D 400 IU, C 60 mg, B_1 1 mg, B_2 1.2 mg, niacinamide 8 mg/0.6 ml. Bot. 50 ml. *otc.*
Use: Vitamin supplement.

•**polybutester.** (PAHL-ee-byoot-ESS-ter) USAN.
Use: Surgical aid (surgical suture material).

•**polybutilate.** (PAHL-ee-BYOO-tih-late) USAN.
Use: Surgical aid (surgical suture coating).

•**polycarbophil.** U.S.P. 23. A synthetic, loosely cross-linked, hydrophilic resin of the polycarboxylic type. Sorboquel.
Use: Laxative.

Polycillin. (Bristol-Myers Squibb) Ampicillin trihydrate. **250 mg/Cap.:** Bot. 100s, 500s, 1000s, UD 100s. **500 mg/Cap.:** Bot. 100s, 500s, UD 100s. **Pediatric Drops:** 100 mg/ml. Dropper bot. 20 ml. *Rx.*
Use: Anti-infective, penicillin.

Polycillin Oral Suspension. (Bristol-Myers Squibb) Ampicillin trihydrate. **125 mg/5 ml:** Bot. 80 ml, 100 ml, 150 ml, 200 ml, UD 5 ml. **250 mg/5 ml:** Bot. 80 ml, 100 ml, 150 ml, 200 ml, UD 5 ml. **500 mg/5 ml:** Bot. 100 ml, UD 5 ml. *Rx.*
Use: Anti-infective, penicillin.

Polycitra K. (Baker Norton Pharmaceuticals, Inc.) Potassium citrate monohydrate 1100 mg, citric acid monohydrate 334 mg, potassium ion 10 mEq/5 ml. Bot. 4 oz, pt. *Rx.*
Use: Alkalinizer, systemic.

Polycitra K Crystals. (Baker Norton Pharmaceuticals, Inc.) Potassium citrate monohydrate 3300 mg, citric acid 1002 mg, potassium ion 30 mEq, equivalent to 30 mEq bicarbonate/UD pkg. Sugar free. Box 100s. *Rx.*
Use: Alkalinizer, systemic.

Polycitra LC. (Baker Norton Pharmaceuticals, Inc.) Potassium citrate monohydrate 550 mg, sodium citrate dihydrate 500 mg, citric acid monohydrate 334 mg, potassium ion 5 mEq, sodium ion 5 mEq/5 ml. Bot. 4 oz, pt. *Rx.*
Use: Alkalinizer, systemic.

Polycitra Syrup. (Baker Norton Pharmaceuticals, Inc.) Potassium citrate monohydrate 550 mg, sodium citrate dihydrate 500 mg, citric acid monohydrate 334 mg, potassium ion 5 mEq, sodium ion 5 mEq/5 ml. Bot. 4 oz, pt. *Rx.*
Use: Alkalinizer, systemic.

Polycose. (Ross Laboratories) **Pow.:** Glucose polymers derived from controlled hydrolysis of corn starch. Calories 380, carbohydrate 94 g, water 6 g, Na 110 mg, K 10 mg, Cl 223 mg, Ca 30 mg, P 5 mg/100 g. Can 12.3 oz. Case 6s. **Liq.:** Calories 200, carbohydrate 50 g, water 70 g, Na 70 mg, K 6 mg, Cl 140 mg, Ca 20 mg, P 3 mg/100 ml. Bot. 4 oz. Case 48s. *otc.*
Use: Nutritional supplement.

•**polydextrose.** (PAH-lee-DEX-trose) USAN.
Use: Food additive.

polydimethylsiloxane (silicone oil).
Use: Ophthalmic.
See: AdatoSil 5000, Inj. (Escalon Ophthalmics, Inc.).

Polydine Ointment. (Century Pharmaceuticals, Inc.) Povidone-iodine in ointment base. Jar 1 oz, 4 oz, lb. *otc.*
Use: Anti-infective, topical.

Polydine Scrub. (Century Pharmaceuticals, Inc.) Povidone-iodine in scrub solution. Bot. 1 oz, 4 oz, 8 oz, pt, gal. *otc.*

Use: Antiseptic.

Polydine Solution. (Century Pharmaceuticals, Inc.) Povidone-iodine solution. Bot. 1 oz, 4 oz, 8 oz, pt, gal. *otc.*
Use: Antiseptic.

•**polydioxanone.** (PAHL-ee-die-OX-ah-nohn) USAN.
Use: Surgical aid (surgical suture material, absorbable).

Poly ENA Test System for RNP and SM. (Wampole Laboratories) Qualitative identification of auto antibodies to extractable nuclear antigens in human serum by gel precipitation technique. Aid in the diagnosis of SLE, MCTD, PSS, SS. Box test 48s.
Use: Diagnostic aid.

Poly ENA Test System for RNP, SM, SSA, and SSB. (Wampole Laboratories) Qualitative identification of auto antibodies to extractable nuclear antigens in human serum by gel precipitation techniques. Aid in the diagnosis of SLE, MCTD, PSS, SS. Box test 96s.
Use: Diagnostic aid.

Poly ENA Test System for SSA and SSB. (Wampole Laboratories) Qualitative identification of auto antibodies to extractable nuclear antigens in human serum by gel precipitation techniques. Aid in the diagnosis of SLE, MCTD, PSS, SS. Box test 48s.
Use: Diagnostic aid.

•**polyethadene.** (PAHL-ee-ETH-ah-DEEN) USAN.
Use: Antacid.

polyethylene excipient. N.F. XVII.
Use: Pharmaceutic aid (stiffening agent).

•**polyethylene glycol.** (poli-eth-uh-leen gli-cawl) N.F. 18.
Use: Pharmaceutic aid (ointment and suppository base, tablet excipient, solvent, tablet and capsule lubricant).

polyethylene glycol 3350 and electrolytes for oral solution. (poli-eth-uh-leen gli-cawl)
Use: Rehydration.

•**polyethylene glycol monomethyl ether.** (PAHL-ee-ETH-ah-LEEN EETH-ehr) N.F. 18.
Use: Pharmaceutic aid (excipient).

•**polyethylene oxide.** (PAHL-ee-ETH-ah-LEEN) N.F. 18.
Use: Pharmaceutic aid (suspending and viscosity agent, tablet binder).

•**polyferose.** (PAHL-ee-feh-rohs) USAN. An iron carbohydrate chelate containing approximately 45% of iron in which the metallic (Fe) ion is sequestered within a polymerized carbohydrate derived from sucrose.
Use: Hematinic.

Poly-F Fluoride Drops. (Major Pharmaceuticals) Fluoride 0.5 mg, vitamins A 1500 IU, D 400 IU, E 5 mg, B_1 0.5 mg, B_2 0.6 mg, B_3 8 mg, B_6 0.4 mg, B_{12} 2 mcg, C 35 mg/ml. Drops. Bot. 50 ml. *Rx.*
Use: Mineral, vitamin supplement.

Polygam S/D. (American Red Cross) Protein 50 mg (90% gamma globulin). Inj. Single-use vials 2.5 g, 5 g, 10 g. *Rx.*
Use: Immunization.

•**polyglactin 370.** (PAHL-ee-GLAHK-tin 370) USAN. Lactic acid polyester with glycolic acid.
Use: Surgical aid (surgical suture coating, absorbable).

•**polyglactin 910.** (PAHL-ee-GLAHK-tin 910) USAN.
Use: Surgical aid (surgical suture coating, absorbable).

•**polyglycolic acid.** (PAHL-ee-glie-KAHL-ik) USAN.
Use: Surgical aid (surgical suture material).
See: Dexone Sterile Suture (David & Geck).

•**polyglyconate.** (PAHL-ee-GLIE-koe-nate) USAN.
Use: Surgical aid (surgical suture material, absorbable).

Poly-Histine. (Sanofi Winthrop Pharmaceuticals) Pheniramine maleate 4 mg, pyrilamine maleate 4 mg, phenyltoloxamine citrate 4 mg, alcohol 4%/5 ml. Elix. Bot. 473 ml. *Rx.*
Use: Antihistamine.

Poly-Histine CS. (Sanofi Winthrop Pharmaceuticals) Brompheniramine maleate 2 mg, phenylpropanolamine HCl 12.5 mg, codeine phosphate 10 mg/5 ml, alcohol 0.95%. Bot. Pt. *c-v.*
Use: Antihistamine, antitussive, decongestant.

Poly-Histine-D Capsules. (Sanofi Winthrop Pharmaceuticals) Phenylpropanolamine HCl 50 mg, phenyltoloxamine citrate 16 mg, pyrilamine maleate 16 mg, pheniramine maleate 16 mg/Cap. Bot. 100s. *Rx.*
Use: Antihistamine, decongestant.

Poly-Histine-D Elixir. (Sanofi Winthrop Pharmaceuticals) Phenylpropanolamine HCl 12.5 mg, phenyltoloxamine citrate 4 mg, pyrilamine maleate 4 mg, pheniramine 4 mg/5 ml. Bot. 473 ml. *Rx.*
Use: Antihistamine, decongestant.

Poly-Histine DM. (Sanofi Winthrop Pharmaceuticals) Dextromethorphan HBr 10 mg, phenylpropanolamine HCl 12.5 mg, brompheniramine maleate 2 mg/5 ml. Bot. Pt. *Rx.*
Use: Antihistamine, antitussive, decongestant.

Poly-Histine-D Ped Caps. (Sanofi Winthrop Pharmaceuticals) Phenylpropanolamine HCl 25 mg, phenyltoloxamine citrate 8 mg, pheniramine maleate 8 mg, pyrilamine maleate 8 mg/Cap. Bot. 100s. *Rx.*
Use: Antihistamine, decongestant.

Poly-Histine Elixir. (Sanofi Winthrop Pharmaceuticals) Phenyltoloxamine citrate 4 mg, pyrilamine maleate 4 mg, pheniramine maleate 4 mg/5 ml, alcohol 4%. Elix. Bot. Pt. *Rx.*
Use: Antihistamine.

poly I; poly C12U.
Use: AIDS, antineoplastic. [Orphan Drug]

•**polymacon.** (PAHL-ee-MAY-kahn) USAN.
Use: Contact lens material (hydrophilic).

polymeric oxygen.
Use: Sickle cell disease. [Orphan Drug]

•**polymetaphosphate p 32.** (pahl-ee-met-ah-FOSS-fate) USAN.
Use: Radiopharmaceutical.

Polymox. (Bristol-Myers Squibb) Amoxicillin trihydrate. **Cap.:** 250 mg. Bot. 100s, 500s, UD 100s; 500 mg. Bot. 50s, 100s, 500s, UD 100s. **Oral Susp.:** 125 mg, 250 mg/5 ml. Bot. 80 ml, 100 ml, 150 ml. **Ped. Drops:** 50 mg/ml. Bot. 15 ml. *Rx.*
Use: Anti-infective, penicillin.

•**polymyxin b.** (Various Mfr.) Antimicrobial substances produced by *Bacillus polymyxa.*

•**polymyxin b sulfate.** (pahl-ee-mix-in) U.S.P. 23.
Use: Anti-infective.
See: Aerosporin, Pow., Soln. (GlaxoWellcome).

polymyxin b sulfate and bacitracin zinc topical aerosol.
Use: Anti-infective, topical.

polymyxin b sulfate and bacitracin zinc topical powder.
Use: Anti-infective, topical.

polymyxin b sulfate and hydrocortisone otic solution.
Use: Anti-infective, anti-inflammatory, otic.

polymyxin b sulfate sterile. (Roerig) Polymyxin B sulfate 500,000 units Ophth Soln. Vial 20 ml for reconstitution. *Rx.*
Use: Anti-infective.

polymyxin b sulfate w/combinations.
See: AK-Poly-Bac Oint. (Akorn, Inc.).
AK-Spore, Preps. (Akorn, Inc.).
Aquaphor, Oint. (Beiersdorf, Inc.).
Clomycin (Roberts).
Cortisporin, Preps. (GlaxoWellcome).
Maxitrol, Oint., Ophthalmic Oint. (Pharmacia & Upjohn).
Mycitracin, Oint., Ophthalmic Oint. (Pharmacia & Upjohn).
Neomixin, Oint. (Roberts Pharmaceuticals).
Neosporin, Preps. (GlaxoWellcome).
Neosporin G.U. Irrigant, Amp. (GlaxoWellcome).
Neotal, Oint. (Roberts Pharmaceuticals).
Neo-Thrycex, Oint. (Del Pharmaceuticals, Inc.).
Ocutricin, Preps. (Bausch & Lomb Pharmaceuticals).
Otobiotic, Soln. (Schering-Plough Corp.).
Polysporin, Oint., Ophthalmic Oint. (GlaxoWellcome).
Polytrim Ophth., Soln. (Allergan, Inc.).
Pyocidin-Otic, Soln. (Berlex Laboratories, Inc.).
Terramycin, Preps w/Oxytetracycline (Pfizer US Pharmaceutical Group).
Tigo, Oint. (Burlington).
Tribiotic Plus, Oint. (Thompson Medical Co.).
Trimixin, Oint. (Hance).

polymyxin-neomycin-bacitracin ointment. (Various Mfr.) *otc.*
Use: Anti-infective, topical.

polynoxylin. Anaflex.

polyoxyethylene 8 stearate. Myrj 45. (Zeneca Pharmaceuticals), Polyoxyl 8 Stearate.

polyoxyethylene 20 sorbitan monoleate.
See: Polysorbate 80, USP 23 (Various Mfr.).

polyoxyethylene 20 sorbitan trioleate. Tween 85. (Zeneca Pharmaceuticals), Polysorbate 85.

polyoxyethylene 20 sorbitan tristearate. Tween 65. (Zeneca Pharmaceuticals), Polysorbate 65.

polyoxyethylene 40 monostearate.
See: Polyoxyl 40 Stearate.
Myrj 52 & Myrj 52S (Zeneca Pharmaceuticals).

polyoxyethylene 50 stearate.
See: Polyoxyl 50 stearate.

polyoxyethylene lauryl ether. W/Benzoyl peroxide, ethyl alcohol.

See: Benzagel, Gel (Dermik Laboratories, Inc.).
Desquam-X, Preps. (Westwood Squibb Pharmaceuticals).
W/Hydrocortisone, sulfur.
See: Fostril HC, Lot. (Westwood Squibb Pharmaceuticals).
W/Sulfur.
See: Fostril, Lot. (Westwood Squibb Pharmaceuticals).

polyoxyethylene nonyl phenol.
W/Sodium edetate, docusate sodium, 9-aminoacridine HCl.
See: Vagisec Plus, Supp. (Durex).

polyoxyethylene sorbitan monolaurate. Polysorbate 20.
W/Ferrous gluconate.
See: Simron, Cap. (Hoechst Marion Roussel).
W/Ferrous gluconate, vitamins.
See: Simron Plus, Cap. (Hoechst Marion Roussel).

•**polyoxyl 8 stearate.** (PAHL-ee-OX-ill 8 STEE-ah-rate) USAN.
Use: Pharmaceutic aid (surfactant).
See: Myrj 45 (Atlas).

•**polyoxyl 10 oleyl ether.** (PAHL-ee-OX-ill 10 EETH-ehr) N.F. 18.
Use: Pharmaceutic aid (surfactant).

•**polyoxyl 20 cetostearyl ether.** (PAHL-ee-OX-ill 20 SEE-toe-STEE-rill EETH-ehr) N.F. 18.
Use: Pharmaceutic aid (surfactant).

•**polyoxyl 35 castor oil.** (PAHL-ee-OX-ill) N.F. 18.
Use: Pharmaceutic aid (surfactant, emulsifying agent).

•**polyoxyl 40 hydrogenated castor oil.** (PAHL-ee-OX-ill 40 high-DRAH-jen-ATE-ehd) N.F. 18.
Use: Pharmaceutic aid (surfactant, emulsifying agent).

•**polyoxyl 40 stearate.** (PAHL-ee-OX-ill 40 STEE-ah-rate) N.F. 18. Macrogic Stearate 2,000 (I.N.N.) Polyoxyethylene 40 monostearate.
Use: Pharmaceutic aid; hydrophilic oint., surfactant; surface-active agent.
See: Myrj 52 (Atlas).
Myrj 52S (Atlas).

•**polyoxyl 50 stearate.** (PAHL-ee-OX-ill 50 STEE-ah-rate) N.F. 18. *Formerly Polyxyethylene 50 stearate.*
Use: Pharmaceutic aid (surfactant, emulsifying agent).

•**polyoxypropylene 15 stearyl ether.** USAN. *Formerly PPG-15 Stearyl Ether.*
Use: Pharmaceutic aid (solvent).

Poly-Pred Suspension. (Allergan, Inc.) Prednisolone acetate 0.5%, neomycin sulfate equivalent to 0.35% neomycin base, polymyxin B sulfate 10,000 units/ml. Dropper bot. 5 ml, 10 ml. *Rx.*
Use: Anti-infective; corticosteroid, ophthalmic.

polypropylene glycol. An addition polymer of propylene oxide and water.
Use: Pharmaceutic aid (suspending agent).

polysaccharide iron complex. (Various Mfr.) Iron 50 mg/Cap. Bot. 100s. *otc.*
Use: Mineral supplement.
See: Hytinic, Preps. (Hyrex Pharmaceuticals).
Niferex, Prods. (Schwarz Pharma, Inc.).
Nu-Iron, Prods. (Merz Pharmaceuticals).

polysonic lotion. (Parker) Multi-purpose ultrasound lotion with high coupling efficiency. Bot. 8.5 oz, gal.
Use: Diagnostic aid, therapeutic aid.

•**polysorbate 20.** (PAHL-ee-SORE-bate 20) N.F. 18.
Use: Pharmaceutic aid (surfactant).

•**polysorbate 40.** (PAHL-ee-SORE-bate 40) N.F. 18.
Use: Pharmaceutic aid (surfactant).

•**polysorbate 60.** (PAHL-ee-SORE-bate 60) N.F. 18.
Use: Pharmaceutic aid (surfactant).

•**polysorbate 65.** (PAHL-ee-SORE-bate 65) USAN.
Use: Pharmaceutic aid (surfactant).

•**polysorbate 80.** (PAHL-ee-SORE-bate 80) N.F. 18.
Use: Pharmaceutic aid (surfactant).

•**polysorbate 85.** (PAHL-ee-SORE-bate 85) USAN.
Use: Pharmaceutic aid (surfactant).

Polysorb Hydrate. (E. Fougera and Co.) Sorbitan sesquinoleate in a wax and petrolatum base. Cream Tube 56.7 g, lb. *otc.*
Use: Emollients.

Polysporin Ointment. (GlaxoWellcome) Polymyxin B sulfate 10,000 units, bacitracin zinc 500 units/g in special white petrolatum base. Tube 3.75 g. *otc.*
Use: Anti-infective, topical.

Polysporin Ophthalmic Ointment. (GlaxoWellcome) Polymyxin B sulfate, 10,000 units, bacitracin zinc 500 units. Tube 3.5 g. *Rx.*
Use: Antibiotic, ophthalmic.

Polysporin Powder. (GlaxoWellcome) Polymyxin B 10,000 units, zinc bacitracin 500 units, lactose base/g. Shaker vial 10 g. *Rx.*
Use: Anti-infective, topical.

polysulfides. Polythionate.

Polytabs-F Chewable Vitamin. (Major Pharmaceuticals) Fluoride 1 mg, vitamins A 2500 IU, D 400 IU, E 15 mg, B_1 1.05 mg, B_2 1.2 mg, B_3 13.5 mg, B_6 1.05 mg, B_{12} 4.5 mcg, C 60 mg, folic acid 0.3 mg/Chew. Tab. Bot. 100s, 1000s. *Rx.*
Use: Mineral, vitamin supplement.

Polytar Shampoo. (Stiefel Laboratories, Inc.) A neutral soap containing 1% Polytar in a surfactant shampoo. Buffered. Plastic Bot. 6 fl oz, 12 fl oz, gal. *otc.*
Use: Antiseborrheic.

Polytar Soap. (Stiefel Laboratories, Inc.) A neutral soap containing 1% Polytar. Cake 4 oz. *otc.*
Use: Dermatologic.

•**polytef.** (PAHL-ee-teff) USAN.
Use: Prosthetic aid.

•**polythiazide.** (PAHL-ee-THIGH-azz-ide) U.S.P. 23.
Use: Antihypertensive, diuretic.
See: Renese, Tab. (Pfizer US Pharmaceutical Group).
W/Prazosin.
See: Minizide, Cap. (Pfizer US Pharmaceutical Group).
W/Reserpine.
See: Renese-R, Tab. (Pfizer US Pharmaceutical Group).

Polytinic. (Pharmics, Inc.) Elemental iron 100 mg, vitamin C 300 mg, folic acid 1 mg/tab. Bot. 100s. *Rx.*
Use: Mineral, vitamin supplement.

Polytrim. (Allergan, Inc.) Polymyxin B sulfate 10,000 units/g or ml, trimethoprim 1 mg/ml. Drop. Bot. 10 ml. *Rx.*
Use: Anti-infective, ophthalmic.

Polytuss-DM. (Rhode) Dextromethorphan HBr 15 mg, chlorpheniramine maleate 1 mg, guaifenesin 25 mg/5 ml. Bot. 4 oz, 8 oz. *otc.*
Use: Antihistamine, antitussive, expectorant.

•**polyurethane foam.** (PAHL-ih-you-ree-thane foam) USAN.
Use: Prosthetic aid (internal bone splint).

polyvidone.
See: Polyvinylpyrrolidone.

Poly-Vi-Flor 0.25 mg. (Bristol-Myers Squibb) **Drops:** Vitamins A 1500 IU, D 400 IU, E 5 IU, C 35 mg, B_1 0.5 mg, B_2 0.6 mg, B_6 0.4 mg, B_3 8 mg, B_{12} 2 mcg, fluoride 0.25 mg/ml. Dropper Bot. 50 ml. **Chew. Tab.:** Vitamins A 2500 IU, D 400 IU, E 15 IU, B_1 1.05 mg, B_2 1.2 mg, B_3 13.5 mg, B_6 1.05 mg, B_{12} 4.5 mcg, C 60 mg, folic acid, 0.3 mg, fluoride 0.25 mg, lactose, sucrose. Bot. 100s. *Rx.*
Use: Mineral, vitamin supplement; dental caries agent.

Poly-Vi-Flor 0.5 mg Chewable Tabs. (Bristol-Myers Squibb) Vitamins A 2500 IU, D 400 IU, E 15 IU, C 60 mg, B_1 1.05 mg, B_2 1.2 mg, B_3 13.5 mg, B_6 1.05 mg, B_{12} 4.5 mcg, fluoride 0.5 mg, folic acid 0.3 mg/Chew. Tab. Bot. 100s. **With Iron:** Above formula plus Fe 12 mg, Cu, Zn 10 mg/Tab. Bot. 100s. *Rx.*
Use: Mineral, vitamin supplement; dental caries agent.

Poly-Vi-Flor 1 mg Chewable Tablets. (Bristol-Myers Squibb) Vitamins A 2500 IU, D 400 IU, E 15 IU, C 60 mg, B_1 1.05 mg, B_2 1.2 mg, B_3 13.5 mg, B_6 1.05 mg, B_{12} 4.5 mcg, fluoride 1 mg, folic acid 0.3 mg, sucrose/Chew. Tab. Bot. 100s, 1000s. **With Iron:** Above formula plus Fe 12 mg, Cu 1 mg, Zn 10 mg/Tab. *Rx.*
Use: Mineral, vitamin supplement; dental caries agent.

Poly-Vi-Flor 0.5 mg Drops. (Bristol-Myers Squibb) Vitamins A 1500 IU, D 400 IU, E 5 IU, C 35 mg, B_1 0.5 mg, B_2 0.6 mg, B_6 0.4 mg, niacin 8 mg, B_{12} 2 mcg, fluoride 0.5 mg/ml. Dropper Bot. 30 ml, 50 ml. *Rx.*
Use: Mineral, vitamin supplement; dental caries agent.

Poly-Vi-Flor 0.25 mg w/Iron. (Bristol-Myers Squibb) **Drops:** Vitamins A 1500 IU, D 400 IU, E 5 IU, C 35 mg, B_1 0.5 mg, B_2 0.6 mg, B_6 0.4 mg, niacin 8 mg, fluoride 0.25 mg, Fe 10 mg/ml. Bot. 50 ml. **Chew. Tab.:** Vitamins A 2500 IU, D 400 IU, E 15 IU, B_1 1.05 IU, B_2 1.2 mg, B_3 13.5 mg, B_6 1.05 mg, B_{12} 4.5 mcg, C 60 mg, folic acid 0.3 mg, fluoride 0.25 mg, Cu, Fe 12 mg, Zn 10 mg, lactose, sucrose. Bot. 100s. *Rx.*
Use: Mineral, vitamin supplement; dental caries agent.

Poly-Vi-Flor 0.5 mg w/Iron. (Bristol-Myers Squibb) **Drops:** Vitamins A 1500 IU, D 400 IU, E 5 IU, C 35 mg, B_1 0.5 mg, B_2 0.6 mg, B_3 8 mg, B_6 0.4 mg, fluoride 0.5 mg, Fe 10 mg/ml. Dropper Bot. 50 ml. **Chew. Tab.:** Vitamins A 2500 IU, D 400 IU, E 15 IU, B_1 1.05 mg, B_2 1.2 mg, $B_3$13.5 mg, B_6 1.05 mg, B_{12} 4.5 mcg, C 60 mg, folic acid 0.3 mg, fluoride 0.5 mg, Fe 12 mg, Cu, Zn 10 mg, lactose, sucrose. Bot. 100s. *Rx.*
Use: Mineral, vitamin supplement; dental caries agent.

Poly-Vi-Flor 0.5 Tabs. (Bristol-Myers

Squibb) Fluoride 0.5 mg, vitamins A 2500 IU, D 400 IU, E 15 mg, B_1 1.05 mg, B_2 1.2 mg, B_3 13.5 mg, B_6 1.05 mg, B_{12} 4.5 mcg, C 60 mg, folic acid 0.3 mg, Cu, Fe 12 mg, Zn 10 mg, sucrose. Tab. Bot. 100s. *Rx.*
Use: Mineral, vitamin supplement; dental caries agent.

•**polyvinyl acetate phthalate.** (pahl-ee-VYE-nil) N.F. 18.
Use: Pharmaceutic aid (coating agent).

•**polyvinyl alcohol.** U.S.P. 23. Ethanol, homopolymer.
Use: Pharmaceutic aid (viscosity-increasing agent).
See: Liquifilm Forte (Allergan, Inc.).
Liquifilm Tears (Allergan, Inc.).
Puralube Tears, Drops (Fougera).
W/Hydroxypropyl methylcellulose.
See: Liquifilm Wetting, Soln. (Allergan, Inc).

polyvinylpyrrolidone vinylacetate copolymers.
See: Ivy-Rid, Spray (Roberts Pharmaceuticals).
W/Benzalkonium.
See: Ivy-Chex, Aer. (Jones Medical Industries, Inc.).

Poly-Vi-Sol Drops. (Bristol-Myers Squibb) Vitamins A 1500 IU, D 400 IU, C 35 mg, B_1 0.5 mg, B_2 0.6 mg, E 5 IU, B_6 0.4 mg, B_3 8 mg, B_{12} 2 mcg/ml. Bot. 50 ml. *otc.*
Use: Vitamin supplement.

Poly-Vi-Sol Tablets. (Bristol-Myers Squibb) Vitamins A 2500 IU, E 15 IU, D 400 IU, C 60 mg, B_1 1.05 mg, B_2 1.2 mg, B_3 13.5 mg, B_6 1.05 mg, B_{12} 4.5 mcg, folic acid 0.3 mg/Chew. Tab. Bot. 100s. **With Iron:** Above formula plus Fe 12 mg, Zn 8 mg/Tab. Bot. 100s. Circus shape Tab. Bot. 100s. *otc.*
Use: Mineral, vitamin supplement.

Poly-Vi-Sol w/Iron Drops. (Bristol-Myers Squibb) Vitamins A 1500 IU, D 400 IU, E 5 IU, C 35 mg, B_1 0.5 mg, B_2 0.6 mg, B_3 8 mg, B_6 0.4 mg, Fe 10 mg/ml. Bot. 50 ml. *otc.*
Use: Mineral, vitamin supplement.

Poly-Vi-Sol w/Iron Tablets, Chewable. (Bristol-Myers Squibb) Fe 12 mg, vitamins A 2500 IU, D 400 IU, E 15 mg, B_1 1.05 mg, B_2 1.2 mg, B_3 13.5 mg, B_6 1.05 mg, B_{12} 4.5 mcg, C 60 mg, folic acid 0.3 mg, Cu, Zn 8 mg, sugar/Chew. Tab. Bot. 100s. *otc.*
Use: Mineral, vitamin supplement.

Poly-Vi-Sol w/Minerals. (Bristol-Myers Squibb) Fe 12 mg, vitamins A 2500 IU, D 400 IU, E 15 mg, B_1 1.05 mg, B_2 1.2 mg, B_3 13.5 mg, B_6 1.06 mg, B_{12} 4.5 mcg, C 60 mg, folic acid 0.3 mg, Cu, Zn 8 mg/Chew. Tab. Bot. 60s, 100s. *otc.*
Use: Mineral, vitamin supplement.

Poly-Vitamin Drops. (Schein Pharmaceutical, Inc.) Vitamins A 1500 IU, D 400 IU, E 5 IU, B_1 0.5 mg, B_2 0.6 mg, B_3 8 mg, B_6 0.4 mg, B_{12} 1.5 mcg, C 35 mg/ml. Dropper. Bot. 50 ml. *otc.*
Use: Vitamin supplement.

Polyvitamin Drops with Iron. (Various Mfr.) Fe 10 mg, vitamins A 1500 IU, D 400 IU, E 5 mg, B_1 0.5 mg, B_2 0.6 mg, B_3 8 mg, B_6 0.4 mg, C 35 mg/ml. Bot. 50 ml. *otc.*
Use: Mineral, vitamin supplement.

Polyvitamin Drops w/Iron and Fluoride. (Various Mfr.) Fluoride 0.25 mg, Vitamins A 1500 IU, D 400 IU, E 5 IU, B_1 0.5 mg, B_2 0.6 mg, B_3 8 mg, B_6 0.4 mg, C 35 mg, Fe 10 mg. Bot. 50 ml. *Rx.*
Use: Mineral, vitamin supplement; dental caries agent.

Polyvitamin Fluoride. (Various Mfr.) Fluoride 0.25 mg, vitamins A 1500 IU, D 400 IU, E 5 IU, B_1 0.5 mg, B_2 0.6 mg, B_3 8 mg, B_6 0.4 mg, B_{12} 2 mcg, C 35 mg/ml. Dropper. Bot. 50 ml. *Rx.*
Use: Mineral, vitamin supplement; dental caries agent.

Poly-Vitamins w/Fluoride 0.5 mg. (Various Mfr.) **Drops:** Fluoride 0.5 mg, vitamins A 1500 IU, D 400 IU, E 5 IU, B_1 0.5 mg, B_2 0.6 mg, B_3 8 mg, B_6 0.4 mg, B_{12} 2 mcg, C 35 mg/ml. Bot. 50 ml. **Tab.:** Fluoride 0.5 mg, vitamins A 2500 IU, D 400 IU, E 15 mg, B_1 1 mg, B_2 1.2 mg, B_3 13.5 mg, B_6 1 mg, B_{12} 4.5 mcg, C 60 mg, folic acid 0.3 mg/Tab. Bot. 100s, 1000s. *Rx.*
Use: Mineral, vitamin supplement; dental caries agent.

Poly-Vitamins w/Fluoride Tablets Chewable. (Various Mfr.) Fluoride 1 mg, vitamins A 2500 IU, D 400 IU, E 15 mg, B_1 1.05 mg, B_2 1.2 mg, B_3 13.5 mg, B_6 1.05 mg, B_{12} 4.5 mcg, C 60 mg, folic acid 0.3 mg. Bot. 100s, 1000s. *Rx.*
Use: Mineral, vitamin supplement; dental caries agent.

Polyvitamin Fluoride w/Iron. (Various Mfr.) Fluoride 1 mg, vitamins A 2500 IU, D 400 IU, E 15 mg, B_1 1.05 mg, B_2 1.2 mg, B_3 13.5 mg, B_6 1.05 mg, B_{12} 4.5 mcg, C 60 mg, folic acid 0.3 mg, Fe 12 mg, Cu, Zn 10 mg/Tab. Bot. 100s, 1000s. *Rx.*
Use: Mineral, vitamin supplement; dental caries agent.

Polyvitamin w/Fluoride. (Rugby Labs, Inc.) Fluoride 0.5 mg, vitamins A 1500 IU, D 400 IU, E 5 mg, B_1 0.5 mg, B_2 0.6 mg, B_3 8 mg, B_6 0.4 mg, B_{12} 2 mcg, C 35 mg/ml. Dropper Bot. 50 ml. *Rx.*
Use: Mineral, vitamin supplement; dental caries agent.

Polyvitamins w/Fluoride 0.5 mg and Iron. (Rugby Labs, Inc.) Fluoride 0.5 mg, vitamins A 2500 IU, D 400 IU, E 15 IU, B_1 1.05 mg, B_2 1.2 mg, B_3 13.5 mg, B_6 1.05 mg, B_{12} 4.5 mcg, C 60 mg, folic acid 0.3 mg, Cu, Fe 12 mg, Zn 10 mg, sucrose/Tab. Bot. 100s. *Rx.*
Use: Mineral, vitamin supplement; dental caries agent.

Polyvite with Fluoride. (Geneva Pharmaceuticals) Fluoride 0.25 mg, vitamins A 1500 IU, D 400 IU, E 5 mg, B_1 0.5 mg, B_2 0.6 mg, B_3 8 mg, B_6 0.4 mg, B_{12} 2 mcg, C 35 mg/ml. Dropper Bot. 50 ml. *Rx.*
Use: Mineral, vitamin supplement; dental caries agent.

•**ponalrestat.** (poe-NAHL-ress-TAT) USAN.
Use: Antidiabetic.

Ponaris. (Jamol Lab Inc.) Nasal emollient of mucosal lubricating and moisturizing botanical oils. Cajeput, eucalyptus, peppermint in iodized cottonseed oil. Bot. 1 oz w/dropper. *otc.*
Use: Moisturizer, nasal.

Ponstel Kapseals. (Parke-Davis) Mefenamic acid 250 mg/Cap. Bot. 100s. *Rx.*
Use: Analgesic, NSAID.

Pontocaine. (Sanofi Winthrop Pharmaceuticals) **Cream:** Tetracaine HCl 1%, glycerin, light mineral oil, methylparaben, sodium metabisulfite. Tube 28.35 g. **Oint.:** Tetracaine 0.5%, menthol, white petrolatum. Tube 28.35 g. *otc.*
Use: Anesthetic, topical.

Pontocaine Hydrochloride. (Sanofi Winthrop Pharmaceuticals) Tetracaine HCl. **Inj. 0.2%:** Dextrose 6%. Amp 2 ml. **0.3%:** Dextrose 6%. Amp 5 ml. **1%:** Acetone sodium bisulfite. Amp 2 ml. **Powd. for reconstitution:** Niphanoid (instantly soluble). Amp 20 mg. *Rx.*
Use: Anesthetic, topical.

Pontocaine Hydrochloride 0.5% Solution for Ophthalmology. (Sanofi Winthrop Pharmaceuticals) Tetracaine HCl 0.5%. Bot. 15 ml, 59 ml. *Rx.*
Use: Anesthetic, local.

Pontocaine Hydrochloride in Dextrose (Hyperbaric). (Sanofi Winthrop Pharmaceuticals) **0.2%:** Tetracaine HCl 2 mg/ml in a sterile solution containing dextrose 6%. Amp. 2 ml, 10s. **0.3%:** Tetracaine HCl 3 mg/ml in a sterile solution containing dextrose 6%. Amp. 5 ml, 10s. *Rx.*
Use: Anesthetic, local.

Pontocaine Ointment. (Sanofi Winthrop Pharmaceuticals) Tetracaine 0.5% and menthol in an ointment consisting of white petrolatum and white wax. Tube 1 oz. *Rx.*
Use: Anesthetic, local.

Pontocaine 2% Aqueous Solution. (Sanofi Winthrop Pharmaceuticals) Tetracaine HCl 20 mg, chlorobutanol 4 mg/ml of 2% soln. Bot. 30 ml, Box 12s. Bot. 118 ml, Box 6s. *Rx.*
Use: Anesthetic, local.

Po-Pon-S. (Shionogi USA) Vitamins A 2000 IU, D 100 IU, E 5 mg, B_1 5 mg, B_2 3 mg, B_3 35 mg, B_5 15 mg, B_6 4 mg, B_{12} 6 mcg, C 100 mg, Ca, P/Tab. Bot. 60s, 240s. *otc.*
Use: Vitamin/mineral supplement.

poppy-seed oil. The ethyl ester of the fatty acids of the poppy w/iodine.

Porcelana Skin Bleaching Agent. (DEP Corp.) **Regular:** Hydroquinone 2%. Jar 2 oz, 4 oz. **Sunscreen:** Hydroquinone 2%, octyl dimethyl PABA 2.5%. Jar 4 oz. *Rx.*
Use: Dermatologic.

porcine islet preparation, encapsulated.
Use: For type I diabetes patients already on immunosuppression. [Orphan Drug]

•**porfimer sodium.** (PORE-fih-muhr) USAN.
Use: Antineoplastic. [Orphan Drug]
See: Photofrin, Inj. (QLT Phototherapeutics, Inc.).

•**porfiromycin.** (par-FIH-row-MY-sin) USAN.
Use: Anti-infective, antineoplastic.

Pork NPH Iletin II. (Eli Lilly and Co.) Purified pork insulin 100 units/ml in isophane insulin suspension (insulin w/protamine and zinc). Inj. Bot. 10 ml.
Use: Antidiabetic.

Pork Regular Iletin II. (Eli Lilly and Co.) Insulin 100 units/ml. Purified pork. Inj. Vial 10 ml.
Use: Antidiabetic.

•**porofocon a.** (PAR-oh-FOE-kahn A) USAN.
Use: Contact lens material (hydrophobic).

•**porofocon b.** (PAR-oh-FOE-kahn B) USAN.
Use: Contact lens material (hydrophobic).

Portabiday. (Washington Ethical) Concentrated soln. of alkylamine lauryl sulfate, a mild detergent with pH approx. 6 for use with Portabiday Vaginal Cleansing Kit. Bot. 3 oz. *otc.*
Use: Vaginal agent.

Portagen. (Bristol-Myers Squibb) A nutritionally complete dietary powder containing as a % of the calories protein 14% as caseinate, fat 41% (medium chain triglycerides 86%, corn oil 14%), carbohydrate 45% as corn syrup solids and sucrose, vitamins A 5000 IU, D 500 IU, E 20 IU, C 52 mg, B_1 1 mg, B_2 1.2 mg, B_6 1.4 mg, B_{12} 4 mcg, niacin 13 mg, folic acid 0.1 mg, choline 83 mg, biotin 0.05 mg, Ca 600 mg, P 450 mg, Mg 133 mg, Fe 12 mg, I 47 mcg, Cu 1 mg, Zn 6 mg, Mn 0.8 mg, Cl 550 mg, Na 300 mg, K 800 mg, pantothenic acid 6.7 mg, K-1 0.1 mg/qt. 20 Kcal/fl oz. Can 1 lb. *otc.*
Use: Nutritional supplement, enteral.

porton asparaginase.
See: Erwinia L-asparaginase.

positive and negative hCG urine controls. (Wampole Laboratories) Positive and negative human urine controls for Wampole urine pregnancy tests. 1 set, 1 vial each.
Use: Diagnostic aid.

Poslam Psoriasis Ointment. (Last) Sulfur 5%, salicylic acid 2%. Jar 1 oz.
Use: Antipsoriatic.

posterior pituitary hormones.
See: Pitressin Synthetic (Parke-Davis).
Pitressin Tannate in Oil (Parke-Davis).
Diapid (Novartis Pharmaceutical Corp.).
Concentraid (Ferring Pharmaceuticals, Inc).
DDAVP (Rhone-Poulenc Rorer Pharmaceuticals, Inc.).

posterior pituitary injection.
Use: Hormone (antidiuretic).

postlobin-o.
See: Pituitary, Posterior, Hormone (b).

postlobin-v.
See: Pituitary, Posterior, Hormone (a).

Posture. (Wyeth-Ayerst Laboratories) Calcium phosphate 300 mg, 600 mg/Tab. Bot. 60s. *otc.*
Use: Mineral supplement.

Posture D 600. (Wyeth-Ayerst Laboratories) Calcium phosphate 600 mg, vitamin D 125 IU/Tab. Bot. 60s. *otc.*
Use: Mineral supplement.

Potaba. (Glenwood, Inc.) Potassium p-aminobenzoate. **Cap.:** 0.5 g. Bot. 250s, 1000s. **Pow.:** 100 g. 1 lb. **Tab.:** 0.5 g. Bot. 100s, 1000s. **Envule:** 2 g. Box 50s. *Rx.*
Use: Nutritional supplement.

Potable Aqua Kit. (Wisconsin Pharmacal Co.) Tetraglycine hydroperiodide 16.7% (6.68% titrable iodine). Tab. Bot. 50s with collapsible gallon container. *otc.*
Use: Water purifier.

Potachlor 10%. (Rosemont Pharmaceutical Corp.) Potassium and chloride 20 mEq/15 ml. Alcohol 5%. Bot. Pt, gal. Alcohol 3.8%. Bot. Pt, gal, UD 15 ml, 30 ml. *Rx.*
Use: Electrolyte supplement.

Potachlor 20%. (Rosemont Pharmaceutical Corp.) Potassium and chloride 40 mEq/15 ml. Alcohol free. Liq. Bot. pt, gal. *Rx.*
Use: Electrolyte supplement.

•**potash, sulfurated.** U.S.P. 23.
Use: Source of sulfide.

potassic saline lactated injection.
Use: Fluid, electrolyte replacement.

•**potassium acetate.** (poe-TASS-ee-uhm ASS-eh-tate) U.S.P. 23. Acetic acid, potassium salt.
Use: Electrolyte replacement; to avoid Cl when high concentration of potassium is needed.

potassium acetate. (Various Mfr.) **Inj.:** 40 mEq, 20 ml in 50 ml Vial.
Use: Electrolyte replacement; to avoid Cl when high concentration of potassium is needed.

potassium acid phosphate.
See: K-Phos, Tab. (Beach Pharmaceuticals).
Uro-K, Tab. (Star Pharmaceuticals, Inc.).

potassium acid phosphate/sodium acid phosphate.
Use: Genitourinary.
See: K-Phos M.F. (Beach Pharmaceuticals).
K-Phos No. 2 (Beach Pharmaceuticals).

•**potassium aspartate and magnesium aspartate.** (poe-TASS-ee-uhm ass-PAR-tates and mag-NEE-zee-uhm ass-PAR-tate) USAN.
Use: Nutrient.

•**potassium benzoate.** (poe-TASS-ee-uhn) N.F. 18.
Use: Pharmaceutic aid (preservative).

•**potassium bicarbonate.** (poe-TASS-ee-uhm) U.S.P. 23.
Use: Pharmaceutic necessity; electrolyte replacement.

potassium bicarbonate effervescent

tablets for oral solution.
Use: Electrolyte supplement.

potassium bicarbonate and potassium chloride for effervescent oral solution.
Use: Electrolyte supplement.

potassium bicarbonate and potassium chloride effervescent tablets for oral solution.
Use: Electrolyte supplement.

potassium bicarbonate and sodium bicarbonate and citric acid effervescent tablets for oral solution.
Use: Electrolyte supplement.

•**potassium bitartrate.** (poe-TASS-ee-uhm bye-TAR-trate) U.S.P. 23.
Use: Cathartic.

•**potassium carbonate.** U.S.P. 23.
Use: Potassium therapy; pharmaceutic aid (alkalizing agent).

•**potassium chloride.** (poe-TASS-ee-uhm KLOR-ide) U.S.P. 23.
Use: Electrolyte replacement, potassium deficiency, hypopotassemia.

potassium chloride. (Abbott Laboratories) **Ampules:** 20 mEq, 10 ml; 40 mEq, 20 ml. **Pintop Vials:** 10 mEq, 5 ml in 10 ml; 20 mEq, 10 ml in 20 ml; 30 mEq, 12.5 ml in 30 ml; 40 mEq, 12.5 ml in 30 ml. **Fliptop Vials:** 20 mEq, 10 ml in 20 ml; 40 mEq, 20 ml in 50 ml. **Univ. Add. Syr.:** 5 mEq/5 ml, 20 mEq/10 ml, 30 mEq/20 ml, 40 mEq/20 ml (Eli Lilly and Co.) Amp. (40 mEq) 20 ml, 6s, 25s.
See: Cena-K, Liq. (Century Pharmaceuticals, Inc.).
Choice 10 and 20, Soln. (Whiteworth Towne).
K+8, ER Tab. (Alra Laboratories, Inc).
Kaochlor, Preps. (Pharmacia & Upjohn).
Kaochlor-Eff, Gran. (Pharmacia & Upjohn).
Kaon, Tab. (Pharmacia & Upjohn).
Kaon-Cl 20%, Liq. (Pharmacia & Upjohn).
Kaon Controlled Release, Tab. (Pharmacia & Upjohn).
Kato, Pow. (Ingram).
Kay Ciel, Elix. (Berlex Laboratories, Inc.).
Kay Ciel, Pow. (Berlex Laboratories, Inc.).
K-Lor, Pow. (Abbott Laboratories).
Klor-Con, Liq. (Upsher-Smith Labs, Inc.).
Klorvess Effervescent Tab. (Novartis Pharmaceutical Corp.).
Klotrix, Tab. (Bristol-Myers Squibb).
Klowess Tab. (Novartis Pharmaceutical Corp.).
K-Lyte/Cl, Pow. (Bristol-Myers Squibb).
K-Lyte/Cl, Tab. (Bristol-Myers Squibb).
K-Lyte/Cl 50, Tab. (Bristol-Myers Squibb).
K-Norm, Cap. (Medeva Pharmaceuticals, Inc.).
K-Tab, Tab. (Abbott Laboratories).
Micro-K Extencaps, Cap. (Wyeth-Ayerst Laboratories).
Pan-Kloride, Liq. (U.S. Products).
Potage, Pow. (Teva Pharmaceuticals USA).
Potassine, Liq. (Recsei Laboratories).
Slow-K, Tab. (Novartis Pharmaceutical Corp.).
Ten-K, Cap. (Novartis Pharmaceutical Corp.).

potassium chloride. (Roxane Laboratories, Inc.) **Oral soln.:** Potassium Cl, sugar free. 40 mEq/30 ml. Bot. 6 oz, 500 ml, 1 L, 5 L 20%. 80 mEq/30 ml. Bot. 500 ml, 1 L, 5 L. **Pow.:** 20 mEq/4 g. Pkt. 30s, 100s. *Rx.*
Use: Electrolyte supplement.

potassium chloride in dextrose and sodium chloride injection.
Use: Electrolyte supplement.

potassium chloride in lactated ringer's and dextrose injection.
Use: Electrolyte supplement.

potassium chloride in sodium chloride injection.
Use: Electrolyte supplement.

•**potassium chloride k 42.** (poe-TASS-ee-uhm KLOR-ide K 42) USAN.
Use: Radiopharmaceutical.

potassium chloride with potassium gluconate.
See: Kolyum, Prods. (Medeva Pharmaceuticals, Inc.).

potassium chloride solution. (ESI Lederle Generics) Potassium Cl 10%, 20%. Sugar free. Bot. 16 oz, gal. *Rx.*
Use: Electrolyte supplement.

•**potassium citrate.** (poe-TASS-ee-uhm SIH-trate) U.S.P. 23. Tripotassium Citrate.
Use: Alkalizer. [Orphan Drug]
See: Urocit-K, Tab. (Mission Pharmacal Co.).
W/Sodium citrate.
See: Bicitra, Liq. (Baker Norton Pharmaceuticals, Inc.).
W/Sodium citrate, citric acid.
See: Cytra, Prods. (Cypress Pharmaceutical, Inc.).
Polycitra K, Crystals, Liq. (Baker Nor-

ton Pharmaceuticals, Inc.).
Polycitra LC, Liq. (Baker Norton Pharmaceuticals, Inc.).

potassium citrate and citric acid oral solution.
Use: Alkalizer, systemic.

potassium clavulanate/amoxicillin.
Use: Anti-infective, penicillin.
See: Amoxicillin and Potassium Clavulanate.
Augmentin (SmithKline Beecham).

potassium clavulanate/ticarcillin.
Use: Anti-infective, penicillin.
See: Ticarcillin and Clavulanate Potassium.

•**potassium glucaldrate.** (poe-TASS-ee-uhm glue-KAL-drate) USAN.
Use: Antacid.

•**potassium gluconate.** U.S.P. 23.
Use: Electrolyte replacement.
See: Kaon, Elix., Tab. (Warren-Teed).

potassium gluconate and potassium chloride oral solution.
Use: Replacement therapy.

potassium gluconate and potassium chloride for oral solution.
Use: Replacement therapy.

potassium gluconate elixir. (Various Mfr.) Potassium 40 mEq provided by potassium gluconate 9.36 g/30 ml, alcohol 5%. Bot. Pt, Patient-Cup 15 ml. *Rx.*
Use: Electrolyte supplement.

potassium gluconate, potassium citrate, and ammonium chloride oral solution.
Use: Electrolyte supplement.

potassium gluconate and potassium citrate oral solution.
Use: Electrolyte supplement.

potassium glutamate. The monopotassium salt of l-glutamic acid.

potassium G penicillin.
See: Penicillin G Potassium, USP 23.

•**potassium guaiacolsulfonate.** (poe-TASS-ee-uhm gwie-ah-kole-SULL-foe-nate) U.S.P. 23. Sulfoguaiacol. Potassium Hydroxymethoxybenzene sulfonate. Used in many cough preps.
Use: Expectorant.
See: Conex, Liq. (Westerfield).
Pinex Regular, Syr. (Pinex).

potassium guaiacolsulfonate w/combinations.
See: Partuss, Liq. (Parmed Pharmaceuticals, Inc.).
Protuss, Liq. (Horizon Pharmaceutical Corp.).
Protuss-D, Liq. (Horizon Pharmaceutical Corp.).
Tusquelin, Syr. (Circle Pharmaceuticals, Inc.).

•**potassium hydroxide.** N.F. 18.
Use: Pharmaceutic aid (alkalinizing agent).

potassium in sodium chloride. (Various Mfr.) Potassium Cl 0.15%, 0.22%, 0.3% in sodium Cl 0.9%. Soln. for Inj. 1000 ml. *Rx.*
Use: Intravenous replenishment solution, nutritional supplement.

•**potassium iodide.** (poe-TASS-ee-uhm EYE-oh-dide) U.S.P. 23.
Use: Expectorant, antifungal, supplement (iodine).
See: Pima Expectorant, Syr. (Fleming & Co.).

potassium iodide w/combinations.
See: Diastix, Reagent Strips (Bayer Corp. (Consumer Div.)).
Elixophyllin-KI, Elix. (Berlex Laboratories, Inc.).
KIE, Syr., Tab. (Laser, Inc.).
Mudrane, Tab. (ECR Pharmaceuticals).
Mudrane-2, Tab. (ECR Pharmaceuticals).

•**potassium metabisulfite.** N.F. 18.
Use: Pharmaceutic aid (antioxidant).

•**potassium metaphosphate.** N.F. 18.
Use: Pharmaceutic aid (buffering agent).

•**potassium nitrate.** (poe-TASS-ee-uhm NYE-trate) U.S.P. 23.

potassium p-aminobenzoate.
See: Potaba, Preps. (Glenwood, Inc.).
W/Potassium salicylate.
See: Pabalate-SF, Tab. (Wyeth-Ayerst Laboratories).
W/Pyridoxine.
See: Potaba Plus 6, Cap., Tab. (Glenwood, Inc.).

potassium penicillin g.
Use: Anti-infective, penicillin.
See: Penicillin G, Potassium, U.S.P. 23.

potassium penicillin v.
Use: Anti-infective, pencillin.
See: Phenoxymethyl Penicillin Potassium, USP 23.

potassium perchlorate.
Use: Radiopaque agent.
See: Perchloracap (Mallinckrodt).

•**potassium permanganate.** (poe-TASS-ee-uhm per-MANG-gah-nate) U.S.P. 23. Permanganic acid, potassium salt.
Use: Anti-infective, topical.

•**potassium phenethicillin.** U.S.P. 23. Phenethicillin Potassium.
Use: Anti-infective.

potassium phenoxymethyl penicillin.
Use: Anti-infective.
See: Penicillin V Potassium, USP 23.

•**potassium phosphate, dibasic.** (poe-TASS-ee-uhm FOSS-fate) U.S.P. 23.
Use: Calcium regulator.

•**potassium phosphate, monobasic.** (poe-TASS-ee-uhm FOSS-fate) N.F. 18. Dipotassium hydrogen phosphate.
Use: Pharmaceutic aid (buffering agent), source of potassium.

potassium phosphate, monobasic. (Abbott Laboratories) 15 mM, 5 ml in 10 ml Vial; 45 mM, 15 ml in 20 ml/Inj. Vial.
Use: Pharmaceutic aid (buffering agent), source of potassium.

potassium reagent strips. (Bayer Corp. (Consumer Div.)) Quantitative dry reagent strip test for potassium in serum or plasma. Bot. 50s.
Use: Diagnostic aid.

potassium-removing resins.
See: Sodium Polystyrene Sulfonate (Various Mfr.).
SPS (Carolina Medical Products Co.).
Kayexalate (Sanofi Winthrop Pharmaceuticals).

potassium rhodanate.
See: Potassium Thiocyanate.

potassium salicylate.
See: Neocylate, Tab. (Schwarz Pharma, Inc.).
W/Potassium bromide, methapyrilene HCl, vitamins.
See: Alva-Tranquil, Cap., Tab., T.D. Tab. (Alva/Amco Pharmacal Cos. Inc.).
W/Potassium p-aminobenzoate.
See: Pabalate-SF, Tab. (Wyeth-Ayerst Laboratories).

potassium salt.
See: Potassium Sorbate, N.F. 18.

•**potassium sodium tartrate.** (poe-TASS-ee-uhm so-dee-uhm TAR-trate) U.S.P. 23.
Use: Laxative.

•**potassium sorbate.** N.F. 18.
Use: Pharmaceutic aid (antimicrobial).

potassium sulfocyanate. Potassium Rhodanate.
See: Potassium Thiocyanate (Various Mfr.).

potassium thiocyanate. Potassium sulfocyanate, Potassium Rhodanate.

potassium thiphencillin. (poe-TASS-ee-uhm thigh-FEN-sill-in)
Use: Anti-infective.

potassium troclosene. (poe-TASS-ee-uhm TROE-kloe-seen) (Monsanto) Potassium dichloroisocyanurate.
Use: Anti-infective.

•**povidone.** (POE-vih-dohn) U.S.P. 23. Formerly Polyvidone, Polyvinylpyrrolidone.
Use: Pharmaceutic aid (dispersing and suspending agent).

•**povidone I 125.** (POE-vih-dohn) USAN.
Use: Radiopharmaceutical.

•**povidone I 131.** (POE-vih-dohn) USAN.
Use: Radiopharmaceutical.

•**povidone-iodine.** (POE-vih-dohn-EYE-uh-dine) U.S.P. 23.
Use: Anti-infective, topical.
See: Betadine, Preps. (Purdue Frederick Co.).
EfoDine, Oint. (E. Fougera and Co.).
Massengill Medicated, Liq. (SmithKline Beecham Pharmaceuticals).

povidone-iodine complex.
See: Betadine, Preps. (Purdue Frederick Co.).

PowerMate. (Green Turtle Bay Vitamin Co.) Vitamins A 5000 IU, E 100 IU, B_3 12.5 mg, C 250 mg, Zn 2.5 mg, Se, n-acetyl-L-cysteine/Tab. Bot. 50s. *otc.*
Use: Mineral, vitamin supplement.

PowerVites. (Green Turtle Bay Vitamin Co.) Vitamin A 2500 IU, D 150 IU, E 12.5 IU, C 125 mg, B_1 6.3 mg, B_2 6.3 mg, B_3 25 mg, B_5 25 mg, B_6 12.5 mg, B_{12} 6.3 mcg, biotin, folic acid 0.15 mg, B, Ca, Mg, Cu, Zn 2.5 mg, Cr, Mn, K, Se, betaine, hesperidin/Tab. Bot. 40s, 100s, 200s. *otc.*
Use: Mineral, vitamin supplement.

Poyaliver Stronger. (Forest Pharmaceutical, Inc.) Liver inj. (equivalent to 10 mcg B_{12}), vitamin B_{12} 100 mcg, folic acid 10 mcg, niacinamide 1%/ml. Vial 10 ml. *Rx.*
Use: Nutritional supplement, parenteral.

Poyamin Jel Injection. (Forest Pharmaceutical, Inc.) Cyanocobalamin 1000 mcg/ml. Vial 10 ml.
Use: Nutritional supplement, parenteral.

Poyaplex. (Forest Pharmaceutical, Inc.) Vitamins B_1 100 mg, niacinamide 100 mg, B_6 10 mg, B_2 1 mg, panthenol 10 mg, B_{12} 5 mcg/ml. Vial 10 ml, 30 ml. *Rx.*
Use: Nutritional supplement, parenteral.

P.P.D. tuberculin.
See: Tuberculin, Purified Protein Derivative, U.S.P. 23. (Various Mfr.).

P.P. factor (pellagra preventive factor).
See: Nicotinic Acid, Preps. (Various Mfr.).

ppg-15 stearyl ether. (PPG-15 STEE-rill EE-ther)
Use: Pharmaceutic aid (surfactant).

PPI-002.
Use: Malignant mesothelioma. [Orphan Drug]

PR-122 (redox-phenytoin). (Pharmos Corp.)

Use: Anticonvulsant. [Orphan Drug]

PR-225 (redox-acyclovir). (Pharmos Corp.)
Use: Treatment of herpes simplex encephalitis in AIDS. [Orphan Drug]

PR-239 (redox-penicillin g). (Pharmos Corp.)
Use: Treatment of AIDS-associated neurosyphilis. [Orphan Drug]

PR-320 (molecusol-carbamazepine). (Pharmos Corp.)
Use: Anticonvulsant. [Orphan Drug]

•**practolol.** (PRAK-toe-lole) USAN.
Use: Antiadrenergic (β-receptor).

•**pralidoxime chloride.** (pra-lih-DOCK-seem) U.S.P. 23.
Use: Cholinesterase reactivator.
See: Protopam Chloride, Tab., Inj. (Wyeth-Ayerst Laboratories).

pralidoxime chloride. (Survival Technology, Inc.) 600 mg. Benzyl alcohol, aminocaproic acid. Inj. Vial 2 ml. *Rx.*
Use: Antidote.

•**pralidoxime iodide.** (pral-ih-DOX-eem EYE-oh-dide) USAN.
Use: Cholinesterase reactivator.
See: Protopam Iodide (Wyeth-Ayerst Laboratories).

•**pralidoxime mesylate.** (pral-ih-DOX-eem) USAN.
Use: Cholinesterase reactivator.

pralidoxime methiodide.
See: Pralidoxime Iodide (Various Mfr.).

pralmorelin dihydrochloride. (pral-more-ELL-in die-HIGH-droe-KLOR-ide) USAN.
Use: Growth hormone-releasing factor.

PrameGel. (Medicis Dermatologicals, Inc.) Pramoxine HCl 1%, menthol 0.5% in base w/benzyl alcohol. Gel Bot. 118 ml. *otc.*
Use: Anesthetic, local.

Pramilet FA. (Ross Laboratories) Vitamins A 4000 IU, B_1 3 mg, B_2 2 mg, B_6 3 mg, B_{12} 3 mcg, C 60 mg, D 400 IU, B_5 1 mg, B_3 10 mg, Ca 250 mg, Cu, I, Fe 40 mg, Mg, Zn, folic acid 1 mg/Filmtab. Bot. 100s. *Rx.*
Use: Mineral, vitamin supplement.

•**pramipexole.** (pram-ih-PEX-ole) USAN. (Pharmacia & Upjohn)
Use: Antidepressant, dopamine agonist; antiparkinsonian; antischizophrenic.
See: Mirapex, Tab. (Pharmacia & Upjohn).

•**pramipexole dihydrochloride.** USAN.
Use: Antiparkisonian; antischizophrenic; antidepressant.

•**pramiracetam hydrochloride.** (PRAM-ih-RASS-eh-tam) USAN. *Formerly Amacetam Hydrochloride.*
Use: Cognition adjuvant.

•**pramiracetam sulfate.** (PRAM-ih-RASS-eh-tam) USAN. *Formerly Amacetam Sulfate.*
Use: Cognition adjuvant.

•**pramlintide.** (PRAM-lin-tide) USAN.
Use: Antidiabetic.

Pramosone Cream 0.5%. (Ferndale Laboratories, Inc.) Hydrocortisone acetate 0.5%, pramoxine HCl 1% in cream base. Tube 1 oz, 4 oz. Jar 4 oz, lb.
Use: Corticosteroid; anesthetic, local.

Pramosone Cream 1%. (Ferndale Laboratories, Inc.) Hydrocortisone acetate 1%, pramoxine HCl 1% in cream base. Tube 1 oz, 4 oz. Jar 4 oz, lb. *Rx.*
Use: Corticosteroid; anesthetic, local.

Pramosone Cream 2.5%. (Ferndale Laboratories, Inc.) Hydrocortisone acetate 2.5%, pramoxine HCl 1% in cream base. Tube 1 oz, 4 oz. Jar lb. *Rx.*
Use: Corticosteroid; anesthetic, local.

Pramosone Lotion 0.5%. (Ferndale Laboratories, Inc.) Hydrocortisone acetate 0.5%, pramoxine HCl 1% in lotion base. Bot. 1 oz, 4 oz, 8 oz. *Rx.*
Use: Corticosteroid; anesthetic, local.

Pramosone Lotion 1%. (Ferndale Laboratories, Inc.) Hydrocortisone acetate 1%, pramoxine HCl 1% in lotion base. Bot. 2 oz, 4 oz, 8 oz. *Rx.*
Use: Corticosteroid; anesthetic, local.

Pramosone Lotion 2.5%. (Ferndale Laboratories, Inc.) Hydrocortisone acetate 2.5%, pramoxine HCl 1% in lotion base. Bot 2 oz, gal. *Rx.*
Use: Corticosteroid; anesthetic, local.

Pramosone Ointment 1%. (Ferndale Laboratories, Inc.) Hydrocortisone acetate 1%, pramoxine HCl 1% in ointment base. Tube 1 oz, 4 oz. Jar 4 oz, lb. *Rx.*
Use: Corticosteroid; anesthetic, local.

Pramoxine HC. (Rugby Labs, Inc.) Pramoxine HCl 1%, hydrocortisone acetate 1%. Aerosol foam. 10 g w/applicator. *Rx.*
Use: Anorectal preparation.

•**pramoxine hydrochloride.** (pram-OX-een) U.S.P. 23.
Use: Anesthetic, topical.
See: Itch-X, Gel, Spray (B.F. Ascher and Co.).
Prax, Cream, Lot. (Ferndale Laboratories, Inc.).
Proctofoam, Aer. (Schwarz Pharma, Inc.).
Tronothane HCl, Cream, Gel (Abbott Laboratories).

pramoxine hydrochloride w/combinations.
See: Anti-Itch, Lot. (Towne).
Caladryl, Prods. (Parke-Davis).
Cortic (Everett Lab).
Gentz, Jelly, Wipes (Roxane Laboratories, Inc.).
1 + 1 Creme (Dunhall Pharmaceuticals, Inc.).
1 +1-F Creme (Dunhall Pharmaceuticals, Inc.).
Oti-Med, Drops (Hyrex Pharmaceuticals).
Otocalm-H Ear Drops (Parmed Pharmaceuticals, Inc.).
Proctofoam-HC, Aer. (Reed-Carnrick).
Sherform-HC, Oint. (Sheryl).
Tri-Otic, Drops (Pharmics, Inc.).
Zoto-HC, Drops (Horizon Pharmaceutical Corp.).

Prandin. (Novo/Nordisk Pharm, Inc.) Repaglinide 0.5 mg, 1 mg, 2 mg. Tab. Bot. 100s, 500s, 1000s. *Rx.*
Use: Antidiabetic.

•**pranolium chloride.** (pray-NO-lee-uhm) USAN.
Use: Cardiovascular agent, antiarrhythmic.

Pravachol. (Bristol-Myers Squibb) Pravastatin sodium 10 mg, 20 mg, 40 mg. Tab. Bot. 90s, 1000s (20 mg only), UD 100s. *Rx.*
Use: Antihyperlipidemic.

•**pravadoline maleate.** (pray-AH-doe-leen) USAN.
Use: Analgesic.

•**pravastatin sodium.** (PRUH-vuh-stuh-tin) USAN.
Use: Antihyperlipidemic.
See: Pravachol, Tab. (Bristol-Myers Squibb).

Prax. (Ferndale Laboratories, Inc.) Pramoxine HCl 1%. **Cream:** Glycerin, cetyl alcohol, white petrolatum. Jar 13.4 g. **Lot.:** Potassium sorbate, sorbic acid, mineral oil, cetyl alcohol, glycerin, lanolin. Bot. 15 ml, 120 ml, 240 ml. *otc.*
Use: Anesthetic, local.

•**prazosin hydrochloride.** (PRAY-zoe-sin) U.S.P. 23.
Use: Antihypertensive.
See: Minipress, Cap. (Pfizer US Pharmaceutical Group).

prazosin hydrochloride. (Various Mfr.) 1 mg, 2 mg, 5 mg. Cap. Bot. 30s, 60s, 90s, 100s, 120s, 250s, 500s, 1000s, UD 100s.
Use: Antihypertensive.

Pre-Attain Liquid. (Sherwood Davis & Geck) Sodium caseinate, maltodextrin, corn oil, soy lecithin, vitamins A, B_1, B_2, B_3, B_5, B_6, B_{12}, C, D, E, K, folic acid, Ca, Cl, Cu, Fe, I, Mg, Mn, P, Zn. Can 250 ml, closed system 1000 ml. *otc.*
Use: Nutritional supplement.

Precef for Injection. (Bristol-Myers Squibb) Ceforanide 500 mg, 1 g/Vial or piggyback. *Rx.*
Use: Anti-infective, cephalosporin.

Precision High Nitrogen Diet. (Novartis Pharmaceutical Corp.) Vanilla flavor: Maltodextrin, pasteurized egg white solids, sucrose, natural and artificial flavors, medium chain triglycerides, partially hydrogenated soybean oil, polysorbate 80, mono- and diglycerides, vitamins, minerals. Pow. Packet 2.93 oz. *otc.*
Use: Nutritional supplement.

Precision LR Diet. (Novartis Pharmaceutical Corp.) Orange flavor: Maltodextrin, pasteurized egg white solids, sucrose, medium chain triglycerides, partially hydrogenated soybean oil with BHA, citric acid, natural and artificial flavors, mono- and diglycerides, polysorbate 80, FD&C Yellow No. 5 and No. 6, vitamins, minerals. Pow. Packet 3 oz. *otc.*
Use: Nutritional supplement.

Precose. (Bayer Corp. (Consumer Div.)) Acarbose 50 mg, 100 mg/Tab. Bot. 100s, UD 100s. *Rx.*
Use: Antidiabetic.

Predalone 50. (Forest Pharmaceutical, Inc.) Prednisolone acetate 50 mg/ml. Vial 10 ml. *Rx.*
Use: Corticosteroid.

Predamide Ophthalmic. (Maurry) Sodium sulfacetamide 10%, prednisolone acetate 0.5%, hydroxyethyl cellulose, polysorbate 80, sodium thiosulfate, benzalkonium Cl 0.025%. Bot. 5 ml, 15 ml. *Rx.*
Use: Anti-infective, corticosteroid, ophthalmic.

Predcor-50 Injection. (Roberts Pharmaceuticals) Prednisolone acetate 50 mg/ml. Vial 10 ml. *Rx.*
Use: Corticosteroid.

Pred Forte. (Allergan, Inc.) Prednisolone acetate 1%. Susp. Bot. 1 ml, 5 ml, 10 ml, 15 ml. *Rx.*
Use: Corticosteroid, ophthalmic.

Pred-G. (Allergan, Inc.) Prednisolone acetate 1%, gentamicin sulfate 0.3%. Bot. 2 ml, 5 ml, 10 ml. *Rx.*
Use: Corticosteroid, anti-infective, ophthalmic.

Pred-G S.O.P. (Allergan, Inc.) Predniso-

lone acetate 0.6%, gentamicin sulfate 0.3%, chlorobutanol 0.5%. Oint. Tube 3.5 g. *Rx.*
Use: Anti-infective, corticosteroid, ophthalmic.

Predicort-AP. (Dunhall Pharmaceuticals, Inc.) Prednisolone sodium phosphate 20 mg, prednisolone acetate 80 mg/ml. Vial 10 ml. *Rx.*
Use: Corticosteroid.

Predicort-RP. (Dunhall Pharmaceuticals, Inc.) Prednisolone sodium phosphate equivalent to prednisolone phosphate 20 mg, niacinamide 25 mg/ml. Vial 10 ml. *Rx.*
Use: Corticosteroid.

Pred Mild. (Allergan, Inc.) Prednisolone acetate 0.12%. Susp. Bot. 5 ml, 10 ml. *Rx.*
Use: Corticosteroid, ophthalmic.

•**prednazate.** (PRED-nah-zate) USAN.
Use: Anti-inflammatory.

•**prednicarbate.** (PRED-nih-CAR-bate) USAN.
Use: Corticosteroid, topical.
See: Dermatop, Cream (Hoechst Marion Roussel).

Prednicen-M. (Schwarz Pharma, Inc.) Prednisone 5 mg/Tab. Bot. 100s, 1000s. *Rx.*
Use: Corticosteroid.

•**prednimustine.** (PRED-nih-MUSS-teen) USAN.
Use: Antineoplastic. [Orphan Drug]

•**prednisolone.** (pred-NISS-oh-lone) U.S.P. 23. Metacortandralone.
Use: Corticosteroid.
See: Cordrol, Tab. (Vita Elixir).
Delta-Cortef, Tab. (Pharmacia & Upjohn).
Fernisolone, Tab., Inj. (Ferndale Laboratories, Inc.).
Orasone, Tab. (Solvay Pharmaceuticals).
Orasone 50, Tab. (Solvay Pharmaceuticals).
Prednis, Tab. (Rhone-Poulenc Rorer Pharmaceuticals, Inc.).
Prelone (Muro Pharmaceuticals).
W/Aluminum hydroxide gel, dried.
See: Predoxide, Tab. (Roberts Pharmaceuticals).
W/Chloramphenicol.
See: Chloroptic-P, Ophth. Oint. (Allergan, Inc.).
Neo-Deltef, Drops (Pharmacia & Upjohn).
W/Sulfacetamide sodium, methylcellulose.
See: Isopto Cetapred, Susp. (Alcon Laboratories, Inc.).
W/Sulfacetamide sodium.
See: Cetapred, Ophth. Oint. (Alcon Laboratories, Inc.).

•**prednisolone acetate.** (pred-NISS-oh-lone ASS-eh-tate) U.S.P. 23.
Use: Corticosteroid, topical.
See: Econopred, Susp. (Alcon Laboratories, Inc.).
Key-Pred, Inj. (Hyrex Pharmaceuticals).
Predicort, Amp. (Dunhall Pharmaceuticals, Inc.).
Pred, Preps. (Allergan, Inc.).
Pred Forte, Ophthalmic Susp. (Allergan, Inc.).
Pred Mild (Allergan).
Sigpred, Inj. (Sigma-Tau Pharmaceuticals, Inc).
Steraject, Vial (Merz Pharmaceuticals).

prednisolone acetate ophthalmic. (Falcon) 1% Susp. Bot. 5 ml, 10 ml. *Rx.*
Use: Corticosteroid, topical.

prednisolone acetate w/combinations.
See: Blephamide Liquifilm, Soln. (Allergan, Inc.).
Blephamide S.O.P., Ophth. Oint. (Allergan, Inc.).
Cetapred, Ophth. Oint. (Alcon Laboratories, Inc.).
Isopto Cetapred Susp. (Alcon Laboratories, Inc.).
Metimyd, Ophth. Susp., Oint. (Schering-Plough Corp.).
Vasocidin, Preps. (Novartis Pharmaceutical Corp.).
Vasocine (Ciba Vision).

prednisolone acetate and prednisolone sodium phosphate. (Various Mfr.) Prednisolone acetate 80 mg, prednisolone sodium phosphate 20 mg/ml. Inj. Vial 10 ml. *Rx.*
Use: Corticosteroid.

prednisolone acetate ophthalmic suspension. (Falcon Ophthalmics, Inc.) Prednisolone 1%, benzalkonium Cl 0.01%, EDTA. Susp. Bot. 5 ml, 10 ml. *Rx.*
Use: Corticosteroid.

prednisolone butylacetate.
Use: Corticosteroid.

prednisolone cyclopentylpropionate.
Use: Corticosteroid.

•**prednisolone hemisuccinate.** U.S.P. 23.
Use: Corticosteroid, topical.

•**prednisolone sodium phosphate.** (pred-NISS-oh-lone So-dee-uhm FOSS-fate) U.S.P. 23.
Use: Corticosteroid, topical.
See: AK-Pred, Soln. (Akorn, Inc.).

Alto-Pred Soluble, Vial (Alto Pharmaceuticals, Inc.).
Hydeltrasol, Inj. (Merck & Co.).
Inflamase Forte, Ophth. Soln. (Novartis Pharmaceutical Corp.).
Inflamase, Ophth. Soln. (Novartis Pharmaceutical Corp.).
Key-Pred SP, Inj. (Hyrex Pharmaceuticals).
Liquid Pred, Inj. (Muro Pharmaceutical, Inc.).
Metreton, Ophth. Soln. Sterile (Schering-Plough Corp.).
Pediapred, Liq. (Medeva Pharmaceuticals, Inc.).
P.S.P. IV (Four), Inj. (Solvay Pharmaceuticals).
Savacort-S, Inj. (Savage Laboratories).

W/Neomycin sulfate.
See: P.SP IV, Inj. (Solvay Pharmaceuticals).

W/Prednisolone acetate.
See: Optimyd, Soln. (Schering-Plough Corp.).
Vasocidin, Liq. (Novartis Pharmaceutical Corp.).

prednisolone sodium phosphate. (Various Mfr.) 0.125%, 1%. Soln. Bot. 5 ml, 10 ml, 15 ml. *Rx.*
Use: Corticosteroid, topical.

•**prednisolone sodium succinate for injection.** (pred-NISS-oh-lone SO-dee-uhm SUCK-sih-nate) U.S.P. 23.
Use: Corticosteroid, topical.

prednisolone tertiary-butylacetate.
See: Prednisolone Tebutate, U.S.P. 23.

Prednisol TBA. (Taylor Pharmaceuticals) Prednisolone tebutate 20 mg/ml. Vial 10 ml. *Rx.*
Use: Corticosteroid.

•**prednisolone tebutate.** U.S.P. 23.
Use: Corticosteroid, topical.
See: Metalone, Vial (Foy Laboratories).

•**prednisone.** (PRED-nih-sone) U.S.P. 23.
Use: Corticosteroid.
See: Delta-Dome, Tab. (Bayer Corp. (Consumer Div.)).
Deltasone, Tab. (Pharmacia & Upjohn).
Keysone, Tab. (Hyrex Pharmaceuticals).
Meticorten, Tab. (Schering-Plough Corp.).
Maso-Pred, Tab. (Mason Pharmaceuticals, Inc.).
Orasone, Tab. (Solvay Pharmaceuticals).
Sterapred, Tab. (Merz Pharmaceuticals).

W/Chlorpheniramine maleate.
See: Histone, Tab. (Blaine Co, Inc.).

prednisone. (Various Mfr.) 1 mg, 5 mg, 20 mg/Tab. Bot. 100s, 1000s, UD 100s. *Rx.*
Use: Corticosteroid, topical.

Prednisone Intensol Oral Solution. (Roxane Laboratories, Inc.) Prednisone concentrated oral solution 5 mg/ml. Bot. 30 ml w/calibrated dropper. *Rx.*
Use: Corticosteroid.

•**prednival.** (PRED-nih-val) USAN.
Use: Corticosteroid.

Predsulfair. (Bausch & Lomb Pharmaceuticals) **Drops:** Prednisolone acetate 0.5%, sodium sulfacetamide 10%, hydroxypropyl methylcellulose, polysorbate 80 0.5%, sodium thiosulfate, benzalkonium Cl 0.01%. Bot. 5 ml, 15 ml. **Oint.:** Prednisolone acetate 0.5%, sodium sulfacetamide 10%, mineral oil, white petrolatum, lanolin, parabens. 3.5 g. *Rx.*
Use: Anti-infective; corticosteroid, ophthalmic.

Preflex Daily Cleaning Especially for Sensitive Eyes. (Alcon Laboratories, Inc.) Isotonic, aqueous solution of sorbic acid, sodium phosphates, sodium Cl, tyloxapol, hydroxyethyl cellulose, polyvinyl alcohol, EDTA. Bot. 30 ml. *otc.*
Use: Contact lens care.

Prefrin Liquifilm. (Allergan, Inc.) Phenylephrine HCl 0.12%. Bot. 20 ml. *otc.*
Use: Mydriatic, vasoconstrictor.

•**pregabalin.** (preh-GAB-ah-lin) USAN.
Use: Anticonvulsant.

Pregestimil. (Bristol-Myers Squibb) Protein hydrolysate formula supplies 640 calories/qt. protein 18 g, fat 26 g, carbohydrate 86 g, vitamins A 2000 IU, D 400 IU, E 15 IU, C 52 mg, folic acid 100 mcg, thiamine HCl 0.5 mg, riboflavin 0.6 mg, niacin 8 mg, B_6 0.4 mg, B_{12} 2 mcg, biotin 0.05 mg, pantothenic acid 3 mg, K-1 100 mcg, choline 85 mg, inositol 30 mg, Ca 600 mg, P 400 mg, I 45 mcg, Fe 12 mg, Mg 70 mg, Cu 0.6 mg, Zn 4 mg, Mn 0.2 mg, Cl 550 mg, K 700 mg, Na 300 mg/Qt. (20 Kcal/fl oz.). Pow. Can lb. *otc.*
Use: Nutritional supplement, enteral.

Pregnaslide Latex hCG Test with Fast Trak Slides. (Wampole Laboratories) Latex agglutination slide test for the qualitative detection of hCG in urine. Test 24s. Test kit 96s.
Use: Diagnostic aid.

pregneninolone.
See: Ethisterone.

pregnenolone. (preg-NEN-oh-lone)

Use: Treatment of rheumatoid arthritis.

•**pregnenolone succinate.** (PREG-neh-no-lone SUCK-sih-nate) USAN.
Use: Non-hormonal sterol derivative.

Pregnosis Slide Test. (Roche Laboratories) Latex agglutination inhibition slide test. 50s, 200s.
Use: Diagnostic aid.

Pregnyl. (Organon Teknika Corp.) hCG 10,000 IU/Vial w/diluent 10 ml, mannitol, benzyl alcohol. Vial 10 ml. *Rx.*
Use: Hormone, chorionic gonadotropin.

Pre-Hist-D. (Marnel Pharmaceuticals, Inc.) Phenylephrine HCl 20 mg, chlorpheniramine maleate 8 mg, methscopolamine nitrate 2.5 mg/SR Tab. or Capl. Bot. 100s. *Rx.*
Use: Anticholinergic, antihistamine, decongestant.

Preject Preinjection Topical Anesthetic. (Colgate Oral Pharmaceuticals) Benzocaine 20% in polyethylene glycol base. Jar 2 oz. *otc.*
Use: Anesthetic, local.

Prelestrin. (Taylor Pharmaceuticals) Conjugated estrogens 0.625 mg, 1.25 mg/Tab. Bot. 100s, 1000s. *Rx.*
Use: Estrogen.

Prelone Syrup. (Muro Pharmaceutical, Inc.) Prednisolone. **5 mg/ml:** alcohol ≤ 0.4%. Plast Bot. 120 ml. **15 mg/5 ml:** alcohol 5% Plast. Bot. 240 ml. *Rx.*
Use: Corticosteroid.

Prelu-2. (Boehringer Ingelheim, Inc.) Phendimetrazine tartrate 105 mg/Cap. Bot. 100s. *c-III.*
Use: Anorexiant.

Premarin. (Wyeth-Ayerst Laboratories) Conjugated estrogens. 0.3 mg, 0.625 mg, 0.9 mg, 1.25 mg, 2.5 mg/Tab. Bot. 100s, 1000s (except 0.9 mg), 5000s (0.625 mg and 1.25 mg only), UD 100s (0.625 mg and 1.25 mg only). *Rx.*
Use: Estrogen.

Premarin Intravenous. (Wyeth-Ayerst Laboratories) Conjugated estrogens 25 mg. Inj. *Secules* each with 5 ml sterile diluent. *Rx.*
Use: Estrogen.

Premarin Vaginal Cream. (Wyeth-Ayerst Laboratories) Conjugated estrogens 0.625 mg/1 g w/ benzyl alcohol, cetyl alcohol, mineral oil. Tube w/applicator 42.5 g. *Rx.*
Use: Estrogen.

Premarin w/Meprobamate.
See: PMB 200 and 400, Tab. (Wyeth-Ayerst Laboratories).

Premarin w/Methyltestosterone. (Wyeth-Ayerst Laboratories) Premarin (Conjugated Estrogens, U.S.P.) 1.25 mg, methyltestosterone 10 mg/Yellow Tab. Premarin 0.625 mg, methyltestosterone 5 mg/Red Tab. Bot. 100s. *Rx.*
Use: Androgen, estrogen combination.

Premate-200. (Major Pharmaceuticals) Meprobamate 200 mg, tridihexethyl Cl 25 mg/Tab. Bot. 100s. *Rx.*
Use: Anticholinergic, anxiolytic.

Premate-400. (Major Pharmaceuticals) Meprobamate 400 mg, tridihexethyl Cl 25 mg/Tab. Bot. 100s. *Rx.*
Use: Anticholinergic, anxiolytic.

Premphase. (Wyeth-Ayerst Laboratories) Conjugated estrogens 0.625 mg/Tab. Medroxyprogesterone acetate 5 mg, conjugated estrogens 0.625 mg/Tab. Blister-card 14s. *Rx.*
Use: Estrogen, progestin combination.

Prempro. (Wyeth-Ayerst Laboratories) Conjugated estrogen 0.625 mg, medroxyprogesterone acetate 2.5 mg or conjugated estrogen 0.625 mg, medroxyprogesterone acetate 5 mg, lactose, sucrose/Tab. Blister-card 14s. *Rx.*
Use: Estrogen, progestin combination.

Premsyn PMS. (Chattem Consumer Products) Acetaminophen 500 mg, pamabrom 25 mg, pyrilamine maleate 15 mg/Capl. Bot. 20s, 40s. *otc.*
Use: Analgesic, antihistamine, diuretic.

•**prenalterol hydrochloride.** (PREE-NAL-teh-role) USAN.
Use: Adrenergic.

Prenatal Folic Acid + Iron. (Everett Laboratories, Inc.) Vitamins, minerals, folic acid 1 mg/Tab. Bot. 100s. *Rx.*
Use: Mineral, vitamin supplement.

Prenatal MR 90. (Ethex Corp.) Ca 250 mg, Fe 90 mg, vitamins A 4000 IU, D 400 IU, E 30 mg, B_1 3 mg, B_2 3.4 mg, B_3 20 mg, B_6 20 mg, B_{12} 12 mcg, C 120 mg, folic acid 1 mg, Zn 25 mg, I, Cu, DSS. Tab. Bot. 100s. *Rx.*
Use: Mineral, vitamin supplement.

Prenatal-S. (Zenith Forest Pharmaceutical) Ca 200 mg, Fe 60 mg, vitamins A 4000 IU, D 400 IU, E 11 mg, B_1 1.5 mg, B_2 1.7 mg, B_3 18 mg, B_6 2.6 mg, B_{12} 4 mcg, C 100 mg, folic acid 0.8 mg, Zn 25 mg/Tab. Bot. UD 100s. *otc.*
Use: Mineral, vitamin supplement.

Prenatal with Folic Acid. (Geneva Pharmaceuticals) Ca 200 mg, Fe 60 mg, vitamins A 4000 IU, D 400 IU, E 11 mg, B_1 1.5 mg, B_2 1.7 mg, B_3 18 mg, B_6 2.6 mg, B_{12} 4 mcg, C 100 mg, folic acid 0.8 mg, Zn 25 mg/Tab. Bot. 100s. *otc.*
Use: Mineral, vitamin supplement.

Prenatal with Folic Acid. (Eon Labs Manufacturing, Inc.) Vitamins A 6000

IU, D 400 IU, E 30 IU, folic acid 1 mg, C 60 mg, B_1 1.1 mg, B_2 1.8 mg, B_6 2.5 mg, B_{12} 5 mcg, niacin 15 mg, Ca 125 mg, Fe 65 mg/Tab. Bot. 100s, 1000s. *Rx.*
Use: Mineral, vitamin supplement.

Prenatal H.P. (Mission Pharmacal Co.) Vitamins A 4000 IU, C 100 mg, D_3 400 IU, B_1 4 mg, B_2 2 mg, B_3 10 mg, B_5 1 mg, B_6 20 mg, B_{12} 2 mcg, folate 0.8 mg, Ca 50 mg, Fe 30 mg, sugar. Tab. Bot. 100s. *otc.*
Use: Mineral, vitamin supplement.

Prenatal Maternal. (Ethex Corp.) Ca 250 mg, Fe 4 mg, B_2 60 mg, vitamins A 5000 IU, D 400 IU, E 30 mg, B_1 2.9 mg, B_2 3.4 mg, B_3 20 mg, B_5 10 mg, B_6 12.2 mg, B_{12} 12 mcg, C 100 mg, folic acid 1 mg, Cr, Cu, I, Mg, Mn, Mo, Zn 25 mg, biotin 30 mcg/Tab. Bot. 100s. *Rx.*
Use: Mineral, vitamin supplement.

Prenatal-1 + Iron. (Various Mfr.) Ca 200 mg, Fe 65 mg, vitamins A 4000 IU, D 400 IU, E 11 mg, B_1 1.5 mg, B_2 3 mg, B_3 20 mg, B_6 10 mg, B_{12} 12 mcg, C 120 mg, folic acid 1 mg, Cu, Zn 25 mg/Tab. Bot. 100s, 500s. *Rx.*
Use: Mineral, vitamin supplement.

Prenatal Plus. (Zenith Forest Pharmaceutical) Vitamins A (as acetate and carotene) 4000 IU, D 400 IU, E 22 mg, C 120 mg, folic acid 1 mg, B_1 1.84 mg, B_2 3 mg, B_3 20 mg, B_6 10 mg, B_{12} 12 mcg, Ca 200 mg, Fe 65 mg, Cu 2 mg, Zn 25 mg/Tab. Bot. 100s. *Rx.*
Use: Mineral, vitamin supplement.

Prenatal Plus-Improved. (Rugby Labs, Inc.) Ca 200 mg, Fe 65 mg, vitamins A 4000 IU, D 400 IU, E 11 mg, B_1 1.5 mg, B_2 3 mg, B_3 20 mg, B_6 10 mg, B_{12} 12 mcg, C 120 mg, folic acid 1 mg, Cu, Zn 25 mg/Tab. Bot. 100s. *Rx.*
Use: Mineral, vitamin supplement.

Prenatal Plus Iron. (Major Pharm) Vitamins A 4000 IU, D 400 IU, E 22 mg, C 120 mg, folic acid 1 mg, B_1 1.84 mg, B_2 3 mg, niacinamide 20 mg, B_6 10 mg, B_{12} 12 mcg, Ca 200 mg, Cu 2 mg, Fe 27 mg, Zn 25 mg. Tab. Bot. 100s. *Rx.*
Use: Vitamin, mineral supplement.

Prenatal Plus with Beta Carotene. (Rugby Labs, Inc.) Ca 200 mg, Fe 65 mg, vitamins A 4000 IU, D 400 IU, E 11 mg, B_1 1.84 mg, B_2 3 mg, B_3 20 mg, B_6 10 mg, B_{12} 12 mcg, C 120 mg, folic acid 1 mg, Cu, Zn 25 mg/Tab. Bot. 100s, 500s. *Rx.*
Use: Mineral, vitamin supplement.

Prenatal Rx. (Mission Pharmacal Co.) Vitamins A 3000 IU (as acetate), D_3 400 IU, C 240 mg (as ascorbic and calcium ascorbate), B_1 4 mg, B_2 2 mg, B_3 20 mg, B_5 10 mg, B_6 20 mg, B_{12} 8 mcg, folic acid 1 mg, Fe 29.5 mg (as ferrous fumarate), Ca 175 mg (as carbonate and ascorbate), I 0.3 mg (as potassium iodide), Zn 15 mg (as dried zinc sulfate), Cu 2 mg (as cupric oxide). Tab. Bot. 100s. *Rx.*
Use: Mineral, vitamin supplement.

Prenatal Rx with Beta Carotene. (Various Mfr.) Ca 200 mg, Fe 60 mg, vitamins A 4000 IU, D 400 IU, E 15 mg, B_1 1.5 mg, B_2 1.6 mg, B_3 17 mg, B_5 7 mg, B_6 4 mg, B_{12} 2.5 mcg, C 80 mg, folic acid 1 mg, biotin 30 mcg, Cu, Mg, Zn 25 mg/Tab. Bot. 100s, 500s. *Rx.*
Use: Mineral, vitamin supplement.

Prenatal Z. (Ethex Corp.) Ca 300 mg, Fe 65 mg, vitamins A 5000 IU, D 400 IU, E 30 mg, B_1 3 mg, B_2 3 mg, B_3 20 mg, B_6 12.2 mg, B_{12} 12 mcg, C 80 mg, folic acid 1 mg, Zn 20 mg, I, Mg/Tab. Bot. 100s. *Rx.*
Use: Mineral, vitamin supplement.

Prenatal Z Advanced Formula. (Ethex Corp.) Vitamin A 3000 IU, ascorbic acid 70 mg, calcium carbonate 200 mg, ferrous fumarate 65 mg, cholecalciferol 400 IU, dl-alpha tocopheryl acetate 10 IU, B_1 1.5 mg, B_2 1.6 mg, B_3 17 mg, B_6 2.2 mg, folic acid 1 mg, B_{12} 2.2 mcg, potassium iodide 175 mcg, magnesium oxide 100 mg, zinc oxide 15 mg. Tab. Bot. 100s. *Rx.*
Use: Mineral, vitamin supplement.

Prenate 90 Tablets. (Sanofi Winthrop Pharmaceuticals) Vitamins A 4000 IU, D 400 IU, E 30 mg, C 120 mg, folic acid 1 mg, B_1 3 mg, B_2 3.4 mg, B_6 20 mg, B_{12} 12 mcg, B_3 20 mg, DSS, Ca 250 mg, I, Fe 90 mg, Cu, Zn 20 mg/FC Tab. Bot. 100s, 1000s. *Rx.*
Use: Mineral, vitamin supplement.

Prenavite. (Rugby Labs, Inc.) Ca 200 mg, Fe 60 mg, vitamins A 4000 IU, D 400 IU, E 11 mg, B_1 1.5 mg, B_2 1.7 mg, B_3 18 mg, B_6 2.6 mg, B_{12} 4 mcg, C 100 mg, folic acid 0.8 mg, Zn 25 mg/Tab. Bot. 100s, 500s. *otc.*
Use: Mineral, vitamin supplement.

•**prenylamine.** (PREH-nill-ah-meen) USAN. Segontin; synadrin lactate.
Use: Coronary vasodilator.

Preparation H. (Whitehall Robins Laboratories) Shark liver oil 3%, cocoa butter 79%, corn oil, EDTA, parabens, tocopherol. Supp. 12s, 24s, 36s, 48s. *otc.*
Use: Anorectal preparation.

Preparation H Cream. (Whitehall Robins Laboratories) Petrolatum 78%, gly-

cerin 12%, shark liver oil 3%, phenylephrine HCl 0.25%, cetyl and stearyl alcohol, EDTA, parabens, lanolin, tocopherol. Tube 27 g, 54 g. *otc.*
Use: Anorectal preparation.

Preparation H Ointment. (Whitehall Robins Laboratories) Petrolatum 71.9%, mineral oil 14%, shark liver oil 3%, phenylephrine HCl 0.25%, corn oil, glycerin, lanolin, lanolin alcohol, parabens, tocopherol. Oint. 30 g, 60 g. *otc.*
Use: Anorectal preparation.

Prepcat. (Lafayette Pharmaceuticals, Inc.) Barium sulfate 1.2% w/w suspension. Bot. 480 ml, Case Bot. 24s.
Use: Radiopaque agent.

Prepcat 2000. (Lafayette Pharmaceuticals, Inc.) Barium sulfate 1.2% w/w suspension. Bot. 2000 ml, Case Bot. 4s.
Use: Radiopaque agent.

Prepcort Cream. (Whitehall Robins Laboratories) Hydrocortisone 0.5%. Tube 0.5 oz, 1 oz.
Use: Corticosteroid.

Pre-Pen. (Schwarz Pharma) Benzylpenicilloyl-polylysine 0.25 ml/Amp. *Rx.*
Use: Diagnostic aid.

Pre-Pen/MDM. (Schwarz Pharma)
See: Benzylpenicillin, Benzylpenicilloic, Benzylpenilloic Acid.

Prepidil. (Pharmacia & Upjohn) Dinoprostone 0.5 mg. Gel. Syringes (with 2 shielded catheters 10 and 20 mm tip) 3 g. *Rx.*
Use: Cervical ripening.

Prepodyne. (West) Titratable iodine. **Soln.:** 1%. Bot. Pt, gal. **Scrub:** 0.75%. Bot. 6 oz, gal. **Swabs:** Saturated with soln. Pkt. 1s, Box 100s. **Swabsticks:** Saturated with soln. Pkt. 1s, Box 50s. Pkt. 3s, Box 75s.
Use: Antiseptic, topical.

Presalin. (Roberts Pharmaceuticals) Aspirin 260 mg, salicylamide 120 mg, acetaminophen 120 mg, aluminum hydroxide 100 mg/Tab. Bot. 50s. *otc.*
Use: Analgesic combination, antacid.

Prescription Strength Desenex. (Novartis Pharmaceutical Corp.) **Spray Liquid:** Miconazole nitrate 2%. 105 ml. **Spray Powder:** Miconazole nitrate 2%. 90 ml. **Cream:** Clotrimazole 1%. Tube 15 g. *otc.*
Use: Antifungal, topical.

Preservative Free Moisture Eyes. (Bausch & Lomb) Propylene glycol 0.95%, boric acid, NaCl, KCl, sodium borate, EDTA. Soln. UD 32s. *otc.*
Use: Artificial tear solution.

pressor agents.
See: Sympathomimetic agents.

Pressorol. (Baxter Pharmaceutical Products, Inc.) Metaraminol bitartrate 10 mg/ml. Inj. Vial 10 ml. *Rx.*
Use: Vasoconstrictor.

PreSun 4 Creamy. (Bristol-Myers Squibb) Padimate O 1.4%, alcohol, titanium dioxide. Waterproof lotion. SPF 4. Bot. 4 oz. *otc.*
Use: Sunscreen.

PreSun 8 Creamy. (Bristol-Myers Squibb) Padimate O 5%, oxybenzone 2%. Waterproof. SPF 8. Bot. 4 oz. *otc.*
Use: Sunscreen.

PreSun 8 Lotion. (Bristol-Myers Squibb) Padimate O 7.3%, oxybenzone 2.3%, SD alcohol 40 60%. SPF 8. Bot. 4 oz. *otc.*
Use: Sunscreen.

PreSun 15 Creamy. (Bristol-Myers Squibb) Padimate O 8%, oxybenzone 3%, benzyl alcohol. Waterproof. SPF 15. Bot. 4 oz. *otc.*
Use: Sunscreen.

PreSun 15 Facial Sunscreen. (Bristol-Myers Squibb) Padimate O (Octyl dimethyl PABA) 8%, oxybenzone 3%. SPF 15. Bot. 2 oz. *otc.*
Use: Sunscreen.

PreSun 15 Facial Sunscreen Stick. (Bristol-Myers Squibb) Octyl dimethyl PABA 8%, oxybenzone 3%. SPF 15. Stick 0.42 oz. *otc.*
Use: Sunscreen.

PreSun 15 Lip Protector. (Bristol-Myers Squibb) Padimate O 8%, oxybenzone 3%. SPF 15. Stick 4.5 g. *otc.*
Use: Sunscreen.

PreSun 15 Lotion. (Bristol-Myers Squibb) Padimate O 5%, PABA 5%, oxybenzone 3%, SD alcohol 40 58%. SPF 15. Bot. 4 oz. *otc.*
Use: Sunscreen.

PreSun 15 Sensitive Skin Sunscreen. (Bristol-Myers Squibb) Octyl methoxycinnamate, oxybenzone, octyl salicylate, cetyl alcohol, PABA free, waterproof, SPF 15. Cream. Bot. 120 ml. *otc.*
Use: Sunscreen.

PreSun 23. (Bristol-Myers Squibb) Padimate O, octyl methoxycinnamate, oxybenzone, octyl salicylate, SD alcohol 40 19%. Waterproof. SPF 23. Spray mist. Bot. 105 ml. *otc.*
Use: Sunscreen.

PreSun 29 Sensitive Skin Sunscreen. (Bristol-Myers Squibb) Octyl methoxycinnamate, oxybenzone, octyl salicylate. Waterproof. SPF 29. Bot. 4 oz. *otc.*
Use: Sunscreen.

PreSun 39 Creamy Sunscreen. (Bristol-

Myers Squibb) Padimate O, oxybenzone, cetyl alcohol. Waterproof. SPF 39. Cream Bot. 120 ml. *otc.*
Use: Sunscreen.

PreSun Active. (Bristol-Myers Squibb) Octyl methoxycinnamate, oxybenzone, octyl salicylate, 69% SD alcohol 40. PABA free. Waterproof. SPF 15, 30. Gel. 120 g. *otc.*
Use: Sunscreen.

PreSun for Kids Cream. (Bristol-Myers Squibb) Octyl methoxycinnamate, oxybenzone, octyl salicylate, cetyl alcohol, PABA free. Waterproof. SPF 29. Cream. Bot. 120 ml. *otc.*
Use: Sunscreen.

PreSun for Kids Spray. (Bristol-Myers Squibb) Padimate O, octyl methoxycinnamate, oxybenzone, octyl salicylate, SD alcohol 40 19%. Waterproof. SPF 23. Liq. Spray Bot. 105 ml. *otc.*
Use: Sunscreen.

PreSun Moisturizing. (Bristol-Myers Squibb) Octyl dimethyl PABA, oxybenzone, cetyl alcohol, diazolidinyl urea. SPF 46. Lot. Bot. 120 ml. *otc.*
Use: Sunscreen.

PreSun Moisturizing Sunscreen with Keri, SPF 15. (Bristol-Myers Squibb) Octyl dimethyl PABA, oxybenzone, cetyl alcohol, diazolidinyl urea. Waterproof. Lot. Bot. 120 ml. *otc.*
Use: Sunscreen.

PreSun Moisturizing Sunscreen with Keri, SPF 25. (Bristol-Myers Squibb) Octyl methoxycinnamate, oxybenzone, octyl salicylate, petrolatum, cetyl alcohol, diazolidinyl urea. Waterproof. Lot. Bot. 120 ml. *otc.*
Use: Sunscreen.

PreSun Spray Mist. (Bristol-Myers Squibb) Octyl dimethyl PABA, octyl methoxycinnamate, oxybenzone, octyl salicylate, 19% SD alcohol 40, C12-15 alcohols benzoate. Waterproof. SPF 23. Liq. Bot. 120 ml. *otc.*
Use: Sunscreen.

PreSun Ultra. (Bristol-Myers Squibb) Avobenzone 3%, octyl methoxycinnamate 7.5%, octyl salicylate 5%, oxybenzone 3%. SPF 30. Lot., Clear Gel Tube. 4 oz. *otc.*
Use: Sunscreen.

Pretend-U-Ate. (Vitalax) Enriched candy-appetite pacifier. Pkg. 20s. *otc.*
Use: Dietary aid.

prethcamide. Mixture of crotethamide and cropropamide.
See: Micoren (Novartis Pharmaceutical Corp.).

Pretts Diet Aid. (Milance Laboratories, Inc.) Alginic acid 200 mg, sodium carboxymethylcellulose 100 mg, sodium bicarbonate 70 mg/Chew. Tab. Bot. 60s. *otc.*
Use: Dietary aid.

Pretty Feet & Hands. (B.F. Ascher and Co.) Paraffin, triethanolamine, parabens. Cream 90 g. *otc.*
Use: Emollient.

PretzPak. (Parnell Pharmaceuticals, Inc.) Benzyl alcohol 3.5%, polyethylene glycols, carboxymethylcellulose, urea, poloxamer, *Mucoprotective Factor* yerba santa, allantoin, aluminum chlorhydroxy allantoin. Oint. Tube 15 g. *otc.*
Use: Operative and postoperative care in intranasal and endoscopic surgery; local anesthetic.

Prevacid. (Tap Pharmaceuticals) Lansoprazole 15 mg, 30 mg/SR Cap. Bot. 100s, 1000s, unit-of-use 30s, UD 100s. *Rx.*
Use: Proton pump inhibitor.

Prevalite. (Upsher-Smith Labs, Inc.) Cholestyramine 4 g, phenylalanine 14.1 mg/Dose. Pow. Box. 5.5 g single-dose packets. 60s. *Rx.*
Use: Antihyperlipidemic agent.

Preven. (Gynetics) Levonorgestrel 0.25 mg, ethinyl estradiol 0.05 mg, lactose, polysorbate 80. Tab. Emergency Contraceptive Kit of 4 pills. *Rx.*
Use: Contraceptive.

Prevident Disclosing Drops. (Colgate Oral Pharmaceuticals) Erythrosine sodium 1%. Bot. 1 oz.
Use: Diagnostic aid, dental plaque.

Prevident Disclosing Tablet. (Colgate Oral Pharmaceuticals) Erythrosine sodium 1%/Tab. UD strip 1000s.
Use: Diagnostic aid, dental plaque.

Prevident Prophylaxis Paste. (Colgate Oral Pharmaceuticals) Sodium fluoride containing 1.2% fluoride ion w/pumice and alumina abrasives. Cup 2 g, Box 200s. Jar 9 oz. *Rx.*
Use: Dental caries agent.

Prevident Rinse. (Colgate Oral Pharmaceuticals) Neutral sodium fluoride 0.2%, alcohol 6%. Sol. Bot. 250 ml, gal (w/ pump dispenser). *Rx.*
Use: Dental caries agent.

Preview. (Lafayette Pharmaceuticals, Inc.) Barium sulfate 60% w/v suspension. Bot. 355 ml, Case 24 bot.
Use: Radiopaque agent.

Preview 2000. Barium sulfate 60% w/v suspension. Bot. 2000 ml, Case 4 Bot.
Use: Radiopaque agent.

Prevision. Mestranol, U.S.P 23.

Prevpac. (TAP Pharmaceuticals) Two

Prevacid (lansoprazole) 30 mg Cap. Four *Trimox* (amoxicillin) 500 mg Cap. Two *Biaxin* (clarithromycin) 500 mg. Tab. Daily administration pack.
Use: *H. pylori* eradication.

Prexonate Tablets. (Tennessee Pharmaceutic) Vitamins A acetate 5000 IU, D 500 IU, B_6 2 mg, B_1 5 mg, B_2 2 mg, C 100 mg, B_{12} 2.5 mcg, calcium pantothenate 1 mg, niacinamide 15 mg, folic acid 1 mg, Fe 45 mg, Ca 500 mg, intrinsic factor 3 mg/Tab. Bot. 100s, 1000s. *Rx.*
Use: Mineral, vitamin supplement.

•**prezatide copper acetate.** (PREH-zat-IDE KAH-per) USAN.
Use: Immunomodulator.

Prid Salve. (Walker Pharmacal) Ichthammol, Phenol, Lead Oleate, Rosin, Beeswax, Lard. Tin 20 g. *otc.*
Use: Drawing salve.

•**pridefine hydrochloride.** (PRIH-deh-FEEN) USAN.
Use: Antidepressant.

•**prifelone.** (PRIH-feh-LONE) USAN.
Use: Anti-inflammatory (dermatologic).

Priftin. (Hoechst Marion Roussel) Rifapentine 150 mg. Tab. Bot. 32s. *Rx.*
Use: Antituberculosal.

•**priliximab.** (prih-LICK-sih-mab) USAN.
Use: Monoclonal antibody (autoimmune lymphoproliferative diseases, organ transplantation).

•**prilocaine.** (PRILL-oh-cane) USAN.
Use: Anesthetic, local.

prilocaine and epinephrine injection.
Use: Anesthetic, local.

•**prilocaine hydrochloride.** (PRILL-oh-cane) U.S.P. 23.
Use: Anesthetic, local.
See: Citanest Hydrochloride, Vial, Amp. (Astra Pharmaceuticals, L.P.).

Prilosec. (Astra Pharmaceuticals, L.P.) Omeprazole 10 mg, 20 mg, lactose/ DR Cap. 100s, 1000s, unit-of-use 30s, UD 100s. *Rx.*
Use: Antiulcerative.

primacaine.
Use: Anesthetic, local.

Primacor. (Sanofi Winthrop Pharmaceuticals) Milrinone lactate. **Inj.:** 1 mg/ml. Single-dose vial 10 ml, 20 ml; Carpuject units 5 ml. **Inj., Premixed:** 200 mcg/ml in dextrose 5%. Vial 100 ml. *Rx.*
Use: Cardiovascular agent.
See: Milrinone.

•**primaquine phosphate.** (PRIM-uh-kween) U.S.P. 23.
Use: Antimalarial.

primaquine phosphate. (PRIM-uh-kween) (Sanofi Winthrop Pharmaceuticals) 26.3 mg/Tab. Bot. 100s.
Use: Antimalarial.

primaquine phosphate. (PRIM-uh-kween) (Sanofi Winthrop Pharmaceuticals)
Use: Treatment of AIDS-associated PCP. [Orphan Drug]

Primatene. (Whitehall Robins Laboratories) Theophylline 130 mg, ephedrine HCl 24 mg, phenobarbital 7.5 mg/Tab. Bot. 24s. *otc.*
Use: Antiasthmatic combination.

Primatene Dual Action. (Whitehall Robins Laboratories) Theophylline 60 mg, ephedrine HCl 12.5 mg, guaifenesin 100 mg/Tab. Bot. 24s. *otc.*
Use: Antiasthmatic combination.

Primatene Mist. (Whitehall Robins Laboratories) Epinephrine 0.2 mg, alcohol 34%. Aer. Bot. 15 ml w/mouthpiece or 15 ml, 22.5 ml refills. *otc.*
Use: Bronchodilator.

Primatene Mist Suspension. (Whitehall Robins Laboratories) Epinephrine bitartrate 0.3 mg. Bot. 10 ml w/mouthpiece. Spray. *otc.*
Use: Bronchodilator.

Primatene M. (Whitehall Robins Laboratories) Theophylline 118 mg, ephedrine HCl 24 mg, pyrilamine maleate 16.6 mg/Tab. Bot. 24s, 60s. *otc.*
Use: Antihistamine, bronchodilator.

Primatene P. (Whitehall Robins Laboratories) Theophylline 118 mg, ephedrine HCl 24 mg, phenobarbital 8 mg/ Tab. Bot. 24s, 60s. *otc.*
Use: Bronchodilator, hypnotic, sedative.

Primatuss Cough Mixture 4 Liquid. (Rugby Labs, Inc.) Doxylamine succinate 3.75 mg, dextromethorphan HBr 7.5 mg/5 ml, alcohol 10%. Liq. Bot. 180 ml. *otc.*
Use: Antihistamine, antitussive.

Primatuss Cough Mixture 4D Liquid. (Rugby Labs, Inc.) Pseudoephedrine HCl 20 mg, dextromethorphan HBr 10 mg, guaifenesin 67 mg/5 ml, alcohol 10%. Liq. Bot. 120 ml. *otc.*
Use: Antitussive, decongestant, expectorant.

Primaxin. (Merck & Co.) Imipenem (anhydrous equivalent), cilastatin w/sodium bicarbonate buffer. **250-250:** *ADD-Vantage* Vial, Tray 10s, 25s. Tray 10 infusion bottles. **500-500:** *ADD-Vantage* Vial, Tray 10s, 25s. Tray 10 infusion bottles. *Rx.*
Use: Anti-infective.

Primaxin I.M. (Merck & Co.) Imipenem 500 mg, cilastatin 500 mg, Na 1. 4

mEq. Imipenem 750 mg, cilastatin 750 mg, Na 2.1 mEq. Pow. for Inj. Vial. *Rx.*
Use: Anti-infective.

Primaxin I.V. (Merck & Co.) Imipenem 250 mg, cilastatin 250 mg, Na 0.8 mEq. Imipenem 500 mg, cilastatin 500 mg, Na 1.6 mEq. Pow. for Inj. Infusion bot., *ADD-Vantage* vial. *Rx.*
Use: Anti-infective.

•**primidolol.** (prih-MID-oh-lahl) USAN.
Use: Antianginal; antihypertensive; cardiovascular agent, antiarrhythmic.

•**primidone.** (PRIM-ih-dohn) U.S.P. 23.
Use: Anticonvulsant.

primidone. (Various Mfr.) 250 mg. Tab. Bot. 100s, 500s, 1000s, UD 100s.
Use: Anticonvulsant.

primostrum. A prep. of primiparous colostrum.

Principen. (Apothecon) Ampicillin trihydrate. **Cap.:** 250 mg, 500 mg. Bot. 100s, 500s, UD 100s. **Pow. for Oral Susp.:** 125 mg/5 ml, 250 mg/5 ml. Bot. 100 ml, 150 ml, 200 ml, UD 5 ml. *Rx.*
Use: Anti-infective, penicillin.

Principen with Probenecid. (Bristol-Myers Squibb) Ampicillin (as trihydrate)3.5 g, probenecid 1 g/regimen. Single-dose Bot., 9s. *Rx.*
Use: Anti-infective, penicillin.

Prinivil. (Merck & Co.) Lisinopril. **2.5 mg/Tab.:** Bot. 30s, 100s, UD 100s. **5 mg/Tab.:** Bot. 1000s, Unit-of-Use 90s, 100s, UD 100s. **10 mg, 20 mg/Tab.:** Bot. 1000s, Unit-of-Use 30s, 90s, 100s, UD 100s. **40 mg/Tab.:** Bot. 100s. *Rx.*
Use: Antihypertensive.

•**prinomide tromethamine.** (PRIH-no-MIDE troe-METH-ah-meen) USAN.
Use: Antirheumatic.

•**prinoxodan.** (prin-OX-oh-dan) USAN.
Use: Cardiovascular agent.

Prinzide. (Merck & Co.) Lisinopril 10 mg, 20 mg, hydrochlorothiazide 12.5 mg/Tab or lisinopril 20 mg, hydrochlorothiazide 25 mg/Tab. Bot. 30s, 100s. *Rx.*
Use: Antihypertensive.

Priscoline. (Novartis Pharmaceutical Corp.) Tolazoline HCl 25 mg/ml, tartaric acid 0.65%, hydrous sodium citrate 0.65%. Vial 4 ml. *Rx.*
Use: Antihypertensive.

Privine. (Novartis Pharmaceutical Corp.) Naphazoline HCl. **Nasal Soln.:** 0.05%. Bot. 20 ml w/dropper. **Nasal Spray:** 0.05%. Bot. 15 ml. *otc.*
Use: Decongestant.

•**prizidilol hydrochloride.** (PRIH-zie-DILL-ole) USAN.
Use: Antihypertensive.

Pro-Acet Douche Concentrate. (Pro-Acet) Lactic, citric, and acetic acids, sodium lauryl sulfate, lactose, dextrose, sodium acetate. Pkg. polyethylene envelope 10 ml. Contents of 1 envelope to be diluted with 2 quarts of water. Douche 6 oz, 12 oz. Travel Packet 10 ml. *otc.*
Use: Vaginal agent.

•**proadifen hydrochloride.** (pro-AD-ih-fen) USAN.
Use: Synergist (non-specific).

ProAmatine. (Roberts Pharmaceuticals) Midodrine HCl 2.5 mg, 5 mg/Tab. Bot. 100s. *Rx.*
Use: Orthostatic hypotension.

Pro-Banthine. (Schiapparelli Searle) Propantheline bromide. **7.5 mg/Tab.:** Bot. 100s. **15 mg/Tab.:** Bot. 100s, 500s, UD 100s.
Use: Anticholinergic, antispasmodic.

Probarbital Sodium. 5-Ethyl-5-isopropylbarbiturate sodium.

Probax. (Fischer Pharmaceuticals, Inc.) Propolis 2%, petrolatum, mineral oil, lanolin. Gel Tube 3.5 g. *otc.*
Use: Mouth and throat preparation.

Probec-T. (Roberts Pharmaceuticals) Vitamins B_1 12.2 mg, B_2 10 mg, B_3 100 mg, B_5 18.4, B_6 4.1 mg, B_{12} 5 mcg, C 600 mg/Tab. Bot. 60s. *otc.*
Use: Mineral, vitamin supplement.

Proben-C. (Rugby Labs, Inc.) Probenecid 500 mg, colchicine 0.5 mg/Tab. Bot. 100s, 1000s. *Rx.*
Use: Antigout agent.

•**probenecid.** (pro-BEN-uh-sid) U.S.P. 23.
Use: Uricosuric.
See: Benemid, Tab. (Merck & Co.).
W/Ampicillin.
See: Amcill-GC, Oral Susp. (Parke-Davis).
Principen w/Probenecid, Cap. (Bristol-Myers Squibb).

probenecid and colchicine. (Various Mfr.) Probenecid 500 mg, colchicine 0.5 mg/Tab. Bot. 100s, 1000s. *Rx.*
Use: Uricosuric combination for chronic gouty arthritis.
See: Col-Probenecid, Tab. (Various Mfr.).

•**probicromil calcium.** (pro-BYE-KROE-mill) USAN.
Use: Antiallergic (prophylactic).

Pro-Bionate. (Natren, Inc.) *Lactobacillus acidophilus* strain NAS 2 billion units/g. **Pow.:** 52.5 g, 90 g. **Cap.:** Bot. 30s, 60s. *otc.*
Use: Antidiarrheal, nutritional supplement.

•**probucol.** (PRO-byoo-kahl) U.S.P. 23.
Use: Antihyperlipidemic.
See: Lorelco, Tab. (Hoechst Marion Roussel).

•**procainamide hydrochloride.** (pro-CANE-uh-mide) U.S.P. 23.
Use: Cardiovascular agent, antiarrhythmic.
See: Procanbid, ER Tab. (Parke-Davis). Pronestyl, Cap., Vial (Bristol-Myers Squibb).

procaine base.
Use: Anesthetic, local.
See: Anucaine, Amp. (Calvin).

•**procaine hydrochloride.** (pro-CANE) U.S.P. 23. Bernocaine, Chlorocaine, Ethocaine, Irocaine, Kerocaine, Syncaine.
Use: Anesthetic, local.
See: Novocain, Inj. (Sanofi Winthrop Pharmaceuticals).

procaine hydrochloride. (Abbott Laboratories) 1%, 2% solution. Multiple-dose Vial 30 ml.
Use: Anesthetic, local.

procaine hydrochloride and epinephrine injection.
Use: Anesthetic, local.

procaine hydrochloride and levonordefrin injection.
Use: Anesthetic, local.

procaine penicillin g suspension, sterile.
Use: Anti-infective, penicillin.
See: Penicillin G, Procaine (Various Mfr.).
Pfizerpen for Injection (Pfizer).

procaine, penicillin g w/aluminum stearate suspension, sterile.
Use: Anti-infective, penicillin.
See: Penicillin G Procaine with Aluminum Stearate, Sterile, U.S.P 23.

procaine and phenylephrine hydrochlorides injection.
Use: Anesthetic, local.

procaine and tetracaine hydrochlorides and levonordefrin injection.
Use: Anesthetic, local.

procaine, tetracaine and nordefrin hydrochlorides injection.
Use: Anesthetic, local.

procaine, tetracaine and phenylephrine hydrochlorides injection.
Use: Anesthetic.

ProcalAmine Injection. (McGaw, Inc.) Injection of amino acid 3%, glycerin 3%, electrolytes. Bot. 1000 ml. *Rx.*
Use: Nutritional supplement, parenteral.

Pro-Cal-Sof. (Vangard Labs, Inc.) Docusate calcium 240 mg/Cap. Bot. 100s, 1000s, UD 100s. *otc.*
Use: Laxative.

Procanbid. (Parke-Davis) Procainamide 500 mg, 1000 mg/SR Tab. Bot. 60s, UD 100s. *Rx.*
Use: Antiarrhythmic.

•**procarbazine hydrochloride.** (pro-CAR-buh-ZEEN) U.S.P. 23. (Roche Laboratories) Natulan.
Use: Cytostatic, antineoplastic.
See: Matulane, Cap. (Roche Laboratories).

Procardia. (Pfizer US Pharmaceutical Group) Nifedipine 10 mg, 20 mg/Cap. Bot. 100s, 300s, UD 100s. *Rx.*
Use: Calcium channel blocker.

Procardia XL. (Pfizer US Pharmaceutical Group) Nifedipine 30 mg, 60 mg, 90 mg/SR Tab. **30 mg or 60 mg:** Bot. 100s, 300s, 5000s, UD 100s. **90 mg:** Bot 100s. *Rx.*
Use: Calcium channel blocker.

•**procaterol hydrochloride.** (PRO-CAT-ehr-ole) USAN.
Use: Bronchodilator.

Proception Sperm Nutrient Douche. (Milex Products, Inc.) Ringer type glucose douche. Bot. sufficient for 10 douches. *otc.*
Use: Vaginal agent.

•**prochlorperazine.** (pro-klor-PURR-uh-zeen) U.S.P. 23.
Use: Antiemetic.
See: Compazine, Preps. (SmithKline Beecham Pharmaceuticals).

prochlorperazine maleate. (Various Mfr.) Prochlorperazine maleate 5 mg, 10 mg, 25 mg. Tab. Bot. 30s (except 25 mg), 100s, 1000s, UD 100s. *Rx.*
Use: Antipsychotic.

prochlorperazine edisylate. (Various Mfr.) Prochlorperazine edisylate 5 mg/ml. Inj. Amp. 2 ml. Vial 10 ml. Tubex 1 ml, 2 ml. *Rx.*
Use: Antipsychotic.

prochlorperazine. (G & W Laboratories) Prochlorperazine 25 mg, coconut oil, palm kernel oil. Supp. 12s. *Rx.*
Use: Antiemetic.

•**prochlorperazine edisylate.** (pro-klor-PURR-uh-zeen) U.S.P. 23.
Use: Antipsychotic, antiemetic.
See: Compazine, Preps. (SmithKline Beecham Pharmaceuticals).

prochlorperazine ethanedisulfonate. Prochlorperazine Edisylate, U.S.P. 23.
Use: Anxiolytic.

prochlorperazine/isopropamide. (Various Mfr.) Isopropamide iodide 5 mg, prochlorperazine maleate 10 mg/Cap. Bot. 100s, 500s, 1000s, UD 100s. *Rx.*

Use: Anticholinergic, antispasmodic, antiemetic, antivertigo.

•**prochlorperazine maleate.** (pro-klor-PURR-uh-zeen) U.S.P. 23.
Use: Antiemetic, antipsychotic.
See: Compazine, Preps. (SmithKline Beecham Pharmaceuticals).

•**procinonide.** (pro-SIN-oh-nide) USAN.
Use: Adrenocortical steroid.

•**proclonol.** (PRO-klah-nole) USAN. Under study.
Use: Anthelmintic, antifungal.

Pro Comfort Athlete's Foot Spray. (Scholl, Inc.) Tolnaftate 1%. Aer. Can 4 oz. *otc.*
Use: Antifungal, topical.

Pro Comfort Jock Itch Spray Powder. (Scholl, Inc.) Tolnaftate 1%. Aer. Can 3.5 oz. *otc.*
Use: Antifungal, topical.

Procort. (Roberts Pharmaceuticals) Hydrocortisone 1%. **Cream:** Tube. 30 g. **Spray:** Can. 45 ml. *otc.*
Use: Corticosteroid, topical.

Procrit. (Ortho Biotech, Inc.) Epoetin alfa 2000, 3000, 4000, 10,000 units. Inj. Vial. 1 ml. *Rx.*
Use: Hematopoietic.

Proctocort. (Monarch Pharmaceuticals) Hydrocortisone Cream 30 g w/rectal applicator. Hydrocortisone acetate 30 mg. Supp. Box. 12s. *Rx.*
Use: Corticosteroid.

ProctoCream-HC. (Schwarz Pharma, Inc.) Hydrocortisone acetate 1%, 2.5%, pramoxine HCl 1%. Cream Jar 30 g. *Rx.*
Use: Corticosteroid; anesthetic, local.

Proctofoam. (Schwarz Pharma, Inc.) Pramoxine HCl 1% in an anesthetic muco adhesive foam base. Foam. Can. 15 g. *otc.*
Use: Anorectal preparation.

ProctoFoam-HC. (Schwarz Pharma, Inc.) Hydrocortisone acetate 1%, pramoxine HCl 1% in hydrophilic foam base. Bot. aerosol container, Aerosol foam 10 g w/applicator. *Rx.*
Use: Corticosteroid, anesthetic, local.

Proctofoam NS. (Schwarz Pharma, Inc.) Pramoxine HCl 1%. Aer. Bot. 15 g w/ applicator. *otc.*
Use: Anesthetic, local.

Pro-Cute Cream. (Ferndale Laboratories, Inc.) Silicone, hexachlorophene, lanolin. 2 oz, lb. *otc.*
Use: Emollient.

ProCycle Gold. (Cyclin Pharmaceuticals, Inc.) Vitamins A 833.3 IU, D 66.7 IU, E 66.7 IU, C 30 mg, B_1 1.7 mg, B_2 1.7 mg, B_3 3.3 mg, B_5 1.7 mg, B_6 3.3 mg, B_{12} 21 mcg, folic acid 66.7 mg, Ca 166.7 mg, Fe 3 mg, Zn 2.5 mg, B, Cu, Cr, I, Mg, Mn, Se, PABA, inositol, rutin, biotin, hesperidin, pancreatin, betaine/ Tab. Sugar free. Bot. 100s. *otc.*
Use: Mineral, vitamin supplement.

•**procyclidine hydrochloride.** (pro-SI-klih-deen) U.S.P. 23.
Use: Muscle relaxant; antiparkinsonian.
See: Kemadrin, Tab. (GlaxoWellcome).

Procysteine. (Free Radical Sciences, Inc.)
See: L_2-Oxothiazolidine$_4$-carboxylic acid.

Proderm Topical Dressing. (Dow B. Hickam) Castor oil 650 mg, peruvian balsam 72.5 mg/0.82 ml. Aer. 4 oz. *otc.*
Use: Dermatologic, wound therapy.

•**prodilidine hydrochloride.** (pro-DIH-lih-deen) USAN.
Use: Analgesic.

Prodium. (Breckenridge Pharmaceuticals, Inc.) Phenazopyramide HCl 90 mg/Tab. Pkg. 12s, Bot. 30s. *otc.*
Use: Analgesic.

•**prodolic acid.** (PRO-dole-ik acid) USAN.
Use: Anti-inflammatory.

Pro-Est. (Burgin-Arden) Progesterone 25 mg, estrogenic substance 25,000 IU, sodium carboxymethylcellulose 1 mg, sodium Cl 0.9%, benzalkonium Cl 1:10,000, sodium phosphate dibasic 0.1% in water. *Rx.*
Use: Estrogen, progestin combination.

•**profadol hydrochloride.** (PRO-fah-dahl) USAN.
Use: Analgesic.

profamina.
See: Amphetamine (Various Mfr.).

Profasi. (Serono Laboratories, Inc.) Chorionic gonadotropin 5000 units or 10,000 units/Vial. 10 ml. *Rx.*
Use: Chorionic gonadotropin.

Profenal. (Alcon Laboratories, Inc.) Suprofen 1%. Soln. Drop-Tainer 2.5 ml. *Rx.*
Use: NSAID, ophthalmic.

Profen LA. (Wakefield Pharmaceuticals, Inc.) Phenylpropanolamine HCl 75 mg, guaifenesin 600 mg/TR Tab. Dye free. Bot. 100s. *Rx.*
Use: Decongestant, expectorant.

Profen II. (Wakefield Pharmaceuticals, Inc.) Phenylpropanolamine HCl 37.5 mg, guaifenesin 600 mg/TR Tab. Dye free. Bot. 100s. *Rx.*
Use: Decongestant, expectorant.

Profen II DM. (Wakefield Pharmaceuticals, Inc.) Phenylpropanolamine HCl

37.5 mg, guaifenesin 600 mg, dextromethorphan HBr 30 mg. TR Tab. Bot. 100s. *Rx.*
Use: Antihistamine, decongestant, expectorant.

Professional Care Lotion, Extra Strength. (Walgreen Co.) Zinc oxide 0.25% in a lotion base. Lot. Bot. 16 oz. *otc.*
Use: Astringent, antiseptic, dermatologic.

Profiber. (Sherwood Davis & Geck) Sodium caseinate, dietary fiber from soy, calcium caseinate, hydrolyzed cornstarch, corn oil, soy lecithin, vitamins A, B_1, B_2, B_3, B_5, B_6, B_{12}, C, D, E, K, folic acid, biotin, choline, Ca, Cl, Cr, Cu, Fe, I, Mg, Mn, Mo, P, Se, Zn. Liq. Can 250 ml, closed system 1000 ml. *otc.*
Use: Nutritional supplement.

Profilnine Heat-Treated. (Alpha Therapeutic Corp.) Dried plasma fraction of coagulation factors II, VII, IX, and X. Heparin free. Vial, single-dose with diluent. *Rx.*
Use: Antihemophilic.

Profilnine SD. (Alpha Therapeutic Corp.) Dried plasma fraction of coagulation factors II, VII, IX, and X. Heparin free. Solvent detergent treated. Inj. Single-dose vials with diluent. *Rx.*
Use: Antihemophilic.

proflavine.
Use: Antiseptic, topical.

proflavine dihydrochloride. 3,6-Diaminoacridine dihydrochloride.

proflavine sulfate. 3,6-Diaminoacridine sulfate.

ProFree/GP Weekly Enzymatic Cleaner. (Allergan, Inc.) Papain, sodium Cl, sodium borate, sodium carbonate, edetate disodium. Kit 16s or 24s with vials. *otc.*
Use: Contact lens care.

•**progabide.** (pro-GAB-ide) USAN.
Use: Anticonvulsant, muscle relaxant.

Progens. (Major Pharmaceuticals) Conjugated estrogens. **0.625 mg/Tab.:** Bot. 100s, 1000s. **1.25 mg/Tab.:** Bot. 1000s. **2.5 mg/Tab.:** Bot. 100s, 1000s. *Rx.*
Use: Estrogen.

Pro-Gesic. (Nastech Pharmaceutical Co., Inc.) Trolamine salicylate 10%, propylene glycol, methylparahydroxybenzoic acid, propyl parahydroxybenzoic acid, EDTA. Liq. Bot. 75 ml. *otc.*
Use: Liniment.

Progestasert. (Alza Corp.) T-shaped intrauterine device (IUD) unit containing a reservoir of progesterone 38 mg with barium sulfate dispersed in medical grade silicone fluid. In 6s w/inserter. *Rx.*
Use: Contraceptive.

•**progesterone.** (pro-JESS-ter-ohn) U.S.P. 23. Flavolutan, Luteogan, Luteosan, Lutren.
Use: Hormone, progestin. [Orphan Drug]
W/Aqueous. Susp.
See: Prorone, Inj. (Sigma-Tau Pharmaceuticals, Inc.).
W/Oil.
See: Crinone 8%, Gel (Wyeth-Ayerst Laboratories).
Femotrone, Inj. (Bluco Inc./Med. Discnt. Outlet).
Lipo-Lutin, Amp. (Parke-Davis).
Progestin, Vial (Various Mfr.).
Prometrium (Solvay).
Prorone, Inj. (Sigma-Tau Pharmaceuticals, Inc.).
W/Estradiol, testosterone, procaine HCl, procaine base.
See: Hormo-Triad, Vial (Bell).

progesterone. (Various Mfr.) Pow. 1 g, 10 g, 25 g, 100 g, 1000 g.
Use: Hormone, progestin.

progesterone in oil. (Various Mfr.) 50 mg/ml. In sesame or peanut oil with benzyl alcohol. Inj. Vial 10 ml. *Rx.*
Use: Hormone, progestin.

progesterone intrauterine contraceptive system.
Use: Contraceptive.

progestin. (Various Mfr.) Progesterone.
See: Hydroxyprogesterone.
Medroxyprogesterone.
Megestrol.
Norethindrone.

•**proglumide.** (pro-GLUE-mid) USAN. (Wallace Laboratories)
Use: Anticholinergic.

Proglycem. (Baker Norton Pharmaceuticals, Inc.) **Cap.:** Diazoxide 50 mg/Cap. Bot. 100s. **Oral Susp.:** Diazoxide 50 mg/ml. Bot. 30 ml w/calibrated dropper. *Rx.*
Use: Hyperglycemic.

Prograf. (Fujisawa USA, Inc.) **Cap.:** Tacrolimus 1 mg, 5 mg. Bot. 100s. **Inj.:** Tacrolimus 5 mg/ml. Amp 1 ml, 10s. *Rx.*
Use: Immunosuppressant.

proguanil hydrochloride.
See: Chloroguanide Hydrochloride.

ProHance. (Bracco Diagnostics) Gadoteridol 279.3 mg, calteridol calcium 0.23 mg, tromethamine 1.21 mg/ml. Inj. Vials. 15 ml, 30 ml. *Rx.*
Use: Radiopaque agent.

ProHIBIT. (Pasteur Merieux Connaught) Purified capsular polysaccharide of

Haemophilus influenzae type b 25 mcg, conjugated diphtheria toxoid protein 18 mcg/0.5 ml dose. Also called PRP-D. Inj. Vial 0.5 ml, 2.5 ml, 5 ml. Syr. 0.5 ml. *Rx.*
Use: Immunization.

•**proinsulin human.** (PRO-in-suh-LIN HYOO-muhn) USAN.
Use: Antidiabetic.

Prolactin RIA. (Abbott Diagnostics) Quantitative measurement of total circulating human prolactin. Test unit 50s, 100s.
Use: Diagnostic aid.

Prolactin RIAbead. (Abbott Diagnostics) Radioimmunoassay for the quantitative measurement of prolactin in human serum and plasma.
Use: Diagnostic aid.

proladyl. Pyrrobutamine.
Use: Antihistamine.

prolase. Proteolytic enzyme from *Carica papaya.*
See: Papain.

Prolastin. (Bayer Corp. (Consumer Div.)) Alpha$_1$-proteinase inhibitor G 20 mg alpha$_1$-PI/ml when reconstituted. W/polyethylene glycol, sucrose and small amounts of other plasma proteins. Inj. Vial, single dose. *Rx.*
Use: Alpha$_1$-proteinase inhibitor.

Proleukin. (Chiron Therapeutics) Aldesleukin, interleukin-2. Pow. for Inj. 22 million IU/Vial (1.1 mg when reconstituted). Single-use Vial. *Rx.*
Use: Antineoplastic.

•**proline.** (PRO-leen) U.S.P. 23.
Use: Amino acid.

•**prolintane hydrochloride.** (pro-LIN-tane) USAN.
Use: Antidepressant.

Prolixin. (Bristol-Myers Squibb) Fluphenazine HCl. **Tab.:** 1 mg, 2.5 mg, 5 mg, 10 mg. Bot. 50s, 100s, 500s, 1000s, UD 100s. **Elixir:** 2.5 mg/5 ml, alcohol 14%. Dropper Bot. 60 ml. Bot. 473 ml. **Conc.:** 5 mg/ml, alcohol 14%, Dropper Bot. 120 ml. **Inj.:** 2.5 mg/ml. Vial 10 ml w/methyl- and propylparabens. *Rx.*
Use: Antipsychotic.

Prolixin Decanoate. (Bristol-Myers Squibb) Fluphenazine decanoate 25 mg/ml (in sesame oil with benzyl alcohol). Unimatic syringe 1 ml. Vial 5 ml. *Rx.*
Use: Antipsychotic.

Prolixin Enanthate. (Bristol-Myers Squibb) Fluphenazine enanthate 25 mg/ml (in sesame oil with benzyl alcohol). Vial 5 ml. *Rx.*
Use: Antipsychotic.

Proloprim. (GlaxoWellcome) Trimethoprim 100 mg/Tab. Bot. 100s, UD 100s (in sesame oil with benzyl alcohol). *Rx.*
Use: Anti-infective, urinary.

Promachlor. (Geneva Pharmaceuticals) Chlorpromazine HCl 10 mg, 25 mg, 50 mg, 100 mg, 200 mg/Tab. Bot. 100s, 1000s. *Rx.*
Use: Antiemetic, antivertigo, antipsychotic.

•**promazine hydrochloride.** (PRO-mahzeen) U.S.P. 23.
Use: Antipsychotic, anticholinergic, ataraxic.

promazine hydrochloride. (Various Mfr.) Promazine HCl 25 mg/ml, 50 mg/ml. Inj. Vial 10 ml. *Rx.*
Use: Antipsychotic.

Promega. (Parke-Davis) Omega-3 (N-3) polyunsaturated fatty acids 1000 mg, containing EPA 350 mg, DHA 150 mg, vitamins E (3% RDA), A, B$_1$, B$_2$, B$_3$, Ca, Fe (< 2% RDA)/Cap., cholesterol and sodium free. Bot. 30s. *otc.*
Use: Mineral, vitamin supplement.

Promega Pearls. (Parke-Davis) EPA 168 mg, DHA 72 mg, < cholesterol 2 mg, E 1 IU, < 2% RDA of A, B$_1$, B$_2$, B$_3$, Fe, Ca. Cap. Bot. 60s, 90s. *otc.*
Use: Vitamin supplement.

Prometa. (Muro Pharmaceutical, Inc.) Metaproterenol sulfate 10 mg/5 ml, with saccharin and sorbitol, strawberry flavor. Syr. Bot. 480 ml. *Rx.*
Use: Bronchodilator.

Promethazine DM. (Various Mfr.) Promethazine HCl 6.25 mg, dextromethorphan HBr 15 mg/5 ml, alcohol. Syr. Bot. 120 ml, pt, gal. *Rx.*
Use: Antihistamine, antitussive.

Prometh VC Plain. (Various Mfr.) Phenylephrine HCl 5 mg, promethazine HCl 6.25 mgm/5 ml. Liq. Bot. 120 ml, 473 ml, gal. *Rx.*
Use: Antihistamine, decongestant.

promethazine. (pro-METH-uh-zeen) **Tab.:** 25 mg, 50 mg. Bot. 100s, 1000s. **Syr.:** 6.25 mg/ 5 ml, alcohol. Bot. 118 ml, pt. **Supp.:** 50 mg, cocoa butter. Pkg. 12s. **Inj.:** 25 mg/ml, 50 mg/ml. Amp. 1 ml, Multi-dose Vial 10 ml. *Rx.*
Use: Antiemetic, antihistamine, sedative.

•**promethazine hydrochloride.** (pro-METH-uh-zeen) U.S.P. 23.
Use: Antiemetic, antihistamine.
See: Pentazine, Expectorant, Vial (Century Pharmaceuticals, Inc.).
Phenergan, Prods. (Wyeth-Ayerst Laboratories).

Sigazine, Inj. (Sigma-Tau Pharmaceuticals, Inc.).

promethazine hydrochloride with codeine. (pro-METH-uh-zeen) (Various Mfr.) Promethazine HCl 6.25 mg, codeine phosphate 10 mg/5 ml, alcohol 7%. Syr. Bot. 120 ml, pt, gal. *c-v.*
Use: Antihistamine, antitussive.

promethazine hydrochloride w/combinations. (pro-METH-uh-zeen)
Use: Antiemetic, antihistamine, antivertigo.
See: Mepergan, Vial, Cap. (Wyeth-Ayerst Laboratories).
Phenergan-D, Tab. (Wyeth-Ayerst Laboratories).
Phenergan VC Expectorant (Wyeth-Ayerst Laboratories).

Promethazine VC. (Various Mfr.) Promethazine HCl 6.25 mg, phenylephrine HCl 5 mg/5 ml. Syr. Bot. 120 ml, 240 ml, 473 ml, gal. *Rx.*
Use: Antihistamine, decongestant.

Promethazine VC with Codeine. (Various Mfr.) Promethazine HCl 6.25 mg, phenylephrine HCl 5 mg, codeine 10 mg/5 ml, alcohol 7%. Syr. Bot. 4 oz, pt, gal. *c-v.*
Use: Antihistamine, antitussive, decongestant.

Promethazine VC Plain. (Various Mfr.) Phenylephrine HCl 5 mg, promethazine HCl 6.25 mg/5 ml. Syr. Bot. 473 ml. *Rx.*
Use: Antihistamine, decongestant.

promethestrol dipropionate.
Use: Estrogen.

Prometol. (Viobin) Concentrated wheat germ oil. **3 min/Cap.:** Bot. 100s, 250s. **10 min/Cap.:** Bot. 100s. *otc.*
Use: Supplement.

Prometrium. (Solvay) Progesterone 100 mg, peanut oil, glycerin. Cap. Bot. 100s. *Rx.*
Use: Progestin.

prominal.
See: Mephobarbital.

Promine. (Major Pharmaceuticals) Procainamide 250 mg, 375 mg, 500 mg/Cap. Bot. 100s, 250s, 1000s, UD 100s (375 mg/Cap. w/500s instead of 250s). *Rx.*
Use: Antiarrhythmic.

Promine S.R. (Major Pharmaceuticals) Procainamide. **SR Tab.:** 250 mg. Bot. 100s, 250s; 500 mg. Bot. 100s, 250s, 1000s; 750 mg. Bot. 100s, 250s. **SR Cap.:** 250 mg, 375 mg, 500 mg. *Rx.*
Use: Antiarrhythmic.

Prominol. (MCR American Pharmaceuticals) Butalbital 50 mg, acetaminophen 650 mg/Tab. Bot. 100s. *Rx.*
Use: Analgesic.

Promist HD. (UCB Pharmaceuticals, Inc.) Hydrocodone bitartrate 2.5 mg, pseudoephedrine HCl 30 mg, chlorpheniramine maleate 2 mg/5 ml, alcohol 5%, menthol, saccharin, sorbitol. Bot. Pt. *c-III.*
Use: Antihistamine, antitussive, decongestant.

Promist LA. (UCB Pharmaceuticals, Inc.) Pseudoephedrine HCl 120 mg, guaifenesin 500 mg/Tab. Bot. 100s. *Rx.*
Use: Decongestant, expectorant.

Promit. (Pharmacia & Upjohn) Dextran 1 150 mg/ml Inj. Vial 20 ml. *Rx.*
Use: Antiallergic.

Pro-Mix R.D.P. (Navaco) Protein 15 g (from whey protein), fat 0.8 g, carbohydrate 1 g, Na 46 mg, K 165 mg, Cl 46 mg, Ca 73.6 mg, P 64.4 mg, Fe 0.3 mg, Cr, Cu, Mg, Mn, Mo, Se, Zn, 72 Cal./5 Tbsp. (20 g). Pow. Packet 20 g, can 300 g. *otc.*
Use: Nutritional supplement.

ProMod. (Ross Laboratories) Protein supplement. Nine scoops provides protein 45 g, 100% US RDA. Pow. Can 9.7 oz. *otc.*
Use: Nutritional supplement.

Promylin Enteric Coated Microzymes. (Shear/Kershman) Enteric-coated pancrelipase. Lipase 4000 units, amylase 20,000 units, protease 25,000 units. *Rx.*
Use: Digestive enzymes.

Pro-Nasyl. (Progonasyl) o-Iodobenzoic acid 0.5%, triethanolamine 5.5% in a special neutral hydrophilic base compounded from oleic acid, mineral oil, vegetable oil. Bot. 15 ml, 60 ml.
Use: Treatment of sinusitis.

Pronemia Hematinic. (ESI Lederle Generics) Iron 115 mg, B_{12} 15 mcg, IFC 75 mg, C 150 mg, folic acid 1 mcg. Cap. Bot. 30s. *Rx.*
Use: Iron w/B_{12} and intrinsic factor.

Pronestyl. (Bristol-Myers Squibb) Procainamide. **Cap.:** 250 mg. Bot. 100s, 1000s; 375 mg. Bot. 100s; 500 mg. Bot. 100s, 1000s. **Inj.:** 100 mg/ml w/benzyl alcohol 0.9%, sodium bisulfite 0.09%. Vial 10 ml; 500 mg/ml w/methylparaben 0.1%, sodium bisulfite 0.2%. Vial 2 ml. **Tab.:** 250 mg. Bot. 100s, 1000s, Unimatic 100s; 375 mg. Bot. 100s; 500 mg. Bot. 100s, 1000s, Unimatic 100s. *Rx.*
Use: Antiarrhythmic.

Pronestyl-SR. (Bristol-Myers Squibb) Procainamide 500 mg/Tab. Bot. UD 100s. *Rx.*

Use: Antiarrhythmic.

pronethelol. (Zeneca Pharmaceuticals) Adrenergic beta-receptor antagonist; pending release.

Pronto Concentrate Lice Killing Shampoo Kit. (Del Pharmaceuticals, Inc.) Pyrethrins 0.33%, piperonyl butoxide technical 4%. Bot. 2 oz, 4 oz. *otc.*
Use: Pediculicide.

Pronto Lice Killing Spray. (Del Pharmaceuticals, Inc.) Spray cans 5 oz. *otc.*
Use: Pediculicide for inanimate objects.

Propac. (Biosearch Medical Products) Protein 3 g (from whey protein), carbohydrate 0.2 g, fat 0.3 g, Cl 3 mg, K 20 mg, Na 9 mg, Ca 24 mg, P 12 mg, 16 Cal./Tbsp. (4 g). Pow. Packet 19.5 g, Can 350 g. *otc.*
Use: Nutritional supplement.

Propacet 100. (Teva Pharmaceuticals USA) Propoxyphene napsylate 100 mg, acetaminophen 650 mg/Tab. Bot. 100s, 500s. *c-IV.*
Use: Analgesic combination, narcotic.

propaesin. (Various Mfr.) Propyl p-Aminobenzoate.

•**propafenone hydrochloride.** (pro-pah-FEN-ohn) U.S.P. 23.
Use: Cardiovascular agent, antiarrhythmic.
See: Rythmol, Tab. (Knoll Pharmaceuticals).

Propagest. (Schwarz Pharma, Inc.) Phenylpropanolamine HCl 25 mg/Tab. Bot. 100s. *otc.*
Use: Decongestant.

Propagon-S. (Spanner) Estrone 2 mg, 5 mg/ml. Vial 10 ml. *Rx.*
Use: Estrogen.

Propain HC. (Springbok) Acetaminophen 500 mg, hydrocodone bitartrate 5 mg/Cap. Bot. 100s, 500s. *c-III.*
Use: Analgesic combination, narcotic.

propamidine isethionate 0.1% ophthalmic soln.
Use: Acanthamoeba keratitis. [Orphan Drug]

•**propane.** N.F. 18.
Use: Aerosol propellant.

propanediol diacetate, 1,2.
See: VoSoL, Liq. (Wampole Laboratories).

1,2,3-propanetriol, trinitrate. Nitroglycerin Tab., U.S.P. 23.

•**propanidid.** (pro-PAN-ih-did) USAN.
Use: Anesthetic (intravenous).

propanolol. Propranolol.

•**propantheline bromide.** (pro-PAN-thuh-leen) U.S.P. 23.
Use: Anticholinergic.
See: Pro-Banthine, Preps. (Searle).
W/Phenobarbital.
See: Probital, Tab. (Searle).
W/Thiopropazate dihydrochloride.
See: Pro-Banthine W/Dartal, Tab. (Searle).

PROPApH Cleansing Lotion for Normal/Combination Skin. (Del Pharmaceuticals, Inc.) Salicylic acid 0.5%, SD alcohol 40, EDTA. Lot. Bot. 180 ml. Pads. 45s. *otc.*
Use: Antiacne.

PROPApH Cleansing for Oily Skin. (Del Pharmaceuticals, Inc.) Salicylic acid 0.6%, SD alcohol 40, EDTA, menthol. Lot. Bot. 180 ml. *otc.*
Use: Dermatologic, acne.

PROPApH Cleansing for Sensitive Skin. (Del Pharmaceuticals, Inc.) Salicylic acid 0.5%, SD alcohol 40, aloe vera gel, EDTA, menthol. Pads. In 45s. *otc.*
Use: Dermatologic, acne.

PROPApH Cleansing Maximum Strength. (Del Pharmaceuticals, Inc.) Salicylic acid 2%, SD alcohol 40, aloe vera gel, EDTA, propylene glycol, menthol. Pads. In 45s. *otc.*
Use: Dermatologic, acne.

PROPApH Cleansing Pads. (Del Pharmaceuticals, Inc.) Salicylic acid 0.5%, SD alcohol 40, EDTA, menthol. Pads. 45s. *otc.*
Use: Dermatologic, ance.

PROPApH Foaming Face Wash. (Del Pharmaceuticals, Inc.) Salicylic acid 2%, aloe vera gel, EDTA, menthol. Alcohol, oil and soap free. Liq. Bot. 180 ml. *otc.*
Use: Dermatologic, acne.

PROPApH Maximum Strength Acne Cream. (Del Pharmaceuticals, Inc.) Salicylic acid 2%, acetylated lanolin alcohol, cetearyl alcohol, stearyl alcohol, EDTA, menthol. Cream Tube 19.5 g. *otc.*
Use: Dermatologic, acne.

PROPApH Medicated Acne Cream with Aloe. (Del Pharmaceuticals, Inc.) Salicylic acid 2%. Tube 1 oz. *otc.*
Use: Dermatologic, acne.

PROPApH Medicated Acne Stick with Aloe. (Del Pharmaceuticals, Inc.) Salicylic acid 2%. Stick 0.05 oz. *otc.*
Use: Dermatologic, acne.

PROPApH Medicated Cleansing Pads with Aloe. (Del Pharmaceuticals, Inc.) Salicylic acid 0.5%, SD alcohol 40 25%, aloe. Jar containing 45 pads. *otc.*
Use: Dermatologic, acne.

PROPApH Peel-Off Acne Mask. (Del

Pharmaceuticals, Inc.) Salicylic acid 2%, tartrazine, parabens, polyvinyl alcohol, vitamin E acetate, SD alcohol 40. Mask. 60 ml. *otc.*
Use: Dermatologic, acne.

PROPApH Skin Cleanser with Aloe. (Del Pharmaceuticals, Inc.) Salicylic acid USP 0.5%, SD alcohol 40 25%. Liq. Bot. 6 oz, 10 oz. *otc.*
Use: Dermatologic, acne.

•**proparacaine hydrochloride.** (pro-PAR-ah-cane) U.S.P. 23.
Use: Anesthetic local, ophthalmic.
See: Alcaine, Ophth. Soln. (Alcon Laboratories, Inc.).
AK-Taine, Soln. (Akorn, Inc.).
Fluoracaine, Soln. (Akorn, Inc.).
Ophthaine HCl, Soln. (Bristol-Myers Squibb).
Ophthetic, Ophth. Soln. (Allergan, Inc.).

proparacaine hydrochloride. (Various Mfr.) 0.5% Soln. Bot. 2 ml, 15 ml, UD 1 ml.
Use: Anesthetic local, ophthalmic.

proparacaine hydrochloride & fluorescein sodium. (Taylor Pharmaceuticals) Proparacaine HCl 0.5%, fluorescein sodium 0.25%, thimerosal 0.01%, EDTA. Soln. Bot. 5 ml. *Rx.*
Use: Anesthetic local, ophthalmic.

proparacaine hydrochloride/procaine hydrochloride.
Use: Anesthetic.
See: Ravocaine and Novocain w/Levophed (Cook-Waite Laboratories, Inc.).
Ravocaine and Novocain w/Neocobefrin (Cook-Waite Laboratories, Inc.).

•**propatyl nitrate.** (PRO-pah-till) USAN. Investigational drug in US but available in England.
Use: Coronary vasodilator.

Propecia. (Merck & Co.) Finasteride 1 mg, lactose. Tab. Unit-of-Use 30s, UD 30s. *Rx.*
Use: Androgen hormone inhibitor, hair growth.

•**propenzolate hydrochloride.** (pro-PEN-zoe-late) USAN.
Use: Anticholinergic.

propesin. Name used for Risocaine.

Prophene 65. (Halsey Drug Co.) Propoxyphene HCl 65 mg/Cap. Bot. 100s, 500s, 1000s. *c-IV.*
Use: Analgesic, narcotic.

prophenpyridamine.
See: Pheniramine (Various Mfr.).

prophenpyridamine maleate.
See: Pheniramine Maleate.

prophenpyridamine maleate w/combinations.
See: Panadyl, Tab., Cap. (Misemer Pharmaceuticals, Inc.).
Trimahist Elix., Liq. (Tennessee Pharmaceutic).
Vasotus, Liq. (Sheryl).

Pro-Phree. (Ross Laboratories) Fat 31 g, carbohydrate 60 g, linoleic acid 2250 mg, Fe 11.9 mg, Na 250 mg, K 875 mg, with appropriate vitamins and minerals, 520 Cal/100 g. Protein free. Pow. Can 350 g. *otc.*
Use: Nutritional supplement.

Prophyllin. (Rystan, Inc.) Sodium propionate 5%, chlorophyll derivatives 0.0125%. Tube 1 oz. *Rx.*
Use: Anti-infective, topical.

•**propikacin.** (PRO-pih-KAY-sin) USAN.
Use: Anti-infective.

Propimex-1. (Ross Laboratories) Protein 15 g, fat 23.9 g, carbohydrate 46.3 g, linoleic acid 1800 mg, Fe 9 mg, Na 190 mg, K 675 mg, with appropriate vitamins and minerals, 480 Cal/100 g. Methionine and valine free. Pow. Can 350 g. *otc.*
Use: Nutritional supplement.

Propimex-2. (Ross Laboratories) Protein 30 g, fat 15.5 g, carbohydrate 30 g, Na 880 mg, K 1370 mg, with appropriate vitamins and minerals, 410 Cal/ml. Methionine and valine free. Pow. Can 325 g. *otc.*
Use: Nutritional supplement for propionic or methylmalonic acidemia.

Propine Sterile Ophthalmic Solution. (Allergan, Inc.) Dipivefrin HCl 0.1%. Soln. Bot. 5 ml, 10 ml, 15 ml. *Rx.*
Use: Antiglaucoma.

propiodal.
See: Entodon.

•**propiolactone.** (PRO-pee-oh-LACK-tone) USAN.
Use: Disinfectant, sterilizing agent of vaccines and tissue grafts.

•**propiomazine.** (PRO-pee-oh-MAY-zeen) USAN.
Use: Sedative (pre-anesthetic).
See: Dorevane; Indorm.
Largon, Amp. (Wyeth-Ayerst Laboratories).

propiomazine. (PRO-pee-oh-MAY-zeen)
Use: Sedative.
See: Largon, Inj. (Wyeth-Ayerst Laboratories).

propiomazine hydrochloride. (PRO-pee-oh-MAY-zeen)
Use: Sedative.
See: Largon, Inj. (Wyeth-Ayerst Laboratories).

Propion, Gel (Wyeth-Ayerst Laboratories).

•**propionic acid.** (pro-pee-AHN-ik) N.F. 18.
Use: Antimicrobial; pharmaceutic aid (acidifying agent).

propionyl erythromycin lauryl sulfate.
See: Erythromycin Propionate Lauryl Sulfate.

•**propiram fumarate.** (PRO-pih-ram) USAN.
Use: Analgesic.

propisamine.
See: Amphetamine (Various Mfr.).

propitocaine. Prilocaine.
See: Citanest, Soln., Vial, Amp. (Astra Pharmaceuticals, L.P.).

Proplex. (Baxter Pharmaceutical Products, Inc.) Factor IX Complex (Human), clotting Factor II (prothrombin), VII (proconvertin), IX (PTC, antihemophilic factor B) and X (Stuart-Porwer Factor) all dried and concentrated. Vial 30 ml w/Diluent. *Rx.*
Use: Antihemophilic.

Proplex T. (Baxter Pharmaceutical Products, Inc.) Factor IX complex, heat treated. W/Factors II, VII, IX and X. W/ heparin. Dried concentrate. Vial w/diluent. *Rx.*
Use: Antihemophilic.

•**propofol.** (PRO-puh-FOLE) USAN.
Use: Anesthetic (intravenous).
See: Diprivan, Inj. (Zeneca Pharmaceuticals).

Proponade Capsules. (Halsey Drug Co.) Chlorpheniramine maleate 8 mg, phenylpropanolamine HCl 50 mg, isopropamide 2.5 mg/Cap. Bot. 100s. *Rx.*
Use: Antihistamine, decongestant.

Propoquin. Amopyroquin HCl.
Use: Antimalarial.

•**propoxycaine hydrochloride.** (pro-POX-ih-cane) U.S.P. 23.
Use: Anesthetic, local.

propoxycaine and procaine hydrochlorides and levonordefrin injection.
Use: Anesthetic, local.

propoxycaine and procaine hydrochlorides and norepinephrine bitartrate injection.
Use: Anesthetic, local.
See: Ravocaine and Novocain w/Levophed, Inj. (Cook-Waite Laboratories, Inc.).

propoxychlorinol. Toloxychlorinol.

•**propoxyphene hydrochloride.** (pro-POX-ih-feen) U.S.P. 23.
Use: Analgesic.
See: Darvon, Pulvules (Eli Lilly and Co.).
Dolene, Cap. (ESI Lederle Generics).
Pro-Gesic, Cap. (Ulmer Pharmacal Co.).

propoxyphene hydrochloride. (Various Mfr.) 65 mg. Cap. Bot. 100s, 500s, 1000s. *c-IV.*
Use: Analgesic, narcotic.

propoxyphene hydrochloride w/combinations.
Use: Analgesic.
See: Darvon Compound, Pulvules (Eli Lilly and Co.).
Darvon Compound-65, Cap. (Eli Lilly and Co.).
Darvon With A.S.A., Cap. (Eli Lilly and Co.).
Dolene, AP-65, Tab. (ESI Lederle Generics).
Dolene Compound-65, Cap. (ESI Lederle Generics).
Wygesic, Tab. (Wyeth-Ayerst Laboratories).

propoxyphene hydrochloride and acetaminophen tablets. (pro-POX-ee-feen HIGH-droe-KLOR-ide & ass-cet-ah-MEE-noe-fen tablets)
Use: Analgesic.

propoxyphene hydrochloride and acetaminophen tablets. (Various Mfr.) Propoxyphene HCl 65 mg, acetaminophen 650 mg/Tab. Bot. 500s. *c-IV.*
Use: Analgesic.

propoxyphene hydrochloride and APC capsules.
Use: Analgesic.

propoxyphene hydrochloride, aspirin and caffeine capsules.
Use: Analgesic.

propoxyphene hydrochloride compound capsules. (Various Mfr.) Propoxyphene HCl 65 mg, aspirin 389 mg, caffeine 32.4/Cap. Bot. 100s, 500s. *c-IV.*
Use: Analgesic.

•**propoxyphene napsylate.** (pro-POX-ih-feen NAP-sill-ate) U.S.P. 23.
Use: Analgesic.
See: Darvocet-N, Tab. (Eli Lilly and Co.).
Darvon-N, Tab. (Eli Lilly and Co.).
W/Acetaminophen.
See: Darvocet-N, Tab. (Eli Lilly and Co.).

propoxyphene napsylate and acetaminophen tablets. (Various Mfr.) Propoxyphene napsylate 50 mg, acetaminophen 325 mg/Tab. Bot. 100s, 500s, 550s, 1000s, UD 100s. Propoxyphene napsylate 100 mg, acetaminophen 650 mg/Tab. Bot. 30s, 50s, 100s, 500s, 1000s, UD 100s. *c-IV.*

Use: Analgesic.

propoxyphene napsylate and aspirin tablets.
Use: Analgesic.

•**propranolol hydrochloride.** (pro-PRAN-oh-lahl) U.S.P. 23.
Use: Cardiovascular agent (antiarrhythmic), antiadrenergic (β-receptor).
See: Betachron E-R, Cap. (Inwood Laboratories, Inc.).
Inderal, Tab., Inj. (Wyeth-Ayerst Laboratories).

proprandol hydrochloride SR capsules. (Various Mfr.) Propranolol HCl 60 mg, 80 mg, 120 mg, 160 mg. Bot. 100s, 250s, 500s, 1000s. *Rx.*
Use: Cardiovascular agent (antiarrhythmic), antiadrenergic (β-receptor).

propanol hydrochloride tablets. (Various Mfr.) Propranolol HCl 10 mg, 20 mg, 40 mg, 60 mg, 80 mg, 90 mg. Bot. 100s, 500s, 1000s, UD 100s. *Rx.*
Use: Cardiovascular agent (antiarrhythmic), antiadrenergic (β-receptor).

propranolol hydrochloride solution. (Roxane Laboratories, Inc.) **Oral Soln.:** 20 mg, 40 mg/5 ml. Patient cups UD 5 ml (10s). **Concentrated Oral Soln.:** 80 mg/ml. Bot. 30 ml w/calibrated dropper.
Use: Cardiovascular agent (antiarrhythmic), antiadrenergic (β-receptor).

propranolol hydrochloride and hydrochlorothiazide tablets. (Various Mfr.) Propanolol HCl 40 mg, 80 mg, hydrochlorothiazide 25 mg/Tab. Bot. 100s, 1000s. *Rx.*
Use: Antihypertensive.
See: Inderide, Tab. (Wyeth-Ayerst Laboratories).

Propranolol Hydrochloride Intensol. (Roxane Laboratories, Inc.) Propranolol HCl 80 mg/ml concentrated oral soln. Bot. 30 ml with dropper. *Rx.*
Use: Beta-adrenergic blocker.

Propulsid. (Janssen Pharmaceutical, Inc.) Cisapride. **Tab.:** 10 mg, 20 mg, lactose. Bot. 100s, 250s (20 mg only), 500s (10 mg only), blister pack 100s. **Susp.:** 1 mg/ml, parabens, sorbitol. Bot. 450 ml. *Rx.*
Use: Gastrointestinal.

•**propyl gallate.** (PRO-pill GAL-ate) N.F. 18.
Use: Pharmaceutic aid (antioxidant).

propyl p-aminobenzoate. (Various Mfr.) Propaesin.
Use: Anesthetic, local.

•**propylene carbonate.** (PRO-pih-leen CAR-boe-nate) N.F. 18.
Use: Pharmaceutic aid (gelling agent).

•**propylene glycol.** U.S.P. 23.
Use: Pharmaceutic aid (humectant, solvent, suspending agent).

•**propylene glycol alginate.** N.F. 18.
Use: Pharmaceutic aid (suspending, viscosity-increasing agent).

•**propylene glycol diacetate.** N.F. 18.
Use: Pharmaceutic aid (solvent).

•**propylene glycol monostearate.** N.F. 18.
Use: Pharmaceutic aid (emulsifying agent).

•**propylhexedrine.** (pro-pill-HEX-ih-dreen) U.S.P. 23.
Use: Adrenergic (vasoconstrictor), appetite suppressant, antihistamine.

•**propyliodone.** (pro-pill-EYE-oh-dohn) U.S.P. 23.
Use: Diagnostic aid (radiopaque medium).
See: Dionosil Oily (GlaxoWellcome).

propylnoradrenaline-iso.
See: Isoproterenol.

•**propylparaben.** (pro-pill-PAR-ah-ben) N.F. 18. Propyl Chemosept (Chemo Puro).
Use: Pharmaceutic aid (antifungal agent).

•**propylparaben sodium.** (pro-pill-PAR-ah-ben) N.F. 18.
Use: Pharmaceutic aid (antimicrobial preservative).

•**propylthiouracil.** (pro-puhl-thigh-oh-YOU-rah-sill) U.S.P. 23.
Use: Antithyroid agent.

propylthiouracil. (Abbott Laboratories) 50 mg/Tab. Bot. 100s, 1000s. (Eli Lilly and Co.) 50 mg/Tab. Bot. 100s, 1000s. (ESI Lederle Generics) 50 mg/Tab. Bot. 100s, 1000s. 50 mg/Tab. Bot. 100s, 1000s, UD 100s.
Use: Antithyroid agent.

•**proquazone.** (PRO-kwah-zone) USAN.
Use: Anti-inflammatory.

•**prorenoate potassium.** (pro-REN-oh-ate) USAN.
Use: Aldosterone antagonist.

Prorone. (Sigma-Tau Pharmaceuticals, Inc.) Progesterone 25 mg/ml. Aqueous or oil susp. Vial 10 ml. *Rx.*
Use: Hormone, progestin.

•**proroxan hydrochloride.** (pro-ROCK-san) USAN. *Formerly Pyrroxane, Pirrousan.*
Use: Antiadrenergic (α-receptor).

Proscar. (Merck & Co.) Finasteride 5 mg/Tab. Unit-of-Use 30s, 100s, UD 100s. *Rx.*

Use: Androgen inhibitor.

•**proscillaridin.** (pro-sih-LARE-ih-din) USAN. Talusin, Tradenal.
Use: Cardiovascular agent.

Prosed/DS. (Star Pharmaceuticals, Inc.) Methenamine 81.6 mg, phenyl salicylate 36.2 mg, methylene blue 10.8 mg, benzoic acid 9 mg, atropine sulfate 0.06 mg, hyoscyamine sulfate 0.06 mg. Tab. Bot. 100s, 1000s. *Rx.*
Use: Anti-infective, urinary.

Pro Skin. (Marlyn Nutraceuticals, Inc.) Vitamins A 6250 IU, E 100 IU, C 100 mg, B_5 10 mg, Zn 10 mg, Se/Cap. Bot, 60s. *otc.*
Use: Mineral, vitamin supplement.

ProSobee. (Bristol-Myers Squibb) Milk free formula supplies 640 cal/qt, protein 19.2 g, fat 34 g, carbohydrate 64 g, vitamins A 2000 IU, D 400 IU, E 20 IU, C 52 mg, folic acid 100 mcg, B_1 0.5 mg, B_2 0.6 mg, niacin 8 mg, B_6 0.4 mg, B_{12} 2 mcg, biotin 50 mg, pantothenic acid 3 mg, K-1 100 mcg, choline 50 mg, inositol 30 mg, Ca 600 mg, P 475 mg, I 65 mcg, Fe 12 mg, Mg 70 mg, Cu 0.6 mg, Zn 5 mg, Mn 1.6 mg, Cl 530 mg, K 780 mg, Na 230 mg/Qt. (20 Kcal/fl oz). Concentrated liq. can 13 fl oz; Ready-to-Use Liq. Can 8 fl oz, 32 fl oz. Pow., Can 14 oz. *otc.*
Use: Nutritional supplement.

ProSobee Concentrate. (Bristol-Myers Squibb) P-soy protein isolate, l-methionine. CHO. corn syrup solids, soy and coconut oil, lecithin, mono- and diglycerides. Protein 20.3 g, CHO 65.4 g, fat 33.6 g, Fe 12 mg, 640 cal./serving. Concentrate 390 ml. *otc.*
Use: Nutritional supplement.

Pro-Sof Plus. (Vangard Labs, Inc.) Docusate sodium 100 mg, casanthranol 30 mg/Cap. Bot. 100s, 1000s, UD 32s, 100s. *otc.*
Use: Laxative.

Pro-Sof w/Casanthranol SG. (Vangard Labs, Inc.) Casanthranol 30 mg, docusate sodium 100 mg/Cap. Bot. 100s, 1000s.
Use: Laxative.

ProSom. (Abbott Laboratories) Estazolam 1 mg, 2 mg/Tab. Bot. 100s, UD 100s. *c-IV.*
Use: Hypnotic, sedative.

prostaglandins.
Use: Abortifacient, agent for impotence, agent for cervical ripening, patent ductus arteriosus.
See: Caverject, Inj. (Pharmacia & Upjohn).
Cervidil, Inj. (Forest Pharmaceutical, Inc.).
Hemabate, Inj. (Pharmacia & Upjohn).
Prepidil, Gel. (Pharmacia & Upjohn).
Prostin E2, Supp. (Pharmacia & Upjohn).
Prostin VR Pediatric, Inj. (Pharmacia & Upjohn).

prostaglandin E_1.
See: Alprostadil.

prostaglandin E_2.
See: Dinoprostone.

•**prostalene.** (PRAHST-ah-leen) USAN.
Use: Prostaglandin.

ProstaScint. (Cytogen) Pendetide 0.5 mg for conjugation w/indium-111. Kit. *Rx.*
Use: Radioimmunoscintigraphy agent.

ProStep. (ESI Lederle Generics) Transdermal nicotine 11 mg, 22 mg/day. Patch 7s. *Rx.*
Use: Smoking deterrent.

Prostigmin. (Zeneca Pharmaceuticals) Injectable neostigmine methylsulfate. **1:1000:** 1 mg/ml w/phenol 0.45%. Vial 10 ml. Box 10s. **1:2000:** 0.5 mg/ml. Amp. 1 ml w/methyl- and propylparabens 0.2%. Box 10s. Vial 10 ml w/phenol 0.45%. Box 10s. **1:4000:** 0.25 mg/ml Amp. 1 ml w/methyl- and propylparabens 0.2%. Box 10s. *Rx.*
Use: Muscle stimulant.

Prostigmin Bromide. (Zeneca Pharmaceuticals) Neostigmine bromide 15 mg/Tab. Bot. 100s, 1000s. *Rx.*
Use: Muscle stimulant.

Prostin E2. (Pharmacia & Upjohn) Dinoprost 20 mg. Supp. Containers of 1 each. *Rx.*
Use: Abortifacient.

Prostin VR Pediatric. (Pharmacia & Upjohn) Alprostadil 500 mcg/ml. Amp. 1 ml. *Rx.*
Use: Arterial patency agent.

Prostonic. (Seatrace Pharmaceuticals, Inc.) Thiamine HCl 10 mg, alanine 130 mg, glutamic acid 130 mg, amino-acetic acid 130 mg/Cap. Bot. 100s. *Rx.*
Use: Palliative relief of benign prostatic hypertrophy.

Protabolin. (Taylor Pharmaceuticals) Methandriol dipropionate 50 mg/ml. Vial 10 ml. *Rx.*
Use: Hormone.

•**protamine sulfate.** (PRO-tuh-meen) U.S.P. 23.
Use: Antidote, heparin.

protamine sulfate. (Eli Lilly and Co.) Amp. 1%, 5 ml; 1s, 25s; 25 ml 6s.
Use: Antidote, heparin.

protargin mild.
See: Silver Protein, Mild (Various Mfr.).

Protargol. (Sterwin) Strong silver protein. Pow. Bot. 25 g. *Rx.*
Use: Antiseptic.

protease.
W/Pancreatin, amylase
See: Dizymes, Cap. (Recsei Laboratories).
W/Vitamins B_1, B_{12}.
See: Arcoret, Tab. (Arco Pharmaceuticals, Inc.).

Protectol Medicated Powder. (Jones Medical Industries, Inc.) Calcium undecylenate 15%. Bot. 2 oz. *otc.*
Use: Diaper rash preparation.

Protegra Softgels. (ESI Lederle Generics) Vitamins E 200 IU, C 250 mg, betacarotene 3 mg, Zn 7.5 mg, Cu, Se, Mn. Cap. Bot. 50s. *otc.*
Use: Vitamin supplement.

proteinase inhibitor, alpha 1.
See: Prolastin (Bayer Corp. (Consumer Div.)).

protein c concentrate.
Use: Protein C deficiency. [Orphan Drug]

•**protein hydrolysate injection.** U.S.P. 23.
Use: Fluid, nutrient replacement.
See: Amigen, Inj. (Baxter Healthcare Hyland/Immuno Division).
Aminogen, Amp., Vial (Christina).
Lacotein, Vial (Christina).

protein hydrolysates oral.
Use: Enteral nutritional supplement.
See: Lofenalac, Pow. (Bristol-Myers Squibb).
Nutramigen, Pow. (Bristol-Myers Squibb).
Pregestimil, Pow. (Bristol-Myers Squibb).
Stuart Amino Acids, Pow. (Zeneca Pharmaceuticals).
W/Vitamin B_{12}.
See: Stuart Amino Acids and B_{12}, Tab. (Zeneca Pharmaceuticals).

Protenate. (Baxter Pharmaceutical Products, Inc.) Plasma protein fraction (Human) 5%. Inj. Vial 250 ml, 500 ml w/ administration set. *Rx.*
Use: Plasma protein fraction.
See: Arco-Lase, Tab. (Arco Pharmaceuticals, Inc.).
Kutrase, Cap. (Schwarz Pharma).
Ku-Zyme, Cap. (Schwarz Pharma).
See: Arco-Lipase Plus, Tab. (Arco Pharmaceuticals, Inc.).

Prothers. (ICN Pharmaceuticals, Inc.) Soap Free. White petrolatum, disodium cocamido MIPA-sulfosuccinate, pentane, ammonium laureth sulfate, PEG-150 distearate, hydroxypropyl methylcellulose, imidazolidinyl urea, parabens, propylene glycol stearate, hydrogenated soy glyceride, sodium stearyl lactylate. Liq. Bot. 180 ml. *otc.*
Use: Dermatologic, cleanser.

prothipendyl hydrochloride.
Use: Sedative.

Proticuleen. (Spanner) Vitamin B_{12} activity 10 mcg, folic acid 10 mg, B_{12} crystalline 50 mcg, niacinamide 75 mg/ml. Multiple-dose vial 10 ml. IM Inj. *Rx.*
Use: Nutritional supplement, parenteral.

•**protirelin.** (PRO-tie-reh-lin) USAN. *Formerly Lopremone.*
Use: Prothyrotropin.
See: Thypinone, Inj. (Abbott Laboratories).

protirelin. (UCB Pharmaceuticals, Inc.)
Use: Diagnostic aid, thyroid. [Orphan Drug]

Protopam Chloride. (Wyeth-Ayerst Laboratories) **Hospital package:** Six 20 ml vials of 1 g each of sterile Protopam Cl powder, without diluent or syringe. *Rx.*
Use: Antidote.

Protosan. (Recsei Laboratories) Protein 87.5%, lactose 0.5%, fat 1.3%, ash 3.5%, Na 0.02%. Jar 1 lb, 5 lb. *otc.*
Use: Nutritional supplement.

Prot-O-Sea. (Barth's) Protein 90%, containing amino acids and minerals. Bot. 100s, 500s. *otc.*
Use: Nutritional supplement.

Protostat. (Ortho McNeil Pharmaceutical) Metronidazole 250 mg, 500 mg/Tab. **250 mg:** Bot. 100s. **500 mg:** Bot. 50s. *Rx.*
Use: Anti-infective.

Protran Plus. (Vangard Labs, Inc.) Meprobamate 150 mg, ethoheptazine citrate 75 mg, aspirin 250 mg/Tab. Bot. 100s. 500s. *Rx.*
Use: Analgesic, anxiolytic combination.

•**protriptyline hydrochloride.** (pro-TRIP-tih-leen) U.S.P. 23.
Use: Antidepressant.
See: Vivactil, Tab. (Merck & Co.).

Protropin. (Genentech, Inc.) Somatrem. Vial 5 mg (13 IU), 10 mg (26 IU). Contains 2 vials somatrem and 2 vials 10 ml diluent. *Rx.*
Use: Hormone, growth.

Protuss. (Horizon Pharmaceutical Corp.) Hydrocodone bitartrate 5 mg, potassium guaiacolsulfonate 300 mg/5 ml, saccharin, sorbitol. Alcohol free. Liq. Bot. 20 ml, 120 ml, 480 ml. *c-III.*
Use: Antitussive, expectorant.

Protuss-D. (Horizon Pharmaceutical Corp.) Hydrocodone bitartrate 5 mg,

pseudoephedrine HCl 30 mg, potassium guaiacolsulfonate 300 mg/5 ml. Alcohol free, dye free. Liq. Bot. 120 ml, 480 ml. *c-III.*
Use: Antitussive, decongestant, expectorant.

Protuss DM. (Horizon Pharmaceutical Corp.) Guaifenesin 600 mg, pseudoephedrine HCl 60 mg, dextromethorphan HBr 30 mg. Tab. and SR Tab. Bot. 14s, 100s. *Rx.*
Use: Antitussive, decongestant, expectorant.

Proval #3. (Horizon Pharmaceutical Corp.) Guaifenesin 600 mg, pseudoephedrine HCl 60 mg, dextromethorphan HBr 30 mg. Tab. Bot. 14s, 100s. *c-III.*
Use: Analgesic combination, narcotic.

Proventil. (Schering-Plough Corp.) Albuterol sulfate 2 mg, 4 mg/Tab. Bot. 100s, 500s. *Rx.*
Use: Bronchodilator.

Proventil HFA. (Key Pharmaceuticals) Albuterol 90 mcg/actuation. Aer. Can. 6.7 g/(200 inhalations). *Rx.*
Use: Bronchodilator.

Proventil Inhaler. (Schering-Plough Corp.) Albuterol 90 mcg/actuation. Aer. Canister 17 (≥ 200 inhalations). *Rx.*
Use: Bronchodilator.

Proventil Repetabs. (Schering-Plough Corp.) Albuterol sulfate 4 mg, lactose/ ER Tab. Bot. 100s, 500s, UD 100s. *Rx.*
Use: Bronchodilator.

Proventil Solution. (Schering-Plough Corp.) Albuterol sulfate 0.083%, 0.5%. Soln. for Inh. Bot. 3 ml (0.083%), 20 ml w/dropper (0.5%). *Rx.*
Use: Bronchodilator.

Proventil Syrup. (Schering-Plough Corp.) Albuterol sulfate 2 mg/5 ml. Bot. 480 ml. *Rx.*
Use: Bronchodilator.

Provera. (Pharmacia & Upjohn) Medroxyprogesterone acetate 2.5 mg, 5 mg, 10 mg/Tab. Bot. 30s, 100s; 500s, UD 10s (10 mg only). *Rx.*
Use: Hormone, progestin.

Provigil. (Cephalon) Modafinil 100 mg, 200 mg. Tab. Bot. 100s. *Rx.*
Use: Analeptic.

Provocholine. (Roche Laboratories) Methacholine Cl for inhalation 100 mg/ 5 ml for reconstitution. Vial 5 ml. *Rx.*
Use: Diagnostic aid.

Prox/APAP. (Forest Pharmaceutical, Inc.) Propoxyphene HCl 65 mg, acetaminophen 650 mg/Tab. Bot. 100s, 500s. *c-IV.*
Use: Analgesic combination, narcotic.

•**proxazole.** (PROX-ah-zole) USAN.
Use: Analgesic, anti-inflammatory, muscle relaxant.

•**proxazole citrate.** (PROX-ah-zole) USAN.
Use: Relaxant (smooth muscle), analgesic, anti-inflammatory.

•**proxicromil.** (prox-ih-KROE-mill) USAN.
Use: Antiallergic.

Proxigel. (Schwarz Pharma, Inc.) Carbamide peroxide 10% in a water-free gel base. Tube 34 g w/applicator. *otc.*
Use: Antiseptic, cleanser.

•**proxorphan tartrate.** (PROX-ahr-fan TAR-trate) USAN.
Use: Analgesic; antitussive.

Proxy 65. (Parmed Pharmaceuticals, Inc.) Propoxyphene HCl 65 mg, acetaminophen 650 mg/Tab. Bot. 100s, 500s. *c-IV.*
Use: Narcotic analgesic combination.

Prozac. (Eli Lilly and Co.) Fluoxetine HCl. **Pulvules:** 10 mg, 20 mg. Bot. 30s (20 mg only), 100s, 2000s, UD 31s, 100s (20 mg only). **Oral Soln.:** 20 mg/5 ml Bot. 120 ml. *Rx.*
Use: Antidepressant.

Prudents. (Bariatric) Acetylphenylisatin 5 mg. Chewable protein and amino acid. Tab. Bot. 30s, 100s. *otc.*
Use: Laxative.

Prulet. (Mission Pharmacal Co.) White phenolphthalein 60 mg/Tab. Strips 12s, 40s. *otc.*
Use: Laxative.

prune powder concentrated dehydrated.
See: Diacetyldihydroxyphenylisatin.

Prurilo. (Whorton Pharmaceuticals, Inc.) Menthol 0.25%, phenol 0.25%, calamine lotion in special lubricating base. Bot. 4 oz, 8 oz. *otc.*
Use: Dermatologic, counterirritant.

Pseudo-Car DM. (Geneva Pharmaceuticals) Pseudoephedrine HCl 60 mg, carbinoxamine maleate 4 mg, dextromethorphan HBr 15 mg/5 ml, alcohol < 0.6%. Bot. Pt, gal. *Rx.*
Use: Antihistamine, antitussive, decongestant.

Pseudo-Chlor. (Various Mfr.) Pseudoephedrine HCl 120 mg, chlorpheniramine maleate 8 mg/Cap. Bot. 100s, 250s. *Rx.*
Use: Antihistamine, decongestant.

•**pseudoephedrine hydrochloride.** (SUE-doe-eh-FED-rin) U.S.P. 23.
Use: Adrenergic (vasoconstrictor).
See: Allerest No Drowsiness, Tab. (Novartis Pharmaceutical Corp.).

Anatuss DM, Syr. (Merz Pharmaceutcials).
Aspirin-Free Cayer Select Head & Chest Cold, Capl. (Bayer Corp. (Allergy Div.)).
Benylin Multi-Symptom, Liq. (GlaxoWellcome).
Bromfenex, ER Cap. (Ethex Corp.).
Cenafed, Tab., Syr. (Century Pharmaceuticals, Inc.).
Children's Silfedrine, Liq. (Silarx Pharmaceuticals, Inc.).
Claritin, Prods. (Schering-Plough Corp.).
Coldrine, Tab. (Roberts Pharmaceuticals).
Cycofed Pediatric, Syr. (Cypress Pharmaceutical, Inc.).
Dynafed Pseudo, Tab. (Novartis Pharmaceutical Corp.).
Efidac/24, Tab. (Novartis Pharmaceutical Corp.).
Iofed, ER Cap. (Iomed).
Mini Thin Pseudo, Tab. (BDI Pharmaceuticals, Inc.).
Pseudo, Tab. (Novartis Pharmaceutical Corp.).
Ornex No Drowsiness, Tab. (Menley & James).
Sildec-DM (Silarx).
Sinufed, Cap. (Roberts Pharmaceuticals).
Sinus Relief, Tab. (Major Pharmaceuticals).
Sudafed, Tab, Syr. (GlaxoWellcome).
Sudafed SA, Cap. (GlaxoWellcome).
Sudal, Prods. (Alley Pharm.).
Triaminic AM Decongestant Formula, Syr. (Novartis Pharmaceutical Corp.).
Ursinus, Inlay Tab. (Novartis Pharmaceutical Corp.).

pseudoephedrine hydrochloride w/ combinations.

See: Actifed, Tab., Syr. (GlaxoWellcome).
Actifed Allergy, Cap. (GlaxoWellcome).
Alka-Seltzer Plus & Sinus (Bayer Corp. (Consumer Div.)).
Allegra-D (Hoechst Marion Roussel).
Allerest No Drowsiness (Norvartis Pharmaceutical Corp.).
Ambenyl-D, Liq. (Hoechst Marion Roussel).
Anatuss DM, Syr., Tab. (Merz Pharmaceuticals).
Aspirin-Free Bayer Select Head & Chest Cold, Capl. (Bayer Corp. (Allergy Div.)).
Atridine, Tab. (Henry Schein, Inc.).
Banophen Decongestant (Major).
Benylin Multi-Symptom, Liq. (GlaxoWellcome).
Biohist-LA (Wakefield).
Brexin, Cap., Liq. (Savage Laboratories).
Bromadine-DM, Syr. (Cypress Pharmaceutical, Inc.).
Bromfenex (Ethex Corp.).
Carbinoxamine, Prods. (Morton Grove Pharmaceuticals, Inc.).
Children's Cēpacol (J.B. Williams).
Children's Tylenol Cold Plus Cough (Ortho McNeil Pharmaceuticals).
Claritin-D (Schering).
Coldrine (Roberts Pharmaceuticals).
Congestac, Tab. (SmithKline Beecham Pharmaceuticals).
Cycofed Pediatric, Syr. (Cypress Pharmaceutical, Inc.).
Deconamine, Cap., Tab., Elix., Syr. (Berlex Laboratories, Inc.).
Deconsal Pediatric, Syr. (Medeva Pharmaceuticals, Inc.).
Defen-LA, SR Tab. (Horizon Pharmaceutical Corp.).
Dimacol, Cap., Liq. (Wyeth-Ayerst Laboratories).
Dorcol, Prods. (Novartis Pharmaceutical Corp.).
Drixomed, SR Tab. (Iomed).
Fedahist Expectorant (Schwarz Pharma, Inc.).
Guaifenesin DAC, Liq. (Cypress Pharmaceutical, Inc.).
Guaifenex Preps. (Ethex Corp.).
Guiatex PSE, Tab. (Rugby Labs, Inc.).
Guaivent, Cap. (Ethex Corp.).
Guaivent PD, Cap. (Ethex Corp.).
Guai-Vent/PSE, SR Tab. (Dura).
Histinex-D (Ethex Corp.).
Histinex PV, Syr. (Ethex Corp.).
Histussin D, Liq. (Sanofi Winthrop Pharmaceuticals).
H-Tuss-D, Liq. (Cypress Pharmaceutical, Inc.).
Hyphed (Cypress Pharm).
Iofed (Iomed).
Iosal II, ER Tab. (Iomed).
Isoclor, Preps. (Du Pont Merck Pharmaceutical Co.).
Kronofed-A, Cap. (Ferndale Laboratories, Inc.).
Mapap Cold Formula, Tab. (Major Pharmaceuticals).
Maximum Strength Dynafed Plus (BDI).
Maximum Strength Tylenol Flu, Tab. (McNeil Consumer Products Co.).
MED-Rx, CR. Tab. (Iomed).
Mescolor (Horizon).

Multi-Symptom Tylenol Cough with Decongestant, Liq. (Ortho McNeil Pharmaceuticals).
Nasabid, PA Cap. (Jones Medical Industries, Inc.).
Nasbid Sr, LA Tab. (Jones Medical Industries, Inc.).
Nasatab LA, LA Tab. (ECR Pharmaceuticals).
Night Time Cold/Flu Relief (Prometic Pharma).
Novahistine Sinus, Tab. (Hoechst Marion Roussel).
Ornex No Drowsiness (Menley & James).
Pancof-HC, Liq. (Pan American Labs).
Panmist JR, LA Tab. (Pan American Labs).
Phenergan-D, Tab. (Wyeth-Ayerst Laboratories).
Protuss-D, Liq. (Horizon Pharmaceutical Corp.).
Protuss DM, Tab. (Horizon Pharmaceutical Corp.).
Respa-1st, SR Tab. (Respa Pharmaceuticals, Inc.).
Robitussin Cold & Cough, Cap. (Wyeth-Ayerst Laboratories).
Robitussin-DAC, Liq. (Wyeth-Ayerst Laboratories).
Robitussin-PE, Liq. (Wyeth-Ayerst Laboratories).
Robitussin Severe Congestion, Cap. (Wyeth-Ayerst Laboratories).
Rondec D (Dura).
Rondec DM, Drops, Syr. (Dura)
Sine-Aid IB, Cap. (McNeil Consumer Products Co.).
Sine-Off, Prods. (SmithKline Beecham Pharmaceuticals).
Sinus Relief (Major Pharmaceuticals).
Sinutab Non-Drying, Cap., Liq. (GlaxoWellcome).
Sudafed Plus, Tab. Syr. (GlaxoWellcome).
Sudal, Prods. (Atley Pharmaceuticals, Inc.).
Syn-Rx, CR Tab. (Medeva Pharmaceuticals, Inc.).
Touro LA, LA Capl. (Dartmouth).
Triaminic AM Cough & Decongestant Formula, Liq. (Novartis Pharmaceutical Corp.).
Tussafed Expectorant Liq. (Cavital).
Tussend, Syr. (Monarch Pharmaceuticals).
Tylenol Cold Night Time, Liq. (McNeil Consumer Products Co.).
Tyrodone, Liq. (Major Pharmaceuticals).
Vicks 44D Cough & Head Congestion, Liq. (Procter & Gamble Pharm.).
Vicks NyQuil Multi-Symptom Cold Flu Relief, Liq. (Procter & Gamble Pharm.).

pseudoephedrine hydrochloride and triprolidine hydrochloride. (Various Mfr.) Pseudoephedrine HCl 60 mg, triprolidine HCl 2.5 mg/Tab. Bot. 100s, 1000s, UD 100s. *Rx.*
Use: Antihistamine, decongestant.

•**pseudoephedrine polistirex.** (sue-doe-ee-FED-rin pahl-ee-STIE-rex) USAN.
Use: Decongestant, nasal.

•**pseudoephedrine sulfate.** (sue-do-eh-FED-rin) U.S.P. 23.
Use: Bronchodilator.
See: Afrinol Repetabs (Schering-Plough Corp.).
W/Chlorpheniramine maleate.
See: Chlor-trimeton Decongestant, Tab. (Schering-Plough Corp.).
W/Dexbrompheniramine.
See: Disophrol Chronotabs, Tab. (Schering-Plough Corp.).
Drixoral S.A., Tab. (Schering-Plough Corp.).
W/Dexchlorpheniramine.
See: Polaramine Expectorant (Schering-Plough Corp.).

pseudoephedrine tannate w/combinations.
See: Tanafed (Horizon).

Pseudo-Gest. (Major Pharmaceuticals) Pseudoephedrine HCl 30 mg, 60 mg/Tab. Bot. 24s, 100s. *otc.*
Use: Decongestant.

Pseudo-Gest Plus. (Major Pharmaceuticals) Pseudoephedrine HCl 60 mg, chlorpheniramine maleate 4 mg/Tab. Bot. 24s, 100s, 200s. *otc.*
Use: Antihistamine, decongestant.

Pseudo-Hist. (Holloway) Pseudoephedrine HCl 30 mg, chlorpheniramine maleate 10 mg/Cap. Bot. 100s. *otc.*
Use: Antihistamine, decongestant.

Pseudo-Hist Expectorant. (Holloway) Pseudoephedrine 15 mg, hydrocodone bitartrate 2.5 mg, guaifenesin 100 mg, alcohol 5%. Bot. 480 ml. *c-III.*
Use: Antitussive, decongestant, expectorant.

pseudomonas hyperimmune globulin (mucoid exopolysaccharide).
Use: Pulmonary infection in cystic fibrosis. [Orphan Drug]

pseudomonas test.
Use: Urine test.
See: Isocult for *Pseudomonas aeruginosa* (SmithKline Diagnostics).

pseudomonic acid A.

Use: Anti-infective, topical.
See: Bactroban (SmithKline Beecham Pharmaceuticals).

Pseudo-Phedrine. (Whiteworth Towne) Pseudoephedrine HCl 30 mg/Tab. Bot. 100s, 1000s. *otc.*
Use: Decongestant.

Pseudo Plus. (Weeks & Leo) Pseudoephedrine HCl 60 mg, chlorpheniramine maleate 4 mg/Tab. Bot. 40s. *otc.*
Use: Antihistamine, decongestant.

Pseudo Syrup. (Major Pharmaceuticals) Pseudoephedrine 30 mg/5 ml. Liq. Bot. 120 ml, pt, gal. *otc.*
Use: Decongestant.

psoralens.
See: Methoxsalen.
Trioxsalen.

Psor-a-set. (Hogil Pharmaceutical Corp.) Salicylic acid 2%. Soap. Bar 97.5 g. *otc.*
Use: Keratolytic.

Psorcon. (Dermik Laboratories, Inc.) Diflorasone diacetate (0.05%) 0.5 mg/g. **Oint.**: Tube 15 g, 30 g, 60 g. **Cream:** Tube 15 g, 30 g, 60 g. *Rx.*
Use: Corticosteroid, topical.

PsoriGel. (Galderma Laboratories, Inc.) Coal tar soln. 7.5%, alcohol 33% in hydroalcoholic gel vehicle. Tube 4 oz. *otc.*
Use: Dermatologic.

Psorinail. (Summers Laboratories, Inc.) Coal tar solution w/isopropyl alcohol 2.5%, 3-butylene glycol I, acetyl mandelic acid. Liq. Bot. 30 ml. *otc.*
Use: Antipsoriatic, topical.

Psorion. (ICN Pharmaceuticals, Inc.) Betamethasone dipropionate 0.05%, mineral oil, white petrolatum, propylene glycol. Cream Tube 15 g, 45 g. *Rx.*
Use: Corticosteroid, topical.

psychotherapeutic agents.
See: Tranquilizers.

psyllium granules.
Use: Laxative.
See: Perdiem Fiber, Gran. (Rhone-Poulenc Rorer Pharmaceuticals, Inc.).
W/Dextrose.
See: Muci-lax, Gran. (Shionogi USA).
W/Senna.
See: Perdiem, Gran. (Rhone-Poulenc Rorer Pharmaceuticals, Inc.).

•**psyllium husk.** (SILL-ee-uhm husk) U.S.P. 23.
Use: Laxative, cathartic.

psyllium hydrocolloid.
Use: Laxative.

psyllium hydrophilic mucilloid for oral suspension.
Use: Laxative.
See: Konsyl, Pow. (Lafayette Pharmaceuticals, Inc.).
Modane Versabran, Pow. (Pharmacia & Upjohn).
Mucillium, Pow. (Whiteworth Towne).
Mylanta Natural Fiber Supplement, Pow. (J & J Merck Consumer Pharm.).
Restore (Inagra).
W/Dextrose.
See: Hydrocil Plain (Solvay Pharmaceuticals).
Konsyl-D Pow. (Lafayette Pharmaceuticals, Inc.).
V-lax, Pow. (Century Pharmaceuticals, Inc.).
W/Dextrose, casanthranol.
See: Hydrocil Fortified (Solvay Pharmaceuticals).
W/Oxyphenisatin acetate.
See: Plova, Pow. (WEL).
W/Standardized senna concentrate.
See: Senokot w/Psyllium, Pow. (Purdue Frederick Co).

psyllium seed gel.
Use: Laxative.

PTE-4. (Fujisawa USA, Inc.) Zn 1 mg, Cu 0.1 mg, CR 1 mcg, Mn 25 mcg/ml. Vial 3 ml. *Rx.*
Use: Mineral supplement.

PTE-5. (Fujisawa USA, Inc.) Zn 1 mg, Cu 0.1 mg, Cr 1 mcg, Mn 25 mcg, Se 15 mcg/ml. Vial 3 ml, 10 ml. *Rx.*
Use: Mineral supplement.

pteroic acid. The compound formed by the linkage of carbon 6 of 2-amine-4-hydroxypteridine by means of a methylene group with the nitrogen of p-aminobenzoic acid.

pteroylglutamic acid.
See: Folic Acid, Preps. (Various Mfr.).

pteroylmonoglutamic acid. Pteroylglutamic acid.
See: Folic Acid, Preps. (Various Mfr.).

PTFE. (Ethicon, Inc.) Polytef.

PTU.
See: Propylthiouracil.

Pulmicort Turbuhaler. (Astra Pharmaceuticals, L.P.) Budesonide 200 mcg (≈ 160 mcg per metered dose). Pow. *Turbuhaler* 200 doses. **:** *Rx.*
Use: Respiratory inhalant.

Pulmocare. (Ross Laboratories) High-fat, low-carbohydrate liquid diet for pulmonary patients containing 1500 calories/L; 1420 calories provides 100% US RDA vitamins and minerals. Cal/Nitrogen ratio is 150:1. Osmolarity: 490 mOsm/kg water. Can 8 fl oz. *otc.*
Use: Nutritional supplement.

pulmonary surfactant replacement. (Scios Nova, Inc.)
Use: Diagnostic aid, thyroid. [Orphan Drug]

pulmonary surfactant replacement, porcine.
Use: Diagnostic aid, thyroid. [Orphan Drug]
See: Curosurf.

Pulmosin. (Spanner) Guaiacol 0.1 g, eucalyptol 0.08 g, camphor 0.05 g, iodoform 0.02 g/2 ml. Multiple-dose vial 30 ml. IM. Inj. *Rx.*

Pulmozyme. (Genentech, Inc.) Dornase alfa 1 mg, calcium chloride dihydrate 0.15 mg, NaCl 8.77 mg/ml. Soln. for Inh. Amps. Single-use 2.5 ml. *Rx.*
Use: Anti-infective.

•**pumice.** (PUM-iss) U.S.P. 23.
Use: Abrasive (dental).

punctum plug. (Eagle Vision, Inc.) Silicone plug. 0.5 mm, 0.6 mm, 0.7 mm, 0.8 mm. Pkg. 2 plugs, one inserter tool. *Rx.*
Use: Punctal plug.

Pura. (D'Franssia Corp.) High-potency vitamin E cream.
Use: Emollient.

Puralube. (E. Fougera and Co.) White petrolatum, light mineral oil. Oint. Tube 3.5 g. *otc.*
Use: Lubricant, ophthalmic.

Puralube Tears. (E. Fougera and Co.) Polyvinyl alcohol 1%, polyethylene glycol 400 1%, EDTA, benzalkonium Cl. Soln. Bot. 15 ml. *otc.*
Use: Lubricant, ophthalmic.

Purebrom Compound Elixir. (Purepac Pharmaceutical Co.) Brompheniramine maleate 4 mg/5 ml, phenylephrine HCl, phenylpropanolamine HCl, alcohol. Bot. Pt, gal. *Rx.*
Use: Antihistamine, decongestant.

Puresept Murine Saline. (Ross Laboratories) **Disinfecting soln.:** Sterile hydrogen peroxide solution 3%, sodium stannate, sodium nitrate, phosphate buffers, thimerosal free. 237 ml. **Murine Saline Soln.:** Buffered isotonic solution w/borate buffers, NaCl, sorbic acid 0.1%, EDTA 0.1%. 60, 237, 355 ml. Includes cups and lens holder. *otc.*
Use: Contact lens care.

Purge Evacuant. (Fleming & Co.) Castor oil 95%. Bot. 1 oz, 2 oz. *otc.*
Use: Laxative.

Puri-Clens. (Sween) UD 2 oz. Bot. 8 oz.
Use: Dermatologic, wound therapy.

purified oxgall.
See: Bile Extract, Ox (Various Mfr.).

purified protein derivative of tuberculin.
Use: Mantoux TB test.
See: Aplisol, Vial (Parke-Davis).
Aplitest, Jar (Parke-Davis).
Tubersol, Vial (Pasteur Merieux Connaught).

purified type II collagen.
Use: Juvenile rheumatoid arthritis. [Orphan Drug]

Purinethol. (GlaxoWellcome) Mercaptopurine 50 mg/Tab. Bot. 25s, 250s. *Rx.*
Use: Antineoplastic.

•**puromycin.** (PURE-oh-MY-sin) USAN.
Use: Antineoplastic; antiprotozoal (trypanosoma).

•**puromycin hydrochloride.** (PURE-oh-MY-sin) USAN.
Use: Antineoplastic; antiprotozoal (trypanosoma).

purple foxglove.
See: Digitalis, Preps. (Various Mfr.).

Purpose Shampoo. (Advanced Care Products) Water, amphoteric-19, PEG-44 sorbitan laurate, PEG-150 distearate, sorbitan laurate, boric acid, fragrance, benzyl alcohol. Bot. 8 oz. *otc.*
Use: Dermatologic.

Purpose Soap. (Johnson & Johnson) Sodium tallowate, sodium cocoate, glycerin, NaCl, BHT, EDTA. Bar 108 g, 180 g. *otc.*
Use: Dermatologic, cleanser.

Pursettes Premenstrual Tablets. (DEP Corp.) Acetaminophen 500 mg, pamabrom 25 mg, pyrilamine maleate 15 mg/Tab. Bot. 24s. *otc.*
Use: Analgesic, antihistamine, diuretic.

P.V. Carpine Liquifilm. (Allergan, Inc.) Pilocarpine nitrate 1%, 2%, 4%, polyvinyl alcohol 1.4%, sodium acetate, sodium Cl, citric acid, menthol, camphor, phenol, eucalyptol, chlorobutanol 0.5%, purified water. Dropper Bot. 15 ml. *Rx.*
Use: Antiglaucoma agent.

PVP-I Ointment. (Day-Baldwin) Povidone-iodine. Tube 1 oz, Jar lb, Foilpac 1.5 g. *otc.*
Use: Antiseborrheic, antiseptic.

P-V-Tussin Syrup. (Solvay Pharmaceuticals) Hydrocodone bitartrate 2.5 mg, pseudoephedrine HCl 30 mg, chlorpheniramine maleate 2 mg/5 ml, alcohol 5%. Bot. Pt, gal. *c-III.*
Use: Antihistamine, antitussive, decongestant.

P-V-Tussin Tablets. (Solvay Pharmaceuticals) Hydrocodone bitartrate 5 mg, phenindamine tartrate 25 mg, guaifenesin 200 mg/Tab. Bot. 100s. *c-III.*
Use: Antihistamine, antitussive, expectorant.

Py-Co-Pay Tooth Powder. (Block Drug Co., Inc.) Sodium Cl, sodium bicarbonate, calcium carbonate, magnesium carbonate, tricalcium phosphate, euge-

nol, methyl salicylate. Can 7 oz. *otc.*
Use: Dentifrice.

9-[3-pydidylmethyl]-9-deazaguanine. (Briocryst Pharm)
Use: Antineoplastic. [Orphan Drug]

Pyma. (Forest Pharmaceutical, Inc.) **TR Cap.:** Pyrilamine maleate 50 mg, chlorpheniramine maleate 6 mg, pheniramine maleate 20 mg, phenylephrine HCl 15 mg. Bot. 30s, 100s, 1000s. **Inj.:** Chlorpheniramine maleate 5 mg, phenylpropanolamine HCl 12.5 mg, atropine sulfate 0.2 mg/ml. Vial 10 ml. *Rx.*
Use: Anticholinergic, antihistamine, antispasmodic, decongestant.

Pyocidin-Otic Solution. (Forest Pharmaceutical, Inc.) Hydrocortisone 5 mg, polymyxin B sulfate 10,000 USP units/ml in a vehicle containing water and propylene glycol. Bot. 10 ml w/sterile dropper. *Rx.*
Use: Anti-infective, corticosteroid, otic.

•**pyrabrom.** (PEER-ah-brahm) USAN.
Use: Antihistamine.

Pyracol. (Davis & Sly) Pyrathyn HCl 0.08 g, ammonium Cl 0.778 g, citric acid 0.52 g, menthol 0.006 g/fl oz. Bot. pt.

pyradone.
See: Aminopyrine (Various Mfr.).

pyraminyl.
See: Pyrilamine Maleate (Various Mfr.).

pyranilamine maleate.
See: Pyrilamine Maleate, Preps. (Various Mfr.).

pyranisamine bromotheophyllinate.
See: Pyrabrom (Various Mfr.).

pyranisamine maleate.
See: Pyrilamine Maleate, Preps. (Various Mfr.).

•**pyrantel pamoate.** (pie-RAN-tell PAM-oh-ate) U.S.P. 23.
Use: Anthelmintic.
See: Antiminth, Oral Susp. (Pfizer US Pharmaceutical Group).
Pin-Rid, Cap., Liq. (Apothecary Products, Inc.).
Pin-X, Liq. (Effcon Labs, Inc).

•**pyrantel tartrate.** (pie-RAN-tell) USAN.
Use: Anthelmintic.

•**pyrazinamide.** (peer-uh-ZIN-uh-mide) U.S.P. 23. Aldinamide, Zinamide.
Use: Anti-infective, tuberculostatic.

pyrazinamide. (ESI Lederle Generics) 500 mg/Tab. Bot. 500s.
Use: Anti-infective, tuberculostatic.

pyrazinecarboxamide. U.S.P. 23. Pyrazinamide.

•**pyrazofurin.** (pihr-AZZ-oh-FYOO-rin) USAN.
Use: Antineoplastic.

pyrazoline.
See: Antipyrine (Various Mfr.).

pyrbenzindole.
See: Benzindopyrine Hydrochloride (Various Mfr.).

•**pyrethrum extract.** U.S.P. 23.
Use: Pediculicide.

pyribenzamine.
See: PBZ, Prods. (Novartis Pharmaceutical Corp.).

Pyridamole. (Major Pharmaceuticals) Dipyridamole 25 mg, 50 mg, 75 mg/Tab. **25 mg:** Bot. 1000s, 2500s. **50 mg, 75 mg:** 100s, 1000s. *Rx.*
Use: Antianginal, antiplatelet.

Pyridate. (Major Pharmaceuticals) Phenazopyridine 100 mg, 200 mg/Tab. Bot. 1000s. *Rx.*
Use: Analgesic, anti-infective, urinary.

Pyridene. (Health for Life Brands, Inc.) Phenylazo Diamino Pyridine HCl 100 mg/Tab. Bot. 24s, 100s, 1000s. *Rx.*
Use: Analgesic, urinary.

Pyridium. (Warner Chilcott Laboratories) Phenazopyridine HCl 100 mg, 200 mg/Tab. Bot. 100s, 1000s, UD 100s. *Rx.*
Use: Analgesic, anti-infective, urinary.
W/Hyoscyamine HBr, butabarbital.
See: Pyridium Plus, Tab. (Parke-Davis).

•**pyridostigmine bromide.** (pihr-id-oh-STIG-meen BROE-mide) U.S.P. 23.
Use: Cholinergic.
See: Mestinon, Tab., Syr., Amp. (Roche Laboratories).
Regonol (Organon Teknika Corp.).

Pyridox. (Oxford) **No. 1:** Pyridoxine HCl 100 mg/Tab. **No. 2:** Pyridoxine HCl 200 mg/Tab. Bot. 100s. *otc.*
Use: Vitamin supplement.

pyridoxal. Vitamin B_6. *otc.*
Use: Vitamin supplement.

pyridoxamine. Vitamin B_6. *otc.*
Use: Vitamin supplement.
See: Pyridoxine.

•**pyridoxine hydrochloride.** (peer-ih-DOX-een) U.S.P. 23.
Use: Enzyme co-factor vitamin.
See: Hexa Betalin, Amp., Tab., Vial (Eli Lilly and Co.).
Pan B_6, Tab. (Panray).

pyridoxol.
See: Pyridoxine, Vitamin B_6.

pyrilamine bromotheophyllinate.
See: Bromaleate.
Pyrabrom.

pyrilamine maleate w/combinations.
See: Iohist D (Iomed).
Statuss Green (Huckaby).
Tri-P Oral Infant Drops (Cypress Pharm.).

Vetuss HC (Cypress Pharm.).

•**pyrimethamine.** (pihr-ih-METH-ah-meen) U.S.P. 23.
Use: Antimalarial.
See: Daraprim, Tab. (GlaxoWellcome).
W/Sulfadoxine.
See: Fansidar, Tab. (Roche Laboratories).

Pyrinex Pediculicide. (Ambix Laboratories, Inc.) Pyrethrins 0.2%, piperonyl butoxide technical 2%, deodorized kerosene 0.8%. Shampoo. Bot. 118 ml. *otc.*
Use: Pediculicide.

•**pyrinoline.** (PIHR-ih-NO-leen) USAN.
Use: Cardiovascular agent, antiarrhythmic.

pyrinyl. (Various Mfr.) Pyrethrins 0.2%, piperonyl butoxide technical 2%, deodorized kerosene 0.8%. Liq. Bot. 60, 120 ml. *otc.*
Use: Pediculicide.

Pyristan. (Arcum) Phenylephrine HCl 8 mg, phenylpropanolamine HCl 15 mg, chlorpheniramine maleate 3 mg, pyrilamine maleate 10 mg/Cap. Bot. 50s, 500s. Elix. Bot. 4 oz, pt, gal. *otc.*
Use: Antihistamine, decongestant.

pyrithen.
See: Chlorothen Citrate (Various Mfr.).

•**pyrithione sodium.** (PEER-ih-THIGH-ohn) USAN.
Use: Antimicrobial, topical.

•**pyrithione zinc.** (PEER-ih-THIGH-ohn zingk) USAN. Zinc Omadine.
Use: Antifungal, anti-infective, antiseborrheic.
See: Zincon Shampoo (ESI Lederle Generics).

Pyrogallic Acid. (Gordon Laboratories) Pyrogallic acid 25%, chlorobutanol. Oint. Jar 1 oz, 1 lb.
Use: Dermatologic, wart therapy.

pyrogallol. Pyrogallic acid.

Pyrohep Tabs. (Major Pharmaceuticals) Cyproheptadine HCl 4 mg/Tab. Bot. 250s, 500s. *Rx.*
Use: Antihistamine.

pyrophenindane. (Bristol-Myers Squibb)

•**pyrovalerone hydrochloride.** (PIE-row-val-EH-rone) USAN.
Use: Central stimulant.

•**pyroxamine maleate.** (pihr-OX-ah-meen) USAN.
Use: Antihistamine.

•**pyroxylin.** (pihr-OX-ih-lin) U.S.P. 23. Soluble gun cotton. Cellulose nitrate.
Use: Pharmaceutic necessity for Collodion.

pyrrobutamine phosphate. U.S.P. XXI.
Use: Antihistamine.
W/Clopane HCl, Histadyl.
See: Co-Pyronil, Preps. (Eli Lilly and Co.).

•**pyrrocaine.** (PIHR-oh-cane) USAN.
Use: Anesthetic, local.

pyrrocaine hydrochloride.
Use: Anesthetic, local.

pyrrocaine hydrochloride and epinephrine inj.
Use: Anesthetic, local.

•**pyrroliphene hydrochloride.** (pihr-OLE-ih-feen) USAN.
Use: Analgesic.

•**pyrrolnitrin.** (pihr-OLE-nye-trin) USAN. Under study.
Use: Antifungal.

Pyrroxate. (Roberts Pharmaceuticals) Chlorpheniramine maleate 4 mg, phenylpropanolamine HCl 25 mg, acetaminophen 650 mg/Cap. Blister pkg. 24s. Bot. 500s. *otc.*
Use: Analgesic, antihistamine, decongestant.

•**pyrvinium pamoate.** (pihr-VIN-ee-uhm PAM-oh-ate) U.S.P. 23.
Use: Anthelmintic.

PYtest. (TRi-Med) 1mCi^{14}-C-urea. Cap. UD 1s, 10s, 100s. *Rx.*
Use: Diagnostic aid.

PYtest Kit. (Tri-Med Specialities, Inc.) Breath test for detecting *H. pylori.* Kit. 1 PYtest Cap. and breath collection equipment. *Rx.*
Use: Diagnostic aid.

Q

QB Liquid. (Major Pharmaceuticals) Theophylline 150 mg, guaifenesin 90 mg. Bot. Pt, gal. *Rx.*
Use: Bronchodilator, expectorant.

Q.T. Quick Tanning Suntan by Coppertone. (Schering-Plough Corp.) Ethylhexyl p-methoxycinnamate, dihydroxyacetone. SPF 2. Lot. Bot. 120 ml. *otc.*
Use: Sunscreen, tanning.

Qua-Bid. (Quaker City Pharmacal) Papaverine HCl 150 mg. TR Cap. Bot. 100s, 1000s. *otc.*
Use: Vasodilator.

•**quadazocine mesylate.** (kwad-AZE-oh-SEEN) USAN.
Use: Opioid antagonist.

Quadramet. (Du Pont Pharma.) Samarium SM 153 lexidronam 1850 MBq/ml (50 mCi/ml) at calibration. Inj. Frozen, single-dose 10 ml vials. In 2 ml fill (3700 MBq) and 3 ml fill (5550 MBq). *Rx.*
Use: Treatment for bone lesions.

quadruple sulfonamides.
See: Sulfonamide.

Quarzan. (Roche Laboratories) Clidinium bromide 2.5 mg or 5 mg. Cap. Bot. 100s. *Rx.*
Use: Anticholinergic, antispasmodic.

•**quazepam.** (KWAY-zuh-pam) USAN.
Use: Hypnotic, sedative.
See: Doral (Baker Norton Pharmaceuticals, Inc.).

•**quazinone.** (KWAY-zih-NOHN) USAN.
Use: Cardiovascular agent.

•**quazodine.** (KWAY-zoe-deen) USAN.
Use: Cardiovascular agent.

•**quazolast.** (KWAY-ZOLE-ast) USAN.
Use: Antiasthmatic mediator release inhibitor.

Quelicin. (Abbott Hospital Products) Succinylcholine Cl. **20 mg/ml:** Fliptop vial 10 ml, Abboject Syringe 5 ml; **50 mg/ml:** Amp. 10 ml; **100 mg/ml:** Amp. 10 ml; **Quelicin-500:** 5 ml in Pintop vial 10 ml; **Quelicin-1000:** 10 ml in Pintop vial 20 ml. *Rx.*
Use: Muscle relaxant.

Quelidrine Cough Syrup. (Abbott Laboratories) Dextromethorphan HBr 10 mg, chlorpheniramine maleate 2 mg, ephedrine HCl 5 mg, phenylephrine HCl 5 mg, ammonium Cl 40 mg, ipecac fluid extract 0.005 ml, ethyl alcohol 2%/5 ml. Bot. 4 oz. *Rx.*
Use: Antihistamine, antitussive, bronchodilator, decongestant, expectorant.

Quercetin. Active constituent of rutin. Quertine.

Quertine.
Use: Bioflavonoid supplement.

Questran. (Bristol-Myers Squibb) Cholestyramine resin 4 g active ingredient/9 g Powder Packet. Box packet 60s. Can 378 g (42 dose). *Rx.*
Use: Antihyperlipidemic, antipruritic.

Questran Light. (Bristol-Myers Squibb) Anhydrous cholestyramine 4 g/Packet or scoopful. Pow. for Oral Susp. Can 210 g (42 doses), carton packet 5 g (60s). *Rx.*
Use: Antihyperlipidemic.

•**quetiapine fumarate.** (cue-TIE-ah-peen) USAN.
Use: Antipsychotic.
See: Seroquel, Tab. (Zeneca Pharmaceuticals).

quetiapine hydrochloride. (cue-TIE-ah-peen)
Use: Antipsychotic.

Quiagel. (Rugby Labs, Inc.) Kaolin 6 g, pectin 142.8 mg, hyoscyamine sulfate 0.1037 mg, atropine sulfate 0.0194 mg, scopolamine HBr 0.0065 mg/30 ml. Susp. Bot. Pt, gal. *Rx.*
Use: Antidiarrheal.

Quibron. (Roberts Pharmaceuticals) Theophylline (anhydrous) 150 mg, guaifenesin 90 mg. Cap. Bot. 100s, 1000s, UD 100s. *Rx.*
Use: Bronchodilator, expectorant.

Quibron-300. (Roberts Pharmaceuticals) Theophylline (anhydrous) 300 mg, guaifenesin 180 mg. Cap. Bot. 100s. *Rx.*
Use: Bronchodilator, expectorant.

Quibron Plus. (Bristol-Myers Squibb) Ephedrine HCl 25 mg, theophylline (anhydrous) 150 mg, butabarbital 20 mg, guaifenesin 100 mg. Cap. Bot. 100s. *Rx.*
Use: Antiasthmatic combination.

Quibron Plus Elixir. (Bristol-Myers Squibb) Theophylline 150 mg, ephedrine HCl 25 mg, guaifenesin 100 mg, butabarbital 20 mg, alcohol 15%. Elix. Bot. Pt. *Rx.*
Use: Antiasthmatic combination.

Quibron-T Dividose Tablets. (Roberts Pharmaceuticals) Theophylline anhydrous 300 mg. Tab. Dividose design breakable into 100, 150, or 200 mg portions. Immediate-release. Bot. 100s. *Rx.*
Use: Bronchodilator.

Quibron-T/SR Dividose Tablets. (Roberts Pharmaceuticals) Theophylline anhydrous 300 mg. Tab. Dividose design breakable into 100 mg, 150 mg, or 200

mg portions. Sustained-release. Bot. 100s. *Rx.*
Use: Bronchodilator.

Quick AC Enema Kit. (LPI Diagnostics) Barium sulfate 150%. Susp. Enema kit. 500 ml. *Rx.*
Use: Radiopaque agent; GI contrast agent.

Quick CARE. (Novartis Pharmaceutical Corp.) **Disinfecting solution:** Isopropanol, sodium Cl, polyoxypropylene-polyoxyethylene block copolymer, disodium lauroamphodiacetate. Bot. 15 ml. **Rinse and neutralizer:** Sodium borate, boric acid, sodium perborate (generating up to 0.006% hydrogen peroxide), phosphoric acid. Bot. 360 ml. *otc.*
Use: Contact lens care.

Quick-K. (Western Research) Potassium bicarbonate 650 mg (6.5 mEq) potassium. Tab. Bot. 30s, 100s. *Rx.*
Use: Electrolyte supplement.

Quick Pep. (Thompson Medical Co.) Caffeine 150 mg, dextrose, sucrose 300 mg. Tab. Bot. 32s. *otc.*
Use: CNS stimulant.

Quiebar. (Nevin) Butabarbital sodium. **Spantab:** 1.5 gr. TR Spantab. Bot. 50s, 500s. **Elix.:** 30 mg/5 ml. Bot. pt, gal. **Tab.:** 15 mg. Bot. 100s, 1000s; 30 mg. Bot. 1000s. **A.C. Cap.:** Bot. 100s, 500s. *c-III.*
Use: Hypnotic, sedative.

Quiebel. (Nevin) Butabarbital sodium 15 mg, belladonna extract 15 mg. Cap. Bot. 100s, 1000s. Elix. Pt, gal. *c-III.*
Use: Anticholinergic, antispasmodic, hypnotic, sedative.

Quiecof. (Nevin) Dextromethorphan HBr 7.5 mg, chlorpheniramine maleate 0.75 mg, guaiacol glyceryl ether 25 mg/5 ml. Bot. 4 oz, pt, gal. *otc.*
Use: Antitussive, antihistamine, expectorant.

Quiet Night. (Rosemont Pharmaceutical Corp.) Pseudoephedrine HCl 10 mg, doxylamine succinate 1.25 mg, dextromethorphan HBr 5 mg, acetaminophen 167 mg/5 ml. Liq. Bot. 180 ml, 300 ml. *otc.*
Use: Analgesic, antihistamine, antitussive, decongestant.

Quiet Time. (Whiteworth Towne) Acetaminophen 600 mg, ephedrine sulfate 8 mg, dextromethorphan HBr 15 mg, doxylamine succinate 7.5 mg, alcohol 25 mg/30 ml. Bot. 180 ml. *otc.*
Use: Analgesic, antihistamine, antitussive, decongestant.

Quiet World. (Whitehall Robins Laboratories) Acetaminophen 2.5 gr, aspirin 3.5 gr, pyrilamine maleate 25 mg. Tab. Bot. 12s, 30s. *otc.*
Use: Analgesic combination, antihistamine.

•**quiflapon sodium.** (KWIH-flap-ahn) USAN.
Use: Antiasthmatic, inflammatory bowel disease suppressant.

Quik-Cept. (Laboratory Diagnostics) Slide test for pregnancy, rapid latex inhibition test. Kit 25s, 50s, 100s.
Use: Diagnostic aid.

Quik-Cult. (Laboratory Diagnostics) Slide test for fecal occult blood. Kit 150s, 200s, 300s, and tape test.
Use: Diagnostic aid.

•**quilostigmine.** (Kwill-oh-STIG-meen) USAN.
Use: Cholinergic (cholinesterase inhibitor); treatment of Alzheimer's disease.

Quinaglute Dura-Tabs. (Berlex Laboratories, Inc.) Quinidine gluconate 324 mg. Tab. Bot. 100s, 250s, 500s, UD 100s. Unit-of-use 90s, 120s. *Rx.*
Use: Antiarrhythmic.

•**quinaldine blue.** (kwin-AL-deen) USAN.
Use: Diagnostic agent (obstetrics).

•**quinapril hydrochloride.** (KWIN-uh-PRILL) USAN.
Use: Antihypertensive, enzyme inhibitor (angiotensin-converting).
See: Accupril, Tab. (Parke-Davis).

•**quinaprilat.** (KWIN-ah-PRILL-at) USAN.
Use: Antihypertensive, enzyme inhibitor (angiotensin-converting).

•**quinazosin hydrochloride.** (kwin-AZZ-oh-sin) USAN.
Use: Antihypertensive.

•**quinbolone.** (KWIN-bole-ohn) USAN.
Use: Anabolic.

•**quindecamine acetate.** (kwin-DECK-ah-meen) USAN.
Use: Anti-infective.

•**quindonium bromide.** (kwin-DOE-nee-uhn) USAN.
Use: Cardiovascular agent (antiarrhythmic).

•**quinelorane hydrochloride.** (kwih-NELL-oh-RANE) USAN.
Use: Antihypertensive, antiparkinsonian.

quinethazone. U.S.P. XXII.
Use: Diuretic.
See: Hydromox, Tab. (ESI Lederle Generics).
W/Reserpine.
See: Hydromox R, Tab. (ESI Lederle Generics).

•**quinetolate.** (Kwin-EH-toe-late) USAN.
Use: Muscle relaxant.

•**quinfamide.** (KWIN-fah-mide) USAN.
Use: Antiamebic.

•**quingestanol acetate.** (kwin-JESS-tan-ahl) USAN.
Use: Hormone, progestin.

•**quingestrone.** (kwin-JESS-trone) USAN.
Use: Hormone, progestin.

Quinidex Extentabs. (Wyeth-Ayerst Laboratories) Quinidine sulfate 300 mg. Tab. Bot. 100s, 250s. Dis-co pack 100s. *Rx.*
Use: Antiarrhythmic.

Quinidex L-A.
See: Quinidex Extentabs (Wyeth-Ayerst Laboratories).

•**quinidine gluconate.** (KWIN-ih-deen) U.S.P. 23.
Use: Cardiovascular agent (antiarrhythmic).
See: Duraquin, Tab. (Parke-Davis).
Quinaglute, Dura-Tab. (Berlex Laboratories, Inc.).

quinidine polygalacturonate.
See: Cardioquin Tab. (Purdue Frederick Co.).

•**quinidine sulfate.** (KWIN-ih-deen) U.S.P. 23.
Use: Cardiovascular agent (antiarrhythmic).
See: Quinidex Extentabs (Wyeth-Ayerst Laboratories).
Quinora, Tab. (Key Pharmaceuticals).

quinidine sulfate. (Various Mfr.) 300 mg. Tab., SR Tab. Bot. 100s, 250s, 1000s. *Rx.*
Use: Cardiovascular agent.

•**quinine ascorbate.** (KWIE-nine ass-CORE-bate) USAN. *Formerly quinine biascorbate.*
Use: Smoking deterrent.

quinine bisulfate. (KWIE-nine)
Use: Analgesic, antimalarial, antipyretic.

quinine dihydrochloride. (KWIE-nine)
Use: Antimalarial.

quinine ethylcarbonate.
See: Euquinine (Various Mfr.).

quinine glycerophosphate. Quinine compound with glycerol phosphate.

•**quinine sulfate.** (KWIE-nine) U.S.P. 23.
Use: Antimalarial.
See: Quinamm, Tab. (Hoechst Marion Roussel).
W/Aminophylline.
See: Strema, Cap. (Foy Laboratories).
W/Atropine sulfate, emetine HCl, aconitine, camphor monobromate.
See: Coryza, Tab. (Jones Medical Industries, Inc.).

quinine and urea hydrochloride.
Use: Sclerosing agent.

quinisocaine.
See: Dimethisoquin HCl.

quinophan.
See: Cinchophen (Various Mfr.).

Quinora. (Key Pharmaceuticals) Quinidine sulfate 300 mg. Tab. Bot. 100s, 1000s, UD 100s. *Rx.*
Use: Antiarrhythmic.

quinoxyl.
See: Chiniofon.

•**quinpirole hydrochloride.** (KWIN-pihr-ole) USAN.
Use: Antihypertensive.

quinprenaline. Quinterenol Sulfate.

Quin-Release. (Major Pharmaceuticals) Quinidine gluconate 324 mg. SR Tab. Bot. 100s, 250s, 500s, UD 100s. *Rx.*
Use: Antiarrhythmic.

Quinsana Plus. (Stephan Company) Tolnafate 1%, cornstarch, talc. Pow. In 90 g. *otc.*
Use: Antifungal, topical.

Quintabs. (Freeda Vitamins, Inc.) Vitamins A 10,000 IU, D 400 IU, E 29 mg, B_1 25 mg, B_2 25 mg, B_3 100 mg, B_5 25 mg, B_6 25 mg, B_{12} 25 mcg, C 300 mg, folic acid 0.1 mg, inositol, PABA/Tab. Bot. 100s, 250s. *otc.*
Use: Vitamin supplement.

Quintabs-M. (Freeda Vitamins, Inc.) Iron 15 mg, Vitamins A 10,000 IU, D 400 IU, E 50 mg, B_1 30 mg, B_2 30 mg, B_3 150 mg, B_5 30 mg, B_6 30 mg, B_{12} 30 mcg, C 300 mg, folic acid 0.4 mg, Ca, Cu, K, Mg, Mn, Se, Zn 30 mg, PABA/Tab. Bot. 100s, 250s, 500s. *otc.*
Use: Mineral, vitamin supplement.

•**quinterenol sulfate.** (kwin-TER-en-ahl) USAN.
Use: Bronchodilator.

•**quinuclium bromide.** (kwih-NEW-klee-uhm) USAN.
Use: Antihypertensive.

•**quinupristin.** (kwih-NEW-priss-tin) USAN.
Use: Anti-infective.

•**quipazine maleate.** (KWIP-ah-zeen) USAN.
Use: Antidepressant, oxytocic.

quipenyl naphthoate.
See: Plasmochin naphthoate.

R

R-3 Screen Test. (Wampole Laboratories) A three-minute latex-eosin slide test for the qualitative detection of rheumatoid factor activity in serum. Kit 100s.
Use: Diagnostic aid.

RabAvert. (Chiron) Rabies antigen 2.5 IU, < 1 mcg neomycin, < 20 ng chlortetracycline, < 2 ng amphotericin B, < 3 ng ovalbumin. Inj. *Rx.*
Use: Immunization.

•**rabeprazole sodium.** (rab-EH-pray-zahl) USAN.
Use: Antiulcerative, gastric acid pump inhibitor.

rabies antigen.
Use: Immunization.

•**rabies immune globulin.** (RAY-beez-ih-MYOON GLAB-byoo-lin) U.S.P. 23.
Use: Immunization.
See: Bayrab (Bayer Corp. (Consumer Div.)).
Imogam Rabies (Pasteur Merieux Connaught)

rabies immune globulin (RIG), human.
See: Rabies immune globulin.

•**rabies vaccine.** (RAY-beez vaccine) U.S.P. 23.
Use: Immunization.
See: Imovax Rabies, Syr. (Pasteur Merieux Connaught).
RabAvert (Chiron).
Rabies Vaccine Adsorbed, Vial (Michigan Department of Health).

rabies vaccine (adsorbed). (Michigan Department of Health) Challenge virus standard (CVS) Kissling/MDPH Strain. Inj. Vial 1 ml. *Rx.*
Use: Immunization.

•**racemethionine.** (RAY-see-meh-THIGH-oh-neen) USAN. U.S.P. XXI *Formerly Methionine.*
Use: Acidifier, urinary.
See: Pedameth., Liq. (Forest Pharmaceutical, Inc.).

racemic amphetamine sulfate.
See: Amphetamine sulfate.

racemic calcium pantothenate.
See: Calcium Pantothenate, Racemic.

racemic desoxynorephedrine.
See: Amphetamine (Various Mfr.).

racemic ephedrine hydrochloride. Racephedrine HCl.

racemic pantothenic acid.
See: Vitamin, Preps.

•**racephedrine hydrochloride.** USAN.
Use: Vasoconstrictor; decongestant, nasal.
See: Ephedrine Combinations.
W/Aminophylline, phenobarbital.
See: Amodrine, Tab. (Searle).

racephedrine hydrochloride. (Pharmacia & Upjohn) **Cap.:** 3/8 gr. Bot. 40s, 250s, 1000s. **Soln.:** 1%. Bot. 1 fl oz, pt, gal.
Use: Vasoconstrictor; decongestant, nasal.

•**racephenicol.** (ray-see-FEN-ih-KAHL) U.S.P. 23.
Use: Anti-infective.

•**racepinephrine hydrochloride.** (race-epp-ih-NEFF-rin) U.S.P. 23.
Use: Bronchodilator.

•**raclopride C11.** (RACK-low-pride) U.S.P. 23.
Use: Radiopharmaceutical.

radioactive isotopes.
See: Albumin, Aggregated Iodinated, Human I-131.
Chlormerodrin Hg-197, Inj.
Chlormerodrin Hg-203, Inj.
Cyanocobalamin Co-57, Cap.
Cyanocobalamin Co-60, Cap.
Gold Au-198, Inj.
Medotope, Prods. (Bristol-Myers Squibb).
Radio-Iodinated Serum Albumin (Human).
Sodium Radio-Chromate, Inj.
Sodium Radio-Iodide, Soln.
Sodium Radio Phosphate, Soln.
Selenomethionine Se-75, Inj.
Sodium Chromate Cr-51, Inj.
Sodium Iodide I-125, Soln, Cap.
Sodium Iodide I-131, Soln, Cap.
Sodium Phosphate P-32, Cap, Inj.
Sodium Rose Bengal I-131, Inj.
Strontium Nitrate Sr-85, Inj.
Technetium Tc-99m, Kit, Inj.
Triolein I-131, Cap, Soln.
Xenon Xe-133, Inj.

radiogold (^{198}Au), solution. Gold Au-198 Injection, U.S.P. XX.
Use: Irradiation therapy.

radio-iodide (^{131}I), sodium.
Use: Radiopharmaceutical.
See: Iodotope (Bristol-Myers Squibb).

radio-iodinated (^{131}I) serum albumin. (Human) Iodinated I-131 Albumin Injection.

radio-iodinated serum albumin (human), (^{125}I).
See: Albumotope (^{125}I) (Bristol-Myers Squibb).

radiopaque polyvinyl chloride.
Use: Radiopaque agent, gastrointestinal.
See: Sitzmarks (Konsyl Pharm.).

radio-phosphate (^{32}P), sodium.
Use: Radiopharmaceutical.

radioselenomethionine 75 Se. Selenomethionine Se 75.

radiotolpovidone I-131. Tolpovidone I-131.

•**rafoxanide.** (ray-FOX-ah-nide) USAN.
Use: Anthelmintic.

Ragus. (Miller Pharmacal Group, Inc.) Mg 27 mg, vitamins C 100 mg, Ca 580 mg, P 450 mg, l-lysine 25 mg, dl-methionine 50 mg, A 5000 IU, D 400 IU, E 10 mg, B_1 20 mg, B_2 3 mg, B_6 5 mg, B_{12} 9 mcg, niacinamide 80 mg, pantothenic acid 5 mg, Fe 20 mg, Cu 1 mg, Mn 2 mg, K 10 mg, Zn 2 mg, I 0.1 mg/3 Tab. Bot. 100s. *otc.*
Use: Mineral, vitamin supplement.

•**ralitoline.** (rah-LIT-oh-leen) USAN.
Use: Anticonvulsant.

R A Lotion. (Medco Lab, Inc.) Resorcinol 3%, alcohol 43%. Plastic Bot. 120 ml, 240 ml, 480 ml. *otc.*
Use: Dermatologic, acne.

•**raloxifene hydrochloride.** (ral-OX-ih-FEEN) USAN. *Formerly Keoxifene hydrochloride.*
Use: Antiestrogen.
See: Evista, Tab. (Eli Lilly and Co.).

•**raltitrexed.** (ral-tih-TREX-ehd) USAN.
Use: Advanced colorectal cancer treatment (thymidylate synthase inhibitor), antineoplastic.

•**raluridine.** (ral-YOUR-ih-deen) USAN.
Use: Antiviral.

•**ramipril.** (ruh-MIH-prill) USAN.
Use: Antihypertensive, enzyme inhibitor (angiotensin-converting), congestive heart failure.
See: Altace, Cap. (Hoechst Marion Roussel, Pharmacia & Upjohn).

•**ramoplanin.** (ram-oh-PLAN-in) USAN.
Use: Anti-infective.

Ramses. (Durex) Nonoxynol-9 5%. Vaginal jelly. 150 g. *otc.*
Use: Contraceptive, spermicide.

Ramses Bendex. (Durex) Flexible cushioned diaphragm; arcing spring. 65 to 90 mm. Pkg. w/Ramses Vaginal Jelly Tube 1 oz, 3 oz. *Rx.*
Use: Contraceptive.

Ramses Diaphragm. (Durex) Flexible cushioned diaphragm 50 to 95 mm. Pkg. diaphragm, tube of Ramses Vaginal Jelly. Pkg. diaphragm alone. *Rx.*
Use: Contraceptive.

Ramses Extra. (Durex) Condom with nonoxynol-9 15%. In 3s, 12s, 24s, 36s. *otc.*
Use: Contraceptive.

Ramses Jelly. (Durex) Nonoxynol-9 5%. Tube w/applicator 150 g. *otc.*
Use: Contraceptive.

Randolectil. (Farbenfabriken Bayer Corp.) Butaperazine. *Rx.*
Use: Psychotherapeutic agent.

ranestol. Triclofenol piperazine.
Use: Anthelmintic.

•**ranimycin.** (ran-ih-MY-sin) USAN.
Use: Anti-infective.

•**ranitidine.** (ran-EYE-tih-DEEN) USAN.
Use: Antiulcerative.
See: Zantac, Tab., Inj., Syr. (Glaxo-Wellcome, Roche Laboratories).

ranitidine. (Zenith Goldline Pharmaceuticals) Ranitidine 150 mg, 300 mg. Tab. Bot. 30s (300 mg only), 60s (150 mg only), 100s, 250s (300 mg only), 500s (150 mg only). *Rx.*
Use: Antiulcerative.

•**ranitidine bismuth citrate.** (ran-EYE-tih-DEEN BIZZ-muth SIH-trate) USAN.
Use: Antiulcerative.
See: Tritec, Tab. (GlaxoWellcome).

•**ranitidine hydrochloride.** (ran-EYE-tih-DEEN) U.S.P. 23.
Use: Antiulcerative.
See: Zantac, Inj., Tab., Syr. (Glaxo-Wellcome).

ranitidine hydrochloride. (UDL Laboratories, Inc.) 15 mg/ml. Syr. Bot. UD 10 ml.
Use: Antiulcerative.

ranitidine hydrochloride in sodium chloride injection.
Use: Antiulcerative.
See: Zantac Inj. Premixed (Glaxo-Wellcome).

•**ranolazine hydrochloride.** (RAY-no-lah-ZEEN) USAN.
Use: Antianginal.

Rapid Test Strep. (SmithKline Diagnostics) Latex slide agglutination test for identification of group A streptococci. Box. 25s, 100s.
Use: Diagnostic aid.

•**rapacuronium bromide.** USAN.
Use: Neuromuscular blocking agent.

•**rasagiline mesylate.** (rass-AH-jih-leen MEH-sih-late) USAN.
Use: Antiparkinsonian.

rastinon. Tolbutamide, U.S.P. 23.
Use: Antidiabetic.

rattlesnake bite therapy.
See: Antivenin (crotalidae) (Wyeth-Ayerst Laboratories).

Rauneed. (Hanlon) Rauwolfia 50 mg, 100 mg/Tab. Bot. 100s. *Rx.*
Use: Antihypertensive.

Raunescine. (Penick) An alkaloid of rau-

wolfia serpentina. Under study.
Use: Antihypertensive.

Raunormine. (Penick) 11-Desmethoxy reserpine. *Rx.*

Raurine. (Westerfield) Reserpine. **Tab.:** 0.1 mg. Bot. 100s. **Delayed Action Cap.:** 0.5 mg. Bot. 100s. *Rx.*
Use: Antihypertensive.

Rauserfia. (New Eng. Phr. Co.) Rauwolfia serpentina 50 mg, 100 mg/Tab. Bot. 100s. *Rx.*
Use: Antihypertensive.

Rautina. (Fellows) Rauwolfia serpentina whole root 50 mg, 100 mg/Tab. Bot. 1000s. *Rx.*
Use: Antihypertensive.

Rauval. (Pal-Pak, Inc.) Rauwolfia whole root 50 mg, 100 mg/Tab. Bot. 100s, 500s, 1000s. *Rx.*
Use: Antihypertensive.

rauwolfia/bendroflumethiazide. (Various Mfr.) Bendroflumethiazide 4 mg, powdered rauwolfia serpentina 50 mg/Tab. Bot. 100s. *Rx.*
Use: Antihypertensive.
See: Rauzide, Tab. (Bristol-Myers Squibb).

rauwolfia serpentina active principles (alkaloids). Deserpidine, Rescinnamone.
See: Reserpine, Inj. (Various Mfr.).

•**rauwolfia serpentina.** (rah-WOOL-fee-ah ser-pen-TEE-nah) U.S.P. 23.
Use: Antihypertensive.
See: Raudixin, Tab. (Bristol-Myers Squibb).
Rauneed, Tab. (Hanlon).
Rauval, Tab. (Pal-Pak, Inc.).
Rawfola, Tab. (Foy Laboratories).
T-Rau, Tab. (Tennessee Pharmaceutic).
Wolfina, Tab. (Westerfield).
W/Bendroflumethiazide.
See: Rauzide, Tab. (Bristol-Myers Squibb).

rauwolscine. An alkaloid of *Rauwolfia canescens.* Under study.
Use: Antihypertensive.

Rauzide. (Bristol-Myers Squibb) Rauwolfia serpentina pow. 50 mg, bendroflumethiazide 4 mg, tartrazine/Tab. Bot. 100s. *Rx.*
Use: Antihypertensive.

Ravocaine. (Cook-Waite Laboratories, Inc.) Propoxycaine HCl 4 mg, procaine 20 mg, norepinephrine bitartrate equivalent to 0.033 mg levophed base, sodium Cl 3 mg, acetone sodium bisulfite not more than 2 mg. Cartridge 1.8 ml. *Rx.*
Use: Anesthetic, local.

Ravocaine and Novocain with Levophed. (Cook-Waite Laboratories, Inc.) Propoxycaine HCl 7.2 mg, procaine 36 mg, norepinephrine 0.12 mg, acetone sodium bisulfite 1.8 ml. Inj. Dental Cartridge. *Rx.*
Use: Anesthetic, local.

Rawfola. (Foy Laboratories) Rauwolfia serpentina 50 mg/Tab. Bot. 1000s. *Rx.*
Use: Antihypertensive.

Rawl Vite. (Rawl) Vitamins A 10,000 IU, D 500 IU, B_1 10 mg, B_2 5 mg, B_6 1 mg, calcium pantothenate 5 mg, nicotinamide 50 mg, C 125 mg, E 2.5 IU/Tab. Bot. 100s. *otc.*
Use: Mineral, vitamin supplement.

Rawl Whole Liver Vitamin B Complex. (Rawl) Whole liver 500 mg, amino acids found in the whole liver, vitamins B_1 1 mg, B_2 2 mg, niacinamide 5 mg, choline Cl 12 mg, B_6 0.2 mg, calcium pantothenate 0.2 mg, inositol 5 mg, biotin 0.6 mcg, B_{12} 0.3 mcg/Cap. Bot. 100s, 500s.
Use: Mineral, vitamin supplement.

Raxar. (GlaxoWellcome) Grepafloxacin HCl 200 mg, 400 mg, 600 mg. Tab. Bot. 60s, UD 10s, 60s. *Rx.*
Use: Anti-infective.

Ray Block. (Del-Ray Laboratory, Inc.) Octyl dimethyl PABA 5%, benzophenone-3 3%, SD alcohol. Lot. Bot. 118.3 ml. *otc.*
Use: Sunscreen.

Ray-D. (Nion Corp.) Vitamin D 400 IU, thiamine mononitrate 1 mg, riboflavin 2 mg, niacin 10 mg, I 0.1 mg, Ca 375 mg, P 300 mg/6 Tab. In base of brewer's yeast. Bot. 100s, 500s. *otc.*
Use: Mineral, vitamin supplement.

Rayderm Ointment. (Velvet Pharmacal) Euphorbia extract, phenyl salicylate, neatsfoot oil, olive oil, lanolin in emulsion base preserved with methyl- and propylparabens. Tube 1.5 oz, Jar lb. *otc.*
Use: Burn therapy.

•**rayon, purified.** (RAY-ahn) U.S.P. 23.
Use: Surgical aid.

raythesin. (Raymer)
See: Propyl p-Aminobenzoate.

Razepam. (Major Pharmaceuticals) Temazepam 15 mg, 30 mg/Cap. Bot. 100s. *c-IV.*
Use: Hypnotic, sedative.

RCF. (Ross Laboratories) Carbohydrate free low iron soy protein formula base. Carbohydrate and water must be added. For infants unable to tolerate the amount or type of carbohydrate in conventional formulas. Can 14 fl oz. (Concentrated liq.). *otc.*

Use: Nutritional supplement.

R & C Shampoo. (Schwarz Pharma, Inc.) Pyrethrin shampoo. Bot. 2 oz, 4 oz. *otc.*
Use: Pediculicide.

R & C Spray III. (Schwarz Pharma, Inc.) Spray containing pyrethroid (sumethrin) 0.382%, other isomers 0.018%, petroleum distillate 4.255%. Aer. Cont. 5 oz. *otc.*
Use: Pediculicide.

Reabilan. (Elan Pharma) Protein 31.5 g, fat 39 g, carbohydrates 131.5 g, Na 702 mg, K 1.252 g/L, lactose free. With appropriate vitamins and minerals. Liq. Bot. 375 ml. *otc.*
Use: Nutritional supplement.

Reabilan HN. (Elan Pharma) Protein 58.2 g, fat 52 g, carbohydrates 158 g, Na 1000 mg, K 1661 mg/L, lactose free. With appropriate vitamins and minerals. Liq. Bot. 375 ml. *otc.*
Use: Nutritional supplement.

Rea-Lo. (Whorton Pharmaceuticals, Inc.) Urea in water-soluble moisturizing oil base. **Lot.:** 15%. Bot. 4 oz, pt. **Cream:** 30%. Jar 2 oz, 16 oz. *otc.*
Use: Emollient.

Rebetron. (Schering Corporation) Interferon Alfa-2b, recombinant 3 million/0.5 ml, ribavirin 200 mg. Inj./Cap. Intron A in single- and multi-dose vials. Rebetol in blister-pack 35s, 42s. *Rx.*
Use: Antineoplastic.

•**recainam hydrochloride.** (reh-CANE-am) USAN.
Use: Cardiovascular agent (antiarrhythmic).

•**recainam tosylate.** (reh-CANE-am TAH-sill-ate) USAN.
Use: Cardiovascular agent (antiarrhythmic).

•**reclazepam.** (reh-CLAY-zeh-pam) USAN.
Use: Hypnotic, sedative.

Reclomide. (Major Pharmaceuticals) Metoclopramide HCl 10 mg/Tab. Bot. 100s, 500s, 1000s, UD 100s. *Rx.*
Use: Antiemetic, gastrointestinal stimulant.

recombinant human insulin-like growth factor I.
Use: Antibody-mediated growth hormone resistance. [Orphan Drug]

recombinant tissue plasminogen activator. *Rx.*
See: Activase (Genentech, Inc.).

recombinant vaccinia (human papillomavirus).
Use: Cervical cancer. [Orphan Drug]

Recombinate. (Hyland Therapeutics) Concentrated recombinant antihemophilic factor, contains albumin (human) 12.5 mg/ml, polyethylene glycol 1.5 mg, Na 180 mEq/L, histidine 55 mm, polysorbate 80 1.5 mcg/AHF IU, Ca 0.2 mg/ml. Pow. for Inj. 250 IU, 500 IU, 1000 IU. Single-dose Bot. *Rx.*
Use: Antihemophilic.

Recombivax HB. (Merck & Co.) Hepatitis B vaccine recombinant. **Pediatric/Adolescent:** 10 mcg/5 ml. Single-dose vial 0.5 ml, prefilled, single-dose syringes 0.5 ml. **Adult:** 10 mcg/ml. Vial 1 ml, 3 ml, prefilled, single-dose syringe 1 ml. **Dialysis:** 40 mcg/ml. Vial 1 ml. *Rx.*
Use: Immunization.

Recortex 10X in Oil. (Forest Pharmaceutical, Inc.) 1000 mcg/ml. Vial 10 ml. *Rx.*

Recover. (Dermik Laboratories, Inc.) Bot. 2.25 oz. *otc.*
Use: Dermatologic.

Rectagene. (Pfeiffer Co.) Live yeast cell derivative supplying 2000 units Skin Respiratory Factor/oz, shark liver oil in a cocoa butter base. Supp. 12s. *otc.*
Use: Anorectal preparation.

Rectagene Medicated Rectal Balm. (Pfeiffer Co.) Live yeast cell derivative that supplies 2000 units Skin Respiratory Factor/30 g, refined shark liver oil 3%, white petrolatum, lanolin, thyme oil, 1:10,000 phenylmercuric nitrate. Oint. 56.7 g. *otc.*
Use: Anorectal preparation.

Rectal Medicone. (Medicore) Benzocaine 2 gr, balsam peru 1 gr, hydroxyquinoline sulfate 0.25 gr, menthol 1/7 gr, zinc oxide 3 gr/Supp. Box 12s, 24s. *otc.*
Use: Anesthetic; antiseptic, topical.

Rectal Medicone Unguent. (Medicore) Benzocaine 20 mg, oxyquinoline sulfate 5 mg, menthol 4 mg, zinc oxide 100 mg, balsam peru 12.5 mg, petrolatum 625 mg, lanolin 210 mg/g. Tube 1.5 oz. *otc.*
Use: Anorectal preparation.

Rectules. (Forest Pharmaceutical, Inc.) Chloral hydrate 10 gr, 20 gr in water-soluble base. Supp. Pkg. 12s.
Use: Hypnotic, sedative.

red blood cells. Human red blood cells given by IV infusion.
Use: Blood replenisher.

red cell tagging solution.
See: A-C-D, Soln. (Bristol-Myers Squibb).

Red Cross Toothache Kit. (Mentholatum Co., Inc.) Eugenol 85%, sesame oil. Drops. Bot. 3.7 ml w/cotton pellets and tweezers. *otc.*

Use: Anesthetic, local.

red ferric oxide.
Use: Pharmaceutic aid (color).

Reditemp-C. (Wyeth-Ayerst Laboratories) Ammonium nitrate, water, and special additives. Pkg. Large and small sizes. 4 × 10s.
Use: Cold compress.

Reducto, Improved. (Arcum) Phendimetrazine bitartrate 35 mg/Tab. Bot. 100s, 1000s. *c-III.*
Use: Anorexiant.

Redutemp. (International Ethical Labs) Acetaminophen 500 mg/Tab. Bot. 60s. *otc.*
Use: Analgesic.

Reese's Pinworm. (Reese Pharmaceutical Co. Inc.) Pyrantel pamoate 144 mg. Liq. 30 ml. *otc.*
Use: Anthelmintic.

Refludan. (Hoechst Marion Roussel) Lepirudin (rDNA) 50 mg, sodium hydroxide, mannitol. Pow. for Inj. Vial 50 mg. Box 10s. *Rx.*
Use: Anticoagulant.

Refresh. (Allergan, Inc.) Polyvinyl alcohol 1.4%, povidone 0.6%, sodium Cl. UD 30s, 50s (0.3 ml single-dose container). *otc.*
Use: Artificial tears.

Refresh Plus. (Allergan, Inc.) Carboxymethylcellulose sodium 0.5%, NaCl. Preservative-free. Soln. 0.3 ml/single-use container 4s, 30s. *otc.*
Use: Artificial tears.

Refresh PM. (Allergan, Inc.) White petrolatum 56.8%, mineral oil 41.5%, lanolin alcohol, sodium Cl. Tube 3.5 g. *otc.*
Use: Lubricant, ophthalmic.

Refresh Tears. (Allergan) Carboxymethylcellulose 0.5%. Drops. Bot. 15 ml w/dropper. *otc.*
Use: Artificial tears.

Regain. (NCI Medical Foods) Protein 15 g, carbohydrates 52 g, fat 7 g, Na 45 mg, K 75 mg, Ca 200 mg, P 100 mg, Ca, Fe, vitamin B_{12}, Mg, folic acid, fructose. With dietary fiber. 300 calories. Lactose free. Vanilla, strawberry, and malt flavors. Bar 85 g. *otc.*
Use: Nutritional supplement.

Regitine. (Novartis Pharmaceutical Corp.) Phentolamine mesylate 5 mg/Vial (w/mannitol 25 mg in lyophilized form). Pkg. 2s, 6s.
Use: Diagnostic aid.

Reglan. (Wyeth-Ayerst Laboratories) Metoclopramide HCl. **Inj.: 10 mg/2 ml:** Amp. 2 ml, 10 ml; **5 mg/ml:** Vial 2 ml, 10 ml, 30 ml. **Syr.:** 5 mg (as monohydrochloride monohydrate)/5 ml. Bot. Pt, Dis-Co Pack 10×10s. **Tab.: 5 mg:** Bot. 100s. **10 mg:** Bot. 100s, 500s, Dis-co Pak 100s. *Rx.*
Use: Antiemetic, gastrointestinal stimulant.

Regonol. (Organon Teknika Corp.) Pyridostigmine bromide 5 mg/ml. Amp 2 ml, Vial 5 ml. *Rx.*
Use: Muscle stimulant.

•**regramostim.** (reh-GRAH-moe-STIM) USAN.
Use: Biological response modifier; antineoplastic adjunct; antineutropenic; hematopoietic stimulant.

Regranex. (Ortho McNeil Pharmaceutical) Becaplermin 100 mcg, parabens. Gel. Tube 2 ml, 7.5 ml, 15 ml. *Rx.*
Use: Diabetic neuropathic ulcers.

Regroton. (Rhone-Poulenc Rorer Pharmaceuticals, Inc.) Chlorthalidone 50 mg, reserpine 0.25 mg/Tab. Bot. 100s. *Rx.*
Use: Antihypertensive.

Regroton Demi. (Rhone-Poulenc Rorer Pharmaceuticals, Inc.) Chlorthalidone 25 mg, reserpine 0.125 mg/Tab. Bot. 100s, 1000s. *Rx.*
Use: Antihypertensive.

Regular Iletin I. (Eli Lilly and Co.) Insulin 100 units/ml. Beef and pork. Inj. Bot. 10 ml. *otc.*
Use: Antidiabetic agent.

regular purified pork insulin. (Novo/Nordisk Pharm., Inc.) Insulin 100 units/ml. Purified pork. Inj. Vial. 10 ml. *otc.*
Use: Antidiabetic.

Regular Strength Bayer Enteric Coated Caplets. (Bayer Corp. (Consumer Div.)) Aspirin 325 mg. Bot. 50s, 100s. *otc.*
Use: Analgesic.

Regular Strength Midol Multisymptom. (Bayer Corp. (Consumer Div.)) Acetaminophen 325 mg, pyrilamine maleate 12.5 mg. Tab. Bot. 30s. *otc.*
Use: Analgesic combination.

Reguloid, Orange. (Rugby Labs, Inc.) Psyllium mucilloid 3.4 g, sucrose 70%/rounded tsp. Pow. 420 g, 630 g. *otc.*
Use: Laxative.

Reguloid Sugar Free. (Rugby Labs, Inc.) Psyllium hydrophilic mucilloid 3.4 g, sodium ≤ 0.01 g, aspartame, phenylalanine 6 mg. Pow. 222, 333 g. *otc.*
Use: Laxative.

Rehydralyte. (Ross Laboratories) Sodium 75 mEq, potassium 20 mEq, chloride 65 mEq, citrate 30 mEq, dextrose 25 g/L, 100 calories/L. Ready-to-use Bot. 8 oz. *Rx.*
Use: Fluid, electrolyte replacement.

Relafen. (SmithKline Beecham Pharma-

ceuticals) Nabumetone 500 mg/Tab. Bot. 100s, 500s, UD 100s. Nabumetone 750 mg/Tab. Bot. 100s, 500s, UD 100s. *Rx.*
Use: Analgesic, NSAID.

relaxin. A purified ovarian hormone of pregnancy (obtained from sows) responsible for pubic relaxation or separation of the symphysis pubis in mammals.

Relenza. (GlaxoWellcome) Zanamivir 5 mg, lactose 20 mg. Pow. for Inh. Rotadisk 4 blisters. *Rx.*
Use: Antiviral.

Relief Eye Drops. (Allergan, Inc.) Phenylephrine HCl 0.12%, antipyrine 0.1%, polyvinyl alcohol 1.4%, edetate disodium. Bot. UD 0.3 ml. *otc.*
Use: Decongestant, ophthalmic.

Relief Solution. (Allergan, Inc.) Phenylephrine HCl 0.12%, antipyrine 0.1%. Soln. Bot. 20 ml. *otc.*
Use: Decongestant combination, ophthalmic.

•**relomycin.** (REE-low-MY-sin) USAN. A macrolide antibiotic produced by a variant strain of *Streptomyces hygroscopicus.*
Use: Anti-infective.

•**remacemide hydrochloride.** (rem-ASS-eh-MIDE) USAN.
Use: Anticonvulsant (neuroprotective).

Rem Cough Medicine. (Last) Dextromethorphan HBr 5 mg/5 ml. Bot. 3 oz, 6 oz. *otc.*
Use: Antitussive.

Remegel Soft Chewable Antacid. (Warner Lambert) Aluminum hydroxide-magnesium carbonate 476.4 mg/Chew. Tab. Pkg. 8s, 24s. *otc.*
Use: Antacid.

Remeron. (Organon Teknika Corp.) Mirtazapine 15 mg, 30 mg, 45 mg, lactose/Tab. Bot. 30s, 100s, UD 100s (15 mg and 30 mg only). *Rx.*
Use: Antidepressant.

Remicade. (Centocor) Infliximab 100 mg. Pow. for Inj. Preservative free. Sucrose. Single-use vial. 20 ml. *Rx.*
Use: Crohn's disease.

•**remifentanil hydrochloride.** (reh-mih-FEN-tah-nill) USAN.
Use: Analgesic.
See: Ultiva, Pow. for Inj. (GlaxoWellcome).

•**remiprostol.** (reh-mih-PROSTE-ole) USAN.
Use: Antiulcerative.

Remivox. (Janssen Pharmaceutical, Inc.) Lorcainide HCl. *Rx.*
Use: Antiarrhythmic.

•**remoxipride.** (reh-MOX-ih-PRIDE) USAN.
Use: Antipsychotic.

•**remoxipride hydrochloride.** (reh-MOX-ih-PRIDE) USAN.
Use: Antipsychotic.

Remular-S. (International Ethical Labs) Chlorzoxazone 250 mg/Tab. Bot. 100s. *Rx.*
Use: Muscle relaxant.

Renacidin. (Guardian Laboratories) The composition of this powder, as manufactured, is in terms of 156 to 171 g citric acid (anhydrous) and 21 to 30 g d-gluconic acid (as the lactone) w/purified magnesium hydroxycarbonate 75 to 87 g, magnesium acid citrate 9 to 15 g, calcium (as carbonate) 2 to 6 g, water 17 to 21 g per 300 g. Bot. 25 g 6s; 150 g, 300 g. *Rx.*
Use: Irrigant, genitourinary.

Renagel. (Genzyme) Sevelamer HCl 403 mg (anhydrous), collodial silicon dioxide, 4.6 mg, stearic acid 4.6 mg. Cap. Bot. 200s. *Rx.*
Use: Urinary tract product.

Renaltabs-S.C. (Forest Pharmaceutical, Inc.) Methenamine 40.8 mg, benzoic acid 4.5 mg, phenyl salicylate 18.1 mg, hyoscyamine sulfate 1/2000 gr, atropine sulfate 0.03 mg, methylene blue 5.4 mg, gelsemium 6.1 mg/Tab. Bot. 1000s. *Rx.*
Use: Anti-infective, urinary.

RenAmin. (Clintec Nutrition) Sterile hypertonic soln. of essential and nonessential amino acids. Bot. 250 ml, 500 ml. *Rx.*
Use: Nutritional supplement, parenteral.

renanolone. *Rx.*
Use: Steroid anesthetic.

Renbu. (Wren) Butabarbital sodium 32.4 mg/Tab. Bot. 100s, 1000s. *c-III.*
Use: Hypnotic, sedative.

Renese. (Pfizer US Pharmaceutical Group) Polythiazide 1 mg, 2 mg, 4 mg/Tab. Bot. 100s, 1000s. *Rx.*
Use: Antihypertensive, duretic.

Renese-R Tablets. (Pfizer US Pharmaceutical Group) Polythiazide 2 mg, reserpine 0.25 mg/Tab. Bot. 100s, 1000s. *Rx.*
Use: Antihypertensive.

Rengasil. (Novartis Pharmaceutical Corp.) Pirprofen. Investigational drug.
Use: Anti-inflammatory.

RenoCal-76. (Bracco Diagnostics) Diatrizoate meglumine 660 mg, diatrizoate sodium 100 mg, iodine 370 mg/ml. Inj. Vial 50 ml. Bot. 100 ml, 150 ml,

200 ml. *Rx.*
Use: Radiopaque agent.

renoform.
See: Epinephrine, Preps. (Various Mfr.).

Renografin-60. (Bracco Diagnositics) Diatrizoate meglumine 520 mg, sodium diatrizoate 80 mg, iodine 292.5 mg/ml. Inj. Vial 10 ml, 30 ml, 50 ml, Bot. 100 ml. *Rx.*
Use: Radiopaque agent.

Reno-M Dip. (Bracco Diagnostics) Diatrizoate meglumine 300 mg, iodine 141 mg/ml. Inj. Bot. 300 ml. *Formerly Renografin-Dip. Rx.*
Use: Radiopaque agent.

Reno-30. (Bracco Diagnostics) Diatrizoate meglumine 300 mg, iodine 141 mg/ml. Inj. Multi-dose Vial 50 ml. *Rx.*
Use: Radiopaque agent.

Reno-60. (Bracco Diagnostics) Diatrizoate meglumine 600 mg, iodine 282 mg/ml. Inj. Vial 10 ml, 30 ml, 50 ml. Bot. 100 ml, 150 ml (w/ and w/o infusion sets). *Rx.*
Use: Radiopaque agent.

Renormax. (Novartis Pharmaceutical Corp.) Spirapril 3 mg, 6 mg, 12 mg, 24 mg/Tab. *Rx.*
Use: ACE inhibitor.

Reno-Sed. (Vita Elixir) Methenamine 2 gr, salol 0.5 gr, methylene blue 1/10 gr, benzoic acid 1/8 gr, atropine sulfate 1/1000 gr, hyoscyamine sulfate 1/2000 gr/Tab. *Rx.*
Use: Anti-infective, urinary.

Renova. (Ortho McNeil Pharmaceutical) Tretinoin 0.05%, water in oil emulsion. Cream 40 g, 60 g. *Rx.*
Use: Dermatologic.

Renovist Inj. (Bracco Diagnostics) Diatrizoate methylglucamine 34.3%, diatrizoate sodium 35%, iodine 37%. Vial 50 ml, Box 25s.
Use: Radiopaque agent.

Renovist II. (Bracco Diagnostics) Diatrizoate sodium 29.1%, meglumine diatrizoate 28.5%, iodine 31%. Inj. Vial 30 ml, 60 ml, Box 25s.
Use: Radiopaque agent.

Renovue-65. (Bracco Diagnostics) Iodamide meglumide 65%, organically bound iodine 30%, edetate disodium. Vial 50 ml.
Use: Radiopaque agent.

Renovue-Dip. (Bracco Diagnostics) Iodamide meglumide 24%, iodine 11.1%. Infusion Bot. 300 ml.
Use: Radiopaque agent.

Renpap. (Wren) Acetaminophen 4 gr, salicylamide 3 gr, caffeine 2/3 gr, allylisobutylbarbituric acid gr/Tab. Bot. 100s, 1000s. *otc.*
Use: Analgesic.

Rentamine Pediatric. (Major Pharmaceuticals) Phenylephrine tannate 5 mg, chlorpheniramine tannate 4 mg, carbetapentane tannate/5 ml, saccharin, sucrose. Bot. Pt. *Rx.*
Use: Antihistamine, antitussive, decongestant.

ReNu Effervescent Enzymatic Cleaner. (Bausch & Lomb Pharmaceuticals) Subtilisin, polyethylene glycol, sodium carbonate, sodium Cl, tartaric acid. Tab. Bot. 10s, 20s, 30s. *otc.*
Use: Contact lens care.

ReNu Liquid. (Biosearch Medical Products) P-Ca and Na caseinates, CHO-maltodextrin sucrose, F-partially hydrogenated soy oil, mono- and diglycerides, soy lecithin, protein 35 g, CHO 125 g, fat 40 g, Na 500 mg, K 1250 mg/L, 1 Cal/ml, 300 mOsm/kg, H_2O. In 250 ml ready to use. *otc.*
Use: Nutritional supplement.

ReNu Multi-Purpose. (Bausch & Lomb Pharmaceuticals) Isotonic soln. w/sodium Cl, sodium borate, boric acid, poloxamine, polyaminopropyl biguanide 0.00005%, EDTA. Soln. Bot. 118 ml, 237 ml, 355 ml. *otc.*
Use: Contact lens care.

ReNu Saline. (Bausch & Lomb Pharmaceuticals) Isotonic buffered soln. of sodium Cl, boric acid, polyaminopropyl biguanide 0.00003%, EDTA. Soln. Bot. 355 ml. *otc.*
Use: Contact lens care.

ReNu Thermal Enzymatic Cleaner. (Bausch & Lomb Pharmaceuticals) Subtilisin, sodium carbonate, sodium Cl, boric acid. Tab. 16s. *otc.*
Use: Contact lens care.

ReoPro. (Eli Lilly and Co.) Abciximab 2 mg/ml. Inj. Vial 5 ml. *Rx.*
Use: Antiplatelet, monoclonal antibody (antithrombotic).

repaglinide.
Use: Antidiabetic.
See: Prandin, Tab. (Novo/Nordisk Pharm, Inc.).

Repan. (Everett Laboratories, Inc.) Butalbital 50 mg, caffeine 40 mg, acetaminophen 325 mg/Tab. Cap. Bot. 100s. *Rx.*
Use: Analgesic, hypnotic, sedative.

Repan CF. (Everett Laboratories, Inc.) Acetaminophen 650 mg, butalbital 50 mg/Tab. Bot. 100s. *Rx.*
Use: Analgesic combination.

•**repirinast.** (reh-PIRE-ih-nast) USAN.
Use: Antiallergic; antiasthmatic.

Replens. (Warner Lambert) Purified wa-

ter, glycerin, mineral oil, methylparaben. Gel. Appl. 3, 8 pre-filled. *otc.*
Use: Vaginal agent.

Replete Liquid. (Clintec Nutrition) K caseinate, Ca caseinate, maltodextrin, sucrose, corn oil, lecithin, vitamins A, B_1, B_2, B_3, B_5, B_6, B_{12}, C, D, E, K, folic acid, biotin, choline, Ca, Cl, Cu, Fe, I, Mg, Mn, P, Zn. Bot. 250 ml. *otc.*
Use: Nutritional supplement.

Reposans-10. (Wesley Pharmacal Co., Inc.) Chlordiazepoxide HCl 10 mg/Cap. Bot. 1000s. *c-IV.*
Use: Anxiolytic.

Reprieve. (Mayer Lab) Caffeine 32 mg, salicylamide 225 mg, vitamin B_1 50 mg, homatropine methylbromide 0.5 mg/Tab. Bot. 8s, 16s. *Rx.*
Use: Analgesic combination.

•**repromicin.** (rep-ROW-MY-sin) USAN.
Use: Anti-infective.

Repronex. (Ferring Pharmaceuticals, Inc.) FSH activity 75 IU or 150 IU, luteinizing hormone (LH) activity 75 IU, 150 IU, lactose. Inj. Box 1 or 5 Vials. *Rx.*
Use: Ovulation inducer.

•**reproterol hydrochloride.** (rep-ROW-TEE-role) USAN.
Use: Bronchodilator.

Reptilase-R. (Abbott Diagnostics) Diagnostic for the investigation of fibrin formation and disturbances in fibrin formation due to causes other than thrombin inhibition.
Use: Diagnostic aid.

Requa's Charcoal Tablets. (Requa, Inc.) Wood charcoal 10 gr/Tab. Pkg. 50s. Can 125s. *otc.*
Use: Antiflatulent.

Requip. (SmithKline Beecham) Ropinirole HCl 0.25 mg, 0.5 mg, 1 mg, 2 mg, 5 mg, lactose. Tab. Bot. 30s, 100s. *Rx.*
Use: Antiparkinson agent.

Resa. (Vita Elixir) Reserpine 0.25 mg/Tab. Bot. *Rx.*
Use: Antihypertensive.

Resaid. (Geneva Pharmaceuticals) Phenylpropanolamine HCl 75 mg, chlorpheniramine maleate 12 mg/Cap. Bot. 100s, 1000s. *Rx.*
Use: Antihistamine, decongestant.

Resaid S.R. (Geneva Pharmaceuticals) Phenylpropanolamine HCl 75 mg, chlorpheniramine maleate 12 mg/SR Cap. Bot. 100s, 1000s. *Rx.*
Use: Antihistamine, decongestant.

Rescaps-D S.R. (Geneva Pharmaceuticals) Phenylpropanolamine HCl 75 mg, caramiphen edisylate 40 mg/Cap. Bot. 100s. *Rx.*
Use: Antitussive, decongestant.

Rescon Capsules. (ION Laboratories, Inc.) Pseudoephedrine 120 mg, chlorpheniramine maleate 12 mg/TR Cap. Bot. 100s. *Rx.*
Use: Antihistamine, decongestant.

Rescon-DM. (ION Laboratories, Inc.) Dextromethorphan HBr 10 mg, pseudoephedrine HCl 30 mg, chlorpheniramine maleate 2 mg/5 ml, sugar free. Liq. Bot. 120 ml. *otc.*
Use: Antihistamine, antitussive, decongestant.

Rescon-ED. (ION Laboratories, Inc.) Chlorpheniramine maleate 8 mg, pseudoephedrine HCl 120 mg/Cap. Bot. 100s. *Rx.*
Use: Antihistamine, decongestant.

Rescon-GG Capsules. (ION Laboratories, Inc.) Pseudoephedrine HCl 120 mg, chlorpheniramine maleate 8 mg/Cap. Bot. 100s. *otc.*
Use: Antihistamine, decongestant.

Rescon-GG Liquid. (ION Laboratories, Inc.) Phenylephrine HCl 5 mg, guaifenesin 100 mg/5 ml Bot. 4 oz. *otc.*
Use: Decongestant, expectorant.

Rescon JR. (ION Laboratories, Inc.) Pseudoephedrine HCl 60 mg, chlorpheniramine maleate 4 mg/SR Cap. Bot. 100s. *Rx.*
Use: Antihistamine, decongestant.

Rescon Liquid. (ION Laboratories, Inc.) Phenylpropanolamine HCl 12.5 mg, chlorpheniramine maleate 2 mg/5 ml. Bot. 120 ml, 473 ml. *otc.*
Use: Antihistamine, decongestant.

Rescriptor. (Pharmacia & Upjohn) Delavirdine mesylate 100 mg, lactose. Tab. Bot. 360s. *Rx.*
Use: Antiviral.

Resectisol. (McGaw, Inc.) Mannitol soln. 5 g/1000 ml in distilled water (275 mOsm/L). In 2000 ml. *Rx.*
Use: Irrigant, genitourinary.

Reserpaneed. (Hanlon) Reserpine 0.25 mg/Tab. Bot. 100s, 1000s. *Rx.*
Use: Antihypertensive.

•**reserpine.** (reh-SER-peen) U.S.P. 23.
Use: Antihypertensive.
See: Arcum R-S, Tab. (Arcum).
Broserpine, Tab. (Brothers).
De Serpa, Tab. (De Leon).
Elserpine, Tab. (Canright).
Raurine, Tab. (Westerfield).
Reserpaneed, Tab. (Hanlon).
Serpasil Preps. (Novartis Pharmaceutical Corp.).
Sertabs, Tab. (Table Rock).
T-Serp, Tab. (Tennessee Pharmaceutic).

Zepine, Tab. (Foy Laboratories).

reserpine w/combinations.
See: Demi-Regroton, Tab. (Rhone-Poulenc Rorer Pharmaceuticals, Inc.).
Harbolin, Tab. (Arcum).
Hydromox R, Tab. (ESI Lederle Generics).
Hydropres-50, Tab. (Merck & Co.).
Hydroserp, Tab. (Zenith Goldline Pharmaceuticals).
Hydroserpine, Tab. (Geneva Pharmaceuticals).
Hydrotensin-50, Tab. (Merz Pharmaceuticals).
Metatensin, Tab. (Hoechst Marion Roussel).
Regroton, Tab. (Rhone-Poulenc Rorer Pharmaceuticals, Inc.).
Renese-R, Tab. (Pfizer US Pharmaceutical Group).
Salutensin, Tab. (Bristol-Myers Squibb).
Salutensin-Demi (Roberts Pharm.).
Ser-Ap-Es, Tab. (Novartis Pharmaceutical Corp.).
Serpasil-Apresoline, Tab. (Novartis Pharmaceutical Corp.).
Serpasil-Esidrix, Tab. (Novartis Pharmaceutical Corp.).

reserpine and chlorothiazide tablets.
Use: Antihypertensive.

reserpine and hydrochlorothiazide tablets. (Various Mfr.) Hydrochlorothiazide 25 mg, 50 mg, reserpine 0.125 mg/Tab. Bot. 100s, 1000s. *Rx.*
Use: Antihypertensive.

reserpine, hydralazine hydrochloride, and hydrochlorothiazide.
Use: Antihypertensive.

Resinol Medicinal Ointment. (Mentholatum Co., Inc.) Zinc oxide 12%, calamine 6%, resorcinol 2% in a lanolin and petrolatum base. Jar 3.5 oz, 1.25 oz. *otc.*
Use: Dermatologic, protectant.

resins, antacid.
See: Polyamine methylene Resins.

•**resocortol butyrate.** (reh-so-CORE-tole BYOO-tih-rate) USAN.
Use: Corticosteroid; anti-inflammatory, topical.

Resol. (Wyeth-Ayerst Laboratories) Na 50 mEq, K 20 mEq, Cl 50 mEq, citrate 34 mEq, Ca 4 mEq, Mg 4 mEq, phosphate 5 mEq, glucose 20 g/L. Contains 80 calories/L. Ctn. 32 fl oz. *Rx.*
Use: Fluid, electrolyte replacement.

Resolve/GP Daily Cleaner. (Allergan, Inc.) Buffered solution with cocoamphocarboxyglycinate, sodium lauryl sulfate, hexylene glycol, alkyl ether sulfate, fatty acid amide surfactant cleaning agents, preservative free. Soln. Bot. 30 ml. *otc.*
Use: Contact lens care.

Resonium-A. (Sanofi Winthrop Pharmaceuticals) Sodium polystyrene sulfonate. *Rx.*
Use: Potassium removing resin.

resorcin.
See: Resorcinol (Various Mfr.).

•**resorcinol.** (reh-SORE-sih-nole) U.S.P. 23.
Use: Keratolytic.

resorcinol and sulfur lotion.
Use: Antifungal, parasiticide, scabicide.

resorcinol w/combinations.
See: Acnomel, Cake, Cream (SmithKline Beecham Pharmaceuticals).
Bicozene, Cream (Ex-Lax).
Black and White, Oint. (Schering-Plough Corp.).
Clearasil, Stick (Procter & Gamble Co.).
Lanacane, Creme (Combe, Inc.).
RA, Lot. (Medco Diagnostic Supply).
Rezamid Lot. (Del Pharmaceuticals, Inc.).

•**resorcinol monoacetate.** U.S.P. 23.
Use: Antiseborrheic, keratolytic.
See: Euresol, Liq. (Knoll Pharmaceuticals).

resorcinolphthalein sodium.
Use: Antiseborrheic, topical.
See: Fluorescein Sodium, U.S.P. 23. (Various Mfr.).

Resource. (Novartis Pharmaceutical Corp.) Ca and Na caseinates, soy protein isolate 37 g, sugar, hydrolyzed cornstarch 140 g, corn oil, soy lecithin 37 g, Na 890 mg, K 1600 mg, A, B_1, B_2, B_3, B_5, B_6, B_{12}, C, D, E, K, Ca, P, I, Fe, Mg, Cu, Zn, Mn, Cl, gluten free, vanilla, chocolate, strawberry flavor. Liq. Bot. 237 ml. *otc.*
Use: Nutritional supplement.

Resource Instant Crystals. (Novartis Pharmaceutical Corp.) Vanilla flavor: maltodextrin, sucrose, hydrogenated soy oil, sodium caseinate, calcium caseinate, soy protein isolate, potassium citrate, polyglycerol esters of fatty acids, artificial flavors, vitamins and minerals. Instant Crystals 1.5 oz., 2 oz. packets. *otc.*
Use: Nutritional supplement.

Resource Plus. (Novartis Pharmaceutical Corp.) Ca and Na caseinates, soy protein isolate 54.9 g, maltodextrin, sucrose 200 g, corn oil, lecithin 53.3 g, Na 899 mg, K 1740 mg, A, B_1, B_2, B_3, B_5, B_6, B_{12}, C, D, E, K, bio-

tin, choline, Ca, P, I, Fe, Mg, Cu, Zn, Cl, Mn, gluten free, vanilla, chocolate, strawberry flavor. Liq. Bot. 8 oz. *otc.*
Use: Nutritional supplement.

Respa-1st. (Respa Pharmaceuticals, Inc.) Pseudoephedrine HCl 60 mg, guaifenesin 600 mg. SR Tab. Bot. 100s. *Rx.*
Use: Decongestant, expectorant.

Respa-DM. (Respa Pharmaceuticals, Inc.) Dextromethorphan HBr 30 mg, guaifenesin 600 mg. SR Tab. Bot. 100s. *Rx.*
Use: Antitussive, expectorant.

Respa-GF. (Respa Pharmaceuticals, Inc.) Guaifenesin 600 mg, lactose. SR Tab. Bot. 100s. *Rx.*
Use: Expectorant.

Respahist. (Respa Pharmaceuticals, Inc.) Pseudoephedrine HCl 60 mg, brompheniramine maleate 6 mg/SR Cap. Bot 100s. *Rx.*
Use: Antihistamine, decongenstant.

Respaire-60 SR. (Laser, Inc.) Pseudoephedrine HCl 60 mg, guaifenesin 200 mg/SR Cap. Bot. 100s, 1000s. *Rx.*
Use: Decongestant, expectorant.

Respaire-120 SR. (Laser, Inc.) Pseudoephedrine HCl 120 mg, guaifenesin 250 mg/SR Cap. Bot. 100s, 1000s. *Rx.*
Use: Decongestant, expectorant.

Respalor. (Bristol-Myers Squibb) Protein 75 g, carbohydrate 146 g, fat 70 g, Na 1248 mg, K 1456 mg, Fe 12.5 mg, cal/L 1498. Lactose free. Vanilla flavor. With appropriate vitamins and minerals. Liq. Bot. 237 ml. *otc.*
Use: Nutritional supplement.

Respbid. (Boehringer Ingelheim, Inc.) Theophylline 250 mg, 500 mg/Tab. Bot. 100s. *Rx.*
Use: Bronchodilator.

RespiGam. (MedImmune, Inc.) RSV immunoglobulin (human) 2500 mg, sucrose 5%, albumin (human) 1% w/sodium 1 to 1.5 mEq/50 ml. Preservative free. IV Vial 2500 mg/50 ml. *Rx.*
Use: Immunization.

Respihaler Decadron Phosphate. (Merck & Co.)
See: Decadron phosphate, Respihaler (Merck & Co.).

Respiracult. (Orion Diagnostica) Culture test for group A beta-hemolytic streptococci. In 10s.
Use: Diagnostic aid.

Respiralex. (Orion Diagnostica) Latex agglutination test to detect group A streptococci in throat and nasopharynx. Kit 1s.
Use: Diagnostic aid.

respiratory syncytial virus immune globulin (human) (RSV-IG).
Use: Prophylaxis against respiratory tract infection. [Orphan Drug]
See: RespiGam, Inj. (MedImmune, Inc.).

respiratory syncytial virus immune globulin intravenous (human) (RSV-IVIG).
Use: Respiratory syncytial virus immune serum.
See: RespiGam (MedImmune, Inc.).

Rest Easy. (Walgreen Co.) Acetaminophen 1000 mg, pseudoephedrine HCl 60 mg, dextromethorphan HBr 30 mg, doxylamine succinate 7.5 mg/30 ml. Bot. 6 oz, 16 oz. *otc.*
Use: Analgesic, antihistamine, antitussive, decongestant.

Restore. (Inagra) Psyllium hydrophilic mucilloid fiber 3.4 g/12 g dose, orange flavor, saccharin, sucrose. Pow. 390 g, 538 g. Also available sugar free with aspartame, phenylalanine 30 mg/tsp, saccharin. Pow. 300 g, 425 g. *otc.*
Use: Laxative.

Restoril. (Novartis Pharmaceutical Corp.) Temazepam 7.5 mg, lactose. Cap. Bot. 100s. ControlPak 25s, UD 100s. *c-IV.*
Use: Hypnotic, sedative.

Retavase. (Boehringer Mannheim Pharmaceuticals) Reteplase 10.8 IU (18.8 mg)/Pow. for Inj. Kit. *Rx.*
Use: Management of acute myocardial infarction.

•**reteplase.** USAN.
Use: Management of acute myocardial infarction, plasminogen activator.
See: Retavase, Pow. for Inj. (Boehringer Mannheim Pharmaceuticals).

Retin-A Cream. (Ortho McNeil Pharmaceutical) Tretinoin 0.1%, 0.05%, 0.025%. Tube 20 g, 45 g. *Rx.*
Use: Dermatologic, acne.

Retin-A Gel. (Ortho McNeil Pharmaceutical) Tretinoin 0.01%, 0.025%, alcohol 90%. Tube 15 g, 45 g. *Rx.*
Use: Dermatologic, acne.

Retin-A Liquid. (Ortho McNeil Pharmaceutical) Tretinoin (retinoic acid, vitamin A acid) 0.05%, polyethylene glycol 400, butylated hydroxytoluene and alcohol 55%. Bot. 28 ml. *Rx.*
Use: Dermatologic, acne.

Retin-A Micro. (Ortho McNeil Pharmaceutical) Tretinoin 0.1%, glycerin, propylene glycol, benzyl alcohol, EDTA. Gel. Tube 20 g, 45 g. *Rx.*
Use: Dermatologic, acne.

retinoic acid. Tretinoin, U.S.P. 23
Use: Keratolytic.

See: Retin A, Prods. (Ortho McNeil Pharmaceutical).

retinoic acid, 9-cis.
Use: Acute promyelocytic leukemia. [Orphan Drug]

retinoin.
Use: Squamous metaplasia of the ocular surface epithelia with mucus deficiency and keratinization. [Orphan Drug]

Retinol. (NBTY, Inc.) Vitamin A 100,000 IU, glycol stearate, mineral oil, propylene glycol, lanolin oil, propylene glycol stearate SE, lanolin alcohol, retinol, parabens, EDTA. Cream Tube 60 g. *otc.*
Use: Emollient.

Retinol-A. (Young Again Products) Vitamin A palmitate 300,000 IU/30 g. Cream Tube 60 g. *otc.*
Use: Emollient.

Retrovir. (GlaxoWellcome) Zidovudine. **Tab.:** 300 mg. Bot. 60s. **Cap:** 100 mg. Bot. 100s. UD 100s. **Syrup:** 50 mg/5 ml. Bot. 240 ml. **Inj:** 10 mg/ml. Vial 20 ml. *Rx.*
Use: Antiviral.

Reversol. (Organon Teknika Corp.) Edrophonium chloride 10 mg/ml. Inj. Vial. 10 ml. *Rx.*
Use: Muscle stimulant.

Revex. (Ohmeda Pharmaceuticals) Nalmefene 100 mcg/ml, 1 mg/ml. **100 mcg/ml:** Amp 1 ml; **1 mg/ml:** Amp 2 ml. *Rx.*
Use: Narcotic antagonist, antidote.

Rev-Eyes. (Storz/Lederle Ophthalmic Pharmaceuticals) Dapiprazole HCl 25 mg. Pow. Vial. 5 ml. *Rx.*
Use: Alpha-adrenergic blocker, ophthalmic.

ReVia. (Du Pont Merck Pharmaceutical Co.) Naltrexone HCl 50 mg/Tab. Bot. 50s. *Rx.*
Use: Antagonist, narcotic.

Revs Caffeine T.D. (Eon Labs Manufacturing, Inc.) Caffeine 250 mg/Cap. Bot. 100s, 1000s. *otc.*
Use: CNS stimulant.

Rexahistine. (Econo Med Pharmaceuticals) Phenylephrine HCl 5 mg, chlorpheniramine maleate 1 mg, menthol 1 mg, sodium bisulfite 0.1%, alcohol 5%/5 ml. Bot. Gal. *otc.*
Use: Antihistamine, decongestant.

Rexahistine DH. (Econo-Rx) Codeine phosphate 10 mg, phenylephrine HCl 10 mg, chlorpheniramine maleate 2 mg, menthol 1 mg, alcohol 5%/5 ml. Bot. Gal. *c-v.*
Use: Antihistamine, antitussive, decongestant.

Rexahistine Expectorant. (Econo-Rx) Codeine phosphate 10 mg, phenylephrine HCl 10 mg, chlorpheniramine maleate 2 mg, guaifenesin 100 mg, menthol 1 mg, alcohol 5%/5 ml. Bot. Gal. *c-v.*
Use: Antihistamine, antitussive, decongestant, expectorant.

Rexigen. (ION Laboratories, Inc.) Phendimetrazine tartrate 35 mg/Tab. Bot. 100s. *c-III.*
Use: Anorexiant.

Rexigen Forte. (ION Laboratories, Inc.) Phendimetrazine tartrate 105 mg/SR Cap. Bot. 100s. *c-III.*
Use: Anorexiant.

Rezamid. (Summers Laboratories, Inc.) Sulfur 5%, resorcinol 2%, SD alcohol 40 28%. Lot. 56.7 ml. *otc.*
Use: Dermatologic, acne.

Rezine. (Marnel Pharmaceuticals, Inc.) Hydroxyzine HCl 10 mg, 25 mg. Tab. Bot. 100s. *Rx.*
Use: Anxiolytic.

Rezulin. (Parke-Davis) Troglitazone 200 mg, 300 mg, 400 mg. Tab. Bot. 30s, 90s, UD 100s (200 mg and 400 mg only); 60s, 120s (300 mg only). *Rx.*
Use: Antidiabetic.

RF Latex Test. (Laboratory Diagnostics) Rapid latex agglutination test for the qualitative screening and semi-quantitative determination of rheumatoid factor. Kit 100s.
Use: Diagnostic aid.

R-Frone. (Serono Laboratories, Inc.)
See: Interferon Beta (Recombinant).

R-Gel. (Healthline Laboratories, Inc.) Capsaicin 0.025%, EDTA. Gel. Tube 15 ml, 30 ml. *otc.*
Use: Analgesic, topical.

R-Gen. (Galderma Laboratories, Inc.) Purified water, amphoteric 2, hydrolyzed animal protein, lauramine oxide, methylparaben, benzalkonium Cl, tetrasodium, EDTA, propylparaben, fragrance. Bot. 8 oz. *otc.*
Use: Dermatologic, hair.

R-Gen. (Zenith Goldline Pharmaceuticals) Iodinated glycerol 60 mg/5 ml, alcohol 21.75%. Elix. Bot. Pt. *Rx.*
Use: Expectorant.

R-Gene 10. (Pharmacia & Upjohn) Arginine HCl 10% (950 mOsm/L) with Cl ion 47.5 mEq/100 ml. Inj. 300 ml. *Rx.*
Use: Diagnostic aid, pituitary (growth hormone) function test.

R-HCTZ-H. (ESI Lederle Generics) Reserpine 0.1 mg, hydrochlorothiazide 15 mg, hydralazine HCl 25 mg/Tab. Bot. 100s, 500s. *Rx.*

Use: Antihypertensive.

Rheaban Maximum Strength. (Pfizer US Pharmaceutical Group) Activated attapulgite 750 mg. Capl. Pkg. 12s. *otc.*
Use: Antidiarrheal.

Rheomacrodex. (Medisan) Dextran 40 10% in sodium Cl 0.9% or in dextrose 5%. Soln. Bot. 500 ml. *Rx.*
Use: Plasma expander.

Rheumatex. (Wampole Laboratories) Latex agglutination test for the qualitative detection and quantitative determination of rheumatoid factor in serum. Kit 100s.
Use: Diagnostic aid.

Rheumaton. (Wampole Laboratories) Two-minute hemagglutination slide test for the qualitative and quantitative determination of rheumatoid factor in serum or synovial fluid. Test kit 20s, 50s, 150s.
Use: Diagnostic aid.

Rheumatrex Dose Pack. (ESI Lederle Generics) Methotrexate 2.5 mg. Tab. Pkg. 5 mg, 7.5 mg, 10 mg, 12.5 mg, 15 mg/week dose packs. *Rx.*
Use: Antipsoriatic.

Rhinall Drops. (Scherer Laboratories, Inc.) Phenylephrine HCl 0.25%, sodium bisulfite. Bot. oz. *otc.*
Use: Decongestant.

Rhinall Spray. (Scherer Laboratories, Inc.) Phenylephrine HCl 0.25%. Bot. oz. *otc.*
Use: Decongestant.

Rhinall 10. (Scherer Laboratories, Inc.) Phenylephrine HCl 0.2%. Drop. Bot. oz. *otc.*
Use: Decongestant.

Rhinatate. (Major Pharmaceuticals) Phenylephrine tannate 25 mg, chlorpheniramine tannate 8 mg, pyrilamine tannate 25 mg/Tab. Bot. 100s, 250s. *Rx.*
Use: Antihistamine, decongestant.

Rhinocort. (Astra Pharmaceuticals, L.P.) Budesonide 32 mcg/actuation. Can 7 g (≥ 200 sprays). *Rx.*
Use: Corticosteroid, nasal.

Rhinolar-EX. (McGregor Pharmaceuticals, Inc.) Phenylpropanolamine HCl 75 mg, chlorpheniramine maleate 8 mg/SR Cap. Dye free. Bot. 60s. *Rx.*
Use: Antihistamine, decongestant.

Rhinolar-EX 12. (McGregor Pharmaceuticals, Inc.) Phenylpropanolamine HCl 75 mg, chlorpheniramine maleate 12 mg/SR Cap. Dye free. Bot. 60s. *Rx.*
Use: Antihistamine, decongestant.

Rhinosyn. (Great Southern Laboratories) Pseudoephedrine HCl 60 mg, chlorpheniramine maleate 4 mg/5 ml, alcohol 0.45%, sucrose. Liq. Bot. 120 ml, 473 ml. *otc.*
Use: Antihistamine, decongestant.

Rhinosyn-DM. (Great Southern Laboratories) Pseudoephedrine HCl 30 mg, chlorpheniramine maleate 2 mg, dextromethorphan HBr 15 mg/5 ml, alcohol 1.4%, sucrose. Liq. Bot. 120 ml. *otc.*
Use: Antihistamine, antitussive, decongestant.

Rhinosyn-DMX. (Great Southern Laboratories) Dextromethorphan HBr 15 mg, guaifenesin 100 mg/5 ml, alcohol 1.4%. Syr. Bot. 120 ml. *otc.*
Use: Antitussive, expectorant.

Rhinosyn-PD. (Great Southern Laboratories) Pseudoephedrine HCl 30 mg, chlorpheniramine maleate 2 mg/5 ml. Liq. Bot. 120 ml. *otc.*
Use: Antihistamine, decongestant.

Rhinosyn-X. (Great Southern Laboratories) Pseudoephedrine HCl 30 mg, dextromethorphan HBr 10 mg, guaifenesin 100 mg/5 ml, alcohol 7.5%. Liq. Bot. 120 ml. *otc.*
Use: Antitussive, decongestant, expectorant.

rhodanate.
See: Potassium Thiocyanate.

rhodanide. More commonly Rhodanate, same as thiocyanate.
See: Potassium thiocyanate.

•**rh$_o$(d) immune globulin.** (RH$_0$D ih-MYOON GLAB-byoo-lin) U.S.P. 23.
Formerly Rh$_o$(D) Immune Globulin
Use: Immunizination.
See: Gamulin Rh, Vial (Centeon).
Mini-Gamulin Rh (Centeon).
MICRh$_o$GAM (Ortho McNeil Pharmaceutical).
BayRh$_o$D (Bayer Corp. (Consumer Div.)).
RhoGAM (Ortho McNeil Pharmaceutical).
WinRho SD (Univax Biologics).

rh$_o$(d) immune globulin. (RH$_0$D ih-MYOON GLAB-byoo-lin) *Formerly RH$_o$ Immune Human Globulin.*
Use: Immune thrombocytopenic purpura, immunizing agent (passive). [Orphan Drug]
See: WinRho SD (Univax Biologics).

RhoGAM. (Ortho Diagnostic Systems, Inc.) Rh$_o$ (D) immune globulin (human). Single-dose vial Pkg. 5s; Prefilled syringe Pkg. 5s, 25s. *Rx.*
Use: Immunization.

Rhuli Gel. (Rydelle Laboratories) Phenylcarbinol 2%, menthol 0.3%, camphor 0.3%, SD alcohol 23A 31%. Gel 60 ml.

otc.
Use: Dermatologic, poison ivy.

Rhuli Spray. (Rydelle Laboratories) Phenylcarbinol 0.67%, calamine 4.7%, menthol 0.025%, camphor 0.25%, benzocaine 1.15%, alcohol 28.8%. Aerosol 120 g. *otc.*
Use: Dermatologic, poison ivy.

Rhythmin. (Sidmak Laboratories, Inc.) Procainamide 250 mg, 500 mg/SR Tab. Bot. 100s, 500s, 1000s. *Rx.*
Use: Antiarrhythmic.

•**ribaminol.** (rye-BAM-ih-nahl) USAN.
Use: Memory adjuvant.

•**ribavirin.** (rye-buh-VIE-rin) U.S.P. 23.
Use: Antiviral. [Orphan Drug]
See: Virazole, Inj. (ICN Pharmaceuticals, Inc.).

ribavirin and interferon alfa-2b, recombinant.
Use: Antineoplastic.
See: Rebetron, Inj./Cap. (Schering Corporation).

•**riboflavin.** (RYE-boh-FLAY-vin) U.S.P. 23. W/Nicotinamide. (Eli Lilly and Co.)
Use: Vitamin (enzyme co-factor).

•**riboflavin 5'-phosphate sodium.** (RYE-boh-FLAY-vin 5'-FOSS-fate so-dee-oum) U.S.P. 23.
Use: Vitamin.

•**riboprine.** (RYE-boe-PREEN) USAN.
Use: Antineoplastic.

Ribozyme Injection. (Fellows) Riboflavin-5-phosphate sodium 50 mg/ml Vial 10 ml. *Rx.*

ricin (blocked) conjugated murine mca. (ImmunoGen)
Use: Antineoplastic. [Orphan Drug]

ricin (blocked) conjugated murine moab.
Use: Antineoplastic. [Orphan Drug]

Ricolon Solution. (Sanofi Winthrop Pharmaceuticals) Ricolon concentrate. *Rx.*
Use: Leucocytotic preparation.

RID. (Pfizer US Pharmaceutical Group) Piperonyl butoxide 3%, pyrethrins 0.3%, petroleum distillate 1.2%, benzyl alcohol 2.4%. Bot. 2 oz, 4 oz. *otc.*
Use: Pediculicide.

Ridaura. (SmithKline Beecham Pharmaceuticals) Auranofin 3 mg/Cap. Bot. 60s. *Rx.*
Use: Antirheumatic.

Ridenol. (R.I.D., Inc.) Acetaminophen 80 mg/5 ml. Syr. Bot. 120 ml. *otc.*
Use: Analgesic.

Rid Lice Control Spray. (Pfizer US Pharmaceutical Group) Synthetic pyrethroids 0.5%, related compounds 0.065%, aromatic petroleum hydrocarbons 0.664%. Can 5 oz. *otc.*
Use: Pediculicide.

Rid Lice Elimination System. (Pfizer US Pharmaceutical Group) Rid lice killing shampoo, nit removal comb, Rid lice control spray and instruction booklet/unit. *otc.*
Use: Pediculicide.

Rid Lice Shampoo-Kit. (Pfizer US Pharmaceutical Group) Pyrethrins 0.3%, piperonyl butoxide 3%. Bot. 2 oz, 4 oz. *otc.*
Use: Pediculicide.

•**ridogrel.** (RYE-doe-grell) USAN.
Use: Thromboxane synthetase inhibitor.

•**rifabutin.** (RIFF-uh-BYOO-tin) U.S.P. 23.
Use: Anti-infective (antimycobacterial), MAC disease. [Orphan Drug]
See: Mycobutin.

Rifadin. (Hoechst Marion Roussel) Rifampin. **150 mg/Cap.:** Bot. 30s. **300 mg/Cap.:** Bot. 30s, 60s, 100s. **600 mg/Inj.:** Vials. *Rx.*
Use: Antituberculous.

•**rifalazil.** (RIFF-ah-lah-zill) USAN.
Use: Antibacterial.

Rifamate. (Hoechst Marion Roussel) Rifampin 300 mg, isoniazid 150 mg/Cap. Bot. 60s. *Rx.*
Use: Antituberculosal.

•**rifametane.** (RIFF-ah-met-ane) USAN.
Use: Anti-infective.

•**rifamexil.** (riff-ah-MEX-ill) USAN.
Use: Anti-infective.

•**rifamide.** (RIFF-am-ide) USAN.
Use: Anti-infective.

•**rifampin.** (RIFF-am-pin) U.S.P. 23.
Use: Anti-infective.
See: Rifadin, Cap, Inj. (Hoechst Marion Roussel).
Rifater, Tab. (Hoechst Marion Roussel).
Rimactane, Cap. (Novartis Pharmaceutical Corp.).

rifampin and isoniazid capsules.
Use: Anti-infective (tuberculostatic).

rifampin, isoniazid, pyrazinamide.
Use: Anti-infective (tuberculostatic). [Orphan Drug]
See: Rifater (Hoechst Marion Roussel).

rifapentine.
Use: Pulmonary tuberculosis; *mycobacterium avium* complex in AIDS patients. [Orphan Drug]

•**rifapentine.** (RIFF-ah-pen-teen) USAN.
Use: Anti-infective.
See: Priftin, Tab. (Hoechst Marion Roussel).

Rifater. (Hoechst Marion Roussel) Rifampin 120 mg, isoniazid 50 mg, pyrazinamide 300 mg. Tab. 60s, UD 100s. *Rx.*
Use: Antituberculosal.

•**rifaximin.** (riff-AX-ih-min) USAN.
Use: Anti-infective.

r-IFN-beta. (Biogen)
See: Interferon Beta (Recombinant).

RIG.
Use: Immunization, rabies.
See: Bayrab (Bayer Corp. (Allergy Div.)).
Imogam (Merieux).

Rilutek. (Rhone-Poulenc Rorer Pharmaceuticals, Inc.) Riluzole 50 mg/Tab. *Rx.*
Use: Amyotrophic lateral sclerosis agent.

•**riluzole.** (RILL-you-zole) USAN.
Use: Amyotrophic lateral sclerosis agent. [Orphan Drug]
See: Rilutek, Tab. (Rhone-Poulenc Rorer Pharmaceuticals, Inc.).

Rimactane. (Novartis Pharmaceutical Corp.) Rifampin 300 mg/Cap. Bot. 30s, 60s, 100s. *Rx.*
Use: Antituberculous.

Rimadyl. (Roche Laboratories) *Rx.*
Use: Analgesic, NSAID.
See: Carprofen.

•**rimantadine hydrochloride.** (rih-MAN-tuh-deen) USAN.
Use: Antiviral.
See: Flumadine, Tab., Syr. (Forest Pharmaceutical, Inc.).

•**rimcazole hydrochloride.** (RIM-kazz-OLE) USAN.
Use: Antipsychotic.

•**rimexolone.** (rih-MEX-oh-lone) USAN.
Use: Anti-inflammatory.
See: Vexol, Susp. (Alcon Laboratories, Inc.).

•**rimiterol hydrobromide.** (RIH-mih-TER-ole) USAN.
Use: Bronchodilator.

Rimso-50. (Research Industries Corp.) Dimethyl sulfoxide in a 50% aqueous soln. Bot. 50 ml. *Rx.*
Use: Urinary tract agent.

Rinade. (Econo Med Pharmaceuticals) Chlorpheniramine maleate 8 mg, phenylephrine HCl 20 mg, methscopolamine nitrate 2.5 mg/Cap. Bot. 120s. *Rx.*
Use: Anticholinergic, antihistamine, decongestant.

Rinade-B.I.D. (Econo Med Pharmaceuticals) Chlorpheniramine maleate 8 mg, pseudoephedrine HCl 120 mg/SR Cap. Bot. 100s. *Rx.*
Use: Antihistamine, decongestant.

ringer's-dextrose injection. (Various Mfr.) Dextrose 50 g/l, Na 147, K 4, C 4.5, Cl 156. 500, 1000 ml. *Rx.*
Use: Nutritional supplement, parenteral.

•**ringer's injection.** U.S.P. 23.
Use: Fluid, electrolyte replacement; irrigant, ophthalmic.

ringer's injection. (Abbott Laboratories) 250 ml, 500 ml, 1000 ml; (Invenex) 250 ml, 500 ml, 1000 ml; Abbo-Vac glass or flexible containers, Vial 50 ml Pkg. 25s. (Eli Lilly and Co.) Amp. 20 ml, Pkg. 6s. (Bayer Corp. (Consumer Div.)) Bot. 500 ml, 1000 ml.
Use: Fluid, electrolyte replacement; irrigant.

ringer's injection, lactated.
Use: Fluid, electrolyte replacement.

ringer's irrigation. (Various Mfr.) Sodium chloride 0.86 g, potassium chloride 0.03 g, calcium chloride 0.033 g/100 ml. Bot. 1 liter. *Rx.*
Use: Irrigant, ophthalmic.

Riopan. (Whitehall Robins Laboratories) Magaldrate 540 mg, Na 0.1 mg/5 ml. Bot. 6 oz, 12 oz. Individual Cup 30 ml each. *otc.*
Use: Antacid.

Riopan Plus Double Strength Suspension. (Whitehall Robins Laboratories) Magaldrate 1080 mg, simethicone 40 mg/5 ml. Bot. 360 ml. *otc.*
Use: Antacid, antiflatulent.

Riopan Plus Double Strength Tablets. (Whitehall Robins Laboratories) Magaldrate 1080 mg, simethicone 20 mg. Chew. Tab. Bot. 60s. *otc.*
Use: Antacid, antiflatulent.

Riopan Plus Tablets. (Whitehall Robins Laboratories) Magaldrate 480 mg, simethicone 20 mg. Chew. Tab. Bot. 50s, 100s. *otc.*
Use: Antacid, antiflatulent.

•**rioprostil.** (RYE-oh-PRAHS-till) USAN.
Use: Gastric antisecretory.

•**ripazepam.** (rip-AZE-eh-pam) USAN.
Use: Anxiolytic.

•**risedronate sodium.** (riss-ED-row-nate) USAN.
Use: Regulator (calcium).

•**rismorelin porcine.** (riss-more-ELL-in PORE-sine) USAN.
Use: Hormone, growth hormone-releasing.

•**risocaine.** (RIZZ-oh-cane) USAN.
Use: Anesthetic, local.

•**risotilide hydrochloride.** (rih-SO-tih-LIDE) USAN.
Use: Cardiovascular agent (antiarrhythmic).

Risperdal. (Janssen Pharmaceutical, Inc.) Risperidone 1 mg, 2 mg, 3 mg, 4 mg. Tab. Bot. 60s, 500s, blister pack 100s. Risperidone 1 mg/ml/Oral Soln. Bot. 100 ml w/calibrated pipette. *Rx.*
Use: Antipsychotic.

•**risperidone.** (RISS-PURR-ih-dohn) USAN.
Use: Antipsychotic, neuroleptic.
See: Risperdal, Oral Soln. (Janssen Pharmaceutical, Inc.).

•**ristianol phosphate.** (riss-TIE-ah-NOLE) USAN.
Use: Immunoregulator.

Ritalin Hydrochloride. (Novartis Pharmaceutical Corp.) Methylphenidate HCl. 5 mg, 10 mg, 20 mg. Tab. Bot. 100s. *c-II.*
Use: CNS stimulant.

Ritalin-SR. (Novartis Pharmaceutical Corp.) Methylphenidate HCl 20 mg/SR Tab. Bot. 100s. *c-II.*
Use: CNS stimulant.

•**ritanserin.** (rih-TAN-ser-in) USAN.
Use: Serotonin antagonist.

•**ritodrine.** (RIH-toe-DREEN) USAN.
Use: Muscle relaxant.
See: Yutopar, Inj. (Astra Pharmaceuticals, L.P.).

•**ritodrine hydrochloride.** (RIH-toe-dreen) U.S.P. 23.
Use: Muscle relaxant.

ritodrine hydrochloride. (Abbott Laboratories) Ritodrine HCl 10 mg/ml, 15 mg/ml, 0.3 mg/ml. **10 mg/ml:** Amp. 5 ml. **15 mg/ml:** Vial 10 ml. **0.3 mg/ml:** In 15% dextrose. LifeCare flexible container 500 ml. *Rx.*
Use: Uterine relaxant.

•**ritolukast.** (rih-tah-LOO-kast) USAN.
Use: Antiasthmatic (leukotriene antagonist).

•**ritonavir.** (rih-TON-a-veer) USAN.
Use: Antiviral.
See: Norvir, Cap., Susp. (Abbott Laboratories).

Rituxan. (IDEC Pharmaceuticals) Rituximab 10 mg/ml. Inj. Single-unit Vial 10 ml, 50 ml. *Rx.*
Use: Antineoplastic.

•**rituximab.** (rih-TUCK-sih-mab) USAN.
Use: Antineoplastic (microtubule inhibitor), monoclonal antibody.
See: Rituxan, Inj. (IDEC Pharmaceuticals).

•**rizatriptan benzoate.** (rye-zah-TRIP-tan BENZ-oh-ate) USAN.
Use: Antimigraine.
See: Maxalt, Tab. (Merck & Co.).
Maxalt-MLT, Tab. (Merck & Co.).

•**rizatriptan sulfate.** (rye-zah-TRIP-tan) USAN.
Use: Antimigraine.

RMS. (Upsher-Smith Labs, Inc.) Morphine sulfate 5 mg, 10 mg, 20 mg, 30 mg/Supp. Box 12s. *c-II.*
Use: Analgesic, narcotic.

Robafen. (Major Pharmaceuticals) Guaifenesin 100 mg/5 ml, alcohol 3.5%. Syr. Bot. 118 ml, 240 ml, pt, gal. *otc.*
Use: Expectorant.

Robafen AC Cough. (Major Pharmaceuticals) Guaifenesin 100 mg, codeine phosphate 10 mg/5 ml, alcohol 3.5%, parabens. Syr. Bot. 473 ml. *c-v.*
Use: Antitussive; expectorant, narcotic.

Robafen CF. (Major Pharmaceuticals) Phenylpropanolamine HCl 12.5 mg, dextromethorphan HBr 10 mg, guaifenesin 100 mg/5 ml, alcohol 4.75%. Liq. Bot. 118 ml. *otc.*
Use: Antitussive, decongestant, expectorant.

Robafen DAC. (Major Pharmaceuticals) Pseudoephedrine 30 mg, codeine phosphate 10 mg, guaifenesin 100 mg/5 ml, alcohol 1.4%. Liq. Bot. Pt. *c-v.*
Use: Antitussive, decongestant, expectorant.

Robafen DM. (Major Pharmaceuticals) Dextromethorphan HBr 10 mg, guaifenesin 100 mg/5 ml, alcohol 1.4%. Syr. Bot. 473 ml. *otc.*
Use: Antitussive, expectorant.

robanul.
See: Robinul, Preps. (Wyeth-Ayerst Laboratories).

RoBathol Bath Oil. (Pharmaceutical Specialties, Inc.) Cottonseed oil, alkyl aryl polyether alcohol. Lanolin free. Bot. 240 ml, 480 ml, gal. *otc.*
Use: Dermatologic.

Robaxin. (Wyeth-Ayerst Laboratories) Methocarbamol. **Tab.:** 500 mg, Bot. 100s, 500s, UD 100s. **Inj.:** 100 mg/ml of a 50% aqueous soln. of polyethylene glycol 300. Vial 10 ml. *Rx.*
Use: Muscle relaxant.

Robaxin-750. (Wyeth-Ayerst Laboratories) Methocarbamol 750 mg/Tab. Bot. 100s, 500s, Dis-Co Pak 100s. *Rx.*
Use: Muscle relaxant.

Robaxisal. (Wyeth-Ayerst Laboratories) Methocarbamol (Robaxin) 400 mg, aspirin 325 mg/Tab. Bot. 100s, 500s, Dis-Co pack 100s. *Rx.*
Use: Muscle relaxant, analgesic.

Robimycin. (Wyeth-Ayerst Laboratories) Erythromycin 250 mg/Tab. Bot. 100s, 500s. *Rx.*
Use: Anti-infective, erythromycin.

Robinul. (Wyeth-Ayerst Laboratories) Glycopyrrolate 1 mg/Tab. Bot. 100s, 500s. *Rx.*
Use: Anticholinergic.

Robinul Forte. (Wyeth-Ayerst Laboratories) Glycopyrrolate 2 mg/Tab. Bot. 100s. *Rx.*
Use: Anticholinergic.

Robinul Injectable. (Wyeth-Ayerst Laboratories) Glycopyrrolate 0.2 mg/ml, benzyl alcohol 0.9%. Vial 1 ml, 2 ml, 5 ml, 20 ml. *Rx.*
Use: Anticholinergic.

Robitussin. (Wyeth-Ayerst Laboratories) Guaifenesin 100 mg/5 ml, alcohol 3.5%. Bot. 1 oz, 4 oz, 8 oz, 1 pt, gal, UD 5 ml, 10 ml, 15 ml. *otc.*
Use: Expectorant.

Robitussin A-C. (Wyeth-Ayerst Laboratories) Guaifenesin 100 mg, codeine phosphate 10 mg/5 ml, alcohol 3.5%, saccharin, sorbitol. Bot. 2 oz, 4 oz, pt, gal. *c-v.*
Use: Antitussive, expectorant.

Robitussin-CF. (Wyeth-Ayerst Laboratories) Guaifenesin 100 mg, phenylpropanolamine HCl 12.5 mg, dextromethorphan HBr 10 mg/10 ml, alcohol 4.75%, saccharin, sorbitol. Syr. Bot. 4 oz, 8 oz, 12 oz, pt. *otc.*
Use: Antitussive, decongestant, expectorant.

Robitussin Cold & Cough Liqui-Gels. (Wyeth-Ayerst Laboratories) Guaifenesin 200 mg, pseudoephedrine HCl 30 mg, dextromethorphan HBr 10 mg, sorbitol. Cap. Bot. 20s. *otc.*
Use: Antitussive, expectorant, decongestant.

Robitussin Cough Calmers. (Wyeth-Ayerst Laboratories) Dextromethorphan HBr 5 mg, corn syrup, sucrose, cherry flavor. Loz. Pkg. 16s. *otc.*
Use: Antitussive.

Robitussin Cough Drops. (Wyeth-Ayerst Laboratories) Menthol 7.4 mg, 10 mg, eucalyptus oil, sucrose, corn syrup. Loz. Pkg. 9s, 25s, menthol 10 mg, eucalyptus oil, sucrose, corn syrup, honey-lemon flavor. Loz. Pkg. 9s, 25s. *otc.*
Use: Antitussive.

Robitussin-DAC. (Wyeth-Ayerst Laboratories) Guaifenesin 100 mg, pseudoephedrine HCl 30 mg, codeine phosphate 10 mg/5 ml, alcohol 1.9%, saccharin, sorbitol. Syr. Bot. 4 oz, pt. *c-v.*
Use: Antitussive, expectorant, decongestant.

Robitussin Dis-Co. (Wyeth-Ayerst Laboratories) Guaifenesin 100 mg/5 ml, alcohol 3.5%. Syr. UD pack 5 ml, 10 ml, 15 ml. *otc.*
Use: Expectorant.

Robitussin-DM. (Wyeth-Ayerst Laboratories) Guaifenesin 100 mg, dextromethorphan HBr 10 mg/5 ml. Syr. Bot. 4 oz, 8 oz, pt, gal, UD 5 ml, 10 ml (100s). *otc.*
Use: Antitussive, expectorant.

Robitussin Liquid Center Cough Drops. (Wyeth-Ayerst Laboratories) Menthol 10 mg, eucalyptus oil, corn syrup, honey, lemon oil, high fructose, parabens, sorbitol, sucrose. Loz. Pkg. 20s. *otc.*
Use: Mouth and throat preparation.

Robitussin Maximum Strength Cough & Cold Formula. (Wyeth-Ayerst Laboratories) Dextromethorphan HBr 15 mg, pseudoephedrine HCl 30 mg/5 ml, alcohol 1.4%, glucose. Liq. Bot. 240 ml. *otc.*
Use: Antitussive, decongestant.

Robitussin Night Relief. (Wyeth-Ayerst Laboratories) Acetaminophen 108.3 mg, pseudoephedrine HCl 10 mg, pyrilamine maleate 8.3 mg, dextromethorphan HBr 5 mg, alcohol-free, saccharin, sorbitol. Bot. 300 ml. *otc.*
Use: Analgesic, antihistamine, antitussive, decongestant.

Robitussin-PE. (Wyeth-Ayerst Laboratories) Guaifenesin 100 mg, pseudoephedrine HCl 30 mg/5 ml, alcohol 1.4%, saccharin. Syr. Bot. 4 oz, 8 oz, pt. *otc.*
Use: Decongestant, expectorant.

Robitussin Pediatric. (Wyeth-Ayerst Laboratories) Dextromethorphan HBr 7.5 mg/5 ml, alcohol free, saccharin, sorbitol, cherry flavor. Liq. Bot. 120 ml, 240 ml. *otc.*
Use: Antitussive.

Robitussin Pediatric Cough & Cold Formula. (Wyeth-Ayerst Laboratories) Dextromethorphan HBr 7.5 mg, pseudoephedrine HCl 15 mg/5 ml. Liq. Bot. 120 ml. *otc.*
Use: Antitussive, decongestant.

Robitussin Severe Congestion Liqui-Gels. (Wyeth-Ayerst Laboratories) Guaifenesin 200 mg, pseudoephedrine HCl 30 mg, sorbitol. Cap. Pkg. 24s. *otc.*
Use: Decongestant, expectorant.

Robomol/ASA. (Major Pharmaceuticals) Methocarbamol w/ASA. Tab. Bot. 100s, 500s. *Rx.*
Use: Muscle relaxant, analgesic.

Rocaltrol. (Roche Laboratories) Calcitriol. **Cap.:** 0.25 mcg, 0.5 mcg. Bot.

30s (0.25 mcg only), 100s. **Oral Soln.:** 1 mcg/ml. Bot. 15 ml. *Rx.*
Use: Antihypocalcemic.

•**rocastine hydrochloride.** (row-KASS-teen) USAN.
Use: Antihistamine.

Rocephin. (Roche Laboratories) Ceftriaxone sodium **Pow. for Inj.:** 250 mg, 500 mg, 1 g, 2 g, 10 g Vial. **250 mg, 500 mg:** Vial. **1 g, 2 g:** Vial, piggyback vial, ADD-Vantage vial. **10 g:** Bulk Containers. **Inj.: 1 g, 2 g, Frozen Premixed:** 50 ml plastic containers. *Rx.*
Use: Anti-infective, cephalosporin.

•**rocuronium bromide.** (row-kuhr-OH-nee-uhm) USAN.
Use: Neuromuscular blocker.

•**rodocaine.** (ROW-doe-cane) USAN.
Use: Anesthetic, local.

roentgenography.
See: Iodine Products, Diagnostic.

•**rofecoxib.** (roe-feh-cox-ib) USAN.
Use: Anti-inflammatory; analgesic.

Roferon-A. (Roche Laboratories) Interferon alfa-2a, recombinant as 3 million, 6 million, 9 million, 36 million IU/ml or 6 million or 9 million IU/0.5 ml. Inj. Soln. Vial. *Rx.*
Use: Antineoplastic agent.

•**roflurane.** (row-FLEW-rane) USAN.
Use: Anesthetic, general.

Rogaine. (Pharmacia & Upjohn) Minoxidil 2% Topical Soln. Bot. 60 ml w/applicator. *otc.*
Use: Antialopecia agent.

•**rogletimide.** (row-GLETT-ih-MIDE) USAN.
Use: Antineoplastic (aromatase inhibitor).

Rolaids Calcium Rich. (Warner Lambert) Calcium carbonate 412 mg, magnesium hydroxide 80 mg. Chew. Tab. 12s, 36s, 75s, 150s. *otc.*
Use: Antacid.

Rolatuss Expectorant. (Huckaby Pharmacal, Inc.) Phenylephrine HCl 5 mg, chlorpheniramine maleate 2 mg, codeine phosphate 9.85 mg, ammonium Cl 33.3 mg/5 ml, alcohol 5%. Bot. 480 ml. *c-v.*
Use: Antihistamine, antitussive, decongestant, expectorant.

Rolatuss w/Hydrocodone. (Major Pharmaceuticals) Phenylpropanolamine HCl 3.3 mg, phenylephrine HCl 5 mg, pyrilamine maleate 3.3 mg, pheniramine maleate 3.3 mg, hydrocodone bitartrate 1.67 mg/5 ml. Liq. Bot. 480 ml. *c-III.*
Use: Antihistamine, antitussive, decongestant.

Rolatuss Plain. (Major Pharmaceuticals) Phenylephrine HCl 5 mg, chlorpheniramine maleate 2 mg/5 ml. Liq. Bot. 473 ml. *otc.*
Use: Antihistamine, decongestant.

•**roletamide.** (row-LET-am-ide) USAN.
Use: Hypnotic, sedative.

•**rolgamidine.** (role-GAM-ih-deen) USAN.
Use: Antidiarrheal.

Rolicap. (Arcum) Vitamins A acetate 5000 IU, D_2 400 IU, B_1 3 mg, B_2 2.5 mg, B_6 10 mg, C 50 mg, niacinamide 20 mg, B_{12} 1 mcg/Chew. Tab. Bot. 100s, 1000s. *otc.*
Use: Vitamin supplement.

•**rolicyprine.** (ROW-lih-SIGH-preen) USAN.
Use: Antidepressant.

•**rolipram.** (ROLE-ih-pram) USAN.
Use: Anxiolytic.

•**rolitetracycline.** (ROW-lee-tet-rah-SIGH-kleen) USAN.
Use: Anti-infective.

•**rolitetracycline nitrate.** (ROW-lee-tet-rah-SIGH-kleen) USAN. Tetrim.
Use: Anti-infective.

•**rolodine.** (ROW-low-deen) USAN.
Use: Muscle relaxant.

Romach Antacid. (Last) Magnesium carbonate 400 mg, sodium bicarbonate 250 mg/Tab. Strip pack 60s, 500s. *otc.*
Use: Antacid.

•**romazarit.** (row-MAZZ-ah-rit) USAN.
Use: Anti-inflammatory, antirheumatic.

Romazicon. (Roche Laboratories) Flumazenil 0.1 mg/ml, parabens, EDTA. Inj. Vials 5 ml, 10 ml. *Rx.*
Use: Antidotes.

Romex Cough & Cold. (APC) Guaifenesin 65 mg, dextromethorphan HBr 10 mg, chlorpheniramine maleate 1.5 mg, pyrilamine maleate 12.5 mg, phenylephrine HCl 5 mg, acetaminophen 160 mg/Cap. Bot. 21s. *otc.*
Use: Antihistamine, antitussive, decongestant, expectorant.

Romex Cough & Cold. (APC) Dextromethorphan HBr 7.5 mg, phenylephrine HCl 2.5 mg, ascorbic acid 30 mg/Tab. Box 15s. *otc.*
Use: Antitussive, decongestant.

Romex Troches & Liquid. (APC) **Troche:** Polymyxin B sulfate 1000 units, benzocaine 5 mg, cetalkonium Cl 2.5 mg, gramicidin 100 mcg, chlorpheniramine maleate 0.5 mg, tyrothricin 2 mg. Pkg. 10s. **Liq.:** Guaifenesin 200 mg, dextromethorphan HBr 60 mg, chlorpheniramine maleate 12 mg, phenylephrine HCl 30 mg/fl oz. Bot. 4 oz. *Rx.*

Use: Antihistamine, anti-infective, antitussive, decongestant, expectorant.

Rondamine-DM. (Major Pharmaceuticals) Pseudoephedrine 25 mg, carbinoxamine maleate 2 mg, dextromethorphan HBr 4 mg/ml. Drop. 30 ml. *Rx.*
Use: Antihistamine, antitussive, decongestant.

Rondec Chewable Tablets. (Dura Pharmaceuticals) Brompheniramine maleate 4 mg, pseudoephedrine HCl 60 mg, aspartame, phenylalanine 30.9 mg. Chew. Tab. Bot. 100s. *Rx.*
Use: Antihistamine, decongestant.

Rondec-DM Oral Drops. (Dura Pharmaceuticals) Carbinoxamine maleate 2 mg, pseudoephedrine HCl 25 mg, dextromethorphan HBr 4 mg/ml, alcohol 6%. Bot. 30 ml w/dropper. *Rx.*
Use: Antihistamine, antitussive, decongestant.

Rondec-DM Syrup. (Dura Pharmaceuticals) Carbinoxamine maleate 4 mg, pseudoephedrine HCl 60 mg, dextromethorphan HBr 15 mg/5 ml, alcohol 6%. Bot. 4 oz, pt. *Rx.*
Use: Antihistamine, antitussive, decongestant.

Rondec Oral Drops. (Dura Pharmaceuticals) Carbinoxamine maleate 2 mg, pseudoephedrine HCl 25 mg/ml. Bot. 30 ml. *Rx.*
Use: Antihistamine, decongestant.

Rondec Syrup. (Dura Pharmaceuticals) Carbinoxamine maleate 4 mg, pseudoephedrine HCl 60 mg/5 ml. Syr. Bot. 120 ml, 473 ml. *Rx.*
Use: Antihistamine, decongestant.

Rondec Tablets. (Dura Pharmaceuticals) Pseudoephedrine HCl 60 mg, carbinoxamine maleate 4 mg, lactose/Tab. Bot. 100s, 500s. *Rx.*
Use: Antihistamine, decongestant.

Rondec-TR. (Dura Pharmaceuticals) Carbinoxamine 8 mg, pseudoephedrine HCl 120 mg/SR Tab. Bot. 100s. *Rx.*
Use: Antihistamine, decongestant.

•**ronidazole.** (row-NYE-dazz-OLE) USAN.
Use: Antiprotozoal.

•**ronnel.** (RAHN-ell) USAN. Fenchlorphos.
Use: Insecticide (systemic).

Ronvet. (Armenpharm Ltd.) Erythromycin stearate 250 mg/Tab. Bot. 100s. *Rx.*
Use: Anti-infective, erythromycin.

•**ropinirole hydrochloride.** (row-PIN-ih-role) USAN.
Use: Antiparkinsonian (D_2 receptor agonist).
See: Requip, Tab. (SmithKline Beecham).

•**ropitoin hydrochloride.** (ROW-pih-toe-in) USAN.
Use: Cardiovascular agent (antiarrhythmic).

ropivacaine HCl.
Use: Anesthetic.
See: Naropin, Inj. (Astra Pharmaceuticals, L.P.).

•**ropizine.** (row-PIH-zeen) USAN.
Use: Anticonvulsant.

•**roquinimex.** (row-KWIH-nih-mex) USAN.
Use: Biological response modifier; immunomodulator; antineoplastic. [Orphan Drug]
See: Linomide.

rosaniline dyes.
See: Fuchsin, Basic (Various Mfr.). Methylrosaniline Cl, Soln., Inj. (Various Mfr.).

•**rosaramicin.** (row-ZAR-ah-MY-sin) USAN. *Formerly Rosamicin.*
Use: Anti-infective.

•**rosaramicin butyrate.** (row-ZAR-ah-MY-sin BYOO-tih-rate) USAN. *Formerly Rosamicin Butyrate.*
Use: Anti-infective.

•**rosaramicin propionate.** (row-ZAR-ah-MY-sin PRO-pee-oh-nate) USAN. *Formerly Rosamicin Propionate.*
Use: Anti-infective.

•**rosaramicin sodium phosphate.** (row-ZAR-ah-MY-sin) USAN. *Formerly Rosamicin Sodium Phosphate.*
Use: Anti-infective.

•**rosaramicin stearate.** (row-ZAR-ah-MY-sin STEE-ah-rate) USAN. *Formerly Rosamicin Stearate.*
Use: Anti-infective.

rose bengal. (Akorn, Inc.) Rose bengal 1%. Bot. 5 ml.
Use: Diagnostic, tissue staining.

•**rose bengal sodium I-125.** (rose BEN-gal) USAN.
Use: Radiopharmaceutical.

•**rose bengal sodium I-131 injection.** U.S.P. 23.
Use: Diagnostic aid (hepatic function), radiopharmaceutical.

rose bengal strips. (PBH Wesley Jessen) Rose bengal 1.3 mg. Strip Box 100s. *otc.*
Use: Diagnostic aid.

Rose-C Liquid. (Barth's) Vitamin C 300 mg, rose hip extract/5 ml. Dropper Bot. 2 oz, 8 oz. *otc.*
Use: Vitamin supplement.

rose hips. (Burgin-Arden) Vitamin C 300 mg, in base of sorbitol. Bot. 4 oz, 8 oz. *otc.*
Use: Vitamin supplement.

rose hips vitamin C. (Kirkman Sales Co., Inc.) Vitamin C. **100 mg/Tab:** Bot. 100s, 250s. **250 mg or 500 mg/Tab:** Bot. 100s, 250s, 500s. *otc.*
Use: Vitamin supplement.

•**rose oil.** N.F. 18.
Use: Pharmaceutic aid, perfume.

Rosets. (Akorn, Inc.) Rose bengal 1.3 mg/Strip. Pkg. 100s. *Rx.*
Use: Diagnostic agent, ophthalmic.

•**rose water, stronger.** N.F. 18.
Use: Pharmaceutic aid, perfume.

rose water ointment.
Use: Emollient, ointment base.

•**rosiglitazone maleate.** (roe-sih-GLIH-tah-sone MAL-ee-ate) USAN.
Use: Antidiabetic.

rosin. U.S.P. XXI.
Use: Stiffening agent, pharmaceutical necessity.

•**rosoxacin.** (row-SOX-ah-sin) USAN.
Use: Anti-infective.
See: Rosoxacin, Pow. (Sanofi Winthrop Pharmaceuticals).

Ross SLD. (Ross Laboratories) Low-residue nutritional supplement for patients restricted to a clear liquid feeding or with fat malabsorption disorders. Packet 1.35 oz. Ctn. 6s. Case 4 ctn. Can 13.5 oz. Case 6s. *otc.*
Use: Nutritional supplement.

Rotalex Test. (Orion Diagnostica) Latex slide agglutination test for detection of rotavirus in feces. Kit 1s.
Use: Diagnostic aid.

RotaShield. (Wyeth-Ayerst) Rotavirus vaccine 2.5 ml (4×10^5 pfu total virus). Oral vac., lyophilized. Preservative free. Single-dose vial w/filled Dispettes 12s, 50s. *Rx.*
Use: Vaccine.

rotavirus vaccine.
Use: Vaccine.
See: RotaShielf, Vac. (Wyeth-Ayerst).

Rotazyme II. (Abbott Diagnostics) Enzyme immunoassay for detection of rotavirus antigen in feces. Test kit 50s.
Use: Diagnostic aid.

•**rotoxamine.** (row-TOX-ah-meen) USAN.
Use: Antihistamine.

Rowasa. (Solvay Pharmaceuticals) **Rectal Susp.:** Mesalamine 4 g/60 ml. Units of 7 disposable Bot. **Supp.:** Mesalamine 500 mg. Box 12s, 24s. *Rx.*
Use: Anti-inflammatory.

•**roxadimate.** (rox-AD-ih-mate) USAN.
Use: Sunscreen.

Roxanol. (Roxane Laboratories, Inc.) Morphine sulfate 20 mg/ml. Bot. 30 ml, 120 ml w/calibrated dropper. *c-II.*
Use: Analgesic, narcotic.

Roxanol 100. (Roxane Laboratories, Inc.) Morphine sulfate 100 mg/5 ml. Soln. Bot. 240 ml. *c-II.*
Use: Analgesic, narcotic.

Roxanol Rescudose. (Roxane Laboratories, Inc.) Morphine sulfate 10 mg/2.5 ml. Soln. UD 2.5 ml. *c-II.*
Use: Analgesic, narcotic.

Roxanol T. (Roxane Laboratories, Inc.) Morphine sulfate 20 mg/ml. Soln. Bot. 30 ml, 120 ml. *c-II.*
Use: Analgesic, narcotic.

Roxandol UD. (Roxane Laboratories, Inc.) Morphine sulfate 10 mg/2.5 ml, UD 2.5 ml; 20 mg/5 ml, UD 5 ml; 30 mg/1.5 ml, UD 1.5 ml. Soln. *c-II.*
Use: Analgesic, narcotic.

•**roxarsone.** (ROX-AHR-sone) USAN.
Use: Anti-infective.

•**roxatidine acetate hydrochloride.** (ROX-ah-tih-DEEN) USAN.
Use: Antiulcer.

Roxicet Oral Solution. (Roxane Laboratories, Inc.) Oxycodone HCl 5 mg, acetaminophen 325 mg/5 ml. Bot. UD 5 ml, 500 ml. *c-II.*
Use: Analgesic combination, narcotic.

Roxicet 5/500. (Roxane Laboratories, Inc.) Oxycodone HCl 5 mg, acetaminophen 500 mg/Cap. Bot. 100s, UD 100s. *c-II.*
Use: Analgesic combination, narcotic.

Roxicet Tablets. (Roxane Laboratories, Inc.) Oxycodone HCl 5 mg, acetaminophen 325 mg, 0.4% alcohol/Tab. Bot. 100s, 500s, UD 100s. *c-II.*
Use: Analgesic combination, narcotic.

Roxicodone. (Roxane Laboratories, Inc.) **Oral Soln.:** Oxycodone HCl 5 mg/5 ml. Bot. 500 ml, UD 5 ml. **Tab.:** Oxycodone HCl 5 mg. Bot. 100s, UD 100s. *c-II.*
Use: Analgesic, narcotic.

Roxicodone Intensol. (Roxane Laboratories, Inc.) Oxycodone HCl 20 mg/ml. Conc. Soln. Bot. 30 ml. *c-II.*
Use: Analgesic, narcotic.

•**roxifiban acetate.** (rox-ih-FIE-ban) USAN.
Use: Antithrombotic, fibrinogen receptor antagonist.

Roxilox. (Roxane Laboratories, Inc.) Oxycodone HCl 5 mg, acetaminophen 500 mg/Cap. Bot. 100s. *c-II.*
Use: Narcotic analgesic combination.

Roxiprin Tablets. (Roxane Laboratories, Inc.) Oxycodone HCl 4.5 mg, oxycodone terephthalate 0.38 mg, aspirin 325 mg/Tab. Bot. 100s, 1000s, UD

100s. *c-II.*
Use: Analgesic combination, narcotic.

•**roxithromycin.** (ROX-ith-row-MY-sin) USAN.
Use: Anti-infective.

R/S Lotion. (Summers Laboratories, Inc.) Sulfur 5%, resorcinol 2%, alcohol 28%. Lot. Bot. 56.7 ml. *otc.*
Use: Dermatologic, acne.

R-S Lotion. (Hill Dermaceuticals, Inc.) No. 2: Sulfur 8%, resorcinol monoacetate 4%. Bot. 2 oz. *otc.*
Use: Drying medication, topical.

R-Tannamine. (Qualitest Products, Inc.) Phenylephrine tannate 25 mg, chlorpheniramine tannate 8 mg, pyrilamine tannate 25 mg/Tab. Bot. 100s. *Rx.*
Use: Antihistamine, decongestant.

R-Tannamine Pediatric. (Qualitest Products, Inc.) Phenylephrine tannate 5 mg, chlorpheniramine tannate 2 mg, pyrilamine tannate 12.5 mg/5 ml, 120 ml, 473 ml. *Rx.*
Use: Antihistamine, decongestant.

R-Tannate. (Various Mfr.) Phenylephrine tannate 25 mg, chlorpheniramine tannate 8 mg, pyrilamine tannate 25 mg. Tab. Bot. 100s. *Rx.*
Use: Antihistamine, decongestant.

R-Tannate Pediatric Suspension. (Various Mfr.) Phenylephrine tannate 5 mg, chlorpheniramine tannate 2 mg, pyrilamine tannate 12.5 mg/5 ml, saccharin. Bot. 473 ml. *Rx.*
Use: Antihistamine, decongestant.

RII Retinamide.
Use: Myelodysplastic syndromes. [Orphan Drug]

rt-PA.
Use: Tissue plasminogen.
See: Activase (Genentech, Inc.).

RU 486.
Use: Antiprogesterone.

Rubacell. (Abbott Diagnostics) Passive hemagglutination (PHA) test for the detection of antibody to rubella virus in serum or recalcified plasma.
Use: Diagnostic aid.

Rubacell II. (Abbott Laboratories) Passive hemagglutination (PHA) test to detect antibody to rubella in serum or recalcified plasma. In 100s, 1000s.
Use: Diagnostic aid.

Rubaquick Diagnostic Kit. (Abbott Diagnostics) Rapid passive hemagglutination (PHA) for the detection of antibodies to rubella virus in serum specimens.
Use: Diagnostic aid.

Ruba-Tect. (Abbott Diagnostics) Hemagglutination inhibition test for the detection and quantitation of rubella antibody in serum. In 100s.
Use: Diagnostic aid.

Rubazyme. (Abbott Diagnostics) Enzyme immunoassay for 1 gG antibody to rubella virus. Test kit 100s, 1000s.
Use: Diagnostic aid.

Rubazyme-M. (Abbott Diagnostics) Enzyme immunoassay for IgM antibody to rubella virus in serum. Test kit 50s.
Use: Diagnostic aid.

rubella & measles vaccine. (Merck & Co.) M-R-VAX II. Inj. Vial. *Rx.*
Use: Immunization.

rubella & mumps virus vaccine, live.
Use: Immunization.
See: Biavax II, Inj. (Merck & Co.).

•**rubella virus vaccine, live.** (roo-BELL-ah) U.S.P. 23.
Use: Immunization.
See: Meruvax II, Inj. (Merck & Co.).
W/Measles vaccine.
See: M-R-Vax II, Inj. (Merck & Co.).
W/Measles vaccine, mumps vaccine.
See: M-M-R Vax II, Inj. (Merck & Co.).

Rubex. (Bristol-Myers Oncology/Immunology) Doxorubicin HCl 50 mg, 100 mg. **50 mg:** w/lactose 250 mg. **100 mg:** w/lactose 500 mg. Pow. for Inj. Vial. *Rx.*
Use: Antibiotic.

•**rubidium chloride Rb 82 injection.** (roo-BIH-dee-uhm) U.S.P. 23.
Use: Diagnostic aid (radioactive, cardiac disease), radiopharmaceutical.

•**rubidium chloride Rb 86.** (roo-BIH-dee-uhm) USAN.
Use: Radiopharmaceutical.

Rubratope-57. (Bristol-Myers Squibb) Cyanocobalamin Co 57 Capsules; Soln U.S.P. 23. *otc.*
Use: Vitamin supplement.

Ru-lets M 500. (Rugby Labs, Inc.) Vitamin C 500 mg, B_3 100 mg, B_5 20 mg, B_1 15 mg, B_2 10 mg, B_6 5 mg, A 10,000 IU, B_{12} 12 mcg, D 400 IU, E 30 mg, Mg, Fe 20 mg, Cu, Zn 1.5 mg, Mn, I. Tab. Bot. 100s. *otc.*
Use: Mineral, vitamin supplement.

Rulox. (Rugby Labs, Inc.) **#1 Tab.:** Aluminum hydroxide 200 mg, magnesium hydroxide 200 mg. **#2 Tab.:** Aluminum hydroxide 400 mg, magnesium hydroxide 400 mg. Bot. 100s, 1000s. *otc.*
Use: Antacid.

RuLox Plus Suspension. (Rugby Labs, Inc.) Aluminum hydroxide 500 mg, magnesium hydroxide 450 mg, simethicone 40 mg/5 ml. Bot. 355 ml. *otc.*
Use: Antacid, antiflatulent.

RuLox Plus Tablets. (Rugby Labs, Inc.) Aluminum hydroxide 200 mg, magnesium hydroxide 200 mg, simethicone 25 mg. Chew. Tab. Bot. 50s. *otc.*
Use: Antacid, antiflatulent.

RuLox Suspension. (Rugby Labs, Inc.) Aluminum hydroxide 225 mg, magnesium hydroxide 200 mg/5 ml. Susp. Bot. 360 ml, 769 ml, gal. *otc.*
Use: Antacid.

Rum-K. (Fleming & Co.) Potassium Cl 10 mEq/5 ml in butter rum flavored base. Bot. Pt, gal. *Rx.*
Use: Electrolyte supplement.

rust inhibitor.
See: Sodium Nitrite, Tab. (Various Mfr.).

•**rutamycin.** (ROO-tah-MY-sin) USAN. From strain of *Streptomyces rutgersensis.* Under study.
Use: Antifungal.

rutgers 612.
See: Ethohexadiol. (Various Mfr.).

rutin. (Various Mfr.) 3-Rhamnoglucoside of 5,7,3',4-tetrahydroxyflavonol. Eldrin, globulariacitrin, myrticalorin, oxyritin, phytomelin, rutoside, sophorin. Tab. 20 mg, 50 mg, 60 mg, 100 mg. *Rx.*
Use: Vascular disorders.

rutoside.
See: Rutin, Tab. (Various Mfr.).

Ru-Tuss DE. (Knoll Pharmaceuticals) Pseudoephedrine HCl 120 mg, guaifenesin 600 mg/Tab. Bot. 100s. *Rx.*
Use: Decongestant, expectorant.

Ru-Tuss II. (Knoll Pharmaceuticals) Phenylpropanolamine HCl 75 mg, chlorpheniramine maleate 12 mg/Cap. Bot. 100s. *Rx.*
Use: Antihistamine, decongestant.

Ru-Tuss Expectorant. (Knoll Pharmaceuticals) Pseudoephedrine HCl 30 mg, dextromethorphan HBr 10 mg, guaifenesin 100 mg/5 ml, alcohol 10%. Bot. Pt. *otc.*
Use: Antitussive, decongestant, expectorant.

Ru-Tuss Liquid. (Knoll Pharmaceuticals) Phenylephrine HCl 5 mg, chlorpheniramine maleate 2 mg/5 ml, alcohol 5%. Bot. 473 ml. *otc.*
Use: Antihistamine, decongestant.

Ru-Tuss w/Hydrocodone. (Knoll Pharmaceuticals) Hydrocodone bitartrate 1.67 mg, phenylephrine HCl 5 mg, phenylpropanolamine HCl 3.3 mg, pheniramine maleate 3.3 mg, pyrilamine maleate 3.3 mg/5 ml, alcohol 5%. Bot. 473 ml. *c-III.*
Use: Antihistamine, antitussive, decongestant.

RVPaque. (ICN Pharmaceuticals, Inc.) Red petrolatum, zinc oxide, cinoxate, in water-resistant base. Tube 15 g, 37.5 g. *otc.*
Use: Sunscreen.

Rymed. (Edwards Pharmaceuticals, Inc.) Pseudoephedrine HCl 30 mg, guaifenesin 250 mg/Cap. Bot. 100s. *otc.*
Use: Decongestant, expectorant.

Rymed Liquid. (Edwards Pharmaceuticals, Inc.) Pseudoephedrine HCl 30 mg, guaifenesin 100 mg/5 ml, alcohol 1.4%. Bot. Pt. *otc.*
Use: Decongestant, expectorant.

Rymed-TR. (Edwards Pharmaceuticals, Inc.) Phenylpropanolamine HCl 75 mg, guaifenesin 400 mg/Tab. Bot. 100s. *otc.*
Use: Decongestant, expectorant.

Ryna. (Wallace Laboratories) Chlorpheniramine 2 mg, pseudoephedrine HCl 30 mg/5 ml. Bot. 118 ml, 473 ml. *otc.*
Use: Antihistamine, decongestant.

Ryna-C. (Wallace Laboratories) Codeine phosphate 10 mg, pseudoephedrine HCl 30 mg, chlorpheniramine maleate 2 mg, saccharin, sorbitol/5 ml. Bot. 4 oz, pt. *c-v.*
Use: Antihistamine, antitussive, decongestant.

Ryna-CX. (Wallace Laboratories) Guaifenesin 100 mg, pseudoephedrine HCl 30 mg, codeine phosphate 10 mg, alcohol 7.5%, saccharin, sorbitol/5 ml. Bot. 4 oz, pt. *c-v.*
Use: Antitussive, decongestant, expectorant.

Rynatan. (Wallace Laboratories) **Tab.:** Phenylephrine tannate 25 mg, chlorpheniramine tannate 8 mg, pyrilamine tannate 25 mg. Bot. 100s, 500s, 2000s. **Pediatric Susp.:** Phenylephrine tannate 5 mg, chlorpheniramine tannate 2 mg, pyrilamine tannate 12.5 mg/5 ml. Bot. 473 ml. *Rx.*
Use: Antihistamine, decongestant.

Rynatan-S Pediatric Suspension. (Wallace Laboratories) Phenylephrine tannate 5 mg, chlorpheniramine tannate 2 mg, pyrilamine tannate 12.5 mg/5 ml. Susp. Bot. 120 ml w/syringe. *Rx.*
Use: Antihistamine, decongestant.

Rynatuss. (Wallace Laboratories) Carbetapentane tannate 60 mg, chlorpheniramine tannate 5 mg, ephedrine tannate 10 mg, phenylephrine tannate 10 mg/Tab. Bot. 100s. *Rx.*
Use: Antihistamine, antitussive, decongestant.

Rynatuss Pediatric Suspension. (Wallace Laboratories) Carbetapentane tan-

nate 30 mg, chlorpheniramine tannate 4 mg, ephedrine tannate 5 mg, phenylephrine tannate 5 mg, saccharin, tartrazine/5 ml. Susp. Bot. 8 oz, pt. *Rx.*
Use: Antihistamine, antitussive, decongestant.

Rythmol. (Knoll Pharmaceuticals) Propafenone HCl 150 mg, 225 mg, 300 mg. Tab. **50 mg or 300 mg:** Bot. 100s, 500s. **225 mg:** Bot. 100s, UD 100s. *Rx.*
Use: Antiarrhythmic.

S

S-2. (Nephron Pharmaceuticals Corp.) Racepinephrine HCl 2.25% (epinephrine base 1.125%). Inh. Soln. Bot. 15 ml. *otc.*
Use: Bronchodilator; sympathomimetic.

Saave+. (NeuroGenesis/Matrix Tech., Inc.) Vitamin D 40 mg, L-phenylalanine, L-glutamine 25 mg, vitamins A 333.3 IU, B_1 2.417 mg, B_2 0.85 mg, B_3 33 mg, B_5 15 mg, B_6 3 mg, B_{12} 5 mcg, folic acid 0.067 mg, C 100 mg, E 5 IU, biotin 0.05 mg, Ca 25 mg, Cr 0.01 mg, Fe 1.5 mg, Mg 25 mg, Zn 2.5 mg/Cap. Yeast and preservative free. Bot. 42s, 180s. *otc.*
Use: Mineral, vitamin supplement.

•**sabcomeline hydrochloride.** (sab-KOE-meh-leen HIGH-droe-KLOR-ide) USAN.
Use: Treatment of Alzheimer's diease.

•**sabeluzole.** (sah-BELL-you-zole) USAN.
Use: Anticonvulsant; antihypoxic.

Sabin vaccine.
Use: Immunization.
See: Orimune (ESI Lederle Generics).

Sac-500. (Western Research) Vitamin C 500 mg/TR Cap. Bot. 1000s. *otc.*
Use: Vitamin supplement.

•**saccharin.** (SACK-ah-rin) N.F. 18.
Use: Pharmaceutic aid (flavor).

saccharin. (Merck & Co.) Pow. Pkg. 1 oz, 0.25 lb, 1 lb. (Bristol-Myers Squibb) Tabs. 0.25 gr, 0.5 gr. Bot. 500s, 1000s; 1 gr. Bot. 1000s.
Use: Pharmaceutic aid (flavor).

•**saccharin calcium.** U.S.P. 23.
Use: Non-nutritive sweetener.

•**saccharin sodium.** U.S.P. 23.
Use: Sweetener (non-nutritive).
See: Ril Sweet, Liq. (Schering-Plough Corp.).
Sweeta (Bristol-Myers Squibb).

saccharin sodium. (Various Mfr.) Pow., Bot. 1 oz, 0.25 lb, 1 lb. Tab.
Use: Sweetener (non-nutritive).

saccharin soluble.
See: Saccharin Sodium, Tab., Pow. (Various Mfr.).

sacrosidase.
Use: Nutritional therapy.
See: Sucraid, Soln. (Orphan Medical, Inc.).

Saf-Clens. (Calgon Vestal Laboratories) Meroxapol 105, NaCl, potassium sorbate NF, DMDM hydantoin/Spray. Bot. 177 ml. *otc.*
Use: Dermatologic, wound therapy.

Safeskin. (C & M Pharmacal, Inc.) A dermatologically acceptable detergent for patients who are sensitive to ordinary detergents. No whiteners, brighteners, or other irritants. Bot. qt.
Use: Laundry detergent for sensitive skin.

Safe Suds. (Ar-Ex) Hypoallergenic, all-purpose detergent for patients whose hands or respiratory membranes are irritated by soaps or detergents. pH 6.8. No enzymes, phosphates, lanolin, fillers, bleaches. Bot. 22 oz.
Use: Detergent.

Safe Tussin 30. (Kramer Laboratories, Inc.) Guaifenesin 100 mg, dextromethorphan HBr 15 mg/5 ml. Liq. Bot. 120 ml. *otc.*
Use: Antitussive, expectorant.

Safety-Coated Arthritis Pain Formula. (Whitehall Robins Laboratories) Enteric coated aspirin 500 mg/Tab. Bot. 24s, 60s. *otc.*
Use: Analgesic.

safflower oil.
Use: Nutritional supplement.
See: Microlipid (Sherwood Davis & Geck).

•**safflower oil.** U.S.P. 23.
Use: Pharmaceutic aid (vehicle, oleaginous).
See: Safflower Oil, Caps. (Various Mfr.).

•**safingol.** (saff-IN-gole) USAN.
Use: Antineoplastic (adjunct); antipsoriatic.

•**safingol hydrochloride.** (saff-IN-gole) USAN.
Use: Antineoplastic (adjunct); antipsoriatic.

Saizeno. (Serono Laboratories, Inc.) Somatropin 5 mg, sucrose. Pow. for Inj., lyophilized. Vial ≈ 15 IU. *Rx.*
Use: Hormone, growth.

SalAc Cleanser. (Medicis Dermatologicals, Inc.) Salicylic acid 2%, benzyl alcohol, glyceryl cocoate. Liq. Bot. 177 ml. *otc.*
Use: Dermatologic, acne.

salacetin.
See: Acetylsalicylic Acid (Various Mfr.).

Sal-Acid. (Pedinol Pharmacal, Inc.) Salicylic acid 40% in collodion-like vehicle. Plaster. Pkg. 14s. *otc.*
Use: Keratolytic.

Salacid 25%. (Gordon Laboratories) Salicylic acid 25% in ointment base. Jar 2 oz, lb. *otc.*
Use: Keratolytic.

Salacid 60%. (Gordon Laboratories) Salicylic acid 60% in ointment base. Jar 2 oz. *otc.*
Use: Keratolytic.

Salactic Film. (Pedinol Pharmacal, Inc.) Salicylic acid 16.7% in flexible collodion w/color. Liq. Applicator Bot. 15 ml. *otc.*
Use: Keratolytic.

Salagen. (SAL-an-tell) (MGI Pharma, Inc.) Pilocarpine HCl 5 mg. Tab. Bot. 100s. *Rx.*
Use: Mouth and throat preparation.

Salazide-Demi Tablets. (Major Pharmaceuticals) Hydroflumethiazide 25 mg, reserpine 0.125 mg/Tab. Bot. 100s. *Rx.*
Use: Antihypertensive combination.

Salazide Tabs. (Major Pharmaceuticals) Hydroflumethiazide 50 mg, reserpine 0.125 mg/Tab. Bot. 100s, 500s, 1000s. *Rx.*
Use: Antihypertensive combination.

salbutamol.
See: Albuterol.

Salcegel. (Apco) Sodium salicylate 5 gr, calcium ascorbate 25 mg, calcium carbonate 1 gr, dried aluminum hydroxide gel 2 gr/Tab. Bot. 100s. *otc.*
Use: Analgesic.

Sal-Clens Acne Cleanser Gel. (C & M Pharmacal, Inc.) Salicylic acid 2%. Gel Tube 240 g. *otc.*
Use: Dermatologic, acne.

•**salcolex.** (SAL-koe-lex) USAN.
Use: Analgesic, anti-inflammatory, antipyretic.

•**salethamide maleate.** (sal-ETH-ah-MIDE) USAN. Under study.
Use: Analgesic.

saletin.
See: Acetylsalicylic Acid (Various Mfr.).

Saleto. (Roberts Pharmaceuticals) Aspirin 210 mg, acetaminophen 115 mg, salicylamide 65 mg, caffeine anhydrous 16 mg/Tab. Bot. 50s, 100s, 1000s, Sani-Pak 1000s. *otc.*
Use: Analgesic.

Saleto-200. (Roberts Pharmaceuticals) Ibuprofen 200 mg/Tab. Bot. 1000s, UD 50s. *otc.*
Use: Analgesic, NSAID.

Saleto-400. (Roberts Pharmaceuticals) Ibuprofen 400 mg/Tab. Bot. 100s, 500s. *Rx.*
Use: Analgesic, NSAID.

Saleto-600. (Roberts Pharmaceuticals) Ibuprofen 600 mg/Tab. Bot. 100s, 500s. *Rx.*
Use: Analgesic, NSAID.

Saleto-800. (Roberts Pharmaceuticals) Ibuprofen 800 mg/Tab. Bot. 100s, 500s. *Rx.*
Use: Analgesic, NSAID.

Saleto CF. (Roberts Pharmaceuticals) Phenylpropanolamine 12.5 mg, dextromethorphan HBr 10 mg, acetaminophen 325 mg/Tab. Bot. UD 8s, 1000s. *otc.*
Use: Analgesic, antitussive, decongestant.

Saleto-D. (Roberts Pharmaceuticals) Acetaminophen 240 mg, salicylamide 120 mg, caffeine 16 mg, phenylpropanolamine HCl 18 mg/Cap. Bot. 50s, 1000s, Sani-Pak 500s. *otc.*
Use: Analgesic, decongestant.

Salflex. (Carnrick Laboratories, Inc.) Salsalate 500 mg, 750 mg/Tab. Bot. 100s. *Rx.*
Use: Analgesic.

•**salicyl alcohol.** (SAL-ih-sill AL-koe-hahl) USAN. *Formerly Saligenin, Saligenol, Salicain.*
Use: Anesthetic, local.

•**salicylamide.** U.S.P. 23.
Use: Analgesic.

salicylamide w/combinations.
See: Anodynos, Tab. (Buffington).
Anodynos Forte, Tab. (Buffington).
Dapco, Tab. (Mericon Industries, Inc.).
Decohist, Cap. (Towne).
Emersal, Liq. (Medco Research, Inc.).
F.C.A.H., Cap. (Scherer Laboratories, Inc.).
Lobac, Cap. (Seatrace Pharmaceuticals, Inc.).
Nokane, Tab. (Wren).
Partuss T.D., Tab. (Parmed Pharmaceuticals, Inc.).
P.M.P. Compound, Tab. (Mericon Industries, Inc.).
Presalin, Tab. (Roberts Pharmaceuticals).
Renpap, Tab. (Wren).
Saleto, Preps (Roberts Pharmaceuticals).
Salipap, Tab. (Freeport).
Salocol, Tab. (Roberts Pharmaceuticals).
Sinulin, Tab. (Schwarz Pharma, Inc).
Sleep, Tab. (Towne).

salicylanilide.
Use: Antifungal.

•**salicylate meglumine.** (suh-LIH-sih-late) USAN.
Use: Antirheumatic, analgesic.

salicylated bile extract. Chologestin.

salicylazosulfapyridine.
See: Sulfasalazine, U.S.P. 23.

•**salicylic acid.** (sal-ih-SILL-ik) U.S.P. 23.
Use: Keratolytic.
See: Calicylic, Creme (Gordon Laboratories).
Clearasil Acne-Fighting Pads (Procter & Gamble).

Fung-O (S.S.S. Company).
Maximum Strength Wart Remover, Liq. (Stiefel Laboratories, Inc.).
OFF-Ezy Corn & Callous Remover, Kit (Del Pharmaceuticals, Inc.).
Psor-a-set (Hogil).
Sal-Acid, Plaster (Pedinol Pharmacal, Inc.).
Salactic Film, Liq. (Pedinol Pharmacal, Inc.).
Salicylic Acid Acne Treatment, Bar (Stiefel Laboratories, Inc.).
Sal-Plant, Gel (Pedinol Pharmacal, Inc.).
Scalpicin (Combe).
Sebulex, Cream (Westwood Squibb Pharmaceuticals).
Wart-Off, Liq. (Pfizer US Pharmaceutical Group).

Salicylic Acid Cleansing Bar. (Stiefel Laboratories, Inc.) Salicylic acid 2%, EDTA. Cake 113 g. *otc.*
Use: Antiseborrheic, keratolytic.

salicylic acid combinations.
See: Acnaveen, Bar (Rydelle Laboratories).
Acno (Baker Norton Pharmaceuticals, Inc.).
Akne Drying Lotion, Liq. (Alto Pharmaceuticals, Inc.).
Bensal HP (7 Oaks Pharmaceutical Corp.).
Clearasil, Preps (Procter & Gamble Pharm.).
Cuticura (Purex).
Duofilm, Liq. (Stiefel Laboratories, Inc.).
Duo-WR, Soln. (Whorton Pharmaceuticals, Inc.).
Fostex, Cream, Liq. (Westwood Squibb Pharmaceuticals).
Ionax, Liq. (Galderma Laboratories, Inc.).
Ionil, Liq. (Galderma Laboratories, Inc.).
Ionil T, Liq. (Galderma Laboratories, Inc.).
Neutrogena T/Sal, Shampoo (Neutrogena).
Occlusal HP, Liq. (Medicis Dermatologicals, Inc.).
Oxy Clean Medicated Pads for Sensitive Skin (SmithKline Beecham Pharmaceuticals).
Oxy Night Watch, Lot. (SmithKline Beecham Pharmaceuticals).
Pernox, Lot. (Westwood Squibb Pharmaceuticals).
Propa pH, Preps (Del Pharmaceuticals, Inc.).
Salicylic Acid Soap (Stiefel Laboratories, Inc.).
Sebucare, Liq. (Westwood Squibb Pharmaceuticals).
Sebulex Shampoo, Liq. (Westwood Squibb Pharmaceuticals).
Therac, Lot. (C & M Pharm.).
Tinver, Lot. (PBH Wesley Jessen).

Salicylic Acid & Sulfur Soap. (Stiefel Laboratories, Inc.) Salicylic acid 3%, sulfur 10%, EDTA. Cake 116 g. *otc.*
Use: Antiseborrheic, keratolytic.

salicylic acid topical foam.
Use: Keratolytic.

salicylsalicylic acid. USAN. Salsalate.
Use: Analgesic.
See: Arcylate, Tab. (Roberts Pharmaceuticals).
Disalcid, Tab. (3M Pharm.).
W/Aspirin.
See: Duragesic, Tab. (Meyer).

salicylsulphonic acid. Sulfosalicylic acid.

Saligenin. (City Chemical Corp.) Salicyl alcohol. Bot. 25 g, 100 g. *otc.*

Saline. (Bausch & Lomb Pharmaceuticals) Buffered isotonic. Thimerosal 0.001%, boric acid, NaCl, EDTA. Soln. Bot. 355 ml. *otc.*
Use: Contact lens care.

Saline Solution. (Americal Pharmaceutical, Inc.) Saline solution, isotonic, preserved. Bot. 12 oz. *otc.*
Use: Contact lens care, soaking.

Saline Spray. (Americal Pharmaceutical, Inc.) Isotonic nonpreserved saline aerosol soln. Bot. 2 oz, 8 oz, 12 oz. *otc.*
Use: Contact lens care.

Salinex Nasal Drops. (Muro Pharmaceutical, Inc.) Buffered nasal isotonic saline drops. Bot. 15 ml w/dropper. *otc.*
Use: Moisturizer, nasal.

Salinex Nasal Mist. (Muro Pharmaceutical, Inc.) Sodium Cl 0.4%. Drops 15 ml, spray 50 ml. *otc.*
Use: Moisturizer, nasal.

Salipap. (Freeport) Salicylamide 5 gr, acetaminophen 5 gr/Tab. Bot. 1000s. *otc.*
Use: Analgesic.

Salithol Liquid. (Madland) Balm of methyl salicylate, menthol, camphor. Bot. Pt, gal. Oint. Jar 1 lb, 5 lb. *otc.*
Use: Analgesic, topical.

Salivart. (Gebauer Co.) Sodium carboxymethylcellulose 1%, sorbitol 3%, NaCl 0.084%, KCl 0.12%, calcium Cl 0.015%, magnesium Cl 0.005%, dibasic potassium phosphate 0.034% and nitrogen (as propellant). Soln. Spray can 25 ml, 75 ml. *otc.*
Use: Mouth preparation.

Saliva Substitute. (Roxane Laborato-

ries, Inc.) Sorbitol, sodium carboxymethylcellulose. Soln. Vial 5 ml, 120 ml. *otc.*
Use: Mouth preparation, saliva substitute.

Salix. (Scandinavian Natural Health & Beauty Products) Sorbitol, dicalcium phosphate, hydroxypropyl methylcellulose, carboxymethylcellulose, malic acid, hydrogenated cottonseed oil, sodium citrate, citric acid, silicon dioxide. Loz. 100s. *otc.*
Use: Saliva substitute.

Salk vaccine.
See: IPOL (Pasteur Merieux Connaught).
Poliovirus vaccine, inactivated.

•**salmeterol.** (sal-MEH-teh-role) USAN.
Use: Bronchodilator.
See: Serevent (GlaxoWellcome).

•**salmeterol xinafoate.** (sal-MEH-teh-role zin-AF-oh-ate) USAN.
Use: Bronchodilator.

•**salnacedin.** (sal-NAH-seh-din) USAN.
Use: Anti-inflammatory, topical.

Salocol. (Roberts Pharmaceuticals) Acetaminophen 115 mg, aspirin 210 mg, salicylamide 65 mg, caffeine 16 mg/Tab. Bot. 1000s. *Rx.*
Use: Analgesic combination.

Salpaba w/Colchicine. (Madland) Sodium salicylate 0.25 g, para-aminobenzoic acid 0.25 g, vitamin C 20 mg, colchicine 0.25 mg/Tab. Bot. 100s, 1000s. *Rx.*
Use: Antigout.

Sal-Plant. (Pedinol Pharmacal, Inc.) Salicylic acid 17% in flexible collodion vehicle. Gel Tube 14 g. *otc.*
Use: Keratolytic.

•**salsalate.** (SAL-sah-late) U.S.P. 23.
Use: Analgesic, anti-inflammatory.
See: Marthritic, Tab. (Marnel Pharmaceuticals, Inc.).

Salsitab. (Upsher-Smith Labs, Inc.) Salsalate 500 mg, 750 mg/Tab. Bot. 100s, 500s, UD 100s. *Rx.*
Use: Analgesic.

Salten. (Wren) Salicylamide 10 gr/Tab. Bot. 100s, 1000s. *otc.*
Use: Analgesic.

Sal-Tropine. (Hope Pharmaceuticals) Atropine sulfate 0.4 mg. Tab. Bot. 100s. *Rx.*
Use: Anticholinergic.

salt replacement products.
See: Slo-Salt (Mission Pharmacal Co.).
Slo-Salt-K (Mission Pharmacal Co.).
Sodium Chloride (Various Mfr.).

•**salts, rehydration, oral.** U.S.P. 23.
Use: Electrolyte combination.

salt substitutes.
Use: Sodium-free seasoning agent.
See: Adolph's Salt Substitute (Adolphs).
Adolph's Seasoned Salt Substitute (Adolphs).
Morton Salt Substitute (Morton Grove Pharmaceuticals, Inc.).
Morton Seasoned Salt Substitute (Morton Grove Pharmaceuticals, Inc.).
NoSalt (SmithKline Beecham Pharmaceuticals).
Nu-Salt (Cumberland Packing Corp.).

salt tablets. (Cross) Sodium Cl 650 mg/Tab. Dispenser 500s. *otc.*
Use: Salt replenisher.

Saluron. (Bristol-Myers Squibb) Hydroflumethiazide 50 mg/Tab. Bot. 100s. *Rx.*
Use: Diuretic.

Salutensin. (Roberts Pharmaceuticals) Hydroflumethiazide 50 mg, reserpine 0.125 mg/Tab. Bot. 100s, 1000s. *Rx.*
Use: Antihypertensive combination.

Salutensin-Demi. (Roberts Pharmaceuticals) Hydroflumethiazide 25 mg, reserpine 0.125 mg/Tab. Bot. 100s, 1000s. *Rx.*
Use: Antihypertensive combination.

Salvarsan.
Use: Antisyphilitic.

Salvite-B. (Faraday) Sodium chloride 7 gr, dextrose 3 gr, vitamin B_1 1 mg/Tab. Bot. 100s, 1000s. *otc.*

•**samarium Sm 153 lexidronam pentasodium.** (sah-MARE-ee-uhm Sm 153 lex-IH-drah-nam pen-tah-SO-dee-uhm) USAN.
Use: Antineoplastic, radiopharmaceutical.
See: Quadramet, Inj. (Du Pont Merck Pharmaceuticals).

Sancura. (Thompson Medical Co.) Benzocaine, chlorobutanol, chlorothymol, benzoic acid, salicylic acid, benzyl alcohol, cod liver oil, lanolin in a washable petrolatum base. Oint. 30 g, 90 g.
Use: Anesthetic, local.

•**sancycline.** (SAN-SIGH-kleen) USAN.
Use: Anti-infective.

Sandimmune. (Novartis Pharmaceutical Corp.) Cyclosporine. **Oral soln.:** 100 mg/ml. Bot. 50 ml with syringe. **IV Soln.:** 50 mg/ml Amp. 5 ml. **Cap.:** 25 mg, 50 mg, 100 mg/Cap. Bot. Sorbitol. UD 30s. *Rx.*
Use: Immunosuppressant.

Sandoglobulin. (Novartis Pharmaceutical Corp.) Reconstitution fluid 1 g, 3 g, 6 g, 12 g NaCl 0.9%/Pow. for Inj., lyophilized. Vials or Kits. Also available

as bulk packs without diluent. *Rx.*
Use: Immunization.

sandoptal. Isobutyl allylbarbituric acid.
See: Butalbital.
W/Caffeine, aspirin, phenacetin.
See: Fiorinal, Tab., Cap. (Novartis Pharmaceutical Corp.).
W/Caffeine, aspirin, phenacetin, codeine phosphate.
See: Fiorinal w/Codeine, Cap. (Novartis Pharmaceutical Corp.).

Sandostatin. (Novartis Pharmaceutical Corp.) Octreotide acetate. **0.05 mg, 0.1 mg, 0.5 mg/ml:** Inj. Amp 1 ml. **0.2 mg, 1 mg/ml:** 5 ml multidose vials. *Rx.*
Use: Antineoplastic, adjunctive.

Sanestro. (Sandia) Estrone 0.7 mg, estradiol 0.35 mg, estriol 0.14 mg/Tab. Bot. 100s, 1000s. *Rx.*
Use: Estrogen.

•**sanfetrinem cilexetil.** (san-FEH-trih-nem sigh-LEX-eh-till) USAN.
Use: Anti-infective.

•**sanfetrinem sodium.** (san-FEH-trih-nem) USAN.
Use: Anti-infective.

SangCya. (SangStat) Cyclosporine 100 mg/ml, alcohol 10.5%. Oral Soln. Bot. 50 ml. *Rx.*
Use: Immunosuppressive.

•**sanguinarium chloride.** (san-gwih-NARE-ee-uhm) USAN. *Formerly Sanguinarine Chloride.*
Use: Antimicrobial, anti-inflammatory, antifungal.

Sanguis. (Sigma-Tau Pharmaceuticals, Inc.) Liver 10 mcg, vitamin B_{12} 100 mcg, folic acid 1 mcg/ml. Vial 10 ml. *Rx.*
Use: Nutritional supplement.

Sanhist T.D. 5. (Sandia) Phenylpropanolamine HCl 50 mg, chlorpheniramine maleate 5 mg, ascorbic acid 100 mg/Tab. Bot. 100s, 1000s. *Rx.*
Use: Decongestant, antihistamine.

Sanhist T.D. 12. (Sandia) Phenylpropanolamine HCl 50 mg, chlorpheniramine maleate 12 mg, ascorbic acid 100 mg, methscopolamine nitrate 4 mg/Tab. Bot. 100s, 1000s. *Rx.*
Use: Decongestant, antihistamine combination.

Sani-Supp. (G & W Laboratories) Glycerin, sodium stearate. Supp. 10s, 12s, 24s, 25s, 48s, 50s, 100s, 1000s. *otc.*
Use: Laxative.

sanluol.
See: Arsphenamine (Various Mfr.).

Sanorex. (Novartis Pharmaceutical Corp.) Mazindol 1 mg, 2 mg/Tab. Bot. 100s. *c-IV.*
Use: Anorexiant.

Sansert. (Novartis Pharmaceutical Corp.) Methysergide maleate 2 mg/Tab. Bot. 100s. *Rx.*
Use: Antimigraine.

Sanstress. (Sandia) Vitamins A 25,000 IU, D 400 IU, B_1 10 mg, B_2 5 mg, niacinamide 100 mg, $B_6$1 mg, B_{12} 5 mcg, C 150 mg, Ca 103 mg, P 80 mg, Fe 10 mg, Cu 1 mg, I 0.1 mg, Mg 5.5 mg, Mn 1 mg, K 5 mg, Zn 1.4 mg/Cap. Bot. 100s, 1000s. *otc.*
Use: Mineral, vitamin supplement.

Santiseptic. (Santiseptic) Menthol, phenol, benzocaine, zinc oxide, calamine. Lot. Bot. 4 oz. *otc.*
Use: Dermatologic, counterirritant.

Santyl. (Knoll Pharmaceuticals) Proteolytic enzyme derived from *Clostridium histolyticum.* 250 units/g Oint. Tube 15 g, 30 g. *Rx.*
Use: Enzyme, topical.

•**saperconazole.** (SAP-ehr-KOE-nah-zole) USAN.
Use: Antifungal.

saponated cresol solution.
See: Cresol (Various Mfr.).

saponins, water soluble.

•**saprisartan potassium.** (sap-rih-SAHR-tan) USAN.
Use: Antihypertensive.

•**saquinavir mesylate.** (sack-KWIN-uh-vihr) USAN.
Use: Antiviral.
See: Invirase, Cap. (Roche Laboratories).
Fortovase (Roche).

•**sarafloxacin hydrochloride.** (sa-rah-FLOX-ah-SIN) USAN.
Use: Anti-infective (DNA gyrase inhibitor).

•**saralasin acetate.** (sare-AL-ah-sin) USAN.
Use: Antihypertensive.

Saratoga. (Blair Laboratories) Boric acid, zinc oxide, eucalyptol, white petrolatum. Oint. Tube 1 oz, 2 oz. *otc.*
Use: Dermatologic, counterirritant.

Sardo Bath Oil Concentrate. (Schering-Plough Corp.) Mineral oil, isopropyl palmitate. Bot. 3.75 oz, 7.75 oz. *otc.*
Use: Emollient.

Sardo Bath & Shower. (Schering-Plough Corp.) Mineral oil, tocopherol. Oil. Bot. 112.5 ml. *otc.*
Use: Emollient.

Sardoettes. (Schering-Plough Corp.) Mineral oil, tocopherol, beta-carotene. Towelettes. Box 25s. *otc.*

Use: Emollient.

Sardoettes Moisturizing Towelettes. (Schering-Plough Corp.) Mineral oil, isopropyl palmitate, impregnated towelling material. Individual packets. Box 25s. *otc.*
Use: Emollient.

•**sargramostim.** (sar-GRUH-moe-STIM) USAN.
Use: Antineutropenic, hematopoietic stimulant, leukopoietic (granulocyte macrophage colony-stimulating factor). [Orphan Drug]
See: Leukine, Preps. (Immunex Corp.).

Sarisol No. 2. (Halsey Drug Co.) Butabarbital sodium 30 mg/Tab. Bot. 100s, 1000s. *c-III.*
Use: Hypnotic, sedative.

•**sarmoxicillin.** (sar-MOX-ih-SILL-in) USAN.
Use: Anti-infective.

Sarna. (Stiefel Laboratories, Inc.) Camphor 0.5%, menthol 0.5%, phenol 0.5% in a soothing emollient base. Bot. 7.4 oz. *otc.*
Use: Emollient.

Sarna Anti-Itch. (Stiefel Laboratories, Inc.) Camphor 5%, menthol 5%, carbomer 940, cetyl alcohol, DMDM hydantoin. Foam. Bot. 105 ml. *otc.*
Use: Emollient.

•**sarpicillin.** (sahr-PIH-SILL-in) USAN.
Use: Anti-infective.

SAStid soap. (Stiefel Laboratories, Inc.) Precipitated sulfur 10%. Bar 116 g. *otc.*
Use: Dermatologic, acne.

satumomab pendetide.
Use: Detection of ovarian cancer. [Orphan Drug]
See: Oncoscint CR/OV.

saxol.
See: Petrolatum, Liq. (Various Mfr.).

scabicides.
See: Benzyl Benzoate (Various Mfr.).
Eurax, Cream, Lot. (Novartis Pharmaceutical Corp.).

Scalpicin. (Combe, Inc.) Salicylic acid 3%, menthol, SD alcohol 40. Shampoo. Bot. 45 ml, 75 ml, 120 ml. *otc.*
Use: Corticosteroid, topical.

Scan. (Parker) Water-soluble gel. Bot. 8 oz, gal.
Use: Ultrasound aid.

Scarlet Red Ointment Dressings. (Sherwood Davis & Geck) 5% scarlet red, lanolin, olive oil, petrolatum. Gauze. 5″ x 9″ strips. *Rx.*
Use: Dermatologic, wound therapy.

Schamberg's. (C & M Pharmacal, Inc.) Menthol 0.15%, phenol 1%, zinc oxide, peanut oil, lime water. Bot. Pt, gal. *otc.*
Use: Antipruritic, counterirritant.

•**schick test control.** U.S.P. 23. *Formerly Diphtheria Toxin, Inactivated Diagnostic.*
Use: Diagnostic aid (dermal reactivity indicator).

Schirmer Tear Test. (Various Mfr.) Sterile tear test strips. 250s. *otc.*
Use: Diagnostic aid, ophthalmic.

Schlesinger's Solution.
See: Morphine HCl (Various Mfr.).

Sclerex. (Miller Pharmacal Group, Inc.) Inositol 2 g, magnesium complex 34 mg, vitamins C 100 mg, calcium succinate 25 mg, A 2500 IU, D 200 IU, E 100 IU, B_1 5 mg, B_2 5 mg, B_6 5 mg, B_{12} 5 mcg, niacin 10 mg, niacinamide 30 mg, pantothenic acid 7.5 mg, folic acid 0.1 mg, Fe 10 mg, Cu 1 mg, Mn 2 mg, Zn 9 mg, I 0.10 mg/3 Tab. Bot. 60s. *otc.*
Use: Mineral, vitamin supplement.

Scleromate. (Palisades Pharmaceuticals, Inc.) Morrhuate sodium 50 mg/ml. Inj. Vial 30 ml. *Rx.*
Use: Sclerosing agent.

sclerosing agents.
See: Morrhuate Sodium (Taylor Pharmaceuticals).
Scleromate (Palisades Pharmaceuticals, Inc.).
Sotradecol (ESI Lederle Generics).

Scopace. (Hope Pharmaceuticals) Scopolamine hydrobromide. 0.4 mg. Tab. Bot. 100s. *Rx.*
Use: Antiparkinson.

•**scopafungin.** (SKOE-pah-FUN-jin) USAN.
Use: Antifungal, anti-infective.

Scope. (Procter & Gamble Pharm.) Cetylpyridinium Cl, tartrazine, saccharin, SD alcohol 38F 67.9%. Liq. Bot. 90 ml, 180 ml, 360 ml, 720 ml, 1080 ml, 1440 ml. *otc.*
Use: Mouthwash.

scopolamine. (skoe-PAHL-uh-meen) Hyoscine, l-Scopolamine, Epoxytropine tropate.
See: Hyoscine, Preps. (Various Mfr.).

•**scopolamine hydrobromide.** (skoe-PAHL-uh-meen) U.S.P. 23. *Formerly Hyoscine Hydrobromide.*
Use: Anticholinergic (ophthalmic), cycloplegic, hypnotic, mydriatic, sedative.
See: Scopace, Tab. (Hope Pharmaceuticals).
W/Atropine and hyoscyamine.
See: Atropine sulfate, Tab.

Belladonna alkaloids.
W/Butabarbital, chlorpheniramine maleate.
See: Pedo-Sol, Elix., Tab. (Warren).
W/Hydroxypropyl methylcellulose.
See: Isopto HBr, Soln. (Alcon Laboratories, Inc.).
W/Hyoscyamine sulfate, atropine sulfate, phenobarbital.
See: Nilspasm, Tab. (Parmed Pharmaceuticals, Inc.).
Sedamine, Tab. (Dunhall Pharmaceuticals, Inc.).
Sedapar, Tab. (Parmed Pharmaceuticals, Inc.).
Spasaid, Cap. (Century Pharmaceuticals, Inc.).
W/Pamabrom, pyrilamine maleate, homatropine methylbromide, hyoscyamine sulfate, methamphetamine HCl.
See: Aridol, Tab. (MPL).

scopolamine hydrobromide. (Invenex) Scopolamine HBr 0.3 mg/ml. Inj. Vial 1 ml. *Rx.*
Use: Amnestic, anxiolytic, sedative.

scopolamine hydrobromide. (Glaxo-Wellcome) Scopolamine HBr 0.86 mg/ml. Inj. amp. 0.5 ml. *Rx.*
Use: Amnestic, anxiolytic, sedative.

scopolamine hydrobromide. (Various Mfr.) Scopolamine HBr 0.4 mg, 1 mg/ml. Inj. Amp., Vial 1 ml. *Rx.*
Use: Amnestic, anxiolytic, sedative.

scopolamine hydrobromide combinations.
See: Belladonna Products.
Hyoscine HBr. (Various Mfr.).

scopolamine methobromide.
See: Methscopolamine Bromide, Preps. (Various Mfr.).

scopolamine methyl nitrate.
See: Methscopolamine Nitrate, Preps. (Various Mfr.).

scopolamine salts.
See: Belladonna Products.
Hyoscine salts.

Scorbex/12. (Taylor Pharmaceuticals) Vitamins B_1 20 mg, B_2 3 mg, B_3 75 mg, B_5 5 mg, B_6 5 mg, B_{12} 1000 mcg, C 100 mg/ml. Vial dual compartment 10 ml. *Rx.*
Use: Vitamin supplement.

Scotavite. (Scott/Cord) Vitamins A 25,000 IU, D 400 IU, B_1 10 mg, B_2 10 mg, B_6 5 mg, B_{12} 5 mcg, niacinamide 100 mg, calcium pantothenate 20 mg, C 200 mg, d-alpha tocopheryl 15 IU, acid succinate iodine 0.15 mg/Tab. Bot. 100s, 500s. *otc.*
Use: Mineral, vitamin supplement.

Scotcil. (Scott/Cord) **Tab.:** Potassium penicillin 400,000 units w/calcium carbonate/Tab. Bot. 100s, 500s. **Pow.:** 80 ml, 150 ml. *Rx.*
Use: Anti-infective; penicillin.

Scotcof. (Scott/Cord) Dextromethorphan HBr 6.85 mg, chlorpheniramine maleate 1.8 mg, phenylephrine HCl 4.4 mg, guaifenesin 66 mg, ammonium Cl 30 mg, chloroform 0.125 mg, alcohol 4.1%/5 ml. Bot. 4 oz, pt, gal. *otc.*
Use: Antihistamine, antitussive, decongestant, expectorant.

Scotnord. (Scott/Cord) Chlorpheniramine maleate 8 mg, phenylephrine HCl 20 mg, methscopolamine nitrate 2.5 mg/Cap. Bot. 100s, 500s. *Rx.*
Use: Anticholinergic, antihistamine, decongestant.

Scotonic. (Scott/Cord) Vitamins B_1 10 mg, B_2 5 mg, B_6 1 mg, niacinamide 50 mg, choline Cl 100 mg, inositol 100 mg, B_{12} 25 mcg, Ca 19 mg, Fe 50 mg, folic acid 0.15 mg, alcohol 15%, sodium benzoate 0.1%/45 ml. Bot. Pt, gal. *otc.*
Use: Mineral/vitamin supplement.

Scotrex. (Scott/Cord) Tetracycline 250 mg/Cap. or 5 ml. Cap. Bot. 16s, 100s, 500s. Syr. 2 oz, pt. *Rx.*
Use: Anti-infective, tetracycline.

Scott's Emulsion. (SmithKline Beecham Pharmaceuticals) Vitamins A 1250 IU, D 1400 IU/4 tsp. Bot. 6.25 oz, 12.5 oz. *otc.*
Use: Vitamin supplement.

Scot-Tussin Allergy. (Scot-Tussin Pharmacal, Inc.) Diphenhydramine HCl 12.5 mg/5 ml, parabens, menthol. Liq. Bot. 120 ml. *otc.*
Use: Antihistamine.

Scot-Tussin Pharmacal Allergy. (Scot-Tussin Pharmacal, Inc.) Diphenhydramine HCl 12.5 mg/5 ml, parabens, menthol. Liq. Dye free, sugar free. Bot. 120 ml. *otc.*
Use: Antihistamine.

Scot-Tussin Pharmacal DM Cough Chasers. (Scot-Tussin Pharmacal, Inc.) Dextromethorphan HBr 2.5 mg, dye free, sorbitol. Loz. Pkg. 20s. *otc.*
Use: Antitussive.

Scot-Tussin Pharmacal DM Liquid. (Scot-Tussin Pharmacal, Inc.) Dextromethorphan HBr 15 mg, chlorpheniramine maleate 2 mg/5 ml, alcohol 10%. Bot. 4 oz, 8 oz. Sugar free. *otc.*
Use: Antihistamine.

Scot-Tussin Pharmacal DM2 Syrup. (Scot-Tussin Pharmacal, Inc.) Dextromethorphan HBr 15 mg, guaifenesin 100 mg, alcohol 1.4%/5 ml. Bot. 120 ml, 240 ml. *otc.*

Use: Antitussive, expectorant.

Scot-Tussin Pharmacal Expectorant. (Scot-Tussin Pharmacal, Inc.) Guaifenesin 100 mg/5 ml, alcohol 3.5%, saccharin, menthol, sorbitol, dye free. Syr. Bot. 120 ml, pt, gal. *otc.*
Use: Expectorant.

Scot-Tussin Pharmacal Original 5-Action. (Scot-Tussin Pharmacal, Inc.) Phenylephrine HCl 4.2 mg, pheniramine maleate 13.33 mg, sodium citrate 83.33 mg, sodium salicylate 83.33 mg, caffeine citrate 25 mg/5 ml, non-alcoholic. Bot. 118 ml, 473 ml, gal. *otc.*
Use: Analgesic combination, antihistamine, decongestant.

Scot-Tussin Pharmacal Original 5-Action Cold Formula. (Scot-Tussin Pharmacal, Inc.) Phenylephrine HCl 4.2 mg, pheniramine maleate 13.3 mg, sodium citrate 83.3 mg, sodium salicylate 83.3 mg, caffeine citrate 25 mg/5 ml, sugar. Alcohol free. Grape flavor. Syr. Bot. 118 ml, 473 ml, gal. *otc.*
Use: Analgesic, antihistamine, decongestant.

Scot-Tussin Pharmacal Senior Clear. (Scot-Tussin Pharmacal, Inc.) Guaifenesin 200 mg, dextromethorphan HBr 15 mg/5 ml, parabens, phenylalanine, menthol, aspartame/Liq. Alcohol and sugar free. Bot 118.3 ml. *otc.*
Use: Antitussive, expectorant.

Scot-Tussin Pharmacal Sugar-Free. (Scot-Tussin Pharmacal, Inc.) Dextromethorphan HBr 15 mg, chlorpheniramine maleate 2 mg/5 ml. Bot. 4 oz, 8 oz, 16 oz, gal. *otc.*
Use: Antitussive, antihistamine.

Scot-Tussin Pharmacal Sugar Free Expectorant. (Scot-Tussin Pharmacal, Inc.) Guaifenesin 100 mg/5 ml w/alcohol 3.5%. Dye free, sodium free, sugar free. *otc.*
Use: Expectorant.

Scot-Tussin Pharmacal with Sugar. (Scot-Tussin Pharmacal, Inc.) Phenylephrine HCl 4.17 mg, pheniramine maleate 13.3 mg, sodium citrate 83.33 mg, sodium salicylate 83.33 mg, caffeine citrate 25 mg/5 ml. Bot. 4 oz, 8 oz, 16 oz, gal. *otc.*
Use: Analgesic combination, antihistamine, decongestant.

Scot-Tussin Senior Clear. (Scot-Tussin Pharmacal, Inc.) Guaifenesin 200 mg, dextromethorphan HBr 15 mg/5 ml, parabens, phenylalanine, aspartame, menthol, alcohol free. Liq. Bot. 118.3 ml. *otc.*
Use: Antitussive, expectorant.

scurenaline.
See: Epinephrine, Prep. (Various Mfr.).

scuroforme.
See: Butyl Aminobenzoate (Various Mfr.).

S.D.M. #5. (Zeneca Pharmaceuticals) Mannitol hexanitrate 7% in lactose. *Rx.*
Use: Vasodilator.

S.D.M.#17. (Zeneca Pharmaceuticals) Nitroglycerin 10% in lactose. *Rx.*
Use: Vasodilator.

S.D.M. #23. (Zeneca Pharmaceuticals) Pentaerythritol tetranitrate 20% in lactose. *Rx.*
Use: Vasodilator.

S.D.M. #27. (Zeneca Pharmaceuticals) Nitroglycerin 10% in propylene glycol. *Rx.*
Use: Vasodilator.

S.D.M. #35. (Zeneca Pharmaceuticals) Pentaerythritol tetranitrate 35% in mannitol. *Rx.*
Use: Vasodilator.

S.D.M. #37. (Zeneca Pharmaceuticals) Nitroglycerin 10% in ethanol. *Rx.*
Use: Vasodilator.

S.D.M. #40. (Zeneca Pharmaceuticals) Isosorbide dinitrate 25% in lactose. *Rx.*
Use: Vasodilator.

S.D.M. #50. (Zeneca Pharmaceuticals) Isosorbide dinitrate 50% in lactose. *Rx.*
Use: Vasodilator.

SDZ MSL-109. (Novartis Pharmaceutical Corp.)
Use: Antiparkinson. [Orphan Drug]

Sea Greens. (Modern Aids Inc.) Iodine 0.25 mg/Tab. Bot. 220s, 460s. *otc.*

Sea Master. (Barth's) Vitamins A 10,000 units, D 400 units/Cap. Bot. 100s, 500s. *otc.*
Use: Vitamin supplement.

Sea-Omega 30. (Rugby Labs, Inc.) N-3 fat content (mg) EPA 180, DHA 140. 100s. *otc.*
Use: Nutritional supplement.

Sea-Omega 50. (Rugby Labs, Inc.) Omega-3 polyunsaturated fatty acid 1000 mg/Cap. containing EPA 300 mg, DHA 200 mg, vitamin E 1 IU. Bot. 30s, 50s. *otc.*
Use: Nutritional supplement.

Sea & Ski Baby Lotion Formula. (Carter Wallace) Octyl-dimethyl PABA. SPF 2. Lot. Bot. 120 ml. *otc.*
Use: Sunscreen.

Sea & Ski Golden Tan. (Carter Wallace) Padimate O. SPF 4. Lot. Bot. 120 ml. *otc.*
Use: Sunscreen.

Seba-Lo. (Whorton Pharmaceuticals, Inc.) Acetone-alcohol cleanser. Bot. 4

oz. *otc.*
Use: Skin cleanser.

Sebana Shampoo. (Myers) Salicylic acid 2%. Bot. 4 oz, 8 oz, pt, qt, 0.5 gal. *otc.*
Use: Antiseborrheic.

Sebanatar. (Myers) Salicylic acid 2%, liquor carbonis detergens 3%. Shampoo. Bot. 4 oz, 8 oz, pt, qt, 0.5 gal, gal. *otc.*
Use: Antiseborrheic.

Seba-Nil Cleansing Mask. (Galderma Laboratories, Inc.) Astringent face mask containing SD alcohol 40, sulfated castor oil, methylparaben. Tube 105 g. *otc.*
Use: Dermatologic, acne.

Seba-Nil Liquid. (Galderma Laboratories, Inc.) Alcohol 49.7%, acetone, polysorbate 20. Liq. Bot. 240 ml, pt. *otc.*
Use: Dermatologic, acne.

Seba-Nil Oily Skin Cleanser. (Galderma Laboratories, Inc.) SD alcohol, acetone. Liq. Bot. 240 ml, 473 ml. *otc.*
Use: Dermatologic, acne.

Sebasorb. (Summers Laboratories, Inc.) Activated attapulgite 10%, salicylic acid 2%. Lot. Bot. 45 ml. *otc.*
Use: Dermatologic, acne.

Sebizon. (Schering-Plough Corp.) Sulfacetamide sodium 100 mg, methylparaben 1 mg w/trisodium edetate, sodium thiosulfate, propylene glycol, isopropyl myristate, propylene glycol monostearate, polyethylene glycol 400 monostearate, water. Lot. Tube 3 oz. *otc.*
Use: Antiseborrheic.

Sebucare Scalp. (Westwood Squibb Pharmaceuticals) Laureth-4, salicylic acid 1.5%, alcohol 61%, PPG-40 butyl ether, dihydroabietyl alcohol, fragrance. Lot. Bot. 4 oz. *otc.*
Use: Antiseborrheic.

Sebulex with Conditioners. (Westwood Squibb Pharmaceuticals) Sulfur 2%, salicylic acid 2%. Bot. 4 oz, 8 oz. *otc.*
Use: Antiseborrheic.

•**secalciferol.** (seh-kal-SIFF-eh-ROLE) USAN.
Use: Regulator (calcium); treatment of familial hypophosphatemic rickets. [Orphan Drug]
See: Osteo-D (Tera, Israel).

•**seclazone.** (SEK-lah-zone) USAN.
Use: Anti-inflammatory; uricosuric.

•**secobarbital.** (see-koe-BAR-bih-tahl) U.S.P. 23.
Use: Hypnotic, sedative.

secobarbital combinations.
See: Efed, Syr., Tab. (Alto Pharmaceuticals, Inc.).
Monosyl, Tab. (Arcum).

secobarbital elixir.
See: Seconal, Elix. (Eli Lilly and Co.).

•**secobarbital sodium.** (see-koe-BAR-bih-tahl) U.S.P. 23.
Use: Hypnotic, sedative.
See: Seconal Sodium, Prep. (Eli Lilly and Co.).

secobarbital sodium. (Wyeth-Ayerst Laboratories) 50 mg/ml. Inj. Tubex 2 ml. *c-II.*
Use: Hypnotic, sedative.

secobarbital sodium and amobarbital sodium capsules.
Use: Hypnotic, sedative.
See: Tuinal, Cap. (Eli Lilly and Co.).

Seconal Sodium Pulvules. (Eli Lilly and Co.) Secobarbital sodium 100 mg. Cap. Bot. 100s, UD 100s. *c-II.*
Use: Hypnotic, sedative.

Secran. (Scherer Laboratories, Inc.) Vitamins B_1 10 mg, B_3 10 mg, B_{12} 25 mcg, alcohol 17%. Liq. Bot. 480 ml. *otc.*
Use: Vitamin supplement.

Secretin Ferring Powder. (Ferring Pharmaceuticals, Inc.) Secretin 75 cu/10 ml Vial. 10 cu/ml when reconstituted with 7.5 ml.
Use: Diagnostic aid.

Sectral. (Wyeth-Ayerst Laboratories) Acebutolol HCl 200 mg, 400 mg/Cap. Bot. 100s, UD 100s. *Rx.*
Use: Antihypertensive.

sedaform.
See: Chlorobutanol (Various Mfr.).

Sedamine. (Health for Life Brands, Inc.) Phosphorated carbohydrate soln. Bot. 4 oz. *otc.*
Use: Antinauseant.

Sedamine. (Dunhall Pharmaceuticals, Inc.) Hyoscyamine sulfate 0.1037 mg, atropine sulfate 0.0194 mg, hyoscine HBr 0.0065 mg, phenobarbital 16.2 mg/Tab. Bot. 100s, 1000s. *Rx.*
Use: Antispasmodic, sedative.

Sedapap. (Merz Pharmaceuticals) Acetaminophen 650 mg, butalbital 50 mg. Tab. Bot. 100s. *Rx.*
Use: Analgesic.

Sedapap#3. (Merz Pharmaceuticals) Acetaminophen 500 mg, butalbital 50 mg, codeine phosphate 30 mg/Cap. Bot. 100s. *c-III.*
Use: Analgesic combination, narcotic.

Sedapap-10. (Merz Pharmaceuticals) Acetaminophen 10 gr, butabarbital 50 mg/Tab. Bot. 100s. *Rx.*
Use: Analgesic, sedative.

Sedapar. (Parmed Pharmaceuticals, Inc.) Atropine sulfate 0.0195 mg, hyoscine HBr 0.0065 mg, hyoscyamine sulfate

0.1040 mg, phenobarbital 0.25 gr/Tab. Bot. 1000s. *Rx.*
Use: Antispasmodic, sedative.

sedative/hypnotic agents.
See: Bromides (Various Mfr.).
Barbiturates (Various Mfr.).
Butisol Sodium (Ortho McNeil Pharmaceutical).
Carbamide (Urea) Compounds (Various Mfr.).
Chloral Hydrate, Preps. (Various Mfr.).
Chlorobutanol (Various Mfr.).
Dalmane, Cap. (Roche Laboratories).
Largon, Inj. (Wyeth-Ayerst Laboratories).
Paraldehyde, Preps. (Various Mfr.).
Phenergan HCl, Preps (Wyeth-Ayerst Laboratories).
Placidyl, Cap. (Abbott Laboratories).
Restoril, Cap. (Novartis Pharmaceutical Corp.).
Triazolam, Tab. (Various Mfr.).

sedeval.
See: Barbital (Various Mfr.).

•**sedoxantrone trihydrochloride.** (sed-OX-an-trone try-HIGH-droe-KLOR-ide) USAN.
Use: Antineoplastic (DNA topoisomerase II inhibitor).

Sedral. (Vita Elixir) Phenobarbital 1/8 gr, theophylline 2 gr, ephedrine gr/Tab. *Rx.*
Use: Bronchodilator, sedative.

•**seglitide acetate.** (SEH-glih-TIDE) USAN.
Use: Antidiabetic.

selegiline hydrochloride.
Use: Antiparkinson agent.
See: Carbex, Tab. (Du Pont Merck Pharmaceuticals).
Eldepryl, Cap. (Somerset Pharmaceuticals).

selegiline hydrochloride. (Various Mfr.) Selegiline HCl 5 mg, lactose. Tab. Bot. 60s, 500s. *Rx.*
Use: Antiparkinson agent.

Selenicel. (Taylor Pharmaceuticals) Selenium yeast complex 200 mcg, vitamins C 100 mg, E 100 mg/Cap. Bot. 90s. *otc.*
Use: Vitamin supplement.

•**selenious acid.** (seh-LEE-nee-us) U.S.P. 23.
Use: Supplement (trace mineral).

selenium. (Nion Corp.) Selenium 50 mcg/Tab. Bot. 100s. *Rx.*
Use: Nutritional supplement, parenteral.

selenium disulfide.
See: Selenium Sulfide, Deterg., Susp. (Various Mfr.).

•**selenium sulfide.** (seh-LEE-nee-uhm SULL-fide) U.S.P. 23.
Use: Antidandruff; antifungal, antiseborrheic.
See: Selsun, Susp. (Abbott Laboratories).

•**selenomethionine Se 75.** (seh-LEE-no-meh-THIGH-oh-neen Se 75) USAN. U.S.P. XXII.
Use: Diagnostic aid (pancreas function determination), radiopharmaceutical.
See: Sethotope, Inj. (Bristol-Myers Squibb).

Sele-Pak. (SoloPak Pharmaceuticals, Inc.) Selenium 40 mcg/ml. Inj. Vial 10 ml, 30 ml. *Rx.*
Use: Nutritional supplement, parenteral.

Selepen. (Fujisawa USA, Inc.) Selenium 40 mcg/ml. Vial 3 ml, 10 ml. *Rx.*
Use: Nutritional supplement, parenteral.

•**selfotel.** (SELL-fah-tell) USAN.
Use: NMDA antagonist.

Selora. (Sanofi Winthrop Pharmaceuticals) Potassium Cl. Pow. *otc.*
Use: Salt substitute.

Selsun Blue. (Ross Laboratories) Selenium sulfide 1% in lotion base. Bot. 4 oz, 7 oz, 11 oz. Dry, oily, normal extra conditioning, and extra medicated (contains 0.5% menthol) formulas. *otc.*
Use: Antiseborrheic.

Selsun Suspension. (Abbott Laboratories) Selenium sulfide 2.5%. Bot. 4 fl oz. *Rx.*
Use: Antiseborrheic.

•**sematilide hydrochloride.** (SEH-may-tih-LIDE) USAN.
Use: Cardiovascular agent (antiarrhythmic).

•**semduramicin.** (sem-DER-ah-MY-sin) USAN.
Use: Coccidiostat.

•**semduramicin sodium.** (sem-DER-ah-MY-sin) USAN.
Use: Coccidiostat.

Semicid. (Whitehall Robins Laboratories) Nonoxynol-9 100 mg/Vag. Supp. Box 9s, 18s. *otc.*
Use: Contraceptive.

Semprex-D. (GlaxoWellcome) Acrivastine 8 mg, pseudoephedrine HCl 60 mg. Cap. Bot. 100s. *Rx.*
Use: Decongestant.

•**semustine.** (SEH-muss-teen) USAN.
Use: Antineoplastic.

Senexon. (Rugby Labs, Inc.) Senna concentrate 5.6 mg/Tab. Bot. 100s, 1000s. *otc.*
Use: Laxative.

Senilavite. (Defco) Vitamins A 5000 IU, C 100 mg, B_1 2.5 mg, B_2 2 mg, nico-

tinamide 10 mg, B_6 1 mg, calcium pantothenate 5 mg, B_{12} w/intrinsic factor concentrate 0.133 IU, ferrous fumarate 150 mg, glutamic acid HCl 150 mg, docusate sodium 50 mg/Cap. Bot. 100s. *otc.*
Use: Nutritional supplement.

Senilezol. (Edwards Pharmaceuticals, Inc.) Vitamins B_1 0.42 mg, B_2 0.42 mg, B_3 1.67 mg, B_5 0.83 mg, B_6 0.17 mg, B_{12} 0.83 mcg, ferric pyrophosphate 3.3 mg/15 ml, alcohol 15%. Liq. Bot. 473 ml. *otc.*
Use: Mineral, vitamin supplement.

•**senna.** (SEN-ah) U.S.P. 23.
Use: Laxative.
See: Senokot (Purdue Frederick Co.).

senna conc., standardized.
Use: Cathartic.
See: Senexon (Rugby).
Senokot, Gran., Tab., Supp. (Purdue Frederick Co.).
X-Prep. Pow. (Gray Pharmaceutical Co.).
W/Docusate sodium.
See: Gentlax S. Tab. (Blair Laboratories).
Senokap-DSS, Cap. (Purdue Frederick Co.).
Senokot S., Tab. (Purdue Frederick Co.).
W/Guar gum.
See: Gentlax B Tab., Gran. (Blair Laboratories).
W/Psyllium.
See: Perdiem, Gran. (Rhone-Poulenc Rorer Pharmaceuticals, Inc.).
Senokot W/Psyllium Pow. (Purdue Frederick Co.).

senna fruit extract, standarized.
Use: Cathartic.
See: Dosaflex (Richwood).
Senokot, Syr. (Purdue Frederick Co.).
X-Prep, Liq. (Gray Pharmaceutical Co.).

Senna-Gen. (Zenith Goldline Pharmaceuticals) Sennosides 8.6 mg, lactose. Tab. Bot. 1000s. *otc.*
Use: Laxative.

•**sennosides.** (SEN-oh-sides) U.S.P. 23.
Use: Laxative.
See: Ex-Lax Chocolated Regular Strength (Novartis Pharmaceutical Corp.).
Ex-Lax Regular Strength (Novartis Pharmaceutical Corp.).
Ex-Lax Maximum Strength (Novartis Pharmaceutical Corp.).
Gentle Nature (Novartis Pharmaceutical Corp.).
Senna-Gen, Tab. (Zenith Goldline Pharmaceuticals).

sennosides a & b.
Use: Laxative.
See: Ex-Lax Gentle Nature (Novartis Pharmaceutical Corp.).

Senokot. (Purdue Frederick Co.) **Gran.:** Standardized senna concentrate. Canister 2 oz, 6 oz, 12 oz. **Tab.:** Bot. 50s, 100s, 1000s, Unit strip pack 100s, Box 20s. *otc.*
Use: Laxative.

Senokot-S Tablets. (Purdue Frederick Co.) Standardized senna concentrate w/docusate sodium. Tab. Bot. 30s, 60s, 1000s. *otc.*
Use: Laxative.

Senokot Suppositories. (Purdue Frederick Co.) Standardized senna concentrate. Pkg. 6s. *otc.*
Use: Laxative.

Senokot Syrup. (Purdue Frederick Co.) Standardized extract senna fruit. Bot. 2 oz, 8 oz. *otc.*
Use: Laxative.

Senokotxtra. (Purdue Frederick Co.) Senna concentrate 374 mg/Tab. Bot. 12s. *otc.*
Use: Laxative.

Sensitive Eyes. (Bausch & Lomb Pharmaceuticals) Sorbic acid 0.1%, EDTA 0.025%, sodium Cl, boric acid, sodium borate. Soln. Bot. 118 ml, 237 ml, 355 ml. *otc.*
Use: Contact lens care.

Sensitive Eyes Daily Cleaner. (Bausch & Lomb Pharmaceuticals) Sorbic acid 0.25%, EDTA 0.5%, sodium Cl, hydroxypropyl methylcellulose, poloxamine, sodium borate. Soln. Bot. 20 ml. *otc.*
Use: Contact lens care.

Sensitive Eyes Drops. (Bausch & Lomb Pharmaceuticals) Isotonic solution, sorbic acid 0.1%, EDTA 0.025%, NaCl, boric acid, sodium borate. Soln. Bot. 30 ml. *otc.*
Use: Contact lens care.

Sensitive Eyes Plus. (Bausch & Lomb Pharmaceuticals) Boric acid, sodium borate, KCl, NaCl, polyaminopropyl biguanide 0.00003%, EDTA 0.025%. Soln. Bot. 118 ml, 355 ml. *otc.*
Use: Contact lens care.

Sensitive Eyes Saline. (Bausch & Lomb Pharmaceuticals) NaCl, borate buffer, sorbic acid 0.1%, EDTA. Soln. Bot. 118 ml, 237 ml, 355 ml. *otc.*
Use: Contact lens care.

Sensitive Eyes Saline/Cleaning Solution. (Bausch & Lomb Pharmaceuticals) Isotonic solution w/borate buffer, NaCl, poloxamine, sorbic acid 0.15%,

sodium borate, boric acid, EDTA 0.1%. Soln. Bot. 237 ml. *otc.*
Use: Contact lens care.

Sensodyne Fresh Mint Toothpaste. (Block Drug Co., Inc.) Potassium nitrate 5%, sodium monofluorophosphate 0.76%, saccharin, sorbitol, mint flavor. Tube 2.4 oz, 4.6 oz. *otc.*
Use: Dentrifice.

Sensodyne-SC Toothpaste. (Block Drug Co., Inc.) Glycerin, sorbitol, sodium methyl cocoyltaurate, PEG-40 stearate, strontium Cl hexahydrate 10%, methyl- and propylparabens. Tinted. Tube 2.1 oz, 4.0 oz. *otc.*
Use: Dentrifice.

SensoGARD. (Block Drug Co., Inc.) Benzocaine 20%. Parabens. Gel Tube 9.4 g. *otc.*
Use: Anesthetic, local.

Sensorcaine. (Astra Pharmaceuticals, L.P.) Bupivacaine HCl 0.25%: w/methylparaben. 50 ml. w/epinephrine 1:200,000 methylparaben. 50 ml. 0.5%: w/methylparaben. 50 ml. w/epinephrine 1:200,000, methylparaben. 50 ml. 0.75%: 30 ml. Inj. Vial 50 ml. *Rx.*
Use: Anesthetic, local.

Sensorcaine MPF. (Astra Pharmaceuticals, L.P.) Bupivacaine HCl. 0.25%. w/ epinephrine 1:200,000, 0.5%. w/epinephrine 1:200,000, 0.75%. w/epinephrine 1:200,000, sodium metabisulfite. Inj. Vial 10 ml, 30 ml. Amp. 5 ml (0.5% only), 30 ml (except 0.25%). *Rx.*
Use: Anesthetic, local.

Sensorcaine MPF Spinal. (Astra Pharmaceuticals, L.P.) Bupivacaine HCl 0.75%, dextrose 8.25%. Inj. 2 ml. Vial. *Rx.*
Use: Anesthetic, local.

Sensorcaine MPF Spinal. (Astra Pharmaceuticals, L.P.) Bupivacaine HCl 0.75%, dextrose 8.25%. Inj. Bot. 2 ml. *Rx.*
Use: Anesthetic, local.

•**sepazonium chloride.** (SEP-ah-ZOE-nee-uhm) USAN.
Use: Anti-infective, topical.

•**seperidol hydrochloride.** (seh-PURR-ih-dahl) USAN.
Use: Neuroleptic, antipsychotic.

•**seprilose.** (SEH-prih-LOHS) USAN.
Use: Antirheumatic.

•**seproxetine hydrochloride.** (sep-ROX-eh-teen) USAN.
Use: Antidepressant.

Septa. (Circle Pharmaceuticals, Inc.) Bacitracin 400 units, neomycin sulfate 5 mg, polymyxin B sulfate 5000 units/g in ointment base. Tube oz. *otc.*
Use: Anti-infective, topical.

Septi-Chek. (Roche Laboratories) Blood culture and simultaneous sub-culture system with three media to support clinically significant pathogens. Quick and easy assembly forms a closed system to protect sub-cultures from contamination.
Use: Diagnostic aid.

Septiphene. (SEP-tih-feen) (Monsanto)
Use: Disinfectant.

Septi-Soft. (SmithKline Beecham Pharmaceuticals) Hexachlorophene 0.25%. Liq. Bot. 240 ml, pt, gal. *otc.*
Use: Antimicrobial, antiseptic.

Septisol. (SmithKline Beecham Pharmaceuticals) **Soln.:** Hexachlorophene 0.25%. Bot. 240 ml, qt, gal. **Foam:** Hexachlorophene 0.23%, alcohol 46%. In 180 ml, 600 ml. *otc.*
Use: Antimicrobial, antiseptic.

Septo. (Vita Elixir) Methylbenzethonium Cl, ethanol 2%, menthol. *otc.*
Use: Antimicrobial, antiseptic.

Septra. (GlaxoWellcome) Sulfamethoxazole 400 mg, trimethoprim 80 mg/Tab. Bot. 100s. *Rx.*
Use: Anti-infective.

Septra DS. (GlaxoWellcome) Trimethoprim 160 mg, sulfamethoxazole 800 mg/Tab. Bot. 100s, 250s, UD 100s. *Rx.*
Use: Anti-infective.

Septra Grape Suspension. (GlaxoWellcome) Trimethoprim 40 mg, sulfamethoxazole 200 mg/5 ml. Bot. 473 ml. *Rx.*
Use: Anti-infective.

Septra I.V. (Monarch) **80/400:** Trimethoprim 80 mg, sulfamethoxazole 400 mg/ 5 ml. Amp. 5 ml, Vial 10 ml, 20 ml, multidose vials 20 ml. *Rx.*
Use: Anti-infective.

Septra Suspension. (GlaxoWellcome) Trimethoprim 40 mg, sulfamethoxazole 200 mg/5 ml. Bot. 20 ml, 100 ml, 150 ml, 200 ml, 473 ml. *Rx.*
Use: Anti-infective.

•**seractide acetate.** (seer-ACK-tide) USAN.
Use: Corticotrophic peptide, hormone (adrenocorticotrophic).

Ser-A-Gen. (Zenith Goldline Pharmaceuticals) Hydrochlorothiazide 15 mg, reserpine 0.1 mg, hydralazine HCl 25 mg/Tab. Bot. 100s, 1000s. *Rx.*
Use: Antihypertensive combination.

Seralyzer. (Bayer Corp. (Consumer Div.)) A system for the measurement of enzymes, potassium levels, blood chemistries and therapeutic drug assays con-

sisting of a reflectance photometer and a series of solid-phase reagent strips.
Use: Diagnostic aid.

Ser-Ap-Es. (Novartis Pharmaceutical Corp.) Reserpine 0.1 mg, hydralazine HCl 25 mg, hydrochlorothiazide 15 mg/Tab. Bot. 100s, 1000s. *Rx.*
Use: Antihypertensive combination.

•**seratrodast.** (seh-RAH-troe-dast) USAN.
Use: Anti-inflammatory (non-antihistaminic), antiasthmatic (thromboxane receptor antagonist).

Serax. (Wyeth-Ayerst Laboratories) Oxazepam. **Cap.:** 10 mg, 15 mg, 30 mg. Bot. 100s, 500s, Redipak 25s, 100s. **Tab.:** 15 mg. Bot. 100s. *c-IV.*
Use: Anxiolytic.

•**serazapine hydrochloride.** (ser-AZE-ah-PEEN) USAN.
Use: Anxiolytic.

Sereen. (Foy Laboratories) Chlordiazepoxide HCl 10 mg/Cap. Bot. 500s, 1000s. *c-IV.*
Use: Anxiolytic.

Sereine Cleaning Solution. (Optikem International, Inc.) Cocoamphodiacetate and glycols, EDTA 0.1%, benzalkonium Cl 0.01%. Soln. Bot. 60 ml. *otc.*
Use: Contact lens care.

Sereine Wetting Solution. (Optikem International, Inc.) EDTA 0.1%, benzalkonium chloride 0.01%. Soln. Bot. 60 ml, 120 ml. *otc.*
Use: Contact lens care.

Sereine Wetting/Soaking Solution. (Optikem International, Inc.) EDTA 0.1%, benzalkonium Cl 0.01%. Soln. Bot. 120 ml. *otc.*
Use: Contact lens care, soaking, wetting.

Serene. (Health for Life Brands, Inc.) Salicylamide 2 gr, scopolamine aminoxide HBr 0.2 mg/Cap. Bot. 24s, 60s. *Rx.*
Use: Analgesic, sedative.

Serentil. (Boehringer Ingelheim, Inc.) Mesoridazine besylate. **Inj.:** 25 mg/ml Amp. 1 ml. **Tab.:** 10 mg, 25 mg, 50 mg, 100 mg. Bot. 100s. **Oral Conc.:** 25 mg/ml dropper. *Rx.*
Use: Antipsychotic.

Serevent. (GlaxoWellcome) Salmeterol xinafoate 25 mcg/actuation. Aerosol. Canister 6.5 g (60 actuations), 13 g (12 actuations), refills 13 g. *Rx.*
Use: Bronchodilator.

Serevent Diskus. (GlaxoWellcome) Salmeterol xinafoate 50 mcg. Inh. Pow. Disp. device blisters 28s, 60s. *Rx.*
Use: Bronchodilator.

•**sergolexole maleate.** (SER-go-LEX-ole) USAN.
Use: Antimigraine.

sericinase. A proteolytic enzyme.

•**serine.** (SER-een) U.S.P. 23.
Use: Amino acid.

•**sermetacin.** (ser-MET-ah-sin) USAN.
Use: Anti-inflammatory.

•**sermorelin acetate.** (SER-moe-REH-lin) USAN.
Use: Growth hormone-releasing factor, diagnostic aid. [Orphan Drug]

Seromycin. (Dura Pharmaceuticals) Cycloserine 250 mg/Pulv. Bot. 40s. *Rx.*
Use: Antituberculosal.

Serophene. (Serono Laboratories, Inc.) Clomiphene citrate 50 mg/Tab. Bot. 10s, 30s. *Rx.*
Use: Ovulation inducer.

Seroquel. (Zeneca Pharmaceuticals) Quetiapine fumarate 25 mg, 100 mg, 200 mg. Tab. 100s, UD 100s. *Rx.*
Use: Antipsychotic.

Serostim. (Serono Laboratories, Inc.) Somatropin 5 mg ($\approx$ 15 IU/Vial), 6 mg ($\approx$ 18 IU/ml). Sucrose. Pow. for Injection, lyophilized. Vial. IV. *Rx.*
Use: Hormone, growth.

serotonin reuptake inhibitors, selective.
Use: Antidepressant.
See: Paxil, Tab. (SmithKline Beecham Pharmaceuticals).
Prozac, Liq., Pulv. (Eli Lilly and Co.).
Zoloft, Tab. (Roerig).

Serpasil-Apresoline. (Novartis Pharmaceutical Corp.) **#1:** Reserpine 0.1 mg, hydralazine HCl 25 mg/Tab. Bot. 100s. **#2:** Reserpine 0.2 mg, hydralazine HCl 50 mg/Tab. Bot. 100s. *Rx.*
Use: Antihypertensive combination.

Serpasil-Esidrix. (Novartis Pharmaceutical Corp.) **#1:** Reserpine 0.1 mg, hydrochlorothiazide 25 mg/Tab. **#2:** Reserpine 0.1 mg, hydrochlorothiazide 50 mg/Tab. Bot. 100s, 1000s. *Rx.*
Use: Antihypertensive combination.

Serpazide Tablets. (Major Pharmaceuticals) Reserpine 0.1 mg, hydralazine HCl 25 mg, hydrochlorothiazide 15 mg. Bot. 100s, 1000s. *Rx.*
Use: Antihypertensive combination.

serratia marcescens extract (polyribosomes).
Use: Primary brain malignancies. [Orphan Drug]

Sertabs. (Table Rock) Reserpine 0.25 mg, 0.5 mg/Tab. Bot. 100s, 500s. *Rx.*
Use: Antihypertensive.

Sertina. (Fellows) Reserpine 0.25 mg/

Tab. Bot. 1000s, 5000s. *Rx.*
Use: Antihypertensive.

•**sertindole.** (ser-TIN-dole) USAN.
Use: Antipsychotic; neuroleptic.

•**sertraline hydrochloride.** (SIR-truh-leen) USAN.
Use: Antidepressant.
See: Zoloft, Tab. (Roerig).

serum, albumin, normal human.
See: Albumin Human, U.S.P. 23 (Various Mfr.).

serum, albumin, human, radioiodinated.
See: Albumin Injection, U.S.P. 23.

serum, globulin (human), immune.
Use: Immunization.

Serutan. (SmithKline Beecham Pharmaceuticals) Psyllium. **Gran.:** Pkg. 6 oz, 18 oz. **Pow.:** 7 oz, 14 oz, 21 oz. Fruit flavored: 6 oz, 12 oz, 18 oz. *otc.*
Use: Laxative.

Serzone. (Bristol-Myers Squibb) Nefazodone 50 mg, 100 mg, 150 mg, 200 mg, 250 mg/Tab. Bot. 60s, blister pack 100s (except 50 mg and 250 mg). *Rx.*
Use: Antidepressant.

•**sesame oil.** N.F. 18.
Use: Pharmaceutic aid (solvent; vehicle, oleaginous).

Sesame Street Complete. (McNeil Consumer Products Co.) Ca 80 mg, Fe 10 mg, vitamins A 2750 IU, D 200 IU, E 10 mg, B_1 0.75 mg, B_2 0.85 mg, B_3 10 mg, B_5 5 mg, B_6 0.7 mg, B_{12} 3 mcg, C 40 mg, folic acid 0.2 mg, biotin 15 mg, Cu, I, Mg, Zn 8 mg, lactose/Tab. Bot. 50s. *otc.*
Use: Mineral, vitamin supplement.

Sesame Street Plus Extra C. (McNeil Consumer Products Co.) Vitamins A 2750 IU, D 200 IU, E 10 IU, B_1 0.75 mg, B_2 0.85 mg, B_3 10 mg, B_5 5 mg, B_6 0.7 mg, B_{12} 3 mcg, C 80 mg, folic acid 0.2 mg/Tab. Bot. 50s. *otc.*
Use: Vitamin supplement.

Sesame Street Plus Iron. (McNeil Consumer Products Co.) Fe 10 mg, vitamins A 2750 IU, D 200 IU, E 10 IU, B_1 0.75 mg, B_2 0.85 mg, B_3 10 mg, B_5 5 mg, B_6 0.7 mg, B_{12} 3 mcg, C 40 mg, folic acid 0.2 mg/Chew. Tab. Bot. 50s. *otc.*
Use: Mineral, vitamin supplement.

Sesame Street Vitamins. (McNeil Consumer Products Co.) **For ages 4 and older:** Vitamins A 5000 IU, B_1 1.5 mg, B_{12} 6 mcg, C 60 mg, D 400 IU, E 30 IU, folic acid 400 mcg, biotin 300 mcg/Chew. Tab. Bot. 60s. **For ages 2-3:** Vitamins A 2500 IU, B_1 0.7 mg, B_2 0.8 mg, B_3 9 mg, B_5 5 mg, B_6 0.7 mg, B_{12} 3 mcg, C 40 mg, D 400 IU, E 10 IU, folic acid 200 mcg, biotin 150 mcg/Chew. Tab. Bot. 60s. *otc.*
Use: Vitamin supplement.

Sesame Street Vitamins and Minerals. (McNeil Consumer Products Co.) **For ages 4 and older:** Vitamins A 5000 IU, B_1 1.5 mg, B_2 1.7 mg, B_3 20 mg, B_5 10 mg, B_6 2 mg, B_{12} 6 mcg, C 60 mg, D 400 IU, E 30 IU, folic acid 400 mcg, biotin 300 mcg, Ca 100 mg, Fe 18 mg, I 150 mcg, Zn 15 mg, Cu 2 mg/Chew. Tab. Bot. 60s. **For ages 2-3:** Vitamins A 2500 IU, B_1 0.7 mg, B_{12} 3 mcg, C 40 mg, D 400 IU, E 10 IU, folic acid 200 mcg, biotin 150 mcg, Ca 80 mg, Fe 10 mg, I 70 mcg, Zn 8 mg, Cu 1 mg/Chew. Tab. Bot. 60s. *otc.*
Use: Mineral, vitamin supplement.

Sethotope. (Bristol-Myers Squibb) Selenomethionine selenium 75; available as 0.25, 1 mCi.

•**setoperone.** (SEE-toe-per-OHN) USAN.
Use: Antipsychotic.

•**sevelamer hydrochloride.** (seh-VELL-ah-mer) USAN.
Use: Antihyperphosphatemic, control of hyperphosphatemia in end-stage renal disease (phophate binder).
See: Renagel (Genzyme).

•**sevirumab.** (seh-VIE-roo-mab) USAN.
Use: Monoclonal antibody (antiviral).

•**sevoflurane.** (SEE-voe-FLEW-rane) USAN.
Use: Anesthetic, general.
See: Ultane, Soln. for Inh. (Abbott Laboratories).

•**sezolamide hydrochloride.** (seh-ZOLE-ah-MIDE) USAN.
Use: Carbonic anhydrase inhibitor.

SFC Lotion. (Stiefel Laboratories, Inc.) Soap free. Stearyl alcohol, PEG-75, sodium cocoyl isethionate, parabens. Bot. 237 ml, 480 ml. *otc.*
Use: Dermatologic, cleanser.

Shade. (Schering-Plough Corp.) SPF 15. Contains one or more of the following ingredients: Padimate O, oxybenzone, ethylhexyl-p-methoxycinnamate. Bot. 118 ml, 120 ml, 240 ml. *otc.*
Use: Sunscreen.

Shade Cream. (O'Leary) Jar 0.25 oz. *otc.*
Use: Contouring cream.

Shade Sunblock Gel, 15 SPF. (Schering-Plough Corp.) Ethylhexyl p-methoxycinnamate, octyl salicylate, oxybenzone, SD alcohol 40. PABA free. SPF 15. Waterproof. Gel Bot. 120 ml. *otc.*

Use: Sunscreen.

Shade Sunblock Gel, 25 SPF. (Schering-Plough Corp.) Ethylhexyl p-methoxycinnamate, octyl salicylate, homosalate, oxybenzone, SD alcohol 40. PABA free. Gel Bot. 120 ml. *otc.*
Use: Sunscreen.

Shade Sunblock Gel, 30 SPF. (Schering-Plough Corp.) Ethylhexyl p-methoxycinnamate, homosalate, oxybenzone, 73% SD alcohol 40. Bot. 120 ml. *otc.*
Use: Sunscreen.

Shade Sunblock Lotion, 15 SPF. (Schering-Plough Corp.) Ethylhexyl p-methoxycinnamate, oxybenzone, benzyl alcohol, phenethyl alcohol. PABA free. Waterproof. Lot. Bot. 120 ml. *otc.*
Use: Sunscreen.

Shade Sunblock Lotion, 30 SPF. (Schering-Plough Corp.) Ethylhexyl p-methoxycinnamate, 2-ethylhexyl salicylate, homosalate, oxybenzone, benzyl alcohol, phenethyl alcohol. PABA free. Waterproof. Lot. Bot. 120 ml. *otc.*
Use: Sunscreen.

Shade Sunblock Lotion, 45 SPF. (Schering-Plough Corp.) Ethylhexyl p-methoxycinnamate, oxybenzone, 2-ethylhexyl salicylate, benzyl alcohol, phenethyl alcohol. PABA free. Waterproof. Lot. Bot. 120 ml. *otc.*
Use: Sunscreen.

Shade Sunblock Stick, 30 SPF. (Schering-Plough Corp.) Ethylhexyl p-methoxycinnamate, oxybenzone, 2-ethylhexyl salicylate, homosalate. PABA free. Waterproof. Stick. 18 g. *otc.*
Use: Sunscreen.

Shade UvaGuard. (Schering-Plough Corp.) Octyl methoxycinnamate 7.5%, avobenzone 3%, oxybenzone 3%. Waterproof. SPF 15. Lot. 120 ml. *otc.*
Use: Sunscreen.

Sheik Elite. (Durex) Condom with nonoxynol-9 15%. 3s, 12s, 24s, 36s. *otc.*
Use: Contraceptive.

•**shellac.** N.F. 18.
Use: Pharmaceutic aid (tablet coating agent).

Shepard's Cream Lotion. (Dermik Laboratories, Inc.) Creamy lotion with no lanolin or mineral oil, for entire body. Scented or unscented. Lot. Bot. 8 oz, 16 oz. *otc.*
Use: Emollient.

Sherform-HC Creme. (Sheryl) Hydrocortisone 1%, pramoxine HCl 0.5%, clioquinol 3%. Oint. Tube 0.5 oz. *Rx.*
Use: Corticosteroid, anesthetic, local, antifungal, topical.

Sherhist. (Sheryl) Phenylephrine HCl, pyrilamine maleate/Tab. 100s. Liq. Bot. Pt.
Use: Decongestant, antihistamine.

Shernatal. (Sheryl) Phosphorus free calcium, non-irritating iron, trace minerals and essential vitamins. Tab. Bot. 100s. *otc.*
Use: Mineral, vitamin supplement.

Shertus. (Sheryl) Dextromethorphan HBr, chlorpheniramine maleate, phenylephrine HCl, ammonium Cl. Liq. Bot. Pt. *otc.*
Use: Antihistamine, antitussive, decongestant, expectorant.

Shohl's Solution. U.S.P. 23. Sodium Citrate and Citric Acid Oral Soln.
Use: Alkalizer, systemic.

short chain fatty acid solution.
Use: Ulcerative colitis. [Orphan Drug]

Shur-Clens. (SmithKline Beecham Pharmaceuticals) Poloxamer 188 20%. Soln. Bot. UD 100 ml, 200 ml. *otc.*
Use: Dermatologic.

Shur Seal Gel. (Milex Products, Inc.) Nonoxynol-9 2. 24 UD gel paks. *otc.*
Use: Contraceptive, spermicide.

Sibelium. (Janssen Pharmaceutical, Inc.) Flunarizine HCl. *Rx.*
Use: Vasodilator.

•**sibopirdine.** (sih-BOE-pihr-deen) USAN.
Use: Nootropic; cognition enhancer (Alzheimer's disease).

•**sibrafran.** (sib-rah-FIE-ban) USAN.
Use: Antithrombotic, fibrinogen receptor antagonist, platelet aggregation inhibitor.

•**sibutramine hydrochloride.** (sih-BYOO-trah-meen) USAN.
Use: Antidepressant, anorexic.
See: Meridia, Cap. (Knoll Pharmaceuticals).

sickle cell test.
Use: Diagnostic aid.
See: Sickledex, Test (Ortho Diagnostic Systems, Inc.).

Sickledex. (Ortho Diagnostic Systems, Inc.) Test kit 12s, 100s.
Use: Diagnostic aid to detect hemoglobin S.

Sigamine. (Sigma-Tau Pharmaceuticals, Inc.) Cyanocobalamin injection 1000 mcg/ml. Vial 10 ml, 30 ml. Also Sigamine L.A. Vial 10 ml. *Rx.*
Use: Vitamin supplement.

Sigazine. (Sigma-Tau Pharmaceuticals, Inc.) Promethazine HCl 50 mg/ml. Vial 10 ml. *Rx.*
Use: Antihistamine.

Signa Creme. (Parker) Conductive cos-

metic quality electrolyte cream. Bot. 5 oz, 2 L, 4 L. *otc.*
Use: Diagnostic aid.

Signa Gel. (Parker) Conductive saline electrode gel. Tube 250 g.
Use: Diagnostic aid, gel.

Signa Pad. (Parker) Premoistened electrode pads.
Use: Diagnostic aid, pad.

Signatal C. (Sigma-Tau Pharmaceuticals, Inc.) Ca 230 mg, Fe 49.3 mg, vitamins A 4000 IU, D 400 IU, B_1 2 mg, B_2 2 mg, B_6 1 mg, B_{12} 2 mcg, folic acid 0.1 mg, niacinamide 10 mg, C 50 mg, I 0.15 mg/SC Tab. Bot. 100s, 1000s. *otc.*
Use: Mineral, vitamin supplement.

Signate. (Sigma-Tau Pharmaceuticals, Inc.) Dimenhydrinate 50 mg, propylene glycol 50%, benzyl alcohol 5%/ml. Vial 10 ml. *Rx.*
Use: Antiemetic, antivertigo.

Signef "Supps". (Fellows) Hydrocortisone 15 mg/Supp. 12s. w or w/out applicator. *Rx.*
Use: Corticosteroid, vaginal.

Sigpred. (Sigma-Tau Pharmaceuticals, Inc.) Prednisolone acetate. Vial 10 ml. *Rx.*
Use: Corticosteroid.

Sigtab. (Roberts Pharmaceuticals) Vitamins A 5000 IU, D 400 IU, B_1 10.3 mg, B_2 10 mg, C 333 mg, B_3 100 mg, B_6 6 mg, B_5 20 mg, folic acid 0.4 mg, B_{12} 18 mcg, E 15 mg/Tab. Bot. 90s, 500s. *otc.*
Use: Vitamin supplement.

Sigtab-M. (Roberts Pharmaceuticals) Vitamins A 6000 IU, D_3 400 IU, E 45 mg, C 100 mg, B_3 25 mg, B_1 5 mg, B_2 5 mg, B_6 3 mg, folic acid 400 mcg, B_5 0.015 mg, biotin 45 mcg, Ca 200 mg, P, Fe 18 mg, Mg, Cu, Zn 15 mg, Mn, K, Cl, Mo, Se, Cr, Ni, Sn, V, Si, B, vitamin K, I/Tab. Bot. 100s. *otc.*
Use: Mineral, vitamin supplement.

Silace. (Silarx Pharmaceuticals, Inc.) Docusate sodium 20 mg/5 ml, alcohol ≤ 1%. Syrup. Bot. 473 ml. *otc.*
Use: Laxative.

Silace-C. (Silarx Pharmaceuticals, Inc.) Docusate sodium 60 mg, casanthranol 30 mg/15 ml, alcohol 10%. Syr. Bot. 473 ml. *otc.*
Use: Laxative combination.

Siladryl. (Silarx Pharmaceuticals, Inc.) Diphenhydramine HCl 12.5 mg/5 ml, alcohol 5.6%. Elix. Bot. 118 ml. *otc.*
Use: Antihistamine.

Silafed. (Silarx Pharmaceuticals, Inc.) Pseudoephedrine HCl 30 mg, triprolidine HCl 1.25 mg/5 ml. Syr. Bot. 120 ml, 240 ml, 473 ml, gal. *otc.*
Use: Antihistamine, decongestant.

•**silafilcon a.** (SIH-lah-FILL-kahn A) USAN.
Use: Contact lens material (hydrophilic).

•**silafocon a.** (SIH-lah-FOH-kahn A) USAN.
Use: Contact lens material (hydrophobic).

Silaminic Cold. (Silarx Pharmaceuticals, Inc.) Phenylpropanolamine HCl 12.5 mg, chlorpheniramine maleate 2 mg/5 ml. 5% alcohol. Bot. 118 ml. *otc.*
Use: Antihistamine, decongestant.

Silaminic Expectorant. (Silarx Pharmaceuticals, Inc.) Phenylpropanolamine HCl 12.5 mg, guaifenesin 100 mg/5 ml, alcohol 5%. Liq. Bot. 118 ml. *otc.*
Use: Decongestant, expectorant.

•**silandrone.** (sil-AN-drone) USAN.
Use: Androgen.

Sildec-DM. (Silarx Pharmaceuticals, Inc.) **Drops, Pediatric:** Carbinoxamine maleate 2 mg, pseudoephedrine HCl 25 mg, dextromethorphan HBr 4 mg/ml. Alcohol and sugar free. Bot. 30 ml. **Syrup:** Carbinoxamine maleate 4 mg, pseudoephedrine HCl 60 mg, dextromethorphan HBr 15 mg/5 ml. Bot. 473 ml. *Rx.*
Use: Antihistamine, antitussive, decongestant.

•**sildenafil citrate.** (sill-DEN-ah-fil SIH-trate) USAN.
Use: Anti-impotence agent.
See: Viagra, Tab. (Pfizer US Pharmaceutical Group).

Sildicon-E. (Silarx Pharmaceuticals, Inc.) Phenylpropanolamine HCl 6.25 mg, guaifenesin 30 mg/ml, alcohol 0.6%. Pediatric drops. Bot. 30 ml. *otc.*
Use: Decongestant, expectorant.

•**silica, dental-type.** (SILL-ih-kah) N.F. 18.
Use: Pharmaceutic aid.

•**siliceous earth, purified.** (sih-LIH-shus) N.F. 18.
Use: Pharmaceutic aid (filtering medium).

•**silicon dioxide.** (SILL-ih-kahn die-OX-ide) N.F. 18. *Formerly Silica Gel.*
Use: Pharmaceutic aid (dispersing and suspending agent).

•**silicon dioxide, colloidal.** N.F. 18.
Use: Pharmaceutic aid (tablet/capsule diluent, suspending and thickening agent).

Silicone. (Dow Chemicals) Dimethicone. Liq., Bot. oz. Bulk Pkg. Oint.
W/Nitro-Cellulose, castor oil.

See: Allergex, Liq., Spray (Bayer Corp. (Consumer Div.)).

silicone oil.
See: polydimethylsiloxane.
Silicone oil.

silicone ointment. Dimethicone Dimethyl Polysiloxane.

Silicone Ointment No. 2. (C & M Pharmacal, Inc.) High viscosity silicone 10% in a blend of petrolatum and hydrophobic starch. Jar 2 oz, lb. *otc.*
Use: Protective agent.

Silicone Powder. (Gordon Laboratories) Talc with silicone. Pkg. 4 oz, 1 lb, 5 lb. *otc.*
Use: Dusting powder.

•**silodrate.** (SILL-oh-drate) USAN.
Use: Antacid.

Silphen Cough. (Silarx Pharmaceuticals, Inc.) Diphenhydramine HCl 12.5 mg/5 ml, alcohol 5%, menthol, sucrose. Syr. Bot. 118 ml. *otc.*
Use: Antihistamine.

Silphen DM. (Silarx Pharmaceuticals, Inc.) Dextromethorphan HBr 10 mg/5 ml, alcohol 5%. Syr. Bot. 118 ml. *otc.*
Use: Antitussive.

Siltapp with Dextromethorphan HBr Cold & Cough. (Silarx Pharmaceuticals, Inc.) Brompheniramine maleate 2 mg, phenylpropanolamine HCl 12.5 mg, dextromethorphan HBr 10 mg/5 ml, alcohol 2.3%, sorbitol, saccharin. Elix. Bot. 118 ml. *otc.*
Use: Antihistamine, antitussive, decongestant.

Sil-Tex. (Silarx Pharmaceuticals, Inc.) Phenylephrine HCl 5 mg, phenylpropanolamine HCl 20 mg, guaifenesin 100 mg/5 ml, alcohol 5%, saccharin, sorbitol, sucrose. Liq. Bot. 473 ml. *Rx.*
Use: Expectorant.

Siltussin. (Silarx Pharmaceuticals, Inc.) Guaifenesin 100 mg/5 ml, alcohol 3.5%. Syr. Bot. 473 ml. *otc.*
Use: Expectorant.

Siltussin-CF. (Silarx Pharmaceuticals, Inc.) Phenylpropanolamine HCl 12.5 mg, dextromethorphan HBr 10 mg, guaifenesin 100 mg/5 ml, alcohol 4.75%. Liq. Bot. 118 ml. *otc.*
Use: Antitussive, decongestant, expectorant.

Siltussin DM. (Silarx Pharmaceuticals, Inc.) Dextromethorphan HBr 10 mg, guaifenesin 100 mg/5 ml, saccharin, sucrose. Alcohol free. Syr. Bot. 118 ml. *otc.*
Use: Antitussive, expectorant.

Silvadene. (Hoechst Marion Roussel) Silver sulfadiazine (10 mg/g) 1%, base w/ white petrolatum, stearyl alcohol, isopropyl myristate, sorbitan monooleate, polyoxyl 40 stearate, propylene glycol, methylparaben. Cream Jar 50 g, 85 g, 400 g, 1000 g. Tube 20 g. *Rx.*
Use: Antimicrobial, topical.

silver compounds.
See: Silver Iodide, Colloidal.
Silver Nitrate, Preps. (Various Mfr.).
Silver Protein, Mild (Various Mfr.).
Silver Protein, Strong (Various Mfr.).

•**silver nitrate.** (SILL-ver NYE-trate) U.S.P. 23.
Use: Anti-infective, topical.

silver nitrate ointment. (Gordon Laboratories) Silver nitrate 1% in ointment base. Jar oz. *Rx.*
Use: Astringent, epithelial stimulant.

silver nitrate ophthalmic solution. Soln. 10%, 25%, 50%. Bot. oz.: (Gordon Laboratories) **Amp 1%, 100s:** (Eli Lilly and Co.) **Cap 1%, 100s:** (Parke-Davis) *Rx.*
Use: Astringent, anti-infective.

silver nitrate topical sticks. (Graham Field) Silver nitrate, potassium nitrate 25%. Appl. 100s. *Rx.*
Use: Cauterizing agent.

•**silver nitrate, toughened.** (SILL-ver NYE-trate) U.S.P. 23.
Use: Caustic.

silver protein, mild. Argentum Vitellinum, Cargentos, Mucleinate Mild, Protargin Mild.

silver protein, strong.
See: Protargol, Pow. (Bayer Corp. (Consumer Div.)).

silver sulfadiazine. (SILL-ver SULL-fah-DIE-ah-zeen)
Use: Anti-infective, topical.
See: Silvadene, Cream (Hoechst Marion Roussel).
SSD, Cream (Knoll Pharmaceuticals).
SSD AF, Cream (Knoll Pharmaceuticals).
Thermazene, Cream (Sherwood Davis & Geck).

Simaal Gel. (Schein Pharmaceutical, Inc.) Aluminum hydroxide 200 mg, magnesium hydroxide 200 mg, simethicone 20 mg/5 ml. Liq. Bot. 360 ml. *otc.*
Use: Antacid, antiflatulent.

Simaal Gel 2. (Schein Pharmaceutical, Inc.) Aluminum hydroxide 500 mg, magnesium hydroxide 400 mg, simethicone 40 mg/5 ml. Liq. Bot. 360 ml. *otc.*
Use: Antacid, antiflatulent.

•**simethicone.** (sih-METH-ih-cone) U.S.P. 23. Mixture of liquid dimethyl polysiloxanes with silica aerogel.

Use: Antiflatulent.
See: Degas, Chew. Tab. (Invamed, Inc.).
Gas-X Extra Strength, Softgel Cap. (Novartis Pharmaceutical Corp.).
Maalox Anti-Gas, Chew. Tab. (Rhone-Poulenc Rorer Pharmaceuticals, Inc.).
Mylicon, Tab., Liq. (J & J Merck Consumer Pharm.).
Mylicon-80, Tab. (J & J Merck Consumer Pharm.).
Mylanta, Tab., Liq. (J & J Merck Consumer Pharm.).
Phazyme, Tab. (Reed & Carnick).

W/Aluminum hydroxide, magnesium hydroxide.
See: Di-Gel, Liq., Tab. (Schering-Plough Corp.).
Gas-Ban (Roberts Med).
Mylanta, Mylanta II, Tab., Liq. (J & J Merck Consumer Pharm.).
Phazyme, Tab. (Schwarz Pharma, Inc.).

W/Hyoscyamine sulfate, atropine sulfate, hyoscine HBr, butabarbital sodium.
See: Sidonna, Tab. (Schwarz Pharma, Inc.).

W/Hyoscyamine sulfate, atropine sulfate, scopolamine HBr, phenobarbital.
See: Maalox Plus, Susp. (Rhone-Poulenc Rorer Pharmaceuticals, Inc.).

W/Magnesium carbonate.
See: Di-Gel, Tab., Liq. (Schering-Plough Corp.).

W/Magnesium hydroxide.
See: Laxsil, Liq. (Schwarz Pharma, Inc.).

W/Magnesium hydroxide, dried aluminum hydroxide gel.
See: Maalox Plus, Tab. (Rhone-Poulenc Rorer Pharmaceuticals, Inc.).

W/Pancreatin.
See: Phazyme-95, Tab. (Reed & Carnrick).
Phazyme, Tab. (Schwarz Pharma, Inc.).

simethicone coated cellulose suspension.
Use: Diagnostic aid.
See: SonoRx, Susp. (Bracco Diagnostics).

Similac 13/Similac 13 with Iron. (Ross Laboratories) Milk-based infant formula ready-to-feed containing 13 calories/fl oz, 1.8 mg Fe/100 calories. Bot. 4 fl. oz. *otc.*
Use: Nutritional supplement.

Similac 20/Similac with Iron 20. (Ross Laboratories) Milk-based infant formula. Standard dilution (20 cal/fl oz). Similac with iron: Fe 1.8 mg/100 cal. **Pow.:** Can lb. **Concentrated Liq.:** Can 13 fl oz. **Ready-to-feed:** Can 8 fl oz, 32 fl oz. Bot. 4 fl oz, 8 fl oz. *otc.*
Use: Nutritional supplement.

Similac 24 LBW. (Ross Laboratories) Low-iron infant formula, ready-to-feed, 24 calories/fl oz. Bot. 4 fl oz. *otc.*
Use: Nutritional supplement.

Similac 24/Similac 24 with Iron. (Ross Laboratories) Milk-based infant formula ready-to-feed (24 cal/fl oz), Fe 1.8 mg/100 calories. Bot. 4 fl oz. *otc.*
Use: Nutritional supplement.

Similac 27. (Ross Laboratories) Milk-based ready-to-feed infant formula (27 cal/fl oz). Bot. 4 fl oz. *otc.*
Use: Nutritional supplement.

Similac Low-Iron Liquid & Powder. (Ross Laboratories) Protein 14.3 g, carbohydrates 72 g, fat 36 g, Fe 1.5 mg, with appropriate vitamins and minerals. **Liq.:** 390 ml concentrate, 240 ml and 1 qt. ready-to-use, 120 ml and 240 ml nursettes. **Pow.:** 1 lb. *otc.*
Use: Nutritional supplement.

Similac Natural Care Human Milk Fortifier. (Ross Laboratories) Liquid fortifier designed to be mixed with human milk or fed alternately with human milk to low-birth-weight infants. Supplied as 24 Cal/fl oz. Bot. 4 fl oz. *otc.*
Use: Nutritional supplement.

Similac PM 60/40. (Ross Laboratories) Milk-based formula ready-to-feed or powder with 60:40 whey to casein ratio (20 Cal/fl oz). **Bot.:** Hospital use 4 fl oz. ready-to-feed. **Pow.:** Can lb. *otc.*
Use: Nutritional supplement.

Similac Special Care 20. (Ross Laboratories) Infant formula ready-to-feed (20 Cal/fl oz). Bot. 4 fl oz. *otc.*
Use: Nutritional supplement.

Similac Special Care 24. (Ross Laboratories) Infant formula ready-to-feed (24 Cal/fl oz). Bot. 4 fl oz. *otc.*
Use: Nutritional supplement.

Simplet. (Major Pharmaceuticals) Pseudoephedrine HCl 60 mg, chlorpheniramine maleate 4 mg, acetaminophen 650 mg/Tab. Bot. 100s. *otc.*
Use: Analgesic, antihistamine, decongestant.

Simron Plus. (SmithKline Beecham Pharmaceuticals) Fe 10 mg, vitamins B_{12} 3.33 mcg, C 50 mg, B_6 1 mg, folic acid 0.1 mg/Cap. Parabens. Bot. 100s. *otc.*
Use: Mineral supplement.

•**simtrazene.** (SIM-trah-seen) USAN.
Use: Antineoplastic.

Simulect. (Novartis Pharmaceutical Co.) Basiliximab 200 mg. Pow. for Inj. Single-use vial. *Rx.*
Use: Immunosuppressant.

•**simvastatin.** (SIM-vuh-STAT-in) U.S.P. 23. *Formerly Synvinolin.*
Use: Antihyperlipidemic.
See: Zocor, Tab. (Merck & Co.).

Sinapils. (Pfeiffer Co.) Phenylpropanolamine HCl 12.5 mg, chlorpheniramine maleate 2 mg, acetaminophen 325 mg, caffeine 32.5 mg/Tab. Bot. 36s. *otc.*
Use: Analgesic, antihistamine, decongestant.

•**sinapultide.** USAN.
Use: Treatment of respiratory distress syndrome (pulmonary surfactant).

Sinarest 12 Hour. (Novartis Consumer Health) Oxymetazoline HCl 0.05%. Spray Bot. 15 ml. *otc.*
Use: Decongestant.

Sinarest Decongestant Nasal Spray. (Novartis Consumer Health) Oxymetazoline HCl 0.05%. Bot. 0.5 oz. *otc.*
Use: Decongestant.

Sinarest Extra-Strength. (Novartis Consumer Health) Acetaminophen 500 mg, chlorpheniramine maleate 2 mg, pseudoephedrine HCl 30 mg/Tab. 24s. *otc.*
Use: Analgesic, antihistamine, decongestant.

Sinarest No Drowsiness. (Novartis Consumer Health) Pseudoephedrine HCl 30 mg, acetaminophen 500 mg/Tab. Pkg. 20s. *otc.*
Use: Analgesic, decongestant.

Sinarest Sinus. (Novartis Consumer Health) Acetaminophen 325 mg, chlorpheniramine maleate 2 mg, pseudoephedrine HCl 30 mg/Tab. Pkg. 20s, 40s, 80s. *otc.*
Use: Analgesic, antihistamine, decongestant.

•**sincalide.** (SIN-kah-lide) USAN.
Use: Choleretic.

Sine-Aid IB. (McNeil Consumer Products Co.) Pseudoephedrine 30 mg, ibuprofen 200 mg. Capl. Pkg. 20s. *otc.*
Use: Analgesic, decongestant.

Sine-Aid Maximum Strength. (McNeil Consumer Products Co.) Pseudoephedrine HCl 30 mg, acetaminophen 500 mg/Tab. or Cap. **Tab.:** Bot. 24s, 100s. **Cap.:** Bot. 24s, 50s. *otc.*
Use: Analgesic, decongestant.

Sine-Aid Sinus Headache Caplets, Extra Strength. (McNeil Consumer Products Co.) Acetaminophen 500 mg, pseudoephedrine HCl 30 mg/Capl. Bot. 24s, 50s. *otc.*
Use: Analgesic, decongestant.

Sine-Aid Sinus Headache Tablets. (McNeil Consumer Products Co.) Acetaminophen 325 mg, pseudoephedrine HCl 30 mg/Tab. Bot. 24s, 50s, 100s. *otc.*
Use: Analgesic, decongestant.

•**sinefungin.** (sih-neh-FUN-jin) USAN.
Use: Antifungal.

Sinemet CR. (Du Pont Merck Pharmaceuticals) Carbidopa 25 mg, 50 mg, levodopa 100 mg, 200 mg/SR Tab. Bot. 100s, UD 100s. *Rx.*
Use: Antiparkinsonian.

Sinemet 10/100. (Du Pont Merck Pharmaceutical Co.) Carbidopa 10 mg, levodopa 100 mg/Tab. Bot. 100s, UD 100s. *Rx.*
Use: Antiparkinsonian.

Sinemet 25/100. (Du Pont Merck Pharmaceutical Co.) Carbidopa 25 mg, levodopa 100 mg/Tab. Bot. 100s, UD 100s. *Rx.*
Use: Antiparkinsonian.

Sinemet 25/250. (Du Pont Merck Pharmaceutical Co.) Carbidopa 25 mg, levodopa 250 mg/Tab. Bot. 100s, UD 100s. *Rx.*
Use: Antiparkinsonian.

Sine-Off Maximum Strength No Drowsiness Formula Caplets. (SmithKline Beecham Pharmaceuticals) Pseudoephedrine HCl 30 mg, acetaminophen 500 mg/Cap. Pkg. 24s. *otc.*
Use: Decongestant, analgesic.

Sine-Off Sinus Medicine. (SmithKline Beecham Pharmaceuticals) Chlorpheniramine maleate 2 mg, pseudoephedrine HCl 30 mg, acetaminophen 500 mg/Cap. Pkg. 24s. *otc.*
Use: Analgesic, antihistamine, decongestant.

Sine-Off Tablets. (SmithKline Beecham Pharmaceuticals) Chlorpheniramine maleate 2 mg, phenylpropanolamine HCl 12.5 mg, aspirin 325 mg. Tab. Pkg. 24s, 48s, 100s. *otc.*
Use: Analgesic, antihistamine, decongestant.

Sinequan. (Roerig) Doxepin HCl. **Cap.:** 10 mg, 25 mg, 50 mg, 75 mg, 100 mg, 150 mg. Bot. 50s (150 mg only), 100s; 500s (150 mg only), 1000s, 5000s. **Oral Concentrate:** 10 mg/ml. Bot. 120 ml. *Rx.*
Use: Antidepressant.

Sinex. (Procter & Gamble Pharm.) Phenylephrine HCl 0.5%, cetylpyridinium Cl 0.04% w/thimerosal 0.001% preservative. Nasal Spray. Bot. 0.5 oz,

1 oz. *otc.*
Use: Decongestant.

Singlet for Adults. (SmithKline Beecham Pharmaceuticals) Pseudoephedrine HCl 60 mg, chlorpheniramine maleate 4 mg, acetaminophen 650 mg/Tab. Bot. 100s. *otc.*
Use: Analgesic, antihistamine, decongestant.

Singulair. (Merck & Co.) Montelukast sodium. **Tab.:** 10 mg, lactose. **Chew. Tab.:** 5 mg, aspartame. Unit-of-use 30s, 90s, UD 100s. *Rx.*
Use: Antiasthmastic.

Sinocon TR. (Vangard Labs, Inc.) Phenylpropanolamine HCl 20 mg, phenylephrine HCl 5 mg, phenyltoloxamine citrate 7.5 mg, chlorpheniramine maleate 2.5 mg/Tab. Bot. 100s, 1000s. *Rx.*
Use: Antihistamine, decongestant.

Sino-Eze MLT. (Global Source) Salicylamide 3.5 gr, acetaminophen 100 mg, phenylephrine HCl 5 mg, chlorpheniramine maleate 2 mg/Tab. Bot. 1000s. *Rx.*
Use: Analgesic, antihistamine, decongestant.

Sinografin. (Bracco Diagnostics) Diatrizoate meglumine 527 mg, iodipamide meglumine 268 mg, iodine 380 mg/ml. Inj. Vial 10 ml. *Rx.*
Use: Radiopaque agent.

Sinucol. (Tennessee Pharmaceutic) Chlorpheniramine maleate 8 mg, phenylephrine HCl 20 mg, methscopolamine nitrate 2.5 mg/Cap. Bot. 100s, 500s. Inj. Vial 10 ml. *Rx.*
Use: Antihistamine, decongestant combination.

Sinufed Timecelle. (Roberts Pharmaceuticals) Pseudoephedrine HCl 60 mg, guaifenesin 300 mg/Cap. Bot. 100s. *Rx.*
Use: Decongestant, expectorant.

Sinulin Tablets. (Carnrick Laboratories, Inc.) Phenylpropanolamine HCl 25 mg, chlorpheniramine maleate 4 mg, acetaminophen 650 mg/Tab. Bot. 20s, 100s. *otc.*
Use: Analgesic, antihistamine, decongestant.

Sinumist-SR. (Roberts Pharmaceuticals) Guaifenesin 600 mg/Tab. Bot. 100s. *Rx.*
Use: Expectorant.

Sinupan. (ION Laboratories, Inc.) Phenylephrine HCl 40 mg, guaifenesin 200 mg/SR Cap. Bot. 100s. *Rx.*
Use: Decongestant, expectorant.

Sinuseze. (Amlab) Acetaminophen 325 mg, phenylpropanolamine HCl 25 mg, phenyltoloxamine citrate 22 mg/Tab. Bot. 36s. *otc.*
Use: Analgesic, antihistamine, decongestant.

Sinus Excedrin Extra Strength. (Bristol-Myers Squibb) Pseudoephedrine HCl 30 mg, acetaminophen 500 mg/Tab or Cap. Bot. 50s. *otc.*
Use: Decongestant, analgesic.

Sinus Headache & Congestion. (Rugby Labs, Inc.) Pseudoephedrine HCl 30 mg, chlorpheniramine maleate 2 mg, acetaminophen 500 mg/Tab. Bot. 100s, 1000s. *otc.*
Use: Decongestant, antihistamine, analgesic.

Sinus Pain Formula Allerest. (Medeva Pharmaceuticals, Inc.) Pseudoephedrine HCl 30 mg, chlorpheniramine maleate 2 mg, acetaminophen 500 mg. **Cap.:** Bot. 24s, 50s. **Gelcap:** Bot. 20s, 40s. *otc.*
Use: Analgesic, antihistamine, decongestant.

Sinus Relief. (Major Pharmaceuticals) Pseudoephedrine HCl 30 mg, acetaminophen 325 mg/Tab. Bot. 24s, 100s, 1000s. *otc.*
Use: Decongestant, analgesic.

Sinus Tablets. (Walgreen Co.) Acetaminophen 325 mg, chlorpheniramine maleate 2 mg, pseudoephedrine HCl mg/Tab. Bot. 30s. *otc.*
Use: Analgesic, antihistamine, decongestant.

Sinutab Maximum Strength Sinus Allergy. (Warner Lambert) Acetaminophen 500 mg, pseudoephedrine HCl 30 mg, chlorpheniramine maleate 2 mg/Tab. or Capl. Blister pack 24s. *otc.*
Use: Analgesic, antihistamine, decongestant.

Sinutab Non-Drying. (Warner Lambert) Pseudoephedrine HCl 30 mg, guiafenesin 200 mg/Cap. (Liq.) Pkg. 24s. *otc.*
Use: Decongestant, expectorant.

Sinutab Sinus Maximum Strength Without Drowsiness Formula. (Warner Lambert) Acetaminophen 500 mg, pseudoephedrine HCl 30 mg/Tab or Cap. Pack 24s. *otc.*
Use: Analgesic, decongestant.

Sinutab Sinus Regular Strength Without Drowsiness. (Warner Lambert) Pseudoephedrine HCl 30 mg, acetaminophen 325 mg/Tab. Bot. 24s. *otc.*
Use: Analgesic, decongestant.

Sinutrol. (Weeks & Leo) Phenylpropanolamine HCl 25 mg, phenyltoloxamine citrate 22 mg, acetaminophen 325 mg/Tab. Bot. 40s, 90s. *otc.*

Use: Analgesic, antihistamine, decongestant.

SINUvent. (WE Pharmaceuticals, Inc.) Phenylpropanolamine 75 mg, guaifenesin 600 mg. LA Tab. Bot. 100s. *Rx.*
Use: Decongestant, expectorant.

Siroil. (Siroil) Mercuric oleate, cresol, vegetable and mineral oil. Emulsion Bot. 8 oz. *otc.*
Use: Antiseptic.

sir-o-lene.
Use: Emollient.

•**sirolimus.** (SER-oh-lih-muss) USAN. *Formerly Rapamycin.*
Use: Immunosuppressant.

•**sisomicin.** (SIS-oh-MY-sin) USAN.
Use: Anti-infective.

•**sisomicin sulfate.** (SIS-oh-MY-sin) U.S.P. 23.
Use: Anti-infective.

Sitabs. (Canright) Lobeline sulfate 1.5 mg, benzocaine 2 mg, aluminum hydroxide--magnesium carbonate codried gel 150 mg/Loz. Bot. 100s. *otc.*
Use: Smoking deterrent.

•**sitogluside.** (SIGH-toe-GLUE-side) USAN.
Use: Antiprostatic hypertrophy.

Sitzmarks. (Konsyl Pharmaceuticals) Radiopaque polyvinyl chloride radiopaque rings 24/Cap. Bot. 10s. *Rx.*
Use: Radiopaque agent, gastrointestinal.

Sixameen. (Spanner) Vitamins B_1 100 mg, B_6 100 mg/ml. Vial 10 ml. *otc.*
Use: Vitamin supplement.

Skeeter Stik. (Outdoor Recreation) Lidocaine 4%, phenol 2%, isopropyl alcohol 45.5% in a propylene glycol base. Stick 1s. *otc.*
Use: Anesthetic, local.

Skelaxin. (Carnrick Laboratories, Inc.) Metaxalone 400 mg/Tab. Bot. 100s, 500s. *Rx.*
Use: Muscle relaxant.

skeletal muscle relaxants.
See: Anectine, Soln., Pow. (Glaxo-Wellcome).
Flexeril, Tab. (Merck & Co.).
Mephenesin (Various Mfr.).
Metubine Iodide, Vial (Eli Lilly and Co.).
Neostig, Tab. (Freeport).
Paraflex, Tab. (Ortho McNeil Pharmaceutical).
Parafon Forte, Tab. (Ortho McNeil Pharmaceutical).
Quelicin, Fliptop & Pintop Vials, Syringe w/lancet, Amp. (Abbott Laboratories).
Rela, Tab. (Schering-Plough Corp.).
Robaxin, Tab, Inj. (Wyeth-Ayerst Laboratories).
Skelaxin, Tab. (Carnrick Laboratories, Inc.).
Soma, Preps. (Wallace Laboratories).
Sucostrin, Vial, Amp. (Bristol-Myers Squibb).
Trancopal, Cap. (Sanofi Winthrop Pharmaceuticals).

Skelid. (Sanofi Winthrop Pharmaceuticals) Tiludronate sodium 240 mg/lactose/Tab. Foil Strips 5s. *Rx.*
Use: Treatment of Paget's disease.

SK& F 110679. (SmithKline Beecham Pharmaceuticals)
Use: Hormone, growth. [Orphan Drug]

Skin Degreaser. (Health & Medical Techniques) Freon 100%. Bot. 2 oz, 4 oz. *otc.*
Use: Dermatologic, degreaser.

Skin Shield. (Del Pharmaceuticals, Inc.) Dyclonine HCl 0.75%, benzethonium Cl 0.2%, acetone, amyl acetate, castor oil, SD alcohol 40 10%. Waterproof. Liq. Bot. 13.3 ml. *otc.*
Use: Dermatologic, protectant.

skin test antigen, multiple.
See: Multitest CMI (Pasteur Merieux Connaught).

Sleep II. (Walgreen Co.) Diphenhydramine HCl 25 mg/Tab. Bot. 16s, 32s, 72s. *otc.*
Use: Sleep aid.

Sleep Cap. (Weeks & Leo) Diphenhydramine HCl 50 mg/Cap. Bot. 25s, 50s. *otc.*
Use: Sleep aid.

Sleep-Eze Tablets. (Whitehall Robins Laboratories) Diphenhydramine HCl 25 mg/Tab. Pkg. 12s, 26s, 52s. *otc.*
Use: Sleep aid.

Sleep-Eze 3. (Whitehall Robins Laboratories) Diphenhydramine HCl 25 mg/Tab. Pkg. 12s, 24s. *otc.*
Use: Sleep aid.

Sleep Tabs. (Towne) Scopolamine aminoxide HBr 0.2 mg, salicylamide 250 mg/Tab. Bot. 36s, 90s. *Rx.*
Use: Sleep aid.

Sleepwell 2-Nite. (Rugby Labs, Inc.) Diphenhydramine HCl 25 mg. Tab. Bot. 72s. *otc.*
Use: Sleep aid.

Slender. (Carnation) Skim milk, vegetable oils, caseinates, vitamins, minerals. **Liq.:** 220 Cal/10 oz. Can. **Pow.:** 173 or 200 Cal mixed w/6 oz skim or low fat milk. Pkg 1 oz. *otc.*
Use: Dietary aid.

Slender-X. (Progressive Drugs) Phenyl-

propanolamine, methylcellulose, caffeine, vitamins/Tab. Pkg. 21s, 42s, 84s. Gum 20s, 60s. *otc.*
Use: Dietary aid.

Slimettes. (Halsey Drug Co.) Phenylpropanolamine HCl 35 mg, caffeine 140 mg/Cap. Box 20s. *otc.*
Use: Dietary aid.

Slim-Fast. (Thompson Medical Co.) Meal replacement powder mixed with milk to replace 1, 2 or 3 meals a day. *otc.*
Use: Dietary aid.

Slim-Line. (Thompson Medical Co.) Benzocaine, dextrose/Chewing gum. Box 24s. *otc.*
Use: Dietary aid.

Slim Plan Plus Without Caffeine. (Whiteworth Towne) Phenylpropanolamine HCl 75 mg/Tab. Box 40s. *otc.*
Use: Dietary aid.

Slim-Tabs. (Wesley Pharmacal Co., Inc.) Phendimetrazine tartrate 35 mg/Tab. Bot. 1000s. *c-III.*
Use: Anorexiant.

Sloan's Liniment. (Warner Lambert) Capsicum oleoresin 0.62%, methyl salicylate 2.66%, oil of camphor 3.35%, turpentine oil 46.76%, oil of pine 6.74%. Bot. 2 oz, 7 oz. *otc.*
Use: Analgesic, topical.

Slo-Niacin. (Upsher-Smith Labs, Inc.) Niacin. **250 mg/Tab.:** Bot. 100s, 1000s. **500 mg/Tab.:** Bot. 100s, UD 100s. **750 mg/Tab.:** Bot. 100s. *otc.*
Use: Vitamin supplement.

Slo-Phyllin 80 Syrup. (Rhone-Poulenc Rorer Pharmaceuticals, Inc.) Theophylline anhydrous 80 mg/15 ml. Nonalcoholic. Bot. 4 oz, pt, gal, UD 15 ml. *Rx.*
Use: Bronchodilator.

Slo-Phyllin GG. (Rhone-Poulenc Rorer Pharmaceuticals, Inc.) Theophylline anhydrous 150 mg, guaifenesin 90 mg/Cap. or 15 ml Syr. **Cap.:** Bot. 100s. **Syr.:** Bot. 480 ml. *Rx.*
Use: Bronchodilator, expectorant.

Slo-Phyllin Gyrocaps. (Rhone-Poulenc Rorer Pharmaceuticals, Inc.) Theophylline anhydrous 60 mg, 125 mg, 250 mg/TR Cap. Bot. 100s, 1000s, UD 100s. *Rx.*
Use: Bronchodilator.

Slo-Phyllin Tablets. (Rhone-Poulenc Rorer Pharmaceuticals, Inc.) Theophylline anhydrous 100 mg, 200 mg/Tab. Bot. 100s, 1000s, UD 100s. *Rx.*
Use: Bronchodilator.

Slo-Salt-K. (Mission Pharmacal Co.) KCl 150 mg, NaCl 410 mg/Tab. Bot. 1000s. Strip 100s. *otc.*
Use: Salt substitute.

Slow Fe. (Novartis Pharmaceutical Corp.) Dried ferrous sulfate 160 mg/Tab. Bot. 30s, 100s. *otc.*
Use: Mineral supplement.

Slow Fe Slow Release Iron With Folic Acid. (Novartis Pharmaceutical Corp.) Fe 50 mg, folic acid 0.4 mg/SR Tab. Bot. 20s. *otc.*
Use: Mineral, vitamin supplement.

Slow-K. (Novartis Pharmaceutical Corp.) Potassium Cl. Bot. 100s, 1000s, Accu-Pak units 100s. Consumer Pack 100s. *Rx.*
Use: Electrolyte supplement.

Slow-Mag. (Searle) Magnesium 64 mg/DR Tab. Bot. 60s. *otc.*
Use: Vitamin supplement.

SLT Tablets. (Western Research) Sodium levothyroxine 0.1 mg, 0.2 mg, 0.3 mg/Tab. Bot. 1000s.
Use: Hormone, thyroid.

SLT Lotion. (C & M Pharmacal, Inc.) Salicylic acid 3%, lactic acid 5%, coal tar soln. 2%. Lot. Bot. 4.3 oz. *otc.*
Use: Antiseborrheic.

Small Fry Chewable Tabs. (Health for Life Brands, Inc.) Vitamins A 5000 IU, D 1000 IU, B_{12} 5 mcg, B_1 3 mg, B_2 2.5 mg, B_6 1 mg, C 50 mg, niacinamide 20 mg, calcium pantothenate 1 mg, E 1 IU, l-lysine 15 mg, biotin 10 mg/Chew. Tab. Bot. 100s, 250s, 365s. *otc.*
Use: Mineral, vitamin supplement.

•**smallpox vaccine.** U.S.P. 23.
Use: Immunization.

smallpox vaccine. (ESI Lederle Generics) Tube 100 vaccinations.
Use: Immunization.

SN-13, 272.
See: Primaquine Phosphate, U.S.P. 23 (Various Mfr.).

snakebite antivenins.
See: Antivenin (Crotalidae) (Wyeth-Ayerst Laboratories).
Antivenin (Micurus fulvius) (Wyeth-Ayerst Laboratories).

snake venom.
Use: SC, IM, orally; trypanosomiasis.

Snaplets-D. (Baker Norton Pharmaceuticals, Inc.) Pseudoephedrine HCl 6.25 mg, chlorpheniramine maleate 1 mg/Pkt., taste free. Granules 30s. *otc.*
Use: Antihistamine, decongestant.

Snaplets-DM. (Baker Norton Pharmaceuticals, Inc.) Phenylpropanolamine HCl 6.25 mg, dextromethorphan HBr 5 mg/Pkt., taste free. Granules. 30s. *otc.*
Use: Antitussive, decongestant.

Snaplets-EX. (Baker Norton Pharmaceuticals, Inc.) Phenylpropanolamine HCl 6.25 mg, guaifenesin 50 mg/Pkt., taste

free. Granules 30s. *otc.*
Use: Expectorant, decongestant.

Snaplets-FR. (Baker Norton Pharmaceuticals, Inc.) Acetaminophen 80 mg/Pkt.. Granules. 32s packets. *otc.*
Use: Analgesic.

Snaplets-Multi. (Baker Norton Pharmaceuticals, Inc.) Phenylpropanolamine HCl 6.25 mg, chlorpheniramine maleate 1 mg, dextromethorphan HBr 5 mg/Pkt., taste free. Granules 30s. *otc.*
Use: Antitussive, decongestant.

Snootie by Sea & Ski. (Carter Wallace) Padimate O. SPF 10. Lot. Bot. 30 ml. *otc.*
Use: Sunscreen.

Snooze Fast. (BDI Pharmaceuticals, Inc.) Diphenhydramine HCl 50 mg. Tab. Bot. 36s. *otc.*
Use: Sleep aid.

Sno-Strips. (Akorn, Inc.) Sterile tear flow test strips, 100s. *otc.*
Use: Diagnostic aid, ophthalmic.

Soac-Lens. (Alcon Laboratories, Inc.) Thimerosal 0.004%, EDTA 0.1%, wetting agents. Soln. Bot. 118 ml. *otc.*
Use: Contact lens care.

Soakare. (Allergan, Inc.) Benzalkonium Cl 0.01%, edetate disodium, NaOH to adjust pH, purified water. Bot. 4 fl oz. *otc.*
Use: Contact lens care.

•**soap, green.** U.S.P. 23.
Use: Detergent.

soaps, germicidal.
See: Dial, Preps. (Centeon).
Fostex, Cake, Cream, Liq. (Westwood Squibb Pharmaceuticals).
pHisoHex, Liq. (Sanofi Winthrop Pharmaceuticals).
Thylox, Shampoo, Soap (C.S. Dent & Co. Division).

soap substitutes.
See: Lowila, Cleanser (Westwood Squibb Pharmaceuticals).
pHisoDerm, Preps. (Sanofi Winthrop Pharmaceuticals).

•**soda lime.** N.F. 18.
Use: Carbon dioxide absorbent.

Soda Mint. (Jones Medical Industries, Inc.) Sodium bicarbonate 5 gr, peppermint oil q.s./Tab. Bot. 100s, 1000s. *otc.*
Use: Antacid.

Soda Mint. (Eli Lilly and Co.) Sodium bicarbonate 5 gr, peppermint oil q.s./Tab. Bot. 100s. *otc.*
Use: Antacid.

Sodasone. (Fellows) Prednisolone sodium phosphate 20 mg, niacinamide 25 mg/ml. Vial 10 ml. *Rx.*
Use: Corticosteroid.

•**sodium acetate.** (SO-dee-uhm ASS-eh-tate) U.S.P. 23.
Use: Pharmaceutic aid (in dialysis solutions).

•**sodium acetate c 11 injection.** (SO-dee-uhm ASS-eh-tate) U.S.P. 23.
Use: Radiopharmaceutical.

sodium acetosulfone. (SO-dee-uhm ah-SEE-toe-sull-FONE)
Use: Leprostatic agent.

sodium acid phosphate.
See: Sodium Biphosphate (Various Mfr.).

sodium actinoquinol. (SO-dee-uhm ack-TIH-no-kwin-OLE)
Use: Treatment of flash burns (ophthalmic).
See: Uviban.

•**sodium alginate.** (SO-dee-uhm AL-jih-nate) N.F. 18.
Use: Pharmaceutic aid (suspending agent).

sodium aminobenzoate.
Use: Dermatomyositis and scleroderma.

sodium aminopterin. Aminopterin sodium.

sodium aminosalicylate.
See: Aminosalicylate Sodium, U.S.P. 23.

sodium amobarbital. Amobarbital Sodium, U.S.P. 23.

•**sodium amylosulfate.** (SO-dee-uhm AM-ill-oh-sull-fate) USAN.
Use: Enzyme inhibitor.

sodium anazolene. (SO-dee-uhm an-AZE-oh-leen)
Use: Diagnostic aid.

sodium antimony gluconate. (Pentostam)
Use: Anti-infective.

•**sodium arsenate As 74.** (SO-dee-uhm AHR-seh-nate) USAN.
Use: Radiopharmaceutical.

•**sodium ascorbate.** (SO-dee-uhm ass-CORE-bate) U.S.P. 23.
Use: Vitamin (antiscorbutic).
See: Cenolate, Inj. (Abbott Laboratories).
Vitac Injection, Vial (Hickman).

sodium aurothiomalate.
See: Gold Sodium Thiosulfate, U.S.P. 23.

•**sodium benzoate.** (SO-dee-uhm BEN-zoe-ate) N.F. 18.
Use: Pharmaceutic aid (antifungal, preservative); antihyperammonemic.

sodium benzoate and sodium phenylacetate.

Use: Antihyperammonemic. [Orphan Drug]

sodium benzylpenicillin. Penicillin G Sodium, U.S.P. 23. Sodium Penicillin G. *Rx.*
Use: Anti-infective, penicillin.

•**sodium bicarbonate.** (SO-dee-uhm by-CAR-boe-nate) U.S.P. 23.
Use: Alkalizer, systemic; antacid; electrolyte replacement.
W/Sodium Bitartrate.
See: Ceo-Two, Supp. (Beutlich, Inc.).
W/Sodium carboxymethylcellulose, alginic acid.
See: Pretts, Tab. (Hoechst Marion Roussel).

sodium bicarbonate. (Abbott Laboratories) Inj.: **4.2%:** (5 mEq) Infant 10 ml Syringe. **7.5%:** (44.6 mEq) 50 ml Syringe or 50 ml Amp. **8.4%:** (10 mEq) Pediatric 10 ml Syringe or (50 mEq) 50 ml Syringe or 50 ml Vial.
Use: Alkalizer, systemic; antacid; electrolyte replacement.

sodium biphosphate.
Use: Cathartic.
See: Sodium Phosphate Monobasic, U.S.P. 23.

sodium biphosphate/ammonium phophate sodium acid.
See: Ammonium biphosphate, sodium biphosphate and sodium acid pyrophosphate.

sodium bismuth tartrate.
See: Bismuth Sodium Tartrate, Preps.

sodium bisulfite. Sulfurous acid, monosodium salt. Monosodium sulfite.
Use: Antioxidant.

•**sodium borate.** N.F. 18.
Use: Pharmaceutic aid (alkalizing agent).

sodium butabarbital.
See: Butabarbital Sodium, U.S.P. 23.

sodium calcium edetate.
See: Calcium Disodium Versenate, Amp., Tab. (3M Pharm.).

•**sodium carbonate.** N.F. 18.
Use: Pharmaceutic aid (alkalizing agent).

sodium carboxymethylcellulose. Carboxymethylcellulose Sodium, U.S.P. 23. CMC. Cellulose Gum.

sodium cellulose glycolate.
See: Carboxymethylcellulose, sodium (Various Mfr.).

sodium cephalothin. (SO-dee-uhm SEFF-ah-low-thin) Cephalothin Sodium, U.S.P. 23.
Use: Anti-infective.

•**sodium chloride.** (SO-dee-uhm KLOR-ide) U.S.P. 23.
Use: Pharmaceutic aid (tonicity agent).
See: Afrin Moisturizing Saline Mist (Schering-Plough).
Broncho Saline (Blairex).

sodium chloride 0.45%. (Dey) 0.45% Soln. Single-use vial 3 ml, 5 ml. *otc.*
Use: Bronchodilator, diluent.

sodium chloride 0.9%. (Dey) 0.9% Soln. Vial 3 ml, 5 ml, 15 ml. *otc.*
Use: Bronchodilator, diluent.

sodium chloride. (Various Mfr.) 0.9%. Inj. Vial 1 ml, 2 ml, 2.5 ml, 5 ml, 10 ml, 30 ml. *Rx.*
Use: Bronchodilator, diluent.

sodium chloride and dextrose tablets.
Use: Electrolyte, nutrient replacement.

sodium chloride injection. U.S.P. 23. (Abbott Laboratories) Normal saline 0.9% in 150 ml, 250 ml, 500 ml, 1000 ml cont. **Partial-fill:** 50 ml in 200 ml, 50 ml in 300 ml, 100 ml in 300 ml. **Flip-top vial:** 10 ml, 20 ml, 50 ml, 100 ml. **Bacteriostatic vial:** 10 ml, 20 ml, 30 ml; 50 mEq, 20 ml in 50 ml fliptop or pintop vial; 100 mEq, 40 ml in 50 ml fliptop vial; 50 mEq, 20 ml univ. add. syr.; sodium Cl 0.45%, 500 ml, 1000 ml; sodium Cl 5%, 500 ml; sodium Cl irrigating solution, 250 ml, 500 ml, 1000 ml, 3000 ml; (Pharmacia & Upjohn) sodium Cl 9 mg/ml w/benzyl alcohol 9.45 mg. Vial 20 ml (Sanofi Winthrop Pharmaceuticals). **Carpuject:** 2 ml fill cartridge, 22-gauge 1 ¼ inch needle or 25-gauge ⅝ inch needle.
Use: Fluid and irrigation, electrolyte replacement, isotonic vehicle.

•**sodium chloride Na 22.** (So-dee-uhm KLOR-ide) USAN.
Use: Radioactive agent.

sodium chloride substitutes.
See: Salt substitute.

sodium chloride tablets. (Parke-Davis) Sodium Cl 15 ½ gr/Tab. Bot. 1000s.
Use: Normal saline.

sodium chlorothiazide for injection. (SO-dee-uhm KLOR-oh-thigh-AZZ-ide) Chlorothiazide Sodium For Injection, U.S.P. 23.
Use: Diuretic.

•**sodium chromate Cr 51 injection.** (So-dee-uhm KROE-mate) U.S.P. 23.
Use: Diagnostic aid (blood volume determination), radiopharmaceutical.
See: Radio Chromate Cr 51 Sodium.

•**sodium citrate.** (SO-dee-uhm SIH-trate) U.S.P. 23.
Use: Alkalizer, systemic.
See: Anticoagulant Citrate Dextrose So-

lution, U.S.P. 23; Anticoagulant Citrate Phosphate Dextrose Solution, U.S.P. 23.

sodium citrate and citric acid oral solution. Shohl's Solution.
Use: Alkalinizer, systemic.

sodium cloxacillin. (SO-dee-uhm CLOX-ah-SILL-in)
See: Cloxacillin Sodium, U.S.P. 23.

sodium colistimethate. Colistimethate Sodium, Sterile, U.S.P. 23. Antibiotic produced by *Aerobacillus colistinus.*

sodium colistin methanesulfonate. Colistimethane Sodium, U.S.P. 23. The sodium methanesulfonate salt of an antibiotic substance elaborated by *Aerobacillus colistinus.*
Use: Anti-infective.

•**sodium dehydroacetate.** N.F. 18.
Use: Pharmaceutic aid (antimicrobial preservative).

sodium dextrothyroxine. (SO-dee-uhm DEX-troe-thigh-ROCK-seen)
Use: Anticholesteremic.

sodium diatrizoate. Diatrizoate Sodium, U.S.P. 23.
Use: Radiopaque medium.

sodium dichloroacetate.
Use: Treatment of lactic acidosis and familial hypercholesterolemia. [Orphan Drug]

sodium dicloxacillin. (SO-dee-uhm die-KLOX-ass-IH-lin) Dicloxacillin Sodium, U.S.P. 23.
Use: Anti-infective.

sodium dicloxacillin monohydrate.
Use: Anti-infective.
See: Pathocil, Prep. (Wyeth-Ayerst Laboratories).

sodium dihydrogen phosphate. Sodium Biphosphate, U.S.P. 23.

sodium dimethoxyphenyl penicillin.
See: Methicillin Sodium (Various Mfr.).

sodium dioctyl sulfosuccinate.
See: Docusate Sodium, U.S.P. 23.

sodium diphenylhydantoin. Phenytoin Sodium, U.S.P. 23. Diphenylhydantoin Sodium.
Use: Anticonvulsant.

sodium edetate. (SO-dee-uhm eh-deh-TATE) Edetate Disodium, U.S.P. 23. Tetrasodium ethylenediaminetetraacetate.
Use: Chelating agent.
See: Vagisec, Preps. (Julius Schmid).

sodium ethacrynate. (SO-dee-uhm ETH-ah-krih-nate) Ethacrynate Sodium for Injection, U.S.P. 23.
Use: Diuretic.

•**sodium ethasulfate.** (SO-dee-uhm ETH-ah-SULL-fate) USAN.
Use: Detergent.

sodium ethyl-mercuri-thio-salicylate.
See: Thimerosal (Various Mfr.).
Merthiolate, Preps. (Eli Lilly and Co.).

sodium ferric gluconate complex.
Use: Iron product.
See: Ferrlecit (Schein).

sodium fluorescein. U.S.P. 23. Fluorescein Sodium, U.S.P. 23; Resorcinolphthalein sodium.
Use: Diagnostic aid (corneal trauma indicator).

•**sodium fluoride.** (SO-dee-uhm) U.S.P. 23.
Use: Dental caries agent.
See: Fluoride, Tab. (Kirkman Sales Co., Inc.).
Fluoride Loz. (Kirkman Sales Co., Inc.).
Flura Drops, Drops (Kirkman Sales Co., Inc.).
Flura-Loz, Loz. (Kirkman Sales Co., Inc.).
Karidium, Liq., Tab. (Young Dental).
Kari-Rinse, Liq. (Young Dental).
Luride, Tab. (Colgate Oral Pharmaceuticals).
Mouthkote F/R, Rinse (Parnell Pharmaceuticals, Inc.).
NaFeen, Tab., Liq. (Pacemaker).
Pediaflor, Drops (Ross Laboratories).
T-Fluoride, Tab. (Tennessee Pharmaceutic).
W/Vitamins.
See: Fluorac, Tab. (Rhone-Poulenc Rorer Pharmaceuticals, Inc.).
Mulvidren-F, Tab. (Zeneca Pharmaceuticals).
So-Flo, Tab, Drops (Professional Pharm.).
W/Vitamins A, D, C.
See: Tri-Vi-Flor, Drops, Tab. (Bristol-Myers Squibb).

sodium fluoride and phosphoric acid gel.
Use: Dental caries agent.

sodium fluoride and phosphoric acid topical solution.
Use: Dental caries agent.

•**sodium fluoride f 18.** (SO-dee-uhm) U.S.P. 23.
Use: Radiopharmaceutical.

sodium folate. Monosodium folate.
Use: Water-soluble, hematopoietic vitamin.

•**sodium formaldehyde sulfoxylate.** (SO-dee-uhm) N.F. 18.
Use: Pharmaceutic aid (preservative).

sodium gamma-hydroxybutyric acid. Under study.

Use: Anesthetic adjuvant, sleep disorders. [Orphan Drug]
sodium gentisate.
See: Gentisate Sodium.
•**sodium gluconate.** (SO-dee-uhm) U.S.P. 23.
Use: Electrolyte, replacement.
sodium glucosulfone inj.
Use: Leprostatic.
sodium glutamate.
See: Glutamate.
sodium glycerophosphate. Glycerol phosphate sodium salt.
Use: Pharmaceutic necessity.
sodium glycocholate, a bile salt.
See: Bile Salts.
W/Phenolphthalein, cascara sagrada extract, sodium taurocholate, aloin.
See: So-Nitri-Nacea, Cap. (Scrip).
sodium heparin. U.S.P. 23. Heparin Sodium.
Use: Anticoagulant.
sodium hexobarbital.
Use: Intravenous general anesthetic.
sodium hyaluronate.
Use: Ophthalmic.
See: Amo Vitrax (Allergan, Inc.).
Amvisc (Chiron Therapeutics).
Amvisc Plus (Chiron Therapeutics).
Healon (Pharmacia & Upjohn).
W/Chondroitin sulfate.
See: Viscoat, Soln. (Alcon Laboratories, Inc.).
sodium hyaluronate and fluorescein sodium.
Use: Surgical aid, ophthalmic.
See: Healon Yellow (Pharmacia & Upjohn).
•**sodium hydroxide.** (SO-dee-uhm) N.F. 18.
Use: Pharmaceutic aid (alkalizing agent).
•**sodium hypochlorite solution.** (SO-dee-uhm high-poe-KLOR-ite) U.S.P. 23.
Use: Anti-infective, local, disinfectant.
See: Antiformin.
Dakin's Soln.
Hyclorite.
sodium hypophosphite. Sodium phosphinate.
Use: Pharmaceutic necessity.
sodium hyposulfite.
See: Sodium Thiosulfate (Various Mfr.).
W/Potassium guaiacolsufonate.
See: Guaiadol Aqueous, Vial (Medical Chem.).
W/Potassium guaiacolsulfonate, chlorpheniramine maleate, sodium bisulfite.
See: Gomahist, Inj. (Burgin-Arden).
sodium iodide. (SO-dee-uhm) U.S.P. 23.
Use: Nutritional supplement.
•**sodium iodide I-123 capsules.** U.S.P. 23.
Use: Diagnostic aid (thyroid function determination), radiopharmaceutical.
•**sodium iodide I-125.** USAN.
Use: Diagnostic aid (thyroid function determination), radiopharmaceutical.
•**sodium iodide I-131 capsules.** U.S.P. 23.
Use: Antineoplastic, diagnostic aid (thyroid function determination), radiopharmaceutical.
See: Iodotope, Cap., Soln. (Bristol-Myers Squibb).
sodium iodide I-131. (Mallinckrodt Chemical) 0.75 to 100 mCi/Cap. 3.5 to 150 mCi/Vial. *Rx.*
Use: Antithyroid agent.
sodium iodipamide.
Use: Radiopaque medium.
sodium iodomethane sulfonate. U.S.P. 23. Methiodal Sodium.
sodium iothalamate. U.S.P. 23. Iothalmate Sodium Inj.
Use: Radiopaque medium.
sodium ipodate. (SO-dee-uhm EYE-poe-date) U.S.P. 23. Ipodate Sodium.
Use: Radiopaque.
See: Oragrafin Sodium, Cap. (Bristol-Myers Squibb).
sodium isoamylethylbarbiturate.
See: Amytal Sodium, Prep. (Eli Lilly and Co.).
•**sodium lactate injection.** (SO-dee-uhm LACK-tate) U.S.P. 23.
Use: Fluid and electrolyte replacement.
sodium lactate injection. (Abbott Laboratories) 1/6 Molar, 250 ml, 500 ml, 1,000 ml; 50 mEq, 10 ml in 20 ml fliptop vial.
Use: Electrolyte replacement.
sodium lactate solution.
Use: Electrolyte replacement.
•**sodium lauryl sulfate.** (SO-dee-uhm LAH-rill SULL-fate) N.F. 18. Sulfuric acid monododecyl ester sodium salt. Sodium monododecyl sulfate.
Use: Pharmaceutic aid (surfactant).
See: Duponol.
W/Hydrocortisone.
See: Nutracort, Cream, Lot. (Galderma Laboratories, Inc.).
sodium levothyroxine. U.S.P. 23. Levothyroxine Sodium.
sodium liothyronine. Liothyronine Sodium, U.S.P. 23.
Use: Hormone, thyroid.
sodium lyapolate. (LIE-app-OLE-ate) Polyethylene sulfonate sodium. Peson

(Hoechst Marion Roussel).
Use: Anticoagulant.

sodium malonylurea.
See: Barbital Sodium (Various Mfr.).

sodium mercaptomerin. Mercaptomerin Sodium, U.S.P. 23.
Use: Diuretic.

•**sodium metabisulfite.** (SO-dee-uhm) N.F. 18.
Use: Pharmaceutic aid (antioxidant).

sodium methiodal. Methiodal Sodium, U.S.P. 23. Sodium monoiodomethanesulfonate. Sodium Iodomethanesulfonate, Inj.
Use: Radiopaque medium.

sodium methohexital for injection. Methohexital Sodium for Injection, U.S.P. 23.
Use: Anesthetic, general.
See: Brevital Sod., Pow. (Eli Lilly and Co.).

sodium methoxycellulose. Mixture of methylcellulose and sodium.

•**sodium monofluorophosphate.** (SO-dee-uhm mahn-oh-flure-oh-FOSS-fate) U.S.P. 23.
Use: Dental caries agent.

sodium morrhuate, inj. Morrhuate Sodium Inj., U.S.P. 23.
Use: Sclerosing agent.

sodium nafcillin. (SO-dee-uhm naff-SILL-in) Nafcillin Sodium, U.S.P. 23.
Use: Anti-infective.

sodium nicotinate. (Various Mfr.).
Use: IV nicotinic acid therapy.

•**sodium nitrite.** (SO-dee-uhm NYE-trite) U.S.P. 23.
Use: Antidote to cyanide poisoning, antioxidant. Vasodilator and antidote-cyanide.
See: Cyanide Antidote Pkg. (Eli Lilly and Co.).

sodium nitrite. (Various Mfr.) Gran., Bot. 0.25 lb, 1 lb.
Use: Antidote, cyanide.

•**sodium nitroprusside.** (SO-dee-uhm NYE-troe-PRUSS-ide) U.S.P. 23.
Use: Antihypertensive.
See: Keto-Diastix (Bayer Corp. (Consumer Div.)).
Nitropress, Vial (Abbott Laboratories).

sodium nitroprusside. (ESI Lederle Generics) 50 mg/Pow. for Inj. 5 ml. *Rx.*
Use: Antihypertensive.

sodium novobiocin. Sodium salt of antibacterial substance produced by *Streptomyces niveus.* Novobiocin monosodium salt.
Use: Anti-infective.
See: Albamycin, Cap., Syr., Vial (Pharmacia & Upjohn).

sodium ortho-iodohippurate. Iodohippurate Sodium, I-131 Injection, U.S.P. 23.
See: Hipputope (Bristol-Myers Squibb).

•**sodium oxybate.** (SO-dee-uhm OX-ee-bate) USAN.
Use: Adjunct to anesthesia.

sodium pantothenate.
Use: Orally, dietary supplement.

sodium para-aminohippurate injection.
Use: IV, to determine kidney tubular excretion function.

sodium penicillin G. Penicillin G Sodium, Sterile, U.S.P. 23. Sodium benzylpenicillin.

sodium pentobarbital. Pentobarbital Sodium, U.S.P. 23.
Use: Hypnotic.

•**sodium perborate monohydrate.** (SO-dee-uhm) USAN.

sodium peroxyborate.
See: Sodium Perborate (Various Mfr.).

sodium peroxyhydrate.
See: Sodium Perborate (Various Mfr.).

•**sodium pertechnetate Tc 99m injection.** (SO-dee-uhm per-TEK-neh-tate) U.S.P. 23. Pertechnetic acid, sodium salt.
Use: Radiopharmaceutical.
See: Minitec (Bristol-Myers Squibb).

sodium phenobarbital. Phenobarbital Sodium, U.S.P. 23.
Use: Anticonvulsant, hypnotic.

•**sodium phenylacetate.** (SO-dee-uhm FEN-ill-ASS-eh-tate) USAN.
Use: Antihyperammonemic.

•**sodium phenylbutyrate.** (SO-dee-uhm fen-ill-BYOOT-ih-rate) USAN.
Use: Antihyperammonemic.
See: Buphenyl (Ucyclyd Pharma, Inc.).

sodium phenylethylbarbiturate. Phenobarbital Sodium, U.S.P. 23.

sodium phosphate. Disodium hydrogen phosphate (Abbott Laboratories). 3 mM P and 4 mEq sodium. 15 ml in 30 ml fliptop vial.
Use: Cathartic, buffering agent, source of phosphate.
W/Gentamicin sulfate, monosodium phosphate, sodium Cl, benzalkonium Cl.
See: Garamycin Ophthalmic, Soln. (Schering-Plough Corp.).
W/Sodium biphosphate.
See: Fleet Enema (C.B. Fleet Co., Inc.).
Phospho-Soda, Liq. (C.B. Fleet Co., Inc.).

sodium phosphate, dibasic. (SO-dee-uhm FOSS-fate) U.S.P. 23.
Use: Laxative.

•**sodium phosphate, dried.** U.S.P. 23.
Use: Cathartic.

•**sodium phosphate, monobasic.** (SO-dee-uhm FOSS-fate) U.S.P. 23.
Use: Cathartic.
W/Gentamicin sulfate, disodium phosphate, sodium Cl, benzalkonium Cl.
See: Garamycin, Ophth. Soln. (Schering-Plough Corp.).
W/Methenamine.
See: Uro-Phosphate, Tab. (ECR Pharmaceuticals).
W/Methenamine mandelate, levo-hyoscyamine sulfate.
See: Levo-Uroquid, Tab (Beach Pharmaceuticals).
W/Methenamine, phenyl salicylate, methylene blue, hyoscyamine, alkaloid.
See: Fleet Enema (C.B. Fleet Co., Inc.).
Phospho-Soda, Liq. (C.B. Fleet Co., Inc).

sodium phosphates enema.
Use: Cathartic.

sodium phosphates oral solution.
Use: Cathartic.

sodium phosphate P 32. (Mallinckrodt Chemical) 0.67 mCi/ml. Vial. 5 mCi Inj. *Rx.*
Use: Antineoplastic.

•**sodium phosphate P 32 solution.** (SO-dee-uhm FOSS-fate) U.S.P. 23.
Use: Antineoplastic; antipolycythemic; diagnostic aid (neoplasm); radiopharmaceutical.

sodium phytate. (SO-dee-uhm FYE-tate) Nonasodium phytate: Sodium cyclohexanehexyl (hexaphosphate).
Use: Chelating agent.

•**sodium polyphosphate.** (SO-dee-uhm pahl-ee-FOSS-fate) USAN.
Use: Pharmaceutic aid.

•**sodium polystyrene sulfonate.** (SO-dee-uhm pah-lee-STYE-reen SULL-fuh-nate) U.S.P. 23.
Use: Ion exchange resin (potassium).
See: Kayexalate, Pow. (Sanofi Winthrop Pharmaceuticals).

sodium polystyrene sulfonate. (Roxane Laboratories, Inc.) 15 g, sorbitol 14.1 g, alcohol 0.1%/60 ml. Susp. Bot. 60 ml, 120 ml, 200 ml, 500 ml. *Rx.*
Use: Ion exchange resin (potassium).

sodium polystyrene sulfonate. (Crookes-Barnes) 5% Soln. Eye drops. Lacrivial 15 ml.
Use: Ion exchange resin (potassium).

•**sodium propionate.** (SO-dee-uhm PRO-pee-oh-nate) N.F. 18.
Use: Pharmaceutic aid (preservative).
W/Chlorophyll "a".
See: Prophyllin, Pow., Oint. (Rystan, Inc.).
W/Neomycin sulfate.
See: Otobiotic, Ear Drops (Schering-Plough Corp.).

sodium psylliate.
Use: Sclerosing agent.

•**sodium pyrophosphate.** (SO-dee-uhm pie-row-FOSS-fate) USAN.
Use: Pharmaceutic aid.

sodium radio chromate inj. Sodium Chromate Cr 51 Inj., U.S.P. 23.

sodium radio iodide solution. Sodium Iodide I-131 Solution, U.S.P. 23.
Use: Thyroid tumors, hyperthyroidism, cardiac dysfunction.

sodium radio-phosphate, P-32. Soln.: Radio-Phosphate P 32 Solution. Sodium phosphate P-32 Solution, U.S.P. 23.

sodium removing resins.
See: Resins.

sodium rhodanate.
See: Sodium Thiocyanate.

sodium rhodanide.
See: Sodium Thiocyanate.

sodium saccharin. Saccharin Sodium, U.S.P. 23.
Use: Noncaloric sweetener.

•**sodium salicylate.** (SO-dee-uhm) U.S.P. 23.
Use: Analgesic; IV, gout.

sodium salicylate, natural.
Use: Analgesic.

sodium salicylate combinations.
See: Apcogesic, Tab. (Apco).
Bisalate, Tab. (Allison).
Bufosal, Gran. (Table Rock).
Corilin, Liq. (Schering-Plough Corp.).
Pabalate, Tab. (Wyeth-Ayerst Laboratories).

sodium secobarbital. Secobarbital Sodium, U.S.P. 23.
Use: Hypnotic.

sodium secobarbital and sodium amobarbital capsules.
Use: Sedative.
See: Tuinal, Cap. (Eli Lilly and Co.).

•**sodium starch glycolate.** (SO-dee-uhm) N.F. 18.
Use: Pharmaceutic aid (tablet excipient).

•**sodium stearate.** (SO-dee-uhm) N.F. 18.
Use: Pharmaceutic aid (emulsifying and stiffening agent).

•**sodium stearyl fumarate.** N.F. 18.
Use: Pharmaceutic aid (tablet/capsule lubricant).

sodium stibogluconate.

Use: CDC anti-infective agent.

sodium succinate.
Use: Alkalinize urine & awaken patients following barbiturate anesthesia.

Sodium Sulamyd Ophthalmic Oint. 10% Sterile. (Schering-Plough Corp.) Sulfacetamide sodium 10%. Tube 3.5 g. *Rx.*
Use: Anti-infective, ophthalmic.

Sodium Sulamyd Ophthalmic Soln. 10% Sterile. (Schering-Plough Corp.) Sulfacetamide sodium 10%. Bot. 5 ml, 15 ml. *Rx.*
Use: Anti-infective, ophthalmic.

Sodium Sulamyd Ophthalmic Soln. 30% Sterile. (Schering-Plough Corp.) Sulfacetamide sodium 30%. Bot. 15 ml. Box 1s. *Rx.*
Use: Anti-infective, ophthalmic.

sodium sulfabromomethazine.
Use: Anti-infective.

sodium sulfacetamide.
See: Sulfacetamide Sodium, Preps. (Various Mfr.).

sodium sulfadiazine.
See: Sulfadiazine Sodium, Preps. (Various Mfr.).

sodium sulfamerazine.
See: Sulfamerazine Sodium, Preps. (Various Mfr.).

sodium sulfapyridine.
See: Sulfapyridine Sodium Pow. (Pfaltz & Bauer).

•**sodium sulfate.** (SO-dee-uhm SULL-fate) U.S.P. 23.
Use: Calcium regulator.

•**sodium sulfate s 35.** (SO-dee-uhm SULL-fate) USAN.
Use: Radiopharmaceutical.

sodium sulfathiazole.
Use: Anti-infective.
See: Sulfathiazole Sodium, Inj. (Various Mfr.).

sodium sulfoacetate.
See: Sebulex, Liq., Cream (Westwood Squibb Pharmaceuticals).

sodium sulfobromophthalein. Sulfobromophthalein Sodium, U.S.P. XXII.
Use: Diagnostic aid (hepatic function determination).

sodium sulfocyanate.
See: Sodium Thiocyanate (Various Mfr.).

sodium sulfoxone. Sulfoxone Sodium, U.S.P. 23. Disodium sulfonyl-bis (p-phenyleneimino) dimethanesulfonate.

sodium suramin.
See: Suramin Sodium.

sodium taurocholate, a bile salt.
See: Bile Salts.

sodium tetradecyl sulfate.
Use: Bleeding esophageal varices. [Orphan Drug]
See: Sotradecol, Inj. (ESI Lederle Generics).

sodium tetraiodophenolphthalein.
See: Iodophthalein Sodium (Various Mfr.).

sodium thiacetphenarsamide. (Abbott Laboratories)

sodium thiamylal for injection. Thiamylal Sodium For Injection, U.S.P. 23.
Use: Anesthetic, general.

sodium thiocyanate. Sodium Sulfocyanate. Sodium Rhodanide.

sodium thiopental.
See: Thiopental Sodium, U.S.P. 23.

•**sodium thiosulfate.** (SO-dee-uhm thigh-oh-SULL-fate) U.S.P. 23.
Use: For argyria, cyanide and iodine poisoning, arsphenamine reactions; prevention of spread of ringworm of feet; antidote to cyanide poisoning.
W/Salicylic acid, hydrocortisone acetate, alcohol.
See: Tinver, Lot. (PBH Wesley Jessen).
Versiclear, Lot. (Hope Pharmaceuticals).
W/Salicylic acid, resorcinol, alcohol.
See: Cyanide Antidote Pkg. (Eli Lilly and Co.).
Mild Komed, Lot. (PBH Wesley Jessen).

sodium thiosulfate. (Various Mfr.) 250 mg/ml. KCl 4.4 mg, boric acid 2.8 mg/Inj. 50 ml. *Rx.*
Use: Antidote.

sodium l-thyroxine.
See: Synthroid, Tab., Inj. (Knoll Pharmaceuticals).

sodium tolbutamide. Tolbutamide Sodium, U.S.P. 23.
Use: Diagnostic aid (diabetes).

sodium triclofos. (SO-dee-uhm TRY-kloe-foss) Sodium trichloroethylphosphate.
Use: Sedative, hypnotic.

•**sodium trimetaphosphate.** (SO-dee-uhm try-met-AH-FOSS-fate) USAN.
Use: Pharmaceutic aid.

sodium valproate.
See: Valproate sodium.

sodium vinbarbital injection.
Use: Sedative.

sodium warfarin. Warfarin Sodium, U.S.P. 23.
Use: Anticoagulant.

Sod-Late 10. (Schlicksup) Sodium salicylate 10 gr/Tab. Bot. 1000s. *otc.*
Use: Analgesic.

Sodol Compound. (Major Pharmaceuticals) Carisoprodol 200 mg, aspirin 325

mg/Tab. Bot. 100s, 500s. *Rx.*
Use: Muscle relaxant.

Sofcaps. (Alton) Docusate sodium 100 mg, 250 mg/Cap. Bot. 100s, 1000s. *otc.*
Use: Laxative.

Sofenol 5. (C & M Pharmacal, Inc.) Moisturizing lotion formulation. Bot. 8 oz. *otc.*
Use: Emollient.

Soflens Enzymatic Contact Lens Cleaner. (Allergan, Inc.) Papain, sodium Cl, sodium carbonate, sodium borate, edetate disodium/Tab. Vial 12s, 24s, 48s, Refill 24s, 36s. *otc.*
Use: Contact lens care.

Sof/Pro Clean SA. (Sherman Pharmaceuticals, Inc.) Hypertonic solution: salt buffers, copolymers of ethylene and propylene oxide, octylphenoxypolyethoxyethanol, lauryl sulfate salt of imidazoline, sodium bisulfite 0.1%, sorbic acid 0.1%, trisodium EDTA 0.25%, thimerosal free. Bot. 30 ml. *otc.*
Use: Contact lens care.

Sof/Pro-Clean. (Sherman Pharmaceuticals, Inc.) Buffered, hypertonic solution with thimerosal 0.004%, EDTA 0.1%, ethylene and propylene oxide, octylphenoxypolyethoxyethanol, lauryl sulfate salt of imidazoline. Bot. 30 ml. *otc.*
Use: Contact lens care.

Soft Mate Comfort Drops for Sensitive Eyes. (PBH Wesley Jessen) Borate buffered, potassium sorbate 0.13%, EDTA 0.1%, sodium Cl, hydroxyethylcellulose, octylphenoxyethanol. Drop. Bot. 15 ml. *otc.*
Use: Contact lens care.

Soft Mate Consept 1. (PBH Wesley Jessen) Hydrogen peroxide 3% w/polyoxyl 40 stearate, sodium stannate, sodium nitrate, phosphate buffer. 240 ml. *otc.*
Use: Contact lens care.

Soft Mate Consept 2. (PBH Wesley Jessen) **Soln:** Isotonic solution of sodium thiosulfate 0.5%, borate buffers, chlorhexidine gluconate 0.001%. Bot. 360 ml. **Spray:** Isotonic sodium thiosulfate 0.5%, borate buffers. Aer. 360 ml. *otc.*
Use: Contact lens care.

Soft Mate Daily Cleaning for Sensitive Eyes. (PBH Wesley Jessen) Isotonic solution w/NaCl, octylphenoxy (oxyethylene) ethanol hydroxyethylcellulose w/potassium sorbate 0.13%, EDTA 0.2%. Soln. Bot. 1 ml, 30 ml. *otc.*
Use: Contact lens care.

Soft Mate Daily Cleaning Solution. (PBH Wesley Jessen) Sterile aqueous isotonic solution w/sodium Cl, octylphenoxy (oxyethylene) ethanol, hydroxyethylcellulose, thimerosal 0.004%, edetate disodium 0.2%. Bot. 30 ml. *otc.*
Use: Contact lens care.

Soft Mate Disinfecting Solution For Sensitive Eyes. (PBH Wesley Jessen) Sterile, aqueous, isotonic solution w/ sodium Cl, povidone, octylphenoxy (oxyethylene) ethanol, chlorhexidine gluconate 0.005%, borate buffer, edetate disodium 0.1%. Thimerosal free. Bot. 240 ml. *otc.*
Use: Contact lens care.

Soft Mate Disinfection and Storage Solution. (PBH Wesley Jessen) Sterile aqueous isotonic solution w/sodium Cl, povidone, octylphenoxl (oxyethylene) ethanol with a borate buffer, thimerosal 0.001%, edetate disodium 0.1%, chlorhexidine gluconate 0.005%. Bot. 8 oz. *otc.*
Use: Contact lens care.

Soft Mate Enzyme Plus Cleaner. (PBH Wesley Jessen) Subtilisin, poloxamer 338, povidone, citric acid, potassium bicarbonate, sodium carbonate, sodium benzoate. Tab. Pkg. 8s. *otc.*
Use: Contact lens care.

Soft Mate Lens Drops. (PBH Wesley Jessen) Sterile aqueous isotonic solution w/sodium Cl, potassium sorbate 0.13%, edetate disodium 0.025%. Thimerosal free. Bot. 2 oz. *otc.*
Use: Contact lens care.

Soft Mate Preservative-Free Saline Solution. (PBH Wesley Jessen) Sterile aqueous isotonic solution w/sodium Cl, borate buffer. Contains no preservatives. Bot. 0.5 oz, 30 single use. *otc.*
Use: Contact lens care.

Soft Mate PS Comfort Drops. (PBH Wesley Jessen) Sterile aqueous isotonic solution w/potassium sorbate 0.13%, edetate disodium 0.1%. Bot. 15 ml. *otc.*
Use: Contact lens care.

Soft Mate PS Daily Cleaning Solution. (PBH Wesley Jessen) Sterile aqueous isotonic solution w/sodium Cl, octylphenoxy (oxyethylene) ethanol, hydroxyethyl cellulose, potassium sorbate 0.13%, edetate disodium 0.2%. Bot. 30 ml. *otc.*
Use: Contact lens care.

Soft Mate PS Saline Solution. (PBH Wesley Jessen) Sterile aqueous isotonic solution w/sodium Cl, potassium sorbate 0.13%, edetate disodium 0.025%. Bot. 8 oz, 12 oz. *otc.*
Use: Contact lens care.

Soft Mate Rinsing Solution. (PBH Wesley Jessen) Sterile aqueous isotonic solution w/sodium Cl, thimerosal 0.001%, edetate disodium 0.1%, chlorhexidine gluconate 0.005%. Bot. 8 oz. *otc.*
Use: Contact lens care.

Soft Mate Saline for Sensitive Eyes. (PBH Wesley Jessen) Isotonic, sorbic acid 0.1%, EDTA 0.1%, NaCl, borate buffer. Bot. 360 (2s), 480 ml. *otc.*
Use: Contact lens care.

Soft Mate Saline Preservative-Free. (PBH Wesley Jessen) Sodium Cl w/borate buffer. Soln. Bot. 15 ml. *otc.*
Use: Contact lens care.

Soft Mate Saline Solution. (PBH Wesley Jessen) Sterile aqueous isotonic solution of sodium Cl. Preservative free. Bot. 8 oz, 12 oz. *otc.*
Use: Contact lens care.

Soft Mate Soft Lens Cleaners. (PBH Wesley Jessen) Kit containing: Soft Mate daily cleaning solution II (4 oz.); Soft Mate weekly cleaning solution (1.2 oz.); Hydra-Mat II cleaning and storage unit. *otc.*
Use: Contact lens care.

Soft'n Soothe. (B.F. Ascher and Co.) Benzocaine, menthol, moisturizers. Tube 50 g. *otc.*
Use: Anesthetic, local.

Soft Sense. (Bausch & Lomb Pharmaceuticals) **Hand Lot.:** Petrolatum, vitamin E, aloe, parabens. Non-greasy. Bot. 444 ml. **Body Lot.:** Petrolatum, vitamin E, parabens. Non-greasy. Bot. 444 ml. *otc.*
Use: Emollient.

SoftWear. (Ciba Vision) Isotonic, sodium Cl, boric acid, sodium borate, sodium perborate (generating up to 0.006% hydrogen peroxide stabilized with phosphoric acid). Soln. Bot. 120 ml, 240 ml, 360 ml. *otc.*
Use: Contact lens care.

Solaneed. (Hanlon) Vitamin A 25,000 units/Cap. Bot. 100s. *Rx.*
Use: Vitamin supplement.

Solaquin. (Zeneca Pharmaceuticals) Hydroquinone 2%, ethyl dihydroxypropyl PABA 5%, dioxybenzone 3%, oxybenzone 2%. Tube oz. *otc.*
Use: Dermatologic.

Solaquin Forte Cream. (Zeneca Pharmaceuticals) Hydroquinone 4%, ethyl dihydroxypropyl PABA 5%, dioxybenzone 3%, oxybenzone 2% in a vanishing cream base. Tube 0.5 oz, 1 oz. *otc.*
Use: Dermatologic.

Solaquin Forte Gel. (Zeneca Pharmaceuticals) Hydroquinone 4%, ethyl dihydroxypropyl PABA 5%, dioxybenzone 3%, oxybenzone 2%. Tube 0.5 oz, 1 oz. *Rx.*
Use: Dermatologic.

Solarcaine. (Schering-Plough Corp.) **Lot.:** Benzocaine, triclosan, mineral oil, alcohol, aloe extract, tocopheryl acetate, menthol, camphor, parabens, EDTA. 120 ml. **Spray (aerosol):** Benzocaine 20%, triclosan 0.13%, SD alcohol 40 35%, tocopheryl acetate. 90 ml, 120 ml. *otc.*
Use: Anesthetic, local.

Solarcaine Aloe Extra Burn Relief. (Schering-Plough Corp.) **Cream:** Lidocaine 0.5%, aloe, EDTA, lanolin oil, lanolin, camphor, propylparaben, eucalyptus oil, menthol, tartrazine. 120 g. **Gel:** Lidocaine 0.5%, aloe vera gel, glycerin, EDTA, isopropyl alcohol, menthol, diazolidinyl urea, tartrazine. 120 g, 240 g. **Spray:** Lidocaine 0.5%, aloe vera gel, glycerin, EDTA, diazolidinyl urea, vitamin E, parabens. 135 ml. *otc.*
Use: Anesthetic, local.

Solar Cream. (Doak Dermatologics) PABA, titanium dioxide, magnesium stearate in a flesh-colored, water-repellent base. Tube oz. *otc.*
Use: Sunscreen.

solargentum.
See: Mild silver protein (Various Mfr.).

Solar Shield 15 SPF. (Akorn, Inc.) Ethylhexyl p-methoxy-cinnamate 7.5%, oxybenzone in a moisturizing base 5%, PABA free. Waterproof. Lot. Bot. 120 ml. *otc.*
Use: Sunscreen.

Solar Shield 30 SPF. (Akorn, Inc.) Ethylhexyl p-methoxycinnamate 7.5%, oxybenzone 6%, 2-ethylhexyl salicylate 5%, 3-diphenylacrylate 7.5%, 2-ethylhexyl-2-cyano-3 in a moisturizing base, PABA free. Waterproof. Lot. Bot. 120 ml. *otc.*
Use: Sunscreen.

SolBar PF Cream 50 SPF. (Person and Covey, Inc.) Oxybenzone, octyl methoxycinnamate, octocrylene, PABA free. Waterproof. Cream Tube. 120 g. *otc.*
Use: Sunscreen.

SolBar PF Liquid. (Person and Covey, Inc.) Octyl methoxycinnamate 7.5%, oxybenzone 6%, SD alcohol 40 76%, PABA free. SPF 30. Liq. Bot. 120 ml. *otc.*
Use: Sunscreen.

SolBar PF 15 Cream. (Person and Covey, Inc.) Octyl methoxycinnamate

7.5%, oxybenzone 5%. SPF 15. Bot. 1 oz, 4 oz. *otc.*
Use: Sunscreen.

SolBar PF 50. (Person and Covey, Inc.) Oxybenzone, octyl methoxycinnamate, octocrylene, PABA free. Waterproof. SPF 50. Cream Tube 120 g. *otc.*
Use: Sunscreen.

SolBar PF Paba Free 15. (Person and Covey, Inc.) Oxybenzone 5%, octyl methoxycinnamate 7.5%. SPF 15. Cream Tube 2.5 oz. *otc.*
Use: Sunscreen.

SolBar Plus 15. (Person and Covey, Inc.) Padimate 6%, oxybenzone 4%, dioxybenzone 2%. SPF 15. Cream Tube 1 oz, 4 oz. *otc.*
Use: Sunscreen.

Solex A15 Clear Lotion Sunscreen. (Dermol Pharmaceuticals, Inc.) Octyl dimethyl PABA 5%, benzophenone 33%, SD alcohol. SPF 15. Lot. Bot. 120 ml. *otc.*
Use: Sunscreen.

Solfoton. (ECR Pharmaceuticals) Phenobarbital 16 mg/Tab. or Cap. Bot. 100s, 500s. *c-IV.*
Use: Hypnotic, sedative.

Solfoton S/C Tabs. (ECR Pharmaceuticals) Phenobarbital 16 mg/SC Tab. Bot. 100s. *c-IV.*
Use: Hypnotic, sedative.

Solganal. (Schering-Plough Corp.) Aurothioglucose 50 mg/ml. Vial 10 ml. *Rx.*
Use: IM, gold therapy, antiarthritic.

Soliwax. Docusate Sodium, U.S.P. 23. Docusate Sodium, Solasulfone (I.N.N.).

Soltice Quick-Rub. (Chattem Consumer Products) Methyl salicylate, camphor, menthol, eucalyptol. Cream Tube 1.33 oz, 3.75 oz. *otc.*
Use: Analgesic, topical.

Solu-Barb 0.25 Tablets. (Forest Pharmaceutical, Inc.) Phenobarbital 0.25 gr/Tab. Bot. 24s. *c-IV.*
Use: Hypnotic, sedative.

soluble complement receptor (recombinant human) type 1.
Use: Prevention or reduction of adult respiratory distress syndrome. [Orphan Drug]

Solu-Cortef. (Pharmacia & Upjohn) **100 mg:** Hydrocortisone sodium succinate, w/benzyl alcohol. Plain vial, 5s, 25s. 100 mg/2 ml Mix-O-Vial. **250 mg:** Hydrocortisone sodium succinate, benzyl alcohol. Mix-O-Vial 2 ml, 5s, 25s. 25-Pack, 25s, 50s. **500 mg:** Hydrocortisone sodium succinate, benzyl alcohol. Mix-O-Vial, 5s, 25s. **1000 mg:** Hydrocortisone sodium succinate, benzyl alcohol. Mix-O-Vial, 5s, 25s. *Rx.*
Use: Corticosteroid.

Solu-Eze. (Forest Pharmaceutical, Inc.) Hydroxyquinoline 0.12%, carbitol acetate 12.10%. Liq. Bot. 3 oz. *Rx.*
Use: Dermatologic.

Solu-Medrol. (Pharmacia & Upjohn) **40 mg:** Methylprednisolone sodium succinate, benzyl alcohol. Univial 1 ml. **125 mg:** Methylprednisolone sodium succinate, benzyl alcohol. Act-O-Vial 2 ml, 5s, 25s. 25-Pack, 25s, 50s. **500 mg:** Methylprednisolone sodium succinate, benzyl alcohol. Vial 8 ml, vials w/diluent 8 ml. **1000 mg:** Methylprednisolone sodium succinate, benzyl alcohol. Vial 16 ml, vial w/diluent 16 ml. **2000 mg:** Methylprednisolone sodium succinate powder for injection, benzyl alcohol. Vial 30.6 ml, vial w/diluent 30.6 ml. *Rx.*
Use: Corticosteroid.

Solumol. (C & M Pharmacal, Inc.) Petrolatum, mineral oil, cetylstearyl alcohol, sodium lauryl sulfate, glycerin, propylene glycol, sorbic acid, purified water. Jar lb. *otc.*
Use: Pharmaceutical aid, ointment base.

Solurex. (Hyrex Pharmaceuticals) Dexamethasone sodium phosphate 4 mg/ml. Methyl- and propylparabens, sodium bisulfite. Liq. Vial 5 ml, 10 ml, 30 ml. *Rx.*
Use: Corticosteroid.

Solurex LA. (Hyrex Pharmaceuticals) Dexamethasone acetate 8 mg/ml w/ polysorbate 80, carboxymethylcellulose, sodium bisulfite, EDTA, benzyl alcohol. Susp. Vial 5 ml. *Rx.*
Use: Corticosteroid.

Soluvite C.T. (Pharmics, Inc.) Vitamins A 2500 IU, D 400 IU, B_1 1.05 mg, B_2 1.2 mg, B_6 1.05 mg, B_{12} 4.5 mcg, C 60 mg, B_3 13.5 mg, E 15 IU, fluoride 1 mg, folic acid 0.3 mg/Tab. Bot. 100s, 1000s. *Rx.*
Use: Mineral, vitamin supplement.

Soluvite-f Drops. (Pharmics, Inc.) Vitamins A 1500 IU, D 400 IU, C 35 mg, fluoride 0.25 mg/0.6 ml. Bot. 57 ml. *Rx.*
Use: Mineral, vitamin supplement.

Solvisyn-A. (Towne) Water-soluble vitamin A 10,000 units, 25,000 units or 50,000 units/Cap. Bot. 100s, 1000s. *Rx-otc.*
Use: Vitamin supplement.

•**solypertine tartrate.** (SAHL-ee-PURR-teen) USAN.
Use: Antiadrenergic.

Soma. (Wallace Laboratories) Carisoprodol 350 mg/Tab. Bot. 100s, 500s, UD

500s. *Rx.*
Use: Muscle relaxant.

Soma Compound Tabs. (Wallace Laboratories) Carisoprodol 200 mg, aspirin 325 mg/Tab. Bot. 100s, 500s, UD 500s. *Rx.*
Use: Muscle relaxant.

Soma Compound w/Codeine. (Wallace Laboratories) Carisoprodol 200 mg, aspirin 325 mg, codeine phosphate 16 mg/Tab. Sodium metabisulfite. Bot. 100s. *c-III.*
Use: Muscle relaxant.

Somagard. (Roberts Pharmaceuticals)
See: Deslorelin.

•**somantadine hydrochloride.** (sah-MAN-tah-deen) USAN.
Use: Antiviral.

somatostatin.
Use: Digestive aid. [Orphan Drug]
See: Zecnil.

•**somatrem.** (so-muh-TREM) USAN.
Use: Hormone, growth.
See: Protropin, Inj. (Genentech, Inc.).

•**somatropin.** (SO-muh-TROE-pin) USAN. Growth hormone derived from the anterior pituitary gland.
Use: Hormone, growth. [Orphan Drug]
See: Humatrope, Inj. (Eli Lilly and Co.).
Norditropin, Pow. for Inj. (Novo/Nordisk Pharm, Inc.).
Nutropin, Inj. (Genentech, Inc.).
Saizen, Inj. (Serono Laboratories, Inc.).
Serostim, Inj. (Serono Laboratories, Inc.).

Sominex. (SmithKline Beecham Pharmaceuticals) Diphenhydramine HCl 25 mg/Tab. Blister pack 16s, 32s, 72s. *otc.*
Use: Sleep aid.

Sominex Caplets. (SmithKline Beecham Pharmaceuticals) Diphenhydramine HCl 50 mg. Tab. Blister pack 8s, 16s, 32s. *otc.*
Use: Sleep aid.

Sominex Pain Relief Formula. (SmithKline Beecham Pharmaceuticals) Diphenhydramine HCl 25 mg, acetaminophen 500 mg/Tab. Blister pack 16s. Bot. 32s. *otc.*
Use: Sleep aid, analgesic.

Sonacide. (Wyeth-Ayerst Laboratories) Potentiated acid glutaraldehyde. Bot. 1 gal, 5 gal. *otc.*
Use: Disinfectant, sterilizing agent.

Sonekap. (Eastwood) Cap. Bot. 100s.

soneryl.
See: Butethal (Various Mfr.).

SonoRx. (Bracco Diagnostics) Simethicone-coated cellulose 7.5 mg/ml. Susp. Glass bot. 400 ml. *Rx.*
Use: Diagnostic aid.

Soothaderm. (Pharmakon Laboratories, Inc.) Pyrilamine maleate 2.07 mg, benzocaine 2.08 mg, zinc oxide 41.35 mg/ml, camphor, menthol. Lot. Bot. 118 ml. *otc.*
Use: Antihistamine, anesthetic, local.

Soothe. (Alcon Laboratories, Inc.) Tetrahydrozoline 0.05%, benzalkonium Cl 0.004%, adsorbobase. Liq. Bot. 15 ml. *otc.*
Use: Decongestant, ophthalmic.

Soothe. (Walgreen Co.) Bismuth subsalicylate 100 mg/Tsp. Bot. 9 oz. *otc.*
Use: Antidiarrheal.

Soquette. (PBH Wesley Jessen) Polyvinyl alcohol w/benzalkonium Cl 0.01%, EDTA 0.2%. Bot. 4 fl oz. *otc.*
Use: Contact lens care.

Sorbase Cough Syrup. (Fort David) Dextromethorphan HBr 10 mg, guaifenesin 100 mg/5 ml in sorbitol base. Bot. 4 oz, pt, gal. *otc.*
Use: Antitussive, expectorant.

•**sorbic acid.** (SORE-bik) N.F. 18.
Use: Pharmaceutic aid (antimicrobial).

Sorbide T.D. (Merz Pharmaceuticals) Isosorbide dinitrate 40 mg/TR Cap. Bot. 100s. *Rx.*
Use: Antianginal.

Sorbidon Hydrate. (Gordon Laboratories) Water-in-oil ointment. Jar 2 oz, 0.5 oz, 1 lb, 5 lb. *otc.*
Use: Emollient.

sorbimacrogol oleate 300.
See: Polysorbate 80.

•**sorbinil.** (SORE-bih-nill) USAN.
Use: Enzyme inhibitor (aldose reductase).

•**sorbitan monolaurate.** (SORE-bih-tan MAHN-oh-LORE-ate) N.F. 18.
Use: Pharmaceutic aid (surfactant).
See: Span 20 (Zeneca Pharmaceuticals).

•**sorbitan monooleate.** (SORE-bih-tan MAHN-oh-OH-lee-ate) N.F. 18.
Use: Pharmaceutic aid (surfactant).
See: Span 80 (Zeneca Pharmaceuticals).

sorbitan monooleate polyoxyethylene derivatives.
See: Polysorbate 80, N.F. 18.

•**sorbitan monopalmitate.** (SORE-bih-tan MAHN-oh-PAL-mih-tate) N.F. 18.
Use: Pharmaceutic aid (surfactant).
See: Span 40 (Zeneca Pharmaceuticals).

•**sorbitan monostearate.** (SORE-bih-tan MAHN-oh-STEE-ah-rate) N.F. 18.

Use: Pharmaceutic aid (surfactant).
See: Span 60 (Zeneca Pharmaceuticals).

•**sorbitan sesquioleate.** (SORE-bih-tan SESS-kwih-OH-lee-ate) N.F. 18.
Use: Pharmaceutic aid (surfactant).
See: Arlacel C (Zeneca Pharmaceuticals).

•**sorbitan trioleate.** (SORE-bih-tan TRY-OH-lee-ate) N.F. 18.
Use: Pharmaceutic aid, surfactant.
See: Span 85 (Zeneca Pharmaceuticals).

•**sorbitan tristearate.** (SORE-bih-tan TRY-STEE-ah-rate) USAN.
Use: Pharmaceutic aid; surfactant.
See: Span 65 (Zeneca Pharmaceuticals).

sorbitans.
See: Polysorbate 80, U.S.P. 23.

•**sorbitol.** N.F. 18.
Use: Diuretic, dehydrating agent, humectant, pharmaceutic aid (sweetening agent, tablet excipient, flavor).
See: Sorbo (Zeneca Pharmaceuticals).
W/Homatropine methylbromide.
See: Probilagol, Liq. (Purdue Frederick Co.).
W/Mannitol.
See: Sorbitol-mannitol Irrigation (Abbott Laboratories).

•**sorbitol solution.** U.S.P. 23.
Use: Pharmaceutic aid (flavor, tablet excipient).

Sorbitol-Mannitol. (Abbott Laboratories) Mannitol 0.54 g, sorbitol 2.7 g. Liq. Bot. 100 ml, 1500 ml, 3000 ml. *Rx.*
Use: Irrigant, genitourinary.

Sorbitrate. (Zeneca Pharmaceuticals) Isosorbide dinitrate. **Tab.:** 5 mg Bot. 100s, 500s, UD 100s; 10 mg Bot. 100s, 500s, UD 100s; 20 mg, 30 mg Bot. 100s, UD 100s. **SA Tab.:** 40 mg Bot. 100s, UD 100s. **Sublingual Tab.:** 2.5 mg, 5 mg, 10 mg Bot. 100s. **Chew. Tab.:** 5 mg Bot. 100s, 500s; 10 mg Bot. 100s. *Rx.*
Use: Antianginal.

Sorbitrate SA. (Zeneca Pharmaceuticals) Isosorbide dinitrite, oral 40 mg/SR Tab. Bot. 100s, UD 100s *Rx.*
Use: Antianginal.

Sorbo. (Zeneca Pharmaceuticals) Sorbitol Solution, U.S.P. 23.

Sorbsan. (Dow B. Hickam, Inc.) Calcium alginate fiber 2 x 2, 3 x 3, 4 x 4, 4 x 8 inch. Box 1s. Wound packing fibers-calcium alginate fiber ¼ x 12 inch. Box 1s. *Rx.*
Use: Dermatologic, wound therapy.

sorethytan (20) monooleate.
See: Polysorbate 80 (Various Mfr.).

Soriatane. (Roche Laboratories) Acitretin 10 mg, 25 mg. Cap. Bot. 30s. *Rx.*
Use: Antipsoriatic.

Sosegon Solution. (Sanofi Winthrop Pharmaceuticals) Pentazocine. *c-IV.*
Use: Analgesic.

Sosegon Suspension. (Sanofi Winthrop Pharmaceuticals) Pentazocine. *c-IV.*
Use: Analgesic.

Sosegon Tablets. (Sanofi Winthrop Pharmaceuticals) Pentazocine. *c-IV.*
Use: Analgesic.

Soss-10. (Roberts Pharmaceuticals) Sodium sulfacetamide 10%. Soln. Bot. 15 ml. *Rx.*
Use: Anti-infective, ophthalmic.

•**sotalol hydrochloride.** (SOTT-uh-lahl) USAN.
Use: Beta-adrenergic blocker.
See: Betapace, Tab. (Berlex Laboratories, Inc.).

•**soterenol hydrochloride.** (so-TER-en-ole) USAN.
Use: Bronchodilator.

Sotradecol. (ESI Lederle Generics) Sodium tetradecyl sulfate 1%, 3%. Inj. Dosette amp. 2 ml. *Rx.*
Use: Sclerosing agent.

Soxa. (Vita Elixir) Sulfisoxazole 0.5 g/Tab. Bot. 100s, 1000s. *Rx.*
Use: Anti-infective.

Soxa-Forte. (Vita Elixir) Sulfisoxazole 0.5 g, phenazopyridine 50 mg/Tab. *Rx.*
Use: Anti-infective.

Soyalac. (Mt. Vernon Foods, Inc.) Infant formula based on an extract from whole soybeans containing all-essential nutrients. **Ready to Serve Liq.:** Can 32 fl oz. **Double Strength Conc.:** Can 13 fl oz. **Pow.:** Can 14 oz. *otc.*
Use: Nutritional supplement.

Soyalac-I. (Mt. Vernon Foods, Inc.) Soy protein isolate infant formula containing no corn derivatives and a negligible amount of soy carbohydrates. Contains all essential nutrients in various forms. **Ready to Serve Liq.:** Can 32 fl oz. **Double Strength Conc.:** Can 13 fl oz. *otc.*
Use: Nutritional supplement.

soya lecithin. Soybean extract. 100s.
Use: Phosphorus therapy.
See: Neo-Vadrin (Scherer Laboratories, Inc.).

•**soybean oil.** U.S.P. 23.
Use: Pharmaceutic necessity.

Spabelin No. 1. (Arcum) Phenobarbital 15 mg, belladonna powdered extract

⅛ gr/Tab. Bot. 100s, 1000s. *Rx.*
Use: Hypnotic, sedative.

Spabelin No. 2. (Arcum) Phenobarbital 30 mg, belladonna powdered extract ⅛ gr/Tab. Bot. 100s, 1000s. *Rx.*
Use: Hypnotic, sedative.

Spabelin Elixir. (Arcum) Hyoscyamine sulfate 81 mcg, atropine sulfate 15 mcg, scopolamine HBr 5 mcg, phenobarbital 16.2 mg/5 ml. Bot. 16 oz, gal. *Rx.*
Use: Anticholinergic, antispasmodic, hypnotic, sedative.

Span 20. (Zeneca Pharmaceuticals) Sorbitan Monolaurate, N.F. 18.

Span 40. (Zeneca Pharmaceuticals) Sorbitan Monopalmitate, N.F. 18.

Span 60. (Zeneca Pharmaceuticals) Sorbitan Monostearate, N.F. 18.

Span 65. (Zeneca Pharmaceuticals) Sorbitan tristearate. Mixture of stearate esters of sorbitol and its anhydrides.
Use: Surface active agent.

Span 80. (Zeneca Pharmaceuticals) Sorbitan monooleate, N.F. 18

Span 85. (Zeneca Pharmaceuticals) Sorbitan trioleate. Mixture of oleate esters of sorbitol and its anhydrides.
Use: Surface active agent.

Span C. (Freeda Vitamins, Inc.) Citrus bioflavonoids 300 mg, rutin 50 mg, vitamin C 200 mg/Tab. Bot. 100s, 250s, 500s. *otc.*
Use: Vitamin supplement.

Span PD. (Lexis Laboratories) Phentermine HCl 37.5 mg/Cap. Bot. 100s. *c-IV.*
Use: Anorexiant.

Span-RD. (Lexis Laboratories) d-methamphetamine HCl 12 mg, dl-methamphetamine HCl 6 mg, butabarbital 30 mg/Tab. Bot. 100s, 1000s. *c-III.*
Use: Amphetamine, hypnotic, sedative.

•**sparfloxacin.** (spar-FLOX-ah-sin) USAN.
Use: Anti-infective.
See: Zagam, Tab. (Rhone-Poulenc Rorer Pharmaceuticals, Inc.).

•**sparfosate sodium.** (spar-FOSS-ate) USAN.
Use: Antineoplastic.

Sparkles Effervescent Granules. (Lafayette Pharmaceuticals, Inc.) Sodium bicarbonate 2000 mg, citric acid 1500 mg, simethicone/pkt. Bot. UD 50s. *otc.*
Use: Antacid.

Sparkles Granules. (Lafayette Pharmaceuticals, Inc.) Effervescent granules 4 g/Packet or 6 g/Packet. Each 6 g produces 500 ml of carbon dioxide gas. Ctn. 25 packets. Pkg. 2.
Use: Diagnostic aid.

Sparkles Tablets. (Lafayette Pharmaceuticals, Inc.) Effervescent tablets. Each 4.3 g of tablets produces 250 ml of carbon dioxide gas. Tab. Bot. 43 g (10 doses).
Use: Diagnostic aid.

•**sparsomycin.** (SPAR-so-MY-sin) USAN.
Use: Antineoplastic.

•**sparteine sulfate.** (SPAR-teh-een SULL-fate) USAN.
Use: Oxytocic.
W/Sodium Cl.
See: Tocosamine sulfate, Amp. (Trent).

Spasmatol. (Pharmed) Homatropine MBr 3 mg, pentobarbital 12 mg, mephobarbital 8 mg/Tab. Bot. 100s, 1000s. *Rx.*
Use: Anticholinergic, antispasmodic, hypnotic, sedative.

Spasmolin. (Global Source) Phenobarbital 16.2 mg, hyoscyamine sulfate 0.1037 mg, atropine sulfate 0.0194 mg, hyoscine HBr 0.0065 mg/Tab. Bot. 1000s. *Rx.*
Use: Anticholinergic, antispasmodic, hypnotic, sedative.

spasmolytic agents.
See: Antispasmodics.

Spasno-Lix. (Freeport) Phenobarbital 16.2 mg, hyoscyamine sulfate 0.1037 mg, atropine sulfate 0.0194 mg, hyoscine HBr 0.0065 mg, alcohol 21% to 23%/5 ml. Bot. 4 oz. *Rx.*
Use: Anticholinergic, antispasmodic, hypnotic, sedative.

S.P.B. (Sheryl) Therapeutic B complex formula with ascorbic acid 300 mg/Tab. Bot. 100s. *otc.*
Use: Vitamin supplement.

SPD. (A.P.C.) Methyl salicylate, methyl nicotinate, dipropylene glycol salicylate, oleoresin capsicum, camphor, menthol. Cream Bot. 4 oz, Tube 1.5 oz. *otc.*
Use: Analgesic, topical.

spearmint. N.F. XVI.
Use: Flavor.

spearmint oil. N.F. XVI.
Use: Flavor.

Special Shampoo. (Del-Ray Laboratory, Inc.) Non-medicated shampoo. *otc.*
Use: Cleanser.

Spectazole. (Ortho McNeil Pharmaceutical) Econazole nitrate 1% in a water-miscible base. Tube 15 g, 30 g, 85 g. *Rx.*
Use: Antifungal, topical.

spectinomycin. (speck-TIN-oh-MY-sin) *Formerly Actinospectocin.* An antibiotic isolated from broth cultures of *Streptomyces spectabilis. Rx.*
Use: Anti-infective.

See: Trobicin, Vial, Amp. (Pharmacia & Upjohn).

•**spectinomycin hydrochloride, sterile.** (speck-TIN-oh-MY-sin) U.S.P. 23.
Use: Anti-infective.
See: Trobicin (Pharmacia & Upjohn).

Spectra 360. (Parker) Salt-free electrode gel. Tube 8 oz.
Use: T.E.N.S. application, ECG pediatric, and long-term procedures.

Spectrobid. (Roerig) Bacampicillin HCl 400 mg/Tab. Bot. 100s. *Rx.*
Use: Anti-infective, penicillin.

Spectro-Biotic. (A.P.C.) Bacitracin 400 units, neomycin sulfate 5 mg, polymyxin B sulfate 5000 units/g Oint. Tube 0.5 oz, 1 oz. *otc.*
Use: Anti-infective, topical.

Spectrocin Plus. (Numark Laboratories, Inc.) Polymyxin B sulfate 5000 units/g or ml, neomycin 3.5 mg/g or ml, bacitracin 400 units/g or ml, lidocaine 5 mg, mineral oil, white petrolatum. Oint. Tube 15 g, 30 g. *otc.*
Use: Anti-infective, topical.

Spectro-Jel. (Recsei Laboratories) Soap free. Iodo-methylcellulose, carboxypolymethylene, cetyl alcohol, sorbitan monooleate, fumed silica, triethanolamine stearate, glycol polysiloxane, propylene glycol, glycerin, isopropyl alcohol 5%. Gel Bot. 127.5 ml, pt, gal. *otc.*
Use: Dermatologic, cleanser.

Spec-T Sore Throat Anesthetic Lozenges. (Apothecon, Inc.) Benzocaine 10 mg/Loz. Box 10s. *otc.*
Use: Anesthetic, local.

Spec-T Sore Throat/Cough Suppressant Lozenges. (Apothecon, Inc.) Benzocaine 10 mg, dextromethorphan HBr 10 mg w/tartrazine. *otc.*
Use: Anesthetic, local; antitussive.

Spec-T Sore Throat/Decongestant Lozenges. (Apothecon, Inc.) Benzocaine 10 mg, phenylephrine HCl 5 mg, phenylpropanolamine HCl 10.5 mg w/ tartrazine. Loz. Pkg. 10s. *otc.*
Use: Anesthetic, local; decongestant.

spermaceti.
Use: Stiffening agent; pharmaceutic necessity for cold cream.

spermine. Diaminopropyltetramethylene.

Sperti Ointment. (Whitehall Robins Laboratories) Live yeast cell derivative supplying 2000 units skin respiratory factor/g w/shark liver oil 3%, phenylmercuric nitrate 1:10,000. Tube oz. *otc.*
Use: Dermatologic, wound therapy.

Spherulin. (ALK Laboratories, Inc.) Coccidioidin: 1:100 equivalent, Vial 1 ml, 1:10 equivalent, Vial 0.5 ml. *Rx.*
Use: Diagnostic aid, skin test.

spider-bite antivenin.
See: Antivenin, Latrodectus Mactans (Merck & Co.).

Spider-Man Children's Chewable Vitamin. (NBTY, Inc.) Vitamins A 2500 IU, D 400 IU, E 15 mg, B_1 1.05 mg, B_2 1.2 mg, B_3 13.5 mg, B_6 1.05 mg, B_{12} 4.5 mcg, C 60 mg, folic acid 0.3 mg/Chew. Tab., xylitol, sorbitol. Bot. 75s, 130s. *otc.*
Use: Vitamin supplement.

•**spiperone.** (spih-per-OHN) USAN.
Use: Antipsychotic.

•**spiradoline mesylate.** (spy-RAH-doe-leen) USAN.
Use: Analgesic.

•**spiramycin.** (SPIH-rah-MY-sin) USAN. Antibiotic substance from cultures of *Streptomyces ambofaciens.*
Use: Anti-infective.

•**spirapril hydrochloride.** (SPY-rah-prill) USAN.
Use: ACE inhibitor.
See: Renormax, Tab. (Novartis Pharmaceutical Corp.).

•**spiraprilat.** (SPY-rah-PRILL-at) USAN.
Use: ACE inhibitor.

•**spirogermanium hydrochloride.** (SPY-row-JER-MAY-nee-uhm) USAN.
Use: Antineoplastic.

•**spiromustine.** (SPY-row-MUSS-teen) USAN. *Formerly spirohydantoin mustard.*
Use: Antineoplastic.

spironazide. (Schein Pharmaceutical, Inc.) Spironolactone 25 mg, hydrochlorothiazide 25 mg/Tab. Bot. 100s, 1000s, UD 100s. *Rx.*
Use: Diuretic combination.

•**spironolactone.** (SPEER-oh-no-LAK-tone) U.S.P. 23.
Use: Diuretic, aldosterone antagonist.
See: Aldactone, Tab. (Searle).
W/Hydrochlorothiazide.
See: Aldactazide, Tab. (Searle).

spironolactone w/hydrochlorothiazide. (Various Mfr.) Spironolactone 25 mg, hydrochlorothiazide 25 mg. Tab. Bot. 30s, 60s, 100s, 250s, 500s, 1000s, UD 32s, 100s. *Rx.*
Use: Diuretic combination.

spiropitan. (SPY-row-PLAT-in) (Janssen Pharmaceutical, Inc.) Spiperone. *Rx.*
Use: Antipsychotic.

•**spiroplatin.** (SPY-row-PLAT-in) USAN.
Use: Antineoplastic.

spirotriazine hydrochloride.
Use: Anthelmintic.

•**spiroxasone.** (spy-ROX-ah-sone) USAN.
Use: Diuretic.

Spirozide. (Rugby Labs, Inc.) Spironolactone 25 mg, hydrochlorothiazide 25 mg/Tab. Bot. 100s, 500s, 1000s. *Rx.*
Use: Diuretic combination.

SPL-Serologic Types I and III. (Delmont Laboratories, Inc.) *Staphylococcus aureus* 120 to 180 million units, *staphylococcus* bacteriophage plaque-forming units 100 to 1000 million/ml. Inj. Amp. 1 ml, Vial 10 ml. *Rx.*
Use: Anti-infective.

Sporanox. (Janssen Pharmaceutical, Inc.) Itraconazole 10 mg/ml, saccharin, sorbitol. Oral Soln. Bot. 150 ml. *Rx.*
Use: Antifungal.

Sportscreme. (Thompson Medical Co.) Triethanolamine salicylate 10% in a nongreasy base. Cream. 37.5 g, 90 g. *otc.*
Use: Analgesic, topical.

Sports Spray Extra Strength. (Mentholatum Co., Inc.) Methyl salicylate 35%, menthol 10%, camphor 5%, alcohol 58%, isobutane. Spray. 90 ml. *otc.*
Use: Analgesic, topical.

Spray Skin Protectant. (Morton International) Isopropyl alcohol, polyvinylpyrrolidone, vinyl alcohol, plasticizer & propellant. Aer. Can 6 oz. *otc.*
Use: Dermatologic, protectant.

Spray-U-Thin. (Caprice-Greystoke) Phenylpropanolamine HCl 6.58 mg, sorbitol, saccharin. Spray. Bot. 44 ml. *otc.*
Use: Dietary aid.

spreading factor.
See: Hyaluronidase (Various Mfr.).

•**sprodiamide.** (sprah-DIE-ah-mide) USAN.
Use: Diagnostic aid (paramagnetic).

SPRX-105. (Reid-Provident) Phendimetrazine tartrate 105 mg/SR Cap. Bot. 28s, 500s. *c-III.*
Use: Anorexiant.

SPS. (Carolina Medical Products) Sodium polystyrene sulfonate 15 g, sorbitol solution 21.5 ml, alcohol 0.3%/60 ml. Susp. Bot. 120 ml, 480 ml, UD 60 ml. *Rx.*
Use: Potassium-removing resin.

S-P-T. (Fleming & Co.) Pork thyroid, desiccated 1 gr, 2 gr, 3 gr, 5 gr/Cap. Bot. 100s, 1000s. *Rx.*
Use: Hypothyroidism.

•**squalane.** (SKWAH-lane) N.F. 18.
Use: Pharmaceutic aid (vehicle, oleaginous).

SRC Expectorant. (Edwards Pharmaceuticals, Inc.) Hydrocodone bitartrate 5 mg, pseudoephedrine HCl 60 mg, guaifenesin 200 mg w/alcohol 12.5%. Bot. Pt. *c-III.*
Use: Antitussive, decongestant, expectorant.

SSD AF. (Knoll Pharmaceuticals) Silver sulfadiazine 1% in a cream base containing white petrolatum, stearyl alcohol, isopropyl myristate, sorbitan monooleate, polyoxyl 40 stearate, sodium hydroxide, propylene glycol, methylparaben 3%. Cream Tube 50 g, 400 g, 1000 g. *Rx.*
Use: Burn therapy.

SSD Cream. (Knoll Pharmaceuticals) Silver sulfadiazine cream 1%. Jar 50 g, 85 g, 400 g, 1000 g. Tube 25 g. *Rx.*
Use: Burn therapy.

SSKI. (Upsher-Smith Labs, Inc.) Potassium iodide 300 mg/0.3 ml. Soln. Dropper Bot. 1 oz, 8 oz.
Use: Expectorant.

S-Spas. (Southern States) Pentobarbital 16.2 mg, atropine sulfate 0.0194 mg, hyoscyamine sulfate 0.1037 mg, hyoscine HBr 0.0065 mg/Tab. or 5 ml. **Liq.:** Bot. Pt. **Tab.:** Bot. 100s, 1000s. *Rx.*
Use: Anticholinergic, antispasmodic, hypnotic, sedative.

S.S.S. High Potency Vitamin. (S.S.S. Company) Vitamins C 300 mg, B_1 7.5 mg, B_2 7.5 mg, B_3 50 mg, Ca 100 mg, Fe 27 mg, E 50 IU, B_6 2.5 mg, folic acid 200 mcg, B_{12} 12.5 mg, Mg 50 mg, Zn 12 mg, Cu 1.5 mg, biotin 22.5 mcg, pantothenic acid 10 mg. Tab. Bot. 20s, 40s, 80s. *otc.*
Use: Vitamin, mineral supplement.

S.S.S. Vitamin and Mineral Supplement. (S.S.S. Company) Vitamins A 833 IU, C 20 mg, E 10 IU, B_1 1.7 mg, B_2 0.57 mg, niacinamide 6.7 mg, B_6 0.67 mg, B_{12} 2 mcg, D_3 133 IU, biotin 100 mcg, pantothenic acid 3 mg, I 50 mcg, Fe 3 mg, Zn 1 mg, Ma 0.8 mg, Cr 8 mcg, Mo 8 mcg/5 ml, alcohol 6.6%, sugar. Liq. Bot. 236 ml. *otc.*
Use: Vitamin, mineral supplement.

Stadol. (Bristol-Myers Squibb) Butorphanol tartrate 1 mg/ml; Vial 1 ml. 2 mg/ml; Vial 1 ml, 2 ml, 10 ml. *c-IV.*
Use: Analgesic.

Staftabs. (Modern Aids Inc.) Fine bone flour containing calcium, phosphorus, iron, iodine, vitamin D, magnesium/Tab. Bot. 85s, 160s. *otc.*
Use: Mineral, vitamin supplement.

Stagesic. (Huckaby Pharmacal, Inc.) Hydrocodone bitartrate 5 mg, acetaminophen 500 mg/Cap. Bot. 100s. *c-III.*
Use: Analgesic combination, narcotic.

Stahist. (Huckaby Pharmacal, Inc.) Phenylpropanolamine HCl 50 mg, phenylephrine HCl 25 mg, chlorpheniramine maleate 8 mg, hyoscyamine sulfate 0.19 mg, atropine sulfate 0.04 mg, scopolamine HBr 0.01 mg/SR Tab. Bot. 100s. *Rx.*
Use: Antihistamine, anticholinergic, decongestant.

stainless iodized ointment. (Day-Baldwin) Jar lb.

stainless iodized ointment with methyl salicylate 5%. (Day-Baldwin) Jar lb.

•**stallimycin hydrochloride.** (stal-IH-MY-sin) USAN.
Use: Anti-infective.

Stamoist E. (Huckaby Pharmacal, Inc.) Pseudoephedrine HCl 120 mg, guaifenesin 500 mg. SR Tab. Bot. 100s. *Rx.*
Use: Decongestant, expectorant.

Stamoist LA. (Huckaby Pharmacal, Inc.) Phenylpropanolamine HCl 75 mg, guaifenesin 400 mg. SR Tab. Bot. 100s. *Rx.*
Use: Decongestant, expectorant.

Stamyl Tablets. (Sanofi Winthrop Pharmaceuticals) Pancreatin.
Use: Digestive aid.

•**stannous chloride.** (STAN-uhs KLOR-ide) USAN.
Use: Pharmaceutic aid.

•**stannous fluoride.** (STAN-uhs FLOR-ide) U.S.P. 23.
Use: Dental caries agent.

•**stannous pyrophosphate.** (STAN-uhs PIE-row-FOSS-fate) USAN.
Use: Diagnostic aid (skeletal imaging).

•**stannous sulfur colloid.** (STAN-uhs SULL-fer KAHL-oyd) USAN.
Use: Diagnostic aid (bone, liver, and spleen imaging).

•**stanozolol.** (STAN-oh-zole-ahl) U.S.P. 23. *Formerly Androstanazole.*
Use: Androgen.
See: Stromba.
Winstrol Tab. (Sanofi Winthrop Pharmaceuticals).

staphage lysate (SPL). (Delmont Laboratories, Inc.) Phage-lysed staphylococci 120-180 million/ml Amp. 1 ml, package 10s for Inj.; Multidose Vial 10 ml for other methods of administration. *Rx.*
Use: Anti-infective.

staphylococcus bacteriophage lysate.
See: Staphage Lysate (Delmont Laboratories, Inc.).

staphylococcus test.
See: Isocult for *Staphylococcus Aureus* (SmithKline Diagnostics).

•**starch.** N.F. 18.
Use: Dusting powder, pharmaceutic aid.

starch glycerite.
Use: Emollient.

•**starch, pregelatinized.** N.F. 18.
Use: Pharmaceutic aid (tablet excipient).

•**starch, topical.** U.S.P. 23.
Use: Dusting powder.

Star-Otic. (Star Pharmaceuticals, Inc.) Burrows soln. 10%, acetic acid 1%, boric acid 1%. Drop Bot. 15 ml. *otc.*
Use: Otic.

Staticin. (Westwood Squibb Pharmaceuticals) Erythromycin 1.5%, alcohol 55%. Soln. Bot. 60 ml. *Rx.*
Use: Dermatologic, acne.

•**statolon.** (STAY-toe-lone) USAN. Antiviral agent derived from *Penicillium stoloniferum.*
Use: Antiviral.

Statomin Maleate II. (Jones Medical Industries, Inc.) Chlorpheniramine maleate 2 mg, acetaminophen 324 mg, caffeine 32 mg/Tab. Bot. 1000s. *Rx.*
Use: Antihistamine, analgesic.

Statuss Expectorant. (Huckaby Pharmacal, Inc.) Phenylpropanolamine HCl 12.5 mg, codeine phosphate 10 mg, guaifenesin 100 mg, alcohol 5%, menthol, saccharin, sorbitol/5 ml. Dye free. Liq. Bot. 473 ml. *c-v.*
Use: Antitussive, decongestant, expectorant.

Statuss Green. (Huckaby Pharmacal, Inc.) Phenylpropanolamine HCl 3.3 mg, phenylephrine HCl 5 mg, pheniramine maleate 3.3 mg, pyrilamine maleate 3.3 mg, hydrocodone bitartrate 1.67 mg/5 ml, alcohol 5%, saccharin, parabens, sorbitol, glucose. Liq. Bot. 480 ml. *c-III.*
Use: Antihistamine, antitussive, decongestant.

•**stavudine.** (STAHV-you-deen) USAN.
Use: Antiviral.
See: Zerit, Preps. (Bristol-Myers Squibb).

Sta-Wake Dextabs. (Health for Life Brands, Inc.) Caffeine 1.5 gr, dextrose 3 gr/Tab. Bot. 36s, 1000s. *otc.*
Use: CNS stimulant.

Stay Awake Capsules. (Whiteworth Towne) Caffeine 250 mg/Cap. Bot. 30s. *otc.*
Use: CNS stimulant.

Stay-Brite. (Sherman Pharmaceuticals, Inc.) EDTA 0.25%, benzalkonium Cl 0.01%. Spray 30 ml. *otc.*
Use: Contact lens care.

Stay Moist Lip Conditioner. Padimate

O, oxybenzone, aloe vera, vitamin E, tropical fruit flavor. SPF 15. Lip Balm 48 g. *otc.*
Use: Emollient.

Stay Trim. (Schering-Plough Corp.) Phenylpropanolamine. **Gum:** 8.33 mg. Pkg. 20s. **Mints:** 12.5 mg. Pkg. 36s. *otc.*
Use: Dietary aid.

Stay-Wet. (Sherman Pharmaceuticals, Inc.) Polyvinyl alcohol, hydroxyethylcellulose, povidone, sodium Cl, potassium Cl, sodium carbonate, benzalkonium Cl 0.01%, EDTA 0.025%. Soln. Bot. 30 ml. *otc.*
Use: Contact lens care.

Stay-Wet 3. (Sherman Pharmaceuticals, Inc.) Sodium and potassium Cl salts containing polyvinyl pyrrolidone, polyvinyl alcohol, hydroxyethylcellulose, sodium bisulfite 0.02%, benzyl alcohol 0.1%, sorbic acid 0.05%, EDTA 0.1%. Soln. 30 ml. *otc.*
Use: Lubricant, ophthalmic.

Stay-Wet 4. (Sherman Pharmaceuticals, Inc.) Benzyl alcohol 0.15%, EDTA 0.1%, NaCl, KCl, polyvinyl alcohol, hydroxyethyl cellulose. Thimerosal free. Soln. 30 ml. *otc.*
Use: Contact lens care (RGP lenses).

Stay-Wet Rewetting. (Sherman Pharmaceuticals, Inc.) Polyvinyl alcohol, hydroxyethycellulose, povidone, NaCl, KCl, sodium carbonate, benzalkonium Cl 0.01%, EDTA 0.025%. Soln. Bot. *otc.*
Use: Lubricant-ophthalmic.

Stay-Wet 3 Wetting. (Sherman Pharmaceuticals, Inc.) Polyvinyl alcohol, hydroxyethycellulose, povidone, sodium Cl, potassium Cl, sodium carbonate, benzalkonium Cl 0.01%, EDTA 0.025%. Soln. 30 ml. *otc.*
Use: Lubricant, ophthalmic.

Staze. (Del Pharmaceuticals, Inc.) Karaya gum. Tube 1.75 oz, 3.5 oz. *otc.*
Use: Denture adhesive.

S-T Cort Cream. (Scot-Tussin Pharmacal, Inc.) Hydrocortisone 0.5%, water-washable base, parabens. 120 g. *Rx.*
Use: Corticosteroid, topical.

S-T Cort Lotion. (Scot-Tussin Pharmacal, Inc.) Hydrocortisone 0.5%, water-washable, lanolin alcohol, mineral oil base. 60 ml, 120 ml. *Rx.*
Use: Corticosteroid, topical.

•**stearic acid.** (STEER-ik) N.F. 18. Octadecanoic acid.
Use: Pharmaceutic aid (emulsion adjunct, tablet/capsule lubricant).

•**stearyl alcohol.** (STEE-rill AL-koe-hahl) N.F. 18.
Use: Pharmaceutic aid (emulsion adjunct).

•**steffimycin.** (steh-fih-MY-sin) USAN.
Use: Anti-infective, antiviral.

Stelazine. (SmithKline Beecham Pharmaceuticals) Trifluoperazine HCl. **Tab.:** 1 mg, 2 mg, 5 mg, 10 mg. Bot. 100s, 500s, 100s, UD 100s. **Inj.:** 2 mg/ml. Vial 10 ml. Box 1s, 20s. **Oral Conc.:** 10 mg/ml. Bot. 60 ml. *Rx.*
Use: Antipsychotic.

•**stenbolone acetate.** (STEEN-bow-lone) USAN.
Use: Anabolic.

Step 2. (Medicis Dermatologicals, Inc.) Benzyl alcohol, cetyl alcohol, formic acid 8%, glyceryl stearate, PEG-100 stearate, polyquaterium-10. Creme rinse. Bot. 60 ml. *otc.*
Use: Pediculicide, nit removal.

Steraject. (Merz Pharmaceuticals) Prednisolone acetate 25 mg, 50 mg/ml. Inj. Vial 10 ml. *Rx.*
Use: Corticosteroid.

Sterapred DS. (Merz Pharmaceuticals) Prednisone 10 mg/Tab. Uni-pak 21s. *Rx.*
Use: Corticosteroid.

Sterapred-Unipak. (Merz Pharmaceuticals) Prednisone 5 mg/Tab. Dosepak 21s. *Rx.*
Use: Corticosteroid.

Sterculia Gum.
See: Karaya Gum (Various Mfr.).
W/Vitamin B_1.
See: Imbicoll W/Vitamin B_1 (Pharmacia & Upjohn).

Stericol. (Alton) Isopropyl alcohol 91%. Soln. Bot. 16 oz, 32 oz, gal. *otc.*
Use: Anti-infective, topical.

sterile aurothioglucose suspension. Aurothioglucose Injection. Gold thioglucose.
Use: Antirheumatic.
See: Solganal, Vial (Schering-Plough Corp.).

sterile erythromycin gluceptate. Erythromycin monoglucoheptonate (salt). Erythromycin glucoheptonate (1:1) (salt).
Use: Anti-infective.

Sterile Lens Lubricant. (Blairex Labs, Inc.) Isotonic w/borate buffer system, sodium Cl, hydroxypropyl methylcellulose, glycerin, sorbic acid 0.25%, EDTA 0.1%, thimerosal free. Soln. Bot. 15 ml. *otc.*
Use: Lubricant, ophthalmic.

Sterile Saline. (Bausch & Lomb Pharmaceuticals) Sodium Cl, borate buffer, EDTA, thimerosal free. Soln. Bot. 60 ml.

otc.
Use: Lubricant, ophthalmic.

sterile thiopental sodium. Thiopental sodium, U.S.P. 23.
See: Pentothal Sodium, Amp. (Abbott Laboratories).

sterile water for irrigation. (Various Mfr.) 0.45%, 0.9%. Soln. Bot. 150 ml, 250 ml, 500 ml, 1000 ml, 1500 ml, 2000 ml, 4000 ml. *Rx.*
Use: Irrigant, genitourinary.

Steri-Unna Boot. (Pedinol Pharmacal, Inc.) Glycerin, gum acacia, zinc oxide, white petrolatum, amylum in an oil base. 10 yds. × 3.5 in. sterilized bandage.
Use: Treatment of leg ulcers, varicosities, sprains, strains & to reduce swelling after surgery.

S-T Forte 2 Liquid. (Scot-Tussin Pharmacal, Inc.) Chlorpheniramine maleate 2 mg, hydrocodone bitartrate 2.5 mg, 99.7% glycerin, menthol, parabens. Alcohol and dye free. Bot. Pt, gal. *c-III.*
Use: Antihistamine, antitussive.

S-T Forte Sugar Free Liquid. (Scot-Tussin Pharmacal, Inc.) Hydrocodone bitartrate 2.5 mg, phenylephrine HCl 5 mg, phenylpropanolamine HCl 5 mg, pheniramine maleate 13.33 mg, guaifenesin 80 mg/5 ml w/alcohol 5%. Bot. 4 oz, 8 oz, pt, gal. *c-III.*
Use: Antitussive, antihistamine, decongestant, expectorant.

S-T Forte Syrup. (Scot-Tussin Pharmacal, Inc.) Hydrocodone bitartrate 2.5 mg, phenylephrine HCl 5 mg, phenylpropanolamine HCl 5 mg, pheniramine maleate 13.33 mg, guaifenesin 80 mg/5 ml, w/alcohol 5%. Bot. 4 oz, 8 oz, pt, gal. *c-III.*
Use: Antitussive, antihistamine, decongestant, expectorant.

stilbamidine isethionate.
Use: Antiprotozoal.

•**stilbazium iodide.** (still-BAY-zee-uhm EYE-oh-dide) USAN.
Use: Anthelmintic.

stilbestrol.
See: Diethylstilbestrol, U.S.P. 23 (Various Mfr.).

stilbestronate.
See: Diethylstilbestrol Dipropionate (Various Mfr.).

stilboestrol.
See: Diethylstilbestrol (Various Mfr.).

Stilboestrol DP.
See: Diethylstilbestrol Dipropionate (Various Mfr.).

•**stilonium iodide.** (STILL-oh-nee-uhm EYE-oh-dide) USAN.
Use: Antispasmodic.

Stilphostrol. (Bayer Corp. (Consumer Div.)) Diethylstilbestrol diphosphate. Amp. (250 mg/5 ml as sodium salt) 5 ml. Box 20s. Tab. 50 mg, Bot. 50s. *Rx.*
Use: Antineoplastic.

Stilronate.
See: Diethylstilbestrol Dipropionate (Various Mfr.).

Stimate. (Centeon) Desmopressin acetate 1.5 mg, chlorobutanol 5 mg, sodium Cl 9 mg/ml. Nasal spray. Vial 2.5 ml. *Rx.*
Use: Hormone.

Sting-Eze. (Wisconsin Pharmacal Co.) Diphenhydramine HCl, camphor, phenol, benzocaine, eucalyptol. Liq. Bot. 15 ml. *otc.*
Use: Antihistamine, topical.

Sting-Kill. (Milance Laboratories, Inc.) Benzocaine 18.9%, menthol 0.9%. Swab 14 ml, 0.5 ml (5s). *otc.*
Use: Anesthetic, local.

•**stiripentol.** (STY-rih-PEN-tole) USAN.
Use: Anticonvulsant.

St. Joseph Adult Chewable Aspirin. (Schering-Plough Corp.) Aspirin 81 mg, saccharin. Chew. Tab. Bot. 36s. *otc.*
Use: Analgesic.

St. Joseph Aspirin for Adults. (Schering-Plough Corp.) Aspirin 5 gr/Tab. Bot. 36s, 100s, 200s. *otc.*
Use: Analgesic.

St. Joseph Aspirin-Free Cold for Children. (Schering-Plough Corp.) Phenylpropanolamine HCl 3.125 mg, acetaminophen 80 mg, fruit flavor. Chew. Tab. Bot. 30s. *otc.*
Use: Decongestant combination.

St. Joseph Aspirin-Free Elixir for Children. (Schering-Plough Corp.) Acetaminophen 160 mg/5 ml. Alcohol free. Elix. Bot. 2 oz, 4 oz. *otc.*
Use: Analgesic.

St. Joseph Aspirin-Free for Children Chewable. (Schering-Plough Corp.) Acetaminophen 80 mg, fruit flavor. Chew. Tab. Bot. 30s. *otc.*
Use: Analgesic.

St. Joseph Aspirin-Free Infant Drops. (Schering-Plough Corp.) Acetaminophen 100 mg/ml. Aspirin and sugar free. Bot. w/dropper. 0.5 oz. *otc.*
Use: Analgesic.

St. Joseph Aspirin-Free Tablets for Children. (Schering-Plough Corp.) Acetaminophen 80 mg/Tab. Bot. 30s. *otc.*
Use: Analgesic.

St. Joseph Cold Tablets for Children. (Schering-Plough Corp.) Aspirin 80

mg, phenylpropanolamine HCl 3.125 mg/Tab. Bot. 30s. *otc.*
Use: Analgesic, decongestant.

St. Joseph Cough Suppressant. (Schering-Plough Corp.) Dextromethorphan HBr 7.5 mg/5 ml, alcohol free, sucrose, cherry flavor. Liq. Bot. 60 ml, 120 ml. *otc.*
Use: Antitussive.

St. Joseph Cough Syrup for Children. (Schering-Plough Corp.) Dextromethorphan HBr 7.5 mg/5 ml. Bot. 2 oz, 4 oz. *otc.*
Use: Antitussive.

Stomal. (Foy Laboratories) Phenobarbital 16.2 mg, hyoscyamine sulfate 0.1037 mg, atropine sulfate 0.0194 mg, scopolamine HBr 0.0065 mg/Tab. Bot. 1000s. *Rx.*
Use: Anticholinergic, antispasmodic, hypnotic, sedative.

ST1-RTA immunotoxin (SR44163).
Use: Leukemia, graft-vs-host disease in bone marrow transplants. [Orphan Drug]

Stool Softener. (Amlab) Docusate sodium 100 mg, 250 mg/Cap. Bot. 100s. *otc.*
Use: Laxative.

Stool Softener. (Weeks & Leo) Docusate sodium 100 mg, 250 mg/Cap. Bot. 30s, 100s. Calcium docusate 240 mg/Cap. Bot. 100s. *otc.*
Use: Laxative.

Stop. (Oral-B Laboratories, Inc.) Stannous fluoride 0.4%. Tube 2 oz. *Rx.*
Use: Dental caries agent.

Stopayne Capsules. (Springbok) Codeine phosphate 30 mg, acetaminophen 357 mg/Cap. Bot. 100s, 500s, UD 100s. *c-III.*
Use: Analgesic, antitussive.

Stopayne Syrup. (Springbok) Acetaminophen 120 mg, codeine phosphate 12 mg/5 ml. Bot. 4 oz, 16 oz. *c-v.*
Use: Analgesic, antitussive.

Stop-Zit. (Purepac Pharmaceutical Co.) Denatonium benzoate in a clear nail polish base. Bot. 0.75 oz. *otc.*
Use: Nail-biting deterrent.

•**storax.** (STORE-ax) U.S.P. 23.
Use: Pharmaceutic necessity for Benzoin Tincture compound.

Stovarsol.
Use: Trichomonas vaginalis vaginitis, amebiasis, Vincent's angina.
See: Acetarsone, Tab.

Strema. (Foy Laboratories) Quinine sulfate 260 mg/Cap. Bot. 100s, 500s, 1000s.
Use: Antimalarial.

Stren-Tab. (Barth's) Vitamins C 300 mg, B_1 10 mg, B_2 10 mg, niacin 33 mg, B_6 2 mg, pantothenic acid 20 mg, B_{12} 4 mcg/Tab. Bot. 100s, 300s, 500s. *otc.*
Use: Vitamin supplement.

Streptase. (Astra Pharmaceuticals, L.P.) Streptokinase IV infusion. Ctn. Vial 10s. 250,000 IU/Vial 6.5 ml; 750,000 IU/Vial 6.5 ml. *Rx.*
Use: Thrombolytic.

streptococcus immune globulin group B.
Use: Immunization. [Orphan Drug]

streptokinase.
Use: Thrombolytic.
See: Kabikinase (SmithKline Beecham).
Streptase (Hoechst Marion Roussel).

Streptolysin O Test. (Laboratory Diagnostics) Reagent 6 x 10 ml, buffer 6 x 40 ml, Control Serum, 6 x 10 ml, or Kit.
Use: Diagnosis of "group A" streptococcal infections.

streptomycin calcium chloride. Streptomycin Calcium Chloride Complex.

Streptonase B. (Wampole Laboratories) Tube test for determination of streptococcal infection by serum DNase-B antibodies. Kit 1.
Use: Diagnostic aid.

•**streptonicozid.** (STREP-toe-nih-KOE-zid) USAN.
Use: Anti-infective.

•**streptonigrin.** (strep-toe-NYE-grin) USAN. Antibiotic isolated from both filtrates of *Streptomyces flocculus.*
Use: Antineoplastic.
See: Nigrin (Pfizer US Pharmaceutical Group).

streptovaricin. An antibiotic composed of several related components derived from cultures of*Streptomyces variabilis.*

•**streptozocin.** (STREP-toe-ZOE-sin) USAN.
Use: Antineoplastic.
See: Zanosar, Powder (Pharmacia & Upjohn).

Streptozyme. (Wampole Laboratories) Rapid hemagglutination slide test for the qualitative detection and quantitative determination of streptococcal extracellular antigens in serum, plasma and peripheral blood. Kit 15s, 50s, 150s.
Use: Diagnostic aid, streptococcus.

Stress "1000". (NBTY, Inc.) Vitamins E 22 mg, B_1 15 mg, B_2 15 mg, B_3 100 mg, B_5 20 mg, B_6 5 mg, B_{12} 12 mcg, C 1000 mg/Tab. Bot. 60s. *otc.*
Use: Vitamin supplement.

Stress B-Complex. (H.L. Moore Drug Exchange Inc.) Vitamins E 30 IU, B_1 15 mg, B_2 15 mg, B_3 100 mg, B_5 20 mg, B_6 20 mg, B_{12} 12 mcg, C 500 mg, folic acid 0.4 mg, Zn 23.9 mg, Cu, biotin 45 mcg/Tab. Bot. 60s. *otc.*
Use: Mineral, vitamin supplement.

Stress B Complex with Vitamin C. (Mission Pharmacal Co.) Vitamins B_1 13.8 mg, B_2 10 mg, B_3 50 mg, B_6 4.1 mg, C 300 mg, Zn 15 mg/Tab. Bot. 60s. *otc.*
Use: Mineral, vitamin supplement.

Stress-Bee Capsules. (Rugby Labs, Inc.) Vitamins B_1 10 mg, B_2 10 mg, B_3 100 mg, B_5 20 mg, B_6 2 mg, B_{12} 6 mcg, C 300 mg/Cap. Bot. 100s. *otc.*
Use: Vitamin supplement.

Stressform "605" With Iron. (NBTY, Inc.) Iron 27 mg, vitamins E 30 mg, B_1 15 mg, B_2 15 mg, B_3 100 mg, B_5 20 mg, B_6 5 mg, B_{12} 12 mcg, C 605 mg, folic acid 0.4 mg, biotin 45 mg/Tab. Bot. 60s. *otc.*
Use: Vitamin supplement.

Stress Formula. (Various Mfr.) Vitamins E 30 mg, B_1 15 mg, B_2 15 mg, B_3 100 mg, B_5 20 mg, B_6 5 mg, B_{12} 12 mcg, C 600 mg, folic acid 0.4 mg, biotin 45 mcg/Cap., Tab. **Cap.:** Bot. 60s, 100s, 1000s. **Tab.:** Bot. 30s, 60s, 100s, 250s, 300s, 400s, 1000s, UD 100s. *otc.*
Use: Vitamin supplement.

Stress Formula 600. (Vangard Labs, Inc.) Vitamins E 30 IU, B_1 15 mg, B_2 10 mg, B_3 100 mg, B_5 20 mg, B_6 5 mg, B_{12} 12 mcg, C 500 mg, folic acid 0.4 mg, biotin 45 mcg/Tab. Bot. UD 100s. *otc.*
Use: Vitamin supplement.

Stress Formula 600 w/Iron. (Halsey Drug Co.)
Use: Vitamin supplement.

Stress Formula 600 Plus Iron. (Schein Pharmaceutical, Inc.) Iron 27 mg, vitamins E 30 IU, B_1 15 mg, B_2 15 mg, B_3 100 mg, B_5 20 mg, B_6 5 mg, B_{12} 12 mcg, C 600 mg, folic acid 0.4 mg, biotin 45 mcg/Tab. Bot. 60s, 250s. *otc.*
Use: Mineral, vitamin supplement.

Stress Formula 600 Plus Zinc. (Schein Pharmaceutical, Inc.) Vitamins E 30 mg, B_1 20 mg, B_2 10 mg, B_3 100 mg, B_5 25 mg, B_6 5 mg, B_{12} 12 mcg, C 600 mg, folic acid 0.4 mg, zinc 23.9 mg, Cu, Mg, biotin 45 mcg/Tab. Bot. 60s, 250s. *otc.*
Use: Mineral, vitamin supplement.

Stress Formula 600 w/Zinc. (Halsey Drug Co.)
Use: Dietary supplement.

Stress Formula "605". (NBTY, Inc.) Vitamins E 30 mg, B_1 15 mg, B_2 15 mg, B_3 100 mg, B_5 20 mg, B_6 5 mg, B_{12} 12 mcg, C 605 mg, folic acid 0.4 mg, biotin 45 mg/Tab. Bot. 60s. *otc.*
Use: Vitamin supplement.

Stress Formula "605" with Zinc. (NBTY, Inc.) Vitamins E 30 mg, B_1 20 mg, B_2 10 mg, B_3 100 mg, B_5 25 mg, B_6 5 mg, B_{12} 12 mcg, C 605 mg, folic acid 0.4 mg, Zn 23.9 mg, Cu, biotin 45 mcg/Tab. Bot. 60s. *otc.*
Use: Mineral, vitamin supplement.

Stress Formula Vitamins. () (Various Mfr.) Vitamins E 30 mg, B_1 10 mg, B_2 10 mg, B_3 100 mg, B_5 20 mg, B_6 5 mg, B_{12} 12 mcg, C 500 mg, folic acid 0.4 mg, biotin 45 mcg. Cap. Bot. 100s/Tab. Bot. 60s. *otc.*
Use: Vitamin supplement.

Stress Formula with Iron. (NBTY, Inc.) Vitamins C 500 mg, B_1 10 mg, B_2 10 mg, B_3 100 mg, B_5 20 mg, B_6 5 mg, B_{12} 12 mcg, E 30 IU, Fe 27 mg, folic acid 0.4 mg, biotin 45 mcg. Tab. Bot. 60s. *otc.*
Use: Mineral, vitamin supplement.

Stress Formula w/Zinc. (Various Mfr.) Vitamins E 30 IU, B_1 10 mg, B_2 10 mg, B_3 100 mg, B_5 20 mg, B_6 5 mg, B_{12} 12 mcg, C 500 mg, folic acid 0.4 mg, biotin 45 mcg, Zn 23.9 mg, Cu/Tab. Bot. 60s. *otc.*
Use: Mineral, vitamin supplement.

Stress Formula with Zinc. (Towne) Vitamins E 45 IU, C 600 mg, folic acid 400 mcg, B_1 20 mg, B_2 10 mg, niacinamide 100 mg, B_6 10 mg, B_{12} 25 mcg, biotin 40 mcg, pantothenic acid 25 mg, Cu 3 mg, Zn 23.9 mg/Tab. Bot. 60s. *otc.*
Use: Mineral, vitamin supplement.

Stress 600 w/Zinc. (Nion Corp.) Vitamins E 45 IU, B_1 20 mg, B_2 10 mg, B_3 100 mg, B_5 25 mg, B_6 10 mg, B_{12} 25 mcg, C 600 mg, folic acid 0.4 mg, Zn 5.5 mg, Cu, biotin 45 mcg/Tab. Bot. 60s. *otc.*
Use: Mineral, vitamin supplement.

Stresstabs. (ESI Lederle Generics) Vitamins E 30 mg, B_1 10 mg, B_2 10 mg, B_3 100 mg, B_5 20 mg, B_6 5 mg, B_{12} 12 mcg, C 500 mg, folic acid 0.4 mg, biotin 45 mcg/Tab. Bot. 60s. *otc.*
Use: Vitamin supplement.

Stresstabs + Iron. (ESI Lederle Generics) Fe 18 mg, E 30 IU, B_1 10 mg, B_2 10 mg, B_3 100 mg, B_5 20 mg, B_6 5 mg, B_{12} 12 mcg, C 500 mg, folic acid 0.4 mg, biotin 45 mcg/Tab. Bot. 60s. *otc.*
Use: Mineral, vitamin supplement.

Stresstabs + Zinc. (ESI Lederle Generics) Vitamins E 30 mg, B_1 10 mg, B_2

10 mg, B_3 100 mg, B_5 20 mg, B_6 5 mg, B_{12} 12 mcg, C 500 mg, folic acid 0.4 mg, Zn 23.9 mg, Cu, biotin 45 mcg/Tab. Bot. 60s. *otc.*
Use: Mineral, vitamin supplement.

Stresstabs 600. (ESI Lederle Generics) Vitamins B_1 15 mg, B_2 10 mg, B_6 5 mg, B_{12} 12 mcg, C 600 mg, niacinamide 100 mg, vitamin E 30 IU, biotin 45 mcg, folic acid 400 mcg, calcium pantothenate 20 mg/Tab. Bot. 30s, 60s, UD 10 x 10s. *otc.*
Use: Vitamin supplement.

Stresstabs 600 with Iron. (ESI Lederle Generics) Ferrous fumarate 27 mg, vitamins E 30 IU, B_1 15 mg, B_2 15 mg, B_3 100 mg, B_5 20 mg, B_6 5 mg, B_{12} 12 mcg, C 600 mg, folic acid 0.4 mg, biotin 45 mcg/Tab. Bot. 30s, 60s. *otc.*
Use: Mineral, vitamin supplement.

Stresstabs 600 with Zinc. (ESI Lederle Generics) Vitamins B_1 15 mg, B_2 10 mg, B_3 100 mg, B_5 20 mg, B_6 5 mg, B_{12} 12 mcg, C 600 mg, E 30 IU, folic acid 0.4 mg, biotin 45 mcg, Cu, Zn 23.9 mg/Tab. Bot. 30s, 60s. *otc.*
Use: Mineral, vitamin supplement.

Stresstein. (Novartis Pharmaceutical Corp.) Maltodextrin, medium chain triglycerides, l-leucine, soybean oil, l-isoleucine, l-valine, l-glutamic acid, l-arginine, l-lysine acetate, l-alanine, l-threonine, l-phenylalanine, l-aspartic acid, l-histidine, l-methionine, glycine, polyglycerol esters of fatty acids, l-serine, l-proline, sodium Cl, l-tryptophan, l-cysteine, sodium citrate, vitamins and minerals. Powder 3.4 oz. packets. *otc.*
Use: High-protein, branched chain enriched tube feeding.

Stri-dex Antibacterial Cleansing. (Bayer Corp. (Consumer Div.)) Triclosan 1%, acetylated lanolin alcohol, EDTA. Bar. 105 g. *otc.*
Use: Dermatologic, acne.

Stri-dex B.P. (Bayer Corp. (Consumer Div.)) Benzoyl peroxide 10%. in greaseless, vanishing cream base. *otc.*
Use: Dermatologic, acne.

Stri-dex Clear. (Bayer Corp. (Consumer Div.)) Salicylic acid 2%, SD alcohol 9.3%, EDTA. Gel: 30 g. *otc.*
Use: Dermatologic, acne.

Stridex Face Wash. (Bayer Corp. (Consumer Div.)) Triclosan 1%, glycerin, EDTA, alcohol free. Soln. Bot. 237 ml. *otc.*
Use: Dermatologic, acne.

Stri-dex Lotion. (Bayer Corp. (Consumer Div.)) Salicylic acid 0.5%, alcohol 28%, sulfonated alkyl benzenes, citric acid, sodium carbonate, simethicone, water. Bot. 4 oz. *otc.*
Use: Dermatologic, acne.

Stri-dex Maximum Strength Pads. (Bayer Corp. (Consumer Div.)) Salicylic acid 2%, SD alcohol 44%, citric acid, menthol. Pads 55s, 90s, dual-textured 32s. *otc.*
Use: Antiacne.

Stri-dex Oil Fighting Formula Pads. (Bayer Corp. (Consumer Div.)) Salicylic acid 2%, citric acid, menthol, SD alcohol 54%. Super Scrub Pads 55s. *otc.*
Use: Dermatologic, acne.

Stri-dex Regular Strength Pads. (Bayer Corp. (Consumer Div.)) Salicylic acid 0.5%, SD alcohol 28%, citric acid, menthol. Pads 55s. *otc.*
Use: Dermatologic, acne.

Stri-dex Sensitive Skin Pads. (Bayer Corp. (Consumer Div.)) Salicylic acid 0.5%, citric acid, aloe vera gel, menthol, SD alcohol 28%. Pads 50s, 90s. *otc.*
Use: Dermatologic, acne.

Stromba Ampules. (Sanofi Winthrop Pharmaceuticals) Stanozolol. *c-III.*
Use: Anabolic steroid.

strong iodine tincture. (Various Mfr.) Iodine 7%, potassium iodide 5%, alcohol 83%. Soln. Bot. 500 ml, 4000 ml. *otc.*
Use: Antimicrobial, antiseptic.

strontium bromide. Cryst. or Granule, Bot. 0.25 lb, 1 lb. Amp. 1 g/10 ml. *Rx.*
Use: Antiepileptic, sedative.

•**strontium chloride Sr 85.** (STRAHN-shee-uhm) USAN.
Use: Radiopharmaceutical.

•**strontium chloride Sr 89 injection.** (STRAHN-shee-uhm) U.S.P. 23.
Use: Antineoplastic; radiopharmaceutical.
See: Metastron, Inj. (Amersham).

•**strontium nitrate Sr 85.** (STRAHN-shee-uhm) USAN.
Use: Radiopharmaceutical.

strontium Sr 85 injection.
Use: Diagnostic aid (bone scanning).

Strovite Forte. (Everett Laboratories) Fe 10 mg, vitamins A 3000 IU (acetate), A 1000 IU (beta-carotene), E 60 IU, D_3 400 IU, folic acid 1 mg, C 500 mg, B_1 20 mg, B_2 20 mg, B_6 25 mg, B_{12} 50 mcg, B_3 100 mg, biotin 0.15 mg, B_5 25 mg, Se 50 mcg, Mg 50 mg, Zn 15 mg, Mo 20 mcg, Cu 3 mg, Cr 0.05 mg. Tab. Bot. 100s. *Rx.*
Use: Vitamin, mineral supplement.

Strovite Plus. (Everett Laboratories, Inc.) Vitamins A 5000 IU, E 30 mg, B_1 20 mg, B_2 20 mg, B_3 100 mg, B_5 25 mg, B_6 25

mg, B_{12} 50 mcg, C 500 mg, Fe 9 mg, folic acid 0.8 mg, Zn 22.5 mg, biotin 150 mcg, Cr, Cu, Mg, Mn. Bot. 100s. *otc.*
Use: Mineral, vitamin supplement.

Strovite Tablets. (Everett Laboratories, Inc.) Vitamins B_1 15 mg, B_2 15 mg, B_3 100 mg, B_5 18 mg, B_6 4 mg, B_{12} 5 mcg, C 500 mg, folic acid 0.5 mg. Bot. 100s. *otc.*
Use: Mineral, vitamin supplement.

S.T. 37. (SmithKline Beecham Pharmaceuticals) Hexylresorcinol 0.1% in glycerin aqueous soln. Bot. 5.5 oz, 12 oz. *otc.*
Use: Antiseptic, topical.

Stuart Formula. (J & J-Merck Consumer Pharm.) Vitamins A 5000 IU, B_1 1.5 mg, B_2 1.7 mg, B_3 20 mg, B_6 1 mg, B_{12} 3 mcg, C 50 mg, D 400 IU, E 10 IU, Fe 5 mg, Cu, folic acid 0.4 mg, Ca, I, P/Tab. Bot. 100s. *otc.*
Use: Mineral, vitamin supplement.

Stuartnatal Plus. (Wyeth-Ayerst Laboratories) Vitamins A 4000 IU, D 400 IU, E 22 mg, C 120 mg, B_1 1.84 mg, B_2 3 mg, B_3 20 mg, B_6 10 mg, B_{12} 12 mcg, Ca 200 mg, folic acid 1 mg, Fe 65 mg, Zn 25 mg, Cu 2 mg. Tab. Bot. 100s. *Rx.*
Use: Mineral, vitamin supplement.

Stuart Prenatal. (Wyeth-Ayerst Laboratories) Vitamins A 4000 IU, B_1 1.8 mg, B_2 1.7 mg, B_6 2.6 mg, B_{12} 4 mcg, C 100 mg, D 400 IU, E 11 mg, B_3 18 mg, Fe 60 mg, Ca 200 mg, Cu 2 mg, Zn 25 mg, folic acid 0.8 mg/Tab. Bot. 100s. *otc.*
Use: Mineral, vitamin supplement.

Stulex. (Jones Medical Industries, Inc.) Docusate sodium 250 mg/Tab. Bot. 100s, 1000s. *otc.*
Use: Fecal softener.

Stye. (Del Pharmaceuticals, Inc.) White petrolatum 55%, mineral oil 32%, boric acid, wheat germ oil, stearic acid. Oint. Bot. 3.5 g. *otc.*
Use: Lubricant, ophthalmic.

Stypt-Aid. (Pharmakon Laboratories, Inc.) Benzocaine 28.71 mg, methylbenzethonium HCl 9.95 mg, aluminum Cl hexahydrate 55.43 mg, ethyl alcohol 70.97%/ml in a glycerin, menthol base. Spray. 60 ml. *otc.*
Use: Anesthetic, local.

styptirenal.
See: Epinephrine (Various Mfr.).

Stypto-Caine. (Pedinol Pharmacal, Inc.) Hydroxyquinoline sulfate, tetracaine HCl, aluminum Cl, aqueous glycol base. Soln. Bot. 2 oz. *Rx.*
Use: Hemostatic solution.

styrene polymer, sulfonated, sodium salt. Sodium Polystyrene Sulfonate, U.S.P. 23.

styronate resins. Ammonium and potassium salts of sulfonated styrene polymers.
Use: Conditions requiring sodium restriction.

Sublimaze. (Taylor) Fentanyl 0.05 mg as citrate/ml. Inj. Amp. 2 ml, 5 ml, 10 ml, 20 ml. *c-II.*
Use: Analgesic, narcotic.

Sublingual B Total Liquid. (Pharmaceutical Labs) Vitamins B_2 1.7 mg, B_3 20 mg, B_5 30 mg, B_6 2 mg, B_{12} 1000 mcg, C 60 mg. Liq. Bot. 30 ml. *otc.*
Use: Vitamin supplement.

Suby's Solution G. (Various Mfr.) Citric acid 3.24 g, sodium carbonate 0.43 g, magnesium oxide 0.38 g/100 ml. Soln. Bot. 1000 ml. *Rx.*
Use: Irrigant, genitourinary.

•**succimer.** (SUX-ih-mer) USAN.
Use: Diagnostic aid; cystine kidney stones, mercury and lead poisoning. [Orphan Drug]
See: Chemet (McNeil Consumer Products Co.).

•**succinylcholine chloride.** (suck-sin-ill-KOE-leen KLOR-ide) U.S.P. 23.
Use: Neuromuscular blocker.
See: Anectine Cl, Amp. (Glaxo-Wellcome).
Quelicin, Amp., Additive Syringes, Fliptop & Pintop Vials (Abbott Laboratories).
Sucostrin, Amp, Vial (Bristol-Myers Squibb).

succinylsulfathiazole.
Use: Anti-infective, intestinal.

Succus Cineraria Maritima. (Walker, Corp & Co., Inc.) Aqueous and glycerin solution of senecio compositae, hamamelis water and boric acid. Soln. Bot. 7 ml. *Rx.*
Use: Ophthalmic.

Sucostrin. (Apothecon, Inc.) Succinylcholine Cl 20 mg/ml Inj. Vial 10 ml. *Rx.*
Use: Neuromuscular blocker.

Sucostrin Chloride. (Marsam Pharmaceuticals, Inc.) Succinylcholine Cl 20 mg/ml w/methylparaben 0.1%, propylparaben 0.01%. Vial 10 ml; High potency 100 mg/ml. Vial 10 ml. *Rx.*
Use: Muscle relaxant.

Sucraid. (Orphan Medical, Inc.) Sacrosidase 8500 IU/ml. Soln. Bot. 118 ml. *Rx.*
Use: Nutritional therapy.

•**sucralfate.** (sue-KRAL-fate) U.S.P. 23.

Use: Antiulcerative, oral complications of chemotherapy. [Orphan Drug]
See: Carafate, Tab., Susp. (Hoechst Marion Roussel).

sucralfate. (Biocraft Laboratories, Inc.) Sucralfate 1 g/Tab. Bot. 30s, 100s, 500s. *Rx.*
Use: Antiulcerative.

Sucrets Children's Sore Throat Lozenges. (SmithKline Beecham) Dyclonine HCl 1.2 mg/Loz. Corn syrup, sucrose, cherry flavor. Tin 24s. *otc.*
Use: Sore throat treatment for children 3 years and over.

Sucrets Cold Decongestant Lozenge. (SmithKline Beecham) Phenylpropanolamine HCl 25 mg/Loz. Box 24s. *otc.*
Use: Decongestant.

Sucrets Cough Control Lozenge. (SmithKline Beecham) Dextromethorphan HBr 5 mg/Loz. Tin 24s. *otc.*
Use: Antitussive.

Sucrets 4-Hour Cough. (SmithKline Beecham) Dextromethorphan 15 mg/ Loz. Menthol, sucrose, corn syrup. Pkg. 20s. *otc.*
Use: Antitussive.

Sucrets Maximum Strength. (SmithKline Beecham) Dyclonine HCl 3 mg/ lozenge. Corn syrup, menthol, sucrose. Tin 24s, 48s, 55s. *otc.*
Use: Mouth and throat preparation.

Sucrets Sore Throat Lozenge. (SmithKline Beecham) Hexylresorcinol 2.4 mg/loz. Tin 24s. *otc.*
Use: Mouth and throat preparation.

Sucrets Sore Throat Spray. (SmithKline Beecham) Dyclonine HCl 0.1%, alcohol 10%, sorbitol spray. Bot. 90 ml, 120 ml. *otc.*
Use: Mouth and throat preparation.

Sucrets Wintergreen. (SmithKline Beecham) Dyclonine HCl 0.1%, alcohol 10%, sorbitol. Spray Bot. 90 ml. *otc.*
Use: Mouth and throat preparation.

•**sucrose.** (SUE-krose) N.F. 18.
Use: IV; diuretic & dehydrating agent; pharmaceutic aid (flavor, tablet excipient).

•**sucrose octaacetate.** N.F. 18.
Use: Pharmaceutic aid (alcohol denaturant).

•**sucrosofate potassium.** (sue-KROE-so-FATE) USAN.
Use: Antiulcerative.

Sudafed 12 Hour. (Warner Lambert) Pseudoephedrine HCl 120 mg/SA Cap. Box 10s, 20s, 40s. *otc.*
Use: Decongestant.

Sudafed Cold & Cough Liquid Caps. (Warner Lambert) Dextromethorphan HBr 10 mg, pseudoephedrine HCl 30 mg, acetaminophen 250 mg, guaifenesin 100 mg. Cap. Pkg. 10s, 20s. *otc.*
Use: Analgesic, antitussive, decongestant, expectorant.

Sudafed Plus. (Warner Lambert) Pseudoephedrine HCl 60 mg, chlorpheniramine maleate 4 mg/Tab. Box 24s, 48s. *otc.*
Use: Antihistamine, decongestant.

Sudafed, Severe Cold. (Warner Lambert) Pseudoephedrine HCl 30 mg, dextromethorphan HBr 15 mg, acetaminophen 500 mg/Tab. Pkg. 10s, 20s. *otc.*
Use: Analgesic, antitussive, decongestant.

Sudafed Sinus Maximum Strength. (Warner Lambert) Pseudoephedrine HCl 30 mg, acetaminophen 500 mg. Capl. 24s. *otc.*
Use: Analgesic, decongestant.

Sudafed Tablets. (Warner Lambert) Pseudoephedrine HCl 30 mg, 60 mg/ Tab. **30 mg:** Box 24s, 48s. Bot. 100s, 1000s. **60 mg:** Bot. 100s, 1000s. *otc.*
Use: Decongestant.

Sudal 60/500. (Atley Pharmaceuticals, Inc.) Pseudoephedrine HCl 60 mg, guaifenesin 500 mg. TR Tab. Bot. 100s. *Rx.*
Use: Decongestant, expectorant.

Sudal 120/600. (Atley Pharmaceuticals, Inc.) Pseudoephedrine HCl 120 mg, guaifenesin 600 mg. SR Tab. Bot. 100s. *Rx.*
Use: Decongestant, expectorant.

Sudanyl. (Dover Pharmaceuticals) Pseudoephedrine HCl/Tab. Sugar, lactose and salt free. UD Box 500s.
Use: Decongestant.

Sudden Tan Lotion. (Schering-Plough Corp.) Padimate O, dihydroxyacetone, Bot. 4 oz. *otc.*
Use: Artificial tanning, moisturizer, sunscreen.

•**sudoxicam.** (sue-DOX-ih-kam) USAN.
Use: Anti-inflammatory.

Sudrin. (Jones Medical Industries, Inc.) Pseudoephedrine HCl 30 mg/Tab. Bot. 100s, 1000s. *otc.*
Use: Decongestant.

Sufenta. (Taylor) Sufentanil citrate 50 mcg/ml. Inj. Amp. 1 ml, 2 ml, 5 ml. *c-II.*
Use: Analgesic, narcotic.

•**sufentanil.** (sue-FEN-tuh-nill) USAN.
Use: Analgesic.

•**sufentanil citrate.** (sue-FEN-tuh-nill SIH-trate) U.S.P. 23.

Use: Analgesic, narcotic.
See: Sufenta (Janssen Pharmaceutical, Inc.).

sufentanil citrate. (ESI Lederle Generics) 50 mcg/ml. Inj. Amp. 1 ml, 2 ml, 5 ml. *c-II.*
Use: Analgesic, narcotic.

•**sufotidine.** (sue-FOE-tih-DEEN) USAN.
Use: Antiulcerative.

Sufrex. (Janssen Pharmaceutical, Inc.) Ketanserin tartrate. *Rx.*
Use: Serotonin antagonist.

•**sugar, compressible.** N.F. 18.
Use: Pharmaceutic aid (flavor; tablet excipient).

•**sugar, confectioner's.** N.F. 18.
Use: Pharmaceutic aid (flavor; tablet excipient).

•**sugar, invert, injection.** U.S.P. 23.
Use: Replenisher (fluid and nutrient).

•**sugar spheres.** N.F. 18.
Use: Pharmaceutic aid (vehicle, solid carrier).

Sulamyd Sodium.
Use: Sulfonamide, ophthalmic.
See: Sodium Sulamyd, Ophth. Soln. (Schering-Plough Corp.).

Sular. (Zeneca Pharmaceuticals) 10 mg, 20 mg, 30 mg, 40 mg nisoldipine, lactose/ER Tab. 100s, UD 100s. *Rx.*
Use: Calcium channel blocker.

•**sulazepam.** (sull-AZE-eh-pam) USAN.
Use: Anxiolytic.

Sulazo. (Freeport) Sulfisoxazole 500 mg, phenylazodiaminopyridine HCl 50 mg/Tab. Bot. 1000s. *Rx.*
Use: Analgesic, anti-infective.

•**sulbactam benzathine.** (sull-BACK-tam BENZ-ah-theen) USAN.
Use: Synergistic (penicillin/cephalosporin), inhibitor (β-lactamase).

•**sulbactam pivoxil.** (sull-BACK-tam pihv-OX-ill) USAN.
Use: Inhibitor (β-lactamase), synergist (penicillin/cephalosporin).

•**sulbactam sodium sterile.** (sull-BACK-tam) U.S.P. 23.
Use: Inhibitor (β-lactamase), synergist (penicillin/cephalosporin).

sulbactam sodium/ampicillin sodium.
Use: Anti-infective, penicillin.
See: Unasyn (Roerig).

•**sulconazole nitrate.** (SULL-CONE-ah-zole) U.S.P. 23.
Use: Antifungal.

•**sulesomab.** (sue-LEH-so-mab) USAN.
Use: Monoclonal antibody (diagnostic aid for detection of infectious lesions).

Sulf-10. (Ciba Vision) Sodium sulfacetamide 10%. Bot. 15 ml; Dropperette 1 ml. *Rx.*
Use: Anti-infective, ophthalmic.

Sulf-15. (Ciba Vision) Sodium sulfacetamide 15%. Soln. Bot. 5 ml, 15 ml. *Rx.*
Use: Anti-infective, ophthalmic.

Sulfa-10 Ophthalmic. (Maurry) Sodium sulfacetamide 10%, hydroxyethylcellulose, sodium borate, boric acid, disodium edetate, sodium metabisulfite, sodium thiosulfate 0.2%, chlorobutanol 0.2%, methylparaben 0.015%. Bot. 15 ml. *Rx.*
Use: Anti-infective, ophthalmic.

•**sulfabenz.** (SULL-fah-benz) USAN.
Use: Anti-infective.

•**sulfabenzamide.** (SULL-fah-BENZ-ah-mid) U.S.P. 23.
Use: Anti-infective.
See: Sultrin, Vag. Tab., Cream (Ortho McNeil Pharmaceutical).

sulfabromethazine sodium.
Use: Anti-infective.

Sulfacet. (Dermik Laboratories, Inc.)
See: Sulfacetamide.

Sulfacet-R. (Dermik Laboratories, Inc.) Sulfur 5%, sulfacetamide sodium 10%, parabens. Lot. Bot. 25 ml. *Rx.*
Use: Dermatologic, acne.

•**sulfacetamide.** (sull-fah-SEE-tah-mide) U.S.P. 23.
Use: Anti-infective.

sulfacetamide w/combinations.
See: Acet-Dia-Mer Sulfonamides.
Cetapred, Oint. (Alcon Laboratories, Inc.).
Chero-Trisulfa (V), Susp. (Vita Elixir).
Sulf-10, Ophth. Soln. (Ciba Vision).
Sulster, Soln. (Akorn, Inc).
Sultrin, Tab, Cream (Ortho McNeil Pharmaceutical).
Triurisul, Tab. (Sheryl).

•**sulfacetamide sodium.** U.S.P. 23.
Use: Anti-infective.
See: AK-Sulf, Preps. (Akorn, Inc.).
Bleph 10, Liquifilm (Allergan, Inc.).
Cetamide, Ophth. Oint. (Alcon Laboratories, Inc.).
Isopto Cetamide, Ophth. Soln. (Alcon Laboratories, Inc.).
Ocusulf-10, Ophth. Soln. (Optopics Laboratories, Corp.).
Sebizon Lotion (Schering-Plough Corp.).
Sodium Sulamyd Ophthalmic Ointment 30% (Schering-Plough Corp.).
Sulf-10, Drops (Maurry).
Sulf-10, Soln., Drops (Ciba Vision).

Sulf-15, Ophth. Soln. (Ciba Vision).
W/Fluorometholone.
See: FML-S Susp. (Allergan, Inc.).
W/Methylcellulose.
See: Sodium Sulamyd Ophth. Soln. 10% (Schering-Plough Corp.).
W/Phenylephrine HCl, methylparaben, propylparaben.
See: Vasosulf, Liq. (Ciba Vision).
W/Prednisolone.
See: Cetapred Ophth. Ointment (Alcon Laboratories, Inc.).
Vasocidin, Soln. (Ciba Vision).
W/Prednisolone acetate.
See: Blephamide S.O.P., Ophth. Oint. and Susp. (Allergan, Inc.).
Metimyd, Ophth. Oint. and Susp. (Schering-Plough Corp.).
W/Prednisolone, methylcellulose.
See: Isopto Cetapred, Susp. (Alcon Laboratories, Inc.).
W/Prednisolone acetate, phenylephrine.
See: Blephamide Liquifilm, Ophth. Susp. (Allergan, Inc.).
Optimyd Soln., Sterile (Schering-Plough Corp.).
W/Prednisolone sodium phosphate, phenylephrine, sulfacetamide sodium.
See: Vasocidin, Ophth Soln. (Ciba Vision).
W/Sulfur.
See: Novacet, Lot. (Medicis Dermatologicals, Inc.).
Sulfacet-R, Lot. (Dermik Laboratories, Inc.).

sulfacetamide sodium. (Various Mfr.) **Soln.: 10%, 30%:** Bot. 15 ml. **Oint.:** 10% Tube 3.5 g.
Use: Anti-infective.

sulfacetamide sodium and prednisolone acetate ophthalmic ointment.
Use: Anti-infective, anti-inflammatory.
See: AK-Cide (Akorn, Inc.).
Blephamide S.O.P. (Allergan, Inc.).
Cetapred (Alcon Laboratories, Inc.).
Metimyd (Schering-Plough Corp.).
Predsulfair (Bausch & Lomb Pharmaceuticals).
Vasocidin (Ciba Vision).

sulfacetamide sodium and prednisolone sodium phosphate. (Schein Pharmaceutical, Inc.) Sulfacetamide sodium 10%, prednisolone sodium phosphate 0.25%. Soln. 5 ml, 10 ml. *Rx.*
Use: Anti-infective, ophthalmic.

Sulfacetamide Sodium 10% and Sulfur 5%. (Glades Pharmaceuticals) Sulfur 5%, sodium sulfacetamide 10%, cetyl alcohol, benzyl alcohol, EDTA. Bot. 25 ml. Tube 30 ml. *Rx.*
Use: Dermatologic, acne.

sulfacetamide, sulfadiazine, & sulfamerazine oral suspension.
See: Acet-dia-mer-sulfonamide.

Sulfacet-R. (Dermik Laboratories, Inc.) Sodium sulfacetamide 10%, sulfur 5%, in flesh-tinted base. Lot. Bot. 25 g. *Rx.*
Use: Dermatologic, acne; seborrhea.

•**sulfacytine.** (SULL-fah-SIGH-teen) USAN.
Use: Anti-infective.

sulfadiasulfone sodium. Acetosulfone sodium.

•**sulfadiazine.** (SULL-fah-DIE-ah-zeen) U.S.P. 23.
Use: Anti-infective. [Orphan Drug]

sulfadiazine. (Various Mfr.) Sulfadiazine 500 mg. Tab. Bot. 100s, 1000s, UD 100s. *Rx.*
Use: Anti-infective.

sulfadiazine combinations. (SULL-fah-DIE-ah-zeen)
See: Acet-dia-mer-sulfonamide (Various Mfr.).
Chemozine, Tab., Susp. (Tennessee Pharmaceutic).
Chero-Trisulfa, Susp. (Vita Elixir).
Meth-Dia-Mer Sulfonamides (Various Mfr.).
Silvadene (Hoechst Marion Roussel).
Triple Sulfa, Tab (Various Mfr.).

sulfadiazine and sulfamerazine. Citrasulfas.

•**sulfadiazine, silver.** (sull-fah-DIE-ah-zeen) U.S.P. 23.
Use: Anti-infective, topical.

•**sulfadiazine sodium.** (SULL-fah-DIE-ah-zeen) U.S.P. 23.
Use: Anti-infective.
See: Sod. bicarbonate: Tab. 5 gr, Bot. 1000s; 2.5 gr, Bot. 100s, 500s, 1000s. (Pitman-Moore).

sulfadiazine, sulfamerazine & sulfacetamide suspension.
See: Acet-dia-mer-sulfonamide.
Coco Diazine (Eli Lilly and Co.).

sulfadimidine.
See: Sulfamethazine.

sulfadine.
See: Sulfadimidine.
Sulfamethazine.
Sulfapyridine, Tab. (Various Mfr.).

•**sulfadoxine.** (SULL-fah-DOX-een) U.S.P. 23.
Use: Anti-infective.
W/Pyrimethamine.
See: Fansidar, Tab. (Roche Laboratories).

sulfadoxine and pyrimethamine tablets.

Use: Anti-infective, antimalarial.

sulfaguanidine.
Use: GI tract infections.

Sulfair 15. (Bausch & Lomb Pharmaceuticals) Sodium sulfacetamide 15%. Soln. Bot. 15 ml. *Rx.*
Use: Anti-infective, ophthalmic.

Sulfalax Calcium. (Major Pharmaceuticals) Docusate calcium 240 mg/Cap. Bot. 500s. *otc.*
Use: Laxative.

•**sulfalene.** (SULL-fah-leen) USAN.
Use: Anti-infective.

•**sulfamerazine.** (sull-fah-MER-ah-zeen) U.S.P. 23.
Use: Anti-infective.

sulfamerazine combinations.
Use: Anti-infective.
See: Chemozine Tab., Susp. (Tennessee Pharmaceutic).
Chero-Trisulfa-V, Susp. (Vita Elixir).
Triple Sulfa, Tab. (Various Mfr.).

sulfamerazine sodium.
Use: Anti-infective.

sulfamerazine, sulfadiazine & sulfamethazine.
Use: Anti-infective.
See: Meth-Dia-Mer Sulfonamides.

sulfamerazine, sulfadiazine & sulfathiazole.
Use: Anti-infective.

•**sulfameter.** (SULL-fam-EE-ter) USAN.
Use: Anti-infective.

•**sulfamethazine.** (sull fa-METH-ah zeen) U.S.P. 23.
Use: Anti-infective.
See: Sulfa-Plex, Vaginal Cream (Solvay Pharmaceuticals).
W/Sulfadiazine, sulfamerazine.
See: Triple Sulfa, Tab. (Various Mfr.).

•**sulfamethizole.** (sull-fah-METH-ih-zole) U.S.P. 23.
Use: Anti-infective.
See: Bursul, Tab. (Burlington).
Sulfurine, Tab. (Table Rock).
Thiosulfil, Forte, Tab. (Wyeth-Ayerst Laboratories).
Urifon, Tab. (T.E. Williams Pharmaceuticals).

sulfamethizole w/combinations.
Use: Anti-infective.
See: Triurisul, Tab. (Sheryl).
Urobiotic, Cap. (Pfizer US Pharmaceutical Group).

sulfamethoprim. (Par Pharmaceuticals) Sulfamethoxazole 400 mg, trimethoprim 80 mg/Tab. Bot. 100s, 500s. *Rx.*
Use: Anti-infective.

•**sulfamethoxazole.** (sull-fah-meth-OX-ah-zole) U.S.P. 23.
Use: Anti-infective.
See: Gantanol, Prep. (Roche Laboratories).
W/Trimethoprim.
See: Bactrim, Prods. (Roche Laboratories).
Septra, Tab. (GlaxoWellcome).
Septra DS, Tab. (GlaxoWellcome).

sulfamethoxazole and phenazopyridine hydrochloride.
Use: Anti-infective, urinary.

sulfamethoxazole and trimethoprim for injection. (SULL-fah-meth-OX-ah-zole and try-METH-oh-prim)
Use: Anti-infective, urinary.

sulfamethoxazole and trimethoprim oral suspension. (Various Mfr.) Trimethoprim 40 mg, sulfamethoxazole 200 mg/5 ml. Bot. 150 ml, 200 ml, 480 ml. *Rx.*
Use: Anti-infective, urinary.

sulfamethoxazole and trimethoprim tablets. (Various Mfr.) Trimethoprim 80 mg, sulfamethoxazole 400 mg/Tab. Bot. 100s, 500s. *Rx.*
Use: Anti-infective, urinary.

sulfamethoxazole/trimethoprim DS. (Various Mfr.) Trimethoprim 160 mg, sulfamethoxazole 800 mg. Tab, double-strength. Bot. 100s, 500s. *Rx.*
Use: Anti-infective.

sulfamethoxydiazine. Sulfameter.
Use: Anti-infective.

sulfamethoxypyridazine acetyl.
Use: Anti-infective.

sulfamethylthiadiazole.
Use: Anti-infective.
See: Sulfamethizole Preps.

sulfametin. *Formerly sulfamethoxydiazine.*
Use: Anti-infective.

sulfamezanthene.
Use: Anti-infective.
See: Sulfamethazine.

Sulfamide Suspension. (Rugby Labs, Inc.) Prednisolone acetate 0.5%, sodium sulfacetamide, hydroxypropyl methylcellulose, polysorbate 80, sodium thiosulfate, benzalkonium Cl 0.01%. Susp. Bot. 5 and 15 ml. *Rx.*
Use: Anti-infective, ophthalmic.

•**sulfamonomethoxine.** (SULL-fah-mahn-oh-meh-THOCK-seen) USAN.
Use: Anti-infective.

•**sulfamoxole.** (sull-fah-MOX-ole) USAN.
Use: Anti-infective.

p-sulfamoylbenzylamine hydrochloride. Sulfbenzamide.

Sulfamylon. (Bertek Pharmaceuticals) Mafenide acetate 5%. Packets containing 50 g of sterile mafenide acetate

to be reconstituted in 1000 ml of sterile water for irrigation or 0.9% Sodium Chloride Irrigation. Top. Soln. Ctn. Pkt. 50 g, 5s. *Rx.*
Use: Burn therapy adjunct.

sulfanilamide. p-Aminobenzene sulfonamide.
Use: Anti-infective.

sulfanilamide. (Various Mfr.) Sulfanilamide 15%. Vaginal Cream. Tube 120 g with applicator. *Rx.*
Use: Anti-infective, vaginal.

sulfanilamide combinations.
Use: Anti-infective.
See: AVC, Cream, Supp. (Hoechst Marion Roussel).
Par Cream (Parmed Pharmaceuticals, Inc.).

2-sulfanilamidopyridine. Sulfadiazine, U.S.P. 23.
Use: Anti-infective.

•**sulfanilate zinc.** (sull-FAN-ih-late) USAN.
Use: Anti-infective.

n-sulfanilylacetamide.
Use: Anti-infective.
See: Sulfacetamide, Tab. (Various Mfr.).

sulfanilylbenzamide.
Use: Anti-infective.
See: Sulfabenzamide.

•**sulfanitran.** (SULL-fah-NYE-tran) USAN.
Use: Anti-infective.

•**sulfapyridine.** (sull-fah-PEER-ih-deen) U.S.P. 23.
Use: Dermatitic herpetiformis suppressant. [Orphan Drug]

•**sulfasalazine.** (SULL-fuh-SAL-uh-zeen) U.S.P. 23. *Formerly Salicylazosulfapyridine.*
Use: Anti-infective.
See: Azulfidine, Preps. (Pharmacia & Upjohn).
Salicylazosulfapyridine.
Sulfapyridine (I.N.N).

sulfasalazine. (Various Mfr.) Sulfasalazine 500 mg. Tab. Bot. 50s, 100s, 500s, 1000s. *Rx.*
Use: Anti-infective.

•**sulfasomizole.** (SULL-fah-SAHM-ih-zole) USAN.
Use: Antibacterial, anti-infective, sulfonamide.

sulfasymasine.
Use: Anti-infective sulfonamide.

Sulfa-Ter-Tablets. (A.P.C.) Trisulfapyrimidines, U.S.P. Bot. 1000s.

•**sulfathiazole.** (sull-fah-THIGH-ah-zole) U.S.P. 23.
Use: Anti-infective.

sulfathiazole combinations.
See: Sultrin, Tab., Cream (Ortho Mc-Neil Pharmaceutical).

sulfathiazole, sulfacetamide, and sulfabenzamide vaginal cream.
See: Dayto Sulf (Dayton Laboratories, Inc.).
Triple Sulfa Vaginal Cream.

sulfathiazole, sulfacetamide, and sulfabenzamide vaginal tablets.
See: Triple Sulfa Vaginal Tablets.

Sulfatrim. (Various Mfr.) Trimethoprim 40 mg, sulfamethoxazole 200 mg/5 ml Susp. Bot. 473 ml. *Rx.*
Use: Anti-infective.

Sulfatrim DS. (Zenith Goldline Pharmaceuticals) Trimethoprim 800 mg, sulfamethoxazole 160 mg/Tab. Bot. 100s, 500s. *Rx.*
Use: Anti-infective.

Sulfatrim SS. (Zenith Goldline Pharmaceuticals) Trimethoprim 400 mg, sulfamethoxazole 80 mg/Tab. Bot. 100s. *Rx.*
Use: Anti-infective.

Sulfa-Trip. (Major Pharmaceuticals) Sulfathiazole 3.42%, sulfacetamide 2.86%, sulfabenzamide 3.7%, urea 0.64%. Cream Tube 82.5 g. *Rx.*
Use: Anti-infective, vaginal.

Sulfa Triple No. 2. (Global Source) Sulfadiazine 162 mg, sulfamerizine 162 mg, sulfamethazine 162 mg/Tab. Bot. 1000s. *Rx.*
Use: Anti-infective.

•**sulfazamet.** (sull-FAZE-ah-MET) USAN.
Use: Anti-infective.

•**sulfinalol hydrochloride.** (SULL-FIN-ah-lahl) USAN.
Use: Antihypertensive.

•**sulfinpyrazone.** (sull-fin-PEER-uh-zone) U.S.P. 23.
Use: Uricosuric.
See: Anturane, Tab., Cap. (Novartis Pharmaceutical Corp.).

•**sulfisoxazole.** (sull-fih-SOX-uh-zole) U.S.P. 23.
Use: Anti-infective.
See: Gantrisin, Preps. (Roche Laboratories).
Soxa, Tab. (Vita Elixir).
Sulfisoxazole, Tab. (Purepac Pharmaceutical Co.).
Sulfizin, Tab. (Solvay Pharmaceuticals).
W/Aminoacridine HCl, allantoin.
See: Azo-Gantrisin, Tab. (Roche Laboratories).
Azo-Soxazole, Tab. (Quality Formulations, Inc.).
Azo-Sulfisoxazole, Tab. (Global Pharm; Century).

sulfisoxazole. (Various Mfr.) Sulfisoxazole 500 mg. Tab. Bot. 100s, 1000s. *Rx.*
Use: Anti-infective.

•**sulfisoxazole, acetyl.** (sull-fih-SOX-uh-zole, ASS-eh-till) U.S.P. 23.
Use: Anti-infective.
W/Erythromycin Ethylsuccinate.
See: Pediazol, Susp. (Ross Laboratories).

sulfisoxazole diethanolamine. Sulfisoxazole Diolamine.

•**sulfisoxazole diolamine.** (sull-fin-SOX-azz-ole die-OLE-ah-meen) U.S.P. 23.
Use: Anti-infective.
See: Gantrisin, Ophth. Soln., Oint. (Roche Laboratories).

Sulfoam Medicated Antidandruff Shampoo. (Kenwood Laboratories) Sulfur 2% with cleansers & conditioners. Bot. 4 oz, 8 oz, 15.5 oz. *otc.*
Use: Control dandruff.

sulfobromophthalein sodium. U.S.P. XXII.
Use: Liver function test.

sulfocarbolates. Salts of Phenolsulfonic Acid, Usually Ca, Na, K, Cu, Zn.

sulfocyanate.
See: Potassium Thiocyanate.

Sulfo-Ganic. (Marcen) Thioglycerol 20 mg, sodium citrate 5 mg, phenol 0.5%, benzyl alcohol 0.5%/ml. Inj. Vial 10 ml, 30 ml.
Use: Antiarthritic.

Sulfoil. (C & M Pharmacal, Inc.) Sulfonated castor oil, water. Oil. Bot. Pt, gal. *otc.*
Use: Dermatologic, hair and skin.

Sulfolax Calcium. (Major Pharmaceuticals) Docusate calcium 240 mg/Cap. Bot. 100s. *otc.*
Use: Laxative.

Sulfo-Lo. (Whorton Pharmaceuticals, Inc.) Sublimed sulfur, freshly precipitated polysulfides of zinc, potassium, sulfate, and calamine in aqueous-alcoholic suspension. **Lotion:** Bot. 4 oz, 8 oz. **Soap:** 3 oz. *otc.*
Use: Dermatologic, acne.

•**sulfomyxin.** (SULL-foe-MIX-in) USAN.
Use: Anti-infective.

sulfonamide preps.
See: Acet-Dia-Mer (Various Mfr.).
Dayto Sulf, Vag. Cream (Dayton Laboratories, Inc.).
Gyne-Sulf, Vag. Cream (G & W Laboratories).
Meth-Dia-Mer, Preps. (Various Mfr.).
Sultrin Triple Sulfa, Vag. Cream, Tab. (Ortho McNeil Pharmaceutical).
Triple Sulfa, Vag. Cream (Various Mfr.).
Trysul, Vag. Cream (Savage Laboratories).
VVS, Vag. Cream (Econo Med Pharmaceuticals).

sulfonamides, triple.
See: Acet-Dia-Mer Sulfonamides.
Meth-Dia-Mer Sulfonamides.

sulfones.
See: Dapsone.
Glucosulfone Sodium.

•**sulfonterol hydrochloride.** (sull-FAHN-teer-ole) USAN.
Use: Bronchodilator.

sulfonylureas.
See: DiaBeta (Hoechst Marion Roussel).
Diabinese, Tab. (Pfizer US Pharmaceutical Group).
Dymelor, Tab. (Eli Lilly and Co.).
Glucotrol (Roerig).
Glynase PresTab. (Pharmacia & Upjohn).
Micronase (Pharmacia & Upjohn).
Orinase, Tab, Vial (Pharmacia & Upjohn).
Tolinase, Tab. (Pharmacia & Upjohn).

Sulforcin Lotion. (Galderma Laboratories, Inc.) Sulfur 5%, resorcinol 2%, SD alcohol 40 11.65%, methylparaben. Bot. 120 ml. *otc.*
Use: Dermatologic.

sulformethoxine. Name used for Sulfadoxine.

sulforthomidine. Name used for Sulfadoxine.

sulfosalicylate w/methenamine.
See: Hexalen, Tab. (PolyMedica Pharmaceuticals).

sulfosalicylic acid. Salicylsulphonic acid.

sulfoxone sodium. U.S.P. XXII.

sulfoxyl regular. (Stiefel Laboratories, Inc.) Benzoyl peroxide 5%, sulfur 2% Bot. 60 ml. *Rx.*
Use: Dermatologic, acne.

sulfoxyl strong. (Stiefel Laboratories, Inc.) Benzoyl peroxide 10%, sulfur 5%. Bot. 60 ml. *Rx.*
Use: Dermatologic, acne.

Sulfur-8 Hair & Scalp Conditioner. (Schering-Plough Corp.) Sulfur 2%, menthol 1%, triclosan 0.1%. Cream Jar 2 oz, 4 oz, 8 oz. *otc.*
Use: Antiseborrheic.

Sulfur-8 Light Formula Hair & Scalp Conditioner. (Schering-Plough Corp.) Sulfur, triclosan, menthol. Cream Jar 2 oz, 4 oz. *otc.*
Use: Antiseborrheic.

Sulfur-8 Shampoo. (Schering-Plough Corp.) Triclosan 0.2%. Bot. 6.85 oz, 10.85 oz. *otc.*
Use: Antiseborrheic.

sulfurated lime topical solution. Vleminckx Lotion.
Use: Scabicide, parasiticide.

sulfur combinations.
See: Acnaveen, Bar (Rydelle Laboratories).
Akne Oral Kapsulets, Cap. (Alto Pharmaceuticals, Inc.).
Acnomel, Cake, Cream (SmithKline Beecham Pharmaceuticals).
Acno, Soln., Lot. (Baker Norton Pharmaceuticals, Inc.).
Acnotex, Liq. (C & M Pharmacal, Inc.).
Akne, Drying Lot. (Alto Pharmaceuticals, Inc.).
Antrocol, Tab., Cap. (ECR Pharmaceuticals).
Bensulfoid, Cream (ECR Pharmaceuticals).
Clearasil, Stick (Procter & Gamble Pharm.).
Fostex, Liq. Cream, Bar (Westwood Squibb Pharmaceuticals).
Fostex, Cream, Liq. (Westwood Squibb Pharmaceuticals).
Fostex CM, Cream (Westwood Squibb Pharmaceuticals).
Fostril, Cream (Westwood Squibb Pharmaceuticals).
Hydro Surco, Lot. (Almo).
Klaron, Lot. (Dermik Laboratories, Inc.).
Liquimat, Liq. (Galderma Laboratories, Inc.).
Neutrogena Disposables (Neutrogena).
Pernox, Lot. (Westwood Squibb Pharmaceuticals).
Rezamid, Lot. (Summers Laboratories, Inc.).
SAStid Soap (Stiefel Laboratories, Inc.).
Sebulex Shampoo, Liq. (Westwood Squibb Pharmaceuticals).
Sulfacet-R, Lot. (Dermik Laboratories, Inc.).
Sulfo-lo, Lot. (Wharton).
Sulforcin, Pow, Lot. (Galderma Laboratories, Inc.).
Sulfur-8, Prods. (Schering-Plough Corp.).
Sulpho-Lac, Cream (Kenwood Laboratories).
Xerac, Oint. (Person and Covey, Inc.).

•**sulfur dioxide.** (SULL-fer die-OX-ide) N.F. 18.
Use: Pharmaceutic aid (antioxidant).

sulfur ointment.
Use: Scabicide, parasiticide.

•**sulfur, precipitated.** U.S.P. 23.
Use: Scabicide; parasiticide.
See: Bensulfoid, Pow., Lot. (ECR Pharmaceuticals).
SAStid Soap, Bar (Stiefel Laboratories, Inc.).
Sulfur Soa (Steifel Labs).

sulfur, salicyl diasporal. (Doak Dermatologics)
See: Diasporal, Cream (Doak Dermatologics).

sulfur soap. (Stiefel Laboratories, Inc.) Precipitated sulfur 10%, EDTA. Cake 116 g. *otc.*
Use: Dermatologic, acne.

•**sulfur, sublimed.** U.S.P. 23. Flowers of Sulfur.
Use: Parasiticide, scabicide.

sulfur, topical.
See: Thylox, Liq., Soap (C.S. Dent & Co. Division).

•**sulfuric acid.** N.F. 18.
Use: Pharmaceutic aid (acidifying agent).

Sulfurine. (Table Rock) Sulfamethizole 0.5 g/Tab. Bot. 100s, 500s. *Rx.*
Use: Anti-infective, urinary.

•**sulindac.** (sull-IN-dak) U.S.P. 23.
Use: Anti-inflammatory.
See: Clinoril, Tab. (Merck & Co.).

•**sulisobenzone.** (sul-EYE-so-BEN-zone) USAN.
Use: Ultraviolet screen.
See: Uval, Lot. (Novartis Pharmaceutical Corp.).
Uvinul MS-40 (General Aniline & Film).

•**sulmarin.** (SULL-mah-rin) USAN.
Use: Hemostatic.

Sulmasque. (C & M Pharmacal, Inc.) Sulfur 6.4%, isopropyl alcohol 15%, methylparaben. Mask 150 g. *otc.*
Use: Dermatologic, acne.

Sulnac. (NMC Laboratories) Sulfathiazole 3.42%, sulfacetamide 2.86%, sulfabenzamide 3.7%, urea 0.64% in cream base. Tube 2.75 oz. *Rx.*
Use: Anti-infective.

•**sulnidazole.** (sull-NIH-dah-zole) USAN.
Use: Antiprotozoal (trichomonas).

•**suloctidil.** (sull-OCK-tih-dill) USAN.
Use: Vasodilator (peripheral).

•**sulofenur.** (SUE-low-FEN-ehr) USAN.
Use: Antineoplastic.

•**sulopenem.** (sue-LOW-PEN-em) USAN.
Use: Anti-infective.

•**sulotroban.** (suh-LOW-troe-ban) USAN.

Use: Treatment of glomerulonephritis.
•**suloxifen oxalate.** (sull-OX-ih-fen OX-ah-late) USAN.
Use: Bronchodilator.
suloxybenzone. (ESI Lederle Generics)
sulphabenzide.
See: Sulfabenzamide.
Sulpho-Lac Acne Medication. (Doak Dermatologics) Sulfur 5%, zinc sulfate 27%, Vleminckx's Soln. 53%. Cream. Tube 28.35 g, 50 g. *otc.*
Use: Dermatologic, acne.
Sulpho-Lac Soap. (Doak Dermatologics) Sulfur 5%, a coconut and tallow oil soap base. Bar 85 g. *otc.*
Use: Dermatologic, acne.
•**sulpiride.** (SULL-pih-ride) USAN.
Use: Antidepressant.
•**sulprostone.** (sull-PRAHST-ohn) USAN.
Use: Prostaglandin.
Sul-Ray Acne Cream. (Last) Sulfur 2% in cream base. Jar 1.75 oz, 6.75 oz, 20 oz. *otc.*
Use: Dermatologic, acne.
Sul-Ray Aloe Vera Analgesic Rub. (Last) Camphor 3.1%, menthol 1.25%. Bot. 4 oz, 8 oz. *otc.*
Use: Analgesic, topical.
Sul-Ray Aloe Vera Skin Protectant. (Last) Zinc oxide 1%, allantoin 0.5%. Cream Jar 1 oz. *otc.*
Use: Dermatologic, protectant.
Sul-Ray Shampoo. (Last) Sulfur shampoo 2%. Bot. 8 oz. *otc.*
Use: Antidandruff.
Sul-Ray Soap. (Last) Sulfur soap. Bar 3 oz. *otc.*
Use: Dermatologic, acne.
Sulster. (Akorn, Inc.) Sulfacetamide sodium 1%, prednisolone sodium phosphate. 0.25% Soln. Bot. 5 ml, 10 ml. *Rx.*
Use: Ophthalmic preparation.
•**sultamicillin.** (SULL-TAM-ih-sill-in) USAN.
Use: Anti-infective.
•**sulthiame.** (sull-THIGH-aim) USAN.
Use: Anticonvulsant.
Sultrin Triple Sulfa Cream. (Ortho McNeil Pharmaceutical) Sulfathiazole 3.42%, sulfacetamide 2.86%, sulfabenzamide 3.7%, urea 0.64%. Tube 78 g. with measured dose applicator. *Rx.*
Use: Treatment of *Gardnerella vaginalis* vaginitis.
Sultrin Triple Sulfa Vaginal Tablets. (Ortho McNeil Pharmaceutical) Sulfathiazole 172.5 mg, sulfacetamide 143.75 mg, sulfabenzamide 184 mg/Vag. Tab. Pkg. 20s w/appl. *Rx.*
Use: Treatment of *Gardnerella vaginalis* vaginitis.
•**sulukast.** (suh-LOO-kast) USAN.
Use: Antiasthmatic (leukotriene antagonist).
Sumacal Powder. (Biosearch Medical Products) CHO 95 g, 380 Cal., Na 100 mg, chloride 210 mg, K < 39 mg, Ca 20 mg/100 g. Pwd. 400 g. *otc.*
Use: Glucose polymer.
•**sumarotene.** (sue-MAHR-oh-teen) USAN.
Use: Keratolytic.
•**sumatriptan succinate.** (SUE-muh-TRIP-tan SOOS-in-ate) USAN.
Use: Antimigraine, treatment of cluster headaches.
See: Imitrex, Preps. (GlaxoWellcome).
Summer's Eve Disposable Douche. (C.B. Fleet Co., Inc.) **Soln.:** Vinegar. 135 ml (1s, 2s). **Soln. Reg.:** Citric acid, sodium benzoate. **Soln. Scented:** Citric acid, sodium benzoate, octoxynol-9, EDTA. 135 ml (1s, 2s, 4s). *otc.*
Use: Douche.
Summer's Eve Disposable Douche Extra Cleansing. (C.B. Fleet Co., Inc.) Vinegar, sodium Cl, benzoic acid. Soln. 135 ml (1s, 2s, 4s). *otc.*
Use: Douche.
Summer's Eve Feminine Bath. (C.B. Fleet Co., Inc.) Ammonium laureth sulfate, EDTA. Liq. Bot. 45 ml, 345 ml. *otc.*
Use: Vaginal preparation.
Summer's Eve Feminine Powder. (C.B. Fleet Co., Inc.) Cornstarch, octoxynol-9, benzethonium chloride. Pow. Bot. 30 g, 210 g. *otc.*
Use: Vaginal preparation.
Summer's Eve Feminine Wash. (C.B. Fleet Co., Inc.) **Wipes:** Octoxynol-9, EDTA. Box 16s. **Liq.:** Ammonium laureth sulfate, PEG-75, lanolin, EDTA. Bot. 60 ml, 240 ml, 450 ml. *Rx.*
Use: Vaginal preparation.
Summer's Eve Medicated Disposable Douche. (C.B. Fleet Co., Inc.) Contains povidone-iodide 0.3%. Single or twin 135 ml disposable units. *otc.*
Use: Temporary relief of minor vaginal irritation and itching.
Summer's Eve Post Menstrual Disposable Douche. (C.B. Fleet Co., Inc.) Sodium lauryl sulfate, parabens, monosodium and disodium phosphates, EDTA. Soln. 135 ml (2s). *otc.*
Use: Douche.
Sumycin. (Apothecon, Inc.) Tetracycline HCl. **Cap.:** 250 mg/Cap. Bot. 100s, 1000s, Unimatic 100s; 500 mg/Cap. Bot. 100s, 500s, Unimatic 100s. **Tab.:** 250 mg/Tab. Bot. 100s, 1000s; 500 mg/

Tab. Bot. 100s, 500s. *Rx.*
Use: Anti-infective, tetracycline.

•**suncillin sodium.** (SUN-SILL-in SO-dee-uhm) USAN.
Use: Anti-infective.

Sundown. (Johnson & Johnson) A series of products marketed under the Sundown name including: **Moderate:** (SPF 4) Padimate O, oxybenzone. **Extra:** (SPF 6) Oxybenzone, padimate O. **Maximal:** (SPF 8) Oxybenzone, padimate O. **Ultra:** (SPF 15, 30) oxybenzone, padimate O, octyl methoxycinnamate. *otc.*
Use: Sunscreen.

Sundown Sport Sunblock. (Johnson & Johnson) Titanium dioxide, zinc oxide. PABA free. Waterproof. SPF 15. Lot. 90 ml. *otc.*
Use: Sunscreen.

Sundown Sunblock Cream Ultra SPF 24. (Johnson & Johnson) Padimate O, oxybenzone. *otc.*
Use: Sunscreen.

Sundown Sunblock Stick SPF 15. (Johnson & Johnson) Octyl dimethyl PABA, oxybenzone. Stick 0.35 oz. *otc.*
Use: Sunscreen.

Sundown Sunblock Stick SPF 20. (Johnson & Johnson) Octyl dimethyl PABA, octyl methoxycinnamate, oxybenzone, titanium dioxide. *otc.*
Use: Sunscreen.

Sundown Sunblock Ultra Lotion 30 SPF. (Johnson & Johnson) Octyl methoxycinnamate, octyl salicylate, oxybenzone, titanium dioxide, cetyl alcohol, PABA free. Waterproof. Lot. Bot. 120 ml. *otc.*
Use: Sunscreen.

Sundown Sunblock Ultra SPF 20. (Johnson & Johnson) Octyl dimethyl PABA, octyl methoxycinnamate, oxybenzone, titanium dioxide. *otc.*
Use: Sunscreen.

Sundown Sunscreen Stick SPF 8. (Johnson & Johnson) Octyl dimethyl PABA, oxybenzone. Stick 0.35 oz. *otc.*
Use: Sunscreen.

Sundown Sunscreen Ultra. (Johnson & Johnson) Octyl methoxycinnamate, octyl salicylate, oxybenzone, titanium dioxide, stearyl alcohol, cetyl alcohol, PABA free. Waterproof. SPF 15. Cream Tube 60 g. *otc.*
Use: Sunscreen.

•**sunepitron hydrochloride.** USAN.
Use: Anxiolytic, antidepressant.

Sunice. (Citroleum) Allantoin 0.25%, menthol 0.25%, methyl salicylate 10%/ Cream Jar 3 oz. *otc.*
Use: Burn therapy.

Sunkist Multivitamins Complete, Children's. (Novartis Pharmaceutical Corp.) Fe 18 mg, vitamin A 5000 IU, D_3 400 IU, E 30 IU, B_1 1.5 mg, B_2 1.7 mg, B_3 20 mg, B_5 10 mg, B_6 2 mg, B_{12} 6 mcg, C 60 mg, folic acid 400 mcg, Ca 100 mg, Cu, I, K, Mg, Mn, P, Zn 10 mg, biotin 40 mcg, K_1 10 mcg, sorbitol, aspartame, phenylalanine, tartrazine. Chew. Tab. Bot. 60s. *otc.*
Use: Mineral, vitamin supplement.

Sunkist Multivitamins + Extra C, Children's. (Novartis Pharmaceutical Corp.) Vitamin A 2500 IU, E 15 IU, D_3 400 IU, B_1 1.05 mg, B_2 1.2 mg, B_3 13.5 mg, B_6 1.05 mg, B_{12} 4.5 mcg, C 250 mg, folic acid 0.3 mg, vitamin K 5 mcg, sorbitol, aspartame, phenylalanine/ Chew. Tab. Bot. 60s. *otc.*
Use: Vitamin supplement.

Sunkist Multivitamins+ Iron, Children's. (Novartis Pharmaceutical Corp.) Fe 15 mg, vitamin A 2500 IU, E 15 IU, D_3 400 IU, E 30 IU, B_1 1.05 mg, B_2 1.2 mg, B_3 13.5 mg, B_6 1.05 mg, B_{12} 4.5 mcg, C 60 mg, folic acid 0.3 mg, K_1 5 mcg, sorbitol, aspartame, phenylalanine, tartrazine. Chew. Tab. Bot. 60s. *otc.*
Use: Vitamin/mineral supplement.

Sunkist Vitamin C. (Novartis Pharmaceutical Corp.) Vitamin C (as ascorbic acid) 500 mg. Capl. Bot. 60s. *otc.*
Use: Vitamin supplement.

Sunkist Vitamin C. (Novartis Pharmaceutical Corp.) Vitamin C (as ascorbic acid) 60 mg, sorbitol, sucrose, lactose. Chew. Tab. Pkg. 11s. *otc.*
Use: Vitamin supplement.

Sunkist Vitamin C. (Novartis Pharmaceutical Corp.) Vitamin C (as sodium ascorbate and ascorbic acid) 250 mg, 500 mg, fructose, sorbitol, sucrose, lactose. Chew. Tab. Bot. 60s. *otc.*
Use: Vitamin supplement.

SUNPRuF 15. (C & M Pharmacal, Inc.) Octyl methoxycinnamate 7.5%, benzopherone-3 5%. PABA free. Waterproof. SPF 15. Lot. Bot. 240 ml. *otc.*
Use: Sunscreen.

SUNPRuF 17. (C & M Pharmacal, Inc.) Octyl methoxycinnamate 7.8%, octyl salicylate 5.2%, oil-free, water-resistant. SPF 17. Lot. Bot. 120 g. *otc.*
Use: Sunscreen.

Sunshine Chewable Tablets. (Fibertone) Fe 5 mg, vitamins A 5000 IU, D 400 IU, E 67 mg, B_1 15 mg, B_2 15 mg, B_3 25 mg, B_5 20 mg, B_6 15 mg, B_{12} 15 mcg, C 150 mg, folic acid 0.1 mg, Ca,

Cu, Mn, Zn, K, iodide, biotin, betaine, PABA, choline bitartrate, inositol, lecithin, hesperidin, rutin, bioflavonoids, sorbitol, aspartame, citrus flavor/Chew. Tab. Bot. 60s. *otc.*
Use: Mineral, vitamin supplement.

Sunstick. (Rydelle Laboratories) Lip and face protectant containing digalloyl trioleate 2.5% in emollient base. Stick Plas. swivel container 0.14 oz. *otc.*
Use: Lip protectant.

SU-101.
Use: Malignant glioma. [Orphan Drug]

Supac. (Mission Pharmacal Co.) Acetaminophen 160 mg, aspirin 230 mg, caffeine 33 mg, calcium gluconate 60 mg/Tab. Bot. 100s. *otc.*
Use: Analgesic.

Super Aytinal Tablets. (Walgreen Co.) Vitamins A 7000 IU, B_1 5 mg, B_2 5 mg, B_5 10 mg, B_6 3 mg, B_{12} 9 mcg, C 90 mg, pantothenic acid 10 mg, D 400 IU, E 30 IU, niacin 30 mg, biotin 55 mcg, folic acid 0.4 mg, Fe 30 mg, Ca 162 mg, P 125 mg, I 150 mcg, Cu 3 mg, Mn 7.5 mg, Mg 100 mg, K 7.7 mg, Zn 24 mg, Cl 7 mg, Cr 15 mcg, Se 15 mcg, choline bitartrate 1000 mcg, inositol 1000 mcg, PABA 1000 mcg, rutin 1000 mcg, yeast 12 mg. Bot. 50s, 100s, 365s. *otc.*
Use: Mineral, vitamin supplement.

Super-B. (Towne) Vitamins B_1 50 mg, B_2 20 mg, B_6 5 mg, B_{12} 15 mcg, C 300 mg, liver desiccated 100 mg, dried yeast 100 mg, niacinamide 25 mg, Ca pantothenate 5 mg, Fe 10 mg/Captab. Bot. 50s, 100s, 150s, 250s. *otc.*
Use: Mineral, vitamin supplement.

Super Calicaps M-Z. (Nion Corp.) Ca 1200 mg, Mg 400 mg, Zn 15 mg, vitamins A 5000 IU, D 400 IU, Se 15 mcg/3 Tabs. Bot. 90s. *otc.*
Use: Mineral, vitamin supplement.

Super Calcium 1200. (Schiff Products) Calcium carbonate 1512 mg (600 mg calcium)/Cap. Bot. 60s, 120s. *otc.*
Use: Mineral supplement.

Super Citro Cee. (Marlyn Nutraceuticals, Inc.) Lemon bioflavonoids 500 mg, rutin 50 mg, ascorbic acid 500 mg, rosehips powder 500 mg. Tab. Bot. 50s, 100s, 200s. *otc.*
Use: Vitamin supplement.

Super Complex C-500. (Health for Life Brands, Inc.) Citrus hesperidin complex 25 mg, citrus bioflavonoid complex 100 mg, rutin 50 mg, ascorbic acid 500 mg, rose hips 100 mg, acerola, green pepper & black currant concentrate, sodium free. Tab. Bot. 100s. *otc.*
Use: Vitamin supplement.

Superdophilus. (Natren, Inc.) *Lactobacillus acidophilus* strain DDS 1.2 billion/g Pow. 37.5 g, 75 g, 135 g. *otc.*
Use: Antidiarrheal, nutritional supplement.

Super D Perles. (Pharmacia & Upjohn) Vitamins A 10,000 IU, D 400 IU/Cap. Bot. 100s. *otc.*
Use: Vitamin supplement.

SuperEPA. (Advanced Nutritional Technology) Omega-3 polyunsaturated fatty acids 1200 mg/Cap. containing EPA 360 mg, DHA 240 mg. Bot. 60s, 90s. *otc.*
Use: Nutritional supplement.

Superepa 2000. (Advanced Nutritional Technology) EPA 563 mg, DHA 312 mg, vitamin E 20 IU. Cap. Bot. 30s, 60s, 90s. *otc.*
Use: Nutritional supplement.

Supere-Pect. (Barth's) Alpha tocopherol 400 IU, apple pectin 100 mg/Cap. Bot. 50s, 100s, 250s. *otc.*
Use: Nutritional supplement.

Super Hi Potency. (Nion Corp.) Vitamins A 10,000 IU, D 400 IU, E 150 IU, B_1 75 mg, B_2 75 mg, B_3 75 mg, B_5 75 mg, B_6 75 mg, B_{12} 75 mcg, C 250 mg, folic acid 0.4 mg, Zn 15 mg, betaine, biotin 75 mcg, Ca, Fe, hesperidin, I, K, Mg, Mn, Se/Tab. Bot. 100s. *otc.*
Use: Mineral, vitamin supplement.

Super Hydramin Protein Powder. (Nion Corp.) Protein 41%, carbohydrate 21.8%, fat 1% in powder form. Cans 1 lb. *otc.*
Use: Nutritional supplement.

superinone. Tyloxapol.

Super Nutri-Vites. (Faraday) Vitamins A 36,000 IU, D 400 IU, B_1 25 mg, B_2 25 mg, B_6 50 mg, B_{12} 50 mcg, niacinamide 50 mg, Ca pantothenate 12.5 mg, choline bitartrate 150 mg, inositol 150 mg, betaine HCl 25 mg, PABA 15 mg, glutamic acid 25 mg, desiccated liver 50 mg, C 150 mg, E 12.5 IU, Mn gluconate 6.15 mg, bone meal 162 mg, Fe gluconate 50 mg, Cu gluconate 0.25 mg, Zn gluconate 2.2 mg, K iodide 0.1 mg, Ca 53.3 mg, P 24.3 mg, Mg gluconate 7.2 mg/Protein Coated Tab. Bot. 60s, 100s. *otc.*
Use: Mineral, vitamin supplement.

superoxide dismutase (human, recombinant human).
Use: Protection of donor organ tissue. [Orphan Drug]

Super Plenamins Multiple Vitamins and Minerals. (Rexall Group) Vitamins A 8000 IU, D_2 400 IU, vitamins B_1 2.5

mg, B_2 2.5 mg, C 75 mg, niacinamide 20 mg, B_6 1 mg, B_{12} 3 mcg, biotin 20 mcg, E 10 IU, pantothenic acid 3 mg, liver conc. 100 mg, Fe 30 mg, Ca 75 mg, P 58 mg, I 0.15 mg, Cu 0.75 mg, manganese 1.25 mg, Mg 10 mg, Zn 1 mg/Tab. Bot. 36s, 72s, 144s, 288s, 365s. *otc.*
Use: Mineral, vitamin supplement.

Superplex T. (Major Pharmaceuticals) Vitamins B_1 15 mg, B_2 10 mg, B_3 100 mg, B_5 20 mg, B_6 5 mg, B_{12} 10 mcg, C 500 mg/Tab. Bot. 100s. *otc.*
Use: Vitamin supplement.

Super Poli-Grip/Wernet's Cream. (Block Drug Co., Inc.) Carboxymethylcellulose gum, ethylene oxide polymer, petrolatum-mineral oil base. Tube 0.7 oz, 1.4 oz, 2.4 oz. *otc.*
Use: Denture adhesive.

Super Quints-50. (Freeda Vitamins, Inc.) Vitamins B_1 50 mg, B_2 50 mg, B_3 50 mg, B_5 50 mg, B_6 50 mg, B_{12} 50 mcg, folic acid 0.4 mg, PABA 30 mg, d-biotin 50 mcg, inositol 50 mg. Tab. Bot. 100s, 250s, 500s. *otc.*
Use: Vitamin supplement.

Super Shade SPF-25. (Schering-Plough Corp.) Ethylhexyl p-methoxycinnamate, padimate O oxybenzone. SPF 25. Lot. Bot. 4 fl. oz. *otc.*
Use: Sunscreen.

Super Shade Sunblock Stick SPF-25. (Schering-Plough Corp.) Ethylhexyl p-methoxycinnamate, oxybenzone, padimate O in stick. SPF 25. Tube 0.43 oz. *otc.*
Use: Sunscreen.

Super Stress. (Towne) Vitamins C 600 mg, E 30 IU B_1 15 mg, B_2 15 mg, niacin 100 mg, B_6 5 mg, B_{12} 12 mcg, pantothenic acid 20 mg/Tab. Bot. 60s. *otc.*
Use: Vitamin supplement.

Super Troche. (Weeks & Leo) Benzocaine 5 mg, cetalkonium Cl 1 mg/lozenge. Bot. 15s, 30s. *otc.*
Use: Mouth and throat preparation.

Super Troche Plus. (Weeks & Leo) Benzocaine 10 mg, cetalkonium Cl 2 mg/Loz. Bot. 12s. *otc.*
Use: Mouth and throat preparation.

Super-T with Zinc. (Towne) Vitamins A 10,000 IU, D 400 IU, E 15 IU, C 200 mg, B_1 10 mg, B_2 10 mg, B_6 5 mg, B_{12} 6 mcg, niacinamide 50 mg, Fe 18 mg, I 0.1 mg, Cu 2 mg, Mn 1 mg, Zn 15 mg/Cap. Bot. 130s. *otc.*
Use: Mineral, vitamin supplement.

Supervim. (U.S. Ethicals) Vitamins and minerals. Tab. Bot. 100s.
Use: Mineral, vitamin supplement.

Super Wernet's Powder. (Block Drug Co., Inc.) Carboxymethylcellulose gum, ethylene oxide polymer. Bot. 0.63 oz, 1.75 oz, 3.55 oz. *otc.*
Use: Denture adhesive.

Suplena. (Ross Laboratories) A vanilla flavored liquid containing 29.6 g protein, 252.5 g carbohydrates, 95 g fat/L. With appropriate vitamins and minerals. Cans 240 ml. *otc.*
Use: Nutritional supplement.

Suplical. (Parke-Davis) Calcium 600 mg/Square. Bot. 30s, 60s. *otc.*
Use: Mineral supplement.

Suppap-120. (Raway Pharmacal, Inc.) Acetaminophen 120 mg/Supp. 12s, 50s, 100s, 500s, 1000s. *otc.*
Use: Analgesic.

Suppap-650. (Raway Pharmacal, Inc.) Acetaminophen 650 mg/Supp. 50s, 100s, 500s, 1000s. *otc.*
Use: Analgesic.

Supprelin. (Roberts Pharmaceuticals) Histrelin acetate 200 mcg, 300 mcg, 600 mcg/ml. Inj. Vials 0.6 ml. *Rx.*
Use: Hormone.

Suppress. (Ferndale Laboratories, Inc.) Dextromethorphan HBr 7.5 mg/Loz. 1000s. *otc.*
Use: Antitussive.

Supra Min. (Towne) Vitamins A 10,000 IU, D 400 IU, E 30 IU, C 250 mg, folic acid 0.4 mg, B_1 10 mg, B_2 10 mg, niacin 100 mg, B_6 5 mg, B_{12} 6 mcg, pantothenic acid 20 mg, I 150 mcg, Fe 100 mg, Mg 2 mg, Cu 20 mg, Mn 1.25 mg/Tab. Bot. 130s. *otc.*
Use: Mineral, vitamin supplement.

Suprane. (Ohmeda Pharmaceuticals) Desflurane. 240 ml. Volatile Liq. Bot. *Rx.*
Use: Anesthetic, general.

Suprarenal. Dried, partially defatted and powdered adrenal gland of cattle, sheep or swine.

Suprax. (ESI Lederle Generics) Cefixime. **Tab.:** 200 mg, Bot. 100s, 400 mg, 50s, 100s UD 10s, unit-of-use 10s. **Pow. for Oral Susp.:** (strawberry flavor) 100 mg/5 ml. Bot. 50 ml, 75 ml, 100 ml. *Rx.*
Use: Anti-infective, cephalosporin.

Suprazine Tabs. (Major Pharmaceuticals) Trifluoperazine 1 mg/Tab. Bot. 100s, 250s, 1000s; 2 mg/Tab. Bot. 100s, 250s, 1000s, UD 100s; 5 mg/Tab. Bot. 100s, 250s, 1000s; 10 mg/Tab. Bot. 100s, 250s, 1000s. *Rx.*
Use: Anxiolytic.

Suprins. (Towne) Vitamins A palmitate

10,000 IU, D 400 IU, B_1 10 mg, B_2 10 mg, B_6 5 mg, B_{12} 6 mcg, C 250 mg, calcium pantothenate 20 mg, niacinamide 100 mg, biotin 25 mcg, E 15 IU, Ca 103 mg, P 80 mg, Fe 10 mg, I 0.1 mg, Cu 1.0 mg, Zn 20 mg, Mn 1.25 mg/Captab. Bot. 100s. *otc.*
Use: Mineral, vitamin supplement.

•**suproclone.** (SUH-pro-klone) USAN.
Use: Sedative, hypnotic.

•**suprofen.** (sue-PRO-fen) U.S.P. 23.
Use: Anti-inflammatory.
See: Profenal (Alcon Laboratories, Inc.).

•**suramin hexasodium.** (SOOR-ah-min hex-ah-SO-dee-uhm) USAN. U.S.P. XVII.
Use: Antineoplastic.

Surbex Filmtab. (Abbott Laboratories) Vitamins B_1 6 mg, B_2 6 mg, B_3 30 mg, B_6 2.5 mg, B_5 10 mg, B_{12} 5 mcg/Filmtab. Bot. 100s. *otc.*
Use: Mineral, vitamin supplement.

Surbex-T Filmtab. (Abbott Laboratories) Vitamins B_1 15 mg, B_2 10 mg, B_3 100 mg, B_6 5 mg, B_{12} 10 mcg, B_5 20 mg, C 500 mg/Filmtab. Bot. 100s. *otc.*
Use: Mineral, vitamin supplement.

Surbex with C Filmtabs. (Abbott Laboratories) Vitamins B_1 6 mg, B_2 6 mg, B_3 30 mg, B_5 10 mg, B_6 2.5 mg, B_{12} 5 mg, C 500 mg/Film coated. Tab. Bot. 100s. *otc.*
Use: Vitamin supplement.

Surbex 750 with Iron. (Abbott Laboratories) Vitamins B_1 15 mg, B_2 15 mg, B_6 25 mg, B_{12} 12 mcg, C 750 mg, B_5 20 mg, E 30 IU, B_3 100 mg, Fe 27 mg, folic acid 0.4 mg/Tab. Bot. 50s. *otc.*
Use: Mineral, vitamin supplement.

Surbex 750 with Zinc. (Abbott Laboratories) B_1 15 mg, B_2 15 mg, B_6 20 mg, B_{12} 12 mcg, C 750 mg, E 30 IU, B_5 20 mg, niacin 100 mg, folic acid 0.4 mg, Zn 22.5 mg/Tab. Bot. 50s. *otc.*
Use: Mineral, vitamin supplement.

Surbu-Gen-T. (Zenith Goldline Pharmaceuticals) Vitamins B_1 15 mg, B_2 10 mg, B_3 100 mg, B_5 20 mg, B_6 5 mg, B_{12} 10 mcg, C 500 mg/Tab. Bot. 100s. *otc.*
Use: Vitamin supplement.

SureCell HCG-Urine Test. (Kodak Dental) Polyclonal/monoclonal antibody sandwich-based ELISA to detect human chorionic gonadotropin in urine. Kit 10s, 25s, 100s.
Use: Diagnostic aid.

SureCell Herpes (HSV) Test. (Kodak Dental) Monoclonal antibody-based ELISA to detect HSV 1 & 2 antigens from lesions. Kit 10s, 25s.
Use: Diagnostic aid.

SureCell Strep A Test. (Kodak Dental) ELISA to detect group A streptococci. Kit 10s, 25s, 100s.
Use: Diagnostic aid.

SureLac. (Caraco Pharmaceutical Labs, Ltd.) 3000 FCC lactase units, sorbitol, mannitol. Chew. Tab. Bot. 60s. *otc.*
Use: Nutritional supplement.

surface active extract of saline lavage of bovine lungs.
Use: Respiratory failure in preterm infants. [Orphan Drug]

surfactant, natural lung.
Use: Surfactant replacement therapy in neonatal respiratory distress syndrome.
See: Survanta (Ross Laboratories).

surfactant, synthetic lung.
Use: Surfactant replacement therapy in neonatal respiratory distress syndrome.
See: Exosurf Neonatal (Glaxo-Wellcome).

Surfak. (Pharmacia & Upjohn) Docusate calcium. 50 mg: 30s, 100s. 240 mg: 30s, 100s, 500s, UD 100s. Cap. *otc.*
Use: Laxative.

•**surfilcon a.** (SER-FILL-kahn A) USAN.
Use: Hydrophilic contact lens material.

Surfol Post-Immersion Bath Oil. (Stiefel Laboratories, Inc.) Mineral oil, isopropyl myristate, isostearic acid, PEG-40, sorbitan peroleate. Bot. 8 oz. *otc.*
Use: Dermatologic.

•**surfomer.** (SER-foe-mer) USAN.
Use: Hypolipidemic.

Surgasoap. (Wade) Castile vegetable oils. Bot. Qt., gal. *otc.*
Use: Dermatologic, cleanser.

Surgel. (Ulmer Pharmacal Co.) Propylene glycol, glycerin. Gel. 120 ml, 240 ml, gal. *otc.*
Use: Lubricant.

Surgel Liquid. (Ulmer Pharmacal Co.) Patient lubricant fluid. Bot. 4 oz, 8 oz, gal.
Use: Lubricant.

•**surgibone.** (SER-jih-bone) USAN. Bone and cartilage obtained from bovine embryos and young calves.
Use: Prosthetic aid (internal bone splint).

Surgical Simplex P. (Howmedica) Methyl methacrylate 20 ml poly 6.7 g, methyl methacrylate-styrene copolymer 33.3 g. **Pow.:** 40 g. **Liq.:** 20 ml.
Use: Bone cement.

Surgical Simplex P Radiopaque. (How-

medica) Methyl methacrylate 20 ml, poly 6 g, methyl methacrylate-styrene copolymer 30 g. **Pow.:** 40 g. **Liq.:** 20 ml.
Use: Bone cement.

Surgicel. (Johnson & Johnson) Sterile absorbable knitted fabric prepared by controlled oxidation of regenerated cellulose. Sterile strips 2 x 14, 4 x 8, 2 x 3, 0.5 x 2 inches. Surgical Nu-knit: 1 x 1, 3 x 4, 6 x 9 inches. 1s.
Use: Hemostatic.

Surgidine. (Continental Consumer Products) Iodine 0.8% in iodine complex. Germicide. Bot. 8 oz, gal. Foot operated dispenser 8 oz, gal. *otc.*
Use: Antiseptic.

Surgi-Kleen. (Sween) Bot. 2 oz, 8 oz, 16 oz, 21 oz, gal, 5 gal, 30 gal, 55 gal.
Use: Dermatologic, cleanser.

Surgilube. (Day-Baldwin) Sterile-bacteriostatic. Foilpac: 3 g, 5 g, Tube: 5 g, 2 oz, 4.5 oz.
Use: Lubricant.

Surgilube. (E. Fougera and Co.) Sterile surgical lubricant. Foilpac: 3 g, 5 g; Tube 5 g, 2 oz, 4.25 oz.
Use: Lubricant.

•**suricainide maleate.** (ser-ih-CANE-ide) USAN.
Use: Cardiovascular agent (antiarrhythmic).

•**suritozole.** (suh-RIH-tah-ZOLE) USAN.
Use: Antidepressant.

Surmontil. (Wyeth-Ayerst Laboratories) Trimipramine maleate 25 mg, 50 mg, 100 mg/Cap. Bot. 100s. Redipaks. *Rx.*
Use: Antidepressant.

surofene. Hexachlorophene.

•**suronacrine maleate.** (SUE-row-NAH-kreen) USAN.
Use: Cholinergic, cholinesterase inhibitor.

Survanta. (Ross Laboratories) Beractant 25 mg/ml. Inj. Vial 8 ml. *Rx.*
Use: Lung surfactant.

Susano Elixir. (Halsey Drug Co.) Phenobarbital 0.25 gr, hyoscyamine sulfate 0.1037 mg, atropine sulfate 0.0194 mg, scopolamine HBr 0.0065 mg/5 ml. 23% alcohol, tartrazine. Bot. 16 oz, gal. *Rx.*
Use: Antispasmodic, sedative.

Suspen. (Circle Pharmaceuticals, Inc.) Penicillin V potassium 250 mg/5 ml. Bot. 100 ml. *Rx.*
Use: Anti-infective, penicillin.

Sus-Phrine. (Forest Pharmaceutical, Inc.) Epinephrine 1:200 Inj. Amp. 0.3 ml, Vial 5 ml. *Rx.*
Use: Bronchodilator, sympathomimetic.

Sustacal Basic. (Bristol-Myers Squibb) A vanilla, strawberry, or chocolate flavored liquid containing 36.6 g protein, 34.6 g fat, 145.8 g carbohydrate, 833 mg Na, 1583 mg K/L. 1.04 Cal/ml, with appropriate vitamin and mineral levels to meet 100% of the US RDAs. Liq. Can 240 ml. *otc.*
Use: Nutritional supplement.

Sustacal HC. (Bristol-Myers Squibb) High calorie nutritionally complete food. Protein 16%, fat 34%, carbohydrate 50%. Can 8 oz. Vanilla, chocolate, or eggnog. *otc.*
Use: Nutritional supplement.

Sustacal Plus. (Bristol-Myers Squibb) A vanilla, eggnog, or chocolate flavored liquid containing 61 g protein, 58 g fat, 190 g carbohydrate, 15.2 mg Fe, 850 mg Na, 1480 mg K, 1520 cal/L, with appropriate vitamin and mineral levels to meet 100% of the US RDAs. Liq. Bot. 237 ml, 960 ml. *otc.*
Use: Nutritional supplement.

Sustacal Powder. (Bristol-Myers Squibb) Caloric distribution and nutritional value when added to milk are similar to that of Sustacal liquid except lactose. Contains vanilla: Pow. 1.9 oz. packets 4s, 1 lb. can; Chocolate 1.9 oz. packets 4s. *otc.*
Use: Nutritional supplement.

Sustacal Pudding. (Bristol-Myers Squibb) Ready-to-eat fortified pudding containing at least 15% of the US RDAs for protein, vitamins and minerals, in a 240 calorie serving. As a % of the calories, protein 11%, fat 36%, carbohydrate 53%. Flavors: Chocolate, vanilla, and butterscotch. Tins, 5 oz, 110 oz. *otc.*
Use: Nutritional supplement.

Sustagen. (Bristol-Myers Squibb) High-calorie, high-protein supplement containing as a % of the calories, 24% protein, 8% fat, 68% carbohydrate. Contains all known essential vitamins and minerals. Prepared from nonfat milk, corn syrup solids, powdered whole milk, calcium caseinate, and dextrose. Vanilla: Can 1 lb, 5 lb. Chocolate: Can 1 lb. *otc.*
Use: Nutritional supplement.

Sustaire. (Pfizer US Pharmaceutical Group) Theophylline 100 mg, 300 mg/ SR Tab. Bot. 100s. *Rx.*
Use: Bronchospasm therapy.

Sustiva. (Du Pont Merck Pharmaceuticalsceuticals) Efavirenz 50 mg, 100 mg, 200 mg. Cap. Bot. 30s, 90s (200 mg only). *Rx.*

Use: Antiviral.

•**suture, absorbable surgical.** U.S.P. 23.
Use: Surgical aid.

•**suture, nonabsorbable surgical.** U.S.P. 23.
Use: Surgical aid.

Suvaplex Tablet. (Tennessee Pharmaceutic) Vitamins A 5000 IU, D 500 IU, B_1 2.5 mg, B_2 2.5 mg, B_6 0.5 mg, B_{12} 1 mcg, C 37.5 mg, Ca pantothenate 5 mg, niacinamide 20 mg, folic acid 0.1 mg/Tab. Bot. 100s. *otc.*
Use: Mineral, vitamin supplement.

•**suxemerid sulfate.** (sux-EM-er-rid) USAN.
Use: Antitussive.

swamp root. Compound of various organic roots in an alcohol base.
Use: Diuretic to the kidney.

Sween-A-Peel. (Sween) Wafer 4 x 4. Box 5s, 20s; Sheets 1212. Box 2s, 12s.
Use: Dermatologic, protectant.

Sween Cream. (Sween) Vitamin A and D cream. Tube 0.5 oz, 2 oz, 5 oz. Jar 2 oz, 9 oz. *otc.*
Use: Dermatologic.

Sween Kind Lotion. (Sween) Bot. 21 oz, gal.
Use: Dermatologic, cleanser.

Sween Prep. (Sween) Box wipes 54s. Dab-o-matic 2 oz. Spray Top 4 oz.
Use: Dermatologic, protectant, medicated.

Sween Soft Touch. (Sween) Bot. 2 oz, 16 oz, 21 oz, 32 oz, 1 gal., 5 gal.
Use: Dermatologic, protectant, medicated.

Sweeta. (Bristol-Myers Squibb) Saccharin sodium, sorbitol. Bot. 24 ml, 2 oz, 4 oz. *otc.*
Use: Sweetening agent.

Sweetaste. (Purepac Pharmaceutical Co.) Saccharin 0.25 g, 0.5 g, 1 g/Tab. w/Sodium bicarbonate. Bot. 1000s. *otc.*
Use: Sugar substitute.

sweetening agents.
See: Saccharin, Preps. (Various Mfr.).
Sweetaste, Tab. (Purepac Pharmaceutical Co.).

Sweet'n Fresh Clotrimazole-7. (Nutra-Max Products) **Cream:** Clotrimazole 1%, benzyl and cetostearyl alcohol. 45 g. **Vaginal inserts:** Clotrimazole 100 mg. 7s. *otc.*
Use: Antifungal, vaginal.

Swim-Ear. (E. Fougera and Co.) 2.75% boric acid in isopropyl alcohol. Bot. 1 oz. *otc.*
Use: Otic.

Swiss Kriss. (Modern Aids Inc.) Senna leaves, herbs. Coarse cut mixture. Can 1.5 oz, 3.25 oz, Tab. 24s, 120s, 250s. *otc.*
Use: Laxative.

Syllact. (Wallace Laboratories) Psyllium seed husks 3.3 g/tsp., saccharin. Pow. Bot. 11 oz. *otc.*
Use: Laxative.

Syllamalt. (Wallace Laboratories) Malt soup extract 4 g, psyllium seed husks 3 g, calories/rounded tsp 13. Pow. 300 g. *otc.*
Use: Laxative.

•**symclosene.** (SIM-kloe-seen) USAN.
Use: Anti-infective, topical.

•**symetine hydrochloride.** (SIM-eh-teen) USAN.
Use: Antiamebic.

Symmetrel. (Du Pont Merck Pharmaceutical Co.) Amantadine HCl. 50 mg/5 ml. Syr. Bot. Pt. *Rx.*
Use: Antiviral, antiparkinsonian, treatment of drug-induced extrapyramidal symptoms.

sympatholytic agents.
See: Adrenergic-Blocking Agents.
D.H.E. 45, Amp. (Novartis Pharmaceutical Corp.).
Dibenzyline, Cap. (SmithKline Beecham Pharmaceuticals).
Dihydroergotamine.
Ergotamine Tartrate.

sympathomimetic agents.
See: Adrenalin (Parke-Davis).
Adrenergic agents.
Aerolate Sr. & Jr., Cap. (Fleming & Co.).
Afrin, Preps. (Schering-Plough Corp.).
Miles Diagnostic, Enseal, Pulvule (Eli Lilly and Co.).
Aramine, Amp., Vial (Merck & Co.).
Brethine, Amp., Tab. (Novartis Pharmaceutical Corp.).
Bronkometer (Sanofi Winthrop Pharmaceuticals).
Bronkosol Soln. (Sanofi Winthrop Pharmaceuticals).
Demazin, Tab., Syr. (Schering-Plough Corp.).
Desoxyn, Gradumet, Tab. (Abbott Laboratories).
Dexedrine, Elix., Spansule, Tab. (SmithKline Beecham Pharmaceuticals).
Didrex, Liq., Tab. (Pharmacia & Upjohn).
Dipivefrin HCl, Soln. (Schein Pharmaceutical, Inc.).
Ephedrine preps.
Epinephrine salts.
Extendryl, Cap., Syr., Tab. (Fleming & Co.).

Fiogesic, Tab. (Novartis Pharmaceutical Corp.).
Isoephedrine HCl.
Isuprel HCl, Preps. (Sanofi Winthrop Pharmaceuticals).
Levophed Bitartrate, Amp. (Sanofi Winthrop Pharmaceuticals).
Metaproterenol Sulfate (Various Mfr.).
Neo-Synephrine HCl, Preps. (Sanofi Winthrop Pharmaceuticals).
Nolamine, Tab. (Carnrick Laboratories, Inc.).
Norisodrine Sulfate, Soln. (Abbott Laboratories).
Orthoxine, Orthoxine & Aminophylline (Pharmacia & Upjohn).
Orthoxine HCl, Tab., Syr. (Pharmacia & Upjohn).
Otrivin, Soln., Spray (Novartis Pharmaceutical Corp.).
Phenylephrine HCl, Preps.
Phenylpropanolamine HCl.
Pseudoephedrine HCl, Syr., Tab. (Various Mfr.).
Rondec DSC & T. (Ross Laboratories).
Sudafed, Tab., Syr. (GlaxoWellcome).
Triaminic, Prep. (Novartis Pharmaceutical Corp.).
Triaminicol, Syr. (Novartis Pharmaceutical Corp.).
Ursinus, Tab. (Novartis Pharmaceutical Corp.).
Vasoxyl HCl, Amp, Vial (GlaxoWellcome).
Wyamine Sulfate, Amp, Vial (Wyeth-Ayerst Laboratories).

Syna-Clear. (Pruvo) Decongestant plus Vitamin C. 25 mg/Tab. Bot. 12s, 30s.
Use: Decongestant.

Synacol CF. (Roberts Pharmaceuticals) Dextromethorphan HBr 15 mg, guiafenesin 200 mg/Tab. Bot. UD 8s, 500s. *otc.*
Use: Antitussive, expectorant.

Synacort. (Roche Laboratories) Hydrocortisone cream. **1%:** Tube 15 g, 30 g, 60 g. **2.5%:** Tube 30 g. *Rx.*
Use: Corticosteroid, topical.

Synagis. (MedImmune) Palivizumab 100 mg, histidine 47 mM, glycine 3 mM, mannitol 5.6%. Inj., lyophilized. Single-use vial 100 mg. *Rx.*
Use: Antibody.

Synalar. (Roche Laboratories) Fluocinolone acetonide. **Cream: 0.01%:** Tube 15 g, 30 g, 45 g, 60 g, 120 g. Jar 425 g. **0.025%:** Tube 15 g, 30 g, 60 g, 120 g. Jar 425 g. **Oint.: 0.025%:** Tube 15 g, 30 g, 60 g, 120 g. Jar 425 g. **Soln. 0.01%:** Bot. 20 ml, 60 ml. *Rx.*
Use: Corticosteroid, topical.

Synalar-HP Cream. (Roche Laboratories) Fluocinolone acetonide 0.2% in water-washable aqueous base. Tube 12 g. *Rx.*
Use: Corticosteroid, topical.

Synalgos-DC Capsules. (Wyeth-Ayerst Laboratories) Dihydrocodeine bitartrate 16 mg, aspirin 356.4 mg, caffeine 30 mg/Cap. Bot. 100s, 500s. *c-III.*
Use: Analgesic combination, narcotic.

Synapp-R. (Halsey Drug Co.) Acetaminophen 325 mg, phenylpropanolamine HCl 25 mg, phenyltoloxamine citrate 22 mg/Tab. Bot. 40s. *otc.*
Use: Analgesic, decongestant.

Synarel. (Roche Laboratories) Nafarelin acetate 2 mg/ ml (as nafarelin base). Nasal solution. Bot. 10 ml with metered pump spray. *Rx.*
Use: Endometriosis.

Synatuss-One. (Freeport) Guaifenesin 100 mg, dextromethorphan HBr. 15 mg, alcohol 1.4%/5 ml. Bot. 4 oz. *otc.*
Use: Antitussive.

Syncaine.
See: Procaine Hydrochloride, Inj., Tab. (Various Mfr.).

Syncort.
See: Desoxycorticosterone Acetate, Inj., Pellets (Various Mfr.).

Syncortyl.
See: Desoxycorticosterone Acetate, Inj., Pellets (Various Mfr.).

Syndolor Capsules. (Knight) Bot. 100s, 1000s.
Use: Analgesic.

Synemol. (Roche Laboratories) Fluocinolone acetonide 0.025% in water-washable aqueous emollient base. Tube 15 g, 30 g, 60 g, 120 g. *Rx.*
Use: Corticosteroid, topical.

synkonin.
See: Hydrocodone (Various Mfr.).

Synophylate. (Schwarz Pharma, Inc.) Theophylline sodium glycinate. **Elix.:** Theophylline 165 mg/15 ml w/alcohol 20%. Bot. Pt, gal. **Tab.:** Theophylline 165 mg/Tab. Bot. 100s, 1000s. *Rx.*
Use: Bronchodilator.

Synophylate-GG. (Schwarz Pharma, Inc.) Theophylline sodium glycinate 300 mg, guaifenesin 100 mg. **Syr.:** 10% alcohol, pt, gal. *Rx.*
Use: Bronchodilator.

Syn-Rx. (Medeva Pharmaceuticals, Inc.) **AM:** Pseudoephedrine HCl 60 mg, guiafenesin 600 mg/CR Tab. Bot. 28s. **PM:** Guaifenesin 600 mg/CR Tab. Bot. 28s. In 14-day treatment regimen of 56 tablets. *Rx.*

Use: Decongestant, expectorant.

Synsorb Pk.
Use: Verocytotoxogenic *E. coli* infections. [Orphan Drug]

Synthaloids. (Buffington) Benzocaine, calcium-iodine complex/Loz. Salt free. Bot. 100s, 1000s. Unit boxes 8s, 16s. Box 24s. Dispens-a-Kit 500s. Aidpaks 100s. Medipaks 200s. *otc.*
Use: Sore throat relief.

synthetic conjugated estrogens, a.
Use: Estrogen.
See: Cenestin (Duramed).

synthetic lung surfactant.
See: Exosurf Neonatal (Glaxo-Wellcome).

synthoestrin.
See: Diethylstilbestrol, Preps. (Various Mfr.).

Synthroid. (Knoll Pharmaceuticals) Sodium levothyroxine 25 mcg, 50 mcg, 75 mcg, 88 mcg, 100 mcg, 112 mcg, 125 mcg, 137 mcg, 150 mcg, 200 mcg, 300 mcg/Tab. Bot. 100s (all), 1000s (except 88 mcg, 200 mcg), UD 100s (except 25 mcg, 88 mcg, 200 mcg). *Rx.*
Use: Hormone, thyroid.

Synthroid Injection. (Knoll Pharmaceuticals) Lyophilized sodium levothyroxine 200 mcg, 500 mcg/vial. (100 mcg/ml when reconstituted.) Vial 10 ml. *Rx.*
Use: Hormone, thyroid.

Synvisc. (Wyeth-Ayerst Laboratories) Sodium hyaluronate/hylan G-F 20 16 mg/2 ml. Glass syringe 2.25 ml. *Rx.*
Use: Antiarthritic.

Syphilis (FTA-ABS) Fluoro Kit. (Clinical Sciences)
Use: Test for syphilis.

Syprine. (Merck & Co.) Trientine HCl 250 mg/Cap. Bot. 100s. *Rx.*
Use: Chelating agent.

Syracol. (Roberts Pharmaceuticals) Phenylpropanolamine HCl 12.5 mg, dextromethorphan 7.5 mg Liq. 60 ml, 120 ml. *otc.*
Use: Antitussive, decongestant.

Syracol CF. (Roberts Pharmaceuticals) Dextromethorphan HBr 15 mg, guaifenesin 200 mg/Tab. Bot. 500s. *otc.*
Use: Antitussive, expectorant.

Syroxine Tabs. (Major Pharmaceuticals) Sodium levothyroxine 0.1 mg, 0.2 mg, 0.3 mg/Tab. Bot. 100s, 250s, 1000s, UD 100s. (3 mg 1000s). *Rx.*
Use: Hormone, thyroid.

Syrpalta. (Emerson Laboratories) Syr. containing comb. of fruit flavors. Bot. Pt, gal.
Use: Pharmaceutical aid.

•**syrup.** N.F. 18.
Use: Pharmaceutic aid (flavor).

Syrvite. (Various Mfr.) Vitamins A 2500 IU, D 400 IU, E 15 mg, B_1 1.05 mg, B_2 1.2 mg, B_3 13.5 mg, B_6 1.05 mg, B_{12} 4.5 mcg, C 60 mg/5 ml Liq. Bot. 480 ml. *otc.*
Use: Vitamin supplement.

T

T-3 RIAbead. (Abbott Diagnostics) Test kit 50s, 100s.
Use: Diagnostic aid, thyroid.

T4.
See: levothyroxine sodium.

T4 endonuclease v, liposome encapsulated.
Use: Xeroderma pigmentosum. [Orphan Drug]

T-4 RIA (PEG). (Abbott Diagnostics) Diagnostic kit 50s, 100s, 500s.
Use: For quantitative measurement of total circulating serum thyroxine.

T4, soluble, human recombinant. (Biogen) Phase I/II HIV.
Use: Antiviral.

TA. (Wampole Laboratories) Antithyroid antibodies by IFA. Test 48s.
Use: Diagnostic aid, thyroid.

Tabasyn. (Freeport) Chlorpheniramine maleate 2 mg, phenylephrine HCl 10 mg, acetaminophen 5 g, salicylamide 5 g/Tab. Bot. 1000s. *Rx.*
Use: Analgesic, antihistamine, decongestant.

Tab-A-Vite. (Major Pharmaceuticals) Vitamins A 5000 IU, D 400 IU, E 30 IU, B_1 1.5 mg, B_2 1.7 mg, B_3 20 mg, B_5 10 mg, B_6 2 mg, B_{12} 6 mcg, C 60 mg, FA 0.4 mg/Tab. Bot. 30s, 100s, 250s, 1000s, UD 100s. *otc.*
Use: Mineral, vitamin supplement.

Tab-A-Vite + Iron. (Major Pharmaceuticals) Fe 18 mg, vitamins A 5000 IU, D 400 IU, E 30 IU, B_1 1.5 mg, B_2 1.7 mg, B_3 20 mg, B_5 10 mg, B_6 2 mg, B_{12} 6 mcg, C 60 mg, FA 0.4 mg, tartrazine/Tab. Bot. 100s. *otc.*
Use: Mineral, vitamin supplement.

Tac-3. (Allergan, Inc.) Triamcinolone acetonide 3 mg/ml. Susp. Vial 5 ml. *Rx.*
Use: Corticosteroid.

Tac-40. (Parnell Pharmaceuticals, Inc.) Triamcinolone acetonide 40 mg/ml. Inj. Susp. Vial 5 ml. *Rx.*
Use: Corticosteroid.

Tacaryl. (Westwood Squibb Pharmaceuticals) Methdilazine 3.6 mg/Chew. Tab. Bot. 100s. *Rx.*
Use: Antipruritic.

tachysterol.
See: Dihydrotachysterol, Tab. (Roxane Laboratories, Inc.).

Tacitin. (Novartis Pharmaceutical Corp.) Under study. Benzoctamine, B.A.N.

•**taclamine hydrochloride.** (TACK-lah-meen) USAN.
Use: Anxiolytic.

TA Cream. (C & M Pharmacal, Inc.) Triamcinolone acetonide 0.025% or 0.05%. Jar 2 oz., 8 oz., 1 lb. *Rx.*
Use: Corticosteroid, topical.

•**tacrine hydrochloride.** (TACK-reen) USAN.
Use: Cognition adjuvant.
See: Cognex, Cap. (Parke-Davis).

•**tacrolimus.** (tack-CROW-lih-muss) USAN.
Use: Immunosuppressant.
See: Prograf (Fujisawa USA, Inc.).

Tagamet. (SmithKline Beecham Pharmaceuticals) Cimetidine. **FC Tab., 200 mg:** Bot. 100s. **300 mg:** Bot. 100s, UD 100s. **400 mg:** Bot. 60s, UD 100s. **800 mg:** Bot. 30s, UD 100s. **Liq.:** 300 mg (as HCl)/5 ml 2.8% alcohol. Bot. 240 ml, UD 5 ml (10s). **Inj., 300 mg:** (as HCl) 2 ml with phenol in an aqueous solution. Single-dose vials, disp. syringes, ADD-Vantage vials, 8 ml Vials. **300 mg:** (as HCl) in 50 ml 0.9% sodium chloride. Single-dose container. *Rx.*
Use: Antiulcerative.

Tagamet HB. (SmithKline Beecham Pharmaceuticals) Cimetidine 100 mg/Tab. Bot. 16s, 32s, 64s. *otc.*
Use: Antiulcerative.

Talacen. (Sanofi Winthrop Pharmaceuticals) Pentazocine HCl 25 mg, acetaminophen 650 mg/Capl. Bot. 100s. UD 250s. (10 x 25s). *c-IV.*
Use: Analgesic combination, narcotic.

•**talampicillin hydrochloride.** (TAL-AM-pih-sill-in) USAN.
Use: Anti-infective.

•**talc.** U.S.P. 23. A native hydrous magnesium silicate.
Use: Dusting powder, pharmaceutic aid (tablet/capsule lubricant).

•**taleranol.** (TAL-ehr-ah-nole) USAN.
Use: Enzyme inhibitor (gonadotropin).

•**talisomycin.** (tal-EYE-so-MY-sin) USAN.
Formerly Tallysomycin A.
Use: Antineoplastic.

•**talmetacin.** (TAL-MET-ah-sin) USAN.
Use: Analgesic, antipyretic, anti-inflammatory.

•**talniflumate.** (tal-NYE-FLEW-mate) USAN.
Use: Anti-inflammatory, analgesic.

Taloin. (Pharmacia & Upjohn) Methylbenzethonium chloride, zinc oxide, calamine, eucalyptol in a water-repellent base. Oint. Tube 2 oz.
Use: Skin protectant & antiseptic.

•**talopram hydrochloride.** (TAY-low-pram) USAN.
Use: Potentiator (catecholamine).

•**talosalate.** (TAL-oh-SAL-ate) USAN.
Use: Analgesic, anti-inflammatory.

•**talsaclidine fumarate.** (tale-SACK-lih-deen) USAN.
Use: Alzheimer's disease treatment (muscarinic $M_{.1}$-agonist).

Talwin Compound. (Sanofi Winthrop Pharmaceuticals) Pentazocine HCl 12.5 mg, aspirin 325 mg/Tab. Bot. 100s. *c-IV.*
Use: Analgesic, narcotic.

Talwin Injection. (Sanofi Winthrop Pharmaceuticals) Pentazocine lactate injection. 30 mg/ml. **Vials:** 10 ml. **Uni-Amps:** 1 ml, 1.5 ml, 2 ml. **Uni-Nest amps:** 1 ml, 2 ml. **Carpujects:** 1 ml, 1.5 ml, 2 ml. *c-IV.*
Use: Analgesic, narcotic.

Talwin NX. (Sanofi Winthrop Pharmaceuticals) Pentazocine HCl 50 mg, naloxone 0.5 mg/Tab. Bot. 100s, UD 250s. *c-IV.*
Use: Analgesic, narcotic.

Tambocor. (3M Pharmaceuticals) Flecainide acetate 50 mg, 100 mg, 150 mg/Tab. Bot. 100s, UD 100s. *Rx.*
Use: Antiarrhythmic.

•**tametraline hydrochloride.** (tah-MET-rah-leen) USAN.
Use: Antidepressant.

Tamine S.R. (Geneva Pharmaceuticals) Phenylpropanolamine HCl 15 mg, phenylephrine HCl 15 mg, brompheniramine maleate 12 mg. Sugar coated. Tab. Bot. 100s, 1000s. *Rx.*
Use: Antihistamine, decongestant.

tamoxifen. (Various Mfr.) Tamoxifen citrate 10 mg, 20 mg. Tab. Bot. 60s, 250s (10 mg only). *Rx.*
Use: Antineoplastic, antiestrogen.

•**tamoxifen citrate.** (ta-MOX-ih-fen) U.S.P. 23.
Use: Treatment of mammary carcinoma, antiestrogen.
See: Nolvadex, Tab. (Zeneca Pharmaceuticals).
Tamoxifen, Tab. (Barr Laboratories, Inc.).

•**tampramine fumarate.** (TAM-prah-MEEN) USAN.
Use: Antidepressant.

Tamp-R-Tel. (Wyeth-Ayerst Laboratories) A tamper-resistant package for narcotic drugs which includes the following: **Codeine phosphate:** 30 mg, 60 mg/ml. **Hydromorphone HCl:** 1 mg, 2 mg, 3 mg, 4 mg/Tubex. **Meperidine HCl:** 25 mg/ml. **Promethazine HCl:** 25 mg/ml, 2 ml. **Meperidine HCl:** 25 mg/ml, 50 mg/ml, 75 mg/ml, 100 mg/ml. **Morphine Sulfate:** 2 mg, 4 mg, 8 mg, 10 mg, 15 mg/ml. **Pentobarbital, Sodium:** 100 mg/2 ml. **Phenobarbital, Sodium:** 30 mg, 60 mg, 130 mg/ml. **Secobarbital, Sodium:** 100 mg/2 ml.

•**tamsulosin hydrochloride.** USAN.
Use: Benign prostatic hyperplasia therapy.
See: Flomax, Cap. (Boehringer Ingelheim, Inc.).

Tanac Gel. (Del Pharmaceuticals, Inc.) Dyclonine HCl 1%, allantoin 0.5%, petrolatum, lanolin. Tube. 9.45 ml. *otc.*
Use: Cold sores, fever blisters, moisturizer.

Tanac Liquid. (Del Pharmaceuticals, Inc.) Benzalkonium Cl 0.12%, benzocaine 10%, tannic acid 6%. Saccharin. Bot. 13 ml. *otc.*
Use: Mouth and throat preparation.

Tanac Stick. (Del Pharmaceuticals, Inc.) Benzocaine 7.5%, tannic acid 6%, octyl dimethyl PABA 0.75%, allantoin 0.2%, benzalkonium Cl. 7.5%. Saccharin. Stick 0.1 oz. *otc.*
Use: Cold sores, fever blisters, moisturizer.

Tanadex. (Del Pharmaceuticals, Inc.) Tannic acid 2.86%, phenol 1.05%, benzocaine 0.47%. Liq. Bot. 3 oz. *otc.*
Use: Throat preparation.

Tan-a-Dyne. (Archer-Taylor) Tannic acid compound w/iodine. Liq. Bot. 4 oz., pt., gal. *otc.*
Use: Gargle.

Tanafed. (Horizon Pharmaceutical Corp.) Chlorpheniramine tannate 4.5 mg, pseudoephedrine tannate 75 mg/5 ml. Susp. Bot. 20 ml, 118 ml, 473 ml. *Rx.*
Use: Antihistamine, decongestant.

tanbismuth.
See: Bismuth Tannate.

•**tandamine hydrochloride.** (TAN-dah-meen) USAN.
Use: Antidepressant.

•**tandospirone citrate.** (tan-DOE-spy-rone) USAN.
Use: Anxiolytic.

•**tannic acid.** U.S.P. 23. Gallotannic acid. Glycerite. Tannin.
Use: Astringent.
See: Zilactin Medicated, Gel (Zila Pharm).
W/Benzocaine, phenol, thymol iodide, ephedrine HCl, zinc oxide, peru balsam.
See: Clysodrast, Packet (PBH Wesley Jessen).
W/Boric acid, salicylic acid, isopropyl alcohol.
See: Sal Dex Boro, Liq. (Scrip).

W/Cyanocobalamin, zinc acetate, glutathione, phenol.
See: Depinar, Amp. (Centeon).

Tannic Spray. (Gebauer Co.) Tannic acid 4.5%, chlorobutanol 1.3%, menthol < 1%, benzocaine < 1%, propylene glycol 33%, ethanol 60%. Liq. Bot. 2 oz, 4 oz. *otc.*
Use: Relief of sunburn and other minor burns.

Tanoral. (Pharmed) Phenylephrine tannate 25 mg, chlorpheniramine tannate 8 mg, pyrilamine tannate 25 mg/Tab. Bot. 100s. *Rx.*
Use: Antihistamine, decongestant.

tanphetamin.
See: Dextroamphetamine tannate.

Tao. (Pfizer) Troleandomycin equivalent to 250 mg oleandomycin/Cap. Bot. 100s. *Rx.*
Use: Anti-infective.

Tapar. (Warner Chilcott Laboratories) Acetaminophen 325 mg/Tab. Bot. 100s. *otc.*
Use: Analgesic.

Tapazole. (Eli Lilly and Co.) Methimazole. 5 mg or 10 mg/Tab. Bot. 100s. *Rx.*
Use: Hyperthyroidism.

•**tape, adhesive.** U.S.P. 23.
Use: Surgical aid.

Ta-Poff. (Ulmer Pharmacal Co.) Adhesive tape remover. Liq. Bot. 1 pt. Aerosol. Can 6 oz.

Tapuline. (Wesley Pharmacal Co., Inc.) Activated attapulgite 600 mg, pectin 60 mg, homatropine methylbromide 0.5 mg/Chew. Tab. Bot. 100s, 1000s. *otc.*
Use: Antidiarrheal.

tar.
See: Coal Tar, Preps.

Tar Distillate. (Doak Dermatologics) Decolorized fractional distillate of crude coal tar. Each ml equiv. to 1 g whole crude coal tar. Bot. 2 oz., 16 oz.
Use: Dermatologic.

Tarka. (Knoll Pharmaceuticals) Trandolapril maleate 2 mg, verapamil HCl 180 mg, or trandolapril 1 mg, verapamil HCl 240 mg, or trandolapril 2 mg, verapamil 240 mg, or trandolapril 4 mg, verapamil 240 mg/Tab. Bot. 100s. *Rx.*
Use: Antihypertensive.

Tarnphilic. (Medco Lab, Inc.) Coal tar 1%, polysorbate 0.5% in aquaphilic base. Jar 16 oz. *otc.*
Use: Dermatologic.

Tarpaste. (Doak Dermatologics) Coal tar distilled 5% in zinc paste. Tube 1 oz, Jar 4 oz, w/Hydrocortisone 0.5%. Tube 1 oz. *otc.*
Use: Dermatitis.

Tarsum Shampoo/Gel. (Summers Laboratories, Inc.) Coal tar 10%, salicylic acid 5% in shampoo base. Bot. 4 oz. *otc.*
Use: Antiseborrheic, dermatologic, hair, and scalp.

tartar emetic.
See: Antimony Potassium Tartrate, U.S.P. 23.

•**tartaric acid.** N.F. 18.
Use: Pharmaceutic aid (buffering agent).

Tashan. (Block Drug Co., Inc.) Skin Cream. Vitamins A palmitate, D_2, D-panthenol, E. Tube 1 oz. *otc.*
Use: Emollient.

Tasmar. (Roche Laboratories) Tolcapone 100 mg, 200 mg, lactose. Tab. Bot. 90s. *Rx.*
Use: Antiparkinson agent.

•**tasosartan.** (tass-OH-sahr-tan) USAN.
Use: Antihypertensive.

Taste Function Test, Accusens T. (Westport Pharmaceuticals, Inc.) Tastant 60 ml. Kit. 15 Bot.
Use: Diagnostic aid.

Ta-Verm. (Table Rock) Piperazine citrate 100 mg/ml Syr. Bot. 1 pt., 1 gal. 500 mg Tab. Bot. 100s, 500s. *Rx.*
Use: Anthelmintic.

Tavilen Plus. (Table Rock) Liver solution 1 g, ferric pyrophosphate soluble 500 mg, vitamins B_1 6 mg, B_2 7.2 mg, B_6 3 mg, B_{12} 24 mcg, panthenol 3 mg, niacinamide 60 mg, l-lysine HCl 300 mg, 5% alcohol/ml. Bot. 16 oz., 1 gal. *otc.*
Use: Hematinic.

Tavist. (Novartis Pharmaceutical Corp.) Clemastine fumarate 2.68 mg/Tab. Bot. 100s. *Rx.*
Use: Antihistamine.

Tavist Syrup. (Novartis Pharmaceutical Corp.) Clemastine fumarate 0.67 mg/5 ml. Bot. 118 ml. *Rx.*
Use: Antihistamine.

Tavist-D. (Novartis Pharmaceutical Corp.) Clemastine fumarate 1.34 mg, phenylpropanolamine HCl 75 mg/SR Tab. Pkg. 8s, 16s. *otc.*
Use: Antihistamine, decongestant.

Taxol. (Bristol-Myers Squibb) Paclitaxel. 30 mg/5 ml. Inj. Vial 5 ml, 16.7 ml. *Rx.*
Use: Antineoplastic.

Taxotere. (Rhone-Poulenc Rorer Pharmaceuticals, Inc.) Docetaxel 20 mg/0.5 ml, 80 mg/2 ml. Inj. Single-dose vial with diluent.
Use: Antineoplastic (breast cancer).

•**tazadolene succinate.** (TAZZ-ah-DOE-leen) USAN.

Use: Analgesic.

•**tazarotene.** (tazz-AHR-oh-teen) USAN.
Use: Keratolytic.
See: Tazorac, Gel (Allergan, Inc.).

Tazicef. (SmithKline Beecham, Bristol-Myers Squibb) Ceftazidime 500 mg, 1 g, 2 g, 6 g. Pow. for Inj. Vial 10 ml (500 mg only), 100 ml (6 g only); *ADD-Vantage* vials 20 ml (1 g only), 50 ml (2 g only), 100 ml (1 g and 2 g only); *Faspaks* (1 g and 2 g only). *Rx.*
Use: Anti-infective, cephalosporin.

Tazidime. (Eli Lilly and Co.) Ceftazidime. **Inj.:** 1 g, 2 g. *Galaxy* cont. **Pow. for Inj.:** 1 g, 2 g, 6 g. Vial, *ADD-Vantage* vials, piggyback vials. Bulk pkg. (6 g only). *Rx.*
Use: Anti-infective, cephalosporin.

•**tazifylline hydrochloride.** (TAY-zih-FIH-lin) USAN.
Use: Antihistamine.

•**tazobactam.** (TAZZ-oh-BACK-tam) USAN.
Use: Inhibitor (beta-lactamase).

•**tazobactam sodium.** (TAZZ-oh-BACK-tam) USAN.
Use: Inhibitor (beta-lactamase).

tazobactam sodium/piperacillin sodium.
See: Piperacillin sodium, sterile w/tazobactam.

•**tazofelone.** (TAY-zah-feh-lone) USAN.
Use: Suppressant (inflammatory bowel disease).

•**tazolol hydrochloride.** (TAY-zoe-lole) USAN.
Use: Cardiotonic.

•**tazomeline citrate.** (tazz-OH-meh-leen SIH-trate) USAN.
Use: Alzheimer's disease treatment (cholinergic agonist).

Tazorac. (Allergan, Inc.) Tazarotene 0.05%, 0.1%. Gel Tube 30 g, 100 g. *Rx.*
Use: Antiacne, antipsoriatic.

TBA-Pred. (Keene Pharmaceuticals, Inc.) Prednisolone tebutate 10 mg/ml Susp. Vial 10 ml. *Rx.*
Use: Corticosteroid.

TC Suspension. (Rhone-Poulenc Rorer Pharmaceuticals, Inc.) Aluminum hydroxide 600 mg, magnesium hydroxide 300 mg/5 ml, sorbitol, sodium 0.8 mg/5 ml Liq. In UD 15 ml, 30 ml (100s). *otc.*
Use: Antacid.

T/Derm Tar Emollient. (Neutrogena) Neutar solubilized coal tar extract 5% in oil base. Bot. 4 oz. *otc.*
Use: Antipsoriatic, antipruritic.

T-Dry. (Jones Medical Industries, Inc.) Pseudoephedrine HCl 120 mg, chlorpheniramine maleate 12 mg/SR Cap. Bot. 100s. *Rx.*
Use: Antihistamine, decongestant.

T-Dry Jr.. (Jones Medical Industries, Inc.) Pseudoephedrine HCl 60 mg, chlorpheniramine maleate 4 mg/SR Cap. Bot. 100s. *otc.*
Use: Antihistamine, decongestant.

TDX Cortisol. (Abbott Diagnostics) Fluorescence polarization immunoassay for the quantitative determination of cortisol in serum, plasma, or urine.
Use: Diagnostic aid.

TDX Thyroxine. (Abbott Diagnostics) Automated assay for quantitation of unsaturated thyroxine-binding sites in serum or plasma.
Use: Diagnostic aid.

TDX Total Estriol. (Abbott Diagnostics) Fluorescence polarization immunoassay for the quantitative determination of total estriol in serum, plasma, or urine.
Use: Diagnostic aid.

TDX Total T3. (Abbott Diagnostics) Automated assay for quantitation of total circulating triiodothyronine (T3) in serum or plasma.
Use: Diagnostic aid.

TDX T-Uptake. (Abbott Diagnostics) Automated assay for the determination of thyroxine-binding capacity in serum or plasma.
Use: Diagnostic aid.

Te Anatoxal Berna. (Berna Products Corp.) Tetanus toxoid adsorbed, 10 Lf units/0.5 ml. Vial 5 ml, Syr. 0.5 ml. *Rx.*
Use: Immunization.

Tear Drop. (Parmed Pharmaceuticals, Inc.) Benzalkonium Cl 0.01%, polyvinyl alcohol, NaCl, EDTA. Soln. Drop. Bot. 15 ml. *otc.*
Use: Artificial tears.

TearGard. (KM Lee) Hydroxyethyl cellulose, sorbic acid 0.25%, EDTA 0.1%. Soln. Bot. 15 ml. *otc.*
Use: Lubricant, ophthalmic.

Teargen. (Zenith Goldline Pharmaceuticals) Benzalkonium Cl 0.01%, EDTA, NaCl, polyvinyl alcohol. Soln. Bot. 15 ml. *otc.*
Use: Artificial tears.

Teargen II. (Zenith Goldline Pharmaceuticals) Hydroxypropyl methylcellulose 0.3%, dextran 70 0.1%, benzalkonium Cl 0.01%, EDTA 0.05%. Bot. 15 ml. *otc.*
Use: Artificial tears.

Tearisol. (Ciba Vision) Hydroxypropyl methylcellulose 0.5%, edetate disodium, benzalkonium chloride 0.01%,

boric acid, potassium chloride. Bot. 15 ml. *otc.*
Use: Artificial tears.

Tears Naturale. (Alcon Laboratories, Inc.) Dextran 70 0.1%, benzalkonium Cl 0.01%, hydroxypropyl methylcellulose 0.3%, sodium Cl, EDTA, hydrochloric acid, sodium HCl, potassium Cl. Soln. Bot. 15 ml, 30 ml. *otc.*
Use: Artificial tears.

Tears Naturale II. (Alcon Laboratories, Inc.) Dextran 70 0.1%, hydroxypropyl methylcellulose 2910 0.3%, polyquaternium-1 0.001%, sodium Cl, potassium Cl, sodium borate. Soln. Drop-tainer 15 ml, 30 ml. *otc.*
Use: Artificial tears.

Tears Naturale Free. (Alcon Laboratories, Inc.) Hydroxypropyl methylcellulose 2910 0.3%, dextran 70 0.1%, NaCl, KCl, sodium borate. Soln. Single-use containers 0.6 ml. *otc.*
Use: Artificial tears.

Tears Plus. (Allergan, Inc.) Polyvinyl alcohol 1.4%, NaCl, povidone 0.6%, chlorobutanol 0.5%. *otc.*
Use: Artificial tears.

Tears Renewed Ointment. (Akorn, Inc.) White petrolatum, light mineral oil. Ophth. Tube 3.5 g. *otc.*
Use: Lubricant, ophthalmic.

Tears Renewed Solution. (Akorn, Inc.) Dextran 70 0.1%, sodium chloride, hydroxypropyl methylcellulose 2906, benzalkonium chloride 0.01%, EDTA. Soln. Bot. 2 ml, 15 ml, 30 ml. *otc.*
Use: Artificial tears.

tea tree oil. (Metabolic Prod.) Australian oil of *Melaleuca alternifolia* 100% pure. Bot. 1 oz, 4 oz, 8 oz, 16 oz. **Cream:** Bot. 8 oz. **Oint.:** Tube 1 oz, 3 oz. *otc.*
Use: Antiseptic, antifungal, topical.

Tebamide. (G & W Laboratories) Trimethobenzamide HCl 100 mg/Supp. In 10s. *Rx.*
Use: Antiemetic, antivertigo.

•**tebufelone.** (teh-BYOO-feh-LONE) USAN.
Use: Analgesic, anti-inflammatory.

•**tebuquine.** (TEH-buh-KWIN) USAN.
Use: Antimalarial.

T.E.C. (Invenex) Zn 1 mg, Cu 0.4 mg, Cr 4 mcg, Mn 0.1 mg. Vial 10 ml. *Rx.*
Use: Trace element supplement.

•**teceleukin.** (teh-see-LOO-kin) USAN.
Use: Immunostimulant.

Technescan MAA. (Mallinckrodt Medical, Inc.) Aggregated albumin (human).
Use: Preparation of Tc 99m Aggregated Albumin (Human).

Techneplex. (Bristol-Myers Squibb) Technetium Tc 99m penetate kit. 10 vials/kit.
Use: Radiopaque agent.

•**technetium Tc 99m albumin aggregated injection.** (tek-NEE-shee-uhm Tc 99m al-BYOO-min AGG-reh-GAY-tuhd) U.S.P. 23.
Use: Diagnostic aid (lung imaging), radioactive agent.

•**technetium Tc 99m albumin colloid injection.** (tek-NEE-shee-uhm Tc 99m al-BYOO-min) U.S.P. 23.
Use: Radiopharmaceutical.

•**technetium Tc 99m albumin injection.** (tek-NEE-shee-uhm Tc 99m al-BYOO-min) U.S.P. 23.
Use: Radiopharmaceutical.

•**technetium Tc 99m albumin microaggregated.** (tek-NEE-shee-uhm Tc 99m al-BYOO-min) USAN.
Use: Radiopharmaceutical.

technetium Tc 99m antimelanoma murine monoclonalantibody. (tek-NEE-shee-uhm)
Use: Diagnostic aid. [Orphan Drug]

•**technetium Tc 99m antimony trisulfide colloid.** (tek-NEE-shee-uhm) USAN.
Use: Radiopharmaceutical.

•**technetium Tc 99m apcitide.** (tek-NEE-shee-uhm APP-sih-tide) USAN.
Use: Radiopharmaceutical.

•**technetium Tc 99m bicisate.** (tek-NEE-shee-uhm Tc 99m bye-SIS-ate) USAN.
Use: Diagnostic aid (brain imaging), radiopharmaceutical.

•**technetium Tc 99m disofenin injection.** (tek-NEE-shee-uhm) U.S.P. 23.
Use: Radiopharmaceutical; diagnostic aid (hepatobiliary function determination).

•**technetium Tc 99m etidronate injection.** (tek-NEE-shee-uhm) U.S.P. 23.
Use: Radiopharmaceutical.

•**technetium Tc 99m exametazime injection.** (tek-NEE-shee-uhm Tc 99m ex-ah-MET-ah-zeem) U.S.P. 23.
Use: Radiopharmaceutical.

technetium Tc 99m ferpentetate injection. (tek-NEE-shee-uhm)
Use: Radiopharmaceutical.

•**technetium Tc 99m furifosmin.** (tek-NEE-shee-uhm Tc 99m fyoor-ih-FOSS-min) USAN.
Use: Diagnostic aid (radioactive, cardiac disease), radiopharmaceutical.

technetium Tc 99m generator solution. (tek-NEE-shee-uhm) (New England Nuclear) Pertechnetate sodium Tc 99m.

Use: Radiopharmaceutical, radiopaque agent.

•**technetium Tc 99m glucepate injection.** (tek-NEE-shee-uhm) U.S.P. 23. *Formerly Technetium Tc 99m Sodium Gluceptate.*
Use: Radiopharmaceutical.

•**technetium Tc 99m lidofenin injection.** (tek-NEE-shee-uhm) U.S.P. 23.
Use: Radiopharamceutical.

•**technetium Tc 99m mebrofenin injection.** (tek-NEE-shee-uhm) U.S.P. 23.
Use: Radiopharmaceutical.

•**technetium Tc 99m medronate injection.** (tek-NEE-shee-uhm) U.S.P. 23.
Use: Diagnostic aid (skeletal imaging), radiopharmaceutical.
See: Macrotec, Inj. (Bristol-Myers Squibb).

•**technetium Tc 99m medronate disodium.** (tek-NEE-shee-uhm) USAN.
Use: Radiopharmaceutical.

•**technetium Tc 99m mertiatide injection.** ((tek-NEE-shee-uhm Tc 99m MEER-TIE-ah-tide)) U.S.P. 23.
Use: Diagnostic aid (renal function); radiopharmaceutical.

technetium Tc 99m murine monoclonal antibody to hCG. (tek-NEE-shee-uhm)
Use: Diagnostic aid. [Orphan Drug]

technetium Tc 99m murine monoclonal antibody to human afp. (tek-NEE-shee-uhm)
Use: Diagnostic aid. [Orphan Drug]

technetium Tc 99m murine monoclonal antibody (IgG2a) to BCE.
Use: Diagnostic aid. [Orphan Drug]

•**technetium Tc 99m oxidronate injection.** (tek-NEE-shee-uhm) U.S.P. 23.
Use: Diagnostic aid (skeletal imaging), radiopharmaceutical.

•**technetium Tc 99m pentetate injection.** (tek-NEE-shee-uhm) U.S.P. 23. *Formerly Technetium Tc 99m Pentetate Sodium.*
Use: Radiopharmaceutical.

•**technetium Tc 99m pentetate calcium trisodium.** (tek-NEE-shee-uhm KAL-see-uhm try-so-dee-uhm) USAN.
Use: Radiopharmaceutical.

•**technetium Tc 99m pyrophosphate injection.** (tek-NEE-shee-uhm) U.S.P. 23.
Use: Radiopharmaceutical.

•**technetium Tc 99m (pyro- and trimetra-) phosphates injection.** (tek-NEE-shee-uhm) U.S.P. 23.
Use: Radiopharmaceutical.

•**technetium Tc 99m red blood cells injection.** (tek-NEE-shee-uhm) U.S.P. 23.
Use: Radiopharmaceutical.

•**technetium Tc 99m sestamibi.** (tek-NEE-shee-uhmTc 99 m SESS-tah-MIH-bih) U.S.P. 23.
Use: Diagnostic aid (radiopaque medium, cardiac perfusion); radiopharmaceutical.

•**technetium Tc 99m siboroxime.** (tek-NEE-shee-uhm Tc 99m sih-boe-ROX-eem) USAN.
Use: Diagnostic aid (brain imaging), radiopharmaceutical.

•**technetium Tc 99m succimer injection.** (tek-NEE-shee-uhm) U.S.P. 23.
Use: Radiopharmaceutical, diagnostic aid (renal function determination).

technetium Tc 99m sulfur colloid kit. (tek-NEE-shee-uhm)
Use: Radiopharmaceutical.
See: Tesuloid (Bristol-Myers Squibb).

•**technetium Tc 99m sulfur colloid injection.** (tek-NEE-shee-uhm) U.S.P. 23.
Use: Radiopharmaceutical.

•**technetium Tc 99m teboroxime.** (tek-NEE-shee-uhm Tc 99m teh-boe-ROX-eem) USAN.
Use: Diagnostic aid (radiopaque medium, cardiac perfusion), radiopharmaceutical.

teclosine. Under study.
Use: Amebicide.

•**teclozan.** (TEH-kloe-zan) USAN.
Use: Antiamebic.
See: Falmonox (Sanofi Winthrop Pharmaceuticals).

Tecnu Poison Oak-N-Ivy. (Tec Laboratories, Inc.) Deodorized mineral spirits, propylene glycol, polyethylene glycol, octylphenoxy-polyethoxyethanol, mixed fatty acid soap. Liq. Bot. 118.3 ml. *otc.*
Use: Dermatologic, poison ivy.

•**tecogalan sodium.** (TEE-koe-gay-lan) USAN.
Use: Antineoplastic adjunct.

Teczem. (Hoechst Marion Roussel) Enalapril maleate 5 mg, diltiazem maleate 180 mg, sucrose/ER Tab. Unit-of-use 100s. *Rx.*
Use: Antihypertensive.

Tedral. (Parke-Davis) **Tab.:** Theophylline 118 mg, ephedrine HCl 24 mg, phenobarbital 8 mg/Tab. Bot. 24s, 100s, 1000s. UD 100s. **Susp. (Pediatric Pharmaceuticals):** Theophylline 65 mg, ephedrine HCl 12 mg, phenobarbital 4 mg/5 ml. Bot. 8 oz. *Rx.*
Use: Antiasthmatic.

Tedral Elixir. (Parke-Davis) Theophylline 32.5 mg, ephedrine HCl 6 mg, pheno-

barbital 2 mg/5 ml. Alcohol 15%. Pediatric. Bot. Pt. *Rx.*
Use: Antiasthmatic.

Tedral-SA. (Parke-Davis) Theophylline 180 mg, ephedrine HCl 48 mg, phenobarbital 25 mg/SA Tab. Bot. 100s, 1000s. *Rx.*
Use: Antiasthmatic.

Tedrigen. (Zenith Goldline Pharmaceuticals) Theophylline 120 mg, ephedrine HCl 22.5 mg, phenobarbital 7.5 mg/Tab. Bot. 100s, 1000s. *otc.*
Use: Antiasthmatic.

Teebacin. (CMC) Sod. p-aminosalicylate. **Tab.:** 0.5 g Bot. 1000s. **Pow.:** Bot. lb. *Rx.*
Use: Antituberculosal.

Teebaconin. (CMC) Isoniazid 50, 100, 300 mg/Tab. Bot. 100s, 1000s. *Rx.*
Use: Antituberculosal.

Teebaconin w/Vitamin B^6. (CMC) Isoniazid 100 mg, 10 mg pyridoxine HCl/Tab. Bot. 100s, 500s, 1000s. Isoniazid 300 mg, 30 mg pyridoxine HCl/Tab. Bot. 100s and 1000s. *Rx.*
Use: Antituberculosal.

Teen Midol. (Bayer Corp. (Consumer Div.)) Acetaminophen 400 mg, pamabrom 25 mg. Cap. Bot. 16s. *otc.*
Use: Analgesic combination.

Teev. (Keene Pharmaceuticals, Inc.) Estradiol valerate 4 mg, testosterone enanthate 90 mg/ml. Inj. Vial 10 ml. *Rx.*
Use: Androgen, estrogen combination.

•**teflurane.** (TEH-flew-rane) USAN.
Use: Anesthetic, general.

tegacid.
See: Glyceryl monostearate.

•**tegafur.** (TEH-gah-fer) USAN.
Use: Antineoplastic.

Tegamide. (G & W Laboratories) Trimethobenzamide HCl 100 mg, 200 mg/Supp. Box. 10s, 50s. *Rx.*
Use: Antiemetic.

Tegretol. (Novartis Pharmaceutical Corp.) Carbamazepine **Tab.:** 200 mg. Bot. 100s, 1000s. UD 100s. **Chew. Tab.:** 100 mg/Tab. Bot. 100s. UD 100s; **Susp.:** 100 mg/5 ml, sorbitol. Sucrose. Bot. 450 ml. *Rx.*
Use: Anticonvulsant.

Tegretol-XR. (Novartis Pharmaceutical Corp.) Carbamazepine 100 mg, 200 mg, 400 mg, mannitol/ER Tab. Bot. 100s, UD 100s. *Rx.*
Use: Anticonvulsant.

Tegrin Cream. (Block Drug Co., Inc.) Allantoin 2%, coal tar extract 5% in cream base. Tube 2 oz, 4.4 oz. *otc.*
Use: Antipsoriatic.

Tegrin Medicated. (Block Drug Co., Inc.)
Shampoo: Crude coal tar 7%, sodium lauryl sulfate, ammonium lauryl sulfate, alcohol 6.4%. Cream 110 ml. *otc.*
Use: Antiseborrheic.

Tegrin Medicated Extra Conditioning. (Block Drug Co., Inc.) Coal tar solution 7%, alcohol 6.4%. Shampoo. Bot. 110 ml, 198 ml. *otc.*
Use: Antiseborrheic.

T.E.H. Compound. (Various Mfr.) Theophylline 130 mg, ephedrine sulfate 25 mg, hydroxyzine HCl 10 mg/Tab. Bot. 100s, 500s. *Rx.*
Use: Antiasthmatic.

•**teicoplanin.** (teh-kah-PLAN-in) USAN.
Use: Anti-infective.

Telachlor TD Caps. (Major Pharmaceuticals) Chlorpheniramine maleate 8 mg, 12 mg/TD Tab. Bot. 1000s. *Rx.*
Use: Antihistamine.

Teldrin Maximum Strength Spansules. (SmithKline Beecham Pharmaceuticals) Chlorpheniramine maleate 12 mg/Cap. Pkg. 12s, 24s, 48s. *otc.*
Use: Antihistamine.

Teldrin Tablets. (SmithKline Beecham Pharmaceuticals) Chlorpheniramine maleate 4 mg/Tab. *otc.*
Use: Antihistamine.

Teldrin 12-Hour Allergy Relief. (SmithKline Beecham Pharmaceuticals) Chlorpheniramine maleate 8 mg, pseudoephedrine HCl 75 mg/Cap. Pkg. 12s, 24s. Bot. 48s. *otc.*
Use: Antihistamine, decongestant.

Telepaque. (Nycomed) Iopanoic acid 500 mg, iodine 333.4 mg. Tab. Pkg. 6s. *Rx.*
Use: Radiopaque agent.

•**telinavir.** (teh-LIN-ah-veer) USAN.
Use: Antiviral.

•**telmisartan.** (tell-mih-SAHR-tan) USAN.
Use: Angiotensin II receptor antagonist; antihypertensive.
See: Micardis (Boehringer Ingelheim).

Telodron. (Norden) Chlorpheniramine maleate.
Use: Antihistamine.

•**teloxantrone hydrochloride.** (teh-LOX-an-trone) USAN.
Use: Antineoplastic.

•**teludipine hydrochloride.** (teh-LOO-dih-peen) USAN.
Use: Antihypertensive, calcium channel antagonist.

•**temafloxacin hydrochloride.** (teh-mah-FLOX-ah-SIN) USAN.
Use: Anti-infective (microbial DNA topoisomerase inhibitor).

•**tematropium methylsulfate.** (teh-mah-TROE-pee-UHM METH-ill-SULL-fate)

USAN.
Use: Anticholinergic.

•**temazepam.** (tem-AZE-uh-pam) U.S.P. 23.
Use: Anxiolytic.
See: Restoril, Cap. (Novartis Pharmaceutical Corp.).

temazepam. (Various Mfr.) 7.5 mg/Cap. 100s, UD 100s. *c-iv.*
Use: Hypnotic, sedative.

•**temelastine.** (teh-mell-ASS-teen) USAN.
Use: Antihistamine.

Temetan. (Nevin) Acetaminophen 324 mg/Tab. Bot. 100s, 500s. Elix. 324 mg/5 ml. Bot. Pt. *otc.*
Use: Analgesic.

•**temocapril hydrochloride.** (teh-MOE-cap-RILL) USAN.
Use: Antihypertensive.

•**temocillin.** (TEE-moe-SIH-lin) USAN.
Use: Anti-infective.

•**temoporfin.** (teh-moe-PORE-fin) USAN.
Use: Antineoplastic.

Temovate Cream. (GlaxoWellcome) Clobetasol propionate 0.05%. Cream Tube 15 g, 30 g, 45 g. *Rx.*
Use: Corticosteroid, topical.

Temovate Emollient. (GlaxoWellcome) Clobetasol propionate 0.05%. Cream Tube 15 g, 30 g, 60 g. *Rx.*
Use: Corticosteroid, topical.

Temovate Gel. (GlaxoWellcome) Clobetasol propionate 0.05%. Gel Tube 15 g, 30 g, 60 g. *Rx.*
Use: Corticosteroid, topical.

Temovate Ointment. (GlaxoWellcome) Clobetasol propionate 0.05%. Oint. Tube 15 g, 30 g, 45 g. *Rx.*
Use: Corticosteroid, topical.

Temovate Scalp. (GlaxoWellcome) **Oint.:** Clobetasol propionate 0.05%, white petrolatum base. 15 g, 30 g, 45 g. **Cream:** Clobetasol propionate 0.03%, 15 g, 30 g, 45 g. **Scalp application:** Clobetasol propionate 0.05%, carbomer 934P. 25 ml, 50 ml. *Rx.*
Use: Corticosteroid, topical.

Tempo. (Thompson Medical Co.) Calcium carbonate 414 mg, aluminum hydroxide 133 mg, magnesium hydroxide 81 mg, simethicone 20 mg. Chew. Tab. Bot. 10s, 30s, 60s. *otc.*
Use: Antacid, antiflatulent.

Temporary Punctal/Canalicular Collagen Implant. (Eagle Vision, Inc.) 0.2 mm, 0.3 mm, 0.4 mm, 0.5 mm, 0.6 mm. Box 72s. *Rx.*
Use: Collagen implant, ophthalmic.

Tempra. (Bristol-Myers Squibb) Acetaminophen. **Drops:** Grape flavor. 80 mg/0.8 ml. Bot. w/dropper 15 ml. **Syrup:** Cherry flavor. 160 mg/5 ml. Bot. 4 oz. **Tab.:** 80 mg/Chewable grape flavor Tab. Bot 30s. 160 mg/Chewable grape flavor Tab. Bot. 30s. *otc.*
Use: Analgesic.

•**temurtide.** (teh-MER-TIDE) USAN.
Use: Vaccine adjuvant.

Tencet. (Robers Pharmaceuticals) Acetaminophen 500 mg, butalbital 50 mg, caffeine 40 mg. Cap. Bot. 100s, UD 1000s. *Rx.*
Use: Analgesic, hypnotic, sedative.

Tencon. (International Ethical Labs) Acetaminophen 650 mg, butalbital 50 mg. Cap. Bot. 100s. *Rx.*
Use: Analgesic, hypnotic, sedative.

Tenex. (Wyeth-Ayerst Laboratories) Guanfacine HCl 1 mg, 2 mg/Tab. Bot. 100s, 500s (1 mg only), UD 100s (1 mg only). *Rx.*
Use: Antihypertensive.

•**tenidap.** (TEH-nih-DAP) USAN.
Use: Anti-inflammatory (osteoarthritis and rheumatoid arthritis).

•**tenidap sodium.** (TEH-nig-DAP) USAN.
Use: Anti-inflammatory (osteoarthritis and rheumatoid arthritis).

•**teniposide.** (TEN-ih-POE-side) USAN.
Use: Antineoplastic. [Orphan Drug]
See: Vumon (Bristol-Myers Oncology/Immunology).

Ten-K. (Novartis Pharmaceutical Corp.) Potassium Cl 750 mg (10 mEq)/CR Cap. Bot. 100s, 500s. UD, blister pak 100s. *Rx.*
Use: Electrolyte supplement.

Tenol. (Vortech Pharmaceuticals) Acetaminophen 325 mg/Tab. Bot. 1000s. *otc.*
Use: Analgesic.

Tenol Liquid. (Vortech Pharmaceuticals) Acetaminophen 120 mg, NAPA alcohol 7%/5 ml. Bot. 3 oz, 4 oz, gal. *otc.*
Use: Analgesic.

Tenol-Plus. (Vortech Pharmaceuticals) Acetaminophen 250 mg, aspirin 250 mg, caffeine 65 mg/Tab. Bot. 1000s. *otc.*
Use: Analgesic.

Tenoretic. (Zeneca Pharmaceuticals) **50 mg:** Atenolol 50 mg, chlorthalidone 25 mg/Tab. Bot. 100s. **100 mg:** Atenolol 100 mg, chlorthalidone 25 mg/Tab. Bot. 100s. *Rx.*
Use: Antihypertensive, diuretic.

Tenormin. (Zeneca Pharmaceuticals) **Oral:** Atenolol 50 mg, 100 mg/Tab. Bot. 100s. UD 100s. **Parenteral:** 5 mg/10 ml. Amp. 10 ml. *Rx.*
Use: Antihypertensive.

•**tenoxicam.** (ten-OX-ih-kam) USAN.
Use: Anti-inflammatory.

Tensilon. (Zeneca Pharmaceuticals) Edrophonium chloride. **Vial:** 10 mg/ml, w/phenol 0.45%, sodium sulfite 0.2% 10 ml. **Amp.:** 10 mg/ml, w/sodium sulfite 0.2%. 1 ml.
Use: Diagnostic aid, myasthenia gravis.

Tensive Conductive Adhesive Gel. (Parker) Non-flammable conductive adhesive electrode gel, eliminates tape and tape irritation. Tube 60 g.
Use: Therapeutic aid.

Tensocaine Tablets. (Sanofi Winthrop Pharmaceuticals) Acetaminophen. *otc.*
Use: Analgesic.

Tensolate. (Apco) Phenobarbital 0.25 g, hyoscyamine sulfate 0.1037 mg, atropine sulfate 0.0194 mg, hyoscine HBr 0.0065 mg/Tab. Bot. 100s. *Rx.*
Use: Antispasmodic.

Tensolax Tablets. (Sanofi Winthrop Pharmaceuticals) Chlormezanone. *Rx.*
Use: Muscle relaxant.

Tensopin. (Apco) Phenobarbital 0.25 g, homatropine methylbromide 2.5 mg/Tab. Bot. 100s. *Rx.*
Use: Antispasmodic.

Tenuate. (Hoechst Marion Roussel) Diethylpropion HCl 25 mg/Tab. Bot. 100s. *c-IV.*
Use: Anorexiant.

Tenuate Dospan. (Hoechst Marion Roussel) Diethylpropion HCl 75 mg/SR Tab. Bot. UD 100s, 250s. *c-v.*
Use: Anorexiant.

T.E.P. (Geneva Pharmaceuticals) Phenobarbital 8 mg, theophylline 130 mg, ephedrine HCl 24 mg/Tab. Bot. 100s. *Rx.*
Use: Antiasthmatic combination.

Tepanil. (3M Pharmaceuticals) Diethylpropion HCl. Tab. 25 mg Bot. 100s. *c-IV.*
Use: Anorexiant.

Tepanil Ten-Tab. (3M Pharmaceuticals) Diethylpropion 75 mg/Tab. Bot. 30s, 100s, 250s. *c-IV.*
Use: Anorexiant.

•**tepoxalin.** (teh-POX-ah-lin) USAN.
Use: Antipsoriatic.

•**teprotide.** (TEH-pro-tide) USAN.
Use: Angiotensin-converting enzyme inhibitor.

tequinol sodium. Name used for Actinoquinol Sodium.

Terak. (Akorn, Inc.) Polymyxin B sulfate 10,000 units/g, oxytetracycline HCl 5 mg/g. Oint. Tube 3.5 g. *Rx.*
Use: Anti-infective, ophthalmic.

Terazol 3. (Ortho McNeil Pharmaceutical) **Cream, Vaginal:** Terconazole 0.8%. Tube 20 g with applicator. **Vaginal Supp.:** Terconazole 80 mg. Pks. 3s with applicator. *Rx.*
Use: Antifungal, vaginal.

Terazol 7. (Ortho McNeil Pharmaceutical) Terconazole 0.4% Cream Tube 45 g. *Rx.*
Use: Antifungal, vaginal.

•**terazosin hydrochloride.** (ter-AZE-oh-sin) USAN.
Use: Antihypertensive.
See: Hytrin, Cap. (Abbott Laboratories).

•**terbinafine.** (TER-bin-ah-feen) USAN.
Use: Antifungal.
See: Lamisil (Novartis Pharmaceutical Corp.).

•**terbutaline sulfate.** (ter-BYOO-tuh-leen) U.S.P. 23.
Use: Bronchodilator.
See: Brethine, Amp., Tab. (Novartis Pharmaceutical Corp.).
Bricanyl (Hoechst Marion Roussel).

Tercodryl. (Health for Life Brands, Inc.) Codeine phos. ¾ g, pyrilamine maleate 25 mg/fl. oz. Bot. 4 oz. *c-v.*
Use: Antihistamine, antitussive.

•**terconazole.** (ter-CONE-uh-zole) USAN.
Formerly Triaconazole.
Use: Antifungal.
See: Terazol 3, Vag. Cream, Supp. (Ortho McNeil Pharmaceutical).
Terazol 7, Vag. Cream. (Ortho McNeil Pharmaceutical).

Terg-a-Zyme. (Alconox) Alconox with enzyme action. Box 4 lb Ctn. 9 x 4 lb, 25 lb, 50 lb, 100 lb, 300 lb. *otc.*
Use: Biodegradable detergent and wetting agent.

Teridol Jr. (Health for Life Brands, Inc.) Terpin hydrate, cocillana, potassium guaiacol sulfonate, ammonium chloride. Bot. 3 oz. *otc.*
Use: Expectorant.

•**teriparatide.** USAN.
Use: Bone resorption inhibitor, osteoporosis therapy adjunct, diagnostic aid, thyroid function. [Orphan Drug]

•**teriparatide acetate.** (TEH-rih-PAR-ah-TIDE) USAN.
Use: Diagnostic aid (hypocalcemia).

•**terlakiren.** (ter-lah-KIE-ren) USAN.
Use: Antihypertensive.

terlipressin.
Use: Treatment of bleeding esophageal varices. [Orphan Drug]
See: Glypressin.

•**terodiline hydrochloride.** (TEH-row-DIE-leen) USAN.
Use: Vasodilator (coronary).

•**teroxalene hydrochloride.** (ter-OX-ah-leen) USAN.
Use: Antischistosomal.

•**teroxirone.** (TER-OX-ih-rone) USAN.
Use: Antineoplastic.

Terpex Jr. (Health for Life Brands, Inc.) d-Methorphan 25 mg, terpin hydrate, potassium guaiacol sulfonate, cocillana, ammonium chloride. Bot. 4 oz. *otc.*
Use: Expectorant.

Terphan Elixir. (Pal-Pak, Inc.) Terpin hydrate 85 mg, dextromethorphan hydrobromide 10 mg/5 ml w/alcohol 40% Bot. Gal. *otc.*
Use: Antitussive, expectorant.

•**terpin hydrate.** (TER-pin HIGH-drate) U.S.P. 23.
Use: Expectorant for chronic cough.
See: Terp, Liq. (Scrip).

terpin hydrate and dextromethorphan hydrobromide elixir.
Use: Antitussive, expectorant.

Terra-Cortril. (Pfizer) Hydrocortisone 1.5%, oxytetracycline HCl 0.5%. Ophth. Susp. Bot. 5 ml. *Rx.*
Use: Anti-infective, corticosteroid, ophthalmic.

Terramycin. (Pfizer US Pharmaceutical Group) Oxytetracycline. **Cap.:** HCl salt 250 mg. Bot. 100s, 500s. **Oint., Ophth.:** Ocytetracycline HCl 5 mg, polymyxin B sulfate 1 mg/g. Tube 3.75 g. **Oint., Topical:** Oxytetracycline HCl 100 mg, polymyxin B sulfate 10,000 units/g. Tube 0.5 oz., 1 oz. **Tab., Oral:** Oxytetracycline HCl 250 mg/Tab. Bot. 100s. **Tab., Vaginal:** Oxytetracycline HCl 100 mg, polymyxin B sulfate 100,000 units/Tab. Box 10s. *Rx.*
Use: Anti-infective.

Terramycin w/Polymyxin B Ointment. (Pfizer) Polymyxin B sulfate 10,000 units/g, oxytetracycline HCl 5 mg/g. Oint. Tube 3.5 g. *Rx.*
Use: Anti-infective.

Tersaseptic. (Doak Dermatologics) DEA-lauryl sulfate, lauramide DEA, propylene glycol, ethoxydiglycol, PEG-12 distearate, EDTA, triclosan, citric acid/ Shampoo/cleanser. Soapless. 473 ml. *otc.*
Use: Dermatologic, acne.

tersavid.
Use: Monoamine oxidase inhibitor.

tertiary amyl alcohol.
See: Amylene Hydrate (Various Mfr.).

Tesamone. (Dunhall Pharmaceuticals, Inc.) Testosterone aqueous suspension. 25 mg/ml, 50 mg/ml, 100 mg/ml. Inj. Amp. 10 ml. *c-III.*
Use: Androgen.

•**tesicam.** (TESS-ih-kam) USAN.
Use: Anti-inflammatory.

•**tesimide.** (TESS-ih-mide) USAN.
Use: Anti-inflammatory.

Teslac. (Bristol-Myers Squibb) Testolactone 50 mg, lactose/Tab. Bot. 100s. *c-III.*
Use: Antineoplastic, androgen.

Teslascan. (Nycomed Inc.) Mangofodipir trisodium 37.9 mg (50 mcmol/ml). Inj. Vial 10 ml. *Rx.*
Use: Diagnostic aid.

Tesogen. (Sigma-Tau Pharmaceuticals, Inc.) Testosterone 25 mg, estrone 2 mg/ml. Vial 10 ml. *c-III.*
Use: Androgen.

Tesogen L.A. (Sigma-Tau Pharmaceuticals, Inc.) Testosterone enanthate 180 mg, 90 mg, 50 mg, estradiol valerate 8 mg, 4 mg, 2 mg, respectively/ml. Vial 10 ml. *Rx.*
Use: Androgen, estrogen combination.

Tesone. (Sigma-Tau Pharmaceuticals, Inc.) Testosterone 25 mg, 50 mg, 100 mg/ml. Vial 10 ml. *c-III.*
Use: Androgen.

Tesone L.A. (Sigma-Tau Pharmaceuticals, Inc.) Testosterone enanthate 200 mg/ml. Vial 10 ml. *c-III.*
Use: Androgen.

tespa.
Use: Antineoplastic.
See: Thiotepa (ESI Lederle Generics).

Tessalon Perles. (Forest Pharmaceutical, Inc.) Benzonatate 100 mg/Cap. Bot. 100s. *Rx.*
Use: Antitussive.

Testamone. (Dunhall Pharmaceuticals, Inc.) Testosterone 100 mg/ml. Inj. Vial 10 ml. *c-III.*
Use: Androgen.

Test-Estro Cypionates. (Rugby Labs, Inc.) Estradiol cypionate 2 mg, testosterone cypionate 50 mg/ml. Inj. Vial 10 ml. *Rx.*
Use: Androgen, estrogen combination.

Testex. (Taylor Pharmaceuticals) Testosterone propionate 50 mg, 100 mg/ml in sesame oil. Vial 10 ml. *c-III.*
Use: Androgen.

Testoderm. (Alza Corp.) Testosterone 10 mg or 15 mg per 40 or 60 cm^2, respectively. Transdermal system. Box 30s. *c-III.*
Use: Hormone, androgen.

Testoderm TTS. (Alza Corp.) Testosterone 4 mg, 5 mg, 6 mg/day. Transdermal system. Pkg. 30s. *c-III.*
Use: Hormone, androgen.

Testoject. (Merz Pharmaceuticals) Testosterone cypionate 100 mg/ml. Vial 10

ml. *c-III.*
Use: Androgen.

Testoject-50. (Merz Pharmaceuticals) Testosterone 50 mg/ml. Vial 10 ml. *c-III.*
Use: Androgen.

Testoject-LA. (Merz Pharmaceuticals) Testosterone cypionate 200 mg/ml in oil. Vial 10 ml. *c-III.*
Use: Androgen.

•**testolactone.** (TESS-toe-LAK-tone) U.S.P. 23.
Use: Antineoplastic.
See: Teslac, Vial, Tab. (Bristol-Myers Squibb).

Testolin. (Taylor Pharmaceuticals) Testosterone suspension 25 mg, 50 mg, 100 mg/ml. Vial 10 ml 25 mg/ml. Vial 30 ml. *c-III.*
Use: Androgen.

Testopel. (Bartor Pharmacal Co.) Testosterone 75 mg, stearic acid 0.2 mg, polyvinyl pyrrolidone 2 mg/pellet. 1 Pellet/Vial. *c-III.*
Use: Androgen.

•**testosterone.** (tess-TAHS-ter-ohn) U.S.P. 23.
Use: Androgen.
See: Androderm, Transderm. Patch (SmithKline Beecham Pharmaceuticals).
Andronaq, Aq. Susp., Vial (Schwarz Pharma, Inc.).
Depotest, Vial (Hyrex Pharmaceuticals).
Homogene-S, Inj., Vial (Spanner).
Malotrone, Aqueous Inj. (Bluco Inc./ Med. Discnt. Outlet).
Tesone, Inj. (Sigma-Tau Pharmaceuticals, Inc.).
Testoderm, Transdermal Patch (Alza Corp.).
Testoderm TTS (Alza Corp.).
Testolin, Vial (Taylor Pharmaceuticals).
Testopel, Pellet (Bartor Pharmacal Co.).

testosterone aqueous. (Various Mfr.) Testosterone (in aqueous suspension) 25 mg, 50 mg, 100/ml. Inj. Vial 10 ml, 30 ml.
Use: Androgen, parenteral.
See: Histerone 100, Inj. (Roberts Pharmaceuticals).
Tesamone, Inj. (Dunhall Pharmaceuticals, Inc.).

testosterone w/combinations.
See: Andesterone, Vial (Lincoln Diagnostics).
Angen, Vial (Davis & Sly).
Depo-Testadiol, Vial (Pharmacia & Upjohn).
Tesogen, Inj. (Sigma-Tau Pharmaceuticals, Inc.).

testosterone cyclopentane propionate. Testosterone Cypionate.

•**testosterone cypionate.** (tess-TAHS-ter-ohn) U.S.P. 23.
Use: Androgen.
See: Andro-Cyp 100, Inj. (Keene Pharmaceuticals, Inc.).
Andro-Cyp 200, Inj. (Keene Pharmaceuticals, Inc.).
depAndro, Inj. (Forest Pharmaceutical, Inc.).
Depo-Testosterone, Inj. (Pharmacia & Upjohn).
Dep-Test, Inj. (Sigma-Tau Pharmaceuticals, Inc.).
Depotest, Vial (Hyrex Pharmaceuticals).
D-Test 100, 200, Inj. (Burgin-Arden).
Durandro, Inj. (B.F. Ascher and Co.).
Duratest, Inj. (Roberts Pharmaceuticals).
Testoject, Vial (Merz Pharmaceuticals).
W/Combinations.
See: D-Diol, Inj. (Burgin-Arden).
Depotestogen, Vial (Hyrex Pharmaceuticals).
Depo-Testadiol, Soln. (Pharmacia & Upjohn).
Duo-Cyp (Keene Pharmaceuticals, Inc.).
Menoject LA (Kay).
TE Ionate PA, Inj. (Solvay Pharmaceuticals).

testosterone cypionate. (Various Mfr.) 100 mg/ml, 200 mg/ml. Inj. Vial 10 ml.
Use: Androgen.

testosterone cypionate/estradiol cypionate.
See: Estradiol cypionate w/testosterone cypionate.

testosterone cypionate and estradiol cypionate. (Schein Pharmaceutical, Inc.) Testosterone cypionate 50 mg, estradiol cypionate 2 mg/ml. Vials 10 ml. *Rx.*
Use: Androgen, estrogen combination.

•**testosterone enanthate.** (tess-TAHS-ter-ohn) U.S.P. 23.
Use: Androgen.
See: Andryl, Inj. (Keene Pharmaceuticals, Inc.).
Andropository-200, Inj. (Rugby Labs, Inc.).
Arderone 100, 200, Inj. (Burgin-Arden).
Delatest, Inj. (Dunhall Pharmaceuticals, Inc.).
Delatestryl, Inj., Vial (Bristol-Myers Squibb).

Everone 200 mg, Vial (Hyrex Pharmaceuticals).
Tesone L. A., Inj. (Sigma-Tau Pharmaceuticals, Inc.).
Testate, Inj. (Savage Laboratories).
Testrin-P.A., Inj. (Taylor Pharmaceuticals).
W/Chlorobutanol.
See: Anthatest, Vial (Kay).
Andro L.A. 200, Inj. (Forest Pharmaceutical, Inc).
Delatestryl, Inj. (Gynex).
Durathate-200, Inj. (Roberts Pharmaceuticals).
W/Estradiol valerate.
See: Everone 200, Inj. (Hyrex Pharmaceuticals).
See: Valertest No 1, Amp, Vial (Hyrex Pharmaceuticals).

testosterone enanthate. (Various Mfr.) 100 mg/ml, 200 mg/ml. Inj. Vial 10 ml.
Use: Androgen.

testosterone heptanoate.
Use: Androgen.
See: Testosterone enanthate.

•**testosterone ketolaurate.** (tess-TAHS-ter-ohn KEY-toe-LORE-ate) USAN.
Use: Androgen.

testosterone ointment 2%.
Use: Vulvar dystrophies. [Orphan Drug]

•**testosterone phenylacetate.** (tess-TAHS-ter-ohn fen-ill-ASS-ah-tate) USAN. Perandren phenylacetate.
Use: Androgen.

•**testosterone propionate.** (tess-TAHS-ter-ohn) U.S.P. 23.
Use: Androgen.

testosterone propionate. (Various Mfr.) Testosterone propionate 100 mg/ml in oil. Inj. Vial 10 ml.
Use: Androgen.

testosterone sublingual.
Use: Delay of growth and puberty in boys. [Orphan Drug]

Testred. (ICN Pharmaceuticals, Inc.) Methyltestosterone 10 mg/Cap. Bot. 100s. *c-III.*
Use: Androgen.

Testred Cypionate.
Use: Androgen inhibitor.
See: Proscar (Merck & Co.).

Testred Cypionate 200. (Zeneca Pharmaceuticals) Testosterone cypionate 200 mg/ml. Vial 10 ml. *c-III.*
Use: Androgen.

Testrin-P.A. (Taylor Pharmaceuticals) Testosterone enanthate 200 mg/ml, in sesame oil with chlorobutanol. Vial 10 ml. *c-III.*
Use: Androgen.

Testuria. (Wyeth-Ayerst Laboratories) Combination kit containing 5 x 20 sterile dip strips and 5 x 20 culture trays of trypticase soy agar.
Use: Diagnostic aid.

Tesuloid. (Bristol-Myers Squibb) Technetium Tc 99m sulfur colloid. 5 Vials/Kit.
Use: Radiopaque agent.

tetanus and diphtheria toxoids adsorbed for adult use. (TET-ah-nus and diff-THEER-ee-uh TOX-oyds) U.S.P. 23.
Use: Immunization.
See: Vial 5 ml for IM use (generic) (Pasteur Merieux Connaught).
Vial 5 ml (generic) (Wyeth-Ayerst Laboratories).

•**tetanus antitoxin.** (TET-n-us) U.S.P. 23.
Use: Immunization.

tetanus, diphtheria toxoids, and aluminum phosphate adsorbed. (Wyeth-Ayerst Laboratories) Vial 5 ml, Tubex 0.5 ml. *Rx.*
Use: Immunization.

tetanus, diphtheria & pertussis vaccine.
Use: Immunization.
See: Acel-Imune, Vial (Wyeth-Ayerst Laboratories).
Certiva (Ross Pediatrics).
Diphtheria and Tetanus Toxoids and Whole Cell Pertussis Vaccine, Vial (Pasteur Merieux Connaught).
Infanrix (SKB).
TriHIBit (Pasteur Merieux Connaught).
Tri-Immunol, Vial (Wyeth-Ayerst Laboratories).
Tripedia, Vial (Pasteur Merieux Connaught).

tetanus and diphtheria toxoids adsorbed purogenated. (Wyeth-Ayerst Laboratories) Adult Lederject disposable syringe 10 x 0.5 ml. Vial 5 ml, new package. *Rx.*
Use: Immunization.

•**tetanus immune globulin.** (TET-ah-nus ih-MYOON GLAH-byoo-lin) U.S.P. 23. *Formerly Tetanus Immune Human Globulin.* Gamma globulin fraction of the plasma of persons who have been hyperimmunized with tetanus toxoid, 16.5%. Vial 250 units.
Use: Prophylaxis of injured, against tetanus (passive immunizing agent).
See: Baytet (Bayer Corp. (Consumer Div.)).

tetanus immune globulin, human. 250 units/Tubex, 1 ml dissolved in glycine 0.3 M; thimerosal 0.01%. *Rx.*
Use: Immunization.

See: Baytet (Bayer Corp. (Allergy Div.)).

•**tetanus toxoid.** (TET-n-us TOX-oyd) U.S.P. 23.
Use: Immunization.

•**tetanus toxoid, adsorbed.** (TET-n-us TOX-oyd) U.S.P. 23.
Use: Immunization.
See: Te Anatoxal Berna, Vial, Syr. (Berna Products Corp.).

tetanus toxoid, adsorbed. (Pasteur Merieux Connaught) 20 Lf purified tetanus toxoid, 0.01% thimerosal as preservative/ml. Box 2 Amp of 0.5 ml. Vial 5 ml, 7.5 ml. Amp. for booster injection 0.5 ml. *Rx.*
Use: Immunization.
W/Te Anatoxal.
See: Vial 5 ml for IM use. (Berna Products Corp.).
Vial 5 ml, disp. syringes 0.5 ml. (Wyeth-Ayerst Laboratories).

tetanus toxoid adsorbed purogenated. (Wyeth-Ayerst Laboratories) Vial 5 ml. Lederject disposable syringe 0.5 ml. Box 10s, 100s. *Rx.*
Use: Immunization.

tetanus toxoid, aluminum phosphate adsorbed. *Rx.*
Use: Immunization.
See: Vial 5 ml 10s. Lederject Disp. Syr. 10 0.5 ml. (Wyeth-Ayerst Laboratories).

tetanus toxoid, fluid. (Pasteur Merieux Connaught) Vial 7.5 ml for IM or SC use. (Wyeth-Ayerst Laboratories) Vial 7.5 ml, Tubex 0.5 ml. *Rx.*
Use: Immunization.

tetanus toxoid, fluid purogenated. (Wyeth-Ayerst Laboratories) Vial 7.5 ml Lederject disposable syringe. 0.5 ml. Box 10s, 100s. *Rx.*
Use: Immunization.

tetanus toxoid purified, fluid. (Wyeth-Ayerst Laboratories) Vial 7.5 ml, Tubex 0.5 ml. *Rx.*
Use: Immunization.

tetiothalein sodium.
See: Iodophthalein Sodium (Various Mfr.).

Tetrabead. (Abbott Diagnostics) Solid phase radioimmunoassay for the quantitative measurement of total circulating serum thyroxine.

Tetrabead-125. (Abbott Diagnostics) T-3 uptake radioassay for the measurement of thyroid function by indirectly determining the degree of saturation of serum thyroxine binding globulin (TBG).

•**tetracaine.** (TEH-trah-cane) U.S.P. 23.
Use: Anesthetic (topical).
See: Pontocaine, Oint., Cream (Sanofi Winthrop Pharmaceuticals).
Viractin, Preps. (J.B. Williams).

tetracaine and menthol ointment.
Use: Anesthetic, local.

•**tetracaine hydrochloride.** U.S.P. 23.
Use: Spinal anesthetic, local.
See: Pontocaine Hydrochloride Inj., Pow. (Sanofi Winthrop Pharmaceuticals).
W/Benzocaine, butyl aminobenzoate.
See: Cetacaine, Liq., Oint., Spray (Cetylite Industries, Inc.).

tetracaine hydrochloride 0.5%. (Alcon Laboratories, Inc.) 0.5%. 1 ml Drop-Tainer, Ophth. 15 ml Steri-Unit, 2 ml (Ciba Vision) Dropperettes 1 ml in 10s. *Rx.*
Use: Anesthetic, ophthalmic.

Tetracap. (Circle Pharmaceuticals, Inc) Tetracycline HCl 250 mg/Cap. Bot. 100s. *Rx.*
Use: Anti-infective, tetracycline.

tetrachlorethylene. U.S.P. XXI. Perchlorethylene, tetrachlorethylene.
Use: Anthelmintic (hookworms and some trematodes).

Tetracon. (Professional Pharmacal) Tetrahydrozoline HCl 0.5 mg, disodium edetate 1 mg, boric acid 12 mg, benzalkonium Cl 0.1 mg, sodium Cl 2.2 mg, sodium borate 0.5 mg/ml w/water. Liq. Bot. 15 ml. *otc.*
Use: Anti-irritant, ophthalmic.

•**tetracycline.** (teh-truh-SIGH-kleen) U.S.P. 23.
Use: Antiamebic, anti-infective, antirickettsial.
See: Sumycin, Syr. (Bristol-Myers Squibb).

tetracycline w/ n-acetyl-para-aminophenol, phenyltoloxamine citrate. (Roberts Pharmaceuticals) Paltet, Cap.
Use: Anti-infective, tetracycline.
See: Telrex, Bid Cap., Cap., Vial (Bristol-Myers Squibb).

tetracycline and amphotericin B. U.S.P. XXI.

•**tetracycline hydrochloride.** (teh-trah-SIGH-kleen) U.S.P. 23.
Use: Anti-infective, antiamebic, antirickettsial.
See: Achromycin, Preps. (Storz/Lederle Ophthalmic Pharmaceuticals).
Bicycline, Caps. (Knight).
Centet 250, Tab. (Schwarz Pharma, Inc.).
Cyclopar, Cap. (Parke-Davis).
G-Mycin, Cap., Syr. (Coast).
Maso-Cycline, Cap. (Mason Pharmaceuticals, Inc.).

Panmycin, Cap. (Pharmacia & Upjohn).
Scotrex, Cap. (Scott/Cord).
Sumycin, Cap., Tab., Syr. (Bristol-Myers Squibb).
Tetracap 250, Cap. (Circle Pharmaceuticals, Inc.).
Tetracyn, Cap. (Pfizer US Pharmaceutical Group).
Tetram, Cap., Syr. (Dunhall Pharmaceuticals, Inc.).

W/Citric Acid.
See: Topicycline, Liq. (Procter & Gamble Pharm.).

W/Nystatin.
See: Achromycin V, Cap., Drop, Susp., Syr. (ESI Lederle Generics).

tetracycline hydrochloride fiber.
Use: Anti-infective, tetracycline.
See: Actisite (Alza Corp.).

tetracycline hydrochloride and nystatin capsules.
Use: Anti-infective, tetracycline.

tetracycline oral suspension.
Use: Anti-infective, tetracycline.

•**tetracycline phosphate complex.** (teh-truh-SIGH-kleen FOSS-fate) U.S.P. 23.
Use: Anti-infective.

Tetracyn. (Pfizer US Pharmaceutical Group) Tetracycline HCl. 250 mg, 500 mg/Cap. **250 mg:** Cap. Bot. 1000s. **500 mg:** Bot. 100s. *Rx.*
Use: Anti-infective, tetracycline.

tetradecyl sulfate, sodium.
Use: Sclerosing agent.
See: Sotradecol (ESI Lederle Generics).

tetraethyl ammonium bromide (teab).
Use: Diagnostic & therapeutic agent in peripheral vascular disorders. Diagnostic in hypertension.

tetraethylammonium chloride.
Use: Ganglionic blocking.

tetraethylthiuram disulfide.
See: Disulfiram.

•**tetrafilcon a.** (teh-trah-FILL-kahn) USAN.
Use: Contact lens material (hydrophilic).

tetrahydroaminoacridine.
Use: Cholinergic agent for Alzheimer's disease.
See: Cognex (Warner Lambert).

tetrahydrophenobarbital calcium.
See: Cyclobarbital Calcium, Prep.

tetrahydroxyquinone. Name used for Tetroquinone.

•**tetrahydrozoline hydrochloride.** (teh-trah-high-DRAHZ-ah-leen) U.S.P. 23.
Use: Adrenergic (vasoconstrictor).
See: Collyrium Fresh Eye Drops (Wyeth-Ayerst Laboratories).
Eyesine, Soln. (Akorn, Inc.).
Geneye Extra, Drops (Zenith Goldline Pharmaceuticals).
Mallazine Eye Drops (Roberts Pharmaceuticals).
Murine Plus (Abbott Laboratories).
Optigene 3, Soln. (Pfeiffer Co.).
Soothe, Soln. (Alcon Laboratories, Inc).
Tetrasine, Soln. (Optopics Laboratories, Corp).
Tyzine, Soln. (Key Pharmaceuticals).
Visine, Soln. (Pfizer US Pharmaceutical Group).

tetraiodophenolphthalein sodium.
See: Iodophthalein Sodium.

tetraiodophthalein sodium.
See: Iodophthalein Sodium.

tetramethylene dimethanesulfonate.
Busulfan.

tetramethylthiuram disulfide. Thiram.
Use: Anti-infective, antifungal.

•**tetramisole hydrochloride.** (teh-TRAM-ih-sole) USAN.
Use: Anthelmintic.

Tetramune. (Wyeth-Ayerst Laboratories) 12.5 Lf units of tetanus toxoid, 5 Lf units of diphtheria toxoid, 4 units of pertussis vaccine and 10 mcg *Haemophilus influenzae* type b oligosaccharide/0.5 ml. Vial 5 ml. *Rx.*
Use: Immunization.

Tetraneed. (Hanlon) Pentaerythritol tetranitrate 80 mg/Time Cap. Bot. 100s. *Rx.*
Use: Antianginal.

tetrantoin.
Use: Anticonvulsant.

Tetrasine. (Optopics Laboratories, Corp.) Tetrahydrozoline HCl 0.05%. Bot. 15 ml, 22.5 ml. *otc.*
Use: Ophthalmic vasoconstrictor/mydriatic.

Tetrasine Extra. (Optopics Laboratories, Corp.) Polyethylene glycol 400 1%, tetrahydrozoline HCl 0.05%. Bot. 15 ml. *otc.*
Use: Mydriatic, vasoconstrictor.

Tetratab. (Freeport) Pentaerythritol tetranitrate 10 mg/Tab. Bot. 1000s. *Rx.*
Use: Antianginal.

Tetratab No. 1. (Freeport) Pentaerythritol tetranitrate 20 mg/Tab. Bot. 1000s. *Rx.*
Use: Antianginal.

•**tetrazolast meglumine.** (teh-TRAZZ-oh-last meh-GLUE-meen) USAN.
Use: Antiallergic, antiasthmatic.

Tetrazyme. (Abbott Diagnostics) Test kit 100s, 500s.
Use: Enzyme immunoassay for quantitative measurement of total circulat-

ing serum thyroxine (free and protein bound).

•**tetrofosmin.** (teh-troe-FOSS-min) USAN.
Use: Diagnostic aid.

•**tetroquinone.** (TEH-troe-kwih-NOHN) USAN.
Use: Treat keloids, keratolytic (systemic).

•**tetroxoprim.** (tet-ROX-oh-prim) USAN.
Use: Anti-infective.

•**tetrydamine.** (teh-TRID-ah-meen) USAN.
Use: Analgesic, anti-inflammatory.

Tetterine. (Shuptrine) **Oint.:** Antifungal agents in green petrolatum base. Tin oz.; Antifungal agents in white petrolatum base. Tube oz. **Powder:** Fungicide, germicide formula powder for heat and diaper rash. Can 2.25 oz. **Soap:** Bar 3.25 oz.
Use: Dermatologic, counterirritant.

Texacort Scalp Lotion. (Medicis Dermatologicals, Inc.) Hydrocortisone 1%, alcohol 33%. Lipid free. Dropper Bot. 1 fl. oz. *Rx.*
Use: Corticosteroid.

T-Fluoride. (Tennessee Pharmaceutic) Sodium fluoride 2.21 mg/Tab. Bot. 100s, 1000s. *Rx.*
Use: Dental caries preventative.

TG.
Use: Antineoplastic.
See: Thioguanine (GlaxoWellcome).

T/Gel Scalp Solution. (Neutrogena) Neutar coal tar extract 2%, salicylic acid 2%. Bot. 2 oz. *otc.*
Use: Antipsoriatic, antiseborrheic.

T/Gel Therapeutic Conditioner. (Neutrogena) Neutar coal tar extract 1.5% in oil free conditioner base. Liq. Bot. 1.4 oz. *otc.*
Use: Antipsoriatic, antiseborrheic.

T/Gel Therapeutic Shampoo. (Neutrogena) Neutar coal tar extract 2% in mild shampoo base. Bot. 4.4 oz., 8.5 oz. *otc.*
Use: Antipsoriatic, antiseborrheic.

T-Gen Suppositories. (Zenith Goldline Pharmaceuticals) Trimethobenzamide HCl 100 mg/Pediatric Supp. or 200 mg/ Adult Supp. Box 10s, 50s. *Rx.*
Use: Antiemetic.

T-Gesic Capsule. (T.E. Williams Pharmaceuticals) Hydrocodone bitartrate 5 mg, acetaminophen 500 mg/Cap. Bot. 100s. *c-III.*
Use: Analgesic combination, narcotic, hypnotic, sedative.

•**thalidomide.** (the-LID-oh-mide) USAN.
Use: Anti-infective; hypnotic, sedative.
See: Thalomid, Cap. (Celgene).

Thalitone. (Horus Therapeutics, Inc.) Chlorthalidone 15 mg, 25 mg, lactose/ Tab. Bot. 100s. *Rx.*
Use: Diuretic.

•**thallous chloride Tl 201 injection.** (THAL-uhs) U.S.P. 23.
Use: Diagnostic aid (radiopaque medium), radioactive agent.

Thalomid. (Celgene) Thalidomide 50 mg. Cap. Box of 6 packs of 14 caps. *Rx.*
Use: Immunosuppressive.

Tham-E. (Abbott Laboratories) Tromethamine 36 g, NaCl 30 mEq/L, KCl 5 mEq/L, Cl 35 mEq/L. Total osmolarity 367 mOsm/L. Single-dose container 150 ml. *Rx.*
Use: Nutritional supplement.

Tham Solution. (Abbott Laboratories) Tromethamine 18 g, acetic acid 2.5 g single-dose container. *Rx.*
Use: Nutritional supplement.

THC.
Use: Antiemetic, antivertigo.
See: Marinol (Roxane Laboratories, Inc.).

theamin. Monoethanolamine salt of theophylline.
W/Amobarbital.
See: Monotheamin, Supp. (Eli Lilly and Co.).

thenalidine tartrate.
Use: Antihistamine, antipruritic.

thenyldiamine hydrochloride.
Use: Antihistamine.

Theo-24. (UCB Pharmaceuticals, Inc.) Theophylline anhydrous 100 mg, 200 mg, 300 mg/CR Cap. **100 mg:** Bot. 100s. UD 100s. **200 mg:** Bot. 100s, 500s. UD 100s. **300 mg:** Bot. 100s, 500s. UD 100s. *Rx.*
Use: Antiasthmatic, bronchodilator.

Theobid Duracap. (Ross Laboratories) Theophylline anhydrous 260 mg/TR Cap. Bot. 60s, 500s. *Rx.*
Use: Antiasthmatic, bronchodilator.

theobroma oil. N.F. 18. Cocoa Butter.
Use: Pharmaceutical aid, suppository base.

theobromine with phenobarbital combinations.
See: Harbolin, Tab. (Arcum).

theobromine calcium gluconate. (Bates) Tab., Bot. 100s, 1000s. Also available w/phenobarbital (Grant). Tab., Bot. 100s, 500s, 1000s.

theobromine sodium acetate. Theobromine calcium salt mixture with calcium salicylate.
Use: Diuretic; muscle relaxant.

theobromine sodium salicylate.
W/Cal. lactate, phenobarbital.
See: Doan's Pills (Purex).

Theochron. (Various Mfr.) Theophylline anhydrous 100 mg, 200 mg, 300 mg. ER Tab. 100s, 500s, 1000s. *Rx.*
Use: Bronchodilator.

Theochron. (Forest Pharmaceutical, Inc.) Theophylline 200 mg/TR Tab. Bot. 100s, 500s, 1000s. 300 mg/TR Tab. Bot. 100s, 500s. *Rx.*
Use: Bronchodilator.

Theoclear 80 Syrup. (Schwarz Pharma, Inc.) Theophylline 80 mg/15 ml. Bot. Pt, gal. *Rx.*
Use: Bronchodilator.

Theoclear L.A.-130 Cenules. (Schwarz Pharma, Inc.) Theophylline 130 mg/Cap. Bot. 100s. *Rx.*
Use: Bronchodilator.

Theoclear L.A.-260 Cenules. (Schwarz Pharma, Inc.) Theophylline 260 mg/Cap. Bot. 100s, 1000s. *Rx.*
Use: Bronchodilator.

Theocolate. (Rosemont Pharmaceutical Corp.) Theophylline 150 mg, guaifenesin 90 mg/15 ml Liq. Bot. Pt., gal. *Rx.*
Use: Antiasthmatic.

Theodrine. (Rugby Labs, Inc.) Theophylline 120 mg, ephedrine HCl 22.5 mg/Tab. Bot. 1000s. *otc.*
Use: Antiasthmatic.

Theo-Dur. (Schering-Plough Corp.) Theophylline 450 mg/SR Tab. Bot. 100s, UD 100s. *Rx.*
Use: Bronchodilator.

Theo-Dur Tablets. (Key Pharmaceuticals) Theophylline 100 mg, 200 mg, 300 mg/SA Tab. Bot. 100s, 500s, 1000s, 5000s. UD 100s. *Rx.*
Use: Bronchodilator.

•**theofibrate.** (THEE-oh-FIH-brate) USAN.
Use: Antihyperlipoproteinemic.

Theogen. (Sigma-Tau Pharmaceuticals, Inc.) Conjugated estrogens 2 mg/ml. Vial 10 ml, 30 ml. *Rx.*
Use: Estrogen.

Theogen I.P. (Sigma-Tau Pharmaceuticals, Inc.) Estrone 2 mg, potassium estrone sulfate 1 mg/ml. Inj. Vial 10 ml. *Rx.*
Use: Estrogen.

Theolair. (3M Pharmaceuticals) Theophylline 125 mg, 250 mg/Tab. Box 100s, 250s as foil strip 10s. Bot. 100s. *Rx.*
Use: Bronchodilator.

Theolair Liquid. (3M Pharmaceuticals) Theophylline 80 mg/15 ml. Bot. Pt. *Rx.*
Use: Bronchodilator.

Theolair-SR 200. (3M Pharmaceuticals) Theophylline 200 mg/Tab. (slow release). Bot. 100s. Box 100s as foil strip 10s. *Rx.*
Use: Bronchodilator.

Theolair-SR 250. (3M Pharmaceuticals) Theophylline 250 mg/Tab. (slow release). Bot. 100s, 250s. *Rx.*
Use: Bronchodilator.

Theolair-SR 300. (3M Pharmaceuticals) Theophylline 300 mg/Tab. (slow release). Bot. 100s. Box 100s as foil strip 10s. *Rx.*
Use: Bronchodilator.

Theolair-SR 500. (3M Pharmaceuticals) Theophylline 500 mg/Tab. (slow release). Bot. 100s, 250s. *Rx.*
Use: Bronchodilator.

Theolate Liquid. (Various Mfr.) Theophylline 150 mg, guaifenesin 90 mg/15 ml. Liq. Bot. 118 ml, pt, gal. *Rx.*
Use: Antiasthmatic.

Theomax DF Syrup. (Various Mfr.) Theophylline 97.5 mg, ephedrine sulfate 18.75 mg, alcohol 5%, hydroxyzine HCl 7.5 mg/15 ml. Bot. Pt. gal. *Rx.*
Use: Antiasthmatic.

Theo-Organidin. (Wallace Laboratories) Theophylline anhydrous 120 mg, iodinated glycerol 30 mg/15 ml w/alcohol 15%, saccharin. Bot. Pt., gal. *Rx.*
Use: Antiasthmatic.

Theophenyllin. (H.L. Moore Drug Exchange, Inc.) Theophylline 130 mg, ephedrine HCl 24 mg, phenobarbital 8 mg/Tab. Bot. 1000s. *Rx.*
Use: Antiasthmatic.

Theophyl-SR. (Ortho McNeil Pharmaceutical) Theophylline 125 mg. Bot. 100s. *Rx.*
Use: Bronchodilator.

•**theophylline.** (thee-AHF-ih-lin) U.S.P. 23.
Use: Bronchodilator; coronary vasodilator, diuretic; pharmaceutic necessity for Aminophylline Injection.
See: Accurbron, Liq. (Hoechst Marion Roussel).
Aerolate, Cap., Elix. (Fleming & Co.).
Aquaphyllin, Syr. (Ferndale Laboratories, Inc.).
Bronkodyl, Cap. (Sanofi Winthrop Pharmaceuticals).
Elixicon, Susp. (Berlex Laboratories, Inc.).
Elixophyllin, Elix., Cap. (Berlex Laboratories, Inc.).
Elixophyllin SR, Cap. (Berlex Laboratories, Inc.).
Lodrane, Cap. (ECR Pharmaceuticals).
Quibron-T Dividose, Tab. (Roberts Pharmaceuticals).

Quibron-T/SR Dividose, Tab. (Roberts Pharmaceuticals).
Slo-Phyllin, Cap., Syr., Tab. (Dooner).
Sustaire, Tab. (Pfizer US Pharmaceutical Group).
Theobid, Cap. (Ross Laboratories).
Theobid Jr, Cap. (Ross Laboratories).
Theochron, ER Tab. (Various Mfr.).
Theoclear 80, Liq. (Schwarz Pharma, Inc.).
Theoclear L.A., Cenule (Schwarz Pharma, Inc.).
Theo-Dur, Tab. (Key Pharmaceuticals).
Theolair, Tab, Liq. (3M Pharmaceuticals).
Theolair SR, Tab. (3M Pharmaceuticals).
Theospan, Cap. (Laser, Inc).
Theostat, Prods. (Laser, Inc).
Theovent Long-Acting, Cap. (Schering-Plough Corp.).
Theo-X, CR Tab. (Schwarz Pharma, Inc.).
Uni-Dur, ER Tab. (Key Pharmaceuticals).
Uniphyl, TR Tab. (Purdue Frederick Co.).

theophylline. (Various Mfr.) 100 mg, 125 mg, 200 mg, 300 mg/ER Cap. Bot. 100s. *Rx.*
Use: Bronchodilator.

theophylline, 8-chloro, diphenhydramine. U.S.P. 23. Dimenhydrinate.
See: Dramamine, Prep. (Searle).

theophylline aminoisobutanol. Theophylline w/2-amino-2-methyl-1-propanol.
See: Butaphyllamine (Various Mfr.).

theophylline choline salt.
See: Choledyl, Tab., Elix. (Parke-Davis).

theophylline and 5% dextrose. (Abbott and Baxter) Inj. 200 mg/Cont.: 50 ml, 100 ml. 400 mg/Cont.: 100 ml, 250 ml, 500 ml, 1000 ml. 800 mg/Cont.: 250 ml, 500 ml, 1000 ml.
Use: Bronchodilator.

theophylline, ephedrine hydrochloride, andphenobarbital tablets.
Use: Bronchodilator, sedative.

theophylline ethylenediamine.
See: Aminophylline, Prep. (Various Mfr.).

theophylline extended release. (Dey Laboratories, Inc.) Theophylline 100 mg, 200 mg, 300 mg. ER Tab. Bot. 100s, 500s, 1000s. *Rx.*
Use: Bronchodilator.

theophylline extended-release. (Sidmak Laboratories, Inc.) Theophylline anhydrous 450 mg, lactose. ER Tab. Bot. 100s, 250s, 500s. *Rx.*
Use: Bronchodilator.

theophylline extended-release capsules.
Use: Bronchodilator.

theophylline w/combinations.
See: B.A. Prods. (Federal).
Bronkaid, Tab. (Brew).
Co-Xan, Liq. (Schwarz Pharma, Inc.).
Elixophyllin-KI, Elix. (Berlex Laboratories, Inc.).
Marax DF, Syr. (Roerig).
Quibron, Cap., Liq. (Bristol-Myers Squibb).
Quibron-300, Cap. (Bristol-Myers Squibb).
Quibron Plus, Cap. (Bristol-Myers Squibb).
Slo-Phyllin GG, Cap., Syr. (Dooner).
Synophylate, Liq. (Schwarz Pharma, Inc.).
Tedral SA, Tab. (Parke-Davis).
Theolair Plus, Tab, Liq. (3M Pharmaceuticals).
Theo-Organidin, Elix. (Wampole Laboratories).

theophylline and guaifenesin capsules.
Use: Bronchodilator, expectorant.

theophylline and guaifenesin oral solution.
Use: Bronchodilator, expectorant.

theophylline KI. (Various Mfr.) Theophylline 80 mg, potassium iodide 130 mg/15 ml. Elix. 480 ml, gal. *Rx.*
Use: Antiasthmatic combination.

theophylline olamine. Theophylline compound with 2-amino-ethanol (1:1).
Use: Bronchodilator.

theophylline with phenobarbital combinations.
See: Ceepa, Tab. (Geneva Pharmaceuticals).

theophylline reagent strips. (Bayer Corp. (Consumer Div.)) Seralyzer reagent strip. Bot. 25s.
Use: Diagnostic aid, theophylline.

•**theophylline sodium glycinate.** (thee-AHF-ih-lin so-dee-uhm) U.S.P. 23.
Use: Bronchodilator.
See: Synophylate, Elix., Tab. (Schwarz Pharma, Inc.).
W/Guaifenesin.
See: Synophylate-GG, Tab., Syr. (Schwarz Pharma, Inc.).
W/Phenobarbital.
See: Synophylate w/Phenobarbital, Tab. (Schwarz Pharma, Inc.).
W/Potassium iodide.
See: TSG-KI, Elix. (Zeneca Pharmaceuticals).

Theo-Sav. (Savage Laboratories) Theophylline 100 mg/Tab. Bot. 100s. 200 mg, 300 mg/Tab. Bot. 100s, 500s, 1000s. *Rx.*
Use: Bronchodilator.

Theospan-SR 130. (Laser, Inc.) Theophylline anhydrous 130 mg/Cap. Bot. 100s, 1000s. *Rx.*
Use: Bronchodilator.

Theospan-SR 260. (Laser, Inc.) Theophylline anhydrous 260 mg/Cap. Bot. 100s, 1000s. *Rx.*
Use: Bronchodilator.

Theostat 80 Syrup. (Laser, Inc.) Theophylline anhydrous 80 mg/15 ml. Bot. Pt, gal. *Rx.*
Use: Bronchodilator.

Theotal. (Major Pharmaceuticals) Theophylline 125 mg, ephedrine HCl 25 mg, phenobarbital 8 mg, lactose. Tab. Bot. 1000s. *Rx.*
Use: Antiasthmatic combination.

Theo-Time. (Major Pharmaceuticals) Theophylline 100 mg, 200 mg, 300 mg/TR Tab. Bot. 100s, 500s. *Rx.*
Use: Bronchodilator.

Theo-Time SR Tabs. (Major Pharmaceuticals) Theophylline 100 mg, 200 mg, 300 mg/SR Tab. Bot. 100s, 500s.
Use: Bronchodilator.

Theovent Long-Acting. (Schering-Plough Corp.) Theophylline anhydrous 125 mg, 250 mg/Cap. Bot. 100s. *Rx.*
Use: Bronchodilator.

Theo-X. (Schwarz Pharma, Inc.) Theophylline anhydrous 100 mg, 200 mg, 300 mg/CR Tab. Dye free, lactose. Bot. 100s, 500s, 1000s (except 100 mg). *Rx.*
Use: Bronchodilator.

Thera Bath. (Walgreen) Mineral oil 90%. Bot. 16 oz. *otc.*
Use: Emollient.

Thera Bath with Vitamin E. (Walgreen) Mineral oil 91%, Vit. E 2000 IU/16 oz. *otc.*
Use: Emollient.

Therabid. (Mission Pharmacal Co.) Vitamins C 500 mg, B_1 15 mg, B_2 10 mg, B_3 100 mg, B_5 20 mg, B_6 10 mg, B_{12} 5 mcg, A 5000 IU, D 200 IU, E 30 mg/Tab. Bot. 60s. *otc.*
Use: Mineral, vitamin supplement.

Therabloat. (Norden) Poloxalene.

Therabrand. (Health for Life Brands, Inc.) Vitamins A 25,000 IU, D 1000 IU, B_1 10 mg, B_2 10 mg, niacinamide 100 mg, C 200 mg, B_6 5 mg, calcium pantothenate 20 mg, B_{12} 5 mcg/Cap. Bot. 100s, 1000s. *otc.*
Use: Mineral, vitamin supplement.

Therabrand-M. (Health for Life Brands, Inc.) Vitamins A 25,000 IU, D 1000 IU, C 200 mg, B_1 10 mg, B_2 10 mg, B_6 5 mg, niacinamide 100 mg, calcium pantothenate 20 mg, E 5 IU, B_{12} 5 mcg, I 0.15 mg, Fe 15 mg, Cu 1 mg, Ca 125 mg, Mn 1 mg, Mg 6 mg, Zn 1.5 mg/Cap. Bot. 100s, 1000s. *otc.*
Use: Mineral, vitamin supplement.

Therac. (C & M Pharmacal, Inc.) Colloidal sulfur 4% in lotion base. Bot. 60 ml. *otc.*
Use: Antiacne.

Theracap. (Arcum) Vitamins A 10,000 IU, D 400 IU, B_1 10 mg, B_2 5 mg, niacinamide 150 mg, C 150 mg/Cap. Bot. 100s, 1000s. *otc.*
Use: Vitamin supplement.

Thera-Combex H-P. (Parke-Davis) Vitamins C 500 mg, B_1 25 mg, B_2 15 mg, B_{12} 5 mcg, niacinamide 100 mg, panthenol 20 mg/Cap. Bot. 100s. *otc.*
Use: Vitamin supplement.

TheraCys. (Pasteur Merieux Connaught) 81 mg dry weight per vial, 1.7 to 19.2 x 10^8 CFU per vial. Vial with 3 ml vial of diluent; 50 ml vials of phosphate-buffered sodium chloride are available for use as final diluent. *Rx.*
Use: Antineoplastic.

TheraFlu, Flu and Cold Medicine. (Novartis Pharmaceutical Corp.) Pseudoephedrine HCl 60 mg, chlorpheniramine maleate 4 mg, acetaminophen 650 mg, sucrose, lemon flavor. Pow. Pks. 6, 12. *otc.*
Use: Analgesic, antihistamine, decongestant.

TheraFlu, Flu Cold & Cough Medicine. (Novartis Pharmaceutical Corp.) Pseudoephedrine HCl 60 mg, chlorpheniramine maleate 4 mg, dextromethorphan HBr 20 mg, acetaminophen 650 mg. Pow. Pks. 6s. *otc.*
Use: Analgesic, antihistamine, antitussive, decongestant.

Thera-Flu Non-Drowsy Flu, Cold & Cough Maximum Strength. (Novartis Pharmaceutical Corp.) Pseudoephedrine HCl 60 mg, dextromethorphan HBr 30 mg, acetaminophen 1000 mg. Pow. 6s, 12s. *otc.*
Use: Analgesic, antitussive, decongestant.

Thera-Flu Non-Drowsy Formula, Maximum Strength. (Novartis Pharmaceutical Corp.) Pseudoephedrine HCl 30 mg, dextromethorphan HBr 15 mg, acetaminophen 500 mg. Capl. Pkg. 24s. *otc.*
Use: Antitussive, decongestant.

Thera-Flur. (Colgate Oral Pharmaceuticals) Fluoride 0.5% (from sod. fluoride 1.1%). pH 4.5. Gel-Drops. Bot. 24 ml, 60 ml. *Rx.*
Use: Dental caries agent.

Thera-Flur-N. (Colgate Oral Pharmaceuticals) Neutral sodium fluoride 1.1% Liq. Bot. 24 ml, 60 ml. *Rx.*
Use: Dental caries agent.

Therafortis. (General Vitamin) Vitamins A 12,500 IU, D 1000 IU, B_1 5 mg, B_2 5 mg, B_6 1 mg, B_{12} 3 mcg, niacinamide 50 mg, pantothenic acid salt 10 mg, C 150 mg, folic acid 0.5 mg/Cap. Bot. 100s, 1000s. *otc.*
Use: Vitamin supplement.

Theragenerix. (Zenith Goldline Pharmaceuticals) Vitamins A 5500 IU, D 400 IU, E 30 mg, B_1 3 mg, B_2 3.4 mg, B_3 30 mg, B_5 10 mg, B_6 3 mg, B_{12} 9 mcg, C 120 mg, folic acid 0.4 mg, biotin 15 mcg, beta-carotene 2500 IU. Tab. Bot. 130s, 1000s. *otc.*
Use: Vitamin supplement.

Theragenerix-H. (Zenith Goldline Pharmaceuticals) Fe 66.7 mg, vitamins A 8333 IU, D 133 IU, E 5 IU, B_1 3.3 mg, B_2 3.3 mg, B_3 33.3 mg, B_5 11.7 mg, B_6 3.3 mg, B_{12} 50 mcg, C 100 mg, folic acid 0.33 mg, Cu, Mg/Tab. Bot. 100s, 1000s. *otc.*
Use: Mineral, vitamin supplement.

Theragenerix-M. (Zenith Goldline Pharmaceuticals) Fe 27 mg, vitamins A 5000 IU, D 400 IU, E 30 mg, B_1 3 mg, B_2 3.4 mg, B_3 30 mg, B_5 10 mg, B_6 3 mg, B_{12} 9 mcg, C 120 mg, folic acid 0.4 mg, Ca, Cl, Cr, Cu, I, K, biotin 15 mcg, Mg, Mn, Mo, P, Se, Zn 15 mg, beta-carotene 2500 IU. Tab. Bot. 130s, 1000s. *otc.*
Use: Mineral, vitamin supplement.

Thera-Gesic. (Mission Pharmacal Co.) Methyl salicylate, menthol. Balm. Tube 90 g, 150 g. *otc.*
Use: Analgesic, topical.

Theragran. (Bristol-Myers Squibb) Vitamins A 5000 IU, D 400 IU, E 30 IU, B_1 3 mg, B_2 3.4 mg, B_3 20 mg, B_5 10 mg, B_6 3 mg, B_{12} 9 mcg, C 90 mg, folic acid 0.4 mg, biotin 30 mcg/Capl. Bot. 100s. *otc.*
Use: Vitamin supplement.

Theragran AntiOxidant. (Bristol-Myers Squibb) Vitamins A 5000 IU, C 250 mg, E 200 IU, Mn, Cu, Zn, Se/Softgel Cap. Bot. 50s. *otc.*
Use: Mineral, vitamin supplement.

Theragran Jr. with Iron. (Bristol-Myers Squibb) Fe 18 mg, vitamins A 5000 IU, D 400 IU, E 30 mg, B_1 1.5 mg, B_2 1.7 mg, B_3 20 mg, B_6 2 mg, B_{12} 6 mcg, C 60 mg, folic acid 0.4 mg w/tartrazine/ Tab. Bot. 75s. *otc.*
Use: Mineral, vitamin supplement.

Theragran Hematinic. (Apothecon, Inc.) Fe 66.7 IU, vitamins A 1400 IU, D 400 IU, E 5 IU, B_1 3.3 mg, B_2 3.3 mg, B_3 33.3 mg, B_5 11.7 mg, B_6 3.3 mg, B_{12} 50 mcg, C 100 mg, folic acid 0.33 mg, Ca, Cu, Mg/Tab. Bot. 90s. *Rx.*
Use: Mineral, vitamin supplement.

Theragran Liquid. (Bristol-Myers Squibb) Vitamins A 5000 IU, D 400 IU, B_1 10 mg, B_2 10 mg, B_3 100 mg, B_5 21.4 mg, B_6 4.1 mg, B_{12} 5 mcg, C 200 mg/5 ml. Liq. Bot. 120 ml. *otc.*
Use: Vitamin supplement.

Theragran-M. (Bristol-Myers Squibb) Ca 40 mg, Fe 27 mg, vitamins A 5000 IU, D 400 IU, E 30 mg, B_1 3 mg, B_2 3.4 mg, B_3 20 mg, B_5 10 mg, B_6 3 mg, B_{12} 9 mcg, C 90 mg, folic acid 0.4 mg, Cl, Cr, Cu, I, K, Mg, Mn, Mo, P, Se, Zn 15 mg, biotin 30 mcg, lactose, sucrose/ Capl. Bot. 90s, 130s, 180s, 200s. *otc.*
Use: Mineral, vitamin supplement.

Theragran Stress Formula. (Bristol-Myers Squibb) Fe 27 mg, vitamins E 30 IU, B_1 15 mg, B_2 15 mg, B_3 100 mg, B_5 20 mg, B_6 25 mg, B_{12} 12 mcg, C 600 mg, folic acid 0.4 mg, biotin 45 mcg/Tab. Bot. 75s. *otc.*
Use: Mineral, vitamin supplement.

Thera Hematinic. (Major Pharmaceuticals) Fe 66.7 mg, A 8333 IU, D 133 IU, E 5 IU, B_1 3.3 mg, B_2 3.3 mg, B_3 33.3 mg, B_5 11.7 mg, B_6 3.3 mg, B_{12} 50 mcg, C 100 mg, folic acid 0.33 mg, Cu, Mg/Tab. Bot. 250s, 1000s. *otc.*
Use: Mineral, vitamin supplements.

Thera-Hist. (Major Pharmaceuticals) Pseudoephedrine HCl 60 mg, chlorpheniramine maleate 4 mg, acetaminophen 500 mg, sucrose. Pow. Pks. 6. *otc.*
Use: Analgesic, antihistamine, decongestant.

Thera-Hist Syrup. (Major Pharmaceuticals) Phenylpropanolamine HCl 12.5 mg, chlorpheniramine maleate 2 mg/5 ml. Syr. Bot. 120 ml. *otc.*
Use: Antihistamine, decongestant.

Thera H Tabs. (Major Pharmaceuticals) Bot. 100s, 250s.
Use: Mineral, vitamin supplement.

Thera-M. (Various Mfr.) Vitamins A 5000 IU, B_1 3 mg, B_2 3.4 mg, B_3 20 mg, B_5 10 mg, B_6 3 mg, B_{12} 9 mcg, C 90 mg, D 400 IU, E 30 IU, Fe 27 mg, folic acid 0.4 mg, biotin 30 mcg, P, Ca, Cu, Cr, Se, Mo, K, Cl, I, Mg, Mn, Zn 15 mg.

Tab. Bot. 130s, 1000s. *otc.*
Use: Mineral, vitamin supplement.

Thera Multi-Vitamin. (Major Pharmaceuticals) Vitamins A 10,000 IU, D 400 IU, B_1 10 mg, B_2 10 mg, B_3 100 mg, B_5 21.4 mg, B_6 4.1 mg, B_{12} 5 mcg, C 200 mg/5 ml. Liq. Bot. 118 ml. *otc.*
Use: Vitamin supplement.

Theramycin Z. (Medicis Dermatologicals, Inc.) Erythromycin 2%, SD alcohol 40-B 81%. Topical Soln. 60 ml. *Rx.*
Use: Dermatologic, acne.

Theraneed. (Hanlon) Vitamins A 16,000 IU, B_1 10 mg, B_2 10 mg, B_6 2 mg, C 300 mg, calcium pantothenate 10 mg, niacinamide 10 mg, B_{12} 10 mcg/Cap. Bot. 100s. *otc.*
Use: Mineral, vitamin supplement.

Therapals. (Faraday) Vitamins A 25,000 IU, D 400 IU, B_1 10 mg, B_2 5 mg, niacinamide 150 mg, B_6 0.5 mg, E 5 IU, C 150 mg, B_{12} 10 mcg, Ca 103 mg, cobalt 0.1 mg, Cu 1 mg, K 0.15 mg, Mg 6 mg, Mn 1 mg, Mo 0.2 mg, P 80 mg, K 5 mg, Zn 1.2 mg/Tab. Bot. 100s, 250s, 1000s. *otc.*
Use: Mineral, vitamin supplement.

Therapeutic B Complex with Vitamin C. (Upsher-Smith Labs, Inc.) Vitamins B_1 15 mg, B_2 10.2 mg, B_3 50 mg, B_5 10 mg, B_6 5 mg, C 300 mg/Cap. Bot. UD 100s. *otc.*
Use: Vitamin supplement.

Therapeutic-H. (Zenith Goldline Pharmaceuticals) Fe 66.7 mg, A 8333 IU, D 133 IU, E 5 IU, B_1 3.3 mg, B_2 3.3 mg, B_3 33.3 mg, B_5 11.7 mg, B_6 3.3 mg, B_{12} 50 mcg, C 100 mg, folic acid 0.33 mg, Cu, Mg/Tab. Bot. 100s. *otc.*
Use: Mineral, vitamin supplement.

Therapeutic-M. (Zenith Goldline Pharmaceuticals) Fe 27 mg, vitamins A 5000 IU, D 400 IU, E 30 IU, B_1 3 mg, B_2 3.4 mg, B_3 20 mg, B_5 10 mg, B_6 3 mg, B_{12} 9 mcg, C 90 mg, folic acid 0.4 mg, Ca, Cl, Cr, Cu, I, K, Mg, Mn, Mo, P, Se, Zn 15 mg, biotin 30 mcg/Tab. Bot. 1000s. *otc.*
Use: Mineral, vitamin supplement.

Therapeutic Mineral Ice. (Bristol-Myers Squibb) Menthol 2%, ammonium hydroxide, carbomer 934, cupric sulfate, isopropyl alcohol, magnesium sulfate, thymol. Gel Tube 105 ml, 240 ml, 480 ml. *otc.*
Use: Liniment.

Therapeutic Tablets. (Zenith Goldline Pharmaceuticals) Vitamins A 5000 IU, D 400 IU, E 30 IU, B_1 3 mg, B_2 3.4 mg, B_3 20 mg, B_5 10 mg, B_6 3 mg, B_{12} 9 mcg, C 90 mg, folic acid 0.4 mg, d-biotin 30 mcg/Tab. Bot. 100s, 130s. *otc.*
Use: Vitamin supplement.

Therapeutic V & M. (Whiteworth Towne) Vitamins A 10,000 IU, D 400 IU, B_1 10 mg, B_2 10 mg, B_6 5 mg, B_{12} 5 mcg, niacinamide 100 mg, calcium pantothenate 20 mg, C 200 mg, E 15 IU, I 0.15 mg, Fe 12 mg, Cu 2 mg, Mn 1 mg, Mg 60 mg, Zn 1.5 mg/Tab. *otc.*
Use: Mineral, vitamin supplement.

Therapeutic Vitamin Formula w/Minerals. (Towne) Vitamins A palmitate 10,000 IU, D 400 IU, B_1 15 mg, B_2 10 mg, B_6 5 mg, B_{12} 12 mcg, C 200 mg, niacinamide 100 mg, calcium pantothenate 20 mg, E 15 IU, Ca 103 mg, Fe 10 mg, Mn 1 mg, K 5 mg, Zn 1.5 mg, Mg 6 mg/Cap. Bot. 30s, 60s, 100s, 250s. *otc.*
Use: Mineral, vitamin supplement.

Therapeutic Vitamin Formula w/Minerals. (Towne) Vitamins A palmitate 25,000 IU, D 1000 IU, B_1 10 mg, B_2 5 mg, B_6 1 mg, B_{12} 5 mcg, C 150 mg, niacinamide 100 mg, Ca 103 mg, P 80 mg, Fe 10 mg, I 0.1 mg, Mn 1 mg, K 5 mg, Cu 1 mg, Zn 1.4 mg, Mg 5.5 mg/Cap. Bot. 100s, 1000s. *otc.*
Use: Mineral, vitamin supplement.

Theraphon. (Health for Life Brands, Inc.) Vitamins A 25,000 IU, D 1000 IU, B_1 10 mg, B_2 5 mg, C 150 mg, niacinamide 150 mg/Cap. Bot. 100s, 1000s. *otc.*
Use: Vitamin supplement.

Theraplex T. (Medicis Dermatologicals, Inc.) Coal tar 1%, benzyl alcohol. Shampoo. Bot. 240 ml. *otc.*
Use: Antiseborrheic.

Theraplex Z. (Medicis Dermatologicals, Inc.) Pyrithione zinc 1%. Shampoo. Bot. 240 ml. *otc.*
Use: Antiseborrheic.

Theravee Hematinic Vitamin. (Vangard Labs, Inc.) Fe 66.7 mg, A 8333 IU, D 133 IU, E 5 IU, B_1 3.3 mg, B_2 3.3 mg, B_3 33.3 mg, B_5 11.7 mg, B_6 3.3 mg, B_{12} 50 mcg, C 100 mg, folic acid 0.33 mg, Cu, Mg/Tab. Bot. UD 100s. *otc.*
Use: Mineral, vitamin supplement.

Theravee-M. (Vangard Labs, Inc.) Fe 27 mg, vitamin A 5000 IU, D 400 IU, E 30 IU, B_1 3 mg, B_2 3.4 mg, B_3 30 mg, B_5 10 mg, B_6 3 mg, B_{12} 9 mcg, C 120 mg, folic acid 0.4 mg, Ca, Cl, Cr, Cu, K, I, Mg, Mn, Mo, Se, Zn 15 mcg, biotin 15 mcg, beta-carotene 2500 IU/Tab. Bot. 100s, 1000s, UD 100s. *otc.*
Use: Mineral, vitamin supplement.

Theravee Vitamin. (Vangard Labs, Inc.) Vitamins A 5500 IU, D 400 IU, E 30 IU, B_1 3 mg, B_2 3.4 mg, B_3 30 mg, B_5 10

mg, B_6 3 mg, B_{12} 9 mcg, C 120 mg, folic acid 0.4 mg, biotin 15 mcg/Tab. Bot. 100s. UD 100s. *otc.*
Use: Vitamin supplement.

Theravim. (NBTY, Inc.) Vitamins A 5000 IU, D 400 IU, E 30 IU, B_1 3 mg, B_2 3.4 mg, B_3 30 mg, B_5 10 mg, B_6 3 mg, B_{12} 9 mcg, C 90 mg, folic acid 0.4 mg, beta-carotene 1250 IU, biotin 35 mcg/Tab. Bot. 130s. *otc.*
Use: Vitamin supplement.

Theravim-M. (NBTY, Inc.) Fe 27 mg, vitamins A 5000 IU, D 400 IU, E 30 mg, B_1 3 mg, B_2 3.4 mg, B_3 20 mg, B_5 10 mg, B_6 3 mg, B_{12} 9 mcg, C 90 mg, folic acid 0.4 mg, Ca, Cl, Cr, Cu, I, K, Mg, Mn, Mo, P, Se, Zn 15 mg, biotin 30 mcg/Tab. Bot. 130s. *otc.*
Use: Mineral, vitamin supplement.

Theravite. (Alpharma USPD Inc.) Vitamins A 10,000 IU, D 400 IU, B_1 10 mg, B_2 10 mg, B_3 100 mg, B_5 21.4 mg, B_6 4.1 mg, B_{12} 5 mcg, C 200 mg/5 ml. Liq. Bot. 118 ml. *otc.*
Use: Vitamin supplement.

Therems. (Rugby Labs, Inc.) Vitamins A 5000 IU, D 400 IU, E 30 mg, B_1 3 mg, B_2 3.4 mg, B_3 30 mg, B_5 10 mg, B_6 3 mg, B_{12} 9 mcg, C 120 mg, folic acid 0.4 mg, beta-carotene 1250 IU, biotin 15 mcg/Tab. Bot. 130s, 1000s. *otc.*
Use: Vitamin supplement.

Therems-M. (Rugby Labs, Inc.) Fe 27 mg, vitamins A 5500 IU, D 400 IU, E 30 mg, B_1 3 mg, B_2 3.4 mg, B_3 20 mg, B_5 10 mg, B_6 3 mg, B_{12} 9 mcg, C 90 mg, folic acid 0.4 mg, Ca, Cl, Cr, Cu, I, K, Mg, Mn, Mo, P, Se, Zn 15 mg, biotin 30 mcg/Tab. Bot. 90s, 100s, 1000s. *otc.*
Use: Mineral, vitamin supplement.

Therevac. (Jones Medical Industries, Inc.) Docusate potassium 283 mg, benzocaine 20 mg w/soft soap in PEG 400 and glycerin base. Unit 4 ml, Cap. Pkgs. 4s, 12s, 50s. *otc.*
Use: Bowel evacuant.

Therevac Plus. (Jones Medical Industries, Inc.) Docusate sodium 283 mg, benzocaine 20 mg in a base of soft soap, PEG 400, glycerin/Cap. 3.9 g. Jar 30s. Disposable enema. *otc.*
Use: Laxative.

Therevac-SB. (Jones Medical Industries, Inc.) Docusate sodium 283 mg in a base of soft soap, PEG 400, glycerin/Cap. 3.9 g Bot. 30s. Disposable enema. *otc.*
Use: Laxative.

Therex No. 1. (Halsey Drug Co.) Vitamins A 10,000 IU, D 400 IU, E 15 IU, C 200 mg, B_1 10 mg, B_2 10 mg, niacinamide 100 mg, B_6 5 mg, B_{12} 5 mcg, calcium pantothenate 20 mg/Tab. Bot. 100s. *otc.*
Use: Vitamin, mineral supplement.

Therex and Zinc. (Halsey Drug Co.)
Use: Dietary supplement.

Therex-M. (Halsey Drug Co.) Vitamins A 10,000 IU, D 400 IU, E 15 IU, C 200 mg, B_1 10 mg, B_2 10 mg, niacinamide 100 mg, B_6 5 mg, B_{12} 5 mcg, calcium pantothenate 20 mg, I 150 mcg, Fe 12 mg, Mg 65 mg, Cu 2 mg, Zn 1.5 mg, Mn 1 mg/Tab. Bot. 100s. *otc.*
Use: Mineral, vitamin supplement.

Therex-Z. (Halsey Drug Co.) Vitamins A 10,000 IU, D 400 IU, E 15 IU, C 200 mg, B_1 10 mg, B_2 10 mg, niacinamide 100 mg, B_{12} 5 mcg, B_6 5 mg, Ca pantothenate 20 mg, I 150 mcg, Cu 2 mg, Fe 12 mg, Zn 22.5 mg/Tab. Bot. 100s. *otc.*
Use: Mineral, vitamin supplement.

Therma-Kool. (Nortech Laboratories) Compresses in following sizes: 3″ x 5″, 4″ x 9″, 8.5″ x 10.5″.
Use: Cold, hot compress.

Thermazene. (Sherwood Davis & Geck) Silver sulfadiazine 1% in white petrolatum. Cream. 50 g, 400 g, 1000 g. *Rx.*
Use: Burn therapy.

Thermodent. (Mentholatum Co., Inc.) Strontium Cl 10%. Tube. *otc.*
Use: Dentrifice.

Theroal. (Vangard Labs, Inc.) Theophylline 24 mg, ephedrine HCl 24 mg, phenobarbital 8 mg/Tab. Bot. 100s, 1000s. *Rx.*
Use: Antiasthmatic combination.

Theroxide Wash. (Medicis Dermatologicals, Inc.) Benzoyl peroxide 10%. Liq. Bot. 120 ml. *Rx.*
Use: Dermatologic, acid.

ThexForte. (KM Lee) Vitamins B_1 25 mg, B_2 15 mg, B_3 100 mg, B_5 10 mg, B_6 5 mg, C 500 mg/Cap. Bot. 75s. *otc.*
Use: Vitamin supplement.

Thia. (Sigma-Tau Pharmaceuticals, Inc.) Thiamine HCl 100 mg/ml. Inj. Vial 30 ml. *Rx.*
Use: Vitamin supplement.

•**thiabendazole.** (THIGH-uh-BEND-uh-zole) U.S.P. 23.
Use: Anthelmintic.
See: Mintezol, Tab., Susp. (Merck & Co.).

thiacetarsamide sodium. Sodium mercaptoacetate S, S-diester with p-carbamoyl dithiobenzene arsonous acid.
Use: Antitrichomonal.

Thia-Dia-Mer-Sulfonamides. Sulfadiazine w/sulfamerazine & sulfathiazole.

thialbarbital.
See: Kemithal.

•**thiamine hydrochloride.** (THIGH-uh-min) U.S.P. 23.
Use: Enzyme co-factor vitamin.
See: Apatate (Kenwood Laboratories).
Betalin S, Amp., Elixir, Tab. (Eli Lilly and Co.).
Thia, Vial (Sigma-Tau Pharmaceuticals, Inc).

•**thiamine mononitrate.** (THIGH-uh-min) U.S.P. 23.
Use: Enzyme cofactor vitamin.

•**thiamiprine.** (thigh-AM-ih-preen) USAN.
Use: Antineoplastic.

•**thiamphenicol.** (THIGH-am-FEN-ih-kahl) USAN.
Use: Anti-infective.

•**thiamylal.** (thigh-AM-ih-lahl) U.S.P. 23.
Use: Anesthetic (intravenous).

•**thiamylal sodium, for injection.** U.S.P. 23.
Use: Anesthetic (intravenous).

thiazesim.
Use: Antidepressant.

•**thiazesim hydrochloride.** (thigh-AZE-eh-sim) USAN.
Use: Antidepressant.

•**thiazinamium chloride.** (THIGH-ah-ZIN-am-ee-uhm) USAN.
Use: Antiallergic.

thiethylene thiophosphoramide.
See: Thiotepa.

•**thiethylperazine.** (THIGH-eth-ill-PURR-ah-zeem) USAN.
Use: CNS depressant; antiemetic.

•**thiethylperazine maleate.** (THIGH-eth-ill-PURR-ah-zeen MAL-ee-ate) U.S.P. 23.
Use: Antiemetic.

•**thiethylperazine maleate.** U.S.P. 23.
Use: Antiemetic.
See: Torecan, Amp., Supp., Tab. (Boehringer Ingelheim, Inc.).

thihexinol methylbromide.
Use: Anticholinergic.

•**thimerfonate sodium.** (thigh-MER-foe-nate) USAN.
Use: Anti-infective, topical.

•**thimerosal.** (thigh-MER-oh-sal) U.S.P. 23.
Use: Anti-infective, topical; pharmaceutic aid (preservative).
See: Aeroaid, Aerosol (Graham Field).
Merphol Tincture 1:1000, Liq. (Jones Medical Industries, Inc.).
Mersol, Liq. (Century Pharmaceuticals, Inc.).
W/Trifluridine.
See: Merthiolate, Prep. (Eli Lilly and Co.).
See: Viroptic, Soln. (Monarch Pharmaceuticals).

thiocarbanidin. Under study.
Use: Tuberculosis.

thiocyanate sodium. Sodium thiocyanate.
Use: Antihypertensive.

thiodinone. Name used for Nifuratel.

thiodiphenylamine.
See: Phenothiazine.

thioglycerol.
W/Sod. citrate, phenol, benzyl alcohol.
See: Sulfo-ganic, Vial (Marcen).

•**thioguanine.** (THIGH-oh-GWAHN-een) U.S.P. 23.
Use: Antineoplastic.

thiohexamide.
Use: Blood sugar-lowering compound.

thioisonicotinamide. Under study.
Use: Antituberculosal.

Thiola. (Mission Pharmacal Co.) Tiopronin 100 mg. Tab. Bot. 100s. *Rx.*
Use: Anticholelithiasis.

•**thiopental sodium.** (thigh-oh-PEN-tahl) U.S.P. 23.
Use: Anesthetic (intravenous), anticonvulsant.
See: Pentothal Sodium, Amp. (Abbott Laboratories).

thiopental sodium. (I.M.S., Ltd.) Thiopental sodium 20 mg/ml, 25 mg/ml. Pow. for Inj. **20 mg/ml:** 400 mg *Min-I-Mix* vial w/ injector. **25 mg/ml:** 250 mg, 500 mg *Min-I-Mix* vials w/ injector; 500 mg, 1 g, 2.5 g, 5 g, 10 g kits. *Rx.*
Use: Anesthetic, general.

thiophosphoramide.
See: Thiotepa, Vial (ESI Lederle Generics).

Thioplex. (Immunex Corp.) Thiotepa 15 mg. Powd. for Inj. Vials. *Rx.*
Use: Antineoplastic.

thiopropazate hydrochloride.
Use: Anxiolytic.

thioproperazine mesylate.
Use: CNS depressant; antiemetic.

•**thioridazine.** (THIGH-oh-RID-uh-zeen) U.S.P. 23.
Use: Antipsychotic; hypnotic, sedative.
See: Mellaril, Preps. (Novartis Pharmaceutical Corp.).

•**thioridazine hydrochloride.** (THIGH-oh-RID-ah-zeen) U.S.P. 23.
Use: Antipsychotic; hypnotic, sedative.
See: Mellaril, Tabs., Soln. (Novartis Pharmaceutical Corp.).

thioridazine hydrochloride concen-

trate. (Various Mfr.) Thioridazine HCl. **30 mg/ml:** Bot. 120 ml. **100 mg/ml:** Bot 120 ml, 3.4 ml (UD 100s). *Rx.*
Use: Antipsychotic.

thioridazine hydrochloride intensol oral solution. (Roxane Laboratories, Inc.) Thioridazine HCl oral concentrated soln. 30 mg/ml, 100 mg/ml. Bot. 120 ml w/calibrated dropper. *Rx.*
Use: Antipsychotic.

thioridazine hydrochloride tablets. (Various Mfr.) 10 mg, 15 mg, 25 mg, 50 mg, 100 mg, 150 mg, 200 mg. Bot. 100s, 500s, 1000s, UD 100s. *Rx.*
Use: Antipsychotic.

•**thiosalan.** (THIGH-oh-sal-AN) USAN.
Use: Disinfectant.

Thiosulfil Forte. (Wyeth-Ayerst Laboratories) Sulfamethizole 500 mg. Tab. Bot. 100s. *Rx.*
Use: Anti-infective.

•**thiotepa.** (thigh-oh-TEP-uh) U.S.P. 23.
Use: Antineoplastic.
See: Thioplex, Pow. for Inj. (Immunex Corp.).

thiotepa. (thigh-oh-TEP-uh) (ESI Lederle Generics) Thiotepa powder 15 mg, sodium chloride 80 mg, sodium bicarbonate 50 mg/Vial. Pow. for Recon. Vial 15 mg. *Rx.*
Use: Antineoplastic.
See: Thioplex, Pow. (Immunex Corp.).

•**thiothixene.** (THIGH-oh-THIX-een) U.S.P. 23.
Use: Antipsychotic.
See: Navane, Cap. (Pfizer).
Navane Concentrate, Soln. (Pfizer).

•**thiothixene hydrochloride.** (THIGH-oh-THIX-een) U.S.P. 23.
Use: Antipsychotic.
See: Navane Cap. (Pfizer US Pharmaceutical Group).

thiothixene. (Various Mfr.) Thiothixene. **Tab.:** 1 mg, 2 mg, 5 mg, 10 mg, 20 mg. Bot. 100s, 500s, 1000s. **Conc.:** 5 mg/ml. Bot. 30 ml, 120 ml. *Rx.*
Use: Antipsycotic.

thiothixene hydrochloride intensol. (Roxane Laboratories, Inc.) Thiothixene HCl 5 mg/ml, EDTA. Alcohol free. Soln. Bot. 30 ml, 120 ml with dropper. *Rx.*
Use: Antipsychotic.

thiouracil. 2-Thiouracil.
Use: Treatment of hyperthyroidism, antianginal, congestive heart failure.

thioxanthenes.
See: Navane (Pfizer).
Thiothixene (Various Mfr.).

•**thiphenamil hydrochloride.** (thigh-FEN-ah-mill) USAN.
Use: Muscle relaxant.

•**thiphencillin potassium.** (thigh-fen-SILL-in) USAN.
Use: Anti-infective.

Thipyri-12. (Sigma-Tau Pharmaceuticals, Inc.) Vitamins B_1 1000 mg, B_6 1000 mg, cyanocobalamin (B_{12}) 10,000 mcg, sodium chloride 0.5%, sodium bisulfite 0.1%, benzyl alcohol (as preservative) 0.9%. Univial 10 ml. *Rx.*
Use: Vitamin supplement.

•**thiram.** (THIGH-ram) USAN.
Use: Antifungal.

Thixo-Flur Topical Gel. (Colgate Oral Pharmaceuticals) Acidulated phosphate sodium fluoride in gel base 1.2%. Bot. 4 oz. 8 oz., 32 oz.
Use: Dental caries agent.

•**thonzonium bromide.** (thahn-ZOE-nee-uhm) USAN. U.S.P. XXII.
Use: Detergent.
W/Colistin base, neomycin base, hydrocortisone acetate, polysorbate 80, acetic acid, sodium acetate.
See: Coly-Mycin-S, Otic, Liq. (Warner Chilcott Laboratories).
Cortisporin-TC (Monarch Pharmaceuticals).
W/Isoproterenol.
See: Nebair, Aerosol (Warner Chilcott Laboratories).

•**thonzylamine hydrochloride.** USAN.
Use: Antihistamine.

Thorazine. (SmithKline Beecham Pharmaceuticals) Chlorpromazine HCl. **Tab.:** 10 mg, 25 mg, 50 mg, 100 mg, 200 mg. Bot. 100s, 1000s. **Amp.:** 25 mg w/ascorbic acid 2 mg, sodium bisulfite 1 mg, sodium sulfite 1 mg, NaCl 6 mg/ml. Vial 1 ml, 2 ml, 10 ml. **Spansule:** 30 mg, 75 mg, 150 mg, 200 mg. Bot. 50s. **Syr.:** 10 mg/5 ml. Bot. 120 ml. **Supp.:** Chlorpromazine base, w/glycerin, glyceryl monopalmitate, glyceryl monostearate, hydrogenated coconut oil fatty acids, hydrogenated palm kernel oil fatty acids. 25 mg, 100 mg Box 12s. **Conc.:** 30 mg/ml. Bot. 120 ml. 100 mg/ml Bot. 240 ml. *Rx.*
Use: Antiemetic, antipsychotic.

Thorets. (Buffington) Benzocaine lozenge. Dispens-A-Kits 500s. Sugar, lactose and salt free. *otc.*
Use: Sore throat relief.

Thor-Prom. (Major Pharmaceuticals) Chlorpromazine 10 mg, 25 mg, 50 mg, 100 mg. Tab. Bot. 100s, 1000s; 200 mg/Tab. Bot. 250s, 1000s.
Use: Antiemetic, antipsychotic.

Thor Syrup. (Towne) Dextromethorphan HBr 90 mg, pyrilamine maleate 22.5 mg, phenylephrine HCl 10 mg, ephedrine sulfate 15 mg, sodium citrate 325 mg, ammonium chloride 650 mg, guaifenesin 50 mg/fl. oz. Bot. 4 oz. *otc.*
Use: Antitussive, antihistamine, decongestant, expectorant.

•**thozalinone.** (thoe-ZAL-ah-nohn) USAN.
Use: Antidepressant.

Threamine DM. (Various Mfr.) Phenylpropanolamine HCl 12.5 mg, chlorpheniramine maleate 2 mg, dextromethorphan HBr 10 mg/5 ml. Syr. Bot. Pt, gal. *otc.*
Use: Antihistamine, antitussive, decongestant.

Three-Amine TD. (Eon Labs Manufacturing, Inc.) Phenylpropanolamine HBr 50 mg, pheniramine maleate 25 mg, pyrilamine maleate 25 mg/TR Cap. *otc.*
Use: Antihistamine, decongestant.

•**threonine.** (THREE-oh-neen) U.S.P. 23.
Use: Amino acid, antispasmodic. [Orphan Drug]
See: Threostat.

threonine. (Various Mfr.) Threonine 500 mg. **Capsules:** 60s, 100s. **Tablets:** 100s, 250s. *otc.*
Use: Nutritional supplement.

Threostat. (Tyson & Associates, Inc.) *Rx.*
Use: Antispasmodic.
See: Threonine.

Throat Discs. (SmithKline Beecham Pharmaceuticals) Capsicum, peppermint, mineral oil, sucrose. Box 60s. *otc.*
Use: Throat preparation.

Throat-Eze. (Faraday) Cetylpyridinium chloride 1:3000, cetyl dimethylbenzyl ammonium chloride 1:3000, benzocaine 10 mg/Wafer. Loz., foil wrapped. Vial 15. *otc.*
Use: Anesthetic, local.

Thrombate III. (Bayer) Antithrombin III (human) 500 IU, 1000 IU. Pow. for Inj., lyophilized. Single-use vial w/10 ml (500 ml IU only), 20 ml (1000 IU only). Sterile water for injection. *Rx.*
Use: Antithrombin.

•**thrombin.** (THRAHM-bin) U.S.P. 23. Thrombin, topical, mammalian origin.
Use: Hemostatic.
See: Thrombinar, Pow. (Jones Medical Industries, Inc.).
Thrombin-JMI, Pow. (Jones Medical Industries, Inc.).
Thrombogen, Pow. (Johnson & Johnson).
Thrombostat, Pow. (Parke-Davis).

Thrombinar. (Jones Medical Industries, Inc.) Thrombin topical. 1000 units: 50% mannitol, 45% NaCl. 5000 units: 50% mannitol, 45% NaCl, sterile water for injection. 50,000 units: 50% mannitol, 45% NaCl. Pow. Vials. Preservative free. *Rx.*
Use: Hemostatic, topical.

Thrombin-JMI. (Jones Medical Industries, Inc.) Pow. 10,000 units, 20,000 units, 50,000 units. *Rx.*
Use: Hemostatic, topical.

Thrombogen. (Johnson & Johnson) Thrombin 1000 units. 5000 units: With isotonic saline diluent and transfer needle. 10,000 units, 20,000 units: Isotonic saline diluent, benzethonium chloride, and transfer needle. Inj. Vial. *Rx.*
Use: Hemostatic, topical.

thrombolytic enzymes.
See: Abbokinase (Abbott Laboratories).
Abbokinase Open-Cath (Abbott Laboratories).
Eminase (SmithKline Beecham Pharmaceuticals).
Kabikinase (Pharmacia & Upjohn).
Streptase (Astra Pharmaceuticals, LP).

thromboplastin.
Use: Diagnostic aid (prothrombin estimation).

Thrombostat. (Parke-Davis) Prothrombin is activated by tissue thromboplastin in the presence of calcium chloride. **1000 U.S. (N.I.H.) units:** Vial 10 ml. **5000 U.S. units:** Vial 10 ml, 5 ml diluent. **10,000 U.S. units:** Vial 20 m, 10 ml diluent. **20,000 U.S. units:** Vial 30 ml, 20 ml diluent. *Rx.*
Use: Hemostatic.

Thylox. (C.S. Dent & Co. Division) Medicated bar soap w/absorbable sulfur. Bar 3.4 oz. *otc.*
Use: Cleanser.

•**thymalfasin.** (thigh-MAL-fah-sin) USAN.
Formerly Thymosin.
Use: Antineoplastic; vaccine enhancement; hepatitis, infectious disease treatment.

•**thymol.** (THIGH-mole) N.F. 18.
Use: Antifungal; anti-infective; anesthetic, local; antitussive; decongestant; pharmaceutic aid (stabilizer).
See: Vicks Regular & Wild Cherry Medicated Cough Drops (Procter & Gamble Pharm.).
Vicks Vaporub, Oint. (Procter & Gamble Pharm.).
W/Combinations.
See: Listerine Antiseptic, Soln. (Warner Lambert).

thymol. (Various Mfr.) 0.25 lb, 1 lb.
Use: Antifungal; anti-infective; anesthetic, local; antitussive; decongestant; pharmaceutic aid (stabilizer).

thymol iodide.
Use: Antifungal, anti-infective.

•**thymopentin.** (THIGH-moe-PEN-tin) USAN. *Formerly Thymopoietin 32-36.*
Use: Immunoregulator.

thymosin alpha-1.
Use: Antiviral, hepatitis B. [Orphan Drug]

thyodatil. Name used for Nifuratel.

Thypinone. (Abbott Diagnostics) Protirelin 500 mcg/1 ml Amp. *Rx.*
Use: Diagnostic aid, thyroid.

Thyrar. (Rhone-Poulenc Rorer Pharmaceuticals, Inc.) Bovine thyroid preparation 0.5 g, 1 g, 2 g/Tab. Bot. 100s. *Rx.*
Use: Thyroid agent.

Thyrel-TRH. (Ferring Pharmaceuticals, Inc.) Protirelin 0.5 mg/ml. Inj. 1 ml. *Rx.*
Use: Diagnostic aid.

Thyro-Block. (Wallace Laboratories) Potassium iodide 130 mg/Tab. 14s. *Rx.*
Use: Antithyroid.

•**thyroid.** (THIGH-royd) U.S.P. 23.
Use: Hormone, thyroid.
See: Arco Thyroid, Tab. (Arco Pharmaceuticals, Inc.).
S-P-T., Cap. (Fleming & Co.).

thyroid combinations.
See: Henydin, Prep. (Arcum).

thyroid desiccated. (THIGH-royd DESS-ih-KATE-uhd)
Use: Hormone, thyroid.
See: S-P-T (Fleming & Co.).
Thyrar (Rhone-Poulenc Rorer Pharmaceuticals, Inc.).
Thyroid Strong (Jones Medical Industries, Inc.).
Thyroid USP (Various Mfr.).

thyroid diagnostic aids.
Use: Diagnostic aid.
See: Sodium Iodide I-123 (Mallinckrodt Diagnostics).
Thypinone (Abbott Laboratories).
Thytropar (Centeon).

thyroid hormones.
See: Liothyronine Sod.
Thyroxin (Various Mfr.).

thyroid preparations.
See: Thyrar, Tab. (Rhone-Poulenc Rorer Pharmaceuticals, Inc.).
Thyroxin, Prep. (Various Mfr.).

thyroid-stimulating hormone (TSH).
Use: Adjunct in diagnosis of thyroid cancer. [Orphan Drug]

Thyroid Strong. (Jones Medical Industries, Inc.) Thyroid desiccated 30 mg, 60 mg, 120 mg/Tab. Bot. 100s, 1000s; 30 mg, 120 mg, 180 mg Tab. Bot. 100s; 60 mg. Sugar coated. Tab. Bot. 100s, 1000s. *Rx.*
Use: Hormone, thyroid.

Thyrolar. (Forest Pharmaceutical, Inc.) Liotrix 0.25 g/Tab. Bot. 100s; 0.5 g, 1 g, 2 g, 3 g/Tab. Bot. 100s, 1000s. *Rx.*
Use: Hormone, thyroid.

•**thyromedan hydrochloride.** (thigh-ROW-meh-dan) USAN.
Use: Thyromimetic.

thyropropic acid. (Warner Chilcott Laboratories) Triopron.
Use: Anticholesteremic.

thyrotropic hormone.
Use: In vivo diagnostic aid.
See: Thytropar (Centeon).

thyrotropic principle of bovine anterior pituitary glands.
See: Thytropar, Vial (Centeon).

thyrotropin.
Use: Diagnostic aid.
See: Thytropar (Centeon).

•**thyrotropin alfa.** USAN.
Use: Thyroid-stimulating hormone.

thyrotropin-releasing hormone.
Use: Diagnostic aid.
See: Thypinone (Abbott Laboratories).

•**thyroxine I 125.** (thigh-ROX-een) USAN.
Use: Radiopharmaceutical.

•**thyroxine I 131.** USAN.
Use: Radiopharmaceutical.

thyrozyme-II A. (Abbott Diagnostics) T-4 diagnostic kit. 100 & 500 test units.
Use: Diagnostic aid, thyroid.

Thytropar. (Centeon) Thyrotropin from bovine anterior pituitary glands. Thyrotropin. Vial 10 IU.
Use: Thyroid agent.

•**tiacrilast.** (TIE-ah-KRILL-ast) USAN.
Use: Antiallergic.

•**tiacrilast sodium.** (TIE-ah-KRILL-ast) USAN.
Use: Antiallergic.

Tiagabine. (Abbott; Novo/Nordisk Pharm.)
Use: Antiepileptic.

•**tiagabine hydrochloride.** USAN.
Use: Anticonvulsant.
See: Gabitril, Tab. (Abbott Laboratories).

Tiamate. (Hoechst Marion Roussel) Diltiazem maleate 120 mg, 180 mg, 240 mg, sucrose/ER Tab. Bot. UD 30s. *Rx.*
Use: Calcium channel blocker.

•**tiamenidine.** (TIE-ah-MEN-ih-DEEN) USAN.
Use: Antihypertensive.

•**tiamenidine hydrochloride.** (TIE-ah-MEN-ih-DEEN) USAN.

Use: Antihypertensive.

•**tiapamil hydrochloride.** (tie-APP-ah-mill) USAN.
Use: Calcium antagonist.

•**tiaramide hydrochloride.** (TIE-ar-ah-MIDE) USAN.
Use: Antiasthmatic.

Tiazac. (Forest Pharmaceutical, Inc.) Diltiazem HCl 120 mg, 180 mg, 240 mg, 300 mg, 360 mg/ER Cap. Bot. 30s, 90s, 1000s (except 120 mg, 360 mg). *Rx.*
Use: Calcium channel blocker.

•**tiazofurin.** (TIE-AZE-oh-few-rin) USAN.
Use: Antineoplastic.

TI-Baby Natural. (Fischer Pharmaceuticals, Inc.) Titanium dioxide 5%. SPF 16. Lot. Bot. 120 ml. *otc.*
Use: Sunscreen.

•**tibenelast sodium.** (TIE-ben-ell-ast) USAN.
Use: Antiasthmatic; bronchodilator.

•**tibolone.** (TIH-bole-ohn) USAN.
Use: Menopausal symptoms suppressant.

•**tibric acid.** (TIE-brick) USAN.
Use: Antihyperlipoproteinemic.

•**tibrofan.** (TIE-broe-fan) USAN.
Use: Disinfectant.

•**ticabesone propionate.** (tie-CAB-eh-sone) USAN.
Use: Corticosteroid, topical.

Ticar. (SmithKline Beecham Pharmaceuticals) Ticarcillin disodium. 1 g, 3 g, 6 g, 20 mg, 30 g. Pow. for Inj. Vial (1 g, 3 g, 6 g only), piggyback and *ADD-Vantage* vial (3 g only), Bulk vial (20 g and 30 g only). *Rx.*
Use: Anti-infective.

•**ticarbodine.** (tie-CAR-boe-deen) USAN.
Use: Anthelmintic.

ticarcillin and clavulanate potassium.
Use: Penicillin.
See: Timentin (SmithKline Beecham Pharmaceuticals).

•**ticarcillin cresyl sodium.** (tie-CAR-SIH-lin KREH-sill) USAN.
Use: Anti-infective.

•**ticarcillin disodium.** (tie-CAR-SIH-lin) U.S.P. 23.
Use: Anti-infective.
See: Ticar, Inj. (SmithKline Beecham Pharmaceuticals).

ticarcillin disodium and clavulanate potassium, sterile.
Use: Anti-infective, inhibitor (β-lactamase).
See: Timentin, Inj. (SmithKline Beecham Pharmaceuticals).

•**ticarcillin monosodium.** (tie-CAR-SIH-lin) U.S.P. 23.
Use: Anti-infective.

TICE BCG Vaccine. (Organon Teknika Corp.) BCG. Intravesical 50 mg/2 ml. Freeze-dried suspension for reconstitution. Inj. Amp. 2 ml. *Rx.*
Use: Antineoplastic.

•**ticlatone.** (TIE-klah-tone) USAN.
Use: Anti-infective, antifungal.

Ticlid. (Syntex) Ticlopidine HCl 250 mg/Tab. Bot. 30s, 60s, 500s. *Rx.*
Use: Antiplatelet.

•**ticlopidine hydrochloride.** (tie-KLOE-pih-DEEN) USAN.
Use: Platelet inhibitor.
See: Ticlid, Tab. (Syntex).

•**ticolubant.** (tih-kahl-YOU-bant) USAN.
Use: Antipsoriatic.

Ticon. (Roberts Pharmaceuticals) Trimethobenzamide HCl 100 mg/ml. Inj. Vial 20 ml. *Rx.*
Use: Antiemetic, antivertigo.

ticonazole.
Use: Antifungal, vaginal.
See: Vagistat-1, Oint. (Bristol-Myers Squibb).

•**ticrynafen.** (TIE-krin-ah-fen) USAN.
Use: Diuretic, uricosuric, antihypertensive.

Tidex. (Allison) Dextroamphetamine sulfate, 5 mg/Tab. Bot. 100s, 1000s. *c-II.*
Use: Antiobesity agent.

Tidexsol Tablets. (Sanofi Winthrop Pharmaceuticals) Acetaminophen. *otc.*
Use: Analgesic.

•**tifurac sodium.** (TIE-fyoor-ak) USAN.
Use: Analgesic.

Tigan. (Roberts Pharmaceuticals) Trimethobenzamide hydrochloride. **Cap.:** 100 mg Bot. 100s, 250 mg Bot. 100s. **Amp.:** (100 mg/ml) 2 ml. Box 10s. Vial 20 ml **Supp.:** 200 mg Box 10s, 50s. **Pediatric Supp.:** 100 mg Box 10s. *Rx.*
Use: Antiemetic.

•**tigemonam dicholine.** (TIE-jem-OH-nam die-KOE-leen) USAN.
Use: Antimicrobial.

•**tigestol.** (tie-JESS-tole) USAN.
Use: Hormone, progestin.

Tigo. (Burlington) Polymyxin B sulfate 5000 units, zinc bacitracin 400 units, neomycin sulfate 5 mg/g Oint. Tube 0.5 oz. *otc.*
Use: Anti-infective, topical.

Tihist-DP. (Vita Elixir) Dextromethorphan HBr 10 mg, pyrilamine maleate 16 mg, sodium citrate 3.3 g/5 ml. *otc.*
Use: Antitussive, antihistamine.

Tihist Nasal Drops. (Vita Elixir) Pyril-

amine maleate 0.1%, phenylephrine HCl 0.25%, sodium bisulfite 0.2%, methylparaben 0.02%, propylparaben 0.01%/30 ml. Bot. *otc.*
Use: Antihistamine, decongestant.

Tija Tablets. (Vita Elixir) Oxytetracycline HCl 250 mg/Tab. *Rx.*
Use: Anti-infective, tetracycline.

Tija Syrup. (Vita Elixir) Oxytetracycline HCl 125 mg/5 ml. *Rx.*
Use: Anti-infective, tetracycline.

Tilade. (Medeva Pharmaceuticals, Inc.) Nedocromil sodium 1.75 mg per actuation. Aerosol Can. 16.2 g with mouthpiece. *Rx.*
Use: Respiratory, anti-inflammatory.

•**tiletamine hydrochloride.** (tie-LET-ah-meen) USAN.
Use: Anesthetic, anticonvulsant.

•**tilidine hydrochloride.** (TIH-lih-DEEN) USAN.
Use: Analgesic.

Tl-lite. (Fischer Pharmaceuticals, Inc.) Ethylhexyl p-methoxycinnamate 7.5%, titanium dioxide 2%, cetyl alcohol, phenethyl alcohol, parabens, EDTA. Cream 60 g. *otc.*
Use: Sunscreen.

•**tilomisole.** (TILL-oh-mih-sahl) USAN.
Use: Immunoregulator.

•**tilorone hydrochloride.** (TIE-lore-ohn) USAN.
Use: Antiviral.

•**tiludronate disodium.** (tie-LOO-droe-nate) USAN.
Use: Paget's disease, osteoporosis.
See: Skelid, Tab. (Sanofi Winthrop Pharmaceuticals).

Timed Reducing Aids-Caffeine Free. (Weeks & Leo) Phenylpropanolamine HCl 75 mg/TR Cap. Bot. 28s, 56s. *otc.*
Use: Dietary aid.

•**timefurone.** (tie-MEH-fyoor-OHN) USAN.
Use: Antiatherosclerotic.

Timentin. (SmithKline Beecham Pharmaceuticals) **Pow. for Inj.:** Ticarcillin disodium 3 g, clavulanic acid (as potassium salt) 0.1 g. Vials 3.1 g. Piggyback bot., *ADD-Vantage* vial, Pharmacy Bulk Pkg. 31 g. **Inj. Soln.:** Ticarcillin disodium 3 g, clavulanic acid (as potassium salt) 0.1 g. Premixed, frozen *Galaxy* Cont. 100 ml. *Rx.*
Use: Anti-infective.

•**timobesone acetate.** (tie-MOE-beh-sone) USAN.
Use: Adrenocortical steroid, topical.

Timolide 10-25. (Merck & Co.) Timolol maleate 10 mg, hydrochlorothiazide 25 mg/Tab. Bot. 100s. *Rx.*
Use: Antihypertensive.

•**timolol.** (TI-moe-lahl) USAN.
Use: Antiadrenergic (β-receptor).
See: Betimol, Soln. (Ciba Vision).

•**timolol maleate.** (TI-moe-lahl) U.S.P. 23.
Use: Treatment of chronic open-angle, aphakic, and secondary glaucoma, antihypertensive, prevention of recurrent MI; antiadrenergic (β-receptor).
See: Blocadren, Tab. (Merck & Co.).
Betimol (Ciba Vision).
Timoptic (Merck & Co.).

timolol maleate. (TI-moe-lahl) (Various Mfr.) **Ophth. Soln.:** 0.25%, 0.5%. Bot. 5 ml, 10 ml, 15 ml. **Gel-forming Soln.:** (Falcon) 0.25%, 0.5%, Bot. 2.5 ml, 5 ml. *Rx.*
Use: Treatment of chronic open-angle, aphakic, and secondary glaucoma, antihypertensive, prevention of recurrent MI; antiadrenergic (β-receptor).

timolol maleate and hydrochlorothiazide tablets.
Use: Antihypertensive combination.
See: Timolide, Tab. (Merck & Co.).

timolol maleate ophthalmic solution. (Various Mfr.) Timolol maleate 3.4 mg/0.25 ml and 6.8 mg/0.5 ml. Soln. Bot. 2.5 ml, 5 ml, 10 ml, 15 ml. *Rx.*
Use: Antiglaucoma agent.

Timoptic. (Merck & Co.) Timolol maleate 0.25%, 0.5%. Soln. Ocumeter Ophthalmic Dispenser 2.5 ml, 5 ml, 10 ml, 15 ml; Ocudose UD 60s. *Rx.*
Use: Antiglaucoma agent.

Timoptic-XE. (Merck & Co.) Timolol maleate 0.25%, 0.5%. Gel-forming Soln. Bot. 2.5 ml, 5 ml. *Rx.*
Use: Antiglaucoma agent.

•**tinabinol.** (tie-NAB-ih-NOLE) USAN.
Use: Antihypertensive.

Tinactin. (Schering-Plough Corp.) **Soln. 1%:** Tolnaftate (10 mg/ml) w/butylated hydroxytoluene, in nonaqueous homogeneous PEG 400. Plastic squeeze bot. 10 ml. **Cream 1%:** Tolnaftate (10 mg/g) in homogeneous, nonaqueous vehicle of PEG-400, propylene glycol, carboxypolymethylene, monoamylamine, titanium dioxide, butylated hydroxytoluene. Tube 15 g, 30 g, UD 0.7 g. **Pow. 1%:** Tolnaftate w/corn starch, talc. Plastic container 45 g, 90 g. **Aerosol Pow. 1%:** Tolnaftate w/butylated hydroxytoluene, talc, polyethylene-polypropylene glycol monobutyl ether, denatured alcohol and inert propellant of isobutane. Spray Can 100 g. **Aerosol Liq. 1%:** Tolnaftate w/butylated hydroxytoluene, polyethylene-polyproply-

ene glycol monobutyl ether, 36% alcohol, and inert propellant of isobutane. Spray Can 120 ml. *otc.*
Use: Antifungal.

Tinastat. (Vita Elixir) Sodium hyposulfite, benzethonium Cl/2 oz. *otc.*
Use: Keratolytic.

Tinaval Powder. (Pal-Pak, Inc.) Tolnaftate 1%. Bot. 45 g. *otc.*
Use: Antifungal for jock itch, athlete's foot.

tine test, old tuberculin. (Wyeth-Ayerst Laboratories) Box of 25, 100, 250 test applicators.
See: Tuberculin Tine Test (ESI Lederle Generics).

tine test, purified protein derivative. (Wyeth-Ayerst Laboratories) Box of 25 or 100 test applicators.
See: Tuberculin Tine Test (ESI Lederle Generics).

tin fluoride. U.S.P. 23. Stannous Fluoride.

•**tinidazole.** (tie-NIH-dah-zole) USAN.
Use: Antiprotozoal.

Tinset. (Janssen Pharmaceutical, Inc.) Oxatomide.
Use: Antiallergic, antiasthmatic.

Tinver Lotion. (PBH Wesley Jessen) Sodium thiosulfate 25%, salicylic acid 1%, isopropyl alcohol 10%, propylene glycol, menthol, disodium edetate, colloidal alumina. Lot. Bot. 4 oz., 6 oz. *Rx.*
Use: Dermatologic.

•**tinzaparin sodium.** (tin-ZAP-ah-rin) USAN.
Use: Anticoagulant; antithrombotic.

•**tioconazole.** (TIE-oh-KOE-nah-zole) U.S.P. 23.
Use: Antifungal.
See: Vagistat (Fujisawa; SmithKline Beecham).

•**tiodazosin.** (TIE-oh-DAY-zoe-sin) USAN.
Use: Antihypertensive.

•**tiodonium chloride.** (TIE-oh-doe-nee-uhm) USAN.
Use: Anti-infective.

•**tioperidone hydrochloride.** (tie-oh-PURR-ih-dohn) USAN.
Use: Antipsychotic.

•**tiopinac.** (tie-OH-pin-ACK) USAN.
Use: Anti-inflammatory, analgesic, antipyretic.

tiopronin.
Use: Homozygous cystinuria. [Orphan Drug]
See: Thiola (Mission Pharmacal Co.).

•**tiospirone hydrochloride.** (tie-OH-spih-rone) USAN.
Use: Antipsychotic.

•**tiotidine.** (TIE-OH-tih-deen) USAN.
Use: Antiulcerative.

•**tioxidazole.** (tie-OX-ih-DAH-zole) USAN.
Use: Anthelmintic.

•**tipentosin hydrochloride.** (TIE-pin-toe-SIN) USAN.
Use: Antihypertensive.

Tipramine Tabs. (Major Pharmaceuticals) Imipramine 10 mg/Tab. Bot. 250s; 25 mg, 50 mg/Tab. Bot. 250s, 1000s. *Rx.*
Use: Antidepressant.

•**tipredane.** (tie-PRED-ANE) USAN.
Use: Adrenocortical steroid, topical.

•**tiprenolol hydrochloride.** (tie-PREH-no-lole) USAN.
Use: Antiadrenergic (β-receptor).

•**tiprinast meglumine.** (TIE-prih-nast meh-GLUE-meen) USAN. Under study.
Use: Antiallergic.

•**tipropidil hydrochloride.** (TIE-PRO-pih-dill) USAN.
Use: Vasodilator.

•**tiqueside.** (TIE-kweh-side) USAN.
Use: Antihyperlipidemic.

•**tiquinamide hydrochloride.** (tie-KWIN-ah-mide) USAN.
Use: Anticholinergic (gastric).

•**tirapazamine.** (tie-rah-PAZZ-ah-meen) USAN.
Use: Antineoplastic.

tiratricol.
Use: Antineoplastic. [Orphan Drug]

•**tirilazad mesylate.** (tie-RIH-lah-zad MEH-sih-late) USAN.
Use: Lipid Peroxidation Inhibitor.
See: Freedox (Pharmacia & Upjohn).

•**tirofiban hydrochloride.** (tie-rah-FIE-ban) USAN.
Use: Treatment of unstable angina.
See: Aggrastat, Inj. (Merck & Co.).

TI-Screen. (Pedinol Pharmacal, Inc.) **Gel:** SPF 20+, ethylhexyl p-methoxycinnamate 7.5%, oxybenzone 5%, 2-ethylhexyl salicylate 5%, SD alcohol 40 71%. 120 g. **Lip Balm:** SPF 8+, ethylhexyl p-methoxycinnamate 7.5%, oxybenzone 5%, petrolatum. 4.5 g. **Lot., SPF 8:** Ethylhexyl p-methoxycinnamate 6%, oxybenzone 2%. Bot. 120 ml **Lot., SPF 15:** Ethylhexyl p-methoxycinnamate 7.5%, oxybenzone 5%. Bot. 120 ml. **Lot., SPF 30:** Octyl methoxycinnamate 7.5%, octyl salicylate 5%, oxybenzone 6%, octocrylene 7.5%. Bot. 120 ml. *otc.*
Use: Sunscreen.

TI-Screen Natural. (Pedinol Pharmacal, Inc.) Titanium dioxide 5%. Lot. Bot. 120

ml. *otc.*
Use: Sunscreen.

TI-Screen Sunless. (Pedinol Pharmacal, Inc.) Octyl methoxycinnamate 7.5%, benzophene-3 3%, mineral oil, alcohols, PEG-100, parabens. SPF 17 or 23. Cream Tube 118 ml. *otc.*
Use: Sunscreen.

•**tisilfocon a.** (tih-sill-FOE-kahn) USAN.
Use: Contact lens material (hydrophobic).

Tisit. (Pfeiffer Co.) Pyrethrins 0.3%, piperonyl butoxide technical 3%, petroleum distillate 1.2%, benzyl alcohol 2.4%. Shampoo. Bot. 118 ml. *otc.*
Use: Pediculicide.

TiSol. (Parnell Pharmaceuticals, Inc.) Benzyl alcohol 1%, menthol 0.04%, isotonic sodium chloride 0.9%, sorbitol, EDTA. Soln. Bot. 237 ml. *otc.*
Use: Throat preparation.

tissue fixative and wash solution. (Wampole Laboratories) A modified Michel's tissue fixative and buffered wash solution.
Use: Tissue specimen fixative.

tissue plasminogen activator, recombinant.
See: Activase (Genentech, Inc.).

tissue respiratory factor (trf). (International Hormone) RSF, SRF, LYCD, PCO, Procytoxid marketed as 2000 units. Supplied as bulk liquid concentrate. *Rx.*
Use: Promotion of cellular oxidation.

Tis-U-Sol. (Baxter Pharmaceutical Products, Inc.) Pentalyte irrigation containing NaCl 800 mg, KCl 40 mg, magnesium sulfate 20 mg, sodium phosphate 8.75 mg, 6.25 mg monobasic potassium phosphate/100 ml. Bot. 250 ml, 1000 ml. *Rx.*
Use: Irrigant.

Titan. (PBH Wesley Jessen) EDTA 2%, nonionic cleaner buffers, potassium sorbate 0.13%. Soln. Bot. 30 ml. *otc.*
Use: Contact lens care.

•**titanium dioxide.** (tie-TANE-ee-uhm die-OX-ide) U.S.P. 23.
Use: Solar ray protectant, topical.

Titralac. (3M Pharmaceuticals) Calcium carbonate 420 mg, saccharin, Na 0.3 mg. Chew. Tab. Bot. 40s, 100s, 1000s. *otc.*
Use: Antacid.

Titralac Extra Strength Tablets. (3M Pharmaceuticals) Calcium carbonate 750 mg, saccharin, Na 0.6 mg. Chew. Tab. Liq. Bot. 100s. *otc.*
Use: Antacid.

Titralac Plus Liquid. (3M Personal Health Care) Calcium carbonate 500 mg, simethicone 20 mg, saccharin, sorbitol, sodium 0.15 mg. Liq. Bot. 360 ml. *otc.*
Use: Antacid.

Titralac Plus Tablets. (3M Pharmaceuticals) Calcium carbonate 420 mg, simethicone 21 mg, saccharin, sodium 1.1 mg. Chew. Tab. Bot. 100s. *otc.*
Use: Antacid.

•**tixanox.** (TIX-ah-nox) USAN.
Use: Antiallergic.

•**tixocortol pivalate.** (tix-OH-kahr-tole PIH-vah-late) USAN.
Use: Anti-inflammatory, topical.

tizanidine hydrochloride. (tie-ZAN-ih-deen)
Use: Antispasmodic.
See: Zanaflex, Tab. (Athena Neurosciences, Inc.).

•**tizanidine hydrochloride.** USAN.
Use: Antispasmodic. [Orphan Drug]

T-Koff. (T.E. Williams Pharmaceuticals) Phenylpropanolamine HCl 20 mg, phenylephrine HCl 20 mg, chlorpheniramine maleate 5 mg, codeine phosphate 10 mg/5 ml Syr. Bot. 480 ml Grape flavor. *c-v.*
Use: Antihistamine, antitussive, decongestant.

t-lymphotropic virus type III gp 160 antigens. *Rx.*
Use: Treatment for AIDS. [Orphan Drug]
See: Vaxsyn HIV-1.

TMP-SMZ. *Rx.*
Use: Anti-infective.
See: Proloprim (GlaxoWellcome).
Trimethoprim (Various Mfr.).
Trimpex (Roche Laboratories).

TOBI. (PathoGenesis Corp.) Tobramycin 300 mg, NaCl 11.25 g/5 ml. Soln for Inhalation. Single-use Amp. *Rx.*
Use: Cystic fibrosis.

•**toborinone.** (toe-BORE-ih-nohn) USAN.
Use: Cardiotonic.

Tobrades Suspension. (Alcon Laboratories, Inc.) Dexamethasone 0.1%, tobramycin 0.3%, thimerosal 0.001%, alcohol 0.5%, propylene glycol, polyoxyethylene, polyoxypropylene. Susp. 2.5 ml, 5 ml. *Rx.*
Use: Anti-infective, corticosteroid.

TobraDex. (Alcon Laboratories, Inc.) . 0.3% tobramycin, 0.1% dexamethasone. Susp. Bot. 2.5 ml, 5 ml. *Rx.*
Use: Anti-infective, corticosteroid, ophthalmic.

TobraDex, Ointment. (Alcon Laboratories, Inc.) Dexamethasone 0.1%, tobramycin 0.3%, chlorobutanol 0.5%, min-

eral oil, white petrolatum. Ophth. Oint. 3.5 g. *Rx.*
Use: Anti-infective, cortiocosteroid, ophthalmic.

•**tobramycin.** (TOE-bruh-MY-sin) U.S.P. 23. An antibiotic obtained from cultures of *Streptomyces tenebrarius.*
Use: Anti-infective, ophthalmic. [Orphan Drug]
See: TOBI, Soln. (PathoGenesis Corp.).
Tobrex, Preps. (Alcon Laboratories, Inc.).

tobramycin. (TOE-bruh-MY-sin) (Bausch & Lomb Pharmaceuticals) Tobramycin 0.3%, benzalkonium Cl 0.01%, boric acid. Soln. 5 ml. *Rx.*
Use: Anti-infective, ophthalmic.

tobramycin and dexamethasone ophthalmic ointment.
Use: Anti-infective, ophthalmic.

tobramycin sulfate. (Various Mfr.) Tobramycin sulfate 40 mg/ml. Inj. Syringes: 1.5 ml, 2 ml. Vial 2 ml. Pediatric Inj. 10 mg/ml. Vial 2 ml. *Rx.*
Use: Aminoglycoside, anti-infective.

•**tobramycin sulfate.** (TOE-bruh-my-sin) U.S.P. 23.
Use: Anti-infective, aminoglycoside.
See: Nebcin, Amp., Hyporet. (Eli Lilly and Co.).

Tobrex Ophthalmic Ointment. (Alcon Laboratories, Inc.) Tobramycin 0.3% in sterile ointment base. Tube 3.5 g. *Rx.*
Use: Anti-infective, ophthalmic.

Tobrex Solution. (Alcon Laboratories, Inc.) Tobramycin 0.3%. Ophth. Soln. Bot. 5 ml Drop-Tainer. *Rx.*
Use: Anti-infective, ophthalmic.

•**tocainide.** (TOE-cane-ide) USAN.
Use: Antiarrhythmic, cardiovascular agent.
See: Tonocard, Tab. (Merck & Co.).

•**tocainide hydrochloride.** U.S.P. 23.
Use: Antiarrhythmic, cardiac depressant.

•**tocamphyl.** (toe-KAM-fill) USAN.
Use: Choleretic.

tocopherol-dl-alpha. Vitamin E.
See: Aquasol E, Soln. (Rhone-Poulenc Rorer Pharmaceuticals, Inc.).
Denamone, Cap. (Vio-Bin).
Ecofrol, Cap. (O'Neal).
Epsilan M, Cap. (Warren-Teed).
Myopone (Drug Prods.).

•**tocopherols excipient.** N.F. 18.
Use: Pharmaceutic aid (antioxidant).

•**tocophersolan.** (toe-KAHF-ehr-SO-lan) USAN.
Use: Vitamin supplement.

tocopheryl acetate-d-alpha. U.S.P. 23. Vitamin E
See: Aquasol E, Prods. (Rhone-Poulenc Rorer Pharmaceuticals, Inc.).
Tocopher, Cap. (Quality Formulations, Inc.).
Vitamins E (Various Mfr.).

tocopheryl acetates, conc. d-alpha. U.S.P. 23. Vitamin E
Use: Treatment of habitual & threatened abortion.

tocopheryl acid succinated d-alpha. U.S.P. 23. Vitamin E
See: E-Ferol Succinate, Tab., Cap. (Forest Pharmaceutical, Inc.).
Vitamins E (Various Mfr.).

Tocosamine. (Trent) Sparteine sulfate 150 mg, sodium chloride 4.5 mg/ml. Amps. 1 ml. Box 12s, 100s. *Rx.*
Use: Oxytocic.

•**tofenacin hydrochloride.** (tah-FEN-ah-sin) USAN.
Use: Anticholinergic.

tofranazine. (Novartis Pharmaceutical Corp.) Combination of imipramine and promazine. Pending release.

Tofranil. (Novartis Pharmaceutical Corp.) Imipramine HCl. **Tab.:** 10 mg. Bot. 100s, 1000s; 25 mg, 50 mg. Bot. 100s, 1000s. UD 100s. Gy-Pak 100s, 1 unit (12 x 100); 6 units (72100). **Amps.:** 25 mg/2 ml w/ascorbic acid 2 mg, sodium bisulfite 1 mg, sodium sulfite 1 mg, and 2 ml amps. *Rx.*
Use: Antidepressant, antienuretic.

Tofranil-PM. (Novartis Pharmaceutical Corp.) Imipramine pamoate 75 mg, 100 mg, 125 mg, 150 mg/Cap. Bot. 30s, 100s. 75 mg/Cap. Bot. 1000s. UD 75 mg, 150 mg. 100s. *Rx.*
Use: Antidepressant.

Tolamide Tabs. (Major Pharmaceuticals) Tolazamide 100 mg/Tab. Bot. 100s, 250s; 250 mg/Tab. 200s, 500s; 500 mg/Tab. Bot. 100s, 500s. *Rx.*
Use: Antidiabetic.

•**tolamolol.** (tahl-AIM-oh-lahl) USAN.
Use: Beta-adrenergic receptor blocker, coronary vasodilator, cardiovascular agent (antiarrhythmic).

•**tolazamide.** (tole-AZE-uh-mid) U.S.P. 23.
Use: Hypoglycemic, antidiabetic.
See: Tolinase, Tab. (Pharmacia & Upjohn).

tolazamide. (Various Mfr.) 100 mg, 250 mg, 500 mg/Tab. Bot. 100s, 200s (250 mg only), 250s (except 250 mg), 500s (except 100 mg). *Rx.*
Use: Antidiabetic.

•**tolazoline hydrochloride.** (tole-AZZ-oh-leen) U.S.P. 23.
Use: Antiadrenergic, antihypertensive,

vasodilator (peripheral).
See: Priscoline, Inj. (Novartis Pharmaceutical Corp.).

•**tolbutamide.** (tole-BYOO-tuh-mide) U.S.P. 23.
Use: Hypoglycemic, antidiabetic.
See: Orinase, Tab. (Pharmacia & Upjohn).

tolbutamide. (Various Mfr.) 500 mg/Tab. 100s, 500s. *Rx.*
Use: Antidiabetic.

•**tolbutamide sodium.** (tole-BYOO-tuh-mide) U.S.P. 23.
Use: Diagnostic aid (diabetes).
See: Orinase Diagnostic (Pharmacia & Upjohn).

•**tolcapone.** (TOLE-kah-pone) USAN. Investigational.
Use: Antiparkinsonian.
See: Tasmar, Tab. (Roche Laboratories).

•**tolciclate.** (tole-SIGH-klate) USAN.
Use: Antifungal.

Tolectin 200. (Ortho McNeil Pharmaceutical) Tolmetin sodium 200 mg/Tab. Bot. 100s. *Rx.*
Use: Analgesic, NSAID.

Tolectin 600. (Ortho McNeil Pharmaceutical) Tolmetin sodium 600 mg/Tab. Bot. 100s. *Rx.*
Use: Analgesic, NSAID.

Tolectin DS. (Ortho McNeil Pharmaceutical) Tolmetin sodium 400 mg/Cap Bot. 100s, 500s, UD 100s. *Rx.*
Use: Analgesic, NSAID.

Tolerex. (Procter & Gamble Pharm.) Protein 20.6 g, carbohydrate 226.3 g, fat 1.45 g, Na 468 mg, K 1172 mg, mOsm/Kg H_2O 550, cal/ml 1, vitamins A, B_1, B_2, B_3, B_5, B_6, B_{12}, C, D, E, K, folic acid, biotin, choline, Ca, P, I, Fe, Mg,Cu, Zn, Mn, Se, Mo, Cr. Assorted flavors Pow. Pkts. 80 g. *otc.*
Use: Mineral, vitamin supplement.

•**tolfamide.** (TAHL-fah-MIDE) USAN.
Use: Enzyme inhibitor (urease).

Tolfrinic. (B.F. Ascher and Co.) Ferrous fumarate 200 mg, vitamins B_{12} 25 mcg, C 100 mg/Tab. Bot. 100s. *otc.*
Use: Mineral, vitamin supplement.

•**tolgabide.** (TOLE-gah-bide) USAN.
Use: Antiepileptic (control of abnormal movements).

•**tolimidone.** (TAHL-IH-mih-dohn) USAN.
Use: Antiulcerative.

Tolinase. (Pharmacia & Upjohn) Tolazamide 100 mg, 250 mg, 500 mg/Tab. Bot. 200s (250 mg only), 1000s (250 mg only), UD 100s (250 mg only), unit-of-use 100s. *Rx.*
Use: Antidiabetic.

•**tolindate.** (TOLE-in-DATE) USAN.
Use: Antifungal.

tolmetin. (TOLE-meh-tin) USAN.
Use: Anti-inflammatory.

•**tolmetin sodium.** (TOLE-meh-tin) U.S.P. 23.
Use: Anti-inflammatory.
See: Tolectin, Tab. (Ortho McNeil Pharmaceutical).
Tolectin DS, Cap. (Ortho McNeil Pharmaceutical).

tolmetin sodium. (Various Mfr.) Tolmetin sodium. **Tab.:** 200 mg, 600 mg. Bot. 100s; 500s, 1000s (600 mg only). **Cap.:** 400 mg. Bot. 100s, 500s, 1000s. *Rx.*
Use: Anti-inflammatory.

•**tolnaftate.** (tahl-NAFF-tate) U.S.P. 23.
Use: Antifungal.
See: Absorbine Prods. (W.F. Young, Inc.).
Blis-To-Sol (Chattem).
Breezee Mist Antifungal (Pedinol).
Dr. Scholl's, Prods. (Schering-Plough Corp.).
Tinactin, Soln., Cream, Pow., Pow. Aer. (Schering-Plough Corp).

•**tolofocon a.** (TOE-low-FOE-kahn A) USAN.
Use: Contact lens material (hydrophobic).

toloxychlorinal.
Use: Sedative.

•**tolpovidone I 131.** (tahl-POE-vih-dohnl 131) USAN.
Use: Diagnostic aid (hypoalbuminemia), radiopharmaceutical.

•**tolpyrramide.** (tahl-PIHR-ah-mid) USAN.
Use: Oral hypoglycemic; antidiabetic.

•**tolrestat.** (TOLE-ress-TAT) USAN.
Use: Inhibitor (aldose reductase).
See: Alredase (Wyeth-Ayerst Laboratories).

•**tolterodine.** (tole-TEH-roe-deen) USAN.
Use: Treatment of urinary incontinence.

tolterodine tartrate.
Use: Urinary tract product.
See: Detrol, Tab. (Pharmacia & Upjohn).

•**tolu balsam.** (toe-LOO BALL-sam) U.S.P. 23. N.F. XVII.
Use: Pharmaceutic necessity for Compound Benzoin Tincture, expectorant.
See: Vicks Regular & Wild Cherry Medicated Cough Drops (Procter & Gamble Pharm.).

tolu balsam syrup. (Eli Lilly and Co.) N.F. XVII. Bot. 16 fl. oz.
Use: Vehicle.

tolu balsam tincture. N.F. XVII.

Use: Flavor.

toluidine blue o chloride.
See: Blutene Chloride.

Tolu-Sed (No Sugar). (Scherer Laboratories, Inc.) Codeine phosphate 10 mg, guaifenesin 100 mg/5 ml w/alcohol 10%. Bot. 4 oz., pt. *c-v.*
Use: Antitussive, expectorant.

Tolu-Sed DM (No Sugar). (Scherer Laboratories, Inc.) Dextromethorphan HBr 10 mg, guaifenesin 100 mg/5 ml w/ alcohol 10%. Bot. 4 oz, pt. *otc.*
Use: Antitussive, expectorant.

•**tomelukast.** (tah-MELL-you-KAST) USAN.
Use: Antiasthmatic (leukotriene antagonist).

Tomocat. (Lafayette Pharmaceuticals, Inc.) Barium sulfate 5%. Conc. Susp. Bot. 145 ml (480 ml for dilution), 225 ml (1000 ml for dilution). *Rx.*
Use: Radiopaque agent.

Tomocat 1000. (Lafayette Pharmaceuticals, Inc.) Barium sulfate suspension concentrate 5% w/v/Bot. for dilution to 1.5% w/v at time of use. Bot. 225 ml w/1000 ml dilution Bot. Case 24 Bot. and 2 Dilution Bot.
Use: Radiopaque medium used to mark the GI tract during CT scans.

•**tomoxetine hydrochloride.** (TOE-MOX-eh-teen) USAN.
Use: Antidepressant.

Tonavite-M Elixir. (Zenith Goldline Pharmaceuticals) Bot. 12 oz, pt., gal.
Use: Dietary supplement.

•**tonazocine mesylate.** (tone-AZE-oh-SEEN) USAN.
Use: Analgesic.

Tono-B Pediatric. (Pal-Pak, Inc.) Fe 5 mg, thiamine HCl 0.167 mg, riboflavin 0.133 mg/Tab. Bot. 1000s. *otc.*
Use: Mineral, vitamin supplement.

Tonocard. (Astra Pharmaceuticals, L.P.) Tocainide HCl 400 mg, 600 mg/Tab. Bot. 100s, UD 100s. *Rx.*
Use: Antiarrhythmic.

Tonojug 2000. (Lafayette Pharmaceuticals, Inc.) Barium sulfate powder 1200 g for suspension to make 2000 ml. Bot. 2000 g Case: 8 Bot.
Use: Radiopaque contrast medium for use during x-ray examination of the GI tract.

Tonopaque. (Lafayette Pharmaceuticals, Inc.) Barium sulfate 95%. Pow. for Susp. Bot. 180 g, 1200 g. UD 25 lb cont. *Rx.*
Use: Radiopaque agent.

Toothache Gel. (Roberts Pharmaceuticals) Benzocaine, oil of cloves, benzyl alcohol, propylene glycol. Tube 15 g. *otc.*
Use: Anesthetic, local.

Toothache Relief-3 in 1. (C.S. Dent & Co. Division) Toothache gum, toothache drops, benzocaine. Lot. *otc.*
Use: Analgesic, topical.

Topamax. (Ortho McNeil Pharmaceutical) Topiramate 25 mg, 100 mg, 200 mg, lactose/Tab. Bot. 60s. *Rx.*
Use: Anticonvulsant.

Top Brass ZP-11. (Revlon) Zinc pyrithione 0.5% in cream base.
Use: Antidandruff.

Top-Form. (Colgate Oral Pharmaceuticals) Topical form-fitting gel applicators. Disposable trays for topical fluoride office treatments, plus permanent trays for topical fluoride home self-treatments. Box 100s. *Rx.*
Use: Topical fluoride applications in home or office.

Topic. (Roche Laboratories) 5% benzyl alcohol in greaseless gel base containing camphor, menthol, w/30% isopropyl alcohol. Tube 2 oz. *otc.*
Use: Antipruritic.

topical anesthetics, miscellaneous.
See: Ethyl Chloride (Gebauer Co.).
Fluro-Ethyl (Gebauer Co.).

Topical Fluoride. (Pacemaker) Acidulated phosphate fluoride. Flavors: Orange, bubble gum, lime, raspberry, grape, cinnamon. Liq. Bot. 4 oz., pt.
Use: Corticosteroid, topical.

Topicort Cream. (Hoechst Marion Roussel) Desoximetasone 0.25% emollient cream consisting of isopropyl myristate, cetyl stearyl alcohol, white petrolatum, mineral oil, lanolin alcohol, purified water. Tubes 15 g, 60 g, 120 g. *Rx.*
Use: Corticosteroid, topical.

Topicort Gel. (Hoechst Marion Roussel) Desoximetasone 0.05% in gel base. 20% alcohol. Tube 15 g, 60 g. *Rx.*
Use: Corticosteroid, topical.

Topicort LP Cream. (Hoechst Marion Roussel) Desoximetasone 0.05%. Tubes 15 g, 60 g. *Rx.*
Use: Corticosteroid, topical.

Topicort Ointment. (Hoechst Marion Roussel) Desoximetasone 0.25% in ointment base. Tube 15 g, 60 g. *Rx.*
Use: Corticosteroid, topical.

Topicycline. (Roberts Pharmaceuticals) Tetracycline HCl 2.2 mg/ml w/sodium bisulfite, ethanol 40%. Bot. 70 ml w/diluent. *Rx.*
Use: Dermatologic, acne.

•**topiramate.** (toe-PIRE-ah-MATE) USAN.
Use: Anticonvulsant.
See: Topamax, Tab. (Ortho McNeil Pharmaceutical).

Toposar. (Pharmacia & Upjohn) Etoposide 20 mg, benzyl alcohol 30 mg, alcohol 30.5%/ml. Inj. 5 ml, 10 ml, 25 ml. *Rx.*
Use: Antineoplastic.

•**topotecan hydrochloride.** (toe-poe-TEE-kan) USAN.
Use: Antineoplastic (DNA topoisomerase I inhibitor).
See: Hycamtin, Pow. for Inj. (SmithKline Beecham Pharmaceuticals).

Toprol XL. (Astra Pharmaceuticals, L.P.) Metoprolol succinate 47.5 mg, 95 mg, 190 mg/ER Tab. Bot. 100s. *Rx.*
Use: Antihypertensive.

•**topterone.** (TOP-ter-ohn) USAN.
Use: Antiandrogen.

TOPV.
Use: Immunization.
See: Orimune (ESI Lederle Generics).

•**toquizine.** (TOE-kwih-zeen) USAN.
Use: Anticholinergic.

Toradol. (Roche Laboratories) Ketorolac tromethamine 15 mg/ml, 30 mg/ ml. Inj. 15 mg/ml in 1 ml Tubex syringes, 30 mg/ml in 1 ml and 2 ml Tubex syringes. Inj. *Rx.*
Use: Analgesic, NSAID.

Toradol Tablets. (Roche Laboratories) Ketorolac tromethamine 10 mg/Tab. Bot. 100s, UD 100s. *Rx.*
Use: Analgesic, NSAID.

Torecan. (Boehringer Ingelheim, Inc.) Thiethylperazine. **Tab.:** 10 mg w/tartrazine. Bot. 100s. **Amp.:** 10 mg/2 ml (w/ sod. metabisulfite 0.5 mg, ascorbic acid 2 mg, sorbitol 40 mg, q.s. carbon dioxide). *Rx.*
Use: Antiemetic, antinauseant.

toremifene. (TORE-EM-ih-feen SIH-trate)
Use: Antineoplastic. [Orphan Drug]
See: Estrinex.

•**toremifene citrate.** (TORE-EM-ih-feen SIH-trate) USAN.
Use: Antiestrogen, antineoplastic.
See: Fareston, Tab. (Schering-Plough Corp.).

Tornalate. (Dura Pharmaceuticals) **Aer.:** Bitolterol mesylate 0.8% (0.37 mg/actuation). Metered dose inhaler 15 ml (≥ 300 inhalations). **Soln. for Inh.:** Bitolterol mesylate 0.2%, alcohol 25%, propylene glycol. Bot. 10 ml, 30 ml, 60 ml w/ dropper. *Rx.*
Use: Bronchodilator, sympathomimetic.

•**torsemide.** (TORE-suh-MIDE) USAN.
Use: Diuretic.
See: Demadex, Tab., Inj. (Boehringer Mannheim Pharmaceuticals).

torula yeast, dried. Obtained by growing *Candida (torulopsis) utilis* yeast on wood pulp wastes (Nutritional Labs.) Conc. 100 lb drums.
Use: Natural source of protein and Vitamin B-complex vitamins.

•**tosifen.** (TOE-sih-fen) USAN.
Use: Antianginal.

•**tosufloxacin.** (toe-SUE-FLOX-ah-sin) USAN.
Use: Anti-infective.

Totacillin. (SmithKline Beecham Pharmaceuticals) Ampicillin trihydrate equivalent to: **Cap.:** 250 mg, 500 mg. Bot. 500s. **Pow. for Oral Susp.:** 125 mg/5 ml, 250 mg/5 ml. Bot. 100 ml, 200 ml. *Rx.*
Use: Anti-infective, penicillin.

Total. (Allergan, Inc.) Polyvinyl alcohol, edetate disodium, benzalkonium chloride in a sterile, buffered, isotonic solution. Soln. Bot. 60 ml, 120 ml. *otc.*
Use: Contact lens care.

Total Eclipse Cooling Alcohol. (Novartis Pharmaceutical Corp.) Padimate O, oxybenzone, glyceryl PABA, alcohol 77%. SPF 15. Lot. Bot. 120 ml. *otc.*
Use: Sunscreen.

Total Eclipse Moisturizing. (Novartis Pharmaceutical Corp.) Padimate O, oxybenzone, octyl salicylate. Moisturizing base. SPF 15. Lot. Bot. 120 ml. *otc.*
Use: Sunscreen.

Total Eclipse Oil & Acne Prone Skin Sunscreen. (Eclipse) Padimate O, oxybenzone, glyceryl PABA, alcohol 77%. SPF 15. Lot. Bot. 120 ml. *otc.*
Use: Sunscreen.

Total Formula. (Vitaline Corp.) Fe 20 mg, vitamins A 10,000 IU, D 400 IU, E 30 IU, B_1 15 mg, B_2 15 mg, B_3 25 mg, B_5 25 mg, B_6 25 mg, B_{12} 25 mcg, C 100 mg, folic acid 0.4 mg, Ca, Cr, Cu, I, K, Mg, Mn, Mo, P, Se, Si, V, vitamin K, biotin 300 mcg, Zn 30 mg, choline, bioflavonoids, hesperidin, inositol, PABA, rutin/Tab. Bot. 90s, 100s. *otc.*
Use: Mineral, vitamin supplement.

Total Formula-2. (Vitaline Corp.) Fe 20 mg, vitamins A 10,000 IU, D 400 IU, E 30 IU, B_1 15 mg, B_2 15 mg, B_3 25 mg, B_5 25 mg, B_6 25 mg, B_{12} 25 mcg, C 100 mg, folic acid 0.4 mg, Ca, Cr, Cu, I, K, Mg, Mn, Mo, P, Se, Si, V, vitamin K, biotin 300 mcg, Zn 30 mg, choline, bioflavonoids, hesperidin, inositol,

PABA, rutin/Tab. with boron. Bot. 60s. *otc.*
Use: Mineral, vitamin supplement.

Total Solution. (Allergan, Inc.) Isotonic, buffered soln. of polyvinyl alcohol, benzalkonium chloride, EDTA. Soln. Bot. 60 ml, 120 ml. *otc.*
Use: Ophthalmic.

totaquine. Alkaloids from *Cinchona* bark, 7% to 12% quinine anhydrous, 70% to 80% total alkaloids (cinchonidine, cinchonine, quinidine & quinine).

totomycin hydrochloride. U.S.P. 23. Tetracycline.

Touro A & D. (Dartmouth Pharmaceuticals) Chlorpheniramine maleate 4 mg, phenyltoloxamine citrate 50 mg, phenylephrine HCl 20 mg/SR Cap. Bot. 100s. *Rx.*
Use: Antihistamine, decongestant.

Touro EX. (Dartmouth Pharmaceuticals) Guaifenesin 600 mg. SR Capl. Bot. 100s. *Rx.*
Use: Expectorant.

Touro LA. (Dartmouth Pharmaceuticals) Pseudoephedrine HCl 120 mg, guaifenesin 500 mg. LA Capl. Bot. 100s. *Rx.*
Use: Decongestant, expectorant.

Toxo. (Wampole Laboratories) *Toxoplasma* antibody test system. Tests 120s.
Use: An IFA test system for the detection of antibodies to *Toxoplasma gondii.*

toxoid, diphtheria.
Use: Immunization.
See: Acel-Imune, Vial (Wyeth-Ayerst Laboratories).
ActHIB/DTP, Set of DTwP vial plus Hib Pow. for Inj. (Pasteur Merieux Connaught).
diphtheria and tetanus toxoids (pediatric strength).
diphtheria and tetanus toxoids with pertussis vaccine, Vial (Various Mfr.).
Infanrix (SKB).
tetanus and diphtheria toxoids (adult strength), Vial.
Tetramune, Vial (Wyeth-Ayerst Laboratories).
Tri-Immunol, Vial (Wyeth-Ayerst Laboratories).
Tripedia, Vial (Pasteur Merieux Connaught).

toxoid, tetanus adsorbed.
Use: Immunization.

toxoid, tetanus. *Rx.*
Use: Immunization.
See: Acel-Imune, Vial (Wyeth-Ayerst Laboratories).
ActHIB/DTP, Set of DTwP vial plus Hib Pow. for Inj. (Pasteur Merieux Connaught).
diphtheria and tetanus toxoids (pediatric strength).
diphtheria and tetanus toxoids with pertussis vaccine, Vial (Various Mfr.).
Infanrix (SKB).
tetanus and diphtheria toxoids (adult strength), Vial.
Tetramune, Vial (Wyeth-Ayerst Laboratories).
Tri-Immunol, Vial (Wyeth-Ayerst Laboratories).
Tripedia, Vial (Pasteur Merieux Connaught).

toxoplasmosis test.
Use: Diagnostic aid.
See: TPM Test (Wampole Laboratories).

t-PA.
Use: Tissue plasminogen activator.
See: Activase (Genentech, Inc.).

T-Phyl. (Purdue Frederick Co.) Theophylline 200 mg/Tab. Bot. 100s. *Rx.*
Use: Bronchodilator.

TPM-Test. (Wampole Laboratories) Indirect hemagglutination test for the qualitative and quantitative determination of antibodies to *Toxoplasma gondii* in serum. Kit 120s.
Use: Diagnostic aid, toxoplasmosis.

TPN Electrolytes. (Abbott Hospital Products) Multiple electrolyte additive: 321 mg NaCl, 331 mg CaCl, 1491 mg KCl, 508 mg MgCl, 2420 mg sodium acetate; 20 ml in 50 ml fliptop and pintop vial, 20 ml Univ. Add. Syr. *Rx.*
Use: Electrolyte supplement.

TPN Electrolytes II. (Abbott Laboratories) Na 15 mEq/L, K 18 mEq/L, Ca 4.5 mEq/L, Mg 5 mEq/L, Cl 35 mEq/L, acetate 7.5 mEq/L. In 20 ml fill in 50 ml fliptop and pintop vials, 20 ml fill syringes. *Rx.*
Use: Nutritional therapy, parenteral.

TPN Electrolytes III. (Abbott Laboratories) Na 25 Eq/L, K 40.6 mEq/L, Ca 5 mEq/L, Mg 8 mEq/L, Cl 33.5 mEq/L, acetate 40.6 mEq/L, gluconate 5 mEq/L. In 20 ml fill in 50 ml fliptop and pintop vials and 20 ml fill syringes. *Rx.*
Use: Nutritional therapy, parenteral.

•**tracazolate.** (track-AZE-oh-late) USAN.
Use: Sedative, hypnotic.

Trace. (Young Dental) Erythrosine conc. soln. Squeeze Bot. 30 ml, 60 ml Dispenser Packets 200s. *otc.*
Use: Diagnostic aid, disclose dental plaque.

Trace 28 Liquid. (Young Dental) FD&C Red No. 28 in aqueous soln. Bot. 30 ml, 60 ml. *otc.*
Use: Diagnostic aid, disclose dental plaque.

Trace 28 Tablets. (Young Dental) FD&C Red No. 28. Tablets. Box 30s, 180s, 700s. *otc.*
Use: Diagnostic aid, disclose dental plaque.

Tracelyte. (Fujisawa USA, Inc.) A combination of electrolytes and trace elements additive. Inj. Vial 20 ml. *Rx.*
Use: Electrolyte, trace element supplement.

Tracelyte-II. (Fujisawa USA, Inc.) A combination of electrolytes and trace elements additive. Inj. Vial 20 ml. *Rx.*
Use: Electrolyte, trace element supplement.

Tracelyte-II with Double Electrolytes. (Fujisawa USA, Inc.) Combination of electrolytes and trace elements additive. Inj. Vial 40 ml. *Rx.*
Use: Electrolyte, trace element supplement.

Tracelyte with Double Electrolytes. (Fujisawa USA, Inc.) A combination of electrolytes and trace elements additive. Inj. Vial 40 ml. *Rx.*
Use: Electrolyte, trace element supplement.

Traceplex. (Enzyme Process) Fe 30 mg, I 0.1 mg, Cu 0.5 mg, Mg 40 mg, Zn 10 mg, B_{12} 5 mcg/4 Tabs. Bot. 100s, 250s. *otc.*
Use: Mineral supplement.

Tracer bG. (Boehringer Mannheim Pharmaceuticals) Reagent strips. Kit. 25s, 50s.
Use: Diagnostic aid.

Tracrium Injection. (GlaxoWellcome) Atracurium besylate 10 mg/ml Amp. 5ml. Box 10s; 10 ml MDV. Box 10s. *Rx.*
Use: Muscle relaxant.

Trac Tabs 2X. (Hyrex Pharmaceuticals) Atropine sulfate 0.06 mg, hyoscyamine sulfate 0.03 mg, methenamine 120 mg, methylene blue 6 mg, phenyl salicylate 30 mg, benzoic acid 7.5 mg/Tab. Bot. 100s, 1000s. *Rx.*
Use: Anti-infective, urinary.

•**trafermin.** (trah-FUR-min) USAN.
Use: Treatment of stroke and coronary artery disease.

•**tragacanth.** (TRAG-ah-kanth) N.F. 18.
Use: Pharmaceutic aid (suspending agent).

•**tralonide.** (TRAY-low-nide) USAN.
Use: Corticosteoid, topical.

•**tramadol hydrochloride.** (TRAM-uh-dole) USAN.
Use: Analgesic.
See: Ultram, Tab. (Ortho McNeil Pharmaceutical).

•**tramazoline hydrochloride.** (tram-AZE-oh-leen) USAN.
Use: Adrenergic.

trancin. Fluphenazine.
Use: Anxiolytic.

Trancopal. (Sanofi Winthrop Pharmaceuticals) Chlormezanone 100 mg w/saccharin/Cap. Bot. 100s. 200 mg/Cap. Bot. 100s, 1000s. *Rx.*
Use: Anxiolytic.

Trandate. (GlaxoWellcome) Labetalol HCl 100 mg. Tab. Bot. 100s, 500s, UD 100s. *Rx.*
Use: Antihypertensive.

Trandate Injection. (GlaxoWellcome) Labetalol HCl 5 mg/ml Amp. 1 ml. Box 1s. Vial 20 ml, 40 ml. Box 1s. Prefilled Syringes 4 ml, 8 ml. *Rx.*
Use: Antihypertensive.

Trandate Tablets. (GlaxoWellcome) Labetalol HCl 100 mg, 200 mg, 300 mg/Tab. Bot. 100s, 500s. UD 100s. *Rx.*
Use: Antihypertensive.

trandolapril.
Use: Antihypertensive.
See: Mavik, Tab. (Knoll Pharmaceuticals).
Tarka, ER Tab. (Knoll Pharmaceuticals).

•**tranexamic acid.** (tran-ex-AM-ik) USAN.
Use: Hemostatic. [Orphan Drug]
See: Cyklokapron, Tab., Inj. (Pharmacia & Upjohn).

•**tranilast.** (TRAN-ill-ast) USAN.
Use: Antiasthmatic.

tranquilizers.
See: Atarax, Prep. (Pfizer).
Compazine, Prep. (SmithKline Beecham Pharmaceuticals).
Equanil, Tab. (Wyeth-Ayerst Laboratories).
Fenarol, Tab. (Sanofi Winthrop Pharmaceuticals).
Haldol, Tab., Inj., Conc. Soln. (Ortho McNeil Pharmaceutical).
Librium, Cap., Inj. (Roche Laboratories).
Loxitane, Prod. (ESI Lederle Generics).
Mellaril, Tab., Soln. (Novartis Pharmaceutical Corp.).
Meprobamate (Various Mfr.).
Miltown, Prep. (Wallace Laboratories).
Permitil, Prep. (Schering-Plough Corp.).

Prolixin, Prep. (Bristol-Myers Squibb).
Stelazine, Prep. (SmithKline Beecham Pharmaceuticals).
Thorazine HCl, Prep. (SmithKline Beecham Pharmaceuticals).
Trancopal, Cap. (Sanofi Winthrop Pharmaceuticals).
Tranxene, Cap. (Abbott Laboratories).
Trilafon, Prep. (Schering-Plough).
Valium, Prep. (Roche Laboratories).
Vesprin, Prep. (Bristol-Myers Squibb).
Vistaril, Prep. (Pfizer US Pharmaceutical Group).

Tranquils Capsules. (Halsey Drug Co.) Pyrilamine maleate 25 mg/Cap. Bot. 30s. *otc.*
Use: Sleep aid.

Tranquils Tablets. (Halsey Drug Co.) Acetaminophen 300 mg, pyrilamine maleate 25 mg/Tab. Bot. 30s. *otc.*
Use: Analgesic, sleep aid.

•**transcainide.** (trans-CANE-ide) USAN.
Use: Antiarrhythmic, cardiovascular agent.

Transderm-Nitro. (Novartis Pharmaceutical Corp.) Nitroglycerin 12.5 mg, 25 mg, 50 mg, 75 mg, 100 mg/patch. **12.5 mg, 25 mg, 50 mg:** Box 30s, UD 30s, 100s. **75 mg:** Box 30s. **100 mg:** Box 30s, UD 30s. *Rx.*
Use: Antianginal.

Transderm-Scop. (Novartis Pharmaceutical Corp.) Scopolamine 0.5 mg per 2-unit blister pkg. (programmed delivery over 3-day period).
Use: Antiemetic, antivertigo.

transforming growth factor-beta 2. (Celtrix Pharmaceuticals, Inc.)
Use: Immunomodulator. [Orphan Drug]

Transthyretin EIA. (Abbott Diagnostics) Test kits 100s.
Use: Diagnostic aid.

Trans-Ver-Sal AdultPatch. (Doak Dermatologics) Salicylic acid 15%/Transdermal patch. 6 mm, 12 mm. 40s. Securing tape and cleaning file. *otc.*
Use: Keratolytic.

Trans-Ver-Sal PediaPatch. (Doak Dermatologics) Salicylic acid 15%/Transdermal patch. 6 mm. 20s. Securing tape and cleaning file. *otc.*
Use: Keratolytic.

Trans-Ver-Sal PlantarPatch. (Doak Dermatologics) Salicylic acid 15%/Transdermal patch. 20 mm patches, 25s. Securing tapes, cleaning file. *otc.*
Use: Dermatologic, wart therapy.

Tranxene Capsules. (Abbott Laboratories) Clorazepate dipotassium 3.75 mg, 7.5 mg, 15 mg/Cap. UD 100s. *c-IV.*
Use: Anxiolytic.

Tranxene-SD. (Abbott Laboratories) Clorazepate dipotassium 11.25 mg, 22.5 mg/Tab. Bot. 100s. *c-IV.*
Use: Anxiolytic.

Tranxene-SD Half Strength Tablets. (Abbott Laboratories) Clorazepate dipotassium 11.25 mg, 22.5 mg/Tab. Bot. 100s. *c-IV.*
Use: Anxiolytic.

Tranxene-T Tablets. (Abbott Laboratories) Clorazepate dipotassium tab. 3.75 mg, 7.5 mg, 15 mg/Tab. Bot. 100s, 500s, UD 100s. *c-IV.*
Use: Anxiolytic.

tranylcypromine sulfate. (tran-ill-SIP-row-meen) U.S.P. XXI.
Use: Antidepressant.
See: Parnate, Tab. (SmithKline Beecham Pharmaceuticals).

Trasicor. (Novartis Pharmaceutical Corp.) Oxprenolol HCl, B.A.N.

trastuzumab.
Use: Antineoplastic.
See: Herceptin (Genentech).

Trasylol. (Bayer Corp. (Consumer Div.)) Aprotinin 1.4 mg/ml. Inj. Vial 100 ml, 200 ml. *Rx.*
Use: Antihemophilic.

TraumaCal. (Bristol-Myers Squibb) Nutritionally complete formula for traumatized patients. Can 8 oz. Vanilla flavor. *otc.*
Use: Specific for nitrogen and energy needs in a limited volume for multiple trauma and major burns.

T-Rau Tablet. (Tennessee Pharmaceutic) Rauwolfia serpentina 50 mg or 100 mg/Tab. Bot. 100s, 1000s. *Rx.*
Use: Hypotensive.

Travamulsion 10% Intravenous Fat Emulsion. 1.1 kcal/ml 270 mOsm/L. Bot. 500 ml. *Rx.*
Use: Nutritional supplement, parenteral.

Travamulsion 20% Intravenous Fat Emulsion. (Baxter Pharmaceutical Products, Inc.) 2 kcal/ml 300 mOsm/L. Bot. 500 ml. *Rx.*
Use: Nutritional supplement, parenteral.

Travasol. (Baxter Pharmaceutical Products, Inc.) Crystalline L-amino acids injection 5.5%, 8.5% (with or without electrolytes). IV Bot. 500 ml, 1000 ml, 2000 ml. *Rx.*
Use: Nutritional supplement, parenteral.

Travasol 3.5% M Injection with Electrolyte #45. (Baxter Pharmaceutical Products, Inc.) Crystalline L-amino acids 3.5% Soln. Bot. IV 500 ml, 1000 ml. *Rx.*
Use: Nutritional supplement, parenteral.

Travasol 3.5% w/Electrolytes. (Clintec

Nutrition) Amino acid concentration 3.5%, nitrogen 0.591 g/100 ml, 500 ml, 1000 ml. *Rx.*
Use: Nutritional supplement, parenteral.

Travasol 10%. (Baxter Pharmaceutical Products, Inc.) Crystalline L-amino acids 10%. Inj. Bot. 200 ml, 500 ml, 1000 ml, 2000 ml. *Rx.*
Use: Nutritional supplement, parenteral.

Travasorb HN Peptide Diet. (Baxter Pharmaceutical Products, Inc.) High-nitrogen defined peptide 333 kcal/Pkt. 6 pkt/Carton. *otc.*
Use: Nutritional supplement.

Travsorb MCT Liquid Diet. (Baxter Pharmaceutical Products, Inc.) Digestible protein medium-chain triglyceride diet. 89 g packets. *otc.*
Use: Nutritional supplement.

Travasorb MCT Powder Diet. (Baxter Pharmaceutical Products, Inc.) Digestible protein medium-chain triglyceride diet 400 kcal/Pkt. 6 pkt./Carton. *otc.*
Use: Nutritional supplement.

Travasorb Renal Diet. (Baxter Pharmaceutical Products, Inc.) 467 kcal/Pkt. 6 pkt/Carton. 112 g packets. *otc.*
Use: Nutritional supplement.

Travasorb Standard Diet. (Baxter Pharmaceutical Products, Inc.) Defined peptide diet, 333 kcal/pkt. 6 packets/Carton. *otc.*
Use: Nutritional supplement.

Travasorb STD. (Clintec Nutrition) Enzymatically hydrolyzed lactalbumin 10 g, glucose oligosaccharides 63.3 g, MCT (fractioned coconut oil) 4.5 g, sunflower oil 4.5 g, Na 307 mg, K 390 mg, mOsm/560 Kg, H_2O, cal 333.3/ml, vitamins A, B_1, B_2, B_3, B_5, B_6, B_{12}, C, D, E, K, Ca, Cl, Cu, Fe, I, Mg, Mn, P, Zn. Gluten free. Pow. Pkts. 83.3 g. *otc.*
Use: Nutritional supplement.

Travasorb Whole Protein Liquid Diet. (Baxter Pharmaceutical Products, Inc.) Lactose free complete nutrition 250 kcal/Can. Cans 8 oz. *otc.*
Use: Nutritional supplement.

Travel Aids. (Faraday) Dimenhydrinate 50 mg/Tab. Bot. 30s. *otc.*
Use: Antiemetic, antivertigo.

Travel-Eze. (Health for Life Brands, Inc.) Pyrilamine maleate 25 mg, hyoscine hydrobromide 0.325 mg/Tab. Pkg. 20s. *otc.*
Use: Antiemetic, antivertigo.

Travel Sickness. (Walgreen) Dimenhydrinate 50 mg/Tab. Bot. 24s. *otc.*
Use: Antiemetic, antivertigo.

Traveltabs. (Armenpharm Ltd.) Dimenhydrinate 50 mg/Tab. Bot. 100s. *otc.*
Use: Antiemetic, antivertigo.

Travert. (Baxter Pharmaceutical Products, Inc.) Invert sugar injection 10% in water or saline. Plastic Bot. 500 ml, 1000 ml, electrolyte No. 2 Bot. 500 ml, 1000 ml, electrolyte No. 4 Bot. 250 ml, 500 ml Soln. (10%). *Rx.*
Use: Fluid, electrolyte replacement.

5% Travert and Electrolyte No. 2. (Baxter Pharmaceutical Products, Inc.) Invert sugar 50 g/L, calories 196 Cal/L, Na 56 mEq/L, K 25 mEq/L, Mg 6 mEq/L, Cl 56 mEq/L, phosphate 12.5 mEq/L, lactate 25 mEq/L, osmolarity 449 mOsm/L. 1000 ml. *Rx.*
Use: Nutritional supplement, parenteral.

10% Travert and Electrolyte No. 2. (Baxter Pharmaceutical Products, Inc.) Invert sugar 100 g/L, calories 384 Cal/L, Na 56 mEq/L, K 25 mEq/L, Mg 6 mEq/L, Cl 56 mEq/L, phosphate 12.5 mEq/L, lactate 25 mEq/L, osmolarity 726 mOsm/L. 1000 ml. *Rx.*
Use: Nutritional supplement, parenteral.

•**trazodone hydrochloride.** (TRAY-zoe-dohn) U.S.P. 23.
Use: Antidepressant.
See: Desyrel (Bristol-Myers Squibb).

trazodone hydrochloride. (Various Mfr.) 50 mg, 100 mg, 150 mg. Tab. Bot. 20s 50s, 100s, 250s, 500s, 1000s; UD 100s, 600s (except 150 mg). *Rx.*
Use: Antidepressant.

•**trebenzomine hydrochloride.** (TRAY-BEN-zoe-meen) USAN.
Use: Antidepressant.

Trecator S.C.. (Wyeth-Ayerst Laboratories) Ethionamide. 2-Ethyl thioisonicotinamide. 250 mg/Tab. Bot. 100s. *Rx.*
Use: Antituberculosal.

•**trecovirsen sodium.** (treh-koe-VEER-sin) USAN.
Use: Antiviral.

•**trefentanil hydrochloride.** (treh-FEN-tah-nill) USAN.
Use: Analgesic.

•**treloxinate.** (trell-OX-ih-nate) USAN.
Use: Antihyperlipoproteinemic.

Trental Tablets. (Hoechst Marion Roussel) Pentoxifylline 400 mg/CR Tab. Bot. 100s. UD 100s. *Rx.*
Use: Hemorrheologic.

Treo. (Bio-Pharm Inc.) **SPF 8:** Octocrylene, octyl methoxycinnamate, benzophenone-3, octyl salicylate, isostearyl alcohol, diazolidinyl urea, propylparabens, citronella oil 0.05% (as insect repellant). Lot. Bot. 118 ml. **SPF 15:** Octocrylene, octyl methoxycinnamate, benzophenone-3, octyl salicylate,

isostearyl alcohol, diazolidinyl urea, propylparaben, citronella oil 0.05% (as insect repellant). Lot. Bot. 118 ml. **SPF 30:** Octocrylene, octyl methoxycinnamate, benzophenone-3, octyl salicylate, isostearyl alcohol, diazolidinyl urea, propylparaben, citronella oil 0.05% (as insect repellant). Lot. Bot. 118 ml. *otc.*
Use: Sunscreen.

treosulfan.
Use: Antineoplastic. [Orphan Drug]
See: Ovastat.

•**trepipam maleate.** (TREH-pih-pam MAL-ee-ate) USAN. *Formerly Trimopam Maleate.*
Use: Sedative, hypnotic.

•**trestolone acetate.** (TRESS-toe-lone) USAN.
Use: Antineoplastic, androgen.

trethocanoic acid.
Use: Anticholesteremic.

•**tretinoin.** (TREH-tih-NO-in) U.S.P. 23.
Use: Keratolytic. [Orphan Drug]
See: Avita, Cream (DPT Laboratories, Inc.).
Retin-A, Cream, Gel, Soln. (Ortho McNeil Pharmaceutical).
Renova, Cream (Ortho McNeil Pharmaceutical).
Vesanoid, Cap. (Roche Laboratories).

tretinoin lf, iv. (Argus Pharmaceuticals, Inc.)
Use: Antineoplastic. [Orphan Drug]

Trexan Cablets. (Du Pont Merck Pharmaceutical Co.) Naltrexone HCl 50 mg/Tab. Bot. 50s. *Rx.*
Use: Opioid antagonist.

Triac. (Eon Labs Manufacturing, Inc.) Triprolidine HCl 2.5 mg, pseudoephedrine HCl 60 mg/Tab. Bot. 100s, 1000s. *Rx.*
Use: Antihistamine, decongestant.

Triacet Cream. (Teva Pharmaceuticals USA) Triamcinolone acetonide 0.1%. Tube 15 g, 80 g. *Rx.*
Use: Corticosteroid, topical.

•**triacetin.** (try-ah-SEE-tin) U.S.P. 23. *Formerly glyceryl triacetate.*
Use: Antifungal, topical.
See: Fungacetin, Oint. (Blair Laboratories).

triacetyloleandomycin. (try-ASS-eh-till-oh-lee-AN-do-MY-sin) Troleandomycin.
Use: Anti-infective.

Triacin C. (Various Mfr.) Pseudoephedrine HCl 30 mg, triprolidine HCl 1.25 mg, codeine phosphate 10 mg/5 ml, alcohol 4.3%. Syr. Bot. Pt., gal. *c-v.*
Use: Antihistamine, antitussive, decongestant.

Triactin. (Prometic Pharma) Phenylpropanolamine HCl 6.25 mg, chlorpheniramine maleate 1 mg/5 ml, EDTA, sorbitol, sucrose. Syr. Bot. 120 ml, 250 ml. *otc.*
Use: Antitussive, decongestant.

Triact Liquid. (Sanofi Winthrop Pharmaceuticals) Aluminum, magnesium hydroxide, simethicone. *otc.*
Use: Antacid, antiflatulent.

Triact Tablets. (Sanofi Winthrop Pharmaceuticals) Aluminum, magnesium hydroxide, simethicone. *otc.*
Use: Antacid, antiflatulent.

Triad. (Forest Pharmaceutical, Inc.) Butalbital 50 mg, acetaminophen 325 mg, caffeine 40 mg. Cap. Bot. 100s. *Rx.*
Use: Analgesic, hypnotic, sedative.

Triafed with Codeine. (Schein Pharmaceutical, Inc.) Pseudoephedrine HCl 30 mg, triprolidine HCl 1.25 mg, codeine phosphate 10 mg/5 ml. Syr. Bot. 473 ml. *c-v.*
Use: Antihistamine, antitussive, decongestant.

•**triafungin.** (TRY-ah-FUN-jin) USAN.
Use: Antifungal.

Triam-A. (Hyrex Pharmaceuticals) Triamcinolone acetonide 40 mg/ml. Inj. Vial 5 ml. *Rx.*
Use: Corticosteroid.

•**triamcinolone.** (TRY-am-SIN-oh-lone) U.S.P. 23.
Use: Corticosteroid, topical.
See: Aristocort, Tab., Syr. (ESI Lederle Generics).
Aristospan, Parenteral (ESI Lederle Generics).

•**triamcinolone acetonide.** (TRY-am-SIN-oh-lone ah-SEE-toe-nide) U.S.P. 23.
Use: Corticosteroid, topical, anti-inflammatory, topical.
See: Aristocort, Cream, Oint. (Fujisawa USA, Inc.).
Aristogel, Gel (ESI Lederle Generics).
Azmacort, Aer. (Rhone-Poulenc Rorer Pharmaceuticals, Inc.).
Delta-Tritex, Cream, Oint. (Dermol Pharmaceuticals, Inc.).
Flutex, Cream, Oint. (Syosset Laboratories Co., Inc.).
Kenalog, Preps. (Westwood Squibb Pharmaceuticals).
Kenonel, Cream (Marnel Pharmaceuticals, Inc.).
Nasacort, Spray (Rhone-Poulenc Rorer Pharmaceuticals, Inc.).
Nasacort AQ, Spray (Rhone-Poulenc Rorer Pharmaceuticals, Inc).

Triacet, Cream (Teva Pharmaceuticals USA).
Triderm, Cream (Del-Ray Laboratory, Inc.).
Tri-Kort, Inj. (Keene Pharmaceuticals, Inc.).
W/Neomycin, gramicidin, Nystatin.
See: Mycolog, Preps (Bristol-Myers Squibb).

triamcinolone acetonide. (Various Mfr.) **Cream: 0.025%, 0.1%:** Tube 15 g, 80 g, 454 g. **0.5%:** 15 g. **Lot.:** 0.025%, 0.1%. Bot. 60 ml. **Oint.: 0.025%, 0.1%:** Tube 15 g, 80 g, 454 g. **Oint.: 0.5%:** Tube 15 g. **Paste:** 0.1%.
Use: Corticosteroid, topical, anti-inflammatory, topical.

•**triamcinolone acetonide sodium phosphate.** (TRY-am-SIN-oh-lone ah-SEE-toe-nide) USAN.
Use: Costicosteroid, topical.

•**triamcinolone diacetate.** (try-am-SIN-oh-lone try-ASS-ah-tate) U.S.P. 23.
Use: Corticosteroid, topical.
See: Amcort, Inj. (Keene Pharmaceuticals, Inc.).
Aristocort Diacetate Forte (ESI Lederle Generics).
Aristocort Diacetate Intralesional, Inj. (ESI Lederle Generics).
Triam Forte, Inj. (Hyrex Pharmaceuticals).

•**triamcinolone hexacetonide.** (TRY-am-SIN-ole-ohn HEX-ah-SEE-tone-ide) U.S.P. 23.
Use: Costiscosteroid, topical.
See: Aristospan, Prep. (ESI Lederle Generics).

Triam Forte. (Hyrex Pharmaceuticals) Triamcinolone diacetate 40 mg/ml. Vial 5 ml. *Rx.*
Use: Corticosteroid.

Triaminic. (Novartis Pharmaceutical Corp.) Pyrilamine maleate 25 mg, pheniramine maleate 25 mg, phenylpropanolamine HCl 50 mg/TR Tab. Bot. 100s, 250s. *otc.*
Use: Antihistamine, decongestant.

Triaminic-12. (Novartis Pharmaceutical Corp.) Phenylpropanolamine HCl 75 mg, chlorpheniramine maleate 12 mg/SR Tab. Pkg. 20s. *otc.*
Use: Antihistamine, decongestant.

Triaminic Allergy. (Novartis Pharmaceutical Corp.) Phenylpropanolamine HCl 25 mg, chlorpheniramine maleate 4 mg/Tab. Blister pk. 24s. *otc.*
Use: Antihistamine, decongestant.

Triaminic AM Cough and Decongestant Formula. (Novartis Pharmaceutical Corp.) Pseudoephedrine HCl 15 mg, dextromethorphan HBr 7.5 mg/5 ml, sorbitol, sucrose, orange flavor. Alcohol and dye free. Liq. Bot. 118 ml, 237 ml. *otc.*
Use: Antitussive, decongestant.

Triaminic AM Decongestant Formula. (Novartis Pharmaceutical Corp.) Pseudoephedrine HCl 15 mg/5 ml, sorbitol, sucrose, orange flavor, alcohol and dye free. Syr. Bot. 118 ml, 237 ml. *otc.*
Use: Decongestant.

Triaminic Chewable Tablets. (Novartis Pharmaceutical Corp.) Phenylpropanolamine HCl 6.25 mg, chlorpheniramine maleate 0.5 mg/Chew. Tab. Blister pkg. 24s. *otc.*
Use: Antihistamine, decongestant.

Triaminic Cold Syrup. (Novartis Pharmaceutical Corp.) Phenylpropanolamine HCl 12.5 mg, chlorpheniramine maleate 2 mg/5 ml. Sorbitol. Syr. Bot. 4 oz., 8 oz. *otc.*
Use: Antihistamine, decongestant.

Triaminic Cold Tablets. (Novartis Pharmaceutical Corp.) Phenylpropanolamine HCl 12.5 mg, chlorpheniramine maleate 2 mg/Tab. Blister pkg. 24s. *otc.*
Use: Antihistamine, decongestant.

Triaminic-DM. (Novartis Pharmaceutical Corp.) Phenylpropanolamine HCl 6.25 mg, dextromethorphan HBr 5 mg/5 ml, sorbitol, sucrose. Alcohol free. Bot. 120 ml, 240 ml. *otc.*
Use: Antitussive, decongestant.

Triaminic Expectorant. (Novartis Pharmaceutical Corp.) Phenylpropanolamine HCl 12.5 mg, guaifenesin 100 mg/5 ml w/alcohol 5%, saccharin, sorbitol. Bot. 4 oz., 8 oz. *otc.*
Use: Decongestant, expectorant.

Triaminic Expectorant w/Codeine. (Novartis Pharmaceutical Corp.) Phenylpropanolamine HCl 12.5 mg, codeine phosphate 10 mg, guaifenesin 100 mg/5 ml w/alcohol 5%, saccharin, sorbitol. Liq. Bot. Pt. *otc.*
Use: Antitussive, decongestant, expectorant.

Triaminic Expectorant DH. (Novartis Pharmaceutical Corp.) Guaifenesin 100 mg, phenylpropanolamine HCl 12.5 mg, pheniramine maleate 6.25 mg, pyrilamine maleate 6.25 mg, hydrocodone bitartrate 1.67 mg/10 ml w/alcohol 5%, saccharin, sorbitol. Bot. Pt. *c-III.*
Use: Antihistamine, antitussive, decongestant, expectorant.

Triaminic Nite Light Liquid. (Novartis

Pharmaceutical Corp.) Pseudoephedrine 15 mg, chlorpheniramine maleate 1 mg, dextromethorphan HBr 7.5 mg/5 ml. Bot. 120 and 240 ml. *otc.*
Use: Antihistamine, antitussive, decongestant.

Triaminic Oral Infant Drops. (Novartis Pharmaceutical Corp.) Phenylpropanolamine HCl 20 mg, pheniramine maleate 10 mg, pyrilamine maleate 10 mg/ml. Dropper bot. 15 ml. *Rx.*
Use: Antihistamine, decongestant.

Triaminic Sore Throat Formula Liquid. (Novartis Pharmaceutical Corp.) Pseudoephedrine HCl 15 mg, dextromethorphan HBr 7.5 mg, acetaminophen 160 mg/5 ml, EDTA, sucrose, alcohol free. Bot. 240 ml. *otc.*
Use: Antitussive, analgesic, decongestant.

Triaminic Syrup. (Novartis Pharmaceutical Corp.) Phenylpropanolamine HCl 6.25 mg, chlorpheniramine maleate 1 mg/5 ml, sorbitol, sucrose, alcohol free. Bot. 120 ml, 240 ml. *otc.*
Use: Antihistamine, decongestant.

Triaminic TR Tablets. (Novartis Pharmaceutical Corp.) Phenylpropanolamine HCl 50 mg, pheniramine maleate 25 mg, pyrilamine maleate 25 mg/TR Tab. 100s, 250s. *otc.*
Use: Antihistamine, decongestant.

Triaminic Cold, Allergy, Sinus Tablets. (Novartis Pharmaceutical Corp.) Phenylpropanolamine HCl 25 mg, acetaminophen 650 mg, chlorpheniramine maleate 4 mg/Tab. Pkg. 12s. *otc.*
Use: Analgesic, antihistamine, decongestant.

Triaminicol Multi Symptom Cold Syrup. (Novartis Pharmaceutical Corp.) Phenylpropanolamine HCl 12.5 mg, chlorpheniramine maleate 2 mg, dextromethorphan HBr 10 mg/5 ml. *otc.*
Use: Antihistamine, antitussive, decongestant.

Triaminicol Multi-Symptom Cough and Cold Tablet. (Novartis Pharmaceutical Corp.) Phenylpropanolamine HCl 12.5 mg, chlorpheniramine maleate 2 mg, dextromethorphan HBr 10 mg/Tab. Blister pkg. 24s. *otc.*
Use: Antihistamine, antitussive, decongestant.

Triaminicol Multi-Symptom Relief. (Novartis Pharmaceutical Corp.) Phenylpropanolamine HCl 6.25 mg, chlorpheniramine maleate 1 mg, dextromethorphan HBr 5 mg/5 ml. Liq. Bot. 120 ml. *otc.*
Use: Antihistamine, antitussive, decongestant.

triaminilone-16,17-acetonide.
See: Triamcinolone acetonide.

Triamolone 40. (Forest Pharmaceutical, Inc.) Triamcinolone diacetate 40 mg/ml. Vial 5 ml. *Rx.*
Use: Corticosteroid.

Triamonide 40. (Forest Pharmaceutical, Inc.) Triamcinolone acetonide 40 mg/ml. Vial 5 ml. *Rx.*
Use: Corticosteroid.

•**triampyzine sulfate.** (TRY-AM-pih-zeen SULL-fate) USAN.
Use: Anticholinergic.

•**triamterene.** (try-AM-tur-een) U.S.P. 23.
Use: Diuretic.
See: Dyrenium, Cap. (SmithKline Beecham Pharmaceuticals).

triamterene/hydrochlorothiazide. (Various Mfr.) **Cap.:** Triamterene 50 mg, hydrochlorothiazide 25 mg. Bot. 100s, 1000s. **Tab.:** Triamterene 37.5 mg, hydrochlorothiazide 25 mg. Bot. 100s, 500s, 1000s; Triamterene 75 mg, hydrochlorothiazide 50 mg. Bot. 100s, 250s, 500s, 1000s. *Rx.*
Use: Diuretic combination.

triamterene and hydrochlorothiazide capsules.
Use: Diuretic.
See: Dyazide, Cap. (SmithKline Beecham Pharmaceuticals).

Trianide. (Seatrace Pharmaceuticals, Inc.) Triamcinolone acetonide 40 mg/ml. Vial 5 ml. *Rx.*
Use: Corticosteroid.

Tri-Aqua. (Pfeiffer Co.) Caffeine 100 mg, extracts of buchu, uva ursi, zea, triticum/Tab. Bot. 50s, 100s. *otc.*
Use: Diuretic.

Tri-A-Vite F. (Major Pharmaceuticals) F[1] 0.5 mg, vitamins A 1500 IU, D 400 IU, C 35 mg/ml Drops. Bot. 50 ml. *Rx.*
Use: Vitamin supplement.

Triaz. (Medicus Dermatologics) **Gel.:** Benzoyl peroxide 6%, 10%, EDTA. Tube 42.5 g. **Cleanser:** Benzoyl peroxide 10%, Menthol. 85.1 g. *Rx.*
Use: Antiacne.

•**triazolam.** (try-AZE-oh-lam) U.S.P. 23.
Use: Hypnotic, sedative.
See: Halcion, Tab. (Pharmacia & Upjohn).

triazolam. (Various Mfr.) Triazolam 0.125 mg, 0.25 mg. Tab. Bot. 10s, 100s, 500s, UD 100s. *c-IV.*
Use: Sedative.

Triban. (Great Southern Laboratories) Trimethobenzamide HCl 200 mg, benzocaine 2%. Supp. Pkg. 10s, 50s. *Rx.*

Use: Antiemetic.

Triban, Pediatric. (Great Southern Laboratories) Trimethobenzamide HCl 100 mg, benzocaine 2%. Supp. Pkg. 10s. *Rx.*
Use: Antiemetic.

•**tribenoside.** (try-BEN-oh-SIDE) USAN. Not available in US.
Use: Sclerosing agent.

Tri-Biocin. (Health for Life Brands, Inc.) Bacitracin 400 units, polymyxin B sulfate 5000 units, neomycin 5 mg/g Tube 0.5 oz. *otc.*
Use: Antibiotic, topical.

Tribiotic Plus. (Thompson Medical Co.) Polymyxin B sulfate 5000 units, neomycin sulfate (equivalent to 3.5 mg neomycin base), bacitracin 500 units, lidocaine 40 mg/g, lanolin, light mineral oil, petrolatum. Oint. Tube 28 g. 35 g. *otc.*
Use: Anti-infective, topical.

tribromoethanol.
Use: Anesthetic (inhalation).

tribromomethane. Bromoform.

•**tribromsalan.** (try-BROME-sah-lan) USAN.
Use: Disinfectant.

tricalcium phosphate.
Use: Electrolytes, mineral supplement.
See: Posture (Whitehall Robins Laboratories).

•**tricetamide.** (TRY-see-tam-id) USAN.
Use: Hypnotic, sedative.

Tri-Chlor. (Gordon Laboratories) Trichloroacetic acid 80%. Bot. 15 ml. *Rx.*
Use: Cauterizing agent.

•**trichlormethiazide.** (try-klor-meth-EYE-ah-zide) U.S.P. 23.
Use: Antihypertensive, diuretic.
See: Metahydrin, Tab. (Hoechst Marion Roussel).
Naqua, Tab. (Schering-Plough Corp.).

trichloroacetic acid. Acetic acid, trichloro.
Use: Topical, as a caustic.

trichlorobutyl alcohol.
See: Chlorobutanol.

•**trichloromonofluoromethane.** (try-klor-oh-mahn-oh-flure-oh-METH-ane) N.F. 18.
Use: Pharmaceutic aid (aerosol propellant).

tricholine citrate.
See: Choline citrate.

trichomonas test.
See: Isocult for *Trichomonas vaginalis.* (SmithKline Diagnostics).

Trichotine. (Schwarz Pharma, Inc.) **Pow.:** Sodium lauryl sulf., sod. perborate, monohydrate silica. Pkg. 150 g, 360 g. **Liq.:** Sodium lauryl sulfate, sodium borate, SD alcohol 40 8%, SD alcohol 23-A, EDTA. Bot. 120 ml, 240 ml. *otc.*
Use: Feminine hygiene.

•**triciribine phosphate.** (TRY-SIH-bean FOSS-fate) USAN. *Formerly Phosphate Salt of Tricyclic Nucleoside.*
Use: Antineoplastic.

•**tricitrates oral solution.** (TRY-SIH-trates) U.S.P. 23.
Use: Alkalizer (systemic, urinary); antiurolithic (cystine calculi, uric acid calculi); buffer (neutralizing).

triclobisonium. (Roche Laboratories) Triburon, Oint.

triclobisonium chloride.
Use: Anti-infective, topical.

•**triclocarban.** (TRY-kloe-CAR-ban) USAN.
Use: Disinfectant.
W/Clofulcarban.
See: Artra Beauty Ban (Schering-Plough Corp.).

•**triclofenol piperazine.** (TRY-kloe-FEE-nole pih-PURR-ah-zeen) USAN.
Use: Anthelmintic.

•**triclofos sodium.** (TRY-kloe-foss) USAN.
Use: Hypnotic, sedative.

•**triclonide.** (TRY-kloe-nide) USAN.
Use: Anti-inflammatory.

•**triclosan.** (TRY-kloe-san) USAN.
Use: Anti-infective; disinfectant.
See: Ambi 10, Bar (Kiwi Brands, Inc.).
Clearasil Daily Face Wash (Procter & Gamble Pharm.).
Clearasil Soap (Procter & Gamble Pharm.).
Oxy ResiDon't, Liq. (SmithKline Beecham Pharmaceuticals)
Stridex Face Wash, Soln. (Bayer Corp. (Consumer Div)).

Tricodene Cough and Cold. (Pfeiffer Co.) Pyrilamine maleate 12.5 mg, codeine phosphate 8.2 mg/5 ml, menthol, honey, glucose, sucrose. Liq. Bot. 120 ml. *c-v.*
Use: Antihistamine, antitussive.

Tricodene Forte. (Pfeiffer Co.) Phenylpropanolamine HCl 12.5 mg, chlorpheniramine maleate 2 mg, dextromethorphan HBr 10 mg/5 ml Liq. Bot. 120 ml. *otc.*
Use: Antihistamine, antitussive, decongestant.

Tricodene Liquid. (Pfeiffer Co.) Chlorpheniramine maleate 0.5 mg, dextromethorphan HBr 10 mg, ammonium Cl

90 mg, sodium citrate, sorbitol, mannitol/5 ml. Liq. Bot. 120 ml. *otc.*
Use: Antihistamine, antitussive, expectorant.

Tricodene NN. (Pfeiffer Co.) Phenylpropanolamine HCl 12.5 mg, chlorpheniramine maleate 2 mg, dextromethorphan HBr 10 mg/5 ml. Syr. Bot. 120 ml. *otc.*
Use: Antihistamine, antitussive, decongestant.

Tricodene Pediatric Cough & Cold Liquid. (Pfeiffer Co.) Phenylpropanolamine HCl 12.5 mg, dextromethorphan HBr 10 mg/5 ml Liq. Bot. 120 ml. *otc.*
Use: Antitussive, decongestant.

Tricodene Sugar Free. (Pfeiffer Co.) Chlorpheniramine maleate, dextromethorphan HBr 10 mg/5 ml, menthol, saccharin, sorbitol, alcohol free. Liq. 120 ml. *otc.*
Use: Antihistamine, antitussive.

Tricodene Syrup. (Pfeiffer Co.) Pyrilamine maleate 4.17 mg, codeine phosphate 8.1 mg, terpin hydrate, menthol/ 5 ml. Syr. Bot. 120 ml. *c-v.*
Use: Antihistamine, antitussive.

Tricomine. (Major Pharmaceuticals) Pseudoephedrine HCl 60 mg, carbinoxamine maleate 4 mg, dextromethorphan HBr 15 mg/5 ml, alcohol 5%. Liq. Bot. 120 ml. *otc.*
Use: Antihistamine, antitussive, decongestant.

Tricor. (Abbott) Fenofibrate 67 mg, lactose. Cap. Bot. 90s. *Rx.*
Use: Antihyperlipidemic.

Tricosal. (Invamed, Inc.) Choline magnesium trisalicylate 500 mg, 750 mg, 1000 mg/Tab. Bot. 100s, 500s. *Rx.*
Use: Salicylate.

Triderm Cream. (Del-Ray Laboratory, Inc.) Triamcinolone acetonide 0.1%. Tube 30 g, 90 g. *Rx.*
Use: Corticosteroid.

Tridesilon Cream. (Bayer Corp. (Consumer Div.)) Desonide 0.05% in vehicle buffered to the pH range of normal skin w/glycerin, methylparaben, sodium lauryl sulfate, aluminum sulfate, calcium acetate, cetyl stearyl alcohol, synthetic bees wax, white petrolatum, mineral oil. Tube 15 g, 60 g. *Rx.*
Use: Corticosteroid.

Tridesilon Otic. (Bayer Corp. (Consumer Div.)) Desonide 0.05%, acetic acid 2% in vehicle. Bot. 10 ml. *Rx.*
Use: Otic.

Tridex Tab., Timed Tridex Cap., Timed Tridex Jr. Cap. (Fellows) Changed to Daro Tab., Daro Timed Cap., Daro Jr. Timed Cap.

tridihexethyl chloride. U.S.P. 23.
Use: Anticholinergic.
W/Phenobarbital.
See: Pathilon w/Phenobarbital Tab., Cap. (ESI Lederle Generics).

Tridil 0.5 mg/ml. (Faulding USA) Nitroglycerin 0.5 mg/ml w/alcohol 10%, water for injection, buffered with sodium phosphate. Amp. 10 ml. Box 20s. *Rx.*
Use: Vasodilator; antianginal, antihypertensive.

Tridil 5 mg/ml. (Faulding USA) Nitroglycerin 5 mg/ml w/alcohol 30%, propylene glycol 30%, water for injection. Amp. 5 ml, 10 ml. Vial 5 ml, 10 ml, 20 ml. Box 20s. Special administration set w/10 ml Amp. *Rx.*
Use: Vasodilator; antianginal, antihypertensive.

Tridione. (Abbott Laboratories) Trimethadione (Troxidone). Cap. 300 mg, Bot. 100s. Dulcet Tab. 150 mg, Bot. 100s. *Rx.*
Use: Anticonvulsant.

Tridrate Bowel Evacuant Kit. (Mallinckrodt) Magnesium citrate soln. 300 ml, bisacodyl 5 mg/Tab. (3s), bisacodyl 10 mg/Supp. (1). Kit. *otc.*
Use: Laxative.

•**trientine hydrochloride.** (TRY-en-TEEN) U.S.P. 23.
Use: Chelating agent; Wilson's disease therapy adjunct. [Orphan Drug]
See: Cuprid, Cap. (Merck & Co.).

triethanolamine.
See: Trolamine.

triethanolamine polypeptide oleate condensate.
See: Cerumenex, Drops (Purdue Frederick Co.).

triethanolamine salicylate.
See: Aspercreme, Cream (Thompson Medical Co.).
Myoflex, Cream (Warren-Teed).

triethanolamine trinitrate biphosphate. Trolnitrate Phosphate.

•**triethyl citrate.** N.F. 18.
Use: Pharmaceutic aid (plasticizer).

triethylenemelamine. Tretamine TEM.
Use: Antineoplastic.

triethylenethiophosphoramide.
See: Thiotepa (ESI Lederle Generics).

Trifed-C. (Geneva Pharmaceuticals) Pseudoephedrine HCl 30 mg, triprolidine HCl 1.25 mg, codeine phosphate 10 mg/5 ml, alcohol 4.3%. Syr. Bot. Pt., gal. *c-v.*
Use: Antihistamine, antitussive, decongestant.

•**trifenagrel.** (try-FEN-ah-GRELL) USAN.

Use: Antithrombotic.

•**triflocin.** (try-FLOW-sin) USAN.
Use: Diuretic.

Tri-Flor-Vite with Fluoride. (Everett Laboratories, Inc.) Fluoride 0.25 mg, vitamin A 1500 IU, D 400 IU, C 35 mg/ml/Drop. 50 ml. *Rx.*
Use: Fluoride, vitamin supplement.

•**triflubazam.** (try-FLEW-bah-zam) USAN.
Use: Anxiolytic.

•**triflumidate.** (try-FLEW-mih-DATE) USAN.
Use: Anti-inflammatory.

•**trifluoperazine hydrochloride.** (try-flew-oh-PURR-uh-zeen) U.S.P. 23.
Use: Antipsychotic, anxiolytic, hypnotic, sedative.
See: Stelazine Inj., Liq., Tab. (SmithKline Beecham Pharmaceuticals).

trifluoperazine hydrochloride. (Various Mfr.) **Tab.:** 1 mg, 2 mg, 5 mg, 10 mg. Bot. 100s, 500s, 1000s, UD 100s. **Conc.:** 10 mg/ml. Bot. 60 ml. **Inj.:** 2 mg/ml. Vial 10 ml. *Rx.*
Use: Antipsychotic.

n-trifluoroacetyladriamycin-14-valerate. (Anthra Pharmaceuticals, Inc.)
Use: Antineoplastic. [Orphan Drug]

trifluorothymidine. *Rx.*
Use: Ophthalmic.
See: Viroptic (GlaxoWellcome).

•**trifluperidol.** (TRY-flew-PURR-ih-dahl) USAN.
Use: Antipsychotic.

•**triflupromazine.** (try-flew-PRO-mah-zeen) U.S.P. 23.
Use: Antipsychotic, anxiolytic.

•**triflupromazine hydrochloride.** U.S.P. 23.
Use: Antipsychotic, anxiolytic.
See: Vesprin Prods. (Bristol-Myers Squibb).

•**trifluridine.** (try-FLEW-RIH-deen) USAN.
Use: Antiviral used to treat herpes simplex eye infections.
See: Viroptic Ophth. Soln., (Monarch).

triglycerides, medium chain.
Use: Nutritional supplement.
See: MCT (Bristol-Myers Squibb).

triglyceride reagent strip. (Bayer Corp. (Consumer Div.)) Seralyzer reagent strip. Bot. 25s.
Use: Diagnostic aid, triglycerides.

Trihemic-600. (ESI Lederle Generics) Vitamins C 600 mg, B_{12} 25 mcg, intrinsic factor conc. 75 mg, folic acid 1 mg, Vitamins E 30 IU, ferrous fumarate 115 mg, dioctyl sodium succinate 50 mg/Tab. Bot. 30s, 500s. *Rx.*
Use: Mineral, vitamin supplement.

Trihexane. (Rugby Labs, Inc.) Trihexyphenidyl 2 mg/Tab. Bot. 100s, 1000s. *Rx.*
Use: Anticholinergic, antiparkinsonian.

Trihexidyl. (Schein Pharmaceutical, Inc.) Trihexyphenidyl 2 mg/Tab. Bot. 100s, 1000s. *Rx.*
Use: Anticholinergic, antiparkinsonian.

Trihexy-2. (Geneva Pharmaceuticals) Trihexyphenidyl 2 mg/Tab. Bot. 100s, 1000s. *Rx.*
Use: Anticholinergic, antiparkinsonian.

Trihexy-5. (Geneva Pharmaceuticals) Trihexyphenidyl 5 mg/Tab. Bot. 100s, 1000s. *Rx.*
Use: Anticholinergic, antiparkinsonian.

•**trihexyphenidyl hydrochloride.** (try-hex-ee-FEN-in-dill) U.S.P. 23.
Use: Anticholinergic, antiparkinsonian.
See: Artane, Elix., Tab. (ESI Lederle Generics).

TriHIBit. (Pasteur Merieux Connaught) Package containing lyophilized vials of ActHIB brand of Hib vaccine and vials of Tripedia brand of DTaP vaccine. *Rx.*
Use: Immunization.
See: ActHIB (Pasteur Merieux Connaught).
Tripedia (Pasteur Merieux Connaught).

Tri-Histin. (Recsei Laboratories) **25 mg Tab.:** Pyrilamine maleate 10 mg, chlorpheniramine maleate 1 mg. **50 mg Tab.:** Pyrilamine maleate 20 mg, methapyrilene HCl 15 mg, chlorpheniramine maleate 2 mg. **100 mg S.A. Cap.:** Pyrilamine maleate 40 mg, pheniramine maleate 25 mg. **Expectorant:** Pyrilamine maleate 5 mg, chlorpheniramine maleate 0.5 mg, guaifenesin 20 mg, phenylpropanolamine 7.5 mg, phenylephrine HCl 2.5 mg, sod. citrate 100 mg/5 ml. Bot. Pt. gal. **Liquid:** Pyrilamine maleate 5 mg, chlorpheniramine maleate 0.5 mg/5 ml. Bot. Pt. gal. **Tab.:** Bot. 100s, 500s, 1000s. 50 mg Bot. 1000s. **Cap.:** Bot. 100s, 500s, 1000s. *Rx-otc.*
Use: Antihistamine combination.

W/Benzyl alcohol, chlorobutanol and isopropyl alcohol.
See: Derma-Pax, Liq. (Recsei Laboratories).

W/Codeine phosphate, guaifenesin, phenylpropanolamine, phenylephrine HCl, sodium citrate.
See: Trihista-Cod., Liq. (Recsei Laboratories).

W/Ephedrine HCl, aminophylline, mephobarbital.

See: Asmasan, Tab. (Recsei Laboratories).

Tri-Hydroserpine. (Rugby Labs, Inc.) Hydrochlorothiazide 15 mg, reserpine 0.1 mg, hydralazine HCl 25 mg. Tab. Bot. 100s, 1000s. *Rx.*
Use: Antihypertensive combination.

Trihydroxyestrine. Trihydroxyestrin.

Trihydroxyethylamine. Triethanolamine.

Tri-Immunol. (Wyeth-Ayerst Laboratories) 12.5 Lf units diphtheria, 5 Lf units tetanus toxoids and 4 units pertussis vaccine combined, aluminum phosphate adsorbed purogenated. Vial 7.5 ml. *Rx.*
Use: Immunization.

Tri-K. (Century Pharmaceuticals, Inc.) Potassium acetate 0.5 g, potassium bicarbonate 0.5 g, potassium citrate 0.5 g/fl. oz. Saccharin. Bot. Pt., gal. *Rx.*
Use: Electrolyte supplement.

•**trikates oral solution.** (TRY-kates) U.S.P. 23.
Use: Replenisher (electrolyte).

Tri-Kort. (Keene Pharmaceuticals, Inc.) Triamcinolone acetonide suspension 40 mg/ml. Vial 5 ml. *Rx.*
Use: Corticosteroid, topical.

Trilafon. (Schering-Plough Corp.) Perphenazine. **Tab.:** 2 mg, 4 mg, 8 mg, 16 mg. Bot. 100s, 500s. **Inj.:** 5 mg/ml, w/disodium citrate 24.6 mg, sod. bisulfite 2 mg, and water for injection/ml. Amp. 1 ml. **Concentrate:** 16 mg/5 ml. Bot. 4 oz. w/dropper. *Rx.*
Use: Anxiolytic.

Tri-Levlen 21. (Berlex Laboratories, Inc.) **Group 1:** Levonorgestrel 0.05 mg, ethinyl estradiol 0.03 mg/Tab. **Group 2:** Levonorgestrel 0.075 mg, ethinyl estradiol 0.04 mg/Tab. **Group 3:** Levonorgestrel 0.125 mg, ethinyl estradiol 0.03 mg/Tab. Slide case 21s. Box 3s. *Rx.*
Use: Contraceptive

Tri-Levlen 28. (Berlex Laboratories, Inc.) **Group 1:** Levonorgestrel 0.05 mg, ethinyl estradiol 0.03 mg/Tab. **Group 2:** Levonorgestrel 0.075 mg, ethinyl estradiol 0.04 mg/Tab. **Group 3:** Levonorgestrel 0.125 mg, ethinyl estradiol 0.03 mg/Tab. **Group 4:** Inert tablets. Slide case 28s Box 3s. *Rx.*
Use: Contraceptive

Trilisate Liquid. (Purdue Frederick Co.) Choline magnesium trisalicylate from choline salicylate 293 mg, magnesium salicylate 362 mg/tsp to provide 500 mg salicylate/tsp. Bot. 8 oz. *Rx.*
Use: Analgesic, NSAID.

Trilisate Tablets. (Purdue Frederick Co.) Choline magnesium trisalicylate. **750 mg:** Salicylate from choline salicylate 400 mg and magnesium salicylate 544 mg Bot. 100s, UD 100s. **1000 mg:** Salicylate from choline salicylate 587 mg, magnesium salicylate 725 mg Bot. 60s. *Rx.*
Use: Analgesic, NSAID.

Trilog. (Roberts Pharmaceuticals) Triamcinolone acetonide 40 mg/ml. Vial 5 ml. *Rx.*
Use: Corticosteroid.

Trilone. (Century Pharmaceuticals, Inc.) Triamcinolone diacetate susp. Amp. 10 ml. *Rx.*
Use: Corticosteroid.

Trilone. (Roberts Pharmaceuticals) Triamcinolone diacetate 40 mg/ml. Vial 5 ml. *Rx.*
Use: Corticosteroid.

•**trilostane.** (TRY-low-stane) USAN.
Use: Adrenocortical suppressant.

Trimahist Elixir. (Tennessee Pharmaceutic) Phenylephrine HCl 5 mg, prophenpyridamine maleate 12.5 mg, l-menthol 1 mg, alcohol 5%/5 ml. Bot. Pt., gal. *Rx.*
Use: Antihistamine, decongestant.

Trimax Gel. (Sanofi Winthrop Pharmaceuticals) Aluminum, magnesium hydroxide, simethicone. *otc.*
Use: Antacid, antiflatulent.

Trimax Tablet. (Sanofi Winthrop Pharmaceuticals) Aluminum, magnesium hydroxide, simethicone. *otc.*
Use: Antacid, antiflatulent.

Trimazide. (Major Pharmaceuticals) **Capsules:** Trimethobenzamide 250 mg/Cap. Bot. 100s. **Suppositories:** 100 mg and 200 mg/Supp. 10s. *Rx.*
Use: Antiemetic.

trimazinol.
Use: Anti-inflammatory.

•**trimazosin hydrochloride.** (try-MAY-zoe-sin) USAN.
Use: Antihypertensive.

•**trimegestone.** (try-meh-JESS-tone) USAN.
Use: Hormone, progestin.

trimetamide. Trimethamide.

•**trimethadione.** (try-meth-ah-DIE-ohn) U.S.P. 23.
Use: Anticonvulsant.
See: Tridione, Prep. (Abbott Laboratories).

trimethamide.
Use: Antihypertensive.

•**trimethaphan camsylate.** (try-METH-ah-fan KAM-sih-late) U.S.P. 23.
Use: Antihypertensive.

•**trimethobenzamide hydrochloride.** (try-

meth-oh-BEN-zuh-mide) U.S.P. 23.
Use: Antiemetic.
See: Tegamide, Supp. (G & W Laboratories).
Tigan, Preps. (SmithKline Beecham Pharmaceuticals).

trimethobenzamide hydrochloride and benzocaine suppositories.
Use: Antiemetic.
See: Pediatric Triban (Great Southern Laboratories).
Triban (Great Southern Laboratories).

•**trimethoprim.** (try-METH-oh-prim) U.S.P. 23.
Use: Anti-infective.
See: Proloprim, Tab. (GlaxoWellcome).
Trimpex, Tab. (Roche Laboratories).
W/Polymyxin B Sulfate.
See: Polytrim Ophth. Soln. (Allergan, Inc.).
W/Sulfamethoxazole.
See: Bactrim, Oral Susp., Ped. Susp., Tab. (Roche Laboratories).
Septra, Tab. (GlaxoWellcome).
Septra DS, Tab. (GlaxoWellcome).

trimethoprim and sulfamethoxazole. (try-METH-oh-prim and suhl-fuh-meth-OX-uh-zole) (Various Mfr.) **Tab:** Trimethoprim 80 mg, sulfamethoxazole 400 mg/Tab. Bot. 100s, 500s. **Susp.:** Trimethoprim 40 mg, sulfamethoxazole 200 mg/5 ml. Bot. 150 ml, 200 ml, 480 ml. **Inj.:** Sulfamethoxazole 80 mg/ml, trimethoprim 16 mg/ml. 5 ml. *Rx.*
Use: Anti-infective combination.

trimethoprim and sulfamethoxazole DS. (Various Mfr.) Trimethoprim 160 mg, sulfamethoxazole 800 mg/Tab. Bot. 100s, 500s. *Rx.*
Use: Anti-infective combination.

•**trimethoprim sulfate.** (try-METH-oh-prim SULL-fate) USAN.
Use: Anti-infective.

trimethylene. Cyclopropane.

•**trimetozine.** (try-MET-oh-zeen) USAN.
Use: Hypnotic, sedative.

•**trimetrexate.** (TRY-meh-TREK-sate) USAN.
Use: Antineoplastic.
See: Neutrexin, Vial (US Bioscience).

•**trimetrexate glucuronate.** (TRY-meh-TREK-sate glue-CURE-uh-nate) USAN.
Use: Antineoplastic. [Orphan Drug]

Triminol. (Rugby Labs, Inc.) Phenylpropanolamine HCl 12.5 mg, chlorpheniramine maleate 2 mg, dextromethorphan HBr 10 mg/5 ml Syr. Bot. 120 ml. *otc.*
Use: Antihistamine, antitussive, decongestant.

•**trimipramine.** (TRY-MIH-prah-meen) USAN.
Use: Antidepressant.

•**trimipramine maleate.** (TRY-MIH-prah-meen) USAN.
Use: Antidepressant.
See: Surmontil (Wyeth-Ayerst Laboratories).

trimipramine maleate. (Various Mfr.) 25 mg, 50 mg, 100 mg. Cap. Bot. 100s, UD 100s.
Use: Antidepressant.

Trimixin. (Hance) Bacitracin 200 units, polymyxin B sulfate 4000 units, neomycin sulfate 3 mg/g Oint. Tube 0.5 oz. *otc.*
Use: Anti-infective, topical.

•**trimoprostil.** (TRY-moe-PRAHS-till) USAN.
Use: Gastric antisecretory.

Trimo-San. (Milex Products, Inc.) Oxyquinoline sulfate 0.025%, boric acid 1%, sodium borate 0.7%, sodium lauryl sulfate 0.1%, glycerin, methylparaben. Jelly. 120 g w/applicator, 120 g refill. *otc.*
Use: Vaginal agent.

Trimox. (Apothecon) Amoxicillin trihydrate. **Cap.:** 250 mg, 500 mg. Bot. 30s, 100s, 500s, UD 100s. **Oral Susp.:** 125 mg/5 ml, 250 mg/5 ml. Bot. 80 ml, 100 ml, 150 ml. *Rx.*
Use: Anti-infective, penicillin.

•**trimoxamine hydrochloride.** (TRY-MOX-am-een) USAN.
Use: Antihypertensive.

Trimox Pediatric Drops. (Apothecon) Amoxicillin trihydrate 50 mg/ml when reconstituted. Pow. for Oral Susp. Bot. 15 ml. *Rx.*
Use: Anti-infective, penicillin.

Trimpex. (Roche Laboratories) Tel-E-Dose 100s. *Rx.*
Use: Anti-infective, urinary.

Trim-Qwik. (Columbia Laboratories, Inc.) Powder-based meal food supplement. Can 10 oz. *otc.*
Use: Nutritional supplement.

Trimstat. (Laser, Inc.) Phendimetrazine tartrate 35 mg/Tab. Bot. 100s, 1000s. *c-III.*
Use: Anorexiant.

Trim Sulf D/S. (Lexis Laboratories) Sulfamethoxazole 800 mg, trimethoprim 160 mg/Tab. Bot. 100s, 500s. *Rx.*
Use: Anti-infective.

Trim Sulf S/S. (Lexis Laboratories) Sulfamethoxazole 400 mg, trimethoprim 80 mg/Tab. Bot. 100s, 500s. *Rx.*
Use: Anti-infective.

Trim-Sulfa. *Rx.*
Use: Anti-infective.
See: Proloprim (GlaxoWellcome).
Trimethoprim (Various Mfr.).
Trimpex (Roche Laboratories).

Trinalin Repetabs. (Key Pharmaceuticals) Azatadine maleate 1 mg, pseudoephedrine sulfate 120 mg/Tab. Bot 100s. *Rx.*
Use: Antihistamine, decongestant.

Trind. (Bristol-Myers Squibb) Phenylpropanolamine HCl 12.5 mg, chlorpheniramine maleate 2 mg/5 ml w/alcohol 5%, sorbitol. Bot. 5 oz. *otc.*
Use: Antihistamine, decongestant.

Tri-Nefrin Extra Strength. (Pfeiffer Co.) Phenylpropanolamine HCl 25 mg, chlorpheniramine maleate 4 mg/Tab. 24s. *otc.*
Use: Antihistamine, decongestant.

trinitrin tablets.
See: Nitroglycerin Tablets, U.S.P. 23.

trinitrophenol.
See: Picric Acid (Various Mfr.).

Tri-Norinyl. (Roche Laboratories) Norethindrone 1 mg with ethinyl estradiol 0.035 mg/Tab. Norethindrone 0.5 mg with ethinyl estradiol 0.035 mg/Tab. 21 and 28 day. (7 inert tabs) Wallette. *Rx.*
Use: Contraceptive.

Trinotic. (Forest Pharmaceutical, Inc.) Secobarbital 65 mg, amobarbital 40 mg, phenobarbital 25 mg/Tab. Bot. 1000s. *c-II.*
Use: Hypnotic.

Trinsicon. (UCB Pharmaceuticals, Inc.) Liver-stomach concentrate 240 mg, Fe 110 mg, vitamin C 75 mg, folic acid 0.5 mg, B_{12} 15 mcg. Cap. Bot. 60s, 500s, UD 100s. *Rx.*
Use: Nutritional supplement.

Trinsicon M. (UCB Pharmaceuticals, Inc.) Formerly listed by Russ.

Triobead-125. (Abbott Diagnostics) T3 diagnostic kit. Test units 50s, 100s, 500s.
Use: T3 uptake radioassay for the measurement of thyroid function by indirectly determining the degree of saturation of serum thyroxine binding globulin (TBG).

Triofed Syrup. (Alpharma USPD Inc.) Pseudoephedrine HCl 30 mg, triprolidine HCl 1.25 mg/5 ml Syr. Bot. 118 ml, 473 ml. *otc.*
Use: Antihistamine, decongestant.

•**triolein I 125.** (TRY-oh-leen) USAN.
Use: Radiopharmaceutical.

•**triolein I 131.** (TRY-oh-leen) USAN.
Use: Radiopharmaceutical.

Triostat. (SmithKline Beecham Pharmaceuticals) Liothyronine 10 mcg/ml, w/ ammonia 2.19 mg/ml, alcohol 6.8%. Vial 1 ml. *Rx.*
Use: Hormone, thyroid.

Triosulfon DMM. (CMC) Tab. Bot. 100s, 250s, 1000s.

Triotann. (Various Mfr.) Phenylephrine tannate 25 mg, chlorpheniramine tannate 8 mg, pyrilamine tannate 25 mg/Tab. Bot. 100s, 500s. *Rx.*
Use: Antihistamine, decongestant.

Triotann Pediatric. (Various Mfr.) Phenylephrine tannate 5 mg, chlorpheniramine tannate 2 mg, pyrilamine tannate 12.5 mg, saccharin, sucrose. Susp. Pt. *Rx.*
Use: Antihistamine, decongestant.

Tri-Otic. (Pharmics, Inc.) Chloroxylenol 1 mg, pramoxine HCl 10 mg, hydrocortisone 10 mg/ml. Drops. Vial 10 ml. *Rx.*
Use: Otic.

trioxane.
See: Trioxymethylene (Various Mfr.).

•**trioxifene mesylate.** (TRY-OX-ih-feen) USAN.
Use: Antiestrogen.

•**trioxsalen.** (TRI-OX-sale-en) U.S.P. 23.
Use: Pigmenting and phototherapeutic agent.
See: Trisoralen, Tab. (Zeneca Pharmaceuticals).

trioxymethylene. Name is incorrectly used to denote paraformaldehyde in some pharmaceuticals.
See: Paraformaldehyde (Various Mfr.).
W/Sodium oleate, triethanolamine, docusate sodium, stearic acid & aluminum silicate.
See: Cooper Creme (Whittaker).

Tri-Pain. (Ferndale Laboratories, Inc.) Acetaminophen 162 mg, aspirin 162 mg, salicylamide 162 mg, caffeine 16.2 mg/Tab. Bot. 100s. *otc.*
Use: Analgesic combination.

•**tripamide.** (TRIP-ah-mide) USAN.
Use: Antihypertensive, diuretic.

Tripedia. (Pasteur Merieux Connaught) Diphtheria 6.7 Lf units, tetanus 5 Lf units and acellular pertussis antigens 46.8 mcg/0.5 ml, aluminum potassium sulfate (alum), thimerosal, gelatin, polysorbate 80/Inj. Vial 7.5 ml. *Rx.*
Use: Immunization.

•**tripelennamine citrate.** (trih-pell-EN-au-meen SIH-trate) U.S.P. 23.
Use: Antihistamine.

•**tripelennamine hydrochloride.** (trih-pell-EN-au-meen) U.S.P. 23.
Use: Antihistamine.
See: PBZ, Prods. (Novartis Pharmaceutical Corp.).

Pyribenzamine Hydrochloride, Preps. (Novartis Pharmaceutical Corp.).

Triphasil-21. (Wyeth-Ayerst Laboratories) Three drug phases in 21-day cycle: **Phase I:** 6 brown tab. Levonorgestrel 0.05 mg, ethinyl estradiol 0.03 mg/Tab. **Phase II:** 5 white tab. Levonorgestrel 0.075 mg, ethinyl estradiol 0.04 mg/Tab. **Phase III:** 10 yellow tab. Levonorgestrel 0.125 mg, ethinyl estradiol 0.03 mg/Tab. *Rx.*
Use: Contraceptive.

Triphasil-28. (Wyeth-Ayerst Laboratories) Three drug phases and one inert phase in 28-day cycle: **Phase I:** 6 brown tab. Levonorgestrel 0.05 mg, ethinyl estradiol 0.03 mg/Tab. **Phase II:** 5 white tab. Levonorgestrel 0.075/mg, ethinyl estradiol 0.04 mg/Tab. **Phase III:** 10 yellow tab. Levonorgestrel 0.125 mg, ethinyl estradiol 0.03 mg/Tab. **Phase IV:** 7 inert green tablets. *Rx.*
Use: Contraceptive.

Tri-Phen-Chlor. (Rugby Labs, Inc.) Phenylpropanolamine HCl 20 mg, phenylephrine HCl 5 mg, chlorpheniramine maleate 2.5 mg, phenyltoloxamine citrate 7.5 mg/5ml Syr. Bot. 473 ml. *Rx.*
Use: Antihistamine, decongestant.

Tri-Phen-Chlor Tabs, Timed Released. (Rugby Labs, Inc.) Phenylpropanolamine HCl 40 mg, phenylephrine HCl 10 mg, chlorpheniramine maleate 5 mg, phenyltoloxamine citrate 15 mg. 100s. *Rx.*
Use: Antihistamine, decongestant.

Tri-Phen-Chlor Pediatric Drops. (Rugby Labs, Inc.) Phenylpropanolamine HCl 5 mg, phenylephrine HCl 1.25 mg, chlorpheniramine maleate 0.5 mg, phenyltoloxamine citrate 2 mg/ml. Bot. w/drop 30 ml. *Rx.*
Use: Antihistamine, decongestant.

Tri-Phen-Chlor Pediatric Syrup. (Rugby Labs, Inc.) Phenylpropanolamine HCl 5 mg, phenylephrine HCl 1.25 mg, chlorpheniramine maleate 0.5 mg, phenyltoloxamine citrate 2 mg/5 ml. Syr. Bot. 118 ml, 473 ml, gal. *Rx.*
Use: Antihistamine, decongestant.

Tri-Phen-Mine Pediatric Drops. (Zenith Goldline Pharmaceuticals) Phenylpropanolamine HCl 5 mg, phenylephrine HCl 1.25 mg, chlorpheniramine maleate 0.5 mg, phenyltoloxamine citrate 2 mg/ml. Drop. Bot. 30 ml. *Rx.*
Use: Antihistamine, decongestant.

Tri-Phen-Mine Pediatric Syrup. (Zenith Goldline Pharmaceuticals) Phenylpropanolamine HCl 5 mg, phenylephrine HCl 1.25 mg, chlorpheniramine maleate 0.5 mg, phenyltoloxamine citrate 2 mg/5 ml. Syr. Bot. 473 ml. *Rx.*
Use: Antihistamine, decongestant.

Tri-Phen-Mine S.R. (Zenith Goldline Pharmaceuticals) Chlorpheniramine maleate 5 mg, pyrilamine maleate 15 mg, phenylpropanolamine HCl 40 mg, phenylephrine HCl 10 mg/SR Tab. Bot. 100s. *Rx.*
Use: Antihistamine, decongestant.

Triphenyl. (Rugby Labs, Inc.) Phenylpropanolamine HCl 12.5 mg, Chlorpheniramine maleate 2 mg/5 ml, alcohol free. Syr. Bot. 118 ml. *otc.*
Use: Antihistamine, decongestant.

Triphenyl Expectorant. (Rugby Labs, Inc.) Phenylpropanolamine HCl 12.5 mg, guaifenesin 100 mg/5 ml, alcohol 5%. Expec. Bot. 120 ml, pt., gal. *otc.*
Use: Decongestant, expectorant.

triphenylmethane dyes.
See: Fuchsin.
Methylrosaniline Chloride.

Triphenyl T.D. (Rugby Labs, Inc.) Phenylpropanolamine HCl 50 mg, pyrilaminemaleate 25 mg, pheniramine maleate 25 mg/Tab. Bot. 100s, 1000s. *Rx.*
Use: Antihistamine, decongestant.

triphenyltetrazolium chloride. TTC.

tripiperazine dicititrate, hydrous.
See: Piperazine Citrate.

triple antibiotic ophthalmics. (Various Mfr.) Polymyxin B sulfate 10,000 units/g or ml, neomycin sulfate 3.5 mg/g or ml, bacitracin 400 units. Oint. 3.5 g. *Rx.*
Use: Anti-infective, ophthalmic.

triple barbiturate elixir. (CMC) Phenobarbital 0.25 g, butabarbital ⅛ g, pentobarbital g/5 ml. Bot. Pt., gal. *c-II.*
Use: Sedative.

Triple Dye. (Kerr Drug) Gentian violet, proflavine, hemisulfate, brilliant green in water. Dispensing Bot. 15 ml. Single-Use Dispos-A-Swab 0.65 ml. Box 10s. Case 10 x 50 Box.
Use: Antiseptic.

Triple Dye. (Xttrium Laboratories, Inc.) Brilliant green 2.29 mg, proflavine hemisulfate 1.14 mg, gentian violet 2.29 mg/ml. Bot. 30 ml.
Use: Disinfectant.

Triple-Gen Suspension. (Zenith Goldline Pharmaceuticals) Hydrocortisone 1%, neomycin sulfate 0.35%, polymyxin B sulfate 10,000 units/ml, benzalkonium chloride, cetyl alcohol, glyceryl monostearate, polyoxyl 40 stearate, propylene glycol, mineral oil. Bot. 7.5 ml. *Rx.*

Use: Anti-infective, corticosteroid, ophthalmic.

Triplen. (Henry Schein, Inc.) Tripelennamine HCl 50 mg/Tab. Bot. 100s, 1000s. *Rx.*
Use: Antihistamine.

triple sulfa tablets. (Century Pharmaceuticals, Inc.; Stanlabs) Sulfadiazine 2.5 g, sulfamerazine 2.5 g, sulfamethazine 2.5 g/Tab. Bot. 100s, 1000s. *Rx.*
Use: Anti-infective, sulfonamide.

•**triple sulfa vaginal cream.** U.S.P. 23.
Use: Anti-infective, vaginal.

triple sulfa vaginal tablets.
Use: Anti-infective, vaginal.

Triple Sulfoid. (Pal-Pak, Inc.) Sulfadiazine 167 mg, sulfamerazine 167 mg, sulfamethazine 167 mg/5 ml or Tab. **Liq.:** Bot. Pt., 2 oz. 12s. **Tab.:** Bot. 100s, 1000s. *Rx.*
Use: Anti-infective, sulfonamide.

triple sulfonamide. Dia-Mer-Thia Sulfonamides. Meth-Dia-Mer Sulfonamides.
Use: Anti-infective, sulfonamide.

Triple Vita. (Rosemont Pharmaceutical Corp.) Vitamins A 1500 IU, D 400 IU, C 35 mg/ml, alcohol free. Drops. Bot. 50 ml. *otc.*
Use: Vitamin supplement.

Triple Vita-Flor. (Rosemont Pharmaceutical Corp.) Fluoride 0.5 mg, vitamins A 1500 IU, D 400 IU, C 35 mg/ml, alcohol free. Drops. Bot. 50 ml. *Rx.*
Use: Dental caries agent, vitamin supplement.

Triple Vitamin ADC w/Fluoride. (Nilor Pharm) Fluoride 0.5 mg, vitamins A 1500 IU, D 400 IU, C 35 mg/ml. Drops. Bot. 50 ml. *Rx.*
Use: Mineral, vitamin supplement; dental caries agent.

Triple Vitamins w/Fluoride. (Major Pharmaceuticals) Vitamin A 2500 IU, D 400 IU, C 60 mg, fluoride 1 mg, dextrose, sucrose/Chew. Tab. Bot. 100s. *Rx.*
Use: Vitamin supplement; dental caries agent.

Triplevite w/Fluoride. (Geneva Pharmaceuticals) Fluoride 0.25 mg/ml, vitamins A 1500 IU, D 400 IU, C 35 mg, alcohol free. Drop. Bot. 50 ml. *Rx.*
Use: Dental caries agent; vitamin supplement.

Triplevite w/Fluoride. (Geneva Pharmaceuticals) Fluoride 0.5 mg/ml, vitamins A 1500 IU, D 400 IU, C 35 mg/ml, alcohol free, cherry flavor. Drop. Bot. 50 ml. *Rx.*
Use: Dental caries agent; vitamin supplement.

Triple X. (Durex) Pyrethrins 0.3%, piperonyl butoxide 3%, petroleum distillate 1.2%, benzyl alcohol 2.4%. Bot. 2 oz, 4 oz. *otc.*
Use: Pediculicide.

Tripodrine. (Schein Pharmaceutical, Inc.) Pseudoephedrine HCl 60 mg, triprolidine HCl 2.5 mg/Tab. Bot. 100s, UD 100s. *Rx.*
Use: Antihistamine, decongestant.

Tri-P Oral Infants Drops. (Cypress Pharm.) Phenylpropanolamine HCl 20 mg, pheniramine maleate 10 mg, pyrilamine maleate 10 mg/ml. Drops Bot. 15 ml w/calibrated dropper. *Rx.*
Use: Antihistamine, decongestant.

Triposed Syrup. (Halsey Drug Co.) Triprolidine HCl 1.25 mg, pseudoephedrine HCl 30 mg/5 ml. Bot. 120 ml, 240 ml, 473 ml, gal. *otc.*
Use: Antihistamine, decongestant.

Triposed Tablets. (Halsey Drug Co.) Triprolidine HCl 2.5 mg, pseudoephedrine HCl 60 mg/Tab. Bot. 100s, 1000s. *otc.*
Use: Antihistamine, decongestant.

tripotassium citrate. U.S.P. 23.
See: Potassium Citrate.

•**triprolidine hydrochloride.** (try-PRO-lih-deen) U.S.P. 23.
Use: Antihistamine.

triprolidine hydrochloride and pseudoephedrine hydrochloride syrup. (Various Mfr.) Triprolidine HCl 1.25 mg, pseudoephedrine HCl 30 mg/5 ml. Syr. Bot. 118 ml, 237 ml. *Rx.*
Use: Antihistamine, decongestant.
See: Actifed, Syr. (GlaxoWellcome).

triprolidine hydrochloride and pseudoephedrine hydrochloride tablets. U.S.P. 23.
Use: Antihistamine, decongestant.
See: Actifed, Tab. (GlaxoWellcome). Atridine, Tab. (Henry Schein, Inc.).

Triptifed. (Weeks & Leo) Triprolidine HCl 2.5 mg, pseudoephedrine HCl 60 mg/Tab. Bot. 36s, 100s. *Rx.*
Use: Antihistamine, decongestant.

Triptone Caplets. (Del Pharmaceuticals, Inc.) Dimenhydrinate 50 mg/Tab. Bot. 12s. *otc.*
Use: Antiemetic, antivertigo.

•**triptorelin.** (TRIP-toe-RELL-in) USAN.
Use: Antineoplastic.

triptorelin pamoate.
Use: Antineoplastic. [Orphan Drug]

trisaccharides a and b.
Use: Hemolytic disease of the newborn. [Orphan Drug]

trisodium citrate concentration.
Use: Leukapheresis procedures. [Orphan Drug]

Trisol. (Buffington) Borax, sodium Cl, boric acid. Irrig. Bot. oz, 4 oz. *otc.*
Use: Artificial tears.

Trisoralen. (Zeneca Pharmaceuticals) Trioxsalen 5 mg/Tab. Tartrazine. Bot. 28s, 100s. *Rx.*
Use: Dermatologic.

Tri-Statin. (Rugby Labs, Inc.) Triamcinolone acetonide 0.1%, neomycin sulfate 0.25%, gramicidin 0.25 mg, nystatin 100,000 units/g Cream. 15 g, 30 g, 60 g, 120 g, 480 g. *Rx.*
Use: Anti-infective; corticosteroid, topical.

Tri-Statin II. (Rugby Labs, Inc.) Triamcinolone acetonide 0.1%, 100,000 units nystatin per g, white petrolatum, parabens. Cream. Tube 15 g, 30 g, 60 g, 120 g, 480 g. *Rx.*
Use: Antifungal, corticosteroid, topical.

Tristoject. (Merz Pharmaceuticals) Triamcinolone diacetate 40 mg/ml. Vial 5 ml. *Rx.*
Use: Corticosteroid.

trisulfapyridmines.
Use: Anti-infective, sulfonamide.
See: Triple Sulfa No. 2 (Rugby Labs, Inc.).

•**trisulfapyrimidines oral suspension.** (try-SOLL-fah-peer-IH-mih-deenz) U.S.P. 23.
Use: Anti-infective.
See: Meth-Dia-Mer Sulfonamides (Various Mfr.).

Tritan. (Eon Labs Manufacturing, Inc.) Phenylephrine tannate 25 mg, chlorpheniramine tannate 8 mg, pyrilamine tannate 25 mg/Tab. Bot. 100s, 250s, 1000s. *Rx.*
Use: Antihistamine, decongestant.

Tritane. (Econo Med Pharmaceuticals) Brompheniramine maleate 2 mg, guaifenesin 100 mg, phenylephrine HCl 5 mg, phenylpropanolamine HCl 5 mg, alcohol 3.5%/5 ml. Bot. Gal. *Rx.*
Use: Antihistamine, decongestant, expectorant.

Tritane DC. (Econo Med Pharmaceuticals) Brompheniramine maleate 2 mg, guaifenesin 100 mg, phenylephrine HCl 5 mg, phenylpropanolamine HCl 5 mg, alcohol 3.5%, codeine phosphate 10 mg/5 ml. Bot. Gal. *c-v.*
Use: Antihistamine, antitussive, decongestant, expectorant.

Tri-Tannate. (Rugby Labs, Inc.) Phenylephrine tannate 25 mg, chlorpheniramine tannate 8 mg, pyrilamine tannate 25 mg. Tab. Bot. 100s, 250s. *Rx.*
Use: Antihistamine, decongestant.

Tri-Tannate Pediatric. (Rugby Labs, Inc.) Phenylephrine tannate 5 mg, chlorpheniramine tannate 2 mg, pyrilamine tannate 12.5 mg. Susp. Bot. 473 ml. *Rx.*
Use: Antihistamine, decongestant.

Tri-Tannate Plus Pediatric Suspension. (Rugby Labs, Inc.) Phenylephrine tannate 5 mg, ephedrine tannate 5 mg, chlorpheniramine tannate 4 mg, carbetapentane tannate 30 mg/5 ml. Bot. 480 ml. *Rx.*
Use: Antihistamine, antitussive, decongestant.

Tritec. (GlaxoWellcome) Ranitidine bismuth citrate 400 mg/Tab. Bot. 100s, UD 100s. *Rx.*
Use: In combination with clarithromycin to treat active duodenal ulcer associated with *H. pylori.*

•**tritiated water.** (TRISH-ee-at-ehd water) USAN.
Use: Radiopharmaceutical.

Tri-Tinic. (Vortech Pharmaceuticals) Liver desiccated 75 mg, stomach 75 mg, Vitamins B_{12} 15 mcg, Fe 110 mg, folic acid 1 mg, ascorbic acid 75 mg/Cap. Bot. 100s. *Rx.*
Use: Mineral, vitamin supplement.

Tritussin Cough Syrup. (Towne) Pyrilamine maleate 40 mg, pheniramine maleate 20 mg, citric acid 100 mg, codeine phosphate 58 mg/fl. oz. w/menthol and glycerin in flavored base. Bot. 4 oz. *c-v.*
Use: Antihistamine, antitussive, expectorant.

Triurisul. (Sheryl) Sulfacetamide 250 mg, sulfamethizole 250 mg, phenazopyridine HCl 50 mg/Tab. Bot. 100s. *Rx.*
Use: Analgesic; anti-infective, urinary.

Tri-Vert. (T.E. Williams Pharmaceuticals) Dimenhydrinate 25 mg, niacin 50 mg, pentylenetetrazol 25 mg/Cap. Bot. 100s. *otc.*
Use: Motion sickness.

Tri-Vi-Flor 0.25 mg Drops. (Bristol-Myers Squibb) Fluoride 0.25 mg, vitamins A 1500 IU, D 400 IU, C 35 mg/1 ml Drop. Bot. 50 ml. *Rx.*
Use: Dental caries agent; nutritional supplement.

Tri-Vi-Flor 0.25 mg with Iron Drops. (Bristol-Myers Squibb) Fluoride 0.25 mg, vitamins A 1500 IU, D 400 IU, C 35 mg, Fe 10 mg/1 ml Drop. Bot. 50 ml. *Rx.*
Use: Dental caries agent; nutritional supplement.

Tri-Vi-Flor 0.5 mg Drops. (Bristol-Myers Squibb) Fluoride 0.5 mg, vitamins A 1500 IU, D 400 IU, C 35 mg/ml. Bot. 50 ml. *Rx.*

Use: Dental caries agent; nutritional supplement.

Tri-Vi-Flor 1.0 mg Tablets. (Bristol-Myers Squibb) Fluoride 1 mg, vitamins A 2500 IU, D 400 IU, C 60 mg, sucrose/ Tab. Bot. 100s, 1000s. *Rx.*
Use: Dental caries agent; nutritional supplement.

Tri-Vi-Sol Drops. (Bristol-Myers Squibb) Vitamin A 1500 IU, D 400 IU, C 35 mg/ 1 ml Drops. Bot. 50 ml with calibrated safety-dropper. *otc.*
Use: Vitamin supplement.

Tri-Vi-Sol with Iron Drops. (Bristol-Myers Squibb) Vitamins A 1500 IU, C 35 mg, D 400 IU, Fe 10 mg/ml. Bot. 50 ml. *otc.*
Use: Mineral, vitamin supplement.

Trivitamin Fluoride. (Schein Pharmaceutical, Inc.) **Drops:** Fluoride 0.25 mg or 0.5 mg, vitamins A 1500 IU, D 400 IU, C 35 mg/ml. Bot. 50 ml. **Chew. Tab.:** Fluoride 0.5 mg, vitamins A 2500 IU, D 400 IU, C 60 mg, sucrose. Bot. 100s. *Rx.*
Use: Fluoride, vitamin supplement; dental caries agent.

Tri-Vitamin with Fluoride. (Rugby Labs, Inc.) Fluoride 0.5 mg, Vitamins A 1500 IU, D 400 IU, C 35 mg/ml Drops. Bot. 50 ml. *Rx.*
Use: Mineral, vitamin supplement.

Tri Vit w/Fluoride 0.25 mg. (Alpharma USPD Inc.) Fluoride 0.25 mg, vitamins A 1500 IU, D 400 IU, C 35 mg/ml. Drops. Bot. 50 ml. *Rx.*
Use: Mineral, vitamin supplement; dental caries agent.

Tri Vit w/Fluoride 0.5 mg. (Alpharma USPD Inc.) Fluoride 0.5 mg, vitamins A 1500 IU, D 400 IU, C 35 mg/ml. Drops. Bot. 50 ml. *Rx.*
Use: Mineral, vitamin supplement; dental caries agent.

Tri-Vite. (Foy Laboratories) Thiamine HCl 100 mg, pyridoxine HCl 100 mg, cyanocobalamin 1000 mcg/ml. Vial 10 ml. *Rx.*
Use: Vitamin supplement.

Trobicin. (Pharmacia & Upjohn) Spectinomycin HCl 400 mg/ml when reconstituted. Pow. for Inj. Vial 2 g w/diluent 3.2 ml. *Rx.*
Use: Anti-infective.

Trocaine. (Roberts Pharmaceuticals) Benzocaine 10 mg. Loz. UD 4s, 500s. *otc.*
Use: Dietary aid.

Trocal. (Roberts Pharmaceuticals) Dextromethorphan HBr 7.5 mg, guaifenesin 50 mg/Loz. 500s. *otc.*
Use: Antitussive, expectorant.

•**troclosene potassium.** (TROE-kloe-seen) USAN.
Use: Anti-infective, topical.

•**troglitazone.** (TROE-glih-tazz-ohn) USAN.
Use: Antidiabetic.
See: Rezulin, Tab. (Parke-Davis).

•**trolamine.** (TROLE-ah-meen) N.F. 18. *Formerly Triethanolamine.*
Use: Pharmaceutic aid (alkalizing agent), analgesic.
See: Ortho-iodobenzoic.

•**troleandomycin.** (troe-lee-AN-doe-MY-sin) U.S.P. 23. *Formerly Triacetyloleandomycin.*
Use: Anti-infective.
See: Tao (Pfizer).

tromal.
Use: Analgesic, antidepressant agent.

•**tromethamine.** (TROE-meth-ah-meen) U.S.P. 23.
Use: Alkalizer.
W/Combinations.
See: Prohance (Bracco Diagnostics).
Ultravist (Berlex).

Tronolane Cream. (Ross Laboratories) Pramoxine HCl 1% in cream base. Tubes 30 g, 60 g. *otc.*
Use: Anorectal preparation.

Tronolane Suppositories. (Ross Laboratories) Zinc oxide 11%, hard fat 95%. Pkg. 10s, 20s. *otc.*
Use: Anorectal preparation.

Tronothane HCl. (Abbott Laboratories) Pramoxine HCl 1%, cetyl alcohol, glycerin, parabens. Cream. 28.4 g. *otc.*
Use: Anesthetic, local.

Tropamine+. (NeuroGenesis/Matrix Tech., Inc.) Vitamins D 250 mg, l-phenylalanine, l-tyrosine 150 mg, l-glutamine 50 mg, B_1 1.67 mg, B_2 2.5 mg, B_3 16.7 mg, B_5 15 mg, B_6 3.3 mg, B_{12} 5 mcg, folic acid 0.067 mg, C 100 mg, Ca 25 mg, Cr 0.01 mg, Fe 1.5 mg, Mg 25 mg, Zn 5 mg, yeast and preservative free. Cap. Bot. 42s, 180s. *otc.*
Use: Nutritional supplement.

•**tropanserin hydrochloride.** (trope-ANE-ser-IN) USAN.
Use: Seratonin receptor antagonist (specific in migraine).

TrophAmine Injection. (McGaw, Inc.) Nitrogen 4.65 g, amino acids 30 g, protein 29 g/500 ml. Bot. 500 ml IV infusion. *otc.*
Use: Nutritional supplement.

Troph-Iron. (SmithKline Beecham Pharmaceuticals) Vitamins B_{12} 25 mcg, B_1 10 mg, Fe 20 mg/5 ml. Saccharin. Bot. 4

fl. oz. *otc.*
Use: Mineral, vitamin supplement.

Trophite (Iron). (Menley & James Labs, Inc.) Fe 60 mg, B_1 30 mg, B_{12} 75 mcg. Liq. Bot. 120 ml. *otc.*
Use: Mineral, vitamin supplement.

Tropicacyl. (Akorn, Inc.) Tropicamide solution 0.5%. 15 ml. 1% tropicamide. 2 ml, 15 ml. *Rx.*
Use: Cycloplegic, mydriatic.

Tropical Blend. (Schering-Plough Corp.) A series of products is marketed under the Tropical Blend name including: Hawaii Blend Oil SPF 2 (Bot. 8 oz.); Hawaii Blend Lotion SPF 2 (Bot. 8 oz.); Rio Blend Oil SPF 2 (Bot. 8 oz.); Rio Blend Lotion SPF 2 (Bot. 8 oz.); Jamaica Blend Oil SPF 2 (Bot. 8 oz.); Jamaica Blend Lotion SPF 2 (Bot. 8 oz.). All contain homosalate in various oil and lotion bases. *otc.*
Use: Sunscreen.

Tropical Blend Dark Tanning. (Schering-Plough Corp.) **SPF 2:** Homosalate. **Oil:** Bot. 180 ml, 240 ml. **Lot.:** Bot. 240 ml. **SPF 4:** Ethylhexyl p-methoxycinnamate, oxybenzone. Bot. 240 ml. **Oil:** Padimate O, oxybenzone. Bot. 240 ml. *otc.*
Use: Sunscreen.

Tropical Blend Dry Oil. (Schering-Plough Corp.) Homosalate, oxybenzone. Oil Bot. 180 ml. *otc.*
Use: Sunscreen.

Tropical Blend Tan Magnifier. (Schering-Plough Corp.) Triethanolamine salicylate. Oil Bot. 240 ml. *otc.*
Use: Sunscreen.

Tropical Gold Dark Tanning Lotion. (Zenith Goldline Pharmaceuticals) SPF 4. Ethylhexyl p-methoxycinnamate, oxybenzone, benzyl alcohol, parabens, aloe extract, jojoba oil, vitamin E, EDTA. PABA free. Waterproof. Lot. Bot. 240 ml. *otc.*
Use: Sunscreen.

Tropical Gold Dark Tanning Oil. (Zenith Goldline Pharmaceuticals) SPF 2. Ethylhexyl p-methoxycinnamate, octyldimethyl PABA, mineral oil, coconut oil, cocoa butter, aloe, lanolin, eucalyptus oil, oils of plumeria, manako (mango), kuawa (guava), mikara (papaya), liliko (passion fruit), taro, kukui. Oil. Bot. 240 ml. *otc.*
Use: Sunscreen.

Tropical Gold Sport Sunblock. (Zenith Goldline Pharmaceuticals) SPF 15. Ethylhexyl p-methoxycinnamate, oxybenzone, diazolidinyl urea, parabens, aloe extract, jojoba oil, vitamin E, EDTA. PABA free. Perspiration-proof. Lot. Bot. 180 ml. *otc.*
Use: Sunblock.

Tropical Gold Sunblock. (Zenith Goldline Pharmaceuticals) **SPF 15:** Ethylhexyl p-methoxycinnamate, oxybenzone, vegetable oil, benzyl alcohol, parabens, imidazolidinyl urea, vitamin E, aloe extract, jojoba oil, EDTA. PABA free. Waterproof. Lot. Bot. 118 ml. **SPF 17:** Ethylhexyl p-methoxycinnamate, 2-ethylhexyl salicylate, homosalate, oxybenzone, aloe extract, vitamin E, vegetable and jojoba oils, benzyl alcohol, imidazolidinyl urea, parabens, EDTA. PAPA free. Waterproof. Lot. Bot. 118 ml. **SPF 30:** Ethylhexyl p-methoxycinnamate, 2-ethylhexyl salicylate, homosalate, oxybenzone, aloe extract, vitamin E, vegetable and jojoba oils, benzyl alcohol, imidizolidinyl urea, parabens, EDTA. PABA free. Waterproof. 118 ml. *otc.*
Use: Sunblock.

Tropical Gold Sunscreen. (Zenith Goldline Pharmaceuticals) SPF 8. Ethylhexyl p-methoxycinnamate, oxybenzone, benzyl alcohol, parabens, aloe extract, jojoba oil, vitamin E, EDTA. PABA free. Waterproof. Lot. Bot. 118 ml. *otc.*
Use: Sunscreen.

•**tropicamide.** (TROP-ik-ah-mid) U.S.P. 23.
Use: Anticholinergic (ophthalmic).
See: Mydriacyl, Drops. (Alcon Laboratories, Inc.).
Opticyl, Soln. (Optopics Laboratories, Corp.).
Tropicacyl, Soln. (Akorn, Inc.).

tropicamide. (Various Mfr.) 0.5%, 1%. Soln. Bot. 2 ml (0.5%), 15 ml.
Use: Anticholinergic (ophthalmic).

tropine benzohydryl ester methanesulfonate. Also named benztropine methane-sulfonate.

•**trospectomycin sulfate.** (TROE-speck-toe-MY-sin) USAN.
Use: Anti-infective.

•**trovafloxacin mesylate.** (TROE-vah-FLOX-ah-sin) USAN.
Use: Anti-infective.
See: Trovan, Tab. (Pfizer US Pharmaceutical Group).

Trovan. (Pfizer US Pharmaceutical Group) Trovafloxacin mesylate 100 mg, 200 mg. Tab. UD 40s. Alatrofloxacin mesylate 5 mg/ml. Inj. Vial. 40 mg (200 dose), 60 ml (300 dose). *Rx.*
Use: Anti-infective.

Trovit. (Sigma-Tau Pharmaceuticals, Inc.) Vitamins B_2 0.3 mg, B_6 1 mg, choline Cl 25 mg, panthenol 2 mg, dl-methionine 10 mg, inositol 20 mg, niacinamide 50 mg, vitamins B_{12} 10 mcg/ml. Vial 30 ml. *Rx.*
Use: Vitamin B supplement.

T.R.U.E. Test. (GlaxoWellcome) Allergens include nickel sulfate, wool alcohols (lanolin), neomycin sulfate, potassium dichromate (chromium), caine mix (benzocaine, dibucaine, tetracaine), fragrance mix, colophony, epoxyresin, quinoline mix, balsam peru, ethylenediamine, cobalt, p-tert-butylphenol formaldehyde, paraben mix, carba mix, black rubber mix, chloromethyl isothiazolinone, Quaternium 15, mercaptobenzothiazole, p-phenylenediamine, formaldehyde, mercaptomix, thimerosal and thiuram mix. Test in multipak cartons (5s). *Rx.*
Use: Diagnostic aid, allergic.

Truphylline. (G & W Laboratories) Aminophylline 250 mg/Supp. (equiv. to theophylline 198 mg) In UD 10s, 25s. *Rx.*
Use: Bronchodilator.

Trusopt. (Merck & Co.) Dorzolamide 2%. Soln. Bot. 5 ml, 10 ml. *Rx.*
Use: Antiglaucoma.

Trynisin Cold Syrup. (Halsey Drug Co.) Bot. 4 oz., 8 oz.
Use: Antihistamine.

•**trypsin, crystallized.** (TRIP-sin) U.S.P. 23.
Use: Proteolytic enzyme.
W/Castor oil.
See: Granulex (Dow B. Hickam).

tryptizol hydrochloride. U.S.P. 23. Amitriptyline HCl.

•**tryptophan.** (TRIP-toe-FAN) U.S.P. 23.
Use: Amino acid.

Trysul. (Savage Laboratories) Sulfathiazole 3.42%, sulfacetamide 2.86%, sulfabenzamide 3.7%, urea 0.64%. Tube 78 g. *Rx*
Use: Anti-infective, vaginal.

T/Scalp. (Neutrogena) Hydrocortisone 1%. Liq. Greaseless. Bot. 60 ml, 105 ml. *otc.*
Use: Antipruritic, corticosteroid, topical.

T-Serp Tablet. (Tennessee Pharmaceutic) Reserpine alkaloid 0.25 mg/Tab. Bot. 100s, 1000s. *Rx.*
Use: Antihypertensive.

TSPA.
Use: Antineoplastic.
See: Thiotepa (ESI Lederle Generics).

T-Stat. (Westwood Squibb Pharmaceuticals) Erythromycin 2% w/alcohol 71.2%. Bot. 60 ml; Pads, disposable premoistened 60s. *Rx.*
Use: Dermatologic, acne.

TTC. Triphenyltetrazolium Chloride.

tuaminoheptane sulfate. U.S.P. 23.
Use: Adrenergic.

•**tuberculin.** (too-BURR-kyoo-lin) U.S.P. 23.
Use: Diagnostic aid (dermal reactivity indicator).
See: Aplisol (Parke-Davis).
Aplitest (Parke-Davis).
Tubersol (Pasteur Merieux Connaught).

Tuberculin, Mono-Vacc Test. (Lincoln Diagnostics) Mono-Vacc test is a sterile, disposable multiple puncture scarifier with liquid Old Tuberculin on the points. Box 25 tests.
Use: Diagnostic aid.

Tuberculin, Old Monovacc Test. (ESI Lederle Generics) 5 TU activity test. Soln. of Old Tuberculin containing acacia 7%, lactose 8.5%. Test. Kits 25s, 100s, 250s.
Use: Diagnostic aid.

Tuberculin, Old, Tine Test. (ESI Lederle Generics) 5 TY activity per test. Soln. of Old Tuberculin, containing acacia 7%, lactose 8.5%. Test. Kits 25s, 100s, 250s.
Use: Diagnostic aid.

tuberculin purified protein derivative. (Bristol-Myers Squibb; Pasteur Merieux Connaught) Concentrated solution for multiple puncture testing. Vial 1 ml.
Use: Diagnostic aid, tuberculosis.

tuberculin tests.
Use: Diagnostic aid.
See: Aplisol (Parke-Davis).
Aplitest (Parke-Davis).
Tine Test PPD (ESI Lederle Generics).
Tuberculin, Old Mono Vacc Test (Pasteur Merieux Connaught).
Tuberculin, Old, Tine Test (ESI Lederle Generics).
Tubersol (Bristol-Myers Squibb; Pasteur Merieux Connaught).

tuberculin tine test. (ESI Lederle Generics) **Old Tuberculin (OT):** Each disposable test unit consists of a stainless steel disc, with four tines (or prongs) 2 millimeters long, attached to a plastic handle. The tines have been dip-dried with antigenic material. The entire unit is sterilized by ethylene oxide gas. The test has been standardized by comparative studies, utilizing 0.05 mg US Standard Old Tuberculin 5 IU or

0.0001 mg US Standard 5 IU by the Mantoux technique. Reliability appears to be comparable to the standard Mantoux. Tests in a jar 25s. Package 100s. Bin Package 250s. **Purified Protein Derivative (PPD):** Equivalent to or more potent than 5 TU PPD Mantoux test. Tests in a jar 25s. Package 100s.
Use: Diagnostic aid.

tuberculosis vaccine.
Use: Immunization.
See: TICE BCG (Organon Teknika Corp.).

Tuberlate. (Heun) Sodium p-aminosalicylate 12 g, succinic acid 4 gr/Tab. Bot. 500s.
Use: Antituberculosis.

Tubersol. (Pasteur Merieux Connaught) Tuberculin purified protein derivative (Mantoux) 1 TU/0.1 ml: Vial 1 ml. 5 TU/0.1 ml: Vial 1 ml, 5 ml. 250 TU/0.1 ml: Vial 1 ml.
Use: Diagnostic aid, tuberculosis.

Tubex. (Wyeth-Ayerst Laboratories) The following drugs are available in various Tubex sizes: Ativan, Bicillin C-R, Bicillin C-R 900/300, Bicillin Long-Acting, Codeine Phosphate, Cyanocobalamin, Digoxin, Dimenhydrinate, Diphenhydramine HCl, Diphtheria and Tetanus Toxoids Adsorbed (Pediatric Pharmaceuticals), Epinephrine, Furosemide, Heparin Flush Kits, Heparin Lock Flush, Heparin Sodium Solution, Hydromorphone HCl, Hydroxyzine HCl, Influenza Virus Vaccine, Trivalent, Mepergan, Meperidine HCl, Morphine Sulfate, Naloxone Injection, Naloxone Injection, Neonatal, Oxytocin, Pentobarbital Sodium, Phenergan, Phenobarbital Sodium, Prochlorperazine Edisylate, Secobarbital Sodium, Sodium Chloride, Bacteriostatic, Tetanus and Diphtheria Toxoids Adsorbed, Adult, Tetanus Immune Globulin, Human, Tetanus Toxoid Alum Phos Ad.; Tetanus Toxoid, Fluid; Thiamine Hydrochloride; Wycillin.

•**tubocurarine chloride.** (too-boe-cure-AHR-een) U.S.P. 23.
Use: Neuromuscular blocker.

tubocurarine chloride. (Eli Lilly and Co.) 3 mg/ml. Amp. 10 ml. (Abbott Laboratories) 3 mg/ml in 10 ml fliptop vials; 15 mg in 5 ml Abboject Syringe.
Use: Neuromuscular blocker.

tubocurarine chloride, dimethyl. Dimethylether of d-tubocurarine chloride.

tubocurarine chloride hydrochloride pentahydrate. Tubocurarine Chloride, U.S.P. 23.

tubocurarine iodide, dimethyl. Dimethyl ether of d-tubocurarine iodide.
Use: Muscle relaxant.
See: Metubine, Vial (Eli Lilly and Co.).

•**tubulozole hydrochloride.** (too-BYOO-lah-ZAHL) USAN.
Use: Antineoplastic (microtubule inhibitor).

Tucks. (Parke-Davis) Pads saturated with solution of witch hazel 50%, glycerin 10%, benzalkonium Cl 0.003%. Jar 40s, 100s. *otc.*
Use: Dermatologic, proctologic.

Tucks Clear Gel. (GlaxoWellcome) Hamamelis water 50%, glycerin 10%, benzyl alcohol, EDTA. Gel. Tube 19.8 g. *otc.*
Use: Anorectal preparation.

Tucks Take-Alongs. (Parke-Davis) Nonwoven wipes saturated with solution of witch hazel 50%, glycerine 10%, benzalkonium chloride 0.003%. Box 12s. *otc.*
Use: Anorectal preparation.

Tuinal. (Eli Lilly and Co.) Equal parts Seconal Sod. & Amytal Sod. Pulvule **100 mg:** Bot. 100s. **200 mg:** Bot. 100s. *c-II.*
Use: Hypnotic, sedative.

tumor necrosis factor-binding protein I and II. Serono Laboratories, Inc. *Rx.*
Use: Treatment of AIDS. [Orphan Drug]

Tums. (SmithKline Beecham Pharmaceuticals) Calcium carbonate 500 mg/Tab. Available in peppermint and assorted flavors in various package sizes. Rolls of 12 singles, 3-roll wraps. Bot. 75s, 150s. *otc.*
Use: Antacid.

Tums 500. (SmithKline Beecham Pharmaceuticals) Calcium carbonate 1250 mg (500 mg calcium), sucrose, Na < 4 mg. Chew. Tab. Bot. 60s. *otc.*
Use: Antacid.

Tums E-X Extra Strength. (SmithKline Beecham Pharmaceuticals) Calcium carbonate 750 mg, wintergreen or fruit flavors. Chew. Tab. 12s, 48s, 96s. *otc.*
Use: Antacid.

Tums Plus. (SmithKline Beecham Pharmaceuticals) Calcium carbonate 500 mg, (elemental calcium 200 mg), simethicone 20 mg, sucrose, sodium ≤ mg, assorted fruit and mint flavors. Chew. Tab. Bot. 48s. *otc.*
Use: Antacid.

Tur-Bi-Kal Nasal Drops. (Emerson Laboratories) Phenylephrine HCl in a saline solution. Dropper Bot. oz., 12s. *otc.*
Use: Decongestant.

Turbilixir. (Burlington) Chlorpheniramine maleate 2 mg, phenylephrine HCl 5 mg, phenylpropanolamine HCl 5 mg/5 ml. Bot. Pt, gal. *otc.*
Use: Antihistamine, decongestant.

Turbinaire.
See: Decadron Phosphate, Preps. (Merck & Co.).

Turbinaire Decadron Phosphate. (Merck & Co.) Each metered spray delivers dexamethasone sodium phosphate equivalent to dexamethasone ≈ 84 mcg (170 sprays per cartridge), alcohol 2%. Aerosol. 12.6 g w/adapter or 12.6 g refill. *Rx.*
Use: Corticosteroid, topical.

Turbispan Leisurecaps. (Burlington) Chlorpheniramine maleate 12 mg, phenylephrine HCl 15 mg, phenylpropanolamine HCl 15 mg/SR Cap. Bot. 30s. *otc.*
Use: Antihistamine, decongestant.

Turgasept Aerosol. (Wyeth-Ayerst Laboratories) Ethyl alcohol 44.25%, essential oils 0.9%, n-alkyl (50% C-4, 40% C-12, 10% C-16) dimethyl benzyl ammonium Cl 0.33%, o-phenylphenol 0.25% w/propellant. Spray can 11.5 oz. in bouquet, fresh lemon, leather, citrus blossom scents.
Use: Deodorizer, disinfectant.

turpentine oil w/combinations.
See: Sloan's Liniment, Liq. (Warner Lambert).

Tusibron. (Kenwood Laboratories) Guaifenesin 100 mg/5 ml. 3.5% alcohol. Liq. Bot. 118 ml. *otc.*
Use: Expectorant.

Tusibron-DM. (Kenwood Laboratories) Guaifenesin 100 mg, dextromethorphan 15 mg/5 ml. Liq. Bot. 118 ml. *otc.*
Use: Antitussive, expectorant.

tusilan. Dextromethorphan HBr.

Tusquelin. (Circle Pharmaceuticals, Inc) Dextromethorphan HBr 15 g, chlorpheniramine maleate 2 mg, phenylpropanolamine 5 mg, phenylephrine HCl 5 mg, fl. ext. ipecac 0.17 min., potassium guaiacolsulfonate 44 mg/5 ml. Alcohol 5%. Syr. Pt. *Rx.*
Use: Antihistamine, antitussive, decongestant, expectorant.

Tussabar. (Tennessee Pharmaceutic) Acetaminophen 400 mg, salicylamide 500 mg, potassium guaiacolsulfonate 120 mg, pyrilamine maleate 30 mg, ammonium chloride 500 mg, sodium citrate 500 mg, phenylephrine HCl 30 mg/oz. Bot. Pt., gal. *Rx.*
Use: Analgesic, antihistamine, decongestant, expectorant.

Tussabid. (ION Laboratories, Inc.) Guaifenesin 200 mg, dextromethorphan HBr 30 mg/Cap. Bot. 24s, 100s. *otc.*
Use: Antihistamine, expectorant.

Tussafed Drops. (Everett Laboratories, Inc.) Carbinoxamine maleate 2 mg, pseudoephedrine HCl 25 mg, dextromethorphan HBr 4 mg/ml. Bot. 30 ml with calibrated dropper. *Rx.*
Use: Antihistamine, antitussive, decongestant.

Tussafed HC. (Everett Laboratories) Hydrocodone bitartrate 2.5 mg, phenylephrine HCl 7.5 mg, guaifenesin 50 mg/5 ml. Syr. Bot. 473 ml. *c-III.*
Use: Decongestant, antitussive, expectorant.

Tussafed Syrup. (Everett Laboratories, Inc.) Dextromethorphan HBr 15 mg, pseudoephedrine HCl 60 mg, carbinoxamine maleate 4 mg/5 ml. Bot. 4 oz., 16 oz. *Rx.*
Use: Antihistamine, antitussive, decongestant.

Tussahist. (Defco) Codeine phosphate 10 mg, phenylpropanolamine HCl 12.5 mg, chlorpheniramine maleate 2 mg, pyrilamine maleate 7.5 mg, guaifenesin 100 mg/5 ml. Bot. 4 oz. Pt, gal. *c-v.*
Use: Antihistamine, antitussive, decongestant, expectorant.

Tuss-Allergine Modified T.D. (Rugby Labs, Inc.) Phenylpropanolamine HCl 75 mg, caramiphen edisylate 40 mg/TR Cap. Bot. 100s. *Rx.*
Use: Antitussive, decongestant.

Tussafin Expectorant Liquid. (Rugby Labs, Inc.) Pseudoephedrine HCl 60 mg, hydrocodone bitartrate 5 mg, guaifenesin 200 mg/5 ml, alcohol 2.5%. Bot. 480 ml. *c-III.*
Use: Antitussive, decongestant, expectorant.

Tussanil DH. (Misemer Pharmaceuticals, Inc.) Phenylpropanolamine HCl 25 mg, guaifenesin 100 mg, hydrocodone bitartrate 1.66 mg, salicylamide 300 g/ Tab. In 100s. *c-III.*
Use: Analgesic, antitussive, decongestant, expectorant.

Tussanil DH Syrup. (Misemer Pharmaceuticals, Inc.) Phenylephrine HCl 10 mg, chlorpheniramine maleate 4 mg, hydrocodone bitartrate 2.5 mg/5 ml w/ alcohol 5%. Bot. Pt. *c-III.*
Use: Antihistamine, antitussive, decongestant.

Tussanil Expectorant Syrup. (Misemer Pharmaceuticals, Inc.) Hydrocodone bitartrate 2.5 mg, phenylephrine HCl 10 mg, guaifenesin 100 mg/5 ml w/alco-

hol 5%. Bot. Pt. *c-III.*
Use: Antitussive, decongestant, expectorant.

Tussanol. (Tyler) Pyrilamine maleate ¾ g, codeine phosphate 1 g, ammonium chloride 7.5 g, sodium citrate 5 g, menthol g/fl. oz. Bot. 4 fl. oz, pt, gal. *c-V.*
Use: Antihistamine, antitussive, expectorant.

Tussanol with Ephedrine. (Tyler) Ephedrine sulfate 2 g, pyrilamine maleate ¾ g, codeine phosphate 1 g, ammonium chloride 7.5 g, sodium citrate 5 g, menthol g/30 ml. Bot. 16 fl. oz. *c-V.*
Use: Bronchodilator, antihistamine, antitussive, expectorant.

Tussar-2 Syrup. (Rhone-Poulenc Rorer Pharmaceuticals, Inc.) Codeine phosphate 10 mg, guaifenesin 100 mg, pseudoephedrine HCl 30 mg/5 ml, alcohol 2.5%. Bot. 473 ml. *c-V.*
Use: Antitussive, expectorant, decongestant.

Tussar DM. (Rhone-Poulenc Rorer Pharmaceuticals, Inc.) Dextromethorphan HBr 15 mg, chlorpheniramine maleate 2 mg, phenylephrine HCl 5 mg/5 ml w/ methylparaben 0.1% Bot. 4 oz., pt. *Rx.*
Use: Antihistamine, antitussive, expectorant.

Tussar SF. (Rhone-Poulenc Rorer Pharmaceuticals, Inc.) Codeine phosphate 10 mg, guaifenesin 100 mg, pseudoephedrine HCl 30 mg/5 ml, alcohol 2.5%. Bot. 120 ml, 473 ml. *c-V.*
Use: Antitussive, decongestant, expectorant.

Tuss-DM. (Hyrex Pharmaceuticals) Dextromethorphan HBr (10 mg), guaifenesin 200 mg, dye free. Tab. Bot. 100s, 1000s. *Rx.*
Use: Antitussive, expectorant.

Tussend. (Monarch Pharmaceuticals) Hydrocodone bitartrate 2.5 mg, pseudoephredrine HCl 30 mg, chlorpheniramine maleate 2 mg/5 ml. 5% alcohol. Syr. Bot. 480 ml. *c-III.*
Use: Antitussive, expectorant combination.

Tussex Cough. (Various Mfr.) Phenylephrine HCl 5 mg, dextromethorphan HBr 10 mg, guaifenesin 100 mg/5 ml Syr. Bot. 120 ml, gal. *Rx.*
Use: Antitussive, decongestant, expectorant.

Tuss-Genade Modified Caps. (Zenith Goldline Pharmaceuticals) Phenylpropanolamine HCl 75 mg, caramiphen edisylate 40 mg. Bot. 100s, 1000s. *Rx.*
Use: Antitussive, decongestant.

Tussgen Expectorant. (Zenith Goldline Pharmaceuticals) Bot. Pt, gal.
Use: Expectorant.

Tussgen Liquid. (Zenith Goldline Pharmaceuticals) Pseudoephedrine HCl 60 mg, hydrocodone bitartrate 5 mg/5 ml. Bot. 100s, 1000s. *c-III.*
Use: Antitussive, decongestant.

Tussi-12. (Wallace Laboratories) Carbetapentane tannate 30 mg, chlorpheniramine tannate 4 mg, phenylephrine tannate 5 mg/ml, glycerin, methylparaben, saccharin, sucrose. Susp. Bot. Pt. *Rx.*
Use: Antihistamine, antitussive, decongestant.

Tussidram. (Dram) Dextromethorphan 10 mg, phenylpropanolamine 12.5 mg, guaifenesin 50 mg, chlorpheniramine maleate 2 mg/5 ml. Bot. Pt. *Rx.*
Use: Antihistamine, antitussive, decongestant, expectorant.

Tussigon. (Jones Medical Industries, Inc.) Hydrocodone bitartrate 5 mg, homatropine methylbromide 1.5 mg/ Tab. Bot. 100s, 500s. *c-III.*
Use: Anticholinergic, antispasmodic, antitussive.

Tussionex. (Medeva Pharmaceuticals, Inc.) Hydrocodone (as polistirex) 10 mg, chlorpheniramine 8 mg. Liq. Bot. 473 ml, 900 ml. *c-III.*
Use: Antihistamine, antitussive.

Tussi-Organidin DM NR. (Wallace Laboratories) Dextromethorphan HBr 10 mg, guaifenesin 100 mg/5 ml. Saccharin, sorbitol. Liq. Bot. 120 ml, pt, gal. *Rx.*
Use: Antitussive, expectorant.

Tussi-Organidin DM-S NR. (Wallace Laboratories) Guaifenesin 100 mg, dextromethorphan HBr 10 mg/5 ml, saccharin, sorbitol. Liq. Sample 30 ml, Unit-of-use cont. 120 ml w/ oral syringe. *Rx.*
Use: Antitussive, expectorant.

Tussi-Organidin NR. (Wallace Laboratories) Codeine phosphate 10 mg, guaifenesin 100 mg/5 ml, saccharin, sorbitol. Liq. Bot. 120 ml, pt, gal. *c-V.*
Use: Antitussive, expectorant.

Tussi-Organidin-S NR. (Wallace Laboratories) Codeine phosphate 10 mg, guaifenesin 100 mg/5 ml, saccharin, sorbitol. Liq. Sample, 30 ml, Unit-of-use cont. 120 ml w/ 10 ml oral syringe. *c-V.*
Use: Antitussive, expectorant.

Tussirex. (Scot-Tussin Pharmacal, Inc.) Phenylephrine HCl 4.2 mg, pheniramine maleate 13.3 mg, codeine phosphate 10 mg, sodium citrate 83.3 mg, sodium salicylate 83.3 mg, caffeine

citrate 25 mg/5 ml. Syr. Bot. 120 ml, 240 ml, pt, gal. *c-v.*
Use: Antihistamine, antitussive, decongestant, expectorant.

Tussirex Sugar Free Liquid. (Scot-Tussin Pharmacal, Inc.) Codeine phosphate 10 mg, pheniramine maleate 13.33 mg, phenylephrine HCl 4.17 mg, sodium citrate 83.33 mg, sodium salicylate 83.33 mg, caffeine citrate 25 mg/5 ml. Bot. 120 ml, pt. gal. *c-v.*
Use: Analgesic, antihistamine, antitussive, decongestant, expectorant.

Tuss-LA. (Hyrex Pharmaceuticals) Pseudoephedrine HCl 120 mg, guaifenesin 500 mg/LA Tab. Bot. 100s. *Rx.*
Use: Decongestant, expectorant.

Tusso-DM. (Everett Laboratories, Inc.) Dextromethorphan HBr 10 mg, iodinated glycerol 30 mg, alcohol free. Liq. Bot. 473 ml.
Use: Cough preparation.

Tussogest. (Major Pharmaceuticals) Phenylpropanolamine HCl 75 mg, caramiphen edisylate 40 mg/TR Cap. Bot. 100s, 500s, 1000s. *Rx.*
Use: Antitussive, decongestant.

Tusstat. (Century Pharmaceuticals, Inc.) Diphenhydramine HCl 12.5 mg/5 ml, alcohol 5%. Syr. Bot. 118 ml, 473 ml, pt. gal. *Rx.*
Use: Antihistamine.

Tusstat Expectorant. (Century Pharmaceuticals, Inc.) Diphenhydramine HCl 80 mg, ammonium chloride 12 g, sodium citrate 5 g, menthol 1/10 g, alcohol 5%/oz. Bot. 4 fl. oz, pt, gal. *Rx.*
Use: Antihistamine, expectorant.

•**tuvirumab.** (tuh-VIE-roo-mab) USAN.
Use: Monoclonal antibody (antiviral).

T-Vites. (Freeda Vitamins, Inc.) Vitamins B_1 25 mg, B_2 25 mg, B_3 150 mg, B_5 25 mg, B_6 25 mg, C 100 mg, biotin 30 mcg, PABA, K, Mg, Mn carbonate 2 mg, Zn gluconate 20 mg/Tab. Bot. 100s. *otc.*
Use: Mineral, vitamin supplement.

tween 20, 40, 60, 80. (Zeneca Pharmaceuticals) N.F. 18. Polysorbates.
Use: Surface active agents.

12-Hour Antihistamine Nasal Decongestant. (United Research Laboratories) Pseudoephedrine sulfate 120 mg, dexbrompheniramine maleate 6 mg, sugar, sucrose. SR Tab. Bot. 10s. *otc.*
Use: Decongestant.

12-Hour Cold Tablets. (Zenith Goldline Pharmaceuticals) Dexbrompheniramine maleate 6 mg, pseudoephedrine sulfate 120 mg/SR Tab. Pkg. 10s, 20s. *otc.*
Use: Antihistamine, decongestant.

20% ProSol. (Baxter Healthcare) Amino acids 20 g, total nitrogen 3.21 g/100 ml, lysine acetate, glacial acetic acid. Sulfite free. Inj. *Vialflex* Cont. 500 ml, 1000 ml, 2000 ml. *Rx.*
Use: Nutritional therapy, intravenous.

Twice-a-Day. (Major Pharmaceuticals) Oxymetazoline 0.05%. Soln. 15 ml, 30 ml. *otc.*
Use: Decongestant.

Twilite. (Pfeiffer Co.) Diphenhydramine HCl 50 mg. Tab. 20s. *otc.*
Use: Sleep aid.

Twin-K Liquid. (Knoll Pharmaceuticals) Potassium ions 20 mEq/15 ml. Bot. Pt. *Rx.*
Use: Treatment of hypokalemia.

2-Tone Disclosing Solution. (Young Dental) Dropper Bot. 2 oz.
Use: Disclosing solution.

2-24. (Walgreen) Belladonna alkaloids 0.2 mg, phenylpropanolamine HCl 50 mg, chlorpheniramine maleate 4 mg/Cap. Bot. 10s. *otc.*
Use: Anticholinergic, antispasmodic, decongestant, antihistamine.

TwoCal HN High Nitrogen Liquid Nutrition. (Ross Laboratories) High-nitrogen liquid nutrition (2 calories/ml). 1900 calories (1 quart), provides 100% US RDA for vitamins and minerals for adults and children over 4 yrs. Can 8 fl. oz. *otc.*
Use: Nutritional supplement.

•**tybamate.** (TIE-bam-ate) USAN.
Use: Anxiolytic.

Ty-Caplets. (Major Pharmaceuticals) Acetaminophen 500 mg/Tab. Bot. 100s. *otc.*
Use: Analgesic.

Ty-Caps. (Major Pharmaceuticals) Acetaminophen 500 mg/Cap. Bot. 100s, 1000s, UD 100s. *otc.*
Use: Analgesic.

Tycodene Sugar Free. (Pfeiffer Co.) Chlorpheniramine maleate 2 mg, dextromethorphan HBr 10 mg/5 ml, menthol, saccharin, sorbitol, alcohol free. Liq. Bot. 120 ml. *otc.*
Use: Antihistamine, antitussive.

Ty-Cold Tablets. (Major Pharmaceuticals) 30 mg pseudoephedrine, 2 mg chlorpheniramine maleate, 15 mg dextromethorphan HBr, 325 mg acetaminophen. Pkg. 24s. *otc.*
Use: Analgesic, antihistamine, antitussive, decongestant.

Tylenol Children's. (McNeil Consumer Products Co.) Acetaminophen 160 mg/5 ml. Butylparaben, corn syrup, sorbitol. Alcohol free. Susp. Bot. 60 ml. *otc.*

Use: Analgesic.

Tylenol Children's Chewable Tablets. (McNeil Consumer Products Co.) Acetaminophen 80 mg/Chew. Tab. Bot. 30s, 48s. Blisters 2s. Hospital pack 250s. *otc.*
Use: Analgesic.

Tylenol Children's Elixir. (McNeil Consumer Products Co.) Acetaminophen 160 mg/5 ml. Bot. 2 oz., 4 oz., pt. UD 100 x 5 ml, 100 x 10 ml. *otc.*
Use: Analgesic.

Tylenol Cold. (McNeil Consumer Products Co.) Pseudoephedrine HCl 30 mg, chlorpheniramine maleate 2 mg, dextromethorphan HBr 15 mg, acetaminophen 325 mg. Tab., Cap. Bot. 24s, 50s. *otc.*
Use: Analgesic, antihistamine, antitussive, decongestant.

Tylenol Cold & Flu Medication. (McNeil Consumer Products Co.) Pseudoephedrine HCl 60 mg, chlorpheniramine maleate 4 mg, dextromethorphan HBr, acetaminophen 650 mg, aspartame, sucrose, phenylalanine 11 mg, lemon flavor. Pow. Pks. 6s, 12s. *otc.*
Use: Analgesic, antihistamine, decongestant.

Tylenol Cold & Flu No Drowsiness. (McNeil Consumer Products Co.) Acetaminophen 650 mg, pseudoephedrine HCl 60 mg, dextromethorphan HBr per packet 30 mg, aspartame (as phenylalanine 11 mg), sucrose, lemon flavor. Pow. Pkt. 6s, 12s. *otc.*
Use: Analgesic, antihistamine, decongestant.

Tylenol Cold Liquid, Children's. (McNeil Consumer Products Co.) Pseudoephedrine 15 mg, chlorpheniramine maleate 1 mg, acetaminophen 160 mg/5 ml, sorbitol, sucrose, alcohol free, grape flavor. Liq. Bot. 120 ml. *otc.*
Use: Analgesic, antihistamine, decongestant.

Tylenol Cold Multisymptom Plus Cough, Children's. (McNeil Consumer Products Co.) Acetaminophen 160 mg, dextromethorphan HBr 5 mg, chlorpheniramine maleate 1 mg, pseudoephedrine 15 mg/5 ml. Liq. Bot. 120 ml. *otc.*
Use: Antihistamine, antitussive, decongestant.

Tylenol Cold Night Time. (McNeil Consumer Products Co.) Pseudoephedrine HCl 10 mg, diphenhydramine HCl 8.3 mg, acetaminophen 108.3 mg/5 ml, alcohol 10%, sucrose, cherry flavor. Liq. Bot. 150 ml. *otc.*
Use: Analgesic, antihistamine, decongestant.

Tylenol Cold No Drowsiness Caplets & Gelcaps. (McNeil Consumer Products Co.) Pseudoephedrine HCl 30 mg, dextromethorphan HBr 15 mg, acetaminophen 325 mg. **Capl.:** Bot. 24s, 50s. **Gel.:** 20s, 40s. *otc.*
Use: Analgesic, antitussive, decongestant.

Tylenol Cold Tablets, Children's. (McNeil Consumer Products Co.) Pseudoephedrine HCl 7.5 mg, chlorpheniramine maleate 0.5 mg, acetaminophen 80 mg, aspartame, sucrose, phenylalanine 4 mg. Chew. Tab. Grape flavor. Bot. 24s. *otc.*
Use: Analgesic, antihistamine, decongestant.

Tylenol Cough. (McNeil Consumer Products Co.) Dextromethorphan HBr, acetaminophen 250 mg/5 ml, saccharin, sorbitol, sucrose. Liq. Bot. 120 ml. *otc.*
Use: Analgesic, antitussive.

Tylenol Cough w/Decongestant. (McNeil Consumer Products Co.) Pseudoephedrine HCl 15 mg, dextromethorphan HBr 7.5 mg, acetaminophen 250 mg, alcohol 10%, saccharin, sobitol, sucrose. Liq. Bot. 120 ml, 240 ml. *otc.*
Use: Analgesic, antitussive, decongestant.

Tylenol Elixir, Children's. (McNeil Consumer Products Co.) Acetaminophen 160 mg/5 ml. Elix. Bot. 60 mg, 120 ml. *otc.*
Use: Analgesic.

Tylenol Extended Relief. (McNeil Consumer Products Co.) Acetaminophen 650 mg/ER Capl. 100s. *otc.*
Use: Analgesic.

Tylenol Extra Strength. (McNeil Consumer Products Co.) Acetaminophen 500 mg/Tab., Capl. **Tab.:** Bot. 30s, 60s, 100s, 200s. **Cap.:** Bot. 24s, 50s, 100s, 175s. *otc.*
Use: Analgesic.

Tylenol Extra Strength Adult Liquid. (McNeil Consumer Products Co.) Acetaminophen 1000 mg/30 ml w/alcohol 8.5%. Bot. 8 oz. Hosp. 8 oz. *otc.*
Use: Analgesic.

Tylenol Extra Strength Caplets. (McNeil Consumer Products Co.) Acetaminophen 500 mg/Capl. Bot. 24s, 50s, 100s, 175s. *otc.*
Use: Analgesic.

Tylenol Extra Strength Gel-Cap. (McNeil Consumer Products Co.) Acetaminophen 500 mg. Gelcap. Bot. 24s,

50s, 100s. *otc.*
Use: Analgesic.

Tylenol Extra Strength Geltabs. (McNeil Consumer Products Co.) Acetaminophen 500 mg, parabens. Tab. Bot. 24s, 50s, 100s. *otc.*
Use: Analgesic.

Tylenol Flu Maximum Strength. (McNeil Consumer Products Co.) Pseudoephedrine HCl 30 mg, dextromethorphan HBr 15 mg, acetaminophen 500 mg. Gelcap. Pkg. 10s, 20s. *otc.*
Use: Analgesic, antitussive, decongestant.

Tylenol Infant's Drops. (McNeil Consumer Products Co.) Acetaminophen 80 mg/0.8 ml. Butylparaben, corn syrup, sorbitol. Alcohol free. Bot. w/dropper 7.5 ml, 15 ml. *otc.*
Use: Analgesic.

Tylenol Junior Strength. (McNeil Consumer Products Co.) Acetaminophen 160 mg, aspartame (6 mg phenylalanine)/Chew. Tab. 24s. *otc.*
Use: Analgesic.

Tylenol Junior Strength Swallowable Tablets. (McNeil Consumer Products Co.) 160 mg/Tab. Box. 30s. Hosp. 250 x 1. *otc.*
Use: Analgesic.

Tylenol Maximum-Strength Allergy Sinus. (McNeil Consumer Products Co.) Pseudoephedrine HCl 30 mg, chlorpheniramine maleate 2 mg, acetaminophen 500 mg, Capl. Bot. 24s, 50s. Gelcap. Bot. 20s, 40s. *otc.*
Use: Analgesic, antihistamine, decongestant.

Tylenol Maximum Strength Sinus Medication. (McNeil Consumer Products Co.) Acetaminophen 500 mg, pseudoephedrine HCl 30 mg/Tab., Capl. **Tab.:** Bot. 24s, 50s. **Cap.:** Bot. 24s, 50s. *otc.*
Use: Analgesic, decongestant.

Tylenol Multi-Symptom Hot Medication. (McNeil Consumer Products Co.) Pseudoephedrine HCl 60 mg, chlorpheniramine maleate 4 mg, dextromethorphan HBr 30 mg, acetaminophen 650 mg. Pow. Pkt. 6s. *otc.*
Use: Analgesic, antihistamine, antitussive, decongestant.

Tylenol No Drowsiness Cold. (McNeil Consumer Products Co.) Pseudoephedrine HCl 30 g, dextromethorphan HBr 15 mg, acetaminophen 325 mg. Cap. Bot. 24s, 50s. *otc.*
Use: Analgesic, antitussive, decongestant.

Tylenol PM, Extra Strength. (McNeil Consumer Products Co.) Acetaminophen 500 mg, diphenhydramine 25 mg. Tab., Cap. Bot. 24s, 50s. *otc.*
Use: Analgesic, antitussive.

Tylenol Regular Strength. (McNeil Consumer Products Co.) Acetaminophen 325 mg/Tab., Capl. **Tab.:** Tin 12s. Vial 12s. Bot. 24s, 50s, 100s, 200s. **Cap.:** Bot. 24s, 50s. *otc.*
Use: Analgesic.

Tylenol Severe Allergy. (McNeil Consumer Products Co.) Diphenhydramine HCl 12.5 mg, acetaminophen 500 mg/Capl. Pkg. 12s, 24s. *otc.*
Use: Analgesic, antihistamine.

Tylenol with Codeine. (Ortho McNeil Pharmaceutical) **Tab.:** Acetaminophen 300 mg with codeine phosphate. **No. 2:** Codeine phosphate 15 mg. Bot. 100s, 500s. **No. 3:** Codeine phosphate 30 mg. Bot. 100s, 500s, 1000s, UD 100s. **No. 4:** Codeine phosphate 60 mg. Bot. 100s, 500s, UD 500s. *c-III.*
Use: Analgesic combination, narcotic.

Tylenol with Codeine Elixir. (Ortho McNeil Pharmaceutical) Acetaminophen 120 mg, codeine phosphate 12 mg/5 ml w/alcohol 7%. Bot. 480 ml. *c-V.*
Use: Analgesic combination, narcotic.

Tylosterone. (Eli Lilly and Co.) Diethylstilbestrol 0.25 mg, methyltestosterone 5 mg/Tab. Bot. 100s. *Rx.*
Use: Androgen, estrogen combination.

Tylox. (Ortho McNeil Pharmaceutical) Oxycodone HCl 5 mg, acetaminophen 500 mg/Cap. Bot. 100s, UD 100s. *c-II.*
Use: Analgesic combination, narcotic.

•**tyloxapol.** (till-OX-ah-pahl) U.S.P. 23.
Use: Detergent, ophthalmic; cystic fibrosis. [Orphan Drug]
See: Enuclene (Alcon Laboratories, Inc.).

Tympagesic. (Pharmacia & Upjohn) Phenylephrine HCl 0.25%, antipyrine 5%, benzocaine 5%, in propylene glycol. Liq. Bot. w/dropper 13 ml. *Rx.*
Use: Antihistamine, otic.

Ty-Pap. (Major Pharmaceuticals) **Elix.:** Acetaminophen 160 mg/5 ml. Bot. Pt., gal. **Supp.:** Acetaminophen 120 mg, 650 mg. 12s. *otc.*
Use: Analgesic.

Typhim Vi. (Pasteur Merieux Connaught) Typhoid Vi polysaccharide vaccine 0.5 ml. Inj. Single-dose syringes and 25 ml, 50 ml vials. *Rx.*
Use: Immunization, typhoid.

•**typhoid vaccine.** (TIE-foyd) U.S.P. 23.
Use: Immunization.

typhoid vaccine. (Wyeth-Ayerst Laboratories) 8 units per ml (not > 1 billion or-

ganisms per ml). Heat-phenol treated vaccine. Vial 5 ml, 10 ml, 20 ml. Acetone-killed and dried vaccine. Pow. for Inj. 50-dose vial. *Rx.*
Use: Immunization.

typhoid vaccine capsule. *Rx.*
Use: Immnization.
See: Vivotif Berna (Berna Products Corp.).

typhoid vaccine polysaccharide. *Rx.*
Use: Immunization.
See: Typhim Vi (Pasteur Merieux Connaught).

Tyrex-2. (Ross Laboratories) Protein 30 g, fat 15.5 g, carbohydrates 30 g, Na 880 mg, K 1370 mg, Cal 410/100 g. With appropriate vitamins and minerals. Phenylalanine and tyrosine free. Pow. Can 325 g. *otc.*
Use: Nutritional supplement.

Tyrodone. (Major Pharmaceuticals) Hydrocodone bitartrate 5 mg, pseudoephedrine HCl 60 mg/5 ml, alcohol 5%. Liq. Bot. 473 ml. *c-III.*
Use: Antitussive, decongestant.

Tyromex-1. (Ross Laboratories) Protein 15 g, fat 23.9 g, carbohydrates 46.3 g, linoleic acid 1800 mg, Fe 9 mg, Na 190 mg, K 675 mg, Cal 480/100 g. With appropriate vitamins and minerals. Phenylalanine, tyrosine, and methionine free. Pow. Can 350 g. *otc.*
Use: Nutritional supplement.

•**tyropanoate sodium.** (TIE-row-PAN-oh-ate) U.S.P. 23.
Use: Diagnostic aid (radiopaque medium, cholecystographic).
See: Bilopaque (Sanofi Winthrop Pharmaceuticals).

tyropaque caps. (Sanofi Winthrop Pharmaceuticals) Tyropanoate sodium. *Rx.*
Use: Oral cholecystographic medium.

•**tyrosine.** (TIE-row-SEEN) U.S.P. 23. L-Tyrosine.
Use: Amino acid.

tyrosine hydroxylase inhibitor.
Use: Antihypertensive.
See: Demser (Merck & Co.).

Tyrosum Skin Cleanser. (Summers Laboratories, Inc.) Isopropanol 50%, polysorbate 80 2%, and acetone 10%. Bot. 120 ml, pt. Towelettes 24s, 50s. *otc.*
Use: Dermatologic, cleanser.

•**tyrothricin.** (tie-roe-THRYE-sin) U.S.P. 23. An antibiotic from *Bacillus brevis.* Tyrodac; Tyroderm.
Use: Antibacterial.

Ty-Tabs. (Major Pharmaceuticals) Acetaminophen with codeine #2, #3, #4. Bot. 100s, 500s, 1000s. *c-III.*
Use: Analgesic combination, narcotic.

Ty-Tabs, Children's. (Major Pharmaceuticals) Acetaminophen 80 mg/Tab. Bot. 30s, 100s. *otc.*
Use: Analgesic.

Ty-Tabs Extra Strength. (Major Pharmaceuticals) Acetaminophen 500 mg/Tab. Bot. 100s, 1000s. *otc.*
Use: Analgesic.

Tyzine Nasal Solution. (Key Pharmaceuticals) Tetrahydrozoline HCl 0.1%. Bot. Pt., oz. *otc.*
Use: Decongestant.

Tyzine Nasal Spray. (Key Pharmaceuticals) Tetrahydrozoline HCl 0.1%. Bot. 0.5 oz. *otc.*
Use: Decongestant.

Tyzine Pediatric Nasal Drops. (Key Pharmaceuticals) Tetrahydrozoline HCl 0.05%. Bot. 0.5 oz. *otc.*
Use: Decongestant.

U

UAA. (Econo Med Pharmaceuticals) Methenamine 40.8 mg, phenyl salicylate 18.1 mg, methylene blue 5.4 mg, benzoic acid 4.5 mg, atropine sulfate 0.03 mg, hyoscyamine 0.03 mg/Tab. Bot. 100s, 1000s. *Rx.*
Use: Anti-infective, urinary.

UAD Cream. (Forest Pharmaceutical, Inc.) Clioquinol 3%, hydrocortisone 1%, ceresin, glyceryl oleate, propylene glycol, parabens, mineral oil, pramoxine HCl. Jar 15 g. *Rx.*
Use: Corticosteroid; anesthetic, local.

UAD Lotion. (Forest Pharmaceutical, Inc.) Clioquinol 0.75%, hydrocortisone 0.25%, cetyl alcohol, glyceryl stearate, lanolin, parabens, mineral oil, pramoxine HCl, propylene glycol. Bot. 20 ml. *Rx.*
Use: Corticosteroid; anesthetic, local.

UAD Otic. (Forest Pharmaceutical, Inc.) Hydrocortisone 1%, neomycin sulfate 5 mg, polymyxin B sulfate 10,000 units/ml, thimerosal 0.01%, cetyl alcohol, propylene glycol, polysorbate 80. Susp. Bot. 10 ml w/dropper. *Rx.*
Use: Otic.

UBT. (Biomerica, Inc.) For detection of blood in the urine.
Use: Diagnostic aid.

UCG-Beta Slide Monoclonal II. (Wampole Laboratories) Two-minute latex agglutination inhibition slide test for the qualitative detection of B-hCG/hCG (sensitivity 0.5 IU hCG/ml) in urine. Kit 50s, 100s, 300s.
Use: Diagnostic aid.

UCG-Beta Stat. (Wampole Laboratories) One-hour passive hemagglutination inhibition tube test for the qualitative detection and quantitative determination of B-hCG/hCG (sensitivity 0.2 IU hCG/ml) in urine. Kit 50s, 300s.
Use: Diagnostic aid.

UCG-Lyphotest. (Wampole Laboratories) One-hour passive hemagglutination inhibition tube test for the qualitative or quantitative determination of hCG (sensitivity: 0.5 to 1 IU hCG/ml) in urine. Kit 10s, 50s, 300s.
Use: Diagnostic aid.

UCG-Slide Test. (Wampole Laboratories) Rapid latex agglutination inhibition slide test for the qualitative detection of hCG (sensitivity: 2 IU hCG/ml) in urine. Kit 30s, 100s, 300s, 1000s.
Use: Diagnostic aid.

UCG-Test. (Wampole Laboratories) Two-hour hemagglutination inhibition tube test for the determination of hCG (sensitivity: 0.5 IU hCG/ml undiluted specimen. 1.5 IU hCG/ml 1:3 diluted specimen) in urine and serum. Kit 10s, 25s, 100s, 300s.
Use: Diagnostic aid.

UCG-Titration Set. (Wampole Laboratories) A two-hour hemagglutination inhibition tube test for the determination of hCG (sensitivity: 1 IU hCG/ml) in urine or serum. Kit 45s.
Use: Diagnostic aid.

Uendex. Dextran sulfate, inhaled, aerosolized.
Use: Cystic fibrosis treatment. [Orphan Drug]

Ulcerease. (Med-Derm Pharmaceuticals) Liquified phenol 0.6%, glycerin, sugar free. Liq. Bot. 180 ml. *otc.*
Use: Anesthetic, local.

Ulcerin P Tablets. (Sanofi Winthrop Pharmaceuticals) Aluminum hydroxide. *otc.*
Use: Antacid.

Ulcerin Tablets. (Sanofi Winthrop Pharmaceuticals) Aluminum hydroxide. *otc.*
Use: Antacid.

•**uldazepam.** (uhl-DAY-zeh-pam) USAN.
Use: Hypnotic, sedative.

Ulpax. (Roche Laboratories) Ablukast sodium.
Use: Antiasthmatic (leukotriene antagonist).

ULR-LA. (Geneva Pharmaceuticals) Phenylpropanolamine HCl 75 mg, guaifenesin 400 mg. Tab. Bot. 100s. *Rx.*
Use: Decongestant, expectorant.

Ultane. (Abbott Laboratories) Sevoflurane. Volatile liquid for inhalation. Bot. 250 ml. *Rx.*
Use: Anesthetic, general.

Ultiva. (GlaxoWellcome) Remifentanil HCl, lyophilized 1 mg/ml (as HCl; after reconstitution). Preservative free. Pow. for Inj. Vial. 3 ml, 5 ml, 10 ml. *c-II.*
Use: Analgesic, narcotic.

Ultra B-50. (NBTY, Inc.) Vitamins B_1 50 mg, B_2 50 mg, B_3 50 mg, B_5 50 mg, B_6 50 mg, B_{12} 50 mcg, folic acid 0.1 mg, PABA 50 mg, inositol 50 mg, biotin 50 mcg, choline 50 mg, lecithin 50 mg. Tab. Bot. 60s, 180s. *otc.*
Use: Vitamin supplement.

Ultra B-100. (NBTY, Inc.) Vitamins B_1 100 mg, B_2 100 mg, B_3 100 mg, B_5 100 mg, B_6 100 mg, B_{12} 100 mcg, folic acid 0.1 mg, PABA 100 mg, inositol 100 mg, biotin 100 mcg, choline bitartrate 100 mg. TR Tab. Bot. 50s. *otc.*
Use: Vitamin supplement.

Ultrabex. (Health for Life Brands, Inc.) Vi-

tamins B_1 20 mg, C 50 mg, B_2 2 mg, B_6 0.5 mg, niacinamide 35 mg, calcium pantothenate 0.5 mg, wheat germ oil 30 mg, B_{12} 20 mcg, liver desiccated 150 mg, Fe 11.58 mg, Ca 29 mg, P 23 mg, dicalcium phosphate 100 mg, Mg 1.11 mg, Mn 1.3 mg, K 2.24 mg, Zn 0.68 mg, choline 25 mg, inositol 25 mg, pepsin 32.5 mg, diastase 32.5 mg, hesperidin 25 mg, biotin 20 mcg, hydrolyzed yeast 81.25 mg, protein digest 47.04 mg, amino acids 34.21 mg/Cap. Bot. 50s, 100s, 1000s. *otc.*
Use: Mineral, vitamin supplement.

ULTRAbrom. (WE Pharmaceuticals, Inc.) Brompheniramine maleate 12 mg, pseudoephedrine HCl 120 mg/SR Cap. Bot. 100s. *Rx.*
Use: Antihistamine, decongestant.

ULTRAbrom PD. (WE Pharmaceuticals, Inc.) Brompheniramine maleate 6 mg, pseudoephedrine 60 mg/SR Cap. Bot. 100s. *Rx.*
Use: Antihistamine, decongestant.

Ultracal. (Bristol-Myers Squibb) Protein 44 g, carbohydrate 123 g, fat 45 g, Na 930 mg, K 1610 mg, mOsm 310 kg H_2O, cal. 1.06/ml, vitamins A, B_1, B_2, B_3, B_5, B_6, B_{12}, C, D, E, K, folic acid, choline, biotin, Ca, P, I, Fe, Mg, Cu, Zn, Mn, Cl, Se, Cr, Mo. Liq. Can. 8 oz. *otc.*
Use: Nutritional supplement.

Ultra Cap. (Weeks & Leo) Acetaminophen 300 mg, guaifenesin 100 mg, chlorpheniramine maleate 4 mg, phenylephrine HCl 10 mg, dextromethorphan HBr 6 mg/Cap. Vial 18s. *Rx.*
Use: Analgesic, antihistamine, antitussive, decongestant, expectorant.

Ultra-Care. (Allergan, Inc.) **Disinfecting Soln.:** Hydrogen peroxide 3%, sodium stannate, sodium nitrate, phosphate buffer. Bot. 120 ml, 360 ml; **Neutralizer Tab.:** Catalase, hydroxypropyl methylcellulose, buffering agents. Pkg. 12s, 36s w/cup. *otc.*
Use: Contact lens care.

Ultracortinol. (Novartis Pharmaceutical Corp.) Agent to suppress overactive adrenal glands. Pending release.

Ultra Derm Bath Oil. (Baker Cummins Dermatologicals, Inc.) Bot. 8 oz. *otc.*
Use: Emollient.

Ultra Derm Moisturizer. (Baker Cummins Dermatologicals, Inc.) Bot. 8 oz. *otc.*
Use: Emollient.

Ultra Freeda. (Freeda Vitamins, Inc.) Vitamins A 4166 IU, D 133 IU, E 66.7 mg, B_1 16.7 mg, B_2 16.7 mg, B_3 33 mg, B_5 33 mg, B_6 16.7 mg, B_{12} 33 mcg, C 333 mg, folic acid 0.27 mg, Fe 2 mg, Ca 27 mg, Zn 1.1 mg, choline, inositol, bioflavonoids, PABA, biotin 100 mcg, Cr, I, K, Mg, Mn, Mo, Se. Tab. Bot. 90s, 180s, 270s. *otc.*
Use: Mineral, vitamin supplement.

Ultra Freeda Iron Free. (Freeda Vitamins, Inc.) Vitamins A 4166 IU, D 133 IU, E 66.7 mg, B_1 16.7 mg, B_2 16.7 mg, B_3 33 mg, B_5 33 ng, B_6 16.7 mg, B_{12} 33 mcg, C 333 mg, FA 0.27 mg, Ca 27 mg, Zn 1.1 mg, choline, inositol, bioflavonoids, PABA, biotin 100 mcg, Cr, I, K, Mg, Mn, Mo, Se. Tab. Bot. 90s, 180s, 270s. *otc.*
Use: Mineral, vitamin supplement.

Ultragesic. (Stewart-Jackson Pharmacal, Inc.) Acetaminophen 500 mg, hydrocodone bitartrate 5 mg/Cap. Bot. 100s. *c-III.*
Use: Analgesic combination, narcotic.

Ultralan. (Elan Pharma) Protein 60 g, fat 50 g, carbohydrates 202 g, Na 1.035 g, K 1.755 g/L. Lactose free. With appropriate vitamins and minerals. Liq. 1000 ml New Pak systems with and without ColorCheck. *otc.*
Use: Nutritional supplement.

Ultralente insulin.
See: Iletin (Eli Lilly and Co.).

Ultram. (Ortho McNeil Pharmaceutical) Tramadol HCl 50 mg/Tab. Bot. 100s, UD 100s. *Rx.*
Use: Analgesic.

Ultra Mide 25. (Baker Cummins Dermatologicals, Inc.) Bot. 8 oz. *otc.*
Use: Emollient.

Ultrapred. (Horizon Pharmaceutical Corp.) Prednisolone acetate 1%. Susp. Bot. 5 ml. *Rx.*
Use: Corticosteroid, ophthalmic.

Ultrasone. (Gordon Laboratories) Ultrasound aid. Liq. Bot. Qt, gal. Plastic Bot. 8 oz.
Use: Ultrasound contact cream.

Ultra Tears. (Alcon Laboratories, Inc.) Hydroxypropyl methylcellulose 2910 1%, benzalkonium Cl 0.01%, NaCl. Soln. Bot. 15 ml. *otc.*
Use: Artificial tears.

Ultravate. (Westwood Squibb Pharmaceuticals) Halobetasol propionate. *Rx.*
Use: Corticosteroid, topical.

Ultravist. (Berlex Laboratories, Inc.) **150 mgI/ml:** (iopromide 311.7 mg, tromethamine 2.42 mg, EDTA 0.1 mg). Preservative free. Inj. Vial 50 ml. **240 mgI/ml:** (iopromide 498.72 mg, tromethamine 2.42 mg, EDTA 0.1 mg). Preservative free, Inj. Vial 50 ml, 100 ml, 200 ml. **300 mgI/ml:** (iopromide 623.4 mg,

tromethamine 2.42 mg, EDTA 0.1 mg). Preservative free. Inj. Vial 50 ml, 100 ml, 150 ml. **370 mgI/ml:** (iopromide 768.86 mg, tromethamine 2.42 mg, EDTA 0.1 mg). Preservative free. Inj. Vial 50 ml, 100 ml, 150 ml, 200 ml. *Rx.*
Use: Diagnostic aid.

Ultra Vitamin A & D. (NBTY, Inc.) Vitamins A 25,000 IU, D 1000 IU. Tab. Bot. 100s. *otc.*
Use: Vitamin supplement.

Ultra Vita Time. (NBTY, Inc.) Fe 6 mg, vitamins A 10,000 IU, D 400 IU, E 13 IU, B_1 25 mg, B_2 25 mg, B_3 50 mg, B_5 12.5 mg, B_6 15 mg, B_{12} 50 mcg, C 150 mg, folic acid 0.4 mg, B, Ca, Cr, Cu, I, K, Mg, Mn, Mo, P, Se, Zn 5 mg, biotin 1 mg, bioflavonoids, bone meal, PABA, choline bitartrate, betaine, inositol, lecithin, desiccated liver, rutin/Tab. Bot. 100s. *otc.*
Use: Mineral, vitamin supplement.

Ultrazyme Enzymatic Cleaner. (Allergan, Inc.) Subtilisin A, effervescing, buffering and tableting agents for dilution in hydrogen peroxide 3%. Tab. Pkg. 5s, 10s, 15s, 20s. *otc.*
Use: Contact lens care.

Ultrum. (Towne) Vitamins A 5000 IU, E 30 IU, C 90 mg, folic acid 400 mcg, B_1 2.25 mg, B_2 2.6 mg, niacinamide 20 mg, B_6 3 mg, B_{12} 9 mcg, biotin 45 mcg, D 400 IU, pantothenic acid 10 mg, Ca 162 mg, P 125 mg, I 150 mcg, Fe 27 mg, Mg 100 mg, Cu 3 mg, Mn 7.5 mg, K 7.5 mg, Zn 22.5 mg/Tab. Bot. 100s. *otc.*
Use: Mineral, vitamin supplement.

Ultrum with Selenium. (Towne) Vitamins A 5000 IU, E 30 IU, C 90 mg, folic acid 2.25 mg, B_1 2.25 mg, B_2 2.6 mg, niacinamide 20 mg, B_6 3 mg, B_{12} 9 mcg, D 400 IU, biotin 45 mcg, pantothenic acid 10 mg, Ca 162 mg, P 125 mg, I 150 mcg, Fe 27 mg, Mg 100 mg, Cu 3 mg, Mn 7.5 mg, K 7.7 mg, Cl 7 mg, Mo 15 mcg, Se 15 mcg, Zn 22.5 mg/Tab. Bot. 130s. *Rx.*
Use: Mineral, vitamin supplement.

Unasyn. (Roerig) Ampicillin sodium 1 g, sulbactam sodium 0.5 g, ampicillin sodium 2 g, sulbactam sodium 1 g; ampicillin sodium 10 g, sulbactam sodium 5 g. Pow. for Inj. Vial, Piggyback vial, *ADD-Vantage* vial, Bulk Pkg. (10 g only). *Rx.*
Use: Anti-infective, penicillin.

10-undecenoic acid. Undecylenic Acid, U.S.P. 23.
Use: Antifungal, topical.

10-undecenoic acid, zinc (2+) salt. Zinc Undecylenate, U.S.P. 23.
Use: Antifungal, topical.

undecoylium chloride-iodine. Virac, Preps. (Ruson).
Use: Anti-infective, topical.

•**undecylenic acid.** (un-deh-sill-EN-ik) U.S.P. 23.
Use: Antifungal, topical.
See: Desenex (Novartis Pharmaceutical Corp.).
Fungoid AF, Sol. Preps (Novartis Pharmaceutical Corp.).
W/Dichlorophene.
See: Fungicidal, Talc (Gordon Laboratories).
Onychomycetin, Liq. (Gordon Laboratories).
W/Salicylic acid.
See: Fungicidal, Oint. (Gordon Laboratories).
W/Zinc undecylenate.
See: Cruex, Cream, Spray Pow. (Novartis Pharmaceutical Corp.).
Desenex, Preps. (Novartis Pharmaceutical Corp.).

undecylenic acid salts. Calcium, copper, zinc.

Undelenic Ointment. (Gordon Laboratories) Undecylenic acid 5%, zinc undecylenate 20%. Jar oz, lb. *otc.*
Use: Antifungal, topical.

Undelenic Tincture. (Gordon Laboratories) Undecylenic acid 10%, chloroxylenol 0.5%. Brush Bot. oz. Bot. Pt. *otc.*
Use: Antifungal, topical.

Unguentine Ointment "Original Formula". (Mentholatum Co., Inc.) Phenol 1% in ointment base. Tube oz. *otc.*
Use: Dermatologic, counterirritant.

Unguentine Plus First Aid Cream. (Mentholatum Co., Inc.) Parachlorometaxylenol 2%, lidocaine HCl 2%, phenol 0.5% in a moisturizing cream base. Tube ½ oz, 1 oz, 2 oz. *otc.*
Use: Dermatologic, counterirritant.

Unguentum Bossi. (Doak Dermatologics) Ammoniated mercury 5%, methamine sulfosalicylate 2%, tar distillate "Doak" 5%, Doak oil 40%, petrolatum, sorbitol sesquioleate, cholesterol derivatives, beeswax. Cream Tube 60 g, 480 g. *Rx.*
Use: Antipsoriatic.

Uni-Ace. (United Research Laboratories) Acetaminophen 100 mg/ml. Alcohol free. Liq. Bot. 15 ml with dropper. *otc.*
Use: Analgesic.

Unibase. (Parke-Davis) Water-absorbing oint. base. Jar lb. *Rx.*
Use: Pharmaceutical aid, ointment base.

Uni-Bent Cough. (United Research

Laboratories) Diphenhydramine HCl 12.5 mg/5 ml, alcohol 5%. Syr. Bot. 118 ml. *Rx.*
Use: Antihistamine.

Unicap Capsules. (Pharmacia & Upjohn) Vitamins A 5000 IU, D 400 IU, E 30 IU, B_1 1.5 mg, B_2 1.7 mg, B_3 20 mg, B_6 2 mg, B_{12} 6 mcg, C 60 mg, FA 0.4 mg/Cap. Bot. 120s. *otc.*
Use: Vitamin supplement.

Unicap Jr. Chewable. (Pharmacia & Upjohn) Vitamins A 5000 IU, D 400 IU, E 15 IU, C 60 mg, folic acid 400 mcg, B_1 1.5 mg, B_2 1.7 mg, B_3 20 mg, B_6 2 mg, B_{12} 6 mcg/Tab. Bot. 120s. *otc.*
Use: Vitamin supplement.

Unicap M. (Pharmacia & Upjohn) Fe 18 mg, vitamins A 5000 IU, D 400 IU, E 30 IU, B_1 1.5 mg, B_2 1.7 mg, B_3 20 mg, B_5 10 mg, B_6 2 mg, B_{12} 6 mcg, C 60 mg, folic acid 0.4 mg, Ca, Cu, I, K, Mn, P, Zn 15 mg, tartrazine/Tab. Bot. 120s. *otc.*
Use: Mineral, vitamin supplement.

Unicap Plus Iron. (Pharmacia & Upjohn) Vitamins A 5000 IU, D 400 IU, E 30 IU, C 60 mg, folic acid 0.4 mg, B_1 1.5 mg, B_2 1.7 mg, B_3 20 mg, B_5 10 mg, B_6 2 mg, B_{12} 6 mcg, Fe 22.5 mg, Ca/Tab. Bot. 120s. *otc.*
Use: Mineral, vitamin supplement.

Unicap Sr. (Pharmacia & Upjohn) Fe 10 mg, vitamins A 5000 IU, D 200 IU, E 15 IU, B_1 1.2 mg, B_2 1.4 mg, B_3 16 mg, B_5 10 mg, B_6 2.2 mg, B_{12} 3 mcg, C 60 mg, folic acid 0.4 mg, Ca, Cu, I, K, Mg, Mn, P, Zn 15 mg/Tab. Bot. 120s. *otc.*
Use: Mineral, vitamin supplement.

Unicap T. (Pharmacia & Upjohn) Fe 18 mg, vitamins A 5000 IU, D 400 IU, E 30 IU, B_1 10 mg, B_2 20 mg, B_3 100 mg, B_5 25 mg, B_6 6 mg, B_{12} 18 mcg, C 500 mg, folic acid 0.4 mg, Cu, I, K, Mn, Se, Zn 15 mg, tartrazine/Tab. Bot. 60s. *otc.*
Use: Mineral, vitamin supplement.

Unicap Tablets. (Pharmacia & Upjohn) Vitamins A 5000 IU, D 400 IU, E 15 IU, B_1 1.5 mg, B_2 1.7 mg, B_3 20 mg, B_6 2 mg, B_{12} 6 mcg, C 60 mg, FA 0.4 mg/Tab. Bot. 120s. *otc.*
Use: Vitamin supplement.

Unicomplex-M. (Rugby Labs, Inc.) Fe 18 mg, vitamins A 5000 IU, D 400 IU, E 15 mg, B_1 1.5 mg, B_2 1.7 mg, B_3 20 mg, B_5 10 mg, B_6 2 mg, B_{12} 6 mcg, C 60 mg, folic acid 0.4 mg, Ca, Cu, I, K, Mn, Zn/Tab. Bot. 90s, 1000s. *otc.*
Use: Mineral, vitamin supplement.

Unicomplex-T with Minerals. (Rugby Labs, Inc.) Fe 10 mg, vitamins A 5000 IU, D 400 IU, E 15 mg, B_1 10 mg, B_2 10 mg, B_3 100 mg, B_5 20 mg, B_6 2 mg, B_{12} 4 mcg, C 300 mg, folic acid 0.4 mg, Ca, Cu, I, K, Mg, Mn/Tab. Bot. 60s. *otc.*
Use: Mineral, vitamin supplement.

Unicomplex-T&M. (Rugby Labs, Inc.) Fe 18 mg, vitamins A 5000 IU, D 400 IU, E 30 mg, B_1 10 mg, B_2 10 mg, B_3 100 mg, B_5 25 mg, B_6 6 mg, B_{12} 18 mcg, C 500 mg, FA 0.4 mg, Ca, Cu, I, K, Mn, Zn 15 mg/Tab. Bot. 60s. *otc.*
Use: Mineral, vitamin supplement.

Uni-Decon. (United Research Laboratories) Phenylpropanolamine HCl 40 mg, phenylephrine HCl 10 mg, chlorpheniramine maleate 5 mg, phenyltoloxamine citrate 15 mg/Tab. Bot. 100s, 500s, 1000s. *Rx.*
Use: Antihistamine, decongestant.

Uni-Dur. (Key Pharmaceuticals) Theophylline 400 mg, 600 mg, sugar, lactose/ER Tab. Bot. 100s. *Rx.*
Use: Bronchodilator.

Unifiber. (Dow B. Hickam, Inc.) Powdered cellulose 3 g/tbsp. < 4 calories per serving. Corn syrup solids, xanthan gum. Pow. Bot. 454 g. *otc.*
Use: Laxative.

•**unifocon a.** (you-nih-FOE-kahn A) USAN.
Use: Contact lens material (hydrophic).

Unilax. (B.F. Ascher and Co.) Docusate 230 mg, phenolphthalein 130 mg, sorbitol. Cap. Bot. 15s, 20s, 60s. *otc.*
Use: Laxative.

Unipen. (Wyeth-Ayerst Laboratories) Nafcillin sodium 250 mg. Cap. Bot. 100s. *Rx.*
Use: Anti-infective, penicillin.

Uniphyl. (Purdue Frederick Co.) Theophylline 200 mg, 400 mg, 600 mg/CR Tab. **200 mg:** Bot. 60s, 100s, UD 100s. **400 mg:** Bot. 60s, 100s, 500s, UD 100s. **600 mg:** Bot. 100s. *Rx.*
Use: Bronchodilator.

Uniretic. (Schwarz Pharma, Inc.) Moexipril HCl 7.5 mg/hydrochlorothiazide 12.5 mg. Moexipril HCl 15 mg/hydrochlorothiazide 25 mg, lactose/Tab. Bot. 100s. *Rx.*
Use: Antihypertensive.

Unisol. (Alcon Laboratories, Inc.) Buffered isotonic solution with sodium Cl, boric acid, sodium borate. Bot. 15 ml (25s), 120 ml (2s, 3s). *otc.*
Use: Contact lens care.

Unisol 4 Sterile Saline. (Alcon Laboratories, Inc.) Buffered isotonic solution with sodium Cl, boric acid, sodium borate.

Bot. 120 ml. *otc.*
Use: Contact lens care.

Unisol Plus. (Alcon Laboratories, Inc.) Buffered isotonic solution w/NaCl, boric acid, sodium borate. Aer. 240 ml, 360 ml. *otc.*
Use: Contact lens care.

Unisom Nighttime Sleep-Aid. (Pfizer US Pharmaceutical Group) Doxylamine succinate 25 mg/Tab. Blister 8s, 16s, 32s, 48s. *otc.*
Use: Sleep aid.

Unisom with Pain Relief. (Pfizer US Pharmaceutical Group) Acetaminophen 650 mg, diphenhydramine HCl 50 mg/Tab. Blister 16s. *otc.*
Use: Analgesic, sleep aid.

Unituss HC. (United Research Laboratories) Hydrocodone bitartrate 2.5 mg, phenylephrine HCl 5 mg, chlorpheniramine maleate 2 mg/5 ml. Saccharin, sorbitol, sugar free. Syr. Bot. 473 ml. *c-III.*
Use: Antihistamine, antitussive, decongestant.

Uni-Tussin DM. (United Research Laboratories) Dextromethorphan HBr 10 mg, guaifenesin 100 mg/5 ml. Syr. Bot. 118 ml. *otc.*
Use: Antitussive, expectorant.

Uni-Tussin Syrup. (United Research Laboratories) Dextromethorphan HBr 15 mg, guaifenesin 100 mg/5 ml, alcohol 1.4%. Bot. 120 ml. *otc.*
Use: Antitussive, expectorant.

Univasc. (Schwarz Pharma, Inc.) Moexipril HCl 7.5 mg, 15 mg, lactose/Tab. Bot. 100s, UD 90s. *Rx.*
Use: Antihypertensive.

unna's boot.
See: Zinc Gelatin, U.S.P. XXI.

Unproco Capsules. (Solvay Pharmaceuticals) Dextromethorphan HBr 30 mg, guaifenesin 200 mg/Cap. Bot. 100s. *otc.*
Use: Antitussive, expectorant.

Uplex. (Arcum) Vitamins A 5000 IU, D 400 IU, B_1 3 mg, B_2 3 mg, B_6 1 mg, B_{12} 2.5 mcg, nicotinamide 20 mg, calcium pantothenate 5 mg, C 50 mg/Cap. Bot. 100s, 1000s. *otc.*
Use: Mineral, vitamin supplement.

Uplex No. 2. (Arcum) Vitamins A palmitate 10,000 IU, D 400 IU, B_1 5 mg, B_2 5 mg, C 100 mg, B_6 2 mg, B_{12} 3 mcg, E 2.5 IU, niacinamide 25 mg, calcium pantothenate 5 mg/Cap. Bot. 100s, 1000s. *otc.*
Use: Mineral, vitamin supplement.

Urabeth Tabs. (Major Pharmaceuticals) Bethanechol 5 mg, 10 mg, 25 mg, 50 mg/Tab. **5 mg:** Bot. 100s. **10 mg:** Bot. 250s. **25 mg:** Bot. 250s, 1000s. **50 mg:** Bot. 100s, UD 100s. *Rx.*
Use: Genitourinary.

Uracid. (Wesley Pharmacal Co., Inc.) dl-methionine 0.2 g/Cap. Bot. 100s, 1000s. *Rx.*
Use: Diaper rash preparation.

•**uracil.** (YOUR-ah-sil) USAN.
Use: Potentiator in tegafur therapy.

uradal.
See: Carbromal (Various Mfr.).

•**urea.** (you-REE-ah) U.S.P. 23.
Use: Topically for dry skin; diuretic.
See: Aquacare, Cream, Lot. (Allergan, Inc.).
Aquacare-HP, Cream, Lot. (Allergan, Inc.).
Artra Ashy Skin, Cream (Schering-Plough Corp.).
Calmurid, Cream (Pharmacia & Upjohn).
Carmol, Cream (Ingram).
Carmol Ten, Lot. (Ingram).
Elaqua 10%, 20%, Cream (ICN Pharmaceuticals, Inc.).
Gormel, Cream (Gordon Laboratories).
Nutraplus, Cream, Lot. (Galderma Laboratories, Inc.).
Rea-lo, Lot. (Whorton Pharmaceuticals, Inc.).

W/Benzocaine, benzyl alcohol, p-chloro-m-xylenol, propylene glycol.
See: Carmol-HC, Cream (Ingram).

W/Glycerin.
See: Akne Drying Lot. (Alto Pharmaceuticals).

urea peroxide.
See: Gly-Oxide, Liq. (Hoechst Marion Roussel).
Proxigel (Schwarz Pharma, Inc.).

Ureacin-10 Lotion. (Pedinol Pharmacal, Inc.) Urea 10%. Bot. 8 oz. *otc.*
Use: Emollient.

Ureacin-20 Creme. (Pedinol Pharmacal, Inc.) Urea 20%. Jar 2.5 oz. *otc.*
Use: Emollient.

Ureaphil. (Abbott Hospital Products) Sterile urea 40 g, citric acid 1 mg/150 ml. Bot. 150 ml. *Rx.*
Use: Diuretic.

Urecholine. (Merck & Co.) Bethanechol Cl. **Inj.:** 5 mg/ml Vial 1 ml, 6s. **Tab.:** 5 mg, 10 mg, 25 mg, 50 mg. Bot. 100s, UD 100s. *Rx.*
Use: Genitourinary.

•**uredepa.** (YOU-ree-DEH-pah) USAN.
Use: Antineoplastic.
See: Avinar (Centeon).

p-ureidobenzenearsonic acid.

See: Carbarsone, U.S.P. XXI.

Urelief. (Rocky Mtn.) Methenamine 2 gr, salol 0.5 gr, methylene blue 1/10 gr, benzoic acid gr, hyoscyamine sulfate gr, atropine sulfate gr/Tab. Bot. 100s. *Rx.*
Use: Anti-infective, urinary.

Urese. (Roerig)
See: Benzthiazide.

urethan. Ethyl Carbamate, Ethyl Urethan, Urethane.
Use: Antineoplastic.

Urex. (3M Pharm.) Methenamine hippurate 1 g/Tab. Bot. 100s. *Rx.*
Use: Anti-infective, urinary.

U.R.I. (Sigma-Tau Pharmaceuticals, Inc.) Atropine sulfate 0.2 mg, chlorpheniramine maleate 5 mg, phenylpropanolamine HCl 12.5 mg/ml. Inj. Vial 10 ml. *Rx.*
Use: Anticholinergic, antihistamine, antispasmodic, decongestant.

Uric Acid Reagent Strips. (Bayer Corp. (Consumer Div.)) Seralyzer reagent strip. For uric acid in serum or plasma. Bot. 25s.
Use: Diagnostic aid.

uricosuric agents.
See: Anturane, Tab., Cap. (Novartis Pharmaceutical Corp.).
Benemid, Tab. (Merck & Co.).

Uricult. (Orion Diagnostica) Urine culture test to detect bacteria and identify uropathogens. Bot. 10s.
Use: Diagnostic aid.

uridine, 2-deoxy-5-iodo-. Idoxuridine, U.S.P. 23.

uridine 5'-triphosphate. (Inspire Pharmaceuticals)
Use: Cystic fibrosis; ciliany dyskinesia. [Orphan Drug]

Uridium. (Ferndale Laboratories, Inc.) Phenylazodiaminopyridine HCl 75 mg, sulfacetamide 250 mg/Tab. Bot. 30s, 100s, 1000s. (Ferndale Laboratories, Inc.) Bot. 100s.
Use: Anti-infective, urinary.

Uridon Modified. (Rugby Labs, Inc.) Methenamine 40.8 mg, phenyl salicylate 18.1 mg, atropine sulfate 0.03 mg, hyoscyamine 0.03 mg, benzoic acid 4.5 mg, methylene blue 5.4 mg/Tab. Bot. 100s, 1000s. *Rx.*
Use: Anti-infective, urinary.

Urifon-Forte. (T.E. Williams Pharmaceuticals) Sulfamethizole 450 mg, phenazopyridine HCl 50 mg/Cap. Bot. 100s, 1000s. *Rx.*
Use: Anti-infective, urinary.

Urigen. (Fellows) Calcium mandelate 0.2 g, methenamine 0.2 g, phenazopyridine HCl 50 mg, sodium phosphate 80 mg/Cap. Bot. 100s, 1000s. *Rx.*
Use: Anti-infective, urinary.

Urimar-T. (Marnel Pharmaceuticals, Inc.) Methenamine 81.6 mg, sodium biphosphate 40.8 mg, phenyl salicylate 36.2 mg, methylene blue 10.8 mg, hyoscyamine sulfate 0.12 mg. Tab. Bot. 100s. *Rx.*
Use: Anti-infective, urinary.

Urinary Antiseptic #2. (Various Mfr.) Atropine sulfate 0.03 mg, hyoscyamine 0.03 mg, methenamine 40.8 mg, methylene blue 5.4 mg, phenyl salicylate 18.1 mg, benzoic acid 4.5 mg/Tab. Bot. 100s, 1000s. *Rx.*
Use: Anti-infective, urinary.

Urinary Antiseptic #2 S.C.T. (Teva Pharmaceuticals USA) Atropine sulfate 0.03 mg, hyoscyamine sulfate 0.03 mg, methenamine 40.8 mg, methylene blue 5.4 mg, phenyl salicylate 18.1 mg, benzoic acid 4.5 mg/Tab. Bot. 100s, 1000s. *Rx.*
Use: Anti-infective, urinary.

Urinary Antiseptic #3 S.C.T.. (Teva Pharmaceuticals USA) Atropine sulfate 0.06 mg, hyoscyamine sulfate 0.03 mg, methenamine 120 mg, methylene blue 6 mg, phenyl salicylate 30 mg, benzoic acid 7.5 mg/Tab. Bot. 100s, 1000s. *Rx.*
Use: Anti-infective, urinary.

urine.
See: Diagnostic agents.

urine glucose tests.
See: Biotel Diabetes (Biotel Corp.).
Clinitest, Tab. (Bayer Corp. (Consumer Div.)).
Chemstrip uG Strips (Boehringer Mannheim Pharmaceuticals).
Clinistix Strips (Bayer Corp. (Consumer Div.)).
Diastix Strips (Bayer Corp. (Consumer Div.)).
Test Tape (Eli Lilly and Co.).

urine sugar test.
See: Clinistix (Bayer Corp. (Consumer Div.)).

urine tests misc.
See: Nitrazine Paper (Apothecon, Inc.).

Urin-Tek. (Bayer Corp. (Consumer Div.)) Tubes, plastic caps, adhesive labels, collection cups, and disposable tube holder. Package 100 × 5.

Urisan-P. (Sandia) Atropine sulfate 0.03 mg, hyoscyamine 0.03 mg, gelsemium 6.1 mg, methenamine 40.8 mg, salol 18.1 mg, benzoic acid 4.5 mg, methylene blue 5.4 mg, phenylazodiaminopyridine HCl 100 mg/Tab. Bot. 100s, 1000s. *Rx.*
Use: Anti-infective, urinary.

Urised. (PolyMedica Pharmaceuticals) Atropine sulfate 0.03 mg, hyoscyamine 0.03 mg, methenamine 40.8 mg, methylene blue 5.4 mg, benzoic acid 4.5 mg, phenyl salicylate 18.1 mg/Tab. Bot. 100s, 500s. *Rx.*
Use: Anti-infective, urinary.

Urisedamine. (PolyMedica Pharmaceuticals) Methenamine mandelate 500 mg, l-hyoscyamine 0.15 mg/Tab. Bot. 100s. *Rx.*
Use: Anti-infective, urinary.

Urispas. (SmithKline Beecham Pharmaceuticals) Flavoxate HCl 100 mg/Tab. Bot. 100s, UD 100s. *Rx.*
Use: Urinary antispasmodic.

Uristix. (Bayer Corp. (Consumer Div.)) Urine test for glucose and protein. Reagent strips. 100s.
Use: Diagnostic aid.

Uristix 4 Reagent Strips. (Bayer Corp. (Consumer Div.)) Urinalysis reagent strip test for glucose, protein, nitrite, leukocytes. Bot. 100s.
Use: Diagnostic aid.

Uristix Reagent Strips. (Bayer Corp. (Consumer Div.)) Urinalysis reagent strip test for protein and glucose. Bot. 100s.
Use: Diagnostic aid.

Uritin. (Global Source) Methenamine 40.8 mg, atropine sulfate 0.03 mg, hyoscyamine sulfate 0.03 mg, salol 18.1 mg, benzoic acid 4.5 mg, methylene blue 5.4 mg, gelsemium 6.1 mg/Tab. Bot. 1000s. *Rx.*
Use: Anti-infective, urinary.

Uritin Formula. (Various Mfr.) Atropine sulfate 0.03 mg, hyoscyamine 0.03 mg, methenamine 40.8 mg, methylene blue 5.4 mg, phenyl salicylate 18.1 mg, benzoic acid 4.5 mg/Tab. Bot. 1000s. *Rx.*
Use: Anti-infective, urinary.

Urobak. (Shionogi USA) Sulfamethoxazole 500 mg/Tab. Bot. 100s, 1000s. *Rx.*
Use: Anti-infective, sulfonamide.

Urocit-K. (Mission Pharmacal Co.) Potassium citrate. **540 mg:** Tab. Bot. 100s; **10 mEq:** Tab. Bot. 100s. *Rx.*
Use: Genitourinary.

•**urofollitropin.** (YOUR-oh-fahl-ih-TROE-pin) USAN.
Use: Hormone (follicle-stimulating). Ovulation. [Orphan Drug]
See: Fertinex, Pow. For Inj. (Serono Laboratories, Inc.).
Metrodin, Inj. (Serono Laboratories, Inc.).

urogastrone. (Chiron Vision)
Use: Corneal transplant surgery. [Orphan Drug]

Urogesic. (Edwards Pharmaceuticals, Inc.) Phenazopyridine HCl 100 mg, hyoscyamine HBr 0.12 mg, atropine sulfate 0.08 mg, scopolamine HBr 0.003 mg/Tab. Bot. 100s, 500s. *Rx.*
Use: Analgesic, urinary.

Urogesic Blue. (Edwards Pharmaceuticals, Inc.) Methenamine 81.6 mg, sodium biphosphate 40.8 mg, phenyl salicylate 36.2 mg, methylene blue 10.8 mg, hyoscyamine (as sulfate) 0.12 mg. Tab. Bot. 100s. *Rx.*
Use: Anti-infective, urinary.

urography agents.
See: Iodohippurate Sodium, Inj.
Iodopyracet.
Iodopyracet Compound.
Methiodal, Inj.
Renografin (Bristol-Myers Squibb).
Renovist (Bristol-Myers Squibb).
Renovue (Bristol-Myers Squibb).
Sodium Acetrizoate, Inj.
Sodium Iodomethamate, Inj.

•**urokinase.** (YOUR-oh-KIN-ace) USAN. Plasminogen activator isolated from human kidney tissue.
Use: Plasminogen activator.

•**urokinase alfa.** USAN.
Use: Thrombolytic (plasminogen activator).

Uro-KP-Neutral. (Star Pharmaceuticals, Inc.) Na (as dibasic sodium phosphate) 1361 mg, K 298.6 mg, P (as dibasic potassium phosphate) 1037 mg/6 Tab. Bot. 100s. *Rx.*
Use: Mineral supplement.

Urolene Blue. (Star Pharmaceuticals, Inc.) Methylene blue 65 mg/Tab. Bot. 100s, 1000s. *Rx.*
Use: Anti-infective, urinary.

Urologic Sol G. (Abbott Hospital Products) Bot. 1000 ml.
Use: Irrigant, ophthalmic.
See: Thiosulfil, Preps. (Wyeth-Ayerst Laboratories).

Uro-Mag. (Blaine Co., Inc.) Magnesium oxide 140 mg/Cap. Bot. 100s, 1000s. *otc.*
Use: Antacid.

uronal.
See: Barbital (Various Mfr.).

Uro-Phosphate. (ECR Pharmaceuticals) Sodium biphosphate 434.78 mg, methenamine 300 mg/Film Coated Tab. Bot. 100s. *Rx.*
Use: Anti-infective, urinary.

Uroplus DS. (Shionogi USA) Trimethoprim 160 mg, sulfamethoxazole 800 mg/Tab. Bot. 100s, 500s. *Rx.*

Use: Anti-infective.

Uroplus SS. (Shionogi USA) Trimethoprim 80 mg, sulfamethoxazole 800 mg/Tab. Bot. 100s, 500s. *Rx.*
Use: Anti-infective.

Uroquid-Acid No. 2. (Beach Pharmaceuticals) Methenamine mandelate 500 mg, sodium acid phosphate monohydrate 500 mg/Tab. Bot. 100s. *Rx.*
Use: Anti-infective, urinary.

urotropin new. (Various Mfr.) Methenamine Anhydromethylene Citrate

Urovist Cysto. (Berlex Laboratories, Inc.) Diatrizoate meglumine 300 mg, edetate calcium disodium 0.05 mg/ml. Dilution Bot. 500 ml w/300 ml Soln.
Use: Radiopaque agent.

Urovist Cysto Pediatric. (Berlex Laboratories, Inc.) Diatrizoate meglumine 300 mg, edetate calcium disodium 0.1 mg/ml. Dilution bot. 300 ml w/100 ml soln.
Use: Radiopaque agent.

Urovist Meglumine DIU/CT. (Berlex Laboratories, Inc.) Diatrizoate meglumine 300 mg, edetate calcium disodium 0.05 mg/ml. Bot. 300 ml. Ctn. 10s.
Use: Radiopaque agent.

Urovist Sodium 300. (Berlex Laboratories, Inc.) Diatrizoate sodium 500 mg, edetate calcium disodium 0.1 mg/ml. Vial 50 ml, Box 10s.
Use: Radiopaque agent.

Ursinus Inlay-Tabs. (Novartis Pharmaceutical Corp.) Pseudoephedrine HCl 30 mg, aspirin 325 mg/Tab. Bot. 24s. *otc.*
Use: Decongestant, analgesic.

URSO. (Novartis Pharmaceutical Corp.) Ursodiol.
Use: Management and treatment of primary biliary cirrhosis. [Orphan Drug]

ursodeoxycholic acid.
Use: Primary biliary cirrhosis. [Orphan Drug]

•**ursodiol.** (ERR-so-DIE-ole) U.S.P. 23. Ursodeoxycholic acid.
Use: Anticholelithogenic, urolithic; management and treatment of primary biliary cirrhosis. [Orphan Drug]
See: Actigall (Axcan Pharma).
URSO (Novartis Pharmaceutical Corp.).

uterine relaxant.
See: Ritodrine HCl, Inj. (Abbott Laboratories).
Yutopar, Inj. (Astra Pharmaceuticals, L.P.).

Utimox. (Parke-Davis) Amoxicillin trihydrate. **Cap.:** 250 mg. Bot. 100s, 500s, UD 100s; 500 mg. Bot. 100s, UD 100s; **Oral susp.:** 125 mg, 250 mg/5 ml. Bot. 80 ml, 100 ml, 150 ml, 200 ml. *Rx.*
Use: Anti-infective, penicillin.

U-Tran. (Scruggs) Atropine sulfate 0.03 mg, hyoscyamine 0.03 mg, methenamine 40.8 mg, benzoic acid 4.5 mg, salol 18.1 mg, methylene blue 5.4 mg/Tab. Bot. 100s, 1000s. *Rx.*
Use: Anti-infective, urinary.

U-Tri Special Formula Ointment. (U-Tri Products, Inc.) Oint. Jar 4 oz, 7 oz.
Use: Analgesic, topical.

Uvadex. (Therakos, Inc.) Methoxsalen 20 mcg/ml. Soln. Vial 10 ml. *Rx.*
Use: Cutaneous T-cell lymphoma; sclerosis treatment; cardiac allograft rejection prevention.
See: 8-Methoxsalen.

Uvasal Powder. (Sanofi Winthrop Pharmaceuticals) Sodium bicarbonate, tartaric acid. *otc.*
Use: Antacid.

uva ursi. (Sherwood Davis & Geck) Leaves. Fluid extract. Bot. pt, gal.

Uviban. Sodium Actinoquinol.
Use: Treatment of flash burns (ophthalmic).

Uvinul MS-40. (General Aniline & Film)
See: Sulisobenzone.

V

vaccine, adenovirus. *Rx.*
Use: Immunization.
See: Adenovirus vaccine (Wyeth-Ayerst Laboratories).

vaccine, anthrax. *Rx.*
Use: Immunization.
See: Anthrax vaccine (Michigan Department of Health).

vaccine, BCG. *Rx.*
Use: Immunization.
See: TheraCys (Pasteur Merieux Connaught).
Tice BCG, Amp. (Organon Teknika Corp.).

vaccine, cholera. *Rx.*
Use: Immunization.
See: Cholera vaccine, Vial (Wyeth-Ayerst Laboratories).

vaccine, Haemophilus influenzae type B. *Rx.*
Use: Immunization.
See: ActHIB (Pasteur Merieux Connaught).
ActHIB/DTP, Set of DTwP vial plus Hib Pow. for Inj. (Pasteur Merieux Connaught).
HibTITER, Vial (Wyeth-Ayerst Laboratories).
OmniHIB, Pow. for Inj. (SmithKline Beecham Pharmaceuticals).
PedvaxHIB, Pow. for Inj. (Merck & Co.).
ProHIBIT, Vial, Syr. (Pasteur Merieux Connaught).
Tetramune, Vial (Wyeth-Ayerst Laboratories).

vaccine, hepatitis A. *Rx.*
Use: Immunization.
See: Havrix (SmithKline Beecham Pharmaceuticals).
Vaqta (Merck & Co.).

vaccine, hepatitis B. *Rx.*
Use: Immunization.
See: Engerix-B (SmithKline Beecham Pharmaceuticals).
Recombivax HB (Merck & Co.).

vaccine, influenza A & B. *Rx.*
Use: Immunization.
See: Fluogen (Parke-Davis).
FluShield (Wyeth-Ayerst Laboratories).
Fluvirin (Medeva Pharmaceuticals, Inc.).
Fluzone (Pasteur Merieux Connaught).

vaccine, Japanese encephalitis. *Rx.*
Use: Immunization.
See: JE-Vax (Pasteur Merieux Connaught).

vaccine, measles. *Rx.*
Use: Immunization.
See: Attenuvax (Merck & Co.).
W/rubella vaccine.
See: M-R II (Merck & Co.).
W/mumps and rubella vaccines.
See: M-M-R II (Merck & Co.).

vaccine, meningococcal. *Rx.*
Use: Immunization.
See: Menomune A/C/Y/W-135, Pow. for Inj. (Pasteur Merieux Connaught).

vaccine, mumps. Mumps Virus Vaccine Live, U.S.P. 23.
Use: Immunization.
See: Mumpsvax (Merck & Co.).

vaccine, pertussis. Pertussis Vaccine.
Use: Immunization.
See: Acel-Imune, Vial (Wyeth-Ayerst Laboratories).
ActHIB/DTP, Set of DTwP vial plus Hib Pow. for Inj. (Pasteur Merieux Connaught).
Diphtheria and Tetanus Toxoids with Pertussis Vaccine (Various Mfr.).
Tetramune, Vial (Wyeth-Ayerst Laboratories).
Tri-Immunol, Vial (Wyeth-Ayerst Laboratories).
Tripedia, Vial (Pasteur Merieux Connaught).

vaccine, plague.
Use: Immunization.
See: Plague vaccine (Greer Laboratories, Inc.).

vaccine, pneumococcal.
Use: Immunization.
See: Pnu-Imune 23 (Wyeth-Ayerst Laboratories).

vaccine, poliovirus.
Use: Immunization.
See: IPOL (Pasteur Merieux Connaught).
Orimune (Wyeth-Ayerst Laboratories).
Poliovirus vaccine, U.S.P. 23.

vaccine, rabies. Rabies Vaccine.
Use: Immunization.
See: Imovax Rabies (Pasteur Merieux Connaught).
RabAvert (Chiron).
Rabies vaccine adsorbed (Michigan Department of Health).

vaccine, smallpox. Smallpox Vaccine.
Use: Immunization.

vaccine, typhoid.
Use: Immunization.
See: Typhim Vi (Pasteur Merieux Connaught).
Typhoid vaccine (Wyeth-Ayerst Laboratories).
Vivotif Berna (Berna Products Corp).

vaccine, varicella.

Use: Immunization.
See: Varivax (Merck & Co.).

vaccine, whooping cough. Pertussis Vaccine, U.S.P. 23.
Use: Immunization.
See: Acel-Imune, Vial (Wyeth-Ayerst Laboratories).
ActHIB/DTP, Set of DTwP vial plus Hib Pow. for Inj. (Pasteur Merieux Connaught).
Diphtheria and Tetanus Toxoids with Pertussis Vaccine (Various Mfr.).
Tetramune, Vial (Wyeth-Ayerst Laboratories).
Tri-Immunol, Vial (Wyeth-Ayerst Laboratories).
Tripedia, Vial (Pasteur Merieux Connaught).

vaccine, yellow fever.
Use: Immunization.
See: YF-Vax (Pasteur Merieux Connaught).

•**vaccinia immune globulin.** (vax-IN-ee-ah) U.S.P. 23. *Formerly Vaccinia Immune Human Globulin.*
Use: Immunization.

vaccinia immune globulin. (Baxter Pharmaceutical Products, Inc.) Gamma globulin fraction of serum of healthy adults recently immunized w/vaccinia virus 16.5%. Vial 5 ml. *Rx.*
Use: Immunization.

vacocin. Under study.
Use: Anti-infective.

Vademin-Z. (Roberts Pharmaceuticals) Vitamin A 12,500 IU, D 50 IU, E 50 mg, B_1 10 mg, B_2 5 mg, B_3 25 mg, B_5 10 mg, B_6 2 mg, C 150 mg, Zn 2.6 mg, Mg, Mn/Cap. Bot. 60s. *otc.*
Use: Mineral, vitamin supplement.

Vagi-Gard Maximum Strength. (Lake Consumer Products) Benzocaine 20%, resorcinol 3%, methylparaben, sodium sulfite, EDTA, mineral oil. Cream 45 g. *otc.*
Use: Vaginal agent.

Vagifem. (Novo Nordisk) Estradiol hemihydrate 25 mcg, lactose. Vaginal Tab. Single-use applicator 15s. *Rx.*
Use: Estrogen.

Vagi-Gard Advanced Sensitive Formula. (Lake Consumer Products) Benzocaine 5%, resorcinol, methylparaben, sodium sulfite, EDTA, mineral oil. Cream 45 g. *otc.*
Use: Vaginal agent.

Vaginex. (Durex) Tripelennamine HCl. Cream Tube 30 g, 300 g. *otc.*
Use: Vaginal agent.

Vagisec Plus Suppositories. (Durex) Polyoxyethylene nonylphenol 5.25 mg, sodium edetate 0.66 mg, docusate sodium 0.07 mg, aminoacridine HCl 6 mg. Box 28s. *Rx.*
Use: Vaginal agent.

Vagisil. (Combe, Inc.) Benzocaine and resorcin with lanolin alcohol, parabens, trisodium HEDTA, mineral oil, sodium sulfite. Creme. 30 g, 60 g. *otc.*
Use: Vaginal agent.

Vagisil Powder. (Combe, Inc.) Cornstarch, aloe, mineral oil, benzethonium chloride, magnesium stearate, silica, fragrance. Pow. 198 g, 312 g. *otc.*
Use: Vaginal agent.

Vagistat-1. (Bristol-Myers Squibb) Tioconazole 6.5%. Vaginal Oint. Prefilled applicator 4.6 g. *otc.*
Use: Antifungal, vaginal.

Valacet. (Pal-Pak, Inc.) Hyoscyamus 10.8 mg, aspirin 259.2 mg, caffeine anhydrous 16.2 mg, gelsemium extract 0.6 mg/Tab. or Cap. Bot. 100s, 1000s, 5000s. *Rx.*
Use: Analgesic, anticholinergic, antispasmodic.

•**valacyclovir hydrochloride.** (val-lay-SIGH-kloe-vihr) USAN.
Use: Antiviral.
See: Valtrex, Tab. (GlaxoWellcome).

Valergen 20. (Hyrex) Estradiol Valerate in oil 20 mg/ml, castor oil, benzyl benzoate, benzyl alcohol. Inj. Multi-dose vial 10 ml. *Rx.*
Use: Estrogen.

Valerian. (Eli Lilly and Co.) Tincture, alcohol 68%. Bot. 4 fl oz, 16 fl oz.

Valertest. (Hyrex Pharmaceuticals) **No. 1:** Estradiol valerate 4 mg, testosterone enanthate 90 mg/ml. Vial 10 ml. **No. 2:** Double strength. Vial 10 ml. Amp. 2 ml, 10s. *Rx.*
Use: Androgen, estrogen combination.

valethamate bromide.
Use: Anticholinergic.

•**valganciclovir hydrochloride.** (val-gan-SIGH-kloe-veer HIGH-droe-KLOR-ide) USAN.
Use: Antiviral.

•**valine.** (VAY-leen) U.S.P. 23.
Use: Amino acid.

valine, isoleucine, and leucine.
Use: Hyperphenylalaninemia. [Orphan Drug]
See: VIL (Leas Research).

Valisone. (Schering-Plough Corp.) Betamethasone valerate. **Cream:** 1 mg/g Hydrophilic cream of water, mineral oil, petrolatum, polyethylene glycol 1000 monocetyl ether, cetostearyl alcohol, monobasic sodium phosphate, phos-

phoric acid, 4-chloro-m-cresol as preservative. Tube 15 g, 45 g, 110 g. Jar 430 g. **Oint.:** 1 mg/g base of liquid and white petrolatum and hydrogenated lanolin. Tube 15 g, 45 g. **Lot.:** 1 mg/g w/isopropyl alcohol 47.5%, water slightly thickened w/carboxyvinyl polymer, pH adjusted w/sodium hydroxide. Bot. 20 ml, 60 ml. **Reduced Strength Cream 0.01%:** Hydrophilic cream of water, mineral oil, petrolatum, polyethylene glycol 1000 monocetyl ether, cetostearyl alcohol, monobasic sodium phosphate, phosphoric acid, 4-chloro-m-cresol as preservative. Tube 15 g, 60 g. *Rx.*
Use: Corticosteroid, topical.

Valium Injection. (Roche Laboratories) Diazepam 5 mg/ml, propylene glycol 40%, ethyl alcohol 10%, sodium benzoate 5%, benzoic acid, benzyl alcohol 1.5%. Amp. 2 ml. Vial 10 ml. *Tel-E-Ject.* (Disposable syringe) 2 ml. *c-IV.*
Use: Anxiolytic; anticonvulsant.

Valium Tablets. (Roche Laboratories) Diazepam 2 mg, 5 mg, 10 mg/Tab. Bot. 100s, 500s, UD 100s. *c-IV.*
Use: Anxiolytic.

vallergine.
See: Promethazine HCl, U.S.P. 23.

Valnac Cream. (NMC Laboratories) Betamethasone valerate 0.1%. Cream Tube 15 g, 45 g. *Rx.*
Use: Corticosteroid, topical.

Valnac Ointment. (NMC Laboratories) Betamethasone valerate 0.1%. Oint. Tube 15 g, 45 g. *Rx.*
Use: Corticosteroid, topical.

•**valnoctamide.** (val-NOCK-tah-mid) USAN.
Use: Anxiolytic.

•**valproate sodium.** (VAL-pro-ate) USAN.
Use: Anticonvulsant.

•**valproic acid.** (VAL-pro-ik acid) U.S.P. 23.
Use: Anticonvulsant, antimigraine.
See: Depakene, Cap., Liq. (Abbott Laboratories).
Depakote (Abbott Laboratories).
Myproic Acid, Syr. (Rosemont Pharmaceutical Corp.).
Valproic acid (Various Mfr.).

valproic acid. (Various Mfr.) **Cap.:** Valproic acid 250 mg. Bot. 100s, 250s, 500s. **Syrup:** 250 mg/5 ml. Cups. 50 ml, 480 ml, UD 5 ml. *Rx.*
Use: Anticonvulsant.

valrubicin.
Use: Antibiotic.
See: ValStar, Soln. (Medeva).

•**valsartan.** (VAL-sahr-tan) USAN.
Use: Antihypertensive.
See: Diovan, Cap. (Novartis Pharmaceutical Corp.).
W/Hydrochlorothiazide.
See: Diovan HCT (Novartis).

Valstar. (Medeva) Valrubicin 40 mg/ml. Soln. for intravesical instillation. Preservative free, in *Cremophor EL*/dehydrated alcohol. Single-use vial. 5 ml. *Rx.*
Use: Antibiotic.

Valtrex. (GlaxoWellcome) Valacyclovir HCl 500 mg/Capl. Bot. 42s, 60s, UD 100s. *Rx.*
Use: Antiviral.

Valuphed. (H.L. Moore Drug Exchange, Inc.) Pseudoephedrine HCl 60 mg, triprolidine HCl 2.5 mg/Tab. Pkg. 24s. *otc.*
Use: Antihistamine, decongestant.

Vamate. (Major Pharmaceuticals) Hydroxyzine pamoate 50 mg/Cap. Bot. 100s, 250s, 500s, UD 100s. *Rx.*
Use: Anxiolytic.

Vanadryx TR. (Vangard Labs, Inc.) Dexbrompheniramine maleate 6 mg, pseudoephedrine sulfate 120 mg/Tab. Bot. 100s, 500s. *Rx.*
Use: Antihistamine, decongestant.

Vancenase. (Schering) Beclomethasone dipropionate. Each actuation delivers 42 mcg. Canister 6.7 g (≥ 80 metered doses per canister), 16.8 g (≥ 200 metered doses per canister) w/nasal adapter. *Rx.*
Use: Corticosteroid, nasal.

Vancenase AQ. (Schering) Beclomethasone dipropionate monohydrate 0.084%, benzalkonium chloride, dextrose, polysorbate 80. Bot. 19 g (≥ 120 metered doses per bot.) w/metered spray pump. *Rx.*
Use: Corticosteroid, nasal.

Vancenase Pockethaler. (Schering) Beclomethasone dipropionate contains ≈ 42 mcg/actuation. Aerosol. 7 g canisters w/adapter (≥ 200 metered doses).
Use: Corticosteroid, nasal.

Vanceril. (Schering) Beclomethasone dipropionate. Metered-dose aerosol unit. Each actuation delivers ≈ 42 mcg. Aerosol. Canister 6.7 g, 16.8 g (200 metered doses) w/adapter. *Rx.*
Use: Corticosteroid.

Vanceril Double Strength. (Schering/Key) Beclomethasone dipropionate. Metered-dose aerosol unit. Each actuation delivers ≈ 84 mcg. Aerosol. Canister 5.4 g (40 metered doses), 12.2 g (120 metered doses). *Rx.*

Use: Corticosteroid.

Vancocin. (Eli Lilly and Co.) Vancomycin. **Pulvules:** 125 mg, 250 mg. *Identi-Dose* 20s. **Pow. for Oral Soln.:** 1 g, 10 g, Bot. **Pow. for Inj.:** 500 g, 1 g, 10 g. Vials 10 ml, *ADD-Vantage* Vial 15 ml (500 mg); Vials 20 ml *ADD-Vantage* Vials 15 ml (1 g only); Vial 100 ml (10 g only). *Rx.*
Use: Anti-infective.

Vancoled. (ESI Lederle Generics) Vancomycin 500, 1 g, 5 g. Vial (500 mg, 1 g only). Bulk pkg. (5 g only). *Rx.*
Use: Anti-infective.

•**vancomycin.** (van-koe-MY-sin) U.S.P. 23.
Use: Anti-infective.

•**vancomycin hydrochloride.** (van-koe-MY-sin) U.S.P. 23. An antibiotic from *Streptomyces orientalis.*
Use: (IV) Gram-positive (staph.) infection; anti-infective.
See: Vancocin, Prods. (Eli Lilly and Co.).
Vancoled, Vial (ESI Lederle Generics).

vancomycin hydrochloride. (Various Mfr.) Vancomycin. **Pow. for Oral Soln.:** 1 g. Bot. **Pow. for Inj.:** 500 mg, 1 g, 5 g, 10 g. Vial. 100 ml Vial (5 g only). *Rx.*
Use: Anti-infective.

Vancor Intravenous. (Pharmacia & Upjohn) Vancomycin HCl 500 mg, 1 g. Pow. for Inj. Vials.
Use: Anti-infective.

Vanex Expectorant Liquid. (Jones Medical Industries, Inc.) Pseudoephedrine HCl 30 mg, hydrocodone bitartrate 2.5 mg, guaifenesin 100 mg/5 ml, alcohol 5%, glucose, saccharin, sorbitol, sucrose, tartrazine. Tropical fruit punch flavor. Liq. Bot. 473 ml. *c-III.*
Use: Antitussive, decongestant, expectorant.

Vanex Forte. (Jones Medical Industries, Inc.) Phenylpropanolamine HCl 50 mg, phenylephrine HCl 10 mg, chlorpheniramine maleate 4 mg, pyrilamine maleate 25 mg/5 ml, lactose, sugar. Cap. Bot. 100s. *Rx.*
Use: Antihistamine, decongestant.

Vanex Forte-R. (Jones Medical) Phenylpropanolamine HCl 75 mg, chlorpheniramine maleate 12 mg/ER Cap. Bot. 100s. *Rx.*
Use: Antihistamine, decongestant.

Vanex-HD. (Jones Medical Industries, Inc.) Phenylephrine HCl 5 mg, chlorpheniramine maleate 2 mg, hydrocodone bitartrate 1.67 mg/5 ml. Liq. Bot. Pt. gal. *c-III.*
Use: Antitussive, decongestant.

Vanicream. (Pharmaceutical Specialties, Inc.) Oil in water vanishing cream containing white petrolatum, cetearyl alcohol, ceteareth-20, sorbitol, propylene glycol, simethicone, glyceryl monostearate, polyethylene glycol monostearate, sorbic acid. Oint. 1 lb. *otc.*
Use: Pharmaceutical aid, ointment base.

vanilla. N.F. XVII.
Use: Pharmaceutic aid (flavor).

vanillal.
See: Ethyl Vanillin.

•**vanillin.** (vah-NILL-in) N.F. 18.
Use: Pharmaceutic aid (flavor).

vanirome.
See: Ethyl Vanillin.

Vanoxide. (Dermik Laboratories, Inc.) Benzoyl peroxide 5%, cetyl alcohol, lanolin alcohol, parabens, EDTA, calcium phosphate 64%, silica 1%, mineral oil. Bot. 25 ml, 50 ml. *otc.*
Use: Dermatologic, acne.

Vanoxide-HC. (Dermik Laboratories, Inc.) Hydrocortisone alcohol 0.5%, benzoyl peroxide 5% in lotion w/same ingredients as Vanoxide. Bot. 25 g. *Rx.*
Use: Dermatologic, acne.

Vanquish. (Bayer Corp. (Consumer Div.)) Aspirin 227 mg, acetaminophen 194 mg, caffeine 33 mg, dried aluminum hydroxide gel 25 mg, magnesium hydroxide 50 mg/Tab. Bot. 30s, 60s, 100s. *otc.*
Use: Analgesic combination, antacid.

Vansil. (Pfizer US Pharmaceutical Group) Oxamniquine 250 mg/Cap. Bot. 24s. *Rx.*
Use: Anthelmintic.

Vantin. (Pharmacia & Upjohn) Cefpodoxime proxetil, lactose. **Tab.:** 100 mg, 200 mg. Bot. 20s, 100s, UD 100s. **Gran. for Susp.:** 50 mg/5 ml, 100 mg/5 ml. Sucrose, lemon creme flavor. Bot. 50 ml, 75 ml, 100 ml. *Rx.*
Use: Anti-infective.

•**vapiprost hydrochloride.** (VAP-ih-prahst) USAN.
Use: Antagonist (thromboxane A_2).

Vapocet Tablets. (Major Pharmaceuticals) Hydrocodone 5 mg, acetaminophen 500 mg/Tab. Bot. 100s. *c-III.*
Use: Analgesic combination, narcotic.

Vaponefrin Solution. (Medeva Pharmaceuticals, Inc.) A 2.25% solution of bioassayed racemic epinephrine as HCl, chlorobutanol 0.5%. Vial 7.5 ml, 15 ml, 30 ml. *otc.*
Use: Bronchodilator.

Vaporizer in a Bottle. (Columbia Laboratories, Inc.) Wick-dispensed medicated vapors.
Use: Cough, cold, sinus, hayfever preparation.

Vapor Lemon Sucrets. (SmithKline Beecham Pharmaceuticals) Dyclonine HCl 2 mg, corn syrup, sucrose. Loz. Pkg. 18s. *otc.*
Use: Mouth and throat preparation.

VapoRub. (Procter & Gamble Pharm.)
See: Vicks Vaporub (Procter & Gamble Pharm).

Vaposteam. (Procter & Gamble Pharm.)
See: Vicks Vaposteam (Procter & Gamble Pharm.).

•**vapreotide.** (vap-REE-oh-tide) USAN.
Use: Antineoplastic.

Vaqta. (Merck & Co.) **Adult:** Hepatitis A antigen 50 U/ml, Inj. Vial. Single-use (1s and 5s). Syringe. Single-use (1s and 5s). **Pediatric/Adolescent:** Hepatitis A antigen 25 U/0.5 ml, Inj. Vial. Single-use (1s and 5s). Syringe. Single-use (1s and 5s). *Rx.*
Use: Immunization, hepatitis A.

varicella virus vaccine.
Use: Immunization.
See: Varivax, Inj. (Merck & Co.).

varicella-zoster IgG IFA test system. (Wampole Laboratories) Test for the qualitative or semi-qualitative detection of VZ IgG antibody in human serum. Test kit 100s.
Use: Diagnostic aid.

•**varicella-zoster immune globulin.** U.S.P. 23.
Use: Immunization.

varicella-zoster immune globulin, human. (Mass. Public Health Bio. Lab.) Varicella-zoster virus antibody 125 units $\leq$ 2.5 ml. Vial, single-dose. *Rx.*
Use: Immunization.

Vari-Flavors. (Ross Laboratories) Flavor packets to provide flavor variety for patients on liquid diets. Dextrose, artificial flavor, artificial color. Packet 1 g, Ctn. 24s. *Rx.*
Use: Flavoring.

Variplex-C. (NBTY, Inc.) Vitamins B_1 15 mg, B_2 10 mg, B_3 100 mg, B_5 20 mg, B_6 5 mg, B_{12} 10 mcg, C 500 mg/Tab. Bot. 100s. *otc.*
Use: Vitamin supplement.

Varivax. (Merck & Co.) Varicella virus vaccine. 1350 PFU of Oka/Merck varicella virus (live). Inj. Single-dose vials (1s, 10s). *Rx.*
Use: Immunization.

Vascor. (Ortho McNeil Pharmaceutical) Bepridil HCl 200 mg, 300 mg, 400 mg/Tab. Bot. 90s, UD 100s. *Rx.*
Use: Antianginal.

Vascoray. (Mallinckrodt Chemical) Iothalamate meglumine 520 mg, iothalamate sodium 260 mg, iodine 400 mg/ml. Vial 50 ml. *Rx.*
Use: Radiopaque agent.

Vascunitol. (Apco) Mannitol hexanitrate 0.5 gr/Tab. Bot. 100s. *Rx.*
Use: Vasodilator.

Vascused. (Apco) Mannitol hexanitrate 0.5 gr, phenobarbital 0.25 gr/Tab. Bot. 100s. *Rx.*
Use: Vasodilator.

Vaseline Dermatology Formula Cream. (Chesebrough-Ponds USA, Inc.) Petrolatum, mineral oil, dimethicone. Jar 3 oz, 5.25 oz. *otc.*
Use: Emollient.

Vaseline Dermatology Formula Lotion. (Chesebrough-Ponds USA, Inc.) Petrolatum, mineral oil, dimethicone. Bot. 5.5 oz, 11 oz, 16 oz. *otc.*
Use: Emollient.

Vaseline First Aid Carboxylated Petroleum Jelly. (Chesebrough-Ponds USA, Inc.) Petrolatum, chloroxylenol. Plastic Jar 1.75 oz, 3.75 oz. Plastic Tube 1 oz, 2.5 oz. *otc.*
Use: Medicated anti-infective.

Vaseline Intensive Care Active Sport. (Chesebrough-Ponds USA, Inc.) Ethylhexyl p-methoxycinnamate, oxybenzone. PABA free. **SPF 8:** Lot. Bot. 120 ml. **SPF 15:** Lot. Bot. 120 ml. *otc.*
Use: Sunscreen.

Vaseline Intensive Care Baby SPF 15. (Chesebrough-Ponds USA, Inc.) Titanium dioxide. PABA free. Waterproof. Lot. Bot. 120 ml. *otc.*
Use: Sunscreen.

Vaseline Intensive Care Baby SPF 30. (Chesebrough-Ponds USA, Inc.) Ethylhexyl p-methoxycinnamate, oxybenzone, 2-ethylhexyl salicylate, titanium dioxide, C12-15 alkyl benzoate, glycerin, aloe vera gel, vitamin E, cetyl alcohol, parabens, EDTA. Lot. Bot. 118 ml. *otc.*
Use: Sunscreen.

Vaseline Intensive Care Blockout SPF 30. (Chesebrough-Ponds USA, Inc.) Ethylhexyl p-methoxycinnamate, oxybenzone, 2-ethylhexyl salicylate, titanium dioxide. Waterproof. Lot. Bot. 120 ml. *otc.*
Use: Sunscreen.

Vaseline Intensive Care Blockout SPF 40+. (Chesebrough-Ponds USA, Inc.) Padimate O, ethylhexyl p-methoxycinnamate, oxybenzone, 2-ethylhexyl

salicylate, titanium dioxide. Waterproof. Lot. Bot. 120 ml. *otc.*
Use: Sunscreen.

Vaseline Intensive Care Moisturizing Sunscreen. (Chesebrough-Ponds USA, Inc.) Ethylhexyl p-methoxycinnamate, oxybenzone, C12-15 alkyl octanoate, glycerin, aloe vera gel, cetyl alcohol, petrolatum, vitamin E, parabens, EDTA. **SPF4, SPF8:** Lot. Bot. 117 ml. *otc.*
Use: Sunscreen.

Vaseline Intensive Care No Burn No Bite SPF 8. (Chesebrough-Ponds USA, Inc.) Ethylhexyl p-methoxycinnamate, oxybenzone. PABA free. Waterproof. Lot. Bot. 180 ml. *otc.*
Use: Sunscreen.

Vaseline Intensive Care Sport Sunblock. (Chesebrough-Ponds USA, Inc.) Ethylhexyl p-methoxycinnamate, oxybenzone, C12-15 alkyl benzoate, aloe vera gel, vitamin E, EDTA. Lot. Bot. 118 ml. *otc.*
Use: Sunscreen.

Vaseline Intensive Care Sunblock. (Chesebrough-Ponds USA, Inc.) Ethylhexyl p-methoxycinnamate, oxybenzone, 2-ethylhexyl salicylate. PABA free. Waterproof. **SPF 4:** Lot. Bot. 180 ml; **SPF 8:** Lot. Bot. 120 ml, 180 ml; **SPF 15:** Lot. Bot. 120 ml, 180 ml; **SPF 25:** Lot. Bot. 120 ml, 180 ml. *otc.*
Use: Sunscreen.

Vaseline Intensive Care Ultra Violet Daily Defense. (Chesebrough-Ponds USA, Inc.) Ethylhexyl p-methoxycinnamate, oxybenzone, vitamin E, cetyl alcohol, acetylated lanolin, alcohol, parabens, EDTA. SPF 15. Lot. Bot. 118 ml. *otc.*
Use: Sunscreen.

Vaseline Pure Petroleum Jelly Skin Protectant. (Chesebrough-Ponds USA, Inc.) White petrolatum. Tube 1 oz, 2.5 oz. Jar 1.75 oz, 3.75 oz, 7.75 oz, 13 oz. *otc.*
Use: Dermatologic, counterirritant.

Vaseretic 10-25. (Merck & Co.) Enalapril maleate 10 mg, hydrochlorothiazide 25 mg. Tab. Bot. 100s. *Rx.*
Use: Antihypertensive.

Vasimid.
See: Tolazoline HCl, U.S.P. 23.

vasoactive intestinal polypeptide. (Research Triangle Pharmaceuticals)
Use: Treatment of acute esophageal food impaction. [Orphan Drug]

Vasocidin Ophthalmic Ointment. (Ciba Vision) Prednisolone acetate 0.5%, sulfacetamide sodium 10%. Tube 3.5 g. *Rx.*
Use: Anti-infective; corticosteroid, ophthalmic.

Vasocidin Ophthalmic Solution. (Ciba Vision) Prednisolone sodium phosphate 0.25%, sulfacetamide sodium 10%. Bot. 5 ml, 10 ml. *Rx.*
Use: Anti-infective; corticosteroid, ophthalmic.

Vasocine. (Ciba Vision) Prednisolone acetate 0.5%, sulfacetamide sodium 10%, mineral oil, white petrolatum, parabens. Oint. Tube 3.5 g. *Rx.*
Use: Ophthalmic.

VasoClear. (Ciba Vision) Naphazoline HCl 0.02%. Bot. 15 ml. *otc.*
Use: Mydriatic, vasoconstrictor.

VasoClear A. (Ciba Vision) Naphazoline HCl 0.02%. Bot. 15 ml. *otc.*
Use: Mydriatic, vasoconstrictor.

Vasocon-A Ophthalmic Solution. (Ciba Vision) Naphazoline HCl 0.05%, antazoline phosphate 0.5%. Bot. 15 ml. *Rx.*
Use: Mydriatic, vasoconstrictor.

Vasocon Regular. (Ciba Vision) Naphazoline HCl 0.1%. Bot. 15 ml. *Rx.*
Use: Mydriatic, vasoconstrictor.

Vasoderm. (Taro Pharmaceuticals USA, Inc.) Fluocinonide 0.05%, anhydrous glycerin base. Cream Tube 15 g, 30 g, 60 g. *Rx.*
Use: Corticosteroid, topical.

Vasoderm-E. (Taro Pharmaceuticals USA, Inc.) Fluocinonide 0.05%, emollient mineral oil and white petrolatum base. Cream Tube 15 g, 30 g, 60 g, 120 g. *Rx.*
Use: Corticosteroid, topical.

Vasodilan. (Bristol-Myers Squibb) Isoxsuprine HCl 10 mg, 20 mg/Tab. **10 mg:** Bot. 100s, 1000s, UD 100s. **20 mg:** Bot. 100s, 500s, 1000s, UD 100s. *Rx.*
Use: Vasodilator.

vasodilators.
See: Amyl Nitrite.
Apresoline, Tab., Amp. (Novartis Pharmaceutical Corp.).
Cardilate, Tab. (GlaxoWellcome).
Erythrityl Tetranitrate, Tab.
Glyceryl Trinitrate Preps.
Isordil, Tab. (Wyeth-Ayerst).
Mannitol Hexanitrate.
Nitroglycerin.
Peritrate, Tab. (Parke-Davis).
Sodium Nitrate.
Sorbitrate, Tab. (Zeneca Pharmaceuticals).
Vasodilan, Tab., Amp. (Bristol-Myers Squibb).

vasodilators, coronary.

See: Glyceryl Trinitrate, Preps. (Various Mfr.).
Isordil, Tab. (Wyeth-Ayerst).
Khellin (Various Mfr.).
Papaverine, Inj., Tab. (Various Mfr.).
Pentaerythritol Tetranitrate, Tab.
Peritrate, Tab. (Parke-Davis).
Sorbitrate, Tab. (Zeneca Pharmaceuticals).

Vasoflo. (Roberts Pharmaceuticals) Papaverine HCl 150 mg/Cap. Bot. 100s. *Rx.*
Use: Vasodilator.

Vasolate. (Parmed Pharmaceuticals, Inc.) Pentaerythritol tetranitrate 30 mg/Cap. Bot. 100s, 1000s. *Rx.*
Use: Antianginal.

Vasolate-80. (Parmed Pharmaceuticals, Inc.) Pentaerythritol tetranitrate 80 mg/Cap. Bot. 100s, 1000s. *Rx.*
Use: Antianginal.

•**vasopressin.** (VAY-so-PRESS-in) U.S.P. 23. Beta-hypophamine. Posterior pituitary pressor hormone.
Use: Hormone (antidiuretic).
See: Pitressin, Amp. (Parke-Davis).

vasopressin. (American Regent) 20 pressor units/ml, chlorobutanol 0.5%. Inj. Vial. 0.5 ml, 1 ml, 10 ml. *Rx.*
Use: Hormone.

Vasosulf. (Ciba Vision) Sulfacetamide sodium 15%, phenylephrine HCl 0.125%. Bot. 5 ml, 15 ml. *Rx.*
Use: Anti-infective; decongestant, ophthalmic.

Vasotec. (Merck & Co.) Enalapril maleate 2.5 mg, 5 mg, 10 mg, 20 mg, lactose/Tab. **2.5 mg:** Bot. 100s, 1000s, 10,000s, UD 100s, unit-of-use 90s, 180s. **5 mg, 10 mg:** 100s, 1000s, 4000s, 10,000s, UD 100s, unit-of-use 90s, 180s. **20 mg:** 100s, 1000s, 10,000s, UD 100s, unit-of-use 90s. *Rx.*
Use: Antihypertensive.

Vasotec I.V. (Merck & Co.) Enalaprilat 1.25 mg/ml, benzyl alcohol 9 mg. Inj. Vial 1 ml, 2 ml. *Rx.*
Use: Antihypertensive.

Vasotus Liquid. (Sheryl) Codeine phosphate 1/6 gr, phenylephrine HCl, prophenpyridamine maleate. Liq. Bot. Pt. *c-v.*
Use: Antihistamine, antitussive, decongestant.

Vasoxyl. (GlaxoWellcome) Methoxamine HCl 0.1%. Inj. 20 mg/ml. *Rx.*
Use: Vasoconstrictor.

Vaxsyn HIV-1. (MicroGeneSys, Inc.) T-Lymphotropic Virus Type III GP 160 Antigen.
Use: AIDS. [Orphan Drug]

Vazosan. (Sandia) Papaverine HCl 150 mg/Tab. Bot. 100s, 1000s. *Rx.*
Use: Vasodilator.

VCF. (Apothecus, Inc.) Contraceptive film: nonoxynol-9 28%, glycerin, and polyvinyl alcohol. Pkg. 3s, 6s, 12s. *otc.*
Use: Contraceptive, spermicide.

V-Cillin K. (Eli Lilly and Co.) Penicillin V potassium 125 mg, 250 mg, 500 mg/Tab. **125 mg:** Bot. 100s. **250 mg:** Bot. 100s, 500s. **500 mg:** Bot. 24s, 100s, 500s. *Rx.*
Use: Anti-infective, penicillin.

V-Cillin K for Oral Solution. (Eli Lilly and Co.) Penicillin V potassium 125 mg, 250 mg/5 ml. **125 mg:** Bot. 100 ml, 150 ml, 200 ml, UD 5 ml. **250 mg:** Bot. 100 ml, 150 ml, 200 ml. *Rx.*
Use: Anti-infective, penicillin.

V-Dec-M. (Seatrace Pharmaceuticals, Inc.) Pseudoephedrine HCl 120 mg, guaifenesin 500 mg/SR Tab. Bot. 100s. *Rx.*
Use: Decongestant, expectorant.

VDRL Antigen. (Laboratory Diagnostics) VDRL antigen with buffered saline. Blood test in diagnosis of syphilis. **Vial:** Sufficient for 500 tests. **Amp.:** 10 × 0.5 ml sufficient for 500 tests.
Use: Diagnostic aid.

VDRL Slide Test. (Laboratory Diagnostics) VDRL antigen. Slide flocculation and spinal fluid test for syphilis. Vial 5 ml Complete kit, reactive control, nonreactive control, 5 ml.
Use: Diagnostic aid.

VE-400. (Western Research) Vitamin E 400 IU/Cap. Bot. 1008s. *otc.*
Use: Vitamin supplement.

Vectrin. (Warner Chilcott Laboratories) Minocycline 50 mg, 100 mg. Cap. Bot. 50s (100 mg only), 100s (50 mg only), 1000s. *Rx.*
Use: Anti-infective.

•**vecuronium bromide.** (veh-CUE-row-nee-uhm) USAN.
Use: Neuromuscular blocker.

vecuronium. (Marsam Pharmaceuticals, Inc.) Vecuronium bromide 10 mg, 20 mg/Inj. Vial 10 ml (with and without diluent), 20 ml (without diluent). *Rx.*
Use: Neuromuscular blocker.

Veetids. (Apothecon) Penicillin-V. **Pow. for Oral Soln.:** 125 mg/5 ml. Bot. 100 ml, 200 ml. **Tab.:** 250 mg, 500 mg. Bot. 100s, 1000s. *Rx.*
Use: Anti-infective, penicillin.

Veetids '250'. (Apothecon) Penicillin V 250 mg/ml, when reconstituted. Pow. for Oral Soln. Bot. 100 ml, 200 ml. *Rx.*
Use: Anti-infective, penicillin.

•**vegetable oil, hydrogenated.** N.F. 18.
Use: Pharmaceutic aid (tablet/capsule lubricant).

vehicle/n and vehicle/n mild. (Neutrogena) Topical vehicle system for compounding. Appliderm Applicator Bot. oz. *otc.*
Use: Pharmaceutical aid.

velacycline.
Use: Anti-infective, tetracycline.

Velban. (Eli Lilly and Co.) Extract from *Vinca rosea* Linn. Vinblastine sulfate, lyophilized. Vial 10 mg. *Rx.*
Use: Antineoplastic.

•**velnacrine maleate.** (VELL-NAH-kreen) USAN.
Use: Inhibitor (cholinesterase).

Velosef. (Bristol-Myers Squibb) Cephradine. **Pow. for Oral Susp.:** 125 mg, 250 mg/5 ml, sucrose, fruit flavor. Bot. 100 ml. **Cap.:** 250 mg, 500 mg. **Pow. for Inj.:** (contains 6 mEq (136 mg) sodium per g) 250 mg, 500 mg, 1 g, 2 g Vial. Infusion Bot. 100 ml (2 g only). *Rx.*
Use: Anti-infective, cephalosporin.

Velosulin Human. (Novo/Nordisk Pharm, Inc.) Human insulin injection 100 IU/ml, Vial 10 ml. *otc.*
Use: Antidiabetic.

Velvachol. (Galderma Laboratories, Inc.) Hydrophilic ointment base petrolatum, mineral oil, cetyl alcohol, cholesterol, parabens, stearyl alcohol, purified water, sodium lauryl sulfate. Jar lb. *otc.*
Use: Pharmaceutical aid, ointment base.

venesetic.
See: Amobarbital Sodium, Preps. (Various Mfr.).

venlafaxine.
Use: Antidepressant.
See: Effexor, Tab. (Wyeth-Ayerst Laboratories).
Effexor XR, ER Cap. (Wyeth-Ayerst Laboratories).

•**venlafaxine hydrochloride.** (VEN-lah-fax-EEN) USAN.
Use: Antidepressant.
See: Effexor, Tab. (Wyeth-Ayerst Laboratories).
Effexor XR, ER Cap. (Wyeth-Ayerst Laboratories).

Venoglobulin-I. (Alpha Therapeutic Corp.) Immune globulin IV (IGIV). Pow. for Inj. 500 mg. Vial 2.5 g, 5 g, 10 g. *Rx.*
Use: Immune globulin.

Venoglobulin-S. (Alpha Therapeutic Corp.) Immune globulin IV (human) 5%: Vial. 2.5 g, 5 g, 10 g. 10%: Vial 5 g, 10 g, 20 g. Solvent detergent treated. Inj. 50 ml, 100 ml, 200 ml w/sterile IV administration set. *Rx.*
Use: Immune globulin.

Venomil. (Bayer Corp. (Consumer Div.)) Freeze-dried venom or venom protein. Vials of 12 mcg or 120 mcg for honey bee, white-faced hornet, yellow hornet, yellow jacket, or wasp. Vials of 36 mcg or 360 mcg for mixed vespids (white-faced hornet, yellow hornet, yellow jacket). Diagnostic 1 mcg/ml. Maintenance 100 mcg/ml. Individual patient kit. *Rx.*
Use: Antivenin.

Venstat. (Seatrace Pharmaceuticals, Inc.) Brompheniramine maleate 10 mg/ml. Vial 10 ml. *Rx.*
Use: Antihistamine.

Ventolin Inhalation Aerosol. (GlaxoWellcome) Albuterol 90 mcg/actuation. Aerosol canister 17 g containing 200 metered inhalations and 6.8 g containing 80 metered inhalations. *Rx.*
Use: Bronchodilator.

Ventolin Inhalation Solution. (GlaxoWellcome) Albuterol sulfate 0.5%. Bot. 20 ml w/calibrated dropper. *Rx.*
Use: Bronchodilator.

Ventolin Nebules. (GlaxoWellcome) Albuterol sulfate 0.083%, sulfuric acid. Soln. for inhalation. In 3 ml unit-dose nebules. *Rx.*
Use: Bronchodilator.

Ventolin Rotacaps. (GlaxoWellcome) Microfine albuterol sulfate 200 mg, lactose. Cap. for Inh. Bot. 100s, UD 24s. For use with the Rotahaler inhalation device. *Rx.*
Use: Bronchodilator.

Ventolin Syrup. (GlaxoWellcome) Albuterol sulfate 2 mg/5 ml, saccharin, strawberry flavor. Bot. 480 ml. *Rx.*
Use: Bronchodilator.

Ventolin Tablets. (GlaxoWellcome) Albuterol sulfate 2 mg, 4 mg/Tab. Bot. 100s, 500s. *Rx.*
Use: Bronchodilator.

VePesid. (Bristol-Myers Oncology/Immunology) Etoposide. **Vial:** 100 mg/Vial. **Cap.:** 50 mg/Cap. Bot. 20s. *Rx.*
Use: Antineoplastic.

Veracolate. (Numark Laboratories, Inc.) Phenolphthalein 32.4 mg, cascara sagrada extract 75 mg, oleoresin capsicum 0.05 min/Tab. Bot. 100s. *otc.*
Use: Laxative.

•**veradoline hydrochloride.** (VEER-aid-OLE-een) USAN.
Use: Analgesic.

•**verapamil.** (veh-RAP-ah-mill) USAN.
Use: Vasodilator (coronary).

•**verapamil hydrochloride.** (veh-RAP-ah-mill) U.S.P. 23.
Use: Antianginal, antiarrhythmic, antihypertensive.
See: Calan, Tab. (Searle).
Calan SR, Capl. (Searle).
Isoptin, Inj. (Knoll Pharmaceuticals).
Isoptin SR, Tab. (Knoll Pharmaceuticals).
Verelan, SR Cap. (ESI Lederle Generics).
W/Trandolapril.
See: Tarka (Knoll).

verapamil hydrochloride. (Various Mfr.) Verapamil HCl. **40 mg/Tab.:** Bot. 100s. **80 mg, 120 mg/Tab.:** 100s, 250s, 500s, 1000s, UD 100s. **180 mg, 240 mg/SR Tab.:** 100s, 500s. **5 mg/2 ml/ Inj.:** 2 ml, 4 ml vials, amps, and syringes and 4 ml fill in 5 ml vials. *Rx.*
Use: Antianginal, antiarrhythmic, antihypertensive.
See: Calan, Tab. (Searle).
Calan SR, Tab. (Searle).
Isoptin SR, Tab. (Knoll Pharmaceuticals).
Verelan, SR Cap. (ESI Lederle Generics).

veratrum alba.
See: Protoveratrines A and B (Various Mfr.).

Verazeptol. (Femco) Chlorothymol, eucalyptol, menthol, phenol, boric acid, zinc sulfate. Pow. Bot. 3 oz, 6 oz, 10 oz. *otc.*
Use: Vaginal agent.

Verazinc. (Forest Pharmaceutical, Inc.) Zinc sulfate 220 mg/Cap. Bot. 100s, 1000s. *otc.*
Use: Mineral supplement.

Verelan. (Schwarz Pharma) Verapamil HCl 120 mg, 180 mg, 240 mg, 360 mg/SR Cap. Bot. 100s. *Rx.*
Use: Calcium channel blocker.

Vergo Ointment. (Daywell Laboratories, Inc.) Calcium pantothenate 8%, ascorbic acid 2%, starch. Tube 0.5 oz. *Rx.*
Use: Keratolytic.

Vergon. (Marnel Pharmaceuticals, Inc.) Meclizine HCl 30 mg. Cap. Bot. 100s. *otc.*
Use: Antiemetic, antivertigo.

•**verilopam hydrochloride.** (veh-RILL-OH-pam) USAN.
Use: Analgesic.

Verin. (Roberts Pharmaceuticals) Aspirin (Acetylsalicylic Acid; ASA) 650 mg/TR Tab. Bot. 100s.
Use: Analgesic.

•**verlukast.** (ver-LOO-kast) USAN.
Use: Antiasthmatic (leukotriene antagonist).

Verluma. (Neorx Corp.; Du Pont Merck Pharmaceuticals) Nofetumomab merpentan 10 mg for conjugation w/technetium 99m. Kit. *Rx.*
Use: Radioimmunoscintigraphy agent.

Vermox. (Janssen Pharmaceutical, Inc.) Mebendazole 100 mg/Tab. Box 12s. *Rx.*
Use: Anthelmintic.

vernamycins. Under study.
Use: Anti-infective.

vernolepin. A sesquiterpene dilactone. Under study.
Use: Antineoplastic.

•**verofylline.** (VER-OH-fill-in) USAN.
Use: Antiasthmatic, bronchodilator.

veronal sodium.
See: Barbital Sodium (Various Mfr.).

Versacaps. (Seatrace Pharmaceuticals, Inc.) Pseudoephedrine HCl 60 mg, guaifenesin 300 mg/Cap. Bot. 100s. *Rx.*
Use: Decongestant, expectorant.

Versal. (Suppositoria Laboratories, Inc.) Bismuth subgallate, balsam peru, zinc oxide, benzyl benzoate/Supp. Box 12s, 100s, 1000s. *otc.*
Use: Anorectal preparation.

Versa-Quat. (Ulmer Pharmacal Co.) Quaternary ammonium one-step cleaner-disinfectant-sanitizer-fungicide-virucide for general housekeeping. Bot. Gal.
Use: Cleanser, disinfectant.

Versed. (Roche Laboratories) Midazolam HCl 1 mg, 5 mg/ml, sodium Cl 0.8%, disodium edetate 0.01%, benzyl alcohol 1%. **1 mg/ml:** Vial 2 ml, 5 ml, 10 ml. Box 10s. **5 mg/ml:** Vial 1 ml, 2 ml, 5 ml, 10 ml. Box 10s. Disposable Syringe 2 ml. Box 10s. *c-IV.*
Use: Anesthetic, general.

versenate, calcium disodium.
See: Calcium Disodium Versenate, Amp. (3M Pharmaceuticals).

versenate disodium.
See: Disodium Versenate, Amp. (3M Pharmaceuticals).

•**versetamide.** (ver-SET-ah-mide) USAN.
Use: Pharmaceutic aid.

Versiclear. (Hope Pharmaceuticals) Sodium thiosulfate 25%, salicylic acid 1%, isopropyl alcohol 10%, propylene glycol, menthol, EDTA. Lot. 120 ml. *Rx.*
Use: Anti-infective, topical.

versidyne.
Use: Analgesic.

Verstran. (Parke-Davis) Prazepam.
Use: Anxiolytic.

Vertab. (Forest Pharmaceutical, Inc.) Dimenhydrinate 50 mg. Tab. Bot. 100s.
Use: Anticholinergic.

•**verteporfin.** (ver-teh-PORE-fin) USAN.
Use: Antineoplastic.

Verukan-20. (Syosset Laboratories Co., Inc.) Salicylic acid 16.7%, lactic acid in flexible collodion 16.7%. Bot. 15 ml. *otc.*
Use: Keratolytic.

Verv Alertness. (APC) Caffeine 200 mg/ Cap. Vial 15s. *otc.*
Use: CNS stimulant.

Vesanoid. (Roche Laboratories) Tretinoin 10 mg. Cap. Bot. 100s. *Rx.*
Use: Antineoplastic.

•**vesnarinone.** (VESS-nah-rih-NOHN) USAN.
Use: Cardiovascular agent.

Vesprin. (Apothecon, Inc.) Triflupromazine HCl 10 mg/ml, 20 mg/ml, benzyl alcohol 1.5%. Inj. Multidose vial. *Rx.*
Use: Antiemetic, antipsychotic.

Vetuss HC. (Cypress) Hydrocodone bitartrate 1.7 mg, phenylephrine HCl 5 mg, phenylpropanolamine HCl 3.3 mg, pyrilamine maleate 3.3 mg, pheniramine maleate 3.3 mg/5 ml, alcohol 5%, strawberry flavor. Syr. Bot. 473 ml. *c-iii.*
Use: Antitussive combination.

Vexol. (Alcon Laboratories, Inc.) Rimexolone 1%. Ophth. Susp. Drop-Tainers. 2.5 ml, 5 ml, 10 ml. *Rx.*
Use: Corticosteroid, ophthalmic.

Viacaps. (Manne) Vitamins A (soluble) 45,000 IU, C 500 mg/Cap. Bot. 60s, 120s, 1000s. *otc.*
Use: Vitamin supplement.

Viagra. (Pfizer US Pharmaceutical Group) Sildenafil citrate 25 mg, 50 mg, 100 mg, lactose/Tab. Bot. 30s, 100s. *Rx.*
Use: Anti-impotence.

Vianain. (Genzyme Corp.) Ananain, comosain.
Use: Burn treatment. [Orphan Drug]

vi antigen.
Use: Immunization.
See: Typhim Vi (Pasteur Merieux Connaught).

vibesate. Polvinate 9.3%, molrosinol 3.1% with propellant.

Vibramycin. (Pfizer US Pharmaceutical Group) Doxycycline. **Cap.:** 50 mg. Bot. 50s, UD pak 100s, X-Pack (10 Cap.) 5s; 100 mg. Bot. 50s, 500s; UD pak 100s, V-Pak (5 Cap) 5s, Nine-Pak 10s. **Pediatric Oral Susp.:** 25 mg/5 ml. Bot. 2 oz. **Syr.:** 50 mg/5 ml. Bot. oz, pt. *Rx.*
Use: Anti-infective, tetracycline.

Vibramycin IV. (Roerig) Doxycycline (as hyclate) 200 mg. Powder for Inj. Vial. *Rx.*
Use: Anti-infective, tetracycline.

Vibra-Tabs. (Pfizer US Pharmaceutical Group) Doxycycline hyclate 100 mg/ Tab. Bot. 50s, 500s, UD Pack 100s. *Rx.*
Use: Anti-infective, tetracycline.

Vicam Injection. (Keene Pharmaceuticals, Inc.) Vitamins B_1 50 mg, B_2 5 mg, B_3 125 mg, B_5 6 mg, B_6 5 mg, B_{12} 1000 mcg, C 50 mg/ml. Inj. Vial 10 ml. *Rx.*
Use: Vitamin supplement.

Vicam IV. (Keene Pharmaceuticals, Inc.) Vitamins B_1 50 mg, B_2 5 mg, B_{12} 1000 mcg, B_6 5 mg, dexpanthenol 6 mg, niacinamide 125 mg, C 50 mg/ml, benzyl alcohol 1% as preservative in water for injection. Vial, multiple-dose. *Rx.*
Use: Nutritional supplement, parenteral.

Vicks Children's Chloraseptic Lozenges. (Procter & Gamble Pharm.) Benzocaine 5 mg, corn syrup, sucrose. Grape flavor. Loz. Pkg. 18s. *otc.*

Vicks Children's Chloraseptic Spray. (Procter & Gamble Pharm.) Phenol 0.5%, saccharin, sorbitol. Alcohol free. Spray. Bot. 177 ml. *otc.*
Use: Anesthetic, antiseptic.

Vicks Children's NyQuil Nighttime Cold/Cough Liquid. (Procter & Gamble Pharm.) Pseudoephedrine HCl 10 mg, dextromethorphan HBr 5 mg, chlorpheniramine maleate 0.67 mg/5 ml, alcohol free. Bot. 120 ml, 240 ml. *otc.*
Use: Antihistamine, antitussive, decongestant.

Vicks Chloraseptic Mouthrinse/Gargle. (Procter & Gamble Pharm.) Phenol 1.4%, saccharin. Alcohol free. Liq. 355 ml. *otc.*
Use: Antiseptic.

Vicks Chloraseptic Sore Throat. (Procter & Gamble Pharm.) Benzocaine 6 mg, menthol 10 mg. Loz. Pkg. 18s. *otc.*
Use: Anesthetic.

Vicks Cough Drops. (Procter & Gamble Pharm.) Menthol. **Menthol flavor:** Benzyl alcohol, camphor, eucalyptus oil, tolu balsam, corn syrup, sucrose, thymol. **Cherry flavor:** Corn syrup, sucrose, citric acid. Box 14. Bag 40. *otc.*
Use: Mouth and throat preparation.

Vicks DayQuil Allergy Relief 4 Hour. (Procter & Gamble Pharm.) Phenylpropanolamine HCl 25 mg, brompheniramine maleate 4 mg. Tab. Pkg. 24s. *otc.*
Use: Antitussive, decongestant.

Vicks DayQuil Allergy Relief 12 Hour. (Procter & Gamble Pharm.) Phenylpropanolamine HCl 75 mg, brompheniramine maleate 12 mg/SR Tab. Pkg. 12s, 24s. *otc.*
Use: Antitussive, decongestant.

Vicks DayQuil Liquicaps. (Procter & Gamble Pharm.) Dextromethorphan HBr 10 mg, pseudoephedrine HCl 30 mg, acetaminophen 250 mg, guaifenesin 100 mg. Softgel Cap. Pkg. 12s, 20s. *otc.*
Use: Analgesic, antitussive, decongestant, expectorant.

Vicks DayQuil Liquid. (Procter & Gamble Pharm.) Pseudoephedrine HCl 60 mg, guaifenesin 200 mg, acetaminophen 650 mg, dextromethorphan HBr 20 mg/30 ml. Bot. 6 oz. *otc.*
Use: Analgesic, antitussive, decongestant, expectorant.

Vicks DayQuil Sinus Pressure & Pain Relief. (Procter & Gamble Pharm.) Pseudoephedrine HCl 30 mg, acetaminophen 500 mg. Cap. Pkg. 24s. *otc.*
Use: Analgesic, decongestant.

Vicks Dry Hacking Cough. (Procter & Gamble Pharm.) Dextromethorphan HBr 30 mg/10 ml, alcohol 10%, invert sugar. Liq. Bot. 4 oz, 8 oz w/Vicks AccuTip Dispenser. *otc.*
Use: Antitussive.

Vicks 44 Non-Drowsy Cold & Cough liquicaps. (Procter & Gamble Pharm.) Dextromethorphan HBr 30 mg, pseudoephedrine HCl 60 mg. Cap. Pkg. 10s. *otc.*
Use: Antitussive, decongestant.

Vicks 44D Cough & Decongestant Liquid. (Procter & Gamble Pharm.) Pseudoephedrine HCl 20 mg, dextromethorphan HBr 10 mg/5 ml, alcohol 10%, saccharin, sucrose. Bot. 120 ml, 240 ml. *otc.*
Use: Antitussive, decongestant.

Vicks 44D Cough & Head Congestion. (Procter & Gamble Pharm.) Dextromethorphan 10 mg, pseudoephedrine HCl 20 mg/5 ml. Liq. Bot. 5 ml. *otc.*
Use: Antitussive, decongestant.

Vicks 44D Dry Hacking-Cough and Head Congestion, Pediatric. (Procter & Gamble Pharm.) Dextromethorphan HBr 15 mg, pseudoephedrine HCl 3 mg/15 ml, alcohol free, sorbitol, sucrose, cherry flavor. Liq. Bot. 120 ml/ Vicks AccuTip Dispenser. *otc.*
Use: Antitussive, decongestant.

Vicks 44D Pediatric Cough & Decongestant Liquid. (Procter & Gamble Pharm.) Pseudoephedrine HCl 10 mg, dextromethorphan HBr 5 mg/5 ml, alcohol free. Bot. 120 ml. *otc.*
Use: Antitussive, decongestant.

Vicks 44E Liquid. (Procter & Gamble Pharm.) Dextromethorphan HBr 6.7 mg, guaifenesin 66.7 mg/5 ml. Bot. 118 ml, 236 ml. *otc.*
Use: Antitussive, expectorant.

Vicks 44E Pediatric Liquid. (Procter & Gamble Pharm.) Dextromethorphan HBr 10 mg, guaifenesin 100 mg/5 ml, sorbitol, sucrose. Alcohol free. Bot. 120 ml w/Vicks AccuTip Dispenser. *otc.*
Use: Antitussive, expectorant.

Vicks 44M Cough, Cold, and Flu Liquid. (Procter & Gamble Pharm.) Dextromethorphan HBr 30 mg, pseudoephedrine HCl 60 mg, chlorpheniramine maleate 4 mg, acetaminophen 650 mg/ 20 ml, alcohol 10%. Bot. 4 oz, 8 oz w/Vicks AccuTip Dispenser. *otc.*
Use: Analgesic, antihistamine, antitussive, decongestant.

Vicks 44M Cold, Flu & Cough Liquicaps. (Procter & Gamble Pharm.) Dextromethorphan HBr 10 mg, pseudoephedrine HCl 30 mg, chlorpheniramine maleate 2 mg, acetaminophen 250 mg. Cap. Pkg. 12s. *otc.*
Use: Analgesic, antihistamine, antitussive, decongestant.

Vicks NyQuil LiquiCaps. (Procter & Gamble Pharm.) Acetaminophen 250 mg, pseudoephedrine HCl 30 mg, dextromethorphan HBr 10 mg, doxylamine succinate 6.25 mg. Pkg. 12s, 20s. *otc.*
Use: Analgesic, antihistamine, antitussive, decongestant.

Vicks NyQuil Liquid Multi-Symptom Cold Flu Relief. (Procter & Gamble Pharm.) Acetaminophen 1000 mg, doxylamine succinate 12.5 mg, pseudoephedrine HCl 60 mg, dextromethorphan HBr 30 mg/30 ml, alcohol 10%. Regular and cherry flavors. Regular contains FD&C Yellow No. 6. Bot. 6 oz, 10 oz, 14 oz. *otc.*
Use: Analgesic, antihistamine, antitussive, decongestant.

Vicks NyQuil Multi-Symptom Cold Flu Relief. (Procter & Gamble Pharm.) Pseudoephedrine HCl 10 mg, doxylamine succinate 2.1 mg, dextromethorphan HBr 5 mg, acetaminophen 167 mg/5 ml. Alcohol 10%, sucrose, regular and cherry flavor. Liq. Bot. 180 ml, 300 ml, 420 ml. *otc.*
Use: Analgesic, antihistamine, antitussive, decongestant.

Vicks Sinex. (Procter & Gamble Pharm.) Phenylephrine HCl 0.5%, camphor,

menthol, eucalyptol, disodium EDTA. Nasal Spray. Plastic Squeeze Bot. 0.5 oz, 1 oz. *otc.*
Use: Decongestant.

Vicks Sinex 12-Hour. (Procter & Gamble Pharm.) Oxymetazoline HCl 0.05%, camphor, menthol, eucalyptol, disodium EDTA. Nasal Spray. Plastic Squeeze Bot. 1 oz, 0.5 oz. *otc.*
Use: Decongestant.

Vicks Vapor Inhaler. (Procter & Gamble Pharm.) l-Desoxyephedrine 50 mg, Special Vicks Vapors (menthol, camphor, bornyl acetate, lavender oil). Inhaler 0.007 oz (198 mg). *otc.*
Use: Decongestant.

Vicks VapoRub. (Procter & Gamble Pharm.) Camphor 4.7%, menthol 2.6%, eucalyptus oil 1.2%, cedar leaf oil, nutmeg oil. **Ointment:** Mineral oil, petrolatum. **Cream:** EDTA, glycerin, imidazolidinyl urea, cetyl alcohol, parabens, stearyl alcohol, spirits of turpentine, titanium dioxide. Cream Jar 56.7 g. *otc.*
Use: Decongestant, vaporizing agent.

Vicks Vaposteam. (Procter & Gamble Pharm.) Eucalyptus oil 1.5%, camphor 6.2%, menthol 3.2%, alcohol 74%, cedar leaf oil, nutmeg oil. Bot. 4 oz, 8 oz. *otc.*
Use: Antitussive, decongestant.

Vicks Vitamin C Drops. (Procter & Gamble Pharm.) Vitamin C 60 mg as sodium ascorbate and ascorbic acid. Orange flavor. Bag. 14s, 30s. *otc.*
Use: Vitamin supplement.

Vicodin. (Knoll Pharmaceuticals) Hydrocodone bitartrate 5 mg, acetaminophen 500 mg/Tab. Bot. 100s, 500s, UD 100s. *c-III.*
Use: Analgesic combination, narcotic.

Vicodin ES. (Knoll Pharmaceuticals) Hydrocodone bitartrate 7.5 mg, acetaminophen 750 mg/Tab. Bot. 100s, UD 100s. *c-III.*
Use: Analgesic combination, narcotic.

Vicodin HP. (Knoll Pharmaceuticals) Hydrocodone bitartrate 10 mg, acetaminophen 660 mg/Tab. Bot. 100s, 500s. *c-III.*
Use: Analgesic combination, narcotic.

Vicon-C. (UCB Pharmaceuticals, Inc.) Vitamins B_1 20 mg, B_2 10 mg, B_3 100 mg, B_5 20 mg, B_6 5 mg, C 300 mg, Mg, zinc sulfate 80 mg/Cap. Bot. 60s, UD 100s. *otc.*
Use: Mineral, vitamin supplement.

Vicon Forte. (UCB Pharmaceuticals, Inc.) Vitamins A 8000 IU, E 50 IU, C 150 mg, B_3 25 mg, B_1 10 mg, B_5 10 mg, B_2 5 mg, B_6 2 mg, B_{12} 10 mcg, folic acid 1 mg, zinc sulfate 18 mg, Mg, Mn, lactose/Cap. Bot. 60s, 500s, UD 100s. *Rx.*
Use: Mineral, vitamin supplement.

Vicon Plus. (UCB Pharmaceuticals, Inc.) Vitamins A 4000 IU, E 50 IU, C 150 mg, B_3 25 mg, B_1 10 mg, B_5 10 mg, B_2 5 mg, zinc sulfate 18 mg, Mg, Mn, lactose, B_6 2 mg/Cap. Bot. 60s. *otc.*
Use: Mineral, vitamin supplement.

Vicoprofen. (Knoll) Hydrocodone bitartrate 7.5 mg, ibuprofen 200 mg. Tab. Bot. 100s, 500s, UD 100s. *c-III.*
Use: Analgesic, narcotic.

Victors. (Procter & Gamble Pharm.) Special Vicks Medication (menthol, eucalyptus oil) in a soothing Vicks sugar base. Regular or Cherry flavor drops. Stick-Pack 10s, Bag 40s. *otc.*
Use: Anesthetic, local.

•**vidarabine.** (vih-DAR-ah-BEAN) U.S.P. 23.
Use: Antiviral.
See: Vira-A, Oint. (Monarch Pharmaceuticals).

•**vidarabine phosphate.** (vih-DAR-ah-BEAN) USAN.
Use: Antiviral.

•**vidarabine sodium phosphate.** (vih-DAR-ah-BEAN) USAN.
Use: Antiviral.

Vi-Daylin ADC Drops. (Ross Laboratories) Vitamins A 1500 IU, C 35 mg, D 400 IU/ml. Bot. 30 ml, 50 ml w/dropper. *otc.*
Use: Vitamin supplement.

Vi-Daylin ADC Vitamin + Iron Drops. (Ross Laboratories) Vitamins A 1500 IU, C 35 mg, D 400 IU, Fe 10 mg/ml, methylparaben, Bot. 50 ml. *otc.*
Use: Mineral, vitamin supplement.

Vi-Daylin Chewable. (Ross Laboratories) Vitamins A 2500 IU, D 400 IU, E 15 IU, C 60 mg, folic acid 0.3 mg, B_1 1.05 mg, B_2 1.2 mg, niacin 13.5 mg, B_6 1.05 mg, B_{12} 4.5 mcg/Tab. Bot. 100s. *otc.*
Use: Vitamin supplement.

Vi-Daylin/F Chewable Multivitamin. (Ross Laboratories) Fluoride 1 mg, vitamins A 2500 IU, D 400 IU, E 15 mg, B_1 1.05 mg, B_2 1.2 mg, B_3 13.5 mg, B_6 1.05 mg, B_{12} 4.5 mcg, C 60 mg, folic acid 0.3 mg, sucrose, cherry flavor. Chew. Tab. Bot. 100s. *Rx.*
Use: Dental caries agent, mineral, vitamin supplement.

Vi-Daylin Chewable w/Fluoride. (Ross Laboratories) Fluoride 1 mg, vitamins B_1 1.05 mg, B_2 1.2 mg, niacinamide

13.5 mg, B_6 1.05 mg, C 60 mg, A 2500 IU, B_{12} 4.5 mcg, E 15 IU, folic acid 0.3 mg, D 400 IU/Tab. Bot. 100s. *Rx.*
Use: Dental caries agent; mineral, vitamin supplement.

Vi-Daylin Drops. (Ross Laboratories) Vitamins A 1500 IU, D 400 IU, E 5 IU, C 35 mg, B_1 0.5 mg, B_2 0.6 mg, niacin 8 mg, B_6 0.4 mg, B_{12} 1.5 mcg/ml. Bot. 50 ml. *otc.*
Use: Vitamin supplement.

Vi-Daylin/F ADC Vitamins Drops. (Ross Laboratories) Vitamins A 1500 IU, D 400 IU, C 35 mg, fluoride 0.25 mg/ml. Alcohol ≈ 0.3%, parabens. Bot. 50 ml. *Rx.*
Use: Dental caries agent, vitamin supplement.

Vi-Daylin/F ADC + Iron Drops. (Ross Laboratories) Vitamins A 1500 IU, C 35 mg, D 400 IU, Fe 10 mg, fluoride 0.25 mg/ml, methylparaben. Bot. 50 ml. *Rx.*
Use: Dental caries agent; mineral, vitamin supplement.

Vi-Daylin/F Drops. (Ross Laboratories) Vitamins A 1500 IU, D 400 IU, E 5 IU, C 35 mg, B_1 0.5 mg, B_2 0.6 mg, B_3 8 mg, B_6 0.4 mg, fluoride 0.25 mg/ml, methylparaben. Bot. 50 ml. *Rx.*
Use: Dental caries agent, vitamin supplement.

Vi-Daylin/F Multivitamin + Iron. (Ross Laboratories) **Drops:** Fluoride 0.25 mg, vitamins A 1500 IU, D 400 IU, E 4.1 mg, B_1 0.5 mg, B_2 0.6 mg, B_3 8 mg, B_6 0.4 mg, C 35 mg, Fe 10 mg/ml, alcohol < 0.1%, methylparaben. Bot. 50 ml. **Chew. Tab.:** Fluoride 1 mg, vitamins A 2500 IU, D 400 IU, E 15 mg, B_1 1.05 mg, B_2 1.2 mg, B_3 13.5 mg, B_6 1.05 mg, B_{12} 4.5 mcg, C 60 mg, folic acid 0.3 mg, Fe 12 mg. Bot. 100s. *Rx.*
Use: Dental caries agent; mineral, vitamin supplement.

Vi-Daylin Liquid. (Ross Laboratories) Vitamins A 2500 IU, B_1 1.05 mg, B_2 1.2 mg, B_6 1.05 mg, B_{12} 4.5 mcg, C 60 mg, D 400 IU, E 20.4 mg (as d-alpha tocopheryl acetate), niacin 13.5 mg/5 ml. Bot. 8 oz, pt. *otc.*
Use: Vitamin supplement.

Vi-Daylin Multivitamin Drops. (Ross Laboratories) Vitamins A 1500 IU, D 400 IU, E 5 mg, B_1 0.5 mg, B_2 0.6 mg, B_3 8 mg, B_6 0.4 mg, B_{12} 1.5 mcg, C 35 mg/ml, < 0.5% alcohol. Bot. 50 ml. *otc.*
Use: Vitamin supplement.

Vi-Daylin Multivitamin Liquid. (Ross Laboratories) Vitamins A 2500 IU, D 400 IU, E 15 mg, B_1 1.05 mg, B_2 1.2 mg, B_3 13.5 mg, B_6 1.05 mg, B_{12} 4.5 mcg, C 60 mg/5 ml, ≤ 0.5% alcohol. Bot. 240, 480 ml. *otc.*
Use: Vitamin supplement.

Vi-Daylin Multivitamin + Iron Drops. (Ross Laboratories) Fe 10 mg, vitamins A 1500 IU, D 400 IU, E 5 mg, B_1 0.5 mg, B_2 0.6 mg, B_3 8 mg, B_6 0.4 mg, C 35 mg, < 0.5% alcohol, methylparaben. Bot. 50 ml. *otc.*
Use: Mineral, vitamin supplement.

Vi-Daylin Multivitamin Plus Iron Chewable. (Ross Laboratories) Vitamins A 2500 IU, D 400 IU, E 15 IU, C 60 mg, folic acid 0.3 mg, B_1 1.05 mg, B_2 1.2 mg, B_3 13.5 mg, B_6 1.05 mg, B_{12} 4.5 mcg, iron 12 mg/Tab. Bot. 100s. *otc.*
Use: Mineral, vitamin supplement.

Vi-Daylin Multivitamin Plus Iron Liquid. (Ross Laboratories) Vitamins A 2500 IU, D 400 IU, C 60 mg, E 15 IU, B_1 1.05 mg, B_2 1.2 mg, B_3 13.5 mg, B_6 1.05 mg, B_{12} 4.5 mcg, Fe 10 mg/tsp. ≤ 0.5% alcohol, glucose, sucrose, parabens. 237 ml, 473 ml. *otc.*
Use: Mineral, vitamin supplement.

Videcon. (Vita Elixir) Vitamin D 50,000 units/Cap. *Rx.*
Use: Vitamin supplement.

Vi-Derm Soap. (Arthrins) Extract of Amaryllis 10%. Cake Pkg. 1s. Bar 3.5 oz. *otc.*
Use: Dermatologic, cleanser.

•**vifilcon a.** (vie-FILL-kahn A) USAN.
Use: Contact lens material (hydrophilic).

•**vifilcon b.** (vie-FILL-kahn B) USAN.
Use: Contact lens material (hydrophilic).

Vifluorineed. (Hanlon) Vitamins A 5000 IU, D 400 IU, C 75 mg, B_1 2 mg, B_2 3 mg, niacinamide 20 mg, fluoride 1 mg/Chew. Tab. Bot. 100s. *Rx.*
Use: Mineral, vitamin supplement.

•**vigabatrin.** (vie-GAB-at RIN) USAN.
Use: Anticonvulsant (tardive dyskinesia).

Vigomar Forte. (Marlop Pharmaceuticals, Inc.) Fe 12 mg, vitamins A 10,000 IU, D 400 IU, E 15 IU, B_1 10 mg, B_2 10 mg, B_3 100 mg, B_5 20 mg, B_6 5 mg, B_{12} 5 mcg, C 200 mg, I, Mg, Mn, Cu, Zn 1.5 mg/Tab. Bot. 100s. *otc.*
Use: Mineral, vitamin supplement.

Vigortol. (Rugby Labs, Inc.) Vitamins B_1 0.8 mg, B_2 0.4 mg, B_3 8.3 mg, B_5 1.7 mg, B_6 0.2 mg, B_{12} 0.2 mcg, Fe 0.3 mg, Zn 0.3 mg, choline, I, Mg, Mn, alcohol 18%, sugar, methylparaben. Liq. Bot. 473 ml. *otc.*
Use: Mineral, vitamin supplement.

VIL. (Leas Research)

Use: Hyperphenylalaninemia. [Orphan Drug]

Vilex. (Dunhall Pharmaceuticals, Inc.) Vitamin B_1 100 mg, riboflavin phosphate sodium 1 mg, B_6 10 mg, panthenol 5 mg, niacinamide 100 mg/ml. Amp. 30 ml. *Rx.*
Use: Vitamin supplement.

Viliva. (Vita Elixir) Ferrous fumarate 3 gr. *otc.*
Use: Mineral supplement.

•**viloxazine hydrochloride.** (vih-LOX-ah-zeen) USAN.
Use: Antidepressant.
See: Catatrol (Zeneca Pharmaceuticals).

Viminate. (Various Mfr.) Vitamins B_1 2.5 mg, B_2 1.25 mg, B_3 25 mg, B_5 5 mg, B_6 0.5 mg, B_{12} 0.5 mcg, Fe 7.5 mg, Zn 1 mg, choline, I, Mg, Mn/5 ml, alcohol 18%. Liq. Bot. 480. *otc.*
Use: Mineral, vitamin supplement.

Vi-Min-for-All. (Barth's) Vitamins A 3 mg, D 10 mcg, C 120 mg, B_1 35 mg, B_{12} 15 mcg, biotin, niacin 2.33 mg, E 30 IU, B_6, pantothenic acid, Ca 375 mg, P 180 mg, Fe 20 mg, I 0.1 mg, rutin 10 mg, hesperidin-lemon bioflavonoid complex 10 mg, choline, inositol 2.4 mg, Cu 10 mcg, Mn 2 mg, Zn 110 mcg, silicone 210 mcg/Tab. Bot. 100s, 500s. *otc.*
Use: Mineral, vitamin supplement.

Vimms-38. (Health for Life Brands, Inc.) Vitamins A 12,500 IU, D 1200 IU, B_1 15 mg, B_2 10 mg, C 75 mg, niacinamide 30 mg, calcium pantothenate 2 mg, B_6 0.5 mg, E 5 IU, Brewer's yeast 10 mg, B_{12} 15 mcg, Fe 11.58 mg, desiccated liver 15 mg, choline bitartrate 30 mg, inositol 30 mg, Ca 59 mg, P 45 mg, Zn 0.68 mg, dicalcium phosphate 200 mg, Mn 1.11 mg, Mg 1 mg, K 0.68 mg, pepsin 16.5 mg, diastase 16.5 mg, yeast 40.63 mg, protein digest 23.52 mg, amino acids 34.22 mg/Cap. Bot. 50s, 100s, 1000s. *otc.*
Use: Mineral, vitamin supplement.

Vinactane Sulfate. (Novartis Pharmaceutical Corp.) Viomycin Sulfate.

•**vinafocon a.** (VIE-nah-FOE-kahn A) USAN.
Use: Contact lens material (hydrophobic).

vinbarbital.
Use: Hypnotic, sedative.

vinbarbital sodium.
Use: Hypnotic, sedative.

•**vinblastine sulfate.** (vin-BLAST-een) U.S.P. 23. Vincaleukoblastine. Alkaloid extracted from *Vinca rosea* Linn.
Use: Antineoplastic.
See: Velban, Vial (Eli Lilly and Co.).

vinblastine sulfate. (Various Mfr.) Vinblastine sulfate 10 mg. Pow. for Inj. *Rx.*
Use: Mitotic inhibitor.

vinblastine sulfate. (Fujisawa USA, Inc.) Vinblastine sulfate 1 mg/ml, 0.9% benzyl alcohol. Pow. for Inj. 10 ml. *Rx.*
Use: Antineoplastic.

vincaleukoblastine, 22-oxo-sulfate (1:1) (salt). Vincristine Sulfate, U.S.P. 23.

Vincasar PFS. (Pharmacia & Upjohn) Vincristine sulfate 1 mg/ml. Vial 1 ml. *Rx.*
Use: Antineoplastic.

•**vincofos.** (VIN-koe-foss) USAN.
Use: Anthelmintic.

•**vincristine sulfate.** (vin-KRISS-teen) U.S.P. 23.
Use: Antineoplastic.
See: Oncovin, Amp. (Eli Lilly and Co.). Vincasar PFS, Vial (Pharmacia & Upjohn).

•**vindesine.** (VIN-deh-seen) USAN.
Use: Antineoplastic.

•**vindesine sulfate.** (VIN-deh-seen) USAN.
Use: Antineoplastic.

•**vinepidine sulfate.** (VIN-eh-pih-DEEN) USAN.
Use: Antineoplastic.

•**vinglycinate sulfate.** (vin-GLIE-sin-ate) USAN.
Use: Antineoplastic.

•**vinleurosine sulfate.** (vin-LOO-row-seen) USAN. Sulfate salt of an alkaloid extracted from *Vinca rosea* Linn. Also see Vinblastine.
Use: Antineoplastic.

•**vinorelbine tartrate.** (vih-NORE-ell-bean) USAN. Sulfate salt of an alkaloid extracted from *Vinca rosea* Linn.
Use: Antineoplastic.
See: Navelbine, Inj. (GlaxoWellcome).

•**vinpocetine.** (VIN-poe-SEH-teen) USAN.
Use: Antineoplastic.

•**vinrosidine sulfate.** (vin-ROW-sih-deen) USAN. Sulfate salt of an alkaloid extracted from *Vinca rosea* Linn.
Use: Antineoplastic.
See: Vinblastine.

vinylacetate-polyvinylpyrrolidone.
See: Ivy-Rid Spray (Roberts Pharmaceuticals).

vinyl ether. U.S.P. XXI.
Use: Anesthetic, general.

vinyzene. Bromchlorenone.

Use: Fungicide.

•**vinzolidine sulfate.** (VIN-ZOLE-ih-deen) USAN.
Use: Antineoplastic.

Vio-Bec. (Solvay Pharmaceuticals) Vitamins B_1 25 mg, B_2 25 mg, niacinamide 100 mg, calcium pantothenate 40 mg, B_6 25 mg, C 500 mg/Cap. Bot. 100s. *otc.*
Use: Mineral, vitamin supplement.

Viodo HC. (NMC Laboratories) Iodochlorhydroxyquin 3%, hydrocortisone 1% in cream base. Tube 20 g. *otc.*
Use: Antifungal; corticosteroid, topical.

Vioform. (Novartis Pharmaceutical Corp.) Clioquinol. **Cream:** 3%. Tube oz. **Oint.:** 3% in petrolatum base. Tube oz. *otc.*
Use: Antifungal, topical.

Viogen-C. (Zenith Goldline Pharmaceuticals) Vitamins B_1 20 mg, B_2 10 mg, B_3 100 mg, B_5 20 mg, B_6 5 mg, C 300 mg, Mg, zinc sulfate 50 mg, tartrazine/Cap. Bot. 100s. *otc.*
Use: Mineral, vitamin supplement.

Viokase. (Wyeth-Ayerst Laboratories) **Tab.:** Lipase 8000 units, protease 30,000 units, amylase 30,000 units/Tab. Bot. 100s, 500s. **Pow.:** Lipase 16,800 units, protease 70,000 units, amylase 70,000 units/0.7 g (0.25 tsp.). *Rx.*
Use: Digestive enzyme.

Viosterol w/Halibut Liver Oil. Vitamins A 50,000 IU, D 10,000 IU/g. (Abbott Laboratories) Bot. 5 ml, 20 ml, 50 ml. Cap.: Vitamins A 5000 IU, D 1000 IU (Ives) Cap.: Vitamins A 5000 IU, D 1700 IU. *otc.*
Use: Vitamin supplement.

•**viprostol.** (vie-PRAHST-ole) USAN.
Use: Hypotensive, vasodilator.

Viquin Forte. (Zeneca Pharmaceuticals) Hydrochloroquine 4%, padimate O 80 mg, dioxybenzone 30 mg, oxybenzone 20 mg, stearyl alcohol, cetearyl alcohol, EDTA, sodium metabisulfite/Cream Tube 28.4 g. SPF 19. PABA free. *Rx.*
Use: Dermatologic.

Vira-A. (Monarch Pharmaceuticals) Vidarabine 3% monohydrate (equivalent to 2.8% vidarabine), liquid petrolatum base. Tube 3.5 g. *Rx.*
Use: Antiviral, ophthalmic.

Virac. (Ruson) Undecoylium Cl-iodine. Iodine complexed with a cationic detergent. Surgical soln. Bot. 2 oz, 8 oz, 1 gal. *otc.*
Use: Antiseptic.

Viracept. (Agouron Pharmaceuticals, Inc.) Nelfinavir mesylate 250 mg/Tab. Bot. 270s. Nelfinavir mesylate 50 mg/g, aspartame (11.2 mg/g phenylanine), sucrose. Pow. Multi-dose bottles. 144 g Pow. w/1 g scoop. *Rx.*
Use: Antiviral.

Viracil. (Health for Life Brands, Inc.) Phenylephrine HCl 5 mg, hesperidin 50 mg, thenylene HCl 12.5 mg, pyrilamine maleate 12.5 mg, vitamin C 50 mg, salicylamide 2.5 gr, caffeine 0.5 gr, sodium salicylate 1.25 gr/Cap. Bot. 16s, 36s. *otc.*
Use: Analgesic, antihistamine, decongestant, vitamin supplement.

Viractin. (J.B. Williams Company Inc.) **Cream:** Tetracaine 2%, hydrochloric acid, methylparaben. Tube 7.1 g. **Gel:** Tetracaine HCl 2%, parabens. Tube 7.1 g. *otc.*
Use: Anesthetic, local.

Viramisol. (Seatrace Pharmaceuticals, Inc.) Adenosine phosphate 25 mg/ml. Vial 10 ml. *otc.*
Use: Relief of varicose vein complications.

Viramune. (Roxane Laboratories, Inc.) Nevirapine. **Tab.:** 200 mg. Bot. 60s, 100s, UD 100s. **Oral Susp.:** 50 mg/ml (as nevirapine hemihydrate), parabens, sorbitol, sucrose. Plastic bot. 240 ml. *Rx.*
Use: Antiviral.

Viranol. (Rhone-Poulenc Rorer Pharmaceuticals, Inc.) Salicylic acid in collodion gel w/lactic acid, camphor, pyroxylin, ethyl alcohol, ethyl acetate. Gel Tube 8 g. *otc.*
Use: Dermatologic, wart therapy.

Virazole. (ICN) Ribavirin 6 g/100 ml. Vial. Contains 20 mg/ml when reconstituted w/300 ml sterile water. *Rx.*
Use: Antiviral.

•**virginiamycin.** (vihr-JIH-nee-ah-MY-sin) USAN. An antibiotic produced by *Streptomyces virgina.*
Use: Anti-infective.

Viridium. (Vita Elixir) Phenylazodiaminopyridine HCl 100 mg/Tab.
Use: Genitourinary.

•**viridofulvin.** (vih-RID-oh-FULL-vin) USAN.
Use: Antifungal.

Virilon. (Star Pharmaceuticals, Inc.) Methyltestosterone 10 mg/SR Cap. Bot. 100s, 1000s. *c-III.*
Use: Androgen.

Virogen Herpes Slide Test. (Wampole Laboratories) Latex agglutination slide test for the detection of herpes simplex virus antigens directly from lesions or cell culture. Test kit 100s.
Use: Diagnostic aid.

Virogen Rotatest. (Wampole Laboratories) Latex agglutination slide test for the qualitative detection of rotavirus in fecal specimens. Test kit 50s.
Use: Diagnostic aid.

Virogen Rubella Microlatex Test. (Wampole Laboratories) Latex agglutination microlatex test for the detection of rubella virus antibody in serum. Test kit 500s, 5000s.
Use: Diagnostic aid.

Virogen Rubella Slide Test. (Wampole Laboratories) Latex agglutination slide test for the detection of rubella virus antibody in serum. Test kit 100s, 500s, 5000s.
Use: Diagnostic aid.

Virogen Rubella Slide Test with Fast Trak Slides. (Wampole Laboratories) Latex agglutination slide test for the detection of rubella virus antibody in serum.
Use: Diagnostic aid.

Viro-Med Tablets. (Whitehall Robins Laboratories) Acetaminophen 500 mg, chlorpheniramine maleate 2 mg, pseudoephedrine HCl 30 mg, dextromethorphan HBr 15 mg/Tab. Bot. 20s, 48s. *otc.*
Use: Analgesic, antihistamine, antitussive, decongestant.

Viroptic. (Monarch Pharmaceuticals) Trifluridine 1%, thimerosal 0.001%. Soln. Drop-Dose 7.5 ml. *Rx.*
Use: Antiviral, ophthalmic.

•**viroxime.** (vie-ROX-eem) USAN.
Use: Antiviral.

Virozyme Injection. (Marcen) Sodium nucleate 2.5%, phenol 0.5%, protein hydrolysate 2.5%, benzyl alcohol 0.2%. Vial 5 ml, 10 ml. *Rx.*
Use: Immunomodulator.

Virugon. Under study. Anhydro bis-(beta-hydroxyethyl) biguanide derivative.
Use: Treatment of influenza, mumps, measles, chickenpox, and shingles.

Viscoat Solution. (Alcon Laboratories, Inc.) Sodium chondroitin sulfate 40 mg, sodium hyaluronate 30 mg, sodium dihydrogen phosphate hydrate 0.45 mg, disodium hydrogen phosphate 2 mg, sodium Cl 4.3 mg/ml. Syringe disposable 0.5 ml. *Rx.*
Use: Viscoelastic.

viscum album, extract. Visnico.
Use: Vasodilator.

Visine Allergy Relief. (Pfizer US Pharmaceutical Group) Tetrahydrozoline HCl 0.05%. Bot. 15 ml, 30 ml. *otc.*
Use: Mydriatic, vasoconstrictor.

Visine Moisturizing. (Pfizer US Pharmaceutical Group) Polyethylene glycol 400 1%, tetrahydrozoline HCl 0.05%. Drop Bot. 15 ml, 30 ml. *otc.*
Use: Mydriatic, vasoconstrictor.

Visine L.R. (Pfizer US Pharmaceutical Group) Oxymetazoline HCl 0.025%. Soln. Bot. 15 ml, 30 ml. *otc.*
Use: Mydriatic, vasoconstrictor.

Vision Care Enzymatic Cleaner. (Alcon Laboratories, Inc.) Highly purified pork pancreatin to be diluted in saline solution. Tab. Pkg. 24s. *otc.*
Use: Contact lens care.

Visipaque 270. (Nycomed Inc.) Iodixanol 550 mg, iodine 270 mg/ml, EDTA, tromethamine. Inj. Vial 50 ml. Bot. 50 ml, 100 ml, 200 ml, 150 ml fill in 200 ml bot. Flexible containers 100 ml, 150 ml, 200 ml. *Rx.*
Use: Radiopaque agent.

Visipaque 320. (Nycomed Inc.) Iodixanol 652 mg, iodine 320 mg/ml, EDTA, tromethamine. Inj. Vial 50 ml. Bot. 50 ml, 100 ml, 200 ml, 150 ml fill in 200 ml bot. Flexible containers 100 ml, 150 ml, 200 ml. *Rx.*
Use: Radiopaque agent.

Visken. (Novartis Pharmaceutical Corp.) Pindolol 5 mg, 10 mg/Tab. Bot. 100s. *Rx.*
Use: Antihypertensive.

Vistacon. (Roberts Pharmaceuticals) Hydroxyzine HCl 50 mg/ml. Vial 10 ml. *Rx.*
Use: Anxiolytic.

Vistaril. (Pfizer US Pharmaceutical Group) Hydroxyzine pamoate equivalent to hydroxyzine HCl. **Cap.:** 25 mg, 50 mg, 100 mg, sucrose. Bot. 100s, 500s, UD 100s. **Oral Susp.:** 25 mg/5 ml, sorbitol, lemon flavor. Bot. 120 ml, 480 ml. *Rx.*
Use: Anxiolytic.

Vistaril I.M. (Roerig) Hydroxyzine HCl, benzyl alcohol 0.9%. **25 mg/ml:** Vial 10 ml, Box 1s. **50 mg/ml:** Vial 10 ml, Box 1s.; Vial 1 ml, 2 ml, 10 ml. *Rx.*
Use: Anxiolytic.

Vistazine 50. (Keene Pharmaceuticals, Inc.) Hydroxyzine HCl 50 mg/ml. Inj. Vial 10. *Rx.*
Use: Anxiolytic.

Vistide. (Gilead Sciences, Inc.) Cidofovir 75 mg/ml/Inj. Amp. 5 ml. *Rx.*
Use: Antiviral.

Visual-Eyes. (Optopics Laboratories, Corp) Sodium Cl, sodium phosphate mono-and dibasic, benzalkonium Cl, EDTA. Soln. Bot. 120 ml. *otc.*
Use: Irrigant, ophthalmic.

Vita-Bee with C Caplets. (Rugby Labs,

Inc.) Vitamins B_1 15 mg, B_2 10.2 mg, B_3 50 mg, B_5 10 mg, B_6 5 mg, C 300 mg/TR Cap. Bot. 100s, 1000s. *otc.*
Use: Vitamin supplement.

Vitabix. (Spanner) Vitamins B_1 100 mg, B_2 2 mg, B_6 5 mg, B_{12} 30 mcg, niacinamide 100 mg, panthenol 10 mg/ml. Vial 10 ml. Multiple-dose vial 30 ml. *Rx.*
Use: Vitamin supplement.

Vita-Bob Softgel Capsules. (Scot-Tussin Pharmacal, Inc.) Vitamins A 5000 IU, D 400 IU, E 30 mg, B_1 1.5 mg, B_2 1.7 mg, B_3 20 mg, B_6 2 mg, B_{12} 6 mcg, C 60 mg, folic acid 0.4 mg/Cap. Bot. 100s. *otc.*
Use: Vitamin supplement.

Vita-C. (Freeda Vitamins, Inc.) Ascorbic acid 4 g/tsp. Crystals 100 g, 500 g, 1000 g. *otc.*
Use: Vitamin supplement.

Vitacarn. (McGaw, Inc.) L-carnitine 1 g/ 10 ml. UD Box 50s, 100s. *Rx.*
Use: L-carnitine supplement.

Vit-A-Drops. (Vision Pharmaceuticals, Inc.) Vitamin A 5000 IU, polysorbate 80. Bot. 10 ml, 15 ml. *otc.*
Use: Lubricant, ophthalmic.

Vitadye. (Zeneca Pharmaceuticals) FD&C yellow No. 5, FD&C red No. 40, FD&C blue No. 1 dyes and dihydroxyacetone 5%. Bot. 0.5 oz, 2 oz. *otc.*
Use: Cosmetic for hyperpigmentation.

Vitafol Caplets. (Everett Laboratories, Inc.) Fe 65 mg, vitamins A 6000 IU, D 400 IU, E 30 mg, B_1 1.1 mg, B_2 1.8 mg, B_3 15 mg, B_6 2.5 mg, B_{12} 5 mcg, C 60 mg, folic acid 1 mg, calcium/Tab. Bot. 100s, 1000s. *Rx.*
Use: Mineral, vitamin supplement.

Vitafol-PN. (Everett Laboratories) Ca 125 mg, Fe 65 mg, vitamin A 1700 IU, D 400 IU, C 60 mg, E 30 IU, folic acid 1 mg, B_1 1.6 mg, B_2 1.8 mg, B_6 2.5 mg, B_{12} 5 mcg, B_3 15 mg, Mg 25 mg, Zn 15 mg. Tab. UD 100s. *Rx.*
Use: Mineral, vitamin supplement.

Vitafol Syrup. (Everett Laboratories, Inc.) Fe 90 mg, B_3 39.9 mg, B_6 6 mg, B_{12} 25.02 mcg, folic acid 0.75 mg. Syr. Bot. 473 ml. *Rx.*
Use: Mineral, vitamin supplement.

Vita-Iron Formula. (Barth's) Fe 120 mg, vitamins B_1 5 mg, B_2 10 mg, C 20 mg, niacin 2 mg, B_{12} 25 mcg, lysine, desiccated liver 200 mg, bromelains/Tab. Bot. 100s, 500s. *otc.*
Use: Mineral, vitamin supplement.

Vita-Kaps Filmtabs. (Abbott Laboratories) Vitamins A 5000 IU, D 400 IU, B_1 3 mg, B_2 2.5 mg, nicotinamide 20 mg, B_6 1 mg, C 50 mg, B_{12} 3 mcg/Filmtab. Bot. 100s, 1000s. *otc.*
Use: Vitamin supplement.

Vitakaps-M. (Abbott Laboratories) Vitamins A 5000 IU, D 400 IU, B_1 3 mg, B_2 2.5 mg, nicotinamide 20 mg, B_6 1 mg, B_{12} 3 mcg, C 50 mg, Fe 10 mg, Cu 1 mg, I 0.15 mg, Mn 1 mg, Zn 7.5 mg/ Filmtab. Bot. 100s. *otc.*
Use: Mineral, vitamin supplement.

Vita-Kid Chewable Wafers. (Solgar Co., Inc.) Vitamins A 10,000 IU, D 400 IU, E 10 mg, B_1 2 mg, B_2 2 mg, B_3 10 mg, B_6 2 mg, B_{12} 5 mcg, C 100 mg, FA 0.3 mg, orange flavor. Bot. 50s, 100s. *otc.*
Use: Vitamin supplement.

Vitalax. (Vitalax) Candy base, gumdrop flavored. Pkg. 20s. *otc.*
Use: Laxative.

Vital B-50. (Zenith Goldline Pharmaceuticals) Vitamins B_1 50 mg, B_2 50 mg, B_3 50 mg, B_5 50 mg, B_6 50 mg, B_{12} 50 mcg, folic acid 0.1 mg, biotin 50 mcg, PABA, choline bitartrate, inositol/TR Tab. Bot 60s. *otc.*
Use: Vitamin supplement.

Vitalets Tablets. (Freeda Vitamins, Inc.) Fe 10 mg, vitamins A 5000 IU, D 400 IU, E 5 mg, B_1 2.5 mg, B_2 0.9 mg, B_3 20 mg, B_5 3 mg, B_6 2 mg, B_{12} 5 mcg, C 60 mg, biotin 25 mcg, Mn, Ca. Chew. Tab. Bot 100s, 250s. *otc.*
Use: Mineral, vitamin supplement.

VitalEyes. (Allergan, Inc.) Vitamins A 10,000 IU, C 200 mg, E 100 IU, Zn 40 mg, Cu, Se, Mn/Cap. Bot. 60s. *otc.*
Use: Mineral, vitamin supplement.

Vital High Nitrogen. (Ross Laboratories) Amino acids, partially hydrolyzed whey, meat, and soy, hydrolyzed corn starch, sucrose, safflower oil, MCT mono- and diglycerides, soy lecithin, vitamins A, B_1, B_2, B_3, B_5, B_6, B_{12}, C, D, E, K, folic acid, biotin, choline, Ca, P, Mg, Fe, Cu, Zn, Mn, I, Cl. Packet 80 g. *otc.*
Use: Nutritional supplement.

Vitalize SF. (Scot-Tussin Pharmacal, Inc.) Fe 66 mg, B_1 30 mg, B_6 15 mg, B_{12} 75 mcg, l-lysine 300 mg. Liq. Bot. 120 ml. *otc.*
Use: Mineral, vitamin supplement.

Vitamel with Iron. (Eastwood) Drops 50 ml. Chew. Tab. Bot. 100s.
Use: Mineral, vitamin supplement.

•**vitamin A.** U.S.P. 23. *Formerly Oleovitamin A.*
Use: Antixerophthalmic vitamin, emollient.
See: Aquasol A, Drops, Cap., Inj. (Astra Pharmaceuticals, L.P.).
Del-Vi-A, Cap. (Del-Ray Laboratory, Inc.).

Palmitate-A 5000, Tab. (Akorn, Inc.).

vitamin A. (Various Mfr.) Cap. 10,000 IU: 100s, 250s, 1000s. *otc.* 25,000 IU: 100s, 250s, 500s, 1000s. *Rx.* 50,000 IU: 100s, 250s, 500s, 1000s. *Rx.*
Use: Antixerophthalmic vitamin, emollient.
See: Retinol, Cream (Natures Bounty, Inc.).

vitamin A acid.
See: Tretinoin.

vitamin A, alphalin. (Eli Lilly and Co.) Vitamin A 50,000 IU/Gelseal. Bot. 100s. *Rx.*
Use: Vitamin supplement.

vitamin A, water miscible, or soluble. Water-miscible vitamin A.
Use: Vitamin supplement.

vitamin A w/combinations.
See: Advanced Formula Zenate, Tab. (Solvay Pharmaceuticals).
Advera, Liq. (Ross Laboratories).
Bonamil Infant Formula with Iron, Conc., Liq. (Wyeth-Ayerst Laboratories).
Boost, Liq. (Mead Johnson Nutritionals).
Choice dm, Liq. (Mead Johnson Pharmaceuticals).
Fosfree, Tab. (Mission Pharmacal Co.).
Neocate One +, Liq. (Scientific Hospital Supplies, Inc.).
Nepro, Liq. (Ross Laboratories).
Ocuvite Extra, Tab. (Storz).
Oncovite, Tab. (Mission Pharmacal Co.).
Prenatal H.P., Tab. (Mission Pharmacal Co.).
Prenatal Plus, Tab. (Zenith Goldline Pharmaceuticals).
Prenatal Plus w/Beta-Carotene, Tab. (Rugby Labs, Inc.).
Prenatal Rx, Tab. (Misson).
Prenatal Z Advanced Formula, Tab. (Ethex Corp.).
Stuartnatal Plus, Tab. (Wyeth-Ayerst Laboratories).
Theragran AntiOxidant, Softgel (Bristol-Meyers Squibb).
Tri-Flor-Vite with Flouride, Drops (Everett).

vitamin Bc.
See: Folic Acid (Various Mfr.).

vitamin B_1. Thiamine HCl, U.S.P. 23.
Use: Vitamin supplement.

vitamin B_1 mononitrate. Thiamine mononitrate.
Use: Vitamin supplement.

vitamin B_1 w/thyroid.
See: T & T, Tab. (Mason Pharmaceuticals, Inc.).

vitamin B_2. Riboflavin.
Use: Vitamin supplement.

vitamin B_3. Niacinamide, Nicotinamide.
Use: Vitamin supplement.

vitamin B_5. Calcium Pantothenate.
Use: Vitamin supplement.

vitamin B_6. Pyridoxine HCl.
Use: Vitamin supplement.
See: Hexa-Betalin, Tab. (Eli Lilly and Co.).

vitamin B_8.
See: Adenosine phosphate.

vitamin B_{12}. Cyanocobalamin. Cobalamine. Vial, Amp.
See: Bedoce (Lincoln Diagnostics).
Betalin-12 (Eli Lilly and Co.).
Cabadon-M (Solvay Pharmaceuticals).
Cobadoce Forte (Solvay Pharmaceuticals).
Crysto-Gel (Solvay Pharmaceuticals).
Cyano-Gel, Liq. (Maurry).
Dodex (Organon Teknika Corp.).
Rubramin (Bristol-Myers Squibb).
Ruvite 1000 (Savage Laboratories).
Sigamine (Sigma-Tau Pharmaceuticals, Inc.).
Vi-Twel, Inj. (Berlex Laboratories, Inc.).

W/Ferrous sulfate, ascorbic acid, folic acid.
See: Intrin, Cap. (Merit).

W/Folic acid, niacinamide, liver.
See: Hepfomin 500, Inj. (Keene Pharmaceuticals, Inc.).

W/Thiamine.
See: Cobalin, Vial (Ulmer Pharmacal Co.).
Cyamine, Vial (Keene Pharmaceuticals, Inc.).

W/Thiamine, vitamin B_6.
See: Orexin, Tab. (Zeneca Pharmaceuticals).

vitamin B_{12}. (Various Mfr.) Cyanocobalamin crystalline 100 mcg/ml, 1000 mcg/ml. **100 mcg/ml:** Vials 30 ml. **1000 mcg/ml:** Multidose vials 10 ml, 30 ml. *Rx.*
Use: Vitamin supplement.

vitamin B_{12}. (Zenith Goldline Pharmaceuticals) Cyanocobalamin crystalline 500 mcg, 1000 mcg. Tab. Bot. 100s. *otc.*
Use: Vitamin supplement.

vitamin B_{12} a & b.
See: Hydroxocobalamin (Various Mfr.).

vitamin B_{15}.
Use: Alleged to increase oxygen supply in blood. Not approved by FDA as a vitamin or drug. Illegal to sell Vitamin B_{15}.

vitamin B complex. Concentrated extract of dried brewer's yeast and extract of corn processed w/*Clostridium acetobutylicum*.
See: Becotin, Pulvules (Eli Lilly and Co.).
Betalin Complex, Amp. (Eli Lilly and Co.).

Vitamin B complex 100. (McGuff Co., Inc.) Vitamin B_1 100 mg, B_2 2 mg, B_3 100 mg, B_5 2 mg, B_6 2 mg/ml. Inj. Vial 10 ml, 30 ml. *Rx.*
Use: Vitamin supplement.

Vitamin B Complex No. 104. (Century Pharmaceuticals, Inc.) Vitamins B_1 100 mg, B_2 2 mg, B_6 2 mg, d-panthenol 10 mg, niacinamide 125 mg/Vial, benzyl alcohol 1%, gentisic acid ethanolamide 2.5%/Vial 30 ml. *Rx.*
Use: Vitamin supplement.

Vitamin B Complex, Betalin Complex, Elixir. (Eli Lilly and Co.) Vitamins B_1 2.7 mg, B_2 1.35 mg, B_{12} 3 mcg, B_6 0.555 mg, pantothenic acid 2.7 mg, niacinamide 6.75 mg, liver fraction 500 mg/5 ml, alcohol 17%. Bot. 16 oz. *otc.*
Use: Vitamin supplement.

Vitamin B Complex w/Vitamin C. (Century Pharmaceuticals, Inc.) Vitamins B_1 25 mg, B_2 5 mg, B_6 5 mg, niacinamide 50 mg, panthenol 5 mg, Ca 50 mg, propethylene glycol 300 10%, gentisic acid ethanolamide 2.5%, benzyl alcohol 2%/Vial 30 ml. *Rx.*
Use: Mineral, vitamin supplement.

Vitamin B Complex, Betalin Complex Pulvules. (Eli Lilly and Co.) Vitamins B_1 1 mg, B_2 2 mg, B_6 0.4 mg, pantothenic acid 3.333 mg, niacinamide 10 mg, B_{12} 1 mcg/Cap. Bot. 100s. *otc.*
Use: Vitamin supplement.
See: Advanced Formula Zenate, Tab. (Solvay Pharmaceuticals).
Advera, Liq. (Scientific Hospital Supplies, Inc.).
B-C-Bid, Capl. (Roberts Pharmaceuticals).
Bonamil Infant Formula with Iron, Conc. Liq. (Wyeth-Ayerst Laboratories).
Boost, Liq. (Mead Johnson Nutritionals).
Choice dm, Liq. (Mead Johnson Nutritionals).
Fosfree, Tab. (Misson).
Neocate One +, Liq. (Scientific Hospital Supplies, Inc.).
Nephplex RX, Tab. (Nephro-Tech, Inc.).
Nephron FA, Tab. (Nephro-Tech, Inc.).
Nepro, Liq. (Ross Laboratories).
Ocuvite Extra, Tab. (Storz).
Oncovite, Tab. (Mission Pharmacal Co.).
Prenatal HP, Tab. (Mission Pharmacal Co.).
Prenatal Plus, Tab. (Zenith Goldline Pharmaceuticals).
Prenatal Plus w/Beta-Carotene, Tab. (Rugby Labs, Inc.).
Prenatal Rx, Tab. (Mission Pharmacal Co.).
Prenatal Z Advanced Formula, Tab. (Ethex Corp.).
Stuartnatal Plus, Tab. (Wyeth-Ayerst Laboratories).

vitamin C.
See: Ascorbic Acid Preps.
One-A-Day Extras Vitamin C, Tab. (Bayer Corp. (Allergy Div.)).

vitamin C, cevalin. (Eli Lilly and Co.) Ascorbic acid 250 mg, 500 mg/Tab. Bot. 100s. *otc.*
Use: Vitamin supplement.

vitamin C w/combinations.
See: Advanced Formula Zenate, Tab. (Solvay Pharmaceuticals).
Advera, Liq. (Ross Laboratories).
Allbee C-800, Prods. (Wyeth-Ayerst Laboratories).
Allbee with C, Cap. (Wyeth-Ayerst Laboratories).
Allbee-T, Tab. (Wyeth-Ayerst Laboratories).
Antiox, Cap. (Merz Pharmaceuticals).
B-C-Bid, Capl. (Roberts Pharmaceuticals).
Bonamil Infant Formula with Iron, Conc. Liq. (Wyeth-Ayerst Laboratories).
Boost, Liq. (Mead Johnson Nutritionals).
Choice dm, Liq. (Mead Johnson Nutritionals).
Chromagen FA, Cap. (Savage Laboratories).
Chromagen Forte, Cap. (Savage Laboratories).
Fosfree, Tab. (Mission Pharmacal Co.).
Neocate One +, Liq. (Scientific Hospital Supplies, Inc.).
Nephplex Rx, Tab. (Nephro-Tech, Inc.).
Nephron FA, Tab. (Nephro-Tech, Inc.).
Nepro, Liq. (Ross Laboratories).
Nialexo-C, Tab. (Roberts Pharmaceuticals).
Ocuvite Extra, Tab. (Storz).
Oncovite, Tab. (Mission Pharmacal Co.).
Prenatal HP, Tab. (Mission Pharmacal Co.).

Prenatal Plus, Tab. (Zenith Goldline).
Prenatal Plus w/Beta-Carotene, Tab. (Rugby Labs, Inc.).
Prenatal Rx, Tab. (Mission Pharmacal Co.).
Protegra Softgels, Cap. (ESI Lederle Generics).
Stuartnatal Plus, Tab. (Wyeth-Ayerst Laboratories).
Theragran Antioxidant, Softgel (Bristol-Myers Squibb).
Thex, Cap. (Ingram).
Thex Forte, Cap. (Ingram).
Tri-Flor-Vite with Flouride, Drops (Everett).
Vicon-C, Cap. (GlaxoWellcome).
Vicon Forte, Cap. (GlaxoWellcome).
Vicon Plus, Cap. (GlaxoWellcome).
Vi-Zac, Cap. (GlaxoWellcome).
Z-BEC, Tab. (Wyeth-Ayerst Laboratories).

vitamin D. Cholecalciferol.
Use: Vitamin D supplement.

Vitamin D. (Various Mfr.) Ergocalciferol (D_2) 50,000 IU/Cap. Bot. 100s, 1000s. *Rx.*
Use: Vitamin supplement.

vitamin D, deltalin. (Eli Lilly and Co.) Vitamin D-250,000 units (1.25 mg)/ Gelseal. Bot. 100s. *Rx.*
Use: Vitamin supplement.

vitamin D, synthetic.
See: Activated 7-Dehydro-cholesterol Calciferol.

vitamin D-1.
See: Dihydrotachysterol.

vitamin D-2. Activated ergasterol, Ergocalciferol.
See: Calciferol, Preps. (Various Mfr.).
Drisdol, Liq. (Sanofi Winthrop Pharmaceuticals).
Viosterol (Various Mfr.).

vitamin D-3.
See: Activated 7-dehydrocholesterol. Calciferol Prep. for related activity.

vitamin D_3. (Freeda Vitamins, Inc.) Cholecalciferol (D_3) 1000 IU/Tab. Bot. 100s, 500s. *otc.*
Use: Vitamin supplement.

vitamin D-3-cholesterol. Compound of crystalline vitamin D-3 and cholesterol.

vitamin D-4.
See: Dihydrotachysterol, Preps. (Various Mfr.).

Vitamin D Oral Drops. (Cypress) Ergocalciferol (D_2) 8000 IU/ ml. Liq. 60 ml. *otc.*
Use: Vitamin supplement.

vitamin D w/combinations.
See: Advanced Formula Zenate, Tab. (Solvay Pharmaceuticals).
Advera, Liq. (Ross Laboratories).
Bonamil Infant Formula with Iron, Conc., Liq. (Wyeth-Ayerst Laboratories).
Boost, Liq. (Mead Johnson Nutritionals).
Caltrate Plus, Tab. (Lederle).
Caltrate 600 + D, Tab. (Lederle).
Choice dm, Liq. (Mead Johnson Nutritionals).
Desert Pure Calcium, Tab. (Cal-White Mineral).
Fosfree, Tab. (Mission Pharmacal Co.).
Neocate One +, Liq. (Scientific Hospital Supplies, Inc.).
Nepro, Liq. (Ross Laboratories).
Oesto-Mins, Pow. (Tyson & Associates, Inc.).
Oncovite, Tab. (Mission Pharmacal Co.).
Prenatal Plus, Tab. (Zenith Goldline Pharmaceuticals).
Prenatal Plus w/Beta-Carotene, Tab. (Rugby Labs, Inc.).
Prenatal Rx, Tab. (Mission Pharmacal Co.).
Stuartnatal Plus, Tab. (Wyeth-Ayerst Laboratories).
Tri-Flor-Vite with Flouride, Drops (Everett).

•**vitamin E.** U.S.P. 23.
Use: Vitamin E supplement.
See: Aquasol E (Rhone-Poulenc Rorer Pharmaceuticals, Inc.).
Lactinol-E, Creme (Pedinol Pharmacal, Inc.).
One-A-Day Extras Vitamin E, Softgel Cap. (Bayer Corp. (Allergy Div.)).
Soft Sense, Lot. (Bausch & Lomb Pharmaceuticals).
Tocopher, Prod. (Quality Formulations, Inc.).
Tocopherol, Preps. (Various Mfr.).
Wheat Germ Oil (Various Mfr.).

vitamin E, eprolin. (Eli Lilly and Co.) Alpha-tocopherol 100 units/Gelseal. Bot. 100s.
Use: Vitamin supplement.

vitamin E w/combinations.
See: Advanced Formula Zenate, Tab. (Solvay Pharmaceuticals).
Advera, Liq. (Ross Laboratories).
Antiox, Cap. (Merz Pharmaceutcials).
Bonamil Infant Formula with Iron, Conc., Liq. (Wyeth-Ayerst Laboratories).
Boost, Liq. (Mead Johnson Nutritionals).
Choice dm, Liq. (Mead Johnson Nutritionals).

Neocate One +, Liq. (Scientific Hospital Supplies, Inc.).
Nepro, Liq. (Ross Laboratories).
Ocuvite Extra, Tab. (Storz).
Oncovite, Tab. (Mission Pharmacal Co.).
Prenatal Plus, Tab. (Zenith Goldline Pharmaceuticals).
Prenatal Plus w/Beta-Carotene, Tab. (Rugby Labs, Inc.).
Stuartnatal Plus, Tab. (Wyeth-Ayerst Laboratories).
Theragran AntiOxidant, Softgels (Bristol-Meyers Squibb).

vitamin G.
See: Riboflavin.

vitamin K.
See: Menadiol, Sodium Diphosphate, Preps. (Various Mfr.).
Menadione, Preps. (Various Mfr.).
Menadione Sodium Bisulfite, Preps. (Various Mfr.).

vitamin K-1.
See: Phytonadione, U.S.P. 23.

vitamin K-3.
See: Menadione, U.S.P. 23.

vitamin K oxide. Not available, but usually K-1 is desired.

vitamin K w/combinations.
See: Advera, Liq. (Ross Laboratories).
Bonamil Infant Formula with Iron, Conc., Liq. (Wyeth-Ayerst Laboratories).
Choice dm, Liq. (Mead Johnson Nutritionals).
Neocate One +, Liq. (Scientific Hospital Supplies, Inc.).

vitamin M.
See: Folic Acid, U.S.P. 23.

vitamin-mineral-supplement liquid. (Morton Grove Pharmaceuticals, Inc.) Vitamins B_1 0.83 mg, B_2 0.42 mg, B_3 8.3 mg, B_5 1.67 mg, B_6 0.17 mg, B_{12} 0.17 mcg, I, Fe 2.5 mg, Mg, Zn 0.3 mg, Mn, choline, alcohol 18%. Liq. 473 ml. *otc.*
Use: Mineral, vitamin supplement.

vitamin P. Citrin.
See: Bio-Flavonoid Compounds (Various Mfr.).
Hesperidin Preps. (Various Mfr.).
Quercetin (Various Mfr.).
Rutin, Preps. (Various Mfr.).

vitamin T. Sesame seed factor, termite factor.
Use: Claimed to aid proper blood coagulation and promote formation of blood platelets. Not approved by FDA as an active vitamin.

vitamin U. Present in cabbage juice.

vitamin, maintenance formula.
See: Stuart Formula, Tab., Liq. (Zeneca Pharmaceuticals).

vitamins: stress formula.
See: Probec-T, Tab. (Zeneca Pharmaceuticals).
StressForm "605" w/Iron, Tab. (NBTY, Inc.).
Stress Formula with Iron, Tab. (NBTY, Inc.).
Stresstabs 600 (ESI Lederle Generics).
Thera-combex Kap. (Parke-Davis).

vitamins w/liver & lipotropic agents.
See: Metheponex, Cap. (Rawl).

Vita Natal. (Scot-Tussin Pharmacal, Inc.) Folic acid 1 mg/Tab. Bot. 100s. *Rx.*
Use: Vitamin supplement.

Vitaneed. (Biosearch Medical Products) P-beef, Ca and Na caseinates, CHO-maltodextrin. F-partially hydrogenated soy oil, mono- and diglycerides, soy lecithin. Protein 35 g, CHO 125 g, fat 40 g, Na 500 mg, K 1250 mg/L, 1 Cal/ml, 375 mOsm/kg H_2O. Liq. Ready-to-use 250 ml. *otc.*
Use: Nutritional supplement.

Vitaon. (Vita Elixir) Vitamin B_{12} 25 mcg, thiamine HCl 10 mg, ferric pyrophosphate 250 mg/5 ml. *otc.*
Use: Vitamin supplement.

Vita-Plus B12. (Scot-Tussin Pharmacal, Inc.) Vitamin B_{12} 1000 mcg/ml. Inj. *Rx.*
Use: Vitamin supplement.

Vita-Plus E. (Scot-Tussin Pharmacal, Inc.) Vitamin E 294 mg as d-alpha tocopheryl acetate/Cap. *otc.*
Use: Vitamin supplement.

Vita-Plus G Softgel. (Scot-Tussin Pharmacal, Inc.) Vitamins A 5000 IU, D 400 IU, E 10 IU, B_1 5 mg, B_2 5 mg, B_3 15 mg, B_5 5 mg, B_6 1 mg, B_{12} 1 mcg, C 50 mg, Fe 3.3 mg, Ca 145 mg, Zn 0.5 mg, K, Mg, Mn, P, I, Cu, choline, l-lysine, inositol/Cap. Bot. 100s. *otc.*
Use: Mineral, vitamin supplement.

Vita-Plus H Softgel. (Scot-Tussin Pharmacal, Inc.) Fe 13.4 mg, vitamins A 5000 IU, D 400 IU, E 3 IU, B_1 3 mg, B_2 2.5 mg, B_3 20 mg, B_5 5 mg, B_6 1.5 mg, B_{12} 2.5 mcg, C 50 mg, Ca, K, Mg, Mn, P, Zn 1.4 mg/Cap. Bot. 100s. *otc.*
Use: Mineral, vitamin supplement.

Vita-Plus H Liquid Sugar Free. (Scot-Tussin Pharmacal, Inc.) Vitamins B_1 30 mg, l-lysine monohydrochloride 300 mg, B_{12} 75 mcg, B_6 15 mg, iron pyrophosphate soluble 100 mg/5 ml. Bot. 4 oz, 8 oz, pt, gal. *otc.*
Use: Mineral, vitamin supplement.

Vita-PMS. (Bajamar Chemical Co., Inc.) Vitamins A 2083 IU, E 16.7 IU, D_3 16.7

IU, folic acid 33 mcg, B_1 4.2 mg, B_2 4.2 mg, B_3 4.2 mg, B_5 4.2 mg, B_6 50 mg, B_{12} 10.4 mcg, biotin, C 250 mg, Ca, Mg, I, Fe, Cu, Zn 4.2 mg, Mn, K, Se, Cr, betaine/Tab. Bot. 100s. *otc.*
Use: Mineral, vitamin supplement.

Vita-PMS Plus. (Bajamar Chemical Co., Inc.) Vitamins A 667 IU, E 16.7 IU, D_3 16.7 IU, folic acid 33 mcg, B_1 4.2 mg, B_2 4.2 mg, B_3 4.2 mg, B_5 4.2 mg, B_6 16.7 mg, B_{12} 10.4 mcg, biotin, C 250 mg, Mg, I, Ca, Fe, Cu, Zn 4.2 mg, Mn, K, Se, Cr, betaine/Tab. Bot. 100s. *otc.*
Use: Mineral, vitamin supplement.

Vita-Ray Creme. (Gordon Laboratories) Vitamins E 3000 IU, A 200,000 IU/oz w/aloe 10%. Jar 0.5 oz, 2.5 oz. *otc.*
Use: Emollient.

Vitarex. (Taylor Pharmaceuticals) Vitamins A 10,000 IU, D 200 IU, B_1 15 mg, B_2 10 mg, B_6 5 mg, B_{12} 5 mcg, C 250 mg, B_3 100 mg, B_5 20 mg, E 15 mg, Fe 15 mg, Ca, Cu, I, K, Mg, Mn, P, Zn 10 mg/Tab. Bot. 100s. *otc.*
Use: Mineral, vitamin supplement.

Vitazin. (Mesemer) Ascorbic acid 300 mg, niacinamide 100 mg, thiamine mononitrate 20 mg, d-calcium pantothenate 20 mg, riboflavin 10 mg, pyridoxine HCl 5 mg, magnesium sulfate 70 mg, Zn 25 mg/Cap. Bot. 100s. *otc.*
Use: Mineral, vitamin supplement.

Vita-Zoo. (Towne) Vitamins A 2500 IU, D 400 IU, E 15 IU, C 60 mg, folic acid 0.3 mg, B_1 1.05 mg, B_2 1.2 mg, niacin 13.5 mg, B_6 1.05 mg, B_{12} 4.5 mcg/Tab. Bot. 100s. *otc.*
Use: Vitamin supplement.

Vita-Zoo Plus Iron. (Towne) Vitamins A 2500 IU, D 400 IU, E 15 IU, C 60 mg, folic acid 0.3 mg, B_1 1.05 mg, B_2 1.2 mg, niacin 13.5 mg, B_6 1.05 mg, B_{12} 4.5 mcg, Fe 15 mg/Tab. Bot. 100s. *otc.*
Use: Mineral, vitamin supplement.

Vitec. (Pharmaceutical Specialties, Inc.) Dl-alpha tocopheryl acetate in a vanishing cream base. Cream. 120 g. *otc.*
Use: Emollient.

Vitormains. (Roberts Pharmaceuticals) Tab. Bot. 100s.
Use: Vitamin supplement.

Vitrasert. (Chiron Vision) Ganciclovir 4.5 mg (released over 5 to 8 months)/Intravitreal implant. Box 1. *Rx.*
Use: Antiviral, cytomegalovirus.

Vitravene. (Isis) Fomivirsen sodium 6.6 mg/ml, sodium bicarbonate, sodium chloride, sodium carbonate. Inj. Single-use vial 0.25 ml. Preservative free. *Rx.*
Use: Antiviral, ophthalmic.

Vitron-C. (Heritage Consumer Products) Ferrous fumarate 200 mg, ascorbic acid 125 mg. Tab. Bot. 60s. *otc.*
Use: Iron-containing product.

Vivactil. (Merck & Co.) Protriptyline HCl 5 mg, 10 mg/Tab. **5 mg:** Bot. 100s. **10 mg:** Bot. 100s, UD 100s. *Rx.*
Use: Antidepressant.

Viva-Drops. (Vision Pharmaceuticals, Inc.) Polysorbate 80, sodium Cl, EDTA, retinyl palmitate, mannitol, sodium citrate, pyruvate. Soln. Bot. 10 ml, 15 ml. *otc.*
Use: Artificial tears.

Vivarin. (SmithKline Beecham Pharmaceuticals) Caffeine alkaloid 200 mg. Tab. Blister Pk. 16s, 40s, 80s. Capl. Pkg. 24s, 48s. *otc.*
Use: CNS stimulant.

Vivelle. (Ciba-Geigy) Estradiol transdermal system 3.28 mg, 4.33 mg, 6.57 mg, 8.66 mg. Calendar pack (8 and 24 systems). *Rx.*
Use: Estrogen.

Vivikon. (Zeneca Pharmaceuticals) Vitamins B_1 5 mg, B_2 2 mg, B_6 10 mg, d-panthenol 5 mg, niacinamide 10 mg, procaine HCl 2%/ml. 100 ml. *otc.*
Use: Vitamin supplement.

Vivonex Flavor Packets. (Procter & Gamble Pharm.) Non-nutritive flavoring for Vivonex diets when consumed orally. Orange-pineapple, lemon-lime, strawberry, and vanilla. Pkg. 60s. *otc.*
Use: Flavoring.

Vivonex, Standard. (Procter & Gamble Pharm.) Free amino acid/complete enteral nutrition. Six packets provide kcal 1800, available nitrogen 5.88 g as amino acids 37 g, fat 2.61 g, carbohydrate 407 g, and full day's balanced nutrition. Calorie:nitrogen ratio is 300:1. Unflavored pow. Packet 80 g. Pkg. 6s. *otc.*
Use: Nutritional supplement.

Vivonex T.E.N. (Procter & Gamble Pharm.) Free amino acid, high nitrogen/high branched chain amino acid complete enteral nutrition. Ten packets provide kcal 3000, available nitrogen 17 g, amino acids 115 g, fat 8.33 g, carbohydrate 617 g and full day's balanced nutrition. Calorie:nitrogen ratio is 175:1. Unflavored pow. Packet 80 g. Pkg. 10s. *otc.*
Use: Nutritional supplement.

Vivotif Berna. (Berna Products Corp.) Typhoid vaccine (oral). *S. typhi* Ty21a (viable) 2 to 6 $\times$ 10^9 colony-forming units and *S. typhi* Ty21a[2] (non-viable) 5 to 50 $\times$ 10^9 colony-forming units/Cap. Single foil blister with 4 doses. *Rx.*

Use: Immunization.

Vi-Zac. (UCB Pharmaceuticals, Inc.) Vitamins A 5000 IU, E 50 IU, C 500 mg, Zn 18 mg, lactose. Bot. 60s. *otc.*
Use: Mineral, vitamin supplement.

V-Lax. (Century Pharmaceuticals, Inc.) Psyllium mucilloid (hydrophilic) 50%, dextrose 50%. Pow. 0.25 lb, 1 lb. *otc.*
Use: Laxative.

Vlemasque. (Dermik Laboratories, Inc.) Sulfurated lime topical solution 6% (Vleminck's Soln.), alcohol 7% in drying clay mask. Jar 4 oz. *otc.*
Use: Dermatologic, acne.

VM. (Last) Vitamins B_1 6 mg, B_2 4 mg, niacinamide 40 mg, Fe 100 mg, Ca 188 mg, P 188 mg, Mn 4 mg, alcohol 12%. Bot. 16 oz. *otc.*
Use: Mineral, vitamin supplement.

V-M Capsules. (Pal-Pak, Inc.) Vitamins A, D, B_1, B_2, B_6, C, niacinamide, Ca, Fe, calcium pantothenate, Mg, Mn, K, Zn, P/Tab. Bot. 100s, 1000s. *otc.*
Use: Mineral, vitamin supplement.

•**volazocine.** (voe-LAY-zoe-SEEN) USAN. Under study.
Use: Analgesic.

Volidan. (British Drug House) Megestrol acetate. *Rx.*
Use: Hormone.

Volitane. (Trent) Parethoxycaine 0.2%, hexachlorophene 0.025%, dichlorophene 0.025%. Aerosol spray can 3 oz. *otc.*
Use: Counterirritant, antiseptic.

Volmax. (Muro Pharmaceutical, Inc.) Albuterol sufate 4 mg, 8 mg/ER Tab. Bot. 100s, 500s. *Rx.*
Use: Bronchodilator.

Voltaren. (Ciba Vision) Diclofenac sodium 0.1% Soln. Dropper bot. 2.5 ml, 5 ml. *Rx.*
Use: NSAID, ophthalmic.

Voltaren. (Novartis Pharmaceutical Corp.) Diclofenac sodium 25 mg, 50 mg, 75 mg, lactose, SR Tab. **25 mg:** Bot. 60s, 100s, UD 100s; **50 mg, 75 mg:** Bot. 60s, 100s, 1000s, UD 100s. *Rx.*
Use: Analgesic, NSAID.

Voltaren-XR. (Novartis Pharmaceutical Corp.) Diclofenac sodium 100 mg, sucrose/ER Tab. 100s, UD 100s. *Rx.*
Use: Analgesic, NSAID.

Voltaren, Ophthalmic Solution. (Ciba Vision) Diclofenac sodium 0.1%. Soln. Bot. 2.5 ml, 5 ml w/dropper. *Rx.*
Use: NSAID, ophthalmic.

vonedrine hydrochloride. Vonedrine (phenylpropylmethylamine) HCl. *otc.*
Use: Decongestant.

•**vorozole.** (VORE-oh-zole) USAN.
Use: Antineoplastic.

Vortel. Clorprenaline HCl.
Use: Bronchodilator.

VoSoL HC Otic Solution. (Wallace Laboratories) Propylene glycol diacetate 3%, acetic acid 2%, benzethonium Cl 0.02%, hydrocortisone 1%. Soln. Bot. 10 ml. *Rx.*
Use: Otic.

VoSoL Otic Solution. (Wallace Laboratories) Propylene glycol diacetate 3%, acetic acid 2%, benzethonium Cl 0.02%, sodium acetate 0.015%. Soln. Bot. 15 ml, 30 ml. *Rx.*
Use: Otic.

•**votumumab.** (vah-TOOM-uh-mab) USAN.
Use: Monoclonal antibody.

Voxsuprine Tabs. (Major Pharmaceuticals) Isoxsuprine HCl 10 m, 20 mg/Tab. Bot. 100s, 250s, 1000s, UD 100s. *Rx.*
Use: Vasodilator.

V-Tuss Expectorant. (Vangard Labs, Inc.) Hydrocodone bitartrate 5 mg, pseudoephedrine HCl 60 mg, guaifenesin 200 mg/5 ml, alcohol 12.5%. *c-III.*
Use: Antitussive, decongestant, expectorant.

Vumon. (Bristol-Myers Oncology/Immunology) Teniposide 10 mg/ml. Inj. Amp. 5 ml. *Rx.*
Use: Antineoplastic.

V.V.S. (Econo Med Pharmaceuticals) Sulfathiazole 3.42%, sulfacetamide 2.86%, sulfabenzamide 3.7%, urea 0.64%. Cream. Tube 90 g w/applicator. *Rx.*
Use: Anti-infective, vaginal.

Vytone Cream. (Dermik Laboratories, Inc.) Hydrocortisone 1%, iodoquinol 1%, greaseless base. Cream Bot. 30 g. *Rx.*
Use: Anti-infective; corticosteroid, topical.

VZIG. (American Red Cross, Mass. Public Health Bio. Lab.) Varicella-Zoster Immune Globulin Human Globulin fraction of human plasma, primarily 1 G/10% to 18% in single-dose vials containing 125 units varicella-zoster virus antibody in 2.5 mg or less. Inj.
Use: Immunization.

W

Wade Gesic Balm. (Wade) Menthol 3%, methyl salicylate 12%, petrolatum base. Tube oz, Jar lb. *otc.*
Use: Analgesic, topical.

Wade's Drops. Compound Benzoin Tincture.

Wakespan. (Weeks & Leo) Caffeine 250 mg/TR Cap. Pkg. 15s. *Rx.*
Use: CNS stimulant.

Wal-Finate Allergy. (Walgreen Co.) Chlorpheniramine maleate 4 mg/Tab. Bot. 50s. *otc.*
Use: Antihistamine.

Wal-Finate Decongestant. (Walgreen Co.) Chlorpheniramine maleate 4 mg, pseudoephedrine sulfate 60 mg/Tab. Bot. 50s. *otc.*
Use: Antihistamine, decongestant.

Wal-Formula Cough Syrup with D-Methorphan. (Walgreen Co.) Dextromethorphan HBr 15 mg, doxylamine succinate 7.5 mg, sodium citrate 500 mg/10 ml. Syr. Bot. 6 oz, 8 oz. *otc.*
Use: Antihistamine, antitussive, expectorant.

Wal-Formula D Cough Syrup. (Walgreen Co.) Dextromethorphan HBr 20 mg, phenylpropanolamine HCl 25 mg, guaifenesin 100 mg/10 ml, alcohol 10%. Syr. Bot. 6 oz, 8 oz. *otc.*
Use: Antitussive, decongestant, expectorant.

Wal-Formula M Cough Syrup. (Walgreen Co.) Dextromethorphan HBr 30 mg, pseudoephedrine HCl 60 mg, guaifenesin 200 mg, acetaminophen 500 mg/20 ml. Syr. Bot. 8 oz. *otc.*
Use: Analgesic, antitussive, decongestant, expectorant.

Wal-Frin Nasal Mist. (Walgreen Co.) Phenylephrine HCl 0.5%, pheniramine maleate 0.2%. Soln. Bot. 0.5 oz. *otc.*
Use: Antihistamine, decongestant.

Walgreen Artificial Tears. (Walgreen Co.) Hydroxypropyl methylcellulose 0.5%. Soln. Bot. 0.5 oz. *otc.*
Use: Artificial tears.

Walgreen's Finest Iron. (Walgreen Co.) Iron 30 mg/Tab. Bot. 100s. *otc.*
Use: Mineral supplement.

Walgreen's Finest Vit B_6. (Walgreen Co.) Pyridoxine HCl 50 mg/Tab. Bot. 100s. *otc.*
Use: Vitamin supplement.

Walgreen Soda Mints. (Walgreen Co.) Sodium bicarbonate 300 mg/Tab. Bot. 100s, 200s. *otc.*
Use: Antacid.

Wal-Minic. (Walgreen Co.) Phenylpropanolamine HCl 12.5 mg, guaifenesin 100 mg/5 ml, alcohol 5%. Bot. 6 oz, 8 oz. *otc.*
Use: Decongestant, expectorant.

Wal-Minic Cold Relief Medicine. (Walgreen Co.) Phenylpropanolamine HCl 12.5 mg, chlorpheniramine maleate 2 mg/5 ml. Bot. 6 oz, 8 oz. *otc.*
Use: Antihistamine, decongestant.

Wal-Minic DM. (Walgreen Co.) Phenylpropanolamine HCl 12.5 mg, dextromethorphan HBr 10 mg/5 ml Bot. 6 oz, 8 oz. *otc.*
Use: Antitussive, decongestant.

Wal-Phed Plus. (Walgreen Co.) Pseudoephedrine HCl 60 mg, chlorpheniramine maleate 4 mg/Tab. Bot. 50s. *otc.*
Use: Antihistamine, decongestant.

Wal-Phed Syrup. (Walgreen Co.) Pseudoephedrine HCl 30 mg/5 ml. Syr. Bot. 4 oz. *otc.*
Use: Decongestant.

Wal-Phed Tablets. (Walgreen Co.) Pseudoephedrine HCl 30 mg/Tab. Bot. 50s, 100s. *otc.*
Use: Decongestant.

Wal-Tap Elixir. (Walgreen Co.) Brompheniramine maleate 2 mg, phenylpropanolamine HCl 12.5 mg/5 ml. Bot. 4 oz. *otc.*
Use: Antihistamine, decongestant.

Wal-Tussin. (Walgreen Co.) Guaifenesin 100 mg/5 ml. Bot. 4 oz. *otc.*
Use: Expectorant.

Wal-Tussin DM. (Walgreen Co.) Guaifenesin 100 mg, dextromethorphan HBr 15 mg/5 ml. Bot. 4 oz, 8 oz. *otc.*
Use: Antitussive, expectorant.

Wampole One-Step hCG. (Wampole Laboratories) For in vitro detection of hCG in serum and urine. Test. In 3, 24, 96, 500 test kits.
Use: Diagnostic aid, pregnancy.

•**warfarin sodium.** (WORE-fuh-rin) U.S.P. 23.
Use: Anticoagulant.
See: Coumadin Sodium, Tab., Inj. (Du Pont Merck Pharmaceutical Co.).

warfarin sodium. (Barr Laboratories) 1 mg, 2 mg, 2.5 mg, 4 mg, 5 mg, 7.5 mg, 10 mg. Tab. Bot. 100s, 500s, 1000s. *Rx.*
Use: Anticoagulant.

Wart Fix. (Last) Castor oil 100%. Bot. 0.3 fl oz. *otc.*
Use: Dermatologic, wart therapy.

Wart-Off. (Pfizer US Pharmaceutical Group) Salicylic acid 17% in flexible collodion, alcohol 20.5%, ether 54.2%. Bot. 0.5 oz. *otc.*
Use: Keratolytic.

wasp vemon. *Rx.*

Use: Immunization.
See: Albay (Bayer Corp. (Consumer Div.)).
Pharmalgen (ALK Laboratories, Inc.).
Venomil (Bayer Corp. (Consumer Div)).

•**water for injection.** U.S.P. 23.
Use: Pharmaceutic aid (solvent).

•**water o 15 injection.** U.S.P. 23.
Use: Diagnostic aid (radioactive, vascular disorders), radiopharmaceutical.

Water Babies Little Licks by Coppertone. (Schering-Plough Corp.) SPF 30, ethylhexyl p-methoxycinnamate, oxybenzone, 2-ethylhexyl salicylate, cherry flavor. Lot. Tube 4.8 g. *otc.*
Use: Sunscreen.

Water Babies Sunblock Cream. (Schering-Plough Corp.) SPF 25, ethylhexyl p-methoxycinnamate, 2-ethylhexyl salicylate, homosalate, oxybenzone, benzyl alcohol. PABA free, waterproof. Cream. Bot. 90 g. *otc.*
Use: Sunscreen.

Water Babies UVA/UVB Sunblock Lotion. (Schering-Plough Corp.) SPF 30 ethylhexyl p-methoxycinnamate, 2-ethylhexyl salicylate, homosalate, oxybenzone, benzyl alcohol. PABA free, waterproof. Lot. Bot. 120 ml, 240 ml. *otc.*
Use: Sunscreen.

Water Babies UVA/UVB Sunblock Lotion. (Schering-Plough Corp.) SPF 45, ethylhexyl p-methoxycinnamate, 2-ethylhexyl salicylate, otocrylene oxybenzone, benzyl alcohol. PABA free, waterproof. Lot. Bot. 120 ml. *otc.*
Use: Sunscreen.

Water Babies UVA/UVB Sunblock Lotion. (Schering-Plough Corp.) Ethylhexyl-p-methoxycinnamate, oxybenzone in lotion base, SPF-15. Bot. 120 ml. *otc.*
Use: Sunscreen.

watermelon seed extract. Citrin (Table Rock).

watermelon seed extract. W/Phenobarbital, theobromine. Cithal (Table Rock).

•**water, purified.** U.S.P. 23.
Use: Pharmaceutic aid (solvent).

•**wax, carnauba.** N.F. 18.
Use: Pharmaceutic aid (tablet coating agent).

•**wax, emulsifying.** N.F. 18.
Use: Pharmaceutic aid (emulsifying, stiffening agent).

•**wax, microcrystalline.** N.F. 18.
Use: Pharmaceutic aid (stiffening, tablet coating agent).

•**wax, white.** N.F. 18.
Use: Pharmaceutic aid (stiffening agent).

•**wax, yellow.** N.F. 18.
Use: Pharmaceutic aid (stiffening agent).

Waxsol. Docusate Sodium.

Wayds. (Wayne) Docusate sodium 100 mg/Cap. Bot. 100s. *otc.*
Use: Laxative.

Wayds-Plus. (Wayne) Docusate w/ casanthranol. Cap. Bot. 50s. *otc.*
Use: Laxative.

Wayne-E. (Wayne) Vitamin E **100 IU or 200 IU/Cap.:** Bot. 1000s. **400 IU/Cap.:** Bot. 100s *otc.*
Use: Vitamin supplement.

Wehless. (Roberts Pharmaceuticals) Phendimetrazine tartrate 35 mg/Cap. Bot. 100s. *c-III.*
Use: Anorexiant.

Wehless-105 Timecelles. (Roberts Pharmaceuticals) Phendimetrazine tartrate 105 mg/SA Cap. Bot. 100s. *c-III.*
Use: Anorexiant.

Wehydryl. (Roberts Pharmaceuticals) Diphenhydramine HCl 50 mg/ml. Vial 10 ml. *Rx.*
Use: Antihistamine.

Welders Eye Lotion. (Weber) Tetracaine, potassium Cl, boric acid, camphor, glycerin, disodium edetate, benzalkonium Cl as preservatives. Bot. oz. *otc.*
Use: Burn therapy.

Wellbutrin. (GlaxoWellcome) Bupropion 75 mg, 100 mg/Tab. Bot. 100s. *Rx.*
Use: Antidepressant.

Wellbutrin SR. (GlaxoWellcome) Bupropion HCl 100 mg, 150 mg/SR Tab. Bot. 60s. *Rx.*
Use: Antidepressant.

Wellcovorin. (GlaxoWellcome) Leucovorin 5 mg, 25 mg as calcium. **Tab.: 5 mg:** Bot. 20s, 100s, UD 50s. **25 mg:** Bot. 25s, UD 10s. **Pow. for Inj.:** 100 mg/vial as calcium. *Rx.*
Use: Hematopoietic. Colorectal cancer; osteosarcoma. [Orphan Drug]

Wellferon. (GlaxoWellcome) Interferon alfa-NL.
Use: Human papillomavirus in severe respiratory (laryngeal) papillomatosis. [Orphan Drug]

Wernet's Adhesive Cream. (Block Drug Co., Inc.) Carboxymethylcellulose gum, ethylene oxide polymer, petrolatum in mineral oil base. Cream. Tube 1.5 oz. *otc.*
Use: Denture adhesive.

Wernet's Powder. (Block Drug Co., Inc.)

Karaya gum, ethylene oxide polymer. Bot. 0.63 oz, 1.75 oz, 3.55 oz. *otc.*
Use: Denture adhesive.

Wes-B/C. (Western Research) Vitamins B_1 15 mg, B_2 10 mg, B_6 5 mg, niacinamide 50 mg, calcium pantothenate 10 mg, C 300 mg/Cap. Bot. 1000s. *otc.*
Use: Mineral, vitamin supplement.

Wesmatic Forte Tablets. (Wesley Pharmacal Co., Inc.) Phenobarbital ⅛ gr, ephedrine sulfate 0.25 gr, chlorpheniramine maleate 2 mg, guaifenesin 100 mg/Tab. Bot. 100s, 1000s. *Rx.*
Use: Antihistamine, decongestant, expectorant, hypnotic, sedative.

Westcort Cream. (Westwood Squibb Pharmaceuticals) Hydrocortisone valerate 0.2% in a hydrophilic base with white petrolatum. Tube 15 g, 45 g, 60 g, 120 g. *Rx.*
Use: Corticosteroid, topical.

Westcort Ointment. (Westwood Squibb Pharmaceuticals) Hydrocortisone valerate 0.2% in hydrophilic base with white petrolatum, mineral oil. Tube 15 g, 45 g, 60 g. *Rx.*
Use: Corticosteroid, topical.

Westhroid. (Western Research) Thyroid 0.5 gr, 1 gr, 2 gr, 3 gr, 4 gr/Tab.; 5 gr/SC Tab. Handicount 28s (36 bags of 28s). *Rx.*
Use: Hormone, thyroid.

Westrim. (Western Research) Phenylpropanolamine HCl 37.5 mg/Tab. Bot. 100s. *otc.*
Use: Dietary aid, decongestant.

Westrim-LA 50. (Western Research) Phenylpropanolamine HCl 50 mg/TR Cap. Bot. 1000s. *otc.*
Use: Dietary aid, decongestant.

Westrim-LA 75. (Western Research) Phenylpropanolamine HCl 75 mg/TR Cap. Bot. 1000s. *otc.*
Use: Dietary aid, decongestant.

Wesvite. (Western Research) Vitamins B_1 10 mg, B_2 5 mg, B_6 2 mg, pantothenic acid 10 mg, niacinamide 30 mg, B_{12} 3 mcg, C 100 mg, E 5 IU, A 10,000 IU, D 400 IU, Fe 15 mg, Cu 1 mg, I 0.15 mg, Mn 1 mg, Zn 1.5 mg/Tab. Bot. 1000s. *otc.*
Use: Mineral, vitamin supplement.

Wet-N-Soak. (Allergan, Inc.) Borate buffered. WSCP 0.006%, hydroxyethylcellulose. Soln. Bot. 15 ml. *otc.*
Use: Contact lens care.

Wet-N-Soak Plus. (Allergan, Inc.) Polyvinyl alcohol, edetate disodium, benzalkonium Cl 0.003%. Soln. Bot. 120 ml, 180 ml. *otc.*
Use: Contact lens care.

Wetting Solution. (PBH Wesley Jessen) Polyvinyl alcohol, benzalkonium Cl 0.004%, EDTA 0.02%. Soln. Bot. 60 ml. *otc.*
Use: Contact lens care.

Wetting and Soaking. (PBH Wesley Jessen) Buffered, isotonic. Chlorhexidine gluconate 0.005%, EDTA 0.02%, NaCl, octylphenoxy (oxyethylene) ethanol, povidone, polyvinyl alcohol, propylene glycol, hydroxyethylcellulose. Soln. Bot. 120 ml. *otc.*
Use: Contact lens care.

Wetting and Soaking Solution. (Bausch & Lomb Pharmaceuticals) Chlorhexidine gluconate 0.006%, EDTA 0.05%, cationic cellulose derivative polymer. Bot. 118 ml. *otc.*
Use: Contact lens care.

wheat germ oil. (Various Mfr.)
Use: Vitamin supplement
See: Natural Wheat Germ Oil, Cap., Oint. (Spirt).
Natural Viobin Wheat Germ Oil, Liq. (Spirt).
Tocopherol Preps. (Various Mfr.)

Wheat Germ Oil Concentrate. (Thurston) Perles. 6 min. Bot. 100s. *otc.*
Use: Cardiovascular agent.

whey protein concentrate (bovine).
See: Bovine Whey Protein Concentrate.

WHF Lubricating Gel. (Lake Consumer Products) Chlorehexidine gluconate, methylparaben, glycerin/Gel. Tube 113.4 g. Ind. packets 3 g. *otc.*
Use: Vaginal dryness relief.

Whirl-Sol. (Sween) Moisturizing bath additive. Bot. 2 oz, 8 oz, 16 oz, 21 oz, gal, 5 gal, 30 gal, 55 gal. *otc.*
Use: Emollient.

white-faced hornet venom. *Rx.*
Use: Immunization.
See: Albay (Bayer Corp. (Consumer Div.)).
Pharmalgen (ALK Laboratories, Inc.)
Venomil (Bayer Corp. (Consumer Div.)).

•**white lotion.** U.S.P. 23. Lotio Alba.
Use: Astringent.

white precipitate.
See: Ammoniated Mercury.

Whitfield's Ointment. (Various Mfr.) Benzoic acid 6%, salicylic acid 3%. *otc.*
Use: Antiinfective, topical.

whooping cough vaccine. U.S.P. 23.
See: Acel-Imune, Vial (Wyeth-Ayerst Laboratories).
ActHIB/DTP, Set of DTwP vial plus Hib Pow. for Inj. (Pasteur Merieux Connaught).
Diphtheria and tetanus toxoids with

pertussis vaccine (Various Mfr).
Infanrix (SKB).
Pertussis Vaccine.
Tetramune, Vial (Wyeth-Ayerst Laboratories).
Tri-Immunol, Vial (Wyeth-Ayerst Laboratories).
Tripedia, Vial (Pasteur Merieux Connaught).

Whorto's Calamine Lotion. (Whorton Pharmaceuticals, Inc.) Calamine, zinc oxide, glycerin (U.S.P. strength) in carboxymethylcellulose lotion vehicle. Bot. 4 oz, gal. *otc.*
Use: Dermatologic, counterirritant.

Wibi Lotion. (Galderma Laboratories, Inc.) Purified water, SD alcohol 40, glycerin, PEG-4, PEG-6-32 stearate, PEG-6-32, glycol stearate, carbomer 940, PEG-75, methylparaben, propylparaben, triethanolamine, menthol, fragrance. Bot. 8 oz, 16 oz. *otc.*
Use: Emollient.

widow spider species antivenin (Latrodectus mactans). (Merck & Co.) Antivenin, *Lactrodectus mactans.*
Use: Immunization.

Wigraine. (Organon Teknika Corp.) Ergotamine tartrate 1 mg, caffeine 100 mg/Tab. **Tab.:** Box 20s, 100s. *Rx.*
Use: Antimigraine.

wild cherry.
Use: Flavored vehicle.

Wilpowr. (Foy Laboratories) Phentermine HCl 30 mg/Cap. Bot. 100s, 500s, 1000s.
Use: Anorexiant.

Wilpor-Clear. (Foy Laboratories) Phentermine HCl 30 mg/Cap. Bot. 1000s. *c-IV.*
Use: Anorexiant.

WinRho SD. (Univax Biologics) RH_o (D) immune globulin IV human. 600 IU, 1500 IU. Vial 2.5 ml (10s). *Rx.*
Use: Prevention of Rh isoimmunization; immune thrombocytopenic purpura.

Winstrol. (Sanofi Winthrop Pharmaceuticals) Stanozolol 2 mg/Tab. Bot. 100s. *c-III.*
Use: Anabolic steroid.

Wintergreen Sucrets. (SmithKline Beecham Pharmaceuticals) Dyclonine HCl 0.1%, alcohol 10%, sorbitol. Spray. Bot. 90 ml. *otc.*
Use: Mouth and throat preparation.

•**witch hazel.** U.S.P. 23.
Use: Astringent.

witch hazel. (Various Mfr.) Hamamelis water (witch hazel). Bot. 120 ml, 240 ml, 280 ml, 480 ml, 960 ml, gal.
Use: Astringent.

Within. (Bayer Corp. (Consumer Div.)) Vitamins A 5000 IU, E 30 IU, C 60 mg, folic acid 0.4 mg, B_1 1.5 mg, B_2 1.7 mg, niacin 20 mg, B_6 2 mg, B_{12} 6 mcg, pantothenic acid 10 mg, D 400 IU, Fe 27 mg, Ca 450 mg, Zn 15 mg/Tab. Bot. 60s, 100s. *otc.*
Use: Mineral, vitamin supplement.

WNS Suppositories. (Sanofi Winthrop Pharmaceuticals) Sulfamylon HCl. *Rx.*
Use: Anorectal preparation.

Wonderful Dream. (Kondon) Phenylmercuric nitrate 1:5000, oils of tar, turpentine, olive and linseed, rosin, burgundy pitch, camphor, beeswax, mutton tallow. Salve. 34 g. *otc.*
Use: Topical.

Wonder Ice. (Pedinol Pharmacal, Inc.) Menthol in a specially formulated base. Gel. Tube 113 ml. *otc.*
Use: Liniment.

Wondra. (Procter & Gamble Pharm.) Petrolatum, lanolin acid, glycerin, stearyl alcohol, cyclomethicone, EDTA, hydrogenated vegetable glycerides phosphate, cetyl alcohol, isopropyl palmitate, stearic acid, PEG-100 stearate, carbomer 934, dimethicone, titanium dioxide, imidazolidinyl urea, parabens. Lot. Bot. 180 ml, 300 ml, 450 ml. *otc.*
Use: Emollient.

wood charcoal tablets. (Cowley) 5 gr, 10 gr/Tab. Bot. 1000s. *otc.*

wood creosote.
See: Creosote (Various Mfr.)

wool fat. Lanolin, Anhydrous.

Wyamine Sulfate Injection. (Wyeth-Ayerst Laboratories) Mephentermine sulfate 15 mg, 30 mg, methylparaben 1.8 mg, propylparaben 0.2 mg/ml. Vial 10 ml. Amp. 2 ml. *Rx.*
Use: Vasopressor.

Wyanoids Relief Factor. (Wyeth-Ayerst Laboratories) Cocoa butter 79%, shark liver oil 3%, corn oil, EDTA, parabens, tocopherol. Supp. 12s. *otc.*
Use: Anorectal preparation.

Wycillin. (Wyeth-Ayerst Laboratories) Penicillin G procaine, 600,000 U/dose. Inj. 1 ml *Tubex*; 1,200,000 U/dose. Inj. 2 ml *Tubex*; 2,400,000 U/dose. Inj. 4 ml Disp. Syringe. Parabens, lecithin, povidone. *Rx.*
Use: Anti-infective; penicillin.

Wydase Lyophilized. (Wyeth-Ayerst Laboratories) Purified bovine testicular hyaluronidase. Vial 150 units/ml, 1500 units/10 ml with lactose and thimerosal. *Rx.*
Use: Absorption facilitator; hypodermoclysis, urography.

Wydase Stabilized Solution. (Wyeth-Ayerst Laboratories) Purified bovine testicular hyaluronidase 150 units/ml in sterile saline soln. with sodium Cl, EDTA, thimerosal. Vial 1 ml, 10 ml. *Rx.*
Use: Absorption facilitator; hypodermoclysis; urography.

Wygesic. (Wyeth-Ayerst Laboratories) Propoxyphene HCl 65 mg, acetaminophen 650 mg/Tab. Bot. 100s, 500s, Redipak 100s. *c-IV.*
Use: Analgesic combination, narcotic.

Wymox. (Wyeth-Ayerst Laboratories) Amoxicillin. **Cap.:** 250 mg Bot. 100s, 500s; 500 mg Bot. 50s, 500s. **Pow. for Oral Susp.:** 125 mg/5 ml (as trihydrate) when reconstituted; 250 mg/5 ml (as trihydrate) when reconstituted. Bot. 100 ml, 150 ml. Sucrose. *Rx.*
Use: Anti-infective, penicillin.

Wytensin. (Wyeth-Ayerst Laboratories) Guanabenz acetate. **4 mg/Tab.:** Bot. 100s, 500s, Redipak 100s. **8 mg/Tab.:** Bot. 100s. **16 mg/Tab.:** Bot. 100s. *Rx.*
Use: Antihypertensive.

X

Xalatan. (Pharmacia and Upjohn) Latanoprost 0.005% (50 mcg/ml), benzalkonium Cl 0.02%. Sol. In 2.5 ml fill dropper bottles.
Use: Agent for glaucoma.

•**xamoterol.** (ZAM-oh-ter-ole) USAN.
Use: Cardiovascular agent.

•**xamoterol fumarate.** (ZAM-oh-ter-ole) USAN.
Use: Cardiovascular agent.

Xanax. (Pharmacia and Upjohn) Alprazolam 0.25 mg, 0.5 mg, 1 mg, 2 mg. Tab. **0.25 mg, 0.5 mg, 2 mg:** 100s, 500s, UD 100s. Visipack 4 × 25s. **1 mg:** 30s, 90s, 100s, 500s, UD 100s. *c-IV.*
Use: Anxiolytic.

•**xanomeline.** (zah-NO-meh-leen) USAN.
Use: Cholinergic agonist (for Alzheimer's disease).

•**xanomeline tartrate.** (zah-NO-meh-leen) USAN.
Use: Cholinergic agonist (for Alzheimer's disease).

•**xanoxate sodium.** (ZAN-ox-ate) USAN.
Use: Bronchodilator.

•**xanthan gum.** N.F. 18.
Use: Pharmaceutic aid, suspending agent.

xanthine derivatives.
See: Caffeine.
Theobromine.
Theophylline.

•**xanthinol niacinate.** (ZAN-thih-nahl NYE-ah-SIN-ate) USAN.
Use: Vasodilator (peripheral).

xanthiol hydrochloride.
Use: Antinauseant.

xanthotoxin. Methoxsalen.

Xeloda. (Roche Laboratories) Capecitabine 150 mg, 500 mg, lactose/Tab. Bot. 120s. *Rx.*
Use: Treatment of metastatic breast cancer.

•**xemilofiban hydrochloride.** (zem-ih-LOW-fih-ban) USAN.
Use: Treatment of unstable angina, prevention of postrecanalization reocclusion of coronary vessels.

•**xenalipin.** (ZEN-ah-LIH-pin) USAN.
Use: Hypolipidemic.

•**xenbucin.** (ZEN-BYOO-sin) USAN.
Use: Antihyperlipidemic.

•**xenon Xe 127.** ((ZEE-nahn)) U.S.P. 23.
Use: Diagnostic aid; medicinal gas; radiopharmaceutical.

•**xenon Xe 133.** U.S.P. 23.
Use: Radiopharmaceutical.

Xerac AC. (Person and Covey, Inc.) Aluminum Cl hexahydrate 6.25% in anhydrous ethanol 96%. Bot 35 ml, 60 ml. *Rx.*
Use: Dermatologic, acne.

Xeroform Ointment 3%. (City, Consolidated) Pow. 0.25 lb, 1 lb. Jar 1 lb, 5 lb.

Xero-Lube. (Scherer Laboratories, Inc.) Monobasic potassium phosphate, dibasic potassium phosphate, magnesium Cl, potassium Cl, calcium Cl, sodium Cl, sodium fluoride, sorbitol soln., sodium carboxymethylcellulose, methylparaben. Bot. 6 oz. *otc.*
Use: Mouth and throat preparation.

•**xilobam.** (ZIE-low-bam) USAN.
Use: Muscle relaxant.

•**xipamide.** (ZIP-ah-mide) USAN.
Use: Antihypertensive, diuretic.

•**xorphanol mesylate.** (ZAHR-fan-ahl) USAN.
Use: Analgesic.

X-Prep Bowel Evacuant Kit-1. (Purdue Frederick Co.) Kit contains Senokot S tab., X-Prep liquid, Rectolax supp. *otc.*
Use: Laxative.

X-Prep Bowel Evacuant Kit-2. (Purdue Frederick Co.) Kit contains Citralax granules, X-Prep liquid, Rectolax supp. *otc.*
Use: Laxative.

X-Prep Liquid. (Gray Pharmaceutical Co.) Senna extract with alcohol 7%, sucrose 50 g. Bot. 2.5 oz. *otc.*
Use: Laxative.

X-Ray Contrast Media.
See: Iodine Products, Diagnostic.

X-Seb Plus. (Baker Norton Pharmaceuticals, Inc.) Pyrithione zinc 1%, salicylic acid 2%. Shampoo. Bot. 120 ml. *otc.*
Use: Antiseborrheic.

X-Seb Shampoo. (Baker Cummins Dermatologicals, Inc.) Salicylic acid 4%, coal tar soln. 10% in a blend of surface-active agents. Bot. 4 oz. *otc.*
Use: Antiseborrheic.

X-Seb T. (Baker Cummins Dermatologicals, Inc.) Coal tar soln. 10%, salicylic acid 4%. Bot. 4 oz. *otc.*
Use: Antiseborrheic.

X-Sep T Plus. (Baker Norton Pharmaceuticals, Inc.) Coal tar solution 10%, salicylic acid, menthol 1%. Shampoo. Bot. 120 ml. *otc.*
Use: Antiseborrheic.

Xtracare. (Sween) Bot. 2 oz, 4 oz, 8 oz, 21 oz, gal. *otc.*
Use: Emollient.

Xtra-Vites. (Barth's) Vitamins A 10,000 IU, D 400 IU, C 150 mg, B_1 5 mg, B_2

1 mg, niacin 3.33 mg, pantothenic acid 183 mcg, B_6 250 mcg, B_{12} 215 mcg, E 15 IU, rutin 20 mg, citrus bioflavonoid complex 15 mg, choline 6.67 mg, inositol 10 mg, folic acid 50 mcg, biotin, aminobenzoic acid/Tab. Bot. 30s, 90s, 180s, 360s. *otc.*
Use: Vitamin supplement.

X-Trozine Capsules. (Rexar Pharmaceuticals) Phendimetrazine tartrate 35 mg/Cap. Bot. 1000s. *c-III.*
Use: Anorexiant.

X-Trozine S.R. Capsules. (Rexar Pharmaceuticals) Phendimetrazine tartrate 105 mg/SR Cap. Bot. 100s, 200s, 1000s. *c-III.*
Use: Anorexiant.

X-Trozine Tablets. (Rexar Pharmaceuticals) Phendimetrazine tartrate 35 mg/Tab. Bot. 1000s. *c-III.*
Use: Anorexiant.

•**xylamidine tosylate.** (zie-LAM-ih-deen TAH-sill-ate) USAN.
Use: Serotonin inhibitor.

•**xylazine hydrochloride.** (ZIE-lih-zeen HIGH-droe-KLOR-ide) USAN.
Use: Analgesic.

•**xylitol.** (ZIE-lih-tahl) N.F. 18.
Use: Pharmaceutic aid (vehicle, sweetened).

Xylocaine Hydrochloride. (Astra Pharmaceuticals, L.P.) Lidocaine HCl. **Amp.:** (1%): 2 ml, 5 ml, 30 ml; w/epinephrine 1:200,000 30 ml. (1.5%): 20 ml; w/epinephrine 1:200,000 30 ml. (2%): 2 ml, 10 ml; w/epinephrine 1:200,000 20 ml. (4%): 5 ml. **Multi-dose Vial:** (0.5%): 50 ml; w/epinephrine 1:200,000 50 ml. (1%): 20 ml, 50 ml; w/epinephrine 1:100,000 20 ml, 50 ml. (2%): 20 ml, 50 ml; w/epinephrine 1:100,000 20 ml, 50 ml. **Single-dose Vial:** (1%): 30 ml. (1.5%) 20 ml; w/epinephrine 1:200,000 10 ml, 30 ml. (2%) w/epinephrine 1:200,000 20 ml. *Rx.*
Use: Anesthetic, local.

Xylocaine Hydrochloride for Cardiac Arrhythmia. (Astra Pharmaceuticals, L.P.) **Intravenous:** Lidocaine 2%. Amp 5 ml, disp. syringe 5 ml. Continuous infusion 1 g/25 ml Vial; 2 g/50 ml Vial. Prefilled syringe 100 mg/5 ml, 12s. Continuous infusion prefilled syringe 1 g, 2 g. **Intramuscular:** Amp. 10%, 5 ml. *Rx.*
Use: Anesthetic, local.

Xylocaine Hydrochloride 4% Solution. (Astra Pharmaceuticals, L.P.) Topical use. Bot. 50 ml. *Rx.*
Use: Anesthetic, local.

Xylocaine Hydrochloride for Spinal Anesthesia. (Astra Pharmaceuticals, L.P.) Lidocaine HCl 1.5%, 5%, glucose 7.5%, sodium hydroxide to adjust pH. Specific gravity 1.028 to 1.034. Amp. 2 ml. Box 10s. *Rx.*
Use: Anesthetic, local.

Xylocaine Hydrochloride w/Dextrose. (Astra Pharmaceuticals, L.P.) Lidocaine HCl 1.5%, dextrose 7.5%. Inj. Amps. 2 ml. *Rx.*
Use: Anesthetic, local.

Xylocaine Hydrochloride w/Epinephrine. (Astra Pharmaceuticals, L.P.) Lidocaine HCl 2% w/epinephrine 1:200,000. Amps w/sodium metabisulfite 20 ml. Inj. Single-dose Vials w/sodium metabisulfite. 20 ml. *Rx.*
Use: Anesthetic, local.

Xylocaine Hydrochloride w/Glucose. (Astra Pharmaceuticals, L.P.) Lidocaine HCl 5%, glucose 7.5%. Inj. Amp. 2 ml. *Rx.*
Use: Anesthetic, local.

Xylocaine Jelly. (Astra Pharmaceuticals, L.P.) Lidocaine HCl 2% in sodium carboxymethylcellulose with parabens. Tube 5 ml, 30 ml. *Rx.*
Use: Anesthetic, local.

Xylocaine Ointment. (Astra Pharmaceuticals, L.P.) Lidocaine 2.5%, water-soluble carbowaxes. 35 g. *otc.*
Use: Anesthetic, local.

Xylocaine MPF Injection. (Astra Pharmaceuticals, L.P.) Lidocaine HCl. **0.5%:** 50 ml. **1%:** 2 ml, 5 ml, 30 ml. **1.5%:** 10 ml, 20 ml. **2%:** 2 ml, 5 ml, 10 ml. **4%:** 5 ml. **1%:** w/ epinephrine 1:200,000, sodium bisulfite. 5 ml, 10 ml, 30 ml. **2%:** w/ epinephrine, sodium bisulfite. 5 ml, 10 ml, 20 ml. **5%:** w/ glucose 7.5%. 2 ml. *Rx.*
Use: Anesthetic, local.

Xylocaine Viscous. (Astra Pharmaceuticals, L.P.) Lidocaine HCl 2%, sodium carboxymethylcellulose, parabens. Bot. 20 ml (25s), 100 ml, 450 ml, UD 20 ml. *Rx.*
Use: Anesthetic, local.

•**xylofilcon a.** (ZILE-oh-FILL-kahn A) USAN.
Use: Contact lens material (hydrophilic).

•**xylometazoline hydrochloride.** (zie-low-met-AZZ-oh-leen) U.S.P. 23.
Use: Adrenergic (vasoconstrictor).
See: Long Acting Neo-Synephrine, Prods. (Sanofi Winthrop Consumer Products).
Otrivin, Spray (Novartis Pharmaceutical Corp.).
Rhinall L.A., Liq. (First Texas).

Sine-Off, Spray (Menley & James Labs, Inc.).
Vicks Sinex Long Acting, Nasal Spray (Procter & Gamble Pharm.).

Xylo-Pfan. (Pharmacia and Upjohn) Xylose 25 g/Bot.
Use: Diagnostic aid.

Xylophan D-Xylose Tolerance Test. (Pfanstiehl) D-xylose 25 g/UD bot.
Use: Diagnostic aid.

•**xylose.** (ZIE-lohs) U.S.P. 23.
Use: Diagnostic aid (intestinal function determination).

Y

Yager's Liniment. (Yager) Oil of turpentine and camphor w/clove oil fragrance, emulsifier, emollient, ammonium oleate (< 0.5% free ammonia) penetrant base. *otc.*
Use: Rubefacient.

yatren.
See: Chiniofon, Tab.

YDP Lice Spray. (Youngs Drug) Synthetic pyrethroid in aerosol. Can 5 oz. *otc.*
Use: Pediculicide, inanimate objects.

yeast adenylic acid. An isomer of adenosine 5-monophosphate, has been found inactive.
See: Adenosine 5-Monophosphate, Preps. for active compounds.

yeast, dried.
Use: Protein and vitamin B complex source.

yeast tablets, dried.
Use: Supplementary source of B complex vitamins.
See: Brewer's Yeast, Tab.

Yeast-Gard. (Lake Consumer Products) Pulsatilla 28x, *Candida albicans:* 28x. Supp. 10s w/applicator. *otc.*
Use: Vaginal agent.

Yeast-Gard Medicated Disposable Douche. (Lake Consumer Products) Povidone-iodine 0.3% when reconstituted. Soln. 180 ml twin-pack w/two 5.4 ml medicated douche concentrate packets. *otc.*
Use: Douche.

Yeast-Gard Medicated Disposable Douche Premix. (Lake Consumer Products) Octoxynol 9, lactic acid, sodium lactate, sodium benzoate, aloe vera. Soln. 180 ml twin-pack. *otc.*
Use: Douche.

Yeast-Gard Medicated Douche. (Lake Consumer Products) Povidone-iodine 10%. Soln. Concentrate. 240 ml. *otc.*
Use: Douche.

yeast, torula.
See: Torula Yeast.

yeast w/iron.
See: Natural Super Iron Yeast Powder (Spirt) Bot. 200s.

Yeast-X. (C. B. Fleet Co., Inc.) **Supp.:** Pulsatilla 28x. Pkg. 12s w/applicator. *otc.*
Use: Vaginal agent.

Yelets. (Freeda Vitamins, Inc.) Iron 20 mg, vitamins A 10,000 IU, D 400 IU, E 10 IU, B_1 10 mg, B_2 10 mg, B_3 25 mg, B_5 10 mg, B_6 10 mg, B_{12} 10 mcg, C 100 mg, folic acid 0.1 mg, PABA, lysine, glutamic acid, Ca, I, Mg, Mn, Se, Zn 4 mg/Tab. Bot. 100s, 250s. *otc.*
Use: Mineral, vitamin supplement.

yellow enzyme.
See: Riboflavin (Various Mfr.).

•**yellow fever vaccine.** U.S.P. 23.
Use: Immunization.
See: YF-Vax, Inj. (Pasteur Merieux Connaught).

yellow hornet venom.
Use: Desensitizing agent
See: Albay (Bayer Corp. (Consumer Div.)).
Pharmalgen (ALK Laboratories, Inc.).
Venomil (Bayer Corp. (Consumer Div.)).

yellow jacket venom.
Use: Desensitizing agent.
See: Albay (Bayer Corp. (Consumer Div.)).
Pharmalgen (ALK Laboratories, Inc.).
Venomil (Bayer Corp. (Consumer Div.)).

yellow mercuric oxide 1%. (Various Mfr.) Oint. Tube 3.5 g, 3.75 g, 30 g. *otc.*
Use: Antiseptic.

yellow mercuric oxide 2%. (Various Mfr.) Oint. Tube 3.5 g, 3.75 g, 30 g. *otc.*
Use: Antiseptic.
See: Stye, Oint. (Del Pharmaceuticals, Inc.).

yellow ointment.
Use: Pharmaceutic aid (ointment base)

yellow wax.
Use: Pharmaceutic aid (stiffening agent).

YF-Vax. (Pasteur Merieux Connaught) Yellow fever vaccine. Inj. Vial 1 dose, 5 dose, 20 dose with diluent. *Rx.*
Use: Immunization.

Yocon. (Palisades Pharmaceuticals, Inc.) Yohimbine HCl 5.4 mg/Tab. Bot. 100s, 1000s. *Rx.*
Use: Antiimpotence agent.

Yodora Deodorant Cream. (SmithKline Beecham Pharmaceuticals) Jar 2 oz. *otc.*
Use: Deodorant.

Yodoxin. (Glenwood, Inc.) Iodoquinol 210 mg, 650 mg/Tab. Bot. 100s, 1000s. Pow. Bot. 25 g. *Rx.*
Use: Amebicide.

yohimbine hydrochloride. Indolalkylamine alkaloid. (Various Mfr.) 5.4 mg/Tab. Bot. 100s, 500s. *Rx.*
Note: Yohimbine has no FDA sanctioned indications.
See: Dayto Himbin (Dayton).

Yohimex. (Kramer Laboratories, Inc.) Yohimbine HCl 5.4 mg/Tab. Bot. 100s. *Rx.*
Use: Anti-impotence agent.

Your Choice Non-Preserved Saline Solution. (Amcon Laboratories) Buffered, isotonic soln. w/ NaCl, boric acid, sodium borate. Bot. 360 ml. *otc.*
Use: Contact lens care.

Your Choice Sterile Preserved Saline Solution. (Amcon Laboratories) Isotonic. Sorbic acid 0.1%, EDTA, NaCl, boric buffer. Bot. 60 ml, 360 ml. *otc.*
Use: Contact lens care.

ytterbium Yb 169 pentetate injection. U.S.P. XXII.
Use: Radiopharmaceutical.

Yutopar. (Astra Pharmaceuticals, L.P.) Ritodrine HCl 10 mg/ml, Amp. 5 ml; 15 mg/ml, Vial 10 ml, inj. syringe 10 ml. *Rx.*
Use: Uterine relaxant.

Z

•**zacopride hydrochloride.** (ZAK-oh-pride) USAN.
Use: Antiemetic, stimulant (peristaltic).

•**zafirlukast.** (zah-FEER-loo-kast) USAN.
Use: Antiasthmatic (leukotriene antagonist).
See: Accolate, Tab. (Zeneca Pharmaceuticals).

Zagam. (Rhone-Poulenc Rorer Pharmaceuticals, Inc.) Sparfloxacin 200 mg/Tab. Bot. *Rx.*
Use: Fluoroquinolone.

•**zalcitabine.** (zal-SITE-ah-BEAN) USAN.
Use: Antiviral.

zalcitabine. ((National Cancer Inst.))
Use: AIDS. [Orphan Drug]
See: Hivid (Roche Laboratories).

•**zaleplon.** (ZAL-eh-plahn) USAN.
Use: Hypnotic, sedative.

•**zalospirone hydrochloride.** (zal-OH-spy-rone) USAN.
Use: Anxiolytic.

•**zaltidine hydrochloride.** (ZAHL-tih-deen) USAN.
Use: Antiulcerative.

Zanaflex. (Athena Neurosciences, Inc.) Tizanidine HCl 4 mg, lactose/Tab. Bot. 150s *Rx.*
Use: Skeletal muscle relaxant.

•**zanamivir.** (zan-AM-ih-veer) USAN.
Use: Antiviral; influenza virus neuraminidase inhibitor.
See: Relenza, Pow. for Inh. (GlaxoWellcome).

zankiren hydrochloride. (zan-KIE-ren) USAN.
Use: Antihypertensive.

Zanosar. (Pharmacia & Upjohn) Streptozocin 1 g. (100 mg/ml) Pow. for Inj. Vial. *Rx.*
Use: Antineoplastic.

•**zanoterone.** (zan-OH-ter-ohn) USAN.
Use: Antiandrogen.

Zantac EFFERdose Effervescent Granules and Tablets. (GlaxoWellcome) Ranitidine HCl 150 mg. **Granules:** 1.44 g packets (30s, 60s). **Tab:** Bot. 30s, 60s. *Rx.*
Use: Antiulcerative.

Zantac GELdose. (GlaxoWellcome) Ranitidine HCl 150 mg, 300 mg/Cap. **150 mg:** Bot. 60s, UD 60s. **300 mg:** Bot. 30s, UD 30s. *Rx.*
Use: Antiulcerative.

Zantac Injection. (GlaxoWellcome) Ranitidine 25 mg HCl/ml. Vial 2 ml, 10 ml, 40 ml, syringe 2 ml. *Rx.*
Use: Antiulcerative.

Zantac Injection Premixed. (GlaxoWellcome) Ranitidine 0.5 mg as HCl/ml. 100 ml Single-dose Plastic Container. *Rx.*
Use: Antiulcerative.

Zantac 75. (GlaxoWellcome) Ranitidine 75 mg/Tab. Pkg. 4s, 10s, 20s. *otc.*
Use: Antiulcerative.

Zantac Syrup. (GlaxoWellcome) Ranitidine 15 mg as HCl/ml, alcohol 7.5%. Bot. 480 ml. *Rx.*
Use: Antiulcerative.

Zantac Tablets. (GlaxoWellcome) Ranitidine 150 mg, 300 mg as HCl/Tab. **150 mg:** Bot. 60s, 500s, UD 100s. **300 mg:** Bot. 30s, 250s, UD 100s. *Rx.*
Use: Antiulcerative.

Zantine. (Lexis Laboratories) Dipyridamole 25 mg, 50 mg, 75 mg/Tab. Bot. 1000s. *Rx.*
Use: Coronary vasodilator.

Zantryl. (ION Laboratories, Inc.) Phentermine HCl 30 mg/Cap. Bot. 100s. *c-IV.*
Use: Anorexiant.

Zarontin. (Parke-Davis) Ethosuximide. **Cap.:** 250 mg. Bot. 100s. **Syr.:** 250 mg/5 ml. Bot. Pt. *Rx.*
Use: Anticonvulsant.

Zaroxolyn. (Medeva Pharmaceuticals, Inc.) Metolazone 2.5 mg, 5 mg, or 10 mg/Tab. Bot. 100s, 500s, 1000s, UD 100s. *Rx.*
Use: Diuretic.

•**zatosetron maleate.** (ZAT-oh-SEH-trahn) USAN.
Use: Antimigraine.

Z-Bec. (Wyeth-Ayerst Laboratories) Vitamins E 45 mg, C 600 mg, B_1 15 mg, B_2 10.2 mg, B_3 100 mg, B_6 10 mg, B_{12} 6 mcg, pantothenic acid 25 mg, Zn 22.5 mg/Tab. Bot. 60s, 100s, 500s. *otc.*
Use: Mineral, vitamin supplement.

ZBT Baby. (Glenwood, Inc.) Talc, mineral oil, magnesium stearate, propylene glycol, BHT. Pow. 120 g. *otc.*
Use: Diaper rash preparation.

Zeasorb-AF. (Stiefel Laboratories, Inc.) Miconazole nitrate 2%. Pow. Can 70 g. *otc.*
Use: Antifungal, topical.

Zeasorb Powder. (Stiefel Laboratories, Inc.) Talc, microporous cellulose, supersorb carbohydrate acrylic copolymer. Sifter-top Can 2.5 oz, 8 oz. *otc.*
Use: Dermatologic.

Zebeta. (ESI Lederle Generics) Bisoprolol fumarate. **5 mg:** Tab/Bot. 14s, 30s, 100s, 500s, 1000s, UD 10s. **10 mg:** Tab/Bot. 14s, 30s, 100s, 500s, 1000s, UD 10s. *Rx.*
Use: Beta-adrenergic blocker.

Ze Caps. (Everett Laboratories, Inc.) Vitamin E 200 mg, Zn 9.6 mg as gluconate/Cap. Bot. 60s. *otc.*
Use: Mineral, vitamin supplement.

Zefazone. (Pharmacia & Upjohn) Cefmetazole sodium. **Pow. for Inj.:** 1 g, 2 g (2 mEq sodium/g). Vial. **Inj.:** 1 g/50 ml or 2 g/50 ml (2.7 mEq sodium/g) in frozen iso-osmotic, premixed solution in single-dose plastic container. *Rx.*
Use: Anti-infective.

•**zein.** (ZEE-in) N.F. 18.
Use: Pharmaceutic aid (coating agent).

Zemalo. (Alpharma USPD Inc.) Sulfur, zinc oxide, camphor, titanium oxide. Bot. 4 oz, pt, gal. *otc.*
Use: Dermatologic, counterirritant.

Zemplar. (Abbott) Paricaltol 5 mcg/ml Inj. Single-dose fliptop vials, 1 ml, 2 ml. *Rx.*
Use: Vitamin.

Zenapax. (Roche Laboratories) Daclizumab 25 mg/5 ml. Preservative free. Inj. Vial. *Rx.*
Use: Prevent organ rejection.

Zenate. (Solvay Pharmaceuticals)
Use: Mineral, vitamin supplement.
See: Advanced Formula Zenate, Tab. (Solvay Pharmaceuticals).

•**zenazocine mesylate.** (zen-AZE-oh-seen MEH-sih-late) USAN.
Use: Analgesic.

Zendium. (Oral-B Laboratories, Inc.) Sodium fluoride 0.22%. Tube 0.9 oz, 2.3 oz.
Use: Dental caries agent.

•**zeniplatin.** (zen-ih-PLAT-in) USAN.
Use: Antineoplastic.

Zentel. (SmithKline Beecham Pharmaceuticals) Albendazole.
Use: Anthelmintic.

Zephiran. (Sanofi Winthrop Pharmaceuticals) **Aqueous soln.:** Benzalkonium Cl 1:750. Bot. 240 ml, gal. **Disinfectant concentrate:** 17% in 120 ml, gal. **Tincture:** 1:750 in gal. **Tincture spray:** 1:750 in 30 g, 180 g, gal. *otc.*
Use: Antiseptic, antimicrobial.

Zephiran Towelettes. (Sanofi Winthrop Pharmaceuticals) Moist paper towels with soln. of zephiran Cl 1:750. Box 20s, 100s, 1000s. *otc.*
Use: Antiseptic, antimicrobial.

Zephrex. (Sanofi Winthrop Pharmaceuticals) Pseudoephedrine HCl 60 mg, guaifenesin 400 mg/SR Tab. Bot. 100s. *Rx.*
Use: Decongestant, expectorant.

Zephrex-LA. (Sanofi Winthrop Pharmaceuticals) Pseudoephedrine HCl 120 mg, guaifenesin 600 mg/Tab. Bot. 100s. *Rx.*
Use: Decongestant, expectorant.

Zepine. (Foy Laboratories) Reserpine alkaloid 0.25 mg/Tab. Bot. 100s, 500s, 1000s. *Rx.*
Use: Antihypertensive.

•**zeranol.** (ZER-ah-nole) USAN.
Use: Anabolic.

Zerit. (Bristol-Myers Squibb) Stavudine 15 mg, 20 mg, 30 mg, 40 mg/Cap. Bot. 60s. Stavudine 1 mg/ml after reconstitution w/ 202 ml purified water, sucrose, parabens, dye free, fruit flavor. Pow. for Oral Sol. Bot. 200 ml. *Rx.*
Use: Antiviral.

Zestoretic. (Zeneca Pharmaceuticals) Lisinopril 10 mg, hydrochlorothiazide 12.5 mg, or lisinopril 20 mg, hydrochlorothiazide 12.5 mg, or lisinopril 20 mg, hydrochlorothiazide 25 mg/Tab. Bot. 100s. *Rx.*
Use: Antihypertensive.

Zestril. (Zeneca Pharmaceuticals) Lisinopril 5 mg, 10 mg, 20 mg, 40 mg/Tab. Bot. 100s, UD 100s. *Rx.*
Use: Antihypertensive.

Zetar Emulsion. (Dermik Laboratories, Inc.) Colloidal whole coal tar 30% (300 mg/ml) in polysorbates. Bot. 6 oz. *otc.*
Use: Antiseborrheic.

Zetar Shampoo. (Dermik Laboratories, Inc.) Colloidal whole coal tar 1% in a shampoo. Bot. 6 oz. *otc.*
Use: Antiseborrheic.

Z-gen. (Zenith Goldline Pharmaceuticals) Vitamins E 45 mg, B_1 15 mg, B_2 10.2 mg, B_3 100 mg, B_5 25 mg, B_6 10 mg, B_{12} 6 mcg, C 600 mg, zinc 22.5 mg/Tab. Bot. 60s, 100s. *otc.*
Use: Mineral, vitamin supplement.

Ziac. (ESI Lederle Generics) Bisoprolol fumarate 2.5 mg, 5 mg, 10 mg; hydrochlorothiazide 6.25 mg. Tab. **2.5 mg or 5 mg:** Bot. 30s, 100s. **10 mg:** Bot. 30s. *Rx.*
Use: Antihypertensive.

Ziagen. (GlaxoWellcome) Abacavir sulfate. **Tab.:** 300 mg. Bot. 60s, 180s, UD 60s. **Oral Soln.:** 20 mg/ml, parabens, saccharin, sorbitol, strawberry-banana flavor. Bot. 240 ml. *Rx.*
Use: Antiviral.

•**zidometacin.** (ZIE-doe-MEH-tah-sin) USAN.
Use: Anti-inflammatory.

•**zidovudine.** (zie-DOE-view-DEEN) USAN. *Formerly azidothymidine, AZT.*
Use: Antiviral, AIDS, HIV infection.
See: Retrovir (GlaxoWellcome).
W/Lamivudine.

See: Combivir, Tab. (GlaxoWellcome).

•**zifrosilone.** (zih-FROE-sih-lone) USAN.
Use: Acetylcholinesterase inhibitor.

Ziks. (Nnodum Corporation) Methyl salicylate 12%, menthol 1%, capsaicin 0.025%, cetyl alcohol. Cream Tube 60 g. *otc.*
Use: Analgesic.

Zilactin-B Medicated. (Zila Pharmaceuticals, Inc.) Benzocaine 10%, alcohol 76%. Gel Tube 7.5 g. *otc.*
Use: Anesthetic, local.

Zilactin-L. (Zila Pharmaceuticals, Inc.) Lidocaine 2.5%, alcohol 79.3%. Liq. Bot. 7.5 ml. *otc.*
Use: Anesthetic, local.

Zilactin Medicated Gel. (Zila Pharmaceuticals, Inc.) Tannic acid 7%, suspended in alcohol 80.8%. Gel Tube 0.25 oz. *otc.*
Use: Cold sores.

ZilaDent. (Zila Pharmaceuticals, Inc.) Benzocaine 6%, alcohol 74.9%. Gel Tube. 7.5 g, single packs. *otc.*
Use: Anesthetic, local.

•**zilantel.** (ZILL-an-tell) USAN.
Use: Anthelmintic.

•**zileuton.** (ZIE-loo-tone) USAN.
Use: Inhibitor (5-lipoxygenase).
See: Zyflo, Tab. (Abbott Laboratories).

zimco. (Sterwin) Vanillin.

•**zimeldine hydrochloride.** (zie-MELL-ih-deen) USAN. *Formerly Zimelidine Hydrochloride.*
Use: Antidepressant.

Zinacef. (GlaxoWellcome) Cefuroxime 750 mg, 1.5 g, 7.5 g as sodium Pow. for Inj. 750 mg, 1.5 g (as sodium)/Inj. **Pow. for Inj.: 750 mg, 1.5 g:** Vials and infusion pack. **7.5 g:** Pharmacy bulk Pkg. **Inj.: 750 mg, 1.5 g, premixed:** 50 ml. *Rx.*
Use: Anti-infective, cephalosporin.

Zinc-220. (Alto Pharmaceuticals, Inc.) Zinc sulfate 220 mg/Cap. Bot. 100s, 1000s, UD 100s. *otc.*
Use: Mineral supplement.

•**zinc acetate.** (zingk) U.S.P. 23. Acetic acid, zinc salt, dihydrate.
Use: Pharmaceutic necessity for Zinc-Eugenol Cement.

zinc acetate. (zingk)
Use: Wilson's disease. [Orphan Drug]
See: Benadryl Itch Relief, Children's, Cream, Spray (GlaxoWellcome).
Benadryl Itch Relief, Maximum Strength, Cream, Stick (GlaxoWellcome).
Benadryl Itch Relief, Spray (GlaxoWellcome).
Benadryl Itch Stopping Maximum Strength, Gel (GlaxoWellcome).
Benadryl Itch Stopping Children's Formula, Gel (GlaxoWellcome).
Galzin (Lemmon Co.).

Zinca-Pak. (SoloPak Pharmaceuticals, Inc.) Zinc 1 mg, 5 mg/ml. Inj. **1 mg:** Vial 10 ml, 30 ml. **5 mg:** Vial 5 ml. *Rx.*
Use: Nutritional supplement, parenteral.

Zincate. (Paddock Laboratories) Zinc sulfate 220 mg (elemental zinc 50 mg)/Cap. Bot. 100s, 1000s. *otc.*
Use: Mineral supplement.

zinc bacitracin. U.S.P. 23. Bacitracin Zinc.
Use: Anti-infective.

•**zinc carbonate.** U.S.P. 23.
Use: Antiseptic, topical; astringent.

•**zinc chloride.** U.S.P. 23.
Use: Astringent, dentin desensitizer.
W/Formaldehyde.
See: Forma Z Concentrate (Ingram).

•**zinc chloride Zn 65.** USAN.
Use: Radiopharmaceutical.

zinc citrate. (Zingk)
See: Zinc Lozenges (Goldline Consumer Products).

zinc-eugenol cement. U.S.P. XXI.
Use: Dental protectant.

Zincfrin. (Alcon Laboratories, Inc.) Zinc sulfate 0.25%, phenylephrine HCl 0.12%. Soln. Drop-Tainer 15 ml, 30 ml. *otc.*
Use: Astringent, decongestant, ophthalmic.

zinc gelatin. U.S.P. XXI. Impregnated gauge, U.S.P. 23.
Use: Topical protectant.

Zinc-Glenwood. (Glenwood, Inc.) Zinc sulfate 220 mg/Cap. Bot. 100s. *otc.*
Use: Mineral supplement.

•**zinc gluconate.** U.S.P. 23.
Use: Supplement (trace mineral).
See: Zinc Lozenges (Goldline Consumer Products).

zinchlorundesal. Zincundesal.

zinc insulin.
See: Insulin Zinc, Preps. (Various Mfr.).

Zincon Shampoo. (ESI Lederle Generics) Pyrithione zinc 1%, sodium methyl cocoyl taurate, sodium Cl, magnesium aluminum silicate, sodium cocoyl isethionate, glutaral, water w/pH adjusted. Bot. 4 oz, 8 oz. *otc.*
Use: Antiseborrheic.

Zinc Lozenges. (Zenith Goldline Pharmaceuticals) Zinc citrate 23 mg, zinc gluconate, fructose, sorbitol/Loz. Bot. 30s. *otc.*

Use: Mineral supplement.
•**zinc oxide.** U.S.P. 23. Flowers of zinc.
Use: Astringent, topical protectant.
See: Calamine Preps.
W/Combinations.
See: Akne, Drying Lot. (Alto Pharmaceuticals, Inc.).
Anusol, Oint., Supp. (Parke-Davis).
Anusol-HC, Supp. (Parke-Davis).
Blis-To-Sol, Pow. (Chattem).
Bonate, Supp. (Suppositoria Laboratories, Inc.).
Calamatum, Preps. (Blair Laboratories).
Desitin, Oint. (Pfizer US Pharmaceutical Group).
Elder Diaper Rash Oint. (Zeneca Pharmaceuticals).
Hemorrhoidal Oint. (Towne).
Hydro Surco, Lot. (Alma).
Medicated Powder (Johnson & Johnson).
Medicated Foot Powder (Pharmacia & Upjohn).
Mexsana, Pow. (Schering-Plough Corp.).
Pazo, Oint., Supp. (Bristol-Myers Squibb).
Rectal Medicone HC, Supp. (Medicore).
RVPaque, Oint. (Zeneca Pharmaceuticals).
Saratoga, Oint. (Blair Laboratories).
Schamberg, Lot. (Paddock Laboratories).
Sebasorb, Lot. (Summers Laboratories, Inc).
Taloin, Tube (Warren-Teed).
Unguentine Oint. "Original Formula" (Procter & Gamble Pharm).
Versal, Supp. (Suppositoria Laboratories, Inc.).
Wyanoids, Preps. (Wyeth-Ayerst Laboratories).
Xylocaine Supp. (Astra Pharmaceuticals, L.P.).
Zinc Boric Lotion, Liq (Emerson Laboratories).
zinc phenolsulfonate.
Use: Astringent.
W/Belladonna leaf extract, kaolin, pectin, sodium carboxymethylcellulose.
See: Diastay, Tab. (Zeneca Pharmaceuticals).
W/Bismuth subsalicylate, salol, methyl salicylate.
See: Pepto-Bismol, Liq. (Procter & Gamble Pharm.).
W/Kaolin, pectin.
See: Pectocel, Liq. (Eli Lilly and Co.).
W/Opium pow., bismuth subgallate, pectin, kaolin.
See: Bismuth, Pectin & Paregoric (Teva Pharmaceuticals USA).
zinc pyrithione.
Use: Bactericide, fungicide, antiseborrheic.
See: Zincon, Shampoo (ESI Lederle Generics).
•**zinc stearate.** U.S.P. 23. Octadecanoic acid, zinc salt.
Use: Dusting powder; pharmaceutic aid (tablet/capsule lubricant).
zinc sulfanilate. Zinc sulfanilate tetrahydrate. Nizin, Op-Isophrin-Z, Op-Isophrin-Z-M (Broemmel).
Use: Anti-infective.
•**zinc sulfate.** U.S.P. 23. Sulfuric acid, zinc salt (1:1), heptahydrate.
Use: Astringent, ophthalmic.
See: Eye-Sed, Soln. (Scherer Laboratories, Inc.).
Op-Thal-Zin Ophth. (Alcon Laboratories, Inc.).
Zinc-Glenwood, Cap. (Glenwood, Inc.).
Zin-Cora, Cap. (Zeneca Pharmaceuticals).
W/Boric acid, phenylephrine HCl.
See: Phenylzin Drops, Ophth. Soln. (Smith & Nephew United).
W/Calcium lactate.
See: Zinc-220, Cap. (Alto Pharmaceuticals, Inc.).
W/Menthol, methyl salicylate, alum, boric acid, oxyquinoline citrate.
See: Maso pH Powder (Mason Pharmaceuticals, Inc.).
W/Phenylephrine HCl, polyvinyl alcohol.
See: Prefrin-Z, Liquifilm (Allergan, Inc.).
W/Piperocaine HCl, boric acid, potassium Cl.
See: M-Z Drops (Smith & Nephew United).
W/Sodium Cl.
See: Bromidrosis Crystals (Gordon Laboratories).
W/Vitamins.
See: Vicon-C, Cap. (GlaxoWellcome).
Vicon Forte, Cap. (GlaxoWellcome).
Vicon Plus, Cap. (GlaxoWellcome).
Vi-Zac, Cap. (GlaxoWellcome).
Z-Bec, Tab. (Wyeth-Ayerst Laboratories).
zinc sulfate. (Various Mfr.) Zinc 5 mg/ml (as sulfate 21.95 mg). Inj. Vial 5, 10 ml.
Use: Nutritional supplement, parenteral.
zinc sulfate. (Various Mfr.) **Cap.:** Zinc sulfate 220 mg, lactose, gelatin. Bot. 100s. **Inj.:** Zinc 1 mg/ml (as sulfate 4.39 mg). Vial 10, 30 ml. *Rx-otc.*
Use: Nutritional supplement, parenteral.

zinc sulfocarbolate.
W/Aluminum hydroxide, pectin, kaolin, bismuth subsalicylate, salol.
See:

zinc trace metal additive. (I.M.S., Ltd.) Zinc 4 mg/ml. Inj. Vial. 10 ml. *Rx.*
Use: Nutritional supplement, parenteral.

zincundesal.
See: Zinchlorundesal.

zinc-10-undecenoate.
See: Zinc Undecylenate, U.S.P. 23.

•**zinc undecylenate.** (zingk uhn-deh-SILL-en-ate) U.S.P. 23.
Use: Antifungal.
See: Blis-To-Sol, Pow. (Chattem).
W/Benzocaine, hexachlorophene.
See: Decyl-Cream LBS (Scrip).
W/Caprylic acid, sodium propionate.
See: Deso-Cream (Quality Formulations, Inc.).
Deso-Talc, Foot Pow. (Quality Formulations, Inc.).
W/Undecylenic acid.
See: Cruex Cream, Spray Pow. (Novartis Pharmaceutical Corp.).
Desenex, Prods. (Novartis Pharmaceutical Corp.).
Quinsana, Med Oint. (Mennen).

Zincvit. (Kenwood Laboratories) Vitamin A 5000 IU, D_3 50 IU, E 50 IU, B_1 10 mg, B_2 5 mg, B_6 2 mg, C 300 mcg, B_3 25 mg, Zn 40 mg, Mg 9.7 mg, Mn 1.3 mg, folic acid 1 mg/Cap. Bot. 60s. *Rx.*
Use: Mineral, vitamin supplement.

Zinecard. (Pharmacia & Upjohn) Dexrazoxane 250 mg, 500 mg. Powd. for Inj. Lyophilized. Vial 25 ml (250 mg) or 50 ml (500 mg) of 0.167 Molar Sodium Lactate Injection. *Rx.*
Use: Antineoplastic, antidote. [Orphan Drug]

•**zindotrine.** (ZIN-doe-TREEN) USAN.
Use: Bronchodilator.

•**zinoconazole hydrochloride.** (zih-no-KOE-nah-zole) USAN.
Use: Antifungal.

•**zinostatin.** (ZEE-no-STAT-in) USAN. *Formerly neocarzinostatin.*
Use: Antineoplastic.

•**zinterol hydrochloride.** (ZIN-ter-ole) USAN.
Use: Bronchodilator.

•**zinviroxime.** (zin-VIE-rox-eem) USAN.
Use: Antiviral.

•**ziprasidone hydrochloride.** (zih-PRAY-sih-dohn) USAN.
Use: Antipsychotic.

zirconium carbonate or oxide.
See: Dermaneed, Lot. (Hanlon).
W/Benzocaine, menthol, camphor.
See: Rhuli Cream, Oint. (ESI Lederle Generics).
W/Benzocaine, menthol, camphor, calamine, pyrilamine maleate.
See: Ivarest, Cream (Carbisulphoil).
W/Benzocaine, menthol, camphor, calamine, isopropyl alcohol.
See: Rhulispray, Aer. (ESI Lederle Generics).

Zithromax. (Pfizer US Pharmaceutical Group) Azithromycin. **Tab.:** 250 mg, 600 mg. Lactose. In 30s, UD 50s (250 mg only), Z-Pak 6s (3) (250 mg only). **Pow. for Inj.:** 500 mg. 10 ml vials. **Pow. for Oral Susp.:** 100 mg/5 ml, sucrose. Bot. 300 mg. 200 mg/5 ml, sucrose, Bot. 600 mg, 900 mg, 1200 mg. 1 g/packet, sucrose, Single-dose pack, 3s, 10s. *Rx.*
Use: Anti-infective, macrolide.

Zixoryn. (Farmacon, Inc.) Flumecinal.
Use: Hyperbilirubinemia.

ZNG. (Western Research) Zinc gluconate 35 mg/Tab. Handicount 28s (36 bags of 28 tab.). *otc.*
Use: Mineral supplement.

ZNP Bar. (Stiefel Laboratories, Inc.) Zinc pyrithione 2%. Bar 4.2 oz. *otc.*
Use: Antiseborrheic.

ZN-Plus Protein. (Miller Pharmacal Group, Inc.) Zinc in a zinc-protein complex made with isolated soy protein 15 mg/Tab. Bot. 100s. *otc.*
Use: Mineral supplement.

Zocor. (Merck & Co.) Simvastatin **5 mg Tab.:** Bot. 60s, 90s, UD 100s. **10 mg Tab.:** Bot. 60s, 90s, 1000s, 10,000s, UD 100s. **20 mg Tab.:** Bot. 60s, 1000s, 10,000s, UD 100s. **40 mg Tab.:** Bot. 60s. **80 mg Tab.:** Bot. 60s, Lactose, talc. *Rx.*
Use: Antihyperlipidemic.

Zodeac-100. (Econo Med Pharmaceuticals) Fe 60 mg, vitamins A 8000 IU, D 400 IU, E 30 IU, B_1 1.7 mg, B_2 2 mg, B_3 20 mg, B_5 11 mg, B_6 4 mg, B_{12} 8 mcg, C 120 mg, folic acid 1 mg, biotin 300 mcg, Ca, Cu, I, Mg, Zn 15 mg/Tab. Bot. 100s. *Rx.*
Use: Mineral, vitamin supplement.

•**zofenopril calcium.** (zoe-FEN-oh-PRILL) USAN.
Use: Enzyme inhibitor (angiotensin-converting).

•**zofenoprilat arginine.** (zoe-FEN-oh-PRILL-at AHR-jih-neen) USAN.
Use: Antihypertensive.

Zofran. (GlaxoWellcome) Ondansetron HCl **Tab.:** 4 mg, 8 mg, lactose Bot. 30s, UD 100s, 1 x 3 UD pack. **Inj.:** 2 mg/ml in 2 ml, 20 ml vials, or 32 mg/50

ml (premixed) parabens (2 mg/ml); preservative free, with dextrose 2500 mg, citric acid 26 mg, sodium citrate 11.5 mg (32 mg/50 ml). 50 ml containers **Oral Sol.:** 4 mg/5 ml (5 mg as HCl), sorbitol, strawberry flavor. Bot. 50 ml. *Rx.*
Use: Antiemetic.

Zofran ODT. (GlaxoWellcome) Ondansetron 4 mg, 8 mg, aspartame, mannitol, parabens. Orally Disintegrating Tab. UD 30s. *Rx.*
Use: Antiemetic, antivertigo.

Zoladex. (Zeneca Pharmaceuticals) Goserelin acetate 3.6 mg, 10.8 mg. Implant. Syringes. *Rx.*
Use: LHRH agonist.

•**zolamine hydrochloride.** (zoe-lah-meen) USAN.
Use: Antihistamine; anesthetic, topical.

zolazepam hydrochloride. (zole-AZE-eh-pam) USAN.
Use: Hypnotic, sedative.

•**zoledronate disodium.** (ZOE-leh-droe-nate) USAN.
Use: Bone resorption inhibitor; osteoporosis treatment and prevention.

•**zoledronate trisodium.** (ZOE-leh-droe-nate) USAN.
Use: Bone resorption inhibitor; osteoporosis treatment and prevention.

•**zoledronic acid.** (ZOE-leh-drah-nik) USAN.
Use: Calcium regulator; osteoporosis treatment and prevention.

•**zolertine hydrochloride.** (ZOE-ler-teen) USAN.
Use: Antiadrenergic, vasodilator.

•**zolimomab aritox.** (zah-LIM-ah-mab a-rih-TOX) USAN.
Use: Monoclonal antibody (antithrombotic).

•**zolmitriptan.** USAN.
Use: Antimigraine.
See: Zomig, Tab. (Zeneca Pharmaceuticals).

Zoloft. (Roerig) Sertraline HCl 25 mg, 50 mg, 100 mg/Tab. Bot. 50s, (25 mg only); 100s, 500s, 5000s, UD 100s (50 mg and 100 mg only). *Rx.*
Use: Antidepressant.

•**zolpidem tartrate.** (ZOLE-pih-dem) USAN.
Use: Hypnotic, sedative.
See: Ambien.

•**zomepirac sodium.** (ZOE-mih-PEER-ack) USAN. U.S.P. XXI.
Use: Analgesic, anti-inflammatory.

•**zometapine.** (zoe-MET-ah-peen) USAN.
Use: Antidepressant.

Zomig. (Zeneca Pharmaceuticals) Zolmitriptan 2.5 mg, 5 mg, lactose/Tab. Blister pack 6s (2.5 mg), 3s (5 mg). *Rx.*
Use: Antimigraine.

Zone-A Forte. (Forest Pharmaceutical, Inc.) Hydrocortisone 2.5%, pramoxine HCl in a hydrophilic base containing stearic acid 1%, forlan-L, glycerin, triethanolamine, polyoxyl 40 stearate, diisopropyl adipate, povidone, silicone fluid-200. Paraben free. Lot. Bot. 60 ml. *Rx.*
Use: Corticosteroid; anesthetic, local.

Zone-A Lotion. (Forest Pharmaceutical, Inc.) Hydrocortisone acetate 1%, pramoxine HCl 1%. Bot. 2 oz. *Rx.*
Use: Corticosteroid; anesthetic, local.

•**zoniclezole hydrochloride.** (zoe-NIH-klih-ZOLE) USAN.
Use: Anticonvulsant.

•**zonisamide.** (zoe-NISS-ah-MIDE) USAN.
Use: Anticonvulsant.

Zonite Liquid Douche Concentrate. (Menley & James Labs, Inc.) Benzalkonium Cl 0.1%, menthol, thymol, EDTA in buffered soln. Bot. 240 ml, 360 ml. *otc.*
Use: Vaginal agent.

•**zopolrestat.** (zoe-PAHL-reh-STAT) USAN.
Use: Antidiabetic, aldose reductase inhibitor.

•**zorbamycin.** (ZAHR-bah-MY-sin) USAN.
Use: Anti-infective.

ZORprin. (Knoll Pharmaceuticals) Aspirin 800 mg/SR Tab. Bot. 100s. *Rx.*
Use: Analgesic.

•**zorubicin hydrochloride.** (zoe-ROO-bih-sin) USAN.
Use: Antineoplastic.

Zostrix. (Medicis Dermatologicals, Inc.) Capsaicin 0.025%. Cream 45 g. *Rx.*
Use: Analgesic, topical.

Zostrix-HP. (Medicis Dermatologicals, Inc.) Formerly called Axsain, formerly marketed by Galen.

Zosyn. (Wyeth-Ayerst Laboratories) Piperacillin sodium/tazobactam sodium. **2 g/0.25 g:** Na 4.69 mEq. Vial 2.25 g, *ADD-Vantage* vial. **3 g/0.375 g:** Na 7.04 mEq. Vial 3.375 g, *ADD-Vantage* vial. **4 g/0.5 g:** Na 9.39 mEq. Vial 4.5 g, *ADD-Vantage* vial. **36g/4.5 g:** Na 84.5 mEq. Vial 40.5 g. Preservative free. *Rx.*
Use: Anti-infective, penicillins.

Zoto-HC. (Horizon Pharmaceutical Corp.) Chloroxylenol 1%, pramoxine HCl 10%, hydrocortisone 10%/ml in non-aqueous vehicle with 3% propylene glycol di-

acetate. Otic Drops. Vial 10 ml. *Rx.*
Use: Otic.

Zovia. (Watson Laboratories) Ethinyl estradiol 35 mcg, 50 mcg, ethynodiol diacetate 1 mg/Tab. 21s, 28s (7 inert tabs in 28s). *Rx.*
Use: Contraceptive.

Zovirax Capsules. (GlaxoWellcome) Acyclovir 200 mg/Cap. Bot. 100s, UD 100s. *Rx.*
Use: Antiviral.

Zovirax Ointment 5%. (GlaxoWellcome) Acyclovir 50 mg/g. Tube 15 g. *Rx.*
Use: Antiviral, topical.

Zovirax Powder. (GlaxoWellcome) Acyclovir sodium 500 mg/vial or 1000 mg/vial. **500 mg:** Vial 10 ml. **1000 mg:** Vial 20 ml. *Rx.*
Use: Antiviral.

Zovirax Suspension. (GlaxoWellcome) Acyclovir 200 mg/5 ml. Susp. Bot. 473 ml. *Rx.*
Use: Antiviral.

Zovirax Tablets. (GlaxoWellcome) Acyclovir 400 mg, 800 mg/Tab. **400 mg:** Bot. 100s. **800 mg:** Bot. 100s, UD 100s, Shingles Relief Pak 35s. *Rx.*
Use: Antiviral.

Z-Pro-C. (Person and Covey, Inc.) Zinc sulfate 200 mg (elemental zinc 45 mg), ascorbic acid 100 mg/Tab. Bot. 100s. *otc.*
Use: Mineral, vitamin supplement.

Z-Tec. (Seatrace Pharmaceuticals, Inc.) Iron equivalent 50 mg/ml from iron dextran complex. Vial 10 ml. *Rx.*
Use: Mineral supplement.

•**zucapsaicin.** (zoo-cap-SAY-sin) USAN.
Use: Analgesic, topical.

•**zuclomiphene.** (zoo-KLOE-mih-FEEN) USAN. *Formerly transclomiphene.*

Zurinol. (Major Pharmaceuticals) Allopurinol. **100 mg/Tab.:** Bot. 100s, 500s, 1000s, UD 100s. **300 mg/Tab.:** Bot. 100s, 500s, UD 100s. *Rx.*
Use: Antigout agent.

Zyban. (GlaxoWellcome) Bupropion HCl 150 mg/SR Tab. In 60s. *Rx.*
Use: Smoking deterrent.

Zyderm I. (Collagen Corp.) Highly purified bovine dermal collagen 35 mg/ml implant. Sterile syringe 0.1 ml, 0.5 ml, 1 ml, 2 ml.
Use: Collagen implant.

Zyderm II. (Collagen Corp.) Highly purified bovine dermal collagen 65 mg/ml implant. Syringe 0.75 ml.
Use: Collagen implant.

Zydone. (DuPont Merck Pharmaceutical Co.) Hydrocodone bitartrate 5 mg, 7.5 mg, or 10 mg, acetaminophen 400 mg. Cap. Bot. 100s, 500s, UD 100s. *c-III.*
Use: Analgesic combination, narcotic.

Zyflo. (Abbott Laboratories) Zileuton 600 mg/Tab. Bot. 120s. *Rx.*
Use: Antiasthmatic.

Zyloprim. (GlaxoWellcome) Allopurinol. **100 mg/Tab.:** Bot. 100s, 1000s, UD 100s. **300 mg/Tab.:** Bot. 30s, 100s, 500s, UD 100s. *Rx.*
Use: Antigout agent.

Zyloprim. (GlaxoWellcome) Allopurinol Sodium. Inj.
Use: Antineoplastic. [Orphan Drug]

Zymacap. (Pharmacia & Upjohn) Vitamins A 5000 IU, D 400 IU, E 15 mg, C 90 mg, folic acid 400 mcg, B_1 2.25 mg, B_2 2.6 mg, niacin 30 mg, B_6 3 mg, B_{12} 9 mcg, pantothenic acid 15 mg/Cap. Bot. 90s, 240s. *otc.*
Use: Vitamin supplement.

Zymase. (Organon Teknika Corp.) Lipase 12,000 units, protease 24,000 units, amylase 24,000 units. Cap. Bot. 100s. *Rx.*
Use: Digestive enzyme.

Zyprexa. (Eli Lilly and Co.) Olanzapine 2.5 mg, 5 mg, 7.5 mg, 10 mg, lactose/Tab. Bot. 60s, UD 100s (except 2.5 mg). *Rx.*
Use: Antipsychotic.

Zyrkamine. (Ilex Oncology Inc.) Mitoguazone.
Use: Non-Hodgkin's lymphoma treatment. [Orphan Drug]

Zyrtec. (Pfizer US Pharmaceutical Group) Cetirizine 5 mg, 10 mg, lactose, povidone. Tab. Bot. 100s. Cetirizine 5 mg/5 ml, parabens, sugar, banana-grape flavor. Syrup. Bot. 120 ml, Pt. *Rx.*
Use: Antihistamine.

Reference Information

Standard Medical Abbreviations

Abbreviation	Meaning
≈	approximately equals
Δ	delta
ε	epsilon; molar absorption coefficient
Ω	omega; ohm
5-HIAA	5-hydroxyindoleacetic acid
5-HT	5-hydroxytryptamine (serotonin)
6-MP	6-mercaptopurine
17-OHCS	17-hydroxycorticosteroids
α	alpha
A	ampere(s)
Å	angstrom(s)
aa	of each (ana)
āā	of each (ana)
AA	Alcoholics Anonymous; amino acid
AACP	American Association of Clinical Pharmacy; American Association of Colleges of Pharmacy
AARP	American Association of Retired Persons
Ab	antibody
ABGs	arterial blood gases
abs feb	when fever is absent (*absente febre*)
ABVD	Adriamycin (doxorubicin), bleomycin, vinblastine, (and) dacarbazine
ac	before meals or food (*ante cibum*)
ACCP	American College of Clinical Pharmacy
ACD	acid-citrate-dextrose
ACE	angiotensin-converting enzyme
ACEI	angiotensin-converting enzyme inhibitor
ACh	acetylcholine
ACIP	Advisory Committee on Immunization Practices
ACLS	advanced cardiac life support
ACPE	American Council on Pharmaceutical Education
ACS	American Chemical Society
ACT	activated clotting time
ACTH	adrenocorticotropic hormone
ad to;	to; up to (*ad*)
a.d.	right ear (*aurio dextra*)
ADE	adverse drug experience
ADH	antidiuretic hormone
adhib	to be administered (*adhibendus*)

Abbreviation	Meaning
ad lib	as desired, at pleasure (*ad libitum*)
ADLs	activities of daily living
ADME	absorption, distribution, metabolism and elimination
admov	apply (*admove*)
ADP	adenosine diphosphate
ADR	adverse drug reaction
ADRRS	Adverse Drug Reaction Reporting System
ad sat.	to saturation (*ad saturatum, ad saturandum*)
adst feb	when fever is present (*adstante febre*)
ad us.	ext for external use (*ad usum externum*)
adv	against (*adversum*)
aer	aerosol
Ag	antigen; silver (*argentum*)
agit. Ante us.	shake before using (*agita ante usum*)
agit. Bene	shake well (*agita bene*)
AHA	American Hospital Association
AID	artificial insemination donor
AIDS	acquired immunodeficiency syndrome
AJHP	*American Journal of Hospital Pharmacy*
al	left ear (*aurio laeva*)
ala	alanine
ALL	acute lymphocytic leukemia
ALT	alanine aminotransferase, serum (previously SGPT)
alt hor.	every other hour (*alternis horis*)
A.M.	before noon; morning (*ante meridiem*)
AMA	American Medical Association
AML	acute myelogenous leukemia
AMP	adenosine monophosphate
ANA	antinuclear antibody(ies)
ANC	acid neutralizing capacity
ANDA	abbreviated new drug application
ANOVA	analysis of variance
ANUG	acute necrotizing ulcerative gingivitis
APA	antipernicious anemia (factor)
APAP	acetaminophen
APC	antigen presenting cell(s)
APhA	American Pharmaceutical Association

aPTT . . . . .activated partial thromboplastin time
aq. . . . . .water (*aqua*)
aq. dest . . . . . . .distilled water (*aqua destillata*)
ARC . . . . .AIDS-related complex
ARDS . . . . .adult respiratory distress syndrome
ARF . . . . .acute renal failure
Arg . . . . .arginine
ARV . . . . .AIDS-related virus
as . . . . .left ear (*aurio sinister*)
ASHD . . . . .arteriosclerotic heart disease
ASHP . . . . .American Society of Hospital Pharmacists
Asn . . . . .asparagine
Asp . . . . .aspartic acid
AST . . . . .aspartate aminotransferase, serum (previously SGOT)
atm . . . . .standard atmosphere
ATN . . . . .acute tubular necrosis
ATP . . . . .adenosine triphosphate
ATPase . . . . . . .adenosine triphosphatase
ATPD . . . . .ambient temperature and pressure, saturated
at wt . . . . .atomic weight
au . . . . .each ear (*aures utrae*)
AU . . . . .gold (*aurum*)
AUC . . . . .area under the plasma concentration-time curve
AV . . . . .atrioventricular
A-V . . . . .arteriovenous; atrioventricular (block, bundle, conduction, dissociation, extrasystole)
AW . . . . .atomic weight
AWP . . . . .average wholesale price
ax. . . . . .axis
β . . . . .beta
BAC . . . . .blood-alcohol concentration
BADL . . . . .basic activities of daily life
BBB . . . . .blood brain barrier
BDZ . . . . .benzodiazepine
bib . . . . .drink (*bibe*)
bid . . . . .twice daily; two times a day (*bis in die*)
bm . . . . .bowel movement
BMR . . . . .basal metabolic rate
bp. . . . . .boiling point
BP . . . . .blood pressure
BPH . . . . .benign prostatic hypertrophy
bpm . . . . .beats per minute
BSA . . . . .body surface area
BT . . . . .bleeding time
BUN . . . . .blood urea nitrogen
C . . . . .centigrade
C. . . . .*clostridium*
c. . . . . .gallon (*cong*)
c̄. . . . . .with (*cum*)
°C. . . . . .degrees Celsius
Ca . . . . .calcium
CA . . . . .cancer; carcinoma; cardiac arrest; chronologic age; croup-associated
CAD . . . . .coronary artery disease
Cal . . . . .Calorie (kilocalorie)
cAMP . . . . .cyclic adenosine monophosphate
caps . . . . .capsule (*capsula*)
CAS . . . . .Chemical Abstracts Service
CAT . . . . .computerized axial tomography
cath . . . . .catheterize
CBA . . . . .cost-benefit analysis
CBC . . . . .complete blood count
CC . . . . .chief complaint
cc . . . . .cubic centimeter
CCBs . . . . .calcium channel blockers
CCU . . . . .coronary care unit; critical care unit
CD4 . . . . .T-helper lymphocytes and macrophages
CDC . . . . .Centers for Disease Control and Prevention
CEA . . . . .cost effectiveness analysis
CF . . . . .cystic fibrosis
CFC . . . . .chlorofluorocarbon
CFU . . . . .colony-forming units
CHD . . . . .coronary heart disease
CHF . . . . .congestive heart failure
Ci . . . . .curie
CK . . . . .creatinine kinase
Cl . . . . .chlorine
Cl_{cr} . . . . .creatinine clearance
cm . . . . .centimeter; cream
Cm . . . . .curium
cm^2 . . . . .square centimeter(s)
cm^3 . . . . .cubic centimeter
CMA . . . . .Certified Medical Assistant
CMC . . . . .carpometacarpal
CMI . . . . .cell-mediated immunity
CML . . . . .chronic myelocytic leukemia
C_{max} . . . . .maximum effective plasma concentration

C_{min} . . . . .minimum effective plasma concentration
CMT. . . . . .Certified Medical Transcriptionist
CMV. . . . . .cytomegalovirus I
CMVIG. . . . . . . .cytomegalovirus immune globulin
CN . . . . .cranial nerve
CNM. . . . . .Certified Nurse Midwife
CNS. . . . . .central nervous system
CO . . . . .cardiac output
CO_2 . . . . .carbon dioxide
CoA . . . . .coenzyme A
COG. . . . . .center of gravity
comp . . . . .compound (*compositus*)
COMT . . . . .catecholamine-o-methyl transferase
cont rem. . . . . . .let the medicine be continued (*continuetur remedium*)
COPD . . . . .chronic obstructive pulmonary disease
CPAP . . . . .continuous positive airway pressure
CPK . . . . .creatine phosphokinase
CPR . . . . .cardiopulmonary resuscitation
CQI . . . . .continuous quality improvement
Cr. . . . . .creatinine; chromium
CrCl . . . . .creatinine clearance
CRD . . . . .chronic respiratory disease
CRF . . . . .chronic renal failure
CRH . . . . .corticotropin-releasing hormone
crm. . . . . .cream
CRNA. . . . . .Certified Registered Nurse Anesthetist
C&S . . . . .culture and sensitivity
CSA . . . . .Controlled Substances Act; cyclosporin A
CSF . . . . .cerebrospinal fluid; colony-stimulating factors
CSP . . . . .cellulose sodium phosphate
ct . . . . .clotting time
CT . . . . .computerized tomography
CTZ . . . . .chemoreceptor trigger zone
cu. . . . . .cubic
Cu . . . . .copper (*cuprum*)
CV . . . . .cardiovascular
CVA . . . . .cerebrovascular accident
CVP . . . . .central venous pressure
CXR . . . . .chest x-ray
cyl . . . . .cylinder; cylindrical (lens)
cys . . . . .cysteine
d. . . . . .day (*dies*)
D5W. . . . . .Dextrose 5% in Water Solution
D10W. . . . . .Dextrose 10% in Water Solution
D&C . . . . .dilation and curettage; designation applied to dyes permitted for use in drugs and cosmetics
D&E . . . . .dilation and evacuation
DC . . . . .Doctor of Chiropractic
DDS . . . . .Doctor of Dental Surgery
DEA . . . . .Drug Enforcement Administration
deglut. . . . . .swallow (*degluttiatur*)
DERM . . . . .dermatologic
det . . . . .give (*detur*)
DHHS. . . . . .Department of Health and Human Services
DIC. . . . . .disseminated intravascular coagulation
dieb alt. . . . . . . .every other day (*diebus alternis*)
dil . . . . .dilute (*dilue*)
dim. . . . . .one-half (*dimidius*)
dir prop . . . . . . .with proper direction (*directione propria*)
div in par aeq. . .divide into equal parts (*divide in partes aequales*)
DIS. . . . . .drug information source
disp . . . . .dispense (*dispensa*)
div . . . . .divide
DJD . . . . .degenerative joint disease
DKA . . . . .diabetic ketoacidosis
dl . . . . .deciliter (100 ml)
DMD. . . . . .Doctor of Dental Medicine
DMSO . . . . .dimethyl sulfoxide
DNA . . . . .deoxyribonucleic acid
DNR. . . . . .do not resuscitate
DNS . . . . .Director of Nursing Service; Doctor of Nursing Services
DO . . . . .Doctor of Osteopathy
DOA. . . . . .dead on arrival
DP . . . . .Doctor of Podiatry
DPH . . . . .Doctor of Public Health; Doctor of Public Hygiene
DPi. . . . . .dry powder inhaler
DPM. . . . . .Doctor of Physical Medicine; Doctor of Podiatric Medicine
DPS . . . . .disintegrations per second
DRG. . . . . .diagnosis-related groups
DRI. . . . . .Dietary Reference Intakes
drp . . . . .drop(s)
DrPh. . . . . .Doctor of Public Health; Doctor of Public Hygiene
DRR. . . . . .Drug Regimen Review
DT . . . . .delirium tremens

dtd . . . . .give of such a dose (*dentur tales doses*)
DTP . . . . .diphtheria, tetanus toxoids & pertussis vaccine
DTRs . . . . .deep tendon reflexes
DUB. . . . . .dysfunctional uterine bleeding
DUE. . . . . .Drug Usage Evaluations
DUR. . . . . .Drug Utilization Review
dur dol . . . . .while pain lasts (*durante dolore*)
DVA . . . . .Department of Veterans Affairs
DVM. . . . . .Doctor of Veterinary Medicine
DVT . . . . .deep venous thrombosis
E. . . . .*Enterococcus; Escherichia*
EBV . . . . .Epstein-Barr virus
EC . . . . .enteric coated
ECG. . . . . .electrocardiogram
ECT . . . . .electroconvulsive therapy
ed. . . . . .editor
ED . . . . .emergency department; effective dose
ED_{50}. . . . . .median-effective dose
EDTA . . . . .ethylenediamine tetraacetic acid
EEG. . . . . .electroencephalogram
EENT. . . . . .eye, ear, nose, and throat
EF . . . . .ejection fraction
eg. . . . . .for example (*exempli gratia*)
EIA. . . . . .enzyme immunoassay
EKG. . . . . .electrocardiogram
el . . . . .elixir
ELISA. . . . . .enzyme-linked immunosorbent assay
elix . . . . .elixir
EMIT . . . . .enzyme-multiplied immunoassay test
emp . . . . .as directed
ENL . . . . .erythema nodosum leprosum
ENT . . . . .ear, nose, throat
EPA . . . . .Environmental Protection Agency
EPAP . . . . .expiratory positive airway pressure
EPO. . . . . .erythropoietin
EPS . . . . .extrapyramidal syndrome (or symptoms)
ER . . . . .emergency room; estrogen receptor; extended release; endoplasmic reticulum
ESR . . . . .erythrocyte sedimentation rate; electron spin resonance
et . . . . .and
ET . . . . .via endotracheal tube
et al.. . . . . .for 3 or more co-authors or coworkers (*et alii*)
ex aq . . . . .in water
ext rel. . . . . .extended release
F . . . . .fluorine
f . . . . .make; let be made (*fac, fiat, fiant*)
°F. . . . . .degrees Fahrenheit
Fab. . . . . .fragment of immunoglobulin G involved in antigen binding
FAO . . . . .Food and Agriculture Organization
FAS . . . . .fetal alcohol syndrome
FBS . . . . .fasting blood sugar
FDA . . . . .Food and Drug Administration
FD&C. . . . . .designation applied to dyes permitted for use in foods, drugs and cosmetics; Food, Drug and Cosmetic Act
Fe . . . . .iron (*ferrum*)
FEF . . . . .forced expiratory flow
FET . . . . .forced expiratory time
FEV_1 . . . . .forced expiratory volume in 1 second
fl oz . . . . .fluid ounce(s)
Fru . . . . .fructose
FSH . . . . .follicle-stimulating hormone
ft. . . . . .make; let be made (*fac, fiat, fiant*)
ft. . . . . .foot (feet)
ft^2. . . . . .square foot (feet)
FTC . . . . .Federal Trade Commission
FTI . . . . .free-thyroxine index
FUO. . . . . .fever of unknown origin
FVC . . . . .forced vital capacity
γ. . . . . .gamma
g. . . . . .gram (*gramma*)
G-6-P glucose-6-phosphate
G-6-PD. . . . . . . .glucose-6-phosphate dehydrogenase
GABA. . . . . .gamma-aminobutyric acid
Gal. . . . . .galactose
gal . . . . .gallon
G-CSF . . . . .granulocyte colony-stimulating factor
GERD . . . . .gastroesophageal reflux disease
GFR. . . . . .glomerular filtration rate
GGTP. . . . . .gamma glutamyl transpeptidase
GH . . . . .growth hormone
GHRF. . . . . .growth hormone-releasing factor
GHRH . . . . .growth hormone-releasing hormone

GI . . . . .gastrointestinal
GLC . . . . .gas-liquid chromatography
gln . . . . .glutamine
glu . . . . .glutamic acid; glutamyl
gly . . . . .glycine
Gm. . . . . .gram (*gramma*)
gr . . . . .grain (*granum*)
grad . . . . .gradually (*gradatim*)
gran . . . . .granule(s)
GRAS. . . . . .generally regarded as safe*
gtt. . . . . .a drop (*gutta*)
GU . . . . .genitourinary
guttat . . . . .drop by drop (*guttatim*)
Gyn . . . . .gynecology
H. . . . .*Haemophilus*; *Helicobacter*
h. . . . . .hour (*hora*)
H_2 . . . . .histamine 2
H_2O . . . . .water
HA . . . . .hyaluronic acid
Hb . . . . .hemoglobin
HbF . . . . .fetal hemoglobin
HBIG . . . . .hepatitis B immune specific globulin
HCFA . . . . .Health Care Financing Administration
HCG. . . . . .human chorionic gonadotropin
HCl. . . . . .hydrochloric acid
HCN. . . . . .hydrogen cyanide
Hct . . . . .hematocrit
hd. . . . . .bedtime (*hora decubitus*)
HDL . . . . .high-density lipoprotein
HEMA . . . . .hematologic
HEME . . . . .hematologic
hep. . . . . .hepatic
HEPA . . . . .high efficiency particulate air
Hg . . . . .mercury (*hydragyrum*)
Hgb . . . . .hemoglobin
HGH. . . . . .human pituitary growth hormone
Hib. . . . .*Haemophilus influenzae*
His.. . . . .*Haemophilus influenzae* type b
HIV. . . . . .human immunodeficiency virus
HLA . . . . .human leukocyte antigen
HMG-CoA . . . . .3-hydroxy-3-methylglutaryl coenzyme A
HMO . . . . .health maintenance organization
hor decub. . . . . .at bedtime (*hora decubitus*)
hor som . . . . . . .at bedtime (*hora somni*)
HPA . . . . .hypothalamic-pituitary-adrenocortical (axis)
HPLC . . . . .high performance liquid chromatography
HPLC/MS. . . . . .high performance liquid chromatography/mass spectrometry
HPMC . . . . .hydroxypropylmethylcellulose
HPV . . . . .human papillomavirus
HR . . . . .heart rate
hr . . . . .hour
hs. . . . . .at bedtime (*hora somni*)
HSA . . . . .human serum albumin
HSV-1 . . . . .herpes simplex virus type 1
HSV-2 . . . . .herpes simplex virus type 2
Hz . . . . .hertz
I . . . . .iodine
IADL. . . . . .instrumental activities of daily living
I/O . . . . .intake/output
IBW . . . . .ideal body weight
IC. . . . . .intracoronary
ICD. . . . . .International Classification of Diseases of the World Health Organization
ICF. . . . . .intracellular fluid
ICP. . . . . .intracranial pressure
ICU. . . . . .intensive care unit
ID . . . . .intradermal; infective dose
IDDM . . . . .insulin-dependent diabetes mellitus (type 1 diabetes)
IDU. . . . . .idoxuridine
IFN. . . . . .interferon
Ig . . . . .immunoglobulin
IL . . . . .interleukin
Ile. . . . . .isoleucine
IM. . . . . .intramuscular
in . . . . .inch(es)
in^2 . . . . .square inch(es)
IND. . . . . .Investigational New Drug
in d. . . . . .daily (*in dies*)
INDA . . . . .Investigational New Drug Application
Inh . . . . .inhaled
INH. . . . . .isoniazid
Inhal. . . . . .inhalation
Inj. . . . . .injection
INR. . . . . .International Normalizing Ratio
int cib . . . . .between meals (*inter cibos*)
IOP . . . . .intraocular pressure
IP . . . . .intraperitoneal(ly)
IPA . . . . .International Pharmaceutical Abstracts

IPPB. . . . . .intermittent positive pressure breathing
IPV. . . . . .poliovirus vaccine inactivated
IQ. . . . . .intelligence quotient
ISA. . . . . .intrinsic sympathomimetic activity
ISF. . . . . .interstitial fluid
ISI . . . . .Institute for Scientific Information
ISO . . . . .International Organization for Standardization
IT . . . . .intrathecal(ly)
IU . . . . .international unit(s)
IUD. . . . . .intrauterine device
IV . . . . .intravenous
IVF. . . . . .intravascular fluid
IVP. . . . . .intravenous piggyback
J. . . . . .joule(s)
JCAH . . . . .Joint Commission on Accreditation of Hospitals
JCAHO. . . . . . . .Joint Commission on Accreditation of Healthcare Organizations
K . . . . .potassium (*kalium*); kelvin
kcal . . . . .kilocalorie(s)
keV . . . . .kiloelectronvolt(s)
kg. . . . . .kilogram
kJ. . . . . .kilojoule(s)
Kleb.. . . . .*Klebsiella*
KVO. . . . . .keep vein open
L. . . . . .liter
L. . . . .*Legionella*; *Listeria*
lb . . . . .pound
LBW. . . . . .low body weight
LD . . . . .lethal dose
LD-50. . . . . .a dose lethal to 50% of the specified animals or microorganisms
LDH . . . . .lactate dehydrogenase
LDL . . . . .low-density lipoprotein
LE . . . . .lupus erythematosus
Leu. . . . . .leucine
LFT . . . . .liver function test
LH . . . . .luteinizing hormone
liq. . . . . .liquid (*liquor*)
LM . . . . .Licentiate in Midwifery
LOC . . . . .level of consciousness
Lot . . . . .lotion
LPN . . . . .Licensed Practical Nurse
Lr . . . . .lawrencium
LSD . . . . .lysergic acid diethylamide
LTCF . . . . .long-term care facility
LTM . . . . .long-term memory
LUQ . . . . .left upper quadrant (of abdomen)
LVEDP . . . . .left ventricular end-diastolic pressure
LVET . . . . .left ventricular ejection time
LVF . . . . .left ventricular function
LVN . . . . .Licensed Visiting Nurse; Licensed Vocational Nurse
LVP . . . . .large-volume parenterals
Lw . . . . .former symbol for lawrencium (see Lr)
Lys . . . . .lysine
μm . . . . .micrometer
μg. . . . . .microgram
m . . . . .meter
M . . . . .mix (*misce*)
M . . . . .molar (strength of a solution)
M.. . . . .*Moraxella*; *Mycobacterium*; *Mycoplasma*
m^2 . . . . .square meter (of body surface area)
m^3 . . . . .cubic meter(s)
MA . . . . .mental age
MAC. . . . . .maximum allowable cost
MADD . . . . .Mothers Against Drunk Drivers
man pr . . . . .early morning; first thing in the morning (*mane primo*)
MAO. . . . . .monoamine oxidase
MAOI . . . . .monoamine oxidase inhibitor
MAP. . . . . .mean arterial pressure
max . . . . .maximum
MBC. . . . . .minimum bactericidal concentration
MBD. . . . . .minimal brain dysfunction
mcg . . . . .microgram
MCH. . . . . .mean corpuscular hemoglobin
MCHC . . . . .mean corpuscular hemoglobin concentration
mCi . . . . .millicurie
MCT. . . . . .medium-chain triglyceride
MCV. . . . . .mean corpuscular volume
MD . . . . .Doctor of Medicine (*Medicinae Doctor*)
MDI . . . . .metered dose inhaler
m dict. . . . . .as directed (*more dictor*)
MDR. . . . . .minimum daily requirements
MEC. . . . . .minimum effective concentration
MEDLARS . . . . .Medical Literature Analysis and Retrieval System
MEDLINE. . . . . .National Library of Medicine medical database

mEq . . . . .milliequivalent
Met. . . . . .methionine
MeV . . . . .megaelectronvolt(s)
Mg . . . . .magnesium
mg . . . . .milligram
MHC. . . . . .major histocompatibility complex
MI. . . . . .myocardial infarction
MIA . . . . .metabolite bacterial inhibition assay
MIC . . . . .minimum inhibitory concentration
MID . . . . .minimal infecting dose
min. . . . . .minute
min. . . . . .minimum
MIP . . . . .maximum inspiratory pressure
mixt . . . . .a mixture (*mixtura*)
MJ . . . . .mejajoule(s)
ml. . . . . .milliliter
mm. . . . . .millimeter
mm^2. . . . . .square millimeter(s)
mm^3. . . . . .cubic millimeter(s)
mmHg . . . . .millimeters of mercury
mmol . . . . .millimole
MMR . . . . .measles, mumps and rubella virus vaccine, live
MMWR. . . . .*Morbidity and Mortality Weekly Report*
Mn . . . . .manganese
Mo . . . . .molybdenum
mo . . . . .month
mol. . . . . .mole(s)
mor dict . . . . . . .in the manner stated (*more dicto*)
mor sol. . . . . . . .as usual; as customary (*more solito*)
mOsm . . . . .milliosmole
MPH. . . . . .Master of Public Health
MRI . . . . .magnetic resonance imaging
mRNA . . . . .messenger RNA
MS. . . . . .mass spectrometry; mitral stenosis; multiple sclerosis
MW . . . . .molecular weight
N . . . . .normal (strength of a solution)
N. . . . .*Neisseria*
Na . . . . .sodium (*natrium*)
NABP. . . . . .National Association of Boards of Pharmacy
NABPLEX . . . . .National Association of Boards of Pharmacy Licensing Exam
NAD. . . . . .nicotinamide-adenine dinucleotide phosphate
NADH. . . . . .reduced form of nicotine adenine dinucleotide
NADP. . . . . .nicotinamide-adenine dinucleotide phosphate
NADPH . . . . . . .nicotinamide-adenine dinucleotide phosphate (reduced form)
NAPA . . . .*N*-acetyl procainamide
NARD. . . . . .National Association of Retail Druggists - Now NCPA; National Assoc. of Community Pharmacists
nb. . . . . .note well (*nota bene*)
nCi . . . . .nanocurie(s)
NCPA. . . . . .National Assoc. of Community Pharmacists
ND . . . . .Doctor of Naturopathic Medicine
NDA. . . . . .new drug application
NF . . . . .National Formulary
ng. . . . . .nanogram
NG. . . . . .nasogastric
NK . . . . .natural killer (cells); killer T cells
NIDDM. . . . . . . .non-insulin dependent diabetes mellitus (type 2 diabetes)
NIH. . . . . .National Institutes of Health
NLM. . . . . .National Library of Medicine
nm . . . . .nanometer(s)
NMS. . . . . .neuroleptic malignant syndrome
NMT. . . . . .not more than (on prescriptions)
no. . . . . .number (*numerus*)
noc. . . . . .in the night (*nocturnal*)
noc maneq. . . . .at night and the morning (*nocte maneque*)
non rep . . . . . . .do not repeat; no refills (*non repetatur*)
NPN. . . . . .nonprotein nitrogen
NPO. . . . . .nothing by mouth
NS . . . . .normal saline (as in solution)
NSAIA . . . . .nonsteroidal anti-inflammatory agent
NSAID . . . . .nonsteroidal anti-inflammatory drug
NTD . . . . .neutral tube defect
O . . . . .a pint (*octarius*)
OB/GYN. . . . . . .obstetrics and gynecology
OBRA. . . . . .Omnibus Budget Reconciliation Act of 1990
OBS. . . . . .organic brain syndrome
OC . . . . .oral contraceptive
Oct. . . . . .a pint (*octarius*)
od. . . . . .right eye (*oculus dexter*)
OD . . . . .Doctor of Optometry; overdose
Oint . . . . .ointment
ol . . . . .left eye (*oculus laevus*)

omn hor . . . . . . .at every hour (*omni hora*)
Ophth. . . . . .ophthalmic
os. . . . . .left eye (*oculus sinister*)
OSHA. . . . . .Occupational Safety and Health Administration
OT . . . . .occupational therapy
otc . . . . .over-the-counter (nonprescription)
OPV. . . . . .oral poliovirus vaccine, live
ou. . . . . .each eye (*oculo uterque*)
o/w. . . . . .oil-in-water (emulsion)
oz. . . . . .ounce
P . . . . .phosphorus
P . . . . .probability
P&T . . . . .pharmacy and therapeutics (committee)
Pa . . . . .pascal(s)
PA . . . . .Physician Assistant; Physician's Assistant
PABA . . . . .para-aminobenzoic acid
PAC . . . . .premature atrial contraction
$PaCO_2$ . . . . .arterial plasma partial pressure of carbon dioxide
PAD . . . . .premature atrial depolarization
PAF . . . . .platelet-activating factor
PaO_2 . . . . .partial alveolar oxygen
part aeq . . . . . . .equal parts/amounts (*partes aequales*)
part vic. . . . . . . .in divided doses (*partitis vicibus*)
PAS . . . . .para-aminosalicylic acid
PAW. . . . . .pulmonary arterial wedge
PAWP. . . . . .pulmonary artery wedge pressure
Pb . . . . .lead (*plumbum*)
PBP . . . . .penicillin-binding protein
pc. . . . . .after meals (*post cibum; post cibos*)
PCA. . . . . .patient-controlled analgesia
pCO_2 . . . . .plasma partial pressure of carbon dioxide
PCP. . . . . .phencyclidine
PCR. . . . . .polymerase chain reaction
PDGF. . . . . .platelet-derived growth factor
PDLL . . . . .poorly differentiated lymphocytic lymphoma
PE . . . . .pulmonary embolism
PEEP. . . . . .positive end expiratory pressure
PEG. . . . . .polyethylene glycol
PERLA. . . . . . . .pupils equal, react to light and accommodation
PET . . . . .positron emission tomography
pg. . . . . .picogram(s)
PG . . . . .prostaglandin
PGA. . . . . .prostaglandin A
PGB. . . . . .prostaglandin B
PGE. . . . . .prostaglandin E
PGF . . . . .prostaglandin F
pH . . . . .the negative logarithm of the hydrogen ion concentration
PharmD . . . . . . .Doctor of Pharmacy (*Pharmaciae Doctor*)
PhD . . . . .Doctor of Philosophy (*Philosophiae Doctor*)
Phe . . . . .phenylalanine
PhG . . . . .German Pharmacopeia (*Pharmacopoeia Germanica*)
PHS. . . . . .Public Health Service
pKa . . . . .the negative logarithm of the dissociation constant
PKU . . . . .phenylketonuria
PMA. . . . . .Pharmaceutical Manufacturers Association
PMN. . . . . .polymorphonuclear leukocyte
PMR. . . . . .patient medication record
PMS. . . . . .premenstrual syndrome
PND . . . . .paroxysmal nocturnal dyspnea
po. . . . . .by mouth; orally (*per os*)
pO_2 . . . . .oxygen pressure (tension)
POR. . . . . .problem-oriented medical record
POS. . . . . .point of service
post cib . . . . . . .after meals (*post cibos*)
PPD . . . . .purified protein derivative of tuberculin
PPI. . . . . .patient package insert
ppm . . . . .parts per million
PPO. . . . . .preferred provider organization
pr . . . . .per rectum
Pr. . . . .*Proteus*
prn . . . . .as needed; when required (*pro re nata*)
Pro . . . . .proline
pro rat. Aet. . . . .According to patient's age (*pro ratione aetatis*)
Ps. . . . .*Pseudomonas*
PSA . . . . .prostate-specific antigen
PSP . . . . .phenolsulfonphthalein
PSVT . . . . .paroxysmal supraventricular tachycardia
pt . . . . .pint
PT . . . . .prothrombin time; pharmacy and therapeutics; physical therapy
PTH . . . . .parathyroid hormone
PTT . . . . .partial thromboplastin time

PUD. . . . . .peptic ulcer disease
pulv . . . . .a powder (*pulvis)*
PUVA . . . . .oral administration of psoralen and subsequent exposure to ultraviolet light of A wavelengths (UVA)
PVC . . . . .premature ventricular contraction; polyvinyl chloride
PVD . . . . .peripheral vascular disease; premature ventricular depolarizations
pwdr. . . . . .powder
q. . . . . .every
Q . . . . .volume of blood flow
QA . . . . .quality assurance
qad. . . . . .every other day (*quoque alternis die*)
QC . . . . .quality control
qd. . . . . .every day (*quaque die*)
qh. . . . . .every hour (*quaque hora*)
q hr . . . . .every hour
qid . . . . .four times daily (*quarter in die*)
ql . . . . .as much as desired (*quantum libet*)
qod. . . . . .every other day
q 2 hr . . . . .every 2 hours
qs. . . . . .a sufficient quantity (*quantum sufficiat*)
qs. . . . . .as much as is enough (*quantum satis*)
qs ad . . . . .a sufficient quantity to make
qt . . . . .quart
qv. . . . . .as much as you wish (*quam volueris*)
R&D . . . . .research and development
RA . . . . .rheumatoid arthritis
RAI. . . . . .radioactive iodine
RAS . . . . .renin-angiotension system; reticular-activating system
RAST . . . . .radioallergosorbent test
RBC . . . . .red blood (cell) count
RDA . . . . .Recommended Dietary (Daily) Allowance
RDS . . . . .respiratory distress syndrome
RDW . . . . .red-cell distribution width
RE . . . . .reticuloendothelial
rem. . . . . .radio equivalent man
REM. . . . . .rapid eye movement
rep . . . . .let it be repeated (*repetatur*)
RES . . . . .reticuloendothelial system
RF . . . . .releasing factor
Rh . . . . .Rhesus (RH blood group)
RIA. . . . . .radioimmunoassay
RN . . . . .Registered Nurse
RNA . . . . .ribonucleic acid
ROM . . . . .range of motion
RPh . . . . .registered pharmacist
rpm. . . . . .revolutions per minute
rps . . . . .revolutions per second
RR . . . . .respiratory rate
RT_3U . . . . .total serum thyroxine concentration
RUL . . . . .right upper lobe (of lung)
RUQ. . . . . .right upper quadrant (of abdomen)
Rx . . . . .prescription only; take; a recipe (*recipe*)
S. . . . .*Salmonella*; *Serratia*
s. . . . . .second
s. . . . . .without (*sine*)
s̄. . . . . .without (*sine*)
S&S . . . . .signs and symptoms
S-A. . . . . .sinoatrial
sa. . . . . .according to art (*secundum artem*)
sat . . . . .saturated (*sataratus*)
Sb . . . . .antimony (*stibium*)
SBE . . . . .self breast examination; subacute bacterial endocarditis
SC . . . . .subcutaneous(ly)
S_{cr} . . . . .serum creatinine
SD . . . . .standard deviation; streptodornase
Se . . . . .selenium
sec. . . . . .second
Ser. . . . . .serine
sf . . . . .sugar free
SGGT. . . . . .serum gamma-glutamyl transferase
SGOT. . . . .(see AST)
SGPT. . . . .(see ALT)
Sh. . . . .*Shigella*
SIADH . . . . .syndrome of inappropriate secretion of antidiuretic hormone
SIDS . . . . .sudden infant death syndrome
Sig . . . . .label; let it be printed (*signa*)
SI units. . . . . . . .International System of Units
SK . . . . .streptokinase
SL . . . . .sublingual(ly)
SLE . . . . .systemic lupus erythematosus
SMA. . . . . .sequential multiple analysis
Sn . . . . .tin (*stannum*)
SNF . . . . .skilled nursing facility
sol . . . . .solution (*solutio*)

soln . . . . .solution
solv . . . . .dissolve
sp. . . . . .species
SPECT. . . . . . . .single photon emission computerized tomography
sp gr. . . . . .specific gravity
SPF . . . . .sun protection factor
sq. . . . . .square
SR . . . . .sedimentation rate; sustained-release
ss. . . . . .one-half (*semis*)
$\bar{s}\bar{s}$ . . . . .one-half (*semis*)
SSRI . . . . .selective serotonin reuptake inhibitors
Staph. . . . .*Staphylococcus*
stat. . . . . .immediately; at once (*statim*)
STM. . . . . .short-term memory
STP . . . . .standard temperature and pressure
Str. . . . .*Streptococcus*
STD . . . . .sexually transmitted disease
supp. . . . . .suppository (*suppositorium*)
suppl . . . . .supplement(s)
susp. . . . . .suspension
SV . . . . .stroke volume
syr . . . . .syrup (*syrupus*)
$t_{1/2}$ . . . . .half-life
T_3. . . . . .triiodothyronine
T_4. . . . . .thyroxine
tab . . . . .tablet (*tabella*)
tal. . . . . .such
tal dos . . . . .such doses
TB . . . . .tuberculosis
TBG . . . . .thyroxine-binding globulin
TBP . . . . .thyroxine-binding proteins
TBPA . . . . .thyroxine-binding pre-albumin
TBW. . . . . .total body weight
TCA . . . . .tricyclic antidepressant
TD_{50}. . . . . .median toxic dose
TEEC. . . . . .transesophageal echocardiography
TEN . . . . .toxic epidermal necrolysis
TENS. . . . . .transcutaneous electrical nerve stimulation
TG . . . . .total triglycerides
THC. . . . . .tetrahydrocannabinol
Thr . . . . .threonine
TIA. . . . . .transient ischemic attack
tid. . . . . .three times daily (*ter in die*)
tbsp . . . . .tablespoonful
tinct . . . . .tincture
TLC . . . . .total lung capacity; thin layer chromatography
T_{max} . . . . .time to maximum concentration
TMJ . . . . .temporomandibular joint
TNF . . . . .tumor necrosis factor
TNM. . . . . .tumor, node, metastasis (tumor staging)
top . . . . .topical(ly)
TOPV. . . . . .trivalent oral polio vaccine
tPA . . . . .tissue plasminogen activator
TPN . . . . .total parenteral nutrition
TPR . . . . .temperature, pulse, respirations
TQM. . . . . .total quality management
tr . . . . .tincture
trit. . . . . .triturate (*tritura*)
tRNA . . . . .transfer RNA
Trp . . . . .tryptophan
TSA . . . . .tumor-specific antigens
TSH . . . . .thyroid-stimulating hormone
tsp . . . . .teaspoonful
TSS . . . . .toxic shock syndrome
TSTA . . . . .tumor-specific transplantation antigen
TT . . . . .thrombin time
TV . . . . .tidal volume
Tyr . . . . .tyrosine
U . . . . .unit
ud. . . . . .as directed
UD . . . . .unit-dose package
UK . . . . .United Kingdom
ung. . . . . .ointment (*unguentum*)
URI. . . . . .upper respiratory infection
USAN. . . . . .United States Adopted Name(s)
USP . . . .*United States Pharmacopeia*
USPHS . . . . . . .United States Public Health Service
ut dict. . . . . .as directed (*ut dictum*)
UTI. . . . . .urinary tract infection
UVA . . . . .ultraviolet A wave
V . . . . .volt
VA . . . . .Veterans Administration
vag. . . . . .vaginal(ly)
Val . . . . .valine
var . . . . .variety
VC . . . . .vital capacity
V_c. . . . . .volume of distribution of the central compartment
V_d. . . . . .volume of distribution (one compartment)
$V_{d\beta}$. . . . . .volume of distribution of the β phase

V_{dss} . . . . .steady-state apparent volume of distribution
VHDL. . . . . .very high density lipoprotein
VLDL . . . . .very low density lipoprotein
VMA. . . . . .vanillylmandelic acid
vol . . . . .volume
VS . . . . .vital signs
v/v . . . . .volume in volume
v/w . . . . .volume in weight
wa . . . . .while awake
WBC . . . . .white blood (cell) count
WBCT . . . . .whole blood clotting time
WDLL. . . . . .well-differentiated lymphocytic lymphoma
WFI . . . . .water for injection
WHO . . . . .World Health Organization
wk . . . . .week
WNL. . . . . .within normal limits
w/o . . . . .water in oil
wt. . . . . .weight
w/v . . . . .weight in volume
w/w. . . . . .weight in weight
yo. . . . . .years old
yr . . . . .year
ZE . . . . .Zollinger-Ellison
Zn . . . . .zinc

Calculations

To calculate milliequivalent weight: $\text{mEq} = \dfrac{\text{gram molecular weight/valence}}{1000}$

$\text{mEq} = \dfrac{\text{mg}}{\text{eq wt}}$ equivalent weight or eq wt $= \dfrac{\text{gram molecular weight}}{\text{valence}}$

Commonly used mEq weights			
Chloride	35.5 mg = 1 mEq	Magnesium	12 mg = 1 mEq
Sodium	23 mg = 1 mEq	Potassium	39 mg = 1 mEq
Calcium	20 mg = 1 mEq		

To convert temperature °C ↔ °F: $\dfrac{°C}{°F - 32} = \dfrac{5}{9}$ *or* $°C = \dfrac{5}{9}(°F - 32)$

$°F = 32 + \dfrac{9}{5}\ °C$

To calculate creatinine clearance (Ccr) from serum creatinine:

Male: $\text{Ccr} = \dfrac{\text{weight (kg)} \times (140 - \text{age})}{72 \times \text{serum creatinine (mg/dl)}}$ Female: Ccr = 0.85 × calculation for males

To calculate ideal body weight (kg):

Male = 50 kg + 2.3 kg (each inch > 5 ft) Female = 45.5 kg + 2.3 kg (each inch > 5 ft)

To calculate body surface area (BSA) in adults and children:

1) *Dubois method:*

$\text{SA (cm}^2) = \text{wt (kg)}^{0.425} \times \text{ht (cm)}^{0.725} \times 71.84$

$\text{SA (m}^2) = K \times \sqrt[3]{\text{wt}^2\ \text{(kg)}}$ (common K value 0.1 for toddlers, 0.103 for neonates)

2) *Simplified method:*

$\text{BSA (m}^2) = \sqrt{\dfrac{\text{ht (cm)} \times \text{wt (kg)}}{3600}}$

To approximate surface area (m^2) of children from weight (kg):

Weight range (kg)	≈ Surface area (m^2)
1 to 5	(0.05 x kg) + 0.05
6 to 10	(0.04 x kg) + 0.10
11 to 20	(0.03 x kg) + 0.20
21 to 40	(0.02 x kg) + 0.40

Suggested Weights for Adults	
Height*	Weight in pounds†
4'10"	91-119
4'11"	94-124
5'0"	97-128
5'1"	101-132
5'2"	104-137
5'3"	107-141
5'4"	111-146
5'5"	114-150
5'6"	118-155
5'7"	121-160
5'8"	125-164
5'9"	129-169
5'10"	132-174
5'11"	136-179
6'0"	140-184
6'1"	144-189
6'2"	148-195
6'3"	152-200
6'4"	156-205
6'5"	160-211
6'6"	164-216

*Without shoes. † Without clothes.

The higher weights in the ranges generally apply to people with more muscle and bone. Source: Nutrition and Your Health: Dietary Guidelines for Americans, 4th ed, 1995. US Department of Agriculture, US Department of Health and Human Services. At press time, these new guidelines had not been officially released. It is possible some changes to this chart will occur.

Common Systems of Weights and Measures*

METRIC SYSTEM

Metric Weight

1 femtogram	fg	=	0.001	pg
1 picogram	pg	=	0.001	ng
1 nanogram	ng	=	0.001	mcg
1 microgram†	μg (mcg)	=	0.001	mg
1 milligram	mg	=	0.001	g
1 centigram	cg	=	0.01	g
1 decigram	dg	=	0.1	g
1 gram	g	=	1.0	g
1 dekagram	dag	=	10.0	g
1 hectogram	hg	=	100.0	g
1 kilogram	kg	=	1000.0	g

Metric Liquid Measure

1 femtoliter	fL	=	0.001	pL
1 picoliter	pL	=	0.001	nL
1 nanoliter	nL	=	0.001	μL
1 microliter	μL	=	0.001	mL
1 milliliter	mL	=	0.001	L
1 centiliter	cL	=	0.01	L
1 deciliter	dL	=	0.1	L
1 liter	L	=	1.0	L
1 dekaliter	daL	=	10.0	L
1 hectoliter	hL	=	100.0	L
1 kiloliter	kL	=	1000.0	L

APOTHECARY SYSTEM

Apothecary Weight

1 grain‡	gr	=	1 gr		
1 scruple	+	=	20 gr		
1 dram	/	=	60 gr	=	3+
1 ounce	0	=	480 gr	=	8/
1 pound	G	=	5760 gr	=	120

Apothecary Liquid Measure

1 minim	.	=	1 .		
1 fluidram	f/	=	60 .		
1 fluidounce	f0	=	480 .	=	8 f/
1 pint	pt or O	=	7680 .	=	16 f0
1 quart	qt	=	15630 .	=	32 f0
1 gallon	gal or cong	=	61440 .	=	8 pt0

AVOIRDUPOIS SYSTEM

Avoirdupois Weight

1 ounce	=	1 oz	=	437.5 grains (gr)		
1 pound	=	1 lb	=	16 ounces (oz)	=	7000 grains (gr)

* The listing of common systems of weights and measures is included to aid the practitioner in calculating dosages.

† The abbreviation μg or mcg is used for microgram in pharmacy rather than gamma (γ) as in biology.

‡ The grain in each of the above systems has the same value, and thus serves as a basis for the interconversion of the other units.

Approximate Practical Equivalents *

Weight Equivalents

1 grain	=	1 gr	=	64.8	milligrams
1 milligram	=	1 mg	=	0.017	grains
1 gram	=	1 g	=	15.432	grains
1 gram	=	1 g	=	0.035	ounces
1 ounce avoirdupois	=	1 oz	=	28.35	grams
1 ounce apothecary	=	1 O	=	31.1	grams
1 pound avoirdupois	=	1 G	=	454.0	grams
1 pound avoirdupois	=	1 lb	=	0.45	kilograms
1 kilogram	=	1 kg	=	2.20	pounds avoirdupois (G)

Measure Equivalents

1 milliliter	=	1 ml	=	16.23	minims (.)
1 cubic centimeter[a]	=	1 cc	=	1.0	ml
1 fluidram†	=	1 f/	=	3.4	ml
1 teaspoonful†	=	1 tsp	=	5.0	ml
1 tablespoonful	=	1 tbsp	=	15.0	ml
1 fluidounce	=	1 fO	=	29.57	ml
1 wineglassful	=	2 fO	=	60.0	ml
1 teacupful	=	4 fO	=	120.0	ml
1 tumblerful	=	8 fO	=	240.0	ml
1 pint	=	1 pt or O or Oct	=	473.0	ml
1 quart	=	1 qt	=	946.0	ml
1 liter	=	1 l	=	33.8	fluidounces (fO)
1 gallon	=	1 gal or C or Cong	=	3785.0	ml

Weight to Volume Equivalents

1 mg/dL	=	10 µg/mL
1 mg/dL	=	1 mg%
1% solution	=	10 mg per mL
1 ppm	=	1 mg/L

Linear Equivalents

1 millimeter	=	1 mm	=	0.04	inches
1 inch	=	1 in	=	25.4	millimeters
1 inch	=	1 in	=	2.54	centimeters
1 meter	=	1 meter	=	39.37	inches
1 inch	=	1 in	=	0.025	meters

Temperature Equivalents

°C = 5÷9 × (°F − 32)

°F = 9÷5 × (°C) + 32

°K = °C + 273

* The listing of approximate practical equivalents is included to aid the practitioner in calculating and converting dosages among the various systems.

† On prescription a fluidram is assumed to contain a teaspoonful, which is 5 ml.

[a] Cubic centimeter and milliliter are equivalent.

International System of Units

The *Système international d 'unités* (International System of Units) or *SI* is a modernized version of the metric system. The primary goal of the conversion to SI units is to revise the present confused measurement system and to improve test-result communications.

The SI has 7 basic units from which other units are derived:

Base Units of SI		
Physical quantity	Base unit	SI symbol
length	meter	m
mass	kilogram	kg
time	second	s
amount of substance	mole	mol
thermodynamic temperature	kelvin	K
electric current	ampere	A
luminous intensity	candela	cd

Combinations of these base units can express any property, although, for simplicity, special names are given to some of these derived units.

Representative Derived Units		
Derived unit	Name and symbol	Derivation from base units
area	square meter	m^2
volume	cubic meter	m^3
force	newton (N)	$kg \cdot m \cdot s^{-2}$
pressure	pascal (Pa)	$kg \cdot m^{-1} \cdot s^{-2}$ (N/m^2)
work, energy	joule (J)	$kg \cdot m^2 \cdot s^{-2}$ ($N \cdot m$)
mass density	kilogram per cubic meter	kg/m^3
frequency	hertz (Hz)	1 cycle/s^{-1}
temperature degree	Celsius (°C)	°C = °K − 273.15
concentration		
mass	kilogram/liter	kg/L
substance	mole/liter	mol/L
molality	mole/kilogram	mol/kg
density	kilogram/liter	kg/L

Prefixes to the base unit are used in this system to form decimal multiples and submultiples. The preferred multiples and submultiples listed below change the quantity by increments of 10^3 or 10^{-3}. The exceptions to these recommended factors are within the middle rectangle.

Prefixes and Symbols for Decimal Multiples and Submultiples		
Factor	Prefix	Symbol
10^{18}	exa	E
10^{15}	peta	P
10^{12}	tera	T
10^{9}	giga	G
10^{6}	mega	M
10^{3}	kilo	k
10^{2}	hecto	h
10^{1}	deka	da
10^{-1}	deci	d
10^{-2}	centi	c
10^{-3}	milli	m
10^{-6}	micro	μ
10^{-9}	nano	n
10^{-12}	pico	p
10^{-15}	femto	f
10^{-18}	atto	a

To convert drug concentrations to or from SI units:

Conversion factor (CF) = $\frac{1000}{\text{mol wt}}$

Conversion *to* SI units: μg/ml x CF = μmol/L

Conversion *from* SI units: μmol/L ÷ CF = μg/ml

Normal Laboratory Values

In the following tables, normal reference values for commonly requested laboratory tests are listed in traditional units and in SI units. The tables are a guideline only. Values are method dependent and "normal values" may vary between laboratories.

Blood, Plasma or Serum		
	Reference Value	
Determination	Conventional Units	SI Units
Ammonia (NH_3) – diffusion	20-120 mcg/dl	12-70 mcmol/L
Ammonia Nitrogen	15–45 μg/dl	11–32 μmol/L
Amylase	35-118 IU/L	0.58-1.97 mckat/L
Anion Gap ($Na^+-[Cl^-+HCO_3^-]$) (P)	7–16 mEq/L	7–16 mmol/L
Antinuclear antibodies	negative at 1:10 dilution of serum	negative at 1:10 dilution of serum
Antithrombin III (AT III)	80-120 U/dl	800-1200 U/L
Bicarbonate: Arterial	21–28 mEq/L	21–28 mmol/L
Venous	22–29 mEq/L	22–29 mmol/L
Bilirubin: Conjugated (direct)	≤ 0.2 mg/dl	≤ 4 mcmol/L
Total	0.1-1 mg/dl	2-18 mcmol/L
Calcitonin	< 100 pg/ml	< 100 ng/L
Calcium: Total	8.6-10.3 mg/dl	2.2-2.74 mmol/L
Ionized	4.4-5.1 mg/dl	1-1.3 mmol/L
Carbon dioxide content (plasma)	21-32 mmol/L	21-32 mmol/L
Carcinoembryonic antigen	< 3 ng/ml	< 3 mcg/L
Chloride	95-110 mEq/L	95-110 mmol/L
Coagulation screen:		
Bleeding time	3-9.5 min	180-570 sec
Prothrombin time	10-13 sec	10-13 sec
Partial thromboplastin time (activated)	22-37 sec	22-37 sec
Protein C	0.7-1.4 μ/ml	700-1400 U/ml
Protein S	0.7-1.4 μ/ml	700-1400 U/ml
Copper, total	70-160 mcg/dl	11-25 mcmol/L
Corticotropin (ACTH adrenocorticotropic hormone) – 0800 hr	< 60 pg/ml	< 13.2 pmol/L
Cortisol: 0800 hr	5-30 mcg/dl	138-810 nmol/L
1800 hr	2-15 mcg/dl	50-410 nmol/L
2000 hr	≤ 50% of 0800 hr	≤ 50% of 0800 hr
Creatine kinase: Female	20-170 IU/L	0.33-2.83 mckat/L
Male	30-220 IU/L	0.5-3.67 mckat/L
Creatine kinase isoenzymes, MB fraction	0-12 IU/L	0-0.2 mckat/L
Creatinine	0.5-1.7 mg/dl	44-150 mcmol/L
Fibrinogen (coagulation factor I)	150-360 mg/dl	1.5-3.6 g/L
Follicle-stimulating hormone (FSH):		
Female	2-13 mIU/ml	2-13 IU/L
Midcycle	5-22 mIU/ml	5-22 IU/L
Male	1-8 mIU/ml	1-8 IU/L
Glucose, fasting	65-115 mg/dl	3.6-6.3 mmol/L
Glucose Tolerance Test (Oral)	mg/dL	mmol/L
	Normal / Diabetic	Normal / Diabetic
Fasting	70-105 / > 140	3.9-5.8 / > 7.8
60 min	120-170 / ≥ 200	6.7-9.4 / ≥ 11.1
90 min	100-140 / ≥ 200	5.6-7.8 / ≥ 11.1
120 min	70-120 / ≥ 140	3.9-6.7 / ≥ 7.8
(γ) - Glutamyltransferase (GGT): Male	9-50 units/L	9-50 units/L
Female	8-40 units/L	8-40 units/L

Blood, Plasma or Serum		
	Reference Value	
Determination	Conventional Units	SI Units
Haptoglobin	44-303 mg/dl	0.44-3.03 g/L
Hematologic tests:		
Fibrinogen	200-400 mg/dl	2-4 g/L
Hematocrit (Hct), female	36%-44.6%	0.36-0.446 fraction of 1
male	40.7%-50.3%	0.4-0.503 fraction of 1
Hemoglobin A_{1C}	5.3%-7.5% of total Hgb	0.053-0.075
Hemoglobin (Hb), female	12.1-15.3 g/dl	121-153 g/L
male	13.8-17.5 g/dl	138-175 g/L
Leukocyte count (WBC)	3800-9800/mcl	3.8-9.8 x 10^9/L
Erythrocyte count (RBC), female	3.5-5 × 10^6/mcl	3.5-5 x 10^{12}/L
male	4.3-5.9 × 10^6/mcl	4.3-5.9 x 10^{12}/L
Mean corpuscular volume (MCV)	80-97.6 mcm^3	80-97.6 fl
Mean corpuscular hemoglobin (MCH)	27-33 pg/cell	1.66-2.09 fmol/cell
Mean corpuscular hemoglobin concentrate (MCHC)	33-36 g/dl	20.3-22 mmol/L
Erythrocyte sedimentation rate (sedrate, ESR)	≤ 30 mm/hr	≤ 30 mm/hr
Erythrocyte enzymes: Glucose-6-phosphate dehydrogenase (G-6-PD)	250-5000 units/10^6 cells	250-5000 mcunits/cell
Ferritin	10-383 ng/ml	23-862 pmol/L
Folic acid: normal	> 3.1-12.4 ng/ml	7-28.1 nmol/L
Platelet count	150-450 × 10^3/mcl	150-450 × 10^9/L
Reticulocytes	0.5%-1.5% of erythrocytes	0.005-0.015
Vitamin B_{12}	223-1132 pg/ml	165-835 pmol/L
Iron: Female	30-160 mcg/dl	5.4-31.3 mcmol/L
Male	45-160 mcg/dl	8.1-31.3 mcmol/L
Iron binding capacity	220-420 mcg/dl	39.4-75.2 mcmol/L
Isocitrate Dehydrogenase	1.2-7 units/L	1.2-7 units/L
Isoenzymes		
Fraction 1	14%-26% of total	0.14-0.26 fraction of total
Fraction 2	29%-39% of total	0.29-0.39 fraction of total
Fraction 3	20%-26% of total	0.20-0.26 fraction of total
Fraction 4	8%-16% of total	0.08-0.16 fraction of total
Fraction 5	6%-16% of total	0.06-0.16 fraction of total
Lactate dehydrogenase	100-250 IU/L	1.67-4.17 mckat/L
Lactic acid (lactate)	6-19 mg/dl	0.7-2.1 mmol/L
Lead	≤ 50 mcg/dl	≤ 2.41 mcmol/L
Lipase	10-150 units/L	10-150 units/L
Lipids:		
Total Cholesterol		
Desirable	< 200 mg/dl	< 5.2 mmol/L
Borderline-high	200-239 mg/dl	< 5.2-6.2 mmol/L
High	> 239 mg/dl	> 6.2 mmol/L
LDL		
Desirable	< 130 mg/dl	< 3.36 mmol/L
Borderline-high	130-159 mg/dl	3.36-4.11 mmol/L
High	> 159 mg/dl	> 4.11 mmol/L
HDL (low)	< 35 mg/dl	< 0.91 mmol/L
Triglycerides		
Desirable	< 200 mg/dl	< 2.26 mmol/L

Blood, Plasma or Serum		
	Reference Value	
Determination	Conventional Units	SI Units
Borderline-high	200-400 mg/dl	2.26-4.52 mmol/L
High	400-1000 mg/dl	4.52-11.3 mmol/L
Very high	> 1000 mg/dl	> 11.3 mmol/L
Magnesium	1.3-2.2 mEq/L	0.65-1.1 mmol/L
Osmolality	280-300 mOsm/kg	280-300 mmol/kg
Oxygen saturation (arterial)	94%-100%	0.94-1 fraction of 1
PCO_2, arterial	35-45 mm Hg	4.7-6 kPa
pH, arterial	7.35-7.45	7.35-7.45
PO_2, arterial: Breathing room air[1]	80-105 mm Hg	10.6-14 kPa
On 100% O_2	> 500 mm Hg	
Phosphatase (acid), total at 37°C	0.13-0.63 IU/L	2.2-10.5 IU/L or 2.2-10.5 mckat/L
Phosphatase alkaline[2]	20-130 IU/L	20-130 IU/L or 0.33-2.17 mckat/L
Phosphorus, inorganic,[3] (phosphate)	2.5-5 mg/dl	0.8-1.6 mmol/L
Potassium	3.5-5 mEq/L	3.5-5 mmol/L
Progesterone		
Female	0.1-1.5 ng/ml	0.32-4.8 nmol/L
Follicular phase	0.1-1.5 ng/ml	0.32-4.8 nmol/L
Luteal phase	2.5-28 ng/ml	8-89 nmol/L
Male	< 0.5 ng/ml	< 1.6 nmol/L
Prolactin	1.4-24.2 ng/ml	1.4-24.2 mcg/L
Prostate specific antigen	0-4 ng/ml	0-4 ng/ml
Protein: Total	6-8 g/dl	60-80 g/L
Albumin	3.6-5 g/dl	36-50 g/L
Globulin	2.3-3.5 g/dl	23-35 g/L
Rheumatoid factor	< 60 IU/ml	< 60 kIU/L
Sodium	135-147 mEq/L	135-147 mmol/L
Testosterone: Female	6-86 ng/dl	0.21-3 nmol/L
Male	270-1070 ng/dl	9.3-37 nmol/L
Thyroid Hormone Function Tests:		
Thyroid-stimulating hormone (TSH)	0.35-6.2 mcU/ml	0.35-6.2 mU/L
Thyroxine-binding globulin capacity	10-26 mcg/dl	100-260 mcg/L
Total triiodothyronine (T_3)	75-220 ng/dl	1.2-3.4 nmol/L
Total thyroxine by RIA (T_4)	4-11 mcg/dl	51-142 nmol/L
T_3 resin uptake	25%-38%	0.25-0.38 fraction of 1
Transaminase, AST (aspartate aminotransferase, SGOT)	11-47 IU/L	0.18-0.78 mckat/L
Transaminase, ALT (alanine aminotransferase, SGPT)	7-53 IU/L	0.12-0.88 mckat/L
Transferrin	220-400 mg/dL	2.20-4.00 g/L
Urea nitrogen (BUN)	8-25 mg/dl	2.9-8.9 mmol/L
Uric acid	3-8 mg/dl	179-476 mcmol/L
Vitamin A (retinol)	15-60 mcg/dl	0.52-2.09 mcmol/L
Zinc	50-150 mcg/dl	7.7-23 mcmol/L

[1] Age dependent
[2] Infants and adolescents up to 104 U/L
[3] Infants in the first year up to 6 mg/dl

Urine		
	Reference Value	
Determination	Conventional Units	SI Units
Calcium[1]	50-250 mcg/day	1.25-6.25 mmol/day
Catecholamines: Epinephrine	< 20 mcg/day	< 109 nmol/day
Norepinephrine	< 100 mcg/day	< 590 nmol/day
Catecholamines, 24-hr	< 110 µg	< 650 nmol
Copper[1]	15-60 mcg/day	0.24-0.95 mcmol/day
Creatinine: Child	8-22 mg/kg	71-195 µmol/kg
Adolescent	8-30 mg/kg	71-265 µmol/kg
Female	0.6-1.5 g/day	5.3-13.3 mmol/day
Male	0.8-1.8 g/day	7.1-15.9 mmol/day
pH	4.5-8	4.5-8
Phosphate[1]	0.9-1.3 g/day	29-42 mmol/day
Potassium[1]	25-100 mEq/day	25-100 mmol/day
Protein		
Total	1-14 mg/dL	10-140 mg/L
At rest	50-80 mg/day	50-80 mg/day
Protein, quantitative	< 150 mg/day	< 0.15 g/day
Sodium[1]	100-250 mEq/day	100-250 mmol/day
Specific Gravity, random	1.002-1.030	1.002-1.030
Uric Acid, 24-hr	250-750 mg	1.48-4.43 mmol

[1] Diet dependent

Drug Levels†			
		Reference Value	
Drug Determination		Conventional Units	SI Units
Aminoglycosides	Amikacin		
	(trough)	1-8 mcg/ml	1.7-13.7 mcmol/L
	(peak)	20-30 mcg/ml	34-51 mcmol/L
	Gentamicin		
	(trough)	0.5-2 mcg/ml	1-4.2 mcmol/L
	(peak)	6-10 mcg/ml	12.5-20.9 mcmol/L
	Kanamycin		
	(trough)	5-10 mcg/ml	nd
	(peak)	20-25 mcg/ml	nd
	Netilmicin		
	(trough)	0.5-2 mcg/ml	nd
	(peak)	6-10 mcg/ml	nd
	Streptomycin		
	(trough)	< 5 mcg/ml	nd
	(peak)	5-20 mcg/ml	nd
	Tobramycin		
	(trough)	0.5-2 mcg/ml	1.1-4.3 mcmol/L
	(peak)	5-20 mcg/ml	12.8-21.8 mcmol/L
Antiarrhythmics	Amiodarone	0.5-2.5 mcg/ml	1.5-4 mcmol/L
	Bretylium	0.5-1.5 mcg/ml	nd
	Digitoxin	9-25 mcg/L	11.8-32.8 nmol/L
	Digoxin	0.8-2 ng/ml	0.9-2.5 nmol/L
	Disopyramide	2-8 mcg/ml	6-18 mcmol/L
	Flecainide	0.2-1 mcg/ml	nd
	Lidocaine	1.5-6 mcg/ml	4.5-21.5 mcmol/L
	Mexiletine	0.5-2 mcg/ml	nd
	Procainamide	4-8 mcg/ml	17-34 mcmol/ml
	Propranolol	50-200 ng/ml	190-770 nmol/L
	Quinidine	2-6 mcg/ml	4.6-9.2 mcmol/L
	Tocainide	4-10 mcg/ml	nd
	Verapamil	0.08-0.3 mcg/ml	nd
Anti-convulsants	Carbamazepine	4-12 mcg/ml	17-51 mcmol/L
	Phenobarbital	10-40 mcg/ml	43-172 mcmol/L
	Phenytoin	10-20 mcg/ml	40-80 mcmol/L
	Primidone	4-12 mcg/ml	18-55 mcmol/L
	Valproic acid	40-100 mcg/ml	280-700 mcmol/L
Antidepressants	Amitriptyline	110-250 ng/ml[3]	500-900 nmol/L
	Amoxapine	200-500 ng/ml	nd
	Bupropion	25-100 ng/ml	nd
	Clomipramine	80-100 ng/ml	nd
	Desipramine	115-300 ng/ml	nd
	Doxepin	110-250 ng/ml[3]	nd
	Imipramine	225-350 ng/ml[3]	nd
	Maprotiline	200-300 ng/ml	nd
	Nortriptyline	50-150 ng/ml	nd
	Protriptyline	70-250 ng/ml	nd
	Trazodone	800-1600 ng/ml	nd
Antipsychotics	Chlorpromazine	50-300 ng/ml	150-950 nmol/L
	Fluphenazine	0.13-2.8 ng/ml	nd
	Haloperidol	5-20 ng/ml	nd
	Perphenazine	0.8-1.2 ng/ml	nd
	Thiothixene	2-57 ng/ml	nd

Drug Levels†			
		Reference Value	
Drug Determination		Conventional Units	SI Units
Miscellaneous	Amantadine	300 ng/ml	nd
	Amrinone	3.7 mcg/ml	nd
	Chloramphenicol	10-20 mcg/ml	31-62 mcmol/L
	Cyclosporine[1]	250-800 ng/ml (whole blood, RIA)	nd
		50-300 ng/ml (plasma, RIA)	nd
	Ethanol[2]	0 mg/dl	0 mmol/L
	Hydralazine	100 ng/ml	nd
	Lithium	0.6-1.2 mEq/L	0.6-1.2 mmol/L
	Salicylate	100-300 mg/L	724-2172 mcmol/L
	Sulfonamide	5-15 mg/dl	nd
	Terbutaline	0.5-4.1 ng/ml	nd
	Theophylline	10-20 mcg/ml	55-110 mcmol/L
	Vancomycin		
	(trough)	5-15 ng/ml	nd
	(peak)	20-40 mcg/ml	nd

† The values given are generally accepted as desirable for treatment without toxicity for most patients. However, exceptions are not uncommon.

[1] 24 hour trough values [2] Toxic: 50-100 mg/dl (10.9-21.7 mmol/L) [3] Parent drug plus N-desmethyl metabolite

nd – No data available

Classification of Blood Pressure*			
	Reference Value		
Category	Systolic (mm Hg)		Diastolic (mm Hg)
Optimal†	< 120	and	< 80
Normal	< 130	and	< 85
High-normal	130-139	or	85-89
Hypertension‡			
Stage 1	140-159	or	90-99
Stage 2	160-179	or	100-109
Stage 3	≥ 180	or	≥ 110

adopted from the Sixth Report of the Joint National Committee on Prevention, Detection, Evaluation, and Treatment of High Blood Pressure, National Institutes of Health

* For adults age 18 and older who are not taking antihypertensive drugs and not acutely ill. When systolic and diastolic blood pressures fall into different categories, the higher category should be selected to classify the individual's blood pressure status. In addition to classifying stages of hypertension on the basis of average blood pressure levels, clinicians should specify presence or absence of target organ disease and additional risk factors.

† Optimal blood pressure with respect to cardiovascular risk is below 120/88 mm Hg. However, unusually low readings should be evaluated for clinical significance.

‡ Based on the average of two or more readings taken at each of two or more visits after an initial screening.

Trademark Glossary

Many companies use trademarks to identify specific dosage forms or unique packaging materials. The following list is provided as a guide to the interpretation ofthese descriptions.

Abbo-Pac (Abbott)
Unit-dose package

Act-O-Vial (Pharmacia & Upjohn)
Vial system

ADD-Vantage (Abbott)
Sterile dissolution system for admixture

ADT (Pharmacia & Upjohn)
Alternate-day therapy

Arm-A-Med (Rhone Poulenc Rorer)
Single-dose plastic vial

bidCAP (Bristol-Myers Squibb)
Double-strength capsule

Bristoject (Bristol-Myers Squibb)
Unit-dose syringe

Caplet (Various)
Capsule-shaped tablet

Comfortip (Fleet)
Special enema tip

Compack (Searle)
Dispenser pack

ControlPak (Novartis)
Unit-dose rolls, tamper-resistant

Detecto-Seal (Sanofi Winthrop)
Tamper-resistant parenteral package

Dialpak (Ortho McNeil)
Compliance package

Dis-Co Pack (Wyeth-Ayerst)
Unit-dose package

Disket (Lilly)
Dispersible tablet

Diskus (GlaxoWellcome)
Double-foil blister strip of powder

Dispenserpak (GlaxoWellcome)
Unit-of-use package

Dispertab (Abbott)
Particles in tablet

Dispette (Wyeth-Ayerst)
Disposable pipette

Divide-Tab (Abbott)
Scored tablet

Dividose (Mead Johnson)
Tablet, bisected/trisected

Dosa-Trol Pack (Bristol-Myers Squibb)
Unit-dose box packaging

Dosepak (Pharmacia & Upjohn)
Unit-of-use package

Dosette (Wyeth-Ayerst)
Single-dose ampule or vial

Drop Dose (Monarch)
Ophthalmic dropper dispenser

Drop-Tainer (Alcon)
Ophthalmic dropper dispenser

Dulcet (Abbott)
Chewable tablet

Dura-Tab (Berlex)
Sustained-release tablet

Efferdose (GlaxoWellcome)
Individual foil packets

EN-tabs (Pharmacia & Upjohn)
Enteric-coated tablet

Extencaps (Ther-Rx)
Continuous-release capsules

Extentab (Wyeth-Ayerst)
Continuous-release tablet

EZ Dial™ (Wyeth-Ayerst)
Dial dispenser

Faspak (Lilly)
Flexible plastic bag

Fast-Trak (Wyeth-Ayerst)
Quick-loading hypodermic syringe

Filmlok (Bristol-Myers Squibb)
Veneer-coated tablet

Filmtab (Abbott)
Film-coated tablet

FlexPak (Lilly)
Flexible blister card

Flo-Pack (GlaxoWellcome)
Vial for preparation of IV drips

Galaxy Container (Baxter Healthcare)
Bag for frozen premixed solutions

Gradumet (Abbott)
Controlled-release tablet

Gyrocap (Rhone-Poulenc Rorer)
Timed-release capsule

Hyporet (Lilly)
Unit-dose syringe

Identi-Dose (Lilly)
Unit-dose package

Infatab (Parke-Davis)
Chewable pediatric tablet

Inject-all (Bristol-Myers Squibb)
Prefilled disposable dilution syringe

Isoject (Pfizer)
Unit-dose syringe

Kapseal (Parke-Davis)
Banded (sealed) capsule

Kronocap (Ferndale)
Sustained-release capsule

Lederject (Wyeth-Ayerst)
Disposable syringe

Lifeshield Syringe (Abbott)
Extended needle shroud plus a Luer adapter

Liquitab (Mission)
Chewable tablet

Lozitabs (Colgate Oral)
Chewable lozenge tablets

Maxivial (American Pharmaceutical Partners)
Multi-dose vial

Mini Pack™ (Wyeth-Ayerst)
Dial dispenser

Mix-O-Vial (Pharmacia & Upjohn)
Two-compartment vial

Mono-Drop (Sanofi Winthrop)
Ophthalmic plastic dropper

Nutrimix (Abbott)
Dual-chamber flexible container

Ocumeter (Merck & Co.)
Ophthalmic dropper dispenser

Penfill (Novo/Nordisk)
For use with NovoPen Insulin Delivery Device

Perle (Forest)
Soft gelatin capsule

Pockethaler (Schering)
Inhaler device

Prestab-Pharmacia & Upjohn (Glynase)
Bisected tablets

ProPak (Merck)
Cartons contain 3 unit-of-use bottles of 30 tablets

PulsePak (Janssen)
Contains 7 blister packs of 4 capsules each

Pulvule (Lilly)
Bullet-shaped capsule

Rax-Pack (GlaxoWellcome)
Unit-dose pack

Redipak (Wyeth-Ayerst)
Unit-dose or unit-of-issue package

Repetabs (Schering)
Extended-release tablet

Rescue Pak (GlaxoWellcome)
Unit-dose packaging

Rotadisk (GlaxoWellcome)
Circular double-foil pack containing 4 blisters of the drug

RxPak (Lilly)
Prescription package

Secule (Wyeth-Ayerst)
Single-dose vial

Sequels (Wyeth-Ayerst)
Sustained-release capsule or tablet

SigPak (Novartis)
Unit-of-use package

Snap Tabs (Novartis)
Tablet with facilitated bisect

Spansule (SmithKline Beecham)
Sustained-release capsule

STATdose (Cerenex/GlaxoWellcome)
Packaging kit

Stat-Pak (Pharmacia & Upjohn)
Unit-dose package

Steri-Dose (Parke-Davis)
Unit-dose syringe

Steri-Vial (Parke-Davis)
Ampule

Supprette (PolyMedica)
Suppository

Tabloid (GlaxoWellcome)
Branded tablet (with raised lettering)

Tamp-R-Tel (Wyeth-Ayerst)
Cartridge-needle unit (Tubex), tamper-resistant

Tel-E-Amp (Roche)
Single-dose ampule

Tel-E-Dose (Roche)
Unit-dose strip package

Tel-E-Ject (Roche)
Unit-dose syringe

Tel-E-Pack (Roche)
Packaging system

Tel-E-Vial (Roche)
Single-dose vial

Tembids (Wyeth-Ayerst)
Sustained-action capsule

Tempule (Centeon)
Timed-release capsule or tablet

Thera-Ject (Roberts)
Unit-dose syringe

Tiltab (SmithKline Beecham)
Tablet shape

Timecap (Schwarz Pharma)
Sustained-release capsule

Timecelle (Roche)
Timed-release capsule

Timespan (Roche)
Timed-release tablet

Titradose (Wyeth-Ayerst)
Scored tablet

Traypak (Lilly)
Multivial carton

T-Tabs (Abbott)
Tablet appearance and shape

Tubex (Wyeth-Ayerst)
Cartridge-needle unit

UDIP (Hoechst Marion Roussel)
Unit-dose identification pack

U-Ject (Pharmacia & Upjohn)
Disposable syringe

ULTRATAB (Warner Lambert Consumer)
Smaller tablet size

UNIBLISTER (Merck)
Unit-dose package

Unimatic (Bristol-Myers Squibb)
Unit-dose syringe

Unisert (Upsher-Smith)
Suppository

Vaporole (GlaxoWellcome)
Crushable ampule for inhalation

Viaflex (Baxter)
Intravenous bag

Viaflex Plus (Baxter)
Intravenous miniature bag

Visipak (Pharmacia & Upjohn)
Reverse-numbered pack

Medical Terminology Glossary

Abduction – the act of drawing away from a center.
Abstergent – a cleansing application or medicine.
Acaricide – an agent lethal to mites.
Achlorhydria – the absence of hydrochloric acid from gastric secretions.
Acidifier, systemic – a drug used to lower internal body fluid pH in patients with systemic alkalosis.
Acidifier, urinary – a drug used to lower the pH of the urine.
Acidosis – an accumulation of acid in the body.
Acne – an inflammatory disease of the skin accompanied by the eruption of papules or pustules.
Addison's Disease – a condition caused by adrenal gland destruction.
Adduction – the act of drawing toward a center.
Adenitis – a gland or lymph node inflammation.
Adjuvant – an agent added to a product formulation which complements or accentuates the active ingredient.
Adrenergic – a sympathomimetic drug that activates organs innervated by the sympathetic branch of the autonomic nervous system.
Adrenocorticotropic Hormone – an anterior pituitary hormone that stimulates and regulates secretion of the adrenocortical steroids.
Adrenocortical steroid, anti-inflammatory – an adrenal cortex hormone that participates in regulation of organic metabolism and inhibits the inflammatory response to stress; a glucocorticoid.
Adrenocortical steroid, salt-regulating – an adrenal cortex hormone that maintains sodium-potassium electrolyte balance by stimulating and regulating sodium retention and potassium excretion by the kidneys.
Adsorbent – an agent that binds chemicals to its surface, thus reducing the bioavailability of toxic substances.
Alkalizer, systemic – a drug that raises internal body fluid pH in patients with systemic acidosis.
Allergen – a specific substance that causes an unwanted reaction in the body.
Amblyopia – pertaining to a dimness of vision.
Amebiasis – an infection with a pathogenic amoeba.
Amenorrhea – an abnormal discontinuation of the menses.
Amphiarthrosis – a joint in which the surfaces are connected by discs of fibrocartilage.
Anabolic – an agent that promotes conversion of simple substance into more complex compounds; a constructive process for the organism.
Analeptic – a potent central nervous system stimulant used to maintain vital functions during severe central nervous system depression.
Analgesic – a drug that selectively suppresses pain perception without inducing unconsciousness.
Ancyclostomiasis – a disease characterized by the presence of hookworms in the intestine.
Androgen – a hormone that stimulates and maintains male secondary sex characteristics.
Anemia – a deficiency of red blood cells.
Anesthetic, general – a drug that eliminates pain perception by inducing unconsciousness.
Anesthetic, local – a drug that eliminates pain perception in a limited area by local action on sensory nerves; a topical anesthetic.
Angina Pectoris – a sharp chest pain starting in the heart, often spreading down the left arm. A symptom of coronary artery disease.
Angiography – visualization of blood vessels upon X-ray following an injection of contrast media.
Anhidrotic – a drug that checks perspiration flow from sweat glands; an antidiaphoretic.
Anodyne – a drug which acts on the sensory nervous system, either centrally or peripherally, to produce relief from pain.
Anorexiant – a drug that reduces appetite.
Anorexigenic – an agent which promotes appetite reduction.
Antacid – a drug that locally neutralizes excess gastric acid secretions.
Antiadrenergic – a drug that prevents response to sympathetic nervous system stimulation and adrenergic drugs; a sympatholytic or sympathoplegic drug.
Antiamebic – a drug that kills or inhibits the pathogenic protozoan *Entamoeba histolytica,* the causative agent of amebic dysentery.
Antianemic – an agent which treats or prevents anemia.
Antiasthmatic – an agent that relieves the symptoms of asthma.
Antibacterial – a drug that kills or inhibits pathogenic bacteria, the causative agents of many systemic gastrointestinal and superficial infections.
Antibiotic – an agent produced by or derived from living cells of molds, bacteria, or other plants, which destroy or inhibit the growth of microbes.
Anticholesteremic – a drug that lowers blood cholesterol levels.
Anticholinergic – a drug that prevents response to parasympathetic nervous system stimulation and cholinergic drugs; a parasympatholytic or parasympathoplegic drug.
Anticoagulant – a drug that inhibits blood clotting.
Anticonvulsant – a drug that selectively prevents epileptic seizures.
Antidepressant – a psychotherapeutic drug that induces mood elevation, useful in treating depressive neuroses and psychoses.
Antidiabetic – a drug used to lower blood sugar or counteract diabetes.

Antidote – a drug that prevents or counteracts the effects of poisons or drug overdoses, by adsorption in the gastrointestinal tract (general antidotes) or by specific systemic action (specific antidotes).
Antieczematic – a topical drug that aids in the control of exudative inflammatory skin lesions.
Antiemetic – a drug that prevents or controls vomiting.
Antifibrinolytic – an agent (drug) that decreases fibrin breakdown.
Antifilarial – a drug that kills or inhibits pathogenic filarial worms of the superfamily Filarioidea, the causative agents of diseases such as loaiasis.
Antiflatulent – an agent inhibiting the excessive formation of gas in the stomach or intestines.
Antifungal – a drug that kills or inhibits pathogenic fungi; antimycotic.
Antihelmintic – a drug that kills or expels worm infestations such as pinworms and tapeworms (nematodes, cestodes, trematodes).
Antihemophilic – a blood derivative containing the clotting factors absent in the hereditary disease hemophilia.
Antihistaminic – a drug that prevents response to histamine, including histamine released by allergic reactions.
Antihypercholesterolemic – a drug that lowers blood cholesterol levels, especially elevated levels sometimes associated with cardiovascular disease.
Antihypertensive – a drug that lowers blood pressure.
Anti-infective, local – a drug that kills a variety of pathogenic microorganisms and is suitable for sterilizing the skin or wounds.
Anti-inflammatory – a drug which counteracts or suppresses inflammation.
Antileishmanial – a drug that kills or inhibits pathogenic protozoa of the genus *Leishmania,* the causative agents of diseases such as kala-azar.
Antileprotic – an agent effective against leprosy.
Antilipemic – an agent reducing the amount of circulating lipids.
Antimalarial – a drug that prevents malaria or inhibits the causative agent (malarial parasites).
Antimetabolite – a substance that competes with or replaces a certain metabolite.
Antimethemoglobinemic – an agent which reduces the production of methemoglobin.
Antimycotic – an agent inhibiting the growth of fungi.
Antinauseant – a drug that suppresses nausea.
Antineoplastic – a drug that is selectively toxic to rapidly multiplying cells and is useful in destroying malignant tumors.
Antioxidant – an agent used to reduce decay or transformation of a material from oxidation.
Antiperiodic – a drug that prevents the regular recurrence of a disease or symptom.
Antiperistaltic – a drug that inhibits intestinal motility, especially for the treatment of diarrhea.
Antipruritic – a drug that prevents or relieves itching.
Antipyretic – a drug used to reduce fever; antifebrile; a febrifugal.
Antirheumatic – a drug that suppresses symptoms of rheumatic disease (eg, reduces the inflammation of rheumatic arthritis).
Antirickettsial – a drug that kills or inhibits pathogenic microorganisms of the genus *Rickettsia,* the causative agents of diseases such as typhus (eg, Chloramphenicol USP).
Antischistosomal – a drug that kills or inhibits pathogenic flukes of the genus *Schistosoma,* the causative agents of schistosomiasis.
Antiseborrheic – a drug that aids in the control of seborrheic dermatitis ("dandruff"); prevents or relieves excessive sebum secretion.
Antiseptic – a substance that will prevent the growth and development of microorganisms which may lead to infection.
Antisialagogue – a drug which diminishes the flow of saliva.
Antispasmodic – an agent used to quiet the spasms of voluntary and involuntary muscles; calmative or antihysteric.
Antisyphilitic – a remedy used in the treatment of syphilis.
Antitoxin – a biological drug containing antibodies against the toxic principles of a pathogenic microorganism, used for passive immunization against the associated disease.
Antitrichomonal – a drug that kills or inhibits the pathogenic protozoan *Trichomonas vaginalis,* the causative agent of trichomonal vaginitis.
Antitrypanosomal – a drug that kills or inhibits pathogenic protozoa of the genus *Trypanosoma,* the causative agents of diseases such as West African trypanosomiasis.
Antitussive – a drug that suppresses coughing; antibechic.
Antivenin – a biological drug containing antibodies against the venom of a poisonous animal or insect; an antidote for a venomous bite.
Anxiety – a feeling of apprehension, uncertainty and fear.
Aperient – a mild laxative.
Aphasia – the inability to use or understand written and spoken words, due to language center injuries in the brain.
Aphonia – loss of voice due to disease of the larynx or its innervation.
Apnea – the absence of breathing.
Areola – a pigmented/depigmented zone surrounding a neoplasm.
Arsenical – containing arsenic.
Arteriosclerosis – hardening of the arteries.
Arthritis – inflammation of a joint.
Ascariasis – a condition caused by roundworms in the intestine.

Ascaricide – an agent that kills roundworms of the genus *Ascaris.*

Aspergillus – a genus of fungi.

Astasia – the inability to stand up without help.

Asthma – a disease characterized by recurring breathing difficulty due to bronchial muscle constriction.

Astringent – an agent which causes tissue contraction, arrests secretion, or controls bleeding.

Ataractic – an agent having a quieting, tranquilizing effect.

Ataxia – incoordination, especially of gait.

Atheroma – lipid deposits on the inner surface of arteries; a characteristic of atherosclerosis.

Atrophy – a wasting away.

Avitaminosis – a pathologic state or dysfunction resulting in the body lacking one or more vitamins.

Axilla – armpit.

Bacteriostatic – an agent that inhibits the growth of bacteria.

Basedow's Disease – a form of hyperthyroidism, also known as Grave's disease and Parry's disease.

Biliary Colic – a sharp pain in the upper right side of the abdomen due to a gallstone impaction.

Bilirubin – a red bile pigment.

Biliuria – the presence of bile in the urine.

Blood Calcium Regulator – a drug that maintains the blood level of ionic calcium, especially by regulating its metabolic disposition elsewhere.

Blood Volume Supporter – an intravenous solution whose solutes are retained in the vascular system to supplement the osmotic activity of plasma proteins.

Bradycardia – a slow heart rate.

Bright's Disease – a disease of the kidneys, including the presence of edema and excessive urine protein formation.

Bromidrosis – foul-smelling perspiration.

Bronchitis – an inflammation of the bronchi.

Bronchodilator – a drug which dilates the bronchus or bronchial tube (air passages of the lung).

Bruit – an abnormal arterial sound audible with a stethoscope.

Buerger's Disease – a thromboanglitis obliterans inflammation of the walls and surrounding rise of the veins and arteries.

Bursitis – an inflammation of the bursa.

Callus – a tissue mass which develops at bone fracture sites.

Calmative – a sedative.

Candidiasis – an infection by the yeastlike genus *Candida*, especially *Candida albicans.*

Carbonic Anhydrase Inhibitor – an enzyme inhibitor, the therapeutic effects of which are diuresis and reduced formation of intraocular fluid.

Carcinoma – a malignant growth.

Cardiac Depressant – a drug that depresses myocardial function so as to suppress rhythmic irregularities characterized by fast rate; antiarrhythmic.

Cardiac Stimulant – a drug that increases the contractile force of the myocardium, especially in weakened conditions such as congestive heart failure; a cardiotonic.

Cardiopathy – a disease of the heart.

Caries – decay of the teeth.

Carminative – an aromatic or pungent drug that mildly irritates the gastrointestinal tract and is useful in the treatment of flatulence and colic. Peppermint Water is a common carminative.

Caruncle – a small fleshy projection on the skin.

Cathartic – an agent having purgative action.

Caudal – pertains to the distal end or tail.

Caustic – an agent whose effect resembles that of a burn; used to remove abnormal skin growths.

Central Depressant – a drug that reduces the functional state of the central nervous system and with increasing dosage may induce sedation, hypnosis, and general anesthesia; degree of respiratory suppression is agent dependent.

Central Stimulant – a drug that increases the functional state of the central nervous system and with increasing dosage may induce restlessness, insomnia, disorientation, and convulsions; degree of respiratory suppression is agent dependent.

Cerebrum – parts of the brain relating to the telecephalon and includes mainly the cerebral cortex and basal ganglia.

Cerumen – earwax.

Chloasma – skin discoloration.

Cholagogue – a drug that stimulates the empty ing of the gallbladder and the flow of bile into the duodenum.

Cholecystitis – an inflammation of the gallbladder.

Cholecystokinetic – an agent that promotes emptying of the gallbladder.

Cholelithiasis – the presence of calculi (stones) in the gallbladder.

Choleretic – a drug that increases the production and secretion of bile by the liver.

Chorea – a disorder, usually of childhood, characterized by uncontrolled spasmotic muscle movements; sometimes referred to as St. Vitus' dance.

Chymotrypsin – a proteinase in the gastrointestinal tract; its proposed use has been the treatment of edema and inflammation.

Claudication – limping.

Climacteric – a time period in women just preceding menopause.

Clonus – movements noted by rapid muscle contraction then relaxation.

Coagulant – an agent which stimulates or accelerates blood clotting.

Coccidiostat – a drug used in the treatment of coccidal (protozoal) infections in animals, especially birds; used in veterinary medicine.
Colitis – an inflammation of the colon.
Colloid – a disperse system of particles larger than those of true solutions but smaller than those of suspensions (1 to 100 millimicrons in size).
Collyrium – an eyewash.
Colostomy – the surgical formation of a cutaneous opening into the colon.
Corticoid – a term applied to hormones of the adrenal cortex or any substance, natural or synthetic, having similar activity.
Corticosteroid – a steroid produced by the adrenal cortex.
Coryza – a headcold; acute rhinitis.
Counterirritant – an agent (irritant) which causes irritation of the part to which it is applied, and draws blood away from a deep seated area.
Cranial – pertaining to the skull.
Crepitation – a crackling sound.
Cryptitis – an inflammation of a follicle or glandular tubule, usually in the rectum.
Cryptococcus – a genus of fungi which does not produce spores, but reproduces by budding.
Cryptorchidism – the failure of one or both testes to descend.
Cutaneous – pertaining to the skin.
Cyanosis – a blue or purple skin discoloration due to oxygen deficiency.
Cycloplegia – the loss of light accommodation due to loss of control in the eye's ciliary muscle.
Cycloplegic – a drug which paralyzes accommodation of the eye.
Cystitis – an inflammation of the bladder.
Cystourethography – the examination by x-ray of the bladder and urethra.
Cytostasis – a slowing of the movement of blood cells at an inflamed area, sometimes causing capillary blockage.
Debridement – the cutting away of dead or excess skin from a wound.
Decongestant – a drug which reduces congestion.
Decubitus – the patient's position in bed; the act of lying down.
Demulcent – an agent used generally internally to sooth and protect mucous membranes.
Dermatitis – an inflammation of the skin.
Dermatomycosis – fungal skin infection caused by dermatophytes, yeasts, and other fungi.
Detergent – a cleansing or purging agent; an emulsifying agent useful for cleansing wounds and ulcers as well as the skin.
Dextrocardia – when the heart is located on the right side of the chest.
Diagnostic Aid – a drug used to determine the functional state of a body organ or the presence of a disease.
Diaphoretic – a drug used to increase perspiration; a hydroticorsudorfice.
Diarrhea – an abnormally frequent defecation of semisolid or fluid fecal matter from the bowels.
Digestive Enzyme – an enzyme used in digestion.
Digitalization – the administration of digitalis to obtain a desired tissue level of drug.
Diplopia – double vision.
Disinfectant – an agent that destroys pathogenic microorganisms on contact and is suitable for sterilizing inanimate objects.
Distal – farthest from a point of reference.
Diuretic – a drug that promotes renal excretion of electrolytes and water, thereby increasing urine volume.
Dysarthria – difficulty in speech articulation.
Dysmenorrhea – pertaining to painful menstruation.
Dysphagia – difficulty in swallowing.
Dyspnea – difficulty in breathing.
Ecbolic – a drug used to stimulate the gravid uterus to the expulsion of the fetus, or to cause uterine contraction; an oxytocic.
Eclampsia – a toxic disorder occurring late in pregnancy involving hypertension, edema, and renal dysfunction.
Ectasia – pertaining to distension or stretching.
Ectopic – out of place; not in normal position.
Eczema – an inflammatory disease of the skin with infiltrations, watery discharge, scales, and crust.
Effervescent – bubbling; sparkling; giving off gas bubbles.
Embolus – a plug (typically a thrombus, bacteria mass, or foreign body) lodged in a vessel; may obstruct circulation.
Emetic – a drug that induces vomiting, either locally by gastrointestinal irritation or systemically by stimulation of receptors in the central nervous system.
Emollient – a topical drug, especially an oil or fat, used to soften the skin and make it more pliable.
Endometrium – the uterine mucous membrane.
Enteralgia – an intestinal pain.
Enterobiasis – a pinworm infestation.
Enuresis – involuntary urination, as in bedwetting.
Epidermis – the outermost layer of the skin.
Episiotomy – a surgical incision of the vulva when deemed necessary during childbirth.
Epistaxis – a nosebleed.
Erythema – redness.
Erythrocyte – a red blood cell.
Escharotic – corrosive.
Estrogen – a hormone that stimulates and maintains female secondary sex characteristics and functions in the menstrual cycle to promote uterine gland proliferation.
Etiology – the cause of a disease.

Euphoria – an exaggerated feeling of well-being.
Eutonic – having normal muscular tone.
Exfoliation – a scaling of the skin.
Exophthalmos – a protrusion of the eyeballs.
Expectorant – a drug that increases secretion of respiratory tract fluid by lowering its viscosity and promoting its ejection.
Extension – movement of a joint that increases the angle between the bones of the limb at the joint.
Exteroceptors – receptors on the exterior of the body.
Fasciculations – the visible twitching movements of muscle bundles.
Fibroid – a tumor of fibrous tissue, resembling fibers.
Filariasis – the condition of having roundworm parasites reproducing in the body tissues.
Fistula – an abnormal opening between one epithelialized surface to another epithelialized body cavity.
Flexion – movement of a joint that decreases the angle between the bones of the limb at the joint.
Fungistatic – inhibiting the growth of fungi.
Furunculosis – a condition marked by the presence of boils.
Gallop Rhythm – a heart condition where three separate beats are heard instead of two.
Gastralgia – a stomach pain.
Gastritis – inflammation of the stomach lining.
Gastrocele – a hernial protrusion of the stomach.
Gastrodynia – pain in the stomach, a stomach ache.
Geriatrics – a branch of medicine caring for medical problems of the aged.
Germicidal – an agent that kills germs or other pathogenic microorganisms.
Gingivitis – an inflammation of the gums.
Glaucoma – a disease of the eye evidenced by an increase in intraocular pressure and resulting in hardness of the eye, atrophy of the retina, and eventual blindness.
Glossitis – an inflammation of the tongue.
Glucocorticoid – a corticoid which increases gluconeogenesis, thereby raising the concentration of liver glycogen and blood sugar.
Glycosuria – an abnormal quantity of glucose and carbohydrates in the urine.
Gout – a disorder which is characterized by a high uric acid level and sudden onset of recurrent arthritis.
Granulation – the formation of small round fleshy granules on a wound as part of the healing process.
Hematemesis – the vomiting of blood.
Hematinic – an agent which improves blood quality by increasing the hemoglobin concentration and/or the number of red blood cells.
Hematopoietic – a drug that stimulates formation of blood cells.
Hemiplegia – a condition in which one side of the body is paralyzed.
Hemoptysis – coughing-up blood.
Hemorrhage – an escape of blood through vessel walls; to bleed.
Hemostatic – a locally acting drug that arrests hemorrhage by promoting clot formation or by serving as a mechanical matrix for a clot.
Hepatitis – an inflammation of the liver.
Histoplasmosis – a lung infection caused by the inhalation of fungus spores, often resulting in pneumonitis.
Hodgkin's Disease – a disease marked by chronic lymph node enlargement which may also include spleen and liver enlargement.
Hydrocholeresis – puffing out a thinner, more watery bile.
Hypercholesterolemia – the condition of having an abnormally large amount of cholesterol in the plasma and cells of circulating blood.
Hyperemia – an excess of blood in any part of the body.
Hyperesthesia – an increase in sensitivity to sensory stimuli.
Hyperglycemic – a drug that increases blood glucose level, especially for the treatment of hypoglycemic states.
Hypertension – blood pressure above the normally accepted limits; high blood pressure.
Hypertriglyceridemia – an increased level of triglycerides in the blood.
Hypnotic – an agent which promotes sleep.
Hypodermoclysis – a subcutaneous injection with a solution.
Hypoesthesia – a diminished sensation of touch.
Hypoglycemic – a drug that lowers blood glucose levels; useful in the control of diabetes mellitus.
Hypokalemia – an abnormally small concentration of potassium ions in the blood.
Hyposensitize – to reduce the sensitivity to an agent, referring to allergies.
Hypotensive – a drug which diminishes tension or pressure to lower blood pressure.
Ichthyosis – an inherited skin disease characterized by dryness and scales.
Idiopathic – denoting a disease of unknown cause.
Ileostomy – the establishment of an opening from the ileum to the outside of the body.
Immune Serum – a biological drug containing antibodies for a pathogenic microorganism, useful for passive immunization against the associated disease.
Immunizing Agent, active – an antigenic preparation (toxoid or vaccine) used to induce formation of specific antibodies against a pathogenic microorganism, which provides delayed but permanent protection against the associated disease.
Immunizing Agent, passive – a biological preparation (antitoxin, antivenin, or immune serum) containing specific antibodies against a patho-

genic microorganism, which provides immediate but temporary protection against the associated disease.

Impetigo – a contagious inflammatory skin infection with isolated pustules, most commonly occurring on the face of young children.

Insulin – a hormone which promotes use of glucose, protein synthesis, and the formation and storage of neutral lipids; used in the treatment of diabetes mellitus.

Inversion – a turning inward.

Irrigating Solution – a solution for washing wounds or various body cavities.

Isoniazid – a compound effective in tuberculosis treatment.

Keratitis – an inflammation of the cornea.

Keratolytic – a topical drug that softens the superficial keratin-containing layer of the skin to promote exfoliation.

Lacrimal – pertaining to tears.

Laxative – a gentle purgative medicine; a mild cathartic.

Leishmaniasis – infections transmitted by sand flies.

Leukocyte – a white blood cell.

Leukocytopenia – a decrease in the number of white cells.

Leukocytosis – an increased white cell count.

Leukoderma – an absence of pigment from the skin.

Libido – sexual desire.

Lipoma – a benign fatty tumor.

Lipotropic – a drug, especially one supplementing a dietary factor, that prevents the abnormal accumulation of fat in the liver.

Lochia – a vaginal discharge of mucus, blood and tissue after childbirth.

Lues – a plague; specifically syphilis.

Macrocyte – a large red blood cell.

Malaise – a general feeling of illness.

Mastitis – an inflammation of the breast.

Melasma – a darkening of the skin.

Melena – black feces or black vomit from altered blood in the higher GI tract.

Meninges – the membranes covering the brain and spinal cord.

Metastasis – the shifting of a disease or its symptoms from one part of the body to another.

Miotics – agents which constrict the pupil of the eye; a myotic.

Moniliasis – an infection with any of the species of monilia types of fungi *(Candida).*

Mucolytic – an agent that can destroy or dissolve mucous membrane secretions.

Myalgia – a pain in the muscles.

Myasthenia Gravis – a chronic progressive muscular weakness caused by myoneural conduction, usually spreading from the face and throat.

Myelocyte – an immature white blood cell in the bone marrow.

Myelogenous – originating in bone marrow.

Myoclonus – involuntary, sudden, and rapid unpredictable jerks.

Mydriatic – a drug that dilates the pupil of the eye, usually by anticholinergic or adrenergic mechanisms.

Myoneural – pertaining to muscle and nerve.

Myopia – nearsightedness.

Narcotic – a drug with effects similar to opium and derivatives which produces analgesic effects and has the potential for dependence and tolerance.

Neonatal – pertaining to the first four weeks of life.

Neoplasm – an abnormal tissue which grows more rapidly than normal and shows a lack of structural organization.

Nephritis – an inflammation of the kidney.

Nephrosclerosis – a hardening of the kidney tissue.

Neuralgia – a pain extending along the course of one or more nerves.

Neurasthenia – a condition accompanying or following depression which is characterized by vague fatique.

Neuroglia – the supporting elements of the nervous system.

Neuroleptic – psychotropic drug used to treat psychosis.

Neurosis – a psychological or behavioral disorder characterized by anxiety.

Nocturia – urination at night.

Normocytic – erythrocytes which are normal in size, shape, and color.

Nuchal – the back of the neck.

Nystagmus – a rhythmic oscillation of the eyes.

Oleaginous – oily or greasy.

Omphalitis – an inflammation of the navel and surrounding area.

Onychomycosis – fungal infection of the nails.

Ophthalmic – pertaining to the eye.

Oral – pertaining to the mouth.

Orthopnea – a discomfort in breathing when lying flat.

Ossification – a formation of, or conversion to, bone.

Osteomyelitis – an inflammation of the marrow of the bone.

Osteoporosis – a reduction in bone quantity; skeletal atrophy.

Otalgia – pain in the ear; an earache.

Otitis – inflammation of the ear.

Otomycosis – an ear infection caused by fungus.

Otorrhea – a discharge from the ear.

Oxytocic – a drug that selectively stimulates uterine motility and is useful in obstetrics, especially in the control of postpartum hemorrhage.

Palpitations – an awareness of one's heart action.

Paget's Disease – a disease characterized by lesions around the nipple and areola found in elderly women.

Pallor – paleness.
Parasympatholytic – See Anticholinergic.
Parasympathomimetic – See Cholinergic.
Parenteral – pertaining to the administration of a drug by means other than through the intestinal tract; subcutaneous, intramuscular, or intravenous drug administration.
Parkinsonism – a group of neurological disorders caused by dopamine deficiency marked by hypokinesia, tremor, and muscular rigidity.
Paroxysm – a sharp spasm or convulsion.
Pathogenic – causing an abnormality or disease.
Pediatrics – a branch of medicine caring for the medical problems of children from birth through adolescence.
Pediculicide – an agent used to kill lice.
Pediculosis – an infestation with lice.
Pellagra – characterized by GI disturbances, mental disorders, skin redness, and scaling due to niacin deficiency.
Pernicious – particularly dangerous or harmful.
Phlebitis – an inflammation of a vein.
Pleurisy – an inflammation of the membrane surrounding the lungs and the thoracic cavity.
Pneumonia – an infection of the lungs.
Poikilocytosis – a condition in which pointed or irregularly shaped red blood cells are found in the blood.
Polydipsia – excessive thirst.
Posology – the science of dosage.
Posterior Pituitary Hormone(s) – a hormone with oxytocic, vasoconstrictor, antidiuretic, and intestinal stimulant properties.
Progestin – a hormone that functions in the menstrual cycle and during pregnancy to promote uterine gland secretion and to reduce uterine motility.
Pronation – the body's position when lying face downward; rotation of the forearm so the palm on the hand faces backward when the arm is in anatomical position.
Prophylactic – a remedy that tends to prevent disease.
Protectant – a topical drug that remains on the skin and serves as a physical, protective barrier to the environment.
Proteolytic Enzyme – an enzyme used to liquify fibrinous or purulent exudates.
Psoriasis – an inflammatory skin disease accompanied with itching.
Psychotherapy – therapy utilizing communication and interventions with the patient instead of chemical or physical treatments.
Ptosis – a drooping or sagging of a muscle or organ.
Pulmonary – pertaining to the lungs.
Purulent – containing or forming pus.
Pyelitis – a local inflammation of renal and pelvic cells due to bacterial infection.
Pylorospasm – a spasmodic muscle contraction of the pyloric portion of the stomach.
Pyoderma – any fever-producing skin infection.
Radiopaque Medium – a diagnostic drug, opaque to X-rays, whose retention in a body organ or cavity makes X-ray visualization possible.
Raynaud's Phenomenon – spasms of the digital arteries with blanching and numbness precipitated by cold.
Reflex Stimulant – a mild irritant suitable for application to the nasopharynx to induce reflex respiratory stimulation.
Rheumatoid – resembling rheumatoid arthritis.
Rhinitis – an inflammation of the mucous membrane of the nose.
Rubefacient – a topical drug that induces mild skin irritation with erythema, sometimes used to relieve the discomfort of deep-seated inflammation.
Rubeola – measles; not to be confused with rubella.
Saprophytic – getting nourishment from dead material.
Sarcoma – a malignant tumor derived from connective tissue.
Scabicide – an insecticide suitable for the erradication of itch mite infestations in humans (scabies).
Schistosomacide – an agent which destroys schistosomes; destructive to the trematodic parasites or flukes.
Schistosomiasis – an infection with *Schistosoma haematobium.*
Scintillation – a visual sensation manifested by an emission of sparks.
Sclerosing Agent – an irritant suitable for injection into varicose veins to induce their fibrosis and obliteration.
Scotomata – an area of varying size and shape within the visual field in which vision is absent or depressed.
Seborrhea – a condition arising from an excess secretion of sebum.
Sebum – the fatty secretions of sebaceous glands.
Sedative – a drug that calms nervous excitement.
Sinusitis – an inflammation of a sinus.
Skeletal Muscle Relaxant – a drug that inhibits contraction of voluntary muscles, usually by interfering with their innervation.
Smooth Muscle Relaxant – a drug that inhibits contraction of involuntary (eg, visceral) muscles, usually by action upon their contractile elements.
Sociopath – a person designated to have an antisocial personality disorder.
Spasmolytic – an agent that relieves spasms and involuntary contractions of a muscle; an antispasmodic.
Sputum – expectorated mucus.
Stenosis – the narrowing of the lumen of a blood vessel.
Stomachic – a drug which is used to stimulate the appetite and gastric secretion.

Stomatitis – an inflammation of the mucous membranes of the mouth.

Subcutaneous – underneath the skin.

Sudorific – causing perspiration.

Superacidity – excessive acidity.

Supination – the body's position when lying face upwards; rotation of the forearm so the palm on the hand faces forward when the arm is in anatomical position.

Suppressant – a drug useful in the control, rather than the cure, of a disease; an agent that stops secretion, excretion, or normal discharge.

Surfactant – a surface active agent that decreases the surface tension between two miscible liquids; used to prepare emulsions, act as a cleansing agent, etc.

Synarthrosis (fibrous joint) – a joint in which the bony elements are united by continuous fibrous tissue.

Syncope – fainting.

Synovia – clear fluid which lubricates the joints; joint oil.

Systole – the ventricular contraction phase of a heartbeat.

Tachycardia – a rapid contraction rate of the heart.

Taeniacide – an agent used to kill tapeworms.

Taeniafuge – agent to expel tapeworms.

Therapeutic – a treatment of disease.

Thoracic – pertaining to the chest.

Thyroid Hormone – a drug containing one or more of the iodinated amino acids that stimulate and regulate the metabolic rate and functional state of body tissues.

Thyroid Inhibitor – a drug that reduces excessive thyroid hormone production, usually by blocking hormone synthesis.

Tics – a repetitive twitching of muscles, often in the face and upper trunk.

Tinea – a fungal infection of the skin, hair, or nails.

Tonic – continuous muscular contraction.

Tonometry – the measurement of tension in some part of the body.

Topical – the local external application of a drug to a particular place.

Toxoid – a modified toxin, less toxic than the original form, used to induce active immunity to bacterial pathogens.

Tranquilizer – a psychotherapeutic drug that induces emotional repose without significant sedation, useful in treating certain neuroses and psychoses.

Tremors – involuntary rhythmic tremulous movements.

Trichomoniasis – an infection with parasitic flagellate protozoa of the genus *Trichomonas.*

Trypanosomiasis – any disease caused by Trypanosomatidae.

Uricosuric – drug that promotes renal uric acid excretion; used to treat gout.

Urolithiasis – a condition marked by the formation of stones in the urinary tract.

Urticaria – a rash or hives.

Vaccine – preparation of live attenuated or dead pathogenic microorganisms, used to induce active immunity.

Vasoconstrictor – an agent used to narrow blood vessels; to constrict blood vessels and reduce tissue congestion in the nose.

Vasodilator – a drug that relaxes vascular smooth muscles, especially for the purpose of improving peripheral or coronary blood flow.

Vasopressor – an adrenergic drug used systemically to constrict blood vessels and raise blood pressure.

Verruca – a wart.

Vertigo – a whirling motion or spinning sensation.

Vesicant – an agent which, when applied to the skin, causes blistering and the formation of vesicles; an epispastic.

Visceral – pertaining to the internal organs.

Vitamin – an organic chemical essential in small amounts for normal body metabolism, used therapeutically to supplement the naturally occurring counterpart in foods.

Container Requirements for U.S.P. 23 Drugs

The listing of container and storage requirements for U.S.P. drugs is included as an aid to the practitioner in storing and dispensing.

Legend:

A	=	Pressurized Container
C	=	Collapsible Tubes
CD	=	Cool, Dry Place
Ch	=	Child-Resistant Packaging
Co	=	Cold Place
F	=	Avoid Freezing
FR	=	Freezer Temp specified
G	=	Glass Specified
H	=	Reduced Moisture
He	=	Protect from Excessive Heat
In	=	Inert Atmosphere
LR	=	Light-Resistant Container
Ox	=	Protect from Oxidation
OT	=	Ophthalmic Tube
P	=	Plastic Specified
R	=	Remote from Fire
S	=	Separate Ingredient Packaging Before Mixing
SC	=	Radioactive Shielding
S/M	=	Single Dose/Multi Dose
SP	=	Special Consideration
Sy	=	Syringes
T	=	Tight Container
TP	=	Tamper-Proof
U	=	Unit Dose
WC	=	Well-Closed Container
WP	=	Well-Filled Container
+	=	Controlled Temperature

a	=	Tablets
b	=	Capsules
c	=	Solution
d	=	Syrup
e	=	Elixir
f	=	Cream
g	=	Ointment/Paste
h	=	Lotion
i	=	Suppository
j	=	Suspension
k	=	Ophthalmic
l	=	Aerosol
m	=	Vaginal
n	=	Lozenges
o	=	Powder
p	=	Enema
r	=	Inhalation
s	=	Nasal
t	=	Gel/Jelly
u	=	Granules
v	=	Otic
w	=	Intraocular Solution
x	=	Veterinary Use
y	=	Emulsion
z	=	Tincture
*	=	Effervescent
♦	=	Sterile if Required

Drugs (Dosage Form)	WC	T	LR
Acebutolol HCl		X[o]	
Acepromazine Maleate	X[ao]		X[ao]
Acetaminophen	X[it]	X[abo]	X[o]
Acetaminophen Oral		X[ej*]	
Acetaminophen & Aspirin (tab)		X	
Acetaminophen, Aspirin & Caffeine	X[a]	X[b]	
Acetaminophen & Caffeine		X[ab]	
Acetaminophen & Codeine Phosphate		X[ab]	X[ab]
Acetaminophen & Codeine Phosphate Oral		X[cj]	X[cj]
Acetaminophen & Diphenhydramine Citrate (tab)		X	
Capsules Containing at least 3 of the following: Acetaminophen & Salts of Chlorpheniramine, Dextromethorphan, & Phenylpropanolamine		X[b]	
Oral Solutions Containing at least 3 of the following: Acetaminophen & Salts of Chlorpheniramine, Dextromethorphan, & Phenylpropanolamine		X[c]	
Capsules Containing at least 3 of the following: Acetaminophen & Salts of Chlorpheniramine, Dextromethorphan, & Pseudoephedrine		X[b]	

Drugs (Dosage Form)	WC	T	LR
Oral Powder Containing at least 3 of the following: Acetaminophen & Salts of Chlorpheniramine, Dextromethorphan, & Pseudoephedrine		X[o]	
Oral Solution Containing at least 3 of the following: Acetaminophen & Salts of Chlorpheniramine, Dextromethorphan, & Pseudoephedrine		X[b]	
Tablets Containing at least 3 of the following: Acetaminophen & Salts of Chlorpheniramine, Dextromethorphan, & Pseudoephedrine		X[a]	
Acetaminophen, Dextromethorphan HBr, Doxylamine Succinate, & Pseudoephedrine HCl Oral		X[c]	
Acetaminophen, Diphenhydramine HCl, & Pseudoephedrine HCl		X[a]	
Acetaminophen & Pseudoephedrine HCl		X[a]	
Acetaminophen for Effervescent Oral Soln.		X	
Acetohydroxamic Acid		X[ao+]	
Acetazolamide	X[ao]		
Acetic Acid Otic Soln.		X	
Acetohexamide	X[ao]		
Acetohydroxamic Acid		X[ao+]	
Acetylcysteine (Soln.)		S/M(In)	
Acyclovir		X[abgo]	
Adenine	X[o]		
Air, Medical			
Alanine	X[o]		
Albendazole	X[o]	X[a]	
Albendazole, Oral		X[j+]	
Albuterol	X[ao]		X[ao]
Albuterol Sulfate	X[o]		X[o]
Alclometasone		X[0]	X[fg]
Alclometasone Dipropionate			X[o]C[fg]
Alcohol		R	
Alcohol, Dehydrated		R	
Alcohol, Rubbing		R	
Alfentanil HCl	X[o]		
Allopurinol	X[ao]		
Aloe	X		
Alprazolam	X[o]	X[a]	X[a]
Alprostadil			X[+]
Alteplase	SP[+]		
Alum	X		
Alum, Ammonium	X		
Alum, Potassium	X		
Alumina & Magnesia	X[a]		
Alumina & Magnesia Oral			X[j+]
Alumina, Magnesia, & Calcium Carbonate Oral	X[a]	F	
Alumina, Magnesia, Calcium Carbonate, & Simethicone (tabs)	X		
Alumina, Magnesia & Simethicone Oral		F[j+]	
Alumina & Magnesium Carbonate Oral	X[a]		F[j+]
Alumina, Magnesium Carbonate, & Magnesium Oxide (tab)		X	
Alumina & Magnesium Triscilicate Oral		X[j+a]	
Aluminum Acetate Topical Soln.		X	
Aluminum Chloride		X[o]	
Aluminum Chlorhydrate	X[co]		
Aluminum Chlorhydrex Polyethylene Glycol	X		
Aluminum Dichlorhydrate	X[co]		
Aluminum Dichlorhydrex Polyethylene Glycol	X		
Aluminum Hydroxide Gel	X[ab]	X[j+]	
Aluminum Hydroxide Gel, Dried	X[ab]	X[o]	
Aluminum Phosphate Gel	F[a]	F[j+]	

Drugs (Dosage Form)	WC	T	LR
Aluminum Sesquichlorhydrate	X[co]		
Aluminum Sesquichlorhydrex Polyethylene Glycol	X		
Aluminum Subacetate Topical Soln.		X	
Aluminum Sulfate	X[o]		
Aluminum Sulfate & Calcium Acetate for Topical Solution		He[a]	
Aluminum Zirconium Octachlorohydrate	X[co]		
Aluminum Zirconium Octachlorhydrex Gly	X[co]		
Aluminum Zirconium Pentachlorohydrate	X[co]		
Aluminum Zirconium Pentachlorohydrex Gly	X[co]		
Aluminum Zirconium Tetrachlorohydrate	X[co]		
Aluminum Zirconium Tetrachlorohydrex Gly	X[co]		
Aluminum Zirconium Trichlorohydrate	X[co]		
Aluminum Zirconium Trichlorohydrex Gly	X[co]		
Amantadine HCl	X[o]	X[bd]	
Amcinonide	X[o]	X[fg]	
Amdinocillin		X[o]	
Amikacin	X[o]		
Amikacin Sulfate	X[o]		
Amiloride HCl	X[ao]		
Amiloride HCl & Hydrochlorothiazide (tab)	X		
Aminobenzoic Acid		X[ct]	X[ct]
Aminobenzoic Acid Topical		X[c]	X[c]
Aminobenzoate Potassium	X[ab]	X[c]	
Aminobenzoate Potassium Oral		X[c]	
Aminobenzoate Sodium	X[o]		
Aminocaproic Acid		X[ad]	
Aminoglutethimide	X[o]	X[a]	X[a]
Aminophylline	X[i+]	X[a]	
Aminophylline Delayed Release		X[a]	
Aminophylline, Oral		X[c]	
Aminosalicylate Sodium		X[ao+]	X[ao+]
Aminosalicylic Acid		X[ao+]	X[ao+]
Amitriptyline HCl	X[ao]		
Ammonia Spirit, Aromatic		X[+]	X[+]
Ammonium Chloride	X[o]		
Ammonium Chloride Delayed Release (tab)		X	
Amobarbital Sodium		X[o]	
Ammonium Molybdate		X[o]	
Amodiaquine		X	
Amodiaquine HCl		X[ao]	
Amoxapine	X[a]	X[o]	
Amoxicillin		X[abot]	
Amoxicillin Intramammary Infusion		Sy[x+]	
Amoxicillin Oral Susp.	M[x+]		
Amoxicillin for Oral Susp.		X[+]	
Amoxicillin & Clavulanate Potassium		X[h+a]	
Amoxicillin & Clavulanate Potassium for Oral Susp.		X[+]	
Amphetamine Sulfate		X[ao]	
Amphotericin B	C[fgh]		
Ampicillin (all dosage forms)		X	
Ampicillin & Probenecid (cap)		X	
Ampicillin & Probenecid for Oral Susp.		U	
Ampicillin Boluses		X[x]	
Ampicillin Sodium		X[o◆]	
Ampicillin Soluble Powder		X[x]	
Amprolium (all dosage forms)		X	
Amrinone	X		X
Amyl Nitrite (inhalant)		UG[+]	UG[+]
Anileridine HCl		X[ao]	X[ao]
Antazoline Phosphate		X[o]	
Anthralin		X[fg+]	X[fg+]
Antimony Potassium Tartrate	X[o]		
Antimony Sodium Tartrate		X	
Antipyrine	X[o]		
Antipyrine & Benzocaine Otic Soln.		X	X
Antipyrine, Benzocaine, & Phenylephrine HCl Otic Soln.		X	X
Apomorphine HCl		X[ao]	X[ao]
Apraclonidine HCl		X[o]	X[o]
Apraclonidine Ophthalmic		X[c]	X[c]
Arginine	X[o]		
Arginine HCl	X[o]		

Drugs (Dosage Form)	WC	T	LR
Arsanilic Acid	X^{o}		
Ascorbate, Calcium		X^{o}	X^{o}
Ascorbic Acid (tab)		X	X
Ascorbic Acid Oral		X^{c}	X^{c}
Aspirin	X^{i+}	X^{abo}	
Aspirin Boluses	X		
Aspirin, Buffered		X^{a}	
Aspirin, Delayed Release		X^{ab}	
Aspirin Effervescent Tablets for Oral Soln.		X	
Aspirin Extended-Release (tab)		X	
Aspirin, Alumina, & Magnesia (tab)		X	
Aspirin, Alumina, & Magnesium Oxide (tab)		X	
Aspirin, Caffeine, & Dihydrocodeine Bitartrate (cap)		X	
Aspirin & Codeine Phosphate (tab)	X		X
Aspirin, Codeine Phosphate, Alumina, & Magnesia (tab)	X		X
Aspirin, Codeine Phosphate, & Caffeine	X^{ab}		
Atenolol	X^{ao}		
Atenolol & Chlorthalidone	X^{a}		
Atropine		X^{o}	X^{o}
Atropine Sulfate	X^{ao}		
Atropine Sulfate Ophthalmic	C^{g}	X^{c}	
Attapulgite, Activated	X		
Attapulgite, Activated Colloidal	X		
Azaperone	X^{o}		
Azatadine Maleate	X^{ao}		
Azathioprine		X^{a}	X^{ao}
Azithromycin	X^{b}	X^{o}	
Azithromycin for Oral		X^{j}	
Azlocillin Sodium		$X^{o\blacklozenge}$	
Azothioprine (tab)			X
Aztreonam		X^{o}	
Bacampicillin HCl		X^{ao}	
Bacampicillin HCl for Oral Susp.		X	
Bacitracin		X^{o+}	
Bacitracin (ointment)	X^{g+}	COT^{k+}	
Bacitracin & Polymixin B Sulfate Topical		A^{l+}	
Bacitracin Methylene Disalicylate, Soluble	X^{x}	X^{ox}	
Bacitracin Zinc Soluble Powder		X^{x}	
Bacitracin Zinc	X^{g+}	X^{o+}	
Bacitracin Zinc & Polymixin B Sulfate (ointment)	X	COT^{k}	X
Baclofen	X^{a}	X^{o}	
Bandage, Adhesive	SP		
Bandage, Gauze	SP		
Barium Hydroxide Lime		X^{o}	
Barium Sulfate	X^{o}		
Barium Sulfate for Suspension	X		
Beclomethasone Dipropionate	X		
Belladonna Extract		X^{ao}	X^{ao}
Belladonna Leaf	X^{o}		X^{o}
Belladonna Tincture		X^{+}	X^{+}
Bendroflumethiazide		X^{ao}	
Benoxinate HCl	X^{o}		
Benoxinate HCl Ophthalmic Soln.		X	
Benzethonium Chloride (Tincture)		X	X
Benzethonium Chloride Topical	X^{c}	X^{c}	
Benzocaine	X^{nt}	X^{fg+}	X^{fg+}
Benzocaine Otic Soln.		X^{+}	X^{+}
Benzocaine Topical		x^{cl+}	X^{c+}
Benzocaine, Butamben, & Tetracaine HCl		F^{gt}	
Benzocaine, Butamben, & Tetracaine HCl Topical	A^{l+}	F^{c}	
Benzocaine & Menthol Topical		AH^{e}	
Benzoic Acid	X^{o}		
Benzoic & Salicylic Acid (ointment)	X^{+}		
Benzoin (Resin)	X		
Benzoin Tincture Compound		X^{+}	X^{+}
Benzonatate		X^{bo}	X^{bo}
Benzoyl Peroxide		X^{ht}	
Benzoyl Peroxide, Hydrous	SP		
Benzthiazide		X^{ao}	
Benztropine Mesylate	X^{a}	X^{o}	
Benzyl Benzoate		X^{ho}	WP^{o+}
Benzylpenicilloyl Polylysine Concentrate		X	
Beta-Carotene		X^{bo}	X^{bo}
Betadex	X^{o}		
Betaine HCl	X^{o}		

Drugs (Dosage Form)	WC	T	LR
Betamethasone	X[ad]	C[f]	
Betamethasone Acetate		X[o]	
Betamethasone Benzoate		X[ko]C[k]	
Betamethasone Dipropionate	XC[g]	X[hi]	C[f]
Betamethasone Dipropionate Topical		A[l+]	
Betamethasone Sodium Phosphate		X[o]	
Betamethasone Valerate	C[fg]	X[fgo]	X[h]
Betaxolol HCl		X[ao]	
Betaxolol HCl Ophthalmic		X[c]	
Bethanechol Chloride		X[ao]	
Biotin		X[o]	
Biperiden	X[o]		X[o]
Biperiden HCl	X[o]	X[a]	X[o]
Bisacodyl	X[io+]		
Biscadoyl (Delayed Release)	RT[a]		
Bisacodyl Rectal Suspension	URT		
Bismuth, Milk of	X[+]		
Bismuth Subcarbonate	X[o]		X[o]
Bismuth Subgallate		X[o]	X[o]
Bismuth Subnitrate	X[o]		
Bismuth Subsalicylate		X[o]	X[o]
Bleomycin Sulfate		X[o]	
Bretylium Tosylate	X[o]		
Bromocriptine Mesylate		X[ao+]	X[ao+]
Bromodiphenhydramine HCl		X[bo]	X[e]
Brompheniramine Maleate	X[e]	X[ao]	X[eo]
Brompheniramine Maleate & Pseudoephedrine Sulfate Syr.	X		X
Bumetanide		X[ao]	X[ao]
Buprenorphine HCl		X[o]	X[o]
Buspirone HCl		X[oa+]	X[oa+]
Busulfan	X[a]	X[o]	
Butabarbital		X[o]	
Butabarbital Sodium	X[ab]	X[eo]	
Butalbital	X[o]		
Butalbital, Acetaminophen, & Caffeine		X[ab]	
Butabital & Aspirin (tab)		X	
Butabital, Aspirin, & Caffeine		X[ab]	
Butalbital, Aspirin, Caffeine & Codeine Phosphate		X[b]	X[b]

Drugs (Dosage Form)	WC	T	LR
Butamben	X		
Butoconazole Nitrate	X[o]	C[f+]	X[o]
Butorphanol Tartrate		X[o]	
Caffeine, anhydrous	X[o]		
Caffeine, hydrous		X[o]	
Calamine	X[o]	X[h]	
Calamine, Phenolated		X[h]	
Calciferol		X[bo+]	X[bo+]
Calcium Acetate	X[a]	X[o]	
Calcium Ascorbate		X[o]	X[o]
Calcium Carbonate	X[aon]		
Calcium Carbonate Oral		F[j]	
Calcium Carbonate & Magnesia (tab)	X		
Calcium & Magnesium Carbonates (tab)	X		
Calcium & Magnesium Carbonates Oral		F[j]	
Calcium Carbonate, Magnesia & Simethicone (tab)	X		
Calcium Chloride		X[o]	
Calcium Citrate	X[o]		
Calcium Glubionate		X[d+]	
Calcium Gluceptate	X[o]		
Calcium Gluconate	X[ao]		
Calcium Hydroxide Topical Soln.		X	
Calcium Lactate	X[a]	X[o]	
Calcium Lactobionate	X[o]		
Calcium Levulinate	X[o]		
Calcium Pantothenate		X[ao]	
Calcium Pantothenate, Racemic		X[o]	
Calcium Phosphate, dibasic	X[ao]		
Calcium Polycarbophil		X[o]	
Calcium Saccharate	X[o]		
Calcium Undecylenate	X[o]		
Camphor		X[o]	
Camphor Spirit		X	
Candicidin	XT[g+]	X[m+]	
Capreomycin Sulfate		X[o]	
Capsaicin		CD	CD
Captopril		X[oa]	
Captopril & Hydrochlorothiazide		X[a]	
Carbachol		X[o]	
Carbachol Soln.		X[kw+]	
Carbamazepine		X[o]GH[a]	
Carbamazepine Oral		F[j+]	F[j+]
Carbamide Peroxide		X[o+]	X[o+]

Drugs (Dosage Form)	WC	T	LR
Carbamide Peroxide Topical Soln.		X[+]	X[+]
Carbenicillin Disodium		X[o]	
Carbenicillin Indanyl Sodium		X[ao+]	
Carbidopa	X[o]		
Carbidopa & Levodopa	X[a]		X[a]
Carbinoxamine Maleate		X[ao]	X[ao]
Carbol-Fuchsin Topical Soln.		X	X
Carbon Dioxide	A		
Carbon Monoxide C-11	(S/M)A[+]		
Carboprost Tromethamine	X[o+]		
Carboxymethylcellulose Sodium		X[ao]	
Carboxymethylcellulose Sodium Paste	X[+]		
Carisoprodol	X[a]	X[o]	
Carisoprodol & Aspirin (tab)	X		
Carisoprodol, Aspirin, & Codeine Phosphate (tab)	X		
Carteolol HCl	X[o]	X[a]	
Carteolol HCl Soln.		X[k]	
Casanthranol		X[o+]	X[o+]
Cascara Sagrada Extract		X[+]	X[+]
Cascara Sagrada Fluid Extract		X[+]	X[+]
Cascara (tab)		X	
Cascara, Aromatic Fluid Extract		X[+]	X[+]
Castor Oil		X[by+]	
Castor Oil, Aromatic		X	
Cefaclor		X[bo]	
Cefaclor for Oral Susp.		X	
Cefadroxil		X[abo]	
Cefadroxil for Oral Susp.		X	
Cefamandol Naftate		X[o◆]	
Cefazolin		X[o]	
Cefazolin Sodium		X[o]	
Cefixime		X[ao]	
Cefixime for Oral Suspension		X[i]	
Cefmenoxime HCl		X[o◆]	
Cefonicid Sodium		X[o◆]	
Cefoperazone Sodium		X[o◆]	
Ceforanide		X[o◆]	
Cefotaxime Sodium		X[o◆]	
Cefotetan		X[o◆]	
Cefotetan Disodium		X[o◆]	
Cefotiam HCl		X[o◆]	
Cefoxitin Sodium		Co[o]	
Cefpiramide		X[o◆]	
Cefprozil		X[ao]	
Cefprozil for Oral Susp.		X[i]	
Ceftazidime		X[o◆]	
Ceftizoxime Sodium		X[o◆]	
Ceftriaxone Sodium		X[o◆]	
Cefuroxime Axetil	X[a]	X[o]	
Cefuroxime Sodium		X[o◆]	
Cellulose Sodium Phosphate	X		
Cephalexin		X[abo]	
Cephalexin for Oral Susp.		X	
Cephalexin HCl		X[o]	
Cephalothin Sodium		X[o◆]	
Cephapirin Benzathine	X[o]		
Cephapirin Benzathine Intramammary Infusion	Sy[+]		
Cephapirin Sodium		X[o◆]	
Cephapirin Sodium Intramammary Infusion	Sy[+]		
Cephradine		X[ab◆]	
Cephradrine for Oral		X[i]	
Cetylpyridinium Chloride	X[no]	X[c]	
Cetylpyridinium Chloride Topical		X[i]	
Charcoal, Activated	X		
Chloral Hydrate		X[bo]	X[d]
Chlorambucil	X[a]	X[o]	X[ao]
Chloramphenicol (all dosage forms)		X[o◆]	X[o◆]
Chloramphenicol Ophthalmic		CTP[cg+]	
Chloramphenicol Palmitate		X[o]	
Chloramphenicol Palmitate Oral Susp.		X	X
Chloramphenicol & Hydrocortisone Acetate for Ophthalmic Susp.		X	
Chloramphenicol, Polymixin B Sulfate, & Hydrocortisone Acetate Ophthalmic Oint.		COT	
Chloramphenicol & Polymixin B Sulfate Ophthalmic Oint.		COT	
Chloramphenicol & Prednisolone Ophthalmic Oint.		COT	

Drugs (Dosage Form)	WC	T	LR
Chloramphenicol Sodium Succinate		X[o◆]	
Chlordiazepoxide		X[ao]	X[ao]
Chlordiazepoxide & Amitriptyline HCl (tab)	X	X	
Chlordiazepoxide HCl		X[bo]	X[bo]
Chlordiazepoxide HCl & Clidinium Bromide (cap)		X	X
Chlorphyllin Copper Complex Sodium		X[o]	X[o]
Chloroprocaine HCl	X[o]		
Chloroquine	X[o]		
Chloroquine Phosphate	X[ao]		
Chlorothiazide	X[ao]		
Chlorothiazide Oral Susp.		X	
Chlorotrianisene	X[bt]		
Chloroxylenol	X[o]		
Chlorpheniramine Maleate		X[ado]	X[do]
Chlorpheniramine Maleate Extended Release (cap)		X	
Chlorpheniramine Maleate & Pseudoephedrine HCl Oral		X[c]	
Chlorpromazine	X[i]	X[o]	X[io]
Chlorpromazine HCl	X[a]	X[do]	X[ao]
Chlorpromazine HCl Oral Concentrate		X	X
Chlorpromazine HCl (supp)	X[+]		X[+]
Chlorpropamide	X[ao]		
Chlorprothixene	X[ao]		X[ao]
Chlorprothixene Oral Susp.		X	X
Chlortetracycline Bisulfate		X[o]	X[o]
Chlortetracycline HCl	C[g]	X[bao◆]	C[g]X[ba]
Chlortetracycline & Sulfamethazine Bisulfates Soluble Pwd.		X[x]	X[x]
Chlortetracycline HCl Ophthalmic Oint.		COT	
Chlortetracycline HCl Soluble Pwd.		X[x]	X[x]
Chlorthalidone	X[ao]		
Chlorzoxazone		X[ao]	
Cholecalciferol		X[c]In[o+]	X[c]In[o+]
Cholestyramine Resin		X[o]	
Cholestyramine for Oral Susp.		X	
Chromic Chloride		X[o]	

Drugs (Dosage Form)	WC	T	LR
Chymotrypsin		X[o+]	
Chymotrypsin for Ophthalmic Soln.		UG[+]	
Ciclopirox Olamine	X[o]C[f+]		
Ciclopirox Olamine Topical		X[j]	
Cimetidine		X[ao+]	X[ao+]
Cinoxacin	X[b]	X[o]	
Cinoxate		X[ho+]	X[ho+]
Ciprofloxacin	X[a]	X[o]	X[o]
Ciprofloxacin HCl	X[a]	X[o]	X[o]
Ciprofloxacin Soln.		RT[k]	X[k]
Ciprofloxacin Ophth.		X[c+]	X[c+]
Cisplatin		X[o]	X[o]
Citric Acid		X[o]	
Clarithromycin		X[ao]	
Clarithromycin for Oral Susp.		X	
Clavulanate Potassium		X[o◆]	
Clemastine Fumarate	X[a]	X[o+]	X[o+]
Clidinium Bromide		X[bo]	X[bo]
Clindamycin HCl		X[bo]	
Clindamycin Palmitate HCl		X[o]	
Clindamycin Palmitate HCl for Oral Soln.		X	
Clindamycin Phosphate		X[ot◆]	
Clindamycin Phosphate Cream	X[m]		
Clindamycin Phosphate Topical		X[cj]	
Clioquinol	X[o]	C[fg]	C[fg]
Clobetasol Propionate		CF[ft]	
Compound Clioquinol Topical		X[o]	
Clioquinol & Hydrocortisone		XC[fg]	X[fg]
Clobetasol Propionate		CF[ft]	
Clocortolone Pivalate		X[o]C[f]	X[o]C[f]
Clofazimine	X[b]	X[o+]	X[o+]
Clofibrate	X[b]	X[o]	X[bo]
Clomiphene Citrate	X[ao]		X[a]
Clonazepam		X[ao+]	X[ao+]
Clonidine HCl	X[ao]		
Clonidine HCl & Chlorthalidone (tabs)	X		
Clorazepate Dipotassium		In[o]	In[o]
Clorsulon	X[o]		
Clotrimazole	X[mo+]	X[h+]	X[+]
Clotrimazole Topical		X[ct]	
Clotrimazole (Cream)		C[+]	

Drugs (Dosage Form)	WC	T	LR
Clotrimazole & Betamethasone Dipropionate (cream)		XC	
Cloxacillin Benzathine		X[ox♦]	
Cloxacillin Sodium		X[bo+♦]	
Cloxacillin Sodium for Oral		X[c]	
Coal Tar		X[g]	
Coal Tar Topical		X[c]	
Cyanocobalamin Co-57	X[b]	X[c]	X[bc]
Cocaine		X[o]	X[o]
Cocaine HCl		X[o]	X[o]
Cocaine HCl Tablets for Topical Soln.	X		
Cocaine, Tetracaine HCl, & Epinephrine Topical		X[ct♦]	X[ct♦]
Cod Liver Oil		In	
Codeine		X[o]	X[o]
Codeine Phosphate	X[a]	X[o]	X[ao]
Codeine Sulfate	X[a]	X[o]	X[o]
Colchicine	X[a]	X[o]	X[ao]
Colestipol HCl		X[o]	
Colestipol HCl for Oral Susp.		XU	
Colistin Sulfate		X[o]	
Colistin Sulfate for Oral Susp.		X	X
Colistin & Neomycin Sulfates & Hydrocortisone Acetate Otic Susp.		X	
Collodion		X	
Collodion, Flexible		X[+]	
Colloidal Oatmeal	X		
Copper Gluconate	X[o]		
Cortisone Acetate	X[ao]		
Cotton, Purified	SP		
Cromolyn Sodium		X[o]	
Cromolyn Sodium Inhalation		S/M	
Cromolyn Sodium for Inhalation		X[+]	X[+]
Cromolyn Sodium Soln.		X[s]	X[s]
Cromolyn Sodium Ophthalmic		S/M[c]	S/M[c]
Croscarmellose Sodium		X	
Crotamiton		X[o]C[f]	C[f]X[o]
Cupric Chloride		X[o]	
Cupric Sulfate		X[o]	
Cyanocobalamin		X[o]	X[o]
Cyclacillin		X[ao]	
Cyclacillin for Oral Susp.		X	
Cyclizine HCl		X[ao]	X[ao]
Cyclobenzaprine HCl	X[ao]		
Cyclopentolate HCl		X[+]	
Cyclopentolate HCl Ophthalmic Soln.		X[+]	
Cyclophosphamide		X[ao+]	
Cyclopropane		A	
Cycloserine		X[bo]	
Cyclosporine		X[bo]	X[o]
Cyclosporine Oral Soln.		X	
Cyproheptadine HCl	X[ao]	X[d]	
Cysteine HCl	X[o]		
Cytarabine		X[o♦]	X[o♦]
Dacarbazine		X[o+]	X[o+]
Dactinomycin		X[o+]	X[o+]
Danazol	X[b]	X[o]	X[o]
Dapsone	X[ao]		X[ao]
Daunorubicin HCl		X[o+]	X[o+]
Decoquinate	PM[x]	X[o]	
Deferoxamine Mesylate		X[o]	
Dehydrocholic Acid	X[ao]		
Demecarium Bromide		X[o]	X[o]
Demecarium Bromide Ophthalmic Soln.		X	X
Demeclocycline		X[o]	X[o]
Demeclocycline Oral Susp.		X	X
Demeclocycline HCl		X[abo]	X[abo]
Demeclocycline HCl & Nystatin		X[ab]	X[ab]
Desipramine HCl		X[ab]	
Deslanoside		X[o]	X[o]
Desoximetasone	C[ftg+]	C[ft+]	C[f]
Desoxycortisone Acetate	X[o]		X[o]
Dexamethasone	X[ao]	X[e]C[t+]	
Dexamethasone Acetate	X[o]		
Dexamethasone Ophth.		X[i]	
Dexamethasone Sodium Phosphate		C[f]X[rt]	C[k]
Dexamethasone Sodium Phosphate Inhalation	A[l+]		
Dexamethasone Sodium Phosphate Ophth.	C[k]	X[c]	X[c]
Dexamethasone Topical	A[l+]		
Dexbrompheniramine Maleate		X[o]	X[o]
Dexbrompheniramine Maleate & Pseudoephedrine Oral		X[c]	
Dexchlorpheniramine Maleate		X[ado]	X[do]
Dexpanthenol		X[o]	
Dexpanthenol Preparation		X	
Dextroamphetamine Sulfate	X[ao]	X[be]	X[e]

Drugs (Dosage Form)	WC	T	LR
Dextromethorphan		X^{o}	
Dextromethorphan HBr		X^{ao}	X^{a}
Dextrose	X^{o}		
Diatrizoate Meglumine	X^{o}		
Diatrizoate Meglumine & Diatrizoate Sodium Solution		X	X
Diatrizoate Sodium	X^{o}		
Diatrizoate Sodium Soln.		X	X
Diatrizoic Acid	X^{o}		
Diazepam		X^{abo}	X^{abo}
Diazepam Extended-Release (cap)		X	X
Diazoxide	X^{bo}		
Diazoxide Oral Susp.		X	X
Dibucaine		$X^{o}C^{fg}$	$X^{o}C^{fg}$
Dibucaine HCl		X^{o}	X^{o}
Dichloralphenazone	X^{o}		
Dichlorphenamide	X^{ao}		
Diclofenac Sodium		X	X
Diclofenac Sodium Delayed Release		X^{a}	X^{a}
Dicloxacillin Sodium		X^{bo}	
Dicloxacillin Sodium for Oral Susp.		X	
Dicyclomine HCl	X^{abo}	X^{d}	
Dienestrol	X^{o}	C^{f}	
Diethylcarbamazine Citrate		X^{ao}	
Diethylpropion HCl	X^{ao}		X^{o}
Diethylstilbestrol	X^{a}	X^{o}	X^{o}
Diethylstilbestrol Diphosphate		X^{+}	
Diethyltoluamide		X^{o}	
Diethyltoluamide Topical Soln.		X	
Diflorasone Diacetate		$X^{o}C^{fg+}$	C^{fg+}
Diflunisal	X^{ao}		
Digitalis		X^{ab}	X^{o}
Digitoxin	X^{a}	X^{o}	
Digoxin		X^{aeo+}	
Dihydrocodeine Bitartrate		X^{o}	
Dihydrostreptomycin Sulfate		X^{ot}◆	
Dihydrostreptomycin Sulfate Boluses		X^{x}	
Dihydroergotamine Mesylate		X^{o}	X^{o}
Dihydrotachysterol	X^{ab}	In^{o}	X^{ab}
Dihydrotachysterol Oral Soln.		X	X
Dihydroxyacetone		X^{ot}	

Drugs (Dosage Form)	WC	T	LR
Dihydroxyaluminum Aminoacetate	X^{abo}		
Dihydroxyaluminum Aminoacetate Magma	F^{+}		
Dihydroxyaluminum Sodium Carbonate	X^{a}	X^{o}	
Diltiazem HCl		X^{ao}	X^{ab}
Diltiazem HCl Extended Release	X^{ab}		
Dimenhydrinate	X^{ao}	X^{d}	
Dimercaprol		X^{+}	
Dimethyl Sulfoxide		X^{+}	X^{+}
Dimethyl Sulfoxide		X^{tx}	X^{tx}
Dimethyl Sulfoxide Topical		X^{cx}	X^{cx}
Dinoprost Tromethamine		X^{o}	
Diphenhydramine Citrate		X^{o}	X^{o}
Diphenhydramine HCl		X^{bo}	X^{eo}
Diphenhydramine & Pseudoephedrine (cap)		X	
Diphenoxylate HCl	X^{o}		
Diphenoxylate HCl & Atropine Sulfate (tab)	X		X
Diphenoxylate HCl & Atropine Sulfate Oral Soln.		X	X
Dipivefrin HCl		X^{o}	X^{o}
Dipivefrin HCl Ophth.		X^{c}	X^{c}
Dipyridamole		X^{ao}	X^{ao}
Disopyramide Phosphate	X^{b}	X^{o}	X^{o}
Disopyramide Phosphate Extended-Release	X^{b}		
Disulfiram		X^{ao}	X^{ao}
Dobutamine HCl		X^{o+}	
Docusate Calcium	X^{o}	X^{b+}	
Docusate Potassium	X^{o}	X^{b+}	
Docusate Sodium	X^{ao}	X^{b+dc}	X^{d}
Dopamine HCl		X^{o}	
Doxapram		X^{o}	
Doxepin HCl	X^{bo}		
Doxepin HCl Oral Soln.		X	X
Doxorubicin HCl		X^{o}	
Doxycycline		X^{bo}	X^{b}
Doxycycline for Oral Susp.		X	X
Doxycycline Calcium Oral Susp.		X	X
Doxycycline Hyclate		X^{abo}◆	X^{abo}◆
Doxycycline Hyclate Delayed-Release (cap)		X	X
Doxylamine Succinate	X^{ao}	X^{d}	X^{ado}

Drugs (Dosage Form)	WC	T	LR
Dronabinol	X[b+]	In[o+]	In[bo+]
Droperidol		In[o+]	In[o+]
Dusting Powder, Absorbable	X		
Dyclonine HCl (gel)		P/G	G
Dyclonine HCl Topical Soln.		X	X
Dydrogestrone	X[ao]		
Dydrogesterone (tab)	X		
Dyphylline		X[aeo]	
Dyphylline & Guaifenesin		X[ac]	
Echothiophate Iodide		X[o]	X[o]
Echothiophate Iodide for Ophthalmic Soln.		G[+]	
Econazole Nitrate	X[o]		X[o]
Edetate Calcium Disodium		X[o]	
Edrophonium Chloride	X[o]		
Elm	CD[o]		
Emetine HCl		X[o]	X[o]
Enalapril Maleate	X[ao]		
Enalapril Maleate & Hydrochlorothiazide	X[a]		
Enalaprilat	X[o]		
Enflurane		X[o+]	X[o+]
Ephedrine		X[o+]	X[o+]
Ephedrine HCl	X[o]		X[o]
Ephedrine Sulfate	X[a]	X[bd]	X[bd]
Ephedrine Sulfate Nasal		X[c]	X[c]
Ephedrine Sulfate & Phenobarbital (cap)	X		
Epinephrine		X[o]	X[o]
Epinephrine Soln.		X[krs]	X[krs]
Epinephrine Inhalation Aerosol		X	X
Epinephrine Bitartrate	X[o]	X[k]	X[k]
Epinephrine Bitartrate Inhalation Aerosol	X	X	
Epinephryl Borate Ophthalmic Soln.		X	X
Epitetracycline HCl		X[o]	X[o]
Equilin		X[o]	X[o]
Ergocalciferol		In[o]X[ab]	In[o]X[ab]
Ergocalciferol Oral Soln.		X	X
Ergoloid Mesylates		X[abo+]	X[abo+]
Ergoloid Mesylates Oral Soln.		X[+]	X[+]
Ergonovine Maleate	X[a]	X[o]	X[o]
Ergotamine Tartrate	X[ao]		X[o]
Ergotamine Tartrate Inhalation Aerosol		A	A
Ergotamine Tartrate & Caffeine	X[a]	X[i+]	X[a]

Drugs (Dosage Form)	WC	T	LR
Diluted Erythrityl Tetranitrate		X[+]	
Erythrityl Tetranitrate (tab)		X[+]	
Erythromycin		X[ao]	
Erythromycin Delayed-Release		X[ab]	
Erythromycin (oint)		CX[+]	
Erythromycin Ophthalmic		COT[g]	
Erythromycin Pledgets		X	
Erythromycin Topical		X[ct]	
Erythromycin & Benzoyl Peroxide Topical		SX[t]	
Erythromycin Estolate		X[abjo]	
Erythromycin Estolate Oral Susp.		X[+]	
Erythromycin Estolate for Oral Soln.		X	
Erythromycin Estolate & Sulfisoxazole Acetyl Oral		X[j]	
Erythromycin Ethylsuccinate		X[ao]	
Erythromycin Ethylsuccinate Oral Susp.	X		
Erythromycin Ethylsuccinate for Oral Susp.		X	
Erythromycin Ethylsuccinate & Sulfisoxazole Acetyl for Oral Susp.	X		
Erythromycin Stearate		X[ao]	
Estradiol		X[ao]	X[ao]
Estradiol, Cream		C[m]	
Estradiol Cypionate		X[o]	X[o]
Estradiol Valerate		X[o]	X[o]
Estriol		X[o]	
Estrogens, Conjugated	X[ao]		
Estrogens, Esterified	X[a]	X[o]	
Estrone		X[o]	X[o]
Estropipate	X[a]	C[mf]X[o]	
Ethacrynic Acid	X[ao]		
Ethambutol HCl	X[ao]		
Ethchlorvynol		X[ab]P[o]	X[abo]
Ether		R[+]	R[+]
Ethinyl Estradiol	X[a]	X[o]	X[o]
Ethionamide		X[ao]	
Ethopropazine HCl	X[a]	X[o]	X[ao]
Ethosuximide		X[bo]	
Ethotoin		X[ao]	
Ethyl Chloride		R[+]	
Ethylene Diamine		WP,G	
Ethynodiol Diacetate	X[o]		

Drugs (Dosage Form)	WC	T	LR
Ethynodiol Diacetate & Ethinyl Estradiol (tab)	X		
Ethynodiol Diacetate & Mestranol (tab)	X		
Etidronate Disodium		X[ao]	
Etoposide		X[bo]	X[bo]
Eucalyptol		X	
Eucatropine HCl		X[o]	X[o]
Eucatropine HCl Ophthalmic Soln.		X	
Eugenol	X	X	
Factor 1X Complex		X[+]	
Famotidine	X[ao]		X[ao]
Fenoprofen Calcium	X[abo]		
Fentanyl Citrate		X[o]	
Ferrous Fumarate		X[o]	X[a]
Ferrous Fumarate & Docusate Sodium Extended-Release (tabs)	X		
Ferrous Gluconate		X[abeo]	X[e]
Ferrous Sulfate		X[acdo]	X[c]
Ferrous Sulfate, Dried	X[o]		
Flecainide Acetate	X[ao]		X[a]
Floxuridine		X[o]	X[o]
Flucytosine		X[bo]	X[bo]
Fluhydrocortisone Acetate	X[ao]		X[o]
Flumethasone Pivalate		X[o]C[f]	X[o]
Flunisolide Nasal Soln.		X[+]	X[+]
Flunixin Meglumine	X[gou]		
Fluocinolone Acetate Topical Soln.		X	
Fluocinolone Acetonide	X[o]	C[fg]	
Fluocinonide	X[o]C[fgt]		
Fluocinonide Topical		X[c]	
Fluorescein		X[o]	
Fluorescein Sodium		X[o]	
Fluorescein Sodium & Benoxinate HCl Ophthalmic		X[c]	X[c]
Fluorescein Sodium & Proparacaine HCl Ophthalmic		G+	G[+]
Fluorometholone		X[o]C[f]	X[o]
Fluorometholone Ophthalmic Susp.		X	
Fluorouracil		X[of+]	X[o]
Fluorouracil Topical		X[c+]	
Fluoxetine HCl		X	
Fluoxymesterone	X[ao]		X[ao]
Fluphenazine Decanoate	X[o]	X[o]	
Fluphenazine Enanthate	X[o]	X[o]	
Fluphenazine HCl		X[aeo]	X[aeo]
Fluphenazine HCl Oral Soln.		X	X
Flurandrenolide		X[fgh]	X[fgh]
Flurandrenolide tape	X[+]		
Flurazepam HCl		X[bo]	X[bo]
Flurbiprofen	X[a]	X[o]	
Flurbiprofen Sodium		X[o]	
Flurbiprofen Sodium Ophthalmic Soln.		X	
Flutamide		X[bo]	X[bo]
Folic Acid	X[ao]		X[o]
Formaldehyde Soln.		X[+]	
Fructose		X[o]	
Fuchsin, Basic	X[o]		
Furazolidone		X[j+o]	X[j+o]
Furosemide	X[a]	X[o+]	X[ao+]
Gallamine Triethiodide		X[o]	X[o]
Gauze (all)	X		
Gemfibrozil		X[ab]	
Gentamicin Sulfate		X[do]◆C[fg]	
Gentamicin Sulfate Ophthalmic	X[c+]	COT[g]	
Gentamicin Sulfate & Betamethasone Acetate Soln.	X[k]		
Gentamicin Sulfate & Betamethasone Valerate		CT[2]	
Gentamicin Sulfate & Betamethasone Valerate Topical		X[cv]	
Gentamicin & Prednisolone Acetate Ophthalmic	OT[g+]	X[j]	
Gentian Violet		X[c]C[ft]	
Gentian Violet Topical		X[c]	
Glipizide		X[o]	
Glucagon		InG[+]	
Gluconolactone	X[o]		
Glucose Enzymatic Test Strip	SP[+]		
Glutaral Concentrate		X[+]	X[+]
Glutethimide	X[abo]		
Glyburide	X[a]	X[o]	
Glycerin		X	
Glycerin Oral Soln.		X	
Glycerin Ophthalmic Soln.		TPG/P	X
Glycerin Suppository	X[+]		
Glycopyrrolate		X[ao]	
Gold Sodium Thiomalate	X[o]	X[o]	
Gonadotropin, Chorionic	G[+]		
Gramicidin		X[o]	
Green Soap Tincture		X	

Drugs (Dosage Form)	WC	T	LR
Griseofulvin		X[abo]	
Griseofulvin Oral Susp.		X	
Griseofulvin, Ultramicro-size (tab)		X	
Guaifenesin		X[abdo]	
Guaifenesin & Codeine Phosphate Syrup		X[+]	X[+]
Guaifenesin & Pseudo-ephedrine HCl		X[b]	X[b]
Guaifenesin, Pseudo-ephedrine HCl, & Dex-tromethorphan HBr		X[b]	X[b]
Guanabenz Acetate		X[ao]	X[ao]
Guanadrel Sulfate	X[o]	X[a]	X[a]
Guanfacine HCl		X[ao]	X[ao]
Gutta Percha	X[o]		X[o]
Halazone		X[o]	X[o]
Halazone Tablets for So-lution		X	X
Halcinonide	X[afgo]		
Haloperidol		X[ao]	X[ao]
Haloperidol Oral Soln.		X	X
Haloprogin		X[+fo]	X[fo]
Haloprogin Topical Soln.		X[+]	X
Halothane		G[+]	X[+]
Helium		A	
Heparin Calcium		X[o]	
Heparin Sodium		X[o+]	
Hetacillin Potassium	X[ao]		
Hetacillin Potassium Oral Susp.		X	
Hexachlorophene		X[o]	X[o]
Hexachlorophene Cleansing Emulsion		X	X
Hexachlorophene Liquid Soap		X	X
Hexylresorcinol		X[no]	X[o]
Histamine Phosphate		X[o]	X[o]
Histidine	X[o]		
Homatropine HBr		X[o]	X[o]
Homatropine Hydrobro-mide Ophthalmic Soln.		X	
Homatropine Methylbro-mide		X[ao]	X[ao]
Hydralazine HCl		X[ao]	X[a]
Hydralazine HCl Oral	Ch		P[c+]
Hydrochlorothiazide	X[ao]		
Hydrocodone Bitartrate		X[ao]	X[ao]
Hydrocodone Bitartrate & Acetaminophen		X[a]	X[a]
Hydrocortisone	X[ag]	X[fhpt]	
Hydrocortisone Acetate	X[fg]	X[h]	
Hydrocortisone Acetate Ophthalmic		X[gk]	
Hydrocortisone & Acetic Acid Otic Soln.		X	X
Hydrocortisone Butyrate	X[fo]		
Hydrocortisone Hemis-uccinate		X[o]	
Hydrocortisone Sodium Phosphate		X[o]	
Hydrocortisone Sodium Succinate		X[o]	X[o]
Hydrocortisone Valerate	X[fo]		
Hydroflumethiazide		X[ao]	
Hydrogen Peroxide Con-centrate	SP[+]		
Hydrogen Peroxide Topi-cal Soln.		X[+]	X[+]
Hydromorphone HCl		X[ao]	X[ao]
Hydroquinone	X[f]	X[o]	X[+o]
Hydroquinone Topical Soln.		X	X
Hydroxocobalamin		X[o]	X[o]
Hydroxyamphetamine HBr	X[o]		X[o]
Hydroxyamphetamine HBr Ophthalmic Solu-tion		X	X
Hydroxychloroquine Sulfate	X[o]	X[a]	X[ao]
Hydroxyprogesterone Caproate	X[o]		X[o]
Hydroxypropyl Cellulose Ocular System		U[+]	
Hydroxypropyl Methyl-cellulose (all grades)	X[o]		
Hydroxypropyl Methyl-cellulose Ophthalmic Soln.		X	
Hydroxypropyl Methyl-cellulose Phthalate	X[o]		
Hydroxyurea		X[bo]	
Hydroxyzine HCl		X[ado]	X[d]
Hydroxyzine Pamoate	X[b]	X[o]	
Hydroxyzine Pamoate Oral Susp.		X	X
Hyoscyamine	X[a]	X[o]	X[ao]
Hyoscyamine HBr		X[o]	X[o]
Hyoscyamine Sulfate		X[aeo+]	X[aeo+]
Hyoscyamine Sulfate Oral Soln.		X[+]	X[+]
Ibuprofen	X[a]	X[o]	
Ibuprofen Oral	X[j+]		
Ibuprofen & Pseudo-ephedrine HCl		X[a]	
Ichthammol	X	C[g+]	
Idarubicin HCl		X[o]	

Drugs (Dosage Form)	WC	T	LR
Idoxuridine		X^{o}	X^{o}
Idoxuridine Ophthalmic	C^{gt}	X^{c}	X^{c}
Ifosfamide		$X^{o+\blacklozenge}$	
Imipramine HCl		X^{ao}	
Indapamide	X^{ao}		
Indigotindisulfonate Sodium		X^{o}	X^{o}
Indium In 111 Oxyquinoline		U^{c+}	
Indocyanine Green	$X^{o\blacklozenge}$		
Indomethacin	X^{bi+o}		
Indomethacin Extended-Release (cap)	X		
Indomethacin Oral		X^{j}	X^{j}
Indomethacin Sodium	$X^{o\blacklozenge}$		X^{o}
Insulin		X^{+}	X
Insulin Human		X^{+}	X
Inulin	X^{o}		
Iocetamic Acid	X^{o}	X^{a}	
Iodine (all Soln. & Tinct.)		X^{+}	X^{+}
Iodide, Sodium, 1-123, 1-131	X^{bc}		
Iodipamide	X^{o}		
Iodoquinol	X^{ao}		
Iohexol	X^{o}		X^{o}
Iopamidol	X^{o}		X^{o}
Iopanoic Acid		X^{ao}	X^{ao}
Iophendylate		X	X
Iothalamic Acid	X^{o}		
Ioversol	X		
Ioxaglic Acid	X^{o}		
Ioxilan	X^{o}		X^{o}
Ipecac		X^{d+o}	
Ipodate Calcium		X^{o}	
Ipodate Calcium for Oral Susp.	X		
Ipodate Sodium		X^{ao}	
Isocarboxazid	X^{ao}		X^{a}
Isoetharine Inhalation Soln.		WF	Ox
Isoetharine HCl		X^{o}	
Isoetharine Mesylate		X^{o}	
Isoetharine Mesylate Inhalation Aerosol			X
Isoflurane		X^{o}	X^{o}
Isoflurophate		G^{+}	
Isoflurophate Ophthalmic		C^{g}	
Isoleucine	X^{o}		
Isometheptene Mucate	X^{o}		
Isometheptene Mucate Dichloralphenazone, & Acetaminophen	X^{b}		

Drugs (Dosage Form)	WC	T	LR
Isoniazid	X^{a}	X^{do}	X^{ado}
Isopropamide Iodide	X^{ao}		X^{o}
Isopropyl Alcohol (all)		X^{+}	
Isoproterenol Inhalation Soln.		WF	Ox
Isoproterenol HCl	X^{a}	X^{arlo}	X^{arlo}
Isoproterenol HCl Inhalation		A^{l}	
Isoproterenol HCl & Phenylephrine Bitartrate Inhalation Aerosol		X	X
Isoproterenol Sulfate		X^{o}	X^{o}
Isoproterenol Sulfate Inhalation		WF^{cl}	Ox^{cl}
Isosorbide Concentrate		X	X
Isosorbide Oral Soln.	X		
Isosorbide Dinitrate, Diluted		X	
Isosorbide Dinitrate (tab)	X		
Isosorbide Dinitrate Chewable (tab)	X		
Isosorbide Dinitrate Extended Release	X^{ab}		
Isosorbide Dinitrate Sublingual (tab)	X		
Isotretinoin		In^{mo}	X^{o}
Isoxsuprine HCl		X^{ao}	
Isradipine	X		X
Juniper Tar		X^{+}	X^{+}
Kanamycin Sulfate		$X^{bo\blacklozenge}$	
Kaolin	X^{o}		
Ketamine HCl	X^{o}		
Ketoconazole	X^{ao}		
Ketoprofen		X^{o}	
Ketorolac Tromethamine	$X^{o}H^{a+}$		$X^{o}H^{a+}$
Krypton Ke 81m		SP^{+}	
Labetalol HCl		X^{aot}	X^{aot}
Lactase	X^{t}		
Lactic Acid		X	
Lactulose (soln/conc)		X^{+}	
Lanolin	X^{+}		
Lanolin, Modified		X^{+}(Rust proof)	
Leucine	X^{o}		
Leucovorin Calcium	X^{a+o}		X^{a+o}
Levamisole HCl	X^{ao}		X^{o}
Levmetamfetamine		X	X
Levobunolol HCl	X^{o}		
Levobunolol HCl Ophthalmic Soln.		X	
Levocarnitine		X^{ao}	
Levocarnitine Oral Soln.		X	
Levodopa		X^{abo+}	X^{abo+}

Drugs (Dosage Form)	WC	T	LR
Levonordefrin	X^{o}		
Levonorgestrel	X^{ao}		X^{ao}
Levonorgestrel & Ethinyl Estradiol (tab)	X		
Levorphanol Tartrate	X^{ao}		
Levothyroxine Sodium		X^{ao}	X^{ao}
Levothyroxine Sodium Oral		X^{o}	X^{o}
Lidocaine	X^{o}	X^{gl}	
Lidocaine Topical		A^{l}	
Lidocaine Oral Topical Soln.		X	
Lidocaine HCl Oral Topical Soln.		X	
Lidocaine Topical Soln.		X	
Lidocaine HCl	$X^{o\blacklozenge}$	X^{t}	
Lime		X	
Lincomycin HCl		$X^{bdo\blacklozenge}$	
Lindane		X^{fho}	
Lindane Shampoo		X	
Liothyronine Sodium		X^{ao}	
Liotrix (tab)		X	
Lisinopril	X^{ao}		
Lithium Carbonate	X^{abo}		
Lithium Carbonate Extended-Release (tab)	X		
Lithium Citrate		X^{do}	
Lithium Hydroxide		X^{o}	
Loperamide HCl	X^{abo}		
Loracarbef	X^{b}	X^{o}	
Loracarbef for Oral Susp.		X	
Lorazepam		X^{ao}	X^{ao}
Lorazepam Oral Conc.	X		X
Lovastatin	X^{a+}	In^{o+}	X^{a+}
Loxapine		X^{bo}	
Loxapine Succinate		X^{o}	
Lypressin Nasal Soln.		P	
Lysine Acetate	X^{o}		
Lysine HCl	X^{o}		
Mafenide Acetate		X^{f+o}	X^{f+o}
Magaldrate	X^{ao}		
Magaldrate Oral Susp.		X	
Magaldrate & Simethicone (tab)	X		
Magaldrate & Simethicone Oral Susp.		X^{+}	
Magnesia, Milk of		F^{+}	
Magnesia (tab)	X		
Magnesium Carbonate	X^{o}		
Magnesium Carbonate & Citric Acid for Oral		X^{c}	

Drugs (Dosage Form)	WC	T	LR
Magnesium Carbonate & Sodium Bicarbonate for Oral Susp.		X	
Magnesium Chloride		X^{o}	
Magnesium Citrate		X	
Magnesium Citrate Oral Soln.		SP^{+}	
Magnesium Gluconate	X^{ao}		
Magnesium Hydroxide		X^{o}	
Magnesium Hydroxide Paste		X	
Magnesium Oxide	X^{abo}		
Magnesium Salicylate		X^{ao}	
Magnesium Sulfate	X^{o}		
Magnesium Trisilicate	X^{ao}		
Malathion		$X^{o}G^{h}$	X^{o}
Maltitol		X^{c}	
Manganese Chloride		X^{o}	
Manganese Gluconate	X^{o}		
Manganese Sulfate		X^{o}	
Mannitol	X^{o}		
Maprotiline HCl	X^{a}	X^{o}	
Mazindol		X^{ao+}	
Mebendazole	X^{ao}		
Mebrofenin		X^{o}	
Mecamylamine HCl	X^{a}	X^{o}	
Mechlorethamine HCl		X	X
Meclizine HCl	X^{a}	X^{o}	
Meclocycline Sulfosalicylate		X^{fo+}	X^{fo+}
Meclofenamate Sodium		X^{bo+}	X^{bo+}
Medroxyprogesterone Acetate	X^{aj}	X^{o}	X^{o}
Mefenamic Acid		X^{ob}	X^{o}
Megestrol Acetate	X^{ao}		X^{o}
Meglumine	X^{o}		
Melphalon	X^{a}	G^{o}	G^{o}
Menadiol Sodium Diphosphate	X^{a}	X^{o+}	X^{ao+}
Menadione	X^{o}		X^{o}
Menotropins		G^{o+}	
Menthol	X^{n}	X^{+}	
Meperidine HCl	X^{a}	X^{d}	X^{ad}
Mephentermine Sulfate	X^{o}		X^{o}
Mephenytoin	X^{ao}		
Mephobarbital	X^{ao}		
Mepivacaine HCl	X^{o}		
Meprednisone		X^{+}	X^{+}
Meprobamate	X^{a}	X^{o}	
Meprobamate Oral Susp.		X	
Mercaptopurine	X^{ao}		
Mercury, Ammoniated	X^{o}		X^{o}

Drugs (Dosage Form)	WC	T	LR
Mercury, Ammoniated (ointment)		C^{k}	
Mesalamine		X^{o}	
Mesoridazine Besylate	$SP^{a}X^{o}$	X^{ao}	
Mesoridazine Besylate Oral Soln.		X^{+}	X^{+}
Mestranol	X^{o}		X^{o}
Metacresol		X^{o}	X^{o}
Metaproterenol Sulfate	X^{a}	X^{do}	X^{ado}
Metaproterenol Sulfate Soln.	A^{r}	WF^{l}	Ox^{l}
Metaraminol Bitartrate	X^{o}		
Methacholine Chloride		X^{o}	
Methacycline HCl		X^{ao}	X^{ao}
Methacycline HCl Oral Susp.		X	X
Methadone HCl	X^{a}	X^{o}	X^{o}
Methadone HCl Oral Concentrate		X^{+}	X^{+}
Methadone HCl Oral Soln.		X^{+}	X^{+}
Methamphetamine HCl	X^{a}	X^{o}	X^{oa}
Methazolamide	X^{ao}		
Methdilazine		X^{ao}	X^{ao}
Methdilazine HCl		X^{ado}	X^{ado}
Methenamine	X^{ao}	X^{e}	
Methenamine & Monobasic Sodium Phosphate (tab)		X	
Methenamine Mandelate (tab)	X		
Methenamine Mandelate Delayed Release	X^{a}		
Methenamine Mandelate for Oral Soln.	X^{c}	X^{j}	
Methicillin Sodium		$X^{+\blacklozenge o}$	
Methimazole	X^{ao}		X^{ao}
Methionine	X^{o}		
Methocarbamol		X^{ao}	
Methohexital		X^{o}	
Methotrexate	U^{a}	X^{o}	X^{o}
Methotrimeprazine	X^{o}		X^{o}
Methoxsalen	X^{o}	X^{b}	X^{bo}
Methoxsalen Topical Solution		X	X
Methoxyflurane		X^{o+}	X^{o+}
Methsuximide		X^{bo+}	
Methylbenzethonium Chloride	X^{e}	$X^{bo}C^{g}$	
Methylbenzethonium Chloride Topical		X^{o}	
Methylcellulose	X^{ao}		
Methylcellulose Ophth Soln.		X	
Methylcellulose Oral Soln.		X^{+}	X^{+}
Methylclothiazide	X^{ao}		
Methyldopa	X^{ao}		X^{o}
Methyldopa Oral Susp.		X^{+}	X^{+}
Methyldopa & Chlorothiazide (tab)	X		
Methyldopa & Hydrochlorothiazide (tab)	X		
Methyldopate HCl	X^{o}		
Methylene Blue	X^{o}		
Methylergonovine Maleate		X^{ao+}	X^{ao+}
Methylphenidate HCl	X^{o}	X^{a}	
Methylphenidate HCl Extended-Release		X^{a}	
Methylprednisolone		X^{ao}	X^{ao}
Methylprednisolone Acetate	X^{p}	$X^{o}C^{f}$	X^{fo}
Methylprednisolone Hemisuccinate		X^{o}	
Methylprednisolone Sodium Succinate		X^{o}	X^{o}
Methyltestosterone	X^{abo}		X^{o}
Methysergide Maleate		X^{ao}	X^{o}
Metoclopramide Oral Soln.		F^{+}	F^{+}
Metoclopramide HCl		X^{ao}	X^{ao}
Metocurine Iodide		X^{o}	
Metolazone		X^{ao}	X^{ao}
Metoprolol Fumarate		X^{o}	X^{o}
Metoprolol Tartrate		X^{ao}	X^{ao}
Metoprolol Tartrate & Hydrochorothiazide (tab)		X	X
Metronidazole	X^{ao}	CP^{t+}	X^{ao}
Metyrapone		X^{ao+}	X^{ao+}
Metyrosine (cap)	X		
Mexiletine HCl		X^{bo}	
Mezlocillin Sodium		$X^{\blacklozenge o}$	
Miconazole	X^{o}		X^{o}
Miconazole Nitrate		$X^{mi}C^{f}$	
Miconazole Nitrate Topical	X^{o}		
Miconazole Nitrate Vaginal (Supp)		X^{+}	
Mineral Oil		X^{py}	
Mineral Oil, Light, Topical		X	
Minocycline HCl		$X^{abo\blacklozenge}$	X^{abo}
Minocycline HCl Oral Susp.		X	X
Minoxidil	X^{o}	X^{a}	
Minoxidil, Topical		X^{c}	
Mitomycin		X^{o}	X^{o}

Drugs (Dosage Form)	WC	T	LR
Mitotane		X[ao]	X[ao]
Mitoxantrone HCl		X[o]	
Molindone HCl		X[ao]	X[ao]
Monensin	X[x+]		
Monensin, Granulated	X[x+]		
Monensin, Premix	X[x+]		
Monensin, Sodium	X[x+]		
Monobenzone	X[fo+]	X[o+]	
Moricizine HCl		X[ao]	
Morphine Sulfate	X[o]	X[o]	
Mupirocin	XC[g]	X[o]	
Nadolol	X[o]	X[a]	
Nadolol & Bendroflume-thiazide (tab)		X	
Nafcillin Sodium		X[abo]	X[a]
Nafcillin Sodium for Oral Soln.		X	
Naftifine HCl		X[oft]	
Nalidixic Acid		X[ao]	
Nalidixic Acid Oral Susp.		X	
Nalorphine HCl		X[o]	X[o]
Naloxone HCl		X[o]	X[o]
Naltrexone HCl		X[ao]	
Nandrolone Decanoate		X[o]	X[o]
Nandrolone Phenpropi-onate		X[o]	X[o]
Naphazoline HCl		X[o]	X[o]
Naphazoline HCl Soln.		X[ks]	X[ks]
Naproxen	X[o]	X[o]	
Naproxen Oral		X[j+]	X[j+]
Naproxen Sodium	X[a]	X[o]	
Narasin Granular	X[x+]		
Narasin Premix	X[x+]		
Natamycin		X[o]	X[o]
Natamycin Ophthalmic Susp.		TP	
Neomycin Sulfate	X[gf+]	X[ao◆]	X[o◆]
Neomycin Sulfate Oph-thalmic Oint.		COT[+]	
Neomycin Sulfate Oral Soln.		X[+]	X[+]
Neomycin Sulfate & Bacitracin		X[g+]	X[g+]
Neomycin Sulfate & Bacitracin Zinc	XC[g]		
Neomycin Sulfate & Dexamethasone So-dium Phosphate		X[f]	
Neomycin Sulfate & Dexamethasone So-dium Phosphate Oph-thalmic	X[c+]	COT[g]	X[c+]
Neomycin Sulfate & Fluocinolone Aceto-nide		XC[f]	
Neomycin Sulfate & Fluorometholone	CX[g]		
Neomycin Sulfate & Flur-andrenolide		CX[fgh]	X[fgh]
Neomycin Sulfate & Gramicidin	CX[g]		
Neomycin Sulfate & Hydrocortisone	CX[fg]		
Neomycin Sulfate & Hydrocortisone Otic Susp.	X	X	
Neomycin Sulfate & Hydrocortisone Ace-tate	CX[fgh]		
Neomycin Sulfate & Hydrocortisone Ace-tate Ophthalmic		X[i]COT[g]	
Neomycin Sulfate & Methylprednisolone Acetate		CX[f]	X[f]
Neomycin Sulfate & Prednisolone Acetate Ophthalmic		COTX[j]	X[h]
Neomycin Sulfate & Prednisolone Sodium Phosphate Ophthalmic Oint.		COT	
Neomycin Sulfate, Sulf-acetamide Sodium, & Prednisolone Acetate Ophthalmic		COT[g]	
Neomycin Sulfate & Tri-amcinolone Acetonide		XCT[f]	
Neomycin Sulfate & Tri-amcinolone Acetonide Ophthalmic Oint.		COT	
Neomycin & Polymyxin B Sulfates	X[g+]		
Neomycin & Polymyxin B Sulfates Ophthalmic	COT[g+]		X[c+]
Neomycin & Polymyxin B Sulfate & Bacitracin Zinc	CX[g]	CX[g]	X[g+]
Neomycin & Polymyxin B Sulfate, & Bacitracin Zinc & Hydrocortisone Acetate Ophthalmic Oint.		COT	
Neomycin & Polymyxin B Sulfate, & Bacitracin Zinc, & Hydrocortisone Acetate Oint.	CX[+]		

Drugs (Dosage Form)	WC	T	LR
Neomycin & Polymyxin B Sulfates, Bacitracin, & Lidocaine	X[g+]		
Neomycin & Polymyxin B Sulfates, Bacitracin Zinc, & Hydrocortisone Acetate Ointment	X[gk+]		
Neomycin & Polymyxin B Sulfate & Hydrocortisone Otic Soln.		X	X
Neomycin & Polymyxin B Sulfates & Dexamethasone Ophthalmic	COT[g]X[j]	X[j]	
Neomycin & Polymyxin B Sulfate & Gramicidin	CX[f]		
Neomycin & Polymyxin B Sulfate & Gramicidin Ophthalmic Soln.		X	
Neomycin & Polymyxin B Sulfates, Gramicidin, & Hydrocortisone Acetate Cream	X		
Neomycin & Polymyxin B Sulfates & Hydrocortisone Susp.		TP[kv]	X[kv]
Neomycin & Polymyxin B Sulfate & Hydrocortisone Soln.		TP[kv]	X[kv]
Neomycin & Polymyxin B Sulfates & Hydrocortisone Acetate Ophthalmic Susp.		X	
Neomycin & Polymyxin B Sulfates & Prednisolone Acetate Ophthalmic Susp.		X	
Neostigmine Bromide		X[ao]	
Neostigmine Methylsalicylate		X[o]	
Netilmicin Sulfate		X[o]	
Niacin	X[ao]		
Niacinamide		X[ao]	
Nicotine	InH[+]		H[+]
Nicotine Polacrilex		X	
Nicotine Polacrilex Gum	SPU		SPU
Nicotine Transdermal System	SPU		SPU
Nifedipine		X[bo+]	X[bo+]
Nitrofurantoin		X[abo]	X[abo]
Nitrofurantoin Oral Susp.		X	X
Nitrofurazone		X[fgo]	X[fgo]
Nitrofurazone Topical Soln.		X	X
Nitroglycerin		G[a+]	X[g]

Drugs (Dosage Form)	WC	T	LR
Nitroglycerin, Diluted		X[+]	X[+]
Nitromersol		X[o]	X[o]
Nitromersol Topical Solution		X	X
Nitrous Oxide		A[+]	
Nizatidine		X[ob+]	X[ob+]
Nonoxynol-9		X[o]	
Norepinephrine Bitartrate		X[o]	X[o]
Norethindrone	X[ao]		
Norethindrone & Ethinyl Estradiol (tab)	X		
Norethindrone & Mestranol (tab)	X		
Norethindrone Acetate	X[ao]		
Norethindrone Acetate & Ethinyl Estradiol (tab)	X		
Norethynodrel	X[o]		
Norfloxacin	X[a]	X[o]	X[o]
Norgestrel	X[ao]		
Norgestrel & Ethinyl Estradiol (tab)	X		
Nortriptyline HCl		X[ao]	X[o]
Nortryptyline HCl Oral		X[c]	X[c]
Noscapine	X[o]		
Novobiocin Sodium		X[bo]	X[b]
Nystatin	X[g+]	X[ah+n]	X[ah+n]
Nystatin Cream		XC[+]	
Nystatin Oral Susp.		X	X
Nystatin for Oral Susp.		X	
Nystatin Vaginal		X[ai+]	X[ai+]
Nystatin, Neomycin Sulfate, Gramicidin, & Triamcinolone Acetonide		X[fg]	
Nystatin, Neomycin Sulfate, Thiostrepton, & Triamcinolone Acetonide		X[fg]	
Nystatin & Triamcinolone Acetonide		X[fg]	
Ofloxacin	X[o]		X[o]
Ointment, White and/or Yellow	X		
Hydrophilic Ointment		X	
Oleovitamin A & D		X[b]In	X[b]In
Omeprazole	CoH[o]		
Ophthalmic, Bland Lubricating	OT[g]		
Opium Powder	X		
Opium Tincture		X[+]	X[+]
Orphenadrine Citrate		X[o]	X[o]
Oxacillin Sodium		X[bo+◆]	
Oxacillin Sodium for Oral Soln.		X[+]	

Drugs (Dosage Form)	WC	T	LR
Oxamniquine	X[o]	X[b]	
Oxandrolone	X[o]	X[a]	X[ao]
Oxazepam	X[abo]		
Oxprenolol HCl	X[o]	X[a]	X[a]
Oxprenolol HCl Extended Release (tab)		X	X
Oxtriphylline	X[o]		
Oxtriphylline Oral		X[c]	
Oxtriphylline Delayed Release (tab)		X	
Oxtriphylline Extended Release (tab)		X	
Oxybenzone		X[o]	X[o]
Oxybutynin Chloride	X[o]	X[ad]	X[ad]
Oxycodone & Acetaminophen		X[ab]	X[ab]
Oxycodone & Aspirin (tab)		X	X
Oxycodone HCl		X[ao]	X[a]
Oxycodone HCl Oral Soln.		X	X
Oxycodone Terephthalate		X[o]	
Oxygen 93 Percent		A[+]	
Oxymetazoline HCl		X[o]	
Oxymetazoline HCl Soln.		X[ks]	
Oxymetholone	X[ao]		
Oxymorphone HCl	X[i+]	X[o]	X[o]
Oxyphenbutazone		X[ao]	
Oxytetracycline		X[ao◆]	X[ao]
Oxytetracycline Calcium	X[o]	X[o]	
Oxytetracycline Calcium Oral Susp.		X	X
Oxytetracycline HCl		X[bo◆]	X[bo]
Oxytetracycline & Nystatin (cap)		X	X
Oxytetracycline & Nystatin for Oral Susp.		X[+]	X[+]
Oxytetracycline HCl & Hydrocortisone Ointment	X		X
Oxytetracycline HCl & Hydrocortisone Acetate Ophthalmic Susp.		X	X
Oxytetracycline & Phenazopyridine Hydrochlorides & Sulfamethizole (cap)		X	X
Oxytetracycline HCl & Polymyxin B Sulfate	X[gom]		X[g]
Oxytetracycline HCl & Polymyxin B Ophthalmic Oint.		COT	
Oxtriphylline		X[a]	
Oxytocin Nasal Soln.	SP		
Padimate O		X[ho]	X[ho]
Pancreatin		X[abo+]	
Pancrelipase		X[abo+]	
Pancrelipase Delayed-Release		X[b+]	
Panthenol		X[o]	
Papain		X[o]	X[o]
Papain Tablets for Topical Soln.		X[+]	X[+]
Papaverine HCl		X[ao]	X[o]
Parachlorophenol		X[o]	X[o]
Parachlorophenol, Camphorated		X	X
Paraldehyde		G,WF[+]	WF[+]
Paramethasone Acetate	X[a]	X[o]	
Paregoric		X[+]	X[+]
Paromomycin Sulfate		X[bdo]	
Pectin	X		
Penbutolol Sulfate	X[a]	X[ao]	X[ao]
Penicillamine		X[abo]	
Penicillin G Benzathine	X[ao◆]		
Penicillin G Benzathine Oral Susp.		X	
Penicillin G Potassium		X[ao◆]	
Penicillin G Potassium Tablets for Oral Soln.		X	
Penicillin G Procaine, Neomycin & Polymyxin B Sulfates, & Hydrocortisone Acetate Topical Susp.	X		
Penicillin G Sodium		X[o+◆]	
Penicillin V		X[ao]	
Penicillin V for Oral Susp.		X	
Penicillin V Benzathine		X	
Penicillin V Benzathine Oral Susp.		X[+]	
Penicillin V Potassium		X[ao]	
Penicillin V Potassium for Oral Soln.		X	
Pentaerythritol Tetranitrate		X[ao+]	
Pentazocine		X[o]	X[o]
Pentazocine HCl		X[ao]	X[ao]
Pentazocine HCl & Aspirin (tab)		X	X
Pentazocine & Naloxone HCl (tab)		X	X
Pentetic Acid	X[o]		
Pentobarbital		X[aeo]	
Pentobarbital Sodium		X[bo]	

Drugs (Dosage Form)	WC	T	LR
Peppermint Spirit		X	
Perflubron		X[o]	X[o]
Perphenazine	X[d]	X[ao]	X[ado]
Perphenazine Oral Soln.	X		X
Perphenazine & Amitriptyline HCl (tab)	X		
Petrolatum (all)	X		
Petrolatum, Hydrophilic	X		
Phenacemide	X[a]	X[o]	
Phenazopyridine HCl		X[ao]	
Phendimetrazine Tartrate	X[a]	X[bo]	
Phenelzine Sulfate		X[ao+]	X[ao+]
Phenmetrazine HCl		X[ao]	
Phenobarbital	X[ao]	X[e]	X[e]
Phenol		X	X
Phenol, Liquified		G	G
Phenolphthalein (all)	X[o]	X[a]	
Phenoxybenzamine HCl	X[bo]		
Phentermine HCl		X[abo]	
Phentolamine Mesylate	X[o]		X[o]
Phenylalanine	X[o]		
Phenylbutazone		X[abo]	
Phenylbutazone Boluses	X[x]		
Phenylephrine HCl		X[o]	X[o]
Phenylephrine HCl Soln.		X[ks]	X[ks]
Phenylephrine HCl Nasal Jelly	X		
Phenylethyl Alcohol		X[+]	X[+]
Phenylpropanolamine HCl		X[oa]	X[oa]
Phenylpropanolamine HCl Extended-Release		X[ba]	X[ba]
Phenytoin	X[a]	X[o]	
Phenytoin Oral Susp.		ChX[+]	
Phenytoin Sodium		X[o]	
Phenytoin Sodium, Extended (cap)		X	
Phenytoin Sodium, Prompt (cap)		X	
Physostigmine		X[o]	X[o]
Physostigmine Salicylate		X[o]	X[o]
Physostigmine Salicylate Ophthalmic Solution		X	X
Physostigmine Sulfate		X[o]	X[o]
Physostigmine Sulfate Ophthalmic Ointment		COT	
Phytonadione	X[a]	X[o]	X[ao]
Pilocarpine		X[o]	X[o]
Pilocarpine HCl		X[o]	X[o]
Pilocarpine HCl Ophthalmic Soln.		X	
Pilocarpine Nitrate		X[o]	X[o]
Pilocarpine Nitrate Ophthalmic		X	X
Pimozide		X[ao]	X[ao]
Pindolol	X[ao]		X[ao]
Piperacillin	X[o♦]		
Piperacillin Sodium		X[o]	
Piperazine		X	X
Piperazine Citrate	X[o]	X[ad]	
Piroxicam		X[bo]	X[bo]
Plantago Seed	X		
Plicamycin		X	X
Podophyllum Resin		X[o]	X[o]
Podophyllum Resin Topical Soln.		X	X
Poloxelene		X	
Polycarbophil		X[o]	
PEG 3350 & Electrolytes for Oral Soln.		X	
Polymixin B Sulfate		X[o♦]	X[o♦]
Polymixin B Sulfate & Bacitracin Zinc Topical	X[o]	A[lt]	
Polymixin B Sulfate & Hydrocortisone Otic Soln.		X	X
Polythiazide		X[ao]	X[ao]
Polyvinyl Alcohol	X[o]		
Potash, Sulfurated		SP	
Potassium Acetate		X[o]	
Potassium Bicarbonate	X[o]		
Potassium Bicarbonate Effervescent Tabs for Oral Soln.		X[+]	
Potassium Bicarbonate & Potassium Chloride for Effervescent Oral Soln.		X[+oa]	
Potassium & Sodium Bicarbonate & Citric Acid Effervescent for Oral Solution (tab)		X	X
Potassium Bitartrate		X[o]	
Potassium Carbonate	X[o]		
Potassium Chloride	X[o]		
Potassium Chloride Extended Release		X[ab+]	
Potassium Chloride Oral Soln.		X	
Potassium Chloride for Oral Soln.		X	
Potassium Chloride, Potassium Bicarbonate, & Potassium Citrate Effervescent Tablets for Oral Soln.		X[+]	

Drugs (Dosage Form)	WC	T	LR
Potassium Citrate		X[o]	
Potassium Citrate Extended-Release (tabs)		X	
Potassium Citrate & Citric Acid Oral Solution		X	
Potassium Gluconate		X[aeo]	X[e]
Potassium Gluconate & Potassium Chloride for Oral Soln.	X		
Potassium Gluconate & Potassium Chloride Oral		X	
Potassium Gluconate & Potassium Citrate Oral Soln.	X		
Potassium Gluconate, Potassium Citrate, & Ammonium Chloride Oral Soln.		X	
Potassium Guaiacolsulfonate	X[o]		X[o]
Potassium Iodide		X[o]	
Potassium Iodide Delayed Release		X[a]	
Potassium Iodide Oral Soln.		X	X
Potassium Nitrate		X[co]	
Potassium Permanganate	X[o]		
Potassium Phosphate, Dibasic	X[o]		
Potassium Sodium Tartrate		X[o]	
Povidone		X[o]	
Povidone-Iodine		X	
Povidone-Iodine Cleansing Soln.		X	
Povidone-Iodine Topical Soln.		X[+]	
Povidone-Iodine Topical Aerosol Solution		A[+]	
Povidone-Iodine Oint.		X	
Pralidoxime Chloride	X[ao]		
Pramoxine HCl		X[ft]C[t]	
Prazepam		X[abo]	X[abo]
Praziquantel	X[o]	X[a]	X[o]
Prazosin HCl	X[b]	X[o]	X[bo]
Prednisolone	X[ao]	X[cdf]	X[d]
Prednisolone Acetate	X[o]		
Prednisolone Acetate Ophthalmic Susp.		X	
Prednisolone Hemisuccinate		X[o]	

Drugs (Dosage Form)	WC	T	LR
Prednisolone Sodium Phosphate		X[o]	
Prednisolone Sodium Phosphate Ophthalmic Solution		X	X
Prednisolone Tebutate		In[+]	
Prednisone	X[ao]	X[d]	
Prednisone Oral Soln.		X	
Prilocaine HCl	X[o]		
Primaquine Phosphate	X[ao]		X[ao]
Primadone	X[a]		
Primadone Oral Susp.		X	X
Probenecid	X[ao]		
Probenecid & Colchicine (tab)	X		X
Probucol	X[ao]		X[ao]
Procaine HCl	X[o]		
Procainamide HCl		X[abo]	
Procainamide HCl Extended Release (tab)		X	
Procarbazine HCl		X[bo]	X[bo]
Prochlorperazine		X[co]	X[o]
Prochlorperazine Oral		X[c]	X[c]
Prochlorperazine Edisylate		X[o]	X[o]
Prochlorperazine Edisylate Oral Soln.		X	X
Prochlorperazine Maleate	X[a]	X[o]	X[ao]
Procyclidine HCl		X[ao+]	X[o+]
Progesterone		X[o]	X[o]
Proline	X[o]		
Promazine HCl		X[ado]	X[ado]
Promazine HCl Oral Soln.		X	X
Promethazine HCl		X[adi+]	X[adi+]
Propafenone HCl		X[o]	X[o]
Propantheline Bromide	X[ao]		
Proparacaine HCl	X[o]		
Proparacaine HCl Ophthaimic Soln.		X	X
Propoxycaine HCl	X[o]		X[o]
Propoxyphene HCl		X[bo]	
Propoxyphene HCl & Acetaminophen (tab)		X	
Propoxyphene HCl, Aspirin, & Caffeine (cap)		X[+]	
Propoxyphene Napsylate		X[ao]	
Propoxyphene Napsylate Oral Susp.		X	X
Propoxyphene Napsylate & Acetaminophen (tab)		X[+]	

Drugs (Dosage Form)	WC	T	LR
Propoxyphene Napsylate & Aspirin (tab)		X	
Propranolol HCl	X[ao]		
Propranolol HCl Extended-Release (cap)	X		
Propranolol HCl & Hydrochlorothiazide (tab)	X		
Propranolol HCl & Hydrochlorothiazide Extended-Release (cap)	X		
Propylene Glycol		X	
Propylhexedrine		X	
Propylhexedrine Inhalant		X[+]	
Propylthiouracil	X[ao]		
Protamine Sulfate		X[+]	X[+]
Protriptyline HCl	X[o]	X[a]	
Pseudoephedrine HCl		X[ado]	X[do]
Pseudoephedrine HCl Extended Release (tabs)		X	
Psyllium Hydrophilic Mucilloid for Oral Susp.		X	
Pumice	X[o]		
Pyrantel Pamoate	X[o]		X[o]
Pyrantel Pamoate Oral Suspension		X	X
Pyrazinamide	X[ao]		
Pyrethrum Extract		X	X
Pyridostigmine Bromide		X[ado]	X[d]
Pyridoxine HCl	X[a]	X[o]	X[ao]
Pyrilamine Maleate	X[a]	X[o]	X[o]
Pyrimethamine		X[ao]	X[ao]
Pyroxylin			SP
Pyrvinium Pamoate		X[ao]	X[ao]
Pyrvinium Pamoate Oral Susp.		X	X
Quazepam	X[ao]		
Quinidine Gluconate	X[o]		X[o]
Quinidine Gluconate Extended-Release	X[a]		X[a]
Quinidine Sulfate	X[ao]	X[b]	X[abo]
Quinidine Sulfate Extended Release (tab)	X		X
Quinine Sulfate	X[ao]	X[b]	X[o]
Racepinephrine		X[o]	X[o]
Racepinephrine Soln.		X[r+]	X[r+]
Racepinephrine HCl		X[o]	X[o]
Ranitidine HCl		X[ao]	X[ao]
Ranitidine Oral Soln.		X[+]	X[+]
Rauwolfia Serpentina	SP	X[a]	X[a]
Rayon, Purified	SP		
Rehydration Salts, Oral		SX[a+]	

Drugs (Dosage Form)	WC	T	LR
Reserpine		X[aeo]	X[aeo]
Reserpine & Chlorothiazide (tab)		X	X
Reserpine, Hydralazine HCl, & Hydrochlorothiazide (tab)		X	X
Reserpine & Hydrochlorothiazide (tab)		X	X
Resorcinol	X[o]		X[o]
Resorcinol, Compound Ointment		X[+]	
Resorcinol & Sulfur Lotion	X		
Resorcinol Monoacetate		X	X
Ribavirin		X[o]	
Ribavirin for Inhalation Soln.		H[+]	
Riboflavin		X[ao]	X[ao]
Riboflavin 5'-Phosphate Sodium		X[o]	X[o]
Rifampin		X[bo+]	X[bo+]
Rifampin Oral		GChP[j+]	GChP[j+]
Rifampin & Isoniazid (cap)		X[+]	X[+]
Rimexolone	X[o]		
Rimexolone Ophthalmic	X[j]		
Ritodrine HCl		X[ao+]	
Rose Water Ointment		X	X
Roxarsone	X[o]		
Saccharin Calcium	X[o]		
Saccharin Sodium	X[ao]		
Saccharin Sodium Oral Solution		X	
Safflower Oil		X	X
Salicylamide	X[o]		
Salicylic Acid	X[o]		
Salicylic Acid Collodion		X[+]	
Salicylic Acid Gel		XC[+]	
Salicylic Acid Plaster	X[+]		
Salicylic Acid Topical Foam		X	
Salsalate		X[abo]	
Sargramostim	U(FR)		
Scopolamine HBr		X[ao]	X[ao]
Scopolamine HBr Ophthalmic		X[c]C[g]	
Secobarbital		X[o]	
Secobarbital Elixir		X	
Secobarbital Sodium		X[bo]	
Secobarbital Sodium & Amobarbital Sodium	X[b]		
Selegiline HCl	X[ao]		X[ao]
Selenious Acid		X[o]	
Selenium Sulfide	X[o]		

Drugs (Dosage Form)	WC	T	LR
Selenium Sulfide Lotion		X	
Selenomethionine	X[o]		
Senna Fluid Extract		X[+]	X[+]
Senna Syrup		X[+]	
Sennosides	X[ao]		
Serine	X[o]		
Silver Nitrate		X[o]	X[o]
Silver Nitrate Ophthalmic Soln.		X	X
Silver Nitrate, Toughened		X	X
Simethicone	X[a]	X[oy]	
Simethicone Oral Susp.		X	X
Simvastatin	In[o]	X[a]	
Sisomicin Sulfate		X[o]	
Sodium Acetate	ChP[j+]	X[o]	
Sodium Acetate Soln.		X	
Sodium Ascorbate		X[o]	X[o]
Sodium Bicarbonate	X[ao]		
Sodium Bicarbonate Oral Powder	X[o]		
Sodium Chloride	X[ao♦]		
Sodium Chloride Inhalation Soln.	S[r]		
Sodium Chloride Ophthalmic		X[c]C[k]	
Sodium Chloride Tablet for Soln.	X		
Sodium Chloride & Dextrose (tab)	X		
Sodium Citrate & Citric Acid Oral Soln.		X	
Sodium Fluoride	X[o]	X[a]	
Sodium Fluoride Oral Soln.		XP	
Sodium Fluoride & Phosphoric Acid		P[t]	
Sodium Fluoride & Phosphoric Acid Topical Soln.		P	
Sodium Gluconate	X[o]		
Sodium Hypochlorite Topical		SP[c+]	SP[c+]
Sodium Iodide		X[o]	
Sodium Lactate Soln.		X	
Sodium Monofluorophosphate	X[o]		
Sodium Nitrate		X[o]	
Sodium Nitroprusside		X[o]	X[o]
Sodium Phosphate, Dibasic		X[o]	
Sodium Phosphate, Monobasic	X[o]		
Sodium Phosphate	X[P]		

Drugs (Dosage Form)	WC	T	LR
Sodium Phosphates Oral Soln.		X	
Sodium Polystyrene Sulfonate	X[o]		
Sodium Polystyrene Sulfonate Susp.	X[+]		
Sodium Salicylate	X[ao]		X[o]
Sodium Sulfate Inj.		X[+]	
Sodium Thiosulfate		X[o]	
Sorbitol Soln.		X	
Soybean Oil		X[+]	X[+]
Spectinomycin HCl		X[o♦]	
Spironolactone (tab)	X[o]	X[a]	X[a]
Spironolactone & Hydrochlorothiazide		X[a]	X[o]
Stannous Fluoride	X[o]		
Stannous Fluoride Gel	X		
Stanozolol		X[ao]	X[ao]
Starch, Topical	X		
Storax	X[o]		
Succinyl Chloride	X[o]		
Sucralfate		X[ao]	
Sufentanil Citrate	X[o]		
Sulbactam Sodium		X[♦]	
Sulconazole Nitrate	X[o]		X[o]
Sulfa Vaginal, Triple	X[a]C[f]		X[a]C[f]
Sulfabenzamide	X[o]		X[o]
Sulfacetamide	X[o]		X[o]
Sulfacetamide Sodium		X[o]	X[o]
Sulfacetamide Sodium Ophthalmic	COT[g]	X[c+]	X[c+]
Sulfacetamide Sodium & Prednisolone Acetate Ophthalmic		TP[j] CTP[g]	
Sulfachlorpyridazine	X[o]	X[o]	
Sulfadiazine	X[ao]	X[ao]	
Sulfadiazine, Silver	X[o]	C[f]	X[fo]
Sulfadoxine	X[o]		X[o]
Sulfadoxine & Pyrimethamine (tab)	X		X
Sulfamerazine	X[ao]		X[o]
Sulfamethazine	X[o]		X[o]
Sulfamethazine Granulated	X[x]		
Sulfamethizole	X[ao]		X[o]
Sulfamethizole Oral Susp.		X	X
Sulfamethoxazole	X[ao]		X[ao]
Sulfamethoxazole Oral Susp.		X	X
Sulfamethoxazole & Trimethoprim	X[a]		X[a]
Sulfamethoxazole & Trimethoprim Oral Susp.		X	X

Drugs (Dosage Form)	WC	T	LR
Sulfapyridine	X[ao]		X[ao]
Sulfaquinoxaline	X[o]		X[o]
Sulfaquinoxaline Oral		X[c]	X[c]
Sulfasalazine	X[a]	X[o]	X[o]
Sulfasalazine Delayed Release	X[a]		
Sulfathiazole	X[o]		X[o]
Sulfinpyrazone	X[ab]		
Sulfisoxazole (tab)	X		X
Sulfisoxazole Acetyl Oral Suspension		X	X
Sulfisoxazole Diolamine		X[o]	X[o]
Sulfisoxazole Diolamine Ophthalmic		C[g]X[c]	X[c]
Sulfur Ointment	X[+]		
Sulfur, Precipitated	X[o]		
Sulfur, Sublimed	X[o]		
Sulindac	X[ao]		
Suprofen	X[o]		
Suprofen Ophthalmic		X[c]	
Sutilains		X[+]	
Sutilains Ointment		CX[+]	
Surgical Suture, Absorbable	SP		
Surgical Suture, Nonabsorbable	SP		
Talc	X		
Tamoxifen Citrate	X[ao]		X[ao]
Tannic Acid		X[o]	X[o]
Tape, Adhesive	X[+]		
Temazepam	X[bo]		X[bo]
Terbutaline Sulfate	X[o+]	X[+]	X[o+]
Terbutaline Sulfate Inhalation		A[l+]	A[l+]
Terfenadine		X[ao]	X[ao]
Terpin Hydrate	X[o]		
Terpin Hydrate & Codeine Elixir		X	
Terpin Hydrate & Dextromethorphan HBr Elixir		X	
Terpin Hydrate Elixir		X	
Testolactone		X[ao]	
Testosterone	X[o]		
Testosterone Cypionate	X[o]		X[o]
Testosterone Enanthate	X[o+]		
Testosterone Propionate	X[o]		X[o]
Tetracaine		X[o]C[f]	X[o]
Tetracaine Ophthalmic Oint.		C	
Tetracaine & Menthol Oint.		C	
Tetracaine HCl		X[o]C[f]	X[o]
Tetracaine HCl Topical Soln.		X	X
Tetracaine HCl Ophthalmic Soln.		X	X
Tetracycline		X[o]	X[o]
Tetracycline Boluses		X[x]	
Tetracycline Oral Suspension		X	X
Tetracycline HCl (tablet/capsule/ophthalmic/suspension/topical/solution)		X	X
Tetracycline HCl Ophthalmic	COT[g]		
Tetracycline HCl Soluble Pwd.		X[x]	
Tetracycline HCl for Topical Soln.		X	X
Tetracycline HCl & Novobiocin Sodium (tab)		X[x]	
Tetracycline HCl & Nystatin (cap)		X	X
Tetracycline Phosphate Complex		X[bo]	X[bo]
Tetracycline Phosphate Complex & Novobiocin Sodium (cap)		X[x]	
Tetrahydrozoline HCl		X[o]	
Tetrahydrozoline HCl Soln.		X[ks]	
Theophylline	X[abo]		
Theophylline Extended Release (cap)	X		
Theophylline, Ephedrine HCl & Phenobarbital (tab)	X		
Theophylline & Guaifenesin		X[b]	
Theophylline Guaifenesin Oral Soln.	X		
Theophylline Sodium Glycinate	X[a]	X[e]	
Thiabendazole	X[o]	X[a]	
Thiabendazole Oral Susp.		X	
Thiacetarsamide	X[o]		
Thiamine HCl		X[aeo]	X[aeo]
Thiamine Mononitrate		X[eo]	X[eo]
Thiamylal	X[o]		
Thiethylperazine Maleate		X[aio+]	X[aio+]
Thimerosal		X[o]	X[o]
Thimerosal Tincture		X[+]	X[+]
Thimerosal Topical		X[cl+]	X[cl+]

Drugs (Dosage Form)	WC	T	LR
Thioguanine		X[ao]	
Thiopental Sodium		X[o]	
Thioridazine	X[o]		X[o]
Thioridazine Oral Susp.		X	X
Thioridazine HCl		X[ao]	X[ao]
Thioridazine HCl Oral Soln.		X[+]	X[+]
Thiostrepton		X[o]	
Thiotepa		X[o]	X[o]
Thiothixene	X[b]	X[o]	X[bo]
Thiothixene HCl		X[o]	X[o]
Thiothixene HCl Oral Solution		X	X
Threonine	X[o]		
Thyroid		X[ao]	
Ticarcillin Monosodium		X[o]	
Tiletamine HCl		X[o]	
Tilmicosin	He[o]		He[o]
Timolol Maleate	X[ao]		X[a]
Timolol Maleate & Hydrochlorothiazide (tab)	X		X
Timolol Maleate Ophthalmic Soln.		X	
Tioconazole		X[afo]	
Titanium Dioxide	X[o]		
Tobramycin		X[o]	
Tobramycin Ophthalmic		X[c]COT[g]	
Tobramycin & Dexamethasone Ophthalmic		X[i]C[g]	
Tobramycin & Fluorometholone Acetate Ophthalmic		X[c]	
Tobramycin Sulfate		X[o]	
Tocainide HCl	X[ao]		
Tolazamide	X[o]	X[a]	
Tolbutamide	X[ao]		
Tolmetin Sodium	X[ao]	X[b]	
Tolnaftate		X[fto]	
Tolnaftate Topical		X[lco+]	
Tolu Balsam		X[+]	
Trazodone HCl		X[ao]	X[ao]
Trenbolone Acetate		Co	
Tretinoin		C[f]X[c]	X[cft]
Triacetin		X	
Triamcinolone	X[ao]		
Triamcinolone Acetonide	X[go]	X[fh]	
Triamcinolone Acetonide Dental Paste		X	
Triamcinolone Acetonide Topical		X[i+]	
Triamcinolone Diacetate	X[o]	X[d]	X[d]
Triamcinolone Hexacetonide	X		
Triamterene		X[bo]	X[bo]
Triamterene & Hydrochlorothiazide		X[ab]	X[ab]
Triazolam		X[ao]	X[ao]
Trichlorfon	X[+]		
Trichlormethiazide	X[o]	X[a]	
Tricitrates Oral Soln.		X	
Triclosan		X[o]	X[o]
Trientine HCl		X[ao+]	In[o]
Trifluoperazine HCl	X[a]	X[do]	X[ado]
Triflupromazine		X[o]	X[o]
Triflupromazine HCl (tab)	X		X
Triflupromazine Oral Suspension		X	X
Trifluridine		X	X
Trihexyphenidyl HCl		X[aeo]	
Trihexyphenidyl HCl Extended-Release (cap)		X	
Trikates Oral Soln.		X	X
Trimeprazine Tartrate	X[a]	X[do]	X[ado]
Trimethadione		X[abco+]	
Trimethaphan Camsylate		X[+]	
Trimethobenzamide HCl	X[bo]		
Trimethoprim		X[ao]	X[ao]
Trioxsalen	X[ao]		X[ao]
Tripelennamine Citrate	X[a]	X[e]	X[e]
Tripelennamine HCl	X[ao]		X[o]
Triprolidine HCl		X[ado]	X[ado]
Triprolidine & Pseudoephedrine Hydrochlorides		X[ad]	X[ad]
Trisulfapyrimidines (tab)	X		
Trisulfapyrimidines Oral Susp.		X[+]	
Tromethamine		X[o]	
Tropicamide		X[o]	X[o]
Tropicamide Ophthalmic Soln.		X[+]	
Trypsin, Crystallized		X[+]	
Tryptophan	X[o]		
Tubocurarine Chloride		X[o]	
Tylosine	HHe[x]		X[x]
Tylosine Granulated	HHeSp[x]		
Tyloxapol		X[o]	
Tyropanoate Sodium		X[bo]	X[bo]
Tyrosine	X[o]		
Tyrothricin		X[o]	
Undecylenic Acid		X[o]	X[o]

Drugs (Dosage Form)	WC	T	LR
Undecylenic Acid, Compound Ointment		X[+]	
Urea	X[o]		
Valine	X[o]		
Valproic Acid		GP[o]X[bd+]	
Vancomycin		X[o]	
Vancomycin HCl		X[bo]	
Vancomycin HCl for Oral Soln.		X	
Verapamil HCl		X[ao]	X[ao]
Verapamil HCl Extended Release		X[a]	X[a]
Vidarabine		X[◆]	
Vidarabine Ophthalmic Ointment		COT[+]	
Vinblastine Sulfate		X[+]	X[+]
Vincristine Sulfate		X[+]	X[+]
Vitamin A		X[bo+]	X[bo+]
Vitamin E		In[o]X	X
Vitamin E Preparation		In	X
Vitamins, Oil-Soluble		X[ab]	X[ab]
Warfarin Sodium	X[o]	X[a]	X[ao]
Water, Purified		X[◆]	
Water, Sterile Purified		X	
White Lotion		X	
Witch Hazel		X	
Xylometazoline HCl		X[o]	X[o]
Xylometazoline HCl Nasal Soln.		X	X
Xylose		X[+]	
Zidovudine		X[bo]	X[bo]
Zidovudine Oral		X[c]	X[c]
Zinc Acetate		X[o]	
Zinc Carbonate		X[o]	
Zinc Chloride		X[o]	
Zinc Gluconate	X[ao]		
Zinc Oxide	X[o]		
Zinc Oxide (oint/paste)	X[+]		
Zinc Oxide & Salicylic Acid Paste	X		
Zinc Stearate	X[o]		
Zinc Sulfate		X[o]	
Zinc Sulfate Ophthalmic Solution		X	
Zinc Undecylenate	X[o]		
Zolazepam HCl		X[o]	

Provided by Dr. Kenneth S. Alexander, Professor of Pharmacy, College of Pharmacy, University of Toledo.
The listing of container and storage requirements for Compendial drugs is included as an aid to the practitioner in storing and dispensing.

Container and Storage Requirements for Sterile U.S.P. 23 Drugs

The listing of container and storage requirements for U.S.P. drugs is included as an aid to the practitioner in storing and dispensing.

Legend:

A	=	Type I Glass
B	=	Type II Glass
C	=	Type III Glass
CP	=	Cool Place
CV	=	Controlled Volume
D	=	Type II or III Glass Depending on Final Soln. pH
DF	=	Do Not Freeze
F	=	Freezer (-4°C)
H	=	Protect From Heat
He	=	Hermetic Container
I	=	Containers for Sterile Solids as Described Under Injections
In	=	Inert Atmosphere
L	=	Protect from Light
LR	=	Light Resistant
M	=	Multiple Dose
Mo	=	Protect from Moisture
N	=	Intact Flexible Container Meeting the General Requirements
O	=	Original Package
P	=	Plastic
PA	=	Does not Adversely Affect Performance
R	=	Refrigerator (2° to 8°C)
RT	=	Controlled Room Temperature
S	=	Single Dose
SC	=	Radioactive Shielding
SS	=	Stated Size Limitation
Sy	=	Syringe
T	=	Avoid Toxic Substances
Ti	=	Tight Container
TP	=	Tamper-Proof
Tr	=	Treated to Prevent Adsorption
U	=	Unspecified
W	=	Transparent
X	=	Colorless
WC	=	Well Closed

Drugs	Container	Glass Type	Storage Conditions
Acepromazine Maleate Inj.	S,M	A	L
Acetazolamide for Inj.	I	C	
Acetic Acid Irrigation	S,P	A,B	
Acetylcholine for Ophthalmic Soln.	I		
Acetylcysteine & Isoproterenol HCl Inhal. Soln.	S,M	A	WC
Acetylcysteine Solution	S,M	A,P	O_2 excluded
Acyclovir for Inj.			Ti
Albumin, Human	S	U	RT
Alcohol in Dextrose Inj.	S	A,B	
Alcohol Inj., Dehydrated	S	A	In (head space)
Alfentanil Inj.	S,M	A	
Alphaprodine HCl Inj.	S,M	A	
Alprostadil Inj.	S	A	R
Alteplase for Inj.			R-RT/L
Amdinocillin for Inj.	I		
Amikacin Sulfate Inj.	S,M	A,C	
Aminoacetic Acid Irrigation	S	A,B	
Aminocaproic Acid Inj.	S,M	A	
Aminohippurate Sodium Inj.	S,M	A	
Aminophylline Inj.	S	A	CO_2 excluded
Amitriptyline HCl Inj.	S,M	A	
Ammonia N 13 Inj.	S,M		SC
Ammonium Chloride Inj.	S,M	A,B	
Ammonium Molybdate Inj.	S,M	A,B	
Amobarbital Sodium for Inj.	I	D	
Amoxicillin for Injectable Suspension	I	I	

Drugs	Container	Glass Type	Storage Conditions
Amphotericin B for Inj.	I		R,L
Ampicillin & Sulbactam for Inj.	I		
Ampicillin for Inj.	I		DF
Ampicillin for Injectable Oil Suspension	S,M	A	
Ampicillin for Injectable Suspension	I		
Amrinone Inj.	S	A	L,RT
Anileridine Inj.	S,M	A	L
Anticoagulant Citrate Dextrose Solution	M	A,B	
Anticoagulant Citrate Phosphate Dextrose Adenine Solution	S,P	A,B	X,W
Anticoagulant Heparin Soln.	S,P	A,B	
Anticoagulant Sodium Citrate Soln.	S	A,B	
Antihemophilic Factor			R
Antihemophilic Factor, Cryoprecipitated			F (-18°C)
Antirabies Serum	U		R
Antivenin (Crotalidae) Polyvalent	S		H
Antivenin (*Latrodectus mactans*)	S		H
Antivenin (*Micrurus fulvius*)	S		H
Arginine HCl Inj.	S	B	
Ascorbic Acid Inj.	S	A,B	LR
Atenolol Inj.	S,M	A	CP,RT,LR,DF
Atropine Sulfate Inj.	S,M	A	
Aurothioglucose Injectable Oil Suspension	S,M	A	L
Aurothioglucose Suspension, Sterile	I		
Azaperone Inj.	S,M	A	L
Azathioprine Sodium for Inj.	I	C	RT
Azlocillin for Inj.	I		
Aztreonam	I		
Aztreonam for Inj.	I		F
Bacitracin for Inj., Sterile	I	D	R
Bacitracin Zinc, Sterile	I		CP
BCG Vaccine	U	A	R
Benztropine Mesylate Inj.	S,M	A	
Benzylpenicilloyl-Polylysine Inj.	S,M	A	R
Betamethasone Sodium Phosphate & Betamethasone Acetate Injectable Suspension	M	A	
Betamethasone Sodium Phosphate Inj.	S,M	A	
Bethanechol Chloride Inj.	S	A	
Biological Indicator for Dry Heat Sterilization, Paper Strip	O		L,H,Mo,PA
Biological Indicator for Ethylene Oxide Sterilization, Paper Strip	O		L,H,Mo,PA
Biological Indicator for Steam Sterilization, Paper Strip	O		L,H,Mo,PA
Biological Indicator for Steam Sterilization, Self-contained	O		L,H,Mo,PA
Biperiden Lactate Inj.	S	A	L
Bleomycin for Inj.	I	B	
Blood Grouping Serums (All)	U		R
Botulism Antitoxin	S		R
Bretylium Tosylate in Dextrose Inj.	S,M	A,B,P	
Bretylium Tosylate Inj.	S	A	

Drugs	Container	Glass Type	Storage Conditions
Brompheniramine Maleate Inj.	S,M	A	L
Bumetanide Inj.	S,M	A	L
Bupivacaine & Epinephrine Inj.	S,M	A	L
Bupivacaine HCl Inj.	S,M	A	
Bupivacaine in Dextrose Inj.	S	A	
Butorphanol Tartrate Inj.	S,M	A	L
Caffeine & Sodium Benzoate Inj.	S	A	
Calcium Chloride Inj.	S	A	
Calcium Gluceptate Inj.	S	A,B	
Calcium Gluconate Inj.	S	A	
Calcium Levulinate Inj.	S	A	
Capreomycin for Inj.	I	B	R
Carbenicillin for Inj.	I	D	
Carboprost Tromethamine Inj.	S,M	A	R
Cefamandole Nafate for Inj.	I	D	
Cefamandole Nafate, Sterile	I		
Cefamandole Sodium for Inj.	I		
Cefamandole Sodium, Sterile	I		
Cefazolin Inj.	I		F
Cefmenoxime for Inj.	I		
Cefonicid for Inj.	I		
Cefoperazone for Inj.	I		
Cefoperazone Inj.	I		F
Ceforanide for Inj.	I		
Cefotaxime Sodium Inj.	S,M		F
Cefotetan Disodium	I		
Cefotetan for Inj.	I		
Cefotetan Inj.	I		F
Cefotiam for Inj.	I	C	
Cefotaxime for Inj.	I		
Cefoxitin Sodium Inj.	I		F
Cefpiramide for Inj.	I		
Ceftazidime for Inj.	I		L
Ceftazidime Inj.	I		F
Ceftazidime, Sterile	I		L
Ceftizoxime for Inj.	I		
Ceftizoxime Inj.	I		F
Ceftriaxone for Inj.	I		F
Ceftriaxone Inj.	I		F
Cefuroxime for Inj.	I		
Cefuroxime Inj.	I		F
Cellulose Oxidized (all)	I		L,R
Cephalothin for Inj.	I		
Cephalothin Inj.	I		F
Cephapirin for Inj.	I		
Cephradine for Inj.	I		
Chloramphenicol Inj.	S,M		
Chloramphenicol Sodium Succinate, Sterile for Inj.	I	B	
Chlordiazepoxide HCl, Sterile	I	B	L
Chloroprocaine HCl Inj.	S,M	A	
Chloroquine HCl Inj.	S	A	

Drugs	Container	Glass Type	Storage Conditions
Chlorothiazide Sodium for Inj.	I	C	
Chlorphenamine Maleate Inj.	S,M	A	L
Chlorpromazine HCl Inj.	S,M	A	L
Chlorprothixene Inj.	S		L
Chlortetracycline HCl	I		L
Cholera Vaccine	U		R
Chromate Cr51 Inj., Sodium	S,M		
Chromic Chloride Inj.	S,M	A,B	
Cilastatin Sod., Sterile	I	C	R
Ciprofloxacin Inj.	S,M	A	R,L
Cisplatin for Inj.	I		
Citric Acid, Magnesium Oxide Sodium Carbonate Irrigation	S	A,B	
Clavulanate Potassium	I		
Clindamycin for Inj.	I		
Clindamycin Inj.	S,M	A,P	
Cloxacillin Benzathine	U (tight)		
Cloxacilllin Benzathine Intramammary Infusion	Sy		
Cloxacillin Sodium	U (tight)		
Cloxacillin Sodium Intramammary Infusion	Sy		TP
Coccidioidin			R
Codeine Phosphate Inj.	S,M	A	L
Colchicine Inj.	S	A	L
Colistimethate for Inj.	I		
Colistimethate Sodium	I		
Corticotropin for Inj.	I	B	
Corticotropin Inj.	S,M	A	R
Corticotropin Inj., Repository	S,M	A	
Corticotropin Zinc Hydroxide Injectable Suspension	S,M	A	RT
Cortisone Acetate Injectable Suspension	S,M	A	
Cromolyn Sodium Inhalation	S (double-ended Ampule)	A,B,P	
Cupric Chloride Inj.	S,M	A,B	
Cupric Sulfate Inj.	S,M	A,B	
Cyanocobalamin Inj.	S,M	A	LR
Cyclizine Lactate Inj.	S	A	
Cyclophosphamide for Inj.	I	B	RT
Cyclosporine for Inj.	S,M		
Cysteine HCl Inj.	S,M	A	
Cytarabine	I		
Cytarabine for Inj.	I		
Dacarbazine for Inj.	S,M or I	A	L
Dactinomycin for Inj.	I	B	LR
Daunorubicin HCl for Inj.	I	B	LR
Deferoxamine Mesylate for Inj.	S,M	A	
Deslanoside Inj.	S	A	
Desoxycorticosterone Acetate Inj.	S,M	A,C	LH
Desoxycorticosterone Acetate Pellets	U (tight)		
Dexamethasone Acetate Injectable Suspension	S,M	A	
Dextrose & Sodium Chloride Inj.	S	A,B,P	

Drugs	Container	Glass Type	Storage Conditions
Dextrose Inj.	S	A,B,P	
Diatrizoate Meglumine & Diatrizoate Sodium Inj.	S	A,C	L
Diatrizoate Meglumine Inj.	S,M	A,C	L
Diatrizoate Sodium Inj.	S,M	A,C	L
Diazepam Inj.	S,M	A	L
Diazoxide Inj.	S	A	L
Dibucaine HCl Inj.	S,M	A	L
Dicyclomine HCl Inj.	S,M	A	
Diethylstilbestrol Diphosphate Inj.	S,M		
Diethylstilbestrol Inj.	S,M	A	LR
Digitoxin Inj.	S,M	A	L
Digoxin Inj.	S	A	LR, H
Dihydroergotamine Mesylate Inj.	S	A	Avoid heat
Dihydrostreptomycin Inj.	S,M		
Dimenhydrinate Inj.	S,M	A,C	
Dimercaprol Inj.	S,M	A,C	
Dimethyl Sulfoxide Irrigation	S		RT,L
Dinoprost Tromethamine Inj.	S,M	A	
Diphenhydramine HCl Inj.	S,M	A	L
Diphtheria & Tetanus Toxoids	U		R
Diphtheria & Tetanus Toxoids/Adsorbed	U		R
Diphtheria & Tetanus Toxoids & Pertussis Vaccine	U		R
Diphtheria & Tetanus Toxoids & Pertussis Vaccine Adsorbed	U		R
Diphtheria Antitoxin	U		R
Diphtheria Toxin for Schick Test	U		R
Diphtheria Toxoid	U		R
Diphtheria Toxoid Adsorbed	U		
Dobutamine Inj.	S,M	A	
Dobutamine for Inj.	I	B	RT
Dopamine HCl Inj.	S	A	
Dopamine HCl & Dextrose Inj.	S	A,B	
Doxapram HCl Inj.	S,M	A	
Doxorubicin HCl for Inj.	I	B	(not to exceed 250 ml if multidose)
Doxorubicin HCl Inj.	S,M	A	LR,R (not to exceed 100 ml if multidose)
Doxycycline for Inj.	I	B	L
Droperidol Inj.	S,M	A	L
Dyphylline Inj.	S,M	A	RT,L
Edetate Calcium Disodium Inj.	S	A	
Edetate Disodium Inj.	S	A	
Edrophonium Chloride Inj.	S,M	A	
Electrolytes & Dextrose Inj. (Type 1), Multiple	S	A,B,P	
Electrolytes & Dextrose Inj. (Type 2), Multiple	S	A,B,P	
Electrolytes & Dextrose Inj. (Type 3), Multiple	S	A,B,P	
Electrolytes & Dextrose Inj. (Type 4), Multiple	S	A,B,P	
Electrolytes & Invert Sugar Inj. (Type 1), Multiple	S	A,B,P	
Electrolytes & Invert Sugar Inj. (Type 2), Multiple	S	A,B,P	
Electrolytes & Invert Sugar Inj. (Type 3), Multiple	S	A,B,P	

Drugs	Container	Glass Type	Storage Conditions
Electrolytes Inj. (Type 1), Multiple	S	A,B,P	
Electrolytes Inj. (Type 2), Multiple	S	A,B,P	
Elements Inj., Trace	S,M	A,B	
Emetine HCl Inj.	S	A	LR
Ephedrine Sulfate Inj.	S,M	A	LR
Epinephrine Bitartrate for Ophthalmic Solution	I		
Epinephrine Inj.	S,M	A	LR
Epinephrine Injectable Oil Susp.	S	A,C	LR
Ergonovine Maleate Inj.	S	A	LR,R
Ergotamine Tartrate Inj.	S	A	LR
Erythromycin Ethylsuccinate Inj.	S,M	A	
Erythromycin Ethylsuccinate, Sterile	I		
Erythromycin Gluceptate, Sterile	I	D	
Erythromycin Lactobionate, Sterile	I		
Erythromycin Lactobionate for Inj.	I	D	
Estradiol Cypionate Inj.	S,M	A	LR
Estradiol Injectable Suspension	S,M	A	
Estradiol Pellets	U		
Estradiol Valerate Inj.	S,M	A,C	LR
Estrone Inj.	S,M	A	
Estrone Injectable Suspension	S,M	A	
Ethacrynate Sodium for Inj.	I	D	
Ethiodized Oil Inj.	S,M		LR
Fentanyl Citrate Inj.	S	A	L
Ferrous Citrate Fe 59 Inj.	S,M		
Floxuridine for Inj.	I		L (discard after 2 wks when reconstituted)
Fludeoxyglucose F 18 Inj.	S,M		SC
Flunixin Meglumine Injection	M		RT
Fluorescein Inj.	S	A	
Fluorescein Sodium Ophth. Strips	S,SS,U		
Fluoride F 18 Inj., Sodium	S,M		SC
Fluorodopa F 18 Inj.	S,M	SC	
Fluorouracil Inj.	S	A	RT,L
Fluphenazine Decanoate Inj.	S,M	A	L
Fluphenazine Enanthate Inj.	S,M	A,C	L
Fluphenazine HCl Inj.	S,M	A	L
Folic Acid Inj.	S,M	A	
Fructose & Sodium Chloride Inj.	S	A,B	
Fructose Inj.	S	A,B	
Furosemide Inj.	S,M	A	LR
Gadopentetate Dimeglumine Inj.	S	A	LR,RT
Gallamine Triethiodide Inj.	S,M	A	L
Gallium Citrate Ga 67 Inj.	S,M		
Gelatin Film, Absorbable	U		
Gelatin Sponge, Absorbable	U		
Gentamicin Inj.	S,M	A	
Gentamicin Sulfate, Sterile	I		
Globulin, Immune	U		R
Globulin, Rho(D) Immune	U		R

Drugs	Container	Glass Type	Storage Conditions
Globulin Serum, Anti-Human	U		R
Glucagon for Inj.	I/S,M w/solvent		
Glycine Irrigation	S	A,B	
Glycopyrrolate Inj.	S,M	A	
Gold Sodium Thiomalate Inj.	S,M	A	L
Gonadotropin for Inj., Chorionic	I	D	
Guaifenesin for Inj.	S,M		RT
Haloperidol Inj.	S,M	A	L
Heparin Calcium Inj.	S,M	A	R
Heparin Lock Flush Solution	S,M	A	
Heparin Sodium Inj.	S,M	A	
Hepatitis B Immune Globulin	U		R
Hepatitis B Virus Vaccine Inactivated	U		R
Hetacillin Potassium Intramammary Infusion	Sy		
Histamine Phosphate Inj.	S,M	A	L
Histoplasmin	U		R
Hyaluronidase for Inj.	I	A,C	RT
Hyaluronidase Inj.	S,M	A	R
Hydralazine HCl Inj.	S,M	A	
Hydrocortisone Acetate Injectable Suspension	S,M	A	
Hydrocortisone Injectable Suspension	S,M	A	
Hydrocortisone Sodium Phosphate Inj.	I	C	
Hydrocortisone Sodium Succinate for Inj.	I	C	
Hydromorphone HCl Inj.	S,M	A	L
Hydroxocobalamin Inj.	S,M	A	L
Hydroxyprogesterone Caproate Inj.	S,M	A,C	
Hydroxyzine HCl Inj.	S,M		L
Hyoscyamine Sulfate Inj.	S,M	A	
Idarubicin HCl for Inj.	I		
Ifosfamide for Inj.	I		RT
Imipenem & Cilastatin Sodium for Inj.	I		RT
Imipenem & Cilastatin Sodium, Sterile	I		RT
Imipenem, Sterile	I		RT
Imipramine HCl Inj.	S	A	LR
Indigotindisulfonate Sodium Inj.	S	A	LR
Indium In 111 Chloride Solution	S		RT
Indium In 111 Pentetate Inj.	S		
Indium In 111 Satumomab Pendetide Inj.	S		SC,RT
Indocyanine Green for Inj.	I		
Indomethacin Sodium for Inj.	I		
Influenza Virus Vaccine	U		R
Insulin & Sodium Chloride Inj.	S	A,B	
Insulin Human Inj.	M		R
Insulin Inj.	M		R
Insulin Zinc Suspension	M		R
Insulin Zinc Suspension, Extended	M		R
Insulin Zinc Suspension, Prompt	M		R
Iobenguane I 123 Injection	S,M		SC,F
Iodinated I 125 Albumin Inj.	S,M		R
Iodinated I 131 Albumin Inj.	U		
Iodinated I 131 Albumin Aggreg. Inj.	S,M		R

Drugs	Container	Glass Type	Storage Conditions
Iodipamide Meglumine Inj.	S	A,C	
Iodohippurate Sodium 1123 Inj.	S,M		SC
Iodohippurate Sodium I 131 Inj.	S,M		
Iohexol Inj. (Intravascular/Intrathecal)	S	A	L
Iopamidol Inj. (Intravascular/Intrathecal)	S	A	L
Iophendylate Inj.	S	A	LR
Iothalamate Meglumine & Sodium Iothalamate Inj.	S	A	L
Iothalamate Meglumine Inj.	S	A	L
Iothalamate Sodium I-125 Inj.	S	A	L
Ioversol Inj.	S	A	L
Ioxaglate Meglumine & Ioxaglate Sodium Inj.	S	A	LR
Ioxilan Inj.	S	A	LR
Iron Dextran Inj.	S,M	A,B	
Iron Sorbitex Inj.	S	A	
Isoniazid Inj.	S,M	A	L
Isophane Insulin Suspension	M		R
Isoproterenol HCl Inj.	S	A	L
Isoxsuprine HCl Inj.	S,M	A	
Kanamycin Inj.	S,M	A,C	
Ketamine HCl Inj.	S,M	A	L,H
Ketorolac Tromethamine Inj.	S	A	LR,RT
Labetalol HCl Inj.	S,M (60 ml max)	A	R,RT,L
Leucovorin Calcium Inj.	S	A	LR
Levocamitine Inj.	S	A	CP
Levorphanol Tartrate Inj.	S,M	A	
Lidocaine & Epinephrine Inj.	S,M	A	LR
Lidocaine HCl & Dextrose Inj.	S	A,B	
Lidocaine HCl Inj.	S,M	A	
Lidocaine HCl, Sterile	I		
Lincomycin Inj.	S,M	A	
Lorazepam Inj.	S,M	A	L
Magnesium Sulfate in Dextrose Injection	S	A,G,P	
Magnesium Sulfate Inj.	S,M	A	
Manganese Chloride Inj.	S,M	A,B	
Manganese Sulfate Inj.	S,M	A,B	
Mannitol & Sodium Chloride Inj.	U	D	LR
Mannitol Inj.	S	A,B,P	
Measles & Mumps Virus Vaccine Live	S,M		LR,R
Measles & Rubella Virus Vaccine Live	S,M		LR,R
Measles, Mumps, & Rubella Virus Vaccine Live	S,M		LR,R
Measles Virus Vaccine Live	S,M		LR,R
Mechlorethamlne HCl for Inj	I	B	
Medroxyprogesterone Acetate Susp., Sterile	S,M	A	
Menadiol Sodium Diphosphate Inj.	S	A	LR
Menadione Inj.	S,M	A	
Meningococcal Polysaccharide Vaccine (Group A)	M		R
Meningococcal Polysaccharide Vaccine (Group C)	M		R
Meningococcal Polysaccharide Vaccine (Groups A and C combined)	M		R
Menotropins for Inj.	S,M	A	

Drugs	Container	Glass Type	Storage Conditions
Meperidine HCl Inj.	S,M	A	
Mephentermine Sulfate Inj.	S,M	A	
Mepivacaine HCl & Levonordefrin Inj.	S,M	A	
Mepivacaine HCl Inj.	S,M	A	
Meprobamate Inj.	S	A	
Mesoridazine Besylate Inj.	S	A	L
Metaraminol Bitartrate Inj.	S,M	A	L
Methadone HCl Inj.	S,M	A	LR
Methicillin for Inj.	I		L,RT
Methionine C II Inj.	S,M		SC
Methocarbamol Inj.	S	A	
Methohexital Sodium for Inj.	I	C	
Methotrexate for Inj.	I		L
Methotrexate Inj.	S,M	A	L
Methotrimeprazine Inj.	S,M	A	L
Methyldopate HCl Inj.	S	A	
Methylene Blue Inj.	S	A	
Methylergonovine Maleate Inj.	S	A	LR
Methylprednisolone Acetate Injectable Suspension	S,M	A	
Methylprednisolone Sodium Succinate for Inj.	I	C	
Metoclopramide Inj.	S,M	A	LR (no antioxidant)
Metocurine Iodide Inj.	S,M	A	
Metoprolol Tartrate Inj.	S	A,B	L
Metronidazole Inj.	S,P	A,B	L
Mezlocillin for Inj.	I		
Miconazole Inj.	S	A	RT
Minocycline HCl for Inj.	I		L
Mitomycin for Inj.	I	D	L
Mitoxantrone Inj.	S	A	
Morphine Sulfate Inj.	S	A	L
Morphine Sulfate Inj. (Preservative Free)	S	A	L
Morrhuate Sodium Inj.	S,M	A	
Moxalactam Disodium for Inj.	I		
Mumps Skin Test Antigen	U		R
Mumps Virus Vaccine Live	S,M		LR,R
Nafcillin Sodium for Inj.	I	D	
Nafcillin Sodium Inj.	I		F
Nafcillin Sodium, Sterile	I		
Nalorphine HCl Inj.	S,M	A	
Naloxone HCl Inj.	S,M	A	L
Nandrolone Decanoate Inj.	S,M	A	L
Nandrolone Phenpropionate Inj.	S,M	A	L
Neomycin & Polymyxin B Sulfates Soln. for Irrigation	U		
Neomycin for Inj.	I		I
Neostigmine Methylsulfate Inj.	S,M		L
Netilmicin Sulfate Inj.	S,M	A	
Niacin Inj.	S,M	A	
Niacinamide Inj.	S,M	A	
Nitroglycerin Inj.	S,M	A,B	
Norepinephrine Bitartrate Inj.	S	A	LR

Drugs	Container	Glass Type	Storage Conditions
Novobiocin Sod. Intramammary Infusion	Sy		WC
Orphenadrine Citrate Inj.	S,M	A	L
Oxacillin for Inj.	I		RT
Oxacillin Inj.	I		F
Oxymorphone HCl Inj.	S,M	A	L
Oxytetracycline for Inj.	I		L
Oxytetracycline HCl	I		L
Oxytetracycline Inj.	S,M		L
Oxytocin Inj.	S,M	A	(do not freeze)
Papaverine HCl Inj.	S,M	A	
Penicillin G Benzathine	I		
Penicillin G Benzathine & Penicillin G Procaine Injectable Susp.	S,M	A,C	
Penicillin G Benzathine Injectable Susp.	S,M	A,B	R
Penicillin G Potassium for Inj.	S	D	F
Penicillin G Procaine	I		
Penicillin G Procaine & Dihydrostreptomycin Sulfate Injectable Suspension	S,M (tight)		
Penicillin G Procaine, Dihydrostreptomycin Sulfate, and Prednisolone Injectable Suspension	S,M (tight)		
Penicillin G Procaine, Dihydrostreptomycin Sulfate, Chlorpheniramine Maleate, & Dexamethasone Injectable Suspension	S,M (tight)		R
Penicillin G Procaine Dihydrostreptomycin Sulfate Intramammary Infusion	Sy (well closed)		
Penicillin G Procaine for Injectable Susp.	S,M	A,C	
Penicillin G Procaine Injectable Susp.	S,M	A,C	R
Penicillin G Procaine Intramammary Infusion	Sy (well closed)		
Penicillin G Procaine w/Aluminum Stearate Injectable Oil Suspension	S,M	A,C	
Penicillin G Sodium for Inj.	I		
Pentazocine Lactate Inj.	S,M	A	
Pentobarbital Sodium Inj.	S,M	A	
Perphenazine Inj.	S,M	A	L
Pertussis Immune Globulin	U		R
Pertussis Vaccine	U		R
Pertussis Vaccine Adsorbed	U		R
Phenobarbital Sodium Inj.	I	D	
Phenobarbital Sodium, Sterile	I	D	
Phentolamine Mesylate for Inj.	I	B	
Phenylbutazone Injection	S,M (vet. use)	A	L,R
Phenylephrine HCl Inj.	S,M	A	L
Phenytoin Sodium Inj.	S,M	A	RT
Phosphate P 32 Soln., Sodium	S,M		
Phosphate P 32 Susp., Chromic	S,M	Tr	
Physostigmine Salicylate Inj.	S	A	L
Phytonadione Inj.	S,M	A	L
Pilocarpine Ocular System	S		R
Piperacillin for Inj.	I		
Pituitary Inj., Posterior	S,M	A	
Plague Vaccine	U		R

Drugs	Container	Glass Type	Storage Conditions
Plasma Protein Fraction	U		(as labeled)
Platelet Concentrate	U	A,B	(as labeled)
Plicamycin for Inj.	I	D	L
Poliovirus Vaccine Inactivated	U		R
Poliovirus Vaccine Live Oral	S,M		F,R
Polymyxin B for Inj.	I		L
Potassium Acetate Inj.	S,M	A,B	
Potassium Chloride for Inj. Conc.	S,M	A,B	
Potassium Chloride in Dextrose & Sodium Chloride Inj.	S	A,B,P	
Potassium Chloride in Dextrose Inj.	S	A,B,P	
Potassium Chloride in Lactated Ringer's & Dextrose Inj.	S	A,B,P	
Potassium Chloride in Sodium Chloride Inj.	S	A,B,P	
Potassium Phosphates Inj.	S	A	
Pralidoxime Chloride, Sterile	I	B	
Prednisolone Acetate Injectable Susp.	S,M	A	
Prednisolone Sodium Phosphate Inj.	S,M	A	L
Prednisolone Sodium Succinate for Inj.	I	D	
Prednisolone Tebutate Injectable Susp.	S,M	A	
Prilocaine & Epinephrine Inj.	S,M	A	L
Prilocaine HCl Inj.	S,M	A	
Procainamide HCl Inj.	S,M	A	
Procaine HCl & Epinephrine Inj.	S,M	A,B	LR
Procaine HCl Inj.	S,M	A,B	
Procaine HCl, Sterile	I	D	
Procaine & Phenylephrine HCl Inj.	S,M	A	
Procaine & Tetracycline Hydrochlorides & Levonordefrin Inj.	S,M	A	
Prochlorperazine Edisylate Inj.	S,M	A	L
Progesterone Inj.	S,M	A,C	
Progesterone Injectable Susp.	S,M	A	
Progesterone Intrauterine Contraceptive Sys.	S		
Promazine HCl Inj.	S,M	A	L
Promethazine HCl Inj.	S,M	A	L
Propantheline Bromide, Sterile	S	D	
Propoxycaine & Procaine Hydrochlorides & Levonordefrin Inj.	S	A	
Propoxycaine & Procaine Hydrochlorides & Norepinephrine Bitartrate Inj.	S,M	A	
Propranolol HCl Inj.	S	A	LR
Propyliodone Injectable Oil Susp.	S		LR
Protamine Sulfate for Inj.	I	D	
Protamine Sulfate Inj.	S	A	R
Protein Hydrolysate Inj.	S	A,B	H
Pyridostigmine Bromide Inj.	S	A	L
Pyridoxine HCl Inj	S,M	A	L
Quinidine Gluconate Inj.	S,M	A	
Rabies Immune Globulin	U		R
Rabies Vaccine	U		R
Raclopeide C II Inj.	S,M		SC
Ranitidine in Sodium Chloride Inj.	N	A,B	LR,R/RT

Drugs	Container	Glass Type	Storage Conditions
Ranitidine Inj.	S,M	I	LR,RT
Reserpine Inj.	S	A	LR
Riboflavin Inj.	S,M	A	LR
Rifampin for Inj.	I		
Ringer's & Dextrose Inj.	S	A,B,P	
Ringer's & Dextrose Inj., Lactated	S	A,B,P	
Ringer's & Dextrose Inj., Half-Strength Lactated	S	A,B,P	
Ringer's & Dextrose Inj., Modified Lactated	S	A,B,P	
Ringer's Inj.	S	A,B,P	
Ringer's Inj., Lactated	S	A,B,P	
Ringer's Irrigation	S,SS	A,B,P	
Ritodrine HCl Inj.	S	A	RT
Rose Bengal Sodium I 131 Inj.	S,M		
Rubella & Mumps Virus Vaccine Live	S,M		LR,R
Rubella Virus Vaccine Live	S,M		LR,R
Rubidium Chloride Rb 82 Inj.			NA
Sargramostim for Inj.	He		R
Schick Test Control			R
Scopolamine Hydrobromide Inj.	S,M	A	LR
Secobarbital Sodium Inj.	S,M	A	L,R
Secobarbital Sodium, Sterile	I	D	
Selenious Acid Inj.	S,M	A,B	
Sisomicin Sulfate Inj.	S,M	A	
Smallpox Vaccine	U		R
Sodium Acetate C II Inj.	S,M		SC
Sodium Acetate Inj.	S	A	
Sodium Bicarbonate Inj.	S	A	
Sodium Chloride Inhalation Soln.	S		
Sodium Chloride Inj.	S	A,B	
Sodium Chloride Inj., Bacteriostatic	S,M	A,B	
Sodium Chloride Irrigation	S,SS	A,B,P	
Sodium Lactate Inj.	S	A,B	
Sodium Nitrite Inj.	S	A	
Sodium Nitroprusside, Sterile	I	D	L
Sodium Pertechnetate Tc 99m Inj.	S,M		R
Sodium Phosphates Inj.	S,M	A	
Sodium Sulfate Inj.	S	A	
Sodium Thiosulfate Inj.	S	A	
Spectinomycin for Injectable Susp.	I		
Spectinomycin HCl, Sterile	I		
Streptomycin Sulfate Inj.	S,M	A	
Streptomycin Sulfate, Sterile	I	D	
Succinylcholine Chloride for Inj.	I	A	
Succinylcholine Chloride Inj.	S,M	A,B	R
Sufentanil Citrate Inj.	S,M	A	
Sugar Inj., Invert	S,P	A,B	
Sulfadiazine Sodium Inj.	S	A	LR
Sulfamethoxazole & Trimethoprim Inj.	S,M (50 mL)	A	L
Sulfisoxazole Diolamine Inj.	S,M	A	L
Technetium Tc 99m Albumin Aggregated Inj.	S,M		R
Technetium Tc 99m Albumin Colloid Inj.	S,M		R

Drugs	Container	Glass Type	Storage Conditions
Technetium Tc 99m Albumin Inj.	S,M		R
Technetium Tc 99m Bicisate Inj.	S,M		RT
Technetium Tc 99m Disofenin Inj.	S,M		In
Technetium Tc 99m Etidronate Inj.	S,M		
Technetium Tc 99m Exametazine Inj.	S,M		RT
Technetium Tc 99m Gluceptate Inj.	S,M		R
Technetium Tc 99m Lidofenin Inj.	S,M		R
Technetium Tc 99m Mebrofenin Inj.	S,M		RT
Technetium Tc 99m Medronate Inj.	S,M		
Technetium Tc 99m Oxidronate Inj.	S,M		
Technetium Tc 99m Pentetate Inj.	S,M		R
Technetium Tc 99m (Pyro- & Trimeta-) Phosphates Inj.	U		D
Technetium Tc 99m Pyrophos. Inj.	S,M		R
Technetium Tc 99m Succimer Inj.	S		RT,L
Technetium Tc 99m Sulfur Colloid Inj.	S,M		
Terbutaline Sulfate Inj.	S	A	L,RT
Testosterone Cypionate Inj.	S,M	A	L
Testosterone Enanthate Inj.	S,M	A	
Testosterone Injectable Susp.	S,M	A	
Testosterone Propionate Inj.	S,M	A	
Tetanus & Diphtheria Toxoids Adsorbed (for adult use)	U		R
Tetanus Antitoxin	U		R
Tetanus Immune Globulin	U		R
Tetanus Toxoid	U		R
Tetanus Toxoid Adsorbed	U		R
Tetracaine HCl in Dextrose Inj.	S,M (up to 100 ml)	A	R,L,RT (tray for 12 months)
Tetracaine HCl for Inj.	S,M	A	R,L
Tetracycline HCl for Inj.	I	B	L
Tetracycline HCl, Sterile	I		L
Tetracycline Phosphate Complex for Inj.	I	B	L
Tetracycline Phosphate Complex, Sterile	I		L
Thallous Chloride Tl 201 Inj.	S,M		
Theophylline in Dextrose Inj.	S	A,B,P	
Thiamine HCl Inj.	S,M	A	L
Thiamylal Sodium for Inj.	I	C	
Thiethylperazine Maleate Inj.	S	A	L
Thiopental Sodium for Inj.	I	C	
Thiotepa for Inj.	I	D	R,L
Thiothixene HCl for Inj.	I		LR
Thiothixene HCl Inj.	S	A	L
Thrombin			R
Ticarcillin Disodium & Clavulanate Potassium Inj.	I		F
Ticarcillin Disodium & Clavulanate Potassium, Sterile	I		
Ticarcillin Disodium, Sterile	I	D	
Tiletamine & Zolazepam for Inj.	I		
Tilmicosin Injection	I		
Tobramycin Sulfate Inj.	S,M	A,P	

Drugs	Container	Glass Type	Storage Conditions
Tobramycin Sulfate, Sterile	I		RT (below 30°C)
Tolbutamide Sodium for Inj.	I		
Triamcinolone Acetonide Injectable Susp.	S,M	A	L
Triamcinolone Diacetate Injectable Susp.	S,M	A	
Triamcinolone Hexacetonide Injectable Susp.	S,M	A	
Trifluoperazine HCl Inj.	M	A	L
Triflupromazine HCl Inj.	S,M	A	L
Trimethaphan Camsylate Inj.	S,M	A	R
Trimethobenzamide HCl Inj.	S,M	A	
Tromethamine for Inj.	S,M	A	C
Trypsin for Inhalation Aerosol, Crystallized	S	A	RT
Tuberculin			R
Tubocurarine Chloride	S,M		
Typhoid Vaccine	U		R
Urea for Inj.	I	D	
Vaccinia Immune Globulin	U		R
Vancomycin HCl for Inj.	I		
Varicella-Zoster Immune Globulin	U		R
Vasopressin Inj.	S,M	A	
Verapamil HCl Inj.	S	A	LR
Vidarabine Concentrate for Inj.	S,M	A	
Vinblastine Sulfate for Inj.	I	D	R
Vincristine Sulfate for Inj.	U		L,R
Vincristine Sulfate Inj.	U	U	L,R
Warfarin Sodium for Inj.	I	D	LR
Water 0-15 Inj.	S		SC
Water for Inhalation, Sterile	S		
Water for Inj.	SP		
Water for Inj., Bacteriostatic	S,M, CV	A,B,P	
Water for Inj., Sterile	S	A,B,P	SS
Water for Irrigation, Sterile	S	A,B	
Water, Sterile Purified	WC	U	
Xenon Xe 127	S (leakproof stoppers)		RT,SC
Xenon Xe 133	S (leakproof stoppers)		RT,SC
Xenon X3 133 Inj.	S (totally filled)		RT,SC
Yellow Fever Vaccine	U (nitrogen filled ampules)		R
Zidovudine Inj.	Ti		LR
Zinc Chloride Inj.	S,M	A,B	
Zinc Sulfate Inj.	S,M		

Provided by Dr. Kenneth S. Alexander, Professor of Pharmacy, College of Pharmacy, University of Toledo.

Oral Dosage Forms That Should Not Be Crushed or Chewed

This listing is included to alert the health care practitioner about oral dosage forms that should not be crushed or chewed and to serve as an aid in consulting with patients. Refer to the end of the table for a complete explanation of all alphabetical references.

Drug Product	Manufacturer	Dosage Form	Reason/Comments
Accutane	Roche	Capsule	Mucous membrane irritant
Actifed 12 Hour	Warner Lambert Consumer Health Products	Capsule	Slow release (i)
Acutrim	Novartis Consumer Health	Tablet	Slow release
Adalat CC	Bayer	Tablet	Slow release
Aerolate SR, JR, III	Fleming & Co.	Capsule	Slow release*(i)
Afrinol Repetabs	Schering-Plough	Tablet	Slow release
Allegra D	Hoechst Marion Roussel	Tablet	Slow release
Allerest 12 Hour	Novartis Consumer Health	Caplet	Slow release
Ammonium Chloride	(Various Mfr.)	Tablet	Enteric-coated extended release
Artane Sequels	Lederle	Capsule	Slow release*(i)
Arthritis Bayer TR	Bayer	Capsule	Slow release
Arthrotec	Searle	Tablet	Enteric-coated
ASA Enseals	Lilly	Tablet	Enteric-coated
Asacol Delayed Release	Procter & Gamble	Tablet	Slow release
Asbron G Inlay	Sandoz	Tablet	Multiple compressed tablet (i)
Ascriptin Enteric	Novartis	Tablet	Enteric-coated
Atrohist LA	Adams	Tablet	Slow release
Atrohist Plus	Adams	Tablet	Slow release
Atrohist Sprinkle	Adams	Capsule	Slow release*
Azulfidine Entabs	Pharmacia & Upjohn	Tablet	Enteric-coated
Baros	Lafayette	Tablet	Effervescent tab (d)
Bayer Extra Strength Enteric 500	Sterling Health	Tablet	Slow release
Bayer Low Adult 81 mg Strength	Sterling Health	Tablet	Enteric-coated
Bayer Regular Strength 325 mg Caplets	Sterling Health	Tablet	Enteric-coated
Bayer Regular Strength EC Caplets	Sterling Health	Caplet	Enteric-coated
Betachron E-R	Inwood	Capsule	Slow release
Betapen-VK	Bristol	Tablet	Taste (c)
Biohist-LA	Wakefield	Tablet	Slow release (h)
Bisacodyl	(Various Mfr.)	Tablet	Enteric-coated (a)
Bisco-Lax	Raway	Tablet	Enteric-coated (a)
Bontril-SR	Carnrick	Capsule	Slow release
Breonesin	Sanofi Winthrop	Capsule	Liquid filled (b)
Brexin LA	Savage	Capsule	Slow release (i)
Bromfed	Muro	Capsule	Slow release (i)
Bromfed-PD	Muro	Capsule	Slow release (i)

Drug Product	Manufacturer	Dosage Form	Reason/Comments
Calan SR	Searle	Tablet	Slow release (h)
Cama Arthritis Pain Reliever	Sandoz Consumer	Tablet	Multiple compressed tablet
Carbatrol	Shire Richwood	Capsule	Slow-release*
Carbiset-TR	Nutripharm	Tablet	Slow release
Cardizem	Hoechst Marion Roussel	Tablet	Slow release
Cardizem CD	Hoechst Marion Roussel	Capsule	Slow release*
Cardizem SR	Hoechst Marion Roussel	Capsule	Slow release*
Carter's Little Pills	Carter-Wallace	Tablet	Enteric-coated
Ceclor CD	Dura	Tablet	Slow release
Cefol Filmtab	Abbott	Tablet	Enteric-coated
Ceftin	GlaxoWellcome	Tablet	Taste (c) Use suspension for children
CellCept	Roche	Capsule, Tablet	Teratogenic potential
Charcoal Plus	Kramer	Tablet	Enteric-coated
Chloral Hydrate	(Various Mfr.)	Capsule	Liquid in capsule (i)
Chlorpheniramine Maleate Time Release	(Various Mfr.)	Capsule	Slow release
Chlor-Trimeton Repetab	Schering-Plough	Tablet	Slow release (i)
Choledyl SA	Parke-Davis	Tablet	Slow release (i)
Cipro	Bayer	Tablet	Taste (c)
Claritin-D	Schering-Plough	Tablet	Slow release
Codimal LA	Schwarz Pharma	Capsule	Slow release
Codimal LA Half	Schwarz Pharma	Capsule	Slow release
Colace	Roberts	Capsule	Taste (c)
Comhist LA	Roberts	Capsule	Slow release*
Compazine Spansule	SmithKline Beecham	Capsule	Slow release (i)
Congess SR, JR	Fleming & Co.	Capsule	Slow release
Contac	SmithKline Beecham	Capsule	Slow release*
Cotazym-S	Organon	Capsule	Enteric-coated*
Covera-HS	Searle	Tablet	Slow release
Creon 10, 20	Solvay	Capsule	Enteric-coated*
Cystospaz-M	PolyMedica	Capsule	Slow release
Cytoxan	Bristol-Myers	Tablet	May be crushed but maker recommends injection.
Cytorene	Roche	Capsule	Skin irritant
D.A. II	Dura	Tablet	Slow release
Dallergy	Laser	Capsule	Slow release
Dallergy-D	Laser	Capsule	Slow release
Dallergy-JR	Laser	Capsule	Slow release
Deconamine SR	Kenwood	Capsule	Slow release (i)
Deconsal II	Adams	Tablet	Slow release
Deconsal Sprinkle	Adams	Capsule	Slow release*
Defen-LA	Horizon	Tablet	Slow release (h)
Demazin Repetabs	Schering-Plough	Tablet	Slow release (i)
Depakene	Abbott	Capsule	Slow release, mucous membrane irritant (i)

Drug Product	Manufacturer	Dosage Form	Reason/Comments
Depakote	Abbott	Capsule	Enteric-coated
Desoxyn Gradumets	Abbott	Tablet	Slow release
Desyrel	Apothecon	Tablet	Taste (c)
Dexatrim, Max. Strength	Thompson Medical	Tablet	Slow release
Dexedrine Spansule	SmithKline Beecham	Capsule	Slow release
Diamox Sequels	Lederle	Capsule	Slow release
Dilacor XR	Watson	Capsule	Slow release
Dilatrate SR	Schwarz Pharma	Capsule	Slow release
Dimetane Extentab	Robins	Tablet	Slow release (i)
Dimetapp Extentab	Robins	Tablet	Slow release
Disobrom	Geneva Pharm.	Tablet	Slow release
Disophrol Chronotab	Schering-Plough	Tablet	Slow release
Dital	UAD	Capsule	Slow release
Dolobid	Merck	Tablet	Irritant
Donnatal Extentab	Robins	Tablet	Slow release (i)
Donnazyme	Robins	Tablet	Enteric-coated
Drisdol	Sanofi Winthrop	Capsule	Liquid filled (b)
Drixoral	Schering-Plough	Tablet	Slow release (i)
Drixoral Plus	Schering-Plough	Tablet	Slow release
Drixoral Sinus	Schering-Plough	Tablet	Slow release
Dulcolax	Boehringer Ingelheim	Tablet	Enteric-coated (a)
Duratuss	UCB Pharma	Tablet	Slow release (h)
Dura-vent	Dura	Tablet	Slow release (h)
Dynabac	Sanofi Winthrop	Tablet	Enteric-coated
DynaCirc CR	Novartis	Tablet	Slow release
Easprin	Parke-Davis	Tablet	Enteric-coated
EC-Naprosyn	Roche	Tablet	Enteric-coated
Ecotrin	SmithKline Beecham	Tablet	Enteric-coated
E.E.S. 400	(Various Mfr.)	Tablet	Enteric-coated (i)
Efidac 24	Hogil Pharmaceutical	Tablet	Slow release
Efidac 24 Chlorpheniramine	Hogil Pharmaceutical	Tablet	Slow release
Effexor XR	Wyeth-Ayerst	Capsule	Slow release
Elixophyllin SR	Forest	Capsule	Slow release*(i)
E-Mycin	Knoll Pharm.	Tablet	Enteric-coated
Endafed	UAD	Capsule	Slow release
Entex LA	Dura	Tablet	Slow release (i)
Entex PSE	Dura	Tablet	Slow release
Entozyme	Robins	Tablet	Enteric-coated
Equanil	Wyeth-Ayerst	Tablet	Taste (c)
Ergomar	Lotus	Tablet	Sublingual form (g)
Eryc	Parke-Davis	Capsule	Enteric-coated*
Ery-Tab	Abbott	Tablet	Enteric-coated
Erythrocin Stearate	Abbott	Tablet	Enteric-coated
Erythromycin Base	(Various Mfr.)	Tablet	Enteric-coated
Eskalith CR	SmithKline Beecham	Tablet	Slow release
Exgest LA	Carnrick	Tablet	Slow release
Extendryl JR	Fleming	Capsule	Slow release
Extendryl SR	Fleming	Capsule	Slow release

Drug Product	Manufacturer	Dosage Form	Reason/Comments
Fedahist Timecaps	Schwarz Pharma	Capsule	Slow release (i)
Feldene	Pfizer	Capsule	Mucous membrane irritant
Feocyte	Dunhall	Tablet	Slow release
Feosol	SmithKline Beecham	Tablet	Enteric-coated (i)
Feosol Spansule	SmithKline Beecham	Capsule	Slow release*(i)
Feratab	Upsher-Smith	Tablet	Enteric-coated (i)
Fergon	Sanofi Winthrop	Capsule	Slow release*
Fero-Grad-500	Abbott	Tablet	Slow release
Fero-Gradumet	Abbott	Tablet	Slow release
Ferralet SR	Mission	Tablet	Slow release
Festal 11	Hoechst Marion Roussel	Tablet	Enteric-coated
Flomax	Boehringer Ingelheim	Capsule	Slow release
Fumatinic	Laser	Capsule	Slow release
Gastrocrom	Medeva	Capsule	Dissolve in water (j)
Geocillin	Roerig	Tablet	Taste
Glucotrol XL	Pratt	Tablet	Slow release
Gris-PEG	Allergan	Tablet	Crushing may precipitate (k)
Guaifed	Muro	Capsule	Slow release
Guaifed-PD	Muro	Capsule	Slow release
Guaifenex LA	Ethex	Tablet	Slow release (h)
Guaifenex PSE 120	Ethex	Tablet	Slow release (h)
Guaimax-D	Schwarz Pharma	Tablet	Slow release
Humibid DM	Adams	Tablet	Slow release
Humibid DM Sprinkle	Adams	Capsule	Slow release*
Humibid LA	Adams	Tablet	Slow release
Humibid Sprinkle	Adams	Capsule	Slow release*
Hydergine LC	Sandoz	Capsule	Liquid in capsule (i)
Hydergine Sublingual	Sandoz	Tablet	Sublingual route (i)
Hytakerol	Sanofi Winthrop	Capsule	Liquid filled (b)(i)
Iberet	Abbott	Tablet	Slow release (i)
Iberet 500	Abbott	Tablet	Slow release (i)
ICaps Plus	LaHaye Labs	Tablet	Slow release
ICaps Time Release	LaHaye Labs	Tablet	Slow release
Ilotycin	Dista	Tablet	Enteric-coated
Imdur	Key	Tablet	Slow release (h)
Inderal LA	Wyeth-Ayerst	Capsule	Slow release
Inderide LA	Wyeth-Ayerst	Capsule	Slow release
Indocin SR	Merck	Capsule	Slow release*(i)
Ionamin	Medeva	Capsule	Slow release
Isoclor Timesule	Medeva	Capsule	Slow release (i)
Isoptin SR	Knoll Pharm.	Tablet	Slow release
Isordil Sublingual	Wyeth-Ayerst	Tablet	Sublingual form (g)
Isordil Tembid	Wyeth-Ayerst	Tablet	Slow release
Isosorbide Dinitrate SR	(Various Mfr.)	Tablet	Slow release
Isosorbide Dinitrate Sublingual	(Various Mfr.)	Tablet	Sublingual form (g)
Isuprel Glossets	Sanofi Winthrop	Tablet	Sublingual form (g)

Drug Product	Manufacturer	Dosage Form	Reason/Comments
K + Care E+	Alra	Tablet	Effervescent tablet (d)(i)
K + 8	Alra	Tablet	Slow release (i)
K + 10	Alra	Tablet	Slow release (i)
Kadian	Faulding	Capsule	Slow release*
Kaon Cl-10	Savage	Tablet	Slow release (i)
K-Dur	Key	Tablet	Slow release
K-Lease	Adria	Capsule	Slow release*(i)
Klor-Con	Upsher-Smith	Tablet	Slow release (i)
Klor-Con/EF	Upsher-Smith	Tablet	Effervescent tablet (d)(i)
Klorvess	Sandoz	Tablet	Effervescent tablet (d)(i)
Klotrix	Mead Johnson	Tablet	Slow release (i)
K-Lyte	Apothecon	Tablet	Effervescent tablet (d)
K-Lyte/Cl 50	Apothecon	Tablet	Effervescent tablet (d)
K-Lyte DS	Apothecon	Tablet	Effervescent tablet (d)
K-Tab	Abbott	Tablet	Slow release (i)
Levbid	Schwarz Pharma	Tablet	Slow release (g)
Levsinex Timecaps	Schwarz Pharma	Capsule	Slow release
Lexxel	Astra Merck	Tablet	Slow release
Lithobid	Solvay	Tablet	Slow release (i)
Lodrane LD	ECR Pharmaceutical	Capsule	Slow release*
Mag-Tab SR	Niche	Tablet	Slow release
Meprospan	Wallace	Capsule	Slow release*
Mestinon Timespan	ICN	Tablet	Slow release (i)
Mi-Cebrin	Dista	Tablet	Enteric-coated
Mi-Cebrin T	Dista	Tablet	Enteric-coated
Micro K	Robins	Capsule	Slow release*(i)
Monafed	Monarch	Tablet	Slow release
Monafed DM	Monarch	Tablet	Slow release
Motrin	Pharmacia & Upjohn	Tablet	Taste (c)
MS Contin	Purdue Frederick	Tablet	Slow release (i)
MSC Triaminic	Sandoz	Tablet	Enteric-coated
Muco-Fen-LA	Wakefield	Tablet	Slow release (h)
Naldecon	Bristol	Tablet	Slow release (i)
Naprelan	Wyeth-Ayerst	Tablet	Slow release
Nasatab LA	ECR Pharmaceutical	Tablet	Slow release (h)
Niaspan	KOS	Tablet	Slow release
Nico-400	Jones Medical	Capsule	Slow release
Nicobid	Rhone-Poulenc Rorer	Capsule	Slow release
Nitro Bid	Hoechst Marion Roussel	Capsule	Slow release*
Nitrocine Timecaps	Schwarz Pharma	Capsule	Slow release
Nitroglyn	Kenwood	Capsule	Slow release*
Nitrong	Rhone-Poulenc Rorer	Tablet	Sublingual route (g)
Nitrostat	Parke-Davis	Tablet	Sublingual route (g)
Nitro-Time	Time-Cap Labs	Capsule	Slow release
Noctec	Apothecon	Capsule	Liquid in capsule (i)
Nolamine	Carnrick	Tablet	Slow release
Nolex LA	Carnrick	Tablet	Slow release

Drug Product	Manufacturer	Dosage Form	Reason/Comments
Norflex	3M Pharmaceuticals	Tablet	Slow release
Norpace CR	Searle	Capsule	Slow release
Novafed A	Hoechst Marion Roussel	Capsule	Slow release
Ondrox	Unimed	Tablet	Slow release
Optilets-500 Filmtab	Abbott	Tablet	Enteric-coated
Optilets-M-500 Filmtab	Abbott	Tablet	Enteric-coated
Oragrafin	Bracco Diagnostics	Capsule	Liquid in capsule
Oramorph SR	Roxane	Tablet	Slow release (i)
Ornade Spansule	SmithKline Beecham	Capsule	Slow release
Oxycontin	Purdue Pharma	Tablet	Slow release
Pabalate	Robins	Tablet	Enteric-coated
Pabalate SF	Robins	Tablet	Enteric-coated
Pancrease	Ortho McNeil	Capsule	Enteric-coated*
Pancrease MT	Ortho McNeil	Capsule	Enteric-coated*
Panmycin	Pharmacia & Upjohn	Capsule	Taste
Papaverine Sustained Action	(Various Mfr.)	Capsule	Slow release
Pathilon Sequeles	Lederle	Capsule	Slow release*
Pavabid Plateau	Hoechst Marion Roussel	Capsule	Slow release*
PBZ-SR	Novartis Pharm	Tablet	Slow release (i)
Pentasa	Hoechst Marion Roussel	Tablet	Slow release
Perdiem	Rhone-Poulenc Rorer	Granules	Wax coated
Peritrate SA	Parke-Davis	Tablet	Slow release (h)
Permitil Chronotab	Schering	Tablet	Slow release (i)
Phenergan	Wyeth-Ayerst	Tablet	Taste (c)(i)
Phyllocontin	Purdue Frederick	Tablet	Slow release
Plendil	Astra Merck	Tablet	Slow release
Pneumomist	ECR Pharmaceutical	Tablet	Slow release (h)
Polaramine Repetabs	Schering-Plough	Tablet	Slow release (i)
Posicor	Roche	Tablet	Mucous membrane irritant
Prelu-2	Boehringer Ingelheim	Capsule	Slow release
Prevacid	TAP Pharmaceutical	Capsule	Slow release
Prilosec	Astra Merck	Capsule	Slow release
Pro-Banthine	Roberts	Tablet	Taste
Procainamide HCL SR	(Various Mfr.)	Tablet	Slow release
Procanbid	Parke-Davis	Tablet	Slow release
Procan SR	Parke-Davis	Tablet	Slow release
Procardia	Pfizer	Capsule	Delays absorption (b)(e)
Procardia XL	Pfizer	Tablet	Slow release, AUC is unaffected
Profen II	Wakefield	Tablet	Slow release (h)
Profen-LA	Wakefield	Tablet	Slow release (h)
Pronestyl SR	Apothecon	Tablet	Slow release
Propecia	Merck	Tablet	Pregnant women should exercise caution (l)
Proscar	Merck	Tablet	Pregnant women should exercise caution (l)

Drug Product	Manufacturer	Dosage Form	Reason/Comments
Proventil Repetabs	Schering-Plough	Tablet	Slow release (i)
Prozac	Dista	Capsule	Slow release*
Quadra Hist	Schein	Tablet	Slow release
Quibron-T/SR	Bristol-Myers Squibb	Tablet	Slow release (i)
Quinaglute DuraTabs	Berlex	Tablet	Slow release
Quinalan Lanatabs	Lannett	Tablet	Slow release
Quinalan SR	Lannett	Tablet	Slow release
Quinidex Extentabs	Robins	Tablet	Slow release
Quin-Release	Major	Tablet	Slow release
Respa-1st	Respa	Tablet	Slow release (h)
Respa-DM	Respa	Tablet	Slow release (h)
Respa-GF	Respa	Tablet	Slow release (h)
Respahist	Respa	Capsule	Slow release*
Respaire SR	Laser	Capsule	Slow release
Respbid	Boehringer Ingelheim	Tablet	Slow release
Ritalin-SR	Novartis	Tablet	Slow release
Robimycin Robitab	Robins	Tablet	Enteric-coated
Rondec TR	Dura	Tablet	Slow release (i)
Roxanol SR	Roxane	Tablet	Slow release (i)
Sinemet CR	DuPont Pharm	Tablet	Slow release (h)
Singlet	SmithKline Beecham	Tablet	Slow release
Slo-Bid Gyrocaps	Rhone-Poulenc Rorer	Capsule	Slow release*
Slo-Niacin	Upsher-Smith	Tablet	Slow release (h)
Slo-Phyllin GG	Rhone-Poulenc Rorer	Capsule	Slow release (i)
Slo-Phyllin Gyrocaps	Rhone-Poulenc Rorer	Capsule	Slow release*(i)
Slow FE	Novartis Consumer Health	Tablet	Slow release (i)
Slow FE with Folic Acid	Novartis Consumer Health	Tablet	Slow release
Slow-K	Summit	Tablet	Slow release (i)
Slow-Mag	Searle	Tablet	Slow release
Sorbitrate SA	Zeneca	Tablet	Slow release
Sorbitrate Sublingual	Zeneca	Tablet	Sublingual route
Sparine	Wyeth-Ayerst	Tablet	Taste (c)
S-P-T	Fleming	Capsule	Liquid gelatin thyroid suspension
Sudafed 12 hour Caplets	Warner Lambert Consumer Health Products	Tablet	Slow release (i)
Sudal 60/500	Atley	Tablet	Slow release
Sudal 120/600	Atley	Tablet	Slow release
Sudex	Atley	Tablet	Slow release (h)
Sular	Zeneca	Tablet	Slow release
Sustaire	Pfizer	Tablet	Slow release (i)
Syn-RX	Adams Lab	Tablet	Slow release
Syn-Rx DM	Adams Lab	Tablet	Slow release
Tavist-D	Novartis Consumer Health	Tablet	Multiple compressed tablet
Teczam	Hoechst Marion Roussel	Tablet	Slow release

Drug Product	Manufacturer	Dosage Form	Reason/Comments
Tedral SA	Parke-Davis	Tablet	Slow release
Tegretol-XR	Novartis	Tablet	Slow release
Teldrin	SmithKline Beecham	Capsule	Slow release*
Tepanil Ten-Tab	3M Pharmaceuticals	Tablet	Slow release
Tessalon Perles	Forest	Capsule	Slow release
Theo-24	UCB Pharma	Tablet	Slow release (i)
Theochron	Forest	Tablet	Slow release
Theo-Dur	Key	Tablet	Slow release (i)
Theo-Dur Sprinkle	Key	Capsule	Slow release*(i)
Theolair SR	3M Pharmaceuticals	Tablet	Slow release (i)
Theo-Sav	Savage	Tablet	Slow release (h)
Theo-Time SR	Major	Tablet	Slow release
Theovent	Schering-Plough	Capsule	Slow release (i)
Theo-X	Carnrick	Tablet	Slow release
Therapy Bayer	Glenbrook	Caplet	Enteric-coated
Thorazine Spansule	SmithKline Beecham	Capsule	Slow release
Toprol XL	Astra	Tablet	Slow release (h)
Touro A & H	Dartmouth	Capsule	Slow release
Touro DM	Dartmouth	Tablet	Slow release
Touro EX	Dartmouth	Tablet	Slow release
Touro LA	Dartmouth	Tablet	Slow release
T-Phyl	Purdue Frederick	Tablet	Slow release
Trental	Hoechst Marion Roussel	Tablet	Slow release
Triaminic	Sandoz	Tablet	Enteric-coated (i)
Triaminic-12	Sandoz	Tablet	Slow release (i)
Triaminic TR	Sandoz	Tablet	Multiple compressed tablet (i)
Trilafon Repetabs	Schering-Plough	Tablet	Slow release (i)
Tri-Phen-Chlor Time Release	Rugby	Tablet	Slow release
Tri-Phen-Mine SR	Goldline	Tablet	Slow release
Triptone Caplets	Del Pharm	Tablet	Slow release
Trovan	Pfizer	Tablet	Slow release
Tuss-LA	Hyrex	Tablet	Slow release
Tuss Ornade Spansule	SmithKline Beecham	Capsule	Slow release
Tylenol Extended Relief	McNeil Consumer Products	Capsule	Slow release
ULR-LA	Geneva Pharmaceutical	Tablet	Slow release
Ultrase	Scandipharm	Capsule	Enteric-coated*
Ultrase MT	Scandipharm	Capsule	Enteric-coated*
Uni-Dur	Key	Tablet	Slow release
Uniphyl	Purdue Frederick	Tablet	Slow release
Urocit-K	Mission	Tablet	Wax-coated
Valrelease	Roche	Capsule	Slow release
Verelan PM	Schwarz Pharma	Capsule	Slow release*
Volmax	Muro	Tablet	Slow release
Wellbutrin	GlaxoWellcome	Tablet	Anesthetize mucous membrane

Drug Product	Manufacturer	Dosage Form	Reason/Comments
Wyamycin S	Wyeth Ayerst	Tablet	Slow release
Wygesic	Wyeth-Ayerst	Tablet	Taste
ZORprin	Knoll Pharm.	Tablet	Slow release
Zyban	GlaxoWellcome	Tablet	Slow release
Zymase	Organon	Capsule	Enteric-coated

Revised by John F. Mitchell, PharmD, FASHP, from an article originally appearing in *Hosp Pharm 1996;* 31:27-37.

* Capsule may be opened and the contents taken without crushing or chewing; soft food such as applesauce or pudding may facilitate administration; contents may generally be administered via nasogastric tube using an appropriate fluid provided entire contents are washed down the tube.

(a) Antacids or milk may prematurely dissolve the coating of the tablet.

(b) Capsule may be opened and the liquid contents removed for administration.

(c) The taste of this product in a liquid form would likely be unacceptable to the patient; administration via nasogastric tube should be acceptable.

(d) Effervescent tablets must be dissolved in the amount of diluent recommended by the manufacturer.

(e) If the liquid capsule is crushed or the contents expressed, the active ingredient will be, in part, absorbed sublingually.

(f) Acid contents of the stomach may prematurely activate the ingredients.

(g) Tablets are made to disintegrate under the tongue.

(h) Tablet is scored and may be broken in half without affecting release characteristics.

(i) Liquid dosage forms of the product are available; however, dose, frequency of administration, and manufacturers may differ from that of the solid dosage form.

(j) Contents may be dissolved in water for administration.

(k) Crushing may result in precipitation of larger particles.

(l) Crushed or broken tablet should not be handled by women who are pregnant or who may become pregnant.

Drug Names That Look Alike and Sound Alike

No drug name is without problems. They all can be written or spoken poorly enough so that they can be mistaken for another drug. Listed below are drug names that can look and/or sound alike. Some are dangerously close whereas others require incomplete prescribing information, poor communication skills, poor listening skills, and/or a lack of knowledge about the drugs to result in error. To reduce error, the practitioners must be active participants in sharing the common goal of drug name safety with the pharmaceutical manufacturers, FDA, WHO, USANC (United States Adopted Name Council) and the USP.

Error potential can be reduced by:

- Pre-testing of proposed names for error potential.
- Careful selection of trademarks and generic names by manufacturers, FDA, WHO and USANC.
- Legible handwriting.
- Clear oral communications.
- Writing complete drug orders:
  - specify dosage form (eg, tablet)
  - specify strength (eg, 100 mg)
  - specify directions (eg, take one daily with breakfast)
  - specify purpose/indication (eg, take one daily with breakfast to control blood pressure).
- Printing orders when they are for new or rarely prescribed drugs.
- Use of computer-generated orders.
- An awareness of the drugs which are available and careful attention to the work at hand by those involved with the drug dispensing and administration.
- Knowing the patient's condition/problems to ascertain if the drug name that has been read or heard is indicated.
- A system of double-checking completed prescriptions in the pharmacy.
- Educating the patient about the drugs they are to receive so that this serves as another check that the prescription was properly read and dispensed and so that the patient can serve as the final check

If prescriptions are not computer generated, they should be formatted so that prescribers must print the name and strength in blocks, such as -

When printed, a 30% tint should be used so that the block lines appear a light, but visible grey. This will prevent the T from looking like an I (top of the T falling on a dark line), an F looking like an E, an L looking like an I, a 7 looking like a 1, and 2 looking like a 7.

This list has been prepared to sensitize health care professionals and their support personnel for the need to properly communicate when writing, speaking, reading, and hearing drug names.

Proprietary names are capitalized, whereas other names are in lower-case letters.

A

1/2 Halprin	Halfprin 81
abciximab	arcitumomab
Accolate	Accupril
Accupril	Accolate
Accurbron	Accutane
Accutane	Accurbron
acetazolamide	acetohexamide
acetohexamide	acetazolamide
acetylcholine	acetylcysteine
acetylcysteine	acetylcholine
Acthar	Acthrel
Acthar	Acular
Acthrel	Acthar
Acular	Acthar
adapalene	Adapin
Adapin	Adapalene
Adderall	Inderal
Adeflor M	Aldoclor
Adriamycin	Idamycin
Afrin	aspirin
Albutein	albuterol
albuterol	atenolol
albuterol	Albutein
Alcaine	Alcare
Alcare	Alcaine
Aldactazide	Aldactone
Aldactone	Aldactazide
Aldoclor	Aldoril
Aldoclor	Adeflor M
Aldomet	Aldoril
Aldomet	Anzemet
Aldoril	Aldoclor
Aldoril	Aldomet
Aleve	Alesse
Alfenta	Sufenta
alfentanil	Anafranil
alfentanil	fentanyl
alfentanil	sufentanil
Alkeran	Leukeran
alprazolam	lorazepam
alprazolam	alprostadil
alprostadil	alprazolam
Altace	alteplase
Altace	Artane
alteplase	anistreplase
alteplase	Altace
Alupent	Atrovent
Amaryl	Amerge
Ambenyl	Aventyl
Ambien	Amen
Amen	Ambien
Amerge	Amaryl
Amicar	Amikin
Amicar	Amikacin
amikacin	Amicar
Amikin	Amicar
amiloride	amiodarone
amiloride	amlodipine
aminophylline	amitriptyline
aminophylline	ampicillin
amiodarone	amiloride
amiodarone	amrinone
Amipaque	Omnipaque
amitriptyline	nortriptyline
amitriptyline	aminophylline
amlodipine	amiloride
amoxapine	amoxicillin
amoxicillin	amoxapine
ampicillin	aminophylline
amrinone	amiodarone
Anafranil	enalapril
Anafranil	nafarelin
Anafranil	alfentanil
Anaprox	Anaspaz
Anaspaz	Anaprox
Ancobon	Oncovin
anisindione	anisotropine
anisotropine	anisindione
anistreplase	alteplase
Antabuse	Anturane
Anturane	Artane
Anturane	Antabuse
Anusol	Aplisol
Anusol	Aquasol
Anzemet	Aldomet
Aplisol	Aplitest
Aplisol	Anusol

Aplisol .... Atropisol
Aplitest .... Aplisol
Apresazide .... Apresoline
Apresoline .... Apresazide
Aquasol .... Anusol
Ara-C .... Arasine
Arasine .... Ara-C
arcitumomab .... abciximab
Aricept .... Ascriptin
Artane .... Altace
Artane .... Anturane
Asacol .... Os-Cal
Ascriptin .... Aricept
Asendin .... aspirin
aspirin .... Asendin
aspirin .... Afrin
Atarax .... Ativan
Atarax .... Marax
atenolol .... timolol
atenolol .... albuterol
Ativan .... Avitene
Ativan .... Atarax
Atropisol .... Aplisol
Atrovent .... Alupent
Aventyl .... Ambenyl
Aventyl .... Bentyl
Aventyl .... Serentil
Avitene .... Ativan
azatadine .... azathioprine
azathioprine .... azidothymidine
azathioprine .... Azulfidine
azathioprine .... azatadine
azidothymidine .... azathioprine
Azulfidine .... azathioprine

B

bacitracin .... Bactrim
bacitracin .... Bactroban
baclofen .... Bactroban
baclofen .... Beclovent
Bactrim .... bacitracin
Bactroban .... bacitracin
Bactroban .... baclofen
Banthine .... Brethine
Beclovent .... baclofen
Beminal .... Benemid
Benadryl .... Bentyl
Benadryl .... Benylin
Benadryl .... benazepril
benazepril .... Benadryl
Benemid .... Beminal
Benoxyl .... PerOxyl
Benoxyl .... Brevoxyl
Bentyl .... Aventyl
Bentyl .... Benadryl
Benylin .... Ventolin
Benylin .... Benadryl
benztropine .... bromocriptine
Bepridil .... Prepidil
Betadine .... betaine
Betagan .... Betagen
Betagen .... Betagan
betaine .... Betadine
Betoptic .... Betoptic S
Betoptic S .... Betoptic
Bicillin .... V-Cillin
Bicillin .... Wycillin
Brethaire .... Brethine
Brethine .... Banthine
Brethine .... Brethaire
Brevoxyl .... Benoxyl
brimonidine .... bromocriptine
bromocriptine .... benztropine
bromocriptine .... brimonidine
Bronkodyl .... Bronkosol
Bronkosol .... Bronkodyl
Bumex .... Buprenex
bupivacaine .... mepivacaine
Buprenex .... Bumex
bupropion .... buspirone
buspirone .... bupropion
butabarbital .... Butalbital
Butalbital .... butabarbital

C

Cafergot .... Carafate
Caladryl .... calamine
calamine .... Caladryl
calcifediol .... calcitriol
calciferol .... calcitriol
calcitonin .... calcitriol
calcitriol .... calcifediol
calcitriol .... calciferol
calcitriol .... calcitonin
calcium glubionate .... calcium gluconate
calcium gluconate .... calcium glubionate
Capastat .... Cepastat

Capitrol ....Captopril
Captopril ....Capitrol
Carafate ....Cafergot
Carbex ....Surbex
Carboplatin ....Cisplatin
Cardene ....Cardura
Cardene ....codeine
Cardene SR ....Cardizem SR
Cardizem SR ....Cardene SR
Cardura ....Coumadin
Cardura ....K-Dur
Cardura ....Cardene
Cardura ....Cordarone
Catapres ....Cetapred
Catapres ....Combipres
cefamandole ....cefmetazole
cefazolin..................cephalothin
cefazolin ....cefprozil
cefmetazole ....cefamandole
Cefobid ....cefonicid
cefonicid ....Cefobid
Cefotan ....Ceftin
cefotaxime ....cefoxitin
cefotaxime ....cefuroxime
cefotaxime ....ceftizoxime
cefotetan ....cefoxitin
cefoxitin ....Cytoxan
cefoxitin ....cefotaxime
cefoxitin ....cefotetan
cefprozil ....cefazolin
ceftazidime ....ceftizoxime
Ceftin ....Cefotan
ceftizoxime ....ceftazidime
ceftizoxime..................cefotaxime
cefuroxime ....cefotaxime
cefuroxime ....deferoxamine
Cefzil ....Kefzol
Celebrex..................Cerebyx
Cepastat ....Capastat
cephalexin ....cephalothin
cephalothin..................cefazolin
cephalothin..................cephalexin
cephradine ....cephapirin
cephapirin ....cephradine
cephradine..................cephapirin
Cerebyx ....Celebrex
Cerebyx ....Cerezyme
Ceredase ....Cerezyme
Cerezyme ....Cerebyx
Cerezyme ....Ceredase
Cetaphil ....Cetapred
Cetapred ....Cetaphil
Cetapred ....Catapres
Chenix ....Cystex
chlorambucil ....Chloromycetin
Chloromycetin ....chlorambucil
chloroxine ....Choloxin
chlorpromazine ....chlorpropamide
chlorpromazine ....clomipramine
chlorpropamide ....chlorpromazine
Choloxin ....chloroxine
Chorex ....Chymex
Chymex ....Chorex
Cidex ....Lidex
Ciloxan ....Cytoxan
Ciloxan ....cinoxacin
cimetidine ....simethicone
cinoxacin ....Ciloxan
Cisplatin ....Carboplatin
Citracal ....Citrucel
Citrucel ....Citracal
Clinoril ....Clozaril
clofazimine ....clozapine
clofibrate ....clorazepate
clomiphene ....clomipramine
clomiphene ....clonidine
clomipramine ....chlorpromazine
clomipramine ....clomiphene
clonidine ....quinidine
clonidine ....clomiphene
clorazepate ....clofibrate
clotrimazole ....co-trimoxazole
Cloxapen ....clozapine
clozapine ....clofazimine
clozapine ....Cloxapen
Clozaril ....Clinoril
co-trimoxazole ....clotrimazole
codeine ....Cardene
codeine ....Lodine
codeine ....Cordran
Combipres ....Catapres
Combivent ....Combivir
Combivir..................Combivent
Compazine ....Copaxone
Comvax ....Recombivax
Copaxone ....Compazine
Cordarone ....Cardura
Cordarone ....Cordran

Cordran . . . . .codeine
Cordran . . . . .Cordarone
Cort-Dome . . . . .Cortone
Cortone . . . . .Cort-Dome
Cortrosyn . . . . .Cotazym
Cotazym . . . . .Cortrosyn
Coumadin . . . . .Kemadrin
Coumadin . . . . .Cardura
Cozaar . . . . .Zocor
cyclobenzaprine . . . . .cycloserine
cyclobenzaprine . . . . .cyproheptadine
cyclophosphamide . . . . .cyclosporine
cycloserine . . . . .cyclosporine
cycloserine . . . . .cyclobenzaprine
cyclosporin . . . . .Cyklokapron
cyclosporine . . . . .cyclophosphamide
cyclosporine . . . . .cycloserine
Cyklokapron . . . . .cyclosporin
cyproheptadine . . . . .cyclobenzaprine
Cystex .Chenix
Cytadren . . . . .cytarabine
cytarabine . . . . .vidarabine
cytarabine . . . . .Cytadren
CytoGam . . . . .Cytoxan
Cytosar U . . . . .Cytovene
Cytosar U . . . . .Cytoxan
Cytotec . . . . .Cytoxan
Cytovene . . . . .Cytosar U
Cytoxan . . . . .Cytotec
Cytoxan . . . . .Cytosar U
Cytoxan . . . . .CytoGam
Cytoxan . . . . .cefoxitin
Cytoxan . . . . .Ciloxan

D

dacarbazine . . . . .Dicarbosil
dacarbazine . . . . .procarbazine
Dacriose . . . . .Danocrine
Dalmane . . . . .Dialume
Dalmane . . . . .Demulen
Danocrine . . . . .Dacriose
Dantrium . . . . .Daraprim
dapsone . . . . .Diprosone
Daranide . . . . .Daraprim
Daraprim . . . . .Dantrium
Daraprim . . . . .Daranide
Darvocet-N . . . . .Darvon-N
Darvon-N . . . . .Darvocet-N
daunorubicin . . . . .doxorubicin
daunorubicin . . . . .dactinomycin
deferoxamine . . . . .cefuroxime
Delsym . . . . .Desyrel
Demerol . . . . .Demulen
Demerol . . . . .Dymelor
Demulen . . . . .Dalmane
Demulen . . . . .Demerol
Depen .Endep
Depo-Estradiol . . . . .Depo-Testadiol
Depo-Medrol . . . . .Solu-Medrol
Depo-Testadiol . . . . .Depo-Estradiol
Dermatop . . . . .Dimetapp
Desferal . . . . .Disophrol
desipramine . . . . .disopyramide
desipramine . . . . .imipramine
desoximetasone . . . . .dexamethasone
Desoxyn . . . . .digitoxin
Desoxyn . . . . .digoxin
Desyrel . . . . .Zestril
Desyrel . . . . .Delsym
dexamethasone . . . . .desoximetasone
Dexedrine . . . . .dextran
Dexedrine . . . . .Excedrin
dextran . . . . .Dexedrine
DiaBeta . . . . .Zebeta
Dialume . . . . .Dalmane
Diamox . . . . .Trimox
diazepam . . . . .diazoxide
diazepam . . . . .Ditropan
diazoxide . . . . .Dyazide
diazoxide . . . . .diazepam
Dicarbosil . . . . .dacarbazine
dichloroacetic acid . . . . .trichloracetic acid
diclofenac . . . . .Diflucan
diclofenac . . . . .Duphalac
dicyclomine . . . . .dyclonine
dicyclomine . . . . .doxycycline
Diflucan . . . . .diclofenac
digitoxin . . . . .digoxin
digitoxin . . . . .Desoxyn
digoxin . . . . .doxepin
digoxin . . . . .Desoxyn
digoxin . . . . .digitoxin
Dilantin . . . . .Dilaudid
Dilaudid . . . . .Dilantin
dimenhydrinate . . . . .diphenhydramine
Dimetane . . . . .Dimetapp
Dimetapp . . . . .Dermatop

Dimetapp	Dimetane
diphenhydramine	dimenhydrinate
Diprosone	dapsone
dipyridamole	disopyramide
Disophrol	Desferal
disopyramide	desipramine
disopyramide	dipyridamole
dithranol	Ditropan
Ditropan	diazepam
Ditropan	dithranol
dobutamine	dopamine
Dolobid	Slo-bid
Donnagel	Donnatal
Donnatal	Donnagel
dopamine	Dopram
dopamine	dobutamine
Dopar	Dopram
Dopram	dopamine
Dopram	Dopar
doxacurium	doxapram
doxacurium	doxorubicin
doxapram	doxepin
doxapram	doxacurium
doxapram	doxazosin
doxapram	doxorubicin
doxazosin	doxapram
doxazosin	doxorubicin
doxazosin	doxepin
doxepin	doxazosin
doxepin	digoxin
doxepin	doxapram
doxepin	Doxidan
Doxidan	doxepin
Doxil	Paxil
Doxinate	doxapram
doxorubicin	idarubicin
doxorubicin	doxapram
doxorubicin	dactinomycin
doxorubicin	daunorubicin
doxorubicin	doxacurium
doxorubicin	doxazosin
doxycycline	doxylamine
doxycycline	dicyclomine
doxylamine	doxycycline
dronabinol	droperidol
droperidol	dronabinol
Duphalac	diclofenac
Dyazide	diazoxide
dyclonine	dicyclomine
Dymelor	Demerol
Dynabac	Dynacin
Dynabac	DynaCirc
Dynacin	DynaCirc
Dynacin	Dynabac
DynaCirc	Dynabac
DynaCirc	Dynacin

E

Ecotrin	Edecrin
Ecotrin	Akineton
Edecrin	Ecotrin
Elavil	Equanil
Elavil	Mellaril
Eldepryl	enalapril
Emcyt	Eryc
enalapril	Anafranil
enalapril	Eldepryl
encainide	flecainide
Enduronyl Forte	Inderal 40 mg
enflurane	isoflurane
Entex	Tenex
ephedrine	epinephrine
epinephrine	ephedrine
Epogen	Neupogen
Equagesic	EquiGesic (Veterinary)
Equanil	Elavil
EquiGesic (Veterinary)	Equagesic
Eryc	Emcyt
Erythrocin	Ethmozine
Esimil	Estinyl
Esimil	Ismelin
Estinyl	Esimil
Estraderm	Testoderm
Ethamolin	ethanol
ethanol	Ethamolin
ethanol	Ethyol
Ethmozine	Erythrocin
ethosuximide	methsuximide
Ethyol	ethanol
etidocaine	etidronate
etidronate	etretinate
etidronate	etidocaine
etidronate	etomidate
etomidate	etidronate
etretinate	etidronate
Eurax	Serax
Eurax	Urex
Excedrin	Dexedrine

F

Factrel .Sectral
fentanyl . . . . .alfentanil
Feosol .Fer-in-Sol
Fer-in-Sol . . . . .Feosol
Feridex . . . . .Fertinex
Ferralyn . . . . .Verelan
Fertinex . . . . .Feridex
Festal. .Feosol
Fioricet . . . . .Fiorinal
Fiorinal . . . . .Florinef
Fiorinal . . . . .Fioricet
Flaxedil . . . . .Flexeril
flecainide . . . . .encainide
Flexeril . . . . .Floxin
Flexon .Floxin
Flomax. . . . . .Fosamax
Flomax. . . . . .Volmax
Florinef . . . . .Fiorinal
Florvite . . . . .Folvite
Floxin .Flexeril
Floxin .Flexon
Fludara . . . . .FUDR
Flumadine . . . . .flunisolide
Flumadine . . . . .flutamide
flunisolide . . . . .fluocinonide
flunisolide . . . . .Flumadine
fluocinolone . . . . .fluocinonide
fluocinonide . . . . .flunisolide
fluocinonide . . . . .fluocinolone
Fluosol . . . . .Feosol
fluoxetine . . . . .fluvastatin
flutamide . . . . .Flumadine
fluvastatin . . . . .fluoxetine
folic acid . . . . .folinic acid
folinic acid . . . . .folic acid
Folvite .Florvite
Fosamax . . . . .Flomax
fosinopril . . . . .lisinopril
FUDR .Fludara
Fulvicin . . . . .Furacin
Furacin . . . . .Fulvicin
furosemide . . . . .Torsemide

G

Gantanol . . . . .Gantrisin
Gantrisin . . . . .Gantanol
Glaucon . . . . .glucagon
glimepiride . . . . .glipizide
glipizide . . . . .glyburide
glipizide . . . . .glimepiride
glucagon . . . . .Glaucon
Glucotrol . . . . .glyburide
glutethimide . . . . .guanethidine
glyburide . . . . .glipizide
glyburide . . . . .Glucotrol
GoLYTELY . . . . .NuLytely
gonadorelin . . . . .gonadotropin
gonadorelin . . . . .guanadrel
gonadotropin . . . . .gonadorelin
guaifenesin . . . . .guanfacine
guanabenz . . . . .guanadrel
guanabenz . . . . .guanfacine
guanadrel . . . . .gonadorelin
guanadrel . . . . .guanabenz
guanethidine . . . . .guanidine
guanethidine . . . . .glutethimide
guanfacine . . . . .guanidine
guanfacine . . . . .guaifenesin
guanfacine . . . . .guanabenz
guanidine . . . . .guanethidine
guanidine . . . . .guanfacine

H

halcinonide . . . . .Halcion
Halcion . . . . .Haldol
Halcion . . . . .Healon
Halcion . . . . .halcinonide
Haldol .Halog
Haldol .Halcion
Halfprin 81 . . . . .1/2 Halprin
Halog . . . . .Haldol
Halotestin . . . . .Halotex
Halotestin . . . . .halothane
Halotex . . . . .Halotestin
halothane . . . . .Halotestin
Healon . . . . .Halcion
Heparin . . . . .Hespan
Hespan . . . . .Heparin
Humalog . . . . .Humulin
Humulin . . . . .Humalog
Hycodan . . . . .Hycomine
Hycodan . . . . .Vicodin
Hycomine . . . . .Hycodan
hydralazine . . . . .hydroxyzine
hydrochlorothiazide . . . . .hydroflumethiazide
hydrocortisone . . . . .hydroxychloroquine

hydroflumethiazide .... hydrochlorothiazide
hydromorphone .... morphine
hydroxychloroquine .... hydrocortisone
hydroxyprogesterone .... medroxyprogesterone
hydroxyurea .... hydroxyzine
hydroxyzine .... hydralazine
hydroxyzine .... hydroxyurea
Hygroton .... Regroton
HyperHep .... Hyperstat
HyperHep .... Hyper-Tet
Hyperstat .... Nitrostat
Hyperstat .... Hyper-Tet
Hyperstat .... HyperHep
Hyper-Tet .... HyperHep
Hyper-Tet .... Hyperstat
Hytone .... Vytone

I

Idamycin .... Adriamycin
idarubicin .... doxorubicin
Iletin .... Lente
Imipenem .... Omnipen
imipramine .... desipramine
Imodium .... Ionamin
Imuran .... Inderal
indapamide .... Iopidine
indapamide .... iodamide
indapamide .... iopamidol
Inderal .... Inderide
Inderal .... Isordil
Inderal .... Adderall
Inderal .... Imuran
Inderal 40 mg .... Enduronyl Forte
Inderide .... Inderal
interferon 2 .... interleukin 2
interferon alfa 2a .... interferon alfa 2b
interferon alfa 2b .... interferon alfa 2a
interleukin 2 .... interferon 2
Intropin .... Isoptin
iodamide .... indapamide
iodine .... Iopidine
iodine .... Lodine
iodapamide .... Iopidine
Ionamin .... Imodium
iopamidol .... indapamide
Iopidine .... Lodine
Iopidine .... indapamide
Iopidine .... iodine
Iopidine .... iodapamide
Ismelin .... Isuprel
Ismelin .... Esimil
isoflurane .... enflurane
Isoptin .... Intropin
Isopto Carbachol .... Isopto Carpine
Isopto Carpine .... Isopto Carbachol
Isordil .... Isuprel
Isordil .... Inderal
Isuprel .... Ismelin
Isuprel .... Isordil

K

K-Dur .... Cardura
K-Lor .... Kaochlor
K-Phos Neutral .... Neutra-Phos-K
Kaochlor .... K-Lor
Kefzol .... Cefzil
Kemadrin .... Coumadin
Klaron .... Klor-Con
Klor-Con .... Klaron

L

lactose .... lactulose
lactulose .... lactose
Lamictal .... Lomotil
Lamictal .... Lamisil
Lamisil .... Lamictal
lamivudine .... lamotrigine
lamotrigine .... lamivudine
Lanoxin .... Levsinex
Lasix .... Lidex
Lasix .... Luvox
Lente .... Iletin
Leukeran .... Leukine
Leukeran .... Alkeran
Leukine .... Leukeran
Leustatin .... lovastatin
Levatol .... Lipitor
Levbid .... Lithobid
levothyroxine .... liothyronine
Levsinex .... Lanoxin
Librax .... Librium
Librium .... Librax
Lidex .... Cidex
Lidex .... Lasix
Lioresal .... lisinopril
liothyronine .... levothyroxine
Lipitor .... Levatol
lisinopril .... fosinopril

lisinopril .... Lioresal
Lithobid .... Lithostat
Lithobid .... Lithotabs
Lithobid .... Levbid
Lithonate .... Lithostat
Lithostat .... Lithobid
Lithostat .... Lithonate
Lithostat .... Lithotabs
Lithotabs .... Lithostat
Lithotabs .... Lithobid
Livostin .... lovastatin
Lodine .... codeine
Lodine .... iodine
Lodine .... lopidine
Lomotil .... Lamictal
Loniten .... Lotensin
Lopurin .... Lopressor
Lopurin .... Lupron
Lorabid .... Lortab
lorazepam .... alprazolam
Lortab .... Lorabid
Lotensin .... Loniten
Lotensin .... lovastatin
lovastatin .... Lotensin
lovastatin .... Leustatin
lovastatin .... Livostin
Luminal .... Tuinal
Lupron .... Nuprin
Lupron .... Lopurin
Luvox .... Lasix

M

Maalox .... Maolate
Maalox .... Marax
magnesium sulfate .... manganese sulfate
manganese sulfate .... magnesium sulfate
Maolate .... Maalox
Marax .... Atarax
Marax .... Maalox
Maxidex .... Maxzide
Maxzide .... Maxidex
Mebaral .... Medrol
Mebaral .... Mellaril
mecamylamine .... mesalamine
Medrol .... Mebaral
medroxyprogesterone .... methyltestosterone
medroxyprogesterone .... hydroxyprogesterone
medroxyprogesterone .... methylprednisolone
Mellaril .... Moderil
Mellaril .... Elavil
Mellaril .... Mebaral
melphalan .... Mephyton
Mephenytoin .... Mephyton
Mephenytoin .... phenytoin
mephobarbital .... methocarbamol
Mephyton .... melphalan
Mephyton .... Mephenytoin
mepivacaine .... bupivacaine
Mesantoin .... Mestinon
Mestinon .... Mesantoin
Mestinon .... Metatensin
metaproterenol .... metoprolol
metaproterenol .... metipranolol
Metatensin .... Mestinon
methazolamide .... metolazone
methenamine .... methionine
methicillin .... mezlocillin
methionine .... methenamine
methocarbamol .... mephobarbital
methsuximide .... ethosuximide
methylprednisolone .... medroxyprogesterone
methyltestosterone .... medroxyprogesterone
metipranolol .... metaproterenol
metolazone .... metoprolol
metolazone .... methazolamide
metoprolol .... metaproterenol
metoprolol .... metolazone
metyrapone .... metyrosine
metyrosine .... metyrapone
Mevacor .... Mivacron
mezlocillin .... methicillin
miconazole .... Micronase
miconazole .... Micronor
Micro-K .... Micronase
Micronase .... Micronor
Micronase .... Micro-K
Micronase .... miconazole
Micronor .... miconazole
Micronor .... Micronase
Midrin .... Mydfrin
Milontin .... Miltown
Milontin .... Mylanta

Miltown . . . . .Milontin
Minocin . . . . .Mithracin
Minocin . . . . .niacin
Mithracin . . . . .Minocin
mithramycin . . . . .mitomycin
mitomycin . . . . .mithramycin
Mivacron . . . . .Mevacor
Moban .Mobidin
Mobidin . . . . .Moban
Modane . . . . .Mudrane
Moderil . . . . .Mellaril
Monopril . . . . .Monurol
Monurol . . . . .Monopril
morphine . . . . .hydromorphone
Mudrane . . . . .Modane
Myambutol . . . . .Nembutal
Mycelex . . . . .Myoflex
Myciguent . . . . .Mycitracin
Mycitracin . . . . .Myciguent
Mydfrin . . . . .Midrin
Mylanta . . . . .Mynatal
Mylanta . . . . .Milontin
Myleran . . . . .Mylicon
Mylicon . . . . .Myleran
Mynatal . . . . .Mylanta
Myoflex . . . . .Mycelex

N

nafarelin . . . . .Anafranil
Naldecon . . . . .Nalfon
Nalfon .Naldecon
naloxone . . . . .naltrexone
naltrexone . . . . .naloxone
Narcan . . . . .Norcuron
Navane . . . . .Nubain
Navane . . . . .Norvasc
Nembutal . . . . .Myambutol
Nephro-Calci . . . . .Nephrocaps
Nephrocaps . . . . .Nephro-Calci
Neumega . . . . .Neupogen
Neupogen . . . . .Nutramigen
Neupogen . . . . .Epogen
Neutra-Phos-K . . . . .K-Phos Neutral
niacin .Minocin
nicardipine . . . . .nifedipine
Nicobid . . . . .Nitro-Bid
Nicoderm . . . . .Nitroderm
Nicorette . . . . .Nordette
nifedipine . . . . .nimodipine
nifedipine . . . . .nicardipine
Nilstat .Nitrostat
Nilstat .Nystatin
nimodipine . . . . .nifedipine
Nitro-Bid . . . . .Nicobid
Nitroderm . . . . .Nicoderm
nitroglycerin . . . . .nitroprusside
nitroprusside . . . . .nitroglycerin
Nitrostat . . . . .Nystatin
Nitrostat . . . . .Hyperstat
Nitrostat . . . . .Nilstat
Norcuron . . . . .Narcan
Nordette . . . . .Nicorette
Norflex . . . . .Noroxin
Norgesic #40 . . . . .Norgesic Forte
Norgesic Forte . . . . .Norgesic #40
Norlutate . . . . .Norlutin
Norlutin . . . . .Norlutate
Noroxin . . . . .Norflex
nortriptyline . . . . .amitriptyline
Norvasc . . . . .Navane
Norvasc . . . . .Vascor
Nubain .Navane
NuLytely . . . . .GoLYTELY
Nuprin .Lupron
Nutramigen . . . . .Neupogen
Nystatin . . . . .Nilstat
Nystatin . . . . .Nitrostat

O

OctreoScan . . . . .octreotide
OctreoScan . . . . .OncoScint
octreotide . . . . .OctreoScan
Ocufen .Ocuflox
Ocuflox . . . . .Ocufen
olanzapine . . . . .olsalazine
olsalazine . . . . .olanzapine
Omnipaque . . . . .Amipaque
Omnipen . . . . .Unipen
Omnipen . . . . .Imipenem
OncoScint . . . . .OctreoScan
Oncovin . . . . .Ancobon
Ophthaine . . . . .Ophthetic
Ophthetic . . . . .Ophthaine
Optimine. . . . . .Optimyd
Optimyd . . . . .Optimine
Oretic .Oreton
Oreton .Oretic
Orex. . . . . .Urex

Orexin .... Ornex
Orinase .... Ornade
Orinase .... Ornex
Ornade .... Orinase
Ornex .... Orexin
Ornex .... Orinase
Os-Cal .... Asacol
Otobiotic .... Urobiotic
oxaprozin .... oxazepam
oxazepam .... oxaprozin
oxymetazoline .... oxymetholone
oxymetholone .... oxymetazoline
oxymetholone .... oxymorphone
oxymorphone .... oxymetholone

P

paclitaxel .... paroxetine
paclitaxel .... Paxil
Panadol .... pindolol
pancuronium .... pipecuronium
Paraplatin .... Platinol
paregoric .... Percogesic
Parlodel .... pindolol
paroxetine .... paclitaxel
Patanol .... Platinol
Pathilon .... Pathocil
Pathocil .... Placidyl
Pathocil .... Pathilon
Pavabid .... Pavatine
Pavatine .... Pavabid
Pavulon .... Peptavlon
Paxil .... Doxil
Paxil .... paclitaxel
Paxil .... Taxol
Pediapred .... Pediazole
Pediazole .... Pediapred
Penetrex .... Pentrax
penicillamine .... penicillin
penicillin .... penicillamine
pentobarbital .... phenobarbital
pentosan .... pentostatin
pentostatin .... pentosan
Pentrax .... Permax
Pentrax .... Penetrex
Peptavlon .... Pavulon
Perative .... Periactin
Percocet .... Percodan
Percodan .... Percogesic
Percodan .... Periactin
Percodan .... Percocet
Percogesic .... paregoric
Percogesic .... Percodan
Periactin .... Persantine
Periactin .... Perative
Permax .... Pentrax
Permax .... Pernox
Pernox .... Permax
PerOxyl .... Benoxyl
Persantine .... Periactin
phenobarbital .... pentobarbital
phentermine .... phentolamine
phentolamine .... phentermine
phenytoin .... Mephenytoin
pHisoDerm .... pHisoHex
pHisoHex .... pHisoDerm
pHisoHex .... Phos-Ex
Phos-Flur .... PhosLo
PhosChol .... PhosLo
PhosChol .... Phosphocol P32
PhosLo .... Phos-Flur
PhosLo .... PhosChol
Phosphocol P32 .... PhosChol
Phrenilin .... Trinalin
physostigmine .... Prostigmin
physostigmine .... pyridostigmine
pindolol .... Parlodel
pindolol .... Panadol
pindolol .... Plendil
pipecuronium .... pancuronium
Pitocin .... Pitressin
Pitressin .... Pitocin
Placidyl .... Pathocil
Platinol .... Paraplatin
Platinol .... Patanol
Plendil .... pindolol
Plendil .... Pletal
Pletal .... Plendil
Polocaine .... prilocaine
Ponstel .... Pronestyl
Posicor .... Proscar
Posicor .... Psorcon
pralidoxime .... Pramoxine
pralidoxime .... pyridoxine
Pramoxine .... pralidoxime
Pravachol .... Prevacid
Pravachol .... propranolol
prednisolone .... prednisone
prednisone .... primidone

prednisone	prednisolone
Premarin	Primaxin
Prepidil	Bepridil
Prevacid	Pravachol
Prevacid	Prevpac
Prevpac	Prevacid
Prilocaine	Prilosec
prilocaine	Polocaine
Prilosec	Prozac
Prilosec	Prilocaine
Prilosec	Prinivil
Primaxin	Premarin
primidone	prednisone
Prinivil	Proventil
Prinivil	Prilosec
ProAmatine	protamine
Probenecid	Procanbid
Procanbid	Probenecid
procarbazine	dacarbazine
Prokine	procaine
Proloprim	Protropin
promazine	promethazine
promethazine	promazine
Pronestyl	Ponstel
propranolol	Pravachol
Proscar	Posicor
Proscar	Psorcon
Proscar	ProSom
Proscar	Prozac
ProSom	Proscar
ProSom	Prozac
ProSom	Psorcon
Prostigmin	physostigmine
protamine	Protopam
protamine	Protropin
protamine	ProAmatine
Protopam	protamine
Protopam	Protropin
Protropin	Protopam
Protropin	Proloprim
Protropin	protamine
Proventil	Prinivil
Prozac	Proscar
Prozac	Prilosec
Prozac	ProSom
Psorcon	Proscar
Psorcon	ProSom
Pyridium	pyridoxine
pyridostigmine	physostigmine
pyridoxine	pralidoxime
pyridoxine	Pyridium

Q

Quarzan	quazepam
Quarzan	Questran
quazepam	Quarzan
Questran	Quarzan
Quinamm	quinidine
quinidine	Quinamm
quinidine	quinine
quinidine	Quinora
quinidine	clonidine
quinine	quinidine
Quinora	quinidine

R

ranitidine	ritodrine
ranitidine	rimantadine
Reglan	Regonol
Regonol	Reglan
Regonol	Regroton
Regroton	Regonol
Regroton	Hygroton
Renacidin	Remicade
reserpine	Risperidone
Restoril	Vistaril
Restoril	Zestril
Retrovir	ritonavir
Revex	ReVia
ReVia	Revex
Ribavirin	riboflavin
riboflavin	Ribavirin
rifabutin	rifampin
Rifadin	Ritalin
Rifamate	rifampin
rifampin	rifabutin
rifampin	Rifamate
rifampin	rifapentine
rimantadine	ranitidine
Risperidone	reserpine
Ritalin	Rifadin
ritodrine	ranitidine
ritonavir	Retrovir
Roxanol	Roxicet
Roxicet	Roxanol

S

salsalate	sucralfate
salsalate	sulfasalazine

Sandimmune	Sandoglobulin
Sandimmune	Sandostatin
Sandoglobulin	Sandostatin
Sandoglobulin	Sandimmune
Sandostatin	Sandimmune
Sandostatin	Sandoglobulin
saquinavir	Sinequan
Sectral	Factrel
Sectral	Septra
selegiline	Stelazine
Septa	Septra
Septra	Sectral
Septra	Septa
Serax	Xerac
Serax	Eurax
Serentil	Serevent
Serentil	Aventyl
Serevent	Serentil
simethicone	cimetidine
Sinequan	saquinavir
Slo-bid	Dolobid
Slow FE	Slow-K
Slow-K	Slow FE
Solu-Medrol	Depo-Medrol
somatrem	somatropin
somatropin	sumatriptan
somatropin	somatrem
sotalol	Statrol
sotalol	Stadol
Stadol	sotalol
Statrol	sotalol
Stelazine	selegiline
sucralfate	salsalate
Sufenta	Alfenta
Sufenta	Survanta
sufentanil	alfentanil
sulfadiazine	sulfasalazine
sulfamethizole	sulfameth-oxazole
sulfamethoxazole	sulfamethizole
sulfasalazine	sulfisoxazole
sulfasalazine	salsalate
sulfasalazine	sulfadiazine
sulfisoxazole	sulfasalazine
sumatriptan	somatropin
Surbex	Surfak
Surbex	Carbex
Surfak	Surbex
Survanta	Sufenta

T

Taxol	Paxil
Tazicef	Tazidime
Tazidime	Tazicef
Tegretol	Toradol
Ten-K	Tenex
Tenex	Xanax
Tenex	Entex
Tenex	Ten-K
terbinafine	terbutaline
terbutaline	tolbutamide
terbutaline	terbinafine
terconazole	tioconazole
Testoderm	Estraderm
testolactone	testosterone
testosterone	testolactone
Theolair	Thyrolar
Thera-Flur	TheraFlu
TheraFlu	Thera-Flur
thiamine	Thorazine
thioridazine	Thorazine
Thorazine	thiamine
Thorazine	thioridazine
Thyrar	Thyrolar
Thyrolar	Theolair
Thyrolar	Thyrar
Ticar	Tigan
Tigan	Ticar
timolol	atenolol
Timoptic	Viroptic
tioconazole	terconazole
TobraDex	Tobrex
tobramycin	Trobicin
Tobrex	TobraDex
tolazamide	tolbutamide
tolbutamide	terbutaline
tolbutamide	tolazamide
tolnaftate	Tornalate
Topic	Topicort
Topicort	Topic
Toradol	Tegretol
Tornalate	tolnaftate
Torsemide	furosemide
tramadol	Toradol
tramadol	Trandate
Trandate	tramadol
Trandate	Trental
Trandate	Tridrate
Trendar	Trental

Trental ....Trendar
Trental ....Trandate
tretinoin ....trientine
triamcinolone ....Triaminicin
triamcinolone ....Triaminicol
Triaminic ....TriHemic
Triaminic ....Triaminicin
Triaminicin ....Triaminic
Triaminicin ....triamcinolone
Triaminicol ....triamcinolone
triamterene ....trimipramine
trichloracetic acid ....dichloroacetic acid
Tridrate ....Trandate
trientine ....tretinoin
trifluoperazine ....triflupromazine
triflupromazine ....trifluoperazine
TriHemic ....Triaminic
trimeprazine ....trimipramine
trimipramine ....triamterene
trimipramine ....trimeprazine
Trimox ....Tylox
Trimox ....Diamox
Trinalin ....Phrenilin
Trobicin ....tobramycin
Tronolane ....Tronothane
Tronothane ....Tronolane
Tuinal ....Tylenol
Tuinal ....Luminal
Tylenol ....Tylox
Tylenol ....Tuinal
Tylox ....Trimox
Tylox ....Tylenol

U

Ultane ....Ultram
Ultram ....Ultane
Unicap ....Unipen
Unipen ....Urispas
Unipen ....Omnipen
Unipen ....Unicap
Urex ....Erex
Urex ....Eurax
Urex ....Orex
Urised ....Urispas
Urispas ....Urised
Urispas ....Unipen
Urobiotic ....Otobiotic

V

V-Cillin ....Bicillin
Vancenase ....Vanceril
Vanceril ....Vansil
Vanceril ....Vancenase
Vansil ....Vanceril
Vantin ....Ventolin
Vascor ....Norvasc
Vasocidin ....Vasodilan
Vasodilan ....Vasocidin
Vasosulf ....Velosef
Velosef ....Vasosulf
Ventolin ....Benylin
Ventolin ....Vantin
VePesid ....Versed
Verelan ....Vivarin
Verelan ....Voltaren
Verelan ....Ferralyn
Verelan ....Virilon
Versed ....VePesid
Vexol ....VoSol
Vicodin ....Hycodan
vidarabine ....cytarabine
vinblastine ....vincristine
vinblastine ....vinorelbine
vincristine ....vinblastine
vinorelbine ....vinblastine
Virilon ....Verelan
Viroptic ....Timoptic
Visine ....Visken
Visken ....Visine
Vistaril ....Restoril
Vivarin ....Verelan
Volmax ....Flomax
Voltaren ....Verelan
VoSol ....Vexol
Vytone ....Hytone

W

Wellbutrin ....Wellcovorin
Wellbutrin ....Wellferon
Wellcovorin ....Wellferon
Wellcovorin ....Wellbutrin
Wellferon ....Wellbutrin
Wellferon ....Wellcovorin
Wyamine ....Wydase
Wycillin ....Bicillin
Wydase ....Wyamine

X

Xanax ....Zantac

Xanax . . . . Tenex
Xanax. . . . . Xopenex
Xerac . . . . Serax
Xopenex. . . . . Xanax

Z

Zantac . . . . Zofran
Zantac . . . . Xanax
Zarontin . . . . Zaroxolyn
Zaroxolyn . . . . Zarontin
Zebeta . . . . DiaBeta
Zestril . . . . Zostrix
Zestril . . . . Desyrel
Zestril. . . . . Restoril
Zocor . . . . Cozaar
Zofran . . . . Zantac
Zofran . . . . Zosyn
ZORprin . . . . Zyloprim
Zostrix . . . . Zovirax
Zostrix . . . . Zestril
Zosyn . . . . Zofran
Zovirax . . . . Zostrix
Zyloprim . . . . ZORprin
Zyprexa . . . . Zyrtec
Zyrtec . . . . Zyprexa

"Look-Alike, Sound-Alike Drugs," was originated and developed by Benjamin Teplitsky, retired Chief Pharmacist of Veterans Administration Hospitals in Albany NY and Brooklyn NY. The assistance of N. Michael Davis, Leslie Kalash, and Dan Sheridan is gratefully acknowledged.

Recommended Childhood Immunization Schedule

Each year, CDC's Advisory Committee on Immunization Practices (ACIP) reviews the recommended childhood immunization schedule to ensure it remains current with changes in manufacturers' vaccine formulations, revised recommendations for the use of licensed vaccines, and recommendations for newly licensed vaccines.

Vaccine Recommended Changes: *Inactivated Poliovirus Vaccine for First Two Doses:* As a result of progress in the global eradication of poliomyelitis, the need for further reductions in the risk for acquiring vaccine-associated paralytic polio, and the acceptance of inactivated poliovirus vaccine (IPV) by parents and physicians, the ACIP, AAFP, and AAP recommend IPV for the first two doses of poliovirus vaccine for routine childhood vaccination. The ACIP continues to recommend a sequential schedule of two doses of IPV administered at ages 2 and 4 months, followed by two doses of oral poliovirus vaccine (OPV) at ages 12-18 months and 4-6 years. IPV for all four poliovirus vaccine doses also is acceptable and is recommended for immunocompromised persons and their household contacts. OPV is no longer recommended for the first two doses of the schedule and is acceptable only for special circumstances (eg, vaccination of children whose parents do not accept the recommended sequential schedule, late initiation of vaccination that would require an unacceptable number of injections, and imminent travel to countries where polio is endemic.

Recombivax HB® Hepatitis B Vaccine for Persons Aged 0-19 years: The Merck Vaccine Division discontinued production and distribution of the 2.5 µg/0.5 mL pediatric dose of Recombivax HB® hepatitis B vaccine, which was licensed by FDA for infants of HBsAg-negative mothers and children aged < 11 years. The 5 µg/0.5 mL dose of Recombivax HB® is now indicated for all vaccinees aged 0-19 years regardless of the mother's HBsAg status. In addition to receiving the hepatitis B vaccine series, infants born to HBsAg-positive mothers also should receive 0.5 mL of hepatitis B immune globulin within 12 hours of birth at separate injection sites. Infants born to HBsAg-negative mothers or children who received one or two doses of the 2.5 µg/0.5 mL dose of Recombivax HB® may complete the hepatitis B vaccination series with either the 2.5g/0.5 mL or the 5.0 µg/0.5 mL dose. Children who have completed the hepatitis B vaccination series with the 2.5 µg/0.5 mL dose do not require revaccination.

Diphtheria and Tetanus Toxoids and Acellular Pertussis Vaccines Preferred: DTaP is the recommended vaccine for primary vaccination against diphtheria, tetanus, and pertussis. This change makes DTaP the preferred vaccine formulation for all doses in the vaccination series. Whole-cell diphtheria and tetanus toxoids and pertussis vaccine remains an acceptable alternative when DTaP is not available. Hib Conjugate and DTaP Combination vaccines not for infants.

References

1. ACIP. Recommended childhood immunization schedule – United States, 1999. *MMWR* 1999; 48:12-15.

Recommended Childhood Vaccination Schedule* – United States, January - December 1999

Vaccine	Age										
	Birth	1 Mo.	2 Mos.	4 Mos.	6 Mos.	12 Mos.	15 Mos.	18 Mos.	4-6 Yrs.	11-12 Yrs.	14-16 Yrs.
Hepatitis B†		Hep B									
			Hep B			Hep B				Hep B	
Diphtheria and tetanus toxoids and pertussis§			DTaP	DTaP	DTaP		DTaP		DTaP	Td	
H. influenzae type b¶			Hib	Hib	Hib	Hib					
Poliovirus**			IPV	IPV		Polio			Polio		
Measles-mumps-rubella§§						MMR			MMR	MMR	
Varicella-zoster virus¶¶							Var			Var	

☐ Range of Acceptable Ages for Vaccination

Vaccines to be Assessed and Administered if Necessary

* This schedule indicates the recommended ages for routine administration of currently licensed childhood vaccines. Any dose not given at the recommended age should be given as a "catch-up" vaccination at any subsequent visit when indicated and feasible. Combination vaccines may be used whenever any components of the combination are indicated and its other components are not contraindicated. Providers should consult then manufacturers' package inserts for detailed recommendations.

† **Infants born to hepatitis B surface antigen (HBsAg)-negative mothers** should receive the second dose of hepatitis B (Hep B) vaccine at least 1 month after the first dose. The third dose should be administered at least 4 months after the first dose and at least 2 months after the second dose, but not before age 6 months. **Infants born to HBsAg-positive mothers** should receive Hep B vaccine and 0.5 mL hepatitis B immune globulin (HBIG) within 12 hours of birth at separate injection sites. The second dose is recommended at 1-2 months and the third dose at 6 months. **Infants born to mothers whose HBsAg status is unknown** should receive Hep B vaccine within 12 hours of birth. Maternal blood should be drawn at the time of delivery to determine the mother's HBsAg status; if the HBsAg test is positive, the infant should receive HBIG as soon as possible (no later than age 1 week). All children and adolescents (through age 18 years) who have not been vaccinated against hepatitis B may begin the series during any visit. Special efforts should be made to vaccinate children who were born in or whose parents were born in areas of the world where hepatitis B virus infection is moderately or highly endemic.

§ Diphtheria and tetanus toxoids and acellular pertussis vaccine (DTaP) is the preferred vaccine for all doses in the vaccination series, including completion of the series in children who have received one or more doses of whole-cell diphtheria and tetanus toxoids and pertussis vaccine (DTP). Whole-cell DTP is an acceptable alternative to DTaP. The fourth dose (DTP or DTaP) may be administered as early as age 12 months, provided 6 months have elapsed since the third dose and if the child is unlikely to return at age 15-18 months. Tetanus and diphtheria toxoids (Td) is recommended at age 11-12 years if at least 5 years have elapsed since the last dose of DTP, DTaP, or DT. Subsequent routine Td boosters are recommended every 10 years.

¶ Three *Haemophilus influenzae* type b (Hib) conjugate vaccines are licensed for infant use. If Hib conjugate vaccine (PRP-OMP) (PedvaxHIB® or ComVax® [Merck]) is administered at ages 2 and 4 months, a dose at age 6 months is not required. Because clinical studies in infants have demonstrated that using some combination products may induce a lower immune response to the Hib vaccine component, DTaP/Hib combination products should not be used for primary vaccination in infants at ages 2, 4, or 6 months unless approved by the Food and Drug Administration for these ages.

** Two poliovirus vaccines are licensed in the United States: Inactivated poliovirus vaccine (IPV) and oral poliovirus vaccine (OPV). The ACIP, AAFP and AAP recommend that the first two doses of poliovirus vaccine should be IPV. The ACIP continues to recommend a sequential schedule of two doses of IPV administered at ages 2 and 4 months followed by two doses of OPV at age 12-18 months and age 4-6 years. Use of IPV for all doses also is acceptable and is recommended for immunocompromised persons and their household contacts. OPV is no longer recommended for the first two doses of the schedule and is acceptable only for special circumstances (eg, children of parents who do not accept the recommended number of injections, late initiation of vaccination that would require an unacceptable number of injections, and imminent travel to areas where poliomyelitis is endemic. OPV remains the vaccine of choice for mass vaccination campaigns to control outbreaks of wild poliovirus.

§§ The second dose of measles, mumps, and rubella vaccine (MMR) is recommended routinely at age 4-6 years but may be administered during any visit provided at least 4 weeks have elapsed since receipt of the first dose and that both doses are administered beginning at or after age 12 months. Those who have not previously received the second dose should complete the schedule no later than the routine visit to a health care provider at age 11-12 years.

¶¶ Varicella (Var) vaccine is recommended at any visit on or after the first birthday for susceptible children (ie those who lack a reliable history of chickenpox [as judged by a health care provider] and who have not been vaccinated). Susceptible persons aged ≥ 13 years should receive two doses given at least 4 weeks apart.

Source: Advisory Committee on Immunization Practices (ACIP), American Academy of Family Physicians (AAFP) and American Academy of Pediatrics (AAP).

FDA Pregnancy Categories

The rational use of any medication requires a risk versus benefit assessment. Among the myriad of risk factors which complicate this assessment, pregnancy is one of the most perplexing.

The FDA has established five categories to indicate the potential of a systemically absorbed drug for causing birth defects. The key differentiation among the categories rests upon the degree (reliability) of documentation and the risk vs benefit ratio. Pregnancy Category X is particularly notable in that if any data exists that may implicate a drug as a teratogen and the risk vs benefit ratio does not support use of the drug, the drug is contraindicated during pregnancy. These categories are summarized below:

FDA Pregnancy Categories	
Pregnancy Category	**Definition**
A	Controlled studies show no risk. Adequate, well-controlled studies in pregnant women have failed to demonstrate risk to the fetus.
B	No evidence of risk in humans. Either animal findings show risk, but human findings do not; or if no adequate human studies have been done, animal findings are negative.
C	Risk cannot be ruled out. Human studies are lacking, and animal studies are either positive for fetal risk or lacking. However, potential benefits may justify the potential risks.
D	Positive evidence of risk. Investigational or post-marketing data show risk to the fetus. Nevertheless, potential benefits may outweigh the potential risks. If needed in a life-threatening situation or a serious disease, the drug may be acceptable if safer drugs cannot be used or are ineffective.
X	Contraindicated in pregnancy. Studies in animals or human, or investigational or post-marketing reports have shown fetal risk which clearly outweighs any possible benefit to the patient.

Regardless of the designated Pregnancy Category or presumed safety, no drug should be administered during pregnancy unless it is clearly needed and potential benefits outweigh potential hazards to the fetus.

Controlled Substances

The Controlled Substances Act of 1970 regulates the manufacturing, distribution and dispensing of drugs that have abuse potential. The Drug Enforcement Administration (DEA) within the US Department of Justice is the chief federal agency responsible for enforcing the act.

DEA Schedules: Drugs under jurisdiction of the Controlled Substances Act are divided into five schedules based on their potential for abuse and physical and psychological dependence. All controlled substances listed in *Drug Facts and Comparisons®* are identified by schedule as follows:

Schedule I *(c-I):* High abuse potential and no accepted medical use (eg, heroin, marijuana, LSD).

Schedule II *(c-II):* High abuse potential with severe dependence liability (eg, narcotics, amphetamines, dronabinol, some barbiturates).

Schedule III *(c-III):* Less abuse potential than schedule II drugs and moderate dependence liability (eg, nonbarbiturate sedatives, nonamphetamine stimulants, limited amounts of certain narcotics).

Schedule IV *(c-IV):* Less abuse potential than schedule III drugs and limited dependence liability (eg, some sedatives, antianxiety agents, nonnarcotic analgesics).

Schedule V *(c-V):* Limited abuse potential. Primarily small amounts of narcotics (codeine) used as antitussives or antidiarrheals. Under federal law, limited quantities of certain *c-v* drugs may be purchased without a prescription directly from a pharmacist if allowed under state statutes. The purchaser must be at least 18 years of age and must furnish suitable identification. All such transactions must be recorded by the dispensing pharmacist.

Registration: Prescribing physicians and dispensing pharmacies must be registered with the DEA, PO Box 28083, Central Station, Washington, DC 20005.

Inventory: Separate records must be kept of purchases and dispensing of controlled substances. An inventory of controlled substances must be made every 2 years.

Prescriptions: Prescriptions for controlled substances must be written in ink and include: Date; name and address of the patient; name, address and DEA number of the physician. Oral prescriptions must be promptly committed to writing. Controlled substance prescriptions may not be dispensed or refilled more than 6 months after the date issued or be refilled more than five times. A written prescription signed by the physician is required for schedule II drugs. In case of emergency, oral prescriptions for schedule II substances may be filled; however, the physician must provide a signed prescription within 72 hours. Schedule II prescriptions cannot be refilled. A triplicate order form is necessary for the transfer of controlled substances in schedule II. Forms are available for the individual prescriber at no charge from the DEA.

State Laws: In many cases state laws are more restrictive than federal laws and therefore impose additional requirements (eg, triplicate prescription forms).

Radio-Contrast Media

Generic Name	Dose Form	Trade Name	Manufacturer
Barium sulfate	Powder	Baroflave	Lannett
Barium sulfate	Powder	various	various
Barium sulfate	Suspension	E-Z-CAT	E-Z-EM
Barium sulfate	Suspension	E-Z-Paque	E-Z-EM
Barium sulfate	Suspension	Intropaque	Lafayette
Barium sulfate	Suspension	Novopaque	Picker
Barium sulfate	Suspension	Polibar-Plus	E-Z-EM
Barium sulfate	Suspension	Preview	Lafayette
Barium sulfate	Suspension	Redi-CAT	E-Z-Em
Barium sulfate	Suspension	Sol-O-Pake	E-Z-EM
Barium sulfate 1.5%	Suspension	Baro-Cat	Lafayette
Barium sulfate 1.5%	Suspension	PrepCat	Lafayette
Barium sulfate 46%	Granules	Baros	Lafayette
Barium sulfate 5%	Suspension	EneCat	Lafayette
Barium sulfate 5%	Suspension	TomoCat	Lafayette
Barium sulfate 50%	Suspension	Entrobar	Lafayette
Barium sulfate 60%	Suspension	Barosperse Liq.	Lafayette
Barium sulfate 85%	Suspension	HD 85	Lafayette
Barium sulfate 91%	Powder	Intropaque	Lafayette
Barium sulfate 92.5%	Powder	Barotrast	Armour
Barium sulfate 92%	Powder	Micropaque	Picker
Barium sulfate 95%	Powder	Barosperse	Lafayette
Barium sulfate 95%	Powder	E-Z-Paque	E-Z-EM
Barium sulfate 95%	Powder	Tonopaque	Lafayette
Barium sulfate 95%	Powder	Ultra-R	E-Z-EM
Barium sulfate 96%	Powder	Baroloid	Lafayette
Barium sulfate 96%	Powder	Mixture III	Picker
Barium sulfate 96%	Powder	Polibar	E-Z-EM
Barium sulfate 97%	Powder	Barodense	Lafayette
Barium sulfate 97%	Powder	Sol-O-Pake	E-Z-EM
Barium sulfate 97%	Suspension	Barobag	Lafayette
Barium sulfate 98%	Powder	Baricon	Lafayette
Barium sulfate 98%	Powder	HD 200 Plus	Lafayette
Barium sulfate 100%	Paste	Anatrast	Lafayette
Barium sulfate 100%	Suspension	Flo-Coat	Lafayette
Barium sulfate 100%	Suspension	Liquipake	Lafayette
Barium sulfate 150%	Suspension	Epi-C	Lafayette
Diatrizoate meglumine	Injection	Angiovist 282	Berlex
Diatrizoate meglumine	Injection	Cystografin	Squibb
Diatrizoate meglumine	Injection	Hypaque Meglumine 30%	Nycomed
Diatrizoate meglumine	Injection	Hypaque Meglumine 60%	Nycomed
Diatrizoate meglumine	Injection	Hypaque-Cysto	Nycomed
Diatrizoate meglumine	Injection	Hypaque-M 18%	Nycomed

Generic Name	Dose Form	Trade Name	Manufacturer
Diatrizoate meglumine	Injection	Hypaque-M 30%	Nycomed
Diatrizoate meglumine	Injection	Hypaque-M 60%	Nycomed
Diatrizoate meglumine	Injection	Reno-Dip	Squibb
Diatrizoate meglumine	Injection	Reno-M-60	Squibb
Diatrizoate meglumine	Injection	Urovist Cysto	Berlex
Diatrizoate meglumine	Injection	Urovist Meglumine DIU/CT	Berlex
Diatrizoate meglumine & Iodipamide meglumine	Injection	Sinografin	Squibb
Diatrizoate meglumine & sodium	Injection	Angiovist 292	Berlex
Diatrizoate meglumine & sodium	Injection	Angiovist 370	Berlex
Diatrizoate meglumine & sodium	Injection	Gastrografin	Squibb
Diatrizoate meglumine & sodium	Injection	Gastrovist	Berlex
Diatrizoate meglumine & sodium	Injection	Hypaque-76	Nycomed
Diatrizoate meglumine & sodium	Injection	Hypaque-M 75%	Nycomed
Diatrizoate meglumine & sodium	Injection	Hypaque-M 76%	Nycomed
Diatrizoate meglumine & sodium	Injection	MD-76	Mallinckrodt
Diatrizoate meglumine & sodium	Injection	MD-Gastroview	Mallinckrodt
Diatrizoate meglumine & sodium	Injection	Renografin-60	Squibb
Diatrizoate meglumine & sodium	Injection	Renografin-76	Squibb
Diatrizoate meglumine & sodium	Injection	Renovist	Squibb
Diatrizoate meglumine & sodium	Injection	Renovist II	Squibb
Diatrizoate sodium	Injection	Hypaque Oral (Canada)	Nycomed
Diatrizoate sodium	Injection	Hypaque Sodium 25%	Nycomed
Diatrizoate sodium	Injection	Hypaque Sodium 50%	Nycomed
Diatrizoate sodium	Injection	Hypaque Sodium Oral Powder	Nycomed
Diatrizoate sodium	Injection	Hypaque Sodium Oral Solution	Nycomed
Diatrizoate sodium	Injection	Urovist Sodium 300	Berlex
Ethiodized oil	Injection	Ethiodol	Savage
Iocetamic acid	Tablets	Cholebrine	Mallinckrodt
Iodamide meglumine	Injection	Renovue-65	Squibb
Iodipamide meglumine	Injection	Cholografin	Squibb
Iodixanol	Injection	Visipaque	Nycomed
Iohexol	Injection	Omnipaque	Nycomed
Iopamidol	Injection	Isovue-128	Squibb
Iopamidol	Injection	Isovue-200	Squibb

Generic Name	Dose Form	Trade Name	Manufacturer
Iopamidol	Injection	Isovue-300	Squibb
Iopamidol	Injection	Isovue-370	Squibb
Iopamidol	Injection	Isovue-M 200	Squibb
Iopamidol	Injection	Isovue-M 300	Squibb
Iopanoic acid	Tablet	Telepaque	Nycomed
Iopental		Imagopaque	Nycomed
Iopromide	Injection	Ultravist	Berlex
Iothalamate meglumine	Injection	Conray	Mallinckrodt
Iothalamate meglumine	Injection	Conray-30	Mallinckrodt
Iothalamate meglumine	Injection	Conray-43	Mallinckrodt
Iothalamate meglumine	Injection	Conray-60	Mallinckrodt
Iothalamate meglumine	Injection	Cysto-Conray	Mallinckrodt
Iothalamate meglumine	Injection	Cysto-Conray II	Mallinckrodt
Iothalamate meglumine & sodium	Injection	Vascoray	Mallinckrodt
Iothalamate sodium	Injection	Angio-Conray	Mallinckrodt
Iothalamate sodium	Injection	Conray-325	Mallinckrodt
Iothalamate sodium	Injection	Conray-400	Mallinckrodt
Ioversol	Injection	Optiray 160	Mallinckrodt
Ioversol	Injection	Optiray 240	Mallinckrodt
Ioversol	Injection	Optiray 320	Mallinckrodt
Ioversol	Injection	Optiray 350	Mallinckrodt
Ioxaglate meglumine & sodium	Injection	Hexabrix	Mallinckrodt
Ioxaglate meglumine & sodium	Injection	Hexabrix 200	Mallinckrodt
Ioxaglate meglumine & sodium	Injection	Hexabrix 320	Mallinckrodt
Ipodate calcium	Granules	Oragrafin	Squibb
Ipodate sodium	Capsules	Bilivist	Berlex
Ipodate sodium	Capsules	Oragrafin Sodi.	Squibb
Isosulfan blue	Injection	Lymphazurin	Hirsch Industries
Metrizamide	Powder for Inj	Amipaque	Nycomed
Polyvinyl chloride	Capsules	Sitzmarks	Konsyl Pharm
Propyliodone in peanut oil	Suspension	Dionosil Oily	Allen & Hanburys
Tyropanoate sodium	Capsules	Bilopaque	Nycomed
nd		Iopamiron	Berlex

nd = No data available.

Radio-Isotopes

Active Isotope	Generic Name	Dose Form or Packaging	Trade Name	Manufacturer
18-F	Fluorine F-18	Injection	nd	Medi-Physics
32-P	Chromic Phosphate P-32	Suspension	Phosphocol P32	Mallinckrodt
		Injection	Phosphotope	Squibb
		Oral Solution	Phosphotope	Squibb
32-P	Sodium Phosphate P-32	Capsules	nd	Mallinckrodt
		Oral Solution	nd	Mallinckrodt
51-Cr	Sodium Chromate Cr-51	Injection	Chromitope	Squibb
		Injection	nd	Mallinckrodt
57-Co	Cyanocobalamin Co-57	Capsules	nd	Mallinckrodt
		Kit	Rubratope-57	Squibb
57&58-Co	Cyanocobalamin Co-57 & Co-58	Kit	Dicopac Kit	Amersham
59-Fe	Ferrous Citrate Fe-59	Injection	nd	Mallinckrodt
60-Co	Cyanocobalamin Co-60	Capsules	Rubratope-60	Squibb
67-Ga	Gallium Citrate Ga-67	Injection	nd	DuPont-Merck
		Injection	nd	Mallinckrodt
		Injection	nd	Medi-Physics
		Injection	Neoscan	Medi-Physics
75-Se	Selenomethionine Se-75	Injection	Sethotope	Squibb
		Injection	nd	Mallinckrodt
		Injection	nd	Medi-Physics
81m-Kr	Krypton Kr-81m	Gas Generator	nd	Medi-Physics
82-Sr&Rb	Strontium Sr-82/Rubidium Rb-82	Generator	Cardiogen-82	Squibb
89-Sr	Strontium Chloride Sr-89	Injection	Metastron	Medi-Physics/ Amersham
99m-Tc	Technetium Tc-99m	Generator	nd	Cintichem
		Generator (fission)	nd	DuPont-Merck
		Generator (neutron)	nd	DuPont-Merck
		Generator	Ultra-TechneKow	Mallinckrodt
		Generator	Minitec II	Squibb
		Generator	Technetope II	Squibb
99m-Tc	Technetium-99m Albumin Aggegated	Kit	AN Stannous Ag.	Benedict Nuclear
		Kit	nd	CIS-US
		Kit	Pulmolite	DuPont-Merck
		Kit	TechneScan MAA	Mallinckrodt
		Kit	Lungaggregate Reagent	Medi-Physics
		Kit	nd	Merck
		Kit	Macrotec	Squibb
99m-Tc	Technetium-99m Albumin Colloid	Kit	Microlite	DuPont-Merck
99m-Tc	Technetium-99m Arcitumomab	Kit	CEA-Scan	Immuno-medics/ Mallinckrodt
99m-Tc	Technetium-99m Serum Albumin	Kit	nd	Medi-Physics

Active Isotope	Generic Name	Dose Form or Packaging	Trade Name	Manufacturer
99m-Tc	Technetium-99m Bicisate	Kit	Neurolite	DuPont-Merck
99m-Tc	Technetium-99m Disofenin	Kit	Hepatolite	DuPont-Merck
99m-Tc	Technetium-99m Etidronate	Kit		
		Kit	Tc-99m Diphos-phonate-Tin	Medi-Physics
		Kit	Tc-99m HEDSPA	Medi-Physics
		Kit	Stannous Diphosphonate	Medi-Physics
99m-Tc	Technetium-99m Exametazime	Kit	Ceretec	Amersham
99m-Tc	Technetium-99m Lidofenin	Kit	TechneScan HIDA	Merck
99m-Tc	Technetium-99m Mebrofenin	Kit	Choletec	Squibb
99m-Tc	Technetium-99m Medronate	Kit	Amer-Scan MDP	Amersham
		Kit	AN-MDP	CIS-US
		Kit	Osteolite	DuPont-Merck
		Kit	nd	Medi-Physics
		Kit	TechneScan MDP	Merck
		Kit	MDP-Squibb	Squibb
99m-Tc	Technetium-99m Mertiatide	Kit	TechneScan MAG3	Mallinckrodt
99m-Tc	Technetium-99m Oxidronate	Kit	Ostescan HDP	Mallinckrodt
99m-Tc	Technetium-99m Pentetate Sodium	Kit	AN-DTPA	CIS-US
		Kit	MPI DTPA Kit	Medi-Physics
		Kit	TechneScan DTPA	Merck
		Kit	Techneplex	Squibb
		Kit	Renotec-Iron	Squibb
			Ascorbate-DTPA	nd
99m-Tc	Tc-99m Pyro- & Trimeta- Phos-phates	Kit	AN-Pyrotec	CIS-US
		Kit	Pyrolite	DuPont-Merck
		Kit	TechneScan PYP	Mallinckrodt
		Kit	Tc-99m Poly-phosphate	Medi-Physics
		Kit	Phosphotec	Squibb
99m-Tc	Technetium-99m Red Blood Cell	Kit	RBC-Scan	Cadema Med.
		Kit	Ultratag	Mallinckrodt
99m-Tc	Technetium-99m Sestamibi	Kit	Cardiolite	DuPont-Merck
99m-Tc	Technetium-99m Sodium Gluceptate	Kit	Glucoscan	DuPont-Merck
		Kit	Technescan Gluceptate	Merck
99m-Tc	Technetium-99m Succimer	Kit	Tc-99m DMSA	Medi-Physics

Active Isotope	Generic Name	Dose Form or Packaging	Trade Name	Manufacturer
99m-Tc	Technetium-99m Sulfur Colloid	Injection	nd	CIS-US
		Injection	nd	Mallinckrodt
		Injection	nd	Medi-Physics
		Inj. & Kit	nd	Medi-Physics
		Kit	nd	CIS-US
		Kit	TSC	Medi-Physics
		Kit	TechneColl	Mallinckrodt
		Kit	Tesuloid	Squibb
99m-Tc	Technetium-99m Teboroxime	Kit	CardioTec	Squibb
99m-Tc	Sodium Pertechnetate Tc-99m	Injection	nd	CIS-US
		Injection	nd	Mallinckrodt
		Injection	nd	Medi-Physics
99m-Tc	Tc-99m Nofetumomab Merpentan	Kit	Verluma	NeoRx/ DuPont Merck
111-In	Indium-111 Capromab Pendetide	Kit	ProstaScint	Cytogen
111-In	Indium-111 Imciromab Pentetate	Kit	Myoscint	Centocor
111-In	Indium-111 Oxine	Solution	nd	Amersham
111-In	Indium-111 Oxyquinoline Sodium	Solution	nd	Amersham
111-In	Indium-111 Pentetate Disodium	Injection	In-111 DTPA	Medi-Physics
111-In	Indium-111 Pentetreotide	Injection	OctreoScan	Mallinckrodt
111-In	In-111 Satumomab Pentetide	Injection	OncoScint CR/OV	Cytogen
123-I	Sodium Iodide-123	Capsules	nd	Benedict Nuclear
		Capsules	nd	Mallinckrodt
		Capsules	nd	Medi-Physics
123-I	Iohippurate Sodium I-123	Injection	Nephroflow	Medi-Physics
123-I	Iofetamine HCl I-123	Injection	Spectamine	Medi-Physics
125-I	Iothalamate Sodium I-125	Injection	Glofil-125	Iso-Tex
125-I	Iodinated Albumin I-125	Injection	Jeanatope 125-I	Iso-Tex
		Injection	nd	Mallinckrodt
125-I	Iodinated Fibrinogen I-125	Injection	Ibrin	Amersham
127-Xe	Xenon Xe-127	Gas	nd	Mallinckrodt
131-I	Iodinated Albumin I-131	Injection	Megatope	Iso-Tex
131-I	Iodinated-131 Albumin Aggegated	Injection	Albumitope L-S.	Squibb
131-I	Iodohippurate Sodium I-131	Injection	nd	CIS-US
		Injection	Hippuran	Mallinckrodt
		Injection	Hipputope	Squibb
131-I	Rose Bengal Sodium I-131	Injection	Robengatope	Squibb
131-I	Sodium Iodide I-131	Capsules	nd	CIS-US
		Capsules	nd	Mallinckrodt
		Capsules	nd	Squibb

Active Isotope	Generic Name	Dose Form or Packaging	Trade Name	Manufacturer
		Capsules	nd	Syncor
		Oral Solution	nd	CIS-US
		Oral Solution	nd	Mallinckrodt
		Oral Solution	nd	Squibb
		Oral Solution	nd	Syncor
133-Xe	Xenon Xe-133	Injection	nd	DuPont-Merck
		Gas	nd	DuPont-Merck
		Gas	nd	General Electric
		Gas	nd	Mallinckrodt
		Gas	nd	Medi-Physics
		Kit (V.S.S.)	nd	Medi-Physics
197-Hg	Chlormerodrin Hg-197	Injection	nd	Squibb
198-Au	Gold Au-198	Injection	Aureotope	Squibb
201-Tl	Thallous Chloride Tl-201	Injection	nd	DuPont-Merck
		Injection	nd	Mallinckrodt
		Injection	nd	Medi-Physics
		Injection	nd	Squibb

nd = No data available.

Agents for Imaging

Agents for MRI Imaging				
Active Isotope	*Generic Name*	*Dose Form*	*Trade Name*	*Manufacturer*
	Gadodiamide & caldiamide sodium	Injection	Omniscan	Sanofi Ny
	Gadopentetate dimeglumine	Injection	Magnevist	Berlex
	Gadoteridol & calteridol calcium	Injection	ProHance	Squibb
	Perflubron	Liquid	Imagent GI	Alliance
	Ferumoxides (investigational)		Feridex	Nycomed
Agents for PET Imaging				
13-N	Nitrogen	nd	nd	nd
15-O	Oxygen	nd	nd	nd
18-F	Fludeoxyglucose [2-fluoro(F-18)-2-deoxyglucose]	nd	nd	nd
82-Rb	Rubidium	nd	nd	nd
Agents for Ultrasonic Imaging				
	Perfluorodecalin & Perfluorotripropylamine		Fluosol-DA	nd
	Investigational		Levovist	Berlex
	Investigational		Cavisomes	Berlex

nd = No data available.

Pharmaceutical Company Labeler Code Index

LISTED IN NUMERICAL ORDER

00002
Eli Lilly and Co.

00003
Apothecon, Inc.
Braccho Diagnostics
Bristol-Myers Squibb
ConvaTec
Westwood Squibb Pharmaceuticals

00004
Roche Laboratories

00005
ESI Lederle Generics
Lederle Laboratories

00006
Merck & Co.

00007
Connetics
SmithKline Beecham Pharmaceuticals

00008
Wyeth-Ayerst Laboratories

00009
Upjohn Co.
See Pharmacia & Upjohn

00011
Becton Dickinson Microbiology Systems

00013
Pharmacia & Upjohn

00014
Searle

00015
Apothecon, Inc.

00016
Pharmacia & Upjohn

00017
Wampole Laboratories

00019
Mallinckrodt Medical, Inc.

00021
Reed & Carnrick
See Schwarz Pharma

00023
Allergan Herbert
Allergan, Inc.

00024
Sanofi Winthrop Pharmaceuticals

00025
Searle

00026
Bayer Corporation (Biological Division and Pharmaceutical Division)

00028
Geigy Pharmactuticals
See Novartis

00029
SmithKline Beecham Pharmaceuticals

00031
A.H. Robins, Inc.
Whitehall Robins Laboratories
Wyeth-Ayerst Laboratories

00032
Solvay
Scherer

00033
Roche Laboratories
Syntex Laboratories

00034
Purdue Frederick Co.

00037
Wallace Laboratories

00039
Hoechst-Marion Roussel

00041
Oral-B Laboratories, Inc.

00043
Sandoz Consumer
See Novartis

00044
Knoll

00045
McNeil Consumer Products Co.

00047
Warner Chilcott Laboratories
Watson Laboratories

00048
Knoll

00049
Roerig
See Pfizer

00052
Organon, Inc.

00053
Centeon

00054
Roxane Laboratories, Inc.

00056
Du Pont Pharma

00062
Advance Biofactures Corp.
Ortho McNeil Corp.

00064
Healthpoint Medical

00065
Alcon Laboratories, Inc.

00066
Dermik Laboratories, Inc.
See Arcola

00067
Novartis Consumer

00068
Hoechst-Marion Roussel

00069
Pfizer US Pharmaceutical Group

00070
Arcola Laboratories

00071
Parke-Davis
Warner Lambert Co.

00072
Westwood Squibb Pharmaceuticals

00074
Abbott Diagnostics
Abbott Hospital Products
Abbott Laboratories
Ross Laboratories

00075
Rhone-Poulenc Rorer Pharmaceuticals, Inc.

00076
Star Pharmaceuticals, Inc.

00078
Sandoz Pharmaceuticals
See Novartis

00081
GlaxoWellcome

00083
Ciba-Geigy Pharmaceuticals
Novartis Consumer
Novartis Pharmaceutical
Rhone-Poulenc Rorer Pharmaceuticals, Inc.

00085
Key Pharmaceuticals
Schering Plough Healthcare Products

00086
Carnrick Laboratories, Inc.

00087
Bristol-Myers Squibb
Mead Johnson Nutritionals

00088
Hoechst-Marion Roussel

00089
3M Personal Healthcare Products
3M Pharmaceutical

00091
Schwarz Pharma

00093
Lemmon Co.
See Teva Pharmaceuticals USA

00094
Du Pont Merck Pharmaceutical

00095
ECR Pharmaceuticals

00096
Person and Covey, Inc.

00108
SmithKline Beecham Pharmaceuticals

00115
Global Pharmaceutical

00116
Xttrium Laboratories, Inc.

00118
Bayer Corporation (Allergy Division)

00121
Pharmaceutical Associates, Inc.

00122
Rexall Group

00127
Ulmer Pharmacal Co.

00128
SmithKline Beecham Pharmaceuticals

00131
Central Pharmaceuticals, Inc.
Schwarz Pharma

00132
C. B. Fleet, Inc.

00137
Johnson & Johnson

00140
Roche Laboratories

00145
Stiefel Laboratories, Inc.

00147
Camall Co., Inc.

00149
Procter & Gamble Pharm.

00150
Murray Drug Corp.

00152
Gray Pharmaceutical Co.
See Purdue Frederick

00154
Blair Laboratories

00161
Bayer Corp. (Biological and Pharmaceutical Div.)

00163
ICN Pharmaceuticals, Inc.
Zeneca Pharmaceuticals

00164
Carter Wallace

00165
Blaine Co., Inc.

00168
E. Fougera and Co.

00169
Novo Nordisk Pharm., Inc.

00172
Zenith Goldline Laboratories, Inc.

00173
Cerenex Pharmaceuticals
GlaxoWellcome

00178
Mission Pharmacal Co.

00182
Goldline Laboratories, Inc.
See Zenith Goldline

00185
Eon Labs Manufacturing, Inc.

00186
Astra USA, Inc.

00187
ICN Pharmaceuticals, Inc.
Zeneca Pharmaceuticals

00192
Bayer Corp. (Biological and Pharmaceutical Div.)

00193
Bayer Corp. (Diagnostic Division)

00205
Immunex Corp.

00209
Marsam Pharmaceuticals, Inc.

00212
Sandoz Nutrition Corp.
See Novartis

00223
Consolidated Midland Corp.

00224
Konsyl Pharmaceuticals

00225
B. F. Ascher and Co.

00228
Purepac Pharmaceutical Co.
See Faulding Purepac Pharmaceutical Co.

00234
Schmid Products Co.
See Durex

00245
Upsher-Smith Labs, Inc.

00252
Jones Medical Industries

00254
Gambro, Inc.

00256
Fleming & Co.

00258
Forest Pharmaceuticals, Inc.
Inwood Laboratories

00259
Mayrand, Inc.
See Merz Pharmaceuticals

00264
McGaw, Inc.

00268
Center Laboratories

00273
Lovvic Co.
See Young Dental

00274
Scherer Laboratories, Inc.

00275
Arco Pharmaceuticals, Inc.

00276
Misemer Pharmaceuticals, Inc.
See Edwards Pharmaceuticals

00277
Laser, Inc.

00281
Savage Laboratories

00283
Beutlich, Inc.

00288
Fluoritab Corp.

00295
Denison Laboratories, Inc.

00299
Galderma Laboratories, Inc.

00300
Tap Pharmaceuticals

00304
J.J. Balan, Inc.

00310
Zeneca Pharmaceuticals

00314
Hyrex Pharmaceuticals

00316
Del-Ray Laboratory, Inc.

00327
United Guardian Laboratories

00332
Teva Pharmaceuticals USA

00346
Ciba Vision Ophthalmics

00348
Medtech Laboratories, Inc.

00349
Parmed Pharmaceuticals, Inc.

00362
Novocol Chemical Mfr. Co.

00364
Schein Pharmaceutical, Inc.

00372
Scot-Tussin Pharmacal, Inc.

00374
Lyne Laboratories

00378
Mylan Pharmaceuticals

00386
Gebauer Co.

00394
Mericon Industries, Inc.

00395
Humco Holding Group, Inc.

00396
Milex Products, Inc.

00398
C & M Pharmacal, Inc.

00402
Steris Laboratories, Inc.

00406
Mallinckrodt Chemical

00407
Nycomed Inc.

00418
Pasadena Research Labs
Taylor Pharmaceuticals

00421
Fielding Co.

00426
Morton Grove Pharmaceuticals

00430
Warner Chilcott Laboratories

00433
Research Industries Corp.

00436
Century Pharmaceuticals, Inc.

00451
Muro Pharmaceutical, Inc.

00456
Forest Pharmaceutical, Inc.

00463
C. O. Truxton, Inc.

00469
Fujisawa USA, Inc.

00482
Kenwood Laboratories
See Doak

00485
Edwards Pharmaceuticals, Inc.

00486
Beach Products

00487
Nephron Pharmaceuticals Corp.

00496
Ferndale Laboratories, Inc.

00501
Warner Lambert Co.

00514
Dow Hickam, Inc.
See Bertek Pharmaceuticals Inc.

00516
Glenwood, Inc.

00517
American Regent

00521
Chesebrough-Pond's USA, Inc.
See Unilever HCP

00524
Knoll

00527
Lannett, Inc.

00535
Forest Pharmaceuticals, Inc.

00536
Eon Labs Manufacturing, Inc.
Rugby Labs, Inc.
See Watson

00537
Spencer Mead, Inc.
See Rugby

00548
I.M.S., Ltd.
See Medeva

00551
Seatrace Pharmaceuticals

00555
Barr Laboratories, Inc.

00563
Bock Pharmacal Co.

00573
Whitehall Robins Laboratories

00574
P&S Laboratories, Inc.

00575
Baker Norton Pharmaceuticals

00576
Medical Products Panamericana

00585
Fisons Corp.
See Medeva Pharmaceuticals

00588
Keene Pharmaceuticals, Inc.

00591
Schein Pharmaceutical, Inc.

00597
Boehringer Ingelheim, Inc.

00598
Health for Life Brands, Inc.

00603
Qualitest Products, Inc.

00615
Vangard Labs, Inc.

00619
Walker Pharmacal Co.

00641
Elkins-Sinn, Inc.
See Wyeth-Ayerst

00642
Everett Laboratories, Inc.

00659
Circle Pharmaceuticals, Inc.

00663
Pfizer US Pharmaceutical Group

00677
Circa Pharmaceuticals, Inc.
United Research Laboratories

00682
Marnel Pharmaceuticals, Inc.
Mikart, Inc.

00684
Primedics Laboratories

00686
Raway Pharmacal, Inc.

00689
Daniels Pharmaceuticals
See Jones Medical

00703
Gensia Sicor Pharmaceuticals, Inc.

00713
G & W Laboratories

00725
Circa Pharmaceuticals, Inc.

00731
Alto Pharmaceuticals, Inc.

00741
Walker, Corp. and, Inc.

00766
SmithKline Beecham Consumer Healthcare

00777
Dista Products Co.
See Eli Lilly

00781
Geneva Pharmaceuticals

00802
Emerson Laboratories

00813
Phamavite

00814
Interstate Drug Exchange
See Henry Schein, Inc.

00832
Morton Grove Pharmaceuticals
Rosemont Pharmaceutical Corp.

00837
Columbia Laboratories, Inc.

00839
H.L. Moore Drug Exchange, Inc.

00879
Halsey Drug Co.

00884
Pedinol Pharmacal, Inc.

00904
Major Pharmaceuticals

00905
SCS Pharmaceuticals

00917
Wesley Pharmacal, Inc.

00918
General Medical Corp.

00927
Pfeiffer Co.

00938
Davis and Geck
See Sherwood Davis and Geck

00944
Baxter Hyland

00978
SmithKline Diagnostics
See Beckman Coulter Primary Diagnostics

00998
Alcon Laboratories, Inc.
PolyMedica Pharmaceuticals

01020
Cumberland Packing Corp.

05745
C.R. Bard, Inc. Urological Div.
Nastech Pharmaceutical, Inc.

05973
Nabi

08026
Smith & Nephew United
See Smith & Nephew Wound Management Inc.

08884
Sherwood Davis & Geck
Sherwood Medical
See Kendall Healthcare

10019
Ohmeda Pharmaceuticals
See Baxter

10038
Ambix Laboratories, Inc.

10106
J.T. Baker, Inc.
See Mallinckrodt-Baker

10116
Bartor Pharmacal Co.

10118
Norstar Consumer Products

10119
Bausch & Lomb Personal Products Division

10157
Blistex, Inc.

10158
Block Drug Co., Inc.

10160
Bluco Inc./Med. Discnt. Outlet

10223
Cetylite Industries, Inc.

10310
Del Pharmaceuticals, Inc.

10331
E. E. Dickinson Co.

10337
Doak Dermatologics

10356
Beiersdorf, Inc.

10432
Freeda Vitamins, Inc.

10481
Gordon Laboratories

10486
C. S. Dent & Co. Division

10651
Lavoptik, Inc.

10706
Manne

10712
Marlyn Neutraceuticals, Inc.

10742
Mentholatum, Inc.

10797
Oakhurst Co.

10812
Neutrogena Corp.

10865
Parthenon, Inc.

10888
Advanced Nutritional Technology

10952
Recsei Laboratories

10956
Reese Pharmaceutical Co., Inc.

10961
Requa, Inc.

10974
Pegasus Medical, Inc.

11012
Schaffer Laboratories

11017
Schering-Plough Corp.
Schering-Plough Healthcare Products

11086
Summers Laboratories, Inc.

41000
Schering-Plough Corp.

41100
Schering-Plough Healthcare Products
Schering-Plough Corp.

41383
AKPharma, Inc.
Lactaid, Inc.

41785
Unimed

42987
Roche Laboratories
Syntex Laboratories

43656
Cambridge Nutraceuticals, Inc.

43786
Consep Inc.

44087
Serono Laboratories, Inc.

44184
Bajamar Chemical, Inc.

44437
Bolan Pharmaceutical, Inc.

44800
Cumberland Packing Corp.

45334
Pharmaceutical Specialties, Inc.

45565
Med-Derm Pharmaceuticals

45617
Breath Asure, Inc.

45802
Clay-Park Labs, Inc.

46287
Carolina Medical Products

46500
Rydelle Laboratories
See S.C. Johnson Wax

46672
Mikart, Inc.

47144
Polymer Technology Corp.

47992
Holles Laboratories, Inc.

48028
Redi-Products Labs
See Aplicare Inc.

48532
Delmont Laboratories, Inc.

48723
Apothecus, Inc.

49072
McGuff, Inc.

49158
Thames Pharmacal, Inc.

49281
Connaught Labs

49336
Den-Mat Corporation

49447
Chattem Consumer Products

49483
Time-Cap Labs, Inc.

49502
Dey Laboratories, Inc.

49669
Alpha Therapeutic Corp.

49727
Vita-Rx Corp.

49730
Hercon Laboratories, Inc.

49884
Par Pharmaceuticals

49938
Jacobus Pharmaceutical Co.

50111
Sidmak Laboratories, Inc.

50242
Genentech, Inc.

50289
Birchwood Laboratories, Inc.

50361
Connaught Labs

50383
Health Care Products
Hi-Tech Pharmacal

50419
Berlex Laboratories, Inc.

50458
Janssen Pharmaceutical, Inc.

50474
Whitby Pharmaceuticals, Inc.
See UCB Pharmaceuticals, Inc.

50486
Blairex Labs, Inc.

50520
Optimox Corp.

50694
Seres Laboratories

50914
Iso Tex Diagnostics, Inc.

50930
Parnell Pharmaceuticals, Inc.

50962
Xactdose, Inc.

51079
UDL Laboratories, Inc.

51201
American Dermal Corp.

51284
Zila Pharmaceuticals, Inc.

51285
Duramed Pharmaceuticals

51301
Great Southern Laboratories

51318
Stellar Pharmacal Corp.

51479
Dura Pharmaceuticals

51641
Alra Laboratories, Inc.

51655
Pharmaceutical Corp.

51662
Healthfirst Corp.

51672
Taro Pharmaceuticals USA, Inc.

51687
Fischer Pharmaceuticals, Inc.

51801
Nomax, Inc.

51875
Royce Laboratories, Inc.
See Watson

51991
Breckenridge Pharmaceutical, Inc.

52041
Dayton Laboratories, Inc.

52152
Amide Pharmaceuticals, Inc.

52189
Invamed, Inc.

52238
Optopics Laboratories, Corp.

52268
Braintree Laboratories, Inc.

52311
Biosearch Medical Products

52512
Harmony Laboratories

52544
Watson Laboratories

52555
Martec Pharmaceutical, Inc.

52584
General Injectables & Vaccines

52604
Jones Medical Industries

52637
Hauser Pharmaceutical Inc.

52747
US Pharmaceutical Corp.

52761
GenDerm Corp.
See Medicis

52769
American Red Cross

53124
Lederle-Praxis Biologicals

53159
Palisades Pharmaceuticals, Inc.
See Glenwood

53169
Boehringer Mannheim Corp., Therapeutics Div.
Monarch Pharmaceuticals

53191
Biostar, Inc.

53258
VHA Co.

53335
Tyson & Associates, Inc.

53385
Standard Drug Co./Family Pharmacy

53489
Mutual Pharmaceutical, Inc.

53905
Behring GmbH & Co.
Chiron Therapeutics

53926
Steris Labs

53978
Med-Pro, Inc.

53983
Natren, Inc.

54022
Vitaline Corp.

54092
Roberts Pharmaceuticals
Schering-Plough Corp.

54129
Immuno U.S., Inc.

54323
Flanders, Inc.

54391
R & D Laboratories, Inc.

54429
Chase Laboratories

54482
Sigma-Tau Pharmaceuticals, Inc.

54569
Allscrips

54627
ValMed, Inc.

54686
Ethitek Pharmaceuticals

54799
Cynacon/OCuSOFT

54807
R.I.D., Inc.

54838
Silarx Pharmaceuticals, Inc.

54891
Vision Pharmaceuticals, Inc.

54921
IPR Pharmaceuticals, Inc.

54964
Murdock, Madaus, Schwabe

55053
Econolab

55299
Kingswood Laboratories, Inc.

55326
3M Personal Healthcare Products
Curatek Pharm.

55390
Bedford Laboratories

55422
Pharmakon Laboratories, Inc.

55499
Numark Laboratories, Inc.

55505
Kramer Laboratories, Inc.

55513
Amgen, Inc.

55515
Oclassen Pharmaceuticals, Inc.
See Watson Laboratories

55553
Clint Pharmaceutical

55559
Calgon Vestal Laboratories

55566
Ferring Laboratories, Inc.
See Ferring Pharmaceuticals

55688
Speywood Pharmaceuticals, Inc.

55806
Effcon Labs, Inc.

55953
Novopharm USA, Inc.

55994
Dakryon Pharmaceuticals

56091
Johnson & Johnson Medical

56146
Nexstar

57145
CNS Inc.

57267
Summit Pharmaceuticals
See Novartis

57317
Fujisawa USA, Inc.

57480
Medirex, Inc.

57506
American Drug Industries, Inc.

57664
Caraco Pharmaceutical Labs

57665
Enzon, Inc.

57706
Storz
See Bausch & Lomb Surgical

57782
Bausch & Lomb Pharmaceuticals

57844
Gate Pharmaceuticals

58174
Baker Cummins Dermatologicals

58177
Ethex Corp.

58178
US Bioscience

58223
Kirkman Sales, Inc.

58281
Medtronic Neuro

58337
Berna Products Corp.

58406
Immunex Corp.

58407
Houba
See Halsey

58468
Genzyme Corp.

58521
Richwood Pharmaceutical
See Shire Richwood

58573
Hogil Pharmaceutical Corp.

58607
ME Pharmaceuticals, Inc.

58869
Dartmouth Pharmaceuticals

58887
Novartis

58914
Scandipharm, Inc.

58980
Stratus Pharmaceuticals, Inc.

59010
ECR Pharmaceuticals

59016
Niche Pharmaceuticals, Inc.

59075
Athena Neurosciences, Inc.
Elan Pharmaceuticals
Eli Lilly and Co.

59081
Lafayette Pharmaceuticals, Inc.

59148
Otsuka America Pharmaceutical

59196
WE Pharmaceuticals, Inc.

59310
Wakefield Pharmaceuticals, Inc.

59366
Glades Pharmaceuticals

59417
Lotus Biochemical

59426
CooperVision

59439
Ascent Pediatrics

59512
Healthline Laboratories, Inc.

59591
West Point Pharma

59630
Horizon Pharmaceutical Corp.

59676
Ortho Biotech, Inc.

59702
Atley Pharmaceuticals, Inc.

59762
Greenstone

59911
ESI Lederle Generics

59930
Warrick Pharmaceuticals, Corp.

60077
Young Dental

60429
Goldenstate Medical Supply

60432
Morton Grove Pharmaceuticals

60505
Apotex Corp.

60574
Medimmune, Inc.

60575
Respa Pharmaceuticals, Inc.

60793
King Pharmaceuticals Inc.

60799
Liposome Co.

60951
Endo Laboratories

60976
Faro Pharmaceuticals, Inc.

61113
Astra Pharmaceuticals, L.P.

61471
Sequus Pharmaceuticals, Inc.

61563
Medisan

61646
Iomed

62037
Andrx Pharmaceuticals, Inc.

62333
EnviroDerm Pharmaceuticals, Inc.

62592
Ucyclyd Pharma, Inc.

62939
Brightstone Pharma Inc.

63010
Agouron Pharmaceuticals

63256
Bryan Corporation

63323
American Pharmaceutical Partners, Inc.

63717
Hawthorn Pharmaceuticals Inc.

63801
7 Oaks Pharmaceutical Corp.

64543
Capellon Pharmaceuticals. Inc.

64855
Young Again Products

70501
Neutrogena Corp.

71114
Circa Pharmaceuticals, Inc.

72363
Brimms, Inc.

72559
NCI Medical Foods

72959
Alva/Amco Pharmacal Inc.

74300
Pfizer US Pharmaceutical Group

74312
NBTY, Inc.

74684
Goody's Manufacturing Corp.
See Block Drug Company, Inc.

75137
Medtech Laboratories

79511
Triton Consumer Products, Inc.

83926
Tec Laboratories, Inc.

87900
New Mark

88395
J. R. Carlson Laboratories

89223
Stockhausen, Inc.

89709
Amcon Laboratories

90605
Amcon Laboratories

93312
Trask Industries, Inc.

94503
Cirrus Healthcare Products, L.L.C.

98318
Genesis Nutrition

99207
Medicis Dermatologicals, Inc.

99766
Faulding USA

Pharmaceutical Manufacturer and Drug Distributor Listing

LISTED IN ALPHABETICAL ORDER

00089, 55298, 55326
3M Personal Healthcare Products
3M Center
Building 275-5W-05
St. Paul, MN 55133
651-737-6501
800-364-3577

00089
3M Pharmaceutical
3M Center
Building 275-3W-01
St. Paul, MN 55133
651-736-4930
800-328-0255
www.mmm.com

63801
7 Oaks Pharmaceutical Corp.
161 Harry Stanley Dr.
Easley, SC 29640
864-850-1700
e-mail: oaks7mfg@aol.com

12463
Abana Pharmaceuticals, Inc.
See Jones Medical

00074
Abbott Diagnostics
Customer Support Center
Dept. 921
Abbott Park, IL 60064
800-323-9100
www.abbott.com

00074
Abbott Hospital Products
100 Abbott Park Rd.
Abbott Park, IL 60064-3500
847-937-6100

00074
Abbott Laboratories
100 Abbott Park Rd.
Abbott Park, IL 60064-3500
800-633-9110

Able Laboratories, Inc.
6 Hollywood Ct.
South Plainfield, NJ 07080
908-754-2253

Academic Pharmaceuticals, Inc.
25720 Saunders Rd. N.
Lake Forest, IL 60045
847-735-1170

Acme United Corp.
75 Kings Hwy. Cutoff
Fairfield, CT 06430
203-332-7330
800-835-2263
www.acmeunited.com

Acute Therapeutics, Inc.
350 S. Main St.
Suite 307
Doylestown, PA 18901
215-340-4699

53014
Adams Laboratories
See Medeva

Adria Laboratories
See Pharmacia & Upjohn

00062
Advance Biofactures Corp.
35 Wilbur St.
Lynbrook, NY 11563
516-593-7000
www.biospecifics.com

Advanced Care Products
199 Grandview Rd.
Skillman, NJ 08558-9418
800-582-6097
www.jnj.com

10888
Advanced Nutritional Technology
6988 Sierra Ct.
Dublin, CA 94568
800-624-6543

Advanced Polymer Systems
123 Saginaw Dr.
Redwood City, CA 94063
650-366-2626
www.advancedpolymer.com

Advanced Tissue Sciences
10933 N. Torrey Pines Rd.
La Jolla, CA 92037-1005
619-713-7300
www.advancedtissue.com

Advanced Vision Research
7 Alfred St.
Suite 330
Woburn, MA 01801
800-979-8327
www.theratears.com

63010
Agouron Pharmaceuticals
10350 N. Torrey Pines
La Jolla, CA 92037-1020
619-622-3000
800-585-6050
www.agouron.com

A.H. Robins Consumer Products
See Wyeth-Ayerst

00031
A.H. Robins, Inc.
See Wyeth-Ayerst

17478
Akorn, Inc.
2500 Millbrook Dr.
Buffalo Grove, IL 60089
800-535-7155
www.akorn.com

41383
AKPharma, Inc.
P.O. Box 111
Pleasantville, NJ 08232
800-994-4711
www.akpharma.com

00065, 00998
Alcon Laboratories, Inc.
6201 S. Freeway
Ft. Worth, TX 76134
817-551-8057
800-862-5266
www.alconlabs.com

Alimenterics Inc.
301 American Rd.
Morris Plains, NJ 07950
973-285-3100

38697
ALK Laboratories, Inc.
27 Village Lane
Wallingford, CT 06492
203-949-2727
800-325-7354
www.alk-abello.net

A.L. Labs
See Alpharma USPD

00173
Allen & Hanburys
See GlaxoWellcome

Allercreme
See Carme, Inc.

11980
Allergan America
See Allergan, Inc.

00023
Allergan, Inc.
2525 DuPont Dr.
P.O. Box 19534
Irvine, CA 92715-9534
800-347-4500
www.allergan.com

Allermed
7203 Convoy Ct.
San Diego, CA 92111
619-292-1060
800-221-2748
www.allermed.com

Alliance Pharmaceuticals
3040 Science Park Rd.
San Diego, CA 92121
619-558-4300
www.allp.com

Allied Pharmacy
801 Stadium Dr.
Suite 111
Arlington, TX 76111
817-226-5050

54569
Allscripts
2401 Commerce Dr.
Libertyville, IL 60048-4464
847-680-3515
800-654-0889
www.allscripts.com

Alpha 1 Biomedicals, Inc.
P.O. Box 34598
West Bethesda, MD 20827-0598
301-564-4400

Alpharma USPD, Inc.
7205 Windsor Blvd.
Baltimore, MD 21244-2654
800-638-9096
www.alpharma.com

49669
Alpha Therapeutic Corp.
5555 Valley Blvd.
Los Angeles, CA 90032
800-421-0008

Almay, Inc.
1501 Williamsboro St.
P.O. Box 6111
Oxford, NC 27565
919-603-2804
800-334-8332

51641
Alra Laboratories, Inc.
3850 Clearview Ct.
Gurnee, IL 60031
800-248-2572

Altana Incorporated
60 Baylis Rd.
Melville, NY 11747
516-454-7677
800-432-6673

AltaRex Corp.
#125, 303 Wyman St.
Waltham, MA 02451
781-672-0138

00731
Alto Pharmaceuticals, Inc.
P.O. Box 1910
Land O'Lakes, FL 34639-1910
800-330-2891

72959
Alva/Amco Pharmacal Inc.
7711 N. Meremac Ave.
Niles, IL 60714-3423
847-663-0700
800-792-2582
www.alva-amco.com

17314
Alza Corp.
950 Page Mill Rd.
P.O. Box 10950
Palo Alto, CA 94303-0802
650-494-5000
800-634-8977
www.alza.com

10038
Ambix Laboratories, Inc.
210 Orchard St.
East Rutherford, NJ 07073
201-939-2200

89709, 90605
Amcon Laboratories
40 N. Rock Hill Rd.
St. Louis, MO 63119
314-961-5758
800-255-6161

Americal Pharmaceutical, Inc.
See Akorn, Inc.

51201
American Dermal Corp.
See Rhone-Poulenc Rorer

57506
American Drug Industries, Inc.
5810 S. Perry Ave.
Chicago, IL 60621
773-667-7070

American Lecithin Company
115 Hurley Rd., Unit 2B
Oxford, CT 06478
800-364-4416

11649
American Medical Industries
28045 Ashley Circle #106
Libertyville, IL 60048
847-918-9449

American Pharmacal
1201 Douglas Ave.
Kansas City, KS 66103
800-349-4923
www.york-inc.com

63323
American Pharmaceutical Partners, Inc.
10866 Wilshire Blvd.
Suite 1270
Los Angeles, CA 90024
310-470-4222

52769
American Red Cross
1616 N. Ft. Myers Dr.
Arlington, VA 22209
800-446-8883
www.redcross.org/plasma

00517
American Regent
1 Luitpold Dr.
Shirley, NY 11967
516-924-4000
800-645-1706
www.luitpold.com

55513
Amgen, Inc.
One Amgen Center Dr.
Thousand Oaks, CA 91320-1789
805-447-3505
800-772-6436
www.amgen.com

52152
Amide Pharmaceuticals, Inc.
101 E. Main St.
Little Falls, NJ 07424
973-890-1440

53926
Amsco Scientific
See Steris Labs.

Anaquest
See Ohmeda Pharmaceuticals

Andrew Jergens
2535 Spring Grove
Cincinnati, OH 45214
513-421-1400
www.biore.com

Andrulis Pharmaceutical Corp.
P.O. Box 2135
Bethesda, MD 20817
301-419-2400

Andrulis Research Corp.
See Andrulis Pharmaceutical Corp.

62037
Andrx Pharmaceuticals Inc.
4001 S.W. 47th Ave.
Ft. Lauderdale, FL 33314
954-581-7500
www.andrx.com

Angelini Pharmaceuticals, Inc.
70 Grand Ave.
River Edge, NJ 07661
201-646-1697
e-mail: dapp@nac.net

Anthra Pharmaceuticals, Inc.
103 Carnegie Center
Suite 102
Princeton, NJ 08540
609-514-1060
www.anthra.com

Antibodies, Inc.
P.O. Box 1560
Davis, CA 95617
530-758-4400
800-824-8540
www.antibodiesinc.com

48028
Aplicare Inc.
P.O. Box 237
Prichard, WV 25555
304-486-5656
800-955-7334
www.aplicare.com

Apollon Inc.
1 Great Valley Pkwy.
Malvern, PA 19355
610-647-9452

Apotex USA, Inc.
1776 Broadway
Suite 1900
New York, NY 10019
212-664-9200
800-967-7427

60505
Apotex Corp.
50 Lakeview Pkwy.
Suite 127
Vernon Hills, IL 60061
847-573-9999
800-248-5210

Apothecary Products, Inc.
11750 12th Ave. S.
Burnsville, MN 55337-1295
612-890-1940
800-328-2742
www.cornerdrug.com

00003, 00015
Apothecon, Inc.
P.O. Box 4500
Princeton, NJ 08543-4500
609-897-2000
800-321-1335

48723
Apothecus, Inc.
20 Audrey Ave.
Oyster Bay, NY 11771
516-624-8200
800-227-2393

Applied Biotech
10237 Flanders Ct.
San Diego, CA 92121
619-587-6771

Applied Genetics
205 Buffalo Ave.
Freeport, NY 11520
516-868-9026

Applied Medical Research
308 15th Ave. N.
Nashville, TN 37203
615-327-0676

Approved Drug
See Health for Life Brands, Inc.

00070
Arcola Laboratories
500 Arcola Rd.
Collegeville, PA 19426
610-454-8000
800-727-6737

00275
Arco Pharmaceuticals, Inc.
90 Orville Dr.
Bohemia, NY 11716
516-567-9500
800-645-5412

Aronex Pharmaceuticals, Inc.
8707 Technology Forest Place
The Woodlands, TX 77381
281-367-1666

Armour Pharmaceutical
See Centeon

59439
Ascent Pediatrics
187 Ballardvale St.
Suite B125
Wilmington, MA 01887
978-658-2500
www.ascentpediatrics.com

61113
Astra Pharmaceuticals, L.P.
725 Chesterbrook Blvd.
Wayne, PA 19087-5677
800-236-9933
www.astrapharmaceuticals.com

00186
Astra USA, Inc.
50 Otis St.
Westborough, MA 01581
508-366-1100
800-225-6333

59075
Athena Neurosciences, Inc.
See Elan Pharmaceuticals

59702
Atley Pharmaceuticals, Inc.
14433 N. Washington Hwy.
Ashland, VA 23005
804-752-8400
www.atley.com

Autoimmune, Inc.
128 Spring St.
Lexington, MA 02173
781-860-0710

44184
Bajamar Chemical, Inc.
9609 Dielman Rock Island
St. Louis, MO 63132
314-997-3414
888-242-3414
http://walden.mvp.net/~bmizes/bcc/BAJAMAR.htm

58174
Baker Cummins Dermatologicals
See Baker Norton

00575, 11414
Baker Norton Pharmaceuticals
4400 Biscayne Blvd.
Miami, FL 33137
800-735-2315
www.ivax.com

00304
J.J. Balan, Inc.
5725 Foster Ave.
Brooklyn, NY 11234
718-251-8663
800-552-2526
www.jjbalan.com

Banner Pharacaps
4125 Premier Dr.
High Point, NC 27265
800-447-1140

00555
Barr Laboratories, Inc.
2 Quaker Rd.
Pomona, NY 01970
914-362-1100
800-222-0190
www.barrlabs.com

10116
Bartor Pharmacal Co.
70 High St.
Rye, NY 10580
914-967-4219

58887
Basel Pharmaceuticals
See Novartis

Bausch & Lomb Eye Care
1 Bausch & Lomb Place
Rochester, NY 14604
800-828-9030

10119
Bausch & Lomb Personal Products Division
1400 N. Goodman St.
P.O. Box 450
Rochester, NY 14692-0450
716-338-6000
800-553-5340
www.bausch.com

24208, 57782
Bausch & Lomb Pharmaceuticals
8500 Hidden River Pkwy.
Tampa, FL 33637
813-975-7700
800-323-0000
www.bausch.com

Bausch & Lomb Surgical
555 W. Arrow Hwy.
Claremont, CA 91711
909-624-2020

BaxaCorp
13760 Arapahoe Rd.
Englewood, CO 80112
800-525-9567
www.baxa.com

Baxter Healthcare
1 Baxter Parkway DF4-1W
Deerfield, IL 60015
847-270-5700
800-422-9837

00944
Baxter Hyland
550 N. Brand Blvd.
Glendale, CA 91203
818-956-3200
800-423-2090
www.baxter.com

00118
Bayer Corp. (Allergy Div.)
P.O. Box 3145
Spokane, WA 99220
509-489-5656
800-992-1120

00026, 00161, 00192
Bayer Corp. (Biological and Pharmaceutical Div.)
400 Morgan Lane
West Haven, CT 06516
203-812-2000
800-288-8371

12843, 16500
Bayer Corp. (Consumer Div.)
36 Columbia Rd.
P.O. Box 1910
Morristown, NJ 07962-1910
800-331-4536
www.bayercare.com

00193
Bayer Corp. (Diagnostic Div.)
430 S. Beiger St.
P.O. Box 2004
Mishawaka, IN 46544-2004
219-256-3390
800-248-2637

BDI Pharmaceuticals, Inc.
P.O. Box 78610
Indianapolis, IN 46278-0610
317-228-0000
800-428-1717
www.bdip.com

00486
Beach Products
5220 S. Manhattan Ave.
Tampa, FL 33681
800-322-8210

Beckman Coulter Primary Diagnostics
1050 Pagemill Rd.
Palo Alto, CA 94304
www.beckman.com

31280
Becton Dickinson & Co.
One Becton Dr.
Franklin Lakes, NJ 07417-1881
201-847-6800
888-237-2762
www.bd.com

00011
Becton Dickinson Microbiology Systems
7 Loveton Circle
Sparks, MD 21152
410-316-4000
800-638-8663
www.ms.bd.com

55390
Bedford Laboratories
300 N. Field Rd.
Bedford, OH 44146
440-232-3320
800-562-4797

10356
Beiersdorf, Inc.
360 Martin Luther King Dr.
S. Norwalk, CT 06856-5529
203-853-8008
800-233-2340
www.beiersdorf.com

50419
Berlex Laboratories, Inc.
300 Fairfield Rd.
Wayne, NJ 07470
888-237-5394
www.berlex.com

58337
Berna Products Corp.
4216 Ponce De Leon Blvd.
Coral Gables, FL 33146
305-443-2900
800-533-5899
www.bernaproducts.com

Bertek Pharmaceuticals, Inc.
P.O. Box 2006
Sugar Land, TX 77478
281-240-1000
800-231-3052
www.dowhickam.com

Best Generics
See Goldline Laboratories, Inc.

00283
Beutlich, Inc.
1541 Shields Dr.
Waukegan, IL 60085-8304
847-473-1100
800-238-8542
www.beutlich.com

00225
B. F. Ascher and Co.
15501 W. 109th St.
Lenexa, KS 66219
913-888-1880
800-324-1880

Biocare International, Inc.
2643 Grand Ave.
Bellmore, NY 11710
516-781-5800
800-224-0001

00332
Biocraft Laboratories, Inc.
See Teva Pharmaceuticals

Biocryst Pharmaceuticals, Inc.
2190 Parkway Lake Dr.
Birmingham, AL 35244
205-444-4600
www.biocryst.com

Biofilm, Inc.
3121 Scott St.
Vista, CA 92083-8323
760-727-9030
800-848-5900
www.astroglide.com

Biogen
14 Cambridge Center
Cambridge, MA 02142
617-679-2000
800-262-4363
www.biogen.com

BioGenex Laboratories
4600 Norris Canyon Rd.
Suite 400
San Ramon, CA 94583
800-421-4149
www.biogenex.com

Bioglan Pharma
4902 Eisenhower Blvd.
Suite 150
Tampa, FL 33634
813-243-8833
888-246-4526
www.bioglanpharma.com

Bioline Labs, Inc.
See Zenith Goldline Laboratories, Inc.

Biomerica, Inc.
1533 Monrovia Ave.
Newport Beach, CA 92663
949-645-2111
800-854-3002
www.biomerica.com

Biomira, USA
1002 East Park Blvd.
Cranbury, NJ 08512
609-655-5300

Biopharmaceutics, Inc.
990 Station Rd.
Bellport, NY 11713
516-286-5900

Biopure Corp.
1100 Hurley
Cambridge, MA 02111
617-234-6500

52311
Biosearch Medical Products
35 Industrial Parkway
Somerville, NJ 08876
908-722-5000
800-326-5976
www.biosearch.com

53191
Biostar, Inc.
6655 Lookout Rd.
Boulder, CO 80301
303-530-3888
800-637-3717
www.biostar.com

Bio-Tech
P.O. Box 1992
Fayetteville, AR 72702
501-443-9148
800-345-1199
www.bio-tech-pharm.com

Bio-Technology General Corp.
70 Wood Ave. S.
Iselin, NJ 08830
732-632-8800
www.btgc.com

BIRA Corp.
2525 Quicksilver
McDonald, PA 15057
724-796-1820

50289
Birchwood Laboratories, Inc.
7900 Fuller Rd.
Eden Prairie, MN 53344
800-328-6156
www.birchlab.com

12136
Bird Corp.
1100 Bird Center Dr.
Palm Springs, CA 92262
619-778-7200
800-328-4139
www.thermoresp.com

00165
Blaine Co., Inc.
1515 Production Dr.
Burlington, KY 41005
606-283-9437
800-633-9353
www.blainepharma.com

00154
Blair Laboratories
100 Connecticut Ave.
Norwalk, CT 06850-3590
203-853-0123
800-877-5666
www.pharma.com

50486
Blairex Labs, Inc.
P.O. Box 2127
Columbus, IN 47202-2127
812-378-1864
800-252-4739
www.blairex.com

10157
Blistex, Inc.
1800 Swift Dr.
Oak Brook, IL 60523
630-571-2870
800-837-1800

10158
Block Drug Co., Inc.
257 Cornelison Ave.
Jersey City, NJ 07302
201-434-3000
800-365-6500
www.blockdrug.com

10160
Bluco Inc./Med. Discnt. Outlet
28350 Schoolcraft
Livonia, MI 48150
734-513-4500
800-832-4464
e-mail: bluco@wwnet.net

00563
Bock Pharmacal Co.
See Eli Lilly

00597
Boehringer Ingelheim, Inc.
900 Ridgebury Rd.
Ridgefield, CT 06877-0368
203-798-9988
800-542-6257

53169
Boehringer Mannheim Corp., Therapeutics Div.
See Roche Diagnostics

Boehringer Mannheim Diags.
See Roche Diagnostics

Boehringer Mannheim Pharmaceuticals
See Roche Diagnostics

44437
Bolan Pharmaceutical, Inc.
See Allied Pharmacy

Boots Pharmaceuticals, Inc.
See Knoll Laboratories

00003
Bracco Diagnostics
P.O. Box 5225
Princeton, NJ 08543
609-514-2200
800-631-5245
www.bracco.com

Bradley Pharmaceutical
See Kenwood Laboratories

52268
Braintree Laboratories, Inc.
P.O. Box 850929
Braintree, MA 02185-0929
781-843-2202
800-874-6756

45617
Breath Asure, Inc.
26025 Mureau Rd.
Calabasas, CA 91302
818-878-0011
800-548-8686
www.breathasure.com

51991
Breckenridge Pharmaceutical, Inc.
P.O. Box 206
Boca Raton, FL 33429
561-367-8512
800-367-3395

62939
Brightstone Pharma Inc.
109 MacKenan Dr.
Cary, NC 27511
619-615-8906
www.brightstonepharma.com

72363
Brimms, Inc.
425 Fillmore Ave.
Tonawanda, NY 14150
716-694-7100
800-828-7669

Bristol Laboratories
See Bristol-Myers Squibb

Bristol-Myers Oncology
P.O. Box 4500
Princeton, NJ 08543
609-897-2000
800-332-2056

19810
Bristol-Myers Products
225 High Ridge Rd.
Stanford, CT 06905
800-468-7746

00003, 00087
Bristol-Myers Squibb
P.O. Box 4500
Princeton, NJ 08543-4500
609-897-2000
800-321-1335

Britannia Pharmaceuticals
Forum Hs Brighton Rd. Redhill
Surrey, UK RH 1 6YS

63256
Bryan Corporation
4 Plympton St.
Woburn, MA 01801
781-935-0004
800-343-7711

Burroughs Wellcome Co.
See GlaxoWellcome

00398
C & M Pharmacal, Inc.
1721 Maplelane Ave.
Hazel Park, MI 48030-1215
248-548-7846
800-423-5173

00132
C.B. Fleet, Inc.
4615 Murray Place
Lynchburg, VA 24506-1349
804-528-4000
800-999-9711

00463
C.O. Truxton, Inc.
P.O. Box 1081
Bellmawr, NJ 08099
609-933-2333
800-257-7704

08011
C.R. Bard, Inc.
Urological Div.
8195 Industrial Blvd.
Covington, GA 30209
800-526-4455

10486
C.S. Dent & Co. Division
1820 Airport Exchange Blvd.
Erlanger, KY 41018
606-647-0777
800-684-1468

CCA Industries, Inc.
200 Murray Hill Pkwy.
E. Rutherford, NJ 07073
201-330-1400
800-524-2720

CIS-US, Inc.
10 DeAngelo Dr.
Bedford, MA 01730
781-275-7120

57145
CNS Inc.
4400 West 78th St.
Minneapolis, MN 55435
612-820-6696
800-441-0417
www.cns.com

COR Therapeutics, Inc.
256 E. Grand Ave.
S. San Francisco, CA 94080
650-244-6800
888-267-4633
www.corr.com

CTEX Pharmaceuticals Inc.
P.O. Box 1549
Madison, MS 39130
601-898-0751
888-898-0751
www.ctex.com

55559
Calgon Vestal Laboratories
5035 Manchester Rd.
St. Louis, MO 63110
314-535-1810
800-325-8005

California Department
Health Service
2151 Berkeley Way
Berkeley, CA 94704

Cal-White Mineral Co.
P.O. Box 7890
Klamath Falls, OR 97602
800-944-8096

00147
Camall Co., Inc.
P.O. Box 307
Romeo, MI 48065-0307
810-752-9683
800-521-6720
www.camall.com

Cambridge Neuroscience, Inc.
1 Kendall Square
Building 700
Cambridge, MA 02139
617-225-0600

43656
Cambridge Nutraceuticals, Inc.
294 Washington St.
Suite 601
Boston, MA 02108
617-695-1255
800-265-2202
www.cambridgenutra.com

Can-Am Care Corp.
Cimetra Industrial Park
P.O. Box 98
Chazy, NY 12921
800-461-7448
www.ffriedberg@canamcare.com

Cangene Corp.
104 Chancellor Matheson Rd.
Winnipeg, R3T 2N2
CANADA
204-989-6850

64543
Capellon Pharmaceuticals, Inc.
300 Steeple Ridge
Ridgeland, MS 39157
601-853-4227
capellon@compuserve.com

Capmed USA
P.O. Box 14
Bryn Mawr, PA 19010

57664
Caraco Pharmaceutical Labs
1150 Elijah McCoy Dr.
Detroit, MI 48202
313-871-8400
www.caraco.com

Care Technologies, Inc.
55 Holly Hill Lane
Greenwich, CT 06830
800-783-1919

Carme, Inc.
See US International Trading Co.

Carnation
800 N. Brand Blvd.
Glendale, CA 91203
800-628-2229
www.carnationbaby.com

00086
Carnrick Laboratories, Inc.
65 Horse Hill Rd.
Cedar Knolls, NJ 07927
973-267-2670
www.elan.ie

46287
Carolina Medical Products
8026 VS 264 Alternate
P.O. Box 147
Farmville, NC 27828-0147
252-753-7111
800-227-6637
www.carolinamedical.com

Carrington Labs
2001 Walnut Hill Lane
Irving, TX 75038
972-518-1300
800-527-5216
www.carringtonlabs.com

00164
Carter Wallace
Half Acre Rd.
P.O. Box 1001
Cranbury, NJ 08512-0181
609-655-6000
www.astelin.com

Celgene Corp.
7 Powder Horn Dr.
Warren, NJ 07059
800-890-4619

Cellegy Pharmaceuticals, Inc.
371 Bel Marin Keys
Suite 210
Novato, CA 94949
650-616-2200

Cell Pathways, Inc.
702 Electronic Dr.
Horsham, PA 19044
215-706-3800

Celtrix Pharmaceuticals, Inc.
3055 Patrick Henry Dr.
Santa Clara, CA 95054
408-988-2500
www.bioportfolio.com

00053
Centeon
1020 First Ave.
King of Prussia, PA 19408-1310
800-504-5434
www.centeon.com/na

Centeon Pharma GmbH
See Centeon

00268
Center Laboratories
3620 Park Central Blvd. N.
Pompano Beach, FL 33064
800-223-6837
www.centerpharm.com

Centers for Disease Control
1600 Clifton Rd.
Mail Stop D-09
Atlanta, GA 30333
404-639-3670
www.cdc.gov

Centocor, Inc.
200 Great Valley Pkwy.
Malvern, PA 19355
610-651-6000
888-874-3083
www.centocor.com

00131
Central Pharmaceuticals, Inc.
See Schwarz Pharma

00436
Century Pharmaceuticals, Inc.
10377 Hague Rd.
Indianapolis, IN 46256-3399
317-849-4210

Cephalon, Inc.
145 Brandywine Pkwy.
West Chester, PA 19380
610-344-0200

00173
Cerenex Pharmaceuticals
See GlaxoWellcome

10223
Cetylite Industries, Inc.
9051 River Rd.
P.O. Box 90006
Pennsauken, NJ 08110
609-665-6111
800-257-7740
www.cetylite.com

54429
Chase Laboratories
See Banner Pharmacap

49447
Chattem Consumer Products
1715 W. 38th St.
Chattanooga, TN 37409
423-821-4571
800-366-6833

Chembiomed, Ltd.
P.O. Box 8050
Edmonton, AB T6H4NP
CANADA

00521
Chesebrough-Ponds USA, Inc.
See Unilever HPC

Cheshire Pharmaceutical Systems
6225 Shiloh Rd.
Alpharetta, GA 30005
800-582-3194

Chiesi Pharmaceuticals, Inc.
150 Danbury Rd.
Ridgefield, CT 06877
203-438-3390

Children's Hospital of Columbus
700 Childrens Dr.
Columbus, OH 43205
614-722-2000

53905
Chiron Behring GmbH & Co.
D-35006 Marburg, Germany

53905
Chiron Therapeutics
4560 Horton St.
Emeryville, CA 94608
510-655-8730
800-244-7668

Chiron Vision
See Bausch & Lomb Surgical

Chronimed Inc.
10900 Red Circle Dr.
Suite 300
Minnetonka, MN 55343
612-979-3600
800-444-5951
www.chronimed.com

00083
Ciba-Geigy Pharmaceuticals
See Novartis

Ciba Self-Medication, Inc.
See Novartis

00346
Ciba Vision Ophthalmics
11460 Johns Creek Pkwy.
Duluth, GA 30136
770-418-4101

00677, 00725, 71114
Circa Pharmaceuticals, Inc.
33 Ralph Ave.
Copiague, NY 11726-0030
516-842-8383
800-331-3623
www.circapharm.com

00659
Circle Pharmaceuticals, Inc.
4136 N. Keystone Ave.
Indianapolis, IN 46256
317-568-0392
email: hbo@netdirect.net

94503
Cirrus Healthcare Products, L.L.C.
98 Forest Ave.
Locust Valley, NY 11560
516-759-6664
800-327-6151
www.earplanes.com

City Chemical Corp.
139 Allings Crossing Rd.
West Haven, CT 06516
203-932-2489
800-248-2436

Claragen
387 Technology Dr.
College Park, MD 20742
301-405-8593

45802
Clay-Park Labs, Inc.
1700 Bathgate Ave.
Bronx, NY 10457
718-901-2800
800-933-5550

55553
Clint Pharmaceutical
1451 Elm Hill Pike
Nashville, TN 37210
615-366-0086
800-677-5022

Clintec Nutrition
3 Pkwy. N.
Suite 500
Deerfield, IL 60015
847-948-2000
800-422-2751

Cocensys, Inc.
201 Technology Dr.
Irvine, CA 92618
949-453-0131

Colgate Oral Pharmaceuticals
1 Colgate Way
Canton, MA 02021
781-821-2880
800-821-2880

Colgate-Palmolive Co.
300 Park Ave.
New York, NY 10022-7499
800-221-4607

Collagen Corp.
1850 Embarcadero Rd.
Palo Alto, CA 94303
650-856-0200
www.collagen.com

27280
CollaGenex Pharmaceuticals, Inc.
301 S. State St.
Newtown, PA 18940
215-579-7388
888-339-5678
www.collagenex.com

00837, 21406
Columbia Laboratories, Inc.
2875 N.E. 191st St.
Suite 400
Aventura, FL 33180
305-933-6089
800-749-1919
www.columbialabs.com

11509
Combe, Inc.
1101 Westchester Ave.
White Plains, NY 10604
914-694-5454
800-873-7400

Complimed Medical Research Group
1441 West Smith Rd.
Ferndale, WA 98248
360-384-5656
888-977-8008

20254
Concord Laboratories
140 New Dutch Lane
Fairfield, NJ 07704
973-227-6757

11793, 49281, 50361
Connaught Labs
See Pasteur-Mérieux- Connaught

00007
Connetics
1135 Heil Quaker Blvd.
Suite 100
Lavergne, TN 37086
615-793-4400
800-280-2879
www.connetics.com

43786
Consep Inc.
213 S.W. Columbia St.
Bend, OR 97702-1013
519-754-1807
800-367-8727
www.consep.com

00223
Consolidated Midland Corp.
20 Main St.
Brewster, NY 10509
914-279-6108

18149
Consumers Choice Systems, Inc.
2370 130th Ave. N.E.
Suite 101
Bellevue, WA 98005
425-883-6310
800-479-5232
www.ccsemporium.com

34044
Continental Consumer Products
770 Forest
Suite B
Birmingham, MI 48009
800-542-5903

33130
Continental Quest Research
220 W. Carmel Dr.
Carmel, IN 46032
800-451-5773

00003
ConvaTec
P.O. Box 5254
Princeton, NJ 08543-5254
908-904-2200
800-422-8811
www.convatec.com

59426
CooperVision
200 Willowbrook Office Park
Fairport, NY 14450
949-597-8130
800-538-7850
www.coopervision.com

38245
Copley Pharmaceutical, Inc.
25 John Rd.
Canton, MA 02021
781-821-6111
800-325-6111

Cord Labs
See Geneva Pharmaceuticals

Coulter Corp.
11800 S.W. 147 Ave.
P.O. Box 169015
Miami, FL 33116
305-380-3800
800-327-6531
www.coulter.com

01020, 44800
Cumberland Packing Corp.
35 Old Ridgefield Rd.
P.O. Box 7688
Willton, CT 06897
203-762-7227
800-287-4955

55326
Curatek Pharmaceuticals
See 3M Pharmaceuticals

Cutter Biologicals
See Bayer Corp. (Biological and Pharmaceutical Div.)

Cyclin Pharmaceuticals Inc.
429 Gammon Place
Madison, WI 53715
608-833-4767
800-982-1186
www.womenshealth.com

54799
Cynacon/OCuSOFT
5311 Ave. N
P.O. Box 429
Richmond, TX 77406-0429
281-342-3350
800-233-5469
www.ocusoft.com

Cypress Pharmaceutical
135 Industrial Blvd.
Madison, MS 39110
800-856-4393
www.cypressrx.com

Cypros Pharmaceutical Corp.
2714 Loker Ave. West
Carlsbad, CA 92008
760-929-9500
www.cypros.com

Cytel Corp.
9393 Towne Centre Dr.
San Diego, CA 92121
619-552-3000
800-576-2985
www.cytelcorp.com

Cytogen
600 College Rd. East
Princeton, NJ 08540
609-987-8200
800-833-3533
www.cytogen.com

23731
Cytosol Laboratories
55 Messina Dr.
Braintree, MA 02184
800-288-3858

55994
Dakryon Pharmaceuticals
See Medco Pharmaceuticals

Danbury Pharmacal
See Schein Pharmaceutical, Inc.

00689
Daniels Pharmaceuticals, Inc.
See Jones Medical

58869
Dartmouth Pharmaceuticals
38 Church Ave.
Wareham, MA 02571
508-295-2200
800-414-3566

00938
Davis and Geck
See Sherwood Davis and Geck

Davol
160 New Boston St.
Woburn, MA 01801
781-932-5900
www.davol.com

52041
Dayton Laboratories, Inc.
3307 N.W. 74th Ave.
Miami, FL 33122
305-594-0988
800-446-0255
www.daytonlab.com

Deacrin Corp. Development
Bldg. 96, 13th St.
Charlestown, MA 02129
617-242-9100

Debio Pharm SA
1747 Pennsylvania Ave. N.W.
Suite 300
Washington, DC 20006
703-751-7777

Degussa Corp.
65 Challenger Rd.
Ridgefield Park, NJ 07660
201-641-6100
800-334-8772
www.degussa.com

48532
Delmont Laboratories, Inc.
P.O. Box 269
Swarthmore, PA 19081
610-543-3365
800-562-5541
www.delmont.com

10310
Del Pharmaceuticals, Inc.
565 Broad Hallow Rd.
Farmingdale, NY 11735
516-844-2020
800-645-9888
www.dellabs.com

00316
Del-Ray Laboratory, Inc.
22 20th Ave. N.W.
Birmingham, AL 35215
205-853-8247

00295
Denison Laboratories, Inc.
60 Dunnell Lane
P.O. Box 1305
Pawtucket, RI 02862
401-723-5500

49336
Den-Mat Corporation
2727 Skyway Dr.
Santa Maria, CA 93455
800-445-0345
www.den-mat.com

Dental Herb Co.
78 Main St.
Suite 311
North Hampton, MA 01060
800-747-4372

DepoTech Corp.
10450 Science Center Dr.
San Diego, CA 92115
619-625-2424
www.skyepharma.com

Derma Science
1065 Hwy. 315
Suite 403
Wilkesbarre, PA 18702
570-824-3605
800-825-4325
www.dermasciences.com

00066
Dermik Laboratories, Inc.
See Arcola

DeRoyal Industries, Inc.
200 DeBusk Lane
Powell, TN 37849
423-938-7828
800-337-6925

49502
Dey Laboratories, Inc.
2751 Napa Valley Corporate Dr.
Napa, CA 94558
707-224-3200
800-755-5560

DiaPharma Group, Inc.
8948 Beckett Rd.
West Chester, OH 45069-2939
800-526-5224
www.diapharma.com

Diatide, Inc.
9 Delta Dr.
Londonderry, NH 03053
603-437-8970

Digestive Care Inc.
1120 Win Dr.
Bethlehem, PA 18017
610-882-5950

Discovery Experimental & Development, Inc.
29949 SR 54 West
Wesley Chapel, FL 33543
813-973-7200

Discus Dental Inc.
8550 Higuera St.
Culver City, CA 90232
800-273-2847
www.discusdental.com

00777
Dista Products Co.
See Eli Lilly

10337
Doak Dermatologics
383 Route 46 West
Fairfield, NJ 07004-2402
201-882-1505
800-405-3625
www.bradpharm.com

25358
Donell DerMedex
342 Madison Ave.
Suite 1422
New York, NY 10173
212-697-3800

00514
Dow Hickam, Inc.
See Bertek Pharmaceuticals Inc.

13723
Dr. Nordyke Footcare Products
1650 Palma Dr.
Suite 102
Ventura, CA 93003
805-650-8333

00514
Dow Hickam, Inc.
See Bertek Pharmaceuticals

00094
The Du Pont Merck Pharmaceutical
P.O. Box 80705
Wilmington, DE 19807
302-992-5000
800-474-2762
www.dupontpharma.com

00056
DuPont Pharma
P.O. Box 80705
Wilmington, DE 19880

51285
Duramed Pharmaceuticals
5040 Duramed Dr.
Cincinnati, OH 45213
513-731-9900
800-543-8338
www.duramed.com

51479
Dura Pharmaceuticals
7475 Lusk Blvd.
San Diego, CA 92121-4202
619-457-2553
800-859-8585
www.durapharm.com

Durex Consumer Products
3585 Engineering Dr.
Suite 200
Noreriss, GA 30092
770-582-2222
888-566-3468
www.durex.com

DynaGen Inc.
840 Memorial Dr.
Cambridge, MA 02139
617-491-2527
www.dynageninc.com

10331
E. E. Dickinson Co.
31 East High St.
East Hampton, CT 06424
860-267-2279

00168
E. Fougera and Co.
60 Baylis Rd.
Melville, NY 11747
516-454-6996
800-645-9833

EM Industries, Inc.
7 Skyline Dr.
Hawthorne, NY 10532
914-592-4660
800-831-3662
www.emindustries.com

Eagle Vision, Inc.
6263 Poplar Ave.
Suite 650
Memphis, TN 38119
901-682-9400
800-393-7584
www.eaglevis.com

The Ear Foundation
2420 Castillo St.
Suite 100
Santa Barbara, CA 93105
805-563-1111

Eastman Kodak Co.
10 Indigo Creek Dr.
Rochester, NY 14650-0862
800-242-2424
www.kodak.com

Eaton Medical Corp.
1401 Heistan Place
Memphis, TN 38104
901-274-0000
800-253-4740

19458
Eckerd Drug Co.
P.O. Box 4689
Clearwater, FL 34618
727-395-6000
800-876-3075
www.eckerd.com

55053
Econolab
P.O. Box 85543
Westland, MI 48185-0543
561-391-5245

38130
Econo Med Pharmaceuticals
4305 Sartin Rd.
Burlington, NC 27217-7522
336-226-1091
800-327-6007

00095, 59010
ECR Pharmaceuticals
3981 Deep Rock Rd.
Richmond, VA 23233
804-527-1950
800-527-1955

00485
Edwards Pharmaceuticals, Inc.
111 Mulberry St.
Ripley, MS 38663
601-837-8182
800-543-9560

55806
Effcon Labs, Inc.
1800 Sandy Plains Pkwy.
Marietta, GA 30066-7499
770-428-7011
800-722-2428
www.effcon.com

Elan Pharmaceuticals
800 Gateway Blvd.
San Francisco, CA 94080
770-877-0900
888-638-7605

Elan Research Co.
1300 Gould Dr.
Gainsville, GA 30504
770-538-6360

00002, 59075
Eli Lilly and Co.
Lilly Corp. Center
Indianapolis, IN 46285
317-276-2000
800-545-5979
www.lilly.com

00641
Elkins-Sinn, Inc.
See Wyeth-Ayerst

00802
Emerson Laboratories
See Humco

60951
Endo Laboratories
223 Wilmington Westchester Pike
Chadds Ford, PA 19347
800-462-4467

62333
EnviroDerm Pharmaceuticals, Inc.
P.O. Box 32370
Louisville, KY 40232-2370
502-634-7700
800-991-3376

57665
Enzon, Inc.
20 Kingsbridge Rd.
Piscataway, NJ 08854-3998
732-980-4500
www.enzon.com

00185, 00536
Eon Labs Manufacturing, Inc.
227-15 N. Conduit Ave.
Laurelton, NY 11413
718-276-8600
800-526-0225

Epitope Inc.
8505 S.W. Creekside Place
Beaverton, OR 97008
503-641-6115
800-234-3786
www.epitope

E.R. Squibb & Sons, Inc.
See Bristol-Myers Squibb

00005, 59911
ESI Lederle Generics
P.O. Box 8299
Philadelphia, PA 19101-8299
610-688-4400
www.ahp.com

58177
Ethex Corp.
10888 Metro Ct.
St. Louis, MO 63043-2413
314-567-3307
800-321-1705
e-mail: ethex@mvp.net

Ethicon, Inc.
Route 22 West
P.O. Box 151
Somerville, NJ 08876-0151
908-218-0707
800-255-2500
www.ethiconinc.com

54686
Ethitek Pharmaceuticals
7701 N. Austin
Skokie, IL 60077
847-675-6611
800-442-5540

00642
Everett Laboratories, Inc.
29 Spring St.
West Orange, NJ 07052
973-324-0200
800-964-9650
www.everettlabs.com

Falcon Ophthalmics, Inc.
6201 S. Freeway
Fort Worth, TX 76134
817-551-8710
800-343-2133
www.alconlabs.com

Farmacon, Inc.
90 Grove St.
Suite 109
Ridgefield, CT 06877-4118
203-431-9989

60976
Faro Pharmaceuticals, Inc.
10607 Haddington #150
Houston, TX 77043
713-461-6206
800-480-1985
www.faropharma.com

99766
Faulding USA
200 Elmora Ave.
Elizabeth, NJ 07207
908-527-9100
800-526-6978
www.faulding.com.au

11423
Female Health Co.
875 N. Michigan Ave.
Suite 3660
Chicago, IL 60611-9267
312-280-1119
800-635-0844
www.femalehealth.com

00496
Ferndale Laboratories, Inc.
780 W. Eight Mile Rd.
Ferndale, MI 48220-1218
248-548-0900
800-621-6003

55566
Ferring Laboratories, Inc.
See Ferring Pharmaceuticals

Ferring Pharmaceuticals
120 White Plains Rd.
Suite 400
Tarrytown, NY 10591
888-793-6367
www.ferringusa.com

31795
Fibertone
14851 N. Scottsdale Rd.
Scottsdale, AZ 85254
800-462-7596
www.naturallyvitamins.com

Fidia Pharmaceutical
2000 K St. N.W.
Washington, DC 20006
202-371-9898

00421
Fielding Co.
11551 Adie Rd.
Maryland Heights, MO 63043
314-567-5462
800-776-3435
www.fieldingco.com

51687
Fischer Pharmaceuticals, Inc.
3707 Williams Rd.
San Jose, CA 95117
408-615-4148
800-782-0222

Fiske Industries
527 Route 303
Orangeburg, NY 10962
914-634-5099
800-248-8033
www.irenegari.com

00585
Fisons Corp.
See Medeva Pharmaceuticals

54323
Flanders, Inc.
P.O. Box 39143
Charleston, SC 29407-9143
843-571-3363

00256
Fleming & Co.
1733 Gilsinn Lane
Fenton, MO 63026
314-343-8200
www.flemingco.com

00288
Fluoritab Corp.
8151 Brentwood Lane
Temperance, MI 48182-0507
734-847-3985

00258, 00456, 00535
Forest Pharmaceutical, Inc.
13600 Shoreline Dr.
St. Louis, MO 63045
314-493-7000
800-678-1605

Forte Pharma
220 Lake Dr.
Newark, DE 19702
877-993-6783

Free Radical Sciences, Inc.
245 First St.
Cambridge, MA 02142
617-374-1200

10432
Freeda Vitamins, Inc.
36 E. 41st St.
New York, NY 10017-6203
212-685-4980
800-777-3737

Fuisz Technologies, Ltd.
14555 Avion at Lakeside
Suite 250
Chantilly, VA 22151
703-803-3260

00469, 57317
Fujisawa USA, Inc.
3 Parkway N. Center
Deerfield, IL 60015-2548
847-317-8800
800-888-7704
800-727-7003
www.fujisawa.com

00713
G & W Laboratories
111 Coolidge St.
S. Plainfield, NJ 07080
908-753-2000
800-922-1038

Galagen, Inc.
P.O. Box 64314
St. Paul, MN 55164-0314
651-634-4233
www.galagen.com

00299
Galderma Laboratories, Inc.
P.O. Box 331329
Ft. Worth, TX 76163
817-263-2600
800-582-8225

00254
Gambro, Inc.
1185 Oak St.
Lakewood, CO 80215
800-525-2623
www.gambro.com

57844
Gate Pharmaceuticals
151 Domorah Dr.
Montgomeryville, PA 18963
800-292-4283
www.tevapharmusa.com

00386
Gebauer Co.
9410 St. Catherine Ave.
Cleveland, OH 44104
216-271-5252
800-321-9348
www.gebauerco.com

00028
Geigy Pharmaceuticals
See Novartis

52761
GenDerm Corp.
See Medicis

50242
Genentech, Inc.
1 DNA Way
S. San Francisco, CA 94080
650-225-1000
800-225-1000
www.gene.com

52584
General Injectables & Vaccines
U.S. Hwy. 52 S.
Bastian, VA 24314
540-688-4121

00918
General Medical Corp.
8741 Landmark Rd.
Richmond, VA 23261
804-264-7500
800-876-0770
www.mckgenmed.com

98318
Genesis Nutrition
2803 Andover Rd.
Florence, SC 29501
843-665-6928
800-451-7933
www.genesisnutrition.com

Genetic Therapy, Inc.
938 Clopper Rd.
Gaithersburg, MD 20878
301-590-2626

Genetics Institute
35 Cambridge Park Dr.
Cambridge, MA 02140
617-503-7332

00781
Geneva Pharmaceuticals
2599 W. Midway Blvd.
P.O. Box 469
Broomfield, CO 80038-0469
800-525-8747
800-622-9191
www.genevarx.com

Gen-King
See Kinray

00703
Gensia Sicor Pharmaceuticals, Inc.
19 Hughes
Irvine, CA 92718-1902
949-445-0218
www.gensiasicor.com

58468
Genzyme Corp.
One Kendall Square
Building 1400
Cambridge, MA 02139
617-252-7500
800-326-7002
www.genzyme.com

Geriatric Pharmaceutical Corp.
See Roberts Pharmaceuticals

Gilead Sciences, Inc.
333 Lakeside Dr.
Foster City, CA 94404
800-445-3235
www.gilead.com

59366
Glades Pharmaceuticals
255 Alhambra Circle
Suite 1000
Coral Gables, FL 33134
305-567-1319
800-452-3371
www.glades.com

00081, 00173
GlaxoWellcome
5 Moore Dr.
Research Triangle Pk., NC 27709
919-248-2100
888-825-5249
www.glaxowellcome.com

00516
Glenwood, Inc.
82 N. Summit St.
P.O. Box 518
Tenafly, NJ 07670
800-542-0772
www.glenwood-llc.com

00115
Global Pharmaceutical
Castor & Kenesington Aves.
Philadelphia, PA 19124
215-289-2220
e-mail: globalphar@aol.com

Global Source
3001 N. 29th Ave.
Hollywood, FL 33020
954-921-0006
800-662-7556
www.lookup.com

60429
Goldenstate Medical Supply
27644 N. Newhall Ranch Rd.
Valencia, CA 91355
800-284-8633

00182
Goldline Laboratories, Inc.
See Zenith Goldline

74684
Goody's Manufacturing Corp.
See Block Drug Company, Inc.

10481
Gordon Laboratories
6801 Ludlow St.
Upper Darby, PA 19082-1694
610-734-2011
800-356-7870
www.gordonlabs.com

12165
Graham Field
81 Spence St.
Bay Shore, NY 11706
516-273-2200
800-645-1023

Grandpa Brands Company
1820 Airport Exchange Blvd.
606-647-0777
800-684-1468

00152
Gray Pharmaceutical Co.
See Purdue Frederick

51301
Great Southern Laboratories
10863 Rockley Rd.
Houston, TX 77099
281-530-3077

Green Turtle Bay Vitamin Co.
56 High St.
P.O. Box 642
Summit, NJ 07901
908-277-2240
800-887-8535

59762
Greenstone
Moors Bridge Rd.
Portage, MI 49002
800-447-3360

22840
Greer Laboratories, Inc.
639 Nuway Circle
P.O. Box 800
Lenoir, NC 28645-0800
828-754-5327
800-438-0088

Guilford Pharmaceuticals, Inc.
6611 Tributary St.
Baltimore, MD 21224
410-631-6302
800-453-3746
www.guilford.com

Gynetics
P.O. Box 8509
Somerville, NJ 08876
908-359-2429

00879
Halsey Drug Co.
695 N. Perryville Rd.
Rockford, IL 61107
815-399-2060
800-336-2750
www.halseydrug.com

Hannan Ophthalmic Marketing Services, Inc.
163 Meetinghouse Rd.
Duxbury, MA 02332
781-834-8111

52512
Harmony Laboratories
1109 S. Main
P.O. Box 39
Landis, NC 28088
800-245-6284
www.harmonylabs.com

52637
Hauser Pharmaceutical Inc.
4401 E. U.S. Hwy. 30
Valparaiso, IN 46383-9573
219-464-2309
800-441-2309

63717
Hawthorn Pharmaceuticals Inc.
135 Industrial Blvd.
P.O. Box 2248
Madison, MS 39110
601-856-4393
800-856-4393
www.cypressrx.com

HDC Corporation
2109 O'Toole Ave.
San Jose, CA 95131
408-954-1909
800-227-8162
www.hdccorp.com

Health & Medical Techniques
See Graham Field

50383
Health Care Products
369 Bayview Ave.
Amityville, NY 11701
516-789-8455
800-899-3116

00598
Health for Life Brands, Inc.
1643 E. Genesee St.
Syracuse, NY 13210
315-478-6303

51662
Healthfirst Corp.
22316 70th Ave. W.
Mountlake Terrace, WA 98043
425-771-5733
800-331-1984

59512
Healthline Laboratories, Inc.
2805 Danbar Dr.
Green Bay, WI 54313
920-434-9620

Health-Mark Diagnostics
3341 S.W. 15th St.
Pompano Beach, FL 33069
954-984-8881

00064
Healthpoint Medical
2600 Airport Freeway
Ft. Worth, TX 76111
817-900-4000
800-441-8227
www.healthpoint.com

Health Products Corp.
1060 Nepperhan
Yonkers, NY 10703
914-423-2900

Helena Laboratories
1530 Lindbergh Dr.
P.O. Box 752
Beaumont, TX 77707
409-842-3714
800-231-5663
www.helena.com

HEM Research
1617 John F. Kennedy Blvd.
Philadelphia, PA 19103
215-988-0080
www.hemispherx.com

Hemacare Corp.
4954 Van Nuys Blvd.
Sherman Oaks, CA 91403
818-986-3883

Hemispherx
1 Penn Center
1617 John F. Kennedy Blvd.
Philadelphia, PA 19103
215-988-8800
www.hemispherx.com

Hemispherx Biopharma, Inc.
1 Penn Center
1617 John F. Kennedy Blvd.
Suite 660
Philadelphia, PA 19103
215-988-0080

Hemotec Medical Products, Inc.
P.O. Box 19255
Johnston, RI 02919
401-934-2571

Henry Schein, Inc.
135 Duryea Rd.
Melville, NY 11747
516-843-5500
800-472-4346
www.henryschein.com

Herald Pharmacal Inc.
See Allergan, Inc.

Herbert Laboratories
See Allergan, Inc.

49730
Hercon Laboratories, Inc.
460 Park Ave.
New York, NY 10022
212-751-5600

Heritage Consumer Products
141 S. Ave., Suite 2
Fanwood, NJ 07023
908-322-9067
800-344-7239
www.cnewsusa.com

28105
Hill Dermaceuticals, Inc.
2650 S. Mellonville Ave.
Sanford, FL 32773
407-896-8280
800-344-5707
e-mail: hillderm@
internetmci.com

17808
Himmel Pharmaceuticals, Inc.
1926 10th Ave. N., Suite 303
Lake Worth, FL 33461
561-585-0070
800-535-3823

Hind Health Care
3707 Williams Rd.
Suite 101
San Jose, CA 96117
408-615-4140

50383
Hi-Tech Pharmacal
369 Bayview Ave.
Amityville, NY 11701
516-789-8228
800-262-9010
www.diabeticproducts.com

00839
H.L. Moore Drug Exchange, Inc.
389 John Downey Dr.
New Britain, CT 06050
860-826-3600
800-444-8765
www.mooremedical.com

00039, 00068, 00088
Hoechst-Marion Roussel
10236 Marion Park Dr.
P.O. Box 9627
Kansas City, MO 64134-0627
816-966-5000
800-362-7466
www.hmri.com

58573
Hogil Pharmaceutical Corp.
2 Manhattanville Rd.
Purchase, NY 10577
914-696-7600

47992
Holles Laboratories, Inc.
30 Forest Notch
Cohasset, MA 02025-1198
800-356-4015

Hollister-Stier
See Bayer Corp. (Allergy Div.)

Home Access Health Corp.
2401 W. Hassell Rd.
Suite 1510
Hoffman Estates, IL 60195-5200
847-781-2500
www.homeaccess.com

Hope Pharmaceuticals
7626 E. Greenway Rd. #101
Scottsdale, AZ 85260
480-607-1970
800-755-9595
www.hopepharm.com

59630
Horizon Pharmaceutical Corp.
660 Hembree Pkwy. #106
Roswell, GA 30076
770-442-9707
800-849-9707

58407
Houba
See Halsey

Huckaby Pharmacal, Inc.
6316 Old La Grange Rd.
Crestwood, KY 40014
502-243-4000
888-206-5525

25077
Hudson Corp.
90 Orville Dr.
Bohemia, NY 11716
516-567-9500

00395
Humco Holding Group, Inc.
7400 Alumax
Texarkana, TX 75501
903-831-7808
800-662-3435

Hybritech
P.O. Box 269006
San Diego, CA 92196-9006
619-455-6700
800-854-1957
www.beckmancoulter.com

Hyland Therapeutics
See Baxter Hyland

Hynson, Westcott & Dunning
See Becton Dickinson Microbiology Systems

00314
Hyrex Pharmaceuticals
3494 Democrat Rd.
P.O. Box 18385
Memphis, TN 38118-0385
901-794-9050
800-238-5282

ICI Pharmaceuticals
See Zeneca Pharmaceuticals

00163, 00187
ICN Pharmaceuticals, Inc.
3300 Hyland Ave.
Costa Mesa, CA 92626
714-545-0100
800-556-1937
www.icnpharm.com

IDEC Pharmaceuticals
11011 Torreyana Rd.
San Diego, CA 92121
619-550-8500

Ilex Oncology Inc.
14960 Omicron Dr.
San Antonio, TX 78245
210-949-8200
www.ilexonc.com

Immcel Pharmaceuticals, Inc.
79-55 Albion Ave.
Elmhurst, NY 11373

Immucell Corp.
56 Evergreen Dr.
Portland, ME 04103
207-878-2770
www.immucell.com

00205, 58406
Immunex Corp.
51 University St.
Seattle, WA 98101
206-587-0430
800-IMMUNEX
www.immunex.com

Immuno Therapeutics
2135 N. Lakeshore Dr.
Moorhead, MN 27514
701-239-3775

54129
Immuno U.S., Inc.
1200 Parkdale Rd.
Rochester, MI 48307-1744
248-652-4760
www.baxter.com
(See Baxter)

Immunobiology Research Inst.
Route 22 East
P.O. Box 999
Annandale, NJ 08801-0999
908-730-1700

ImmunoGen
148 Sidney St.
Cambridge, MA 02139
617-497-1113

Immunomedics
300 American Rd.
Morris Plains, NJ 07950
973-605-8200
www.immunomedics.com

00548
I.M.S., Ltd.
See Medeva

imx Pharmaceuticals, Inc.
2295 Corporate Blvd.
Boca Raton, FL 33431

Infusaid, Inc.
1400 Providence Hwy.
Norwood, MA 02062
781-769-8330
800-523-8446

Inspire Pharmaceuticals, Inc.
4222 Emperor Blvd.
Suite 470
Durham, NC 27703
919-941-9777
www.inspirepharm.com

Interchem Corp.
120 Route 17 N.
P.O. Box 1579
Paramus, NJ 07653
201-261-7333
800-261-7332
www.interchem.com

Interfalk U.S., Inc.
25 Margaret
Plattsburgh, NY 12901

Interferon Sciences
783 Jersey Ave.
New Brunswick, NJ 08901
732-249-3250
888-728-4372
www.interferonsciences.com

11584
International Ethical Labs
Reparto Metropolitano
Rio Piedras, PR 00921
787-765-3510

Interneuron Pharmaceuticals, Inc.
1 Ledgemont Center
99 Hayden Ave.
Lexington, MA 02421
781-861-8444
www.interneuron.com

00814
Interstate Drug Exchange
See Henry Schein, Inc.

Intramed
102 Tremont Way
Augusta, GA 30907

52189
Invamed, Inc.
2400 Route 130N
Dayton, NJ 08810
732-274-2400

Inveresk Research
4470 Redwood Hwy.
Suite 101
San Rafael, CA 94903
415-491-6460
www.inveresk-research.com

00258
Inwood Laboratories
321 Prospect St.
Inwood, NY 11096
516-371-1155
800-284-6966

Iolab Pharmaceuticals
See Ciba Vision Ophthalmics

61646
Iomed
7425 Pebble Dr.
Fort Worth, TX 76118
817-589-7257
www.iomed.com

11808
ION Laboratories, Inc.
7431 Pebble Dr.
Ft. Worth, TX 76118
817-589-7257

IOP, Inc.
3151 Airway Ave.
Suite I-1
Costa Mesa, CA 92626
714-549-1185
800-535-3545

54921
IPR Pharmaceuticals, Inc.
P.O. Box 6000
Carolina, PR 00984
800-477-6385

Isis Pharmaceuticals
Carlsbad Research Center
2292 Farady Ave.
Carlsbad, CA 92008
760-931-9200
www.isip.com

50914
Iso Tex Diagnostics, Inc.
1511 County Rd. 129
Friendswood, TX 77546
281-482-1231
800-631-0600

Ivax Corporation
4400 Biscayne Blvd.
Miami, FL 33137
305-575-6000
www.ivax.com

16837
J & J Merck Consumer Pharm.
Camp Hill Rd.
Ft. Washington, PA 19034
215-273-7000
800-523-3484
www.jnj-merck.com

J.B. Williams Company, Inc.
65 Harristown Rd., 3rd Floor
Glen Rock, NJ 07452-3317
201-251-8100
800-254-8656

88395
J. R. Carlson Laboratories
15 College Dr.
Arlington Heights, IL 60004-1985
847-255-1600
800-323-4141
www.carlsonlabs.com

49938
Jacobus Pharmaceutical Co.
P.O. Box 5290
37 Cleveland Lane
Princeton, NJ 08540
609-921-7447

50458
Janssen Pharmaceutical, Inc.
P.O. Box 200
Titusville, NJ 08560-0200
609-730-2000
800-526-7736
www.us.janssen.com

Janssen Research Foundation
1125 Trenton Harvourton Rd.
Titusville, NJ 08560
609-730-2000

JMI-Canton Pharmaceuticals
See Jones Medical Industries

56091
Johnson & Johnson Medical
P.O. Box 90130
Arlington, TX 76004-0130
800-433-5009
800-423-5850
www.jnjmedical.com

00137
Johnson & Johnson
Grandview Rd.
Skillman, NJ 08558-9418
800-635-6789
www.jnj.com

00252, 52604, 00689
Jones Medical Industries
P.O. Box 46903
St. Louis, MO 63146-6903
314-576-6100
800-525-8466

10106
J.T. Baker, Inc.
See Mallinckrodt-Baker

KabiVitrum, Inc.
See Pharmacia & Upjohn

Kanetta
90 Park Ave.
New York, NY 10016
212-907-2690
800-372-6634

00588
Keene Pharmaceuticals, Inc.
P.O. Box 7
Keene, TX 76059-0007
817-645-8083
800-541-0530

28851
Kendall Health Care Products
15 Hampshire St.
Mansfield, MA 02048
800-962-9888
www.kendallhq.com

Kendall-McGaw Labs, Inc.
See McGaw, Inc.

00482
Kenwood Laboratories
See Doak

00085
Key Pharmaceuticals
See Schering-Plough

60793
King Pharmaceuticals Inc.
501 Fifth St.
Bristol, TN 37620
423-989-8000
800-336-7783

55299
Kingswood Laboratories, Inc.
10375 Hague Rd.
Indianapolis, IN 46256
317-849-9513
800-968-7772

Kinray
152-35 10th Ave.
Whitestone, NY 11357
718-767-1234

58223
Kirkman Sales, Inc.
P.O. Box 1009
Wilsonville, OR 97070-1009
503-694-1600
800-245-8282

31600
Kiwi Brands, Inc.
447 Old Swede Rd.
Douglassville, PA 19518-1239
610-385-3041

KLI Corp.
1119 Third Ave. S.W.
Carmel, IN 46032
317-846-7452
800-308-7452
www.entertainers-secret.com

00044, 00048, 00524
Knoll
3000 Continental Dr. N.
Mt. Olive, NJ 07828-1234
973-426-2600
800-526-0221
www.basf.com

Kodak Dental
343 State St.
Rochester, NY 14650
800-933-8031
www.lannett.com

00224
Konsyl Pharmaceuticals
4200 S. Hulen
Suite 513
Ft. Worth, TX 76109
817-763-8011
www.konsyl.com

KOS Pharm
2 Oakwood Blvd.
Suite 140
Hollywood, FL 33020
954-920-7200
www.kos.com

55505
Kramer Laboratories, Inc.
8778 S.W. 8th St.
Miami, FL 33174-9990
305-223-1287
800-824-4894
www.kramerlabs.com

Kremers Urban
9428 Baymeadows Rd.
Suite 250
Jacksonville, FL 32256
800-625-5710

K.V. Pharmaceutical Co.
2503 S. Hanley Rd.
St. Louis, MO 63144
314-645-6600

La Haye Laboratories, Inc.
2205 152nd Ave. N.E.
Redmond, WA 98052
425-644-2020

Lacrimedics, Inc.
190 N. Arrowhead Ave.
Suite B
Rialto, CA 92376
800-367-8327
www.lacrimedics.com

41383
Lactaid, Inc.
7050 Camp Hill Rd.
Ft. Washington, PA 19034
215-273-7000
800-522-8243
www.jnj.com

59081
Lafayette Pharmaceuticals, Inc.
526 N. Earl Ave.
Lafayette, IN 47904-4499
765-447-3129
800-428-7843

Lake Consumer Products
625 Forest Edge Dr.
Vernon Hills, IL 60061
847-793-0230
800-739-9883

00527
Lannett, Inc.
9000 State Rd.
Philadelphia, PA 19136
215-333-9000
800-325-9994
www.lannett.com

00277
Laser, Inc.
2200 W. 97th Place
P.O. Box 905
Crown Point, IN 46307
219-663-1165
800-325-0925

10651
Lavoptik, Inc.
661 Western Ave.
St. Paul, MN 55103
651-489-1351

Leas Research
78 Fallon Dr.
N. Haven, CT 05473
203-239-2021

00005
Lederle Laboratories
401 N. Middletown Rd.
Pearl River, NY 10965-1299
914-732-5000
800-395-9938

53124
Lederle-Praxis Biologicals
N. Middletown Rd.
Pearl River, NY 10965
800-820-2815

23558
Lee Pharmaceuticals
1434 Santa Anita Blvd.
S. Elmonte, CA 91733
626-442-3141
800-950-5337

Leeming
See Pfizer US Pharmaceutical Group

25332
Legere Pharmaceuticals, Inc.
7326 E. Evans Rd.
Scottsdale, AZ 85260
602-991-4033
800-528-3144

19200
Lehn & Fink
See Reckitt & Coleman

Leiner Health Products
901 East 233rd St.
Carson, CA 90745
310-835-8400
800-421-1168

Leiras Pharmaceuticals, Inc.
2345 Waukegan Rd.
Suite N-135
Bonnockburn, IL 60015

00093, 00332
Lemmon Co.
See Teva Pharmaceuticals

Lifescan
1000 Gibraltar
Milpitas, CA 95035-6312
408-263-9789
800-227-8862
www.lifescan.com

LifeSign LLC
71 Veronica Ave.
P.O. Box 218
Somerset, NJ 08875-0218
908-246-3366
800-526-2125
www.lifesignmed.com

Ligand Pharmaceuticals, Inc.
10275 Science Center Dr.
San Diego, CA 92121
619-550-7506
www.ligand.com

00002, 59075
Eli Lilly and Co.
Lilly Corp. Center
Indianapolis, IN 46285
317-276-2000
www.elililly.com

Lincoln Diagnostics
P.O. Box 1128
Decatur, IL 62525
217-877-2531
800-537-1336

Lipha Pharmaceuticals, Inc.
9 W. 57th St., Ste. 3825
New York, NY 10019-2701
212-223-1280

60799
Liposome Co.
One Research Way
Princeton, NJ 08540
609-452-7060
www.liposome.com

Lobana Laboratories
2440 Fernbrook Lane
Plymouth, MN 55447
612-559-0601
800-848-5637

Loch Pharmaceuticals
See Bedford Laboratories

00273
Lorvic Corp.
See Young Dental

59417
Lotus Biochemical
7335 Lee Hwy.
P.O. Box 3586
Radford, VA 24141-3586
703-633-3500
800-455-5525

LSI America Corp.
4732 Twin Valley Dr.
Austin, TX 78731-3537
512-451-3738
800-720-5936
www.ondrox.com

00374
Lyne Laboratories
10 Burke Dr.
Brockton, MA 02301
508-583-8700
800-525-0450

00904
Major Pharmaceuticals
31778 Enterprise Dr.
Livonia, MI 48150
734-525-8700
800-688-9696

10106
Mallinckrodt-Baker
222 Red School Lane
Phillipsburg, NJ 08865
908-859-2151
www.mallinckrodt.com

00406
Mallinckrodt Chemical
16305 Swingley Ridge Dr.
Chesterfield, MO 63017
314-654-2000
800-325-8888
www.mallinckrodt.com

00019
Mallinckrodt Medical, Inc.
675 McDonnell Blvd.
P.O. Box 5840
St. Louis, MO 63134
314-895-2000
888-744-1414
www.mallinckrodt.com

Manloe Labs, Inc.
See Skinvisible, Inc.

10706
Manne
P.O. Box 825
Johns Island, SC 29457
803-768-4080
800-517-0228

Marlin Industries
P.O. Box 560
Grover Beach, CA 93483-0560
805-473-2743
800-423-5926

12939
Marlop Pharmaceuticals, Inc.
230 Marshall St.
Elizabeth, NY 07206
908-355-8854
718-796-1570
800-345-7192

10712
Marlyn Neutraceuticals, Inc.
14851 N. Scottsdale Rd.
Scottsdale, AZ 85254
800-462-7596

00682
Marnel Pharmaceuticals, Inc.
206 Luke Dr.
Lafayette, LA 70506
318-232-1396

00209
Marsam Pharmaceuticals, Inc.
24 Olney Ave., Bldg. 31
P.O. Box 1022
Cherry Hill, NJ 08034
609-424-5600
800-883-2600
www.schein-rx.com

52555
Martec Pharmaceutical, Inc.
P.O. Box 33510
Kansas City, MO 64120-3510
816-241-4144
800-822-6782

11845
Mason Distributors, Inc.
5105 N.W. 159th St.
Hialeah, FL 33014-6370
305-624-5557
800-327-6005

12758
Mason Pharmaceuticals, Inc.
4425 Jamboree
Suite 250
Newport Beach, CA 92660
714-851-6860
800-366-2454

14362
Mass. Public Health Bio. Lab.
305 South St.
Jamaica Plains, MA 02130
617-522-3700

Matrix Laboratories, Inc.
34700 Campus Dr.
Fremont, CA 94555
510-742-9900
www.matx.com

Mayo Foundation
200 1st St. S.W.
Rochester, MN 55905
507-284-2511

00259
Mayrand, Inc.
See Merz Pharmaceuticals

00264
McGaw, Inc.
P.O. Box 19791
Irvine, CA 92713-9791
949-660-2000
800-854-6851

11089
McGregor Pharmaceuticals, Inc.
8420 Ulmenton Rd.
Suite 305
Largo, FL 34641
727-530-4361

49072
McGuff, Inc.
3524 W. Lake Center Dr.
Santa Ana, CA 92704
800-854-7220

00045
McNeil Consumer Products Co.
Camp Hill Rd.
Mail Stop 278
Ft. Washington, PA 19034-2292
215-273-7000

MCR American Pharmaceuticals
120 Summit Parkway,
Suite 101
Birmingham, AL 35209
205-942-6415

58607
ME Pharmaceuticals, Inc.
2800 Southeast Pkwy.
Richmond, IN 47374
800-637-4276

Mead Johnson Laboratories
See Bristol-Myers Squibb

00087
Mead Johnson Nutritionals
2400 W. Lloyd Expressway
Evansville, IN 47721
812-429-5000
www.meadjohnson.com

Mead Johnson Oncology
See Bristol-Myers Oncology

Mead Johnson Pharmaceuticals
See Bristol-Myers Squibb

Medac GmbH c/o Princeton Regulatory Assoc.
65 S. Main St.
Pennington, NJ 08534
609-951-9596

Medarex
1545 Rte. 22E
P.O. Box 953
Annandale, NJ 08801
908-713-6001
www.medarex.com

11940
Medco Lab, Inc.
P.O. Box 864
Sioux City, IA 51102-0864
712-255-8770
www.medcolab.com

Medco Pharmaceuticals
2015 Hwy. 190 Bypass
Covington, LA 70433
800-793-8740

Medco Research, Inc.
P.O. Box 13886
Research Triangle Park, NC 27709
919-549-8117

45565
Med-Derm Pharmaceuticals
524 Suncrest Dr.
Gray, TN 37615
423-477-3991
800-334-4286

Medea Research Laboratories
200 Wilson St.
Port Jefferson, NY 11776
516-331-7718

00585
Medeva Pharmaceuticals
755 Jefferson Rd.
Rochester, NY 14623-0000
800-932-1950
www.mdvroc.com

00576
Medical Products Panamericana
647 W. Flagler St.
Miami, FL 33130
305-545-6524

99207
Medicis Pharmaceutical Corp.
4343 E. Cambelback Rd.
Suite 150
Phoenix, AZ 85018
602-808-8800
800-845-1313

60574
Medimmune, Inc.
35 W. Watkins Mill Rd.
Gaithersburg, MD 20878
301-417-0770
800-934-7426
www.medimmune.com

Medi-Plex Pharm., Inc.
See ECR Pharmaceuticals

Medique Products
7701 N. Austin Ave.
Skokie, IL 60077
800-634-7680

57480
Medirex, Inc.
20 Chapin Rd.
Pine Brook, NJ 07058
973-227-4774
800-343-3848
www.medirex.com

61563
Medisan
400 Lanidex Plaza
Parsippany, NJ 07054
973-515-5300
800-763-3472

MediSense, Inc.
4A Crosby Dr.
Bedford, MA 01730
781-276-6000
800-527-3339

Medix Pharmaceuticals Americas, Inc.
6301 Ivy Lane, Ste. 510
Greenbelt, MD 20770
301-479-1717
888-BIAFINE
www.biafine.com

53978
Med-Pro, Inc.
210 E. 4th St.
Lexington, NE 68850
308-324-4571
800-477-6060

00348, 75137
Medtech Laboratories, Inc.
3510 N. Lake Creek
P.O. Box 1108
Jackson, WY 83011-1108
307-733-1680
800-443-4908

58281
Medtronic Neuro
800 53rd Ave. N.E.
Minneapolis, MN 55421
612-572-5000
800-328-0810

Melville Biologics
155 Duryea Rd.
Melville, NY 11747
516-752-7339

Menicon USA
333 W. Pontiac Way
Clovis, CA 93612
800-MENICON
www.menicon.com

22200
Mennen Co.
See Colgate Palmolive

10742
Mentholatum Co.
707 Sterling Dr.
Orchard Park, NY 14127
716-677-2500
800-688-7660

00006
Merck & Co.
P.O. Box 4
West Point, PA 19486
800-672-6372
www.merck.com

00394
Mericon Industries, Inc.
8819 N. Pioneer Rd.
Peoria, IL 61615
309-693-2150
800-242-6464

Meridian Medical Technologies
10240 Old Columbia Rd.
Columbia, MD 21046
410-309-6830
800-638-8093
www.meridianmeds.com

Merieux Institute, Inc.
See Pasteur-Mérieux-Connaught

30727
Merit Pharmaceuticals
2611 San Fernando Rd.
Los Angeles, CA 90065
323-227-4831
800-421-9657

Merz Pharmaceuticals
4215 Tudor Lane
Greensboro, NC 27419
336-856-2003
800-334-0514
www.merzusa.com

MGI Pharma, Inc.
9900 Bren Rd. E.
Ste. 300E, Opus Center
Minnetonka, MN 55343-9667
612-935-7335
800-562-0679
www.mgipharma.com

Michigan Department of Health
P.O. Box 30035
Lansing, MI 48909
517-373-3740

MicroGeneSys, Inc.
1000 Research Pkwy.
Meriden, CT 06450
203-686-0800
800-488-7099
www.proteinsciences.com

00682, 46672
Mikart, Inc.
1750 Chattahoochee Ave.
Atlanta, GA 30318
404-351-4510
www.mikart.com

Miles, Inc.
See Bayer Corp. (Consumer Div.)

Miles, Inc.
See Bayer Corp. (Diagnostic Div.)

00396, 34567
Milex Products, Inc.
4311 N. Normandy
Chicago, IL 60634
800-621-1278

17204
Miller Pharmacal Group, Inc.
350 Randy Rd., Unit #2
Carol Stream, IL 60188
630-871-9557
800-323-2935

00276
Misemer Pharmaceuticals, Inc.
See Edwards Pharmaceuticals

00178
Mission Pharmacal Co.
1325 E. Durango Blvd.
P.O. Box 786099
San Antonio, TX 78278-6099
800-531-3333
www.missionpharmacal.com

53169
Monarch Pharmaceuticals
355 Beecham St.
Bristol, TN 37620
800-776-3637
www.monarchpharm.com

Monticello Drug Co.
1604 Stockton Co.
Jacksonville, FL 32204
800-735-0666
www.monticellocompanies.com

00426, 00832, 60432
Morton Grove Pharmaceuticals
6451 W. Main St.
Morton Grove, IL 60053
847-967-5600
800-346-6854

Morton International
1275 Lake Ave.
Woodstock, IL 60098-7499
815-338-1800
www.morton.com

Morton Salt
100 N. Riverside Plaza
Chicago, IL 60606-1597
312-807-2000

Mova Pharmaceutical
214 Carnegie Center
Ste. 106
Princeton, NJ 08540
800-542-MOVA
www.movalabs.com

MSD
See Merck & Co.

Mt. Vernon Foods, Inc.
13246 Wooster Rd.
Mt. Vernon, OH 43050-9726
740-397-7077

54964
Murdock, Madaus, Schwabe
P.O. Box 4000
Springvale, UT 84663
801-489-1500
ww.naturesway.com

00451
Muro Pharmaceutical, Inc.
890 East St.
Tewksbury, MA 01876-9987
978-851-5981
800-225-0974

00150
Murray Drug Corp.
1103 N. Wood
Murray, KY 42071
502-753-6654

53489
Mutual Pharmaceutical, Inc.
1100 Orthodox St.
Philadelphia, PA 19124
215-288-6500
800-523-3684
www.urlmutual.com

00378
Mylan Pharmaceuticals
P.O. Box 4310
Morgantown, WV 26504
304-599-2595
800-826-9526
www.mylan.com

05973
Nabi
5800 Park of Commerce Blvd. N.W.
Boca Raton, FL 33487
561-989-5800
800-642-8874
www.nabi.com

NAPA of the Bahamas
3560 Pennsylvania Ave.
Dubuque, IA 52002
319-557-9684

05745
Nastech Pharmaceutical, Inc.
45 Davids Dr.
Hauppauge, NY 11788
516-273-0101
www.nastech.com

53983
Natren, Inc.
3105 Willow Lane
Westlake Village, CA 91361
805-371-4737
800-992-3323
www.natren.com

Naturally Vitamins Co.
14851 N. Scottsdale Rd.
Scottsdale, AZ 85254
602-991-0200
www.naturallyvitamins.com

Natures Bounty, Inc.
See NBTY, Inc.

74312
NBTY, Inc.
105 Orville Dr.
Bohemia, NY 11716
516-567-9500
800-645-5412
www.nbty.com

72559
NCI Medical Foods
5801 Ayala Ave.
Irwindale, CA 91706
626-812-6522
800-869-1515

NeoPharm, Inc.
100 Corporate North
Suite 215
Bannockburen, IL 60015
847-295-8678

Neorx Corp.
410 W. Harrison
Seattle, WA 98119
206-281-7001
www.neorx.com

00487
Nephron Pharmaceuticals Corp.
4121 34th St.
Orlando, FL 32811
407-246-1389
800-443-4313
www.nephronpharm.com

Nephro-Tech, Inc.
P.O. Box 14703
Lenexa, KS 66285
913-248-8808
800-879-4755

Nestle Clinical Nutrition
3 Parkway N., Ste. 500
Deerfield, IL 60015
847-317-2800
800-388-0300

Neurex Corporation
See Elan

NeuroGenesis
2045 Space Park Dr.
Suite 132
Houston, TX 77058
281-333-2153
800-345-8912
www.neurogenesis.com

10812, 70501
Neutrogena Corp.
5760 W. 96th St.
Los Angeles, CA 90045-5595
310-647-1150
800-421-6857
www.neutrogena.com

Neuromuscular Adjuncts
University Hospital
Orthopedic Center
HSCT-18020
Stony Brook, NY 11790
516-444-7830

Neutron Technology Corp.
1205 N. 11th
Boise, ID 83702
208-863-4847

New Halsey Drug Co.
1827 Pacific St.
Brooklyn, NY 11233
718-467-7500

87900
New Mark
P.O. Box 6321
Edison, NJ 08818
800-338-8079

New World Trading Corp.
P.O. Box 952
DeBary, FL 32713
407-668-7520

56146
Nexstar Pharmaceuticals, Inc.
2860 Wilderness Place
Boulder, CO 80301
303-444-5893
800-403-3945
www.nexstar.com

59016
Niche Pharmaceuticals, Inc.
200 N. Oak St.
P.O. Box 449
Roanoke, TX 76262
817-491-2770
www.niche-inc.com

Nnodum Corporation
886 Clinton Springs Ave.
Cincinnati, OH 45229
513-861-2329
888-301-ZIKS
www.zikspain.com

51801
Nomax, Inc.
40 N. Rock Hill Rd.
St. Louis, MO 63119
314-961-2500
www.nomax.com

Norcliff Thayer
See SmithKline Beecham Consumer Healthcare

10118
Norstar Consumer Products
206 Pegasus Ave.
North Vale, NJ 07647
201-784-8155
800-897-5050

North American Biologicals, Inc.
See Nabi

North American Vaccine
10150 Old Columbia Rd.
Columbia, MD 21046
410-309-7100
888-628-2829
ww.nava.com

00028, 00067, 00083, 58887
Novartis
59 Route 10
East Hanover, NJ 07936
908-277-5000
888-344-8585
www.us.novartis.com

Novartis Consumer Health
560 Morris Ave., Bldg. F
Summit, NJ 07901
908-598-7600
800-452-0051
www.us.novartis.com

Novartis Nutrition Corp.
5100 Gamble Dr.
St. Louis Park, MN 55416
612-925-2100
800-999-9978
www.us.novartis.com

Novartis Pharmaceutical Corp.
59 Route 10
East Hanover, NJ 07936
973-781-8300
888-669-6682
www.us.novartis.com

Noven
11960 S.W. 144th St.
Miami, FL 33186
305-253-5099

00362
Novocol Chemical Mfr. Co.
P.O. Box 11926
Wilmington, DE 19850
302-328-1102
800-872-8305
www.septodontinc.com

00169
Novo Nordisk Pharm., Inc.
100 Overlook Center
Suite 200
Princeton, NJ 08540
800-727-6500
www.novo-nordisk.com

55953
Novopharm USA, Inc.
165 E. Commerce
Schaumberg, IL 60173-5326
847-882-4200
800-426-0769
www.novopharmusa.com

55499
Numark Laboratories, Inc.
P.O. Box 6321
Edison, NJ 08818
800-338-8079
www.numarklabs.com

NutraMax
208 Lakeside Blvd.
Edgewood, MD 21040
410-776-4000
800-925-5187
www.nutramaxlabs.com

Nutricept Inc.
11220 Grader
Suite 100
Dallas, TX 75238
214-221-3400
800-535-0631
www.nutricept.com

Nutricia, Inc.
See Mt. Vernon Foods, Inc.

Nutrition Medical, Inc.
1275 Red Fox Rd.
Arden Hills, MN 55112
800-569-7828
www.galagen.com

00407
Nycomed Inc.
101 Carnegie Center
Princeton, NJ 08540-6231
609-514-6000
800-332-6334
www.nycomed-amersham.com

10797
Oakhurst Co.
3000 Hempstead Turnpike
Levittown, NY 11756
516-731-5380
800-831-1135

55515
Oclassen Pharmaceuticals, Inc.
See Watson Laboratories

O'Connor, Inc.
See Columbia Laboratories, Inc.

51944
Ocumed, Inc.
119 Harrison Ave.
Roseland, NJ 07068
973-226-2330
800-288-3179

OHM Laboratories, Inc.
P.O. Box 7397
North Brunswick, NJ 08902
732-418-2235
800-527-6481

10019
Ohmeda Pharmaceuticals
See Baxter

OncoRx, Inc
See Vion Pharmaceuticals

OncoTherapeutics, Inc.
1002 East Park Blvd.
Cranbury, NJ 08512
609-655-5300

ONY, Inc.
1576 Sweet Home Rd.
Amherst, NY 14228
716-636-9096

Optikem International, Inc.
2172 S. Jason St.
Denver, CO 80223
303-936-1137

50520
Optimox Corp.
2720 Monterey
Suite 406
Torrance, CA 90503
310-618-9370
800-223-1601
www.optimox.com

52238
Optopics Laboratories Corp.
40 Main St.
P.O. Box 210
Fairton, NJ 08320-0210
508-283-1800

00041
Oral-B Laboratories, Inc.
600 Clipper Dr.
Belmont, CA 94002-4119
650-598-5000
800-446-7252
www.oralb.com

00052
Organon, Inc.
375 Mt. Pleasant Ave.
West Orange, NJ 07052
973-325-4500
800-241-8812

Organon Teknika Corp.
100 Akzo Ave.
Durham, NC 27712
919-620-2000
800-682-2666

Orion Diagnostica
See LifeSign LLC

Orphan Europe
1101 Kermit Dr.
Suite 600
Nashville, TN 37217
615-399-0700

Orphan Medical
13911 Ridgedale Dr.
Minnetonka, MN 55305
612-513-6900
888-867-7426
www.orphan.com

59676
Ortho Biotech, Inc.
Route 202 S.
P.O. Box 670
Raritan, NJ 08869-0670
800-325-7504
www.procrit.com

00062
Ortho McNeil Pharmaceutical
Route 202
P.O. Box 600
Raritan, NJ 08869-0600
908-218-6000
800-682-6532
www.ortho-mcneil.com

Osterreichisches Baxter Healthcare
550 N. Brand Blvd.
Glendale, CA 91203
818-507-5523

59148
Otsuka America Pharmaceutical
2440 Research Blvd.
Suite 250
Rockville, MD 98101
301-990-0030
800-562-3974
www.otsuka.com

Owen/Galderma
See Galderma Laboratories, Inc.

Oxford Pharmaceutical Services, Inc.
1425 Broad Street
Clifton, NJ 07013
973-777-3327
877-284-9120
www.oxfordpharm.com

Oxis International
6040 N. Cutter Circle
Suite 317
Portland, OR 97212
503-283-3911
800-547-3686
www.oxis.com

Oxypure Inc.
3550 Morris St. N.
St. Petersburg, FL 33713
727-522-8490

00574
P&S Laboratories, Inc.
210 W. 131st St.
Los Angeles, CA 90061
800-624-9659
www.hylands.com

Paddock Laboratories
3490 Quebec Ave. N.
Minneapolis, MN 55427
612-546-4676
800-328-5113
www.paddocklabs.com

53159
Palisades Pharmaceuticals, Inc.
See Glenwood

Pan American Labs
P.O. Box 8950
Mandeville, LA 70470-8950
504-893-4097
888-829-4097
www.panamericanlabs.com

49884
Par Pharmaceuticals
1 Ram Ridge Rd.
Spring Valley, NY 10977
914-425-7100
800-828-9393
www.parpharm.com

00071
Parke-Davis
201 Tabor Rd.
Morris Plains, NJ 07950
973-540-2000
800-223-0432
www.parke-davis.com

00349
Parmed Pharmaceuticals, Inc.
4220 Hyde Park Blvd.
Niagara Falls, NY 14305
716-284-5666
800-727-6331

50930
Parnell Pharmaceuticals, Inc.
P.O. Box 5130
Larkspur, CA 94977
415-256-1800
800-457-4276
www.parnellpharm.com

10865
Parthenon, Inc.
3311 W. 2400 S.
Salt Lake City, UT 84119
801-972-5184
800-453-8898

00418
Pasadena Research Labs
See Taylor Pharmaceuticals

11793, 49281, 50361
Pasteur-Mérieux-Connaught Labs
Discovery Dr.
Swiftwater, PA 18370-0187
570-839-7187
800-822-2463

PathoGenesis Corp.
201 Elliott Ave. W.
Seattle, WA 98119
206-467-8100
www.pathogenesis.com

Pediatric Pharmaceuticals
120 Wood Ave. S.
Suite 300
Iselin, NJ 08830
732-603-7708

00884
Pedinol Pharmacal, Inc.
30 Banfi Plaza N.
Farmingdale, NY 11735
516-293-9500
800-733-4665

10974
Pegasus Medical, Inc.
1 Technology Dr.
Building C523
Irvine, CA 92618-2325
949-823-9636

Penederm, Inc.
320 Lakeside Dr.
Suite A
Foster City, CA 94404
650-358-0100
www.penederm.com

Pennex Pharmaceutical, Inc.
See Morton Grove Pharmaceuticals

Pentech Pharmaceuticals, Inc
417 Harvester Ct.
Wheeling, IL 60090
847-459-9122

Permeable Technologies, Inc.
712 Ginesi Dr.
Morganville, NJ 07751
732-972-8585
800-622-7376
www.lifestylecompany.com

00096
Person and Covey, Inc.
616 Allen Ave.
P.O. Box 25018
Glendale, CA 91221-5018
818-240-1030
800-423-2341

00927
Pfeiffer Co.
71 University Ave.
P.O. Box 4447
Atlanta, GA 30302
404-614-0255
800-342-6450

Pfipharmecs
See Pfizer US Pharmaceutical Group

Pfizer Consumer Health
235 E. 42nd St.
New York, NY 10017
212-573-5656
800-332-1240
www.pfizer.com

00069, 00663, 74300
Pfizer US Pharmaceutical Group
235 E. 42nd St.
New York, NY 10017-5755
800-438-1985

39822
Pharmanex, Inc.
75 W. Center
Provo, UT 84601
801-345-9800
800-800-0260
www.pharmanex.com

Pharmascience Laboratories, Inc.
175 Rano St.
Buffalo, NY 14207
716-871-9376
800-207-4477

Pharma-Tek, Inc.
P.O. Box 1920
Huntington, NY 11743-0568
516-757-5522
800-645-6655

00121
Pharmaceutical Associates, Inc.
P.O. Box 128
Conestee, SC 29636
864-277-7282
800-845-8210

Pharmaceutical Basics, Inc.
See Rosemont Pharmaceutical

51655
Pharmaceutical Corp.
12348 Hancock St.
Carmel, IN 46032
317-573-8000
800-722-0772

21659
Pharmaceutical Labs, Inc.
1170 W. Corporate Dr.
Suite 102
Arlington, TX 76006
817-633-1461
800-338-4788
www.phlb.com

45334
Pharmaceutical Specialties, Inc.
P.O. Box 6298
Rochester, MN 55903
507-288-8500
800-325-8232

Pharmaceuticals, Inc.
See Gensia Sicor Pharmaceuticals Inc.

Pharmachemie USA, Inc.
P.O. Box 145
Oradell, NJ 07049
201-265-1942

00013, 00016
Pharmacia & Upjohn
7000 Portage Rd.
Kalamazoo, MI 49001
616-833-4000
800-253-8600
www.pnu.com

Pharmadigm, Inc.
2401 Foothill Dr.
Salt Lake City, UT 84109
650-562-1428

Pharmafair
See Bausch & Lomb Pharmaceuticals

55422
Pharmakon Laboratories, Inc.
6050 Jet Port Industrial Blvd.
Tampa, FL 33634
813-886-3216
800-888-4045

Pharmaquest Corp.
See Inveresk Research

Pharmascience Laboratories, Inc.
175 Rano St.
Buffalo, NY 14207
716-871-9376
800-207-4477

00813
Pharmavite
15451 San Fernando Mission Blvd.
Mission Hills, CA 91345
818-837-3633
800-423-2405
www.pharmavite.com

Pharmics, Inc.
2350 S. Redwood Rd.
Salt Lake City, UT 84119
801-972-4138
800-456-4138
www.pharmics.com

Phillips Gulf Corporation
P.O. Box 270692
Tampa, FL 33688
800-729-8466
www.phillipsgulf.com

Pilkington Barnes Hind-Wesley Jessen
See Wesley Jessen

Playtex. Co
75 Commerce Dr.
Allendale, NJ 07401-1600
201-785-8000
800-816-5742
www.playtex.com

Plough, Inc.
See Schering-Plough Healthcare Products

Poly Pharmaceuticals, Inc.
P.O. Box 93
Quitman, MS 39355
800-882-1041

00998
PolyMedica Pharmaceuticals
11 State Street
Woburn, MA 01801
781-933-2020
www.polymedica.com

47144
Polymer Technology Corp.
100 Research Dr.
Wilmington, MA 01887
978-658-6111
www.polymer.com

Porton Product Limited
See Speywood Pharmaceuticals, Inc.

59012
Pratt Pharmaceuticals
See Pfizer US Pharmaceutical Group

Premier
See Advanced Polymer Systems

00684
Primedics Laboratories
14131 S. Avalon
Los Angeles, CA 90061
323-770-3005

Princeton Pharm. Products
See Bristol-Myers Squibb

37000
Procter & Gamble Co.
1 Procter & Gamble Plaza
Cincinnati, OH 45202
513-983-1100
800-543-7270
www.pg.com

00149
Procter & Gamble Pharm.
P.O. Box 231
Norwich, NY 13815-0191
607-335-3321
800-448-4878
www.pg.com

ProCyte Corporation
8511 154th Ave. N.E.
Bldg. A
Redmond, WA 98052-3557
425-869-1239
www.procyte.com

ProMetic Pharma USA, Inc.
5436 W. 78th St.
Indianapolis, IN 46268
317-334-5600
888-313-2520

Protein Design Labs, Inc.
34801 Campus Dr.
Fremont, CA 94555
510-574-1400
www.pdl.com

Psychemedics Corp.
1280 Massachusetts Ave.
Cambridge, MA 02138
617-868-7455
800-628-8073

00034
Purdue Frederick Co.
100 Connecticut Ave.
Norwalk, CT 06850-3590
203-853-0123
www.pharma.com

00228
Purepac Pharmaceutical Co.
See Faulding Purepac Pharmaceutical Co.

Q-Pharma, Inc.
190 W. Dayton St.
Suite 101-A
Edmonds, WA 98020
425-778-5404
888-742-7687
www.q-pharma.com

QLT Phototherapeutics, Inc.
520 W. 6th Ave.
Vancover, BC V5Z 4H5
604-872-7881
800-663-5486
www.qlt-pdt.com

00603
Qualitest Products, Inc.
1236 Jordan Rd.
Huntsville, AL 35811
256-859-4011
800-444-4011

12225
Quality Formulations, Inc.
P.O. Box 827
Zachary, LA 70791-0827
225-654-6880

Quality Health Products
P.O. Box 31
Yaphank, NY 11980
800-233-7672

Quidel Corp.
10165 McKellar Ct.
San Diego, CA 92121
619-552-1100
800-874-1517
www.quidel.com

54391
R & D Laboratories, Inc.
4640 Admiralty Way,
Suite 710
Marina Del Rey, CA 90292-5608
310-305-8053
800-338-9066

R & R Registrations
P.O. Box 262069
San Diego, CA 92196-2069
619-586-0751

R.P. Scherer-North America
2725 Scherer Dr. N.
St. Petersburg, FL 33716-1016
813-572-4000
www.rpscherer.com

Ranbaxy Pharmaceuticals Inc.
600 College Rd. E.
Suite 2100
Princeton, NJ 08540
609-720-9200
888-726-2299

30103
Randob Laboratories, Ltd.
P.O. Box 440
Cornwall, NY 12518
914-699-3131

00686
Raway Pharmacal, Inc.
15 Granit Rd.
Accord, NY 12404-0047
914-626-8133

12496
Reckitt & Colman
1909 Huguenot Rd.
Suite 300
Richmond, VA 23235
804-379-1090
800-444-7599
www.reckitt.com

10952
Recsei Laboratories
330 S. Kellogg
Building M
Goleta, CA 93117-3875
805-964-2912

48028
Redi-Products Labs, Inc.
See Aplicare, Inc.

00021
Reed & Carnrick
See Schwarz Pharma

10956
Reese Pharmaceutical Co., Inc.
10617 Frank Ave.
Cleveland, OH 44106
216-231-6441
800-321-7178
www.reesechemical.com

Regeneron Pharmaceuticals
777 Old Saw Mill River Rd.
Tarrytown, NY 10591-6707
914-347-7000
800-NERVE22
www.regeneron.com

Reid Rowell
See Solvay

Remel, Inc.
12076 Santa Fe Dr.
Shawnee Mission, KS 66215
913-888-0939
800-225-6730
www.remelinc.com

Republic Drug Co.
175 Great Arrow
Buffalo, NY 14207
716-874-5060
800-828-7444

10961
Requa, Inc.
1 Seneca Place
P.O. Box 4008
Greenwich, CT 06830
203-869-2445
800-321-1085

00433
Research Industries Corp.
6864 S. 300 West
Midvale, UT 84047
801-565-6100
800-453-8432

Research Triangle Pharmaceuticals
13018 Odyssey Dr.
Durham, NC 27713
919-544-4029

60575
Respa Pharmaceuticals, Inc.
P.O. Box 88222
Carol Stream, IL 60188
630-462-9986

00122
Rexall Group
4031 N.E. 12th Terrace
Ft. Lauderdale, FL 33334
800-255-7399

RH Pharmaceuticals, Inc.
See Cangene Corp.

Rhone-Poulenc Rorer Consumer, Inc.
See Novartis

00075, 00083
Rhone-Poulenc Rorer Pharmaceuticals, Inc.
500 Arcola Rd.
P.O. Box 1200
Collegeville, PA 19426
610-454-8110
800-340-7502
www.rp-rorer.com

Ribi Immunochem Research
553 Old Corvallis Rd.
Hamilton, MT 59840-3131
406-363-6214
800-548-7424
www.ribi.com

Richardson-Vicks, Inc.
See Procter & Gamble Co.

12071
Richie Pharmacal, Inc.
119 State Ave.
P.O. Box 460
Glasgow, KY 42141
502-651-6159
800-627-0250

58521
Richwood Pharmaceutical, Inc.
See Shire Richwood

54807
R.I.D., Inc.
609 N. Mednik Ave.
Los Angeles, CA 90022-1320
213-268-0635

54092
Roberts Pharmaceuticals
4 Industrial Way West
Eatontown, NJ 07724
732-676-1200
800-828-2088

A.H. Robins Consumer Products
See Wyeth-Ayerst

00031
A.H. Robins, Inc.
See Wyeth-Ayerst

Roche Diagnostic Systems, Inc.
1080 U.S. Hwy. 202
Somerville, NJ 08876-3771
908-253-7200
800-428-5074
www.rocheusa.com

00004, 00033, 00140, 18393, 42987
Roche Laboratories
340 Kingsland St.
Nutley, NJ 07110-1199
973-235-5000
800-526-6367
www.rocheUSA.com

00049
Roerig
See Pfizer

00832
Rosemont Pharmaceutical Corp.
301 S. Cherokee St.
Denver, CO 80223
303-733-7207
800-445-8091

00074
Ross Laboratories
6480 Busch Blvd.
Columbus, OH 43229
614-624-3333
800-624-7677

00054
Roxane Laboratories, Inc.
P.O. Box 16532
Columbus, OH 43216-6532
614-276-4000
800-848-0120
www.roxane.com

51875
Royce Laboratories, Inc.
See Watson

00536
Rugby Labs, Inc.
See Watson

Russ Pharmaceuticals
See UCB Pharmaceuticals

46500
Rydelle Laboratories
See S.C. Johnson Wax

S.S.S. Company
65-71 University Ave. S.W.
Atlanta, GA 30315
404-521-0857
800-237-3843

Salix Pharmaceuticals, Inc.
3600 W. Bayshore Rd. #205
Palo Alto, CA 94303-4237
650-856-1550

00043
Sandoz Consumer
See Novartis

00212
Sandoz Nutrition Corp.
See Novartis

00078
Sandoz Pharmaceuticals
See Novartis

SangStat
1505 Adams Dr.
Menlo Park, CA 94025
650-328-0300
877-264-7828
www.sangstat.com

00024
Sanofi Winthrop Pharmaceuticals
90 Park Ave.
New York, NY 10016
212-551-4000
800-223-1062

00281
Savage Laboratories
60 Baylis Rd.
Melville, NY 11747-2006
516-454-9071
800-231-0206

Scandinavian Natural Health & Beauty Products
13 N. 7th St.
Perkasie, PA 18944
215-453-2505
800-288-2844

58914
Scandipharm, Inc.
22 Inverness Center Pkwy.
Suite 310
Birmingham, AL 35242
800-950-8085

11012
Schaffer Laboratories
1058 N. Allen Ave.
Pasadena, CA 91104
818-798-0628
800-231-6725

00364, 00591
Schein Pharmaceutical, Inc.
100 Campus Dr.
Florham Park, NJ 07932
800-356-5790
www.schein-rx.com

00274, 00032
Scherer Laboratories, Inc.
2301 Ohio Dr.
Suite 234
Plano, TX 75093
800-449-8290

00085, 11017, 41100, 54092
Schering-Plough Corp.
2000 Galloping Hill Rd.
Kenilworth, NJ 07033-0530
908-298-4000
800-526-4099

00085, 11017, 41000, 41100
Schering-Plough Healthcare Products
110 Allen Rd.
Liberty Corner, NJ 07938
908-604-1995
800-842-4090

Schiapparelli Searle
See SCS Pharmaceuticals

20525
Schiff Products/Weider Nutrition Intl.
2002 S. 5070 West
Salt Lake City, UT 84104
801-975-5000

00234
Schmid Products Co.
See Durex

Scholl, Inc.
See Schering-Plough Healthcare Products

00021, 00091, 00131, 62175
Schwarz Pharma
6140 W. Executive Dr.
Mequon, WI 53092
800-558-5114
www.schwarzusa.com

Schwarzkopf & Dep Inc.
2101 E. Via Arado
Rancho Diminguez, CA 90220
800-326-2855

SciClone Pharmaceuticals, Inc.
901 Mariner's Island Blvd.
San Mateo, CA 94404
650-358-3456
www.sciclone.com

Scios
2450 Bayshore Pkwy.
Mountain View, CA 94043
650-966-1550
Effective 9/99:
820 W. Maude Ave.
Sunnyvale, CA 94086
www.sciosinc.com

S.C. Johnson Wax
1525 Howe St.
Racine, WI 53403-5011
414-631-2000
800-494-4855
www.scjohnsonwax.com

00372
Scot-Tussin Pharmacal, Inc.
50 Clemence St.
P.O. Box 8217
Cranston, RI 02920-0217
800-638-7268
www.scottussin.com

00905
SCS Pharmaceuticals
P.O. Box 5110
Chicago, IL 60680
800-323-1603
www.monsanto.com

00014, 00025
Searle
Box 5110
Chicago, IL 60680-5110
847-982-7000
www.searlehealthnet.com

00551
Seatrace Pharmaceuticals
P.O. Box 363
Gadsden, AL 35902-0363
256-442-5023

Selfcare, Inc.
200 Prospect St.
Waltham, MA 02154
800-899-7353
www.invernessmedical.com

Sepracor
111 Locke Drive
Marlborough, MA 01752
877-SEPRACOR
www.sepracor.com

Septodent, Inc.
P.O. Box 11926
Wilmington, DE 19850
800-872-8305

61471
Sequus Pharmaceuticals, Inc.
960 Hamilton Ct.
Menlo Park, CA 94025
800-323-9051

Seragen, Inc.
97 South Street
Hopkinton, MA 01748
508-435-2331

50694
Seres Laboratories
3331B Industrial Dr.
Santa Rosa, CA 95403
707-526-4526
www.sereslabs.com

44087
Serono Laboratories, Inc.
100 Longwater Circle
Norwell, MA 02061
781-982-9000
800-283-8088

08884
Sherwood Davis & Geck
See Kendall Healthcare

08884
Sherwood Medical
See Kendall Healthcare

58521
Shire Richwood Pharmaceutical, Inc.
P.O. Box 6497
Florence, KY 41022
800-974-4700
www.shiregroup.com

SHS N. America/Scientific Hospital Supplies
9600 Medical Center Dr., Suite 102
Rockville, MD 20850
800-636-2283
www.SHSNA.com

50111
Sidmak Laboratories, Inc.
17 West St.
East Hanover, NJ 07936
800-922-0547
www.sidmaklab.com

54482
Sigma-Tau Pharmaceuticals, Inc.
800 S. Frederick Ave.
Suite 300
Gaithersburg, MD 20877
301-948-1041
800-447-0169
www.sigma-tau.it

54838
Silarx Pharmaceuticals, Inc.
19 West St.
Spring Valley, NY 10977
914-352-4020

Skinvisible, Inc.
6320 S. Sandhill Rd.
Suite 10
Las Vegas, NV 89120
702-433-7154
877-925-6000
ww.skinvisible.com

08026
Smith & Nephew United
See Smith & Nephew Wound Management Inc.

08026
Smith & Nephew Wound Management Inc.
11775 Starkey Rd.
Largo, FL 33773
800-876-1261
www.smithnephew.com

00766
SmithKline Beecham Consumer Healthcare
1500 Littleton Rd.
Parsippany, NJ 07084
973-889-2100

00007, 00029, 00108, 00128
SmithKline Beecham Pharmaceuticals
1 Franklin Plaza
P.O. Box 7929
Philadelphia, PA 19101
215-751-4000
800-366-8900
www.sb.com

00978
SmithKline Diagnostics
See Beckman Coulter Primary Diagnostics

Sola/Barnes-Hind
See PBH Wesley Jessen

33984
Solgar Co., Inc.
500 Willow Tree Rd.
Leonia, NJ 07605
201-944-2311
800-645-2246
www.solgar.com

00032
Solvay Pharmaceuticals
901 Sawyer Rd.
Marietta, GA 30062-2224
770-578-9000
800-354-0026
www.solvay.com

39506
Somerset Pharmaceuticals
777 S. Harbor Island Blvd.
Suite 880
Tampa, FL 33602
727-892-8889

Sparta Pharmaceuticals
111 Rock Rd.
Horsham, PA 19044-2310
215-442-1700
www.spartapharma.com

38137
Spectrum Chemical Mfg. Corp.
See Spectrum Quality Products

38137
Spectrum Quality Products
14422 S. San Pedro St.
Gardena, CA 90248-9985
800-772-8786
www.spectrumchemical.com

00537
Spencer Mead, Inc.
See Rugby

55688
Speywood Pharmaceuticals, Inc.
27 Maple St.
Milford, MA 01757-3650
508-478-8900

Sphinx Pharmaceutical Corp.
P.O. Box 52330
Durham, NC 27717
919-489-0909

Stanback Co.
P.O. Box 1669
Salisbury, NC 28145-1669
704-633-9231
800-338-5428

53385
Standard Drug Co./Family Pharmacy
1279 N. 7th St.
Riverton, IL 62561
217-629-9884
Std. Drug only: 800-632-9884

Standard Homeopathic Co.
P.O. Box 61067
210 W. 131st St.
Los Angeles, CA 90061
800-624-9659

00076
Star Pharmaceuticals, Inc.
1990 N.W. 44th St.
Pompano Beach, FL 33064-1278
954-971-9704
800-845-7827
www.starpharm.com

51318
Stellar Pharmacal Corp.
1990 N.W. 44th St.
Pompano Beach, FL 33064-1278
954-971-9704
800-845-7827

Stephan Company
1850 W. McNab Rd.
Ft. Lauderdale, FL 33300
800-327-4963

St. Jude Medical
1 Lillehei Plaza
St. Paul, MN 55117-1761
651-483-2000

00402
Steris Laboratories, Inc.
620 N. 51st Ave.
Phoenix, AZ 85043
602-278-1400
800-692-9995

Sterling Health
See Bayer Corp. (Consumer Div.)

Sterling Winthrop
See Sanofi Winthrop Pharmaceuticals

00145
Stiefel Laboratories, Inc.
255 Alhambra Circle
Coral Gables, FL 33134
800-327-3858
www.stiefel.com

89223
Stockhausen, Inc.
2401 Doyle St.
Greensboro, NC 27406
336-333-3500
800-334-0242
www.stockhausen-inc.com

57706
Storz
See Bausch & Lomb Surgical

58980
Stratus Pharmaceuticals, Inc.
14377 S.W. 142nd St.
P.O. Box 4632
Miami, FL 33186
800-442-7882
www.stratuspharmaceuticals.com

Stuart Pharmaceuticals
See Zeneca Pharmaceuticals

Sublingual Products International
See Pharmaceutical Labs, Inc.

Sugen Inc.
515 Galveston Dr.
Redwood City, CA 94063-4720
603-433-6288
www.informagen.com

11086
Summers Laboratories, Inc.
103 G.P. Clement Dr.
Collegeville, PA 19426
610-454-1471
800-533-7546
www.sumlab.com

57267
Summit Pharmaceuticals
See Novartis

SuperGen, Inc.
2 Annabel Lane
Suite 220
San Ramon, CA 94583
925-327-0200
www.supergen.com

11704
Survival Technical, Inc.
See Meridian Medical Technologies

Synergen, Inc.
See Amgen

00033, 18393, 42987
Syntex Laboratories
See Roche

Syntex-Synergen Neuroscience
See Roche

Syva Co.
929 Queensbridge
St. Louis, MO 63021
800-227-9948

Tanning Research Labs, Inc.
1190 U.S. 1 N.
Ormond Beach, FL 32174
904-677-9559
www.htropic.com

00300
Tap Pharmaceuticals
2355 Waukegan Rd.
Deerfield, IL 60015
800-621-1020
800-348-2779
www.tapholdings.com

Targeted Genetics Corp.
1100 Olive Way, Ste. 100
Seattle, WA 98101
206-623-7612
www.targen.com

Targon Corp.
See Elan Research Co.

51672
Taro Pharmaceuticals USA, Inc.
5 Skyline Dr.
Hawthorne, NY 10532-9998
914-345-9001
800-544-1449
www.taropharma.com

00418
Taylor Pharmaceuticals
P.O. Box 5136
San Clemente, CA 92674-5136
714-492-4030
800-223-9851

83926
Tec Laboratories, Inc.
615 Water Ave. N.E.
P.O. Box 1958
Albany, OR 97321-0512
541-926-4577
800-482-4464
www.teclabsinc.com

Telluride Pharm. Corp.
146 Flanders Dr.
Hillsborough, NJ 08876-4656
908-359-1375

Teva Marion Partners
See Hoechst

00093, 00332
Teva Pharmaceuticals USA
10236 Marion Park Dr.
Kansas City, MO 64137
888-838-2872
800-867-2444

49158
Thames Pharmacal, Inc.
2100 Fifth Ave.
Ronkonkoma, NY 11779-6906
516-737-1155
800-225-1003

Ther-Rx Corporation
13622 Lakefront Dr.
Earth City, MO 63045
314-209-1517
877-859-9361

Therapeutic Antibodies, Inc.
1207 17th Ave. S.
Suite 103
Nashville, TN 37212
615-327-1027
888-327-1027

11290
Thompson Medical Co.
777 S. Flagler
West Palm Beach, FL 33401
561-820-9900
800-521-7857

T/I Pharmaceuticals, Inc.
See Fischer Pharmaceuticals

49483
Time-Cap Labs, Inc.
7 Michael Ave.
Farmingdale, NY 11735
516-753-9090

Titan Pharmaceuticals, Inc.
50 Division St.
Suite 503
Somerville, NJ 08876
908-429-9880

Transkaryotic Therapies
See Genzyme Corp.

93312
Trask Industries, Inc.
163 Farrell St.
Somerset, NJ 08873
800-579-3131

Triage Pharmaceuticals
See Health for Life Brands, Inc.

Triangle Labs, Inc.
See Tri Tec Laboratories

Tri-Med Specialties, Inc.
16309 W. 108th Circle
Lenexa, KS 66219-1372
800-874-6331
800-528-5591
www.trimed.com

Tri Tec Laboratories
1000 Robins Rd.
Lynchburg, VA 24506-3558
804-845-7073

79511
Triton Consumer Products, Inc.
561 West Golf
Arlington Heights, IL 60005
847-228-7650
800-942-2009

Tsumura Medical
1000 Valley Park Dr.
Shakopee, MN 55379
612-496-4700
800-424-2133

Tweezerman
55 Sea Cliff Ave.
Glen Cove, NY 11542-3695
516-676-7772
800-645-3340

53335
Tyson & Associates, Inc.
12832 S. Chadron Ave.
Hawthorne, CA 90250-5525
310-675-1080

UAD Laboratories, Inc.
See Forest Pharmaceutical, Inc.

UCB Pharmaceuticals, Inc.
1950 Lake Park Dr.
Atlanta, GA 30080
800-477-7877
www.ucb.be

62592
Ucyclyd Pharma, Inc.
500 McCormic Dr., Suite J
Glen Burnie, MD 21061
410-768-5993
www.ucyclyd.com
Oct. 1, 1999 - moving to Phoenix, AZ

51079
UDL Laboratories, Inc.
P.O. Box 2629
Loves Park, IL 61132-2629
815-282-1201
800-435-5272

Ueno Fine Chemicals Industry
31 Koraibashi
Osaka 541, Japan
06-203-0761

00127
Ulmer Pharmacal Co.
2440 Fernbrook Lane
Plymouth, MN 55447-9987
800-848-5637

Unico Holdings, Inc.
1830 2nd Ave. N.
Lake Worth, FL 33461
800-367-4477

Unilever HPC
33 Benedict Place
Greenwich, CT 06830
203-661-2000
800-243-5320
www.unilever.com

Unilever
75 Merritt Blvd.
Trumbull, CT 06611
203-381-3500

41785
Unimed
2150 E. Lake Cook Rd.
Buffalo Grove, IL 60089
847-541-2525
800-541-3492
www.unimed.com

Unipath Diagnostics Co.
47 Hulfish St.
Suite 400
Princeton, NJ 08542
609-430-2727
www.unipath.com

00327
United Guardian Laboratories
230 Marcus Blvd.
Hauppauge, NY 11788
800-645-5566

00677
United Research Laboratories
1100 Orthodox St.
Philadelphia, PA 19124
215-288-6500
800-523-3684
www.urlmutual.com

Univax Biologics
See North American Biologicals, Inc.

University of Georgia College of Veterinary Medicine
Athens, GA 30602
706-542-3221

00009
Upjohn Co.
See Pharmacia & Upjohn

00245
Upsher-Smith Labs, Inc.
14905 23rd Ave. N.
Minneapolis, MN 55447-4709
800-328-3344
www.upsher-smith.com

Urologix
14405 21st Ave. N.
Minneapois, MN 55447
888-229-0772
www.urologix.com

58178
US Bioscience
One Tower Bridge
100 Front St;. Ste. 400
West Conshohocken, PA 19428
800-447-3969
www.usbio.com

US International Trading Co.
5585 S.W. Artic Dr.
Beaverton, OR 97005
503-646-7828
www.millcreekbotanicals.com

52747
US Pharmaceutical Corp.
2401-C Mellon Ct.
Decatur, GA 30035
800-330-3040

US Surgical
150 Glover Ave.
Norwalk, CT
203-845-1000
www.ussurg.com

54627
ValMed, Inc.
100 Otis St.
Suite 4A
Northboro, MA 01532
508-393-1599
800-477-0487

00615
Vangard Labs, Inc.
P.O. Box 1268
Glasgow, KY 42142-1268
800-825-4123

Vertex Pharmaceuticals, Inc.
130 Waverly St.
Cambridge, MA 02139-4211
617-577-6000
www.vpharm.com

53258
VHA Inc.
220 E. Las Colinas Blvd.
Irving, TX 75039
800-842-7587

23900
Vicks Health Care Products
See Procter & Gamble

25866
Vicks Pharmacy Products
See Procter & Gamble

Vintage Pharmaceuticals, Inc.
3241 Woodpark Blvd.
Charlotte, NC 28256
704-596-0516
800-873-6333

Vion Pharmaceuticals, Inc.
4 Science Park
New Haven, CT 06511
203-498-4210
www.vionpharm.com

Viratek
See Zeneca

54891
Vision Pharmaceuticals, Inc.
P.O. Box 400
Mitchell, SD 57301-0400
605-996-3356
800-325-6789

VistaPharm
4647 T Hwy. 280 E.
Suite 145
Birmingham, AL 35242
205-981-1387
www.vistapharm.com

54022
Vitaline Corp.
385 Williamson Way
Ashland, OR 97520
503-482-9231
800-648-4755
ww.vitaline.com

49727
Vita-Rx Corp.
P.O. Box 8229
Columbus, GA 31908
706-568-1881
800-241-8276

Vivus Inc.
605 E. Fairchild Dr.
Mountain View, CA 94043
650-934-5200
www.vivus.com

11444
W. F. Young, Inc.
111 Lyman St.
Springfield, MA 01102
413-737-0201
800-628-9653
www.absorbine.com

59310
Wakefield Pharmaceuticals, Inc.
310 Maxwell Rd.
Suite 100
Alpharetta, GA 30004
770-664-1661

00741
Walker, Corp. and, Inc.
P.O. Box 1320
Syracuse, NY 13201
315-463-4511

00619
Walker Pharmacal Co.
4200 Laclede Ave.
St. Louis, MO 63108
314-533-9600
800-325-8080
www.1800homeopathy.com

00037
Wallace Laboratories
Half Acre Rd.
Cranbury, NJ 08512
609-655-6000
www.astelin.com

00017
Wampole Laboratories
Half Acre Rd.
P.O. Box 1001
Cranbury, NJ 08512-0181
800-257-9525
www.wampolelabs.com

00047, 00430
Warner Chilcott Laboratories
100 Enterprise Dr.
Suite 280
Rockaway, NJ 07866
800-521-8813

11370, 12546, 12547, 00071, 00501
Warner Lambert Co.
201 Tabor Rd.
Morris Plains, NJ 07950
800-223-0182
www.warner-lambert.com

59930
Warrick Pharmaceuticals, Corp.
1095 Morris Ave.
Union, NJ 07083
800-526-4099
800-222-7579

00047, 52544, 51875, 55515
Watson Laboratories
311 Bonnie Circle Dr.
Corona, CA 91720
909-270-1400
800-272-5525
www.watsonpharm.com

59196
WE Pharmaceuticals, Inc.
P.O. Box 1142
Ramona, CA 92065
619-788-9155
800-262-9555

Wendt Laboratories
P.O. Box 128
Belle Plaine, MN 56011
800-328-5890

Wesley Jessen
333 E. Howard
Des Plains, IL 60018
800-854-2790
www.wesley-jessen.com

00917
Wesley Pharmacal, Inc.
114 Railroad Dr.
Ivyland, PA 18974
215-953-1680
800-634-4922

59591
West Point Pharma
See Endo

00003, 00072
Westwood Squibb Pharmaceuticals
100 Forest Ave.
Buffalo, NY 14213
800-333-0950

50474
Whitby Pharmaceuticals, Inc.
See UCB Pharmaceuticals, Inc.

00031, 00573
Whitehall Robins Laboratories
5 Giralda Farms
Madison, NJ 07940-0871
800-322-3129
www.whitehallrobins.com

Willen Pharmaceuticals
See Baker Norton Pharmaceuticals

Winthrop Consumer
See Bayer Corp. (Consumer Div.)

Winthrop Pharmaceuticals
See Sanofi Winthrop Pharmaceuticals

12120
Wisconsin Pharmacal Co.
1 Repel Rd.
Jackson, WI 53037
414-677-4121
800-558-6614

11428
Wonderful Dream Salve Corp.
18546 Old Homestead
Harper Woods, MI 48225
313-521-4233

Woodward Laboratories, Inc.
11132 Winners Circle #100
Los Alamitos, CA 90720
www.woodwardlabs.com

00008, 00031
Wyeth-Ayerst Laboratories
P.O. Box 8299
Philadelphia, PA 19101
610-688-4400
800-934-5556
www.ahp.com/wyeth

50962
Xactdose, Inc.
722 Progressive Lane
South Beloit, IL 61080
815-624-8523
800-397-9228

Xoma
2910 Seventh St.
Berkeley, CA 94710
510-644-1170
800-544-9662
www.xoma.com

00116
Xttrium Laboratories, Inc.
415 W. Pershing Rd.
Chicago, IL 60609
773-268-5800
800-587-3721

64855
Young Again Products
3608-B Oleander Dr. #310
Wilmington, NC 28403
910-392-6775

60077, 00273
Young Dental
13705 Shoreline Ct. E.
Earth City, MO 63045
314-344-0010
800-325-1881
www.youngdental.com

00310, 00163, 00187
Zeneca Pharmaceuticals
1800 Concord Pike
Wilmington, DE 19897
302-886-3000
800-456-3669
www.zeneca.com

00172, 00182
Zenith Goldline Pharmaceuticals
4400 Biscayne Blvd.
Miami, FL 33137
800-327-4114
www.zenithgoldline.com

51284
Zila Pharmaceuticals, Inc.
5227 N. 7th St.
Phoenix, AZ 85014-2817
602-266-6700
800-922-7887
www.zila.com

Zonagen, Inc.
2408 Timberloch Pl., B-4
The Woodlands, TX 77380
281-367-5892
www.zonagen.com

ZymeTx, Inc.
800 Research Parkway
Suite 100
Oklahoma City, OK 73104
405-271-1314
888-817-1314
ww.zymetx.com

Zymogenetics, Inc.
1201 Eastlake Ave. E.
Seattle, WA 98102
206-547-8080
www.bio.com

ISBN 1-57439-051-1